OCTOBER 1997 Volume 205 Number 1

A monthly journal devoted to clinical radiology and allied sciences owned and published by THE RADIOLOGICAL SOCIETY OF NORTH AMERICA, INC.

Radiology

RSNA

October 1997 • Volume 205, Number 1

A monthly journal devoted to clinical radiology and allied sciences owned and published by The Radiological Society of North America, Inc.

Radiology

Radiology is published monthly by the Radiological Society of North America, Inc, 2021 Spring Rd, Suite 600, Oak Brook, IL 60523 (ISSN 0033-8419). Printed in USA. Periodical class postage paid at Oak Brook, IL, and additional mailing offices. The nonmember subscription rate for the USA, Canada, and Mexico is $205.00 per year (add $45.00 for postage to Canada and Mexico). The resident subscription rate is $75.00 per year (foreign residents add $45.00 for postage). The foreign and Pan-American subscription rate is $205.00 per year (add $45.00 for surface mail postage). (Air freight is available; rates are furnished on request.) Single copies are $25.00 each (foreign add $11.00 for postage). Notice of missing issues or change of address (include old mailing label and new address) should be sent to RSNA Subscriptions Department, 2021 Spring Rd, Suite 600, Oak Brook, IL 60523. POSTMASTER: Send address correction "changes" to: *Radiology*, RSNA, 2021 Spring Rd, Suite 600, Oak Brook, IL 60523.

Claims for copies lost in the mail are allowed within 90 days of the date of issue. Claims are not allowed for issues lost as a result of insufficient notice of change of address.

Membership in the Radiological Society of North America is by formal application. Membership information should be secured from the Executive Director, the Radiological Society of North America, Inc, 2021 Spring Rd, Suite 600, Oak Brook, IL 60523. Dues are payable annually in January. In accordance with U.S. postal regulations, $102.50 of active membership dues and $37.50 of members-in-training dues are allocated to a subscription of *Radiology*.

State of the Art

1 **Primer on Medical Device Regulation Part I. History and Background**
Lee H. Monsein

10 **Primer on Medical Device Regulation Part II. Regulation of Medical Devices by the U.S. Food and Drug Administration**
Lee H. Monsein

19 **Primer on Medical Device Regulation Part III. Regulatory Mechanisms and Import/Export Regulation**
Lee H. Monsein

Health Policy and Practice

27 **U.S. Food and Drug Administration and Regulation of Medical Devices in Radiology**
William F. Pritchard, Jr, and Ronald F. Carey

Editorials

37 **Increased CT Contrast Enhancement of "Normal" Hepatic Parenchyma May Herald "Occult" Metastases**
James A. Brink

39 **Limitations of Tried-and-True Imaging Signs with New Modalities**
Richard L. Ehman

41 **An Inflamed Appendix at Sonography When Symptoms Are Improving: To Operate or Not to Operate?**
Julien B. C. M. Puylaert and Arie M. Rijke

Devil's Advocate

43 **Unenhanced Helical CT for Evaluating Acute Abdominal Pain: A Little More Cost, a Lot More Information**
Robert E. Mindelzun and R. Brooke Jeffrey

45 **Unenhanced Helical CT versus Plain Abdominal Radiography: A Dissenting Opinion**
Stephen R. Baker

Abdominal and Gastrointestinal Radiology

49 **Liver Metastases: Early Detection Based on Abnormal Contrast Material Enhancement at Dual-Phase Helical CT**
Joel F. Platt, Isaac R. Francis, James H. Ellis, and Karen A. Reige

55 **Spontaneously Resolving Acute Appendicitis: Clinical and Sonographic Documentation**
Sylvain Migraine, Mostafa Atri, Patrice M. Bret, John O. Lough, and John E. Hinchey

59 **Detection of Colorectal Polyps with CT Colography: Initial Assessment of Sensitivity and Specificity**
Amy K. Hara, C. Daniel Johnson, Judd E. Reed, David A. Ahlquist, Heidi Nelson, Robert L. MacCarty, W. Scott Harmsen, and Duane M. Ilstrup

67 **Early Nonpolypoid Colorectal Cancer: Radiographic Diagnosis of Depth of Invasion**
Jiro Watari, Yusuke Saitoh, Takeshi Obara, Takanori Fujiki, Masato Taniguchi, Masafumi Nomura, Tokiyoshi Ayabe, Tomoyuki Ohta, Yutaka Orii, and Yutaka Kohgo

75 **Hepatocellular Carcinoma: The Role of Helical Biphasic Contrast-enhanced CT versus CT during Arterial Portography**
Masayuki Kanematsu, James H. Oliver III, Brian Carr, and Richard L. Baron

81 **Hepatic Tumor Invasion of Bile Ducts: Wedge-shaped Sign on MR Images**
Yukio Muramatsu, Kenichi Takayasu, Yoshihiro Furukawa, Kunihisa Miyakawa, Ryoko Iwata, Kyosuke Ushio, Junji Yamamoto, and Yukihiro Nakanishi

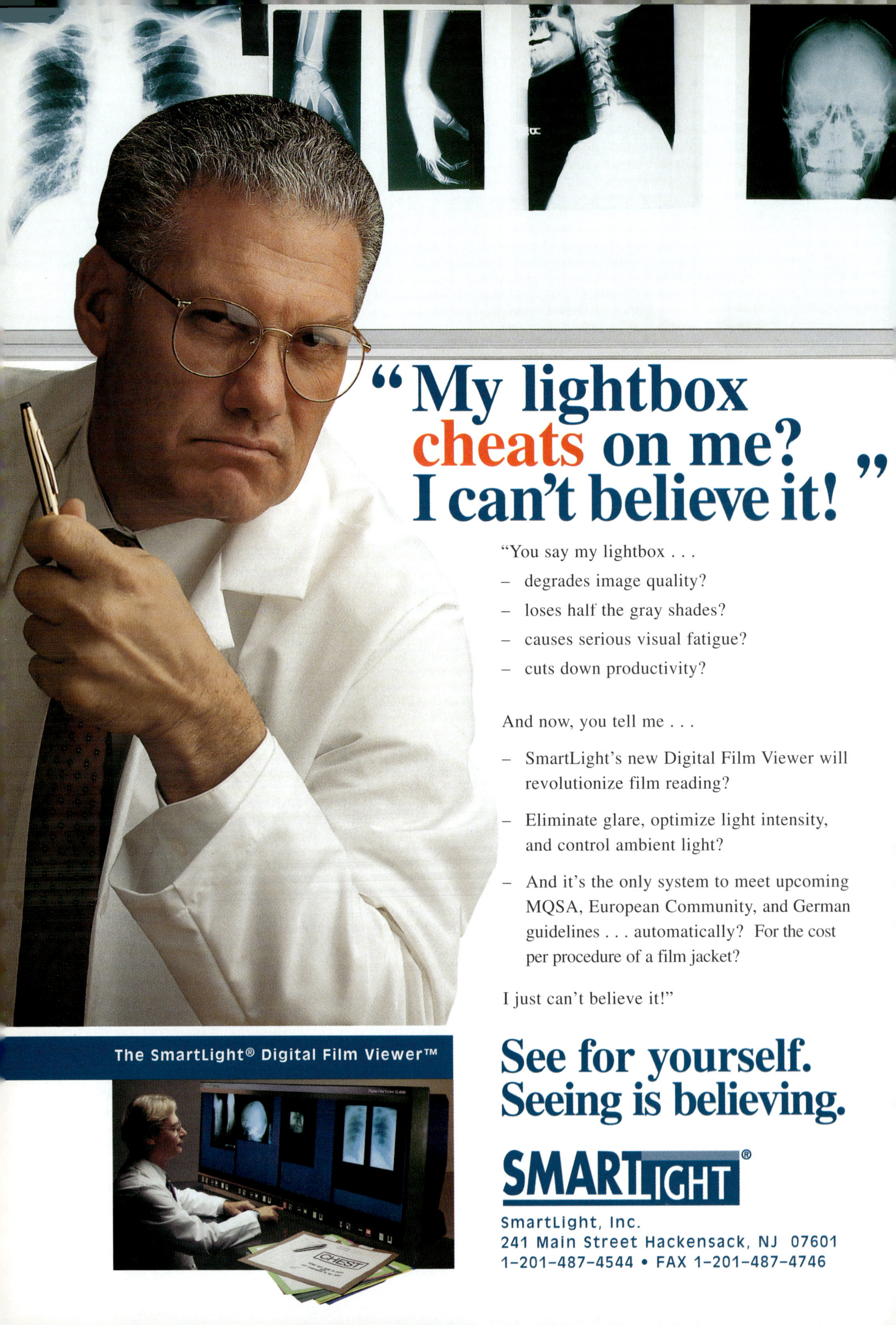
"My lightbox cheats on me? I can't believe it!"
"You say my lightbox . . .
– degrades image quality?
– loses half the gray shades?
– causes serious visual fatigue?
– cuts down productivity?
And now, you tell me . . .
– SmartLight's new Digital Film Viewer will revolutionize film reading?
– Eliminate glare, optimize light intensity, and control ambient light?
– And it's the only system to meet upcoming MQSA, European Community, and German guidelines . . . automatically? For the cost per procedure of a film jacket?
I just can't believe it!"
The SmartLight® Digital Film Viewer™
CHEST
See for yourself. Seeing is believing.
SMARTLIGHT®
SmartLight, Inc.
241 Main Street Hackensack, NJ 07601
1-201-487-4544 • FAX 1-201-487-4746

Pediatric Radiology

87 **Necrotizing Enterocolitis: Diagnosis with CT Examination of Urine after Enteral Administration of Iodinated Water-soluble Contrast Material**
Ingo O. Rencken, Augusto Sola, Firaz Al-Ali, Juan P. Solano, Henry I. Goldberg, Pierre-Alain Cohen, and Charles A. Gooding

Contrast Media

91 **Abdominal Trauma: Use of Oral Contrast Material for CT Is Safe**
Michael P. Federle, Neda Yagan, Andrew B. Peitzman, and James Krugh

95 **Liver Metastases from Colorectal Cancer: Drug Delivery with Liposome-encapsulated Doxorubicin**
Osman Cay, Jonathan B. Kruskal, Imad Nasser, Peter Thomas, and Melvin E. Clouse

Genitourinary Radiology

103 **Lipid in Renal Clear Cell Carcinoma: Detection on Opposed-Phase Gradient-Echo MR Images**
Eric K. Outwater, Manoj Bhatia, Evan S. Siegelman, Melissa A. Burke, and Donald G. Mitchell

109 **Early Systole in the Healthy Kidney: Variability of Doppler US Waveform Parameters**
Mark A. Kliewer, Barbara S. Hertzberg, Mary T. Keogan, Erik K. Paulson, Kelly S. Freed, David M. DeLong, and Barbara A. Carroll

Cardiovascular Radiology

115 **Renal Artery Origins: Best Angiographic Projection Angles**
Evert-Jan Verschuyl, Robert Kaatee, Frederik J. A. Beek, Nilesh H. Patel, Arthur B. Fontaine, Charles P. Daly, Douglas M. Coldwell, William H. Bush, and Willem P. T. M. Mali

121 **Renal Artery Stenosis: Detection and Quantification with Spiral CT Angiography versus Optimized Digital Subtraction Angiography**
Robert Kaatee, Frederik J. A. Beek, Eduard E. de Lange, Maarten S. van Leeuwen, Henk F. M. Smits, Peter J. G. van der Ven, Jaap J. Beutler, Willem P. T. M. Mali

128 **Hemodynamically Significant Atherosclerotic Renal Artery Stenosis: MR Angiographic Features**
Martin R. Prince, Stefan O. Schoenberg, Jennifer S. Ward, Frank J. Londy, Thomas W. Wakefield, and James C. Stanley

137 **Fluoroscopically Triggered Contrast-enhanced Three-dimensional MR Angiography with Elliptical Centric View Order: Application to the Renal Arteries**
Alan H. Wilman, Stephen J. Riederer, Bernard F. King, Josef P. Debbins, Phillip J. Rossman, and Richard L. Ehman

147 **Ability of a Phase Shift US Contrast Agent to Improve Imaging of the Main Renal Arteries**
Michelle L. Melany, Edward G. Grant, André J. Duerinckx, Tina M. Watts, and Barton S. Levine

153 **Spiral CT Artifact That Simulates Aortic Dissection: Image Reconstruction with Use of 180° and 360° Linear-Interpolation Algorithms**
Pierre Loubeyre, Emmanuelle Angelie, Florence Grozel, Hassan Abidi, and Van André Tran Minh

159 **Posterior Aspect of Hepatic Segment IV: Patterns of Portal Venule Branching at Helical CT during Arterial Portography**
Osamu Matsui, Masumi Kadoya, Jun Yoshikawa, Toshifumi Gabata, Yasuhiro Kawamori, Kazuhiko Ueda, Kouji Nobata, and Tsutomu Takashima

163 **Peripheral Vascular Disease Evaluated with Reduced-Dose Gadolinium-enhanced MR Angiography**
Neil M. Rofsky, Glyn Johnson, Mark A. Adelman, Robert J. Rosen, Glenn A. Krinsky, and Jeffrey C. Weinreb

170 **Cardiac Perforation Due to Wallstent Embolization: A Fatal Complication of the Transjugular Intrahepatic Portosystemic Shunt Procedure**
Joseph A. Prahlow, Timothy J. O'Bryant, and Jeffrey J. Barnard

Interventional Radiology

173 **Refractory Ascites: Midterm Results of Treatment with a Transjugular Intrahepatic Portosystemic Shunt**
Gwen K. Nazarian, Haraldur Bjarnason, Charles A. Dietz, Jr, Casandra A. Bernadas, Mary C. Foshager, Hector Ferral, and David W. Hunter

181 **Transjugular Intrahepatic Portosystemic Shunt with Silicone-covered Wallstents: Results in a Swine Model**
Hirohiko Tanihata, Richard R. Saxon, Yasushi Kubota, Dusan Pavcnik, Barry T. Uchida, Josef Rosch, Frederick S. Keller, Ryusaku Yamada, and Morio Sato

185 **Small Lymph Nodes of the Abdomen, Pelvis, and Retroperitoneum: Usefulness of Sonographically Guided Biopsy**
Andrew J. Fisher, Erik K. Paulson, Douglas H. Sheafor, Constance M. Simmons, and Rendon C. Nelson

Neuroradiology

191 **Basilar Tip Aneurysm: Endovascular Treatment with Guglielmi Detachable Coils–Midterm Results**
Guenther E. Klein, Dieter H. Szolar, Klaus A. Leber, Radenko Karaic, and Klaus A. Hausegger

197 **Hippocampal Transverse Relaxation Times in Patients with Alzheimer Disease**
Norbert G. Campeau, Ronald C. Petersen, Joel P. Felmlee, Peter C. O'Brien, and Clifford R. Jack, Jr

Breast Imaging

203 **Evaluation of 14- and 11-gauge Directional, Vacuum-assisted Biopsy Probes and 14-gauge Biopsy Guns in a Breast Parenchymal Model**
Wendie A. Berg, Thorsten L. Krebs, Cristina Campassi, Laurence S. Magder, and Chen-Chih J. Sun

209 **Peripheral Washout Sign on Contrast-enhanced MR Images of the Breast**
Hanan Sherif, Ahmed-Emad Mahfouz, Hans Oellinger, Jose Hadijuana, Jens-Uwe Blohmer, Matthias Taupitz, Roland Felix, and Bernd Hamm

214 **Benign versus Malignant Breast Disease: Comparison of Contrast-enhanced MR Imaging and Tc-99m Tetrofosmin Scintimammography**
Helen M. Fenlon, Niall C. Phelan, Phyllis O'Sullivan, Sean Tierney, Thomas Gorey, and Joseph T. Ennis

221 **Syndrome of Spotty Skin Pigmentation, Myxomas, Endocrine Overactivity, and Schwannomas (Carney Complex): Breast Imaging Findings**
Nikos A. Courcoutsakis, Catherine K. Chow, Thomas H. Shawker, J. Aidan Carney, and Constantine A. Stratakis

Thoracic Radiology

229 **Diffuse Lung Disease: Diagnostic Accuracy of CT in Patients Undergoing Surgical Biopsy of the Lung**
Stephen J. Swensen, Gregory L. Aughenbaugh, and Jeffrey L. Myers

235 **Pulmonary Emphysema: Comparison of Preoperative Quantitative CT and Physiologic Index Values with Clinical Outcome after Lung-Volume Reduction Surgery**
David S. Gierda, Richard M. Slone, Kyongtae T. Bae, Roger D. Yusen, Stephen S. Lefrak, and Joel D. Cooper

243 **Perfusion Scintigraphy in the Evaluation for Lung Volume Reduction Surgery: Correlation with Clinical Outcome**
Samuel C. Wang, Keith C. Fischer, Richard M. Slone, David S. Gierada, Roger D. Yusen, Stephen S. Lefrak, Thomas K. Pilgram, and Joel D. Cooper

249 **Outpatient Treatment of Iatrogenic Pneumothorax after Needle Biopsy**
Karen T. Brown, Lynn A. Brody, George I. Getrajdman, and Tracy E. Napp

Musculoskeletal Radiology

253 **Lumbosacral Junction Injury Associated with Unstable Pelvic Fractice: Classificaton and Diagnosis**
Antonio Leone, Alfonso Cerase, Francesco Priolo, and Pasquale Marano

260 **Extensive Intraosseous Gas Associated with Lymphangiomatosis of Bone: Report of Three Cases**
Robert R. Brown, Mini N. Pathria, Paul M. Ruggieri, Jon A. Jacobson, Joseph G. Craig, and Donald Resnick

Therapeutic Radiology

263 **Quantification of Tumor Reoxygenation during Accelerated Radiation Therapy**
Martin Kocher, Harald Treuer, and Rolf-Peter Müller

Special Report

114 **Jeffrey R. Galvin, MD**
Armed Forces Institute of Pathology 1997–1998 Distinguished Scientist
Melissa L. Rosado-de-Christenson

Technical Developments and Instrumentation

269 **Thoracic Spiral CT: Delivery of Contrast Material Pushed with Injectable Saline Solution in a Power Injector**
Kenneth D. Hopper, Timothy J. Mosher, Claudia J. Kasales, Thomas R. TenHave, Danielle A. Tully, and Jill S. Weaver

272 **Virtual Cystoscopy: Early Clinical Experience**
Helen M. Fenlon, Timoth V. Bell, Heideh K. Ahari, and Sarwat Hussain

276 **Transrectal US-guided Seminal Vesiculography**
Thomas R. Jones, Ronald J. Zagoria, and Jonathan P. Jarow

278 **Pathologic Conditions in the Small Bowel: Findings at Fat-suppressed Gadolinium-enhanced MR Imaging with an Optimized Suspension of Oral Magnetic Particles**
Sonja C. Faber, Michael K. Stehling, Nicolaus Holzknecht, Jörg Gauger, Thomas Helmberger, and Maximilian Reiser

Letters to the Editor

283 **Differentiation between Benign and Malignant Breast Lesions with MR Imaging and Scintimammography**
Fabienne Servais, Didier C. Blocklet, Alain E. Seret, Andre Lenaers, and Andre C. Schoutens

283 E. S. Delpassand and Edward F. Jackson
284 Iraj Khalkhali
285 **Reply**
Thomas H. Helbich, Alexander Becherer, Thomas Leitha, and Gerhard H. Mostbeck

286 **Popliteal Vascular Disease: MR Imaging and MR Angiography**
Mathias Goyen

286 **Postmyelographic Headaches**
Charles E. Seibert

287 **Barium Sulfate versus Water-Soluble, Low-Osmolarity Contrast Medium in Esophageal Examinations**
Abida Z. Ginai

287 **Reply**
Marc J. Gollub and Manjit S. Bains

In Memoriam

289 **Michael J. Feinberg, MD**
Olle Ekberg, MD

289 **Fazlur R. Khan, MD**
Bhogaraju S. Devi, MD

290 **Robert E. L. Stuart, Jr, MD**
John P. Miller, MD

290 **Karl H. Ueberschar, MD**
Karl H. Ficke, MD

Book Reviews

26 **Interpretation of ERCP with Associated Digital Imaging Correlation**
66 **Atlas of Nuclear Medicine**
94 **Imaging of Soft Tissue Tumors**
94 **Imaging of Soft Tissue Tumors**
102 **Biliary Tract Radiology**
158 **Arthritis in Black and White**

Sum & Substance

48 **Innervation of the Liver: Morphology and Function**

Interludes

54 **Ray's Days**
86 **Discography How To**
108 **Satellite Sea Urchin**

Modalities

MR: 81, 103, 128, 137, 163, 209, 214, 278
US: 55, 109, 147, 185
NM: 214, 243

Departments

291 **Abstracts of Current Literature**
288 **Errata**
12A **Advertisers' Index**
41A **RSNA Quick Reference**
55A ***Radiology* Business Information**
25A **Announcements and Books, Audiovisual Materials, and Software Received**
30A **Continuing Medical Education**
49A **Publication Information for Authors**
53A ***Radiology* Manuscript Categorization Terms**
48A **Copyright and Certifications Agreement**
61A **Classified Services**
76A **RSNA Bulletin Board**
74A **RSNA Proposed Amendment to the Bylaws**

November 1997 • Volume 205, Number 2

Radiology

A monthly journal devoted to clinical radiology and allied sciences owned and published by The Radiological Society of North America, Inc.

Radiology is published monthly by the Radiological Society of North America, Inc, 2021 Spring Rd, Suite 600, Oak Brook, IL 60523 (ISSN 0033-8419). Printed in USA. Periodical class postage paid at Oak Brook, IL, and additional mailing offices. The nonmember subscription rate for the USA, Canada, and Mexico is $215.00 per year (add $45.00 for postage to Canada and Mexico). The resident subscription rate (includes both *Radiology* and *RadioGraphics*) is $80.00 per year (foreign residents add $60.00 for postage). The foreign and Pan-American subscription rate is $215.00 per year (add $45.00 for surface mail postage). (Air freight is available; rates are furnished on request.) Single copies are $25.00 each (air freight, $11.00). Notice of missing issues or change of address (include old mailing label and new address) should be sent to RSNA Subscriptions Department, 2021 Spring Rd, Suite 600, Oak Brook, IL 60523. POSTMASTER: Send address correction "changes" to: *Radiology*, RSNA, 2021 Spring Rd, Suite 600, Oak Brook, IL 60523.

Claims for copies lost in the mail are allowed within 90 days of the date of issue. Claims are not allowed for issues lost as a result of insufficient notice of change of address.

Membership in the Radiological Society of North America is by formal application. Membership information should be secured from the Executive Director, the Radiological Society of North America, Inc, 2021 Spring Rd, Suite 600, Oak Brook, IL 60523. Dues are payable annually in January. In accordance with U.S. postal regulations, $107.50 of active membership dues is allocated to a subscription of *Radiology*.

State of the Art

297 **CT of Blunt Abdominal Trauma in Adults**
William P. Shuman

307 **Treatment of Peripheral Vascular Disease with Stent-Grafts**
Andrew H. Cragg and Michael D. Dake

Perspectives

83A **Accountability in Managed Health Care**
Richard M. Friedenberg

Editorials

315 **Diagnosis of Hyperacute Ischemic Infarct with CT: Key to Improved Clinical Outcome after Intravenous Thrombolysis?**
Eric J. Russell

319 **Liver-Specific Contrast Media: A Magic Bullet or a Weapon for Dedicated Targets?**
Michael Laniado and Andreas F. Kopp

Devil's Advocate

323 **A Second Look at the Second-Look Angiogram in Cases of Subarachnoid Hemorrhage**
Harry J. Cloft, David F. Kallmes, and Jacques E. Dion

324 **Reply**
Richard du Mesnil de Rochemont and Walter Heindel

Neuroradiology

327 **Acute Stroke: Usefulness of Early CT Findings before Thrombolytic Therapy**
Rüdiger von Kummer, Kathryn L. Allen, Rolf Holle, Luigi Bozzao, Stefano Bastianello, Claude Manelfe, Erich Bluhmki, Peter Ringleb, Dieter H. Meier, and Werner Hacke

335 **Intracranial Aneurysm: Anatomic Factors That Predict the Usefulness of Intraoperative Angiography**
Colin P. Derdeyn, Christopher J. Moran, DeWitte T. Cross III, Eric W. Sherburn, and Ralph G. Dacey, Jr

Cardiovascular Radiology

341 **Evaluation of Abdominal Aortic Aneurysm for Stent-Graft Placement: Comparison of Gadolinium-enhanced MR Angiography versus Helical CT Angiography and Digital Subtraction Angiography**
Siegfried A. Thurnher, Roland Dorffner, Majda M. Thurnher, Friedrich W. Winkelbauer, Georg Kretschmer, Peter Polterauer, and Johannes Lammer

353 **US-based Evaluation of Hemodynamic Parameters in the Common Carotid Artery: A Nomogram Trial**
Hans Peter Weskott and Kerstin Holsing

Contrast Media

361 **Gd-EOB-DTPA and Yb-EOB-DTPA: Two Prototypic Contrast Media for CT Detection of Liver Lesions in Dogs**
Stephan A. Schmitz, Susanne Wagner, Gabriele Schuhmann-Giampieri, Werner Krause, Matthias Bollow, and Karl-Jürgen Wolf

Interventional Radiology

367 **Hepatic Metastases: Percutaneous Radio-Frequency Ablation with Cooled-Tip Electrodes**
Luigi Solbiati, S. Nahum Goldberg, Tiziana Ierace, Tito Livraghi, Franca Meloni, Marina Dellanoce, Sandro Sironi, and G. Scott Gazelle

375 **Femoropopliteal Artery Stent Placement: Evaluation of Long-term Success**
Ernst-Peter K. Strecker, Irene B. L. Boos, and Dieter Göttmann

Medical Physics

385 **Patient Dose in Radiologically Guided Interventional Vascular Procedures: Conventional versus Digital Systems**
Rafael Ruiz-Cruces, Manuel Pérez-Martínez, Alberto Martín-Palanca, Alberto Flores, Javier Cristófol, Manuel Martínez-Morillo, and Antonio Díez de los Ríos

395 **Entrance Skin Exposure and Mean Glandular Dose: Effect of Scatter and Field Gradient at Mammography**
Kwan H. Ng, Robert J. Aus, Larry A. DeWerd, and John R. Vetter

Breast Imaging

399 **Digital Tomosynthesis in Breast Imaging**
Loren T. Niklason, Bradley T. Christian, Laura E. Niklason, Daniel B. Kopans, Donald E. Castleberry, Beale Opsahl-Ong, Cynthia E. Landberg, Priscilla J. Slanetz, Angela A. Giardino, Richard Moore, Douglas Albagli, Michael C. DeJule, Paul F. Fitzgerald, David F. Fobare, Brian W. Giambattista, Robert F. Kwasnick, Jianqiang Liu, Stanley J. Lubowski, George E. Possin, James F. Richotte, Ching-Yeu Wei, and Reinhold F. Wirth

407 **Tissue Marking Clip for Stereotactic Breast Biopsy: Initial Placement Accuracy, Long-term Stability, and Usefulness as a Guide for Wire Localization**
Fred Burbank and Nancy Forcier

417 **Clip Placement after Stereotactic Vacuum-assisted Breast Biopsy**
Laura Liberman, D. David Dershaw, Elizabeth A. Morris, Andrea F. Abramson, Cynthia M. Thornton, and Paul Peter Rosen

423 **Canceled Stereotactic Core-Needle Biopsy of the Breast: Analysis of 89 Cases**
Liane E. Philpotts, Carol H. Lee, Laura J. Horvath, and Irena Tocino

429 **Breast Carcinoma: MR Imaging before Reexcisional Biopsy**
Susan G. Orel, Carol Reynolds, Mitchell D. Schnall, Lawrence J. Solin, Douglas L. Fraker, and Daniel C. Sullivan

437 **MR Imaging of the Breast in Patients with Occult Primary Breast Carcinoma**
Elizabeth A. Morris, Lawrence H. Schwartz, D. David Dershaw, Kimberly J. Van Zee, Andrea F. Abramson, and Laura Liberman

441 **Screening Mammography: Experience in a Health Maintenance Organization**
Nicholas A. Hanchak, Howard B. Kessler, Shawn MacPherson, Sherry Xuan, and Lawrence J. Solin

Thoracic Radiology

447 **Pulmonary Embolism: Prospective Comparison of Spiral CT with Ventilation-Perfusion Scintigraphy**
John R. Mayo, Martine Remy-Jardin, Nestor L. Müller, Jacques Remy, Daniel F. Worsley, Claude Hossein-Foucher, J. Stephen Kwong, and Maura J. Brown

453 **Acute Pulmonary Embolism: Role of Helical CT in 164 Patients with Intermediate Probability at Ventilation-Perfusion Scintigraphy and Normal Results at Duplex US of the Legs**
Gilbert R. Ferretti, Jean-Luc Bosson, Pierre-Denis Buffaz, David Ayanian, Christophe Pison, François Blanc, Françoise Carpentier, Patrick Carpentier, and Max Coulomb

459 **HIV-associated Human Herpesvirus 8–Positive Primary Lymphomatous Effusions: Radiologic Findings in Six Patients**
Sandro Morassut, Emanuela Vaccher, Luca Balestreri, Annunziata Gloghini, Gianluca Gaidano, Rachele Volpe, Umberto Tirelli, and Antonino Carbone

465 **Mosaic Attenuation Pattern on Thin-Section CT Scans of the Lung: Differentiation among Infiltrative Lung, Airway, and Vascular Diseases as a Cause**
Sylvia A. Worthy, Nestor L. Müller, Thomas E. Hartman, Stephen J. Swensen, Simon P. G. Padley, and David M. Hansell

471 **Solitary Pulmonary Nodules: Evaluation of Blood Flow Patterns with Dynamic CT**
Minming Zhang and Michio Kono

Health Policy and Practice

479 **Hiring by Radiology Groups in 1996**
Rajiv Mallick, Shelah G. Leader, Jonathan H. Sunshine, and Katherine A. Shaffer

Genitourinary Radiology

487 **Ureteropelvic Junction Injuries Secondary to Blunt Abdominal Trauma**
Akira Kawashima, Carl M. Sandler, Joseph N. Corriere, Jr, Brian M. Rodgers, and Stanford M. Goldman

493 **Normal Placenta: Gadolinium-enhanced, Dynamic MR Imaging**
Hani B. Marcos, Richard C. Semelka, and Suvipapun Worawattanakul

497 **Renal Angiomyolipoma: Imaging Findings in Lesions with Minimal Fat**
Masahiro Jinzaki, Akihiro Tanimoto, Yoshiaki Narimatsu, Kiyoshi Ohkuma, Tadayoshi Kurata, Hiroshi Shinmoto, Kyoichi Hiramatsu, Makio Mukai, and Masaru Murai

Abdominal and Gastrointestinal Radiology

503 **Acute Colonic Diverticulitis: Prospective Comparative Evaluation with US and CT**
Jean A. Pradel, Jean-François Adell, Patrice Taourel, Mounir Djafari, Elisabeth Monnin-Delhom, and Jean-Michel Bruel

513 **Pancreatic Malignancy: Effect of Dual-Phase Helical CT in Tumor Detection and Vascular Opacification**
Mary T. Keogan, Vincent G. McDermott, Erik K. Paulson, Douglas H. Sheafor, M. Gena Frederick, David M. DeLong, and Rendon C. Nelson

519 **Intestinal Ischemia in Patients in Whom Small Bowel Obstruction Is Suspected: Evaluation of Accuracy, Limitations, and Clinical Implications of CT in Diagnosis**
Emil J. Balthazar, Marc E. Liebeskind, and Michael Macari

523 **Choledocholithiasis and Bile Duct Stenosis: Diagnostic Accuracy of MR Cholangiopancreatography**
Christoph D. Becker, Marianne Grossholz, Minerva Becker, Gilles Mentha, Raymond de Peyer, and François Terrier

531 **Aplasia or Hypoplasia of the Pancreatic Uncinate Process: Comparison in Patients with and Patients without Intestinal Nonrotation**
Yutaka Inoue and Hironobu Nakamura

Therapeutic Radiology

535 **Primary Non-Hodgkin Lymphoma of the Large Bowel**
Moon-June Cho, Chul S. Ha, Pamela K. Allen, Lillian M. Fuller, Fernando Cabanillas, and James D. Cox

Musculoskeletal Radiology

541 **The Shoulder: Adaptive Motion Correction of MR Images**
Kiaran P. McGee, Roger C. Grimm, Joel P. Felmlee, John R. Rydberg, Stephen J. Riederer, and Richard L. Ehman

546 **Spatial Variation of T2 in Human Articular Cartilage**
Bernard J. Dardzinski, Timothy J. Mosher, Shizhe Li, Mark A. Van Slyke, and Michael B. Smith

551 **Glycosaminoglycan in Articular Cartilage: In Vivo Assessment with Delayed Gd $(DTPA)^{2-}$-enhanced MR Imaging**
Adil Bashir, Martha L. Gray, Robert D. Boutin, and Deborah Burstein

559 **Sciatic Nerve: Paradoxic Hypertrophy after Amputation in Young Patients**
Suvimol Chirathivat Hill, Alan R. Baker, Norman W. Barton, Leonard H. Wexler, and Leland J. C. Scott

Pediatric Radiology

563 **Impaired Cerebrovascular Autoregulation after Hypoxic-Ischemic Injury in Extremely Low-Birth-Weight Neonates: Detection with Power and Pulsed Wave Doppler US**
Francis G. Blankenberg, Nyu-Nyu Loh, Alexander M. Norbash, Judith A. Craychee, Daniel M. Spielman, Brenda L. Person, C. Angela Berg, and Dieter R. Enzmann

Obstetrical Ultrasound

569 **Treatment of Ectopic Pregnancy: Is a Human Chorionic Gonadotropin Level of 2,000 mIU/mL a Reasonable Threshold?**
Tejas S. Mehta, Deborah Levine, and Bruce Beckwith

Technical Developments and Instrumentation

574 **Gel Tubes: A Method of Core-Specimen Retrieval and Transport**
Kenneth D. Hopper and Thomas R. TenHave

Letters to the Editor

577 **Endovascular Therapy for Intracranial Aneurysms**
David M. Pelz, Allan J. Fox, and Stephen P. Lownie

577 **Reply**
Alain Tournade, Patrick Courtheoux, Christian Sengel, Sebnem Ozgulle, and Taghi Tajahmady

577 **Extreme Variability of Cerebrovascular US Results and Some Solutions**
J. Jay Crittenden

579 **Future of Teleradiology**
John S. Wills

579 **Reply**
Peter Dure-Smith and Alain L. Fymat

580 **Enhancement Velocity Not Necessarily Reflective of Contrast Material Uptake in Breast MR Imaging**
Markus Pedevilla

580 **Reply**
Christiane K. Kuhl, Juergen Gieseke, and Hans H. Schild

581 **Vascular Rings and the Straight Trachea**
Alan E. Oestreich

582 **Reply**
Perry J. Pickhardt, Marilyn J. Siegel, and Fernando R. Gutierrez

582 **Percutaneous US-guided Ablation of Liver Metastases**
Alighieri Mazziotti and Antonino Cavallari

583 **Reply**
Luigi Solbiati, Nahum Goldberg, Tito Livraghi, and G. Scott Gazelle

In Memoriam

585 **Ramón Barreda, MD**
Pablo R. Ros, MD

585 **Harold L. Shinall, MD**
William E. Cooley, Jr, MD

586 **Cesar H. Carrasco, MD**
Sidney Wallace, MD, Thomas S. Harle, MD, and William A. Murphy, Jr, MD

Book Reviews

326 **Intramedullary Spinal Cord Tumors**
340 **3D Contrast MR Angiography**
360 **Imaging in Obstetrics and Gynecology**
374 **MRI of the Knee. 2nd ed.**
394 **Diagnostic Breast Imaging**
446 **Differential Diagnosis in Conventional Gastrointestinal Radiology. Excerpt from Differential Diagnosis in Conventional Radiology. 2nd ed.**
446 **Differential Diagnosis in Chest X-rays. Excerpt from Differential Diagnosis in Conventional Radiology. 2nd ed.**
464 **Kinderradiologie [Pediatric Radiology]**

Sum & Substance

534 **Polyposis: The Peutz-Jeghers Syndrome**
540 **Fibrous Dysplasia**

Interludes

334 **Saga of a Driver, a Snake, and a Fish**
384 **Ray's Days**

Modalities

MR: 341, 429, 437, 493, 497, 523, 541, 546, 551
US: 353, 503, 563

Departments

587 **Abstracts of Current Literature**
71A **Research Information Page**
584 **Erratum**
10A **Advertisers' Index**
16A **RSNA Quick Reference**
19A **Announcements and Books, Audiovisual Materials, and Software Received**
28A **Continuing Medical Education**
87A **Publication Information for Authors**
91A ***Radiology* Manuscript Categorization Terms**
86A **Copyright and Certifications Agreement**
103A **Classified Services**
117A **RSNA Bulletin Board**

Part 2 of this issue is the RSNA Scientific Program

December 1997 • Volume 205, Number 3

A monthly journal devoted to clinical radiology and allied sciences owned and published by The Radiological Society of North America, Inc.

Radiology

Contents of *Radiology* copyrighted 1997 by the Radiological Society of North America, Inc. Society Office, 2021 Spring Rd, Suite 600, Oak Brook, IL 60523.

Radiology is published monthly by the Radiological Society of North America, Inc, 2021 Spring Rd, Suite 600, Oak Brook, IL 60523 (ISSN 0033-8419). Printed in USA. Periodical class postage paid at Oak Brook, IL, and additional mailing offices. The nonmember subscription rate for the USA, Canada, and Mexico is $215.00 per year (add $45.00 for postage to Canada and Mexico). The resident subscription rate (includes both *Radiology* and *RadioGraphics*) is $80.00 per year (foreign residents add $60.00 for postage). The foreign and Pan-American subscription rate is $215.00 per year (add $45.00 for surface mail postage). (Air freight is available; rates are furnished on request.) Single copies are $25.00 each (air freight, $11.00). Notice of missing issues or change of address (include old mailing label and new address) should be sent to RSNA Subscriptions Department, 2021 Spring Rd, Suite 600, Oak Brook, IL 60523. POSTMASTER: Send address correction "changes" to: *Radiology*, RSNA, 2021 Spring Rd, Suite 600, Oak Brook, IL 60523.

Claims for copies lost in the mail are allowed within 90 days of the date of issue. Claims are not allowed for issues lost as a result of insufficient notice of change of address.

Membership in the Radiological Society of North America is by formal application. Membership information should be secured from the Executive Director, the Radiological Society of North America, Inc, 2021 Spring Rd, Suite 600, Oak Brook, IL 60523. Dues are payable annually in January. In accordance with U.S. postal regulations, $107.50 of active membership dues is allocated to a subscription of *Radiology*.

State of the Art

593 High-Resolution Imaging of the Musculoskeletal System
Scott J. Erickson

619 Human Immunodeficiency Virus Infection and Hepatitis: Biosafety in Radiology
Susan D. Wall, J. Michael Howe, and Rajiv Sawhney

629 Imaging Squamous Cell Carcinomas of the Upper Aerodigestive Tract: What Clinicians Need to Know
Suresh K. Mukherji, Harold R. Pillsbury, and Mauricio Castillo

Editor's Page

647 Valediction: Sweet Sorrow
Stanley S. Siegelman

Editorial

649 Duplex Sonography: Can It Be Used to Evaluate Carotid Artery Stents?
Joseph F. Polak

Special Report

651 Improving Radiology Research Methods: What Is Being Asked and Who Is Being Studied?
John Eng and Stanley S. Siegelman

Interventional Radiology

657 Traumatic Thoracic Aortic Aneurysm: Treatment with Endovascular Stent-Grafts
Noriyuki Kato, Michael D. Dake, D. Craig Miller, Charles P. Semba, R. Scott Mitchell, Mahmood K. Razavi, and Stephen T. Kee

663 Percutaneous Biliary Drainage: Clinical Trial of Analgesia with Interpleural Block
Eric Therasse, Manon Choinière, Gilles Soulez, Vincent L. Oliva, Pierre Rousseau, François Fugère, Daniel Boudreault, and Jean R. Cusson

669 Radiologically Guided Placement of Pull-type Gastrostomy Tubes
George X. Szymski, Alexandra N. Albazzaz, Brian Funaki, Jordan D. Rosenblum, Craig A. Hackworth, Brian W. Zernich, and Jeffrey A. Leef

675 Rapid Thrombectomy with a Hydrodynamic Catheter: Results from a Prospective, Multicenter Trial
Hans-Joachim Wagner, Stefan Müller-Hülsbeck, Michael B. Pitton, Wolfgang Weiss, and Marcus Wess

682 PTFE-encapsulated Endovascular Stent-Graft for Transjugular Intrahepatic Portosystemic Shunts: Experimental Evaluation
Ziv J. Haskal, Andrew Davis, Ashford McAllister, and Emma E. Furth

Cardiovascular Radiology

689 Renal Artery Stenosis: Evaluation with Breath-hold, Three-dimensional, Dynamic, Gadolinium-enhanced versus Three-dimensional, Phase-Contrast MR Angiography
Francesco De Cobelli, Angelo Vanzulli, Sandro Sironi, Renata Mellone, Enzo Angeli, Massimo Venturini, Maria Paola Garancini, Rita Quartagno, Giuseppe Bianchi, and Alessandro Del Maschio

Cardiac Radiology

697 **Coronary Artery Calcification in Women with Syndrome X: Usefulness of Double-Helical CT for Detection**
Joseph Shemesh, Enrique Z. Fisman, Alexander Tenenbaum, Sara Apter, Liviu Leibovitch, Samuel Rath, Yacov Itzchak, and Michael Motro

Abdominal and Gastrointestinal Radiology

701 **Visualization of Colorectal Polyps with Spiral CT Colography: Evaluation of Processing Parameters with Perspective Volume Rendering**
Elizabeth G. McFarland, James A. Brink, John Loh, Ge Wang, Vincent Argiro, Dennis M. Balfe, Jay P. Heiken, and Michael W. Vannier

709 **Hypervascular Liver Metastases: Do Unenhanced and Hepatic Arterial Phase CT Images Affect Tumor Detection?**
James H. Oliver III, Richard L. Baron, Michael P. Federle, Brian C. Jones, and Reuben Sheng

716 **Colorectal Cancer: Diagnostic Potential of CT Measurements of Hepatic Perfusion and Implications for Contrast Enhancement Protocols**
David A. C. Leggett, Benjamin B. Kelley, Ian H. Bunce, and Kenneth A. Miles

721 **Hepatocellular Carcinoma: Evaluation with Dynamic and Static Gadobenate Dimeglumine–enhanced MR Imaging and Histopathologic Correlation**
Thomas J. Vogl, Andrej Stupavsky, Wassilios Pegios, Renate Hammerstingl, Martin Mack, Thomas Diebold, Klaus-Peter Lodemann, Peter Neuhaus, and Roland Felix

729 **Small (1.5 cm or Less) Liver Metastases: US-guided Biopsy**
William D. Middleton, Stephanie K. Hiskes, Sharlene A. Teefey, and Leslie D. Boucher

733 **Gastrointestinal Submucosal Tumors: Evaluation with Endoscopic US**
Kenji Kawamoto, Yoshio Yamada, Takashi Utsunomiya, Hitoshi Okamura, Masanobu Mizuguchi, Makoto Motooka, Nobuaki Hirata, Hideyuki Watanabe, Kenji Sakai, Shinji Kitagawa, Naoko Kinukawa, and Kouji Masuda

741 **Cystic Dystrophy of the Duodenal Wall: Radiologic Findings**
Carlo Procacci, Rossella Graziani, Giuseppe Zamboni, Giorgio Cavallini, Paolo Pederzoli, Alessandro Guarise, Giuseppe Bogina, Carlo Biasiutti, Giovanni Carbognin, Ivo A. Bergamo-Andreis, and Gian F. Pistolesi

Ultrasound

749 **Carotid Artery Stents: Early and Intermediate Follow-up with Doppler US**
Michelle L. Robbin, Mark E. Lockhart, Therese M. Weber, Jiri J. Vitek, J. Kevin Smith, Jay Yadav, Atul Mathur, Sriram S. Iyer, and Gary S. Roubin

757 **Normalizing Fractional Moving Blood Volume Estimates with Power Doppler US: Defining a Stable Intravascular Point with the Cumulative Power Distribution Function**
Jonathan M. Rubin, Ronald O. Bude, J. Brian Fowlkes, R. Steven Spratt, Paul L. Carson, and Ronald S. Adler

Genitourinary Radiology

767 **Renal Cancer: Preoperative Evaluation with Dual-Phase Three-dimensional MR Angiography**
Peter L. Choyke, McClellan M. Walther, Joseph R. Wagner, Walter Rayford, John C. Lyne, and W. Marston Linehan

773 **Placenta Accreta: Evaluation with Color Doppler US, Power Doppler US, and MR Imaging**
Deborah Levine, Carol A. Hulka, Jack Ludmir, Wei Li, and Robert R. Edelman

777 **The Medial Border of the Perirenal Space: CT and Anatomic Correlation**
Vassilios Raptopoulos, Paula Touliopoulos, Qing F. Lei, Thomas G. Vrachliotis, and Sandy C. Marks, Jr

Head and Neck Radiology

785 **Balloon Dacryocystoplasty: Indications and Contraindications**
Joachim Berkefeld, Johannes Kirchner, Hans Michael Müller, Ullrich Fries, and Jürgen Kollath

791 **Obstructed Nasolacrimal Duct System in Epiphora: Long-term Results of Dacryocystoplasty by Means of Balloon Dilation**
Alfred G. Janssen, Khaled Mansour, Johanna J. Bos

Neuroradiology

797 **Brain Capillary Telangiectasia: MR Imaging Appearance and Clinicohistopathologic Findings**
Roland R. Lee, Mark W. Becher, Mark L. Benson, and Daniele Rigamonti

807 **Intracranial Tumor in Children: MR Imaging Findings within 24 Hours of Craniotomy**
Allen B. Oser, Christopher J. Moran, Bruce A. Kaufman, and Tae S. Park

Obstetrical Ultrasound

813 **Fetal Cerebral Ventriculomegaly: Misidentification of the True Medial Boundary of the Ventricle at US**
Barbara S. Hertzberg, Mark A. Kliewer, and James D. Bowie

Pediatric Radiology

817 **Pneumonia in Children: Decreased Parenchymal Contrast Enhancement–CT Sign of Intense Illness and Impending Cavitary Necrosis**
Lane F. Donnelly and Lance A. Klosterman

821 **Vesicoureteral Reflux in Older Children: Concordance of US and Voiding Cystourethrographic Findings**
Michael A. DiPietro, Caroline E. Blane, and J. Michael Zerin

Breast Imaging

823 **Detection of Malignant and Benign Breast Lesions with an Automated US System: Results in 120 Cases**
Kari Richter, Sylvia Helen Heywang-Köbrunner, Klaus-Jürgen Winzer, Karl-Jürgen Schmitt, Heinz Prihoda, Hans D. Frohberg, Hans Guski, Peter Gregor, Jens-Uwe Blohmer, Franz Fobbe, Karin Döinghaus, Gisela Löhr, and Bernd Hamm

831 **Metastatic Breast Carcinoma in Axillary Lymph Nodes: In Vitro US Detection**
Jaime Feu, Francisco Tresserra, Rafael Fábregas, Beatriz Navarro, Pedro J. Grases, Joan Carles Suris, Alfonso Fernández-Cíd, and Xavier Alegret

837 **Dynamic Echo-Planar Imaging of the Breast: Experience in Diagnosing Breast Carcinoma and Correlation with Tumor Angiogenesis**
Carol A. Hulka, Whitney B. Edmister, Barbara L. Smith, Lujian Tan, Dennis C. Sgroi, Terrance Campbell, Daniel B. Kopans, and Robert M. Weisskoff

Thoracic Radiology

843 **Functional Anatomy of the Thoracic Outlet: Evaluation with Spiral CT**
Martine Remy-Jardin, Jacques Doyen, Jacques Remy, Dominique Artaud, Marc Fribourg, and Alain Duhamel

853 **The Breast: In-plane X-ray Protection during Diagnostic Thoracic CT–Shielding with Bismuth Radioprotective Garments**
Kenneth D. Hopper, Steven H. King, Mark E. Lobell, Thomas R. TenHave, and Jill S. Weaver

859 **Accuracy of Bedside Chest Hard-Copy Screen-Film versus Hard- and Soft-Copy Computed Radiographs in a Medical Intensive Care Unit: Receiver Operating Characteristic Analysis**
Harold L. Kundel, Warren Gefter, Judith Aronchick, Wallace Miller, Jr, Hiroto Hatabu, Charlene H. Whitfill, and Wallace Miller, Sr

Musculoskeletal Radiology

865 **Scaphopisocapitate Alignment: Criterion to Establish a Neutral Lateral View of the Wrist**
Zhiyun Yang, Frederick A. Mann, Louis A. Gilula, Carolyn Haerr, and C. Falck Larsen

871 **Soft-Tissue Sarcoma Involving Bone or Neurovascular Structures: MR Imaging Prognostic Factors**
David M. Panicek, Stephen D. Go, John H. Healey, Denis H. Y. Leung, Murray F. Brennan, and Jonathan J. Lewis

Special Communication

876 **David B. Fraser, MD, President, Radiological Society of North America, 1998**
D. R. Campbell

878 **Farewell to *Radiology* Editor: Stanley S. Siegelman, MD**
R. Nick Bryan

880 **A Note of Thanks**
Michael A. Sullivan and Stanley S. Siegelman

656 **Abstractors of Current Literature 1997**
Stanley S. Siegelman

674 **Book Reviewers 1997**
Stanley S. Siegelman and Harry J. Griffiths

696 **Research Trainee Prizes from the 1997 RSNA Scientific Assembly and Annual Meeting**

Book Reviews

772 **Genitourinary Radiology: The Requisites**
852 **Spiral CT of the Chest**
870 **Ultrasonografia del Ginocchio in Età Pediatrica [Ultrasound imaging of the pediatric knee]**

Sum & Substance

708 **Whipple's Disease**
864 **The Fasciitis-Panniculitis Syndromes: Clinical and Pathologic Features**

Interludes

748 **(Preview of) "A Modest Proposal"**
Richard J. Steckel

766 **Turkey Lionfish and Flying Gurnard**
David Hall

806 **Ray's Days**
Steven J. Perlman

Modalities

MR: 689, 721, 767, 797, 817, 837, 871
US: 733, 749, 757, 773, 821, 823, 831

Departments

885 **Abstracts of Current Literature**
16A **Advertisers' Index**
21A **RSNA Quick Reference**
43A ***Radiology* Business Information**
22A **Announcements and Books, Audiovisual Materials, and Software Received**
28A **Continuing Medical Education**
55A **Publication Information for Authors**
59A ***Radiology* Manuscript Categorization Terms**
54A **Copyright and Certifications Agreement**
87A **Classified Services**
140A **RSNA Bulletin Board**
61A **Publisher's Row**
83A **Book Review Index**
103A **1997 RSNA Research and Education Fund Annual Report**

Lee H. Monsein, MD, MPH

Primer on Medical Device Regulation
Part I. History and Background[1]

BEFORE the 1930s, the medical device industry was practically nonexistent. Many medical devices were sold directly to the public. With the explosion of medical technology after World War II, several intermediaries evolved between the medical device industry and the public. Various local, state, and federal regulatory agencies are now ultimately responsible for the medical technology that reaches consumers. It therefore behooves physicians and health care providers to be knowledgeable about medical device regulation. The following review draws on a number of recent essays on the subject (1–5).

This article is the first of a three-part series reviewing medical device regulation. Part I provides an overview and history of medical device regulation and the U.S. Food and Drug Administration (FDA) and discusses government document nomenclature (Fig 1). Part II details current medical device regulation. Part III describes regulatory mechanisms and enforcement of medical device regulation. It also reviews the regulation of imported and exported medical devices, as well as foreign medical device regulation.

510(k)	Premarket Notification
CBER	Center for Biologics Evaluation and Research
CDER	Center for Drug Evaluation and Research
CDRH	Center for Devices and Radiological Health
CFR	Code of Federal Regulations
DA of 1962	Drug Amendments of 1962
DHEW	Department of Health, Education and Welfare
DHHS	Department of Health and Human Services
DSMA	Division of Small Manufacturers Assistance
EPA	Environmental Protection Agency
F&D Act	Food and Drug Act
FCC	Federal Communications Commission
FD&C Act	Food, Drug and Cosmetic Act
FDA	Food and Drug Administration
FTC	Federal Trade Commission
GPO	Government Printing Office
HCFA	Health Care Financing Administration
IDE	Investigational Device Exemption
MDA of 1976	Medical Device Amendments of 1976
MDA of 1992	Medical Device Amendments of 1992
NIH	National Institutes of Health
NRC	Nuclear Regulatory Commission
ODE	Office of Device Evaluation
OSHA	Occupational Safety and Health Administration
PHS	Public Health Service
PL	Public Law
PMA	Premarket Approval
SR	Senate Resolution
HR	House Resolution
SMDA of 1990	Safe Medical Devices Act of 1990
Stat	Statute at Large
USC	United States Code

Figure 1. Abbreviations used in the area of medical device regulation.

DEFINITIONS

A "medical device" is defined by U.S. statute (Section 201[h] of the Food, Drug and Cosmetic [FD&C] Act, Title 21 USC [United States Code] §321;) (see Appendix for explanation of government document nomenclature) as

> an instrument, apparatus, implement, machine, contrivance, implant, in vitro reagent, or other similar or related article, including any component, part, or accessory, which is: (1) recognized in the official National Formulary, or the U.S. Pharmacopeia, or any supplement to them, (2)

Radiology 1997; 205:1–9

Index terms: Radiology and radiologists • State-of-art reviews • U.S. Food and Drug Administration

[1] From the Department of Radiology, Washington Hospital Center, 110 Irving St NW, #BA60, Washington, DC 20010-2975. Received March 27, 1997; revision requested May 19; revision received June 4; accepted June 9. **Address reprint requests to** the author.

Abbreviations: CBER = Center for Biologics Evaluation and Research, CDER = Center for Drug Evaluation and Research, CDRH = Center for Devices and Radiological Health, CFR = Code of Federal Regulations, DHEW = Department of Health, Education and Welfare, DHHS = Department of Health and Human Services, FDA = Food and Drug Administration, FD&C = Food, Drug and Cosmetic, PHS = Public Health Service, USC = United States Code.

intended for use in the diagnosis of disease or other conditions, or in the cure, mitigation, treatment, or prevention of disease in man or other animals, or (3) intended to affect the structure or any function of the body of man or other animals, and which does not achieve its primary intended purposes through chemical action within or on the body of man or other animals and which is not dependent upon being metabolized for the achievement of any of its primary intended purposes.

Confusion sometimes exists between unregulated consumer products and medical devices. Products are not considered medical devices if they have general utility but are neither dedicated to, nor intended or promoted for, medical applications. They are subject to the Consumer Product Safety Act rather than the FD&C Act. For example, a screw is considered a medical device if it is promoted for holding bones together rather than holding pieces of wood together.

Distinguishing between drugs and devices is also sometimes difficult. Medical devices, unlike drugs, do not achieve their principal action through chemical action or metabolization in or on the body. Drugs are also regulated by the FD&C Act but by a different center within the FDA. For example, plaster cast used for bone healing is considered a device, whereas a topical ointment used to promote bone healing is considered a drug. Combination products have both drug and device components. The mechanism of principal action determines which center regulates it. Bone cement with an antibiotic, for example, is considered a device.

Simple "medical devices," such as splints, crutches, stretchers, and dental devices, existed before recorded history and were initially homemade articles constructed for personal use (1). They later became items for barter and commercialization and provided the basis for a medical device industry that has evolved into a global $129.5 billion business. In 1996, the U.S. medical device industry accounted for roughly $61.2 billion in production (47% of global total) and $54.6 billion in consumption (42% of global total); it employed 280,760 people (6). It consisted of 3,000 product lines and 84,000 individual products, of which an estimated 24% were imaging systems (7).

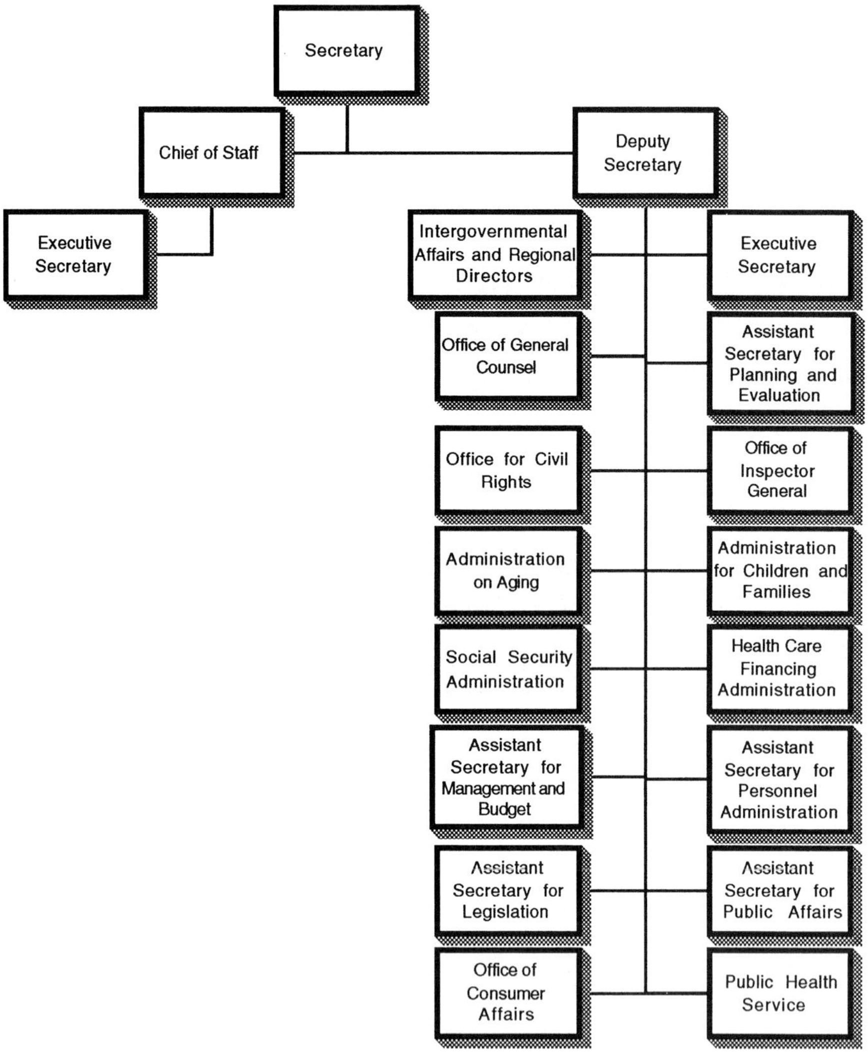

Figure 2. Organization of the DHHS.

OVERVIEW OF MEDICAL DEVICE REGULATION

Various local, state, and federal agencies regulate medical devices. The U.S. Constitution designates three branches of government: executive, legislative, and judicial. By enacting the FD&C Act, Congress has vested federal authority to regulate medical devices to the secretary of the Department of Health and Human Services (DHHS) (Fig 2), one of 15 cabinet-level departments in the executive branch of government. The secretary of the DHHS delegates authority to the assistant secretary of the DHHS, who is the head of the Public Health Service (PHS) (Fig 3). This individual redelegates authority to the commissioner of the FDA. The secretary of the DHHS, nevertheless, reserves the authority to approve regulations of the FDA that "establish procedural rules applicable to a general class of...medical devices" or "present highly significant public issues involving the quality, availability, marketability, or cost of...medical devices" (21 CFR §5.11).

The FDA was originally an executive branch initiative; it was not until congressional legislation in 1988 that it was established by statute (FD&C Act, section 903; 21 USC §393). The legislative branch maintains oversight of the FDA through the Senate Committee on Labor and Human Resources and the House Committee on Energy and Commerce. Furthermore, the Senate must confirm the president's appointment of the FDA commissioner. The judicial branch maintains important judicial checks and balances on the FDA's operations and interpretations of law. The FDA's encounters with the courts are usually screened through the Department of Justice and the U.S. Attorneys.

The major goal of the FD&C Act is to prohibit "the introduction or de-

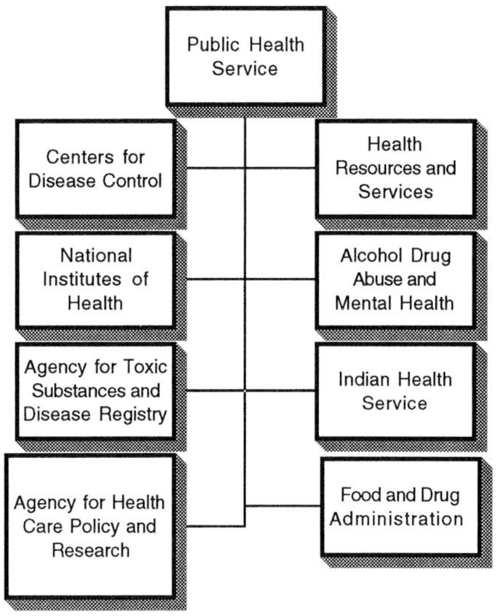

Figure 3. Organization of the PHS.

livery for introduction into interstate commerce of any food, drug, device, or cosmetic that is adulterated or misbranded" (FD&C Act, section 301; 21 USC §331). Therefore, the FD&C Act does not apply to food, drugs, and cosmetics that are manufactured, marketed, and used within an individual state's borders and whose components are from within that state's borders. It is presumed, however, that "a connection with interstate commerce...shall be presumed to exist" for all medical devices (FD&C Act, section 709; 21 USC §379[a]). It is presumed that every device or its components or raw materials eventually cross a state's borders and are therefore subject to federal regulation.

In addition to the authority given by the FD&C Act, the FDA derives authority for regulating medical devices from other federal legislation. Since 1971, the FDA has administered the Radiation Control for Health and Safety Act of 1968. This act gives the FDA authority to establish performance standards and use inspection and recall mechanisms to protect the public from the dangers of electronic products that emit radiation, including ionizing or nonionizing electromagnetic or particulate radiation and sonic, infrasonic, and ultrasonic waves. Provisions of this act were transferred to the FD&C Act in 1990. Other legislation includes the Fair Packaging and Labeling Act of 1966, which concerns standards for the content, form, and placement of product labeling; the Drug Price Competition and Patent Term Restoration Act of 1984, which allows up to 5 years of patent time restoration for a medical device that is subject to a regulatory review period that would otherwise reduce its effective patent life; the Cardiac Pacemaker Registry Act of 1984, which required the FDA to develop a national registry of all cardiac pacemakers and leads implanted or removed with Medicare funds (repealed); and the Orphan Drug Act of 1983, which amended the FD&C (sections 525–528, 21 USC §360[aa–dd]) and the Public Health Service Acts (section 27, 42 USC § 236) to encourage the development of products that are used for treating rare diseases or conditions. The Orphan Drug Act, as amended in 1988, included specific provisions primarily related to grants for research and development for medical devices.

A number of other federal authorities also regulate medical devices with or without collaboration from the FDA. The Nuclear Regulatory Commission has dual responsibility with the FDA in regulating radiologic products. The Office of Export Licensing, in the Department of Commerce, and the Office of Trade, in the Department of State, work with the FDA in overseeing the export of medical devices. The U.S. Customs Service, in the Department of Treasury, works with the FDA to control the import of medical devices. The Federal Trade Commission, operating under the Federal Trade Commission Act of 1938, regulates the advertising of nonrestricted devices. The Federal Communications Commission, directed by the Communications Act of 1934, regulates devices that emit frequencies of electromagnetic energy within the radio-frequency spectrum. The Consumer Product Safety Commission, through its enforcement of the Federal Hazardous Substances Act of 1960, has jurisdiction over medical devices that may be toxic, flammable, corrosive, sensitizers, or irritants.

The Occupational Safety and Health Administration, under the Occupational Safety and Health Act of 1970, and the Environmental Protection Agency, enforcing the Clean Air Act of 1967, the Clean Water Act of 1977, and the Solid Waste Disposal Act of 1965, regulate the conditions under which medical devices are manufactured. They also have dual responsibility with the FDA in regulating ozone-emitting products and germicides, respectively. The National Institutes of Health and the Health Care Financing Administration indirectly regulate medical devices by guiding how federal dollars are used in the development of and reimbursement for new medical technologies.

The FD&C Act prohibits any state from creating or enforcing medical device regulations different from, or in addition to, federal requirements. States may, however, petition the FDA for a federal exemption based on local conditions or special circumstances (FD&C Act, section 521; 21 USC §360[k]). State and local medical device–related requirements are not preempted when they are equal or substantially similar to those of the FD&C Act or when specific federal provisions do not exist. Other state and local requirements may not be preempted by the FD&C Act if they involve practice licensing, contracts, Medicaid and other government-sponsored health program payments, general enforcement of business practices, delegations of authority, generation of revenue, and radiation control (21 CFR §808).

HISTORY OF MEDICAL DEVICE REGULATION

The earliest involvement of the federal government in the regulation of food and drugs involved only imports and therefore did not deal with interstate shipping. An example was the Import Drug Act of 1848. In the late 1800s, it became clear that some form of national legislation was required to prevent the interstate shipment of undesirable food and drugs.

The initial federal regulation of food and drug shipments was under the authority of the U.S. Post Office with enactment of the Postal Fraud Statutes in 1872. They provided criminal penalties for mail fraud and stipulated that mail containing false or fraudulent representations could be declared unmailable by the Postmaster General. Nevertheless, these statutes did not deal specifically with medical devices, and, as a result, fraudulent devices flourished. Enforcement of these statutes has continued to the present.

In 1879, Dr E. R. Squibb, in an address to the Medical Society of the State of New York, proposed the enactment of a national statute to regulate food and drugs. It was not until 27 years later that the Food and Drug Act of 1906 was introduced into Congress and signed into law by President Theodore Roosevelt (Table). Noticeably absent from legislative debates and the Food and Drug Act itself was any mention of medical devices.

The problem of fraudulent medical devices started to gain attention in the early 1900s. By 1917, the administrators of the Food and Drug Act stated in their annual report that it had severe limitations with regard to the control of medical devices. They continued to monitor these products and assisted the U.S. Post Office with their regulatory actions but could take no action of their own.

The shortcomings of the Food and Drug Act with respect to food and drugs, as well as its failure to deal with medical devices, were major reasons for the passage of the FD&C Act in 1938. The bill was created by Agriculture Undersecretary Rexford Tugwell; introduced in 1933 by Senator Royal Copeland, a physician and former New York City health commissioner; and signed into law by President Franklin D. Roosevelt.

The FD&C Act expanded on the framework of the Food and Drug Act and remedied many of its shortcomings. Cosmetics and devices became regulated by the FDA. The FDA had to be notified before the marketing of "new" drugs. Standards of identity for most foods were authorized, and nonstandardized foods with two or more ingredients were required to list all ingredients. The enforcement power of the FDA broadened as the number and type of offenses increased and as injunction became an enforcement mechanism. The FDA no longer had to prove that a therapeutic claim was knowingly falsified or fraudulent to stop its marketing.

The FD&C Act defined medical devices as "instruments, apparatus and contrivances, including their components, parts and accessories, intended (1) for use in diagnosis, cure, mitigation, treatment, or prevention of diseases in man or other animals; or (2) to affect the structure as any function of the body of man or other animals." It provided the FDA with statutory authority to take formal or informal regulatory action against the adulteration or misbranding of medical devices.

Nevertheless, the FD&C Act had certain limitations. Manufacturers were required to notify the FDA only before marketing what they determined to be "new" drugs. Before marketing, the FDA could consider only the safety of a drug. Regulation of medical devices was limited to challenging products that were adulterated or misbranded after marketing through injunction, seizure, or criminal prosecution mechanisms.

For the next several decades, FDA enforcement resources were strained to handle the plethora of fraudulent medical devices being introduced. Furthermore, the revolution in biomedical technology following World War II resulted in the introduction of a wide variety of devices that also demanded attention from the agency. Concerns about medical devices were of low priority in the FDA's Bureau of Drugs, which also regulated medical devices.

In 1955, a Citizen's Advisory Committee of the FDA appointed by the secretary of the Department of Health, Education, and Welfare (DHEW), Oveta B. Hobby, concluded that false claims were frequently being made for medical devices and that additional resources were required by the FDA to deal with the problem. Furthermore, the limitations of the FDA's regulation of medical devices were brought to the attention of Congress when they were debating passage of the Drug Amendments of 1962. To ensure rapid passage of these amendments, however, provisions dealing with medical devices, in particular premarket notification, were omitted from the final legislation. Nevertheless, the Drug Amendments of 1962 became the foundation for modern medical device regulation. Manufacturers of new drugs were then required to receive premarket approval by the FDA before marketing. Previously, manufacturers provided the FDA with notification before marketing. Approval was no longer based solely on the safety of a new drug but also on its effectiveness. After the Drug Amendments of 1962, the FDA successfully sought to regulate certain medical devices by defining them as "drugs."

Between 1962 and 1969 many bills were introduced into Congress to address many of the perceived shortcomings regarding the regulation of medical devices. In 1969 a national conference was convened in Washington, DC, on the subject of medical device regulation, the results of which were published in the *Journal of the American Medical Association* (8). In his October 1969 consumer message, President Richard M. Nixon endorsed medical device legislation and promised that a thorough study would be undertaken before any legislative action was taken. The secretary of the DHEW, Elliott Richardson, soon thereafter formed a study group on medical devices. It was chaired by Dr Theodore Cooper, the director of the National Heart and Lung Institute.

The Cooper committee consisted of two government officials from the FDA, five from the National Institutes of Health, and three from other parts of the DHEW. Their report, issued in September 1970, concluded that it was not acceptable to treat medical devices as new drugs. It documented at least 10,000 injuries from medical devices, including 731 deaths (512 from defective heart valves). It recommended a regulatory system with requirements calibrated to the issues of safety and effectiveness of the specific medical device. All medical devices already on the market were to be inventoried and classified into a three-tiered system. It also detailed requirements for records and reports, registration and inspection of establishments, and uniform quality assurance programs called good manufacturing practices.

Legislative and administrative action commenced on receipt of the Cooper report. The DHEW prepared legislation based on the Cooper committee recommendations, and it was introduced in 1971. The FDA created a medical device advisory panel, performed an inventory of devices already on the market, and started the process of their classification. Fourteen panels of experts were established to classify the devices. Preliminary classification reports were issued before final legislation was completed in 1976.

Senate bill SR 510, which was introduced by Senator Edward M. Kennedy, was passed by the Senate in 1975, and House bill HR 11124, which was introduced by Representative Paul Rogers, was passed by the House in 1976. These bills eventually became the Medical Device Amendments of 1976, which were signed into law by President Nixon. The Medical Device Amendments of 1976 expanded the length of the FD&C Act by about one-third and became the basis for current medical device regulation in the United States.

The Medical Device Amendments of 1976 broadened the definition of a "medical device." They authorized the FDA to categorize all medical devices into a three-tiered classification and regulatory system based on their risk. It specified two types of premarketing procedures. A detailed submission, called a premarket approval or "PMA," was implemented for new and high-risk devices. A less thorough submission was implemented for devices that were "substantially equivalent" to those that

History of Medical Device Regulation

Legislation	Date Signed	President Signing	Legal Reference	Comment
Food and Drug Act	June 30, 1906	Theodore Roosevelt	Pub L no. 59-384, 34 Stat 768, 21 USC §1-15	No mention of medical devices; postmarketing enforcement authority over food and drugs
Food, Drug and Cosmetic Act	June 25, 1938	Franklin D. Roosevelt	Pub L no. 75-717, 52 Stat 1040, 21 USC §301-394	Postmarketing enforcement authority over adulterated and misbranded devices, premarketing enforcement authority over food and drugs
New Drug Amendments	October 10, 1962	John F. Kennedy	Pub L no. 87-781, 76 Stat 780, 21 USC §301-394	No mention of medical devices; premarketing approval of new drugs
Medical Device Amendments of 1976	May 28, 1976	Richard M. Nixon	Pub L no. 94-295, 90 Stat 539, 21 USC §301-394	Premarketing enforcement authority over devices, three-tiered classification and control of devices, substantial equivalency, investigational device exemption, registration and listing, good manufacturing practices, manufacturer medical device reporting, banning authority, notification, and repair, replacement, or refund authority
Safe Medical Devices Act of 1990	November 28, 1990	George H. W. Bush	Pub L no. 101-629, 104 Stat 4511, 21 USC §301-394	User facility and distributor medical device reporting, postmarketing surveillance and tracking, safety and effectiveness summaries in 510(k) submissions, substantial equivalency to postamendment devices and based on improved safety and effectiveness, civil penalties, recalls, humanitarian exemptions
Medical Device Amendments	June 16, 1992	George H.W. Bush	Pub L no. 102-300, 106 Stat 238, 21 USC §301-394	Broadened medical device reporting, postmarket surveillance enforcement authority, delay of tracking regulations, and enhanced repair, replace or refund authority

Note.—Pub L = Public law (Pub L No. Congress number-slip number), Stat = Statute at large (volume number "Stat" page number), USC = U.S. Code (title or volume number "USC" section number).

had been marketed before enactment of the Medical Device Amendments of 1976. This was called a premarket notification or "510(k)" because it was detailed in section 510(k) of the FD&C Act (21 USC §360[k]).

Other provisions of the Medical Device Amendments of 1976 dealt with good manufacturing practices; the authority to ban dangerous products and to require notification, recall, repair, or refund by manufacturers of defective devices; investigational device exemptions; the listing of all medical devices and the registration of establishments responsible for their manufacture; and manufacturer medical device reporting for adverse events related to medical devices.

Congress conducted several major oversight hearings or investigations of the medical device industry and FDA regulation between 1982 and 1988. In 1983, the General Accounting Office issued a report entitled *Federal Regulation of Medical Devices: Problems Still to Be Overcome.* In 1985 the Office of Technology Assessment issued a report concluding that strong reliance on demonstration of substantial equivalence to previously marketed products to expedite regulatory approval would stifle innovation. Problems with heart valves, injectable collagen, intrauterine devices, and intraocular lenses also focused public attention on the regulation of medical devices. These events led to the Safe Medical Devices Act of 1990.

The primary intention of the Safe Medical Devices Act of 1990 was to strengthen the FDA's authority to monitor marketed products, thereby expediting the review process because of less rigid premarketing review criteria. Provisions of the Safe Medical Devices Act of 1990 concerned user and distributor medical device reporting, postmarketing surveillance and tracking, civil penalties, recall authority, humanitarian device exemptions, allowing "substantial equivalency" to postamendment devices, allowing "substantial equivalency" based on enhanced safety and effectiveness, and safety and effectiveness summaries in 510(k) submissions. The Safe Medical Devices Act of 1990 also substituted the word "primary" for "principal" and removed the restriction that a drug could not be considered a device in the definition of a medical device (see Introduction).

To clarify the Safe Medical Devices Act of 1990, the Medical Device Amendments of 1992 were passed. This legislation broadened the indications for medical device reporting, provided enforcement authority for postmarket surveillance, delayed tracking regulations, and enhanced authority for requiring repair, replacement, or refund. Minor adjustments in the medical device regulatory process have continued through administrative and legislative activities since implementation of the Medical Device Amendments of 1992.

THE FDA

Creation

The Food and Drug Act was designed by Dr Harvey Wiley, who was the chief chemist in the Department of Agriculture. When the Bureau of Chemistry was created in 1907 in the Department of Agriculture, he became its director. The Bureau of Chemistry became the initial administrator of the Food and Drug Act and the progenitor of the modern FDA. The Food and Drug Act and subsequent amendments gave the Bureau of Chemistry the authority to stop the sale of food and drugs that it could prove were adulterated (unsafe) or misbranded (bearing misleading claims of effectiveness) but only after they were marketed (Fig 4). Enforcement was by criminal penalties and seizure power. Initially, "misbranding" referred only to false or fraudulent claims regarding the identity of a product's ingredients. In 1911, the Sherley Amendment expanded the definition of "misbranded" to include knowingly false and fraudulent claims about curative or therapeutic effects. No provisions were made for the review, testing, or approval of food and drugs before they were sold. This resulted in the potential exposure of the public to fraud and serious injury before unsatisfactory products could be removed from the market.

The Bureau of Chemistry closed in 1927 with the creation of the Food, Drug and Insecticide Administration. The name was shortened to the Food and Drug Administration in 1931. In 1940 the FDA was transferred from the Department of Agriculture to the Federal Security Agency, which became the DHEW in 1953. In 1968 the FDA became part of the PHS. The DHEW became the DHHS in 1979 with the transfer of educational issues to the new Department of Education.

1798	The Public Health Service is created.
1862	The Department of Agriculture is created.
1907	The Bureau of Chemistry is created in Department of Agriculture and becomes the administrator of the Food and Drug Act of 1906.
1927	The Bureau of Chemistry closes, and the Food, Drug and Insecticide Administration is formed.
1931	The name is shortened to the Food and Drug Administration (FDA).
1939	The Federal Security Agency (FSA) is created.
1940	The FDA is transferred from the Department of Agriculture to the FSA.
1953	The FSA becomes the Department of Health, Education and Welfare (DHEW).
1968	The FDA becomes part of the Public Health Service in the DHEW.
1971	The Office of Medical Devices is transferred from the FDA's Bureau of Drugs to the Office of the Associate Commissioner.
1973	The FDA Bureau of Product Safety becomes the Consumer Product Safety Commission.
1974	The Office of Medical Devices is transferred out of FDA's Office of the Associate Commissioner to create the Bureau of Medical Devices and Diagnostic Products.
1979	With creation of the Department of Education, the DHEW becomes the Department of Health and Human Services.
1982	The FDA Bureau of Radiological Health combines with the Bureau of Medical Devices and Diagnostic Products to form the Center for Devices and Radiological Health.
1982	FDA Bureau of Biologics combines with Bureau of Drugs to form the Center for Drugs and Biologics.
1987	Center for Drugs and Biologics separates into the Centers for Biologics Evaluation and Research (CBER) and Drug Evaluation and Research (CDER).
1988	Congress passes legislation establishing FDA by statute.

Figure 4. History of the FDA.

Current Structure

The FDA is a federal agency of the PHS in the DHHS, which is a cabinet-level department in the executive branch of government (Fig 5). It is headed by the commissioner of Food and Drugs. A number of offices and deputy commissioners report to the commissioner of the FDA. The deputy commissioner for operations is the second in command and is the top enforcement manager on matters of compliance, court enforcement, and field operations. A number of associate commissioners and center directors report to the deputy commissioners.

Office of Regulatory Affairs.—The Office of Regulatory Affairs oversees the Offices of Criminal Investigations, Resource Management, Enforcement, and Regional Operations and a field force. It is responsible for evaluating and coordinating all proposed compliance efforts and legal actions. The field force consists of six regional offices (in San Francisco, Calif; Dallas, Tex; Chicago, Ill; Atlanta, Ga; Philadelphia, Pa; and New York, NY) and 21 district offices. The district offices schedule and perform routine inspections, do complaint investigations and directed inspections as requested by the centers, investigate complaints by patients or hospitals, perform or arrange for laboratory testing of devices, and decide on the appropriate FDA response to the findings of its investigations. Inspections can also be made by resident post inspectors based in smaller towns. Before granting premarket approval of class III medical devices, the FDA sends a field investigator to audit the manufacturing site. Furthermore, once a device is cleared for marketing, the primary FDA contact for a manufacturer is with the district offices.

Center for Devices and Radiological Health.—The Center for Devices and Radiological Health (CDRH) has the primary responsibility for regulating medical devices. It consists of six offices (Fig 6). The CDRH develops, administers, and ensures compliance with programs designed to ensure the safe and effective use of medical devices.

The Office of Device Evaluation consists of six divisions, which are further divided into branches and groups. This office classifies devices; reviews and evaluates medical device premarket approvals, product development protocols, investigational device exemptions, and 510(k) submissions; and monitors the performance of devices once used.

The Office of Health and Industry Programs consists of four divisions (Fig 6). The Division of Small Manufacturers Assistance was created in response to the Medical Device Amendments of 1976, which directed the FDA to establish an office to provide technical and regulatory assistance to small manufacturers in complying with the requirements for medical devices. In reality, information can be obtained by anyone by means of personal visits, mail, telephone, fax, or computer on-line service. This division also conducts regional educational seminars for the medical device industry.

The Office of Surveillance and Biometrics designs surveillance programs and activities, collects and analyzes data (such as adverse event reports collected under medical device reporting regulations), and provides expertise regarding biostatistics, health economics, and methods for ensuring cost-effectiveness. The Office of Compliance designs, develops, and implements programs for compliance, establishment registra-

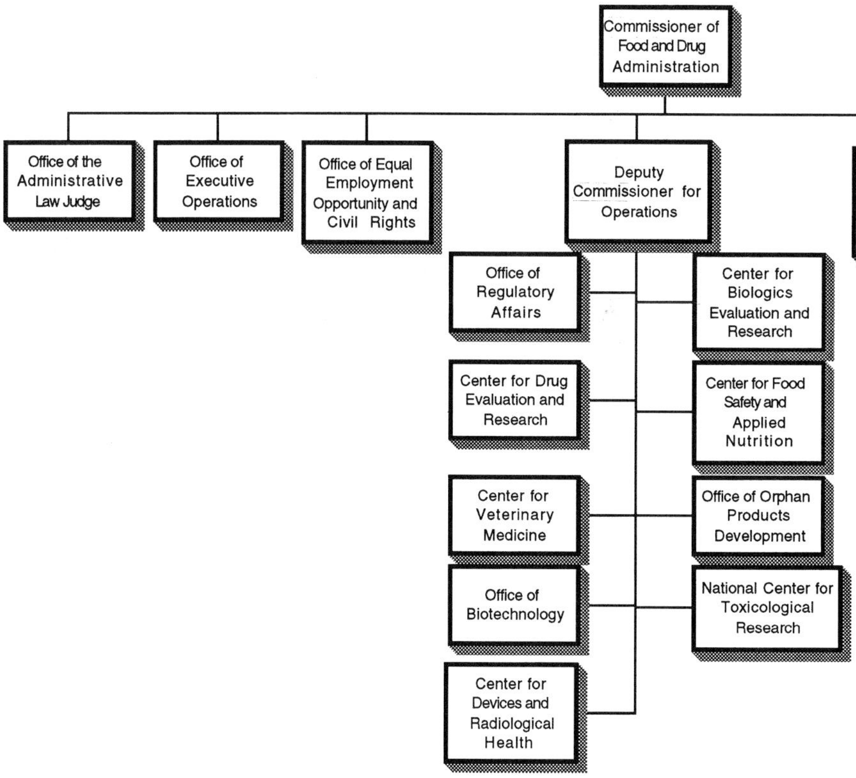

Figure 5. Organization of the FDA.

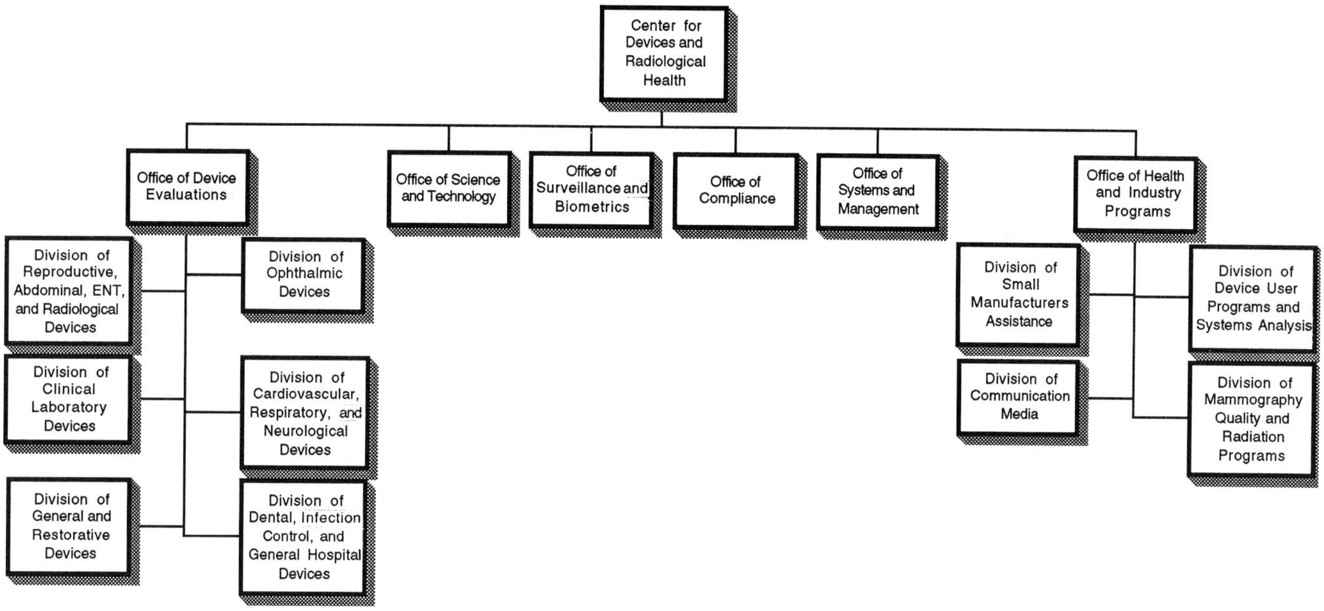

Figure 6. Organization of the CDRH.

tion, and device listing. The Office of Science and Technology provides scientific support and laboratory analysis for the rest of the Center and the FDA. The Office of Systems and Management provides administrative management support for the Center.

Center for Biologics Evaluation and Research.—The Center for Biologics Evaluation and Research (CBER) (Fig 5) works with the CDRH to regulate medical devices used for the collection, processing, or administration of biologic products. An intercenter agreement details the jurisdiction of the CBER and CDRH. The CBER has primary regulatory responsibility for medical devices that are used for the collection, processing, storage, or administration of blood products, blood components, and bone marrow or analogous products unless they are intended for direct therapeutic action in a particular patient. For example, plasmapheresis machines are regulated by the CBER, whereas blood administration sets are regulated by the

CDRH. The CBER also is responsible for in vitro reagents that use various antibody products and all in vitro tests and any other medical devices related to the human immunodeficiency virus.

Center for Drug Evaluation and Research.—The Center for Drug Evaluation and Research (CDER) (Fig 5) works with the CDRH to regulate medical devices that have some drug action. An intercenter agreement details the jurisdiction of the CDER and CDRH. Since imaging agents and radiopharmaceuticals interact with the body, they are considered drugs and are regulated by the Office of Drug Evaluation III in the CDER. For a product that is a combination of a device and a drug, its primary mode of action dictates whether CBER or CDRH will have primary jurisdiction. For example, a polymer wafer designed to release a chemotherapeutic agent would be regulated by the CDER, whereas a bone cement with impregnated antibiotic is regulated by the CDRH.

APPENDIX: PRINCIPLES OF GOVERNMENT DOCUMENT NOMENCLATURE

"Laws" or "statutes" are defined as "rules of conduct or procedures established by custom, agreement, or authority." There are two types of laws: statutory or quasistatutory laws and case laws (9). Statutory laws are original laws that relate to civil or criminal matters that are enacted by a body legally authorized to pass laws. Congress enacts federal laws, state legislatures enact state laws, and city councils enact municipal ordinances.

Case laws are usually derived from the precedent-setting opinions and decisions of appellate courts, which are binding on lower courts. Appellate cases are decided by federal and state appellate judges. Appellate courts hear cases that are appealed from the lower trial courts. Agencies also have the authority to conduct hearings, decide enforcement cases, and hear appeals and therefore establish orders that are applied as laws.

Federal laws enacted by Congress are introduced into either of the two houses of Congress: the Senate or House of Representatives. Bills are read by title and assigned a number, for example, bill SR 510 or bill HR 11124. Bills then go to committees, where over 85% of them never receive consideration and die. If a bill dies, it can be reintroduced in subsequent congressional sessions. SR 510 went initially to the Senate Committee on Commerce and then to the Committee on Labor and Public Welfare. HR 11124 went to the House Committee on Interstate and Foreign Commerce.

In committee there may be hearings, the findings of which can be published. After hearings, study, and investigation, the committee submits a report stating whether the bill should be passed. These reports are numbered. For example, the senate report on SR 510 was S Rep 94-33 and the house report on HR 11124 was HR Rep 94-853. These refer to the 33rd Senate and 853rd House Committee reports of the 94th Congress. When the bill is reported out of committee it is put on a calendar and eventually read. Debates then take place; these are usually published in the *Congressional Record*, and then the bill is voted on.

If a bill is passed in one house it is referred to as an *act*, and it goes on to the other house. The act may be passed, rejected, or amended and returned to the originating house by the second house. If the other house passes a different version of the bill, a Committee of Conference is formed to resolve the differences between the two. In the case of the Medical Device Amendments of 1976, the Committee of Conference submitted a compromise bill on May 6, 1976 (HR Rep 94-1090).

Once the two houses pass a single uniform version of the act it is signed by the head of the Senate, who is the vice president, and the head of the House of Representatives, who is the House Speaker, and sent to the president for consideration. The act becomes law if the president signs it or if it is not vetoed within 10 days.

At this point the law is referred to as a public law or statute and is published in various sets. Initially it is published by the Government Printing Office as a *slip law*, which is an individual publication in pamphlet form. The Office of the Federal Register of the General Services Administration assigns it a public law number. These numbers run in sequence and start anew each congressional year. For example, the Medical Device Amendments of 1992 are referred to as Pub L no. 102-300, June 16, 1992 (Public Law, 102nd Congress, Slip Law 300, enacted on June 16, 1992).

Within 2–3 years of enactment, slip laws are compiled by the Government Printing Office into a set of volumes referred to as *The United States Statutes at Large*. These volumes are arranged in chronological order and contain all public laws followed by private laws, presidential proclamations, reorganization plans, and constitutional amendments. Approximately five additional volumes are produced for each congressional session. Individual volumes have a subject index. Citations are by volume and page number. For example, the Medical Device Amendments of 1992 are cited as 106 Stat 238 (vol 106, Statutes at Large, p 238).

To allow for easier access to laws, the federal government has "codified" or arranged laws into a systematic, classified order. This compilation is referred to as the USC. The USC is divided into 50 "titles" or subject areas and is published by the Government Printing Office every 6 years. Matters dealing with food, drugs, and medical devices are included in Title 21. Citations are by title and section number. For example, details regarding premarket notification that are found in section 510(k) of the FD&C Act can be found in 21 USC §360(k), or title 21, United States Code, section 360(k).

Two annotated sets of the USC are published by private firms that use the same numbering system. The *United States Code Annotated* is published by West Publishing Company. The *United States Code Service* is published by Lawyers Cooperative Publishing Company.

Quasistatutory laws are rules (same as regulations) written by federal, state, county, and city agencies. These agencies issue orders (final disposition of matters before them), issue licenses or permits to operate under agency control, issue advisory opinions about their regulations, and conduct hearings. Hearings arise from violations or controversies over interpretations of their regulations. These are conducted by administrative law judges or review boards.

Federal agencies get their regulation making and enforcing authority from federal statutes and from presidential executive orders. Proposed rules are published in the *Federal Register* with notices of pertinent public hearings and comment periods. After the hearings and comments, necessary changes are made and the final regulations are published in the *Federal Register* with effective dates. The *Federal Register* is published daily by the Government Printing Office and is arranged chronologically, as is the *Statutes at Large.* Citations are by volume number, page number, and date. For example, regulations concerning informed consent for clinical investigations are found in 46 FR 8942, January 27, 1981 (vol 46, *Federal Register,* page 8942, appearing on January 27, 1981).

Current, general, and permanent regulations of federal agencies are codified annually in the *Code of Federal Regulations* (CFR). The CFR is to the *Federal Register* what the USC is to the Statutes at Large. Similar to the USC, the CFR is divided into 50 "titles" representing different broad subject areas. Approximately half of these "titles" correspond to the same subject areas as the USC titles of the same number. For example, 21 CFR and 21 USC both deal with food, drug, and medical device issues. Citations are by title number and part or section number. Medical device—related issues are found in parts 800–1299. For example, medical device reporting requirements are found in 21 CFR 803 (title 21, Code of Federal Regulations, part 803). One fourth of the CFR is published by the Government Printing Office every quarter (Title 21 usually by April 1). ■

Acknowledgments: I thank Stacey J. Ackerman, MSE, PhD (Covance, Inc), Richard P. Kidwell, JD (Johns Hopkins University), and Marlene K. Tandy, MD, JD (Health Industry Manufacturers Association), for reviewing the manuscript.

References

1. Hutt P. A history of government regulation of adulteration and misbranding of medical devices. In: Estrin N, ed. The medical devices industry: science, technology, and regulation in a competitive environment. New York, NY: Dekker, 1990; 17–33.
2. Wholey M, Haller J. An introduction to the Food and Drug Administration and how it evaluates new devices: establishing safety and efficacy. Cardiovasc Intervent Radiol 1995; 18:72–76.
3. O'Reilly J. Food and Drug Administration. Colorado Springs, Colo: Shepard's/McGraw-Hill, 1993.
4. Merrill RA. Regulation of drugs and devices: an evolution. Health Aff 1994; 13:47–69.
5. Kaufman J. Medical device regulation in the United States: protecting the public or impeding progress. Semin Intervent Radiol 1995; 12:277-283.
6. Gallivan M. The 1997 global medical technology update: the challenges facing U.S. industry and policy makers. Washington, DC: Health Industry Manufacturers Association, 1997; 37–51.
7. Forces reshaping the performance and contribution of the U.S. medical device industry. New York, NY: Wilkerson Group, 1995; 3–31.
8. Harkin D, Beall A. Excerpts and summary of a National Conference on Medical Devices: Bethesda, Md, September 6–7, 1969. JAMA 1969; 210:1745–1751.
9. Coco A. Finding the law: a workbook on

Lee H. Monsein, MD, MPH

Primer on Medical Device Regulation
Part II. Regulation of Medical Devices by the U.S. Food and Drug Administration[1]

THIS article is the second in a three-part series reviewing medical device regulation. Part I provided an overview and history of medical device regulation and the Food and Drug Administration (FDA) and discussed government document nomenclature; part II details current medical device regulation. Part III describes regulatory mechanisms and enforcement of medical device regulation; it also reviews the regulation of imported and exported medical devices, as well as foreign medical devices.

CLASSIFICATION OF MEDICAL DEVICES

The regulation of medical devices in the United States is based on a three-tiered classification system. Products are categorized as class I, II, or III devices: The higher the class, the greater the risk and degree of regulation (Table). Class I, II, and III devices are associated with general controls. In addition, class II and III devices are also associated with (*a*) performance standards or special controls and (*b*) PMA, respectively.

"Preamendment" devices, those that were legally marketed before enactment of the Medical Device Amendments (MDA) of 1976 on May 28, 1976, were classified by 19 "classification panels" organized by the FDA. Preliminary classification commenced 5 years before and was largely completed by the time the MDA of 1976 were enacted. To aid in classification, panels were given a list of 18 yes-or-no questions. Final classifications of approximately 1,700 generic product categories were codified as regulations in title 21 of the *Code of Federal Regulations* (21 CFR) in the 1970s and 1980s. The generic categories, classification numbers, classes, and relevant regulation numbers also are found in the book *Classification Names for Medical Devices and in Vitro Diagnostics*, available from the Division of Small Manufacturers Assistance.

In 1990, the original classification panels were replaced by a medical devices advisory committee, which consists of 16 panels, each concerned with a different medical specialty, including Anesthesiology and Respiratory Therapy; Circulatory System; Clinical Chemistry and Clinical Toxicology; Dental Products; Ear, Nose and Throat; Gastroenterology-Urology; General and Plastic Surgery; General Hospital and Personal Uses; Hematology and Pathology; Immunology; Microbiology; Neurological; Obstetrics-Gynecology; Ophthalmology; Orthopedics and Rehabilitation; and Radiological Devices. Each panel consists of six professional voting members, one nonvoting consumer member, and one nonvoting industry member, each serving a 4-year term. Several nonvoting consultants may be used. The panels provide guidance to the respective branch of the Office of Device Evaluations on a number of issues, including device classification; however, their decisions are not binding (Fig 1). Meetings are open to the public, and interested persons are allowed to make statements to the panels. Portions of meetings that relate to trade secrets or confidential information may be closed to the public. Transcripts and executive summaries are available from the FDA staff who respond to Freedom of Information requests, from Freedom of Information Services (Rockville, Md) or similar businesses, or from private transcription companies hired to transcribe specific meetings. Tentative schedules for all panel meetings are published in the *Federal Register* at the beginning of the year. Final schedules for meetings are published in the *Federal Register* at least 15 days before the meeting and are available by calling the FDA Advisory Committee Information Line (1-800-741-8138).

So that it would have the least commercial and medical effect on devices already in use, the MDA of 1976 allowed for the continued distribution or reintroduction of most unchanged "preamendment" devices subject to all relevant controls of their class, with the exception that a premarketing notification (510[k]; described later) submission is not required. The FDA will eventually call for PMA submissions for all preamendment class III devices. All postamendment devices require a 510(k) or PMA.

As set forth in the MDA of 1976, all postamendment devices were automatically placed in class III unless they were substantially equivalent to a preamendment device, in which case they were placed in the same class as their predicate device. They may later be reclassified to class I or II. The Safe Medical Devices Act (SMDA) of 1990 allowed demonstra-

Radiology 1997; 205:10–18

Index terms: Radiology and radiologists • State-of-art reviews • U.S. Food and Drug Administration

[1] From the Department of Radiology, Washington Hospital Center, 110 Irving St NW, #BA68, Washington, DC 20010-2975. Received March 27, 1997; revision requested May 19; revision received June 13; accepted June 23. **Address reprint requests to** the author.

Abbreviations: FDA = Food and Drug Administration, FD&C = Food, Drug and Cosmetic, GMP = good manufacturing practice, HUD = humanitarian-use device, IDE = investigational device exemption, IRB = investigational review board, MDA = Medical Device Amendments, MDR = medical device report, PDP = product development protocol, PMA = premarket approval, SMDA = Safe Medical Devices Act.

Classification of Medical Devices

			Product Approval		
				Post-1976 Devices	
Class	Examples	Controls	Pre-1976 Devices	Substantially Equivalent	Not Substantially Equivalent
I	Tongue depressors, gauze	General	Continued marketing of devices already on market	510(k) submission required*†	510(k) submission required
II	Physiologic monitors, angiography catheters	General and special	Continued marketing of devices already on market	510(k) submission required*	510(k) submission required
III	Heart valves, coronary angioplasty catheters	General and PMA	Continued marketing of devices already on market until PMA called for	510(k) submission required until PMA called for, then PMA required	PMA required unless reclassified as a class I or II device‡

Note.—PMA = premarket approval.
* If the predicate device was cleared through the PMA process, a PMA is required.
† Some class I devices are exempt from 510(k) requirements (eg, cotton tip applicators).
‡ All new devices that are not substantially equivalent are automatically considered class III devices and therefore require a PMA. The FDA or manufacturer may, however, petition to reclassify the device as a class I or class II device, making the 510(k) process applicable.

tion of substantial equivalence to any legally marketed device, regardless of its date of introduction, as long as it does not require a PMA. "Transitional" devices, those that were regulated as drugs before the MDA of 1976, are also assigned automatically to class III but may be reclassified.

The FDA may reclassify a device, either on its own initiative or on the basis of a petition of the manufacturer or any interested person. Reclassification of a device affects all devices in the same category. Thus, a petition for reclassification of a specific device is considered to be a petition to reclassify all devices within that device category. Informal inquiries about the present classification of a device can be made to the Division of Small Manufacturers Assistance. As directed by section 513(g) of the FD&C Act, formal determinations are initiated by filing a written "513(g)" request.

1. Review and evaluate available data concerning the safety and effectiveness of marketed and investigational devices
2. Advise the Commissioner of Food and Drugs regarding recommended classification of these devices into one of three regulatory categories
3. Recommend the assignment of a priority for the application of regulatory requirements for devices classified in the standards or premarket approval category.
4. Advise on any possible risks to health associated with the use of devices
5. Advise on formulation of product development protocols and review PMA applications for those devices classified in the PMA category.
6. Review classification as appropriate
7. Recommend exemptions to certain devices from the application of portions of the Food, Drug and Cosmetic (FD&C) Act
8. Advise on the necessity to ban a device
9. Respond to requests from the agency to review and make recommendations on specific issues or problems concerning the safety and effectiveness of a device.

Figure 1. Responsibilities of medical device advisory panels.

Class I

Class I devices are those that are adequately regulated by "general controls." Similar controls have been present since enactment of the FD&C Act in 1938. Section 513(a)(1)of the FD&C Act(21 USC §360c[a][1]) of the FD&C Act defines a class I device as one for which general controls "are sufficient to provide reasonable assurance of the safety and effectiveness of the device." Alternatively, there may not be enough evidence that general controls will "provide reasonable assurance of the safety and effectiveness of the device." However, a class I device "is not purported or represented to be for use in supporting or sustaining human life or for a use which is of substantial importance in preventing impairment of human health, and does not present a potential unreasonable risk of illness or injury."

A safe device is defined in 21 CFR §860.7(d) as one for which "the probable benefits from health from use of the device for its intended uses and conditions of use, when accompanied by adequate directions and warnings against unsafe use, outweigh any probable risks." An effective device is defined in 21 CFR §860.7(e) as one for which "in a significant portion of the target population, the use of the device for its intended uses and conditions of use, when accompanied by adequate directions for use and warnings against unsafe use, will provide clinically significant results."

General controls are largely postmarketing in nature and are aimed at ensuring that products are pure and safe (without adulteration) and that the labeling is informative and not misleading (without misbranding). Section 501 of the FD&C Act (21 USC §351) provides lengthy and detailed definitions of "adulteration," and section 502 of the FD&C Act (21 USC §352) defines "misbranding" (Fig 2). In addition to general guidelines concerning adulteration and misbranding, general controls in-

Devices are considered "adulterated" if they
1. include any filthy, putrid, or decomposed substance or are prepared, packed, or held under unsanitary conditions;
2. are in a container composed, in whole or part, of any poisonous or deleterious substance;
3. contain, for the purpose of coloring only, an unsafe color additive;
4. differ in strength from, or their purity or quality falls below, that which they claim to represent;
5. do not comply with the requirements for an approved PMA application or product development protocol;
6. are banned devices;
7. were designed or produced under conditions that violate good manufacturing practice (GMP) regulations; or
8. fail to comply with the investigational devices exemption regulation.

A device is considered "misbranded" if
1. its labeling is false or misleading in any particular;
2. it is in package form and its label fails to contain the name and place of business of the manufacturer, packer, or distributor and an accurate statement of the quantity of contents in terms of weight, measure, or numerical count;
3. any required wording is not prominently displayed as compared with any other wording on the device or is not clearly stated;
4. its label does not bear adequate directions for use, including warnings against use in certain pathologic conditions or by children, where its use may be dangerous to health; or against unsafe dosage or methods or duration of administration or application;
5. it is dangerous to health when used in the dosage or manner or with the frequency or duration prescribed, recommended, or suggested in the labeling; or
6. it does not comply with the color additives provisions under section 706 of the FD&C Act.

Figure 2. Definitions from the FD&C Act.

clude requirements for premarket notification, GMPs, registration and listing, restrictions (on the sale, distribution, or use of a device only upon authorization of a licensed practitioner), and records and reporting. Regulatory mechanisms, such as banning and notifications, recalls, repairs, replacements, or refunds for defective devices, also apply.

General controls are required for all devices except when they are inconsistent with performance standards or special control requirements for class II devices or PMA requirements for class III devices. Class I devices are subject to general controls only. The FDA may exempt a product from one or more of these general controls. For example, tongue blades are exempt from GMP and 510(k) requirements. Stethoscopes are exempt from GMP requirements.

Premarket notification.—Section 510(k) of the FD&C Act (21 USC §360[k]) describes the "premarket notification" or "510(k)" process. Companies are required to file a 510(k) application 90 days before anticipated marketing of postamendment class I and class II devices. They also may choose to file a 510(k) application instead of a PMA before marketing postamendment class III devices when they are substantially equivalent to a previously legally marketed "predicate" class III device for which a PMA has not yet been requested by the FDA, submitted, or approved. A new device that is not substantially equivalent is considered a class III device, which requires a PMA.

The purposes of a 510(k) are to identify new devices that must be placed automatically into class III and undergo PMA or reclassification before they are marketed; help classify new devices; and achieve marketing equity by allowing manufacturers of most new devices that are substantially equivalent to preamendment devices to market their devices without facing any greater regulatory burdens than faced by manufacturers of preamendment devices.

A 510(k) is required when a device is introduced into the market for the first time; a new device or product line is being introduced by a manufacturer that may already be marketed by another manufacturer; a device currently in, or being reintroduced into, commercial distribution is about to be substantially changed or modified in a way that could markedly affect the safety or effectiveness of the device; or there is a major change in the indication statement for the device.

The MDA of 1976 allowed demonstration of substantial equivalence to preamendment devices only. This policy was modified by the SMDA of 1990, which allows demonstration of substantial equivalence to any legally marketed device, regardless of its date of introduction, as long as it does not require a PMA. If a PMA has been submitted or approved for the predicate device or requested by the FDA, then the device requires a PMA. A device is considered substantially equivalent to a predicate device if it has the same intended use and technologic characteristics. It also may have the same intended use, but different technologic characteristics, if it can be demonstrated that the device is as safe and effective and does not raise different questions regarding safety and effectiveness.

The content of a 510(k) is specified in 21 CFR §807.81. If an application is incomplete, the FDA can refuse to accept the submission for substantive review. The review process is summarized in Figure 3. There is no time limit for the review process. The FDA may request further information during the review process; it must be submitted within 30 days unless an extension is obtained (1).

Under most circumstances, the FDA will not publicly disclose the existence of a 510(k) for up to 90 days after a submission for a device not on the market and for which the intent to market has not been publicly disclosed (21 CFR §807.95). The period of nondisclosure can be extended under certain circumstances. At the completion of the review process the FDA issues a "substantially equivalent letter" or a "not substantially equivalent letter." A substantially equivalent letter allows immediate marketing of a device. The FDA will make a 510(k) summary of the safety and effectiveness data available to the public within 30 days of the issuance of a determination that the device is substantially equivalent. Confidentiality cannot be granted beyond 30 days after the FDA issues a determination of equivalency. If a "not substantially equivalent letter" is issued, the manufacturer may appeal, file a reclassification petition, or submit a PMA.

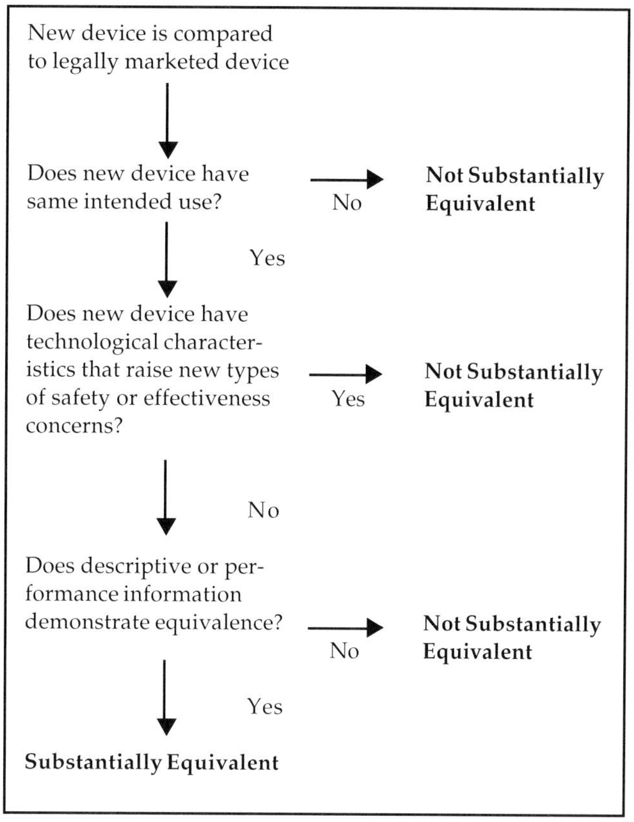

Figure 3. Substantial equivalence determination.

GMP.—The medical device industry consists of manufacturers whose devices and manufacturing processes differ greatly. It would therefore be inappropriate for the FDA to design one specific quality assurance program that would ensure that all finished medical devices are safe and effective. The FDA has thus identified the essential elements that a quality assurance program for any manufacturing operation must embody, without prescribing specific ways in which to establish them. These essential elements were meant to encompass all aspects of a product's life cycle, including customer requirements, development and production, and customer use and feedback. These requirements, referred to as GMPs, were set forth in 21 CFR §820 under authority of section 520 of the FD&C Act (21 USC §360[j]). They were recently revised and renamed Quality System Regulations. Most provisions became effective June 1, 1997. They provide details regarding quality assurance programs; organization and personnel; buildings; equipment; components; production and process controls; packaging and labeling control; holding, distribution, and installation; device evaluation; and records. Design control provisions also become effective sometime after June 1998.

To ensure conformity to GMP regulations, inspections are performed by the FDA district office personnel in the following order of priority: devices for which the last GMP inspection was violative without evidence of correction; critical devices for which a 510(k) was received without an inspection in the past 2 years for a similar device; class II or III devices with no record of a GMP inspection; all other critical risk devices beginning with the "oldest" GMP inspection; and other inspections (initial, PMA, reinspections). If FDA inspections reveal violations of the GMP requirements, companies may receive warning letters or be subject to other enforcement actions. Violations relevant to a specific product with a pending 510(k) or PMA may result in delay of its marketing application.

Registration and listing.—Section 510 of the FD&C Act (21 USC §360) authorized regulations (21 CFR §807) requiring domestic firms to register with the FDA before initially engaging in the manufacture, preparation, propagation, compounding, assembly, or processing of medical devices (form 2891) and annually thereafter (form 2891a). Registration requirements apply to firms that develop specifications for a device, distributors of domestic and imported products, repackagers, relabelers, and manufacturers. They also apply when a manufacturer produces a device for itself or another firm but not when the device is produced to the other firm's specifications and is to be marketed by the other firm. A company must register all establishments where the devices are manufactured or processed. Registrants receive a permanent registration number from the FDA.

Until recently, foreign manufacturers were requested, but not required, to register. New regulations (21 CFR §807.40) issued by the FDA on December 11, 1995 (effective on April 11, 1996, extended until July 31, 1996, and stayed on July 23, 1996)(61 FR 38346, July 23, 1996), required that foreign manufacturers that export devices into the United States designate an agent in the United States to be responsible for registering its establishments (similar to the requirement for a domestic firm). The U.S. designated agent is responsible for submitting medical device reports (MDRs) and annual certifications; acting as the official correspondent; and submitting registration information, device listing information, and marketing applications.

Section 510 of the FD&C Act (21 USC §360) requires domestic and foreign manufacturers to list their devices in commercial distribution with the FDA on form 2892. Manufacturers are also required (21 CFR §807.31) to maintain a historic listing file of labeling and advertisements. Manufacturers must report changes in listing on a new form 2892 when the change occurs or by June or December of each year, whichever comes first. Distributors are required to provide the FDA, by letter, with the manufacturer's name and address for each device they distribute.

Registration and listing requirements do not apply to manufacturers of raw materials; manufacturers of veterinary products; manufacturers of general-purpose articles like chemical reagents; licensed practitioners; pharmacies and other retail outlets; persons who make devices for use in teaching, research, or analysis; wholesalers and warehousers; common carriers; and dispensers of devices to the ultimate consumers such as opticians.

Restrictions.—Section 520(e)(1) of the FD&C Act (21 USC §360[j][e]) authorizes the FDA to establish regulations that may restrict the sale, distribution, or use of a device only on the written or oral authorization of a practitioner licensed by law to administer or use such a device or on other conditions it may specify. This may occur when the safety and effectiveness of a device may be affected greatly by its potentially harmful effects or the collateral measures needed for its use. The FDA has not implemented specific regulations regarding "restricted" devices; however, it derives authority from the requirements pertaining to misbranding. All devices must bear a statement on the label giving adequate directions for use. If a device cannot be properly used by laypersons, no directions can be adequate, and therefore the use of the device must be restricted.

Section 520(e)(1) of the FD&C Act (21 USC §360j[e]) also stipulates that the FDA may not restrict the use of a device to a person with specific training or experience in its use or to persons for use in facilities unless the FDA determines that such a restriction is required for the safe and effective use of the device. In addition, no person can be prevented from using a device solely because he or she does not have the training or experience required for board certification by a certifying board recognized by the American Board of Medical Specialties or because he or she has not been certified by such a board.

Records and reporting.—To ensure that medical devices are safe and effective and are not adulterated or misbranded, the FDA has established record-keeping and reporting requirements for manufacturers, importers, and distributors of medical devices, as well as for user facilities (2,3). These requirements specify mechanisms by which certain adverse events related to medical devices are reported to the FDA (21 CFR §803 and 21 CFR §804) and other device-related events are recorded; they also require implementation of tracking systems for patients who receive certain devices (21 CFR §821).

Under authority of section 519 of the FD&C Act (21 USC §360[i]) and the MDA of 1976, the FDA issued MDR regulations for manufacturers in 1984. To correct weaknesses in these reporting requirements and to better protect the public health, Congress enacted the SMDA of 1990. This act required distributors and user facilities to report certain adverse events related to medical devices. In response, the FDA issued temporary final rules, which became effective by operation of law for user facilities on November 28, 1991, and for distributors on May 28, 1992. Modifications in reporting requirements for manufacturers and user facilities were mandated by the MDA of 1992 and incorporated in a final rule issued on December 11, 1995, effective on April 11, 1996, and extended until July 31, 1996 (21 CFR §803).

Under the new regulations, user facilities must submit an MDR to the device manufacturer within 10 work days after "becoming aware of information from any source that reasonably suggests that a device has or may have caused or contributed to the death or serious injury of a patient of the facility." If the event involves a device-related death, or if the identity of the device manufacturer is unknown, the report must be sent to the FDA. User facilities must also submit semiannual reports on FDA form 3419 or its electronic equivalent to the FDA by January 1 and July 1. These reports summarize all MDR reportable events at that facility during the preceding 6 months.

Device manufacturers are required to submit MDRs to the FDA within 30 calendar days whenever the manufacturer "becomes aware" of information from any source that reasonably suggests that a device marketed by the manufacturer may have caused or contributed to a death or serious injury, or that such a device has malfunctioned and it or a similar device marketed by the manufacturer would be likely to cause or contribute to a death or serious injury (21 CFR §803.20). On receiving information about an MDR event, device manufacturers must also submit a "5-day report" to the FDA within 5 work days of becoming aware that (*a*) a reportable MDR event or events, from any information source, including a trend analysis, necessitates remedial action to prevent an unreasonable risk of substantial harm to the public health or (*b*) an MDR reportable event has prompted the FDA to make a written request for such a report (21 CFR §803.53). New regulations, effective May 19, 1997 (62 FR 13302), require manufacturers (21 CFR §803.57) and distributors (21 CFR §804.30) to certify the number of MDRs filed with the FDA during the preceding year on form 3381 or its electronic equivalent.

Device manufacturers are responsible for submitting MDRs related to their devices, whether or not they are still marketing the devices. If a manufacturer receives information about a reportable event involving a device incorrectly identified as one they marketed, the information must be forwarded to the FDA with a cover letter explaining that the device in question was not manufactured by that firm.

Terms relating to MDRs are detailed in 21 CFR §803.3. A device "user facility" means a hospital, ambulatory surgical facility, nursing home, outpatient diagnostic facility, or outpatient treatment facility that is not a physician's office. A physician's office means a facility that operates as the office of a physician or other health care professional (eg, a dentist, chiropractor, optometrist, nurse practitioner, or school nurse, as well as school clinics, employee health clinics, or free-standing care units) for the primary purpose of examination, evaluation, and treatment or referral of patients.

"Become aware" means that an employee of the entity required to report has acquired information reasonably suggesting a reportable adverse event has occurred. Device user facilities are considered to have become aware when medical personnel employed or otherwise formally affiliated with the facility acquire such information about a reportable event. Manufacturers are considered to have become aware when any employee becomes aware of a reportable event that is required to be reported within 30 days or that is required to be reported within 5 days pursuant to a written request from the FDA under 21 CFR §803.53(b). Manufacturers are also considered to have become aware when any employee with (*a*) management or supervisory responsibilities over persons with regulatory, scientific, or technical responsibilities or (*b*) duties related to the collection and reporting of adverse events becomes aware of a reportable MDR event or events (from any source of information, including trend analysis) that necessitate remedial action to prevent an unreasonable risk of substantial harm to the public health.

"Serious injury" means an injury or illness that is life threatening, results in permanent impairment of a body function or permanent damage to body structure, or necessitates medical or surgical intervention to preclude permanent impairment of a body function or permanent damage to a body structure.

User facilities and manufacturers must submit all reports of individual adverse events on FDA form 3500A (MedWatch form) or in an electronic equivalent as approved under 21 CFR §803.14. FDA form 3500A is the mandatory reporting form to be used by user facilities and manufacturers for submitting reports of FDA-regulated products.

The reports are confidential as long as they are not falsified. Any report, including any FDA record of a telephone report, submitted under 21 CFR §803 is available for public disclosure in accordance with 21 CFR §20. Before public disclosure of a report, the FDA will delete any information that constitutes a trade secret or confidential information (including serial number of implanted devices) or that constitutes an invasion of personal privacy (21 CFR §20.63), as well as any names and other identifying information of a third party voluntarily submitting an adverse event report.

In June 1993, a voluntary reporting program for health care professionals, the FDA Medical Product Reporting Program (MedWatch), was initiated. Serious adverse events and problems with marketed prescription and over-the-counter medications (except vaccines), medical devices, and special nutritional or other medical products regulated by the FDA can be reported with a single form (FDA form 3500). Voluntary reports can also be reported by means of telephoning 1-800-FDA-1088 (1-800-332-1088). Voluntary reporting does not obviate mandatory reporting obligations for manufacturers, distributors, and device user facilities.

Under authority of the MDA of 1992, the FDA will also eventually issue regulations requiring user facilities, manufacturers, importers, and distributors to report "significant adverse device experiences" that might otherwise not fall within the "reportable" categories (ie, death, serious injury, or serious illness).

Section 519(e) of the FD&C Act (21 USC §360i[e]; 21 CFR §821) requires manufacturers and distributors of permanently implantable, life-sustaining, or life-supporting devices used outside a health facility to adopt a system for tracking their devices through the chain of distribution to the patient to ensure that the device may be swiftly recalled if necessary. A manufacturer is required to provide the FDA with the distributor's name, address, and telephone number and the location of the tracked device, within 3 days of a request from the agency if prior to distribution of the device to a patient and within 10 days if already distributed to the patient. Distributors are required to submit information to the manufacturer within 5 days of a request and to the FDA within 10 days of a request. All records must be maintained for the useful life of each tracked device.

Postmarket surveillance.—Section 522 of the FD&C Act (21 USC §360[l]) requires postmarket surveillance for any device that was introduced into interstate commerce for the first time after January 1, 1991, and is (*a*) a permanently implantable device whose failure may cause serious adverse health consequences (not including temporary or reversible non–life-threatening injuries) or death, (*b*) a life-supporting or life-sustaining device, or (*c*) a device that potentially presents a serious risk to health. The FDA may also require postmarket surveillance of any other device it deems necessary to protect the public health.

Within 30 days after introduction of a device requiring postmarket surveillance into interstate commerce, the manufacturer must submit a protocol for this surveillance to the FDA. The FDA must determine whether the protocol is satisfactory within 60 days, during which time it must be reviewed by an appropriately qualified scientific and technical review committee established by the agency. If postmarket surveillance is called for by the FDA, a protocol must be submitted within 30 days.

Class II

Before enactment of the SMDA of 1990, devices were placed in class II if "performance standards" could be developed to provide reasonable assurance of their safety and effectiveness. According to section 514 of the FD&C Act (21 USC §360[d]), performance standards for a class II device "include provisions to provide reasonable assurance of its safe and effective performance"; when necessary, include provisions concerning "the construction, components, ingredients, and properties of the device and its compatibility with power systems," conformity to test results, and measurement of the performance characteristics; and "where appropriate, require the use and prescribe the form and content of the labeling for the proper installation, maintenance, operation, and use of the device."

Between the enactment of the MDA of 1976, in which the performance standard–based definition of class II devices was set forth, and enactment of the SMDA of 1990, the FDA did not issue any performance standards. This led to the expansion of the definition of class II devices in the SMDA of 1990 to include other mechanisms in addition to performance standards to provide reasonable assurance of safety and effectiveness. These "special controls" can include performance and design standards, postmarket surveillance, patient registries, guidelines, recommendations, and other actions. The SMDA of 1990 also simplified the procedures for establishing performance standards. The first performance standards were recently adopted and became effective August 7, 1997. They pertain to lead wires and cables that connect patients to medical devices.

Until special controls take effect for preamendment class II devices, they are subject to the general controls of a class I device and are therefore essentially regulated like a class I device. Class II devices are also subject to the gneral controls of a class I device. Therefore, pending the additional special controls to be developed, class II devices are essentially regulated like a class I device. All class II devices that are life sustaining or life supporting ("critical") require the FDA to examine and identify the special controls necessary to provide adequate assurance of safety and effectiveness.

Class III

In order to have the least commercial and medical effect on devices already in use, the MDA of 1976 allowed the continued distribution of most preamendment devices. Postamendment devices were to be placed automatically in class III and, if not reclassified into class I or II on initiation of the manufacturer or FDA, to undergo a rigorous PMA before marketing.

Section 515(b)(1) of the FD&C Act requires that a preamendment device that the FDA has put into class III is subject to submission of a PMA. A PMA or notice of completion of a product development protocol (PDP) is not required until 90 days after the FDA promulgates a final rule requiring a PMA for the device or 30 months after final classification of the device, whichever occurs later. The FDA finished classification of devices in June 1988, and therefore the grace period ran out as of 1990. The FDA has chosen not to enforce the 30-month requirement.

The SMDA of 1990 added a new section, 515(i), to the FD&C Act (21 USC §360e[i]). It required the FDA, by December 1, 1995, to order manufacturers of preamendment class III devices that had not yet been required to undergo a PMA, to submit to the FDA summaries of, and citations to, any information known about their devices. This was to allow the FDA to review the classification of preamendment devices and enable them to publish final regulations concerning the class of these devices by December 1, 1995. Within 1 year of final review and regulation requiring a device to remain in class III, the FDA was to call for a PMA for the device and those substantially equivalent to it. As of August 14, 1995, however, the FDA had issued final rules for only nine preamendment class III devices and proposed rules for 10 other devices (60 FR 41984, August 14, 1995). There were 116 additional preamendment class III devices for which the FDA had not initiated action.

In August 1995, the FDA called for the summary data to enable review of the classification of the remaining 116 preamendment devices. Devices were divided into three groups. Forty-two devices that were likely to remain in class III were placed in group 3. Thirty-one devices likely to be reclassified into class II were placed in group 2. Forty-three devices that are rarely used and for which PMA submissions were not expected were placed in group 1. Fifteen of the group 3 devices were categorized as "high-priority" devices for which the FDA has "proposed" requesting PMAs. The FDA has ordered summary classification data to be submitted for the remaining 27 group 3 (60 FR 41984, August 14, 1995) and all group 2 (60 FR 41986, August 14, 1995) devices between August 14, 1996, and August 14, 1998. The FDA called for PMAs for 41 group 1 devices; these were to be submitted by December 26, 1996 (61 FR 50704, September 27, 1996).

PMA application.—Section 515 of the FD&C Act (21 USC §360e) describes the PMA process. A PMA includes all known published or unpublished information regarding the safety and effectiveness of a device; a full description of the device; a complete report of manufacturing methods; references to relevant performance standards; samples if feasible; specimens of proposed labeling; and other information as requested by the FDA with concurrence of the advisory panel. The PMA review process includes five steps: administrative and limited scientific review by the FDA staff to determine completeness (filing review); in-depth scientific and regulatory review by appropriate FDA scientific and compliance personnel (in-depth review); review and recommendation by appropriate advisory panel (panel review); an FDA GMP inspection; and final deliberations, documentations, and notification of the FDA decision.

During the "filing review" phase of a PMA, the FDA determines whether the PMA is suitable for filing. If the information presented is unclear or incomplete or not capable of withstanding a rigorous scientific review, the FDA may consider the PMA not suitable for filing. Within 45 days, the FDA reports the filing status of the PMA to the applicant. A 180-day review period commences on the date a PMA is received by the FDA that the FDA subsequently considers to be suitable for filing. Within this period, the FDA completes the review and issues an approval, a denial, or an approvable or not-approvable order. However, since most applications usually require substantial deliberations with the FDA and submission of supplementary information, the total review process is usually longer. An applicant that receives an approvable or nonapprovable order has the option to amend or withdraw the submission or request administrative review.

An approved PMA is, in effect, a private license granted to the applicant for marketing a particular medical device. Data from other PMAs cannot be used to support a PMA without the express consent of the manufacturers who submitted them. This does not include generally acknowledged data such as that in the published literature. The SMDA of 1990 modified this policy; after approval of the fourth PMA of a kind, the FDA can use information contained in the prior PMAs to support subsequent PMAs for similar devices.

The existence of a PMA, unless already known, cannot be acknowledged by the FDA until a final denial or approval letter has been issued. At this time, the application is referred back to the submitter, who has the opportunity to purge it of confidential or proprietary information. The application is then available under freedom of information statutes. A statement of approval or denial is published in the *Federal Register*.

Section 515(f)(1)(21 USC §360[f][1]) authorizes a modified PMA process, a PDP, for certain devices, although it is rarely used. In recognition of the fact that many medical devices are frequently modified during their development, Congress authorized the PDP process. The PDP essentially combines the investigational and PMA processes. The FDA must decide within 30 days of receiving a proposed PDP whether it is an appropriate substitute for a conventional PMA. If so, the FDA will submit the protocol to an advisory panel for recommendations concerning its approvability. The FDA has 120 days to approve or disapprove the proposed PDP protocol. As stated in 21 CFR §814.19, successful completion of a PDP constitutes approval of a PMA.

ALTERNATIVES TO PMA OR PREMARKET NOTIFICATION

A successful 510(k) or PMA is normally required before marketing and interstate commerce of medical devices in the United States. Medical devices may also be obtained through investigational device exemption (IDE), humanitarian device exemption, custom device, and emergency use mechanisms.

IDEs

Section 520(g)(1) of the FD&C Act (21 USC §360j[g][1]; 21 CFR §812) describes the IDE process (1). The purpose of the IDE provisions is to encourage the development of medical devices by suspending certain requirements of the FD&C Act while the safety and effectiveness of the device are being investigated. The requirements that are suspended are those for misbranding, registration, listing, performance standards, premarket notifications, banning devices, premarket approval, records and reports, color additives, restricted devices, and current GMPs. Failure to abide by the terms of the IDE provisions will render a device adulterated.

For IDE purposes, the FDA defines as the sponsor the individual or firm who initiates, but does not actually conduct, an investigation. Investigations are usually referred to as physician sponsored or manufacturer sponsored. The individual under whose immediate direction an investigation is performed is defined as an investigator. If an individual initiates and conducts an investigation, he or she is referred to as a sponsor-investigator.

An institutional review board (IRB) is any group formally designated by a medical institution to review biomedical research involving human subjects. The FDA has established regulations regarding the composition, operation, and responsibilities of IRBs (21 CFR §56). If an IRB does not exist or the FDA finds that an IRB's review is inadequate, a sponsor may submit the application for an investigation directly to the FDA.

The IDE regulations describe significant- and nonsignificant-risk devices. A significant-risk device is one that presents a potential for serious risk to the health, safety, or welfare of a subject and (*a*) is intended as an implant; (*b*) is for use in supporting or sustaining human life; (*c*) is for a use of substantial importance in diagnosing, curing, mitigating, or treating disease or otherwise preventing impairment of human health; or (*d*) otherwise presents a potential for serious risk to the health, safety, or welfare of a subject. A nonsignificant-risk device does not pose a significant risk.

The IDE process is used to conduct research with significant-risk medical devices that are not yet cleared for marketing by the FDA. The IDE process may also be used to collect data about different indications for medical devices than those for which they were originally cleared. In addition to requiring a successful IDE application, IRB approval is required. To conduct research with insignificant-risk devices, only IRB approval is required. If a medical device is already cleared for marketing for any indication, it can be used for other indications or in an "off-label" manner by any licensed physician as long as it is not being used for research purposes and is not being promoted for the unapproved indications.

Humanitarian-Use Devices

Certain products, commonly referred to as orphan devices, are useful in the treatment of rare diseases and conditions but lack committed commercial sponsorship because they are not considered to have significant marketing potential. Section 5 (21 USC §360ee) of the Orphan Drug Act describes the use of these devices in "any disease or condition that occurs so infrequently in the United States that there is no reasonable expectation that a medical device for such disease or condition will be developed."

To assist in bringing these products to market, the FDA set up the Office for Orphan Products Development in 1982; in addition, in 1983 Congress passed the Orphan Drug Act, which amended sections 525–528 of the FD&C Act (21 USC §360aa–§360dd). Although medical devices were not specifically included in the scope of the law, the FDA defined such orphan products as including medical devices in addition to drugs, biologics, in vitro diagnostics, foods for medical purposes, and veterinary products (48 FR 20993, May 10, 1983). The Orphan Drug Amendments of 1988 added medical devices to the provision of the Orphan Drug Act of 1983 that allows financial assistance to defray the cost of developing products for rare diseases or conditions. They also directed the FDA to conduct a study to determine whether the other incentives applicable to orphan drugs should be applied to orphan medical devices. Final regulations were published on December 29, 1992 (21 CFR §316).

Incentives for drug products provided by the Orphan Drug Act include tax credits for clinical research undertaken by a sponsor to generate required data for marketing approval, as well as 7 years of marketing exclusivity for a product approved by the FDA. The FDA also provides protocol assistance and grants to facilitate the development of drug and device products. Requests for protocol assistance are directed to the relevant center in the FDA. Requests for applications for grants are published in the *Federal Register* each summer, and the deadlines for submission of applications are during the following October and January.

Congress also enacted legislation specifically pertaining to medical devices. Section 520(m) of the FD&C Act (21 USC §360j[m]; 21 CFR §814, subpart H) implemented by the SMDA of 1990 authorized the FDA to grant requests to exempt humanitarian-use devices (HUDs) from the effectiveness requirements of performance standards and premarket approval. To qualify as an HUD the device must (*a*) be designed for treatment or diagnosis of diseases or conditions that affect fewer than 4,000 persons per year in the United States; (*b*) be otherwise unavailable if an exemption were not granted; and (*c*) not expose patients to unreasonable or substnatial risks of illness or injury and have probable health benefits that outweigh the risks.

Before submission of an application for an HUD exemption, the device must be designated as an HUD by the Office of Orphan Product Development. An approved exemption permits the marketing of an HUD in the United States for 18 months, which may be extended for additional periods of 18 months.

The HUD may not be sold for an amount that exceeds the cost of research and development, fabrication, and distribution. It can be used only in a facility having an institutional review committee that approves and supervises clinical testing of devices.

Final regulations for HUDs went into effect on January 22, 1997 (62 FR 3297). In February 1997, the first HUD exemption was granted for a medical device, a fetal bladder stent.

Custom Devices

Certain devices referred to as custom devices are exempted from formal marketing clearance from the FDA. According to section 520(b) of the FD&C Act (21 USC §360[j][b]; 21 CFR §812.3[b]), such a designation is appropriate if (*a*) the device is not generally available in finished form for purchase or for dispensing by prescription and is not offered through labeling or advertising by the manufacturer, importer, or distributor thereof for commercial distribution and (*b*) such a device is either intended for use by an individual patient named in such order of such physician or dentist (or other specially qualified person so designated) and is made in a specific form for such patient *or* is intended to meet the special needs of such physician or dentist in the course of the professional practice of such physician or dentist, and the device is not generally available to, or generally used by, other physicians or dentists.

No specific guidance exists regarding how many of a particular type of custom device may be manufactured before that device becomes generally available or generally used and therefore subject to premarketing clearance regulation.

Emergency Devices

An emergency need to use an unapproved device may occur when an IDE for the device does not exist, when a physician wants to use the device in a way not approved under the IDE, or when a physician or institution is not approved under the IDE. Each of the following conditions should exist for a situation to be considered an emergency: (*a*) the patient is in a life-threatening condition that needs immediate treatment, (*b*) no generally acceptable alternative for treating the patient is available, and (*c*) because of the immediate need to use the device, there is no time to use existing procedures to get FDA approval.

In the event that a device is used in emergency circumstances, the "FDA would expect the physician to follow as many patient protection procedures as possible." These include (*a*) an independent assessment by an uninvolved physician, (*b*) informed consent from the patient or legal representative, (*c*) institutional clearance as specified by institutional policies, (*d*) the IRB chairperson's concurrence, and (*e*) authorization from the sponsor, if an unapproved IDE for the device exists.

After an unapproved device is used in an emergency, the physician should (*a*) notify the IRB and otherwise comply with provisions of the IRB and informed consent regulation; (*b*) evaluate the likelihood of a similar need for the device in the future and if it is likely, immediately initiate efforts to obtain IRB approval and an approved IDE for the device's subsequent use; (*c*) if an IDE exists, provide notification of the emergency use of the device to the sponsor, who must comply with the reporting requirements of the IDE regulations; and (*d*) if an IDE does not exist, notify the FDA of the emergency use of the device and provide FDA with a written summary of the conditions constituting the emergency, patient protection measures, and any scientific results.

Subsequent use of the device in an emergency situation may not occur unless an approved IDE is obtained. If an IDE application for subsequent use has been filed and been disapproved, the device may not be used even if the circumstances constituting an emergency exist. ■

Acknowledgments: I thank Stacey J. Ackerman, MSE, PhD (Covance, Inc), Richard P. Kidwell, JD (Johns Hopkins University), and Marlene K. Tandy, MD, JD (Health Industry Manufacturers Association), for reviewing the manuscript.

References

1. Division of Small Manufacturers Assistance Office of Training and Assistance. Regulatory requirements for medical devices: a workshop manual. Rockville, Md: Food and Drug Administration, 1992; 4-4.
2. Office of Surveillance and Biometrics, Systems Division of Surveillance. Medical device reporting: an overview. Rockville, Md: Food and Drug Administration, 1996.
3. Office of Health and Industry Programs, Lowe N, Scott WL. Medical device reporting for user facilities. Rockville, Md: Food and Drug Administration, 1996.

Lee H. Monsein, MD, MPH

Primer on Medical Device Regulation
Part III. Regulatory Mechanisms and Import/Export Regulation[1]

THIS article is the third in a three-part series reviewing medical device regulation. Part I provided an overview and history of medical device regulation and the U.S. Food and Drug Administration (FDA). It also discussed government document nomenclature. Part II detailed current medical device regulation in the United States. Part III describes regulatory mechanisms and enforcement of medical device regulation. Part III also reviews the regulation of imported and exported medical devices and foreign medical device regulation.

REGULATORY MECHANISMS

General

The FDA regulates medical devices through mechanisms that may or may not be binding and enforceable by law. Legal requirements are set forth in statutory and case law through legislative and court action, respectively, or through regulations that are written by the FDA and are, therefore, binding and enforceable by law. Other mechanisms such as guidelines, recommendations, agreements, and informal guidance are nonbinding and unenforceable by law. Regulations may contain provisions that will be enforced as legal requirements, that are intended only as guidelines and recommendations, or both (21 CFR §10.90).

The primary legal requirements for medical devices are detailed by the Food, Drug and Cosmetic (FD&C) Act of 1938. In general, it prohibits the following: the introduction or delivery for introduction of an adulterated or misbranded product into interstate commerce; adulteration or misbranding of a product in interstate commerce; receipt or delivery in interstate commerce of an adulterated or misbranded product; and adulteration or misbranding of a product while it is held for sale after having been in interstate commerce. Performing a "prohibited act" is a violation of the law, which is subject to FDA action including monetary and other penalties.

The FDA has many tools to ensure compliance with legal requirements. Traditional actions applicable to all regulated products include warning letters, seizures, injunctions, and criminal prosecutions. Device-specific actions include civil penalties; administrative detention; mandatory notification or safety alert; repair, replace, or refund; mandatory recalls; reports of removal and correction; temporary premarket approval (PMA) suspension; and PMA withdrawal. Each week the FDA issues "The FDA Enforcement Report," which contains information on enforcement actions taken.

Enforceable Regulatory Mechanisms

The FDA becomes aware of noncompliance with the provisions of the FD&C Act from consumer complaints, trade complaints, and recall actions. They can also become aware of noncompliance from inspections of medical device establishments. Inspections of a facility may take place on a regular basis, as part of a follow-up to previous action, on the basis of budget allocations, or because of complaint letters sent to the FDA or state officials. During the course of the inspection, the inspector may obtain a sample of a product. After completing the inspection and before leaving the premises, the inspector must provide a receipt for the sample and also a written report of conditions that violate the FD&C Act. What follows depends on the seriousness of the violation and the urgency to correct it. In general, the following procedures are followed (1):

1. The inspector completes an inspection report.
2. The inspector's district office supervisor must concur and initiate the recommendation process for bringing action.
3. The district compliance officer must give approval after reviewing the inspection report, recommendation for action, and any other available data.
4. The district director must approve the recommended action. The approval of the regional director is also needed for criminal prosecutions and some injunction actions. The district director may issue a "warning letter."
5. The compliance unit in the FDA center responsible for the product receives, reviews for technical issues, and approves the recommendation.
6. The regulatory management staff of the associate commissioner for regulatory affairs receives, reviews for legal issues, and approves the recommendation.
7. The recommendation goes to the deputy chief counsel for litiga-

Radiology 1997; 205:19–25

Index terms: Radiology and radiologists • State-of-art reviews • U.S. Food and Drug Administration

[1] From the Department of Radiology, Washington Hospital Center, 110 Irving St NW, #BA68, Washington, DC 20010-2975. Received March 27, 1997; revision requested May 19; revision received June 24; accepted June 27. **Address reprint requests to** the author.

Abbreviations: EN = European National, EU = European Union, FDA = Food and Drug Administration, FD&C = Food, Drug and Cosmetic, GMP = good manufacturing practices, ISO = International Organization for Standardization, PMA = premarket approval, USCS = U.S. Customs Service.

tion in the Office of the Chief Counsel. In relatively easy seizure cases, the district may go directly to the Office of the Chief Counsel and then to the U.S. Attorney.

8. The commissioner's office may review criminal cases.

9. The Justice Department's Civil Division, Consumer Affairs Section, reviews all criminal and injunction cases.

10. A request to take action against a product, facility, or persons is made to the U.S. Attorney and/or U.S. Marshal in the federal judicial district where the violation occurred. There is a U.S. Attorney and U.S. Marshal, appointed by the president with confirmation of the Senate, in each of 94 federal judicial districts.

Warning letters are usually issued by the FDA district directors for violations of regulatory importance (ie, those violations that may actually lead to enforcement action if not promptly and adequately corrected), although certain problems require FDA center concurrence. They replaced *notices of adverse findings* and *regulatory letters*, which were used until 1991. They are issued for the purposes of achieving voluntary compliance with the provisions of the FD&C Act and for establishing prior notice. They do not contain a commitment to take enforcement action, but they do contain a specific warning that failure to take prompt corrective action may result in enforcement action. They are issued within 15 days after an inspection if center concurrence is not required and within 30 days if it is. Generally, a response is requested within a certain period of time, usually 15 days. Warning letters are a part of the public record and may be obtained through the Freedom of Information Act and other sources.

Seizures are directed toward violative products, not establishments. The FD&C Act permits the seizure of any adulterated or misbranded device at any time. Unlike drugs, food, and cosmetics, a device does not have to be introduced into interstate commerce to be subject to seizure. The FDA can order an administrative detention of a product before seizure. It can require condemnation and reconditioning or condemnation and destruction of a product once seized. Proceedings are initiated by the U.S. Attorney on behalf of the FDA by filing a complaint in U.S. District Court against the product. The U.S. District Judge then issues a judicial warrant, which is served by the U.S. Marshal who takes custody of the product. Seizures are advantageous for the FDA because they get products off the market quickly and effectively. They are less effective, however, in shutting down an establishment and when products are in multiple locations.

Injunctions are directed toward establishments and personnel rather than violative products. Most violations of the FD&C Act can be enjoined by the FDA through court action. The FDA initiates an injunction by filing a request with the U.S. Attorney, who files an action in federal district court. Injunctions are used when the violations pose a serious health hazard or there is gross consumer deception that requires immediate action to stop a history of uncollected violations, when multiple seizures are impractical, or when the FDA wants to shut down an establishment to prevent future violations.

Administrative detention is intended to protect the public by preventing distribution or use of medical devices encountered during inspections that may be adulterated or misbranded, until the FDA has had time to consider what action it should take concerning the devices and initiate legal action, if appropriate (21 CFR §800.55). An administrative detention is initiated following inspection of a facility and must be approved by the FDA district director and the director of the Office of Compliance. With few exceptions, devices that have been ordered detained may not be used, moved, altered, or tampered with in any way. Detentions can be for up to 20 calendar days; however, the FDA district director can authorize an additional 10 days if necessary. A label or marking, or segregation, serves as notice of the detention.

Mandatory notification can be initiated by the FDA if a product "presents an unreasonable risk of substantial harm to the public health, and notification...is necessary to eliminate the unreasonable risk of such harm and no more practicable means is available...to eliminate such risk" (FD&C Act, section 518(a); 21 USC §360h[a]). Notification refers to the act of making past or potential users aware of the facts discovered relating to the risk. Depending on the situation, patients may be notified directly or indirectly through their physicians. Manufacturers, importers, distributors, and retailers may also be contacted if this will help eliminate the risk. Notifications are issued at the request of the FDA, whereas *safety alerts* are voluntarily issued.

Repair, *replace*, or *refund* remedies are used when notification alone is not sufficient to eliminate the unreasonable risk of substantial harm to the public. They are used when reasonable grounds exist to believe that a device was not properly designed or manufactured with reference to the state of the art as it existed at the time of design or manufacture and the unreasonable risk is not caused by the failure of someone else to exercise due care with respect to the device. Through informal hearings, the FDA can order the device company to submit a plan: "to repair the device so that it does not present the unreasonable risk of substantial harm," "to replace the device with a like or equivalent device which is in conformity with all applicable requirements", or "to refund the purchase price of the device (less a reasonable allowance for use if such device has been in the possession of the device user for one year or more)" (FD&C Act, section 518[b][1]; 21 USC §360h[b][1]). The FDA can impose its own plan if the company's plan is not acceptable.

If the FDA determines that "there is reasonable probability that the continuation of distribution of a device...would cause serious, adverse health consequences or death," the FDA can temporarily suspend its PMA (FD&C Act, section 515[e][3]; 21 USC §360e[e][3]). A *temporary PMA suspension* is used by the FDA as a quick method of removing a dangerous device from the market while pursuing permanent withdrawal. The FDA must provide an opportunity for an informal hearing before an order is issued and must proceed expeditiously to a *PMA withdrawal*. PMAs may be withdrawn at any time "on the basis of new information" that becomes known to the FDA. Withdrawal need not be preceded by a temporary suspension.

Recalls may be voluntary or mandatory. Voluntary recalls may be undertaken by a firm either on its own initiative or in response to a request from the FDA. *Mandatory recalls* can be ordered by the FDA if "there is a reasonable probability that a device intended for human use would cause serious, adverse health consequences or death" (FD&C Act, section 518[e][1]; 21 USC §360h[e]). The FDA issues an order to the firm to immediately cease distribution of the device and to immediately notify health professionals and device user facilities to cease use of the device. An informal hearing may be requested within 10 days. The FDA may then vacate the order or amend it to include a recall. If the FDA orders a recall it will "not include recall of a device from individuals" and will "not include recall of a device from device user facilities if the Secretary determines the risk of recalling such device from the facilities presents a greater health risk than the health risk of not recalling the device from use" (FD&C Act section 519[e][2][B]). Individuals, however, will be notified of potential risks. In order to notify these individuals, the FDA "may use the assistance of health professionals who prescribed or used such a device." If a substantial number of such individuals cannot be identified, they may be reached through use of public media.

Reports of removal and correction are scheduled to go into effect on November 17, 1997 (the final rule was issued on May 19, 1997). These reports will be generated and sent to the FDA whenever a device correction or removal occurs in order to reduce the risk to health posed by the device or to remedy a violation of the FD&C Act caused by the device that may present a risk to health.

The use of a reference list to track companies that have had prior good manufacturing practices (GMP) violations has been eliminated. Being on the reference list could have potentially delayed a firm's future applications for unrelated devices. GMP compliance, however, continues to be checked prior to clearance of class III and PMA devices.

Unenforceable Regulatory Mechanisms

A *guideline* represents the formal position of the FDA on a subject. Guidelines "establish principles or practice of general applicability and do not include decisions or advice on particular situations" (21 CFR §10.90). Except in an emergency situation, the FDA must follow the guideline until it is amended or revoked. Guidelines may be used in administrative and court proceedings to demonstrate acceptable and unacceptable practices but cannot be used as a legal requirement. Action cannot be taken against a manufacturer or product that is in conformity with the guideline. Finalized guidelines can be obtained by the public from the Dockets Management Branch and other sources after the publication of a notice of availability in the *Federal Register*.

The FDA often formulates and disseminates written opinions about matters over which it does not have direct regulatory authority. These are referred to as *recommendations*. Examples include state and local ordinances or personnel practices for reducing radiation exposure. Finalized recommendations can be obtained by the public from the Dockets Management Branch and other sources after the publication of a notice of availability in the *Federal Register*.

Agreements can include formal agreements, memoranda of understanding, or other similar written documents. Finalized agreements can be obtained by the public from the Dockets Management Branch and other sources after publication of a notice of availability in the *Federal Register*.

Informal guidance refers to an oral or written statement made by an employee of the FDA that represented the best judgment at that time but does not constitute a guideline or does not necessarily represent the formal position of the FDA. Examples include guidance documents, policy statements, compliance policy guides, manuals, memoranda, points to consider, bluebook memos, letters, and speeches. They do not bind the FDA to the views expressed and are not subject to federal notice-and-comment rules.

PENALTIES

Violations of the FD&C Act can be considered misdemeanors or felonies and can result in criminal prosecution. Felonies represent more severe crimes, which include acts that are so offensive to morals as to be obviously criminal. They are usually punishable by more than a year of imprisonment in a federal or state facility. They reflect intent to defraud or mislead or a violation after a previous conviction. Misdemeanors are less severe crimes that are violations of specific regulatory statutes which would not be punishable in the absence of statutory enactments prohibiting the commission of the acts. They are usually punishable by a fine and less than 1 year imprisonment. No intent to defraud or mislead is required.

When a corporation violates the provisions of the FD&C Act, the corporation and all involved persons can be found guilty. The FD&C Act imposes a responsibility to seek out and remedy violations and to implement measures to ensure violations will not occur. Corporate officers can be held liable without proof they knew or performed the violative act if they had the responsibility to either prevent or correct it and failed to do so.

The FD&C Act stipulates penalties for individuals of up to 1 year in prison and/or up to $1,000 for the first offense, which is considered a misdemeanor, and up to 3 years in prison and/or up to $10,000 for the second offense or with intent to defraud or mislead, which is considered a felony (FD&C Act, section 303; 21 USC §333). The Sentencing Reform Act of 1984 stipulates individual fines of up to $25,000 and $250,000 for each misdemeanor and felony violation of the FD&C Act, respectively. It stipulates corporate fines of up to $100,000 and $500,000 for each misdemeanor and felony violation, respectively. This act also provides for restitution to identifiable victims of the criminal conduct and payment for the FDA's cost of investigation. Corporations cannot pay the fines of individuals from corporate funds unless permitted under state law. There is a 5-year statute of limitations.

The Safe Medical Devices Act of 1990 also allowed the FDA to pursue civil penalties for certain violations of the FD&C Act. Such administrative civil penalties are fines levied by the FDA after the opportunity for a hearing before an Administrative Law Judge. They are not to be confused with money judgments awarded by courts after civil court proceedings. The maximum penalty is $15,000 per violation with a cumulative cap of $1 million for all violations in a single proceeding. The statute of limitations is 10 years or a maximum of 6 years after the violation should have been discovered. Accused parties are entitled to judicial review in the Federal Court of Appeals. There is one Court of Appeals in each of 11 regions, or "circuits," in the United States.

HEALTH CARE PROVIDERS

General

Most provisions of medical device regulation guide the conduct of the medical device industry and not health care providers. Nevertheless, user facilities, investigational review boards, and physicians have certain responsibilities with respect to medical devices. Potential penalties can be incurred if these duties are neglected.

The FD&C Act only allows medical devices to be introduced into interstate commerce that have approved premarket notification (510[k]), PMA, or investigational device exemption applications; are used on an emergency basis; or are custom made. One may interpret an institution or physician charging a patient for an unallowed device or the procedure in which it was used as "the receipt in interstate commerce of any food, drug, device or cosmetic that is adulterated or misbranded, and the delivery or proffered delivery for pay or otherwise," which is a prohibited act under section 301(c) of the FD&C Act (21 USC §331[c]). The action could, therefore, be subject to enforcement remedies. Health care providers have not yet been subjected to criminal and civil penalties; however, seizures have occurred.

Investigational Devices

Clinical investigators, investigational review boards, and institutions that deal with devices that are under an investigational device exemption are subject to various federal regulations. Failure to comply with these regulations can result in disqualification of investigators, investigational review boards, and institutions from current or future research. This may lead the FDA to "disqualify" the investigator, investigational review board, or institution from investigational device exemption investigations. The FDA may then withhold approval for new studies, halt new subjects from being added to ongoing studies, terminate ongoing studies, or refuse to consider data collected in support of a PMA or 510(k) application. The FDA may also take additional actions, including institution of judicial proceedings through the Department of Justice or referral to other federal, state, and local agencies for appropriate action (21 CFR §56.120-124; 21 CFR §813.119).

Problem Medical Device Reporting

Section 17(b)(1) of the Safe Medical Devices Act of 1990, which deals with "medical device reporting," required the FDA to "conduct a study to determine whether there has been substantial compliance with the requirements of section 519(b) of the FD&C Act (21 USC §360i[b]) by device user facilities." If the results of this study demonstrated substantial noncompliance or the results were not reported to Congress by November 28, 1994, then civil penalties authorized by section 303(f) of the FD&C Act (21 USC §333[f]) were to become applicable. The results of such a study were never submitted to Congress. Civil penalties are, therefore, presumably applicable to noncompliance with user medical device reporting requirements. Civil penalties may not exceed $15,000 per violation or $1 million for all violations adjudicated in a single proceeding.

Criminal penalties may be a fine of up to $1,000 and 1 year imprisonment for the first offense if the offense was unintentional and of up to $10,000 and 3 years imprisonment for subsequent offenses or for intentional offense.

Off-Label Uses

The FDA gives marketing clearance to products based on review of safety and effectiveness data for specific intended uses that are detailed in their labeling. Uses of products for indications that are not detailed in their labeling are referred to as "unapproved" or "off-label" uses. The FDA addressed off-label uses of drugs in the *FDA Drug Bulletin* (2): "Once a product has been approved for marketing, a physician may prescribe it for uses or in treatment regimens or patient populations that are not included in approved labeling. Such 'unapproved' or, more precisely, 'unlabeled' uses may be appropriate and rational in certain circumstances, and may, in fact, reflect approaches to drug therapy that have been extensively reported in medical literature." The FDA has not specifically addressed the off-label use of medical devices. However, prior to being appointed commissioner of the FDA, David Kessler, who recently resigned as commissioner, said, "Use of an approved device for an unapproved use in a nonemergency situation represents a complex legal issue....The FDA will intervene if the device is being commercially promoted for an unapproved use. If the device is to be used in part of a research endeavor, the FDA will require a formal investigation trial. However, a physician who uses a device in an unapproved manner to treat a particular patient, without promoting it for such use, is unlikely to be in violation of the statute. The amendments focus on products, not procedures" (3).

The FDA does not prohibit the sharing of information regarding unapproved products or uses among scientists, clinicians, and industry. Investigators and publishers are not prohibited from describing unapproved products or uses. It is, therefore, the responsibility of investigators and publishers to ensure that their audience understands the marketing status of these products. Companies, however, are prohibited from using these communications for the promotion of unapproved products or uses. Under new guidelines, the FDA has proposed that companies be allowed to disseminate this information as long as their actions are not intended for promotion. In documents entitled "Guidance for Industry-Funded Dissemination of Reference Texts" and "Guidance to Industry on Dissemination of Reprints of Certain Published, Original Data" released in final form on October 8, 1996, the FDA has attempted to ease restrictions on dissemination of data on off-label uses (61 FR 52800-52801, October 8, 1996).

Reimbursement

Although the FDA does not seek to regulate medical practice, the nature of a regulatory scheme that allows marketing of only specific products directly influences how medicine is practiced. Furthermore, reimbursement and medical malpractice issues, associated with unapproved products or use, are powerful indirect influences on the practice of medicine (4,5).

For many years, the Health Care Finance Administration, under Medicare law, knowingly reimbursed for only devices that were cleared by the FDA and related medical services. Devices undergoing investigational device exemption studies were considered experimental and were, therefore, not covered. If this policy had been fully enforced, Medicare beneficiaries would have been excluded from the potential benefits of new medical devices undergoing investigational device exemption clinical trials. On November 1, 1995, the Health Care Finance Administration announced a new policy that would ensure new technologies would be accessible to Medicare recipients (6). Two classes of devices were created. Category A devices are novel, first-of-a-kind products whose safety and effectiveness have not been established. These devices are still considered experimental and are not covered. Category B devices are those products that are newer generations of proved technologies. Safety and effectiveness have been preliminarily established. These devices are considered reasonable and necessary by Medicare and, therefore, reimbursable. The FDA will assist the Health Care Finance Administration in categorizing devices undergoing investigational device exemption trials.

Liability

The FD&C Act does not provide a separate and private right of action to enforce its provisions. Therefore, one cannot bring a suit against a party because of a medical device strictly on the basis that it violated provisions of the FD&C Act. In other words, one cannot bring a private suit against a firm or health care provider solely on the basis that a device was not allowed by the FDA. Nevertheless, it does not prevent product liability suits. Product liability suits can be based on issues of negligence, strict liability, or breach of warranty. *Negligence* refers to conduct that fails to meet reasonable standards to protect people against risks and can apply to manufacturers, sellers, hospitals, and physicians. The use of an unallowed device can make the defense of a medical negligence case difficult for a hospital or physician.

Strict liability refers to products or activities that are unreasonably dangerous, does not depend on how carefully the defendant acted, and does not apply to health care providers. *Breach of warranty* is based on principles of contracts in which the defendant, usually a manufacturer or seller, violates explicit or implicit claims about its product. It can apply to hospitals and physicians if the sale of a product is involved.

IMPORT AND EXPORT OF MEDICAL DEVICES

As of 1996, U.S.–owned companies were responsible for 70% of the U.S. markets of medical devices, 47% of the global markets, 44% of the European Union (EU) markets, and 28% of the Japanese markets (6). The U.S. market accounts for $54.6 billion (42%), the EU market accounts for $36 billion (28%), and the Japanese market accounts for $19.2 billion (15%) of the total global market, which is estimated to be $129.5 billion. The U.S. trade surplus in medical devices has grown at a rate approaching 25% per year since 1988 and reached $6.5 billion in 1996. An understanding of U.S. and foreign medical device regulation is, therefore, very important for the domestic and foreign health care communities.

Imported Medical Devices

Before importing a medical device into the United States, the manufacturer or importer must have previously satisfied all of the same provisions of the FD&C Act that relate to domestic medical devices. Clinical data collected in foreign countries can be used to support a marketing application in the United States as long as the data meet the same requirements as domestic investigations. In addition, the import of medical devices into the United States is specifically covered by two laws. They are section 801(a), (b), and (c) of the FD&C Act (21 USC), which contains special requirements for the import of medical devices, and section 536, which contains special requirements for the import of radiation-emitting electronic products; and sections 418-521 of the Tariff Act of 1930 as amended (19 USC §1521), enforced by the U.S. Customs Service (USCS) of the Department of Treasury, which sets the entry requirements for all imports into the United States.

The primary duties of the USCS include assessment and collection of all duties, taxes, and fees on imported merchandise; administration and review of import entry forms; enforcement of U.S. Customs and related laws; and administration of certain navigation laws and treaties. The FDA and USCS have a working agreement for the cooperative enforcement of section 801 of the FD&C Act. Most cooperative actions involve violations of the FD&C Act, particularly noncompliance with FDA import requirements, or when the FDA determines it necessary to sample imported devices.

The process of importing a medical device into the United States starts when the importer or broker submits the necessary forms to the local USCS district office. The USCS forwards copies of the documents to the local FDA district office. The FDA district office determines if the product complies with FDA import requirements. If the FDA district office determines that the device, manufacturer, or importer has not complied with FDA import requirements, the device will be detained at the port of entry. Recently, the FDA has put in place an electronic entry processing system at over 250 ports of entry in the United States. Importers transmit their entry data to FDA electronically at the same time they are transmitting their required electronic data to the USCS. Within 15 minutes of keying in the data, the importer should receive a computerized response stating whether the entry requires further FDA review or if it can move immediately into domestic commerce.

New regulations (21 CFR §807.40) issued by the FDA on December 11, 1995, effective on April 11, 1996, extended until July 31, 1996, and stayed on July 23, 1996 (61 FR 38346, July 23, 1996), required that a mandatory U.S.–designated agent of a foreign device manufacturer that exports devices into the United States be responsible for registering the foreign manufacturer's establishments (similar to the requirement for a domestic firm). The U.S.–designated agent was responsible for submitting medical device reports, submitting annual certifications, acting as the official correspondent, submitting registration information, submitting device listing information, and submitting marketing applications.

Section 801(d) of the FD&C Act allows unapproved finished products or components to enter the United States for further processing as long as they are ultimately exported.

Exported Medical Devices

Sections 801(e)(1), (e)(2), and 802 of the FD&C Act are concerned with the export of medical devices from the United States. FDA permission is not required to export a medical device that is legally marketed in the United States.

Devices that would be considered adulterated or misbranded if they were sold or offered for sale in commercial distribution in the United States can be exported if they are (*a*) in accordance with the specifications of the foreign purchaser, (*b*) not in conflict with the laws of the country to which it is intended for export, (*c*) labeled on the outside of the shipping package that it is intended for export, and (*d*) not sold or offered for sale in domestic commerce. If a device (*a*) does not comply with performance standards of the FD&C Act, (*b*) lacks a required PMA or 510(k), (*c*) is undergoing clinical investigation, or (*d*) is banned from the U.S. market, it cannot be exported unless the FDA determines in writing that the export (*a*) is not contrary to public health and safety and (*b*) has approval of the recipient country, or unless it has received approval in one of several designated countries or listed countries (Australia; Canada; Israel; Japan; New Zealand; Switzerland; South Africa; members of the EU: Austria, Belgium, Denmark, France, Germany, Greece, Finland, Ireland, Italy, Luxembourg, Netherlands, Portugal, Spain, Sweden, and the United Kingdom; or members of the European Economic Area: the EU countries plus Liechtenstein, Iceland, and Norway). Any device that is approved in one of these countries can be exported anywhere in the world (section 802, FD&C Act). Transshipments (finished devices for which there was no further processing), however, are not permitted to be held over in the United States pending shipment to foreign countries.

Once an adulterated or misbranded device is sold or offered for sale in commercial distribution in the United States, it cannot be exported as an alternative to bringing the device into compliance with the FD&C Act.

Foreign Medical Device Regulation

Europe.—A new system for the regulation of medical devices in the EU countries has been implemented recently. The system allows manufacturers to self-certify that relatively low-risk devices meet European requirements (which are based on compliance with objective international standards) and to utilize third-party bodies for the review and approval of higher risk devices. It is based on three legislative directives, or sets of regulations, which define procedures for reviewing and approving new products: an Active Implantable Medical Device Directive; a Medical Device Directive; and an In Vitro Diagnostic Directive. The first two directives have already been implemented. It is expected that the In Vitro Diagnostic Directive will be finalized in late 1997 and implemented by late 1999. These directives define premarket review procedures, classify devices based on risk, and impose quality assurance and testing requirements for new products.

Devices are divided into five groups: active implantable in vitro diagnostics and four classes of medical devices. Class I medical devices are noninvasive devices that do not deliver energy. Class IIa devices are nonactive, invasive short-term devices or those that deliver energy at nonhazardous levels. They correspond to some class I and II devices in the United States. Class IIb devices are nonactive, invasive, long-term devices that are not used in the heart or central nervous system, or those that deliver energy at potentially hazardous levels. They correspond to some class II and III devices in the United States. Class III devices are those that are invasive and in contact with the circulatory system or central nervous system, or those that contain biologically active components. They correspond to some class III devices in the United States.

The Active Implantable Medical Device Directive became effective on January 1, 1993, and compliance was mandatory on January 1, 1995. It covers permanently implanted medical devices that depend on electricity or some other source of power to function. To obtain a product approval, referred to as a "CE mark" (see below), manufacturers must meet certain essential requirements, such as standards for quality assurance, sterility, and biocompatibility. The purpose is to ensure that the product is safe and performs as intended by the manufacturer. The manufacturer must then engage a private-sector test house, referred to as a *Notified Body*, to test their products and certify that they meet the relevant EU standards. This can be done through product testing or through inspections of a manufacturer's quality assurance system. Notified Bodies are appointed by the member states. As of January 1997, approximately 55 of such organizations were currently authorized to carry out the approval procedures.

The Medical Device Directive became effective on January 1, 1995, but will not be mandatory until June 14, 1998. Until that time, companies will be able to meet either the specific country requirements or the new EU-wide rules. Class I devices are not subject to third-party approval process unless the devices are sterilized or are measuring instruments. In these cases there is a limited examination of manufacturing processes similar to but less comprehensive than that required for class IIa devices.

Class IIa devices require approval of a quality system corresponding to ISO (International Organization for Standardization) 9001 plus EN46001 or to ISO 9002 plus EN46002 (see below). Once given such an approval, the manufacturer can self-certify the devices without further delay. Requirements for class IIb devices are similar to those for class IIa devices. An approval may be also be obtained if the individual product is tested and the manufacturer has an approved quality system corresponding to ISO 9002 plus EN46002. Class III device requirements are similar to those of class IIb devices except that a quality system (ISO 9001 plus EN46001) approval must be supplemented by a design dossier approval, and that both the design dossier and type examination must include clinical data.

The ISO, a worldwide federation of national standards bodies, has produced a series of quality management and quality assurance standards for general manufacturing processes. This set of five international quality assurance standards, known as the ISO 9000 series (ISO 9000 to 9004), attempts to blend the many national approaches to quality management and quality assurance.

ISO 9002, "Quality Systems: Model for Quality Assurance in Production and Installation," is closest in comparison to current FDA GMP regulations. ISO 9001, "Specification for Design/Development, Production, Installation, and Servicing," is essentially ISO 9002 with the addition of design and development quality assurance controls. ISO 9001 specifications are to the CE mark what GMP specifications are to 510(k) approval in the United States. When preproduction design validation requirements are added to the GMP regulations in the near future, a manufacturer complying with the modified GMP regulations should comply with most of the ISO 9001 standards. A manufacturer complying with the ISO 9001 standards may, however, not comply with all provisions of the modified GMP regulations. The GMP regulations require more extensive controls for product labeling, complaint processing, and traceability.

ISO 8042, "Quality Vocabulary," defines the quality terms used in the ISO 9000 series of standards. The European Committee for Standardization has created the European National (EN) standards EN46001 and EN46002, which adapt the ISO series to medical devices. Technical Committee 210 of the ISO is currently working on a new set of international standards based on the EN46001 and EN46002, which are expected to be finished in mid-1996.

A U.S.–based firm anywhere in the United States can work with a Notified Body to secure a "CE" mark for its products without ever traveling to Europe. Notified Bodies can provide U.S.–based firms with the expertise on identifying the essential requirements that must be met to secure European product approval.

The EU regulatory system used an adverse event reporting system referred to as a "Medical Devices Vigilance System." A final draft of guidelines for this system was published in May 1993. It requires that certain types of events be reported to the Member States health officials (*Competent Authorities*). These events are those that led to death; led to serious deterioration in the state of health of a patient, user, or other person; or might have led to death or serious deterioration in health. Manufacturers are to report incidents to Competent Authorities in the country of occurrence within 10 days and near incidents within 30 days of first being informed of the incidents. Competent Authorities record and evaluate information, make recommendations to manufacturers, and make information available to other Member States.

Japan.—The regulatory system for medical devices in Japan is currently being revised. Medical devices must have a "shonin," or product approval, from the Medical Device Division at the Pharmaceutical Affairs Bureau of the Ministry of Health and Welfare before marketing, except those specified by the Ministry of Health and Welfare. A comprehensive assessment of the quality, safety, and effectiveness of a new product is done by the Central Pharmaceutical Affairs Council, which reports its recommendations to the Medical Device Division. Once review of the application is complete, the Ministry of Health and Welfare decides whether to grant approval of the product.

As of July 1997, the Ministry of Health and Welfare has decided to dismantle the Pharmaceutical Affairs Bureau and begin registering medical devices with a new Pharmaceutical Safety Bureau. This bureau will manage evaluation and registration of medical products. Much of the work related to the evaluation of new medical devices will be transferred to a national institute created by reorganizing the existing National Institute of Health Sciences. The new institute will probably be named the National Drug and Food Evaluation Research Institute, which will contain a division temporarily named the Drugs and Medical Devices Evaluation Center (7).

Recently, Japan instituted a mechanism for third-party review of product approval applications for "me-too" (similar to substantially equivalent devices in the United States). The official third-party review organization is the Japan Association for the Advancement of Medical Equipment.

Japan maintains a medical device adverse event reporting system in which designated hospitals are expected to report information about device problems. Manufacturers are also expected to carry out postmarket studies of new devices. ■

Acknowledgments: The author thanks Stacey J. Ackerman, MSE, PhD (Covance, Inc), Richard P. Kidwell, JD (Johns Hopkins University), and Marlene K. Tandy, MD, JD (Health Industry Manufacturers Association), for reviewing the manuscript.

References

1. O'Reilly J. Food and Drug Administration. Colorado Springs, Colo: Shepard's/McGraw-Hill, Inc, 1993.
2. FDA Drug Bull, April 1982.
3. Kessler DA, Pape SM, Sundwall DN. The federal regulation of medical devices. N Engl J Med 1987; 317:357–366.
4. McGivney WT, Hendee WR. Regulation, coverage, and reimbursement of medical technologies. Int J Radiat Oncol Biol Phys 1990; 18:697–700.
5. Sisk JE. The financing and regulation of medical devices in the United States. Med Prog Technol 1982; 9:181–186.
6. Vladeck B. Medicare expands coverage of investigational devices. JAMA 1995; 274:1186.
7. Gallivan M. The 1997 global medical technology update: the challenges facing U.S. industry and policy makers. Washington, DC: Health Industry Manufacturers Association, 1997.

Book Review

Interpretation of ERCP with Associated Digital Imaging Correlation

Andrew J. Taylor, MD, and Anthony G. Bohorfoush III, MD

Philadelphia, Pa: Lippincott-Raven Publishers, 1996. ISBN 0-397-51579-0. Cloth, $95.00; pp 327; 276 figures; tables.

Drs Taylor and Bohorfoush have edited an excellent book, which clearly illustrates the cooperation and interdependence that exist between endoscopists and abdominal radiologists in everyday practice. Endoscopic retrograde cholangiopancreatography (ERCP) is the primary topic of the book, but it also covers imaging of the biliary tract and pancreas (including spiral computed tomography [CT] and magnetic resonance [MR] cholangiography) that is performed by radiologists. However, I believe this book is more appropriate for endoscopists who want to become more familiar with radiology than radiologists who want to learn ERCP.

The book is subdivided into 14 well-constructed chapters. The text is easy to read and well organized. One of the greatest contributions this book provides is excellent photoreproductions.

The first and second chapters discuss technical considerations, causes of technical failure, and possible pitfalls in ERCP. Also complications that are due to ERCP are addressed. However, technical considerations concerning sonography, CT, and MR imaging are only briefly described. The third and fourth chapters cover imaging of congenital abnormalities and the normal anatomic structure of the biliary tree. The fifth chapter presents inflammatory diseases of the biliary tract. The sixth chapter presents neoplasms of the biliary tract; several conditions that uncommonly involve the biliary tract (eg, hepatocellular carcinoma and metastatic disease) are well described. The seventh chapter covers choledocholithiasis. Regrettably, in this chapter, the important function of endoscopic sonography is not addressed. Also, the important function of MR cholangiography in the case of a stone in the main bile duct is not highlighted at all (for some reason there is no illustration that provides a correlation between ERCP and MR cholangiographic findings). The eighth chapter addresses various pathologic conditions such as liver transplantation, biliary tract trauma, and postoperative changes. The ninth and 10th chapters cover imaging of congenital abnormalities and the normal anatomic structure of the pancreatic ducts. The 11th chapter presents inflammatory diseases of the pancreas that may affect the pancreatic duct. The 12th chapter deals with neoplasms of the pancreatic duct, and the 13th chapter covers various pancreatic conditions such as pancreatic trauma, cystic fibrosis, and postoperative changes. The final chapter provides a guide to the differential diagnosis of disorders of the pancreatic and bile ducts.

I found two major limitations of the book. First, as I said, the important function of MR cholangiography in the exploration of jaundiced patients is not stressed. Second, endoscopic sonography—an examination that has been proved to be very sensitive for detecting small stones in the main bile duct—is not addressed in any chapter.

In summary, this book is very well priced at $95.00 and contains an easy-to-read integrated approach to ERCP and imaging of the biliary tract and pancreas. The book would be especially appropriate for residents, radiologists, and gastroenterologists.

Reviewed by Philippe Soyer, MD, PhD

William F. Pritchard, Jr, MD, PhD • Ronald F. Carey, PhD

U.S. Food and Drug Administration and Regulation of Medical Devices in Radiology[1]

The recent decision by the U.S. Food and Drug Administration (FDA) to approve one ultrasound imaging system for use in making breast biopsy decisions prompted considerable interest in the radiology community about the regulatory process and the associated implications for the practice of medicine. In this report, the concepts and statutory authority guiding the FDA in the regulation of medical devices are summarized and discussed, including the device classification scheme, premarket approval, premarket notification, and investigational device exemptions. Also, the critical concepts of safety and effectiveness for a given indication for use, the roles of advisory panels, and examples of imaging and interventional devices are described to shed light on the approval process.

Index terms: Breast, US, 00.1298 • Diagnostic radiology • Radiology and radiologists, socioeconomic issues • U.S. Food and Drug Administration

Radiology 1997; 205:27–36

[1] From the Office of Science and Technology, Center for Devices and Radiological Health, U.S. Food and Drug Administration (HFZ-132), 12721-A Twinbrook Pkwy, Rockville, MD 20852. Received March 4, 1997; revision requested April 21; revision received June 18; accepted June 23. **Address reprint requests to** W.F.P.

The mention of commercial products, their source, or their use in connection with material reported herein is not to be construed as either an actual or implied endorsement of such products by the Department of Health and Human Services.

W.F.P. is a diagnostic radiologist and a medical officer in the Food and Drug Administration's Center for Devices and Radiological Health.

Almost every item used in a department of radiology is regulated by the U.S. Food and Drug Administration (FDA). The FDA operates under a congressional mandate to ensure that medical devices are both reasonably safe and effective, before commercial distribution. Given the broad authority and effect the FDA has over the devices used by physicians, it is unfortunate that most physicians are unfamiliar with the details of the FDA's role in the regulation of medical devices. The decisions of the FDA may seem arbitrary if one is not acquainted with the approval processes and their rationale, particularly when apparently promising devices are not made available, demanding requirements are imposed on an innovative device, or decisions are made that appear to contradict common sense. An example may be the recent approval of one specific diagnostic ultrasound (US) device for the analysis of breast lesions, an issue that is discussed at the end of this article as one of several examples of the device approval process. The controversy aroused by that decision has led radiologists to be more interested in the approval processes and the regulation of devices by the FDA (1–3).

The FDA has considerable responsibility and influence because of its role in the protection of the public health and the sheer size of the health-related manufacturing industry it regulates. In regulating medical devices and in vitro diagnostic products, the FDA oversees an industry that had U.S. consumption (sales) of $54.6 billion in 1996 (4). The FDA regulates approximately 1,700 types of devices with more than 23,000 registered manufacturers. In the 1996 fiscal year, the FDA received 20,236 device-related submissions.

This article explores the concepts guiding the FDA in device regulation, the laws providing the FDA with its regulatory authority over devices, the events that led Congress to enact those laws, the structure of the FDA, and the processes through which devices are approved for marketing. It is not intended to represent a comprehensive policy statement by the FDA. Rather, it is aimed at providing radiologists with a better understanding of how medical devices are approved for sale, what is involved in the process, and the rationale for the process.

CONCEPTS AND REGULATORY FOUNDATION

The primary role of the FDA in the regulation of medical devices is the protection of the public health by ensuring that such devices are reasonably "safe and effective," before commercial marketing. Before 1976, the FDA was effectively limited to reacting to hazardous devices already on the market and, then, only after patient injuries occurred. In 1976, Congress fundamentally changed the FDA's regulatory authority over devices from one of reacting to hazardous devices to one of ensuring device safety and effectiveness before commercial distribution.

Individual users of a device, whether that individual is a patient, physician, or other health care professional, have neither the time nor the scientific and engineering expertise to independently evaluate the safety and effectiveness of every device they use nor should they rely on their own or their colleagues' experiences to detect uncommon adverse events or complications. Therefore, the sponsor (ie, the persons or manufacturer developing a device) is required by law to demonstrate the safety and effectiveness of the device through valid scientific evidence before any commercial distribution. "Safe" means that the probable benefits to health for its intended use outweigh any probable risks of harm

Abbreviations: FD&C = Food, Drug, and Cosmetic, FDA = Food and Drug Administration, IDE = investigational device exemptions, PMA = premarket approval, 510(k) = premarket notification, on the basis of section 510(k) of the FD&C Act.

or injury by the device. "Effective" means that the device does what it is supposed to do in a reliable fashion. For a manufacturer to receive marketing approval for a device, the device must have a useful purpose in medical practice. It is not sufficient to demonstrate that the device is effective if it accomplishes no medical benefit. For example, if a radioactive endovascular stent were shown to be effective in delivering a prescribed radiation dose to the vascular wall with the intention of reducing restenosis but did not actually result in improved patency rates, then it may not be approved. The FDA conducts an independent scientific evaluation of the data provided by the sponsor and makes decisions about marketing and labeling approvals on the basis of these evaluations. The FDA will actively assist sponsors as they navigate through the regulatory pathway, an interaction that may begin early in the development of a product.

The regulatory authority of the FDA was established by the federal Food, Drug, and Cosmetic Act (FD&C Act) in 1938; the FD&C Act addressed devices only to the extent that it prohibited the marketing of adulterated or misbranded devices. Devices that proved to be hazardous after they were on the market were subject to seizure and the manufacturer could be prevented by injunction from further marketing, but the FDA had little premarket role in the evaluation of medical devices. Under the FD&C Act, the FDA had authority in the premarket regulation of medical devices only to the extent that certain devices might be construed to be drugs.

Regulation of radiation-emitting devices began in 1968 with the enactment of the Radiation Control for Health and Safety Act. Congress was responding to concerns about the possibility of excess radiation exposure from color television sets, microwave ovens, and other items. This law was designed to protect the public from unintended or unnecessary exposures to radiation produced by electronic products, whether the devices are consumer items, industrial tools, or medical devices. Under the Radiation Control for Health and Safety Act, the FDA developed and enforces performance standards for diagnostic x-ray equipment, medical lasers, and US therapy equipment.

At the same time, there were rising concerns about the safety of non–radiation-emitting medical devices. At the direction of President Nixon, the Cooper Committee was established and instructed to recommend a procedure for the premarket regulation of devices and to consider the need for new legislation. In its 1970 report, the committee noted the contribution of user error to device hazards and was "distressed by the lack of data in many areas related to the interaction of medical devices with the human body, and by the seeming unquestioning acceptance of claims for medical device safety and performance unsubstantiated or inadequately supported by scientific fact" (5). Among the many examples cited were prosthetic cardiac ball-valves in which the ball escaped from the cage after a decrease in size and weight following implantation. Public awareness increased after the Dalkon shield intrauterine device was withdrawn from the market in June 1974, following reports associating the device with 209 septic midtrimester abortions and 11 maternal deaths (6,7).

In response to these concerns, Congress enacted the Medical Device Amendments of 1976 to the FD&C Act, providing the FDA with explicit authority to regulate medical devices. The legislation was patterned after the recommendations of the Cooper Committee report and designed a regulatory framework tailored for devices, recognizing that existing drug laws were unsuitable for the regulation of devices. The 1976 Amendments broadly defined a "device" as follows (8):

> an instrument, apparatus, implement, machine, contrivance, implant, in vitro reagent, or other similar or related article, including any component, part, or accessory, which is—
>
> (1) recognized in the official National Formulary, or the United States Pharmacopeia, or any supplement to them,
>
> (2) intended for use in the diagnosis of disease or other conditions, or in the cure, mitigation, treatment, or prevention of disease, in man or other animals, or
>
> (3) intended to affect the structure or any function of the body of man or other animals, and which does not achieve its primary intended purposes through chemical action within or on the body of man or other animals and which is not dependent upon being metabolized for the achievement of its primary intended purposes.

This definition excludes drugs but encompasses a wide range of items including tongue depressors, gloves, wheelchairs, in vitro diagnostics, surgical equipment, implants, radiographic film, therapeutic devices, and radiographic imaging systems. The mandate of the 1976 Amendments provided the FDA with the explicit authority to ensure that devices were safe and effective before they could be marketed. This represented a fundamental change in the regulatory authority from one of reacting to hazardous devices already on the market to a proactive review before products could be distributed. The Amendments also strengthened postmarket controls through the definition of explicit device-related prohibited acts within the broader categories of adulteration and misbranding, remedies for violation (recall, seizure, injunction), and establishment of good manufacturing practice requirements.

In 1988, after 12 years of experience with device regulation under the Amendments, Congress and the FDA began to study changes in the Amendments. This was a response, in part, to the fractures of the outlet struts of the Bjork-Shiley 60° convexo-concave heart valves, an event that has occurred in 435 cases of a total of 81,709 valves implanted (Shiley Heart Valve Research Center, Irvine, Calif, written communication to the FDA on outlet strut valve fractures, September 9, 1996) and has a reported mortality rate of 59% (9). The valve was withdrawn from the market in 1986, but Congress believed there was a delayed regulatory response to the failures, resulting from inadequate postapproval follow-up. These concerns led Congress to enact the Safe Medical Devices Act of 1990 and the Medical Device Amendments of 1992, which added, among other things, greater postmarket controls, such as user reporting of device-related deaths or serious injuries to provide an "early warning system" for device complications or failures.

ORGANIZATION OF THE FDA

The FDA is organized into six centers (Fig 1) that have specific responsibilities and report to the commissioner. Radiopharmaceuticals and radiographic contrast agents are regulated as drugs by the Center for Drug Evaluation and Research and are beyond the scope of this article. The regulation of medical devices and radiation-emitting products is the responsibility of the Center for Devices and Radiological Health.

The Center for Devices and Radiological Health is organized into six offices (Fig 1) under the Office of the Center Director. The Office of Device Evaluation has the responsibility for evaluating the safety and effectiveness of medical devices before they are approved or cleared for clinical research or marketing and evaluates related manufacturing and labeling information. The decision to approve or disapprove an application for the commercial distribution of a device for use in humans rests with the Office of Device

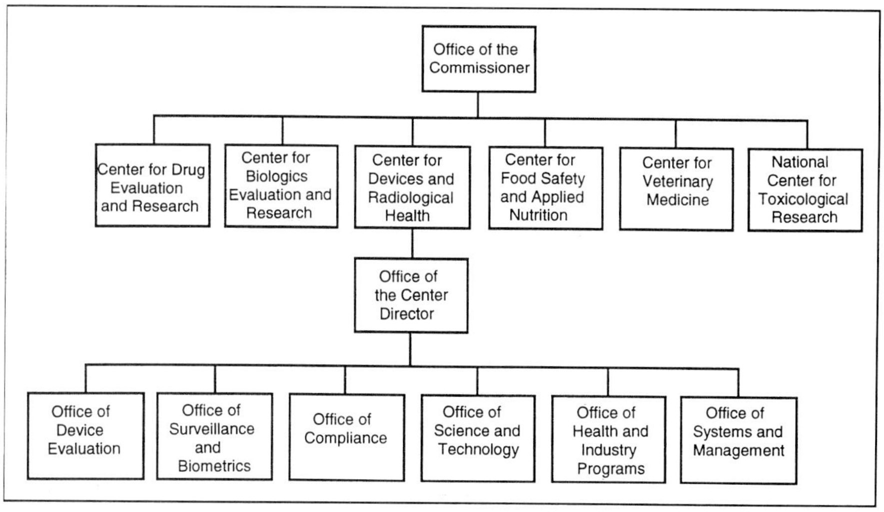

Figure 1. Organizational structure of the FDA and the Center for Devices and Radiological Health.

Class I
- Cardiopulmonary resuscitation board (exempt)
- Nuclear flood source phantom (exempt)
- Radiographic film (exempt)
- Radiographic grid
- Radiographic intensifying screen

Class II
- Automatic contrast medium injector
- Automatic radiographic film processor
- Barium enema retention catheter with bag
- Digital image storage device
- Imaging systems
  - Angiographic x-ray
  - Computed tomographic (CT)
  - Mammographic x-ray
  - Nuclear Magnetic Resonance (MR) imaging and spectroscopy*
  - US (pulsed echo and pulsed Doppler)*
- Interventional radiology
  - Catheter guide wires
  - Diagnostic intravascular catheters
  - Nephrostomy catheter
  - Transluminal peripheral angioplasty catheter
- Nasogastric tube
- Radiographic collimator
- Spinal needle

Class III
- Therapeutic devices
  - Carotid atherectomy system
  - Extracorporeal shock wave lithotriptor
  - Laser angioplasty device, peripheral or coronary
  - Transluminal coronary angioplasty catheter
- Vascular implants
  - Balloon for cerebrovascular occlusion
  - Cardiovascular stent
  - Endovascular graft system (aortic aneurysm treatment)
  - Injectable embolic agent
  - Portosystemic shunt endoprosthesis

Figure 2. Examples of device classifications. * = if operating within specified parameters.

Evaluation. The application review teams may include medical professionals, engineers, scientists, and statisticians with skills appropriate for the device being evaluated. The Office of Surveillance and Biometrics provides biostatistics support for the Office of Device Evaluation and monitors the safety of medical devices by reviewing adverse event information and conducting statistical, epidemiologic, and postmarket surveillance studies. Device problems detected by the Office of Device Evaluation or by the Office of Surveillance and Biometrics may be referred to the Office of Compliance, which is responsible for taking action against firms that have violated the FD&C Act. Inspections of laboratories, corporate and manufacturing sites, and sites of clinical trials are conducted by the FDA's regional offices. The Office of Compliance then reviews and acts on the results of those inspections and the regional offices' recommendations for enforcement actions. The Office of Compliance also administers the Radiation Control for Health and Safety Act of 1968.

The Office of Science and Technology provides broad scientific and engineering support to the other offices, including independent laboratory evaluation of products, development of test methods, and provision of technical expertise in the development of standards. The Office of Health and Industry Programs is responsible for many of the educational programs directed at device problems associated with the users of medical devices as well as programs to educate and assist device manufacturers in complying with the regulatory requirements. The Office of Health and Industry Programs also has responsibility for the administration of the Mammography Quality Standards Act of 1992, which requires accreditation of all facilities performing mammography. The Office of Systems and Management conducts internal ethical oversight and coordinates responses to requests filed under the Freedom of Information Act, in addition to providing overall business management of the Center for Devices and Radiological Health.

DEVICE CLASSIFICATION

Since medical devices vary widely in their complexity and degree of potential risk, they are classified into one of three categories on the basis of the nature of the device and the extent of FDA control required to ensure the device's safety and effectiveness (Fig 2). Class I devices pose the least risk to patients, whereas class III devices pose the greatest risk. The classification of each type of device is determined with the assistance of external advisory panels. Preamendments devices, those devices that were on the market at the time of enactment of the 1976 Amendments, were classified according to this scheme. Devices subsequently introduced are similarly classified.

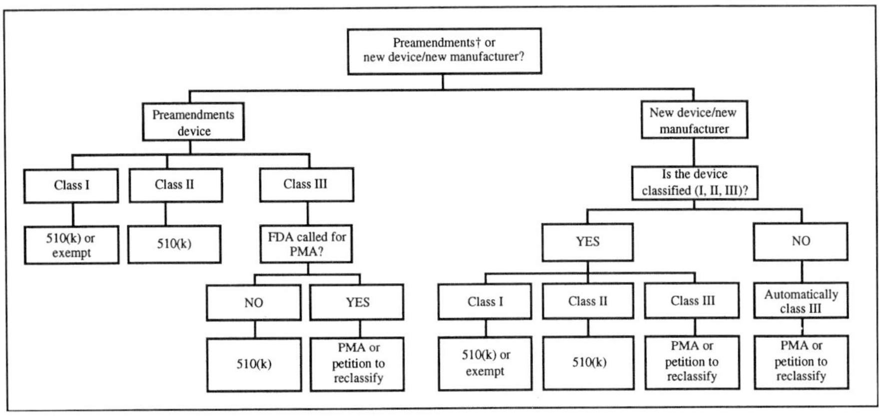

Figure 3. Overview of decision tree for determination of approval mechanism: PMA versus 510(k). † = Preamendments devices are those legally marketed before May 28, 1976, the effective date of the 1976 Amendments to the FD&C Act

Total Submissions to the Office of Device Evaluation for the 1995 and 1996 Fiscal Years

	Submissions Received	
Type of Submission	1995 Fiscal Year	1996 Fiscal Year
PMA		
Original	39	44
Amendments, supplements, and reports	2,736	2,645
510(k)		
Original	6,056	5,297
Amendments and supplements	9,564	8,589
IDE		
Original	214	253
Amendments and supplements	3,381	3,408

Source.—Reference 12.

Class I: General Controls

Class I devices are subject to general controls that include prohibition of adulterated or misbranded devices; good manufacturing practices; registration by manufacturers, importers, and distributors; and authority to ban devices or place restrictions on the sale, distribution, or use of products. Lead shields and radiographic grids are class I devices. These general controls also apply to class II and class III devices.

Class II: General Controls and Special Controls

If general controls are not sufficient, then the device is class II and subject to additional special controls. Special controls may include conformance to mandatory or voluntary performance standards, use of patient registries, requirements for postmarket surveillance, development of guidance documents for in vivo and/or in vitro testing of the device, or other mechanisms that provide additional assurance of safety and effectiveness. Only general controls apply until a special control is established by regulation. The process of development of a regulation provides opportunities for input and comment by industry and consumer groups. Most imaging systems and diagnostic angiography catheters are class II devices.

Class III: General Controls and Premarket Clearance

Class III devices are those for which the general and special controls cannot provide reasonable assurance of safety and effectiveness or those for which there is insufficient information to make that assessment. Typically, a class III device is "represented to be for a use in supporting or sustaining human life or for a use which is of substantial importance in preventing impairment of human health, or presents a potential unreasonable risk of illness or injury" (10). In addition to being subject to the general controls, class III devices also require an approved premarket approval (PMA) application before commercial distribution. In the PMA application, the manufacturer of the device must demonstrate that the device is safe and effective through design validation, manufacturing control and results of performance tests, animal studies, and usually, clinical trials. Cardiovascular stents and endovascular grafts are class III devices.

Class III devices that were on the market before the effective date of the 1976 Amendments were accorded special treatment by a grandfather clause in the Amendments, with a provision that FDA would call for PMA applications at a future date. At present, some of these preamendments devices remain in commercial distribution without an approved PMA application; however, these devices are being reevaluated, as discussed below.

FDA APPROVAL FOR MARKETING

FDA clearance is necessary before commercial distribution of medical devices. This may be accomplished in one of three ways: (*a*) approval of a PMA application; (*b*) clearance of a premarket notification submission, on the basis of section 510(k) of the FD&C Act; or (*c*) approval of a Humanitarian Device Exemption application. The Humanitarian Device Exemption is reserved for devices designed to treat rare conditions and is discussed in a separate section. Most marketing approvals are achieved by means of the PMA application or 510(k) submission.

For devices subject to the PMA or 510(k) regulations, the type of application required is a crucial distinction and depends on the device classification, whether there are similar devices classified as class I or class II approved for use, and the date at which the device was first marketed (Fig 3). In the absence of other information, devices are presumed to be class III requiring an approved PMA application before distribution. If the sponsor can identify a similar legally marketed class I or class II device and document that their device is substantially equivalent to the existing device, then they may prepare a 510(k) submission. In addition, if the device is a preamendments class III device for which FDA has not yet called for PMA applications, then a 510(k) submission may be used. The advantage to the sponsor is that the 510(k) route is generally faster and less costly than the PMA application. The Office of Device Evaluation reviews the submission and makes the determination as to substantial equivalence. In evaluating each application, the reviewing staff members must base their decisions on scientific analysis of the infor-

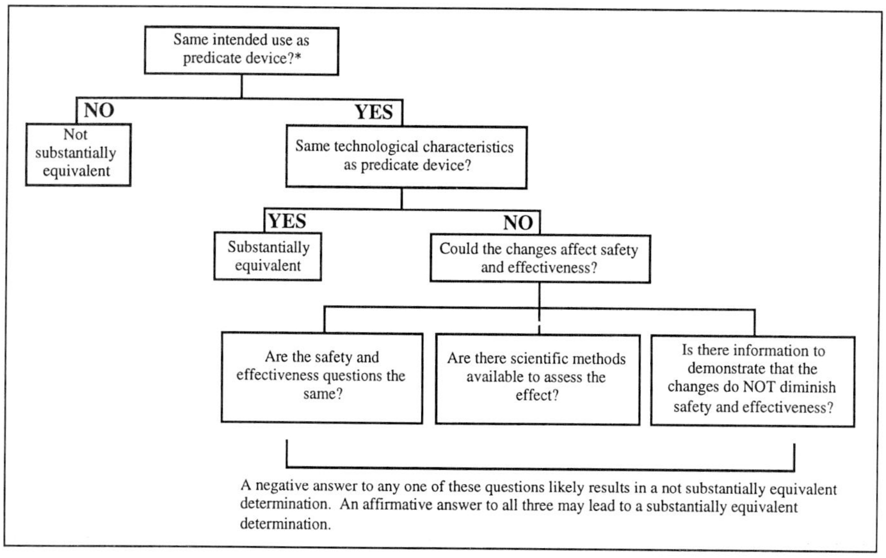

Figure 4. Determination of substantial equivalence. * = A predicate device is one that is legally marketed in the United States as class I or class II or a preamendments device for which the FDA has not yet called for premarket approval applications.

mation and data contained in the submission. The device may be distributed only if a PMA application is approved or a 510(k) submission is cleared by the FDA. Approval of a PMA application is a finding that the device is safe and effective. In contrast, clearance of a 510(k) submission is only a finding that the device is as safe and effective as the existing device with which it is compared.

The approval of marketing applications and follow-up procedures are interactive processes between the sponsor and the FDA, in that presubmission meetings are often arranged to make clear the FDA's expectations for the contents of a particular application and whether a PMA application is needed. In addition, the FDA meets with its medical devices advisory panels and with industry and professional groups to discuss the development of guidance documents for device testing and approval, to consider the concerns of manufacturers and the medical community.

PMA Application

All new class III devices introduced since the effective date of the 1976 Amendments are subject to the PMA requirements. The PMA application may not be approved unless it contains the information and data necessary to establish the safety and effectiveness of the device. A new class III device that does not have an approved PMA application may not be marketed.

The requirements for the PMA application are mandated by statute. The PMA application must include full reports of all information known to the sponsor concerning investigations to show safety and effectiveness; detailed description of all components, ingredients, properties, and principles of operation; detailed manufacturing data; samples of the device, where applicable; and the proposed labeling (11). The application is subjected to an in-depth scientific and regulatory review. After the FDA review, the application may be referred to the appropriate medical devices advisory panel, predominantly composed of practicing physicians, which makes a recommendation for action to the FDA. If recommended for approval, the FDA conducts a manufacturing site inspection, followed by final deliberations, documentation, and notification of the FDA decision.

Premarket Notification or 510(k)

The premarket notification or 510(k) submission is the most common mechanism by which devices are cleared for commercial distribution in the United States (Table)(12). The key feature is that the manufacturer must establish that the new device is "substantially equivalent" to another device that is legally marketed in the United States as class I or class II; this other device is known as the predicate device. A substantially equivalent device shares the same indications for use and is judged to be as safe and effective as the predicate device. Premarket notification is required when a device is introduced or if an existing device is significantly modified in such a way as to affect its safety and effectiveness or if there is a change in the indications for use of the device. Devices for which there is no substantially equivalent predicate device are termed "not substantially equivalent" and are placed by statute into class III and require a PMA application.

The 510(k) submission notifies the FDA of the sponsor's intention to market the device and contains the information required for the FDA to make the determination of substantial equivalence. The submission must include detailed descriptive data about the new device and the predicate device. There may also be a requirement for performance testing, including bench, animal, or clinical studies.

In determining if a new device is substantially equivalent to a predicate device (Fig 4), the key questions are whether the two devices have the same intended use or indications and the same technologic characteristics. The intended use refers to the objective intent of the person legally responsible for the labeling of the device. Such intent may be determined by statements regarding the intent or by the labeling and advertising (13). If the new device has different technologic characteristics, could the differences affect the device's safety and effectiveness or are there new questions of safety and effectiveness that differ from those posed by the predicate device? The 510(k) submission must adequately address these questions. If the device is determined to be substantially equivalent, then a 510(k) submission may be cleared. If the device is determined to be not substantially equivalent to the predicate device, then it is a class III device requiring a PMA application.

Certain class I devices have been exempted from some of the 510(k) requirements on the basis of stable technologic characteristics of commercially available devices within a generic type. These devices do not require premarket notification of the FDA unless there is a new intended use, a device modification, or a fundamentally new technologic change. The FDA retains the authority to withdraw exempt status from a group of devices. For example, medical examination gloves were exempted from 510(k) requirements until the crisis with the acquired immunodeficiency virus developed, at which time the exemption was withdrawn so that the FDA could take measures to ensure product quality.

Preamendments Devices

Devices that were in commercial distribution before May 28, 1976, the effective date of the Amendments, are commonly referred to as "preamendments devices." Class III preamendments devices were not initially subject to the PMA requirements and were cleared for marketing by means of 510(k) submissions. The FDA is engaged in an ongoing process to evaluate which preamendments class III devices should be reclassified as class I or II or remain in class III on the basis of any additional information that has accrued about the device over the past 20 years. In addition, the FDA is in the process of calling for studies of safety and effectiveness on those preamendments devices that remain in class III. All manufacturers of these devices will then be subject to the PMA requirements.

Most of the current radiologic imaging modalities are class I or class II devices and were available before the effective date of the 1976 Amendments. These devices, including x-ray equipment and CT and US devices, are preamendments devices. However, they were subject to regulation under the Radiation Control for Health and Safety Act as radiation-emitting devices before the 1976 Amendments. They are now generally cleared through the 510(k) process.

HUMANITARIAN DEVICE EXEMPTIONS

To encourage the discovery and use of devices that benefit only a small patient population each year, the FDA may grant an exemption from the effectiveness requirements of the FD&C Act, requiring only a safety evaluation. The approach is to regard the Humanitarian Device Exemption application as a PMA application without requiring effectiveness data. Approval is subject to the following requirements: (*a*) The device is designed to treat or diagnose a disease or condition that affects fewer than 4,000 individuals in the United States per year, (*b*) the device would not otherwise be available without the exemption, (*c*) no comparable device is available (other than another device with an approved Humanitarian Device Exemption application or one that is being studied under an approved ivestigational device exemptions [IDE] application), and (*d*) patients will not be exposed to an unreasonable or significant risk of illness or injury by the device. The probable benefits must outweigh the risks, taking into account the probable risks and benefits of currently available devices or forms of treatment. The devices may only be used at facilities with an established Institutional Review Board that has approved the humanitarian use of the device. The exemption is for a period of 18 months and may be renewed. These regulations became effective October 24, 1996, but are scheduled to expire after 5 years due to a sunset provision in the law (14, 15). The first approval of a Humanitarian Device Exemption application was granted early this year for a fetal bladder stent that is placed percutaneously with US guidance to relieve bladder outlet obstruction (16).

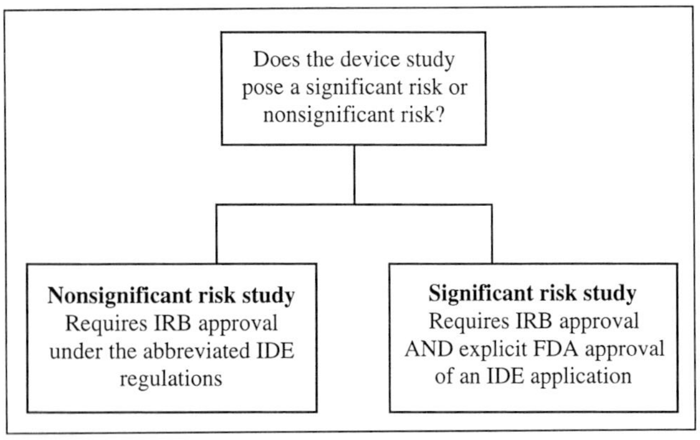

Figure 5. Required approvals for an IDE application.

INVESTIGATIONAL DEVICES AND FDA APPROVAL FOR CLINICAL TRIALS

A clinical trial may be required before marketing approval, whether the device is going through the 510(k) or PMA process. Unlike the drug approval process, which entails phase I, II, and III clinical trials, a single, well-controlled clinical trial of a device may be sufficient to support a marketing application. Approval for the initiation of clinical trials in humans under the IDE regulation is required. The "exemption" is from the restraint on commercial distribution of unapproved devices. In evaluating an IDE application, the FDA is cognizant of the investigational nature of the work. Serious safety issues, however, must be addressed by the bench and preclinical testing before the initiation of testing in human subjects, and due care in the device design, investigational planning, and protection of human subjects is required. In that regard, all protocols must meet the regulatory requirements for adequate informed consent from the study subjects. These requirements adhere to the ethical guidelines of the World Medical Association Declaration of Helsinki.

The type of approval required depends on the level of risk involved with the study (ie, whether it is a significant risk or nonsignificant risk study)(Fig 5)(17,18). If the local Institutional Review Board determines that the study is a nonsignificant risk study, then the Institutional Review Board acts as FDA's surrogate and may approve the study without direct FDA involvement under the abbreviated IDE regulation. If an Institutional Review Board finds that a study constitutes a significant risk, the sponsor must explicitly apply to the FDA for an IDE. If the IDE application is approved, the study sponsor gains permission to distribute a stated number of devices for the purpose of the clinical trial. The FDA has 30 days in which to make a determination whether to approve or disapprove the IDE application. That decision is based on the design information, the results of bench testing and any in vivo animal testing provided by the sponsor, and reports of any previous human experience. If the FDA fails to make a determination within 30 days, the IDE application is approved automatically.

There are two relatively common misunderstandings by device sponsors and Institutional Review Boards in the determination of nonsignificant risk status. One is the distinction that it is the risk of the study, not the device, that is the issue. For example, if general anesthesia were required for a study of a simple low-risk device, the study may still be considered a significant risk study. In addition, the risk should be determined on the basis of absolute risks, not risk relative to an existing device. It would be inappropriate to categorize a study of a new endovascular stent as a nonsignificant risk study on the basis of common usage of existing stents or perceived advantages over current stents. The absolute risk (ie, that failure could be life-threatening or injurious) dictates that it is a significant risk study. Examples of nonsignificant risk devices are MR imaging devices and diagnostic US devices, if the systems are operating within specified parameters. Significant risk devices include cardiovascular intravascular filters, arterial embolization devices, and laser angioplasty devices.

Individual radiologists may be involved in the investigational use of a device provided by a manufacturer or sponsor under an approved IDE application. In that case, the device is not legally marketed for that indication but is undergoing a clinical trial for the evaluation of its safety and effectiveness, usually to collect data to support a marketing application to the FDA. The device is available only for use un-

Anesthesiology and Respiratory Devices Panel
Circulatory System Devices Panel
Clinical Chemistry and Clinical Toxicology Devices Panel
Dental Products Panel
Ear, Nose and Throat Devices Panel
Gastroenterology and Urology Devices Panel
General and Plastic Surgery Devices Panel
General Hospital and Personal Use Devices Panel
Hematology and Pathology Devices Panel
Immunology Devices Panel
Microbiology Devices Panel
Neurological Devices Panel
Obstetrics and Gynecology Devices Panel
Ophthalmic Devices Panel
Orthopedic and Rehabilitation Devices Panel
Radiological Devices Panel

Figure 6. Medical Devices Advisory Committee panels.

der the supervision of designated investigators, and its use is restricted to the terms of the approved IDE application. Briefly, the investigator is responsible for (*a*) ensuring that the investigation is conducted according to the signed agreement, the investigational plan, applicable FDA regulations, and any conditions of approval imposed by an Institutional Review Board and the FDA; (*b*) protecting the rights, safety, and welfare of subjects; and (*c*) control of the devices under investigation. The investigator is also responsible for obtaining informed consent and maintaining records of use of the devices, including each study subject's case history and exposure to the device, documentation of each deviation from the study protocol, and any records required for a particular investigation.

DEVICE LABELS AND LABELING

The labeling of a device conveys the indications and directions for usage. The "label" is the written information on the device itself or its packaging, whereas "labeling" refers to this label and any descriptive or informational literature accompanying the device, as well as any advertising promoting the device. A particular claim may not be included in the labeling if there is no study to support that claim. The device may not be promoted by the manufacturer for an unapproved indication. Thus, the FDA is concerned with the contents of the labeling, including the possibilities for misbranding and inadequate labeling. Misbranding includes false or misleading labeling, inadequate directions, and failure to include applicable warnings such as warnings against use in children or in certain pathologic states or against unsafe methods of use. False and misleading labeling is not limited to misstatement of fact but may also include the omission of important information, such as complications, or creation of a false impression by deceptive statements, ambiguity, or misdirection. Misbranding is a clearly defined legal violation. Inadequate labeling refers to labeling that could be improved to prevent misuse or mishandling of the device. The usage instructions should be directed to the intended use and will differ depending on the skill level of the expected user.

ADVISORY PANELS

The FDA employs a system of external experts to review critical issues and serve in an advisory role. The Medical Devices Advisory Committee is composed of experts in a broad range of medical specialties. The committee is subdivided into 16 panels according to clinical area and device specialty (Fig 6). Each panel includes at least one consumer representative and one industry representative, both nonvoting members. In addition, consultants who are experts in the specific questions being considered by a panel may be added. To ensure an unbiased panel, all panel members must clear an FDA conflict-of-interest review. The Radiological Devices Panel is currently composed of diagnostic radiologists, radiation oncologists, and one health physicist, in addition to the consumer and industry representatives.

A major role of the panel is the review of PMA applications and the recommendation to the FDA for either approval, approval with conditions, or disapproval. In the course of the deliberations, the panel members may review all aspects of the PMA application. They conduct a public hearing in which the sponsor and any interested parties may make presentations of their views and data. Proprietary data and manufacturing information may be discussed in closed session. The FDA is not required to follow the recommendations of the panels, although it generally does.

The panels also provide advice on device classification, potential risks, development of study protocols, and the content of guidelines or guidance documents. For example, with the advent of fast gradient MR imaging capabilities, the risk of neural or cardiac stimulation has become a safety concern. In response to this concern, the Radiological Devices Panel met to discuss the FDA's proposed "Draft MRI Guidance Update for Fast Gradient Procedures." The theoretic foundations and experimental data on stimulation of excitable tissues as well as a review of clinical applications of fast gradient imaging techniques were presented by experts in the fields. Presentations were also made by company representatives, FDA staff members involved in MR imaging review, and the National Electrical Manufacturers Association. The panel made recommendations to the FDA regarding limitations on gradients, operator warning methods, further clinical trials needed, and indications for terminating a patient study. As another example, the Circulatory System Devices Panel evaluated the requirement for cardiac catheterization for obtaining transvalvular pressure drop data in heart valve patients in clinical trials. They considered the state of the art in Doppler cardiac examination to be sufficient to replace the catheterization requirement, a recommendation subsequently adopted by the FDA. Thus, advisory panels provide the FDA with scientific and medical expertise from the user community, which helps to ensure that the FDA's decision making reflects the state of the art.

MEDICAL DEVICE REPORTING

Medical Device Reporting is a system by which the FDA and device manufacturers may detect device-related problems in a timely manner. New regulations, which became effective July 31, 1996, implement the reporting requirements of the Safe Medical Devices Act of 1990 and should provide the FDA with more reliable and higher quality data than were previously available. The regulations apply to user facilities, including hospitals and outpatient diagnostic and treatment centers. Specifically, serious injuries or deaths that may have been caused by or related to a medical device must be reported to the manufacturer of the device within 10 days. Deaths must also be reported to the FDA within 10 days. Serious injuries include life-threatening injuries, injuries that result in permanent damage or impairment, or injuries that require medical or surgical intervention to prevent permanent damage or impairment (19). In the 1995 fiscal year, the Office of Surveillance and Biometrics reviewed 98,915 initial Medical Device Reporting reports.

RESPONSES TO CRITICISMS OF THE FDA

The FDA is frequently criticized for delaying the introduction of new devices and, hence, delaying progress in medical technology. Beginning in the 1992 fiscal year, a substantial backlog in the review of device submissions developed during a period of rapid increase in the number of premarket submissions and intense oversight of the Center for Devices and Radiological Health by Congress and the General Accounting Office. This delay led to widespread criticism of the FDA review times. The Center for Devices and Radiological Health made a concerted effort to eliminate the backlog, including the reallocation of internal resources and enlargement of the review staff. By the end of the 1995 fiscal year, the backlog had been largely eliminated.

During this time and continuing at present, the FDA began instituting changes in the administrative and review processes for devices; these changes are decreasing some sources of delay. For example, by emphasizing presubmission meetings with sponsors regarding IDE and PMA applications, the approval rate for these applications has risen. An internal effort is underway to reclassify certain class III devices as class II and to exempt certain class I devices from the 510(k) requirements. Administrative changes now allow the FDA to promptly determine if a submission is incomplete or contains substantial errors and to return the documents to the sponsor with a deficiency letter. Also, pilot programs are underway for third party review of 510(k) submissions and for streamlining the processing and requirements for certain PMA supplements.

EXAMPLES OF DEVICE APPROVALS

Spiral or Helical CT

The FDA recognizes the dynamic nature of medical technology development and, through the 510(k) process, accommodates it so that not all changes require a PMA application. The 510(k) regulation allows a device to be cleared if it is substantially equivalent to its predicate device, providing the FDA with great latitude in the approval of new features. CT is a good example.

CT was invented in the late 1960s and was marketed before 1976. Thus, CT was a preamendments device placed in class II and was subject to marketing clearance with the 510(k) process. Over time, many technologic advances were made including mechanical operation of the scan head, reconstruction algorithms, and computational equipment. Most recent, helical or spiral scanning was introduced; this technique represents a considerable change from the earlier section-by-section scanning method. It was cleared, however, by using the 510(k) process (Fig 4). The new device did not involve a change in the intended use (imaging). The safety and effectiveness questions raised by the new technologic characteristics were similar to those already asked for previous devices, and there were scientific means available to answer the questions. By using laboratory studies (section width, resolution, contrast, etc) and clinical trials, the device was shown to be substantially equivalent to existing devices.

MR Imaging Systems

A new device without a substantially equivalent predicate device is a class III device and requires an approved PMA application before marketing; however, devices may be reclassified as class II. MR imaging devices were first introduced in 1981. These class III devices were investigated for several years in studies considered nonsignificant risk. The first of several PMA applications for MR imaging devices was approved in 1984. In 1989, after several years of experience, enough was known about MR imaging systems operating within specified parameters to allow reclassification as class II. Since then, most changes have been cleared through the 510(k) process. However, with the advent of high-field-strength systems, the risk of neural or cardiac stimulation is of concern. Such devices raise new questions of safety that may place them in class III.

Diagnostic US Systems

Diagnostic US is similar to CT in that most systems are cleared through the 510(k) process. The performance requirements to establish substantial equivalence for diagnostic US are limited to the acoustic output (to establish equivalent safety) and the accuracy and sensitivity of the Doppler capability (to establish equivalent effectiveness if Doppler capability is included). Historically, the FDA has not considered the system resolution or image quality in evaluating the application. The FDA, however, does examine any claims the sponsor makes in the proposed labeling (including advertising) regarding imaging, all comparative claims, and other issues. As is the case with MR imaging and CT, substantial equivalence of US imaging quality has never been addressed. Generally, imaging device manufacturers follow the 510(k) process and show substantial equivalence to a predicate device without making specific claims regarding imaging capabilities in a particular pathologic process.

US Evaluation of Breast Lesions

A device is not considered separately from its indications for use. Hence, a new indication for a device for which there is no substantially equivalent predicate device with the same indication places the device in class III and requires a PMA application. Advanced Technology Laboratories, or ATL (Bothell, Wash), the manufacturer of the Ultramark 9 Ultrasound System with High Definition Imaging (HDI), submitted a PMA application to the FDA with the claim that examination of solid breast lesions with their device with use of their L10-5 Scanhead provided information that could aid in deciding if a biopsy is needed, an application that was subsequently approved (20). This represented a new intended use, specifically a new indication for the use of a marketed device that presented the risk of harm to patients in case of misdiagnosis. Since this was the first such claim of this indication presented to the FDA by a manufacturer of US devices, there was no predicate device. The device with this new intended use was therefore class III requiring a PMA application. The FDA distinguishes here between explicit claims in the labeling, which ATL was requesting, and the practice of medicine in which such uses of US devices may be ongoing.

After internal review of the application, the FDA sought external advice and referred the PMA application to the Radiological Devices Panel. The advisory panel reviewed the submission and heard testimony from representatives of ATL, including radiologists who participated in the clinical trial, and members of the FDA engineering and medical staffs. In addition, a representative of Acuson (Mountain View, Calif), a competing manufacturer, provided comments regarding ATL's application. The panel recommended "approval with conditions," specifically, that the claim is applicable only to lesions at least 1 cm in diameter. The FDA has agreed with the panel's recommendations. The approved new indication for use is "as an adjunct to mammography and physical breast examination to provide a high degree of physician confidence in differentiating benign from malignant or suspicious breast lesions. This device provides the physician with additional information to guide a biopsy decision. Utility of this system has been demonstrated for lesions with an indeterminate level of suspicion (LOS 2–4) by conventional diagnostic modalities. Using the HDI™ system in the evaluation of solid mass characteristics can reduce the number of biopsies performed on indeterminate lesions" (20). (The scale for the level of suspicion ranged from 1 to 5, where 1 was thought to be definitely benign and 5 was thought to be definitely malignant. LOS 2, 3, and 4 were considered indeterminate.)

These decisions raise pertinent issues for other manufacturers with similar devices and for off-label use by physicians. For another manufacturer to make the same claim in its labeling, it would also have to conduct a clinical trial and submit a complete and approvable PMA application. It would not suffice to demonstrate technical equivalence or comparable imaging capability to the ATL machine. Since the FDA classified the device as class III for this intended use, each manufacturer's device, its performance, and its particular manufacturing process must be reviewed independently through the PMA process. This also follows from the secondary goal of maintaining a balanced regulatory environment in which each sponsor is subject to the same regulatory hurdles as a sponsor of a similar product. A petition for reclassification to class II may be considered if data exist to demonstrate that safety and effectiveness data for individual devices are not needed and that the general or specific controls are sufficient.

The effect of the approval is that ATL has earned the right to promote the sale of its Ultramark 9 Ultrasound System with HDI for this purpose. Any use of other US systems by physicians for this indication represents "off-label" use. Such use is considered a part of the practice of medicine by individuals and is not regulated by the FDA. The FDA's articulated policy states, "Good medical practice and patient interests require that physicians be free to use commercially available drugs, devices and biologics according to their best knowledge and judgment. If a physician uses a product for an indication not in the approved labeling, he or she has the responsibility to be well informed about the product and to base its use on a firm scientific rationale and on sound medical evidence, and to maintain records of the product's use and effects" (21).

Vena Cava Filters

Some preamendments class III devices are cleared for marketing through the 510(k) process; however, the FDA is in the process of evaluating these devices and may either reclassify the devices to class II or call for PMA applications for those devices that remain in class III. Intravascular filters, devices placed in the inferior vena cava for the prevention of recurrent pulmonary embolism, which were marketed before 1976, are preamendments devices. The devices were placed in class III but are cleared for marketing by means of the 510(k) process. New filters may be cleared by demonstration of substantial equivalence to a legally marketed predicate filter if the predicate is a preamendments device or is one that has been cleared through the 510(k) process (Fig 4). In general, clinical trials are required for marketing clearance of these filters. As part of the reclassification effort of class III preamendments devices, preamendments intravascular filters may be reclassified as class II. If that were to occur, there would be no immediate practical effect on the approval process, but it would mean that the FDA would not be calling for PMA applications for these devices.

Stents for Transjugular Intrahepatic Portosystemic Shunts

A new indication for the Wallstent endoprosthesis (Schneider [USA], Plymouth, Minn), a class II device that had been cleared through the 510(k) process for biliary applications, required submission of a PMA application. Although most PMA applications are reviewed by the appropriate medical devices advisory panel, such a review was not required for this PMA application. Schneider, the manufacturer of the Wallstent transjugular intrahepatic portosystemic shunt (TIPS) endoprosthesis, received approval of its PMA application to the FDA for the indication of "creation of intrahepatic shunt connections between the portal venous system and the hepatic vein for prophylaxis of variceal bleeding in the treatment of portal hypertension and its complications in patients who have previously failed conventional treatment techniques" (22). At the time of the PMA application, the Wallstent endoprosthesis was a legally marketed class II device for use as a biliary stent. The proposed labeling change represented a new indication for the Wallstent. Since there were no devices cleared by the FDA for use in TIPS, the device with this new indication was class III and a PMA application was required (Fig 4). The PMA application was granted expedited review status, since the TIPS procedure offered an alternative to surgery or sclerotherapy in some patients with portal hypertension who had failed conventional therapy for variceal hemorrhage.

The FDA reviewed the application, which included the results of prior in vitro testing of the device and the results of a prospective clinical trial conducted under an approved IDE application. The FDA elected not to submit the PMA application to the Circulatory System Devices Panel for its review, in part because the National Institutes of Health's National Digestive Diseases Advisory Board had recently reviewed the available data on TIPS and made recommendations regarding the safety, effectiveness, and indications for TIPS (23). In addition, TIPS had been the subject of a study by the American Medical Association's Department of Technology Assessment (24). The PMA application was subsequently approved (22).

SUMMARY

The FDA operates under the mandate of Congress to ensure that medical devices are reasonably safe and effective before commercial distribution for human use. The FDA's authority to regulate medical devices was principally established by the Medical Device Amendments of 1976 to the FD&C Act. The 1976 Amendments provided a regulatory framework specifically designed for devices. In addition, radiation-emitting devices are regulated under the Radiation Control for Health and Safety Act. Within the FDA, the responsibility for the regulation of devices falls to the Center for Devices and Radiological Health.

The device classification scheme and regulatory requirements for the PMA, 510(k), and IDE are delineated in the FD&C Act, as amended in 1976. Medical devices are classified according to the degree of regulatory control needed to ensure safety and effectiveness, with class I and class II being lesser degrees and class III being the greatest. Manufacturers require FDA approval or clearance before commercial distribution of devices. There are three mechanisms by which such authority may be attained: (*a*) PMA application, (*b*) premarket notification, or 510(k), submission, and (*c*) Humanitarian Device Exemption application. The PMA application is for class III devices and for devices or indications that are not substantially equivalent to a legally marketed class I or class II device. There remain some preamendments class III devices for which the FDA has not yet called for safety and effectiveness data. These devices may continue to be marketed under the 510(k) provisions. Class I and class II devices require a 510(k) submission in which the sponsor demonstrates that the new device is substantially equivalent to a legally marketed device. The Humanitarian Device Exemption is for devices designed to treat rare disorders.

The approval of ATL's application to change the labeling for its Ultramark 9 Ultrasound System with HDI to include a new indication for the evaluation of breast lesions has caused some concern within the radiology community. Although the FDA does not regulate the practice of medicine, it does carefully regulate what manufacturers may claim regarding their products (labeling) and bases its decisions on the scientific evidence presented to it. To promote this claim, FDA clearance or approval was needed. Since no one had previously made nor substantiated a claim of this indication for a US device to the FDA, there was no substantially equivalent predicate device. The device with this new indication was therefore class III, even though the device as it was currently marketed was class II. A PMA application with a clinical trial was required. ATL conducted a well-controlled clinical trial that defined the target population and the effectiveness of the device. The application was reviewed by the FDA, considered by the Radiological Devices Panel, and subsequently approved. ■

Acknowledgments: The authors thank Susan Alpert, Lillian L. Yin, Robert A. Phillips, Dorothy B. Abel, Earl W. Robinson, and Richard G. Stiles for their editorial contributions to the preparation of this manuscript.

References

1. Shawker TH. FDA issues premarket approval. In: Society of Radiologists in Ultrasound Newsletter. Philadelphia, Penn: Society of Radiologists in Ultrasound 1996; 4(4):4–5.
2. Kopans DB. Recent issues in breast cancer detection and the premarket approval by the Food and Drug Administration of a US system for breast lesion evaluation: what happened to science? Radiology 1997; 202:315-316.
3. Schultz DG, Wagner RF, Campbell G. Science is alive and well at the Food and Drug Administration. Radiology 1997; 202:317–318.
4. U.S. Medical Technology Industry Fact Sheet, 1996. Washington, DC: Health Industry Manufacturers Association, 1997.
5. Study Group on Medical Devices, Cooper T (chairman). Medical devices: a legislative plan. Rockville, Md: U.S. Department of Health, Education and Welfare, 1970.
6. Christian CD. Maternal deaths associated with an intrauterine device. Am J Obstet Gynecol 1974; 119:441–444.
7. Culliton BJ, Knopman DS. Dalkon shield affair: a bad lesson in science and decision-making. Science 1974; 185:839–841.
8. Federal Food, Drug, and Cosmetic Act, §201(h).
9. Hendel PN. Bjork-Shiley strut fracture and disc escape: literature review and a method of disc retrieval. Ann Thorac Surg 1989; 47:436–440.
10. Federal Food, Drug, and Cosmetic Act, §513(a)(1)(C)(ii).
11. Federal Food, Drug, and Cosmetic Act, §515(c).
12. Office of Device Evaluation annual report fiscal year 1996. Washington, DC: U.S. Department of Health and Human Services, Public Health Service, Food and Drug Administration, 1997.
13. 21 CFR §801.4.
14. Federal Food, Drug, and Cosmetic Act of 1938, §520(m).
15. 21 CFR §814, subpart H.
16. 62 Federal Register 16593 (1997).
17. Sheretz RJ, Streed SA. Medical devices: significant risk vs nonsignificant risk. JAMA 1994; 272:955-956.
18. Less JR, Alpert S, Nightingale SL. Institutional Review Boards and medical devices. JAMA 1994; 272:968-969.
19. 21 CFR §803.3(aa).
20. 61 Federal Register 60712-60713 (1996).
21. Nightingale SL. Investigational use of marketed products. Rockville, Md: U.S. Food and Drug Administration, 1982.
22. 61 Federal Register 37277-37278 (1996).
23. Shiffman ML, Jeffers L, Hoofnagle JH, Tralka TS. The role of transjugular intrahepatic portosystemic shunt for treatment of portal hypertension and its complications: a conference sponsored by the National Digestive Diseases Advisory Board. Hepatology 1995; 22:1591-1597.
24. Miller-Catchpole R. Transjugular intrahepatic portosystemic shunt (TIPS): diagnostic and therapeutic technology assessment (DATTA). JAMA 1995; 273:1824-1830.

James A. Brink, MD

Increased CT Contrast Enhancement of "Normal" Hepatic Parenchyma May Herald "Occult" Metastases[1]

SINCE their inception, cross-sectional imaging techniques have remained far from ideal for the detection of hepatic neoplasms, particularly small or early lesions. Investigators have performed innumerable studies to improve detection of liver tumors with computed tomography (CT) and magnetic resonance (MR) imaging. To some degree, lesion detection has been augmented by the use of contrast media administered intravascularly, with a wide variety of techniques for contrast material delivery and the timing of scanning.

Helical dual-phase contrast-enhanced CT represents an important addition to the hepatic imaging armamentarium (1). When the hepatic arterial phase is added to the portal venous phase of contrast enhancement, hepatocellular carcinoma may be detected in 8%–11% more patients (2,3). In addition to improved depiction of hypervascular tumors, dual-phase helical CT may be useful for improving detection of hypovascular tumors as well (4,5).

In this issue of *Radiology*, Platt and colleagues (6) look beyond improvements in hepatic lesion detection with dual-phase helical CT to indirect evidence of occult metastases in the liver. By measuring the enhancement of the "normal" hepatic parenchyma, they found that increased hepatic enhancement during the arterial phase may signify the presence of underlying metastases. The authors have quantified several CT parameters of hepatic arterial enhancement, including the ratio of hepatic enhancement at 25 and 40 seconds after initiation of injection to peak hepatic enhancement. All measured CT parameters were statistically significantly higher in patients who developed detectable liver metastases within 18 months of imaging compared with those who did not develop detectable metastases.

By testing several thresholds for their enhancement measures, Platt et al (6) determined that occult metastases were best identified when at least 40% of maximum hepatic contrast enhancement was achieved by 40 seconds after initiation of injection of 150 mL of contrast material at 3 mL/sec. With this criterion, they computed, retrospectively, 75% sensitivity, 96% specificity, and 89% accuracy for determination of patients who did or did not develop hepatic metastases within 18 months. The authors suggest that results may be improved by combining multiple enhancement criteria.

Increased hepatic enhancement during the arterial phase is proposed to result from an increase in hepatic arterial blood flow relative to portal venous blood flow. The authors hypothesize that this increase in hepatic arterial blood flow reflects small, early hepatic metastases that are not visible during either the hepatic arterial or portal venous phases of contrast enhancement.

Several of the authors' ideas have grown from their previous work in which they compared similar measures of hepatic enhancement in patients with visible hepatic metastases to enhancement measures in healthy subjects (7). In the June issue of the *Journal of Computer Assisted Tomography* (7), the authors reported these findings and emphasized that the greatest increase in hepatic arterial enhancement was present in patients with breast carcinoma, compared with that in patients with other primary neoplastic foci.

The authors of various studies have measured hepatic arterial and portal venous perfusion with CT and Doppler sonography. Although increased hepatic arterial perfusion has been shown in patients with cirrhosis or detectable hepatic metastases (8,9), Leen and colleagues (10) also demonstrated an increase in hepatic arterial flow in patients who developed hepatic metastases within 1 year after undergoing duplex and color Doppler sonography. By measuring the angle-corrected velocity and cross-sectional area of the common hepatic artery and the portal vein, the Doppler perfusion index (ratio of hepatic arterial flow to total liver blood flow) was computed; values greater than 0.30 were considered to be abnormal. With this threshold, the authors reported, retrospectively, 100% sensitivity, 57% specificity, and 72% accuracy for the detection of colorectal cancer metastases to the liver.

These works represent an exciting frontier for hepatic imaging and may have an enormous effect on the care of oncology patients suspected of having hepatic metastases. As Leen et al (10) suggested, increased hepatic arterial perfusion, whether measured in terms of hepatic enhancement during arterial-phase helical CT or in terms of the Doppler perfusion index at duplex and color Doppler sonography, may be used to triage patients for more or less aggressive chemotherapeutic regimens and may encourage continued therapy in those with unwanted side effects.

The use of hepatic enhancement during arterial-phase helical CT for this purpose is not without limitations. Platt et al (6) addressed several limitations in their article, including the well-documented increase in arterial perfusion associated with cirrhosis, which may result in false-positive diagnosis of occult metastases. They did not mention, however, that in patients with decreased cardiac output, a false-negative diagnosis may be expected owing to delayed hepatic enhancement at specific time points after initiation of contrast material injection. Use of an absolute threshold of enhancement at fixed time points after initiation of injection will likely result in errors of underestimation of hepatic arterial perfusion in patients with poor cardiac output and occult hepatic metastases. Although the authors found no statistically significant difference in the weight distribution between their two patient groups, patient weight is also an important factor that affects the degree of hepatic enhancement for a given injection of contrast material and may be expected to affect the degree of

Index terms: Computed tomography, helical, 761.12115 • Editorials • Liver, CT, 761.12111, 761.12113, 761.12115 • Liver, blood supply • Liver neoplasms, 761.323 • Liver neoplasms, secondary, 761.332

Radiology 1997; 205:37–38

[1] From the Department of Diagnostic Radiology, Yale University School of Medicine, 333 Cedar St, New Haven, CT 06510. Received and accepted July 28, 1997. **Address reprint requests to** the author.

See also the article by Platt et al (pp 49–53) in this issue.

hepatic enhancement achieved at fixed intervals after initiation of injection, particularly for those at the extreme ends of the weight spectrum.

In these respects, duplex and color Doppler sonography may be superior to dual-phase helical CT insofar as sonography provides direct evidence of increased hepatic arterial perfusion. Dual-phase helical CT provides indirect evidence of increased arterial perfusion on the basis of the degree of early contrast enhancement, the effectiveness of which is related to patient-specific variables such as weight and cardiac output. However, precise and accurate measurement of the Doppler perfusion index depends on a skilled ultrasonographer and is likely subject to greater interobserver variability than the helical CT technique.

In the present study reported by Platt and colleagues (6), the fact that a high percentage of patients had breast carcinoma should not be trivialized. Breast carcinoma, when metastatic to liver, is known to be hypervascular and is frequently infiltrative. It is possible that regions of interest for attenuation measurements at initial helical CT may be established to interrogate directly small or infiltrative metastases that are unrecognized. The authors have emphasized, in their previous work (7), that the greatest discrimination between tumorous and nontumorous livers with arterial-phase helical CT occurred in patients with breast carcinoma rather than other primary neoplasms. The influence of the primary neoplasm on the success of this technique for detecting occult hepatic metastases will need to be better defined in future studies in patients with various primary malignancies. In addition, prospective studies of diagnostic performance will be needed before clinical application.

Regardless, the results of these investigations introduce a new chapter in the continuing saga of hepatic imaging in the oncology patient. Prediction of occult metastases based on direct or indirect evidence of increased hepatic arterial perfusion may become an important tool for evaluating these patients in years to come. ■

References

1. Oliver JH III, Baron RL. Helical biphasic contrast-enhanced CT of the liver: technique, indications, interpretation, and pitfalls. Radiology 1996; 201:1–14.
2. Oliver JH III, Baron RL, Federle MP, Rockette HE Jr. Detecting hepatocellular carcinoma: value of unenhanced or arterial phase CT imaging or both used in conjunction with conventional portal venous phase contrast-enhanced CT imaging. AJR 1996; 167:71–77.
3. Baron RL, Oliver JH III, Dodd GD III, Nalesnik M, Holbert BL, Carr B. Hepatocellular carcinoma: evaluation with biphasic, contrast-enhanced, helical CT. Radiology 1996; 199:505–511.
4. Hollett MD, Jeffrey RB Jr, Nino-Murcia M, Jorgensen MJ, Harris DP. Dual-phase helical CT of the liver: value of arterial phase scans in the detection of small (≤1.5 cm) malignant hepatic neoplasms. AJR 1995; 164:879–884.
5. Bonaldi VM, Bret PM, Reinhold C, Atri M. Helical CT of the liver: value of an early hepatic arterial phase. Radiology 1995; 197:357–363.
6. Platt JF, Francis IR, Ellis JH, Reige KA. Liver metastases: early detection based on abnormal contrast material enhancement at dual-phase helical CT. Radiology 1997; 205:49–53.
7. Platt JF, Francis IR, Ellis JH, Reige KA. Difference in global hepatic enhancement assessed by dynamic CT in normal subjects and patients with hepatic metastases. J Comput Assist Tomogr 1997; 21:348–354.
8. Blomley MJK, Coulden R, Kormano M, Donlan P, Bufkin C, Lipton MJ. Liver perfusion studied with ultrafast CT. J Comput Assist Tomogr 1995; 19:424–433.
9. Miles KA, Hayball MP, Dixon AK. Functional images of hepatic perfusion obtained with dynamic CT. Radiology 1993; 188:405–411.
10. Leen E, Angerson WJ, Wotherspoon H, Moule B, Cook TG, McArdle CS. Detection of colorectal liver metastases: comparison of laparotomy, CT, US, and Doppler perfusion index and evaluation of postoperative follow-up results. Radiology 1997; 195:113–116.

Richard L. Ehman, MD

Limitations of Tried-and-True Imaging Signs with New Modalities[1]

THE ongoing development of medical imaging takes place in at least three distinct areas. Perhaps the most visible of these is technical research, which has yielded a series of increasingly powerful diagnostic imaging tools during the past decades. A second area of endeavor is concerned with the science of interpretation—attempting to understand the meaning of specific imaging findings. A third branch of effort is concerned with defining appropriate and effective applications of the medical imaging tools in clinical practice.

Progress in any one of these three areas often provides impetus for related efforts in the other two. Indeed, such parallel progress is vital. For example, early advances in magnetic resonance (MR) imaging technology made it feasible to delineate the global anatomic structure of joints, such as the knee, in unprecedented detail. Unfortunately, the appearance on MR images of even common lesions, such as meniscal tears, was unknown. Therefore, research efforts were made to define the diagnostic importance of various imaging findings such as abnormal intrameniscal signal intensity and bone marrow edema (1). These accomplishments, in turn, provided motivation for investigators of later studies who defined MR imaging as an appropriate, cost-effective, and now widely used modality for evaluating the knee.

The art and science of image interpretation in diagnostic radiology relies on the knowledge of the anatomic, histologic, and functional effects of various disease processes. Many diagnostic imaging signs are universal: These signs are valid regardless of the imaging technique used because they reflect the underlying pathophysiologic process of the disease. Pancreatic cancer, for instance, may manifest as a local mass, regional adenopathy, and liver metastases. These findings have the same diagnostic importance if they are identified with ultrasound, computed tomography, or MR imaging.

In some cases, however, there are pitfalls in the casual application of traditional diagnostic criteria with new imaging tests. Outwater and colleagues describe such a circumstance in this issue (2). The characterization of renal masses with cross-sectional imaging has become a common task in clinical radiology. Radiologists have long accepted that fat demonstrated in a renal mass is virtually diagnostic of angiomyolipoma, and indeed fat is present in approximately 95% of such lesions (3). Conversely, fat within the tumor is extremely rare in renal carcinoma (4). The few reported exceptions to this rule appear to represent engulfed renal-sinus fat or osteoid metaplasia within necrotic tumor (5).

Macroscopic fat in tissue may be identified with conventional MR imaging; however, a special MR technique, known as "opposed-phase" imaging, is exquisitely sensitive for the detection of minute quantities of lipid. Spin-echo and gradient-echo versions of the technique have been described (6,7). Opposed-phase MR imaging is readily accomplished with most conventional MR systems, and a number of applications—such as discriminating benign adrenocortical masses (which often contain small amounts of lipid) and other adrenal lesions—are well established (8).

Given the dictum that angiomyolipomas often contain demonstrable fat and renal carcinomas rarely do, it may seem attractive to use opposed-phase MR imaging to improve the classification of renal masses. Indeed, this concept has been proposed in the literature (9). With their study, Outwater and colleagues provide a timely service to the clinical community by showing that this approach could lead to an incorrect diagnosis. In fact, they show that many renal carcinomas appear to contain fat when these masses are assessed with opposed-phase imaging. They indicate, from a histologic standpoint, that renal carcinomas often contain intracellular lipid, which (along with glycogen) accounts for the "clear cell" description of many of these tumors (10).

Opposed-phase imaging is one example of an interesting group of diagnostically useful MR imaging techniques that provide contrast among tissues by a phenomenon known as "intravoxel phase dispersion." This phenomenon occurs because the intensity of MR image pixels is determined by a vector average (instead of a scalar average as with CT) of signals from within the corresponding object voxels. Properly understood, this extra complexity provides radiologists with additional capabilities for characterizing tissues. Properties that can be sensitively assessed with such intravoxel-phase-dispersion techniques include the lipid to water ratio (with in-phase and opposed-phase imaging), intravoxel magnetic heterogeneity (with T2-weighted imaging), water diffusion (with diffusion-weighted imaging), fluid shear (with most imaging sequences), and intravoxel T1 dispersion (with inversion-recovery imaging).

The results of the study by Outwater et al suggest that if MR imaging is to be used to characterize renal masses, we may need to refine the diagnostic criteria used to identify fat within lesions so that these criteria are more specific about the quantity of lipid and its macroscopic distribution. The study of Outwater et al illustrates that caution is warranted when even tried-and-true diagnostic criteria are used with sensitive, new imaging tests. Their results also underscore the need for adequate research efforts to ensure that progress in understanding the interpretation and appropriate application of new imaging technology keeps pace with its introduction. ■

Index terms: Editorials • Fat, MR • Kidney neoplasms, diagnosis, 81.121419, 81.3141, 81.324 • Magnetic resonance (MR), tissue characterization, 81.121419 • Kidney neoplasms, MR, 81.121412, 81.3141, 81.324 • Lipoma and lipomatosis, 81.3141

Radiology 1997; 205:39–40

[1] From the Department of Diagnostic Radiology, Mayo Clinic, 200 First Street SW, Rochester, MN 55902. Received and accepted July 17, 1997. **Address reprint requests to** the author.

See also the article by Outwater et al (pp 103–107) in this issue.

References

1. Crues JV III, Mink JH, Levy TL, Lotysch M, Stoller DW. Meniscal tears of the knee: accuracy of MR imaging. Radiology 1987; 164:445–448.

2. Outwater EK, Bhatia M, Siegelman ES, Burke MA, Mitchell DG. Lipid in renal clear cell carcinoma: detection on opposed-phase gradient-echo MR images. Radiology 1997; 205:103–107.
3. Wagner BJ, Wong-You-Cheong JJ, Davis CJ. Adult renal hamartomas. RadioGraphics 1997; 17:155–169.
4. Davidson AJ, Hartman DS, Choyke PL, Wagner BJ. Radiologic assessment of renal masses: implications for patient care. Radiology 1997; 202:297–305.
5. Helenon O, Merren S, Paraf F, et al. Unusual fat-containing tumors of the kidney: a diagnostic dilemma. RadioGraphics 1997; 17:129–144.
6. Dixon WT. Simple proton spectroscopic imaging. Radiology 1984; 153:189–194.
7. Wehrli FW, Perkins TG, Shimakawa A, Roberts F. Chemical shift-induced amplitude modulations in images obtained with gradient refocusing. Magn Reson Imaging 1987; 5:157–158.
8. Mitchell DG, Crovello M, Matteucci T, Peterson RO, Miettinen MM. Benign adrenocortical masses: diagnosis with chemical shift MR imaging. Radiology 1992; 185:345–351.
9. Kido T, Yamashita Y, Sumi S, et al. Chemical shift GRE MRI of renal angiomyolipoma. J Comput Assist Tomogr 1997; 21: 268–270.
10. Rosai J. Ackerman's surgical pathology. Vol 1. St Louis, Mo: Mosby–Year Book, 1996; 1146–1153.

Julien B. C. M. Puylaert, MD, PhD • Arie M. Rijke, MD, PhD

An Inflamed Appendix at Sonography When Symptoms Are Improving: To Operate or Not to Operate?[1]

In 1886, Sir Reginald Fitz presented his classic description of appendicitis. In that first publication he had already recognized the clinical entity of recurrent acute appendicitis (1). Typically, attacks occur only to subside spontaneously in the course of a few hours and usually well within 48 hours after the first onset of symptoms. Intervals between attacks may vary from weeks to years and are essentially free of symptoms. The incidence of these attacks is, in fact, quite high: As many as 13%–25% of patients with surgically proved appendicitis have experienced one or more previous attacks (2,3).

The above findings have been traditionally interpreted as part of the symptomatology of spontaneously resolving appendicitis with recurrent acute appendicitis at a later time. Presumably, there are also patients who experience only one attack and remain symptom free thereafter, but there are no data to substantiate this.

Because of its easy accessibility and noninvasiveness, sonography provides a unique tool to examine the abdomen in patients with suspected appendicitis. As could be expected, many articles about sonography in cases of acute appendicitis have mentioned unequivocal inflammation of the appendix in the presence of improving clinical symptoms. Subsequent analysis in five studies showed this to occur in 9% of patients with suspected appendicitis who underwent sonography (4–8). Patients in this category, who underwent surgery in spite of their improving symptoms, invariably had an acutely inflamed appendix; in others who were treated conservatively, however, symptoms resolved spontaneously. If and how often appendicitis recurred was not mentioned by these authors.

In this issue of *Radiology*, Migraine et al (9) report another nine patients with both sonographic and clinical documentation of spontaneously resolving appendicitis. Recurrent right lower quadrant pain was observed in two of these patients, which eventually led to surgical intervention in one of them. The authors also discuss the mechanism of spontaneously resolving appendicitis. They emphasize that the cause of appendicitis is obstruction of the lumen with subsequent high intraluminal pressure, vascular compromise, and, eventually, infection (10). Therefore, they argue, the most plausible explanation for spontaneously resolving appendicitis—which is supported by the speedy resolution of the clinical symptoms—is relief of obstruction. The authors presume that the obstruction is less likely to resolve spontaneously in the presence of a fecalith than in the presence of lymphoid hyperplasia or soft fecal material.

The management of sonographically confirmed spontaneously resolving appendicitis is the concern of all surgeons. Conceivably, those surgeons who have relied on findings at sonography for the confirmation of their clinical diagnosis in the past may be prompted to perform immediate appendectomy. In that event, the pathologist is likely to justify that decision by reporting acute appendicitis indistinguishable from ordinary acute appendicitis. Alternatively, surgeons who are reluctant to operate on patients with improving symptoms will see their conservative approach justified by a spontaneously recovering patient, an approach that may also have been favored before the advent of sonography. In case surgery is considered, there is no advantage of elective over immediate appendectomy other than a more convenient time for the operation.

A number of considerations are important in surgical decision making. A history of one or more earlier attacks may prompt the surgeon to perform immediate appendectomy despite improving symptoms. Another consideration may be the age of the patient: The history may be very atypical and the initial clinical signs quite mild in the elderly who nonetheless experience progression toward perforation.

A third consideration is the presence of a fecalith in the appendiceal lumen at sonography, which suggests an increased chance of recurrence. This is supported by the work of Eriksson and Granström, who performed a prospective study in 40 patients with sonographically confirmed appendicitis (11). Although this study was directed at determining the effect of antibiotic treatment on the course of acute appendicitis, the results show nonetheless that the presence of a fecalith in the lumen predisposes the patient to recurrent attacks and therefore may constitute an independent risk factor. The fact that the presence of a fecalith in cases of appendicitis is associated with a higher chance of perforation may also be an influence (12).

In summary, spontaneously resolving appendicitis is a clinically recognized entity that is by no means rare. The recurrence rate is uncertain, and performance of a prospective study with sonography is necessary for further evaluation. Until more understanding of this entity is gained, the preferred treatment of patients with clinical and sonographic evidence of spontaneously resolving appendicitis is conservative. Patients should be instructed to report to the hospital without delay in case of recurrent symptoms. Performance of immediate appendectomy in cases of spontaneously resolving appendicitis can be considered (*a*) when there is a history of one or more previous attacks, (*b*) in elderly patients, (*c*) when an obstructing fecalith is present, and (*d*) in patients who frequently travel to underdeveloped countries or who for one reason or another temporarily have no access to advanced health care. ■

Index terms: Appendicitis, 751.291 • Appendix, US, 751.1298 • Editorials

Radiology 1997; 205:41–42

[1] From the Department of Radiology, Westeinde Hospital, Lijnbaan 32, 2512 VA The Hague, The Netherlands, and University Hospital Leiden, Leiden, The Netherlands (J.B.C.M.P.); and the Department of Radiology, Health Sciences Center, University of Virginia, Charlottesville (A.M.R.). Received July 14, 1997; accepted, July 22. **Address reprint requests to** J.B.C.M.P.

See also the article by Migraine et al (pp 55–58) in this issue.

References

1. Fitz HR. Perforating inflammation of the vermiform appendix with special reference to its early diagnosis and treatment. Am J Med 1886; 92:321–346.
2. Lewis FR, Holcroft JW, Boey J, Dunphy JE. Appendicitis: a critical review of diagnosis

and treatment in 1000 cases. Arch Surg 1975; 110:677–681.
3. Ferrier PK. Acute appendicitis in university students: a twenty year study of 1028 cases. Am Coll Health Assoc J 1972; 20:287–290.
4. Amland PF, Skaane P, Ronningen H, Nordshus T, Solheim K. Ultrasonography and parameters of inflammation in acute appendicitis. Acta Chir Scand 1989; 155:185–189.
5. Jeffrey RB Jr, Laing FC, Townsend RR. Acute appendicitis: sonographic criteria based on 250 cases. Radiology 1988; 167:327–329.
6. Ooms HWA, Koumans RMJ, Ho Kang You PJ, Puylaert JBCM. Ultrasonography in the diagnosis of acute appendicitis. Br J Surg 1991; 78:315–318.
7. Rioux M. Sonographic detection of the normal and abnormal appendix. AJR 1992; 158:773–778.
8. Puylaert JBCM, Rutgers PH, Lalisang RI, et al. A prospective study of ultrasonography in the diagnosis of appendicitis. N Engl J Med 1987; 317:666–669.
9. Migraine S, Abri M, Bret PM, Lough JO, Hinchey JE. Spontaneously resolving acute appendicitis: clinical and sonographic documentation. Radiology 1997; 205:55–58.
10. Wangensteen OH, Bowers WF. Significance of the obstructive factor in the genesis of acute appendicitis: experimental study. Arch Surg 1937; 34:496–526.
11. Eriksson S, Granström L. Randomized controlled trial of appendectomy versus antibiotic therapy for acute appendicitis. Br J Surg 1995; 82:166–169.
12. Fagenberg D. Fecaliths of the appendix: incidence and significance. AJR 1963; 89:752–759.

Robert E. Mindelzun, MD • R. Brooke Jeffrey, MD

Unenhanced Helical CT for Evaluating Acute Abdominal Pain: A Little More Cost, a Lot More Information[1]

THE introduction of new imaging techniques and the pressures of the marketplace have challenged the appropriateness of many diagnostic studies currently in use. In no situation is this more dramatically illustrated than in the imaging of the acute abdomen. An acute abdomen is an acute abdominal disorder of uncertain cause that necessitates immediate medical or surgical attention. As physicians well know, there are literally hundreds of diseases that may manifest initially with acute abdominal pain (1). In a 1988 review by the Research Committee of the World Organization of Gastroenterology, de Dombal (2) evaluated 10,682 cases of acute abdominal pain. This review followed studies in 1978 and 1982 in which (for all practical purposes) an unchanged frequency of presenting diagnoses was found. In the large group of patients studied by de Dombal, the cause of abdominal pain was never established in a substantial percentage (34.0%) of cases. Among the other patients, 28.0% had appendicitis, 9.7% had acute cholecystitis, 4.1% had small-bowel obstruction, 4.0% had acute gynecologic disease, 2.9% had acute pancreatitis, 2.9% had renal colic, 2.5% had a perforated peptic ulcer, 1.5% had cancer, and 1.5% had diverticular disease. An analysis of these data suggests that approximately two-thirds of patients with acute abdominal pain have a disease that may be diagnosed on the basis of imaging findings. With cost in mind, use of imaging must enable triage of these patients rapidly, safely, and decisively toward optimal therapy.

Index terms: Abdomen, acute conditions, 70.11, 70.12111, 70.12112, 70.12118 • Abdomen, CT, 70.12111, 70.12112, 70.12118 • Abdomen, radiography, 70.11 • Devil's Advocate

Radiology 1997; 205:43–47

[1] From the Department of Radiology, Stanford University School of Medicine, 300 Pasteur Dr, Stanford, CA 94305-5105. Received May 9, 1997; accepted July 22. **Address reprint requests to** R.E.M.

The traditional approach to evaluating the patient with acute abdominal pain has been immediate plain radiography. The introduction of unenhanced (no oral or intravenous administration of contrast material) helical computed tomography (CT), however, challenges this well-established algorithm. Helical CT provides the combined advantages of speed and a seamless coverage of the abdomen with outstanding spatial resolution of and contrast between tissues. Helical CT can be performed in many patients during one breath-holding interval.

An analysis of the role of abdominal radiography suggests that there are two urgent conditions—pneumoperitoneum and intestinal obstruction—that are best evaluated with this modality (3). The diagnostic evaluation of both conditions merits further scrutiny.

Although plain radiography can be exquisitely sensitive for detecting small amounts of free air (4), a number of authors have shown that abdominal CT is clearly superior to plain radiography for diagnosing free air (5,6). While this is true in all patients, it is especially evident in the evaluation of the very ill or obese patient or the patient who is unable to cooperate with examination (6). Although a high-quality series of abdominal radiographs has been shown to demonstrate 1–2 mL of free air, this situation probably represents an ideal examination of a patient who has not undergone abdominal surgery. In patients with a localized or "walled-off" perforation or in those who have undergone surgery, plain radiography is less sensitive; even large amounts of air can be loculated and difficult to discern on plain radiographs (6). In addition to the increased sensitivity of CT for detecting free air, this modality has been shown to be superior for identifying extraluminal air in the bowel wall or within the mesenteric or portal venous systems. In mesenteric ischemia, mesenteric and portal venous air are important findings because they suggest an unfavorable prognosis (7).

The second entity traditionally evaluated with abdominal radiography has been intestinal obstruction. There is considerable controversy about the best approach for evaluating intestinal obstruction: Some investigators favor abdominal radiography followed with contrast material–enhanced studies, and others tout the superiority of CT (8–10). Both approaches have merit; however, if plain abdominal radiography and CT are evaluated separately, it appears that CT is superior for detecting an obstruction and its location and cause (11–13). On occasion, CT may also enable the distinction of ileus from mechanical obstruction (14).

What about the most common causes of the acute abdomen that were elucidated by de Dombal? Abdominal radiography in patients suspected to have appendicitis is of limited value (15). By contrast, CT performed with oral or intravenous contrast material has been shown to be exquisitely sensitive for diagnosing appendicitis. Balthazer et al (16) achieved a sensitivity of 98%, a specificity of 88%, and an overall accuracy of 95% with use of oral and intravenous contrast material during CT. Malone et al (17), with use of unenhanced nonhelical CT, achieved a sensitivity of 87%, a specificity of 97%, and an accuracy of 93% for the diagnosis of acute appendicitis. In a study of 109 patients, Lane et al (18), with unenhanced helical CT (ie, without oral or intravenous contrast material), achieved a sensitivity of 90%, a specificity of 97%, and an accuracy of 94%. In this group of patients, an alternative diagnosis was correctly established in 22%; these diagnoses included right-sided diverticulitis, ureteral calculi, malignancies, and gynecologic disorders. A similar frequency and range of diagnoses were noted in a recent study by Rao et al (19). One must conclude from these studies that CT, with or without administration of contrast material, is far superior to abdominal radiography for the evaluation of appendicitis.

Abdominal radiographs are often helpful for evaluating renal colic, but they must be acquired with contrast material for the optimal evaluation of ureteral calculi. Unenhanced helical CT for the evaluation of renal colic was first investigated by Smith et al (20,21).

An overall accuracy of 97% for diagnosing ureteral stones was reported. This finding was corroborated by Sommer et al (22). On the basis of their data, both groups indicated that, at their institutions, unenhanced helical CT has completely replaced other techniques (such as excretory urography) for the initial evaluation of renal colic. The impression that unenhanced CT is superior to abdominal radiography for identifying ureteral calculi was corroborated by Carpenter et al (23) in a study of 112 patients. When unenhanced helical CT was used as the standard of reference, they showed that radiography of the kidneys, ureters, and bladder (KUB) had a sensitivity of 84%, a specificity of only 64%, and an accuracy of 74%.

The diagnosis of diverticular disease has not been studied with unenhanced CT alone, although evaluation with contrast-enhanced CT (ie, with use of oral and intravenous contrast material) has shown great promise (24). Many of the findings in diverticular disease are related to diverticular perforation and inflammation of the adjacent mesentery; these findings are readily appreciated on unenhanced CT scans. With CT, the diagnosis of cholecystitis has not improved to the same extent as that of many other entities. At present, the enhanced CT images of a substantial number of patients with acute cholecystitis do not demonstrate sufficient findings to establish a definitive diagnosis (25). Nonetheless, findings such as gallstones, distention of the gallbladder, pericholecystic fluid, pericholecystic stranding, and wall thickening can be readily appreciated on enhanced and unenhanced CT scans. In patients who show strong clinical evidence of acute cholecystitis, sonography remains the initial imaging method of choice.

With unenhanced CT, pancreatitis can be suggested with findings of an enlarged pancreas and infiltration of the anterior pararenal space, small-bowel mesentery, and transverse mesocolon. Findings associated with pancreatitis—such as pancreatic lithiasis, pancreatic hemorrhage, and emphysematous pancreatitis—are readily appreciated on unenhanced scans.

In addition, unenhanced CT provides definitive information in the (*a*) evaluation of intra- and extraperitoneal hemorrhage, (*b*) identification of coproliths, and (*c*) characterization of extraluminal air.

If the information provided with unenhanced CT is indeed considerably superior to that provided with abdominal radiography, then the major obstacle to replacing abdominal radiography with unenhanced CT appears to be its cost and availability. A survey of several local institutions revealed that a two-view abdominal radiographic series costs from $136 to $184; our institution charges $521 for an unenhanced abdominal CT scan. Contrast enhancement can be very helpful for evaluating multiple intraabdominal diseases such as ischemia, pancreatitis, and aneurysms. We hypothesize that, in many situations, administration of contrast material is not necessary. An unenhanced CT examination does not preclude subsequent contrast-enhanced examinations for resolving specific diagnostic questions. When there are unexplained or incompletely explained findings on the unenhanced CT images or when therapy decisions necessitate further information, then contrast material can be administered and another scan can be acquired with little time lost. A number of investigators have suggested that, in the patient with acute abdominal pain, the increased sensitivity and specificity of CT reduce the overall cost of care (26–30).

What about the availability of CT? It is currently estimated that there are 6,500 installed CT systems in the United States (31) and more than 15% of these systems are helical units. The helical CT market is expected to grow slowly for a number of years (32). With the current number of available CT scanners in this country, however, the few patients who present each day with acute abdominal pain could be examined easily. Although we have directed our comments to helical CT, one could arrive at similar conclusions for dynamic CT.

In conclusion, the patient with *acute* abdominal pain needs to be evaluated with a rapid, accurate, and reasonably priced imaging modality. It is our belief that unenhanced helical CT provides clinically relevant information in most patients at a reasonable cost.

References

1. Sleisenger MH, Fordtrau JS. Gastrointestinal disease. Philadelphia, Pa: Saunders, 1989.
2. de Dombal FT. Diagnosis of acute abdominal pain. 2nd ed. New York, NY: Churchill Livingstone, 1 991.
3. Baker SR. Plain film radiography of the acute abdomen. In: Thrall J, ed. Current practice of radiology. St Louis, Mo: Mosby, 1994; 112–114.
4. Miller RE, Nelson SW. The roentgenographic demonstration of tiny amounts of free intraperitoneal gas: experimental and clinical studies. AJR 1971;112:574–585.
5. Stapakis JC, Thickman D. Diagnosis of pneumoperitoneum: abdominal CT vs upright chest film. J Comput Assist Tomogr 1992; 16:713–716.
6. Earls JP, Dachman AH, Colon E, Garrett MG, Molloy M. Prevalence and duration of postoperative pneumoperitoneum: sensitivity of CT vs left lateral decubitus radiography. AJR 1993; 161:781–785.
7. Scheidler J, Stabler A, Kleber G, Neidhardt D. Computed tomography in pneumatosis intestinalis: differential diagnosis and therapeutic consequences. Abdom Imaging 1995; 20:523–528.
8. Fukuya T, Hawes DR, Lu CC, Chang PJ, Barloon TJ. CT diagnosis of small-bowel obstruction: efficacy in 60 patients. AJR 1992; 158:765–769.
9. Maglinte DD, Reyes BL, Harmon BH, et al. Reliability and role of plain film radiography and CT in the diagnosis of small-bowel obstruction. AJR 1996; 167:1451–1455.
10. Mindelzun RE, Vierra M. Role of imaging in the evaluation of small-bowel obstruction. AJR 1995; 164:255–256.
11. Taourel PG, Fabre JM, Pradel JA, Seneterre EJ, Megibow AJ, Bruel JM. Value of CT in the diagnosis and management of patients with suspected acute small-bowel obstruction. AJR 1995; 165:1187–1192.
12. Balthazar EJ, George W. Holmes lecture: CT of small-bowel obstruction. AJR 1994; 162:255–261.
13. Megibow AJ. Bowel obstruction: evaluation with CT. Radiol Clin North Am 1994; 32:861–870.
14. Frager DH, Baer JW, Rothpearl A, Bossart PA. Distinction between postoperative ileus and mechanical small-bowel obstruction: value of CT compared with clinical and other radiographic findings. AJR 1995; 164:891–894.
15. Yacoe ME, Jeffrey RB Jr. Sonography of appendicitis and diverticulitis. Radiol Clin North Am 1994; 32:899–912.
16. Balthazar EJ, Birnbaum BA, Yee J, Megibow AJ, Roshkow J, Gray C. Acute appendicitis: CT and US correlation in 100 patients. Radiology 1994; 190:31–35.
17. Malone AJ Jr, Wolf CR, Malmed AS, Melliere BF. Diagnosis of acute appendicitis: value of unenhanced CT. AJR 1993; 160:763–766.
18. Lane MJ, Katz DS, Ross BA, Clautice-Engle TL, Mindelzun RE, Jeffrey RB Jr. Unen-hanced helical CT for suspected acute appendicitis. AJR 1997; 168:405–409.
19. Rao PM, Rhea JT, Noveline RA,et al. Helical CT technique for the diagnosis of appendicitis: prospective evaluation of a focused appendix CT examination. Radiology 1997; 202:139–144.
20. Smith RC, Rosenfield AT, Choe KA, et al. Acute flank pain: comparison of non-contrast-enhanced CT and intravenous urography. Radiology 1995; 194:789–794.
21. Smith RC, Verga M, McCarthy S, Rosenfield AT. Diagnosis of acute flank pain: value of unenhanced helical CT. AJR 1996; 166:97–101.
22. Sommer FG, Jeffrey RB Jr, Rubin GD, et al. Detection of ureteral calculi in patients with suspected renal colic: value of reformatted noncontrast helical CT. AJR 1995; 154:509–513.
23. Carpenter K, Talner L, Bush W, Schmutz F, Mann F. KUB vs helical CT in patients with acute flank pain. Presented at the Fifth European Symposium, International Society of Urorad-iology and 15th Annual Postgraduate Course, Society of Uroradiology, Zurich, Switzerland, June 14–20, 1996.
24. Padidar AM, Jeffrey RB Jr, Mindelzun RE, Dolph JF. Differentiating sigmoid diverticulitis from carcinoma on CT scans: me-

senteric inflammation suggests diverticulitis. AJR 1994; 163:81–83.
25. Fidler J, Paulson EK, Layfield L. CT evaluation of acute cholecystitis: findings and usefulness in diagnosis. AJR 1996; 166:1085–1088.
26. Simeone JF, Novelline RA, Ferrucci JT Jr, et al. Comparison of sonography and plain films in evaluation of the acute abdomen. AJR 1985; 144:49–52.
27. Siewert B, Raptopoulos V, Mueller MF, Rosen MP, Steer M. Impact of CT on diagnosis and management of acute abdomen in patients initially treated without surgery. AJR 1997; 168:173–178.
28. Johnson GL, Johnson PT, Fishman EK. CT evaluation of the acute abdomen: bowel pathology spectrum of disease. Crit Rev Diagn Imaging 1996; 37:163–190.
29. Siewert B, Raptopoulos V. CT of the acute abdomen: findings and impact on diagnosis and treatment. AJR 1994; 163:1317–1324.
30. Taourel P, Baron MP, Pradel J, Fabre JM, Seneterre E, Bruel JM. Acute abdomen of unknown origin: impact of CT on diagnosis and management. Gastrointest Radiol 1992; 17:287–291.
31. Bieze T, Casey B, Freiherr G, et al. The U.S. diagnostic imaging market: global perspective. San Francisco, Calif: Miller Freeman, 1994.
32. Lindahl RM, Stephens T, Bieze T, Casey B. Computed tomography: analysis of market status and industry trends. San Francisco, Calif: Miller Freeman, 1994.

Stephen R. Baker, MD

Unenhanced Helical CT versus Plain Abdominal Radiography: A Dissenting Opinion[2]

The advent of helical computed tomography (CT) and its widening dissemination in hospitals and clinics throughout the United States have substantially advanced our ability to diagnose abdominal diseases rapidly and comprehensively. This technique is not merely complementary and supplemental, but in some acute conditions, helical CT is competitive and even superior to the traditional, initial imaging approach with plain radiography. Therefore, it is logical to propose, as Mindelzun and Jeffrey have done forcefully, that unenhanced CT should supplant conventional radiography in this setting.

No doubt, on its face, the argument for CT has obvious attractions. CT is "high tech," whereas plain radiography is "old hat." Moreover, helical CT provides much more information about abdominal spaces, organs, and conduits than that provided with conventional radiography. To be sure, CT enables a detailed delineation of the extent and configuration of expected pathologic features and makes possible the recognition of unsuspected treatable conditions. Yet, radiologists must be careful about changing policy solely on the basis of the incisiveness and clarity of a particular new modality. The issue is not just the quality of pictorial display but the cost-effectiveness of substituting a traditional technique with a new modality.

"Acute abdomen" is a broad and even pejorative term that encompasses many diverse functional and anatomic abnormalities. The clinical manifestation must be refined further before CT and plain radiography can be compared. Many such patients do not need to undergo imaging despite their discomfort. The radiographic investigation of mild to moderate pain is usually fruitless. Also, a short history of crampy diarrhea without other symptoms rarely merits radiographic or sonographic assessment. Moreover, most sufferers of an acute abdomen do not come to the radiology department before a preliminary history is obtained and a physical examination and initial laboratory tests are performed. When a patient reaches the general radiography room or CT suite, the diagnostic possibilities usually have been reduced to just a few likely entities. For instance, the differing nature of viscus perforation and intestinal obstruction are almost always evident with careful questioning and expert physical examination. Acute pancreatitis can be diagnosed (even without radiographic confirmation) with a combination of history, pertinent physical findings, and an elevated serum amylase level. Thus, only a subset of patients with acute pain would benefit from a mandated switch from plain radiography to unenhanced helical CT.

Causes of an acute abdomen must be disaggregated further into specific categories of disease before distinctions can be drawn about the relative merits of these two imaging techniques and, consequently, their respective clinical efficacies. First consider two common situations in which plain radiography still has clinical pertinence if not dominance. There is no doubt that abdominal CT is the standard of reference for recognizing tiny amounts of free air. Yet, most recent studies that compare conventional radiography with CT are limited because the two imaging studies were not performed simultaneously (1,2). The time between initial abdominal radiography and cross-sectional imaging raises uncertainty about the different volumes and configurations of pneumoperitoneum observed with each method.

The two modalities can be compared only when they are performed simultaneously—this situation occurs when a digital scout image is acquired as part of the CT study. In this way, we readily reproduced the pioneering finding of Miller and Nelson (3): With plain radiography, 1–2 mL of free air can be recognized (4). In fact, even smaller quantities of extraluminal air can be detected when the entire abdomen, including all of the right upper quadrant, is seen on a single supine view or series of supine views (5). Thus, one can maintain that CT may be superior to plain radiography—but not by very much. Certainly CT is not sufficiently superior to justify the automatic bypassing of conventional radiography in all patients. One may contend that adhesions hinder the upward percolation of air below the diaphragm and thereby limit the sensitivity of plain radiography. This notion has a certain allure, but it is an impression

[2] From the Department of Radiology, Rm C320, New Jersey Medical School, 150 Bergen St, Newark, NJ 07103. Received July 10, 1997; accepted July 22. **Address reprint requests to** the author.

only and not substantiated with any prospective or retrospective clinical data (6).

Free air is often missed on plain radiographs of the abdomen. The detection of free air may be a function of a general laxness of test performance instead of an intrinsic physical limitation of the technique. In many institutions, a radiograph of the kidneys, ureters, and bladder, or KUB, is considered equivalent to a plain radiograph of the abdomen with the patient in a supine position. However, the uppermost portion of the peritoneal cavity, which extends from above the kidneys to the apex of the higher diaphragmatic dome, is excluded from view. Unfortunately, small amounts of intraperitoneal air commonly collect in the right upper quadrant (7). If plain radiography is performed with rigorous attention to patient position (and with sometimes two views—one of the lower abdomen and one of the upper abdomen to the diaphragmatic level), most cases of free air will likely be detected with plain radiography, and routine CT will be avoided.

In the diagnosis of intestinal obstruction, plain radiography still has value even if its primacy has been questioned. In simple mechanical obstruction of the small or large bowel, three questions may be posed: (*a*) Does an obstruction exist? (*b*) Where is it located? (*c*) What is its cause? Plain radiography can really provide an answer only to the first question; with CT, the location and, in some cases, a cause for the blockage can be determined (8–10). In recent studies, the sensitivity of unenhanced radiography for detecting obstruction has ranged from 44% to 88% (11–13). This wide variance results from several factors. The cause and site of luminal occlusion may not be similar among disparate populations. Intermittent obstruction is more difficult to appreciate than complete blockage. Also, on plain radiographs, proximal jejunal obstruction is less often revealed than distal ileal obstruction; in the former condition, fewer dilated gas-filled loops exist proximal to the site of luminal closure. Swallowed air functions as lucent contrast material so that obstruction is discerned. The volume air in the intestine is in part culturally or ethnically influenced and related to differing affective responses to colicky pain. The vigor of air swallowing, in turn, may influence the varying sensitivity of plain radiography. Finally, the emphasis in radiologic training on cross-sectional imaging over the past 15 years has deflected interest away from mastering the subtleties of conventional radiographic interpretation. With greater attention to the signs of accumulated air due to obstruction, the overall effectiveness of plain radiography could be improved.

Nevertheless, does conventional radiography fare badly against CT? Maglinte et al (13) demonstrated that plain radiography was actually superior to CT for the detection of obstruction. Other contemporary investigators who have touted CT used a protocol in which contrast material was administered intravenously in nearly all individuals and oral contrast material was used liberally (8,10). Clearly, there will be patients with sufficient intraluminal fluid so that use of oral contrast material is avoided. Yet, there will be many other patients to whom oral contrast material must be given, and therefore, the cost-effectiveness of helical CT will be diminished.

Furthermore, although CT images can often demonstrate the site and cause of a luminal occlusion, these determinations are not critical for many surgeons. The decision to proceed to surgery may be based solely on the demonstration of an obstruction. When characterizing obstruction, there is no consensus whether expedience or comprehensiveness is more important. Therefore, it seems premature to advocate unenhanced helical CT as the first imaging test when plain radiography still enables the diagnosis in most affected individuals.

A second category of acute abdominal conditions includes diseases for which plain radiography has little value, unenhanced abdominal CT images are more revealing, and other imaging studies enable a definitive diagnosis. Plain radiographs demonstrate gallstones in approximately 15% of patients with cholelithiasis and show acute gallbladder inflammation only in the rare case of emphysematous cholecystitis. Wall thickening, nonopaque calculi, and pericholecystic fluid can all be imaged with CT (14). However, sonography should be the procedure of choice in those patients with acute pain in the right upper quadrant. Thus, the distinct advantage of CT over plain radiography has little meaning in the screening of acute liver, biliary, and gallbladder diseases.

The plain radiographic findings of acute pancreatitis are meager and often nonspecific. For instance, the demonstration of stones indicates only chronic pancreatitis and does not provide any evidence about acute inflammation. Unenhanced helical CT images show pancreatic contours and dimensions and can readily reveal peripancreatic collections, pseudocysts, and abscesses. Do these demonstrations confer a considerable advantage to CT in the initial evaluation of most patients with acute pancreatic inflammation?

Not really. Most individuals with pancreatitis have mild to moderate forms of the disease. There are two schools of thought about how to proceed with imaging studies at admission. One opinion is that radiographic studies are of minimal value because therapy is merely supportive. However, if pain or other indexes of risk persist or worsen, then enhanced CT could be performed later to evaluate better for abscess, pseudocyst, or extension of fluid. An alternative view is that all patients with pancreatitis should be assessed promptly for pancreatic necrosis. This assessment, with CT, requires the administration of contrast material for distinguishing areas of decreased vascularity, which indicate cell death (15). Neither opinion about imaging of acute pancreatitis champions unenhanced helical CT: With use of one technique, information not really needed early is provided; the other technique is inadequate for determining the critical diagnostic issue—the superimposition of necrosis. Hence, notwithstanding its advantages over plain radiography, unenhanced helical CT is not the most appropriate test for acute pancreatitis regardless of which sentiment is adopted.

Colonic diverticulitis can almost never be diagnosed with plain radiography. In this case, CT has become the procedure of choice. CT not only allows recognition of an inflammatory mass with greater sensitivity than barium studies; CT images show the extent of disease and depict other conditions. In diverticulitis, however, CT examination is performed with intravenous, oral, and sometimes rectal contrast material (16). Therefore, unenhanced helical CT images often will not show adequately the appearance and extent of a suspected diverticular abscess.

On the other hand, unenhanced helical CT is certainly superior to plain radiography for the evaluation of acute appendicitis (17–19). Moreover, unenhanced helical CT may also exceed sonography because CT is at least equally sensitive and is not operator dependent. For detecting appendicitis, the limitation of CT, however, is not its inability to show pathologic findings. In the case of appendicitis, most patients are evaluated clinically, and the decision to operate is made frequently on the basis of laboratory findings, an evolving pattern of pain, and abnormal physical examination results. For many surgeons, imaging is required only in a minority of cases in which the diagnosis is unclear with other means of investigation. Hence, CT—although a real improvement over plain radiography—is a crucial test only in a minority of these patients.

Unenhanced helical CT will probably become the technique of choice in the diagnosis of ureteral calculi. CT has been shown to be better and perhaps less costly than the combination of plain radiography and sonography (20–22). However, there are clinical conditions that Mindelzun and Jeffrey did not cite that could nevertheless be included in the differential diagnosis of an acute abdomen. Especially in elderly patients, constipation alone may manifest with acute pain. There is no doubt that this diagnosis can be rapidly achieved with plain radiography. CT provides no additional advantage.

A clear-cut case for the replacement of conventional radiography with helical CT can be made in those instances in which a large percentage of patients with acute abdominal pain have ureteral calculi. To this argument may be added the small number of individuals with appendicitis in whom clinical assessment is not conclusive enough to make a determination about surgery. Yet, when these situations do not occur in a large portion of a population, the increased expense of unenhanced helical CT may not justify its blanket substitution for traditional abdominal radiography.

An innovation, such as helical CT, in radiologic practice brings with it other, less obvious diseconomies. If unenhanced helical CT does not enable a conclusive diagnosis, then an enhanced study may need to be performed. The charge for such a biphasic examination would have to be increased considerably above the baseline price to recoup the expense of injected and/or ingested contrast material. If a large percentage of cases require enhanced studies, the putative cost-effectiveness of the initial "simple" CT examination vanishes very quickly.

There are important management issues to be considered as well. Let us accept the number quoted by Mindelzun and Jeffrey of 6,500 CT scanners in the United States (23). These scanners have been deployed for the care of inpatients, patients in the emergency department, and those in the clinic. Among the approximately 6,000 hospitals in this country, there must be some acute-care institutions that do not have a CT scanner on site. Moreover, in many other facilities, the scanner is operated only during weekday working hours and is unavailable at night and during weekends, when patients with an acute abdomen often present. Furthermore, patients who are acutely ill may first undergo chest radiography, which is often performed in the same room or on the same table where a series of abdominal radiographs is acquired. To undergo helical CT, the patient may have to be transferred to another location within the radiology department or at a distance from it; this is a maneuver that frail and confused patients may not tolerate or need.

A further confounding variable is the capability of selected technologists. Some can perform plain radiography and CT competently, and others can perform conventional studies only. Thus, one cannot conclude that the existing number of CT scanners adequately justifies a nationwide change in standards. All facilities do not have the equipment and personnel to accomplish CT examinations in all patients at all times.

In conclusion, I do not believe it is currently practical or clinically necessary to promote helical CT as a replacement for plain radiography in patients with an acute abdomen. The singular value of CT is well established for some indications but uncertain or controversial for others. The preferential use of CT, as advocated by Mindelzun and Jeffrey, may be easy in certain hospitals but very difficult or impossible in many others. Would the failure to use CT preferentially be malpractice? For the foreseeable future, plain radiography will be with us; we cannot avoid its use for conditions in which it is helpful. Hence, despite the enticements of new imaging techniques, we should not arbitrarily displace or neglect plain radiography because the consequences and costs of change are still problematic. ■

References

1. Markowitz SK, Ziter FMA Jr. The lateral chest film and pneumoperitoneum. Ann Emerg Med 1986; 15:425–426.
2. Stapakis JC, Thickman D. Diagnosis of pneumoperitoneum: abdominal CT vs upright chest film. J Comput Assist Tomogr 1992; 16:713–716.
3. Miller RE, Nelson SW. The roentgenographic demonstration of tiny amounts of free intraperitoneal gas: experimental and clinical studies. AJR 1971; 112:574–585.
4. Baker SR. Imaging of pneumoperitoneum. Abdom Imaging 1996; 21:413–414.
5. Cho KC, Baker SR. Extraluminal air: diagnosis and significance. Radiol Clin North Am 1994; 32:829–844.
6. Earls JP, Dachman AH, Colon E, Garrett MG, Molloy M. Prevalence and duration of postoperative pnueumoperitoneum: sensitivity of CT vs left lateral decubitus radiography. AJR 1993; 161:781–785.
7. Levine MS, Scheiner JD, Rubesin SE, et al. Diagnosis of pneumoperitoneum on supine abdominal radiographs. AJR 1991; 156:731–735.
8. Taourel PG, Fabre JM, Pradel JA, Seneterre EJ, Megibow AJ, Bruel JM. Value of CT in the diagnosis and management of patients with suspected acute small-bowel obstruction. AJR 1995; 165:1187–1192.
9. Balthazar EJ, George W. Holmes lecture: CT of small-bowel obstruction. AJR 1994; 162:255–261.
10. Megibow AJ. Bowel obstruction: evaluation with CT. Radiol Clin North Am 1994; 32:861–870.
11. Fukuya T, Hawes DR, Lu CC, Chang PJ, Barloon TJ. CT diagnosis of small-bowel obstruction: efficacy in 60 patients. AJR 1992; 158:765–769.
12. Frager DH, Baer JW, Rothpearl A, Bossart PA. Distinction between postoperative ileus and mechanical small-bowel obstruction value of CT compared with clinical and other radiographic findings. AJR 1995; 164:891–894.
13. Maglinte DD, Reyes BL, Harmon BH, et al. Reliability and role of plain film radiography and CT in the diagnosis of small-bowel obstruction. AJR 1996; 167:1451–1455.
14. Fidler J, Paulson EK, Layfield L. CT evaluation of acute cholecystitis: findings and usefulness in diagnosis. AJR 1996; 166:1085–1088.
15. Kivisaari L, Somer K, Standertskjold-Nordenstaum CG, et al. A new method for the diagnosis of acute hemorrhagic-necrotizing pancreatitis using contrast-enhanced CT. Gastrointest Radiol 1984; 9:27–30.
16. Cho KC, Morehouse HT, Alterman DD, Thornhill BA. Sigmoid diverticulitis: diagnostic role of CT—comparison with barium enema studies. Radiology 1990; 176:111–115.
17. Yacoe ME, Jeffrey RB Jr. Sonography of appendicitis and diverticulitis. Radiol Clin North Am 1994; 32:899–912.
18. Lane MJ, Katz DS, Ross BA, Clautice-Engle TL, Mindelzun RE, Jeffrey RB Jr. Unenhanced helical CT for suspected acute appendicitis. AJR 1997; 168:405–409.
19. Balthazar EJ, Birnbaum BA, Yee J, Megibow AJ, Roshkow J, Gray C. Acute appendicitis: CT and US correlation in 100 patients. Radiology 1994; 190:31–35.
20. Smith RC, Rosenfield AT, Choe KA, et al. Acute flank pain: comparison of noncontrast-enhanced CT and intravenous urography. Radiology 1995; 194:789–794.
21. Smith RC, Verga M, McCarthy S, Rosenfeld AT. Diagnosis of acute flank pain: value of unenhanced helical CT. AJR 1996; 166:97–101.
22. Sommer FG, Jeffrey RB Jr, Rubin GD, et al. Detection of ureteral calculi in patients with suspected renal colic: value of reformatted noncontrast helical CT. AJR 1995; 154:509–513.
23. Bieze T, Casey B, Freiherr G, et al. The U.S. diagnostic imaging market: global perspective. San Francisco, Calif: Miller Freeman, 1994.

Sum & Substance

Innervation of the Liver: Morphology and Function.
D. G. Tiniakos, J. A. Lee, A. D. Burt. *Liver* 1996; 16:151–160. (A.D.B., Department of Pathology, University of Newcastle upon Tyne, Royal Victoria University, Newcastle upon Tyne, NE1 4LP, England.)

Recently, with the advent of immunohistochemistry, the intricacies of hepatic innervation have begun to be uncovered. The results of multiple animal and human studies have indicated that hepatic efferent innervation plays an active role in regulating portal blood flow, bile flow regulation, parenchymal regeneration, and the metabolism of carbohydrates, lipids, and plasma proteins. Hepatic afferent innervation is less well understood and may be involved in osmoreception and baroreception and in the control of hepatic metabolic receptors.

Anatomic studies have demonstrated nerve bundles in the porta hepatis that are composed of sympathetic fibers from T-7 to T-10 via the celiac ganglion and parasympathetic fibers from the vagus nerve. Nerve bundles travel in close proximity to the portal vein and hepatic artery. Intrasinusoidal nerves also have been demonstrated with electron microscopy studies in humans. Nerve fibers within the sinusoids allow for the direct innervation of hepatic parenchymal cells.

Most neuronal fibers in mammalian livers are adrenergic as evidenced by a high frequency of tyrosine hydroxylase (TH) positivity. While less well understood, the presence of intrahepatic and intrasinusoidal parasympathetic fibers has also been suggested by the demonstration of acetylcholinesterase-containing fibers within portal tracts and hepatic sinusoids.

In addition to classical neurotransmitters, several regulatory peptides have been demonstrated in human livers. One such peptide, neuropeptide tyrosine (NPY), has been identified in nerves associated with the extrahepatic biliary tract as well as intrahepatic and intrasinusoidal nerve fibers. NPY has been shown to have direct vasoconstrictive properties on its target tissue. In addition, the distribution of NPY-positive fibers appears to correlate with that of TH-positive fibers, which raises the possibility of NPY acting as a co-transmitter to potentiate the effects of noradrenaline and adenosine triphosphate released from sympathetic fibers.

Studies of the diseased liver have shown increased numbers of myelinated nerve fibers in fibrotic regions of the cirrhotic liver. Further examination shows this increase in nerve fiber density to be isolated to the developing fibrous septa with an actual paucity of nerve fibers in the developing cirrhotic nodules. Additional studies have demonstrated near complete absence of intrasinusoidal nerve fibers in established cirrhosis.

While the exact importance of hepatic innervation has not been delineated, hepatic nerve fibers do not appear to be necessary for life as demonstrated by the changes found after orthotopic liver transplantation. In the transplanted human liver, the degeneration of parenchymal nerve fibers occurs shortly after transplantation, whereas portal nerve fibers are gone by 6 weeks. Studies have shown the reappearance of some nerve fibers in the portal triads by 32 weeks after transplantation. The extent of the reinnervation, however, is minimal, and there has been no demonstration of reinnervation of the hepatic parenchyma after transplantation. Despite the lack of hepatic innervation in the transplanted liver, there appear to be no directly related ill effects. However, an overall increase in hepatic flow after transplantation has been demonstrated, which may be due to a loss of vasomotor tone.

The fluctuations of extrahepatic splanchnic blood flow were once thought to be the principal means of regulating intrahepatic blood flow. Now the active role the liver plays in regulating its own hemodynamic homeostasis is supported by studies demonstrating that the stimulation of nerve bundles in the portal region causes the release of noradrenaline. This in turn results in a decrease in hepatic blood flow and an increase in portal pressure. Further support is supplied by studies showing that the isolated and perfused liver can support portal pressure oscillations. This is thought to be in part related to hepatic stellate cells, which are fat-containing cells located at various points along the sinusoidal lumen. Stellate cells have been shown to undergo contraction in the presence of several vasoactive agonists. In addition, studies of stellate cells in vitro show that noradrenaline causes the release of prostaglandin F_2 and prostaglandin D_2, which are prostanoids that are known to stimulate glycogenolysis. Thus, sympathetic innervation may aid not only in the regulation of hepatic blood flow but also in hepatic metabolism.

In summary, it is clear that there is extensive hepatic innervation. The liver, once considered a relatively passive organ, is now believed to play an active role in most, if not all, of its functions. The advent of advanced immunohistochemical techniques has provided a means for a basic understanding of the details of intrahepatic neural subtypes, nerve fiber distribution, and general function. Hepatic efferent innervations that aid in regulating portal blood flow are perhaps best understood.

Julie K. Shaffrey, MD
The Johns Hopkins Hospital
Baltimore, Md

Joel F. Platt, MD • Isaac R. Francis, MD • James H. Ellis, MD • Karen A. Reige, BS, RT

Liver Metastases: Early Detection Based on Abnormal Contrast Material Enhancement at Dual-Phase Helical CT[1]

PURPOSE: **To assess whether contrast material enhancement findings on computed tomographic (CT) scans are useful in determination of the risk for development of hepatic metastases.**

MATERIALS AND METHODS: **Dual-phase helical CT scans were obtained in 80 patients with nonhepatic cancer and no hepatic metastases visible at CT. Attenuation was measured on scans obtained at 25 and 40 seconds. Peak liver attenuation was determined in all cases. Unenhanced scans were obtained in 35 patients. The ratio of liver attenuation at 25 and 40 seconds to peak liver attenuation, liver enhancement values at 25 and 40 seconds, and ratio of liver enhancement at 25 and 40 seconds to peak liver enhancement were determined.**

RESULTS: **Liver metastases developed during 18-month follow-up in 22 patients. The 25- and 40-second liver enhancement values and the liver enhancement and attenuation ratios were higher in these patients than in those who did not develop metastases ($P < .01$). Enhancement values and ratios were more accurate than densitometric measurements for predicting development of metastases. Use of an optimal threshold (0.40 or greater) for the 40-second enhancement ratio resulted in a sensitivity of 75%, specificity of 96%, and overall accuracy of 89%.**

CONCLUSION: **CT measurements may help in the prediction of risk for subsequent development of hepatic metastases.**

Computed tomography (CT) is commonly used in the detection of hepatic metastases in patients with an underlying primary neoplasm (1–6). The authors of previous reports (2,3) have shown that although CT is an excellent technique for detection of hepatic metastases, it is less optimal in the detection of smaller (diameter < 1 cm) lesions.

Hepatic metastases are known to receive a much greater proportion of their blood supply from the hepatic artery than from the portal venous system (7–9). Therefore, the presence of hepatic metastases may alter global hepatic hemodynamics (7–9). The results of previous studies (8–12) with dynamic scintigraphy and duplex Doppler ultrasound (US) have shown a generalized increase in hepatic arterial flow relative to portal venous flow in patients with hepatic metastases. Furthermore, these results suggested that the presence of small or occult liver metastases can result in altered liver blood flow. Therefore, it is possible that analysis of differential blood flow in the liver could lead to the determination of patients with small or early hepatic metastases.

The authors of two previous studies (13,14) in which hepatic CT was used suggested that altered hepatic hemodynamics could be detected in the neoplastic liver on the basis of relative contrast enhancement observed at different phases of CT scanning. Helical CT technology facilitates the analysis of hepatic enhancement because it is now possible to scan the liver routinely at many different phases of contrast enhancement.

The goal of our study was to assess differential densitometric and contrast-enhancement patterns in the liver in patients with nonhepatic cancer in whom no hepatic metastases could be visually detected on CT scans. Follow-up CT was performed to determine subsequent development of hepatic metastases. We also sought to identify specific hepatic CT contrast-enhancement characteristics that could be used to distinguish patients with a higher risk of developing liver metastases.

MATERIALS AND METHODS

Study Population

During an 18-month period from January 1994 to June 1995, 100 patients with a known nonhepatic primary neoplasm and no previous CT evidence of hepatic metastases were prospectively evaluated. All patients underwent dual-phase helical CT of the liver. Five patients were excluded from the study because the standardized dual-phase CT scan was not properly obtained, usually because of a CT scanner malfunction. Five patients were excluded because they had evidence of hepatic metastases on the initial dual-phase helical CT scans. Another 10 patients were excluded because of inadequate follow-up CT scans. The remaining 80 patients constituted our study population. There were 55 women and 25 men with a mean age ± 1 standard deviation of 54 years ± 11 (range, 31–81 years). Mean patient weight ± 1 standard deviation was 65 kg ± 19 (range,

Index terms: Computed tomography (CT), helical, 761.12115 • Liver, blood supply • Liver, CT, 761.12111, 761.12113, 761.12115 • Liver neoplasms, secondary, 761.33

Radiology 1997; 205:49–53

[1] From the Department of Radiology, University of Michigan Hospital, 1500 E Medical Center Dr, Ann Arbor, MI 48109-0030. Received March 27, 1997; revision requested May 7; revision received June 2; accepted June 5. **Address reprint requests to** J.F.P.

See also the editorial by Brink (pp 37–38) in this issue.

50–110 kg). For these 80 patients, the most common primary tumors were breast tumor ($n = 44$), melanoma ($n = 11$), carcinoid tumor ($n = 6$), and colon tumor ($n = 6$).

CT Protocol

Helical CT scans were obtained in all patients with the same protocol and similar scanners (HiSpeed Plus; GE Medical Systems, Milwaukee, Wis). All patients received 150 mL of iohexol (300 mg iodine per milliliter) (Omnipaque; Nycomed, Princeton, NJ) administered intravenously at a rate of 3 mL/sec with a power injector. Dual-phase CT of the liver was performed in each patient. Acquisition of the early-phase images began 20 seconds after initiation of contrast material injection, and the later-phase images were obtained 70 seconds after initiation of the contrast material injection. Scanning was performed at 120 kV and 220–250 mA. Contiguously reconstructed sections (pitch of 1:1) were obtained through the liver with 7-mm collimation. In the last 35 patients, a unenhanced scan of the liver was obtained, as well.

CT Densitometry

Absolute liver densitometric measurements (in Hounsfield units) were obtained from those CT images obtained 25 and 40 seconds after the initiation of contrast material injection by using a region-of-interest cursor (55 mm^2). The two sections obtained at 25 and 40 seconds were chosen to represent early and late time points in the first (arterial) phase of dual-phase hepatic helical CT. For each sampling time, three region-of-interest attenuation measurements were recorded from three distinct regions of the liver and were then averaged. Care was taken to exclude hepatic vessels from all region-of-interest placements in the liver. Region-of-interest measurements were obtained in the remaining liver images as well (ie, all early- and late-phase images) to determine a peak liver densitometric value for each patient. All densitometric measurements were performed by one experienced CT technologist (K.A.R.).

CT Densitometric Ratios

The absolute attenuation values of the liver were used to calculate the following densitometric ratios: For each sampling time (25 and 40 seconds), the ratio of liver attenuation at that time point to the peak liver attenuation was determined.

CT Enhancement Data

In the group of patients who underwent both unenhanced and contrast-enhanced CT ($n = 35$), it was possible to analyze true hepatic enhancement. For each time point (25 and 40 seconds), the attenuation value of the liver on corresponding (on the basis of table position) unenhanced CT scans was subtracted from the contrast-enhanced CT attenuation value to yield a liver enhancement value. Peak liver enhancement was also determined, for each patient, by calculating the difference between the peak liver attenuation value and the unenhanced liver attenuation value (the average of values from scans obtained at the table positions that corresponded to the 25- and 40-second sections).

Table 1
Comparison of CT Densitometric Characteristics in Patients Who Did and Did Not Develop Hepatic Metastases

Densitometric Measure	Patients with Metastases	Patients without Metastases
Ratio of liver attenuation to peak liver attenuation		
25 sec	0.52 ± 0.03	0.41 ± 0.04
40 sec	0.67 ± 0.05	0.51 ± 0.06
Liver enhancement (HU)		
25 sec	13 ± 7	2 ± 2
40 sec	35 ± 15	13 ± 8
Ratio of liver enhancement to peak liver enhancement		
25 sec	0.19 ± 0.06	0.04 ± 0.03
40 sec	0.51 ± 0.13	0.17 ± 0.08

Note.—Data are mean ± 1 standard deviation. Differences between groups were statistically significant ($P < .01$) for all CT characteristics.

CT Enhancement Ratios

The CT enhancement data for the liver were used to calculate enhancement ratios. For each sampling time (25 and 40 seconds), the ratio of liver enhancement to peak liver enhancement was determined.

Follow-up Examinations

Follow-up examinations were performed after the initial dual-phase CT examination to assign patients to one of two groups: (*a*) patients with no evidence of hepatic metastases 18 months after the initial CT examination and (*b*) patients who developed hepatic metastases within 18 months. Obviously, if patients developed hepatic metastases, less follow-up time was necessary. In our study, 22 patients developed hepatic metastases, and 58 had no liver tumor on follow-up scans.

In 13 patients, proof of hepatic metastases was obtained by examining surgical specimens or biopsy specimens obtained with CT guidance. In the other nine patients, proof was based on the development, at serial CT, of liver lesions that were clinically considered to indicate obvious hepatic spread of tumor. An average of eight lesions (range, one to 50 lesions) were detected in each of the 22 patients who developed metastases. The average diameter of these lesions was 25 mm (range, 10–50 mm). No patient underwent biopsy or surgery solely for the purpose of this study.

The group of 58 patients without hepatic metastases comprised 39 women and 19 men (mean age ± 1 standard deviation, 53 years ± 11 [range, 31–75 years]; mean weight ± 1 standard deviation, 67 kg ± 17 [range, 50–100 kg]). The group of 22 patients with liver metastases comprised 16 women and six men (mean age, 57 years ± 13 [range, 32–81 years]; mean weight, 60 kg ± 21 [range, 52–110 kg]).

Of the subset of 35 patients who underwent unenhanced hepatic CT before dual-phase CT, 12 patients developed hepatic metastases, and 23 patients did not.

Data Analysis

The Student *t* test was used to compare follow-up CT densitometric and enhancement measures in the two patient groups. Multiple discriminatory ratio levels were analyzed for the 25- and 40-second liver attenuation–to–peak attenuation ratio, the 25- and 40-second liver enhancement values, and the 25- and 40-second liver enhancement–to–peak liver enhancement ratio in the appropriate study groups. A P value of less than .05 was considered to indicate a statistically significant difference.

RESULTS

There were no statistically significant differences in age, sex, or weight between patients who developed liver metastases and those who did not. There was also no statistically significant difference between the two groups in terms of hepatic attenuation on unenhanced CT scans.

CT hepatic densitometric measurements were also analyzed for differences between the two patient groups (Table 1). Both the ratio of hepatic attenuation at 25 seconds to peak liver attenuation and the ratio of hepatic attenuation at 40 seconds to peak liver attenuation were statistically significantly elevated in the patients who developed metastases compared with those who did not develop liver metastases ($P < .01$).

Enhancement measurements were statistically significantly different in the subgroup of 35 patients in whom unenhanced hepatic CT scans were

Table 2
Usefulness of CT Densitometric Characteristics and Optimum Threshold Values for Predicting the Likelihood of Hepatic Metastases

Densitometric Measure	Threshold Value	Sensitivity (%)	Specificity (%)	Positive Predictive Value (%)	Negative Predictive Value (%)	Accuracy (%)
Ratio of liver attenuation to peak liver attenuation						
25 sec	≥0.50	62	85	62	85	78
40 sec	≥0.60	77	75	55	90	76
Liver enhancement						
25 sec	≥10*	67	96	89	85	86
40 sec	≥25*	75	91	82	87	85
Ratio of liver enhancement to peak liver enhancement						
25 sec	≥0.15	67	100	100	85	89
40 sec	≥0.40	75	96	90	88	89

* Data are Hounsfield units.

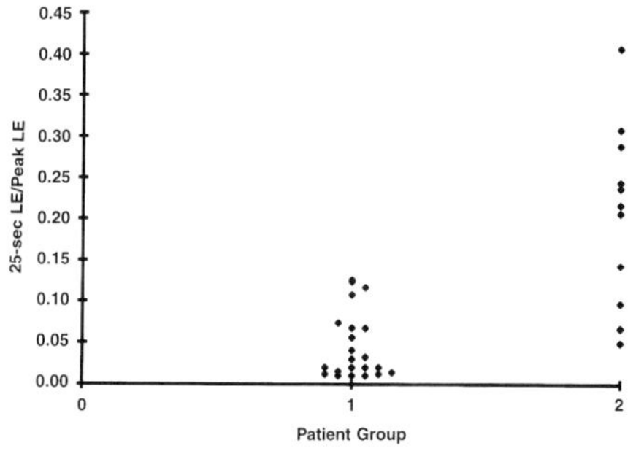

1.

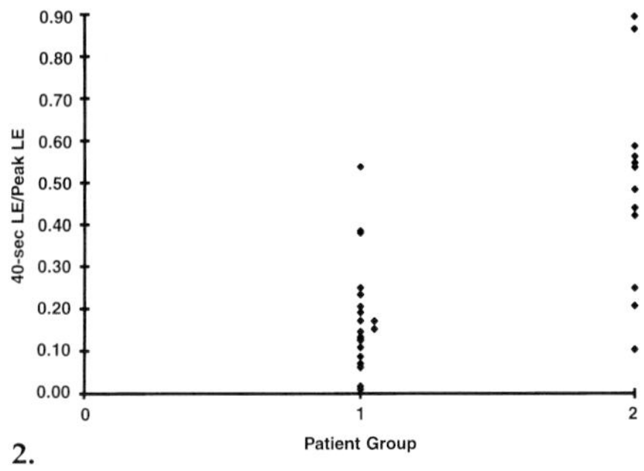

2.

Figures 1, 2. **(1)** Scatterplot shows the relationship between the ratio of liver enhancement (*LE*) to peak liver enhancement at 25 seconds and the development of hepatic metastases during follow-up. Patients in group 1 did not develop hepatic metastases; those in group 2 did develop metastases. **(2)** Scatterplot shows the relationship between the ratio of liver enhancement (*LE*) to peak liver enhancement at 40 seconds and the development hepatic metastases during follow-up. Patients in group 1 did not develop hepatic metastases; those in group 2 did develop metastases.

obtained. Absolute liver enhancement at 25 and 40 seconds was statistically significantly higher (Table 1) in the patients who developed metastases ($P < .01$).

The differences between the two patient groups were even more striking for the ratio of liver enhancement at 25 and 40 seconds to peak liver enhancement. These values were statistically significantly higher in patients who developed hepatic metastases than in those with no metastases ($P < .001$) (Table 1).

We analyzed multiple discriminatory threshold values for the six CT measures discussed. Optimal threshold values were derived on the basis of a receiver operating characteristic analysis to maximize the sensitivity and specificity of each measure. These threshold values and the resultant accuracy data are listed in Table 2. As can be seen in Table 2, measures that incorporated true enhancement (ie, liver enhancement value, liver enhancement–to–peak liver enhancement ratio) yielded greater accuracy than those that did not.

Although the results in Table 2 indicate reasonable accuracy when using a single discriminatory threshold value for enhancement parameters, clinical usefulness may be improved by using more than one threshold value. For example, with regard to the 25-second liver enhancement ratio, values of 0.15 or greater (ie, more than 15% of maximal liver enhancement present by 25 seconds) indicated development of hepatic metastases in all patients ($n = 8$). In contrast, only one of 18 patients with a ratio 0.07 or less developed liver metastases. Ratios of 0.08–0.14 were less helpful: Three patients developed liver metastases, and six did not. Figure 1 shows the relationship between the 25-second liver enhancement ratio and whether or not hepatic metastases were present at follow-up.

With regard to the 40-second liver enhancement ratio, nine of 10 patients with a ratio of 0.40 or greater developed metastases, and only two of 20 patients with a ratio of 0.25 or less developed metastases. Values of 0.26–0.39 were less helpful: One patient developed liver metastases, and four did not. Figure 2 shows the relationship between the 40-second liver enhancement ratio and the presence of hepatic metastases on follow-up scans.

DISCUSSION

CT is commonly used for the detection of liver metastases in patients who are known to have or are suspected of having a primary malignancy (1–6). Hepatic metastases are known to receive blood flow primarily from the hepatic arterial system rather than the portal vein (7–12). With helical CT, it is possible to perform imaging in the arterial (early) and venous (later) phases of liver enhancement in an attempt to improve the sensitivity of standard portal venous–phase CT in the detection of liver lesions (3,4). However, these previous investigators (3,4) who used helical CT to improve lesion detection focused on improvements in the visualization of tumor features rather than on detection of global changes in hepatic parenchymal enhancement due to relative flow disturbances. The authors of previous studies (8–14) with dynamic scintigraphy, duplex Doppler US, and contrast-enhanced CT have reported increased hepatic arterial flow relative to portal venous flow in livers with metastases.

We found altered hepatic enhancement on CT scans in patients who developed hepatic metastases within 18 months of the initial CT examination. These patients had statistically significantly greater early hepatic enhancement in both absolute terms and as a percentage of total liver enhancement.

We evaluated several CT densitometric and enhancement values. The 25- and 40-second liver attenuation–to–peak attenuation ratio, 25- and 40-second liver enhancement values, and 25- and 40-second liver enhancement ratios were all statistically significantly elevated in subjects who later developed hepatic metastases compared with those who did not ($P < .01$) (Table 1). These data suggest that patients who subsequently develop hepatic metastases often already have altered hepatic hemodynamics before tumors can be visualized on helical CT scans.

The altered hepatic hemodynamics we observed manifested as statistically significantly greater liver enhancement on scans obtained at the earlier phases of CT. The absolute and relative increases in early hepatic enhancement we observed in patients who later developed hepatic metastases suggest that hepatic arterial flow was increased relative to portal venous flow. We hypothesize that this shift to greater hepatic arterial flow reflects small or early metastatic disease in patients who have developed detectable liver metastases at follow-up CT. Our findings of altered hepatic hemodynamics in patients who subsequently develop obvious hepatic metastases are strikingly similar to the findings of Leen et al (8). Their duplex Doppler US results, which also included long-term follow-up findings, showed that initial detection of altered hepatic hemodynamics helped predict subsequent development of an obvious hepatic tumor. Leen et al (8) also found an increase in hepatic arterial flow relative to portal venous flow.

Of the CT measures we analyzed, the enhancement values (liver enhancement and its ratio to peak liver enhancement, determined by using unenhanced CT data) appear to have greater potential than the absolute densitometric measurements (liver attenuation at 25 and 40 seconds vs peak liver attenuation). Overall accuracy tended to be higher for the liver enhancement values and the liver enhancement ratios (Table 2). When a single threshold level was used, the simpler absolute enhancement values (25- and 40-second liver enhancement) had accuracies comparable with those of the more complex ratios (25- and 40-second liver enhancement ratios). This finding indicates that a simple analysis of an unenhanced image and an early-phase scan would suffice to obtain the needed data. Our patient group was too small, however, for us to state with confidence that the liver enhancement–to–peak liver enhancement ratio was of no benefit. In fact, further analysis of these ratios yielded interesting results.

It is likely that the clinical utility of the 25- and 40-second liver enhancement ratios can be improved by using more than one threshold value. Use of multiple threshold values would exclude a small subset of borderline patients and would allow more accurate prediction of the risk of imminent development of liver metastases in the remaining majority of patients. For the 40-second liver enhancement ratio, the use of two threshold levels appeared to be helpful with the patient population in our study. A ratio of 0.40 or greater indicated high risk for development of metastases (nine of 10 patients), and a ratio of less than 0.25 implied a low risk of subsequent hepatic metastases (two of 20 patients). Values for the 40-second enhancement ratio that were between these two thresholds (0.26–0.39) were indeterminate: One patient in this small group developed metastases, and four did not. Similarly, for the 25-second liver enhancement ratio, a ratio of 0.15 or greater helped in the determination of patients with a high risk for liver metastases, and values of 0.07 or less helped in the determination of patients with a low risk. Values of 0.08–0.14 were less helpful. Use of multiple thresholds for the liver-enhancement value was not helpful in improving predictive value, as was the case with the liver enhancement ratio. Therefore, it is possible that the extra time needed to obtain the liver enhancement ratio is clinically worthwhile as opposed to simple reliance on absolute hepatic contrast enhancement. Further study with a larger number of patients is needed to better define the best CT measurements for prediction of metastases, as well as optimal threshold levels for these measurements.

The good agreement between our hepatic enhancement values and those of other studies suggests that the technique may be reproducible. For example, we observed mean liver enhancement ± 1 standard deviation of 13 HU ± 8 at 40 seconds in the group that had no liver metastases at follow-up. In another study (15) of liver enhancement, mean attenuation values of 13–18 HU at 40 seconds were reported. The number of patients who had or developed liver metastases was not reported in that study, however, which limited further comparison with our data.

We also compared our data with those of a recent study (14) in which absolute and relative hepatic enhancement were evaluated in healthy subjects and in patients with hepatic metastases that were detectable on CT scans. Similar to our results, a 25-second liver attenuation–to–peak liver attenuation ratio of 0.50 and a 40-second liver attenuation–to–peak liver attenuation ratio of 0.60 were found to be optimal discriminatory levels in that study. Also in agreement with our results was the finding that enhancement measurements (liver enhancement, liver enhancement–to–peak liver enhancement ratio) were potentially more clinically useful than the liver attenuation–to–peak liver attenuation ratios calculated without the use of data from unenhanced CT. The values in patients who did or did not develop metastases in our study were similar to the values in patients with liver metastases and in healthy subjects, respectively, in the previous study (14). It is interesting to note that the enhancement values in patients in our study who developed liver metastases tended to be even more elevated than the values in patients in the other study who already had liver metastases. We hypothesize that the presence of metastases with necrosis together with treatment of liver metastases may, to some degree, reduce the altered hepatic hemodynamics and CT enhancement.

Several potential limitations of our study are important to consider. Some variables can affect liver densitometric measurements on scans obtained before and after intravenous administration of contrast material. Patient weight can affect the degree of liver enhancement, especially if a standard amount of contrast material is used at clinical CT, as is standard practice at our institution (16). In our study, however, there was no statistically significant difference in patient weight between the two groups. Fatty infiltration of the liver or cirrhosis can certainly affect baseline liver densitometric measurements. When unenhanced baseline liver values are taken into account, values such as the liver enhancement ratio should be more useful in this clinical setting. A standardized CT protocol for the contrast material dose and injection rate was used in this study. We hypothesize that overall findings similar to ours should be observed with different amounts and types of contrast material and different injection rates; the optimal threshold values, however, may be different. Further study is needed to address these issues, but we suspect that the liver enhancement ratio may be less variable than the absolute enhancement values. It would certainly be prudent to include both measurements in any future studies.

We chose 18 months as a reasonable period for determining whether a patient would develop hepatic metastases. Given a longer follow-up, it is possible that additional patients may develop metastases. We cannot know, however, whether initial CT scans would show normal or abnormal hepatic enhancement in these patients. Also, further studies would be needed to define whether the site of primary tumor has any major effect on the utility of this CT analysis.

Finally, metabolic hepatocellular disease (eg, cirrhosis) may produce alterations in liver blood flow that simulate the metastatic pattern. These alteration is due to the well-documented decrease in portal venous flow and the relative increase in arterial flow that develop in cirrhotic patients (12,13). This effect could result in false-positive examinations. The patient with the most elevated 25- and 40-second liver enhancement ratios in our series who did not develop hepatic metastases had underlying hepatocellular disease. Because only three patients in our series had known cirrhosis, we cannot comment further on how this disease affects hepatic enhancement. This potential limitation of our technique was also reported as a limitation in the work of Leen et al (8,9). Patients with known cirrhosis may need to be excluded from future attempts to identify occult hepatic metastatic disease.

There has been speculation that CT numbers obtained with some helical scanners may be unreliable (17). In investigations with phantoms at our institution, CT attenuation values were found to be consistent among our scanners and among all modes of operation of those scanners. In addition, use of enhancement ratios (corrected for unenhanced liver data) should also reduce any errors due to densitometric measurements obtained with helical CT data.

In conclusion, the results of our analysis of simple CT attenuation measurements indicate increased absolute and relative liver enhancement in the early phase of scanning after intravenous administration of contrast material in patients without liver cancer who subsequently develop hepatic metastases. Presumably this finding reflects the increased arterial flow associated with liver metastases that occurs even when the tumors are small or occult. These preliminary results suggest that specific CT measurements can help in the identification of patients with much higher or lower risk for subsequent development of hepatic metastases. If these findings are confirmed by the results of further studies, this technique may increase the sensitivity of CT for detection of hepatic metastatic disease and affect oncologic management. ■

Acknowledgment: The authors thank Barbara Poore for her assistance in the preparation of the manuscript.

References

1. Chezmar JL, Rumancik WM, Megibow AJ, Hulnick DH, Nelson RC, Bernardino ME. Liver and abdominal screening in patients with cancer: CT versus MR imaging. Radiology 1988; 168:43–47.
2. Heiken JP, Weyman PJ, Lee JKT, et al. Detection of focal hepatic masses: prospective evaluation with CT, delayed CT during arterial portography, and MR imaging. Radiology 1989; 171:47–51.
3. Hollett MD, Jeffrey RB Jr, Nino-Murcia M, Jorgensen MJ, Harris DP. Dual-phase helical CT of the liver: value of arterial phase scans in the detection of small (≤1.5 cm) malignant hepatic neoplasms. AJR 1995; 164:879–884.
4. Bonaldi VM, Bret PM, Reinhold C, Atri M. Helical CT of the liver: value of an early hepatic arterial phase. Radiology 1995; 197: 357–363.
5. Nelson RC, Chezmar JL, Sugarbaker PH, Bernardino ME. Hepatic tumors: comparison of CT during arterial portography, delayed CT, and MR imaging for preoperative evaluation. Radiology 1989; 172:27–34.
6. Ward BA, Miller DL, Frank JA, et al. Prospective evaluation of hepatic studies in the detection of colorectal metastases: correlation with surgical findings. Surgery 1989; 105:180–187.
7. Ridge JA, Bading JR, Gelbard AS, Benua RS, Daly JM. Perfusion of colorectal liver metastases: relative distribution from the hepatic artery and portal vein. Cancer 1987; 59:1547–1553.
8. Leen E, Angerson WJ, Wotherspoon H, Moule B, Cook TG, McArdle CS. Detection of colorectal liver metastases: comparison of laparotomy, CT, US, and Doppler perfusion index and evaluation of postoperative follow-up results. Radiology 1995; 195:113–116.
9. Leen E, Goldberg JA, Robertson J, et al. Detection of hepatic metastases using duplex/color Doppler sonography. Ann Surg 1991; 214:599–604.
10. Leveson SH, Wiggins PA, Giles GR, Parkin A, Robinson PJ. Deranged liver blood flow patterns in the detection of liver metastases. Br J Surg 1985; 72:128–130.
11. Fleming JS, Ackery DM, Walmsley BH, Karran SJ. Scintigraphic estimate of arterial and portal blood supply to the liver. J Nucl Med 1983; 24:1108–1113.
12. Robertson J, Leen E, Goldberg JA, Angerson WJ, Sutherland GR, McArdle CS. Flow measurement using duplex Doppler ultrasound: hemodynamic changes in patients with colorectal liver metastases. Clin Phys Physiol Meas 1992; 13:299–310.
13. Miles KA, Hayball MP, Dixon AK. Functional images of hepatic perfusion obtained with dynamic CT. Radiology 1993; 188:405–411.
14. Platt JF, Francis IR, Ellis JH, Reige KA. Difference in global hepatic enhancement assessed by dynamic CT in normal subjects and patients with hepatic metastases. J Comput Assist Tomogr 1997; 21:348–354.
15. Chambers TP, Baron RL, Lush RM, Dodd GD III, Miller WJ, Confer SR. Hepatic CT enhancement: a method to demonstrate reproducibility. Radiology 1993; 188:627–631.
16. Heiken JP, Brink JA, McClennan BL, Sagel SS, Crowe TM, Gaines MV. Dynamic incremental CT: effect of volume and concentration of contrast material and patient weight on hepatic enhancement. Radiology 1995; 195:353–357.
17. Bosniak MA, Rofsky NM. Problems in the detection and characterization of small renal masses. Radiology 1996; 198:638–641.

Ray's Days

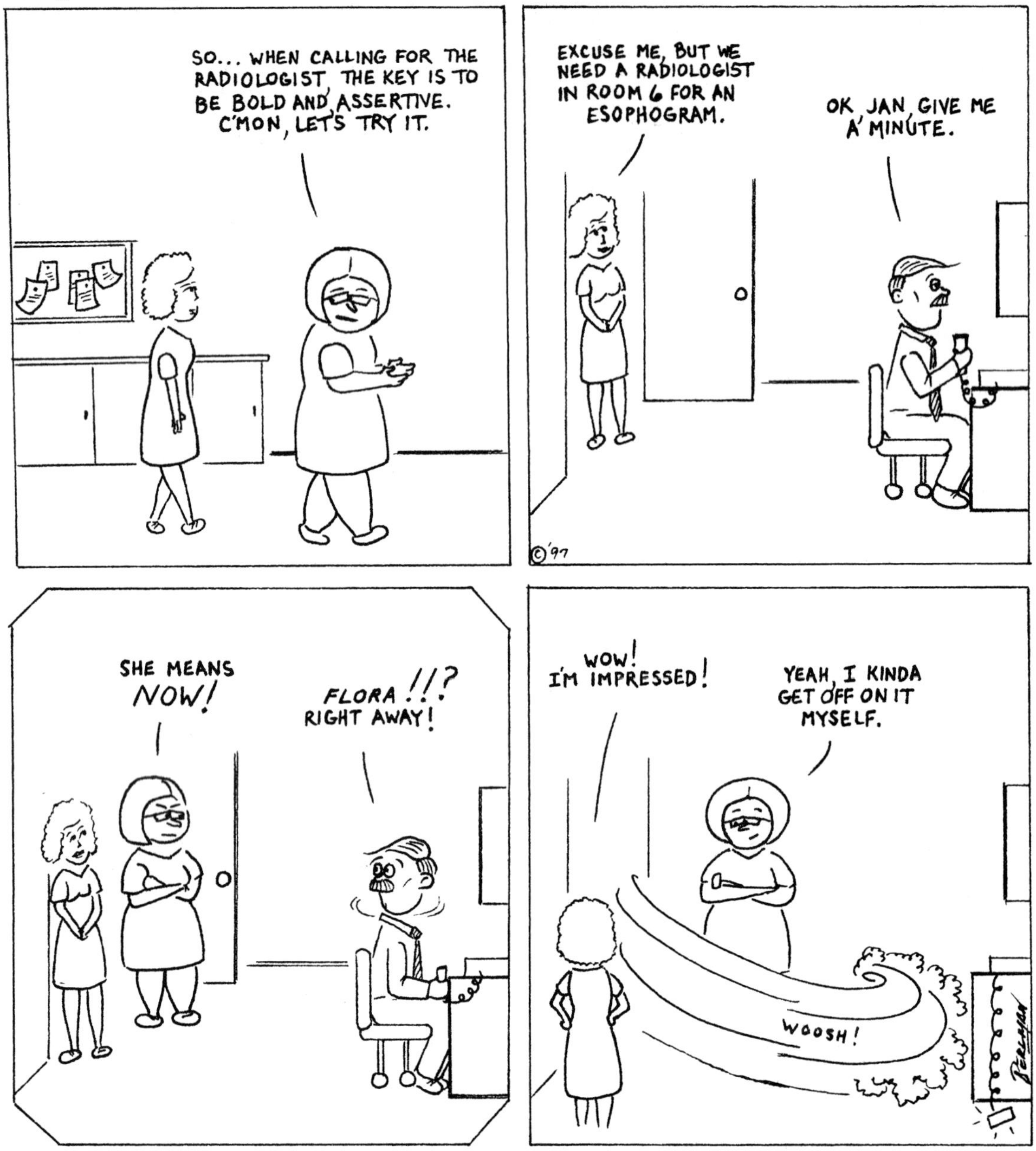

Steven J. Perlman, MD, Cincinnati, Ohio

Sylvain Migraine, MD • Mostafa Atri, MD • Patrice M. Bret, MD • John O. Lough, MD
John E. Hinchey, MD

Spontaneously Resolving Acute Appendicitis: Clinical and Sonographic Documentation[1]

PURPOSE: To document findings in a subgroup of patients with acute appendicitis that spontaneously resolved.

MATERIALS AND METHODS: From February 1989 through December 1995, nine patients were seen with a diagnosis of acute appendicitis that did not necessitate immediate surgery. Clinical, ultrasound (US), and pathologic findings were retrospectively reviewed.

RESULTS: Four of the nine patients underwent elective appendectomy 15–84 days (mean, 52 days) after initial presentation, and five did not undergo surgery. Seven patients experienced spontaneous pain relief before admission to the hospital, and two improved within a few hours of being admitted. No patient had an indication of peritoneal irritation at physical examination. Four patients had a normal white blood cell count, and five had leukocytosis. Maximum appendiceal diameter was 9–12 mm. Five patients had inflamed periappendiceal fat. No patient had abscess or appendicolithiasis shown at US. A normal appendix was identified at follow-up (mean, 40 months; range, 1–60 months) in four of five patients who did not undergo elective appendectomy. Two patients experienced recurrent bouts of pain, and one of these patients underwent appendectomy before the planned elective procedure.

CONCLUSION: On the basis of clinical, US, and pathologic findings, mild acute appendicitis spontaneously resolved in a subgroup of patients.

Appendicitis is the most common cause of an acutely painful abdomen in industrialized countries (1). The treatment for acute appendicitis has remained the same for the past 50 years. Early surgery before appendiceal rupture is considered the best treatment (2) because the chance of appendiceal rupture is high and its occurrence is unpredictable in the course of the inflammatory process (2,3). The spontaneous resolution of acute appendicitis and recurrent appendicitis has been denied by many surgeons (3). However, the concepts of spontaneous resolution of acute appendicitis, with or without antibiotics (4–6), and of recurrent appendicitis have been reported both clinically (5–11) and sonographically (4,12–15). Ultrasound (US) examination allows direct visualization of an inflamed appendix (13,16) and confirmation of the clinical diagnosis. US also can be used to determine whether complications have occurred (14,16) and, potentially, to follow up these patients if appendectomy is not performed immediately (4).

In this article we present the clinical (n = 9) and sonographic (n = 5) findings that document the resolution of unequivocal sonographically diagnosed acute appendicitis in nine patients.

MATERIALS AND METHODS

Patients

From October 1989 through December 1995, a total of 116 patients were seen at our institution with acute appendicitis without a periappendiceal abscess diagnosed at US. Their cases were retrospectively reviewed. One hundred seven of these patients had undergone immediate surgery. Nine patients (one woman, eight men, aged 21–42 years) had not undergone surgery, however, because their clinical condition had improved within a few hours before or after they were seen in the emergency room. Of these nine patients, four later underwent elective appendectomy and five had not undergone surgery as of November 1996.

Clinical and Laboratory Findings

All nine patients experienced pain in the right lower quadrant, and three patients experienced vomiting. The duration of pain ranged from 4 to 120 hours (mean, 44 hours). Seven patients had experienced spontaneous pain relief by the time they came to the hospital, and two improved rapidly during the few hours after admission to the hospital. No patient reported a history of a previous attack. In two patients, test results were positive for the human immunodeficiency virus (HIV), and one of these patients was a hemophiliac. Physical examination revealed voluntary guarding (n = 5), focal tenderness (n = 3), normal findings (n = 1), and the absence of rebound (n = 9) in the right lower abdomen. Six patients had a fever (<38°C), and

Index terms: Appendicitis, 751.291 • Appendix, US, 751.1298

Abbreviation: HIV = human immunodeficiency virus.

Radiology 1997; 205:55–58

[1] From the Departments of Diagnostic Radiology (S.M., M.A., P.M.B.), Pathology (J.O.L.), and General Surgery (J.E.H.), Montreal General Hospital, McGill University, 1650 Cedar Ave, Montreal, Quebec, Canada H3G 1A4. Received February 3, 1997; revision requested March 24; revision received May 12; accepted May 19. **Address reprint requests to** M.A.

See also the editorial by Puylaert and Rijke (pp 41–42) in this issue.

three were afebrile. The white blood cell count was normal in four patients, moderately increased (10,700–15,000 cells per cubic millimeter [10.7–15.0 × 10^{-9}/L]) in three patients, and markedly elevated (16,900–25,600 cells per cubic millimeter [16.9–25.6 × 10^{-9}/L]) in two patients.

US Examination

US examinations were performed by a sonographer and reviewed on-site by a radiologist on a commercially available system (model SSA90 or SS270, Toshiba, Markham, Ontario, Canada; or model 128, Acuson, Mountain View, Calif) with 3.5–7.5-MHz transducers. Color and pulsed-wave Doppler US were performed in two patients.

The criteria for diagnosis of appendicitis at US were the presence of a noncompressible, thickened (at least 7-mm maximal outer diameter) appendix with or without loss of layers, the presence of appendicolithiasis, and/or the presence of periappendiceal inflammatory changes (17,18). All US examinations were videotaped. The videotapes were reviewed by one radiologist (M.A.), and the diagnosis of acute appendicitis based on the stated criteria was reconfirmed.

The four appendiceal pathologic specimens from the four patients who underwent elective appendectomy were reviewed by the same pathologist (J.O.L.).

RESULTS

Patient Treatment

Four patients underwent elective appendectomy within a mean 52 days (range, 15–84 days) of the initial episode of right lower quadrant pain. In one patient, the appendectomy was performed earlier than scheduled because of recurrent right lower quadrant pain. Elective appendectomy was performed owing to patient preference in two cases and to surgeon preference in the other two cases.

Five patients were treated clinically (without surgery), with a mean follow-up of 40 months (range, 1–60 months). In two such cases, the patients were HIV positive. Another patient refused surgery, and two patients were not treated surgically because of the surgeon's decision. One of the HIV-positive patients experienced recurrent right lower quadrant pain 8 months later.

One patient in the group that underwent elective appendectomy and one in the group treated clinically received antibiotics at the time of initial admission to the hospital.

Initial US Findings

The appendix was located adjacent to the cecum in three patients, in the pelvis in five patients, and retrocecally in one patient. The maximum diameter of the appendix ranged from 9 to 12 mm (mean, 10.5 mm). The appendiceal layers were intact in seven patients (Fig 1) and disrupted in two patients (Fig 2). Doppler US performed in two patients showed increased vascularity in the appendiceal wall and in the surrounding fat. The periappendiceal fat was inflamed in five patients (Figs 2, 3). No patient was found to have mesenteric lymph nodes, thickening of the terminal ileum or cecum, periappendiceal abscess or fluid collection, or appendicolithiasis. A small quantity of interloop ascites was seen, however, in the right lower quadrant in five patients.

Follow-up US Findings

Six patients underwent follow-up US (range, 4 days to 5 years; mean, 21 months). In one patient who later underwent elective appendectomy, the appendix was found to have decreased in diameter from 11.7 to 7 mm at follow-up US performed 4 days after the initial US examination (Figs 3, 4). Among the remaining five patients, follow-up US (range, 1–60 months; mean, 40 months) showed a normal appendix in four (Fig 5), and the appendix could not be identified in one patient.

Pathologic Findings

The results of pathologic analysis in the four patients who underwent elective appendectomy were as follows: eosinophilic cells and distal appendiceal fibrosis ($n = 1$), focal distal acute appendicitis as indicated by the presence of eosinophilic and polymorphonuclear inflammatory cells ($n = 1$), and appendiceal fibrosis ($n = 2$). In addition, lymphoid hyperplasia was identified in all four appendiceal pathologic specimens.

DISCUSSION

In 1886, Fitz (19) described the relationship between inflammation of the appendix and subsequent peritonitis

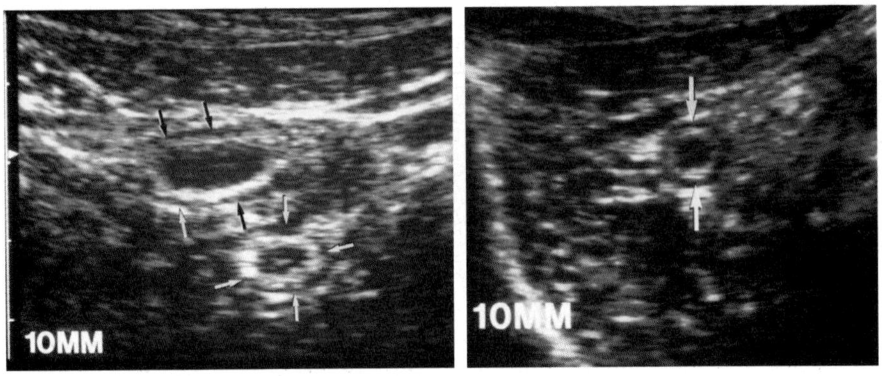

a. b.

Figure 1. Acute appendicitis. **(a)** Longitudinal and **(b)** transverse US scans show a noncompressible, folded appendix (arrows) that is 10 mm in maximum thickness. Notice preservation of layers and lack of periappendiceal fat changes.

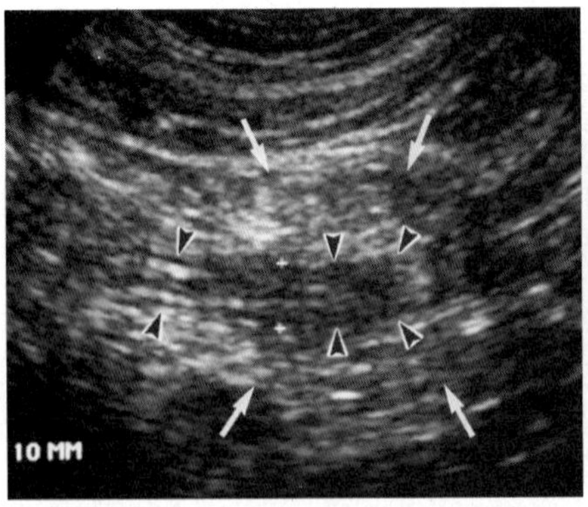

2.

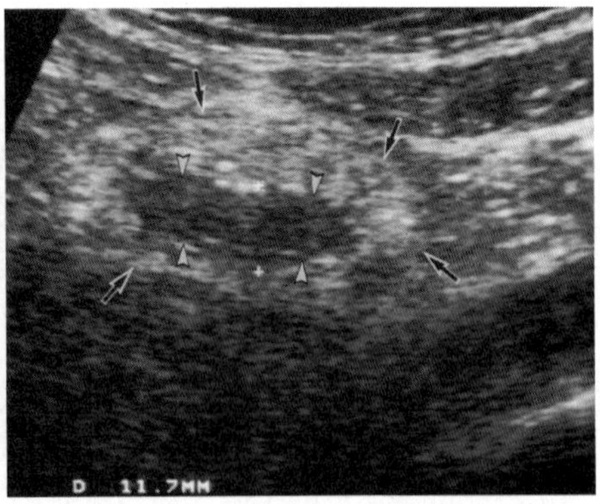

3.

Figures 2, 3. **(2)** Longitudinal US scan of an inflamed appendix (arrowheads) that is 10 mm in diameter. Notice loss of layers of the distal end of the appendix and echogenic inflamed periappendiceal fat (arrows). **(3)** US scan of inflamed appendix (arrowheads) 11.7 mm in diameter. Note the loss of wall layers and inflammation of the echogenic periappendiceal fat (arrows).

or abscess formation, and he outlined the importance of early diagnosis and treatment. He also reported recurrent forms of appendicitis.

Inflammation of the appendix may not be accompanied by clinical symptoms (20) or clinical symptoms may be present but the pain attacks may resolve; 20%–30% of patients who undergo appendectomy have a history of episodes of right lower quadrant pain (9,11,19,21).

Recurrent appendicitis is an entity recognized by most surgeons, and many of them warn that a history of similar attacks is suspect for appendicitis (8,9). The recognition of recurrent appendicitis suggests that spontaneous healing of appendicitis occurs as Fitz (19) reported. In our study, only two patients experienced previous or recurrent pain: One patient underwent appendectomy for recurrent right lower quadrant pain 43 days after the initial attack, and one HIV-positive patient in the group followed up clinically experienced another attack.

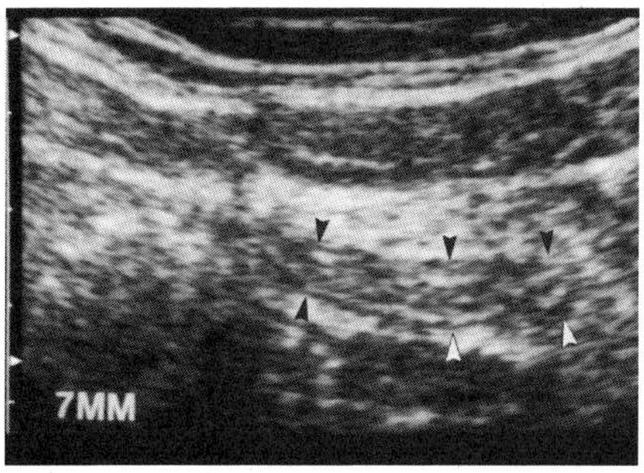

Figure 4. US scan of the same appendix as in Figure 3 obtained 4 days later. Notice the substantial decrease in the thickness of the inflamed appendix (arrowheads), which now measures 7 mm in diameter.

All nine patients with US documentation of acute appendicitis experienced a mild form of acute appendicitis (without anorexia, peritoneal irritation, or moderate fever; with or without leukocytosis) and pain of long duration (average time, 44 hours) before they came to the emergency room. The rapid decrease in the intensity of pain with normalization of the physical examination findings made the need for immediate appendectomy questionable. Ikard (7) described four patients with recurrent acute appendicitis and noticed that each bout of inflammation resolved quickly rather than causing progressive pain.

In a study of 250 patients with right lower abdominal pain, Jeffrey et al (13) described six patients with sonographic evidence of appendicitis in whom symptoms resolved spontaneously without antibiotic therapy and without surgery. This "lowered" the specificity of US to 93% for the diagnosis of acute appendicitis in their series. Heller and Skolnick (4) also described a patient with clinical findings suggestive of acute appendicitis associated with the presence of a noncompressible, thick appendix at US. The patient's treatment consisted of clinical observation only, and follow-up US performed 2 weeks later did not show a thick appendix (4). Spontaneous resolution of US-diagnosed appendicitis is also suggested in two of 30 cases of appendicitis reported by Amland et al (12), in 24 of 231 cases reported by Ooms et al (14), and in four of 49 cases reported by Rioux (15). Appendiceal pathologic specimens in four patients were unequivocally abnormal, with the appendiceal diameter at least 9 mm (normal limit, 6 mm). Therefore, the possibility that the diagnoses of acute appendicitis were false-positive is unlikely. Although the appendiceal wall was partially disrupted in two patients, none of our patients had findings that strongly suggested perforation of the appendix. Also, lack of appendicolithiasis or inflammation of the adjacent cecum or terminal ileum suggests the presence of mild appendicitis.

In one of the four patients who underwent elective appendectomy after resolution of their clinical symptoms of appendicitis, the appendix was found to have diminished in thickness from 11.7 to 7 mm in 4 days (Figs 3, 4). Heller and Skolnick (4) also reported such a rapid decrease in inflammation of the appendix in a patient with spontaneously resolving appendicitis.

The probable sequence of events that lead to acute appendicitis has not been questioned since the original description of this entity by Wangensteen and Bowers (22) in 1937 and by Bowers (5) in 1939. Obstruction of the lumen of the appendix produces distal luminal distention with accumulation of mucin. As intraluminal pressure increases, ischemia, congestion, and polymorphonuclear infiltration of the wall occur. If appendiceal peristalsis cannot overcome the obstruction, which is due to the presence of a fecalith in 90% of cases (2), wall necrosis and perforation follow. On the contrary, if obstruction is relieved (presumably because either the fecalith is soft or lymphoid hyperplasia is present), appendicitis may resolve spontaneously.

All four appendiceal pathologic specimens obtained in this study were found to contain lymphoid hyperplasia, and there was no appendicolithiasis. These findings suggest that the mechanism of appendicitis may be partial obstruction due to infection. Two specimens showed fibrotic changes.

The decision to perform surgery in a patient whose appendix appears abnormal at sonography should be based primarily on the clinical status of the patient. If a surgeon elects not to perform surgery, performance of repeat sonography may be useful to help confirm that the appendix has returned to a normal size or is no longer sonographically visible.

In summary, we have described clinical and US findings in nine patients with a mild form of acute appendicitis that spontaneously resolved. US was performed to help confirm the diagnosis and did not

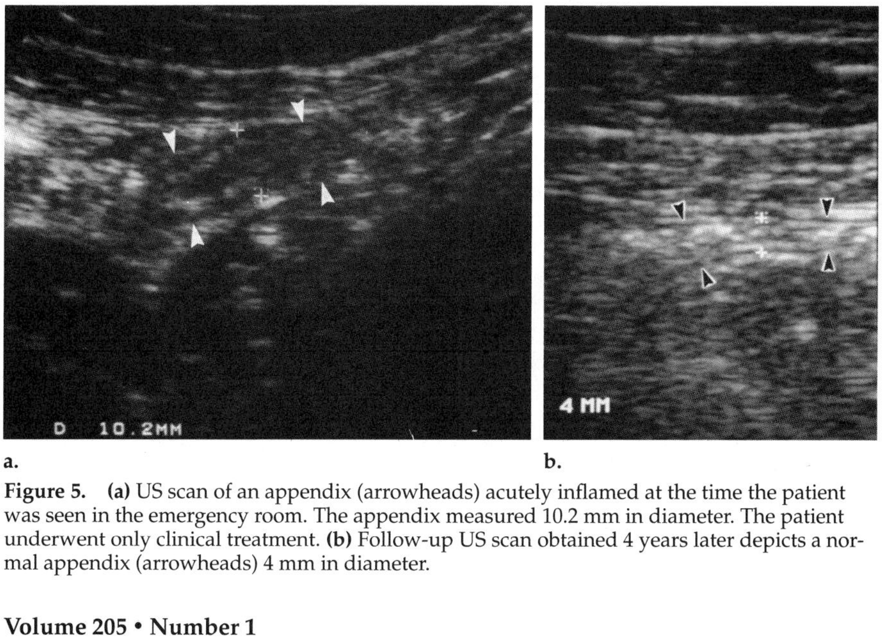

a. b.

Figure 5. **(a)** US scan of an appendix (arrowheads) acutely inflamed at the time the patient was seen in the emergency room. The appendix measured 10.2 mm in diameter. The patient underwent only clinical treatment. **(b)** Follow-up US scan obtained 4 years later depicts a normal appendix (arrowheads) 4 mm in diameter.

show appendicolithiasis or any indication of perforation. In this small series, we have documented the existence of a subgroup of patients with acute appendicitis that spontaneously resolved. ■

References

1. Berry J Jr, Malt RA. Appendicitis near its centenary. Ann Surg 1984; 200:567–575.
2. Schwartz SI. Appendix. In: Schwartz SI, ed. Principles of surgery. 6th ed. New York, NY: McGraw-Hill, 1994.
3. Waxman K, Mason GR. Appendicitis and appendiceal abscess. In: Nyhus LM, Baker RJ, eds. Master of surgery. 2nd ed. Toronto, Ontario, Canada: Little, Brown, 1992.
4. Heller MB, Skolnick ML. Ultrasound documentation of spontaneously resolving appendicitis. Am J Emerg Med 1993; 11:51–53.
5. Bowers WF. Appendicitis, with special reference to pathogenesis, bacteriology and healing. Arch Surg 1939; 39:362–422.
6. Butsch DW, Jothi R, Butsch WL, Butsch JL. Recurrent appendicitis: fact not fallacy. Postgrad Med 1973; 54:132–137.
7. Ikard RW. Recurrent appendicitis: a valid disease. J Tenn Med Assoc 1992; 85:105–106.
8. Mattei P, Sola JE, Yeo CJ. Chronic and recurrent appendicitis are uncommon entities often misdiagnosed. J Am Coll Surg 1994; 178:385–389.
9. Hawes AS, Whalen GF. Recurrent and chronic appendicitis: the other inflammatory conditions of the appendix. Am Surg 1994; 60:217–219.
10. Savrin RA, Clausen K, Martin EW, et al. Chronic and recurrent appendicitis. Am J Surg 1979; 137:355–357.
11. Befeler D. Recurrent appendicitis: incidence and prophylaxis. Arch Surg 1964; 89:666–668.
12. Amland PF, Skaane P, Ronningen H, Nordshus T, Solheim K. Ultrasonography and parameters of inflammation in acute appendicitis. Acta Chir Scand 1989; 155:185–189.
13. Jeffrey RB Jr, Laing FC, Townsend RR. Acute appendicitis: sonographic criteria based on 250 cases. Radiology 1988; 167: 327–329.
14. Ooms HWA, Koumans RMJ, Ho Kang You PJ, Puylaert JBC. Ultrasonography in the diagnosis of acute appendicitis. Br J Surg 1991; 78:315–318.
15. Rioux M. Sonographic detection of normal and abnormal appendix. AJR 1992; 158: 773–778.
16. Yacoe ME, Jeffrey RB Jr. Sonography of appendicitis and diverticulitis. Radiol Clin North Am 1994; 32:899–911.
17. Puylaert JBCM, Rutgers PH, Lalisang RI, et al. A prospective study of ultrasonography in the diagnosis of appendicitis. N Engl J Med 1987; 317:666–669.
18. Puylaert JBCM. Acute appendicitis: US evaluation using graded compression. Radiology 1986; 158:355–360.
19. Fitz RH. Perforating inflammation of the vermiform appendix, with special reference to its early diagnosis and treatment. Trans Assoc Am Physicians 1886; 1:107–144.
20. Pieper R, Kager L, Näsman P. Clinical significance of mucosal inflammation of the vermiform appendix. Ann Surg 1983; 197: 368–374.
21. Lewis FR, Holcroft JW, Bey J, et al. Appendicitis: a critical review of diagnosis and treatment in 1000 cases. Arch Surg 1975; 110:677–684.
22. Wangensteen OH, Bowers WF. Significance of the obstructive factor in the genesis of acute appendicitis: experimental study. Arch Surg 1937; 34:496–526.

Amy K. Hara, MD • C. Daniel Johnson, MD • Judd E. Reed • David A. Ahlquist, MD
Heidi Nelson, MD • Robert L. MacCarty, MD • W. Scott Harmsen, MS • Duane M. Ilstrup, MS

Detection of Colorectal Polyps with CT Colography: Initial Assessment of Sensitivity and Specificity[1]

PURPOSE: To estimate the sensitivity and specificity of computed tomographic (CT) colography in detection of colorectal polyps and to compare these findings with those at axial CT.

MATERIALS AND METHODS: In 70 consecutive patients, CT colography and colonoscopy were performed. Helical axial CT images and CT colographic images (multiplanar two- and three-dimensional endoluminal images) were evaluated separately by two radiologists blinded to results from colonoscopy and other imaging studies. Findings were compared with those at colonoscopy, which was the standard.

RESULTS: The sensitivity and specificity for the two observers with CT colography averaged 75% and 90% in patients with adenomas 10 mm in diameter or larger, 66% and 63% in patients with adenomas 5 mm in diameter or greater, and 45% and 80% for patients with adenomas less than 5 mm in diameter, respectively. Sensitivity and specificity with axial CT were lower than those with CT colography (58% and 74%, respectively) in patients with adenomas 10 mm in diameter or larger.

CONCLUSION: Compared with axial CT, CT colography appears to have superior sensitivity and specificity in detection of clinically important colorectal adenomas. Early performance of CT colography seems promising for detection of colorectal polyps 5 mm and larger.

Computed tomographic (CT) colography represents a promising approach to colorectal cancer screening with potential advantages in sensitivity, specificity, safety, and patient acceptability. This technique uses standard helical CT images of the colon and advanced imaging software to produce reformatted two- and three-dimensional–rendered views of the entire colorectum. Computer-rendered three-dimensional images simulate the endoluminal image seen at colonoscopy but in a minimally invasive manner and without the risks associated with sedation of the patient.

Advanced three-dimensional imaging applications such as CT colography have been made possible with high-speed scanners which, unlike conventional CT scanners, can obtain contiguous volumetric data sets with minimal respiratory artifacts. Although three-dimensional colon imaging has been investigated repeatedly with this technology (1–5), to our knowledge, the axial images that are also available have not been studied similarly. A thorough study of axial images could be important because if axial CT images can be used for polyp detection, time-consuming and expensive advanced imaging may not be necessary. The purpose of this study was to estimate the sensitivity and specificity of CT colography in detection of colorectal polyps and to compare these findings with those of axial CT and colonoscopy. To our knowledge, this study represents the largest (70 patients) clinical study to date and the first blinded evaluation to assess sensitivity and specificity.

MATERIALS AND METHODS

From November 1995 through February 1996, CT colography followed by colonoscopy was performed in 35 patients in whom findings from a barium enema study (n = 31) or flexible sigmoidoscopy (n = 4) were positive for one or more polyps and in 35 additional patients who were being followed up after removal of polyps 1–5 years earlier. The follow-up group was recruited to serve as the control group. The 50 men and 20 women ranged in age from 43 to 80 years (mean, 66.3 years ± 9.0 [standard deviation]). Selection criteria included age of 40–80 years and ability to give written consent. Exclusion criteria included presence of a colostomy, inflammatory bowel disease, acute diverticulitis, pregnancy, colon biopsy performed within 72 hours, polypectomy in the past 6 weeks, or severe claustrophobia. The study was approved by our institutional review board.

All patients underwent standard oral colonoscopy preparation (polyethyleneglycol electrolyte solution [Golytely; Braintree Laboratories, Braintree, Mass] and bisacodyl tablets) before CT colography. All CT colographic examinations were performed immediately before colonoscopy with a helical CT scanner (HiSpeed Advantage; GE Medical Systems, Milwaukee, Wis) with 180° linear interpolation and a standard reconstruction kernel. Insufflation of the colon was performed with approxi-

Index terms: Colon, CT, 75.12115, 75.12117 • Colon, neoplasms, 75.311 • Computed tomography (CT), image processing, 75.12117 • Computed tomography (CT), three-dimensional, 75.12117 • Images, analysis

Radiology 1997; 205:59–65

[1] From the Departments of Diagnostic Radiology (A.K.H., C.D.J., R.L.M.), Information Services (J.E.R.), Gastroenterology (D.A.A.), Colorectal Surgery (H.N.), and Biostatistics (W.S.H., D.M.I.), Mayo Clinic, 200 First St SW, Rochester, MN 55905. From the 1996 RSNA scientific assembly. Received February 11, 1997; revision requested April 8; revision received June 9; accepted June 16. **Address reprint requests to** A.K.H.

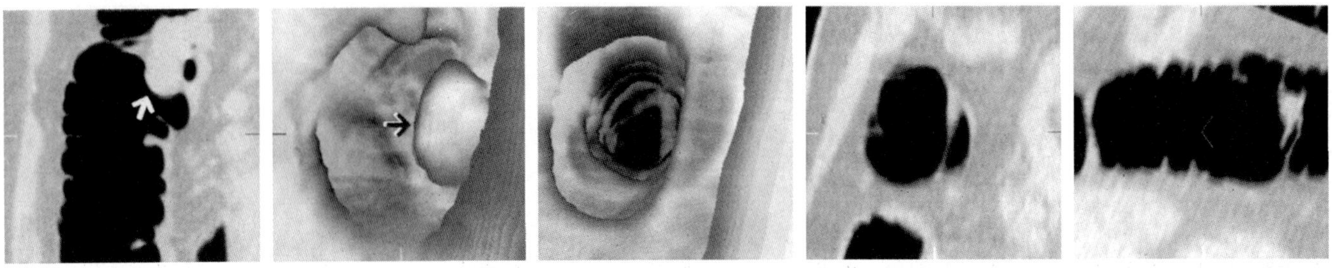

b. c. d. e. f.

Figure 1. Multiple image display screen. Evaluation of a CT colographic examination is performed with this screen, which simultaneously updates all images to any specified colonic location. Images displayed include **(a)** axial CT image, **(b)** two-dimensional CT colographic orthogonal image, **(c)** three-dimensional CT colographic caudal image, **(d)** three-dimensional CT colographic cephalic image, **(e)** two-dimensional CT colographic cross section, and **(f)** two-dimensional CT colographic orthogonal image. Note the 2-cm adenoma on multiple images (arrow).

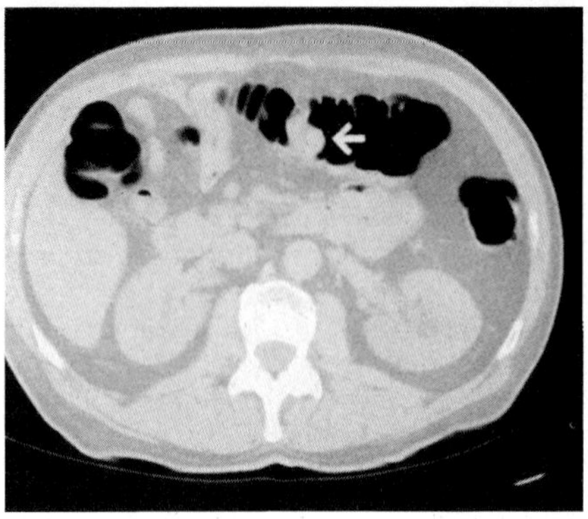

a.

mately 2 L of carbon dioxide gas. Glucagon was not used. Air was used in 10 patients when carbon dioxide was not available; no difference in image quality was noted between patients in whom air was used and patients in whom carbon dioxide was used. Adequacy of distention was assessed with review of the anteroposterior scout image obtained before axial CT data acquisition.

After insufflation of the colon with air or carbon dioxide, images were obtained with the patient in a supine position with a collimation of 5 mm, a table speed of 6.5 mm/sec (pitch of 1.3), reconstruction intervals of 3 mm, matrix of 512 × 512, field of view to fit (range, 35–49 cm²), 140 mA, 120 kVp, and 20-second breath holds. Three to four breath holds were performed within 2 minutes, enabling acquisition of approximately 150 axial images per examination. The rationale for this scanning protocol has been reported previously (1).

Image processing was performed with a computer workstation (SPARC20; Sun Microsystems, San Jose, Calif) and customized software developed at our institution (6,7). Image processing first involved semiautomatic definition of the colon centerline with automatic generation of three-dimensional and multiple reformatted two-dimensional images (perpendicular to the colon lumen with two orthogonal views in observer-specified orientations). All centerline definitions were performed within 10 minutes by one observer (A.K.H.) with a previously described method (1–3,6,7). A multiple image display program was then used for interactive evaluation of the two- and three-dimensional reformatted images for polyp detection (Fig 1). The six simultaneously displayed, high-resolution images included three two-dimensional images (cross section of the colon and two orthogonal views), two three-dimensional images (cephalic and caudal intraluminal views), and nonreformatted axial CT images. Except for axial CT images, all images were centered on the colon midline and interpolated to 1-mm pixel size. If the examiner specified a course off the midline tracing, images would simultaneously center on the new region of interest. Variables that could be altered during evaluation included step length along the midline (1–10 mm and larger), two-dimensional window width and level, three-dimensional field of view (range, 30°–180° with a default setting of 110°), three-dimensional opacity mapping function, and three-dimensional resolution (number of pixels per cast ray). Three-dimensional display used a custom volume-rendering algorithm for rapid display.

Image Analysis

Images from the 70 studies were evaluated with two methods. First, two radiologists (C.D.J., R.L.M.) independently reviewed the axial CT images of each patient on an interactive CT workstation, without knowledge of indications for examination or colonoscopy results. The axial section number and location for each polyp was recorded to enable comparison with colonoscopy results. Observers ranked their level of confidence for diagnosis of each polyp on a scale of 1 to 5, with 1 = least confident and 5 = most confident.

To avoid learning bias, an interval of at least 2 months was established between interpretation of the axial images and interpretation of the CT colographic images. CT colographic images were evaluated independently and randomly by two radiologists (A.K.H., C.D.J.) seated at a comfortable viewing distance from the interactive computer workstation. Both observers were trained in the CT colography technique with a study database of 30 patients with 80 endoscopically proved polyps. Both radiologists were unaware of indications for examination, results of previous studies, colonoscopy results, or axial CT results. For each polyp, the raw axial CT section number, approximate size, confidence level, and distance from the beginning of the tracing were recorded. Polyps identified at CT colography were matched to those identified at colonoscopy by reviewing the dictated colonoscopic report for lesion location and number, correlating distance from the cecum or rectum measured at videotaped endoscopy and CT colography, and comparison of lesion morphology at CT colography with morphology demonstrated on endoscopic images.

All colonoscopy examinations were performed after CT colography on the same day, and 60 of the 70 colonoscopy examinations were recorded on videotape. Results of the imaging studies were compared with colonoscopy findings, which served as the standard. Polyp size was determined from ex vivo pathology specimens or, when whole polyps were not available, from colonoscopic estimates. Colonoscopic estimation was performed by endoscopically placing an open biopsy forceps with a known width of 8 mm next to the polyp. Whole polyps were available for pathologic measurement in 19 (53%) of 36 polyps 5 mm and larger. Since the primary goal of the study did not include assessment of the current standard (colonoscopy), only a single, nonblinded colonoscopic examination was performed in each patient.

All CT colography and videotaped colonoscopy examinations with diagnostic discrepancies involving lesions 5 mm and larger were analyzed further to determine the cause of error. Adenomas identified at CT colography and not reported at colonoscopy were reevaluated by reviewing the colonoscopy videotapes with an experienced endoscopist (D.A.A.). If the polyp was identified retrospectively on the videotape, it was considered a colonoscopic error.

In an effort to compare results of CT colography with those of established radiologic colon examinations, we retrospectively reviewed available barium enema study results in all patients. Indications for barium enema study included colorectal cancer screening and a history of adenomatous polyps. The inclusion criterion consisted of single-contrast, fluoroscopic barium examinations performed at our institution within 1 year before CT colography and colonoscopy. The single-contrast barium enema technique has been

Table 1
Diagnostic Performance of the Two Observers with CT Colography

	Lesion Size (mm)					
	≥10		≥5		<5	
	A	B	A	B	A	B
Adenoma diagnosis*						
TP	11	10	25	20	21	20
FN	4	5	11	16	58	59
FP	5	8	38	37	21	10
Sensitivity (%)	73	67	69	56	27	25
95% confidence interval	45, 92	38, 88	52, 84	38, 72	17, 38	16, 36
Patient identification†						
TP	9	9	17	16	13	12
FN	3	3	8	9	17	18
FP	5	6	19	15	10	6
TN	53	52	26	30	30	34
Sensitivity (%)	75	75	68	64	43	40
95% confidence interval	43, 95	43, 95	47, 85	43, 82	26, 63	23, 59
Specificity (%)	91	90	58	67	75	85
95% confidence interval	81, 97	79, 96	42, 72	51, 80	59, 87	70, 94

Note.—A = observer A, B = observer B, FN = false-negative, FP = false-positive, TP = true-positive.
* In Tables 1 and 2, 15 lesions were ≥10 mm, 36 were 5–9 mm, and 79 were <5 mm.
† In Tables 1 and 2, 12 lesions were ≥10 mm, 25 were 5–9 mm, and 30 were <5 mm.

Table 2
Diagnostic Performance of the Two Observers with Axial CT

	Lesion Size (mm)					
	≥10		≥5		<5	
	A	B	A	B	A	B
Adenoma diagnosis						
TP	7	7	13	16	7	7
FN	8	8	23	20	72	72
Sensitivity (%)	47	47	36	44	9	9
95% confidence interval	21, 73	21, 73	21, 54	28, 62	4, 17	4, 17
Patient identification						
TP	7	7	13	16	3	3
FN	5	5	12	9	27	27
FP	16	14	15	14	12	9
TN	42	44	30	31	28	31
Sensitivity (%)	58	58	52	64	10	10
95% confidence interval	28, 85	28, 85	31, 72	43, 82	2, 27	2, 27
Specificity (%)	72	76	67	69	70	70
95% confidence interval	59, 83	63, 86	51, 80	53, 82	53, 83	62, 89

Note.—A = observer A, B = observer B, FN = false-negative, FP = false-positive, TP = true-positive.

shown to be as accurate as the double-contrast barium enema technique (8–10) when vigorous manual palpation is used (the technique we use most commonly). The preparation for barium enema studies included ingestion of 300 mL of magnesium citrate and bisacodyl the day before the examination, and high-volume tap water enemas the day of the barium enema examination. Reviewers consisted of eight staff radiologists, one radiologist per examination. Results from barium enema studies were compared with those from colonoscopy, which was the standard.

Statistical Analysis

Each diagnostic test was evaluated with colonoscopy results as the standard for the presence of polyps. Only polyps determined to be adenomatous at histopathologic examination were considered for analysis. For calculation of sensitivity and the exact 95% binomial confidence interval, the patient or each adenoma was considered the experimental unit. The patient was considered positive if the imaging modality depicted any adenomas of that size category in the patient. Specificity and the associated 95% confidence interval were also calculated when considering the patient but not when assessing each adenoma. Receiver operating characteristic curves were generated for each observer to examine the efficacy of identification of patients with adenomas 10 mm in diameter or larger, 5 mm in diameter and larger, and less than 5 mm in diameter.

RESULTS

A total of 161 polyps were identified at colonoscopy, and the histopathologic diagnosis was adenoma in 115 lesions and benign in 46 lesions (hyperplastic polyps, normal colonic tissue, and lipomas). Of the 115 adenomas, 15 (13%) were 10 mm in diameter or larger, 21 (18%) were 5–9 mm in diameter, and 79 (69%) were less than 5 mm in diameter. Of 70 studies, 54 (77%) revealed findings positive for adenomas.

The sensitivity and specificity of CT colography in diagnosis of adenoma and patient identification are summarized in Table 1. The sensitivity of identification of patients with adenomas 10 mm in diameter or larger was 75% (nine of 12), with a specificity of 91% for both observers. For patients with adenomas 5 mm in diameter or greater, the sensitivity and specificity averaged 66% and 63%, respectively. Patients with adenomas smaller than 5 mm in diameter were identified less than 45% of the time, with an average specificity of 80%. With CT colography, 11 (73%) of 15 adenomas 10 mm in diameter or larger were identified correctly by observer A and 10 (67%) of 15 by observer B. The sensitivity of CT colography in diagnosis of adenomas 5 mm in diameter or greater averaged 63% and decreased to less than 30% for adenomas smaller than 5 mm in diameter. Results were not statistically significantly different between observers for adenomas of any size.

The receiver operating characteristic curves did not differ statistically significantly between the observers (11). For patients with adenomas 10 mm in diameter or larger, the receiver operating characteristic areas were 0.83 ± 0.08 for observer A and 0.81 ± 0.08 for observer B. For patients with adenomas 5 mm in diameter or greater, the receiver operating characteristic areas were 0.63 ± 0.06 for observer A and 0.69 ± 0.06 for observer B. For patients with adenomas less than 5 mm in diameter, the ROC areas were 0.58 ± 0.07 for observer A and 0.63 ± 0.07 for observer B.

At CT colography, four adenomas 10 mm in diameter or larger were missed by observer A. Of these four adenomas, two were missed due to inadequate insufflation of the colon and retained fluid (technical errors), one was identified retrospectively (perceptive error), and one was a 3-cm flat polyp in the cecum not identified retrospectively. Of the five adenomas 10 mm in diameter or larger missed by observer B, two were missed due

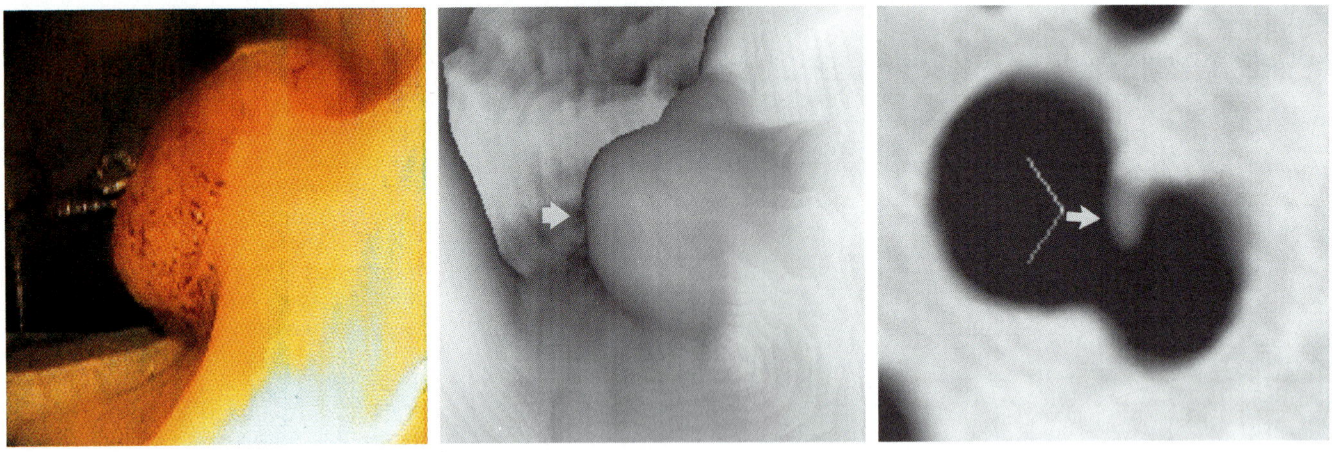

a. b. c.

Figure 2. True positive adenoma (1 cm) at CT colography. Adenoma was seen on **(a)** image obtained at colonoscopy, **(b)** three-dimensional CT colographic image, and **(c)** two-dimensional CT colographic image.

to technical errors (same adenomas as observer A), two were identified retrospectively (different adenomas than those identified retrospectively by observer A), and one was the same flat polyp missed by observer A.

Findings from all CT colographic and videotaped colonoscopy examinations in which false-positive lesions 5 mm in diameter or greater were found were reviewed retrospectively to determine the cause of error. Observer A identified a total of 59 false-positive lesions: 8% (five of 59) were 10 mm in diameter or larger and were in six patients, 56% (33 of 59) were 5–9 mm in diameter and were in 18 patients, and 36% (21 of 59) were smaller than 5 mm in diameter and were in 17 patients. Three (60%) of five false-positive lesions 10 mm in diameter or larger were identified as perceptive errors, with one of the three caused by breath-hold image artifact (a truncated colonic fold that simulated a polyp) and the other two by retained fecal material. By consensus of an endoscopist and radiologist, the remaining two lesions were classified as indeterminate because they were located in areas of the colon that were poorly visualized at colonoscopy. Areas that were generally difficult to evaluate at colonoscopy included the proximal sides of major flexures and haustrations, the medial wall of the cecum, and any surface covered by stool or barium residue.

Observer B identified 47 false-positive lesions: 17% (eight of 47) were 10 mm in diameter or larger and were in six patients, 62% (29 of 47) were 5–9 mm in diameter and were in 15 patients, and 21% (10 of 47) were smaller than 5 mm in diameter and were in nine patients. Of the eight false-positive lesions 10 mm in diameter or larger, three (38%) were perceptive errors caused by stool (n = 2) and a prominent rectal fold (n = 1). The remaining five (62%) lesions were indeterminate because the questionable areas were not well seen on the videotape of the colonoscopy examination due to location, peristaltic contractions, or insufficient insufflation.

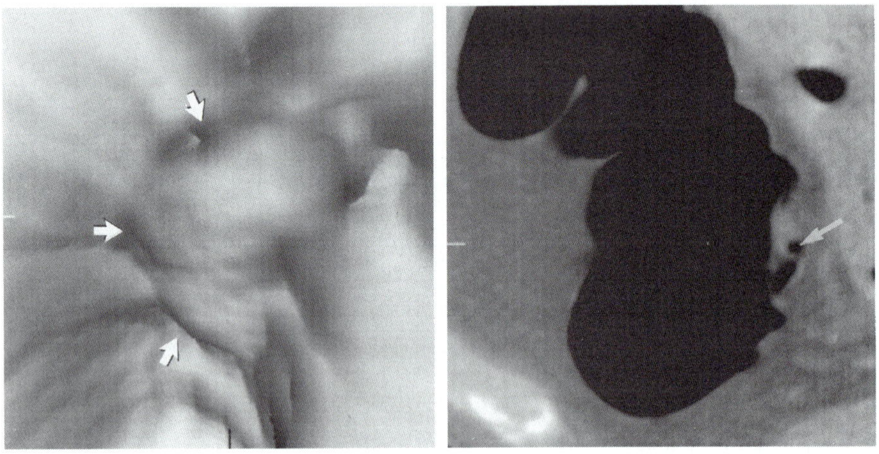

a. b.

Figure 3. Typical appearance of stool at CT colography. **(a)** Three-dimensional CT colographic image shows a lobulated appearance (arrows) suggestive of fecal material. **(b)** Two-dimensional CT colographic image shows the presence of air within the mass (arrow); the presence of air confirms that this is fecal material and not adenomatous tissue.

Of the false-positive lesions 5–9 mm in diameter identified by observer A, 33% (11 of 33) were perceptive errors and 66% (22 of 33) were indeterminate. For false-positive lesions 5–9 mm in diameter identified by observer B, 41% (12 of 29) were perceptive errors and 59% (17 of 29) were indeterminate. Two patients had substantial residual fecal material reported at colonoscopy and at CT colography. These patients accounted for 30% of the total false-positive lesions detected by observer A (18 of 59) and B (14 of 47).

Colonoscopic errors, those discovered at CT colography and confirmed on videotape, were excluded from false-positive analysis. Six colonoscopic errors in six patients were identified. As estimated at CT colography, one was 10 mm in diameter, four were 5–9 mm in diameter, and one was smaller than 5 mm in diameter.

Axial CT was less sensitive than CT colography in adenoma diagnosis and patient identification, as summarized in Table 2. When axial CT was used, the sensitivity for adenomas 10 mm in diameter or larger was 47% (seven of 15) for both observers and averaged 36% (observer A) and 44% (observer B) for adenomas 5 mm in diameter or greater. For adenomas smaller than 5 mm in diameter, sensitivity decreased to less than 10%, significantly lower

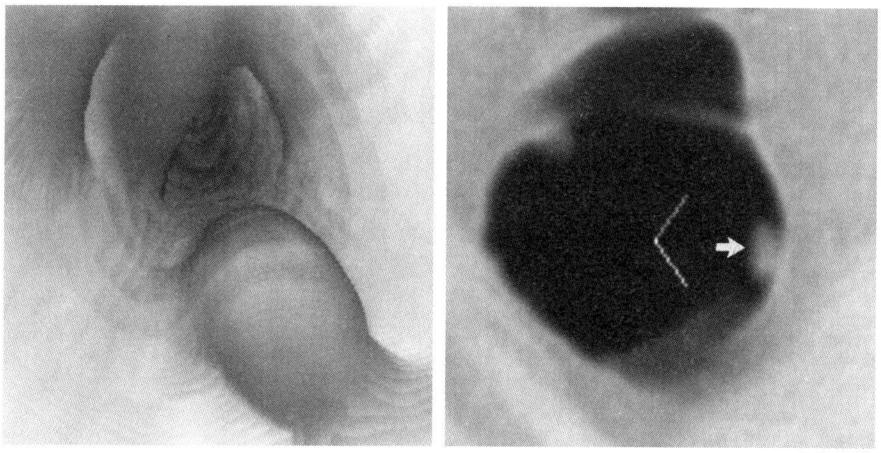

a. b.

Figure 4. False-positive CT colographic findings attributable to stool. **(a)** Three-dimensional CT colographic image shows the morphology of this mass is suggestive of adenoma. **(b)** Two-dimensional CT colographic image shows that without the presence of air or stool marking with orally administered contrast material (arrow), these lesions can be challenging to differentiate from adenomatous adenomas. At colonoscopy, multiple foci of residual stool were noted in the area of this mass.

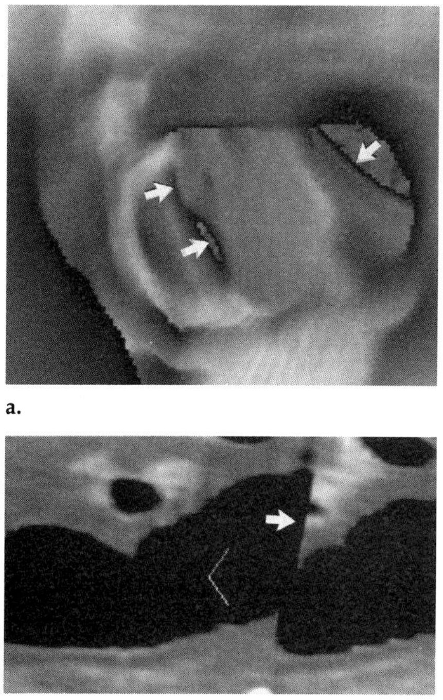

a. b.

Figure 5. False-positive CT colographic findings attributable to a truncated fold between breath holds. **(a)** Three-dimensional CT colographic image shows the truncated fold (arrows) can simulate an obstructing mass. **(b)** Two-dimensional CT colographic image demonstrates the discontinuity between breath-hold images (arrow) to help differentiate truncated folds from true adenomas.

than that for CT colography ($P < .01$). Sensitivity for adenomas 5 mm in diameter or greater was not statistically significantly different between CT colography and axial CT. Observer A identified 26 false-positive lesions in 15 patients, while observer B reported 36 false-positive lesions in 20 patients. For both observers, the sensitivity of identification of patients with adenomas 10 mm in diameter or larger was 58% (seven of 12), while the specificity was 72% (observer A) and 76% (observer B). The sensitivity of patient diagnosis was not significantly different between CT colography and axial CT except for adenomas smaller than 5 mm in diameter ($P < .01$).

One observer (C.D.J.) evaluated CT colographic and axial CT images. For the 15 polyps 10 mm in diameter or larger at endoscopy, six were identified with both techniques, four were identified with CT colography only, and one was identified with axial CT only. Of the 36 polyps 5 mm in diameter or greater at endoscopy, 11 were identified with both techniques, nine were identified with CT colography only, and two were identified with axial CT only. Finally, of the 79 polyps 5 mm in diameter or greater at endoscopy, six were identified with both techniques, 14 were identified with CT colography only, and one was identified with axial CT only.

Nineteen (27%) of 70 patients underwent a single-contrast fluoroscopic barium enema study, which revealed at least one adenoma within a median of 15 days before CT colography and colonoscopy. In these patients, 36 adenomas were subsequently found at colonoscopy. All of the 11 adenomas 5 mm in diameter or greater seen at barium enema examination were also detected at CT colography; furthermore, CT colography depicted nine additional adenomas 5 mm in diameter or larger. Compared with colonoscopy in this subset of patients, false-positive lesions 10 mm in diameter or larger were present at barium enema examination in three cases and at CT colography in none.

DISCUSSION

An acceptable goal of a colorectal screening examination is correct identification of patients with lesions who need to proceed to colonoscopy. Lesions 10 mm in diameter or larger are clinically important because the risk of malignancy is 10% for adenomas 10–20 mm in diameter and increases to at least 30% in adenomas larger than 20 mm in diameter (12–16). The detection of tubular adenomas smaller than 10 mm in diameter is much less crucial, since they have less than a 1% risk of being cancerous (17). In our study, CT colography enabled correct identification of 75% of patients with adenomas 10 mm in diameter or larger (Fig 2). Patients with smaller adenomas were identified less frequently (66% for patients with adenomas 5 mm in diameter or greater and 42% for patients with adenomas less than 5 mm in diameter). Results from analysis that included benign lesions were not statistically significantly different.

Adenomas missed at CT colography were attributable to three types of errors: (*a*) perceptive (adenoma identified in retrospect), (*b*) suboptimal patient preparation (inadequate colon insufflation or retained fecal material), and (*c*) insufficient image resolution (adenomas smaller than 5 mm, flat adenomas). Perceptive errors accounted for 55% (averaged between both observers) of false-negative lesions 5 mm in diameter or greater and can be attributed largely to a previous lack of available training cases and limited knowledge concerning this imaging technique. The majority of training occurred during the course of the study by means of retrospective review of scored CT colographic images along with endoscopic reports and photographs. Characterization of normal anatomic variations and imaging artifacts delineated during the course of our study will undoubtedly help reduce this type of error in the future.

Suboptimal patient preparation also accounted for all but one of the remaining false-negative lesions at CT colography. Currently, retained stool from poor colon cleansing can be differentiated from adenomas most confidently by means of presence of air within the mass on axial or two-dimensional CT

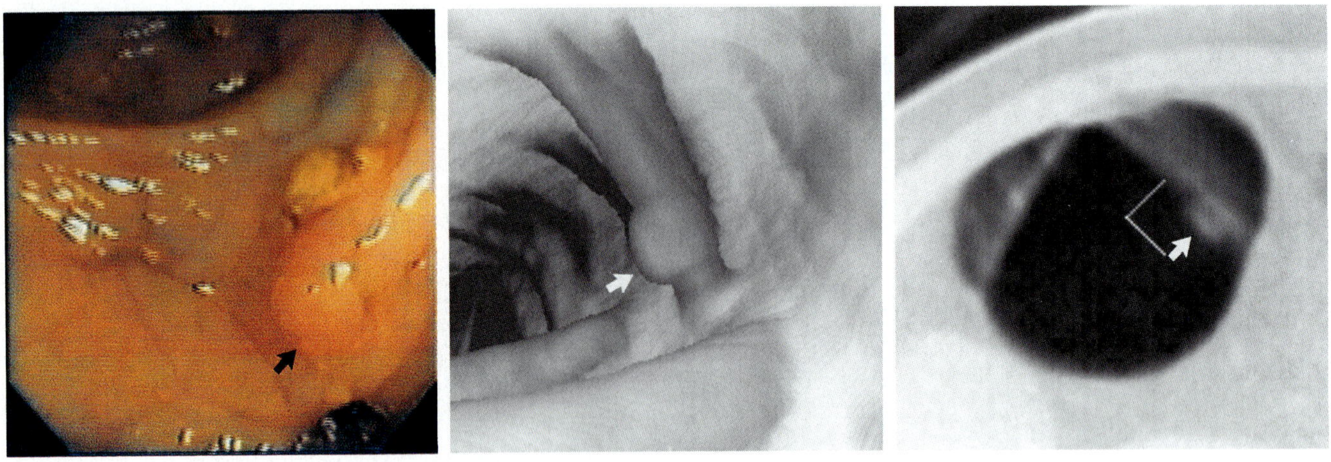

a. b. c.

Figure 6. False-negative colonoscopic findings. **(a)** Colonoscopic image shows a 5–6-mm polyp (arrow) that was seen retrospectively on the videotape but was overlooked at endoscopy. **(b)** Three-dimensional CT colographic image shows a polyp (arrow) clearly. **(c)** Two-dimensional CT colographic image shows the same polyp (arrow).

colographic images (Fig 3), clear separation of the lesion from the colon wall, movement of a nonpedunculated mass, and less confidently by observing unusually lobulated or angular morphology. Marking of stool with an oral radiopaque contrast material, improving software to analyze lesion composition, or scanning in different positions to distend collapsed colon segments or induce stool movement could help reduce these errors.

In all but one case, adenomas 5 mm in diameter or greater missed at CT colography were attributed to correctable causes as described previously. The exception was a 3-cm flat (18) adenoma located at the base of a clean, well-distended cecum that could not be identified even in retrospect. It appears that flat lesions (ie, lesions elevated 2 mm or less from the colon surface) are presently as difficult to diagnose with CT colography as with a barium enema study. Further investigation is needed to improve detection of these difficult lesions.

A high specificity is clinically important to avoid costly and unnecessary colonoscopy. CT colography showed a moderately high specificity of 90% for adenomas 10 mm in diameter or larger. The majority of pseudolesions 10 mm in diameter or larger were attributed to correctable perceptive errors such as misidentification of stool (Fig 4), breath-hold artifacts (Fig 5), and normal anatomic structures. Thus, with experience and technical refinements the specificity should improve eventually. Five false-positive lesions were of indeterminate cause and may represent colonoscopic errors (Fig 6) because colon segments containing the lesion in question were poorly visualized at colonoscopy. Biopsy sites from 1–5 years earlier in follow-up patients were not likely to have caused false-positive lesions, since polypectomy generally heals without residue in 3–4 weeks.

Although axial CT is appealing for colorectal evaluation because of availability, familiar image display, and capacity to enable evaluation of other intraabdominal structures, the sensitivity of axial CT was poor (58%) even in adenomas 10 mm in diameter or larger. Limitations of axial CT include a noncontiguous colon display and partial voluming of small adenomas, which are not imaged in the cross section. CT colography enhances colorectal polyp detection by displaying the colon sequentially from cecum to rectum and by providing a multiplanar two-dimensional image display. Although CT colography enables superior lesion detection, we did find axial CT useful as a familiar reference to determine colon location. Axial CT may eventually attain a more important, complementary role in a nonscreening population. For example, CT colography and standard CT (standard radiation exposure with intravenous administration of contrast material) could be performed simultaneously to evaluate intra- and extracolonic structures (eg, the liver) in patients with colorectal cancer or nonspecific abdominal illnesses.

Clinical acceptance of CT colography among radiologists relies largely on the ability of this technique to depict lesions as well as or better than barium enema examination, the only other radiologic test for colorectal disease. The sensitivity of barium enema examination for colorectal neoplasia varies among examiners (9,19–20), and recent prospective blinded comparisons with colonoscopy suggest that detection rates may be lower than previously assumed. On the basis of a preliminary report of the National Polyp Study in which more than 3,000 adults underwent air-contrast barium enema study and colonoscopy (21), double-contrast barium enema examination depicted only 44% of adenomas 10 mm in diameter or larger compared with colonoscopy. In our patient subgroup, CT colography identified more adenomas 10 mm in diameter or greater and revealed fewer false-positive lesions than single-contrast fluoroscopic barium enema study. Despite the fact that recruitment bias favored barium enema examination in our study, CT colography still showed superior diagnostic results.

CT colography has several inherent advantages over barium enema examination, including imaging of a colonic region in multiple planes, no restrictions from body habitus (ie, overlapping ribs, redundant and overlapping bowel loops), no superimposed radiographic lines or structures, no requirements for mucosal coating, and no need for manual compression. Larger prospective trials are needed, however, to confirm these preliminary results.

Our initial study suggests that CT colography has important potential and may more closely approach an ideal screening test than other currently available choices. Although conclusions concerning the screening applications for CT colography are limited (since we evaluated only high-risk patients), our study provides important data to warrant further investigation. Future studies should be focused on performance in a screening population, prospective comparison of CT colography with barium enema examination, determination of the most efficient display method, evaluation of cost, and assessment of patient acceptability. In addition, other problems aside from perceptive and technical issues already addressed will need to be resolved before CT colography is a viable clinical tool. For example, interpretation time, currently 30–60 minutes of radiologist time per examination, is clearly unacceptable in the currently cost-conscious environment. Experience and more efficient display techniques are necessary to reduce this time.

In conclusion, currently available CT colography performs at a sensitivity and specificity that are attractive for colorectal screening applications. The majority of false-negative and false-positive lesions may be reduced with experience and improved scanning techniques. Current diagnostic limitations of CT colography include flat adenomas and adenomas smaller than 5 mm in diameter. On the basis of study comparisons, CT colography appears to enable more accurate polyp detection compared with axial CT and single-contrast barium enema examination. These findings support further development of CT colography as a promising radiologic approach for detection of colorectal neoplasia. ■

References

1. Hara AK, Johnson CD, Reed JE, et al. Reducing data size and radiation dose for CT colography. AJR 1997; 168:1181–1184.
2. Hara AK, Johnson CD, Reed JE, et al. Detection of colorectal adenomas by computed tomographic colography: feasibility of a novel technique. Gastroenterology 1996; 110:290–294.
3. Hara AK, Johnson CD, Reed JE, Ehman RL, Ilstrup DM. Colorectal polyp detection using computed tomographic colography: two- versus three-dimensional techniques. Radiology 1996; 200:49–54.
4. Vining DJ, Teigen EL, Stetts D, Vanderwerken B, Kopecky KK, Rex D. Virtual colonoscopy: a 60-second colon examination (abstr). Radiology 1995; 197(P):281.
5. Rubin GD, Beaulieu CF, Argiro V, et al. Perspective volume rendering of CT and MR images: applications for endoscopic imaging. Radiology 1996; 199:321–330.
6. Reed JE, Hara AK, Johnson CD. Interpretation of image sets containing convoluted tubular structures via transluminal sections and steerable intraluminal perspective views. Proc SPIE 1996; 2710:1009–1019.
7. Reed JE, Hara AK, Johnson CD. CT colography combines virtual colonoscopy and transluminal cross sections. Paris, France: Excerpta Medical International Congress 1996; 1124:171–176.
8. Ott DJ, Chen YM, Gelfand DW, Wu WC, Munitz HA. Single-contrast vs double-contrast barium enema in the detection of colonic polyps. AJR 1986; 146:993–996.
9. Johnson CD, Carlson HC, Taylor WF, Weiland LP. Barium enemas of carcinoma of the colon: sensitivity of double- and single-contrast studies. AJR 1983; 140:1143–1149.
10. Teefey SA, Carlson HC. The fluoroscopic barium enema in colonic polyp detection. AJR 1983; 141:1279–1281.
11. Hanley JA, McNeil BJ. The meaning and use of the area under a receiver operating characteristic (ROC) curve. Radiology 1982; 143:29–36.
12. Muto T, Bussey HJR, Morson BC. The evolution of cancer of the colon and rectum. Cancer 1975; 36:2251–2270.
13. Stryker SJ, Wolff BG, Culp CE, Libbe SD, Ilstrup DM, MacCarty RL. Natural history of untreated colonic adenomas. Gastroenterology 1987; 93:1009–1013.
14. Simons BD, Morrison AS, Lev R, Verhoek-Oftendahl W. Relationship of adenomas to cancer of the large intestine. J Natl Cancer Inst 1992; 84:962–966.
15. Atkin WS, Morson BC, Cuzick J. Long-term risk of colorectal cancer after excision of rectosigmoid adenomas. N Engl J Med 1992; 326:658–662.
16. O'Brien MJ, Winawer SJ, Zauber AG. The national polyp study: patient and polyp characteristics associated with high-grade dysplasia in colorectal adenomas. Gastroenterology 1990; 98:371–379.
17. Waye JD, Lewis BS, Frankel A, Geller SA. Small colon adenomas. Am J Gastroenterol 1988; 83:120–122.
18. Muto T, Kamiya J, Sawada T, et al. Small flat elevation of the large bowel with special reference to its clinico-pathological features. Stomach Intest 1984; 19:1359–1366.
19. Fork FT. Double contrast enema and colonoscopy in polyp detection. Gut 1981; 22:971–977.
20. Steine S, Stordahl A, Lunde OC, et al. Double-contrast barium enema versus colonoscopy in the diagnosis of neoplastic disorders: aspects of decision-making in general practice. Fam Prac 1993; 10:288–291.
21. Ott DJ. Analysis of accuracy, complications, and cost of barium enema for CRC diagnosis. Bethesda, Md: National Institutes of Health, 1994.

Book Review

Atlas of Nuclear Medicine

Marc Coel, MD, and Jimmy Leung, MD

Philadelphia, Pa: W.B. Saunders & Co, 1996. ISBN 0-7216-3578-4. Cloth, $225.00; pp 749; 2,622 figures; tables.

I enjoyed reading this book! Generally, the comprehensive atlas format makes this book difficult to read cover-to-cover; however, this book provides excellent examples of classic cases and their variations, which are all relayed in a readable, straightforward style. In addition, the authors include notes ("pearls"), differential diagnostic lists, gamuts, and algorithms or flow diagrams to summarize points. Extensive cross-references are used, which assist pattern recognition. These features make the textbook an excellent choice for residents and fellows; thus, reading this textbook in the months before the written and oral radiology boards would be useful.

There are 17 major sections, such as those on the liver, bone, spleen, and hepatobiliary system. In the section on bone, there are 11 individual subchapters; in the section on the lung, there are 10. Strong sections include those on bone, the lung, the gastrointestinal tract, and the kidney. Tumor imaging and a section on the breast are also included. In each section, cases are presented as a series of images, notes, and captions. At times, the cases are presented over several pages or in nonstandard sequences on pages. This presentation can be difficult to follow. A standard pattern or a more spacious sequence would be easier to read; however, these kinds of presentations would necessitate more pages and, consequently, greater expense. The current price of this textbook ($225) is enough.

This atlas competes well with other established nuclear medicine atlases. This atlas is less bulky than most and offers many more useful notes, lists, and gamuts. Drs Coel and Leung designed the book for residents, fellows, and specialists in nuclear medicine, and the text will be a useful addition to the personal libraries of many of these physicians and to department teaching libraries for residents in the United States and overseas.

Reviewed by S. Horatio Slawson, MD

Jiro Watari, MD • Yusuke Saitoh, MD • Takeshi Obara, MD • Takanori Fujiki, MD
Masato Taniguchi, MD • Masafumi Nomura, MD • Tokiyoshi Ayabe, MD
Tomoyuki Ohta, MD • Yutaka Orii, MD • Yutaka Kohgo, MD

Early Nonpolypoid Colorectal Cancer: Radiographic Diagnosis of Depth of Invasion[1]

PURPOSE: **To diagnose depth of invasion of early flat and depressed nonpolypoid colorectal cancers with double-contrast barium enema examination.**

MATERIALS AND METHODS: **Ninety-seven early nonpolypoid colorectal cancers, initially identified with colonoscopy, were investigated with double-contrast barium enema examination. Depth of invasion in resected specimens obtained with endoscopic mucosal or surgical resection was determined. Cancer confined to the mucosal layer or with focal extension to the submucosal layer was defined as Ca-m; moderate to massive extension of cancer into the submucosal layer was classified Ca-sm.**

RESULTS: **In flat elevated and depressed cancers, converging folds and semilunar deformity were observed significantly more frequently in Ca-sm than in Ca-m tumors ($P <$ .05 and $P <$ .01, respectively). Sensitivities and specificities of these findings for Ca-sm tumor were 42%, 93% and 86%, 85%, respectively. Deep depression, irregular surface of the depression, and tumor size larger than 20 mm were also predictive findings for depressed Ca-sm tumors ($P <$ .05); the specificity of each was 100%. With use of these radiographic predictors, overall accuracy for diagnosing depth of invasion was 85%.**

CONCLUSION: **Findings on double-contrast barium enema study are highly predictive of depth of invasion of early nonpolypoid colorectal cancer. Radiographic findings of converging folds, semilunar deformity, deep depression, irregular surface of the depression, and tumor size are predictors of Ca-sm tumor.**

Adenomas and early cancers of the colon manifest most often as polypoid lesions, and it is assumed that most colorectal cancers develop from preexisting adenomas (1,2). However, the concept of flat and depressed nonpolypoid tumor types has been proposed by Muto et al (3), Wolber and Owen (4), Kudo et al (5), and Stolte and Bethke (6). These types of tumors have been detected increasingly in Japan with colonoscopy and appear as small plaquelike lesions with a vague redness or discoloration (7–12). On radiographs, both types of nonpolypoid colon cancer appear as radiolucent areas with a round or irregular margin; in depressed lesions, there is a central barium collection (13,14). Nonpolypoid cancer is more likely than polypoid cancer to invade beyond the mucosa, where lesions are small (3–5,15–17). Lymph node metastases from flat and depressed nonpolypoid types of moderately and massively invasive submucosal cancers are frequent (18–20); however, lymph node metastases from intramucosal and focally invasive submucosal cancers are extremely rare (18,20–22). More advanced lesions are more effectively treated with surgery, and intramucosal cancers may be treated suitably with endoscopic mucosal resection (11,23). Therefore, diagnosis of the depth of cancer invasion is clinically of primary importance.

Generally, barium enema study is considered less sensitive than colonoscopy for the initial detection of colorectal cancer (13,14,24–26). The overall accuracy of colonoscopy for identifying depth of invasion of early colorectal cancers was reported to be 58%–80% by experienced observers (27,28). With radiography, however, some minute nonpolypoid tumors less than 5 mm in diameter can be depicted (13,14,21), and the natural history of superficial depressed cancer may be determined with cautious, retrospective radiographic analysis (29). Accordingly, detailed radiography may be a useful diagnostic modality for detection of minute flat and depressed types of early colorectal tumors. Moreover, barium enema study is more versatile and cost-effective than colonoscopy. Therefore, it is important to evaluate the radiographic findings that enable diagnosis of the depth of invasion of early nonpolypoid colorectal cancers so that diagnostic specificity and sensitivity may be increased and treatment may be optimized.

Double-contrast barium enema examination is the principal diagnostic radiographic procedure for detailed study of the colon; however, to our knowledge, there has been no detailed study of the radiographic findings of depth of invasion of nonpolypoid cancers in the colon. The purpose of this retrospective study was to elucidate

Index terms: Barium enema examination, 75.1282 • Colon, neoplasms, 75.32, 75.3292 • Colon, radiography, 75.1282

Abbreviations: Ca-m = cancer in mucosal layer or extending focally into submucosal layer, Ca-sm = moderate to massive extension of cancer into submucosal layer.

Radiology 1997; 205:67–74

[1] From the Third Department of Internal Medicine, Asahikawa Medical College, Nishikagura 4-5, Asahikawa 078, Japan (J.W., Y.S., T.O., T.F., M.T., M.N., T.A., Y.K.); and the Department of Gastroenterology, Asahikawa Kosei General Hospital, Asahikawa, Japan (T.O., Y.O.). Received April 7, 1997; revision requested May 9; revision received June 9; accepted June 16. **Address reprint requests to** J.W.

the findings on double-contrast barium enema radiographs that enable (*a*) prediction of depth of invasion of early nonpolypoid colorectal cancer and (*b*) choice of therapy.

MATERIALS AND METHODS

Patients and Examinations

Between January 1990 and July 1996, 206 early nonpolypoid colorectal cancers were identified in 185 patients with colonoscopy. Cancers fulfilled the criteria of general rules for clinical and pathologic studies on cancer of the colon, rectum, and anus of the Japanese Research Society for Cancer of the Colon and Rectum (30). Detailed examination with double-contrast barium enema was performed in 96 patients with 99 nonpolypoid cancers. Of 99 lesions, 97 (98%) lesions in 94 patients were demonstrated with double-contrast barium enema, and their radiographic findings were studied. There were 68 men and 26 women; patient ages ranged from 36 to 85 years (mean, 65.4 years). All 94 patients were examined with double-contrast barium enema before tumors were resected with endoscopic mucosal resection or surgery; in this study, therapy was chosen on the basis of tentative colonoscopic diagnosis. Patients were prepared for double-contrast barium enema in the routine way (low residual diet, 7.5 mg sodium picosulfate, and 34 g magnesium citrate the day before examination and 10 mg bisacodyl suppository 2 hours before examination); the double-contrast method was performed with 67%–70% wt/vol barium sulfate (Baroject Sol 100; Horii Pharm, Osaka, Japan).

All resected histologic specimens were examined at the Department of Surgical Pathology of Asahikawa Medical College Hospital. The histologic type and grade of atypia were classified according to the World Health Organization classification (31). Intramucosal epithelial neoplasms with an architectural abnormality with back-to-back glands were diagnosed as intramucosal cancer. The submucosal cancers were classified into three subtypes (11) as follows: sm1, focally extended; sm2, moderately extended; and sm3, massively extended. Depth of invasion of all cancers was confirmed with histologic examination. Intramucosal and sm1 cancers were treated with endoscopic mucosal resection, and these tumors were termed Ca-m; sm2 and sm3 cancers must be resected surgically, and these tumors were termed Ca-sm.

The radiographic findings examined of tumors were the following: (*a*) maximum diameter in millimeters; (*b*) shape, irregular (Fig 1a) or round (Figs 2a, 3a, 4a); (*c*) converging folds, present (Fig 2a) or absent (Figs 1a, 3a, 4a); (*d*) central depression, deep (Fig 4a) or shallow (Fig 3a); (*e*) depression surface, irregular (Fig 4a) or smooth (Fig 3a); and (*f*) semilunar deformity on profile view (Ushio classification) (32), present (Figs 2b, 4b) or absent (Fig 1b).

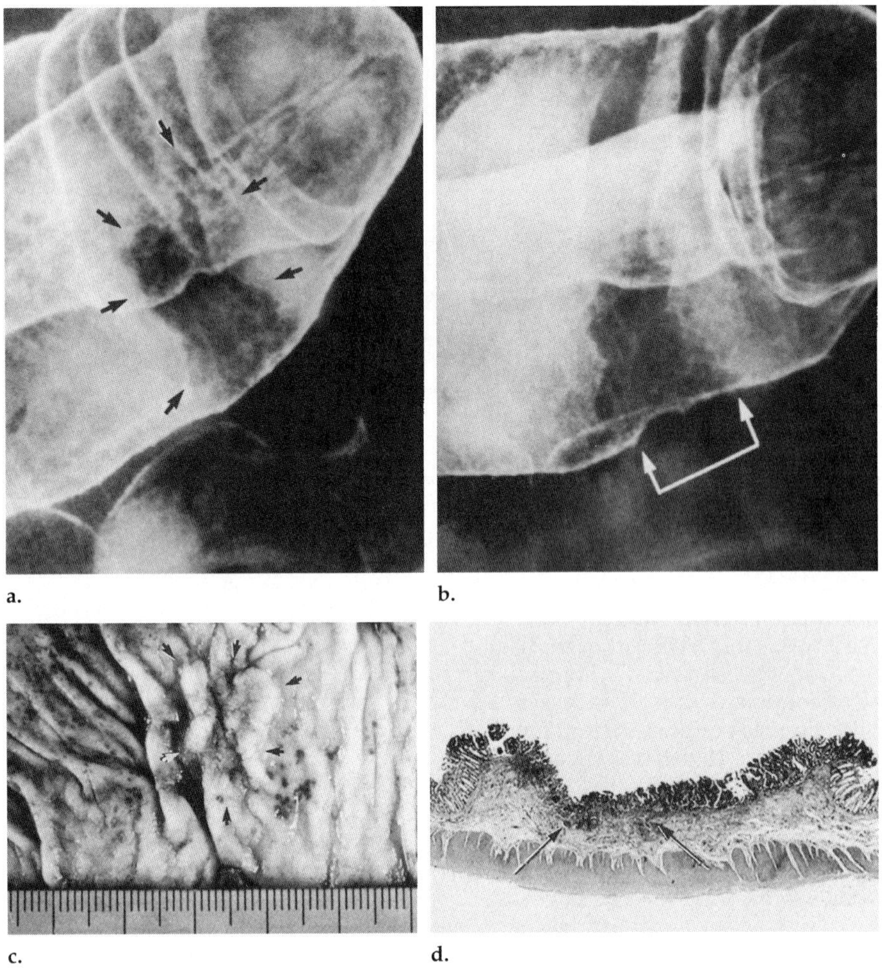

Figure 1. Flat elevated Ca-m tumor. **(a)** Barium enema radiograph with en face view shows an irregularly shaped radiolucent area (arrows) without converging mucosal folds. **(b)** Barium enema radiograph with profile view shows the wedge-shaped deformity (arrows) but not the semilunar deformity. **(c)** Photograph of the resected specimen of colon shows a flat elevated lesion (arrows) with an irregular margin. **(d)** Histologic specimen reveals that the lesion (arrows) extends focally to the submucosal layer. (Hematoxylin-eosin stain; original magnification, ×12.)

We defined converging mucosal folds as two or more mucosal folds converging toward the lesion. Deep depression and irregular surface of the depression were defined as a thick and a rough-appearing barium collection, respectively, on the depression surface. Shallow depression and smooth surface of the depression were defined as a thin and a homogeneous barium collection, respectively.

The incidences of radiographic findings on en face and profile views were statistically evaluated.

Statistical Analysis

Statistical analysis was performed with the Mann-Whitney *U* test and the χ^2 test. A *P* value of less than .05 was considered statistically significant.

RESULTS

Macroscopic and Histologic Findings

Of 97 colorectal cancers of flat and depressed nonpolypoid types, 41 (42%) lesions were resected with endoscopic muscosal resection and 56 (58%) lesions were resected surgically. Table 1 summarizes the distribution of 97 nonpolypoid cancers according to the criteria of macroscopic type (11,33) and the histologic classification of depth of invasion. Macroscopically, 58 (60%) lesions were a flat elevated type and 39 (40%) lesions were a depressed type. Of the 39 depressed cancers, 15 (38%) were slightly depressed and 24 (62%) were flat and elevated with depression.

At histologic classification of depth of invasion, 41 (71%) of the 58 flat elevated cancers were classified Ca-m and 17 (29%) were classified Ca-sm. Mean maximum diameters of Ca-m and Ca-sm tumors were 20.7 mm ± 12.1 and 25.5 mm ± 26.6, respectively; these measures were not statistically significantly different. Of 39 depressed cancers, 13 (33%) were classified Ca-m and 26 (67%) were classified Ca-sm. The mean maximum diameter (9.6 mm ± 5.5) of Ca-m tumors was significantly less than that (15.9 mm ±

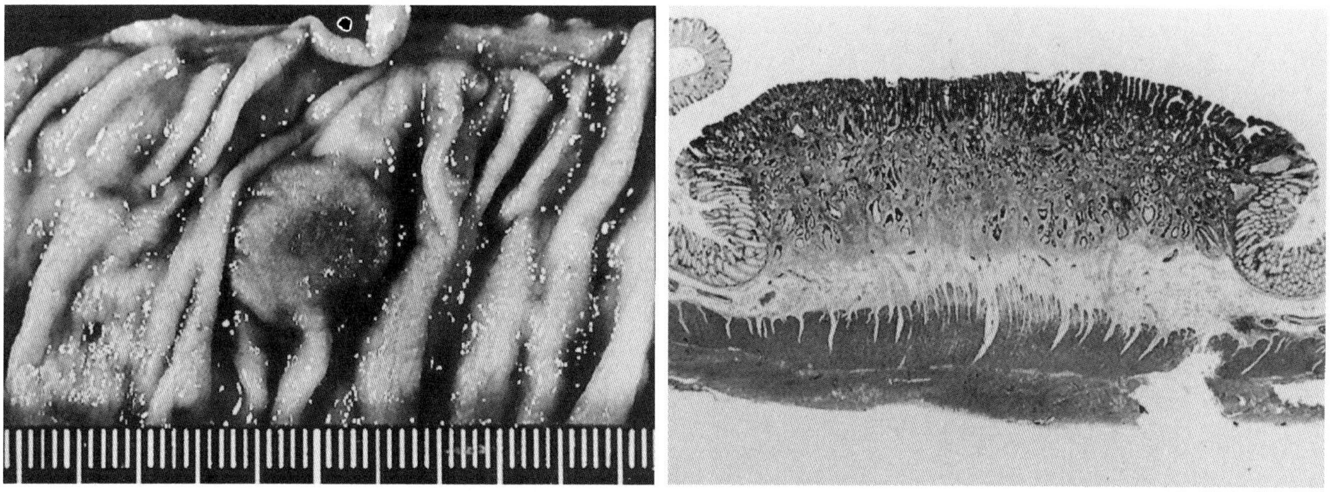

c. d.

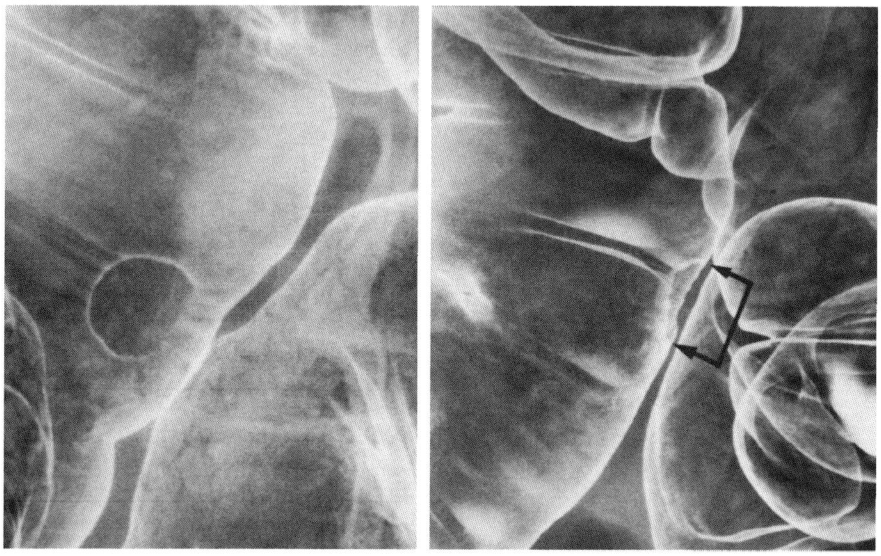

a. b.

Figure 2. Flat elevated Ca-sm tumor. **(a)** Barium enema radiograph with en face view demonstrates a round radiolucent area with converging mucosal folds. **(b)** Barium enema radiograph with profile view shows a semilunar deformity (arrows). **(c)** Photograph of the resected specimen of colon shows a flat elevation with a round margin. **(d)** Histologic specimen reveals massive extension of the lesion to the submucosal layer with fibrotic change. (Hematoxylin-eosin stain; original magnification, ×12.)

7.8) of Ca-sm tumors ($P < .05$). Although all tumors larger than 20 mm ($n = 7$) were Ca-sm tumors, the maximum diameter of 19 (73%) of 26 Ca-sm tumors was 20 mm or less.

Radiographic Findings of Nonpolypoid Colorectal Cancers

Tables 2 and 3 summarize the findings on barium enema radiographs with en face and profile views of flat elevated and depressed cancers. Flat elevated cancer appeared as a radiolucent area, which was sometimes demarcated with a thin white line (Figs 1a, 2a). In depressed cancers, these radiolucent areas were accompanied by a round barium fleck or an irregularly shaped barium collection in the center of the depression (Figs 3a, 4a).

Radiographic Findings of Flat Elevated Cancers

Findings on barium enema radiographs with en face and profile views of flat elevated cancers are summarized in Table 2. En face radiographic views were examined in all 58 flat elevated lesions. Fourteen (34%) of 41 flat elevated Ca-m tumors appeared as round radiolucent areas, and the other 27 (66%) flat elevated Ca-m tumors appeared as radiolucent areas with irregular margins. Eight (47%) of 17 flat elevated Ca-sm tumors appeared as round radiolucent areas, and the other nine (53%) flat elevated Ca-sm tumors had irregular margins. Converging mucosal folds were seen in two (5%) of 41 flat elevated Ca-m tumors and five (29%) of 17 flat elevated Ca-sm tumors. Converging mucosal folds were seen significantly more often in flat elevated Ca-sm tumors than in flat elevated Ca-m tumors ($P < .05$).

A profile view was obtained in 51 (88%) of 58 studies of flat elevated cancers; profile views were available of 38 (93%) of 41 flat elevated Ca-m tumors and 13 (76%) of 17 flat elevated Ca-sm tumors. The profile views of seven lesions (three in the sigmoid colon, one in the transverse colon, and three in the ascending colon) were not obtained. Maximum diameter of these lesions ranged from 8 to 17 mm (mean, 14 mm). Semilunar deformity was found in 11 (85%) of 13 flat elevated Ca-sm tumors and in only three (8%) of 38 flat elevated Ca-m tumors. The semilunar deformity was observed significantly more often in Ca-sm tumors than in Ca-m tumors ($P < .0001$).

Sensitivity and specificity of converging folds and semilunar deformity for Ca-sm tumors were 29%, 95% and 85%, 92%, respectively. Positive predictive values of these findings for Ca-sm tumors were 71% and 79%, respectively. Among the radiographic findings studied, converging folds and semilunar deformity were useful for predicting moderate to massive submucosal invasion (ie, Ca-sm) of flat elevated cancers.

Radiographic Findings of Depressed Cancers

Table 3 summarizes the results of findings on barium enema radiographs with en face and profile views of depressed cancers. En face radiographic views were examined in all 39 depressed lesions. Of 13 depressed Ca-m tumors, nine (69%) appeared as round radiolucent areas and the other

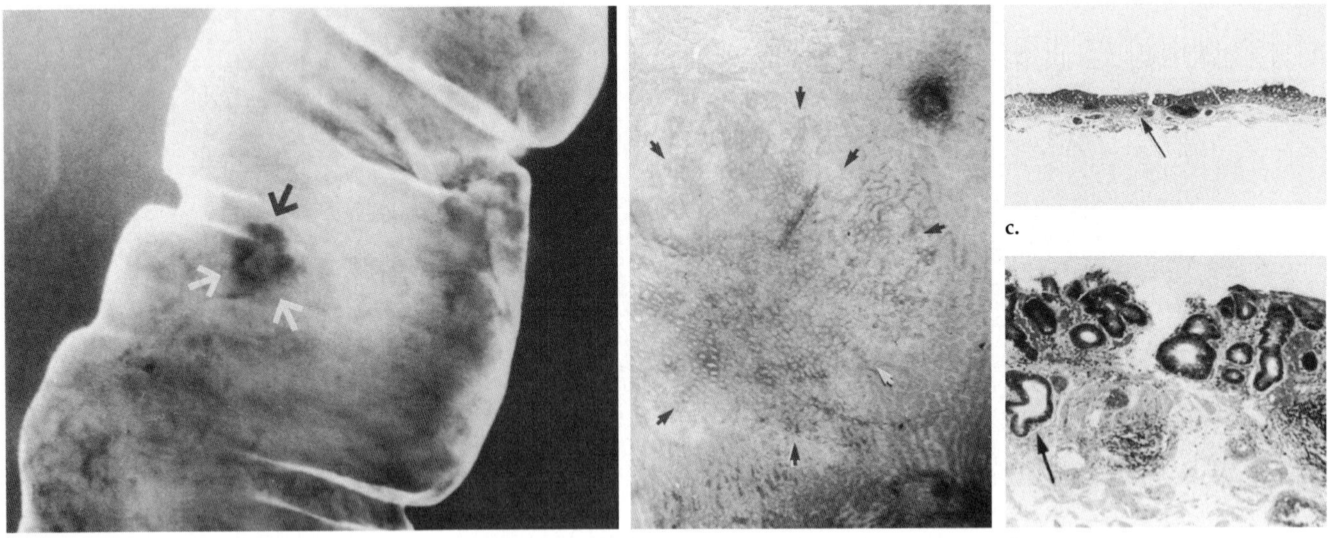

a. b. c. d.

Figure 3. Depressed Ca-m tumor. **(a)** Barium enema radiograph demonstrates a radiolucent lesion (arrows) with a thin, homogeneous barium collection. A deformity in profile view was not seen. **(b)** Photograph obtained with a dissecting stereomicroscope shows an irregular, shallow depression (arrows) in the lesion. **(c, d)** Histologic specimen of the lesion shows focally invasive cancer (arrow) to the submucosal layer. (Hematoxylin-eosin stain; original magnification, ×12 **[c]**, ×84 **[d]**.)

four (31%) lesions appeared as radiolucent areas with an irregular margin. Seventeen (65%) of the 26 depressed Ca-sm tumors appeared as round radiolucent areas, and the other nine (35%) depressed Ca-sm tumors appeared as radiolucent areas with an irregular margin. Converging folds were demonstrated in two (15%) of 13 depressed Ca-m and 13 (50%) of 26 depressed Ca-sm tumors; converging folds were seen in depressed Ca-sm tumors significantly more often than in depressed Ca-m tumors ($P < .05$). The barium collection in the center of tumor that corresponded to a central depression was seen in 32 (82%) of the 39 depressed cancers; nine of these tumors were Ca-m and 23 were Ca-sm. Four Ca-m tumors and three Ca-sm tumors did not demonstrate a barium collection. Of these seven cancers, two were in the rectum, three were in the sigmoid colon, one was in the descending colon, and one was in the transverse colon. Maximum diameters of these seven tumors ranged from 5 to 25 mm (mean, 15 mm). Radiographs of these seven tumors were excluded from further analysis.

Among the 32 depressed cancers that showed a barium collection, all nine of the depressed Ca-m tumors showed a shallow, smooth depression. Seven (30%) of 23 depressed Ca-sm tumors showed a deep depression, and 16 (70%) showed a shallow depression. An irregular surface of the depression was seen in 12 (52%) depressed Ca-sm tumors; a smooth depression was seen in the other 11 (48%) depressed Ca-sm tumors. All depressed Ca-m tumors showed a smooth depression. Thus, a deep depression and an irregular surface of the depression were observed exclusively in depressed Ca-sm tumors.

Precise profile views were obtained of 12 (92%) of 13 depressed Ca-m and 20 (77%) of 26 depressed Ca-sm tumors. The profile views of seven lesions (one in the rectum, two in the sigmoid colon, two in the transverse colon, one in the ascending colon, and one in the cecum) were not demonstrated. Maximum diameters of these seven lesions ranged from 12 to 35 mm (mean, 18 mm). Among the profile views obtained of the 12 depressed Ca-m tumors, semilunar deformity was seen only in one (8%) case. By contrast, semilunar deformity was seen in 14 (70%) of 20 depressed Ca-sm tumors.

Therefore, the sensitivities, specificities, and positive predictive values of converging folds and semilunar deformity for depressed Ca-sm tumors were 50%, 85%, 87% and 70%, 92%, 93%, respectively. Moreover, the sensitivities, specificities, and positive predictive values of a deep depression and an irregular surface of the depression were 30%, 100%, 100% and 52%, 100%, 100%, respectively. Deep depression and irregular surface of the depression each had a specificity of 100% for depressed Ca-sm tumors; thus, these radiographic findings were defined as characteristic of a depressed Ca-sm tumor.

Accuracy for Radiographic Diagnosis of Depth of Invasion

On the basis of the radiographic results described, early nonpolypoid cancers were considered to be Ca-sm tumors if they exhibited at least one of the following radiographic findings: converging folds and semilunar deformity in a flat elevated tumor; and maximum diameter greater than 20 mm, converging folds, deep depression, irregular surface of the depression, and semilunar deformity in a depressed tumor. Tumors were considered to be Ca-m tumors if none of these radiographic findings were demonstrated. The accuracy of double-contrast barium enema radiographs to depict depth of invasion with use of the radiographic findings is shown in Table 4. Overall accuracy of the diagnosis of depth of invasion was 85% (82 of 97 lesions). In 58 cases of flat elevated tumors, 48 (83%) were correctly diagnosed as Ca-m or Ca-sm. In 39 cases of depressed tumors, 34 (87%) were correctly diagnosed as Ca-m or Ca-sm.

DISCUSSION

Colonoscopy has been the primary method used to detect colorectal cancers (34); however, barium enema study still serves a major function in the diagnosis of colorectal cancers because the study is (*a*) used on a widespread basis, (*b*) cost-effective (35), and (*c*) uniquely advantageous (36). To our knowledge, however, only a few investigations have determined the efficacy of barium enema study to enable diagnosis of depth of invasion in colorectal cancers (32,37). In addition to the cost benefit and feasibility in clinical practice of barium enema

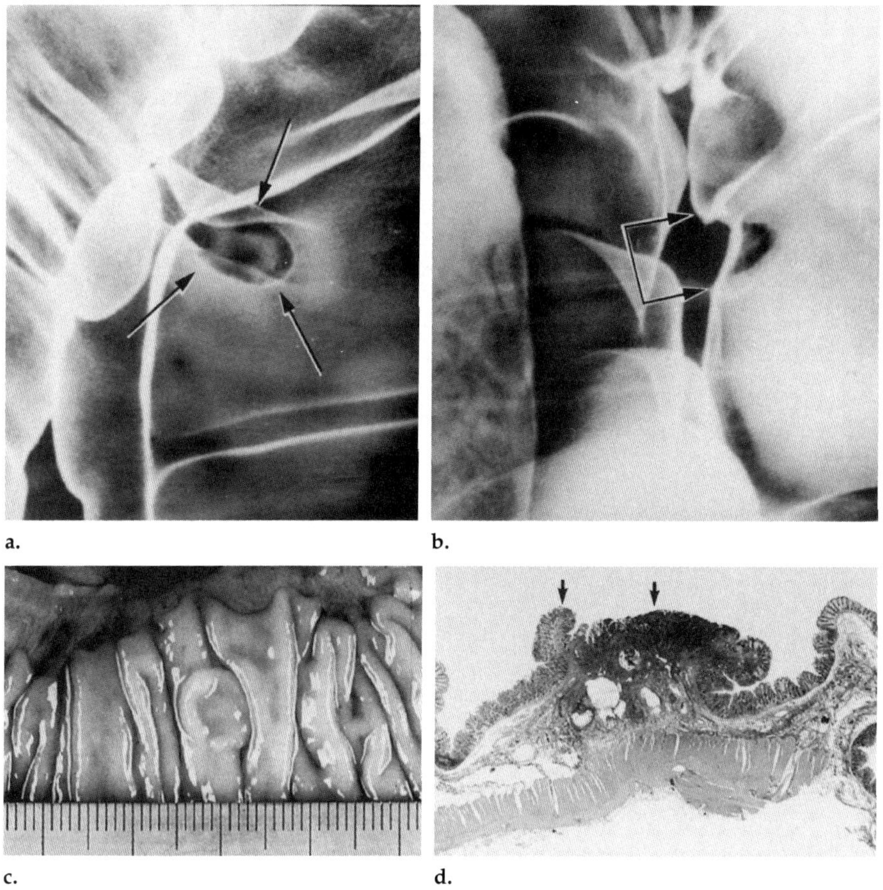

Figure 4. Depressed Ca-sm tumor. **(a)** Barium enema radiograph demonstrates a radiolucent lesion (arrows) with a thick, irregular barium collection. The bottom of the depression appears irregular. **(b)** Barium enema radiograph with profile view shows a semilunar deformity (arrows). **(c)** Photograph of the resected specimen of colon shows a central depression with marginal elevation. **(d)** Histologic specimen of the lesion shows that cancer massively invades the submucosal layer. There is an erosive depression (arrows) in the left side of the tumor. (Hematoxylin-eosin stain; original magnification, ×8.)

Table 1
Macroscopic and Histologic Findings of Resected Nonpolypoid Colorectal Cancers

Macroscopic Classification	No. of Lesions	Histologic Classification of Depth of Invasion*		Maximum Diameter† (mm)	
		Ca-m	Ca-sm	Ca-m	Ca-sm
Flat elevated type	58	41 (20:21)	17 (1:16)	20.7 ± 12.1	25.5 ± 26.6
Depressed type	39	13 (8:5)	26 (2:24)	9.6 ± 5.5‡	15.9 ± 7.8‡
Slightly depressed	15	9 (8:1)	6 (1:5)	7.6 ± 4.3	14.0 ± 9.4
Flat and elevated with depression	24	4 (0:4)	20 (1:19)	14.0 ± 5.9	16.6 ± 7.4

* Numbers are numbers of lesions. Numbers in parentheses are ratios of numbers of lesions treated with endoscopic mucosal resection to those treated with surgery.
† Numbers are mean ± standard deviation.
‡ $P < .05$ for comparison of mean maximum diameter of depressed Ca-m tumors with that of depressed Ca-sm tumors.

study, it can provide information that is not obtained with colonoscopy, such as presence or absence of lateral deformity. Thus, barium enema study is versatile and useful not only for colon cancer screening but for detailed examination of colorectal cancer. We believe efforts should be made to determine the usefulness of barium enema study for assessing the depth of invasion of colorectal cancer.

Recently, early nonpolypoid colorectal cancer has been detected with increasing frequency, and diagnosis of depth of invasion is essential for determining therapy. In the English-language literature, reports on the radiographic diagnosis of depth of invasion of early nonpolypoid colorectal cancer are scarce because this tumor is relatively infrequent in western countries. Therefore, we conducted this retrospective study to elucidate radiographic findings that are useful for predicting depth of invasion of early nonpolypoid colorectal cancer and to clarify the diagnostic function of barium enema study.

In our study, double-contrast barium enema examination proved useful for diagnosing depth of invasion of early nonpolypoid cancer; radiographic predictors of Ca-sm tumor were (*a*) converging folds, (*b*) semilunar deformity, (*c*) deep depression, and (*d*) irregular appearance of the depression surface.

Converging folds and semilunar deformity were highly predictive radiographic findings of flat elevated and depressed Ca-sm tumors. Overall, the sensitivities, specificities, and positive predictive values of converging folds and semilunar deformity for Ca-sm were 42%, 93%, 82% and 76%, 92%, 86%, respectively. The converging fold appeared as a narrow (about 1-mm wide) fold that extended toward the cancer. At histologic examination, converging folds were associated with cancers in which there was submucosal fibrosis and/or moderate to massive cancer invasion in the submucosal layer. Frequency of converging folds increased as cancer invaded deeper into the submucosal layer. All of the Ca-m tumors with converging folds showed fibrosis in the submucosal layer, and the incidence of converging folds in Ca-m tumors was 7% (four of 54 lesions). The pathogenesis of submucosal fibrosis in intramucosal cancer has not been fully clarified. Ozeki et al (38) reported a case of an intramucosal depressed-type cancer that showed converging mucosal folds; on the basis of histologic findings, they suggested that converging folds were caused by submucosal fibrosis.

On profile views, only 8% (four of 50 lesions) of Ca-m tumors showed semilunar deformity; however, this deformity was seen in 76% (25 of 33 lesions) of Ca-sm tumors. Consequently, semilunar deformity on profile view is an indicator of a Ca-sm tumor in flat elevated and depressed tumors because of a high sensitivity (76%) and specificity (92%). To our knowledge, we are the first to show that semilunar deformity is a radiographic predictor of Ca-sm tumor in nonpolypoid colorectal cancer. In polypoid colorectal cancer, semilunar deformity on profile views indicates massive cancer invasion of the submucosal to proper muscular layers (32). Our results in nonpolypoid cancer agree with those of a previous study (32). Ushio et al investigated the correlation between depth of invasion and lateral deformity by subtyping deformity into no deformity, wedge-shaped deformity, and semilunar deformity. Wedge-shaped deformity was observed mainly in intramucosal cancers, although its statistical significance was not determined. In our study, wedge-shaped deformity was an equivocal radiographic finding for the diagnosis of depth of invasion (data not shown); thus, the presence or absence of semilunar deformity was determined to be useful for diagnosing depth of invasion.

In depressed cancers, a deep depression and irregular surface of the depression were observed exclusively in Ca-sm tumors; thus, these two radiographic findings each had a specificity of 100%. However, because it is technically difficult to demonstrate the central depression of the tumor as a barium collection, seven (18%) of the 39 depressed tumors could not be depicted as having the depression, and this finding had a relatively low sensitivity. Failure to demonstrate a barium collection was possibly the result of the following: (*a*) The lesion on double-contrast barium enema study was in a nondependent bowel wall. (*b*) There was poor mucosal coating owing to poor preparation. (*c*) There were technical difficulties similar to those faced in demonstrating lateral deformity. To increase the rate at which these radiographic findings are depicted, double-contrast barium enema images of each segment of the lesion should be obtained from many directions with the patient in the supine and prone positions (13). In our experience, it has been difficult to demonstrate the lateral deformity and barium collection in cancer, especially in the sigmoid colon. Most of the missed polyps on double-contrast barium enema study have been near the sigmoid colon (39). Therefore, much care should be taken to visualize the sigmoid colon in detail. Generally, cancers in which the lateral deformity and central depression were not demonstrated were 10 mm in diameter or larger. It has been reported that the sensitivity of barium enema study for detecting colonic lesions 1 cm or larger is higher than that for detecting 5–9-mm polyps (40). In our study, tumor size was not a major reason for failing to demonstrate detailed features on double-contrast barium enema studies.

Table 2
Radiographic and Histologic Findings in Flat Elevated Cancers

Radiographic Findings	No. of Lesions*	Histologic Classification of Depth of Invasion† Ca-m	Ca-sm	Statistical Calculations for Ca-sm: Sensitivity (%)	Specificity (%)	Positive Predictive Value (%)
Shape‡ (round:irregular)	58 (100)	14:27	8:9	47	66	36
Converging folds§ (present: absent)	58 (100)	2:39	5:12	29	95	71
Semilunar deformity‖ on profile view (present:absent)	51 (88)	3:35	11:2	85	92	79

* Numbers in parentheses are percentages.
† Numbers are numbers of lesions with or without the radiographic findings.
‡ Round radiolucent area was seen significantly more often in depressed tumors than in flat elevated tumors (χ^2 test, $P < .05$).
§ Converging folds were seen significantly more often in flat elevated Ca-sm tumors than in flat elevated Ca-m tumors ($P < .05$).
‖ Semilunar deformity was seen significantly more often in flat elevated Ca-sm tumors than in flat elevated Ca-m tumors ($P < .0001$).

Table 3
Radiographic and Histologic Findings in Depressed Cancers

Radiographic Findings	No. of Lesions*	Histologic Classification of Depth of Invasion† Ca-m	Ca-sm	Statistical Calculations for Ca-sm: Sensitivity (%)	Specificity (%)	Positive Predictive Value (%)
Shape‡ (round:irregular)	39 (100)	9:4	17:9	65	31	65
Converging folds§ (present:absent)	39 (100)	2:11	13:13	50	85	87
Central depression‖ (deep: shallow)	32 (82)	0:9	7:16	30	100	100
Irregularity in depression# (irregular:smooth)	32 (82)	0:9	12:11	52	100	100
Semilunar deformity# on profile view (present: absent)	32 (82)	1:11	14:6	70	92	93

* Numbers in parentheses are percentages.
† Numbers are numbers of lesions with or without the radiographic finding.
‡ Round radiolucent area was seen significantly more often in depressed tumors than in flat elevated tumors (χ^2 test, $P < .05$).
§ Converging folds were seen significantly more often in depressed Ca-sm tumors than in depressed Ca-m tumors ($P < .05$).
‖ $P < .1$ for comparison of central depression in depressed Ca-sm tumors with that in depressed Ca-m tumors.
\# Irregularity in depression and semilunar deformity were each seen significantly more often in depressed Ca-sm tumors than in depressed Ca-m tumors ($P < .01$).

Table 4
Radiographic Diagnosis versus Histologic Diagnosis of Depth of Invasion

Radiographic Diagnosis	Histologic Diagnosis* Ca-m	Ca-sm	Accuracy (%)	Overall Accuracy (%)
Flat elevated type ($n = 58$)				
Ca-m	36	5	88	83
Ca-sm	5	12	71	
Depressed type ($n = 39$)				
Ca-m	12	4	75	87
Ca-sm	1	22	96	
All nonpolypoid cancers ($n = 97$)				
Ca-m	48	9	84	85
Ca-sm	6	34	85	

* Numbers are numbers of lesions.

On double-contrast barium enema studies, deep depression and irregular surface of the depression were observed only in Ca-sm tumors; thus, these two radiographic findings were characteristic of Ca-sm tumors. A thick barium collection that corresponded to the deep central depression of the cancer and an irregular surface of the depression's center reflected histologically the erosions associated with cancer invasion into the submucosa and the irregular growth of the tumor in the submucosa. Consequently, on en face views, converging folds, a deep depression, and an irregular surface of the depression are strongly suggestive of a depressed Ca-sm tumor.

By contrast, the tumor shape on double-contrast barium enema radiographs was not an indicator that enabled differentiation of Ca-m from Ca-sm tumors—although round radiolucent areas were seen in depressed cancers more frequently than in flat elevated cancers ($P < .05$). Moreover, tumor size was not useful for predicting depth of invasion in flat elevated cancers; however, in depressed cancers, Ca-sm tumors were significantly larger than Ca-m tumors. The reason for this difference between flat elevated and depressed cancers may be partly due to the fact that these flat elevated tumors include the so-called "carpetlike lesion" (41) or "flat elevation with conglomerated nodular surfacc" (42); in our study, almost all of these lesions were limited within the mucosal layer despite their large size. In depressed cancers, however, Ca-sm tumors (mean maximum diameter, 15.9 mm) were significantly larger than Ca-m tumors (mean maximum diameter, 9.6 mm). Furthermore, the depressed cancers larger than 20 mm were all Ca-sm tumors in our series. Kudo (11) reported that the frequency of intramucosal invasion of depressed colorectal cancers that were smaller than 10 mm was 82% (94 of 114 lesions); however, among those lesions larger than 15 mm, 73% (11 of 15 lesions) invaded the submucosa. Thus, in depressed cancers, tumor size is predictive of invasion depth.

With use of these findings on double-contrast barium enema radiographs as criteria for diagnosing Ca-sm tumors, overall accuracy for diagnosing depth of invasion was 85% (82 of 97 lesions). In flat elevated cancer, 48 (83%) of 58 lesions were correctly diagnosed; in depressed cancer, 34 (87%) of 39 lesions were correctly diagnosed.

Our study proved that double-contrast barium enema study is useful for diagnosing depth of invasion of early nonpolypoid cancers. However, should barium enema study be used routinely to diagnose depth of invasion of nonpolypoid cancers? Double-contrast barium enema study, a skill-dependent examination, may be performed differently in general clinical practice. Generally, colonoscopy is regarded as superior to barium enema examination for the depiction of nonpolypoid tumors—although some lesions are found at initial double-contrast barium enema examination (13,14). By contrast, colonoscopic criteria for diagnosis of depth of invasion of nonpolypoid cancers has not been determined. Our study clarified the useful radiographic predictors for diagnosis of depth of invasion. Semilunar deformity had a high sensitivity and specificity for Ca-sm, and diagnosis of depth of invasion with the deformity on profile views is available only with barium enema examination. Therefore, depth of invasion of early nonpolypoid cancers may be more accurately diagnosed with double-contrast barium enema study than colonoscopy. Furthermore, for surgical planning, the location of cancer along the colon is sometimes more clearly appreciated on barium enema radiographs than during colonoscopy. We agree with Stevenson (43) and other investigators (44–46) that barium enema examination and colonoscopy are complementary screening and diagnostic tests for colorectal cancer and diminutive polyps. Moreover, Laufer et al (47) emphasized the complementary nature of radiologic studies and endoscopy because polyps were missed at endoscopic "blind spots" such as in the rectum behind the valve of Houston or in any area of the colon where there is a sharp angulation. Both modalities should be used in combination rationally; each modality should be studied prospectively for aiding the diagnosis of depth of invasion.

The distinction between Ca-m and Ca-sm tumors is important clinically for the indication of endoscopic surgery. If a Ca-sm tumor is diagnosed preoperatively, surgery (not treatment such as endoscopic mucosal resection) should be performed. Morbidity and mortality rates for elective colorectal surgery have been reported to be about 20.0%–57.7% and 3%–6%, respectively (48–50); these rates are decreasing with the development of surgical techniques and improved perioperative treatment. The mortality of endoscopic resection, such as endoscopic mucosal resection and polypectomy, is 0.016% (51). The morbidity, such as bleeding and perforation, associated with endoscopic resection is 0.6%–0.8% (51,52); however, the morbidity with lesions larger than 21 mm is reported to be 62.5% (52). Therefore, we choose surgery instead of endoscopic mucosal resection for treatment of large tumors even if we suspect that these tumors are intramucosal or invading the submucosa focally.

In conclusion, this retrospective study of nonpolypoid colorectal cancers provided evidence of five findings on barium enema radiographs that are highly predictive of Ca-sm tumors: converging folds, a deep depression, an irregular surface of a central depression, tumor size on en face views, and semilunar deformity on profile views. These radiographic findings proved to be useful for determining depth of invasion and therapy in early nonpolypoid colorectal cancer. ■

Acknowledgment: The authors thank the late Hikoo Shirakabe, MD, PhD, for his helpful support and encouragement.

References

1. Morson BC. The polyp cancer sequence in the large bowel. Proc R Soc Med 1974; 67: 451–457.
2. Muto T, Bussey HJR, Morson BC. The evolution of cancer of the colon and rectum. Cancer 1975; 36:2251–2270.
3. Muto T, Kamiya J, Sawada T, et al. Small "flat adenoma" of the large bowel with special reference to its clinicopathologic features. Dis Colon Rectum 1985; 28:847–851.
4. Wolber RA, Owen DA. Flat adenoma of the colon. Hum Pathol 1991; 22:70–74.
5. Kudo S, Hayashi S, Miura K, et al. The clinicopathological features of flat and depressed type of early colorectal cancer. Stomach Intestine 1989; 24:317–329.
6. Stolte M, Bethke B. Colorectal mini-de novo carcinoma: a reality in Germany too. Endoscopy 1995; 27:286–290.
7. Kuramoto S, Ihara O, Sakai S, Shimazu R, Kaminishi M, Oohara T. Depressed adenoma in the large intestine: endoscopic features. Dis Colon Rectum 1990; 33:108–112.
8. Hunt DR, Cherian M. Endoscopic diagnosis of small flat carcinoma of the colon: report of three cases. Dis Colon Rectum 1990; 33:143–147.
9. Iishi H, Tatsuta M, Tsutsui S, et al. Early depressed adenocarcinomas of the large intestine. Cancer 1992; 69:2406–2410.
10. Matsumoto T, Iida M, Kuwano Y, Tada S, Yao T, Fujishima M. Minute non-polypoid adenoma of the colon detected by colonoscopy: correlation between endoscopic and histologic findings. Gastrointest Endosc 1992; 38:645–650.
11. Kudo S. Endoscopic mucosal resection of flat and depressed types of early colorectal cancer. Endoscopy 1993; 25:455–461.
12. Jaramillo E, Watanabe M, Slezak P, Rubio C. Flat neoplastic lesions of the colon and rectum detected by high-resolution video endoscopy and chromoscopy. Gastrointest Endosc 1995; 42:114–122.
13. Watari J, Shirakabe H, Ikenobe H, et al. Diagnostic basis and analysis of x-ray examination on early superficial colorectal neoplasms. Stomach Intestine 1992; 27:889–901.
14. Matsumoto T, Iida T, Kohrogi N, et al. Minute nonpolypoid adenomas of the co-

lon depicted with barium enema examination. Radiology 1993; 187:377–380.
15. Muto T, Masaki T, Suzuki K. DNA ploidy pattern of flat adenomas of the large bowel. Dis Colon Rectum 1990; 33:814.
16. Adachi M, Muto T, Okinaga K, Morioka Y. Clinicopathologic features of the flat adenoma. Dis Colon Rectum 1991; 34:981–986.
17. Minamoto T, Sawaguchi K, Ohta T, Itoh T, Mai M. Superficial-type adenomas and adenocarcinomas of the colon and rectum: a comparative morphological study. Gastroenterology 1994; 106:1436–1443.
18. Mochizuki H, Hase K, Yagyu T. The significance of histopathologic findings in the submucosal invasive front of early colorectal carcinoma in terms of regional lymph node metastasis and tumor recurrence. Stomach Intestine 1994; 29:1143–1150.
19. Muto T. Analysis of the data of invasive carcinoma removed by colonoscopic polypectomy. Stomach Intestine 1983; 18:851–855.
20. Kobayashi M, Watanabe H, Maeo S, et al. Correlation of histological atypia and cancer sprouting with vascular permeation and lymph nodal metastasis by our new histological classification of submucosal invasion by colorectal carcinomas. Stomach Intestine 1994; 29:1151–1160.
21. Hirakawa M, Fuchigami T, Iwashita A, Daimaru Y, Matsuzaka T. Diagnosis of the depth of invasion in early colorectal cancer: differential diagnosis between m, sm1 and sm2,3 from the roentgenographic point of view. Stomach Intestine 1994; 29:1249–1259.
22. Haggitt RC, Glotzbach RE, Soffer EE, et al. Prognostic factors in colorectal carcinomas arising in adenomas: implications for lesions removed by endoscopic polypectomy. Gastroenterology 1985; 89:328–336.
23. Karita M, Tada M, Okita K, Kodama T. Endoscopic therapy for early colon cancer: the strip biopsy resection technique. Gastrointest Endosc 1991; 37:128–132.
24. Brady AP, Stevenson GW, Stevenson I. Colorectal cancer overlooked at barium enema examination and colonoscopy: a continuing perceptual problem. Radiology 1994; 192:373–378.
25. Gelfand DW, Ott DJ. Limitations of combined flexible sigmoidoscopy and double-contrast barium enema in patients with rectal bleeding. Eur J Radiol 1990; 11:230–231.
26. Glick SN, Teplick SK, Balfe DM, et al. Large colonic neoplasms missed by endoscopy. AJR 1989; 152:513–517.
27. Shimizu S, Tada M, Ohtomo H, et al. Evaluation of the depth of colorectal cancers using endoscopic ultrasonography in comparison with barium enema and colonoscopic examinations. Stomach Intestine 1993; 28:1183–1189.
28. Yokota T, Matsui T, Fukuda H, et al. Evaluation of the depth of early colorectal cancers by endoscopy. Stomach Intestine 1994; 29:1261–1269.
29. Matsui T, Yao T, Yao K, et al. Natural history of superficial depressed colorectal cancer: retrospective radiographic and histologic analysis. Radiology 1996; 201:226–232.
30. Japanese Research Society for Cancer of the Colon and Rectum. General rules for clinical and pathological studies on cancer of the colon, rectum and anus. II. Histopathological classification. Jpn J Surg 1983; 13:574–598.
31. Jass JR, Sobin LH. WHO histological typing of the intestinal tumors. Berlin, Germany: Springer-Verlag, 1989.
32. Ushio K, Gotoh H, Matsumura Y, et al. Significance of the profile view in the x-ray diagnosis of cancer of the digestive tract: diagnosis of depth invasion by double contrast study. Stomach Intestine 1986; 21:27–41.
33. Saitoh Y, Obara T, Einami K, et al. Efficacy of high-frequency ultrasound probe for the preoperative staging of invasion depth in flat and depressed colorectal tumors. Gastrointest Endosc 1996; 44:34–39.
34. Schrock TR. Colonoscopy versus barium enema in the diagnosis of colorectal cancers and polyps. Gastrointest Endosc Clin North Am 1993; 3:585–610.
35. Karasick S, Ehrlich SM, Levin DC, et al. Trends in use of barium enema examination, colonoscopy, and sigmoidoscopy: is use commensurate with risk of disease? Radiology 1995; 195:777–784.
36. Ferrucci JT. Colonoscopy and barium enema: radiologist's response. Gastroenterology 1997; 112:294–297.
37. McCarthy PA, Rubesin SE, Levine MS, et al. Colon cancer: morphology detected with barium enema examination versus histopathologic stage. Radiology 1995; 197:683–687.
38. Ozeki Y, Saiga T, Matsubara N, Koyama A, Honma M, Koyama N. Depressed type mucosal cancer of large intestine with converging mucosal folds. Dig Endosc 1992; 4:153–158.
39. Skucas J, Spataro R. The radiographic features of small colonic cancers. Radiology 1982; 143:335–340.
40. Ott DJ, Scharling ES, Chen YM, Wu WC, Gelfand DW. Barium enema examination: sensitivity in detecting colonic polyps and carcinomas. South Med J 1989; 82:197–200.
41. Rubesin SE, Saul SH, Laufer I, et al. Carpet lesions of the colon. RadioGraphics 1985; 5:537–552.
42. Iwashita A, Yamada Y, Yao T, et al. Clinicopathological study on colorectal flat elevation with conglomerated nodular surface. Stomach Intestine 1992; 27:409–419.
43. Stevenson GW. Medical imaging in the prevention, diagnosis, and management of colon cancer. In: Herlinger H, Megibow AJ, eds. Advances in gastrointestinal radiology. Vol 1. St Louis, Mo: Mosby–Year Book, 1991; 1–20.
44. Wolff WI, Shinya H, Geffen A, Ozoktay S, DeBeer R. Comparison of colonoscopy and the contrast enema in five hundred patients with colorectal disease. Am J Surg 1975; 129:181–186.
45. Thoeni RF, Menuck L. Comparison of barium enema and colonoscopy in the detection of small colonic polyps. Radiology 1977; 124:631–635.
46. Miller RE, Lehman G. Polypoid colonic lesions undetected by endoscopy. Radiology 1978; 129:295–297.
47. Laufer I, Smith NCW, Mullens JE. The radiological demonstration of colorectal polyps undetected by endoscopy. Gastroenterology 1976; 70:167–170.
48. Irvin GL, Horsley JS, Caruana JA Jr. The morbidity and mortality of emergent operations for colorectal disease. Ann Surg 1984; 199:598–603.
49. Scott-Conner CE, Scher KS. Implications of emergency operations on the colon. Am J Surg 1987; 153:535–540.
50. Nwiloh J, Dardik H, Dardik M, Aneke L, Ibrahim IM. Changing patterns in the morbidity and mortality of colorectal surgery. Am J Surg 1991; 162:83–85.
51. Namiki M. Complications of digestive endoscopy included of endoscopic surgery: the present status and prevention. Gastroenterol Endosc 1984; 26:2439–2455.
52. Okamoto T, Tanaka S, Haruma K, et al. Complications of colonoscopic resection and its prevention. J Hiroshima Med Assoc 1996; 49:585–591.

Masayuki Kanematsu, MD[2] • James H. Oliver III, MD • Brian Carr, MD, PhD • Richard L. Baron, MD

Hepatocellular Carcinoma: The Role of Helical Biphasic Contrast-enhanced CT versus CT during Arterial Portography[1]

PURPOSE: **To assess the role of helical biphasic computed tomography (CT) versus CT during arterial portography (CTAP) in the detection of hepatocellular carcinoma (HCC).**

MATERIALS AND METHODS: **Helical biphasic CT and CTAP examinations were performed in 33 patients with biopsy-proved HCC. Three blinded radiologists retrospectively evaluated portal venous phase images, portal venous phase plus hepatic arterial phase images (helical biphasic CT), and CTAP plus portal venous phase images at separate sittings. In 23 patients with pathologic proof of total tumor burden, the readers conducted a consensus matched-pair reading to determine the sensitivity of each method.**

RESULTS: **In the 23 patients with a proved tumor burden of 100 HCC lesions, the observers detected 74 tumors on portal venous phase images, 82 tumors on hepatic arterial phase images, 87 tumors on CTAP images, 87 tumors on helical biphasic CT images, and 96 tumors on portal venous phase plus CTAP images. Hepatic arterial phase images and CTAP images, respectively, depicted 13 and 23 tumors not seen on portal venous phase images in eight (35%) and 13 (56%) of 23 patients. Ten tumors were seen on portal venous phase images but not on CTAP images owing to the presence of central tumors or segmental portal venous thrombi that obstructed the flow of contrast material to more peripheral portions of the liver.**

CONCLUSION: **The addition of hepatic arterial phase imaging to portal venous phase imaging (helical biphasic CT) provided an incrementally increased yield in HCC tumor detection. Helical biphasic CT should be used as the initial screening examination in patients with suspected or known HCC.**

More than a decade has passed since computed tomography (CT) during arterial portography (CTAP) was first introduced (1). To our knowledge, findings in all subsequent reports have corroborated the high sensitivity of CTAP in the detection of liver tumors (1–6). Its sensitivity has exceeded that of conventional contrast material–enhanced CT. Recently, advances in helical CT technology have allowed imaging of the entire liver during both the hepatic arterial phase and the portal venous phase of contrast enhancement (dual-phase or biphasic contrast-enhanced CT) during intravenous infusion of a single bolus of contrast material (7). Findings in several studies have shown a significant increase in the detection of hypervascular liver neoplasms with this biphasic contrast-enhanced technique (8 12). Hepatocellular carcinoma (HCC) is the neoplasm that has been most thoroughly evaluated in most of the previously published studies. It remains to be determined whether the increased sensitivity of helical biphasic CT for hypervascular neoplasms is sufficient to obviate the very sensitive but invasive CTAP examination in patients in whom documentation of the total liver tumor burden will affect therapeutic decisions. We undertook this study to compare the sensitivity of helical biphasic CT with that of CTAP in the detection of HCC tumor foci to determine the relative roles of these techniques in the evaluation of disease in such patients.

MATERIALS AND METHODS

During an 18-month period from June 1993 through November 1994, 33 patients with HCC (24 men and nine women aged 42–83 years [mean, 58 years]) were referred to undergo both helical biphasic CT and CTAP at our institution. Eight patients had type C viral hepatitis, six had type B viral hepatitis, 14 had cryptogenic cirrhosis, and 11 had no concomitant liver disease. The time between helical biphasic CT and CTAP examinations in these patients ranged from 1 to 70 days (mean, 16.4 days).

All CT examinations were performed with commercially available scanners (HiSpeed Advantage; GE Medical Systems, Milwaukee, Wis). Helical biphasic CT was performed with 7 mm/sec table speed, 1:1 pitch, 120 kVp, and 220–280 mAs. One or two breath-hold spiral acquisitions were obtained during each pass through the liver, depending on the size of the liver and the ability of each patient to suspend respirations. If two acquisitions were necessary to image the entire liver during either the hepatic arterial phase or the portal-venous phase of enhancement, an 8-second breathing interval was used between acquisitions. A 150-mL dose of 60% contrast material was administered at a rate of 2.5–5.0 mL/sec by using an automated power injector (Medrad, Pittsburgh, Pa). Slower injection rates (2.5–3.0 mL/sec) were used in patients who received ionic contrast material, and faster rates (4–5 mL/sec) were used in those who received nonionic contrast material. Hepatic arte-

Index terms: Computed tomography (CT), comparative studies • Computed tomography (CT), technology • Liver, CT, 761.12113, 761.12114 • Liver neoplasms, diagnosis, 761.323

Abbreviations: CTAP = CT during arterial portography, HCC = hepatocellular carcinoma.

Radiology 1997; 205:75–80

[1] From the Departments of Radiology (M.K., J.H.O., R.L.B.) and Surgery (B.C.), University of Pittsburgh Medical Center, 200 Lothrop St, Pittsburgh, PA 15213-2582. From the 1995 RSNA scientific assembly. Received January 22, 1997; revision requested March 11; revision received June 23; accepted June 25. **Address reprint requests to** J.H.O.

[2] Current address: Department of Radiology, School of Medicine, Gifu University, Gifu City, Japan.

rial phase images were obtained in a craniocaudal direction beginning 20–28 seconds after initiation of injection of contrast material (20 seconds for a 5 mL/sec infusion and 28 seconds for a 2.5 mL/sec infusion). Portal venous phase images were obtained in a craniocaudal direction beginning 60–70 seconds after initiation of injection of contrast material (60 seconds for a 5 mL/sec infusion and 70 seconds for a 2.5–3.0 mL/sec infusion) with the same parameters that were used to obtain hepatic arterial phase images. Contiguous 7-mm-thick axial sections were reconstructed from the volumetric data. Overlapping reconstructions were occasionally used but only when clarification was needed of subtle findings seen on the original images.

CTAP images were obtained with helical acquisition techniques in a caudocranial direction with 7 mm/sec table speed, 1:1 pitch, 120 kVp, and 220–280 mAs. One or two breath-hold spiral acquisitions were obtained, depending on the size of the liver. Data acquisition was started 25 seconds after initiation of a transcatheter (5-F catheter) splenic or superior mesenteric arterial injection of 90–150 mL of 60% nonionic contrast material administered at 2.5–3.0 mL/sec with an automated power injector. Contiguous 7-mm-thick axial sections were reconstructed from the volumetric data, with overlapping reconstructions performed only to clarify subtle or confusing imaging findings.

CT scans obtained in all 33 patients were retrospectively reviewed in a blinded fashion at separate sittings by three radiologists experienced in abdominal imaging. Each reader first scored the portal venous phase images for the number of lesions believed to be HCC foci and the range of their size, as well as tumor enhancement characteristics (hypoattenuation, hyperattenuation, or mixed attenuation relative to liver). Each reader then reviewed hepatic arterial phase plus portal venous phase images or CTAP plus portal venous phase images at separate sittings to determine how many additional lesions not seen on portal venous phase images were seen on hepatic arterial phase or CTAP images. During these later readings, the reviewers were always given their original score sheets for the portal venous phase images. The number of lesions detected on the portal venous phase plus hepatic arterial phase (helical biphasic CT) images and on the portal venous phase plus CTAP images were recorded separately. The three readers also subjectively evaluated the conspicuity of lesions on helical biphasic CT images versus portal venous phase plus CTAP images in each case.

When 10 or more lesions of similar appearance were seen in one patient, the patient was considered to have a maximum of 10 lesions. Ten or more lesions were counted as 10 lesions unless more lesions were seen during matched-pair analysis of one set of images. In that event, that particular set of images was scored as showing 11 lesions to document the superiority of that imaging sequence in the quantitative data analysis. This type of scoring was used to prevent the results from being biased by data obtained in a few patients with many lesions. In clinical practice, there should be no difference in the treatment of patients with more than 10 lesions. In our study population, seven patients had 10 or more HCC lesions.

All patients had biopsy-proved HCC within the liver. In our study population, lesions were diagnosed as HCC if they had an appearance similar to lesions sampled at biopsy and if they did not meet the CT criteria for liver cyst, cavernous hemangioma (13,14), or focal fibrosis (15). In addition, known perfusion defects seen during CTAP (including peripheral wedge-shaped lesions and flat lesions in the posterior aspect of segment IV that are caused by benign processes [16–18]) were not considered HCC foci.

Six of the 33 patients subsequently underwent definitive surgery (transplantation in two patients, partial hepatectomy in three patients, and exploration with surgical wedge biopsy in one patient). Surgery was performed between 1 and 141 days (mean, 31.4 days) after the last imaging examination was performed that provided proof of the exact number of lesions within the liver. In a seventh patient with only a single lesion shown on any of the images, a needle core biopsy provided documentation for comparative results of imaging tests. Follow-up imaging in 16 patients showed an interval increase or decrease in the diameter of lesions after chemotherapy or the development of lesions seen on all images; in light of biopsy proof of HCC elsewhere within the liver, this change in diameter was considered proof that these lesions represented HCC. These 23 patients were considered to have proof of all lesions initially seen (100 lesions), and they formed a subset of our total study population.

For the 23-patient subset, the three readers conducted consensus matched-pair readings after they completed the individualized, blinded readings to determine the number of proved lesions detected on hepatic arterial phase images, portal venous phase images, CTAP images, helical biphasic CT images, and portal venous phase plus CTAP images.

A nonparametric one-way analysis of variance was performed to determine whether any statistically significant ($P < .05$) interobserver variation existed for each set of images. P values of .9348, .8438, and .8947 were obtained for the portal venous phase images, helical biphasic CT images, and portal venous phase plus CTAP images, respectively; these findings indicated that there was no statistically significant variation among reviewers for each set of images. Once this lack of variation was determined, the three readers' scores for each image set were averaged to create a single set of data for analysis and presentation. To test whether there was any statistically significant difference in lesion detection between portal venous phase images, helical biphasic CT images, and portal venous phase plus CTAP images, a nonparametric one-way analysis of variance was used; a significant difference ($P = .0321$) was found for the combined data sets. The Duncan multiple range test was used to identify when these significant differences ($P < .05$) in lesion detection occurred.

Table 1
Total Number of Lesions Detected in All 33 Patients

Finding	Reader 1	Reader 2	Reader 3
Lesions at PVP imaging	108	115	118
Additional lesions at HAP imaging	44	31	50
Additional lesions at CTAP	56	59	70
Lesions at HBCT (PVP + HAP)	152	146	168
Lesions at PVP + CTAP	164	174	188

Note.—HAP = hepatic arterial phase, HBCT = helical biphasic CT, PVP = portal venous phase.

RESULTS

The detection rates with each imaging technique are shown in Table 1. For portal venous phase images, the number of lesions detected by each of the three readers ranged from 108 to 118 lesions, and the lesion diameters ranged from 2 to 190 mm. The lesions on portal venous phase images were judged to be hypoattenuating compared with liver in 19–21 patients, hyperattenuating compared with liver in two to three patients, and mixed in 10–11 patients. The number of additional lesions detected on hepatic arterial phase images that were not seen on portal venous phase images by each of the three readers ranged from 31 to 50 lesions in nine to 12 patients. The lesions on hepatic arterial phase images were judged to be hypoattenuating compared with liver in six to eight patients, hyperattenuating in 11–18 patients, and mixed in seven to 14 patients. The total number of lesions detected on portal venous phase plus hepatic arterial phase (helical biphasic CT) images was 146–168 lesions. The three readers rated the conspicuity of lesions on hepatic arterial phase images as better than that on portal venous phase images in 13–17 patients, equal in two to seven patients, and worse in nine to 15 patients.

For the three readers, the number of additional lesions detected on CTAP images that were not seen on portal venous phase images ranged from 56 to 70 lesions in 19–22 patients (Table

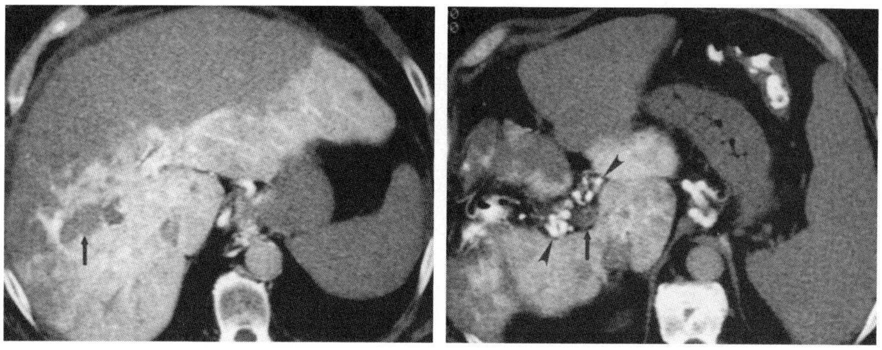

a. b.

Figure 1. **(a, b)** CTAP images obtained in a 62-year-old man with cirrhosis and HCC show large portions of the liver that are not enhanced because of the unsuspected presence of thrombus in the portal vein (arrow in **a** and **b**). Note the enhancing collateral vessels in the porta hepatis (arrowheads in **b**). The unenhanced regions of the liver cannot be accurately evaluated for the presence of HCC.

Table 2
Detection of HCC in the 23 Patients with Proof of Total Tumor Burden

Imaging Method	No. of Tumors Detected (N = 100)
PVP	74 (74)
HAP	82 (82)
HBCT	87 (87)
CTAP	87 (87)
PVP + CTAP	96 (96)

Note.—Percentages are given in parentheses. HAP = hepatic arterial phase, HBCT = helical biphasic CT, PVP = portal venous phase.

1). Lesions on CTAP images were judged to be hypoattenuating in all cases. The number of lesions detected on portal venous phase plus CTAP images for the three readers ranged from 164 to 188 lesions. Insufficient hepatic parenchymal enhancement during CTAP was seen in five patients (three with portal venous thrombosis and two with severe cirrhosis) and precluded the detection of some HCC foci by all three readers (Fig 1).

A significant increase (P = .0145) in lesion detection was seen with helical biphasic CT images compared with portal venous phase images alone. Likewise, portal venous phase plus CTAP images helped detection of significantly more (P = .0096) lesions than portal venous phase images alone. When findings on helical biphasic CT images were compared with those on portal venous phase plus CTAP images, however, there was no statistically significant difference in lesion detection.

In the 23 patients with a proved tumor burden of 100 lesions, the consensus reading by the three readers resulted in detection of 74 lesions on portal venous phase images, 82 lesions on hepatic arterial phase images, 87 lesions on CTAP images, 87 lesions on helical biphasic CT images, and 96 lesions on portal venous phase plus CTAP images (Table 2). Compared with portal venous phase images, an additional 13 lesions were seen with hepatic arterial phase imaging in eight (35%) of 23 patients, and an additional 23 lesions were seen with CTAP in 13 (56%) of 23 patients. Hepatic arterial phase images allowed detection of 13 additional lesions not seen on portal venous phase images, but five lesions were seen on the portal venous phase images that were not seen on the hepatic arterial phase images. Similarly, 10 lesions were seen on portal venous phase images that could not be identified on CTAP images. The reason that CTAP did not depict these 10 lesions is that the lesions were all in a location peripheral to a more centrally located tumor that obstructed portal venous flow, and therefore they were hidden by the perfusion defect caused by the more central tumor (Fig 2) or they were downstream from thrombus in a branch of the portal vein.

The consensus of the three readers was that the conspicuity of the tumor on the portal venous phase plus CTAP images was superior to that on the helical biphasic CT images in 17 patients, equal in one patient, and worse in five patients. Attenuation of liver parenchyma was insufficient to allow detection of tumor in one of 23 patients owing to thrombosis in the main portal vein.

Table 3 shows the number of patients in whom each reader detected lesions on hepatic arterial phase images, CTAP images, or both but not on portal venous phase images. Although some variance existed among readers, approximately half of the additional lesions detected (beyond those seen on portal venous phase images) were seen on hepatic arterial phase images, and nearly all lesions were detected with CTAP. Table 4 delineates the number of patients in whom hepatic arterial phase or CTAP images failed to depict lesions seen on portal venous phase images.

DISCUSSION

The sensitivity of angiographically assisted CT techniques in the detection of liver tumors is reported to be 80%–95% when contrast material is selectively delivered directly to either the liver parenchyma or the tumors (1–6). Such detection rates exceed those for any other imaging method except intraoperative ultrasound (US). Some authors have proposed that CTAP be part of the preoperative imaging required before resection of liver tumors (19,20). CTAP is an invasive procedure, however, and is complicated by false-positive results and technical failures (6,16,21,22). Flow-related artifacts and difficulties in enhancement of the liver parenchyma caused by hepatofugal portal venous flow in patients with cirrhosis (a patient group at high risk for HCC) may cause the quality of CTAP images to deteriorate (23). Also, small, well-differentiated HCC may not be depicted at CTAP presumably because of the presence of portal venous perfusion (24,25). Because these pitfalls can preclude accurate diagnosis of liver tumors, CTAP cannot be used alone for detection and characterization of hepatic lesions, and physicians have been obliged to use conventional CT, US, magnetic resonance imaging, biopsy, and serial imaging examinations to confirm the diagnosis of HCC.

The development of slip-ring technology and high-speed helical CT techniques has allowed the use of multiphasic contrast-enhanced CT, which can help evaluation of the liver at different phases of contrast enhancement during a single examination. Ohashi et al (10) and Honda et al (26) reported the usefulness of biphasic CT examination of the liver with use of an incremental CT technique. Owing to the limitations of their nonhelical CT equipment, however, their scanning-time parameters did not allow acquisition of purely hepatic arterial phase or portal venous phase helical images. Rather, mixed hepatic arterial phase and portal venous phase images were followed by early equilibrium-phase images. Recent reports (8,9,11,12) have shown that combined hepatic arterial phase plus portal venous phase images increase the rate of detection of hypervascular liver tumors. We have optimized our CT protocol so hepatic arterial phase and portal venous phase scanning should occur from 20 to 50 seconds and from 60 to 95 seconds, respectively, after the initiation of contrast material infusion.

In our study population, hepatic arterial phase and CTAP images depicted 31–50 and 56–70 additional lesions, respectively, not seen on portal venous phase images. The number of additional lesions depicted with CTAP was substantially greater than that depicted with hepatic arterial phase imaging, but the number of lesions detected with helical biphasic CT was not statistically significantly different from that detected with portal venous phase imaging plus CTAP. This finding may, in part, be due to the small sample size, as there were several patients in whom findings with CTAP were considerably better than findings with helical biphasic CT (Fig 3). Also, inclusion of findings in the five patients with poor or no liver enhancement at CTAP decreased the overall tumor detection rate for CTAP. Results in our subset of 23 patients with pathologic proof of tumor were virtually the same as those for the entire study population and thus confirmed the validity of the sample as a whole. In the subset of patients with proved lesions, consensus reading determined that hepatic arterial phase images showed 13 more lesions than portal venous phase images in eight (35%) of 23 patients. Findings with CTAP were even better, however, allowing detection of 23 additional lesions in 13 (56%) of 23 patients. Despite the development of helical biphasic contrast-enhanced CT techniques, CTAP still seems to be the most sensitive nonsurgical imaging technique for the detection of liver tumor foci.

The superiority of CTAP may partly be due to its ability to depict tumors regardless of their inherent vascularity, whereas hepatic arterial phase imaging is useful for detection of hypervascular tumors. Nonetheless, in our study, findings with CTAP were found to be superior to those with hepatic arterial phase imaging, even though patients had the predominately hypervascular lesions typical of HCC. Two-thirds of the patients in our series had cirrhosis, which should maximize the impact of hepatic arterial phase imaging (owing to the known hypertrophy of the hepatic arterial system in patients with cirrhosis and portal hypertension) and should decrease the ability of CTAP to help evaluation of the liver (23).

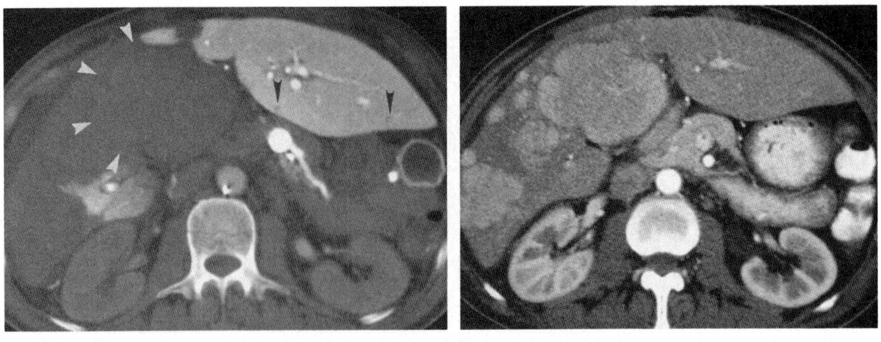

a. b.

Figure 2. **(a)** CTAP image shows no enhancement within the right hepatic lobe owing to a large central HCC lesion (white arrowheads) that has obstructed the portal venous flow of contrast material to the more peripheral portions of the right lobe. This perfusion defect hides many more foci of HCC that are well depicted on **(b)** the hepatic arterial phase image. Two tiny foci of HCC (black arrowheads in **a**) are seen in the left lateral segment in **a** but not in **b**.

Table 3
Detection of Additional Lesions with Hepatic Arterial Phase Imaging Only, CTAP Only, or Both

	Findings for Entire Population (n = 33)			Consensus Reading for Patients with Proved Lesions (n = 23)
Imaging Method	Reader 1	Reader 2	Reader 3	
HAP	5	1	2	1
CTAP	12	13	13	6
HAP and CTAP	7	9	7	7

Note.—Numbers are number of patients. HAP = hepatic arterial phase.

The results given in Table 3 illustrate the importance of CTAP in the evaluation of HCC. In more than one-third of patients, CTAP depicted additional lesions not seen at portal venous phase or hepatic arterial phase imaging. Nonetheless, hepatic arterial phase images helped detection of additional lesions beyond those shown on portal venous phase images in approximately one-third of the patients. Therefore, helical biphasic CT should be used as the initial CT examination in patients with known or suspected HCC. Even though CTAP images may depict additional lesions not shown on helical biphasic CT images, findings at helical biphasic CT may preclude surgical intervention and obviate CTAP in a large number of patients.

As Table 4 shows, hepatic-arterial-phase and CTAP images failed to depict all lesions shown on portal venous phase images in some patients. These observations indicate that either hepatic arterial phase or CTAP images alone are not sufficient to allow detection of all tumor foci and that these images should be combined with portal venous phase images. It is reasonable to assume that hepatic arterial phase images fail to delineate iso- or hypovascular HCC as well as small hypervascular tumor foci. CTAP is limited in its ability to depict tumor foci that lie within regions of the liver that do not receive portal venous flow. Such situations obviously occur in patients with portal venous thrombosis or severe portal hypertension and hepatofugal flow (Fig 1). In addition, large central lesions obscured the detection of more distal peripheral lesions owing to proximal obstruction of portal venous blood flow. These peripheral lesions are not usually clinically important, however, because the presence of the more central tumor already forces the surgeon to resect the liver parenchyma "downstream" from the obstructed portal vein.

Although sensitivity is high with CTAP, specificity is low because all lesions in the liver will have the same appearance on CTAP images. A small cyst, a hemangioma, and a malignant neoplasm cannot be accurately differentiated by means of CTAP alone, and this is another reason why CTAP images should not be read in isolation. Use of portal venous phase images combined with either hepatic arterial phase or CTAP images affords optimal detection and characterization of HCC.

Table 4
Number of Patients in Whom Hepatic Arterial Phase or CTAP Images Failed to Depict All Lesions Shown on Portal Venous Phase Images

Imaging Method	Findings for Entire Population (n = 33) Reader 1	Reader 2	Reader 3	Consensus Reading for Patients with Proved Lesions (n = 23)
HAP	11	6	5	2
CTAP	8	3	2	2*

Note.—HAP = hepatic arterial phase.
* In each patient, lesions were not seen due to insufficient parenchymal hyperattenuation due to portal venous tumor thrombus.

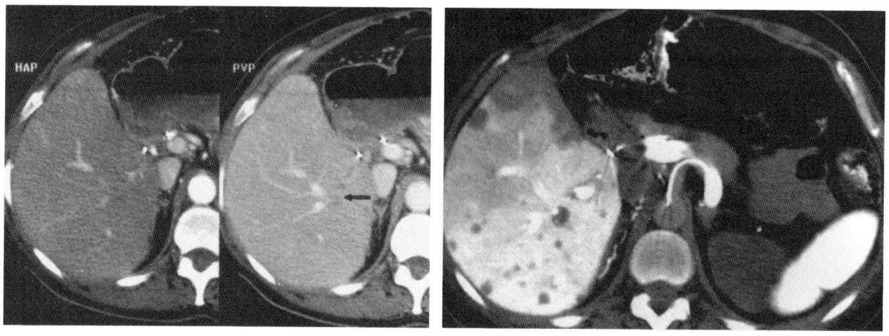

a. b.

Figure 3. **(a)** Hepatic arterial phase (*HAP*) and portal venous phase (*PVP*) images show one questionable focus of tumor (arrow). **(b)** CTAP image obtained the next day clearly depicts multiple foci of HCC, which were confirmed at biopsy.

The three readers rated the relative conspicuity of lesions on hepatic arterial phase and portal venous phase images as generally equal and on CTAP images as better than that of lesions on portal venous phase images. Further, in the consensus reading for patients with proved lesions, the readers found that the portal venous phase plus CTAP images provided greater tumor conspicuity than the helical biphasic CT images.

Our results for HCC do not have indications for the relative accuracy of these tests in the detection of metastatic disease in the liver. In our experience, detection rates with CTAP are higher for metastatic tumor than for HCC. This difference is partly due to the fact that metastatic deposits are not generally substantially perfused by portal blood flow. The quality of CTAP images is also generally better in patients with metastatic liver disease because the majority of these patients do not have cirrhosis, so portal perfusion is usually normal. Further, morphologic changes due to regenerating nodules or fibrosis, causes of false-positive findings at CTAP in cirrhotic patients, are absent. Although findings at CTAP could be expected to be better in these situations, findings at helical biphasic CT may also be less useful because the vast majority of metastatic lesions are hypovascular.

Some recent reports that focused on the vascularity of HCC smaller than 20–30 mm in diameter suggest that an interaction between hepatic arterial flow and portal venous flow determines the vascularity of HCC (24,25,27). These investigators believe that most dysplastic nodules (adenomatous hyperplasia) and some of the small, well-differentiated HCCs are initially perfused with substantial portal venous flow. In the course of the growth of these lesions, however, hepatic arterial flow becomes more dominant and eventually overcomes the portal venous flow; this change results in an obvious portal perfusion defect at CTAP. These alterations in tumor vascularity are believed to take place when the lesion diameter is approximately 12–15 mm (25). Because 24 of 33 patients evaluated in our study had multifocal HCCs 10–190 mm in diameter, we did not focus our evaluation on small HCC lesions, and this selective focus may be one of the limitations of our study. Detection rates need to be determined for helical biphasic CT and portal-venous-phase imaging plus CTAP in patients with only small HCC lesions.

Since the time of this study, we have recognized that use of slower rates of intravenous infusion (2.5–3.0 mL/sec) of contrast material results in a lower sensitivity for tumor detection than use of faster rates (5 mL/sec). It is possible that if all patients had received infusions at a rate of 5 mL/sec, the data for helical biphasic CT would have been better.

Although not statistically significant, minor interobserver variability existed in our data as exhibited by the differences in tumor detection rates among the three readers. Such differences exist for several reasons. First, there will always be differences in readers' ability to detect lesions as there is a rate of perception failure on any given reading that may not occur with subsequent rereading. Second, readers have a different threshold for detecting lesions based on diameter or degree of contrast between liver and tumor foci. Probably the most important reason for the difference in the number of lesions detected is related not to readers actually missing tumors but rather to their personal preference for categorizing clusters of tumor as either one large lesion or several abutting smaller lesions. Therefore, such variability in detection of HCC is to be expected. Evidence of the validity of our conclusions, despite the differences in observer detection rates, lies in the consistent trends for tumor detection seen throughout Tables 1 and 3, irrespective of the reader. For all readers the relative incremental rate of detection of lesions was similar with hepatic-arterial-phase imaging, CTAP, helical biphasic CT, and portal venous phase imaging plus CTAP.

In summary, our findings indicate that the addition of hepatic arterial phase imaging to portal venous phase imaging (helical biphasic CT) provides an incremental increased yield in HCC tumor detection. Biphasic helical CT should be routinely used as the initial examination in patients with HCC and patients with cirrhosis who are suspected of having HCC. Despite the increased rate of tumor detection with biphasic helical CT techniques, CTAP can help detect additional HCCs not seen with helical biphasic CT. Therefore, if a patient with HCC has undergone helical biphasic CT and is still believed to be a candidate for surgery and if that patient does not have severe cirrhosis or thrombosis of the portal vein, performance of CTAP should be considered to obtain the most accurate determination of tumor load within the liver. ■

References

1. Matsui O, Takashima T, Kadoya M, et al. Dynamic computed tomography during arterial portography: the most sensitive examination for small hepatocellular carcinomas. J Comput Assist Tomogr 1985; 9:19–24.

2. Matsui O, Takashima T, Kadoya M, et al. Liver metastases from colorectal cancers: detection with CT during arterial portography. Radiology 1987; 165:65–70.
3. Nelson RC, Chezmar JL, Sugarbaker PH, Bernardino ME. Hepatic tumors: comparison of CT during arterial portography, delayed CT, and MR imaging for preoperative evaluation. Radiology 1989; 172:27–34.
4. Heiken JP, Weyman PJ, Lee JKT, et al. Detection of focal hepatic masses: prospective evaluation with CT, delayed CT, CT during arterial portography, and MR imaging. Radiology 1989; 171:47–51.
5. Soyer P, Levesque M, Elias D, Zeitoun G, Roche A. Preoperative assessment of resectability of hepatic metastases from colonic carcinoma: CT portography vs sonography and dynamic CT. AJR 1992; 159:741–744.
6. Soyer P, Lacheheb D, Levesque M. False-positive CT portography: correlation with pathologic findings. AJR 1993; 160:285–289.
7. Baron RL. Understanding and optimizing use of contrast material for CT of the liver. AJR 1994; 163:323–331.
8. Bonaldi VM, Bret PM, Reinhold C, Atri M. Helical CT of the liver: value of an early hepatic arterial phase. Radiology 1995; 197: 357–363.
9. Hollett MD, Jeffrey RB Jr, Nino-Murcia M, Jorgensen MJ, Harris DP. Dual-phase helical CT of the liver: value of arterial phase scans in the detection of small (≤ 1.5 cm) malignant hepatic neoplasms. AJR 1995; 164:879–884.
10. Ohashi I, Hanafusa K, Yoshida T. Small hepatocellular carcinomas: two-phase dynamic incremental CT in detection and evaluation. Radiology 1993; 189:851–855.
11. Baron RL, Oliver JH, Dodd GD, Nalesnik M, Holbert BL, Carr BI. Hepatocellular carcinoma: evaluation with biphasic, contrast-enhanced, helical CT. Radiology 1996; 199:505–511.
12. Oliver JHI, Baron RL, Federle MP, Rockette HP. Detecting hepatocellular carcinoma: the relative added value of using noncontrast and/or arterial phase imaging in conjunction with conventional portal venous phase contrast CT. AJR 1996: 167:71–77.
13. Quinn SF, Benjamin GG. Hepatic cavernous hemangiomas: simple diagnostic sign with dynamic bolus CT. Radiology 1992; 182:545–548.
14. Gaa J, Saini S, Ferrucci JT. Perfusion characteristics of hepatic cavernous hemangioma using intravenous CT angiography (IVCTA). Eur J Radiol 1991; 12:228–233.
15. Ohtomo K, Baron RL, Dodd GD III, et al. Confluent hepatic fibrosis in advanced cirrhosis: appearance at CT. Radiology 1993; 188:31–35.
16. Peterson MS, Baron RL, Dodd GD III, et al. Hepatic parenchymal perfusion defects detected with CTAP: imaging-pathologic correlation. Radiology 1992; 185:149–155.
17. Matsui O, Takahashi S, Kadoya M, et al. Pseudolesion in segment IV of the liver at CT during arterial portography: correlation with aberrant gastric venous drainage. Radiology 1994; 193:31–35.
18. Fernandez MP, Bernardino ME. Hepatic pseudolesions: appearance of focal low attenuation in the medial segment of the left lobe at CT arterial portography. Radiology 1991; 181:809–811.
19. Langmo LS, Dagher AP, Mehard WB, et al. Does CTAP prior to hepatic resection improve patient survival rates? Abdom Imaging 1994; 19:317–319.
20. Small WC, Mehard WB, Langmo LS, et al. Preoperative determination of the resectability of hepatic tumors: efficacy of CT during arterial portography. AJR 1993; 161: 319–322.
21. Nelson RC, Thompson GH, Chezmar JL, Harned RKD, Fernandez MP. CT during arterial portography: diagnostic pitfalls. RadioGraphics 1992; 12:705–720.
22. Paulson EK, Baker ME, Hilleren DJ, et al. CT arterial portography: causes of technical failure and variable liver enhancement. AJR 1992; 159:745–749.
23. Oliver JH III, Baron RL, Dodd GD III, Peterson MS, Carr BI. Does advanced cirrhosis with portosystemic shunting affect the value of CT arterial portography in the evaluation of the liver? AJR 1995; 164:333–337.
24. Saitoh S, Ikeda K, Koida I, et al. Small hepatocellular carcinoma: evaluation of portal blood flow with CT during arterial portography performed with balloon occlusion of the hepatic artery. Radiology 1994; 193:67–70.
25. Matsui O, Kadoya M, Kameyama T, et al. Benign and malignant nodules in cirrhotic livers: distinction based on blood supply. Radiology 1991; 178:493–497.
26. Honda H, Matsuura Y, Onitsuka H, et al. Differential diagnosis of hepatic tumors (hepatoma, hemangioma, and metastasis) with CT: value of two-phase incremental imaging. AJR 1992; 159:735–740.
27. Winter TC, Takayasu K, Muramatsu Y, et al. Early advanced hepatocellular carcinoma: evaluation of CT and MR appearance with pathologic correlation. Radiology 1994; 192: 379–387.

Yukio Muramatsu, MD • Kenichi Takayasu, MD • Yoshihiro Furukawa, MD
Kunihisa Miyakawa, MD • Ryoko Iwata, MD • Kyosuke Ushio, MD
Junji Yamamoto, MD • Yukihiro Nakanishi, MD

Hepatic Tumor Invasion of Bile Ducts: Wedge-shaped Sign on MR Images[1]

PURPOSE: **To clarify the diagnostic importance of wedge-shaped areas of increased signal intensity that surround liver tumors on T1-weighted magnetic resonance (MR) images.**

MATERIALS AND METHODS: **In five patients with hepatic tumors, T1-weighted MR images that demonstrated wedge-shaped areas of increased signal intensity in the liver were reviewed; findings were compared with those at surgical and histologic examinations.**

RESULTS: **MR images showed localized intrahepatic bile duct dilatation lateral (three patients) and medial (two patients) to liver tumors within the wedge-shaped areas. At histopathologic examination, intraductal tumor growth was seen in local bile ducts in the same areas in five patients, and lipofuscin deposits were seen in the cytoplasm of atrophic hepatocytes in three patients.**

CONCLUSION: **On T1-weighted images, wedge-shaped areas of increased signal intensity associated with liver tumors indicate intraductal tumor extension in intrahepatic bile ducts. T1 shortening is possibly caused by lipofuscin deposits in atrophic hepatocytes.**

WEDGE-SHAPED areas of increased signal intensity that surround liver tumors on T2-weighted magnetic resonance (MR) images have been reported (1–4). These MR imaging findings do not indicate direct tumor invasion of surrounding liver tissues. To our knowledge, however, wedge-shaped areas of increased signal intensity on T1-weighted MR images—except for those related to focal fatty liver (5), hepatic infarction (6), and hemorrhage (7)—have not been investigated. The purpose of this study was to clarify the diagnostic importance of wedge-shaped areas of high signal intensity that are associated with liver tumors on T1-weighted MR images.

MATERIALS AND METHODS

Between March 1994 and August 1996, areas of increased signal intensity that were associated with liver tumors in five patients were detected on T1-weighted images. Four patients had metastatic colorectal cancer, and one patient had cholangiocarcinoma. Two patients were women and three were men; patient ages ranged from 41 to 65 years. Diagnosis of liver tumors (size, 0.8–6.5 cm) was achieved with partial hepatic resection. In all patients, findings on MR images were correlated with those at pathologic examination.

MR imaging was performed with a 1.5-T superconducting magnet (MRT200FX; Toshiba, Tokyo, Japan). T1-weighted spin-echo (SE) (500–600/15 [repetition time msec/echo time msec]) MR images were obtained with a 256 × 256 matrix with no phase wrap and two signals acquired. T2-weighted fast SE (4,000–6,000/112) MR images were obtained with a 256 × 256 matrix with no phase wrap and two signals acquired. Dynamic MR imaging was performed with the field-echo (FE) (60–80/6, 60° flip angle) technique in the axial or sagittal planes with a 256 × 256 matrix with 50% encode reduction and two signals acquired. This pulse sequence enabled us to image three to five sections in 15–20 seconds during a single breath hold. Before administration of gadopentetate dimeglumine (Magnevist; Schering, Berlin, Germany), axial or sagittal T2-weighted fast SE, T1-weighted SE, and FE MR images were obtained. Contrast material was administered intravenously to all patients by rapid manual injection (2 mL/sec) at a dose of 0.1 mmol/kg body weight. Images were obtained at the following times after injection began: 20 seconds (arterial phase), 60 seconds (portal phase), and 2–3 minutes (venous phase). Section thickness was 8–10 mm with a 0–2-mm intersection gap.

Tumors and wedge-shaped areas were examined histologically with conventional hematoxylin-eosin stain in all cases. The specimens of three patients were treated with Prussian blue stain (iron stain, Berlin blue method) and Schmorl ferric-ferricyanide reduction stain (waste pigment stain).

RESULTS

MR Imaging Findings

On the T2-weighted fast SE images, the signal intensity of wedged-shaped

Index terms: Bile ducts, MR, 765.121411, 765.121412, 765.12143 • Bile ducts, stenosis or obstruction, 765.363 • Gadolinium • Liver neoplasms, MR, 761.32, 761.33

Abbreviations: FE = field echo, SE = spin-echo.

Radiology 1997; 205:81–85

[1] From the Departments of Diagnostic Radiology (Y.M., K.T., Y.F., K.M., R.I., K.U.), Surgery (J.Y.), and Pathology (Y.N.), National Cancer Center Hospital, Tsukiji 5-1-1, Chuo-ku, Tokyo 104, Japan. Received January 27, 1997; revision requested March 11; revision received May 12; accepted May 19. Supported in part by Grant-in-Aid for Cancer Research 8-25 from the Ministry of Health and Welfare. **Address reprint requests to** Y.M.

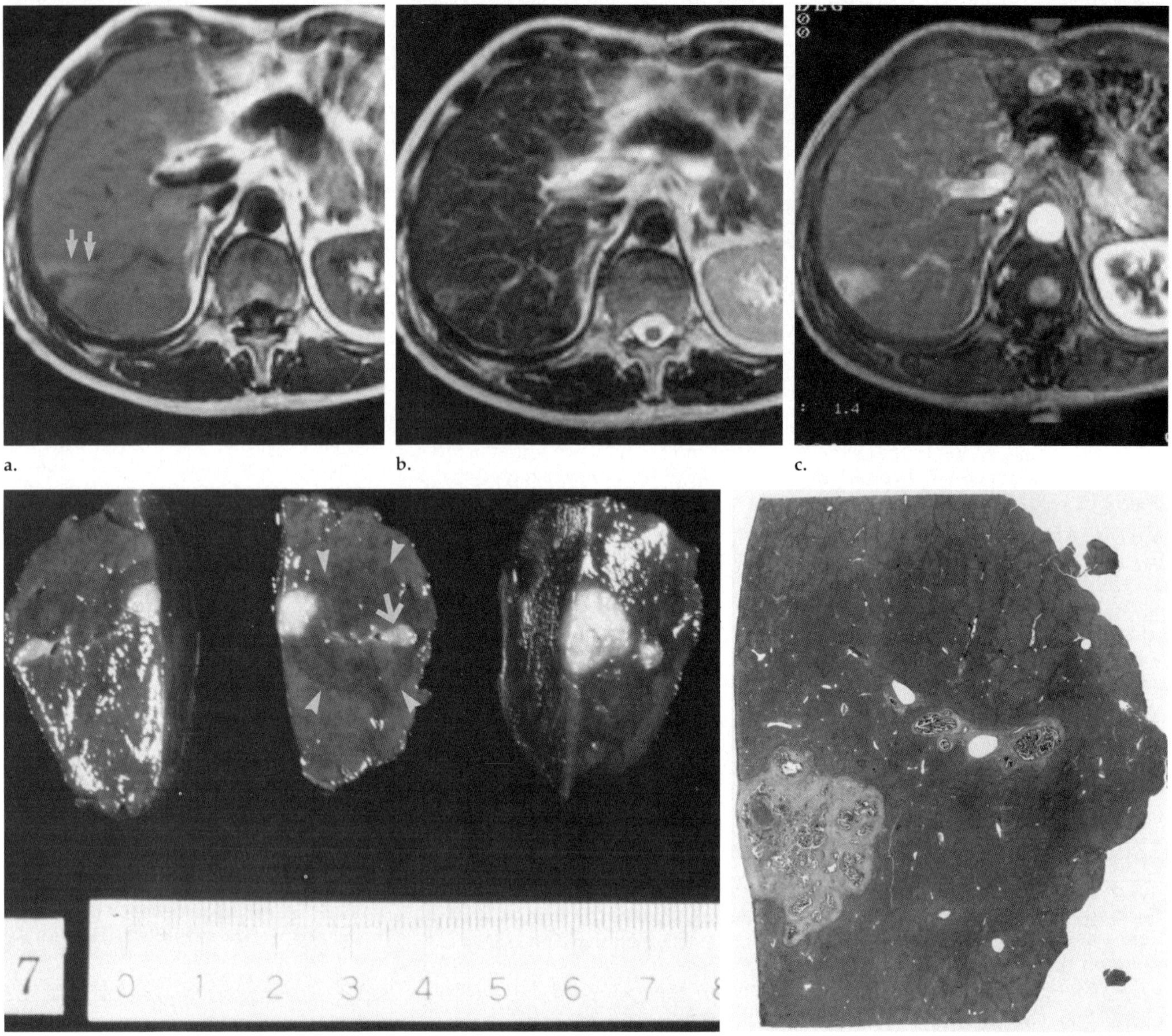

Figure 1. Liver metastases from sigmoid colon cancer in a 53-year-old man. **(a)** T1-weighted SE (600/15) MR image shows a wedge-shaped area of high signal intensity that surrounds a metastatic lesion in segment VII (classification of Couinaud; posterior superior segment of the right hepatic lobe). Intrahepatic bile duct dilatation (arrows) is seen medial to the primary tumor. **(b)** T2-weighted fast SE (6,000/112) MR image shows the same area with less prominent high signal intensity around the ring-shaped metastasis. **(c)** T1-weighted FE (80/6, 60° flip angle) MR image obtained 20 seconds after administration of gadopentetate dimeglumine shows enhancement of the same area. **(d)** Photograph of resected specimens shows wedge-shaped discolored areas (arrowheads) with the primary tumor and evidence of biliary spread (arrow). Scale is in centimeters. **(e)** Photomicrograph shows no fatty deposits or hemorrhage in this area. (Hematoxylin-eosin stain; original magnification, ×2.)

areas was high in four patients (Fig 1) and isointense in one patient. In two of five patients, the wedge-shaped areas were seen more clearly on FE images (Fig 2) than SE images. In four patients, the liver tumors (three metastases and one cholangiocarcinoma) with the wedge-shaped areas showed low signal intensity on T1-weighted SE images and high signal intensity on T2-weighted fast SE images. One metastatic tumor showed low signal intensity on both T1- and T2-weighted images. In addition to these findings, ring-shaped high signal intensity was seen around tumors on FE images (Fig 2). During the arterial phase of enhancement, wedge-shaped enhancement was seen clearly in the same areas that showed high signal intensity on T1-weighted SE and/or FE images (Figs 1, 2). In all patients, enhancement persisted from the arterial to the venous phase. Intrahepatic bile duct dilatation was identified within wedge-shaped areas on T2-weighted fast SE images (Fig 1) and/or enhanced FE images (Figs 1, 2). Duct dilatation was seen on the lateral side (Fig 2) of tumors away from the hepatic portal on the images of three patients. On these images, wedge-shaped areas were mainly seen around the enlarged ducts; intraluminal tumor extension was next to the lateral side of the tumor. In the other two patients, tumors were located near the liver surface, and localized bile duct dilatation was seen medial (Fig 1) to the tumors; wedge-shaped areas that surrounded liver tumors were also recognized. On T2-weighted fast SE images, it was difficult to differentiate these enlarged bile ducts from portal vein branches; however, on enhanced MR images these ducts showed moderately low signal intensity (Figs 1, 2).

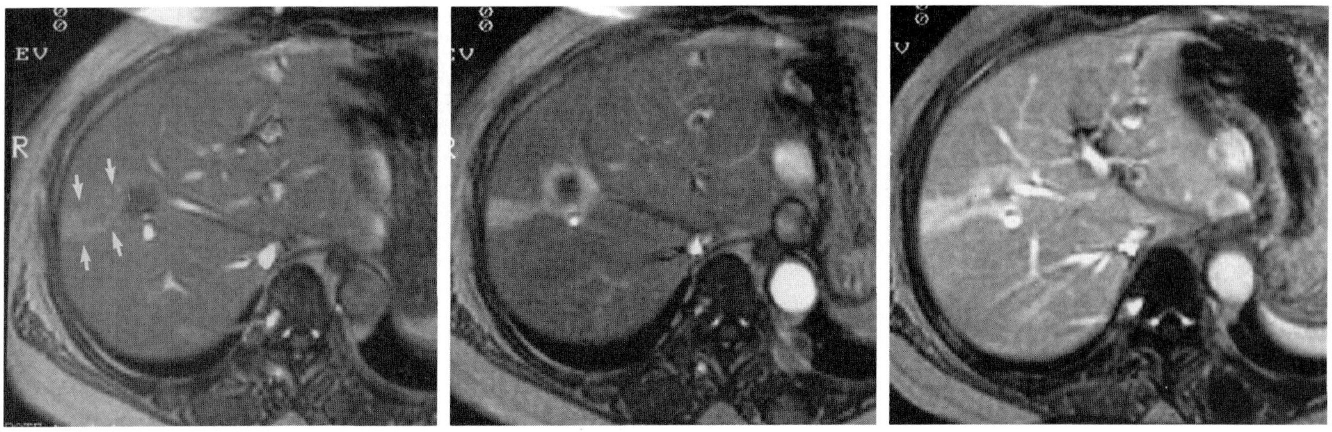

a. b. c.

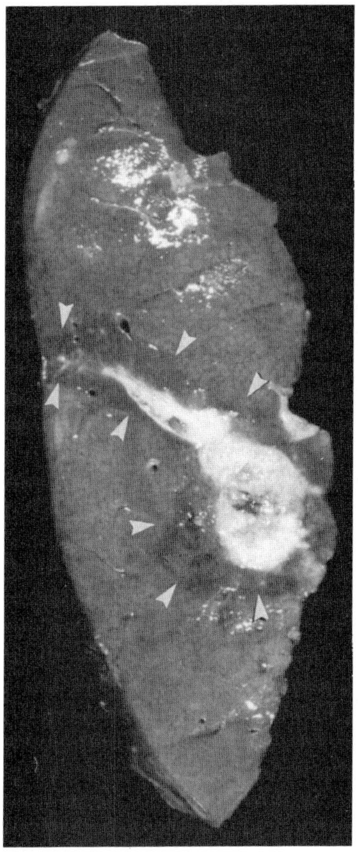

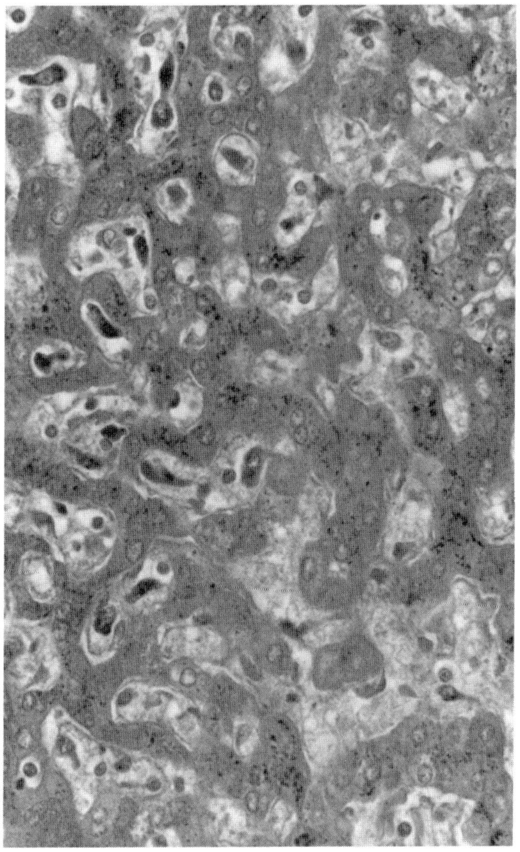

d. e.

Figure 2. Liver metastasis from rectal cancer in a 65-year-old woman. **(a)** Unenhanced FE (80/6, 60° flip angle) MR image shows the wedge-shaped area of increased signal intensity (arrows) around the enlarged intrahepatic bile duct that is next to the lateral portion of the tumor. The ring-shaped area around the tumor shows similar signal intensity. **(b)** FE MR image obtained 20 seconds after administration of gadopentetate dimeglumine shows enhancement of the wedge-shaped and ring-shaped areas. **(c)** FE MR image one section caudal to that in **b** shows intrabiliary tumor spread on the lateral side of the primary tumor. **(d)** Photograph of resected specimen shows wedge-shaped discolored areas (arrowheads) around the enlarged intrahepatic bile duct with intraluminal tumor spread. There are ring-shaped discolored areas (arrowheads) around the tumor; cancerous extension cannot be seen in these areas. **(e)** Photomicrograph of histologic specimen clearly shows granular lipofuscin in the cytoplasm of atrophic liver cells. (Schmorl stain; original magnification, ×400.)

Histopathologic Findings

At macroscopic examination, wedge-shaped areas associated with liver tumors appeared dark red-brown in all patients (Figs 1, 2). Moreover, similarly colored areas were seen around a metastatic tumor in one patient (Fig 2). There was intraductal tumor extension in the adjacent bile ducts within these wedge-shaped areas (Figs 1, 2). Three cases of biliary tumor extension were lateral to the tumor, and two were medial.

At microscopic examination, the wedge-shaped areas revealed liver cell atrophy (Fig 2), sinusoidal dilatation, inflammation of the perivascular fibrous areas, and intraluminal tumor in the bile ducts with papillary growth extending from the main tumor. There was microscopic evidence of tumor thrombus in the portal vein branches in three patients. The liver tumor that showed ring-shaped high signal intensity on FE images (Fig 2) was in the perivascular fibrous capsule of segment VIII (classification of Couinaud; anterior superior segment of the right hepatic lobe). In addition, the tumor was predominantly fibrous, and cancerous tissue was recognized mainly in the bile ducts. Cancerous extension was not seen in the ring-shaped high-signal-intensity areas. Hemorrhage, fatty change, and iron deposits were not recognized in the ring-shaped or wedge-shaped areas either (Figs 1, 2). In three patients, however, moderate to severe deposits of waste pigments or lipofuscin were seen in the atrophic hepatocytes within the wedge-shaped areas (Fig 2).

DISCUSSION

Many MR imaging studies have reported the high signal intensity of wedge-shaped areas that surround liver masses (1–4). These findings have been seen mainly on T2-weighted MR images and have been attributed to sinusoidal congestion and edema around tumors, bile stasis, parenchymal compression (1–4), and infiltrating tumor (8). However, wedge-shaped areas of increased signal intensity on T1-weighted MR images of the liver have not been reported—except in cases of focal fatty infiltration (5), infarction (6), and tumor hemorrhage (7). Among our cases, there were two types of wedge-shaped areas. One type was seen around the enlarged intrahepatic bile ducts with extension of tumor next to the lateral portion of the tumor mass. The configuration of this type of wedge-shaped area was variable because of tumor mass effect. The other type of wedge-shaped area was seen around the tumor mass. The tip of the wedge-shaped area was separate from the tumor mass and located medially next to the enlarged intrahepatic bile duct; this configuration was useful for recognizing intraductal tumor spread toward the hepatic portal. Itai et al (1,9) reported that signal intensity differences were caused by interruption of intrahepatic portal flow as a result of tumor thrombus in the portal vein or compression or ligation of the portal vein branches. These causes, however, do not explain the mechanism of increased signal intensity on T1-weighted images.

Because of respiratory motion artifacts on SE images, FE images were more useful than SE images for evaluating wedge-shaped areas. Possible mechanisms of increased signal intensity of wedge-shaped areas associated with malignant liver tumors on T1-weighted MR images include concentrated bile (10) and deposits of a T1-shortening substance (6,11,12). In our study, no concentrated bile stasis was detected microscopically. Ferric (Fe^{3+}), cupric (Cu^{2+}), and manganous (Mn^{2+}) ions are paramagnetic, and they have the potential to influence relaxation times (11–14). Honda et al (11) reported that signal intensity of hepatocellular carcinoma on T1-weighted images reflected iron and copper concentrations and that iron in hepatocellular carcinoma and the liver has a greater effect on signal intensity patterns than copper. Kadoya et al (13), however, reported that intrahepatic segmental areas of low signal intensity on both T1- and T2-weighted SE and gradient-echo MR images that are associated with decreased portal perfusion are the result of iron deposition in hepatocytes. Nevertheless, iron deposition was not seen in our study. Therefore, we conclude that the T1-shortening effect of iron was weak or even negligible in our patients.

In three of our patients, however, waste pigments or lipofuscin deposits could be seen clearly in the cytoplasm of atrophic hepatocytes within the wedge-shaped areas. Generally, lipofuscin is a waste pigment that appears in several conditions. The relaxation time of lipofuscin is not known. Lipofuscin consists of polymerized phospholipids and polymerized unsaturated fatty acids that are mixed with neutral lipids and protein (15). Some lipofuscins show positive fat-type reactions; others show positive reducing reactions (16). If the lipofuscin type was the former in our patients, a T1-shortening effect of lipofuscin was possible; we believe that lipofuscin contributed more to T1 shortening than iron. Splenic parenchyma in Niemann-Pick disease type C showed increased signal intensity on T1-weighted images because of lipid accumulation (17); this observation supports our theory. Lipofuscin, however, is not a pure substance, and its staining properties are not constant (16). Therefore, further examination is needed.

Dynamic FE images were more useful than SE images for recognizing the wedge-shaped areas. The diagnostic importance of enhancement, however, is not specific; many causes of enhancement have been reported. Arterioportal shunts (18) and interruption of intrahepatic portal flow (1) can increase arterial blood flow. In our series, there were two causes of wedge-shaped enhancement: tumor thrombus in the portal vein branches and portal vein branch compression by the expanding tumor-filled intrahepatic bile duct. Liver cell atrophy and sinusoidal dilatation, however, were recognized in the dark red wedge-shaped areas despite increased arterial blood flow in all patients. Takayasu et al (19) reported that lobar atrophy was caused by bile duct obstruction, and subsequent obstruction of the portal vein branches promoted further atrophic change. Therefore, we speculate that liver cell atrophy and sinusoidal dilatation were caused by reduction of portal flow as a result of portal vein branch compression and tumor thrombus in the portal vein branches.

Malignant liver tumors usually show invasion of the perivascular fibrous capsule. Hepatocellular carcinomas commonly are associated with tumor thrombus in the portal vein, but occlusion of the intrahepatic bile ducts with tumor rarely occurs (20). Others have reported that 60% of liver metastases from colorectal cancer showed intrahepatic bile duct invasion, and some of these tumors were not resected completely because tumor extension in the intrahepatic bile duct was overlooked (21). Therefore, when hepatic surgery is scheduled, preoperative diagnosis of tumor invasion of intrahepatic bile ducts with imaging is very important. Generally, computed tomography and MR imaging are useful for detecting intrahepatic bile duct dilatation (22,23); however, when intraductal tumor spreads medially from the primary tumor, recognition is not easy for two reasons. First, on T2-weighted fast SE images, intrahepatic bile ducts that are filled with tumor instead of bile show intermediate signal intensity. In this instance, it was difficult for us to differentiate the enlarged intrahepatic bile duct from a portal vein branch. Second, there was relative lack of bile in the intrahepatic ducts, and recognition of duct dilatation was somewhat difficult on enhanced images. In fact, medial spread of intraductal tumor in two patients could not be detected preoperatively with MR imaging, but intraductal tumor was recognized with ultrasound during surgery.

One of our cases was especially atypical; the ring-shaped area of high signal intensity could be seen around the tumor on T1-weighted images. Cancerous invasion, however, could not be recognized in the same area. This ring-shaped hyperintense area was due to mass effects or compression of bile duct branches. Therefore, the sign of ring-shaped high signal intensity around the tumor was not useful for evaluating biliary tumor spread.

In summary, we believe the wedge-shaped increased signal intensity on T1-weighted images of liver tumors is caused by lipofuscin. This MR finding was one manifestation of intraductal tumor spread in the intrahepatic bile ducts. ■

Acknowledgment: We are grateful to Isamu Hayashi, MT, for his invaluable suggestion to use the Schmorl stain in this study.

References

1. Itai Y, Ohtomo K, Kokubo T, et al. Segmental intensity differences in the liver on MR images: a sign of intrahepatic portal flow stoppage. Radiology 1988; 167:17–19.
2. Rummeny E, Weisslender R, Stark D, et al. Primary liver tumor: diagnosis by MR imaging. AJR 1989; 152:63–72.
3. Lee MJ, Saini S, Compton CC, et al. MR demonstration of edema adjacent to a liver metastasis: pathologic correlation. AJR 1991; 157:499–450.
4. Giovagnoni A, Terilli F, Ercolani P, et al. MR imaging of hepatic masses: diagnostic significance of wedge-shaped areas of increased signal intensity surrounding the lesion. AJR 1994; 163:1093–1097.
5. Mitchell DG. Focal manifestations of diffuse liver disease at MR imaging. Radiology 1992; 185:1–11.
6. Lee MJ, Hahn PF, Saini S, et al. Differential diagnosis of hyperintense liver lesion on T1-weighted MR images. AJR 1992; 159: 1017–1020.
7. Bradley WG, Schmidt PC. Effect of methemoglobin formation on the MR appearance of subarachnoid hemorrhage. Radiology 1985; 156:99–103.
8. Wachsberg RH, Levine CD, Simmons MZ, et al. Wedge-shaped intrahepatic cholan-

giocarcinoma: MRI-pathologic correlation. Abdom Imaging 1996; 21:219–221.
9. Itai Y, Ohtomo K, Furui S, et al. Lobar intensity differences of the liver on MR imaging. J Comput Assist Tomogr 1986; 10:236–241.
10. Demas BE, Hricak H, Moseley M, et al. Gallbladder bile: an experimental study in dogs using MR imaging and proton MR spectroscopy. Radiology 1985; 157:453–455.
11. Honda H, Onitsuka T, Kanazawa T, et al. MR imaging of hepatocellular carcinoma: correlation of metal content and signal intensity. Acta Radiol 1995; 36:163–167.
12. Ebara M, Watanabe S, Kita K, et al. MR imaging of hepatocellular carcinoma: effect of intratumoral copper content on signal intensity. Radiology 1991; 180:617–621.
13. Kadoya M, Matsui O, Kitagawa K, et al. Segmental iron deposition in the liver due to decreased intrahepatic portal perfusion: findings at MR imaging. Radiology 1994; 193:671–676.
14. Elidondo G, Fretz CJ, Stark DD, et al. Preclinical evaluation of MnDPDP: new paramagnetic hepatobiliary contrast agent for MR imaging. Radiology 1991; 178:73–78.
15. Constantinides P. Ultrastructual pathology. Amsterdam, The Netherlands: Elsevier, 1984; 331.
16. Culling CF, Allison RT, Barr WT. Cellular pathology technique. 4th ed. London, England: Butterworths, 1985; 285.
17. Omarini LPA, Frank-Burkhardt SE, Seemayer TA, et al. Niemann-Pick type C: nodular splenomegaly. Abdom Imaging 1995; 20:157–160.
18. Nakayama T, Hiyama Y, Ohnishi K, et al. Arterioportal shunts on dynamic computed tomography. AJR 1983; 140:953–957.
19. Takayasu K, Muramatsu Y, Shima Y, et al. Hepatic lobar atrophy following obstruction of the ipsilateral portal vein from hilar cholangiocarcinoma. Radiology 1986; 160: 389–393.
20. Nakashima T, Okuda K, Kojiro M, et al. Pathology of hepatocellular carcinoma in Japan: 232 consecutive cases autopsied in ten years. Cancer 1983; 51:863–877.
21. Yamamoto J, Sugihara K, Kosuge T, et al. Pathologic support for limited hepatectomy in the treatment of liver metastases from colorectal cancer. Ann Surg 1995; 221:74–78.
22. Teefey SA, Baron RL, Schulte SJ, et al. Patterns of intrahepatic bile duct dilatation at CT: correlation with obstructive disease processes. Radiology 1992; 182:139–142.
23. Dooms GC, Fisher MR, Higgins CB, et al. MR imaging of the dilated biliary tract. Radiology 1986; 158:337–341.

Discography How To

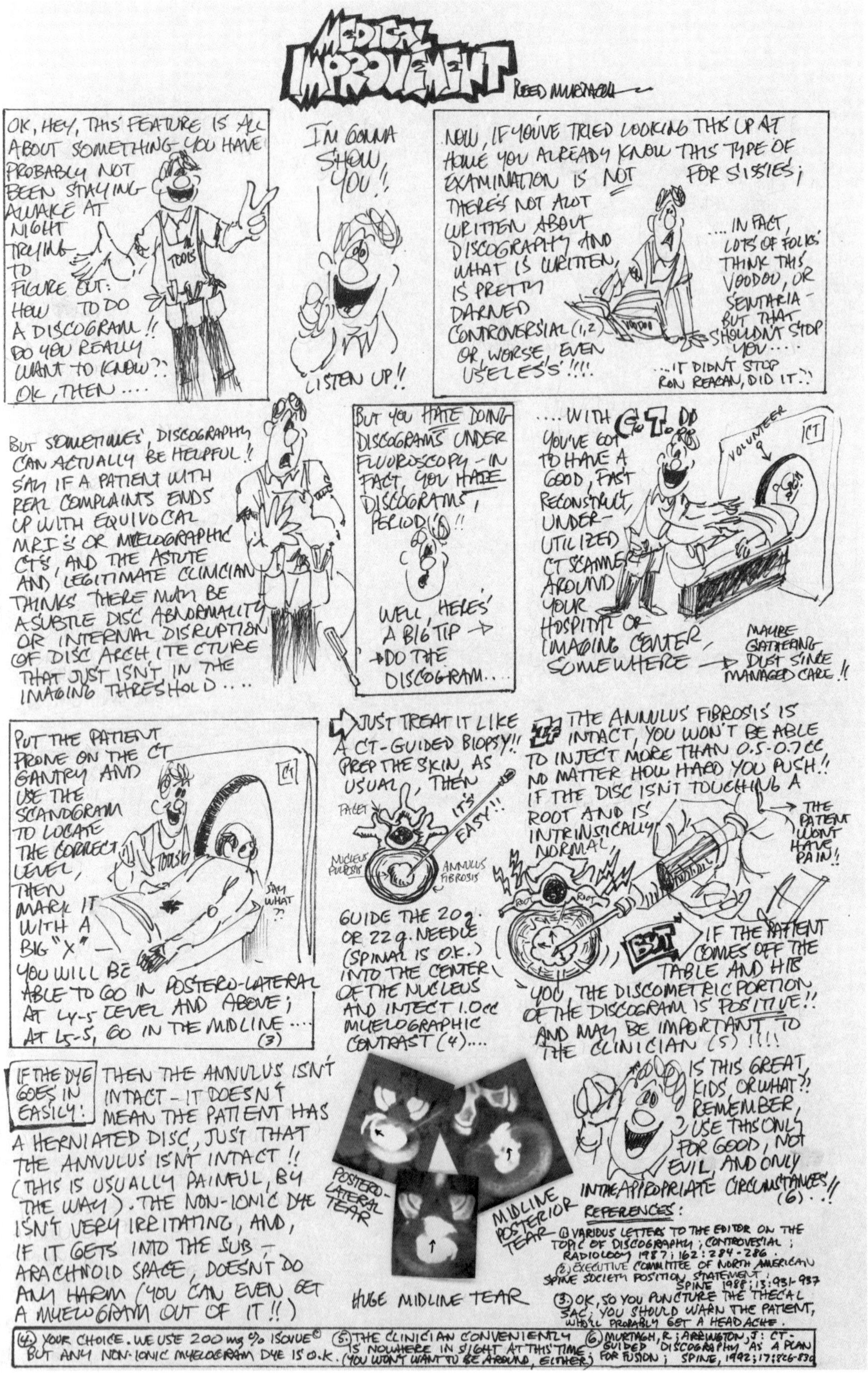

Courtesy of F. Reed Murtaugh, MD, Tampa, Fla

Ingo O. Rencken, MB, ChB • Augusto Sola, MD • Firaz Al-Ali, MD • Juan P. Solano, MD
Henry I. Goldberg, MD • Pierre-Alain Cohen, MD • Charles A. Gooding, MD

Necrotizing Enterocolitis: Diagnosis with CT Examination of Urine after Enteral Administration of Iodinated Water-soluble Contrast Material[1]

PURPOSE: **To develop a new method for diagnosing necrotizing enterocolitis with use of computed tomography (CT).**

MATERIALS AND METHODS: **Urine specimens from 22 neonates were obtained 8–12 hours after iohexol was administered enterally. Twelve neonates had suspected (n = 5) or definite (n = 7) necrotizing enterocolitis, and 10 neonates without necrotizing enterocolitis underwent routine upper gastrointestinal study. Urine from another 13 neonates without necrotizing enterocolitis who did not receive iohexol was collected. The attenuation coefficient of each urine specimen was determined with CT.**

RESULTS: **The mean CT attenuation coefficient of urine from neonates who did not receive iohexol was 5.6 HU ± 3.9, and that from neonates without necrotizing enterocolitis who underwent upper gastrointestinal study was 6.7 HU ± 3.2. The mean CT attenuation coefficient of urine from patients with suspected necrotizing enterocolitis was 26.0 HU ± 3.4, and that in patients with definite necrotizing enterocolitis was 71.0 HU ± 18.8. The mean CT attenuation coefficients in neonates with necrotizing enterocolitis were significantly different from that in patients without necrotizing enterocolitis who underwent upper gastrointestinal study.**

CONCLUSION: **Urine from neonates with necrotizing enterocolitis show significantly higher CT attenuation coefficients than those from patients without necrotizing enterocolitis. CT examination of urine may allow early detection of necrotizing enterocolitis.**

Necrotizing enterocolitis is a disease of unknown cause that occurs predominantly in premature neonates. Necrotizing enterocolitis manifests as gastrointestinal and systemic signs, which include abdominal distention, increasing gastric food residuals, occult or frank blood in the stool, and respiratory distress. Advanced cases are associated with bacteremia, acidosis, and shock. The incidence in the United States is estimated to be between 1,200 and 9,600 cases annually, and the mortality rate varies between 9% and 28% (1). The diagnosis depends on the demonstration of intramural air in the bowel, portal venous air, or pneumoperitoneum on abdominal radiographs in the appropriate clinical setting (2). At times, however, intramural air on radiographs can be difficult to discriminate from overlying bowel segments or intraluminal air mixed with stool. In addition, detection of this finding is subject to interobserver variability (3). Moreover, extensive necrotizing enterocolitis may not demonstrate intestinal pneumatosis, and pneumoperitoneum is not always seen in neonates with bowel-wall perforation (2). Similarly, clinical signs may not be specific or sensitive, particularly in early necrotizing enterocolitis.

The purpose of this study was to develop a safe and objective test that enables the confident and expeditious diagnosis of necrotizing enterocolitis. Such a test would reduce mortality and morbidity of the disease and prevent unnecessary treatment: Many patients suspected to have necrotizing enterocolitis do not; nevertheless, they are treated for the disease.

The test would depend on a constant finding of the disease (ie, gastrointestinal mucosal injury). In animal studies, investigators have shown that water-soluble iodinated contrast material administered into the lumen of ischemic bowel permeates through the bowel wall; contrast material is then absorbed by the peritoneum and excreted by the kidneys into the bladder (4). This process does not occur with normal bowel. We attempted to discriminate patients with from those without necrotizing enterocolitis by measuring in vitro the computed tomographic (CT) attenuation coefficient (in Hounsfield units) of imaged excreted urine after enteral administration of water-soluble contrast material.

MATERIALS AND METHODS

We studied the in vitro CT attenuation coefficients of imaged urine samples from 35 neonates who were divided into four groups. Group 1 consisted of 13 premature neonates who received no contrast material; their gestational ages ranged from 28 to 40 weeks (mean, 36.2 weeks). Group 2 consisted of 10 neonates who underwent upper gastrointestinal studies for diagnostic purposes (eg, to rule out tracheoesophageal fistula); their gestational ages ranged from 26 to 40 weeks (mean, 35.5 weeks). No patient in group 1 or 2 showed clinical evidence of necrotizing enterocolitis at the

Index terms: Colitis, 74.267, 75.267 • Computed tomography (CT), contrast media • Computed tomography (CT), quantitative • Urine

Radiology 1997; 205:87–90

[1] From the Departments of Radiology (I.O.R., F.A., H.I.G., P.A.C., C.A.G.) and Pediatrics (A.S., J.P.S., C.A.G.), University of California at San Francisco, 505 Parnassus Ave, San Francisco, CA 94143. Received March 11, 1997; revision requested April 23; final revision received June 13; accepted June 19. Supported in part by National Institutes of Health grant N01RR01271 awarded to the Pediatric Clinical Research Center. **Address reprint requests to** C.A.G.

time these studies were performed. Neonates suspected to have necrotizing enterocolitis were closely monitored. These neonates formed groups 3 and 4. Group 3 consisted of five neonates with stage I (suspected) necrotizing enterocolitis according to the staging criteria of Bell (5) (Table 1); their gestational ages ranged from 33 to 37 weeks (mean, 34.5 weeks). Group 4 consisted of seven neonates with stage II (definite) necrotizing enterocolitis; their gestational ages ranged from 26 to 37 weeks (mean, 34.2 weeks).

The study was performed with the approval of the Human Research Committee at the University of California at San Francisco. This committee recommended that neonates who weighed less than 500 g be excluded from the study. Also, patients with renal failure or dehydration were excluded. Dehydration was defined as follows: (*a*) weight loss greater than 12%; (*b*) blood urea nitrogen level greater than 10.7 mmol/L; (*c*) serum sodium level greater than 148 mmol/L; and (*d*) urine output greater than 1 mL/kg per hour. Informed consent was obtained from the parents or legal guardians of the neonates after explanation of the procedure and possible complications.

Neonates in groups 2, 3, and 4 who weighed more than 1,000 g each received an oral solution of 5 mL of iohexol (Omnipaque 300; Nycomed, Princeton, NJ) diluted with 7 mL of sterile water; the resulting 12-mL solution had an osmolarity of approximately 240 mOsm/L and was hypotonic when compared with human plasma (osmolarity, 285 mOsm/L). Neonates who weighed less than 1,000 g received 8 mL of the same solution. The solution was administered by means of an indwelling orogastric tube over 30 minutes, and gastric suction was discontinued for 2 hours after administration to allow passage of the solution into the bowel. No patients vomited; however, vomiting was a distinct possibility and could have led to false-negative results. Passage of the solution into the small and large bowel was confirmed with routinely acquired abdominal radiographs. Some patients demonstrated clinical and radiographic features of ileus; however, on abdominal radiographs obtained 8–12 hours after administration of the contrast material solution, all patients showed passage of the solution into at least the distal small bowel.

Urine from all neonates was collected serially at 4-hour intervals after administration of the contrast solution. Urine was collected from a urine bag or squeezed out from a diaper, and a 2-mL aliquot was placed into a small cylindrical plastic vial that measured 1 cm in length and 5 mm in diameter. All vials containing urine were placed into the same CT scanner (HiSpeed Advantage; GE Medical Systems, Milwaukee, Wis) and imaged with use of set parameters: 120 kVp, 80 mA, 1-second scanning time, 15-cm field of view, and 3-mm section thickness. The CT attenuation coefficient of the urine was measured from a central region of interest that equaled 50% of the diameter of the vial. The effect of urine specific gravity on the CT attenuation coefficient was also determined with control samples.

Statistical analyses were performed with the unpaired Student *t* test. A *P* value less than .05 was considered statistically significant.

Table 1
Clinical Staging of Necrotizing Enterocolitis with the Criteria of Bell

Stage	Clinical Signs	Radiographic Findings
I (suspected)	Abdominal distention, poor feeding, and vomiting	Ileus
II (definite)	Abdominal distention, poor feeding, vomiting, and gastrointestinal bleeding	Intestinal pneumatosis and portal venous air
III (advanced)	Abdominal distention, poor feeding, vomiting, gastrointestinal bleeding, and septic shock	Ileus, intestinal pneumatosis, portal venous air, and pneumoperitoneum

Note.—From Bell (5).

RESULTS

Cases are depicted in Figures 1–3. Results are presented in Figure 4. The CT attenuation coefficients increased slightly with increasing specific gravity of urine (Table 2). The maximum CT attenuation coefficients were measured from urine obtained 8–12 hours after administration of the contrast solution. The urine of neonates who did not receive contrast solution (group 1) showed a mean CT attenuation coefficient of 5.6 HU ± 3.9. The urine of patients without necrotizing enterocolitis who underwent upper gastrointestinal study (group 2) showed a mean CT attenuation coefficient of 6.7 HU ± 3.2. The mean CT attenuation coefficient of urine from group 3 patients (with stage I necrotizing enterocolitis) was 26.0 HU ± 3.4. The urine from group 4 patients (with stage II necrotizing enterocolitis) showed a mean CT attenuation coefficient of 71.0 HU ± 18.8. The mean CT attenuation coefficient in group 2 was statistically significantly different from that in group 3 ($P < .01$) and that in group 4 ($P < .01$). As well, the mean CT attenuation coefficient in group 3 was significantly different from that in group 4 ($P < .01$). Although the CT attenuation coefficient increased with increasing specific gravity of urine, these CT attenuation coefficients were significantly below those of groups 3 and 4 (Table 2).

No radiograph showed opacification of the bladder with contrast material. No side effects from enteral administration of contrast material were observed. Two patients underwent surgical exploration; one patient was in group 4, and the other patient was in group 3. These patients are presented as case reports because they demonstrate in detail the clinical circumstances of necrotizing enterocolitis and the potential value of CT examination of urine.

Table 2
CT Attenuation Coefficients of Distilled Water and Urine with Different Specific Gravities

Specific Gravity	CT Attenuation Coefficient (HU)*
1.000†	−2.0 ± 2.6
1.010‡	5.0 ± 2.1
1.015‡	6.0 ± 2.9
1.030‡	14.0 ± 3.0

* Data are the mean ± standard deviation.
† Specific gravity of distilled water.
‡ Specific gravity of urine from control subjects.

Case 1.—A male neonate (gestational age, 37 weeks) who weighed 2,500 g developed abdominal distention and passed frankly bloody stool. The initial abdominal radiograph demonstrated no intestinal pneumatosis. The CT attenuation coefficient of his urine after administration of contrast solution was 68.0 HU. An abdominal radiograph obtained 48 hours later demonstrated pneumoperitoneum. Surgery performed 4 hours after this abdominal radiograph was obtained confirmed extensive necrotizing enterocolitis.

Case 2.—A male neonate (gestational age, 26 weeks) who weighed 800 g developed acidosis and increasing gastric residuals and passed blood-stained stools on two occasions. The CT attenuation coefficient of his urine after administration of contrast solution was 32.0 HU. Surgery performed 24 hours later revealed an 8-cm segment of necrotic bowel, which was resected.

The urine of both patients demonstrated high CT attenuation coefficients; these numbers, according to our results, indicated necrotizing en-

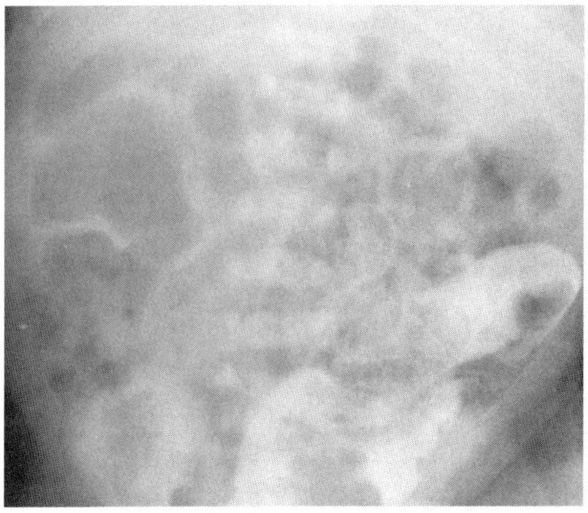

1.

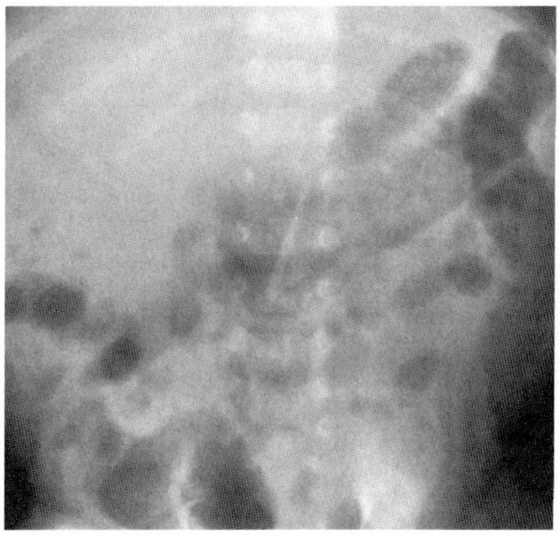

2.

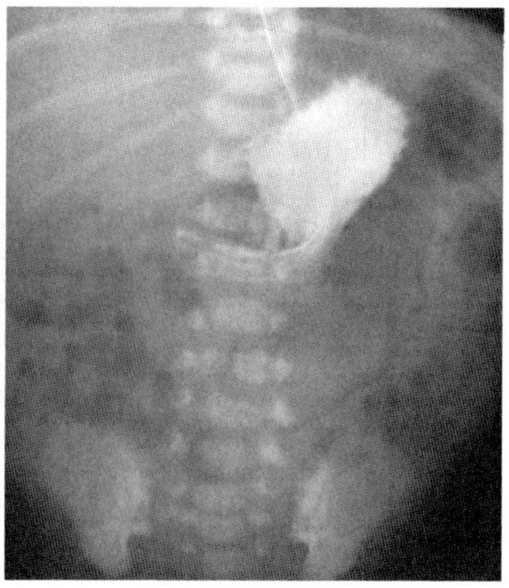

3.

Figures 1–3. **(1)** Neonate without necrotizing enterocolitis who underwent routine upper gastrointestinal study for tracheoesophageal fistula. Abdominal radiograph after oral administration of contrast solution shows water-soluble contrast material in the bowel. The CT attenuation coefficient of urine was 6.0 HU. **(2)** Neonate with stage I necrotizing enterocolitis. Abdominal radiograph shows a segment of bowel, which had been distended for 2 days, in the right lower quadrant. No intestinal pneumatosis is seen. The CT attenuation coefficient of urine was 30.0 HU. **(3)** Neonate with stage II necrotizing enterocolitis. Abdominal radiograph shows water-soluble contrast material in the stomach and intestinal pneumatosis in left upper, left lower, and right upper quadrants. The CT attenuation coefficient of urine was 70.0 HU.

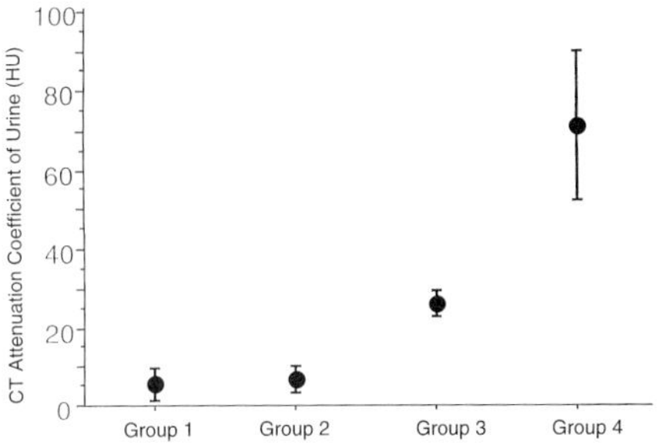

Figure 4. Mean CT attenuation coefficients of urine with 95% confidence intervals in four groups of neonates. Group 1 = neonates who did not receive contrast solution (n = 13), group 2 = neonates without necrotizing enterocolitis who underwent upper gastrointestinal study (n = 10), group 3 = neonates with stage I necrotizing enterocolitis (n = 5), group 4 = neonates with stage II necrotizing enterocolitis (n = 7).

terocolitis. CT examination of both urine samples enabled positive prediction of necrotizing enterocolitis at least 24 hours before surgery (which enabled confirmation of necrotizing enterocolitis). In the first case, the high CT attenuation coefficient was obtained 36 hours before the first radiographic abnormality—extraluminal air—was seen. In the second case, no radiographic abnormality was seen. Thus, in these cases, a high CT attenuation coefficient of imaged urine was measured not only before a radiographic abnormality was seen but in the absence of a radiographic abnormality.

DISCUSSION

On abdominal radiographs, the hallmark of necrotizing enterocolitis is abnormal air distribution such as occurs with intestinal pneumatosis, portal venous air, or pneumoperitoneum (6–8). The presence or extent of abnormal air on radiographs does not always predict the severity of necrotizing enterocolitis (2). The appearance of intestinal pneumatosis may be confused with the bubbly appearance of intraluminal air in the bowel mixed with meconium or feces; blood mixed with intraluminal air may produce a similar appearance. Intestinal pneumatosis appears as a variable-length linear pattern of air outside of the bowel lumen on radiographs with anteroposterior and cross-table lateral views. On radiographs, portal venous air in the liver appears as a linear branching lucency, which may be a very subtle finding. Pneumoperitoneum also can be very difficult to detect on radiographs if only a small amount of free air is present.

Early diagnosis of necrotizing enterocolitis is essential. Neonates with a mild form of the disease who do not receive therapy and continue to receive enteric feedings may develop a severe form of the disease and even bowel perforation. Early radiographic signs of necrotizing enterocolitis are often absent. Kliegmann and Fanaroff (8) demonstrated that among patients with documented necrotizing enterocolitis only 45% showed intestinal pneumatosis and only 17% showed portal venous air. They also found that 14% of patients with documented necrotizing enterocolitis did not show positive radiographic signs (9). Furthermore, when necrotizing enterocolitis is suspected, there is often disagreement among observers about the presence or absence of intestinal pneumatosis on radiographs (3). As a result, early clinical findings and plain radiographic interpretations do not enable a thoroughly reliable diagnosis of necrotizing enterocolitis.

Because of the variability of clinical and radiographic findings, the use of contrast material enemas has been advocated to improve the specificity of diagnosis (10–12). Although use of barium enemas has improved the specificity of diagnosis in some ambiguous cases, the procedure in sick neonates is relatively invasive and requires transfer of the patient to the fluoroscopic unit. Cohen et al (13) studied 28 neonates with suspected necrotizing enterocolitis with metrizamide-enema examination of the small bowel. Four of these patients showed abnormalities, which included separation of bowel segments and irregular, shaggy, and spiculated mucosal margins. Pathologic confirmation was available in two of these patients. The other 24 examinations were negative, and these neonates did not exhibit signs of necrotizing enterocolitis during hospitalization. With metrizamide-enema examination, however, the need to obtain multiple radiographs and differences in interobserver interpretation make standardization of this examination in every suspected case difficult. Small-bowel follow-through examination may not always provide adequate study of the terminal ileum and colon, where necrotizing enterocolitis occurs predominantly.

Several investigators have attempted to diagnose gastrointestinal perforation with use of contrast material. Mori and Barrett (14) found that most gastrointestinal perforations were demonstrated radiographically with opacification of the bladder 2–3 hours after oral ingestion of diatrizoate. McGraw et al (15) looked for diatrizoate, after enteric administration, in the blood or urine to substantiate intestinal perforation. Stordahl (16) and Schwartzentruber et al (17) measured the serum and urinary levels of iohexol (Omnipaque 300) in rats after injecting contrast material directly into closed small-bowel segments. Stordahl found that urinary levels of iohexol were 27 times higher in rats with a ligated mesenteric artery and vein (which induced bowel ischemia) than those in rats without vascular occlusion. He concluded that measuring urinary iohexol levels may aid the evaluation of mucosal injury from bowel ischemia.

In human neonates, there are no data regarding intestinal absorption of contrast material with regard to gestational age. Stordahl (18), in another rat study, concluded that contrast material passes transmurally from the ischemic bowel lumen and then transperitoneally before it is excreted by the kidneys. Stordahl used the urinary excretion of water-soluble contrast material as a measure of intestinal mucosal injury and as a way to discriminate between simple obstruction and ischemia. He found that (*a*) irrespective of the duration of contrast material in the bowel, bladder opacity and the urinary iohexol level varied nearly proportionally to the length of ischemic bowel and (*b*) urinary iohexol levels varied directly with the extent of morphologic changes in the mucosa (caused by different modes of ischemia) in closed intestinal loops.

In rats, Linkous et al (19) developed a noninvasive method for detecting bowel ischemia by examining urine with CT to detect absorption of iohexol after enteric administration. This method was practical and sensitive for detecting urinary levels of iodinated contrast material; there was a high linear correlation (r = .98) between the CT attenuation coefficient (in Hounsfield units) and the in vitro iohexol concentration in urine. Another method for measuring iohexol is an electrophoretic iohexol assay; however, this method is available at a limited number of centers only and not on an immediate basis. CT, by comparison, is widely available. Measurement of the CT attenuation coefficient of urine is a simple procedure that necessitates only approximately 5 minutes of scanner time; it is not necessary to photograph images.

Because necrotizing enterocolitis shows coagulation necrosis and ischemia of bowel wall at pathologic examination (20), we hypothesized, with use of the method of Linkous et al (19), that there would be an increase in the CT attenuation coefficient of imaged urine from patients with necrotizing enterocolitis after enteric administration of iohexol. We used iohexol because it is nonionic, well tolerated, and readily absorbed if leakage into the peritoneal cavity occurs. When perforation cannot be excluded, iohexol is a safe agent to use. Furthermore, orally administered iohexol is very poorly absorbed from the normal gastrointestinal tract (manufacturer's information, Nycomed) (17). This finding was confirmed in our group 2 patients who did not have necrotizing enterocolitis but underwent upper gastrointestinal studies with use of iohexol. The mean CT attenuation coefficient of their urine (6.7 HU) was approximately the same as that (5.6 HU) in patients who did not receive any contrast material. By contrast, patients in group 4 (stage II necrotizing enterocolitis) had a significantly higher mean CT attenuation coefficient of urine (71.0 HU) than that of the control group or that (6.7 HU) of group 2. Other water-soluble contrast material, such as diatrizoate meglumine and diatrizoate sodium, are ionic and absorbed to a much greater extent in normal bowel; thus, these agents were not well suited for use in this study.

The mean CT attenuation coefficient of urine (26.0 HU) from group 3 patients (with stage I necrotizing enterocolitis) was statistically significantly different from those in groups 1 and 2. Because stage II necrotizing enterocolitis represents a more advanced state of the disease and presumably greater ischemic change in bowel, our results supported the finding of Stordahl that urinary iohexol levels after enteric administration vary directly with the degree of morphologic change in the mucosa.

On the basis of our results in this preliminary study, we conclude that, after enteral administration of iohexol, CT attenuation coefficients of imaged urine are statistically higher in neonates with necrotizing enterocolitis than in those without necrotizing enterocolitis. Furthermore, the CT attenuation coefficient of imaged urine (which reflects urinary iohexol levels) is dependent on the extent of bowel ischemia; the urine of patients with more advanced necrotizing enterocolitis showed higher CT attenuation coefficients.

We observed no adverse effects of enterally administered iohexol in any of the neonates studied. We plan to determine the sensitivity and predictive values of this test in another study of patients with clinical signs of necrotizing enterocolitis and normal radiographic studies. If the results of this study are corroborated, this diagnostic test will be performed routinely to evaluate neonates suspected to have necrotizing enterocolitis. ■

Acknowledgments: We thank Cory Fergus, BA, for providing statistical analyses and Liv Cann, CRT, for assisting in the measurement of CT attentuation coefficients.

References

1. Stoll BJ. Epidemiology of necrotizing enterocolitis. Clin Perinatol 1994; 21:205–218.
2. Morrison SC, Jacobson JM. The radiology of necrotizing enterocolitis. Clin Perinatol 1994; 21:347–363.
3. Mata AG, Rosengert RM. Interobserver variability in the radiographic diagnosis of necrotizing enterocolitis. Pediatrics 1980; 66:68–71.
4. Stordahl A. Urinary excretion of iohexol administered enterally in rats with intestinal ischemia: a transmural and transperitoneal route of transport. Scand J Gastroenterol 1988; 23:751–754.
5. Bell MJ. Perforation of the gastrointestinal tract and peritonitis in the neonate. Surg Gynecol Obstet 1985; 160:20–26.
6. Santuli TV, Schullinger JN, Heird WC, et al. Acute necrotizing enterocolitis in infancy: a review of 64 cases. Pediatrics 1975; 55:376–387.
7. Keyting WS, McCarver RR, Kovarik JL, et al. Pneumatosis intestinalis: a new concept. Radiology 1961; 76:733–741.
8. Kliegman RM, Fanaroff AA. Neonatal necrotizing enterocolitis: a nine year experience. II. Outcome assessment. Am J Dis Child 1981; 135:608–611.
9. Kliegmann RM, Fanaroff AA. Neonatal necrotizing enterocolitis in the absence of pneumatosis intestinalis. Am J Dis Child 1982; 136:618–620.
10. Leonadis JC, Bhan I, Leappe LL. Barium enema in suspected necrotizing enterocolitis: is it ever indicated? Clin Radiol 1980; 31:587–590.
11. Negrette J, Ziervogel MA, Young DG, Azmy AF. Barium enema examination in neonates with suspected necrotizing enterocolitis. Z Kinderchir 1986; 41:19–21.
12. Uken P, Smith W, Franken JR, Frey E, Sato Y, Ellerbroek C. Use of barium enema in the diagnosis of necrotizing enterocolitis. Pediatr Radiol 1988; 18:24–27.
13. Cohen MD, Smith JA, Slabaugh RD, Rust RJ. Neonatal necrotizing enterocolitis shown by oral metrizamide (Amipaque). AJR 1982; 138:1019–1023.
14. Mori PA, Barrett HA. A sign of intestinal perforation. Radiology 1962; 79:401–407.
15. McGraw J, McCleod R, McDonald W, Stephenson HF Jr. A rapid bedside test for intestinal perforation. JAMA 1965; 191:939–941.
16. Stordahl A. Urinary excretion of iohexol after intestinal administration in rats with bowel ischemia: the effects of mesenteric arterial and/or venous occlusion. Acta Radiol 1989; 30:87–92.
17. Schwarzentruber DJ, Billmire DF, Cohen M, Block T, Gunter M, Grosfeld JL. Use of iohexol in the radiographic diagnosis of ischemic bowel. J Pediatr Surg 1986; 21:525–529.
18. Stordahl A. Water-soluble contrast media in obstructed and in ischemic small intestine. J Oslo City Hosp 1989; 39:3–22.
19. Linkous MD, Nelson MT, Mulvihull SJ, Goldberg HI. Noninvasive method for the detection of bowel ischemia: CT detection of iodinated contrast material. Acad Radiol 1994; 1:15–20.
20. Ballance WA, Dahms BB, Shenker N, Kliegmann R. Pathology of neonatal necrotizing enterocolitis: a ten year experience. J Pediatr 1992; 117(suppl):6–13.

Michael P. Federle, MD • Neda Yagan, MD • Andrew B. Peitzman, MD • James Krugh, MD

Abdominal Trauma: Use of Oral Contrast Material for CT Is Safe[1]

PURPOSE: **To determine the potential risk of aspiration pneumonitis associated with use of oral contrast material in computed tomography (CT) performed for evaluation of abdominal trauma.**

MATERIALS AND METHODS: **In 510 consecutive adult patients, a dilute 2.5% solution of diatrizoate meglumine and sodium was administered orally or by means of a nasogastric tube as part of a routine protocol for CT evaluation of acute abdominal trauma. A retrospective review of medical records was performed to determine evidence of aspiration pneumonitis occurring before or after CT.**

RESULTS: **None of the patients had aspiration of contrast material or gastric contents attributable to the CT examination.**

CONCLUSION: **Use of contrast material for stomach and bowel opacification during CT for evaluation of abdominal trauma appears to be safe. Proper preparation and administration of contrast material and control of the patient's airway are essential to ensure the safety of this procedure.**

Computed tomography (CT) is used extensively for evaluation of blunt abdominal trauma and is effective in demonstrating injuries of the liver, spleen, or kidneys. Although injuries of the pancreas and bowel are more difficult to diagnose with CT, several investigators have reported excellent results and have stressed the value of enteric (orally administered) contrast material (1–6). Opacification of the bowel lumen aids identification of extravasation of enteric contents, bowel wall thickening, and distinction of hematomas from nonopacified bowel loops. Despite the advantages associated with opacification, some radiologists, surgeons, and anesthesiologists remain reluctant to use oral contrast material in CT performed for assessment of abdominal trauma because it is believed that use of contrast material may increase the occurrence of aspiration of gastric contents in obtunded patients or in patients in whom general anesthesia is administered for surgery soon after CT examination.

To our knowledge, there has been no systematic evaluation of the potential risks of use of oral contrast material in CT performed for assessment of abdominal trauma other than a study we reported in the *Journal of Trauma* in 1995 (7). That investigation included 506 consecutive patient studies from 1993 and 1994. The purpose of this study was to assess the potential risks of occurrence of aspiration pneumonitis before or after CT performed with oral contrast material for evaluation of blunt abdominal trauma.

MATERIALS AND METHODS

During an 8-month period (January to August 1995), 510 consecutive patients underwent CT within several hours of abdominal trauma for evaluation of injuries. The 361 male and 149 female patients ranged in age from 14 to 90 years (mean, 37 years). The mechanism of injury was motor vehicle accident (including pedestrian injury) in 367 patients, fall in 86 patients, assault in 29 patients, and miscellaneous causes in 28 patients.

In all patients, contrast material was administered intravenously with a mechanical injector at an injection rate of 2 mL/sec, with injection of a total volume of 2 mL/kg to a maximum of 150 mL. The contrast agents used were iothalamate meglumine (Conray 60; Mallinckrodt Medical, St Louis, Mo) in 306 patients and ioversol (Optiray 300; Mallinckrodt Medical) in 204 patients.

After intravenous administration of contrast material, a dilute solution of diatrizoate meglumine and sodium (Gastroview; Mallinckrodt Medical) was administered orally. This solution was prepared as a mixture of 6 mL of diatrizoate meglumine and sodium per 240 mL of tap water, yielding a 2.5% solution. Patients who were awake and alert were asked to drink 450 mL of the solution with a straw. In patients with altered sensorium, a nasogastric or orogastric tube was inserted for administration of contrast material. After stomach contents were aspirated with a syringe, the same 450-mL solution was administered by means of the tube. When possible, the patients were encouraged to lie on their

Index terms: Abdomen, CT, 70.12112 • Abdomen, injuries, 70.41 • Computed tomography (CT), contrast media, 70.1211 • Contrast media, complications, 60.4126, 70.99

Radiology 1997; 205:91–93

[1] From the Departments of Radiology (M.P.F., N.Y.), Surgery (A.B.P.), and Anesthesia (J.K.), University of Pittsburgh Medical Center, 200 Lothrop St, Pittsburgh, PA 15213. Received May 20, 1997; accepted June 24. **Address reprint requests to** M.P.F.

right side to facilitate gastric emptying. Initial administration of the oral contrast material was observed or performed by the nursing staff in the emergency department. If more than 30 minutes elapsed from the initial administration of oral contrast material until the beginning of the CT examination, an additional 240 mL of the solution was administered orally in the CT suite.

We reviewed the medical records and computer files of the 510 patients who were entered prospectively into our trauma registry. All radiologic reports were reviewed for evidence of pulmonary infiltration or consolidation. Progress notes and surgical notes by the anesthesiologist and surgeon and all discharge summaries were reviewed for any reports of occurrence of aspiration. We also reviewed the records for reports of fever, with 38.5 °C as a threshold.

We accepted without further investigation the clinical diagnosis of the presence of aspiration pneumonitis or other acute pulmonary pathologic process. Criteria for diagnosis of aspiration pneumonitis typically included the presence of pulmonary infiltration and fever along with vomiting or aspiration observed by medical personnel. Suctioning of gastric contents or recovery of multiple oropharyngeal flora from the tracheobronchial tree also constituted definite proof. Aspiration observed during a fluoroscopic modified barium swallow examination was considered definitive if aspiration was accompanied by fever and infiltration. At least one of these objective criteria was met in all patients who developed aspiration pneumonitis before or after arrival at the hospital.

Traumatic lung injury was diagnosed when at least one of the following abnormalities was observed in the absence of persistent fever: peripheral nonsegmental infiltrates (contusion), lung laceration, or hematoma or traumatic lung cyst. Postoperative atelectasis was diagnosed when fever and infiltration developed in the period immediately after surgery. Atelectasis typically resolved rapidly with incentive spirometry and antibiotics.

RESULTS

Of the 510 patients, 178 (35%) had obtundation or altered mentation caused by head trauma or intoxication, and in 63 (35%) of these patients, airway protection was achieved with endotracheal intubation. Among the 510 patients, endotracheal intubation was performed in 100 (20%) and nasogastric or orogastric intubation was performed in 95 (19%). In 180 (35%) patients, surgery was performed with use of general anesthesia within 24 hours of the CT examination. Types of surgery performed included orthopedic in 108 patients, neurologic (including surgery of the spine) in 48 patients, laparotomy in 20 patients, and thoracotomy in four patients. Some patients underwent multiple surgical procedures.

In 13 (3%) patients, postoperative atelectasis or pneumonia was diagnosed, while the acute lung disease was attributed to congestive heart failure and diffuse respiratory distress syndrome in one patient each. In 18 (4%) patients, confirmed or clinically diagnosed aspiration pneumonitis was present. In 13 (72%) of these 18 patients, the aspiration event preceded hospitalization and CT examination, and all of these patients underwent endotracheal and nasogastric intubation before they arrived at the hospital. In five patients, aspiration pneumonitis occurred at some interval after CT, but in none of these patients was the pneumonitis related to the CT procedure. In one patient, cardiopulmonary deterioration occurred 5 days after CT, and fatal aspiration of gastric contents occurred during attempted emergency resuscitation. In another patient, documented aspiration of gastric contents occurred 7 days after CT, attributable to progressive hepatic encephalopathy. In the other three patients, traumatic brain injuries were present and documented episodes of aspiration occurred at attempted feeding at intervals of days to weeks after CT; these patients were treated with gastrostomy tubes and tracheostomy.

In many additional patients, pulmonary abnormalities were noted on CT scans or chest radiographs. None of these patients had documented fever, clinical suspicion of aspiration, or a temporal relationship between aspiration and oral administration of contrast material for CT. Most radiologic abnormalities were attributable to traumatic lung injury or atelectasis related to splinting of the diaphragm. None of these patients required antibiotic therapy, supplemental oxygen, or other specific pulmonary care.

Bowel injuries were confirmed surgically in 10 patients, and preoperative CT findings were definitive or strongly suggestive of bowel injury in seven of these patients.

DISCUSSION

Opacification of the bowel lumen with radiopaque contrast material is an important technical aid in diagnosis of traumatic injuries to the bowel or pancreas. Extravasation of enteric contrast material is an unequivocal sign of bowel laceration, and intramural hematoma is more easily recognized when the bowel lumen is opacified. Peripancreatic edema or hemorrhage is an important sign of pancreatic trauma but can be simulated by unopacified bowel loops (1). The use of oral contrast material is a standard and accepted part of the CT protocol for diagnosis of other pathologic conditions of the pancreas and bowel and should be part of the trauma CT protocol as well.

Bowel and mesenteric injuries are found in only about 5% of all patients who undergo laparotomy after blunt abdominal trauma (2); however, these injuries can cause life-threatening bleeding or peritonitis. During the 8-month period of our investigation, bowel injuries were confirmed surgically in 10 patients, and preoperative CT findings were definitive or strongly suggestive of bowel injury in seven of these patients. Because bowel injuries are uncommon, a much larger interval and number of patients would be necessary to evaluate the sensitivity and specificity of CT; this study is currently under way.

Other than anecdotal and speculative reports (8,9), to our knowledge there have been no investigative reports published that have demonstrated adverse effects from the use of oral contrast material for CT performed for evaluation of abdominal trauma. Conversely, we studied extensively a total of 1,016 patients in our current investigation combined with our previous study and have documented the safety of oral contrast material used in CT.

In our previous study (7) of 506 patients in whom CT was performed for assessment of abdominal trauma, there was only one case of aspiration pneumonitis attributable to CT. Aspiration pneumonitis occurred in a patient in whom inadvertent insertion of the nasogastric tube into the right mainstem bronchus rather than the stomach was not detected, and a small amount of the oral contrast material was administered accidentally into the lung by means of the tube. The patient developed acute lung infiltration that cleared rapidly over the course of 1 week. Antibiotics were administered parenterally, the fever subsided in 5 days, and the patient was discharged in good condition from the hospital.

Part of the controversy with regard to the use of oral contrast material for trauma patients may be due to a misperception about the nature of the contrast material. We use an undiluted preparation of diatrizoate meglumine and sodium for fluoroscopic upper gastrointestinal series and enema examinations. Gastroview and Gastrografin (Squibb, Princeton, NJ) are essentially identical preparations of iodinated diatrizoate salts. Even in the undiluted form, these preparations have a neutral pH. A 1.0:4.6 dilution is an isotonic preparation containing 16.5% diatrizoate salts. We use a 1:40 dilution of diatrizoate meglumine and sodium solution, which has a neutral pH and is nonhypertonic, as an oral contrast material for CT. Aspiration of the undiluted hypertonic solution is unquestionably harmful, leading to serious pulmonary complications including pulmonary edema or pulmonitis and osmotic effusion. Although aspiration is always a concern, the diluted solution used as an oral contrast material for CT is much less likely to be harmful. The one patient in our previous series in whom contrast material was administered directly into the right lung by means of a misplaced nasogastric tube probably represents a "worst case scenario." Despite this event, the patient had a rapid and uneventful recovery within 5 days.

Although the order "nulla per os," or NPO, has been a standard in preoperative preparation, the wisdom of this order has been questioned recently. The ingestion of clear liquids even shortly before surgery does not appear to alter the volume or pH of gastric contents when anesthetic agents are administered, and many institutions have now changed their policies to allow patients to ingest clear fluids up to 2 hours before elective surgery (10,11).

An alternative oral contrast agent for CT is a dilute suspension of barium. We routinely use these commercially available products in elective CT of the abdomen and pelvis because they provide consistent and persistent opacification of the bowel lumen. Potential disadvantages in the trauma setting include the theoretical risk of introducing barium into the peritoneal cavity through a lacerated bowel and the tendency of barium to become inspissated in the colon in patients who have delayed transit time of contrast material in the bowel. This delayed transit time is encountered frequently in trauma patients.

For elective abdominal CT, we use a large volume of oral contrast material, up to 1,200 mL administered over a 60–90-minute period before initiation of scanning. Such a large volume is unnecessary and contraindicated in the acutely ill patient in need of urgent evaluation. Opacification of the stomach and proximal small bowel is the most important objective because the duodenum and proximal jejunum are the most commonly injured segments of the bowel from blunt trauma and because unopacified jejunal loops may simulate pathologic conditions of the pancreas (1–6). One advantage of the iodinated diatrizoate preparations is that they stimulate bowel peristalsis to a mild degree. Stimulation of bowel peristalsis results in better opacification of more segments of bowel than would be achievable with the barium sulfate preparations when only a short interval is available between oral administration of contrast material and initiation of CT. We do not find it necessary to delay the CT examination to achieve more complete opacification of bowel. When the contrast agent is administered while the patient is still in the emergency department, the CT examination can be completed as soon as the initial evaluation and resuscitation are completed.

The low occurrence of aspiration in our current series may be attributable to the care the patients received outside the radiology department rather than any special techniques used by the radiologic technologists or radiologists. In the prehospital phase of care, paramedics routinely intubate the trachea of patients with decreased sensorium, substantial chest trauma, difficulty in maintaining an open airway, or difficulty in breathing. Despite this aggressive prehospital care, 13 (3%) cases of aspiration occurred in the prehospital phase.

As part of the standard airway evaluation (according to the Advanced Trauma Life Support protocol) (12) in our emergency department, intubation is performed to protect the airway and support ventilation in all patients with a decreased level of consciousness or difficulty with breathing. In addition, if the patient is agitated and requires an emergent CT examination, the trachea is intubated and a muscle relaxant is used to control agitation while the patient is in the scanner and to allow rapid evaluation of the patient. Our protocol for rapid sequence intubation is described in standard trauma anesthesia textbooks and articles (13,14). After endotracheal intubation is performed, a nasogastric or orogastric tube is placed to enable assessment for bleeding and decompression of the stomach. This tube may then be used to administer the oral contrast material. If the patient requires emergency surgery, maintenance of the airway is of the utmost concern to the anesthesiologist. Regional anesthesia, conscious endotracheal intubation, or rapid-sequence induction and intubation as described previously are used. This aggressive airway control in the emergency department and operating room helped account for the low occurrence of aspiration in our current and previous series.

In conclusion, use of contrast material for stomach and bowel opacification during CT for assessment of abdominal trauma appears to be safe. Alert, cooperative patients may drink the diluted aqueous preparation, while in obtunded or uncooperative patients contrast material is administered by means of a nasogastric tube after the airway is controlled with endotracheal intubation. Proper preparation and administration of contrast material and control of the patient's airway are essential to ensure the safety of this procedure. ■

References

1. Jeffrey RB Jr, Federle MP. Computed tomography of pancreatic trauma. Radiology 1983; 147:491–494.
2. Rizzo MJ, Federle MP, Griffiths GB. Bowel and mesenteric imaging following blunt abdominal trauma: evaluation with CT. Radiology 1989; 173:143–148.
3. Donohue JH, Federle MP, Griffiths BG, et al. Computed tomography in the diagnosis of blunt intestinal and mesenteric injuries. J Trauma 1987; 27:11–17.
4. Nghiem HV, Jeffrey RB Jr, Mindelzun RE. CT of blunt trauma to the bowel and mesentery. AJR 1993; 160:53–58.
5. Kunin JR, Korobkin M, Ellis JH, et al. Duodenal injuries caused by blunt abdominal trauma: value of CT in differentiating perforation from hematoma. AJR 1993; 160: 1221–1223.
6. Mirvis S, Gens D, Shanmuganathan K. Rupture of the bowel after blunt abdominal trauma: diagnosis with CT. AJR 1992; 159: 1217–1221.
7. Federle MP, Peitzman A, Krugh J. Use of oral contrast material in abdominal trauma CT scans: is it dangerous? J Trauma 1995; 38:57–53.
8. Trulzsch DV, Penmesta A, Karim A, Evans DA. Gastrografin-induced aspiration pneumonia: a lethal complication of computed tomography. South Med J 1992; 85: 1255–1256.
9. Clancy TV, Ragozzino MW, Ramshaw D, Churchill MP, Covington DL, Maxwell JG. Oral contrast is not necessary in the evaluation of blunt abdominal trauma by computed tomography. Am J Surg 1993; 166: 680–685.
10. Goodwin AP, Rowe WL, Ogg TW, Samaan A. Oral fluids prior to day surgery: the effect of shortening the preoperative fluid fast on postoperative morbidity. Anesthesia 1991; 46:1066–1068.
11. Phillips S, Hutchinson S, Davidson T. Preoperative drinking does not affect gastric contents. Br J Anaesth 1991; 38:425–429.
12. American College of Surgeons. Advanced trauma life support. Chicago, Ill: American College of Surgeons, 1993.
13. Grande CM, ed. Textbook of trauma anesthesia and critical care. St Louis, Mo: Mosby, 1993.
14. Sellick BA. Cricoid pressure to control regurgitation of stomach contents during induction of anaesthesia. Lancet 1961; 2:404.

Book Review

Imaging of Soft Tissue Tumors

Mark Kransdorf, MD, and Mark D. Murphey, MD

Philadelphia, Pa: W.B. Saunders & Co, 1997. ISBN 0-7216-6069-X. Cloth, $145.00; pp 436; 1,109 figures; tables.

Imaging of Soft Tissue Tumors

Edited by Arthur M. De Schepper, MD, PhD, Paul M. Parizel, MD, PhD, Frank Ramon, MD, Luc De Beuckeleer, MD, and Jan E. Vandevenne, MD

Brooklyn, NY: Springer-Verlag New York, Inc, 1997. ISBN 3-540-61392-7. Cloth, $198.00; pp 390; 285 figures; tables.

When it rains, it pours. The drought in the literature on soft-tissue tumor imaging has been lengthy; therefore, I was pleasantly stunned by the arrival of not one, but two marvelous textbooks with identical titles that address the subject. The only other comprehensive textbook that deals with the imaging of soft-tissue tumors is *Soft Tissue Tumors*, 3rd ed by Franz M. Enzinger, MD, and Sharon E. Weiss, MD, eds (St Louis, Mo:Mosby–Year Book, 1994), which is a heavy and dated tome that includes extensive pathologic correlation and is not at all a radiologist's delight. This book is only a reference guide for those who seek the optimal approach to identification of a soft-tissue tumor.

The biggest problem I faced during my review of the two books was deciding which was better. Determining which book was really suited to my needs was like looking through the graduated lenses at the optometrist's office.

The textbook of Drs Kransdorf and Murphey presents over 31,000 soft-tissue tumors that have been seen during 10 years at the Armed Forces Institute of Pathology. These cases are heavily annotated and meticulously organized no doubt by contributing guest residents. This textbook is thus statistically superior, more academic, and comprehensive than the textbook of De Schepper et al. After a singular introductory chapter, the authors expound on various soft-tissue tumors that are classified in the usual fashion. There is an immensely helpful table (3-1) featuring specific diagnoses that can be made with MR imaging. Coccidioidomycosis of the ankle is amusingly referred to as "desert rheumatism," and the function of sonography in the diagnosis of adventitial cystic disease is not mentioned; however, these are minor criticisms of an excellent book.

The book of De Schepper et al is based on the limited pool of a thousand contributions from 29 coinvestigators at the European Congress of Radiology in 1993. The continental imaging approach is refreshing (only four of the textbook's contributors are American) and is especially obvious in the chapters, "Color Doppler Sonography" and "Dynamic Contrast-enhanced MR Imaging." Less than half of the book deals with introductory and general remarks about the imaging approach advocated. I fail to understand why so many authors routinely review MR physics but uniformly ignore the principles of Doppler sonography and computed tomography. All categories of soft-tissue tumors are dealt with in the standard fashion. There are unique, although brief, closing chapters entitled "Soft Tissue Metastasis" and "Imaging after Treatment."

Neither book is rich in algorithms, flow charts, tables, or lists of differential diagnoses, which is disappointing only because we like our information in the form of familiar little aliquots. All modalities are fairly represented, including isotope studies. The photoreproductions are of a consistently high quality in both textbooks. Usually the tumors are fairly obvious so that even my mother could identify them, and subtle soft-tissue pathologic findings have been annotated as needed. The authors of both books have wisely avoided padding their pages with too many photographs of pathologic slides; their relative absence, in my eyes, is most enjoyable.

The textbook of Drs Kransdorf and Murphey is definitely recommended to fill the void in the soft-tissue imaging section of the departmental library—although, both books cover that dusty, empty space on the shelf nearly equally well.

Reviewed by Sundeep M. Nayak, MD

Osman Cay, MD • Jonathan B. Kruskal, MD, PhD • Imad Nasser, MD • Peter Thomas, PhD
Melvin E. Clouse, MD

Liver Metastases from Colorectal Cancer: Drug Delivery with Liposome-encapsulated Doxorubicin[1]

PURPOSE: To evaluate the intratumoral distribution of liposome-encapsulated doxorubicin.

MATERIALS AND METHODS: Tumor-bearing livers of 24 mice were studied with in vivo fluorescence and electron microscopy after injection of liposomal doxorubicin in the hepatic artery, portal vein, or tail vein. Distribution and uptake of liposomes and doxorubicin in tumors were compared at 5, 30, and 60 minutes after injection. In vitro evaluation of uptake of doxorubicin in Kupffer cells and in human colorectal cancer cells incubated under normoxic and hypoxic conditions for 5, 30, and 60 minutes was performed with fluorescence microscopy.

RESULTS: Doxorubicin autofluorescence was seen in tumors 30 minutes after intraarterial and intraportal injection and was statistically significantly greater at 60 minutes ($P <$ .001). Liposomes were observed in small tumors (diameter < 300 μm) and were trapped in Kupffer cells around larger, hypovascular tumors. Electron microscopy findings confirmed intracytoplasmic, perinuclear uptake of liposomes in tumor cells. In vitro, a higher proportion of doxorubicin was seen in cancer cells (92%) than in Kupffer cells (75%) after 60 minutes incubation.

CONCLUSION: Liposomal doxorubicin can be reliably delivered to liver metastases via the hepatic artery, eliminating need for tumor embolization. Further evaluation is warranted, and the drug may be useful for treating patients with unresectable liver metastases.

Liposomes have long been used for the intravascular transport of pharmacologically active agents (1). These vesicles, which range in diameter from 25 Å (2.5 nm) to 20 μm, are composed of phospholipid bilayers surrounding an aqueous compartment. Depending on the hydrophilic or hydrophobic nature of the liposomes, drugs, contrast agents, virus particles, genes, or even plasmids can be trapped in the aqueous or membrane phases for delivery to various sites throughout the body (2–8). The majority of conventional liposomes are rapidly cleared from the blood by means of reticuloendothelial cells in the lungs, spleen, and other solid organs such as the liver and bone marrow (9–11). This clearance, which occurs in minutes, limits the number of liposomes and thus the amount of the drug that reaches specific target sites beyond those of primary reticuloendothelial surveillance.

Recently, a new polymer-coated, sterically stabilized liposome formulation has been synthesized (12–14), the so-called "stealth" liposome (15), which has a prolonged retention within the vascular pool, due partly to reduced reticuloendothelial uptake of the liposomes. The polyethylene glycol coating on these liposomes inhibits or at least reduces phagocytosis of liposomes in the liver and spleen. In addition, this stabilized formulation demonstrates increased uptake in solid tumors (16–18), which is believed to result in part from reduced phagocytosis of the liposomes.

Doxorubicin can be encapsulated in these stabilized liposomes, which have been used as an anticancer delivery system for targeting various tumors in experimental animal models (18–20). Provisional results from these studies demonstrated enhanced uptake of liposomes in and around solid animal tumors, as well as antitumor activity, indicated by both reduction in tumor size and prolonged animal survival. Moreover, and more important, targeting of liposomes to the tumor site was associated with a concomitant decrease in systemic toxicity (16,21), which is a favorable characteristic given the side effects associated with systemic or intraarterial doxorubicin administration. Because these liposomes appear to offer several advantages over currently used transcatheter tumor targeting and drug-delivery techniques (such as intraarterial chemoembolization techniques that use ethiodol-doxorubicin mixtures), we explored the feasibility of using liposomal doxorubicin for this purpose.

The purpose of this study was to evaluate and compare the intrahepatic and intratumoral biologic distribution of stabilized doxorubicin-encapsulated liposomes (DOX-SL; Sequus Pharmaceuticals, Menlo Park, Calif) after intravenous, intra–portal venous, and intraarterial administration, by using our established mouse model of hepatic colorectal cancer metastases (22).

Index terms: Liposomes • Liver neoplasms, chemotherapeutic infusion, 761.1266 • Liver neoplasms, secondary, 761.3327

Radiology 1997; 205:95–101

[1] From the Departments of Radiological Sciences (O.C., J.K., P.T., M.E.C.) and Pathology (I.N.), Beth Israel Deaconess Medical Center and Harvard Medical School, 1 Deaconess Rd, Boston MA 02215. From the 1996 RSNA scientific assembly. Received February 10, 1997; revision requested March 26; revision received June 13; accepted June 19. **Address reprint requests to** O.C. O.C. supported in part by a grant from the Cardiovascular and Interventional Radiology Research Foundation.

This study differs from previous studies (23–25) in that we directly imaged liver tumors and tumor microcirculation with in vivo video microscopy of exteriorized tumor-bearing livers, which took advantage of the autofluorescent properties of doxorubicin. Dynamic in vivo observations were compared with electron microscopy findings in the same tumors and with liposome-uptake studies in normoxic and hypoxic in vitro cultures of CX-1 colorectal cancer cells and Kupffer cells.

MATERIALS AND METHODS

Animal Studies

Experiments were performed with adult athymic nude mice (mean weight, 20 g) according to a protocol approved by our institutional animal care and use committee. Animals were housed under conditions of controlled temperature and humidity and were allowed ad libitum access to water and laboratory chow.

Animal Tumor Model

Human CX-1 colorectal cancer cells (5×10^6 cells in a solution of 0.5 mL phosphate buffered saline, pH 7.4), a moderately to well-differentiated human colorectal cancer line, were derived from the HT-29 cell line and were provided by L. B. Chen, PhD (Dana-Farber Institute, Boston, Mass). These cells were maintained in RPMI 1640 medium (Gibco Laboratories Life Technologies, Grand Island, NY) with 10% fetal bovine serum (Sigma Chemical, St Louis, Mo), 1% L-glutamine (Gibco Laboratories Life Technologies), 100 U of penicillin-G (Gibco Laboratories Life Technologies) per milliliter, and 100 mg of streptomycin (Gibco Laboratories Life Technologies) per milliliter. After induction of anesthesia (intraperitoneal injection of 30 mg of sodium pentobarbital per kilogram of body weight [mg/kg]), a small, left subcostal incision was performed, and 0.1 mL of a solution that contained 1×10^6 CX-1 cells was injected into the spleen of the mice.

In Vivo Video Microscopy

Seven days after the intrasplenic inoculation of tumor cells, anesthesia was induced by using sodium pentobarbital (30 mg/kg delivered intraperitoneally) and a midline abdominal wall incision was performed. The falciform ligament was dissected to avoid excessive movement of the liver lobes during respiration. Mice were placed on their left side on a modified microscopy stage, and the liver was carefully placed on an angled quartz crystal (Precision Instruments, Wakefield, Mass), as we have previously described (22,26). A standard compound binocular microscope (Optiphot; Nikon, Tokyo, Japan) was modified for in vivo microscopy and was equipped for transillumination and fluorescence microscopy. The periphery of the left lateral liver lobe was transilluminated with a 50-W monochromatic halogen lamp bulb with filters that prevent transmission of heat to the exposed liver. By using ×10 and ×40 water-immersion objectives (Nikon) and a zoom lens, images of different periportal, centrilobular, and pericentral regions within peripheral and central hepatic lobules were directly observed and were recorded on video tape. A combination epifluorescence filter (excitation level of 510–560 nm and emission level of more than 580 nm) (G1-B; Nikon) was used to visualize the location and distribution of liposome-encapsulated autofluorescent doxorubicin in each region.

Images were continuously recorded (CCD-72 video camera, DAGE/MTI, Michigan City, Ind) on SVHS video tape by using an SVHS video tape recorder (Panasonic, Tokyo, Japan) for subsequent data and image analysis and reformation. From these video tapes, images were captured with a computer (Power Mac 6400; Apple Computer, Cupertino, Calif) equipped with real-time video frame-grabbing and processing hardware (Pixelpipe; Perceptics, Knoxville, Tenn) for subsequent analysis with image analysis software (NIH Image 1.60; National Institutes of Health, Bethesda, Md).

In Vivo Biologic Distribution of Doxorubicin

Twenty-four mice (eight mice per group) were randomly assigned to receive either an intraarterial, intraportal, or tail vein injection of liposomal doxorubicin (20 mg doxorubicin in a 10 mL solution of sodium chloride [NaCl]). The dose level was 8 mg/kg and was diluted to a constant volume of 200 mL/kg with 0.9% sodium chloride.

For intraarterial injections, the gastroduodenal artery was exposed and dissected. By using a fine silicone elastomer cannula (PE Rose TPE 020x033; Balt Extrusion), the gastroduodenal artery was cannulated hepatopetally, as described previously (27). The catheter tip was positioned below the bifurcation of the gastroduodenal and proper hepatic arteries. Intraportal and tail vein injections were performed with a 30-gauge needle inserted directly in the vein. Immediately after the intraportal injection, a cotton-tipped applicator stick was gently applied to the puncture site until hemostasis was complete.

By using our established high-resolution in vivo microscopic techniques (22,26), microvascular flow patterns, tumor vasculature, and the distribution and behavior of liposomal doxorubicin in and around tumors and normal liver parenchyma were evaluated and compared in different periportal, centrilobular, and pericentral regions within peripheral and central hepatic lobules. Data were continuously recorded for the duration of each experiment and images were captured and analyzed 5, 30, and 60 minutes after doxorubicin injection.

Each microscopy field was first transilluminated and observed under direct light; next, epifluorescence imaging of the same field was performed to correlate tumor location and microvasculature with the presence of autofluorescent liposomal doxorubicin in and around the tumors. Images were then analyzed with the image analysis software. The autofluorescent light intensity of the encapsulated doxorubicin in tumors was measured and compared in terms of mean light intensity (mean value from four regions in each tumor nodule) relative to adjacent, equal-sized non–tumor-containing parenchyma. These measurements were obtained 5, 30, and 60 minutes after injection.

In Vitro Uptake of Doxorubicin in Isolated CX-1 Tumor Cells and in Kupffer Cells

Tumor cell preparations.—The CX-1 human colon carcinoma cell line, prepared similarly to the suspension administered to the mice, was incubated and grown in flasks until the cells became confluent. Growth medium (RPMI 1640 with 10% fetal calf serum, supplemented with L-glutamine, penicillin, and streptomycin) was removed from the flasks, and the cells were washed once with a solution of phosphate-buffered saline with calcium and magnesium. Cells were dissociated in a cell-dissociation solution (Sigma Chemical) and were incubated for 10 minutes at 37°C. Thereafter, cells were removed by flushing with a 10-cm^3 syringe and were centrifuged at 1,100 revolutions per minute for 5 minutes. Supernatant fluid was removed from the centrifuge tube, and the pellet was dispersed. Growth medium was added, and 50 µL of the tumor cell solution was placed on a Petri dish. Four milliliters of medium were added to the Petri dish, and cells were incubated for 2 hours at 37°C. At the end of the incubation period, the cells were washed with phosphate-buffered saline, and growth medium was added before liposomes were added to the Petri dishes.

Normoxic incubation of tumor cells with doxorubicin.—A 0.2-mL solution of liposomal doxorubicin (20 mg doxorubicin hydrochloride in 10 mL NaCl) was incubated with CX-1 tumor cells at 37°C for 5, 30, or 60 minutes. After the respective incubation periods, the Petri dishes were removed from the incubator, and tumor cells were directly observed microscopically. Tumor cells were first transilluminated with direct light in 10 randomly selected microscopy fields. Next, the liposomal autofluorescent doxorubicin uptake in tumor cells in each field was visualized with the epifluorescence filter combination. Tumor cells observed with direct light were counted and compared with the number of fluorescent tumor cells in the same field. The rate of autofluorescent doxorubicin uptake was determined in relation to the incubation period of tumor cells treated with liposomal doxorubicin.

Hypoxic incubation of tumor cells with doxorubicin.—Petri dishes that contained single and confluent CX-1 tumor cells were transferred to an oxygen depleted chamber. Growth medium (RPMI 1640 with 10% fetal calf serum, supplemented with L-glutamine, penicillin, and streptomycin) in Petri dishes was exchanged with an identical but oxygen-depleted medium. Hypoxia (approximately 100 ppm oxygen) was achieved by using an anaerobic chamber (Bactron IV; Sheldon Enterprises, Clearwater, Fla) with a self-contained incubator unit that uses an injected atmosphere of 5% hydrogen-2, 5% carbon dioxide, 90% nitrogen-2 and a palladium catalyst. A 0.2 mL solution of liposomal doxorubicin (20 mg doxorubicin hydrochloride in 10 mL NaCl) was added to Petri dishes, and tumor cells were incubated for 5, 30, and 60 minutes in the hypoxic chamber. After each incubation period, tumor cells were located and counted in 10 randomly selected microscopy fields, as described earlier in this section. The rate of uptake (in terms of percentage) of liposomal doxorubicin under normoxic conditions was compared with that under hypoxic conditions.

Incubation of Kupffer cells with doxorubicin.—Male Sprague-Dawley rats (weight, 300–400 g) were food deprived overnight, and the livers were perfused and incubated with 0.05% collagenase (Sigma Chemical); the livers were minced by means of three centrifugations (50 *g* for 5 minutes each) to remove hepatocytes. The supernatant was retained, and the isolation of Kupffer cells was achieved by means of centrifugation at 1,400 *g* for 5 minutes at room temperature in a 17.5% solution of metrizamide (Accurate Chemicals and Scientific, Westbury, NY) in a Gey balanced-salt solution (Gibco Laboratories Life Technologies). Cell suspensions were incubated with liposomal doxorubicin for 5, 30, and 60 minutes. Uptake of liposomes by Kupffer cells was measured in 10 randomly selected microscopy fields, as described earlier. The rate of uptake of liposomes in the Kupffer cells and in the CX-1 tumor cells was compared for the three incubation periods.

Electron Microscopy

Tumor tissue samples were submitted fresh in Karnovsky fixative (2% paraformaldehyde and 1% glutaraldehyde [Ted Pella, Redding, Calif] with 0.2 M [mol/L] cacodylate [Ted Pella] buffer). After fixation, tissue was embedded in plastic blocks (Eponate; Ted Pella), and 90–100-nm-thick sections were cut. The sections were stained with lead citrate and uranyl acetate for transmission electron microscopy.

Statistical Analyses

The Student *t* test was used to compare the groups of mice in terms of fluorescent activity in tumors. Statistically significant differences were inferred at an overall confidence level of 95%.

RESULTS

Animal Tumor Studies

Intrasplenic injection of 2×10^6 CX-1 human colorectal cancer cells into athymic nude mice resulted in the spontaneous growth of multiple hypo- or avascular metastatic tumors in all livers within 7 days of injection. These spontaneous metastases were distributed throughout the liver and were dispersed equally between the periportal, centrilobular and pericentral zones of each peripheral lobule studied. Data from each inoculated mouse were included in this study, and each mouse liver had tumors in peripheral lobules that could easily be exteriorized (to permit microscopic observation) without any resulting alterations in hepatic and, specifically, intratumoral microvascular blood flow. In addition, microsurgical manipulations such as hepatic artery or portal vein cannulation were performed before liver exteriorization to prevent local microvascular alterations or intrahepatic shunting. In each mouse liver, direct in vivo microscopic observations of at least four tumors (mean, 5 tumors per mouse; range, 3–6 tumors) located in the exteriorized left lateral peripheral lobules were performed in each mouse.

Route of Injection of Doxorubicin

Five minutes after injection into the hepatic artery, the portal vein, or the tail vein, no visible fluorescent activity was observed in the hepatic intravascular or parenchymal compartment; no fluorescent accumulation was observed in tumors, hepatocytes, Kupffer cells, sinusoidal endothelial cells, or the subendothelial spaces of Disse.

Thirty minutes after intraarterial or intraportal injection, focal spots of fluorescence activity ($n = 50$) were observed in exteriorized livers; the areas of activity corresponded to the tumor nodules and to the peritumoral vasculature immediately adjacent to the tumors. These observations were confirmed with contemporaneous dual-phase light (transillumination) and fluorescent microscopic observation. Fluorescence activity in the peritumoral vessels arose from distended portovenous collateral channels and neovessels that supplied the tumor nodules. Accumulation of fluorescence activity was observed in all peripheral tumors larger than 0.1 mm in diameter that were seen at light microscopy.

The zonal biologic distribution of liposomes was evaluated. Uptake of liposomal doxorubicin by multiple tumor nodules (Fig 1) was observed in both the periportal and centrilobular zones, with accumulation in tumors in or around terminal portal venules and in the centrilobular sinusoids, respectively. No focal accumulation of liposomal doxorubicin was observed in nontumorous, normal liver parenchyma.

The mean fluorescent intensity ± 1 standard error of the mean in tumor nodules (81 ± 27) that took up liposomes ($n = 50$) was statistically significantly higher ($P < .03$) than that in adjacent non–tumor-containing liver parenchyma (62 ± 20) at 30 minutes after intraarterial or intraportal administration of liposomes (Table). Conversely, no fluorescent activity was observed in tumors or in normal liver parenchyma 30 minutes after systemic (tail vein) administration of the drug.

Sixty minutes after intraarterial or intraportal injection, fluorescent spots ($n = 50$), which represented accumulation of liposomal doxorubicin, were observed in all microscopy fields. These spots corresponded to metastatic tumors ($n = 50$) in the periportal (Fig 2), centrilobular (Fig 3), and pericentral regions. The mean fluorescent light intensity ± 1 standard error of the mean of tumors (119 ± 28) was statistically significantly higher ($P < .0001$) than that of nontumorous areas (82 ± 23), even when tumors were compared in terms of size and zonal distribution (Table). The rate of liposomal doxorubicin uptake in tumors was rapid after both intraarterial and intraportal injection.

The intratumoral distribution of fluorescence was evaluated and was correlated with tumor size and blood supply. There was a homogeneous distribution of fluorescence in small tumor nodules that had a diameter of 100–300 µm (Fig 2). Conversely, tumors larger than 300 µm in diameter were surrounded by a ring of fluorescent activity that arose from liposomes (Fig 4) in peritumoral portovenous collateral shunts, peripheral intratumoral neovessels, and activated phagocytic Kupffer cells in the sinusoids and portovenous collateral channels that surrounded tumors. In these larger metastases, intratumoral fluorescent activity was identified peripherally, with no accumulation in the central hypovascular or avascular regions.

No differences were observed when the intra- and peritumoral biologic distribution of fluorescent liposomes

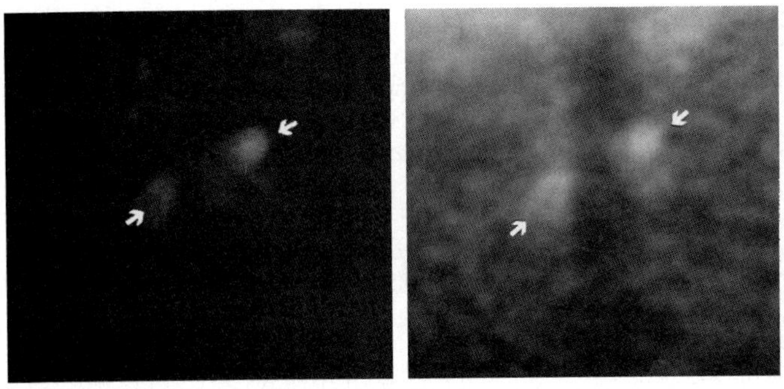

1a. 1b.

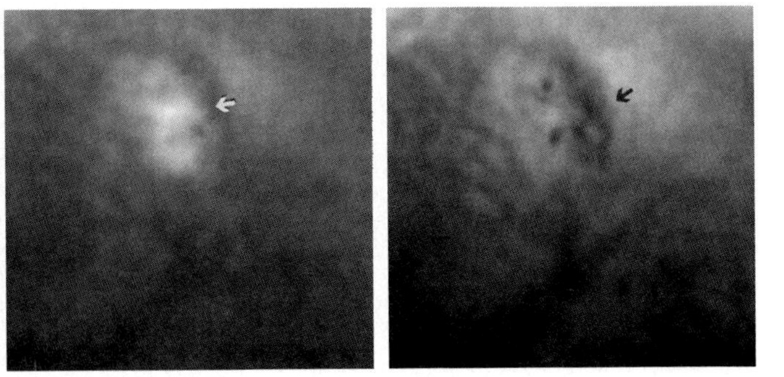

2a. 2b.

Figures 1, 2. **(1a)** In vivo video microscopy image of two colorectal cancer metastatic nodules (arrows) in a mouse liver at 60 minutes after the intraarterial injection of liposome-encapsulated doxorubicin. An epifluorescence filter was used to visualize liposomal autofluorescent doxorubicin as fluorescein spots. (Original magnification, ×150.) **(1b)** In vivo microscopy image of the same colorectal cancer metastatic nodules (arrows) as in **1a**. Transillumination of the same microscopy field in combination with the same epifluorescence filter that was used in **1a** showed that the location of the tumors was periportal. (Original magnification, ×150.) **(2a)** Photomicrograph obtained in vivo 60 minutes after intraarterial injection. Transillumination and the epifluorescence filter were used to visualize preferential uptake of liposome-encapsulated doxorubicin in the colorectal cancer metastatic nodule (arrow), as is evidenced by a homogeneous, diffuse fluorescein spot detected in the tumor. Focal fluorescein uptake was not observed in normal tissue. **(2b)** Transilluminated in vivo photomicrograph of the same field as in **2a** shows that the colorectal cancer metastatic tumor (arrow) is located periportally. (Original magnification, ×150.)

were compared after intraarterial and intraportal administration of doxorubicin. No differences were observed in comparisons among tumors of different sizes and in different zones of the peripheral lobules. Similarly, no difference in delivery or uptake of fluorescent activity was observed in normal liver parenchyma for these two routes of administration.

Within 60 minutes after the systemic (tail vein) administration of doxorubicin, only minimal accumulation was noted in normal livers and in liver tumors. No statistically significant differences were observed between tumor and background liver fluorescent activity after tail vein injection. When all microscopy fields were evaluated for the uptake of liposomes in tumor nodules, the accumulation of fluorescence in livers was not sufficient for evaluation of fluorescein intensity.

In Vitro Uptake of Doxorubicin in Metastatic CX-1 and Kupffer Cells

In vitro analysis of the uptake of liposomal doxorubicin by CX-1 cells and Kupffer cells was performed. Because we have previously demonstrated enhanced retention in tumors of doxorubicin-lopiodol mixtures under hypoxic conditions (26), these experiments were performed under normoxic and hypoxic conditions.

In vitro uptake of doxorubicin in CX-1 cells under hypoxic and normoxic conditions.—The density and percentage of cells that contained fluorescent spots gradually increased after the 5-minute time point in a constant linear relationship with the duration of incubation (Fig 5). At 30 minutes, 75% and 78% of fluorescent activity seen in 10 randomly selected microscopy fields was localized to the tumor cells under hypoxic and normoxic conditions, respectively, compared with 72% and 75% after 5 minutes of incubation under hypoxic and normoxic conditions, respectively. The percentage of tumor cells that contained fluorescent spots was highest (92%) in tumor cells incubated under normoxic conditions for 60 minutes. Sixty minutes of incubation of tumor cells with liposomal doxorubicin under hypoxic conditions did not result in increased uptake of liposomes by tumor cells (82%).

In vitro uptake of doxorubicin in CX-1 cells and Kupffer cells.—As was the case with the tumor cells, the accumulation of liposomes in or on the surface of Kupffer cells was correlated with the duration of incubation (Fig 5). The lowest percentage (61%) accumulation of liposomal doxorubicin in Kupffer cells was observed at 5 minutes incubation. Maximum accumulation of fluorescent spots within Kupffer cells (75%) was observed at 60 minutes incubation. The percentage of Kupffer cells that showed uptake of liposomal doxorubicin was less than the percentage of uptake in tumor cells (92%) for each corresponding incubation time.

Electron Microscopy Findings in Metastases after Liposome Delivery

Electron microscopy was performed with livers after intraarterial and intraportal delivery of liposomes. Intracytoplasmic, perinuclear, small vesicles, which corresponded to liposomes, were observed in CX-1 metastatic tumors after both intraarterial and intraportal (Fig 6) injections of liposomal doxorubicin.

Fluorescein Intensity after Intraarterial or Intraportal Injection of Doxorubicin in Mice

Liver Tissue	Time Point: 30 Minutes	60 Minutes
Tumorous ($n = 50$)	81 ± 27*	119 ± 28†
Nontumorous ($n = 50$)	62 ± 20	82 ± 23

Note.—Data are means ± 1 standard error of the mean.

* Fluorescein intensity in tumors was statistically significantly higher than that in nontumorous parenchyma ($P < .03$).

† Fluorescein intensity measured in tumorous tissue at 60 minutes was statistically significantly greater than that measured in nontumorous tissue ($P < .0001$) at 60 minutes and in tumorous tissue at 30 minutes ($P < .0001$).

DISCUSSION

Local-regional intraarterial administration of chemotherapeutic agents has long been used in patients with primary or metastatic liver tumors who were considered unsuitable candidates for surgery or as adjuvant therapy before surgery (28–32). Regional arterial delivery of anticancer drugs exploits a pathologic feature of certain metastatic liver tumors, namely, that such tumors derive the majority of their blood supply from neovessels arising from the hepatic artery (33). In addition, some drugs and delivery vehicles undergo substantial first-pass metabolism or extraction in the liver, which results in the local deposition of greater concentrations of these drugs than is possible with systemic administration.

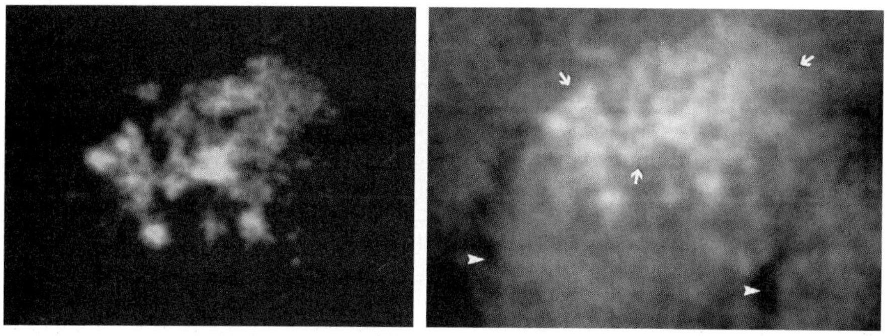

a. b.

Figure 3. **(a)** In vivo photomicrograph shows multiple colorectal cancer metastatic nodules. This image was obtained 60 minutes after portal venous injection by using the epifluorescence filter combination. (Original magnification, ×150.) **(b)** Transilluminated in vivo photomicrograph of the same field as in **a**. Multiple tumors, which appeared as fluorescein spots when the epifluorescence filter combination was used in **a**, were located in the centrilobular region of mouse liver. The colorectal cancer metastatic nodules (arrows) were located between two portal vein branches (arrowheads). There was no visible vascular structure observed in the tumors. The nodules preferentially took up the liposomal autofluorescent doxorubicin, whereas there was no detectable fluorescence observed in the normal liver parenchyma. (Original magnification, ×150.)

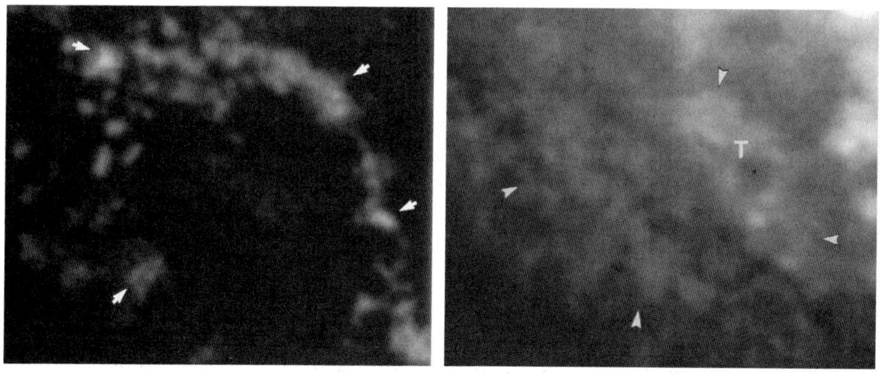

a. b.

Figure 4. **(a)** In vivo photomicrograph obtained with the epifluorescence filter 60 minutes after portal venous injection shows liposome-encapsulated autofluorescent doxorubicin, which is visualized as fluorescent spots in a circular form (arrows) in the microscopy field. (Original magnification, ×150.) **(b)** Transilluminated image of the same field as in **a** with no epifluorescence filter shows that the fluorescent spots (arrowheads) surround a colorectal cancer metastatic nodule (*T*). The tumor nodule, which is 520 μm in diameter, is located periportally and is surrounded by dilated portocentral vessels. (Original magnification, ×150.)

In the current study, we evaluated the intratumoral biologic distribution of a novel drug-delivery system whereby doxorubicin encapsulated in sterically stabilized liposomes was delivered to metastatic liver tumors. Unlike conventional liposomes, which are rapidly phagocytosed by reticuloendothelial cells throughout the body, these so-called stealth liposomes have a methoxy–polyethylene glycol coating attached to the outer membrane; the coating confers prolonged intravascular residence by means of reduction or inhibition of uptake by resident phagocytes in the body. In addition, these liposomes have enhanced transmembrane permeability, especially in tumors where neoangiogenesis has resulted in the formation of vessels with an abnormal endothelial lining. The combination of these two characteristics of prolonged intravascular residence and increased transendothelial permeability suggest, in theory, that these liposomes may provide an effective and novel delivery system for the targeting of hepatic metastases.

Indeed, we have demonstrated that sterically stabilized liposomes rapidly accumulate in and around hepatic metastases from colorectal cancer after intraarterial or intraportal injection with no substantial accumulation in normal liver parenchyma. Our data have demonstrated an additional mechanism that contributes to this localization: Liposomes are trapped by activated Kupffer cells in the peritumoral regions and within tumors.

Another form of local therapy for liver neoplasms is selective chemoembolization. With this technique, a mixture of iodized oil and a chemotherapeutic agent is selectively injected into the hepatic segment that contains a metastatic nodule. Treatment efficacy with this method depends largely on a rich tumor vascularity and focal deposition of emulsion in vessels at the tumor site. Dearterilization produces tumor necrosis, whereas a considerably high drug concentration is achieved in the tumor. In addition, we have previously demonstrated (26) that hypoxia further serves to localize drug deposition in the tumor cells. In this study, no differences were observed when liposome uptake in tumor cells was compared in vitro under hypoxic and normoxic conditions. These data suggest that an alternate mechanism or mechanisms may be involved in delivery of liposomes to tumor cells.

Sterically stabilized liposome–encapsulated doxorubicin has recently emerged as a promising antitumor drug-delivery system owing to the prolonged circulation time and high affinity for a variety of human tumor subtypes. Enhanced therapeutic indexes have been demonstrated with this drug-delivery system in a number of experimental tumor models (12,14, 16,19,21) and in studies with human subjects (10,25), compared with the therapeutic indexes demonstrated with the use of free doxorubicin or doxorubicin encapsulated in conventional liposomes. The liver is also a promising site for liposome delivery because a large percentage of liposomes administered intraarterially can become sequestered in the liver (8) and can reach targets outside the vasculature via the fenestrated sinusoidal endothelium; moreover, the reticuloendothelial cells of the liver can act as a reservoir for drug delivery to tumor cells.

In this study, we investigated selective targeting of liposomal doxorubicin to hepatic metastases from colorectal cancer in mice. Doxorubicin is an autofluorescent agent; therefore, there is no additional need for labeling of the liposomal doxorubicin for visualization in the livers when fluorescein microscopy is used. Our method permits a biologically compatible, realtime assessment in which other substances (eg, dyes, radioisotopes) do not interfere with drug-cell interactions.

In this study, liposomal doxorubicin was preferentially taken up by the tumor cells and nodules, relative to the uptake in normal liver tissue, after administration of the agent via the hepatic artery or the portal vein. Accumulation of the agent in and around the tumors was represented as fluorescent spots. The route of administration (hepatic artery or portal vein) had no effect on uptake of the liposomes by tumors. This finding is not surprising because the results of our previous studies (22,26) and of others' studies (34) have suggested that agents administered via the hepatic artery will eventually end up in the portal venous circulation by way of arterioportal shunts. In our earlier study (22), we demonstrated that intraarterial or intraportal injections of ethiodized oil–doxorubicin mixtures (with oil droplets smaller than 20 μm in diameter) resulted in similar patterns of oil-droplet accumulation in the centers of the tumors. In the present study, the liposomes we used had a diameter that was markedly smaller than 20 μm (80 nm to 2 μm).

We also performed systemic (tail vein) injections of liposomal doxorubicin in mice. In terms of the uptake of the liposomes by the tumor nodules, however, this method did not seem to be as effective as the local-regional administration of the agent. There were not enough fluorescent spots to determine the biologic distribution pattern of the agent in the mouse livers in this group. It is possible that after intravenous injection, the agent reaching the liver is less concentrated and therefore needs a longer period of time than 60 minutes, which was the cutoff point for our observations.

As is the case with the other liposomes, sterically stabilized liposomes are also taken up by the reticuloendothelial cells, especially in the liver (Kupffer cells). However, this uptake has been reported (15,16) to be lower compared with the uptake of conventional liposomes. This is consistent with the findings in our study that the percentage uptake in Kupffer cells (61%, 68%, and 75% at 5, 30, and 60 minutes incubation, respectively) was less than the uptake in CX-1 cells (75%, 78%, and 92% for the same incubation times under the same conditions).

In both the in vivo and the in vitro experiments, liposomes accumulated gradually in the tumor cells and nodules. The maximum accumulation rate of liposomes in tumor nodules, tumor cells, and Kupffer cells was reached within 60 minutes after injection in mice or incubation of the agent in vitro. Although we did not observe fluorescent spots 5 minutes after injection in our in vivo experiments, incubation of CX-1 cells under normoxic conditions at 37°C for 5 minutes with the same dose of the agent resulted in uptake of liposomes in 75% of the tumor cells. It is possible that after local-regional administration, liposomes were taken up in Kupffer cells around the tumor nodules and were then slowly released to the tumor interstitium, where fluorescent spots formed in the centers of the tumor nodules. This suggestion is also supported by our finding that within 30 minutes after injection via the hepatic artery or the portal vein, fluorescent spots that represented liposomal doxorubicin were first observed in the dilated portocentric vessels around the tumor nodules, with no or minimal liposomal accumulation in the tumor centers. Sixty minutes after injection, liposomes had accumulated in the nodules.

Another possible mechanism for the extravasation of liposomes into the tumor interstitium is leakage through the large gaps between endothelial cells (35,36). Tumor vessels generally have wide interendothelial junctions, large numbers of fenestrae and transendothelial channels, and a discontinuous or absent basement membrane (35,36), which may allow liposomes to extravasate through these channels and accumulate in the tumor interstitium. It is not known, however, if these extravasated liposomes are taken up in the tumor cells or stay within the extracellular space of tumor cells and release their contents. In our in vitro experiments, we observed fluorescent spots at microscopy, which indicated that liposomal doxorubicin incubated with CX-1 cells under normoxic or hypoxic conditions was indeed taken up in the tumor cells.

We recognize that fluorescence activity arises from the autofluorescent properties of doxorubicin, and not from the liposomes that encapsulate the aqueous drug. Because the ultimate goal of this project is to deliver high concentrations of drug to liver tumors, direct in vivo evaluation of the biologic distribution of doxorubicin is more relevant than determination of the ultimate deposition of the liposomes. An obvious limitation to this study is the use of animal models for studying targeted drug delivery to human tumor xenografts. Safety and efficacy experiments have been completed in animal and human studies, and the use of these liposomes has received U.S. Food and Drug Administration approval for treatment of certain malignancies, such as Kaposi sarcoma. To our knowledge, our results are the first to demonstrate intraarterial delivery of these liposomes to liver tumors. Consideration should now be given to the use of these liposomes for the targeting of liver tumors via the arterial route.

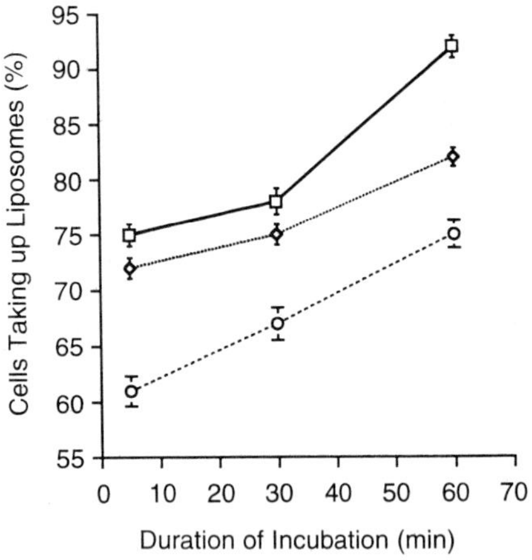

Figure 5. Graph shows the percentage uptake of liposome-encapsulated doxorubicin in CX-1 cells under normoxic (□) and hypoxic (◇) conditions and in Kupffer cells (○) under normoxic conditions. There was a gradual uptake of liposomes in tumor cells and in Kupffer cells, regardless of the availability of oxygen in the environment. Maximum uptake was achieved in tumor cells at 60 minutes incubation. The rate of uptake in Kupffer cells was less than that in the tumor cells.

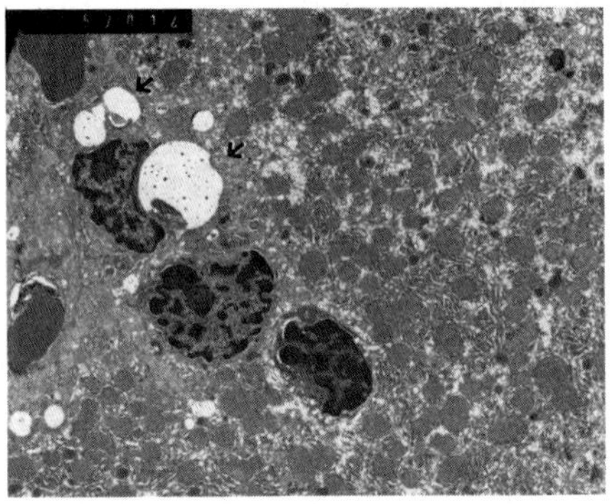

Figure 6. Electron photomicrograph of a metastatic tumor in the liver was obtained 60 minutes after intraportal administration of liposome-encapsulated doxorubicin. Vesicles that corresponded to liposomes (arrows) were observed in the cytoplasm and adjacent to the nucleus of a CX-1 cell. (Lead citrate and uranyl acetate stain; original magnification, ×12,500.)

We have demonstrated the utility of sterically stabilized liposomes in the delivery of drugs to tumor cells in vivo. Other potential diagnostic and therapeutic uses of these liposomes may include transcatheter delivery of radiologic contrast agents or even genes to tumors.

In conclusion, doxorubicin can be selectively targeted to hepatic metastases from colorectal cancer via the hepatic artery or the portal vein by using a novel delivery vector, the sterically stabilized liposome. These liposomes have a prolonged intravascular phase, due to reduced phagocytosis, and increased transendothelial permeability. These characteristics serve to increase the rate and extent of local liposomal uptake in tumors, which permits the delivery of high concentrations of doxorubicin. This results in a peak concentration of the drug in the tumor environment, with less accumulation in other organs, which thereby reduces systemic toxicity. Because our results are from an experimental animal tumor model, further clinical trials with local-regional administration of sterically stabilized liposomes encapsulating doxorubicin is a logical next step in the evaluation of the efficacy of this agent in the treatment of hepatic metastases from colorectal cancer in humans. ■

References

1. Bangham AD, Standish MM, Watkins JC. Diffusion of univalent ions across the lamellae of swollen phospholipids. J Mol Biol 1965; 13:238–252.
2. Sugerman MS, Perez-Soler R. Liposomes in the treatment of malignancy: a clinical perspective. Crit Rev Oncol Hematol 1992; 12:231–242.
3. Weinstein JN, Leserman LD. Liposomes as drug carriers in cancer therapy. Pharmacol Ther 1984; 24:207–233.
4. Vaage J, Mayhew E. Immunotherapy of a mouse mammary carcinoma by sustained release of IL-2. Int J Cancer 1991; 47:582–585.
5. Unger E, Cardenas D, Zerella A, Fajardo LL, Tilcock C. Biodistribution and clearance of liposomal gadolinium-DTPA. Invest Radiol 1990; 25:638–644.
6. Ostro MJ, Cullis PR. Use of liposomes as injectable-drug delivery systems. Am J Hosp Pharm 1989; 46:1576–1587.
7. Kim S. Liposomes as carriers of cancer chemotherapy: current status and future prospects. Drugs 1993; 46:618–638.
8. Wright KC, Kasi LP, Jahns MS, Hashimoto S, Wallace S. Liposome distribution after intravenous and selective intraarterial infusion in dogs. Radiology 1990; 176:691–694.
9. Hwang KJ, Luk KK, Beaumier PL. Hepatic uptake and degradation of unilamellar sphingomyelin/cholesterol liposomes: a kinetic study. Proc Natl Acad Sci USA 1980; 77:4030–4034.
10. Gabizon A, Chisin R, Amselem S, et al. Pharmacokinetic and imaging studies in patients receiving a formulation of liposome-associated adriamycin. Br J Cancer 1991; 64:1125–1132.
11. Papahadjopoulos D, Gabizon A. Targeting of liposomes to tumor cells in vivo. Ann NY Acad Sci 1983; 507:64–74.
12. Gabizon A, Papahadjopoulos D. Liposome formulations with prolonged circulation time in blood and enhanced uptake by tumors. Proc Natl Acad Sci USA 1988; 85: 6949–6953.
13. Lasic DD, Martin FJ, Gabizon A, Huang SK, Papahadjopoulos D. Sterically stabilized liposomes: a hypothesis on the molecular origin of the extended circulation times. Biochim Biophys Acta 1991; 1070:187–192.
14. Mayhew EG, Lasic D, Babbar S, Martin FJ. Pharmacokinetics and antitumor activity of epirubicin encapsulated in long-circulating liposomes incorporating a polyethylene glycol–derivatized phospholipid. Int J Cancer 1992; 51:302–309.
15. Allen TM. Stealth liposomes: avoiding reticuloendothelial uptake. In: Lopez-Berestein G, Fidler IJ, eds. Liposomes in the therapy of infectious diseases and cancer. New York, NY: Liss, 1989; 405–415.
16. Papahadjopoulos D, Allen D, Gabizon A, et al. Sterically stabilized liposomes: improvements in pharmacokinetics and antitumor efficacy. Proc Natl Acad Sci USA 1991; 88:11460–11464.
17. Working PK, Newman MS, Huang SK, et al. Pharmacokinetics, biodistribution and therapeutic efficacy of doxorubicin encapsulated in stealth liposomes (DOXIL). J Lipid Res 1994; 4:667–687.
18. Huang SK, Martin FJ, Jay G, Vogel J, Papahadjopoulos D, Friend DS. Extravasation and transcytosis of liposomes in Kaposi's sarcoma–like dermal lesions of transgenic mice bearing the HIV *TAT* gene. Am J Pathol 1993; 143:10–14.
19. Vaage J, Barbera-Guillem E, Abra R, Huang A, Working P. Tissue distribution and therapeutic effect of intravenous free or encapsulated liposomal doxorubicin on human prostate carcinoma xenografts. Cancer 1994; 73:1478–1483.
20. Vaage J, Donovan D, Mayhew E, Abra R, Huang A. Therapy of human ovarian carcinoma xenografts using doxorubicin encapsulated in sterically stabilized liposomes. Cancer 1993; 72:3671–3675.
21. Gabizon A, Shiota R, Papahadjopoulos D. Pharmacokinetics and tissue distribution of doxorubicin encapsulated in stable liposomes with long circulating times. J Natl Cancer Inst 1989; 81:1484–1488.
22. Cay O, Kruskal J, Thomas P, Clouse ME. Targeting of different ethiodized oil–doxorubicin mixtures to hypovascular hepatic metastases with intraarterial and intraportal injections. JVIR 1996; 7:409–417.
23. Zuo Y, Horikoshi I, Kasagi T, Gu X, Perez-Soler R. Organ distribution and antitumor activity of free and liposomal doxorubicin injected into the hepatic artery. Cancer Chemother Pharmacol 1993; 31:313–318.
24. Zuo Y, Horikoshi I, Ueno M, Gu X, Perez-Soler R. Targeting liver tumors by administering liposomal doxorubicin into hepatic artery. Int J Cancer 1992; 51:232–237.
25. Konno H, Maruo Y, Matsuda I, Nakamura S, Baba S. Intra-arterial liposomal adriamycin for metastatic adenocarcinoma of the liver. Eur Surg Res 1995; 27:301–306.
26. Kruskal JB, Hlatky L, Hahnfeldt P, Teramoto K, Stokes KS, Clouse ME. In vivo and in vitro analysis of the effectiveness of doxorubicin combined with temporary arterial occlusion in liver tumors. JVIR 1993; 4:741–747.
27. Cay O, Radnell O, Jeppsson B, Ahren B, Bengmark S. Inhibitory effect of 2-deoxy-D-glucose on liver tumor growth in rats. Cancer Res 1992; 52:5794–5796.
28. Clouse ME, Perry L, Stuart K, Stokes KR. Hepatic arterial chemoembolization for metastatic neuroendocrine tumors. Digestion 1994; 55(suppl 3):92–97.
29. Clouse ME, Stokes KR, Kruskal JB, et al. Chemoembolization for hepatocellular carcinoma: epinephrine followed by a doxorubicin–ethiodized oil emulsion and gelatin sponge powder. JVIR 1993; 4:717–725.
30. Kobayashi H, Inoue H, Shinohara S, et al. Intra-arterial injection of adriamycin/mitomycin C Lipiodol suspension in liver metastases. Acta Radiol 1987; 28:275–280.
31. Soulen MC. Chemoembolization of hepatic malignancies. Oncology 1994; 8:77–84.
32. Borener M, Castiglione M, Triller J, et al. Considerable side effects of chemoembolization for colorectal carcinoma metastatic to the liver. Ann Oncol 1992; 3:113–115.
33. Ackerman NB, Sien WM, Silverman NA. The blood supply of experimental liver metastases. Surgery 1972; 71:636–641.
34. Kan Z, Ivancev K, Lunderquist A. Peribiliary plexa: important pathways for shunting of iodized oil and silicon rubber solution from the hepatic artery to the portal vein. Invest Radiol 1994; 29:671–676.
35. Leunig M, Yuan F, Menger MD, et al. Angiogenesis, microvascular architecture, microhemodynamics, and interstitial fluid pressure during early growth of human adenocarcinoma LS174T in SCID mice. Cancer Res 1992; 52:6553–6560.
36. Jain RK. Transport of molecules across tumor vasculature. Cancer Metastasis Rev 1987; 6:559–593.

Book Review

Biliary Tract Radiology

Plinio Rossi, MD, and Mario Bezzi, MD

Brooklyn, NY: Springer-Verlag New York, Inc, 1997. ISBN 3-540-58776-4. Cloth, $236.00; pp 427; 362 figures; tables.

Drs Rossi and Bezzi, with the help of an impressive international group of well-known American and European experts, have edited a superb, up-to-date book that contains an almost unique comprehensive approach to imaging of the gallbladder and biliary ducts. The book provides in-depth coverage of diagnostic and interventional imaging of the biliary tract, including percutaneous and endoscopic techniques. The book is subdivided into three sections and 31 chapters; every chapter presents a well-balanced combination of personal experience and an academic review of the literature. The illustrations are of optimal quality, and drawings are used when necessary. The text is concise and well organized. Recent (up to 1995), relevant references are included.

The first section includes four chapters, which cover the surgical and radiologic anatomic structure of the biliary tree. In this first section, variations of biliary anatomic structures that may have surgical or endoscopic implications are well described with use of well-established imaging techniques, such as percutaneous cholangiography and the most recent imaging techniques (including magnetic resonance [MR] cholangiography and computed tomographic [CT] cholangiography).

In the second section, diagnostic imaging of the biliary duct is discussed. In this section, imaging findings on sonograms, CT scans, MR images, and hepatobiliary scintigraphy studies of various diseases of the bile duct and gallbladder are nicely described. Addressed is the relatively new indication of color sonographic imaging for the accurate diagnosis of acute cholecystitis. The topics of MR imaging of the gallbladder and MR cholangiography are well presented with superb illustrations in two chapters. In this section, I especially enjoyed reading the two chapters on the use of uncommon techniques such as endoluminal sonography of the biliary tree and laparoscopic sonography.

The third section deals with interventional radiology of the biliary tree. In this section, surgical considerations with respect to benign biliary diseases and hilar cholangiocarcinoma, which may be useful to the radiologist, are provided in two separate chapters. Various percutaneous techniques such as percutaneous cholecystectomy, percutaneous treatment of benign and malignant biliary tract obstruction, percutaneous biliary endoscopy, and percutaneous drainage of pyogenic cholangitis are appropriately covered. The important function of interventional radiology in the treatment of bile duct injury after laparoscopic surgery or orthotopic hepatic transplantation is well described in two other chapters. The imaging features of recurrent pyogenic cholangitis (also called "oriental" cholangitis) and the role of percutaneous treatment of this somewhat rare condition in Western countries are extensively addressed. The relative merits of metallic and plastic stents in the palliation of bile duct obstruction are discussed in three very interesting chapters. Endoscopic management of biliary strictures, including endoscopic recanalization of an occluded metallic stent, is fully described. Intraluminal radiation therapy of malignant biliary diseases is described in a complete chapter.

In general, every area of the diagnostic and interventional imaging of the biliary tract is appropriately covered. The overall quality of the book is excellent; the presentation is homogeneous, and there is little overlap between the different chapters. I actually could not find any limitation of the book; however, the price ($236.00) is relatively high. Because of its comprehensive nature, this book would be especially appropriate for radiologists, gastroenterologists, and abdominal surgeons.

Reviewed by Philippe Soyer, MD, PhD

Eric K. Outwater, MD • Manoj Bhatia, MD • Evan S. Siegelman, MD
Melissa A. Burke, MD • Donald G. Mitchell, MD

Lipid in Renal Clear Cell Carcinoma: Detection on Opposed-Phase Gradient-Echo MR Images[1]

PURPOSE: **To determine if comparison of in-phase and opposed-phase gradient-echo magnetic resonance (MR) images enables detection of lipid in renal clear cell carcinoma.**

MATERIALS AND METHODS: **A retrospective search of MR and pathologic records identified 43 patients with biopsy-proved renal masses who underwent in-phase and opposed-phase MR imaging. Thirty-three patients had renal cell carcinoma (27 with clear cell carcinoma), and 10 patients had other renal tumors. With MR images, a region-of-interest measurement of signal intensity of the renal mass was divided by that of reference tissue. In each patient, a ratio of these region-of-interest measurements on the opposed-phase images to those on the in-phase images was calculated and termed the opposed-phase/in-phase signal intensity ratio (OIR).**

RESULTS: **The mean OIR of clear cell carcinomas was significantly different from that of other renal masses ($P <$ .0002); in 16 (59%) of 27 patients with clear cell carcinoma, the OIR was less than 2 standard deviations below the mean OIR of other masses. In cases of clear cell carcinoma, focal signal intensity on opposed-phase images was less than that on in-phase images.**

CONCLUSION: **On opposed-phase images, some clear cell carcinomas show relative focal and diffuse loss of signal intensity. In renal masses, this signal intensity loss—which is consistent with lipid—does not necessarily indicate angiomyolipoma.**

Gradient-echo (GRE) magnetic resonance (MR) images can be acquired with an echo time so that signals from fat and water are not in phase, and the resulting signal intensity can reflect the relative proportion of water and lipid in the voxel. Opposed-phase and in-phase imaging can be performed with parameters that differ only in echo time by approximately 2.1 msec (with use of a 1.5-T imager); differences in tissue signal intensity between the two images are largely because of this chemical-shift effect (1). Quantitative or qualitative comparison of such opposed-phase and in-phase T1-weighted images allows accurate distinction of adrenal adenomas from other adrenal masses because of the lipid content in adrenal adenomas (2–8). This imaging technique has also enabled detection of lipids in tissue or fluid in mature cystic teratomas (9,10), hepatic steatosis (1), and liver tumors (11,12).

Renal carcinoma cells frequently contain intracellular lipid, which contributes to the histologic appearance of the clear cell in the most common type of these tumors (13–17). At cytologic examination of urine, intracellular lipid has been used to distinguish renal cell carcinomas from other masses (18,19). To our knowledge, it has not been shown that this lipid can be seen on opposed-phase MR images. If this lipid appears as relatively decreased signal intensity on opposed-phase images, several diagnostic implications become apparent. First, the identification of lipid in a renal mass may result in an erroneous diagnosis of angiomyolipoma. Second, identification of lipid in a solid renal mass may enable diagnosis of clear cell carcinoma (which may be distinguished from other masses such as lymphoma or oncocytoma if it can be determined that the mass is not an angiomyolipoma). Finally, if adrenal metastases from clear cell carcinoma show lipid on MR images, these metastases may be confused with adrenal adenomas on opposed-phase images.

The purpose of this study was to examine quantitatively findings on in-phase and opposed-phase GRE MR images of renal tumors and determine if there is relative loss of signal intensity, consistent with lipid, in clear cell carcinomas on opposed-phase images.

MATERIALS AND METHODS

MR records from January 1995 to December 1996 at two tertiary-care institutions were searched. MR records documenting a renal mass were cross-referenced with pathologic records, and patients who underwent MR examination and biopsy of a solid renal mass or its metastases were identified. Patients were excluded if *(a)* MR studies did not include T1-weighted in-phase and opposed-phase GRE images in

Index terms: Kidney neoplasms, diagnosis, 81.121412, 81.324 • Kidney neoplasms, MR, 81.121412, 81.324 • Lipoma and lipomatosis, 81.3141

Abbreviations: GRE = gradient echo, OIR = opposed-phase/in-phase signal intensity ratio, ROI = region of interest.

Radiology 1997; 205:103–107

[1] From the Departments of Radiology (E.K.O., M.B., D.G.M.) and Pathology (M.A.B.), Thomas Jefferson University Hospital, 132 S 10th St, 1096 Main, Philadelphia, PA 19107-5244; and the Department of Radiology, Hospital of the University of Pennsylvania, Philadelphia (E.S.S.). Received January 16, 1997; revision requested March 4; revision received March 28; accepted May 12. **Address reprint requests to** E.K.O.

See also the editorial by Ehman (pp 39–40) in this issue.

the axial plane or *(b)* MR studies could not be recovered from digital archive media.

Forty-three patients with renal masses were identified. There were 16 women and 27 men. Patient ages ranged from 33 to 81 years (mean, 60 years). Patients underwent surgery or biopsy 0–130 days (mean, 32 days) after MR examination. Pathologic records were reviewed for diagnosis, histologic features, grade, and color of the renal mass.

Diagnosis of the renal mass was made with partial or total nephrectomy in 37 patients and renal biopsy in two patients. Four other patients had large renal masses with metastases; histologic examination of biopsy specimens of metastases showed clear cells, consistent with primary clear cell carcinoma of the kidney. Although these four patients did not undergo biopsy of the renal mass, their renal masses were considered to be clear cell carcinoma.

Of the 43 patients, 33 (77%) had renal cell carcinoma. At histologic examination, 27 of these tumors showed exclusively or predominantly clear cells. Four other patients had granular cell carcinoma, and two other patients had sarcomatoid carcinoma. Of the 33 renal cell carcinomas, five were grade 1 or 1–2, 19 were grade 2, and four were a higher grade; tumor grade was not documented in five tumors. Ten (23%) patients had other renal masses, including transitional cell carcinoma ($n = 5$), oncocytoma ($n = 3$), angiomyolipoma ($n = 1$), and metastasis from lung carcinoma ($n = 1$).

MR imaging was performed with a 1.5-T system (Signa; GE Medical Systems, Milwaukee, Wis) in all patients. For signal reception, the body coil was used in two patients; in 41 patients, the phased-array multicoil was used. In-phase and opposed-phase T1-weighted imaging was performed with breath-hold fast multiplanar spoiled GRE sequences in all patients. Repetition time was 100–220 msec, depending on the patient's ability to suspend respiration. Other parameters were as follows: flip angle, 90°; matrix, 256 × 128–192; signal acquired, one; field of view, sized to the patient; section thickness, 4–9 mm; and section interval, 0–2 mm with a bandwidth of ±16 or ±32 kHz. In-phase and opposed-phase imaging was performed with echo times of 4.2 and 1.6–3.1 msec, respectively. Transmit and receiver gain were not kept constant for in-phase and opposed-phase imaging.

Region-of-interest (ROI) measurements were made of the renal mass, spleen, renal cortex, and noise. In patients with more than one mass, the lesion that underwent biopsy or excision was used for the ROI measurement. If more than one mass was excised, the largest lesion was used for measurement. The radiologist (M.B.) performing the ROI measurements was blinded to the pathologic diagnosis. ROI measurements were made from the T1-weighted in-phase and opposed-phase images; the same location on the images was used for all three measurements.

ROI measurements of the renal mass were made in two ways. First, the largest

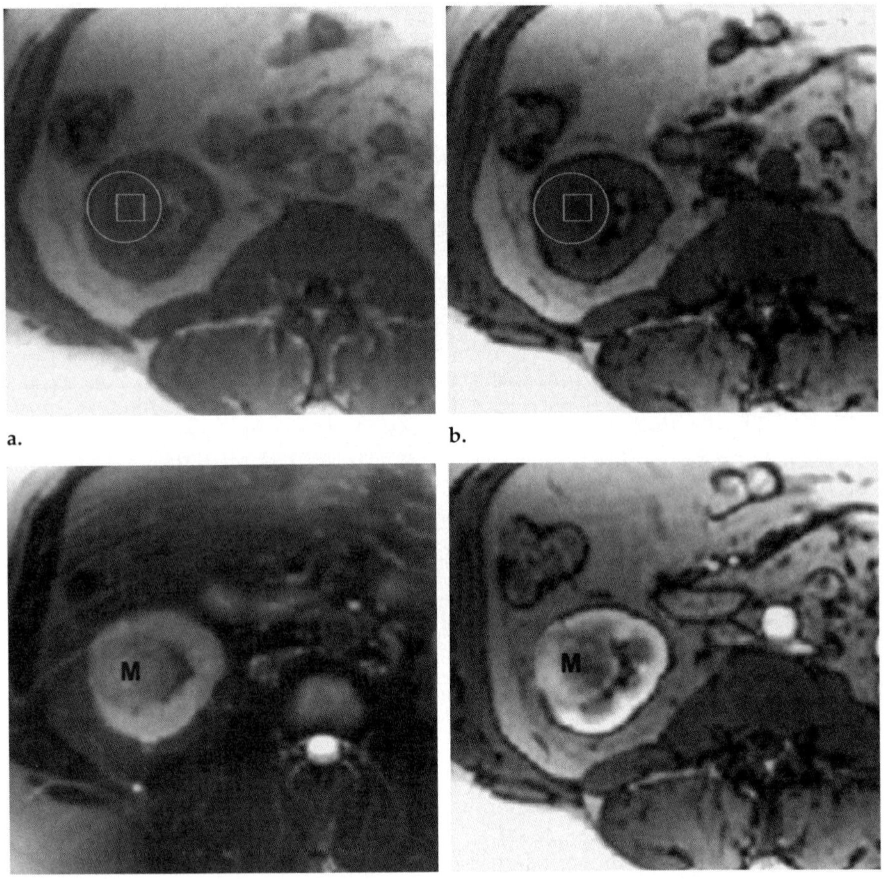

a. b. c. d.

Figure 1. ROI measurements of a clear cell carcinoma in a 42-year-old man. **(a)** In-phase T1-weighted breath-hold spoiled GRE (115/4.2 [repetition time msec/echo time msec]) image shows total (circle) and focal (square) ROIs in a right renal mass. **(b)** On the opposed-phased (145/2.3) image, ROI markers are placed in identical locations; there is relative loss of signal intensity in portions of the tumor. Because the tumor limits were not evident on the T1-weighted images, the T2-weighted fast spin-echo (5,100/96) image **(c)** and gadolinium-enhanced T1-weighted breath-hold (145/2.3) image **(d)** were used to define the limits of the mass (*M*) and place the ROI markers.

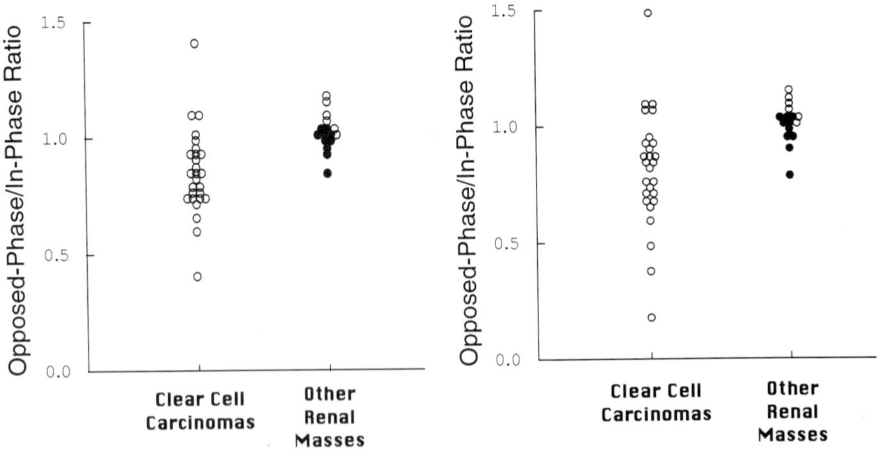

a. b.

Figure 2. Scatterplots of OIRs by diagnosis. **(a)** The OIR was measured with use of the whole-tumor cross section as the ROI. **(b)** To detect focal lipid deposition, the ROI was a 1-cm^2 portion of the tumor. With use of both ROI measurements, OIR values were lower in clear cell carcinoma. In column 1, ○ = clear cell carcinomas; in column 2, ○ = other renal carcinomas (eg, granular cell and sarcomatoid carcinomas), ● = other renal masses (eg, oncocytoma, transitional cell carcinoma, angiomyolipoma, and metastasis).

ROI, which did not include partial-volume effects from adjacent fat, was indicated (Fig 1). Because the edges of the mass were not always apparent on T1-weighted images, gadolinium-enhanced T1- and T2-weighted images were used to assess the

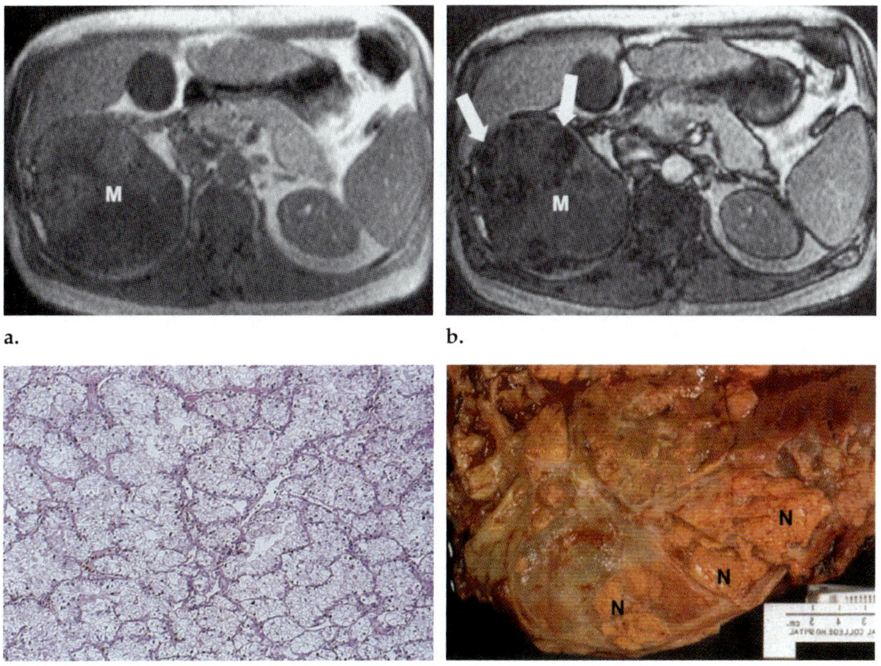

a. b. c. d.

Figure 3. Clear cell carcinoma in a 52-year-old man. **(a)** In-phase T1-weighted breath-hold spoiled GRE (180/4.2) image shows a large right renal mass (*M*). **(b)** Opposed-phased fast multiplanar spoiled GRE (110/2.3) image shows relative loss of signal intensity (arrows) in portions of the tumor (*M*). **(c)** Photomicrograph of the tumor shows clear cells throughout the field. (Hematoxylin-eosin stain; original magnification, ×100.) **(d)** Photograph of gross bisected tumor shows yellow tumor nodules (*N*) at the periphery of the mass.

edges of the mass for ROI measurements (Fig 1); otherwise, these images were not used for data collection. Second, a 1-cm² ROI was indicated on the portion of the mass that appeared to show a possible loss of relative signal intensity on opposed-phase images. This was done in an attempt to detect a focal area of lipid-containing tissue in the larger mass. A measure of the decrease in signal intensity was obtained from the in-phase and opposed-phase images. The ratio of signal intensity of the lesion to that of the reference tissue on the opposed-phase images was determined. This number was divided by the ratio of signal intensity of the lesion to that of the reference tissue on the in-phase images (3). The final ratio was called the opposed-phase/in-phase signal intensity ratio (OIR). Spleen was used as the reference tissue in 41 patients. In two patients who underwent splenectomy, renal cortex was used as the reference tissue.

All Student *t* test comparisons were two-tailed with separate variances.

RESULTS

The mean OIR of clear cell carcinomas (0.84 ± 0.19) was significantly different from that of other renal masses (1.02 ± 0.08) (P = .0002) (Fig 2). Relative loss of signal intensity on opposed-phase images occurred in a heterogeneous and focal distribution in some clear cell carcinomas (Fig 3). The 1-cm² ROIs—which at blinded analysis most likely represented focal signal intensity loss—revealed a mean OIR of 0.81 ± 0.25 in clear cell carcinoma and a mean OIR of 1.01 ± 0.09 in other renal masses (P = .0006). In these other renal tumors (four cases of granular cell carcinoma, two cases of sarcomatoid carcinoma, and 10 other renal masses), there was no change in relative signal intensities between in-phase and opposed-phase images (Fig 4). In many clear cell carcinomas, a loss of signal intensity on the opposed-phase images was either subtle or not visible (Fig 1). Necrotic areas did not show loss of signal intensity (Fig 5). In one patient with an angiomyolipoma, analysis revealed an OIR of 0.97. In one clear cell carcinoma, the OIR was 1.40 (Fig 2); this outlying value was

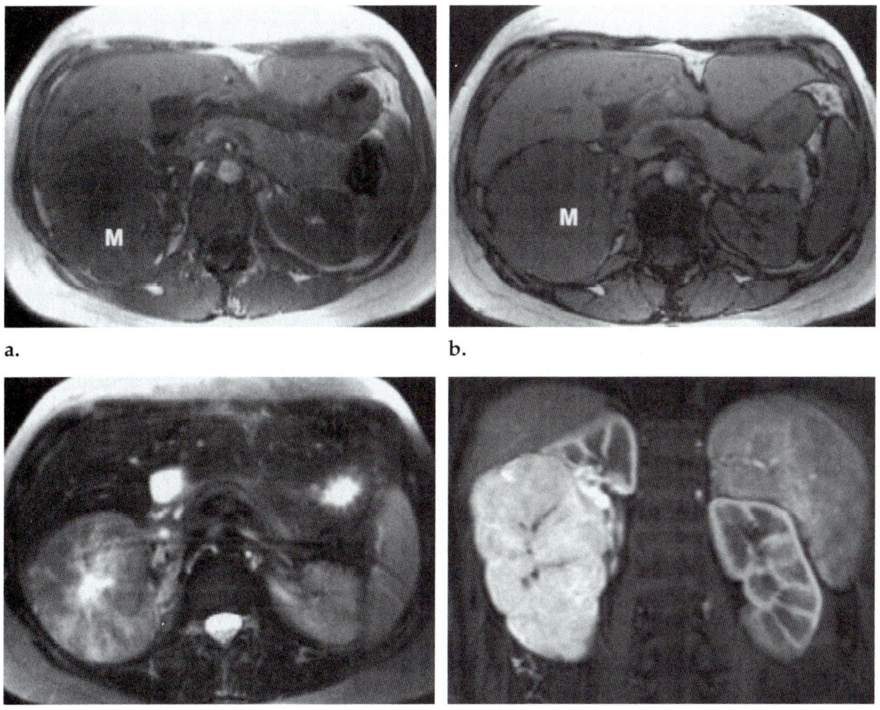

a. b. c. d.

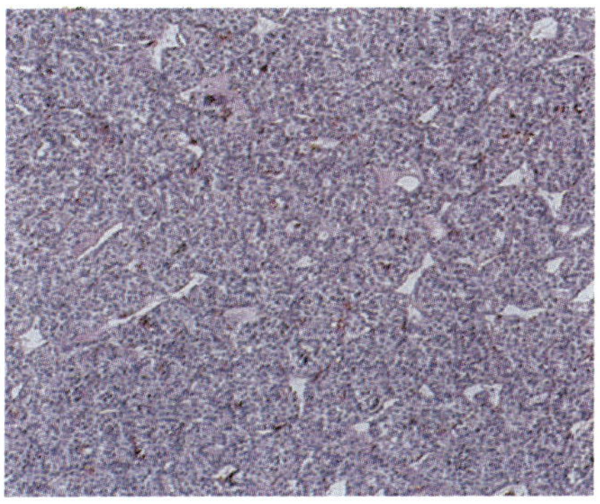

e.

Figure 4. Absence of observable lipid in a renal oncocytoma in a 45-year-old woman. **(a)** In-phase T1-weighted breath-hold GRE (120/4.2) image shows a large right renal mass (*M*). **(b)** Opposed-phase GRE (120/2.5) image shows no change in the signal intensity of the renal mass (*M*) relative to that of the spleen. **(c)** Axial T2-weighted fast spin-echo (7,000/96 [effective]) image and **(d)** coronal breath-hold GRE (100/2.1) image after administration of gadopentetate dimeglumine demonstrate that areas in **a** and **b** are vascularized by the tumor and do not represent necrosis. **(e)** Photomicrograph of histologic tumor section shows oncocytic cells; no clear cells are present. (Hematoxylin-eosin stain; original magnification, ×100.)

due to extensive hemosiderin, which resulted in lower signal intensity on the in-phase (120/4.2) image compared with that on the opposed-phase (120/2.1) image.

Clear cell carcinomas that showed loss of signal intensity on opposed-phase images (OIR less than 2 standard deviations below the mean OIR of other renal tumors) were usually yellow at gross examination (Fig 5). The mean OIR (0.80 ± 0.18) of tumors that were yellow at gross examination (n = 16 renal cell carcinomas) was significantly lower than the mean OIR (1.01 ± 0.13) of hemorrhagic or tan, white, brown, or red tumors (n = 20) (P = .0007). Descriptions of gross features were not available for seven tumors.

The mean signal intensity relative to that of reference tissue on in-phase images of clear cell carcinomas (1.01 ± 0.35) was higher than that of other renal tumors (0.91 ± 0.24); however, this difference was not significant (P = .29).

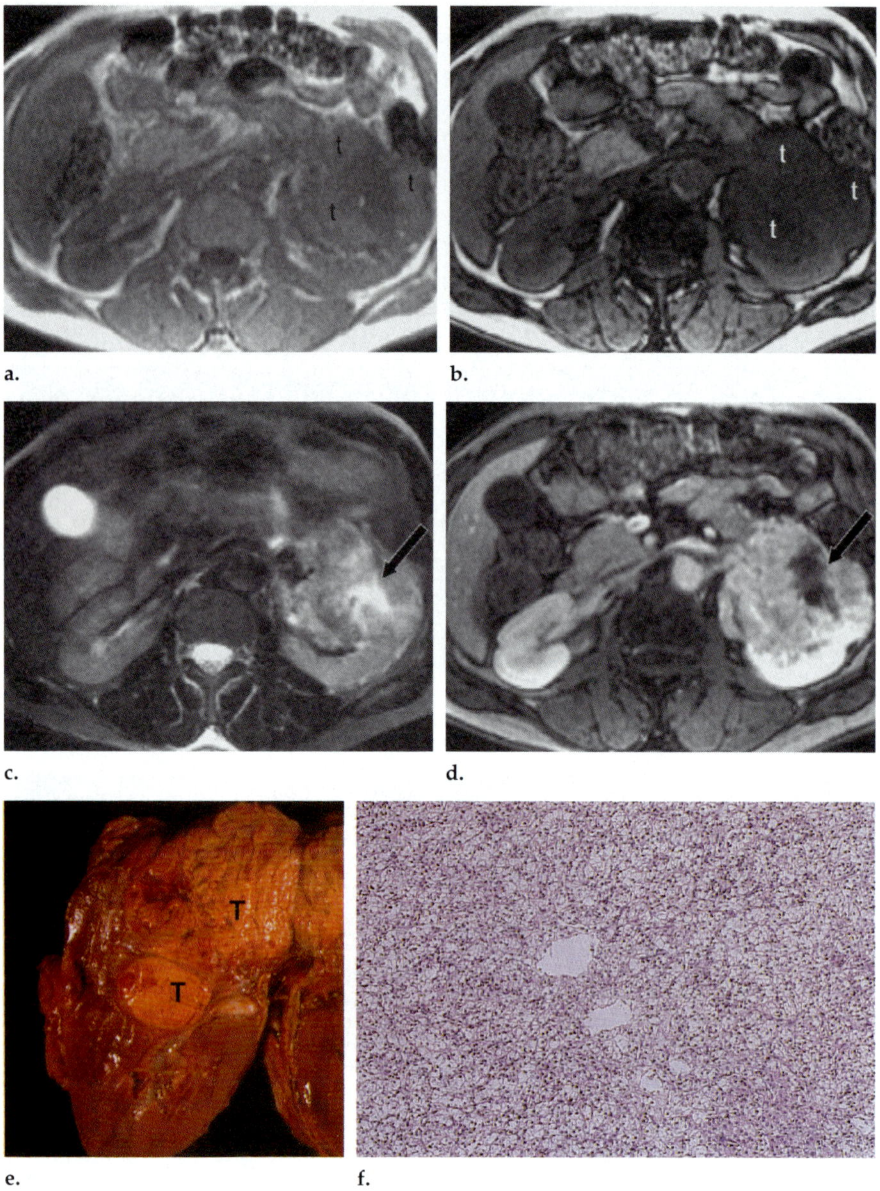

Figure 5. Clear cell carcinoma in a 78-year-old man. **(a)** In-phase (100/4.2) and **(b)** opposed-phase (120/2.2) T1-weighted breath-hold GRE images show a large left renal mass. Areas of slightly higher signal intensity (t in **a**) are seen on the in-phase image; these areas are slightly hypointense (t in **b**) on the opposed-phase image. The total and focal OIRs of this tumor were 0.72 and 0.48, respectively. **(c)** T2-weighted fast spin-echo (5,166/144 [effective]) image and **(d)** gadolinium-enhanced T1-weighted fast multiplanar GRE (120/2.2) image show that the tumor areas without loss of signal intensity on the opposed-phase image in **b** represent necrosis (arrow). **(e)** Photograph of the gross tumor (T) shows characteristic yellow color of clear cell carcinoma. **(f)** Photomicrograph of histologic tumor section shows abundant clear cells. (Hematoxylin-eosin stain; original magnification, ×100.)

DISCUSSION

The histologic appearance of the clear cell in clear cell carcinoma is caused by intracellular accumulation of lipid and glycogen (13–17). Our study demonstrated that clear cell carcinoma, when compared with other renal masses, shows a relative loss of signal intensity on opposed-phase images compared with that on in-phase images. Our methodology did not allow direct proof with specific histologic correlation that this effect is caused by lipid in clear cells. However, similar imaging techniques have been used to detect hepatic steatosis and intracellular lipid in adrenal adenomas, and results have been confirmed with quantitative histologic measurements (1,5,20,21). Because of the marked heterogeneity in renal cell carcinoma (necrosis, hemorrhage, fibrosis, and varied cell types) direct correlation between findings in vivo and at histologic examination is difficult and was not performed in this study.

Three implications of our MR imaging finding of observable lipid in clear cell carcinoma can be advanced. First, lipid is not diagnostic of angiomyolipoma. With computed tomographic or MR imaging, angiomyolipomas usually show focal fat (22–24). By contrast, focal fat in renal cell carcinoma is rarely seen with imaging (22–27). The lipid described in this study did not appear as focal fat in the renal masses (ie, high signal intensity [approximating that of subcutaneous fat] on T1-weighted images and low signal intensity on fat-saturated T1-weighted images). The opposed-phase images—which are more sensitive than frequency-selective fat-saturated images for the detection of relatively small proportions of lipid in a voxel—showed this lipid. Therefore, angiomyolipoma should not be diagnosed with use of opposed-phase imaging alone, which has been used by some authors for this purpose (28,29). Fat-saturated T1-weighted images may be more appropriate for identifying focal fat and thus diagnosing angiomyolipoma.

Second, identification of diffuse lipid in a renal tumor may allow differentiation of clear cell carcinoma from other renal masses, such as oncocytoma and transitional cell carcinoma—which do not show diffuse lipid at pathologic examination and did not reveal diffuse lipid in this study. The converse is not true, however. If a renal mass shows little or no evidence of lipid, clear cell carcinoma is not excluded. The OIRs of 11 (41%)

of 27 clear cell carcinomas were within 2 standard deviations of the mean OIR of other renal tumors. Also, the OIRs of renal carcinomas with histologic cell types other than clear cell (six patients in this study) were similar to those of oncocytoma and other renal masses. Therefore, in-phase and opposed-phase MR imaging does not reliably enable diagnosis of all renal carcinomas; however, MR imaging enables identification of lipid in some clear cell carcinomas.

Third, if a primary clear cell carcinoma shows lipid with MR imaging, then metastases may show lipid as well. It is possible that metastases from clear cell carcinoma to the adrenal gland may show lipid on opposed-phase images; therefore, these metastases may be confused with adrenal adenomas. To our knowledge, studies of metastases with in-phase and opposed-phase imaging have not demonstrated false-positive diagnoses of adrenal adenomas (3,4,8). These studies, however, have included only seven patients with renal cell carcinoma (3,4,8). For these three reasons, the detection of diffuse lipid in renal tumors with MR imaging has diagnostic importance.

Previous descriptions of renal masses on MR images have not revealed specific features of clear cell carcinoma. Choyke et al (30), however, noted that the signal intensity of clear cell carcinoma tends to be slightly high on T1-weighted images compared with that of renal cortex; the signal intensity difference was ascribed to the presence of lipid in these tumors. This signal intensity difference also has been noted by others in a larger series (31). In our study, clear cell carcinoma tended to show higher signal intensity than other masses; however, this difference was not statistically significant.

Our study has several limitations. The MR imaging parameters differed between patients, and greater variance in measures may have resulted. More standardized measures may have resulted in smaller standard deviations, and greater separation between measurements in clear cell carcinoma and other renal masses may have been shown. To some extent, the variability was caused by the individual tailoring of each examination; field of view, repetition time (for a viable breath hold), and echo time (which was dependent on the section thickness and field of view) were affected. A second limitation was the relatively small numbers of masses other than clear cell carcinoma that were studied. Although there is little reason to believe that other malignant lesions show lipid at histologic examination, larger populations of renal tumors other than clear cell carcinoma need to be studied to confirm this assumption. A third limitation was that we did not determine that angiomyolipoma can be differentiated reliably from renal cell carcinomas that show lipid. Presumably, angiomyolipoma shows focal fat on T1-weighted and fat-saturated images. Given our results, however, we caution against diagnosing angiomyolipoma on the primary basis of signal intensity loss on opposed-phase images. Finally, we were not able to evaluate metastases of clear cell carcinoma to the adrenal glands.

In conclusion, there is a subset of clear cell carcinomas that show qualitative and quantitative evidence of lipid on opposed-phase MR images; this finding must be considered when evaluating renal masses. ■

References

1. Mitchell DG, Kim I, Chang TS, et al. Fatty liver: chemical shift phase-difference and suppression magnetic resonance imaging techniques in animals, phantoms, and humans. Invest Radiol 1991; 26:1041–1052.
2. Korobkin M, Lombardi TJ, Aisen AM, et al. Characterization of adrenal masses with chemical shift and gadolinium-enhanced MR imaging. Radiology 1995; 197:411–418.
3. Bilbey JH, McLoughlin RF, Kurkjian PS, et al. MR imaging of adrenal masses: value of chemical-shift imaging for distinguishing adenomas from other tumors. AJR 1995; 164:637–642.
4. Mayo-Smith WW, Lee MJ, McNicholas MM, Hahn PF, Boland GW, Saini S. Characterization of adrenal masses (<5 cm) by use of chemical shift MR imaging: observer performance versus quantitative measures. AJR 1995; 165:91–95.
5. Mitchell DG, Crovello M, Matteucci T, Petersen RO, Miettinen MM. Benign adrenocortical masses: diagnosis with chemical shift MR imaging. Radiology 1992; 185:345–351.
6. Tsushima Y, Dean PB. Characterization of adrenal masses with chemical shift MR imaging: how to select echo times (letter). Radiology 1995; 195:285–286.
7. McNicholas MM, Lee MJ, Mayo-Smith WW, Hahn PF, Boland GW, Mueller PR. An imaging algorithm for the differential diagnosis of adrenal adenomas and metastases. AJR 1995; 165:1453–1459.
8. Outwater EK, Siegelman ES, Radecki PD, Piccoli CW, Mitchell DG. Distinction between benign and malignant adrenal masses: value of T1-weighted chemical-shift MR imaging. AJR 1995; 165:579–583.
9. Yamashita Y, Torashima M, Hatanaka Y, et al. Value of phase-shift gradient-echo MR imaging in the differentiation of pelvic lesions with high signal intensity at T1-weighted imaging. Radiology 1994; 191: 759–764.
10. Yamashita Y, Hatanaka Y, Torashima M, Takahashi M, Miyazaki K, Okamura H. Mature cystic teratomas of the ovary without fat in the cystic cavity: MR features in 12 cases. AJR 1994; 163:613–616.
11. Mitchell DG, Palazzo J, Hann HW, Rifkin MD, Burk DL Jr, Rubin R. Hepatocellular tumors with high signal on T1-weighted MR images: chemical shift MR imaging and histologic correlation. J Comput Assist Tomogr 1991; 15:762–769.
12. Martin J, Falco J, Donoso L, Puig J, Zidan A, Sentis M. Hepatic angiomyolipoma: value of proton (fat/water) chemical shift fast low angle shot (FLASH) MR imaging technique in detecting fatty tissue content. Magn Reson Imaging 1995; 13:903–906.
13. Rosai J. Ackerman's surgical pathology. Vol 1. St Louis, Mo: Mosby–Year Book, 1996; 1146–1153.
14. Thoenes W, Storkel S, Rumpelt HJ. Histopathology and classification of renal cell tumors (adenomas, oncocytomas and carcinomas): the basic cytological and histopathological elements and their use for diagnostics. Pathol Res Pract 1986; 181:125–143.
15. Weiss LM, Gelb AB, Medeiros LJ. Adult renal epithelial neoplasms. Am J Clin Pathol 1995; 103:624–635.
16. Motzer RJ, Bander NH, Nanus DM. Renal-cell carcinoma. N Engl J Med 1996; 335: 865–875.
17. O'Toole KM, Brown M, Hoffmann P. Pathology of benign and malignant kidney tumors. Urol Clin North Am 1993; 20:193–205.
18. Hajdu SI, Savino A, Hajdu EO, Koss LG. Cytologic diagnosis of renal cell carcinoma with the aid of fat stain. Acta Cytol 1971; 15:31–33.
19. Milsten R, Frable WJ, Texter JH Jr, Paxson L. Evaluation of lipid stain in renal neoplasms as adjunct to routine exfoliative cytology. J Urol 1973; 110:169–171.
20. Korobkin M, Giordano TJ, Brodeur FJ, et al. Adrenal adenomas: relationship between histologic lipid and CT and MR findings. Radiology 1996; 200:743–747.
21. Leroy-Willig A, Bittoun J, Luton JP, et al. In vivo MR spectroscopic imaging of the adrenal glands: distinction between adenomas and carcinomas larger than 15 mm based on lipid content. AJR 1989; 153:771–773.
22. Bosniak MA, Megibow AJ, Hulnick DH, Horii S, Raghavendra BN. CT diagnosis of renal angiomyolipoma: the importance of detecting small amounts of fat. AJR 1988; 151:497–501.
23. Helenon O, Merran S, Paraf F, et al. Unusual fat-containing tumors of the kidney: a diagnostic dilemma. RadioGraphics 1997; 17:129–144.
24. Wagner BJ, Wong-You-Cheong JJ, Davis CJ. Adult renal hamartomas. RadioGraphics 1997; 17:155–169.
25. Radin DR, Chandrasoma P. CT demonstration of fat density in renal cell carcinoma. Acta Radiol 1992; 33:365–367.
26. Strotzer M, Lehner KB, Becker K. Detection of fat in a renal cell carcinoma mimicking angiomyolipoma. Radiology 1993; 188: 427–428.
27. Hélénon O, Chrétien Y, Paraf F, Melki P, Denys A, Moreau JF. Renal cell carcinoma containing fat: demonstration with CT. Radiology 1993; 188:429–430.
28. Rofsky NM, Bosniak MA. MR imaging in the evaluation of small (<3.0 cm) renal masses. Magn Reson Imaging Clin N Am 1997; 5:67–82.
29. Kido T, Yamashita Y, Sumi S, et al. Chemical shift GRE MRI of renal angiomyolipoma. J Comput Assist Tomogr 1997; 21: 268–270.
30. Choyke PL, Kressel HY, Pollack HM, Arger PM, Axel L, Mamourian AC. Focal renal masses: magnetic resonance imaging. Radiology 1984; 152:471–477.
31. Hricak H, Thoeni RF, Carroll PR, Demas BE, Marotti M, Tanagho EA. Detection and staging of renal neoplasms: a reassessment of MR imaging. Radiology 1988; 166:643–649.

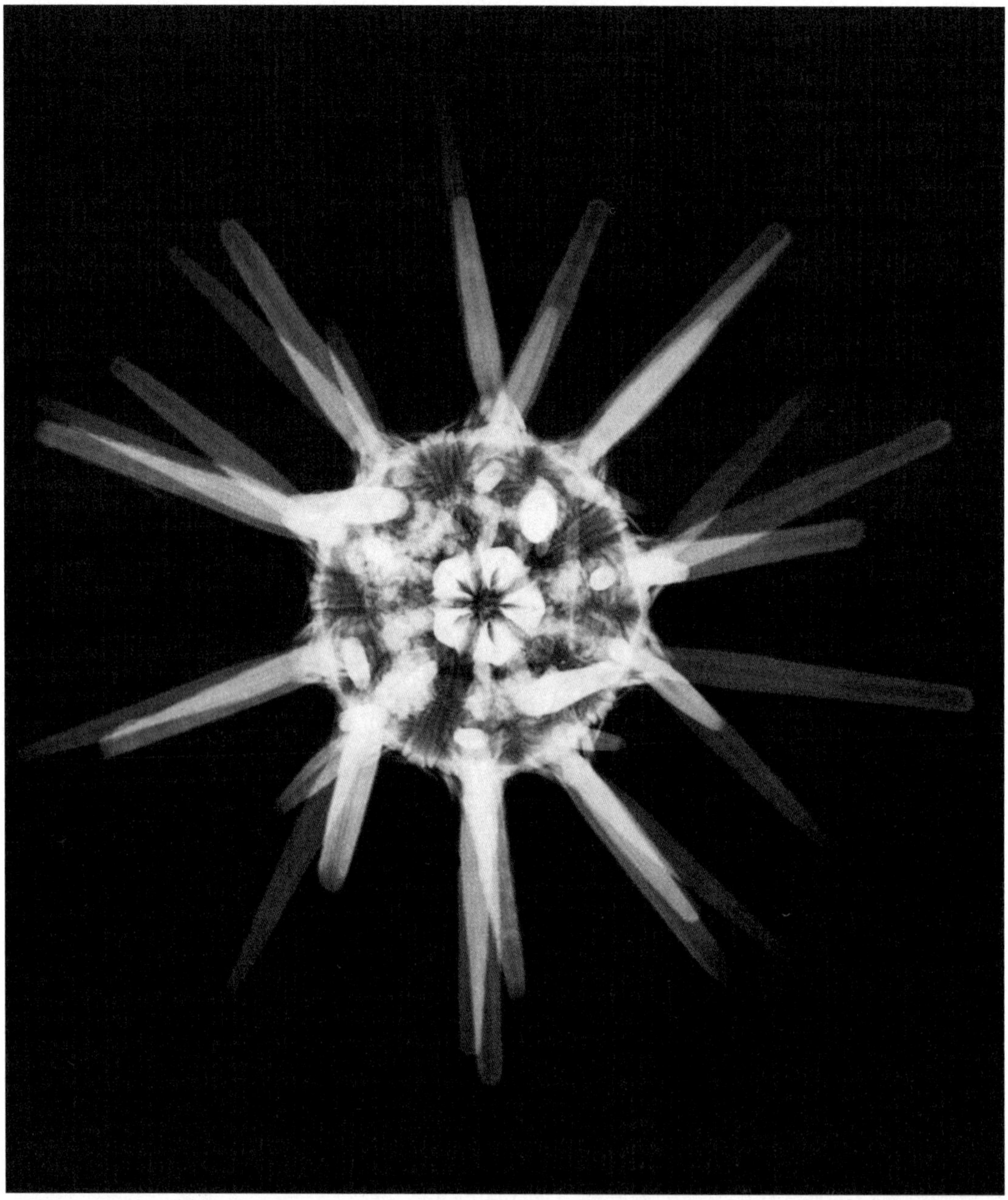

Eucidaris tribuloides
Satellite Sea Urchin

Courtesy of William A. Conklin, RT (FASRT), Inner Dimmension, 1571 Marshall Avenue, Orangeburg, SC 29115

Mark A. Kliewer, MD • Barbara S. Hertzberg, MD • Mary T. Keogan, MD • Erik K. Paulson, MD
Kelly S. Freed, MD • David M. DeLong, PhD • Barbara A. Carroll, MD

Early Systole in the Healthy Kidney: Variability of Doppler US Waveform Parameters[1]

PURPOSE: **To determine the sampling variability of intrarenal Doppler ultrasound (US) indexes of early systole in a screened population of healthy individuals.**

MATERIALS AND METHODS: **Doppler US measurements were obtained in the superior, middle, and inferior regions of 132 kidneys in 66 healthy, potential kidney donors. All individuals subsequently underwent angiography. Systematic measurement differences and random effects were estimated for sampling from a particular parenchymal region, from a kidney in a subject, from an individual in a population, and from a vascular territory.**

RESULTS: **Coefficients of variations ranged from 20% to 30%. Most (55%–66%) of the observed variation was attributable to random differences between repeated measurements in the same kidney. No systematic variations attributable to kidney region, vascular territory, right versus left kidney, or subject age were found for acceleration time, acceleration, or waveform shape. Some evidence of fixed variation between kidneys and between regions was found for peak systolic velocity, but the magnitude of this variation was small. Averages of repeated measurements may decrease the probability of exceeding the normal threshold for acceleration but not for acceleration time.**

CONCLUSION: **Measurements of Doppler parameters of the early systole have substantial intrinsic variability. Thus, caution is needed when interpreting small changes in these measurements within a kidney or between individuals.**

During the past several years, a growing number of investigators (1–10) have examined the morphology of Doppler ultrasound (US) waveforms obtained in intrarenal arteries. The impetus for much of this work is the proposition that definite, measurable waveform changes that reflect upstream stenosis of the extrarenal artery are evident at the early systole. Such changes—often referred to as tardus-parvus changes—have been characterized in terms of a set of measured parameters and a classification of waveform contours. Inherent in this approach is the assumption that intrarenal Doppler indexes are amenable to reliable and reproducible measurement and that the defined normal ranges are sufficiently coherent and distinct from the abnormal ranges. To our knowledge, however, the validity of this assumption has not been rigorously tested.

The tardus-parvus phenomenon results in a prolonged early systole and diminished peak velocities (11,12). On the pulse profile, this phenomenon is seen as a more gradual incline in the upstroke of the early systole and a blunting of the otherwise sharp early systolic peak. The duration of the early systole is increased, the acceleration of blood flow is decreased, and the envelope of peak systolic velocities describes an arc that is smoother and smaller than normal. The pathophysiologic mechanisms that underlie these changes and the diagnostic efficacy of this approach for the evaluation of renal artery stenosis have been the subjects of considerable controversy. In the literature about diagnosis, for example, there is virtual polarization between enthusiastic support (1–5) and deep skepticism (6–10).

Part of this inconsistency of results between laboratories may derive from fundamental problems with the measurements themselves. The purpose of this study was to determine and analyze the sampling variability of the Doppler parameters for the early systole—acceleration time, acceleration, peak velocity, and waveform shape—in healthy kidneys in individuals who had been rigorously screened to ensure the absence of both intrinsic renal disease and systemic illness.

MATERIALS AND METHODS

Color Doppler and duplex Doppler US examinations were performed in 132 kidneys in 66 individuals (39 women, 27 men) referred to our laboratory for evaluation as potential kidney donors. The subjects were aged 24–64 years (mean, 41 years). Before referral, all subjects underwent comprehensive screening by the transplantation service. Screening included a detailed medical history, physical examination, and laboratory tests to detect evidence of current or past renal disease and of systemic illness. All subjects had normal physical examination results, an unremarkable medical history, and normal blood pressure. In addition, all subjects had normal results from a battery of laboratory tests, including serum protein and electrolyte profiles, serum creatinine level, liver function tests, viral serologic evaluation, 24-hour urinary protein and creatinine excretion measurement, and a glucose tolerance test.

Index terms: Renal arteries, angiography, 961.1221, 961.1222 • Renal arteries, flow dynamics, 961.139 • Renal arteries, US, 961.12981, 961.12983 • Ultrasound (US), Doppler studies, 961.12983

Radiology 1997; 205:109–113

[1] From the Department of Radiology, Duke University Medical Center, Box 3808, Durham, NC 27710. Received February 27, 1997; revision requested April 2; revision received May 15; accepted May 19. **Address reprint requests to** M.A.K.

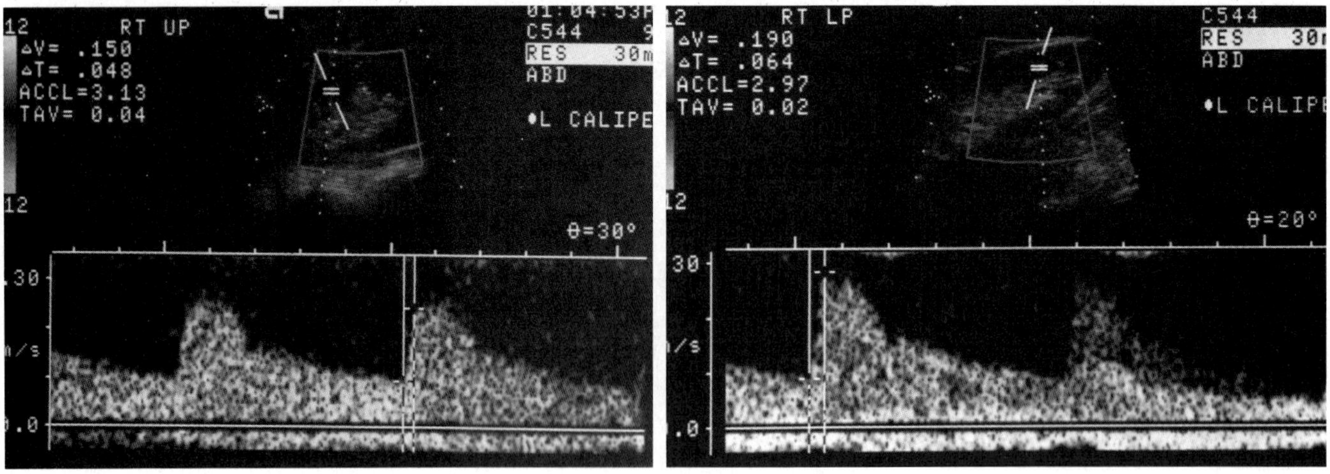

a. b.

Doppler US tracings obtained in the **(a)** upper and **(b)** lower poles of a healthy kidney. Measurement of the acceleration time is demonstrated with calipers placed at the end of the diastole and at the first systolic peak. Note the differences in the measured acceleration time (ΔT) and in the calculated systolic acceleration over this same period (*ACCL*). *TAV* = time-averaged velocity, ΔV = change in velocity.

All US examinations were performed with standard equipment (XP; Acuson, Mountain View, Calif; and HDI 3000; Advanced Technology Laboratories, Bothell, Wash) equipped with a phased-array sector transducer that operated at Doppler center frequencies of 2.00, 2.25, and 3.50 MHz. Doppler waveforms were obtained with the smallest possible velocity scale, the lowest possible wall-filter settings, and a sample gate width of 3–5 mm. Pulsed Doppler waveforms were displayed at sweep speeds of 40–50 mm/sec.

All subjects initially underwent real-time, gray-scale US to detect structural abnormalities in the kidneys. The subjects were positioned to optimize gray-scale imaging and Doppler tracings. Color Doppler sonography was used to determine the course of the interlobar arteries in the superior, middle, and inferior portions of the kidney. At least three similar, sequential Doppler waveforms were obtained at measured angles of insonation of less than 60° while the subject suspended respiration. The single best tracing obtained in each of the three renal regions was selected for analysis.

Systolic acceleration time was measured from the end of the diastole to the first systolic peak (Figure). Systolic acceleration was calculated by dividing the change in peak systolic velocity during this same interval by the acceleration time value. Peak systolic velocity was measured at the apex of the first systolic peak. Finally, the waveform profile of the early systole (the incline of the systolic upstroke and the sharpness of the early systolic peak) was categorized according to previously proposed criteria (13). Specifically, the waveform was considered to be (*a*) normal if the slope of the systolic upstroke was unvarying and the peak formed an acute angle, (*b*) equivocal if the slope curved but the peak formed an acute angle, and (*c*) abnormal if the early systolic peak formed an obtuse angle.

All subjects underwent angiography within 24 hours of the sonographic examination. Angiography was performed by using a femoral artery approach and standard Seldinger techniques. Digital subtraction images were obtained in anteroposterior and oblique projections during aortic injection of iopamidol (Isovue; Bracco Diagnostics, Princeton, NJ) through a 5-F pigtail catheter (Angio Dynamics, Queensbury, NY). When an individual was suspected of having a supernumerary renal artery or renal arterial disease, selective catheter placement in the renal arteries was performed, as necessary, with a 5.5-F, preformed, end-hole catheter (Mikkaelson; Angio Dynamics).

Statistical analyses included calculation of the population means and standard deviations for the three numeric variables (acceleration time, systolic acceleration, and peak systolic velocity). Coefficients of variation were calculated by dividing the standard deviation by the mean and then multiplying that result by 100. Correlations among the variables—acceleration time, systolic acceleration, and peak systolic velocity—were characterized with the Pearson product-moment correlation coefficient. To compare differences in the rates of normal, equivocal, and abnormal waveforms, Rao score tests were used for the early systolic peak variable.

By using mixed linear models with a repeated-measures analysis of variance, systematic measurement differences between kidneys and between sites within a single kidney, as well as random effects that resulted from the intrinsic sampling variability of repeated measurements, were quantified, as were the components of the variance. For each variable, the data were stratified according to subject age and sex to determine any systematic effects governed by these factors. Differences between renal regions supplied by the main renal artery and those supplied by accessory arteries were evaluated with approximate Student *t* tests.

The variance components that were estimated with the linear models were then used to stratify the total variability according to three levels: (*a*) variation between subjects, (*b*) variation between the right and left kidney in the same individual, and (*c*) variation between different sites in the same kidney. The standard deviations of measurements at each level were derived, and the potential utility of averaging more than one measurement of these variables was explored. The standard deviation of a single measurement was determined by calculating the square root of the estimated variance. The standard deviation of the mean of two or more measurements was determined by dividing the variance estimate by the number of averages and calculating the square root of that number as the result. These calculations were compared with published (2,14) threshold values purported to demarcate the boundary between normal and abnormal values for these variables. The probability that a single reading or that an average of several readings would exceed a threshold value was then calculated for increasing numbers of averages. Results were considered to be statistically significant when *P* values were less than .05.

RESULTS

At gray-scale US, all 132 kidneys were normal in terms of sonographic appearance, echogenicity, location, and size. No kidney had evidence of pyelocaliectasis or stones.

At angiography, we found that 103 (78%) of 132 kidneys were supplied by a single renal artery, 23 (17%) kidneys were supplied by two renal arteries, and four (3%) kidneys were supplied by three arteries. Renal arteries in the other two kidneys showed changes related to fibromuscular dysplasia and were excluded from the

Table 1
Summary Statistics Based on Raw Means and Ranges

Variable	Mean	Standard Deviation	Coefficient of Variation (%)	Range of 2 Standard Deviations
Acceleration time	0.08 sec	0.02	25	0.04–0.12
Acceleration	1.88 m/sec^2	0.56	30	0.76–3.00
Peak systolic velocity	0.24 m/sec	0.05	21	0.14–0.34

Note.—Statistics do not account for possible correlation within a subject or for interaction of effects.

Table 2
Variance Estimates Stratified according to Sampling Level

Parameter	Sampling Level		
	Kidney	Patient	Population
Acceleration time	0.00046 (55)	0.00011 (13)	0.00027 (32)
Acceleration	0.50100 (65)	0.08300 (11)	0.18600 (24)
Peak systolic velocity	0.00350 (66)	0.00028 (5)	0.00150 (28)

Note.—Numbers in parentheses are percentages of the total variability.

analysis. Therefore, a total of 390 renal regions were studied.

Table 1 lists summary statistics based on raw averages for the variables of acceleration time, systolic acceleration, and peak systolic velocity. These statistics include means, standard deviations, coefficients of variation, and 2-standard-deviation ranges. Although these statistics are intended to provide an overview of the data, these values do not account for possible correlation of variables within a subject or for the interaction of effects. (Such an accounting was performed with the mixed linear models, however.) Coefficients of variation indicated that 1 standard deviation in the measurement of these three variables was large, relative to the mean, and represented 20%–30% of the mean value.

These three variables were highly intercorrelated: The variables are intimately related conceptually, as well as mathematically. The Pearson product-moment correlation coefficient for acceleration time and acceleration was −.57 (P = .0001). For acceleration time and peak systolic velocity, the correlation coefficient was .36 (P = .003). For acceleration and peak systolic velocity, the correlation coefficient was .41 (P = .0007).

Modeling of the response variables of acceleration time, systolic acceleration, and peak systolic velocity resulted in little evidence for systematic effects due to sampling. By using the linear model for acceleration time, there was no statistically significant systematic difference attributable to sampling between kidneys (P = .85), to sampling between different regions of the same kidney (P = .87), or to subject age (P = .60).

Measurements of systolic acceleration showed equivocal evidence for systematic variation between kidneys (P = .04) and within a kidney (P = .05), but this variation attained only marginal statistical significance. Importantly, the magnitude of this potential difference was small: The acceleration in the lower pole was approximately 0.16 m/sec^2 less than that in other regions, and the acceleration in the right kidney was 0.19 m/sec^2 less than that in the left. These values represent only 8% and 10%, respectively, of the mean value of the measurement. In addition, the peak systolic velocity variable seemed to vary between kidneys (P = .01) and between regions in a single kidney (P = .01). The velocity tended to be 0.02 m/sec slower in the lower pole relative to the velocity in other regions; in the right kidney, the velocity was 0.02 m/sec slower than that in the left kidney. As with systolic acceleration, the magnitude of this potential variation was small and was, therefore, unlikely to be of clinical importance.

For the early systolic peak, there was no statistically significant difference in the rating of waveform category attributable to kidney side (P = .45) or renal region (P = .59). In addition, there was no evidence of a statistically significant effect attributable to sampling according to subject age, sex, or vascular territory (accessory or main arterial supply) for any variable.

The data distributions for acceleration time, acceleration, and peak systolic velocity were skewed to larger values. Therefore, we performed log transformations with these variables so that the underlying distributions better approximated a normal distribution. The models were then refitted with the transformed data. This transformation did not substantially change the calculated P values, and the attribution of statistical significance determined with the untransformed variables was affirmed.

Estimates of variance components are presented in Table 2. For all the variables under study, the largest percentage of total variability was attributable to the intrinsic sampling variability in repeated measurements in the same kidney. Variance estimates attributable to differences between the right and left kidneys of an individual subject and between subjects in a given population were of much smaller magnitude. Indeed, the intrinsic sampling variability in repeated measurement in the same kidney constituted fully 55% of the total variability in the acceleration time measurement, 65% of the total variability in the systolic acceleration measurement, and 66% of the total variability in the peak systolic velocity measurement.

The absolute magnitude of the variation in these parameters was impressive, as well (Table 3). On the basis of these variance estimates, the standard deviation of a single acceleration time measurement in one kidney in one subject was the square root of 0.00046, or 0.02 seconds. The magnitude of this estimate increased, as expected, when accounting for the additional variation that exists between the two kidneys in a single individual and between individuals in a healthy population. For this analysis, variance estimates were summed because kidneys are "nested" in a subject and subjects are nested in a population. Therefore, as we ascended from the level of a single kidney to that of a population of individuals, the standard deviation of the acceleration time increased to 0.03 second. Similar stepwise increases in variance were seen for acceleration and peak systolic velocity.

On the basis of these variance estimates, the standard deviation of the averages of repeated measurements was also calculated (Table 4). In addition, the probability of exceeding a discriminatory threshold value was calculated for acceleration time and for systolic acceleration. By using the published (2) discriminatory threshold of 0.07 second for acceleration time, our data indicated a 69% probability of exceeding this value in a normal kidney at a single reading. This probability did not improve when two, three, or even 1,000 such averaged measurements were used.

Sensitivity and specificity could be estimated when higher threshold levels were used for the upper limit of the normal range (Table 5); these values were optimized at a threshold value of 0.12 second. In contrast, a comparison of the systolic acceleration measurement with the threshold value of 3.0 m/sec^2 suggested that averaging may improve precision. We found a probability of approximately 10% of exceeding this discriminatory threshold in a normal kidney with a single reading, and this percentage decreased steadily for two, three, four, and more readings. In similar fashion, we found that the averaging of multiple readings of peak systolic velocity also produced stepwise increases in precision.

Table 3
Variance Estimates and Standard Deviations for Ascending Levels of Sampling

Source of Variation	Acceleration Time: Variance Estimate	Acceleration Time: Standard Deviation	Acceleration: Variance Estimate	Acceleration: Standard Deviation	Peak Systolic Velocity: Variance Estimate	Peak Systolic Velocity: Standard Deviation
Kidney	0.00046	0.02	0.50	0.71	0.0035	0.06
Kidney and patient	0.00057	0.02	0.59	0.77	0.0038	0.06
Kidney and patient and population	0.00085	0.03	0.77	0.88	0.0053	0.07

DISCUSSION

The results of this study indicate that there is considerable variability in the Doppler parameters of the early systole, even in a population that has been rigorously screened for the absence of renal disease. By determining the components of the total variability—that is, the variability between subjects, between the two kidneys in a single subject, and between the different regions of a single kidney—we found that, for all variables, most of the total variation occurred with repeated measurements obtained in a single kidney. In fact, more than half of the variability in these parameters resulted from random, rather than systematic, effects.

This is not good news: This result suggests that the intrinsic sampling variability in these measurements (somewhat analogous to random background noise) may overwhelm real differences between individuals or between kidneys. The ultimate consequence is a compromised ability to distinguish normal from abnormal kidneys, so that a disease state would need to produce a drastic shift in the magnitude of these variables to be detected amid the "noise." Large deviations from the broad normal ranges of these parameters could still feasibly indicate true disease, but small changes could be due entirely to random variation in these measurements.

One potential strategy to mitigate the variability between single readings is to obtain an average value for multiple readings. The averages of larger numbers of measurements would be more likely to approximate the true parameter value for a kidney; however, we found that repeated sampling did not decrease the probability of obtaining an acceleration time value greater than 0.07 second, which is one proposed upper limit of the normal range (Table 4). Our model suggests that 0.12 second may be a more optimal upper limit of the normal range and that averaging appears to improve sensitivity and specificity estimates at this level (Table 5). For acceleration measurements, an average of three to four samples tended to decrease the likelihood of obtaining an abnormal value. Even so, the skew and spread of the distributions of these parameters will tend to undermine the utility of repeated sampling. Indeed, calculated coefficients of variation reveal that the standard deviation of the measurements represented fully 20%–30% of the population mean values.

On a more hopeful note, our results demonstrate that the parameters of the early systole are not influenced by subject age or the particular pattern of vascular supply to the kidney. An individual kidney can be supplied by any of several patterns of main arterial branches and accessory arteries (15,16). Nonetheless, we could attribute no systematic variation in the parameters of the early systole to accessory or main renal arterial supply.

Several explanations for why these parameters can be so different from one reading to the next are possible. First, we suspect part of the problem may be the difficulty in defining landmarks for the early systole. The first systolic peak, in particular, may be difficult to resolve with clarity, although greater clarity might be achieved by increasing sweep speeds and by maximizing the size of the Doppler spectra. Second, determinations of peak systolic velocity and acceleration depend on an accurate measurement of the angle of insonation, which can be difficult to ascertain in small intrarenal arteries, even with use of sensitive, color Doppler techniques. Third, these parameters could vary depending on the arterial level being sampled (segmental, interlobar, arcuate), just as other Doppler parameters seem to do (17). If the branching pattern of intrarenal arteries is not clearly discerned, different arterial levels could be sampled in different regions of the kidney.

Table 4
Effect of Averaging Multiple Measurements

No. of Averages	Standard Deviation of the Average	Probability of Exceeding a Normal Threshold (%)*
Acceleration time		
1	0.03	69
2	0.03	73
3	0.02	74
4	0.02	75
10	0.02	77
1,000	0.02	78
Acceleration		
1	0.88	10
2	0.72	6
3	0.66	5
4	0.63	4
10	0.56	3
1,000	0.52	2
Peak systolic velocity		
1	0.07	NA
2	0.06	NA
3	0.05	NA
4	0.05	NA
10	0.05	NA
1,000	0.04	NA

* Normal threshold value for acceleration time was 0.07 second; normal threshold value for acceleration was 3.0 m/sec^2. NA = not applicable.

Our findings with regard to the variability of these parameters of the early systole are in agreement with those of studies of arteries elsewhere in the body (17,18). For example, an analysis (18) of the variability components performed with these same parameters measured in the hepatic artery resulted in a similar pattern of estimated variance components, in

Table 5
Predicted Sensitivity and Specificity with Higher Threshold Values of the Normal Range for Acceleration Time

No. of Averages	Upper-Limit Threshold (sec)	Sensitivity	Specificity
1	0.07	0.99	0.25
	0.09	0.98	0.51
	0.11	0.92	0.76
	0.12	0.85	0.86
	0.13	0.75	0.92
2	0.07	0.99	0.22
	0.09	0.99	0.52
	0.11	0.95	0.80
	0.12	0.89	0.89
	0.13	0.79	0.95
3	0.07	0.99	0.20
	0.09	0.99	0.52
	0.11	0.96	0.82
	0.12	0.90	0.91
	0.13	0.81	0.96

which the contribution of the intrinsic sampling variability to the overall variability far outweighed the contributions of other factors. This result suggests that the problems we encountered with these measurements are not limited to the evaluation of the kidney.

In conclusion, measurement of Doppler waveform parameters of the early systole in intrarenal vessels is an approach that is fraught with substantial measurement variability at routine clinical examination. Of the many obstacles to successful application of this approach in the diagnosis of renal artery stenosis, the most formidable may be the disproportionately large amount of variability that is attributable to repeated measurements in the same healthy kidney—that is, the intrinsic background noise of the measurements. Averages of repeated measurements may be partly corrective, at least for measurements of systolic acceleration and peak systolic velocity. Our results call into question the precision and reproducibility of these measurements, however, and we recommend caution when interpreting small changes in these measurements. Those who would make use of this approach must establish for themselves that measurements of these parameters in stenotic renal arteries sufficiently exceed the normal range of variation in their laboratory. ■

Acknowledgment: The authors thank Susan Murray for assistance in preparing this manuscript.

References

1. Handa N, Fukunaga R, Etani H, et al. Efficacy of echo-Doppler examination for the evaluation of renovascular disease. Ultrasound Med Biol 1988; 14:1–5.
2. Stavros AT, Parker SH, Yakes WF, et al. Segmental stenosis of the renal artery: pattern recognition of tardus and parvus abnormalities with duplex sonography. Radiology 1992; 184:487–492.
3. Lafortune M, Patriquin H, Demeule E, et al. Renal arterial stenosis: slowed systole in the downstream circulation—experimental study in dogs. Radiology 1992; 184:475–478.
4. Patriquin HB, Lafortune M, Jéquier JC, et al. Stenosis of the renal artery: assessment of slowed systole in the downstream circulation with Doppler sonography. Radiology 1992; 184:479–485.
5. Burdick L, Airoldi F, Marana I, et al. Superiority of acceleration and acceleration time over pulsatility and resistance indices as screening tests for renal artery stenosis. J Hypertens 1996; 14:1229–1235.
6. Kliewer MA, Tupler RH, Carroll BA, et al. Renal artery stenosis: analysis of Doppler waveform parameters and tardus-parvus pattern. Radiology 1993; 189:779–787.
7. van der Hulst VPM, van Baalen J, Kool LS, et al. Renal artery stenosis: endovascular flow wire study for validation of Doppler US. Radiology 1996; 200:165–168.
8. Postma CT, Bijlstra PJ, Rosenbusch G, Thien T. Pattern recognition of loss of early systolic peak by Doppler ultrasound has a low sensitivity for the detection of renal artery stenosis. J Hum Hypertens 1996; 10:181–184.
9. Gottlieb RH, Hartley DF, Rubens DJ, et al. Effect of a main renal artery stenosis on the downstream Doppler waveform in dogs. Acad Radiol 1995; 2:768–775.
10. Lucas P, Blome S, Roche J. Intra-renal Doppler wave-form analysis as a screening test for renal artery stenosis. Australas Radiol 1996; 40:276–282.
11. Kotval PS. Doppler waveform parvus and tardus: a sign of proximal flow obstruction. J Ultrasound Med 1989; 8:435–440.
12. Bude RO, Rubin JM, Platt JF, Fechner KP, Adler RS. Pulsus tardus: its cause and potential limitations in detection of arterial stenosis. Radiology 1994; 190:779–784.
13. Kliewer MA, Tupler RH, Hertzberg BS, et al. Doppler evaluation of renal artery stenosis: interobserver agreement in the interpretation of waveform morphology. AJR 1994; 162:1371–1376.
14. Ioannou G, Thorpe RJ, MacKechnie SG, Hobbs JM, Williams KM. Duplex sonography in detection of renal artery stenosis: a simplified approach using new parameters. Australas Radiol 1993; 37:386–388.
15. Ajmani ML, Ajmani K. To study the intrarenal vascular segments of human kidney by corrosion cast technique. Anat Anz 1983; 154:293–303.
16. Graves FT, ed. The arterial anatomy of the kidney. Bristol, England: Wright, 1971; 33–34.
17. Knapp R, Plötzeneder A, Frauscher F, et al. Variability of Doppler parameters in the healthy kidney: an anatomic-physiologic correlation. J Ultrasound Med 1995; 14:427–429.
18. Paulson EK, Kliewer MA, Frederick MG, Keogan MT, DeLong DM, Nelson RC. Hepatic artery: variability in measurement of resistive index and systolic acceleration time in healthy volunteers. Radiology 1996; 200:725–729.

Special Report

Melissa L. Rosado-de-Christenson, Lt Col, USAF, MC[2]

Jeffrey R. Galvin, MD
Armed Forces Institute of Pathology 1997–1998 Distinguished Scientist[1]

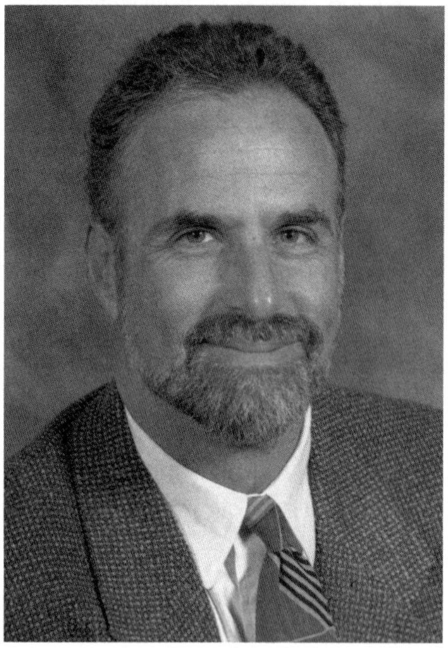

Index terms: Armed Forces Institute of Pathology • Radiology and radiologists • Special reports

Radiology 1997; 205:114

[1]The opinions and assertions contained herein are the private views of the author and are not to be construed as official or as reflecting the views of the Department of the Air Force or the Department of Defense.

[2]Chairman and Registrar, Department of Radiologic Pathology, Armed Forces Institute of Pathology, Bldg 54, Rm M-121, Alaska Ave and Fern St, Washington, DC 20306-6000. Received June 11, 1997; accepted June 12. **Address reprint requests to** the author.

JEFFREY R. Galvin, MD, will serve as Distinguished Scientist in the Department of Radiologic Pathology at the Armed Forces Institute of Pathology (AFIP) from July 1, 1997, to June 30, 1998. Dr Galvin is a professor of radiology and internal medicine at the University of Iowa College of Medicine, Iowa City, and his area of expertise is thoracic radiology. He obtained his medical degree from Northwestern University, Chicago, Ill, in 1975 and completed his residency training in internal medicine at Butterworth Hospital in Grand Rapids, Mich, in 1978. In 1981 he completed fellowship training in pulmonary medicine at the University of Iowa Hospitals and Clinics, and served as director of the Medical Intensive Care Unit at that institution from 1981 to 1984. From 1984 to 1988 he completed a residency in diagnostic radiology at the University of Iowa, where he has since served as director of the Division of Chest Imaging.

Dr Galvin is active in several national and international societies, including the Radiological Society of North America, the American College of Radiology, the American College of Chest Physicians, the American Thoracic Society, and the Society of Thoracic Radiology, where he serves as chairman of the Electronic Education Committee. He is a reviewer for the *American Journal of Roentgenology* and the *Journal of Thoracic Imaging*.

Dr Galvin is the author or coauthor of 60 original publications. His special interests include the study of physiologic imaging and function in thoracic diseases and medical informatics. He is well known for his interest in electronic education and currently has grants from the National Library of Medicine, one of which is entitled "Biomedical Applications of High-Performance Computing", and the other is entitled "Integrated Advanced Information Management Systems (IAIMS)". His expertise in electronic education and information management will greatly enhance the research, education, and consultation missions of the AFIP.

As Distinguished Scientist, Dr Galvin will participate in the education and research programs of the Department of Radiologic Pathology at the AFIP, thus making a major contribution toward the education of radiology residents and practicing radiologists in the United States and throughout the world.

The Distinguished Scientist program was established in 1983 and is now an integral part of the Department of Radiologic Pathology. The position is federally funded through the American Registry of Pathology but is generously supported by contributions from the American College of Radiology, the Radiological Society of North America, the American Roentgen Ray Society, the Association of University Radiologists, and the American Osteopathic College of Radiology. Representatives from each of these organizations, together with a representative from the Association of Program Directors in Radiology, form the Conjoint Committee for Radiologic Pathology at the AFIP and are responsible for selecting the Distinguished Scientist each year.

Any established academic radiologist interested in spending a year studying the correlation between abnormal radiologic images and underlying pathologic processes is welcome to apply. Those who are interested should submit a letter of interest that outlines the projects they would pursue and a copy of their curriculum vitae to Dr Rosado-de-Christenson at the address listed herein. Applications for the Distinguished Scientist position for the 1999–2000 academic year must be received by December 15, 1997. ■

Evert-Jan Verschuyl, MD • Robert Kaatee, MD • Frederik J. A. Beek, MD
Nilesh H. Patel, MD • Arthur B. Fontaine, MD • Charles P. Daly, MD
Douglas M. Coldwell, MD • William H. Bush, MD • Willem P. T. M. Mali, MD

Renal Artery Origins: Best Angiographic Projection Angles[1]

PURPOSE: **To determine the best projection angles for imaging the renal artery origins in profile.**

MATERIALS AND METHODS: **A mathematical model of the anatomy at the renal artery origins in the transverse plane was used to analyze the amount of aortic lumen that projects over the renal artery origins at various projection angles. Computed tomographic (CT) angiographic data about the location of 400 renal artery origins in 200 patients were statistically analyzed.**

RESULTS: **In patients with an abdominal aortic diameter no larger than 3.0 cm, approximately 0.5 mm of the proximal part of the renal artery and origin may be hidden from view if there is a projection error of ±10° from the ideal image. A combination of anteroposterior and 20° and 40° left anterior oblique projections resulted in a 92% yield of images that adequately profiled the renal artery origins. Right anterior oblique projections resulted in the least useful images.**

CONCLUSION: **An error in projection angle of ±10° is acceptable for angiographic imaging of the renal artery origins. Patient sex, site of interest (left or right artery), and local diameter of the abdominal aorta are important factors to consider.**

The origin and proximal portion of the renal artery is a prime target area for atherosclerosis. In a study (1) of autopsy specimens, 136 (87%) of 157 single renal artery stenoses were found in the proximal one-third of the trunk. According to McCormack et al (2,3), the atheroma was usually found in the first 2 cm of the main renal artery and was only occasionally found in a main branch that supplied one renal pole. The renal artery ostium may be involved exclusively, or atherosclerosis may extend from the ostium into the proximal part of the renal artery. This pathologic feature and its appearance on images obtained with different imaging modalities have resulted in many definitions for the term "ostial stenosis" (4). In general, atheroma confined to the aortic wall can be considered truly "ostial." This type of stenosis tends to respond poorly to treatment with percutaneous transluminal angioplasty because of elastic recoil (5,6). This anatomic region is, therefore, the main focus of diagnostic angiography and therapeutic intervention, particularly with regard to deployment of endovascular prostheses for renal artery atherosclerosis.

When renal artery stenosis must be excluded in patients with hypertension and/or renal insufficiency, the number of false-negative diagnostic renal artery angiograms should be reduced to a minimum. Optimal accuracy is important in the deployment of endovascular stents for treatment of atherosclerotic ostial renal artery stenosis because improper positioning may cause higher restenosis rates (6–10). At our institutions, we perform angiography in two or more oblique planes, with injection of contrast material into the abdominal aorta, to determine the optimal angle necessary to evaluate the ostia and proximal aspects of the renal arteries or to determine the projection angle to be used at therapeutic interventions such as percutaneous transluminal angioplasty or endovascular stent deployment.

The purpose of this study was to attempt to answer the following questions: (*a*) At what point, as one rotates away from the true profile angle, is information about the origin and proximal part of the renal artery hidden behind the contrast material–filled abdominal aorta, and what variables play a role in this process? (*b*) What degree of variation is acceptable at diagnostic angiography and during stent deployment at the renal artery origin? (*c*) What is the minimum useful increment of change in x-ray tube angulation at which subsequent projections and injections of contrast material should be performed? (*d*) What are the best projections for imaging the renal artery origin, and is there a sex difference? (*e*) Is there a satisfactory sequence to use when one of the renal artery origins is considered, or

Index terms: Aorta, arteriosclerosis, 981.721 • Computed tomography (CT), helical, 961.12915, 961.12916 • Renal angiography, 961.1211, 961.12916 • Renal arteries, CT, 961.12915, 961.12916

Abbreviations: AP = anteroposterior, LAO = left anterior oblique, RAO = right anterior oblique.

Radiology 1997; 205:115–120

[1] From the Department of Radiology, University of Washington Medical Center, Box 357115, 1959 NE Pacific St, Seattle, WA 98195 (E.J.V., N.H.P., A.B.F., C.P.D., W.H.B.); the Department of Radiology, Utrecht University Hospital, The Netherlands (R.K., F.J.A.B., W.P.T.M.M.); and the Department of Medical Imaging, University of Colorado, Denver (D.M.C.). Received March 4, 1997; revision requested April 29; revision received June 4; accepted June 9. **Address reprint requests to** E.J.V.

when either or both of the renal artery origins are of interest?

MATERIALS AND METHODS

Spiral computed tomographic (CT) angiograms in 70 patients were retrospectively reviewed by two radiologists (F.J.A.B., R.K). The length of the ostial renal artery stenosis was measured with an Easy-Vision postprocessing unit (Philips Medical Systems, Best, The Netherlands). All patients were undergoing treatment at the University of Utrecht, The Netherlands, and were participants in a prospective trial that compared spiral CT angiographic findings with digital substraction angiographic findings in terms of the accuracy of detection of renal artery stenosis. All patients had marked aortic atherosclerotic disease and were evaluated because of renal insufficiency and/or uncontrollable arterial hypertension. Intraarterial digital subtraction angiography was performed with a commercially available system (Integris V 3000; Philips Medical Systems). Spiral CT angiography was performed with a Tomoscan SR 7000 (Philips Medical Systems).

To assess how much of the origin and proximal part of the renal artery is hidden behind the contrast material–filled aorta at various projection angles, a mathematical model of a simplified abdominal aorta with the proximal part of the renal arteries was constructed (Fig 1). In this model, x rays through the aorta and renal arteries were assumed to be parallel, and no corrections were made for beam divergence, parallax, and magnification. Although Rose et al (11) demonstrated substantial and predictable magnification differences between the proximal and the distal portions of the renal artery during angiography, it appears unlikely that appreciable magnification differences are present between the renal artery origins (11). In Figure 1, the renal artery origin is represented as a point on the circle, with a location determined by the angle (α) between a line from the origin to the center of the circle and the horizontal axis. The proximal renal artery is represented by a half circle, y (with radius $x/2$, where x is the horizontal length of the column of contrast material that may block the proximal renal artery from view), or a quarter circle, y' (with radius x). Both y and y' can be expressed as $\pi x/2$. Alternatively, x can be expressed as $r - b \cap \cos \alpha = b/r$, in which case $x = r - (r \cos \alpha)$, and $x = r(1 - \cos \alpha)$, where r is the radius of the aorta and $b = r \cos \alpha$.

Although the length of x itself could be used as a measure of the length of renal artery obscured by the aorta, this would likely underestimate the true length. Because the proximal renal artery tends to be more curvilinear, we considered the quarter- or half-circle representation to be a more conservative estimate. On the basis of our equations, it follows that the length of proximal renal artery hidden behind the aorta can be expressed as $y = y' = (\pi r[1 - \cos \alpha])/2$. The length of the proximal renal artery that is hidden depends, therefore, on the radius of the abdominal aorta and on the location of the renal artery origin. Figure 2 depicts this relationship for aortas with various diameters.

To calculate the average abdominal aortic diameter at the level of the renal arteries in patients with minimal aortic atherosclerotic disease, the AP and transverse diameters were retrospectively measured on spiral CT angiograms in 59 patients with minimal atherosclerotic disease. The average abdominal aortic diameter at the level of the renal artery D was calculated as follows: (average AP diameter + average transverse diameter)/2.

Atherosclerosis in the aorta was graded as mild, moderate, or severe (12,13). Absence of aortic atherosclerosis was defined as grade 0. A mild degree of atherosclerosis (grade 1) was characterized by a regular lumen with noncircumferential thrombus and/or calcification. A moderate degree (grade 2) was characterized by an irregular lumen with circumferential thrombus and/or calcification at different, noncontinuous levels. A severe degree (grade 3) was characterized by an irregular lumen with continuous circumferential thrombus and/or calcification. Only images in patients with grade 0 or 1 aortic atherosclerosis were included in the analysis.

We recently published (14) our data about the location and distribution of the renal artery origins. The main paired renal arteries in 200 patients, many of whom were included in the present study, were retrospectively identified on spiral CT angiograms, and the location of the arteries, defined in terms of the optimal projection angles, was recorded. With these data and the results of our mathematical model, we were able to create distribution graphs, which demonstrated the number of adequately profiled renal artery origins for a given projection angle in our series of 200 patients (Table 1, Fig 3). Analysis of the distribution graphs has led us to insights and recommendations, which may be clinically useful, regarding the best projections to image the renal artery origins.

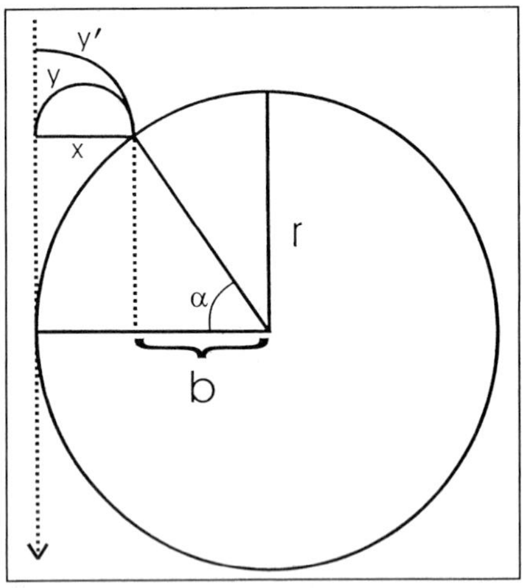

Figure 1. Schematic shows our model of the relationship between the abdominal aorta (circle) and renal artery origin (α) in the transverse plane. The model is used to approximate the various lengths (x, y, y') of the artery that may be obscured by the contrast material–filled aorta. $b = r \cos \alpha$, r = radius of the abdominal aorta, arrow = path of the incident anteroposterior (AP) x-ray beam.

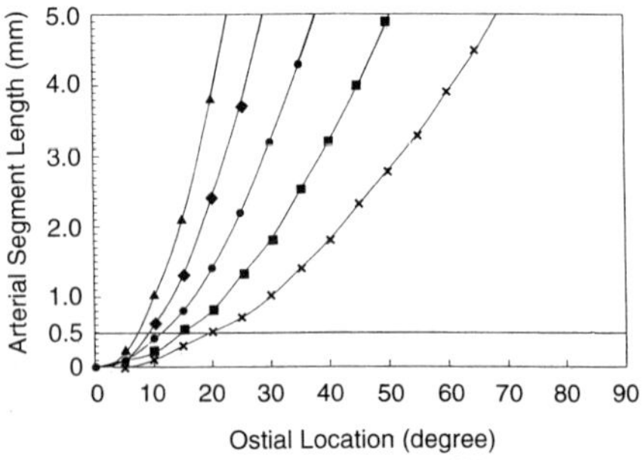

Figure 2. Graph shows the length of the proximal part of the renal artery obscured by a contrast material–filled abdominal aorta with a diameter of 8.00 cm (▲), 5.00 cm (◆), 3.00 cm (●), 1.75 cm (■), or 1.00 cm (×) versus the location of the renal artery origin at AP imaging.

RESULTS

On the basis of our model and the resultant graph, it was evident that the location of the renal artery origin with respect to the x-ray beam and the diameter of the aorta at the level of the renal arteries were important variables for determining the length of the proximal renal artery obscured by contrast material in the abdominal aorta (Figs 1, 2). First, for a given location of the renal artery origin, the length of the proximal renal artery segment hidden behind the aorta increased exponentially as the diameter of the aorta increased. Second, for a given aortic diameter viewed with an AP x-ray beam, there was an exponential increase in the length of the hidden renal artery segment as the location of the renal artery origin changed from 0° to 90° (eg, lateral to anterolateral location of the right renal artery). Conversely, for a given lateral location of the renal artery origin in a given patient, the length of the hidden segment increased exponentially as the x-ray beam angle was changed from the profiled AP projection to incremental LAO or RAO projections.

From a clinical point of view, a conservative estimate of the maximum allowable length of proximal renal artery that may be hidden behind the aorta at digital subtraction angiography is probably approximately 0.5 mm. This is based on the fact that the shortest length of a proximal atherosclerotic renal artery stenosis found in our series of 70 patients at Utrecht University Hospital, The Netherlands,

Table 1
Distribution of Renal Artery Origins Imaged in Profile

Renal Artery Origin	Projection Angle −90° to −71°	−70° to −51°	−50° to −31°	−30° to −11°	−10° to 9°	10° to 29°	30° to 49°	50° to 69°	70° to 89°	Total No. of Arteries*
All patients (n = 200)										
Left	1	1	4	15	94	78	7	0	0	200/200
Right	0	0	0	2	31	100	57	9	1	200/200
Left and right	0	0	0	1	16	38	3	0	0	58/200
Left and/or right	1	1	4	17	125	178	64	9	1	400/400
Male patients (n = 89)										
Left	0	1	3	10	47	27	1	0	0	89/89
Right	0	0	0	1	8	50	25	5	0	89/89
Left and right	0	0	0	0	3	14	1	0	0	18/89
Left and/or right	0	1	3	11	55	77	26	5	0	178/178
Female patients (n = 111)										
Left	1	0	1	5	47	51	6	0	0	111/111
Right	0	0	0	1	23	50	32	4	1	111/111
Left and right	0	0	0	1	13	24	2	0	0	40/111
Left and/or right	1	0	1	6	70	101	38	4	1	222/222

Note.—Data are number of renal artery origins profiled. With our model, a projection error of ±10° was considered to be sufficiently accurate.
* Data are number of renal artery orgins profiled/total number of renal artery origins.

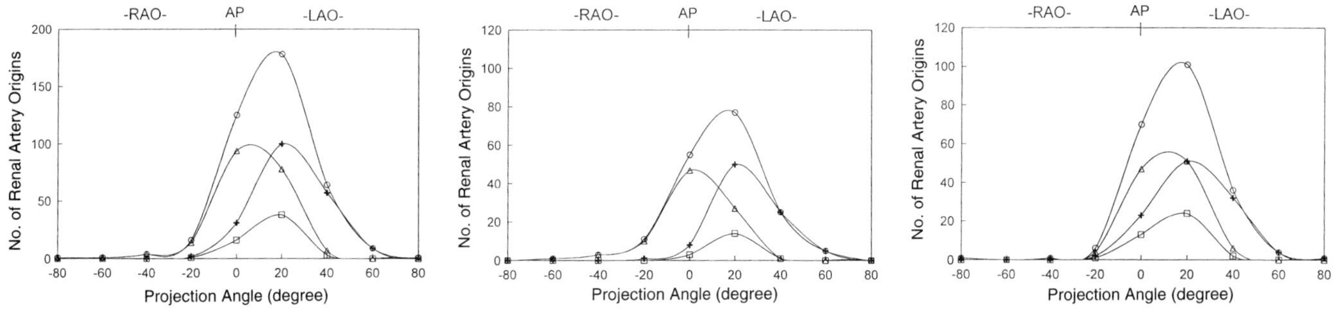

a. b. c.

Figure 3. Graphs show the distribution of profiled arteries at different angles of projection. On the basis of our model, a projection error of ±10° was considered to be sufficiently accurate. *LAO* = left anterior oblique, *RAO* = right anterior oblique, △ = left renal artery origin, □ = left and right renal artery origins, ○ = left and/or right renal artery origin, + = right renal artery origin. **(a)** Graph shows the distribution of profiled artery origins in all 200 patients. **(b)** Graph shows the distribution of profiled artery origins in 89 male patients. **(c)** Graph shows the distribution of profiled artery origins in 111 female patients.

was 1 mm (range, 1–30 mm). By using proper window settings, a stenosis of 1 mm in length or longer should be visible if a projection that results in a length of hidden renal artery of 0.5 mm or less is used. The same argument can be applied for accurate deployment of ostial renal artery stents, which, according to several authors (6,7), should be placed flush with or within 1 mm of the contrast material–filled aortic lumen.

Figure 2 shows that, given a 0.5-mm maximum allowable length of the hidden segment, the associated maximum allowable error in projection was 10°–15° for an abdominal aorta with a diameter that ranged from 3.00 (borderline aneurysmal aorta) to 1.75 cm (average diameter in minimally diseased aorta). Therefore, in a patient with an abdominal aortic diameter (at the level of the renal artery origins) of 3 cm or smaller, an image obtained at a projection angle within 10° of the perfect profile angle may be accurate enough for diagnostic and therapeutic purposes. In a patient with an aortic diameter larger than 3 cm, a projection error of less than 10° is likely to be acceptable.

With the assumption that a projection error of ±10° is allowable during angiography of the renal artery origins, we reevaluated the data obtained at our anatomic study (14) of the location and distribution of the renal artery origins. When constructing the distribution graphs (Fig 3), we took into consideration the ±10° projection error; the graphs show the number of renal artery origins in which an adequate angiographic profile could be obtained with projection angles that ranged from the steep RAO (−75°) to the steep LAO (75°) (Table 1).

Distribution graphs were constructed for the study population as a whole, for male patients, and for female patients. The following observations, which are summarized in Table 2, were made on the basis of the distribution graphs.

Left Renal Artery Origin

Because of the lateral or posterolateral location of the left renal artery origin, AP and 20° LAO projections tended to be most helpful for imaging of the left renal artery origin. Regardless of sex, 94 (47%) of 200 left renal arteries were imaged in profile on an AP projection (Fig 3a, Table 1). If the origin is not visible with an AP projection, a 20° LAO projection may suffice: 78 (39%) of 200 left renal arteries were imaged in profile with this view. After this, 20° RAO and 40° LAO projections can be obtained, although both resulted in low success with regard to imaging of the left renal artery origin (15 [8%] and seven [4%] left renal artery origins imaged in profile, respectively). A combination of the AP and 20° LAO views, therefore, resulted in the accurate profiling of 172 (86%) left renal artery origins.

In male patients, the AP projection resulted in the largest number of left renal artery origins profiled (47 [53%] of 89), whereas the 20° LAO projection resulted in only 25 (28%) origins profiled (Fig 3b, 3c; Table 1). In female patients, profiling of the origin was similar with the 20° LAO view (51 [46%] of 111) and the AP projection (47 [42%] of 111). The LAO projection is more likely to be useful in female patients than in male patients because a posterolateral location of the left renal artery origin is more prevalent in female patients. This is reflected by the fact that, on average, the angle between the renal artery origins (Fig 3) is greater in female patients (165°) than in male patients (155°) (14). The number of left renal artery origins profiled with the AP and 20° LAO projections combined was 74 (83%) of 89 in male patients and 98 (88%) of 111 in female patients.

Table 2
Angiographic Projections That Provide the Best Profiles of Renal Artery Origins

Projection	Renal Artery Origin: Right	Left	Left and/or Right
All patients (n = 200)			
20° RAO	16 (8)		8 (4)
AP	94 (47)	32 (16)	62 (31)
20° LAO	78 (39)	100 (50)	90 (45)
40° LAO	8 (4)	58 (29)	32 (16)
60° LAO		10 (5)	
Male patients (n = 89)			
40° RAO	3 (3)		
20° RAO	10 (11)		5 (6)
AP	47 (53)	8 (9)	28 (31)
20° LAO	25 (28)	50 (56)	38 (43)
40° LAO		27 (30)	13 (15)
60° LAO		5 (6)	
Female patients (n = 111)			
20° RAO	6 (5)		3 (3)
AP	47 (42)	23 (21)	36 (32)
20° LAO	51 (46)	50 (45)	50 (45)
40° LAO	6 (5)	32 (29)	19 (17)
60° LAO		4 (4)	

Note.—Numbers in parentheses are percentages.

Right Renal Artery Origin

Because of the anterolateral location of the right renal artery, the 20° LAO projection tends to be most helpful at imaging of the right renal artery origin. Regardless of sex, 100 (50%) of 200 right renal artery origins were imaged in profile with a 20° LAO projection. If the origin is not visible with this projection in a given patient, the next best projections were the 40° LAO projection, which resulted in profiling of 57 (28%) of 200 origins, followed by the AP view, which resulted in profiling of 31 (16%) origins. These three projections together resulted in the imaging of 188 (94%) of the 200 right renal artery origins.

Regardless of sex, the LAO projections were helpful in profiling the right renal artery origin; in contrast, the AP projection was more helpful in profiling the left renal artery. Imaging of the right renal artery was best with the 20° LAO projection, regardless of sex (50 [56%] of 89 origins in male patients, and 50 [45%] of 111 origins in female patients) (Fig 3b, 3c; Table 1). Overall, the 20° LAO, 40° LAO, and AP projections resulted in adequate depiction of 83 (93%) of 89 origins in male patients and of 105 (95%) of 111 origins in female patients.

Left and/or Right Renal Artery Origin

Regardless of sex, the 20° LAO projection resulted in depiction of the largest number of origins (178 [45%] of 400), when either or both of the renal artery origins composed the site of interest (Table 1). Overall, the AP, 20° LAO, and 40° LAO projections yielded adequate depiction of 367 (92%) of 400 renal artery origins. For the greatest possible efficiency, the 20° LAO view should be obtained first, followed by the AP view and, finally, the 40° LAO projection. Not until these three projections fail to demonstrate the renal artery origins in profile should RAO projections be considered.

Similar results in both male (77 [43%] of 178 origins) and female (101 [45%] of 222 origins) patients were obtained for the 20° LAO view, which was best for adequate depiction of the renal artery origins (Table 1). A combination of AP and 20° and 40° LAO projections resulted, in male patients, in the depiction of 158 (89%) of 178 renal arteries. In female patients, the same combination resulted in the depiction of 209 (94%) of 222 renal artery origins. Regardless of sex, the best results were obtained with, in order, the 20° LAO, the AP, and the 40° LAO projections.

Left and Right Renal Artery Origins

The left and right renal arteries were depicted simultaneously with a single projection in 58 (29%) of 200 patients. Because the angle between the renal artery origins is, on average, greater in female than in male patients, more left and right renal artery origins were depicted simultaneously in female patients (40 of 111 origins [36%]) than in male patients (18 of 89 origins [20%]). Successful depiction of both renal artery origins was most likely with the use of the 20° LAO projection, regardless of the sex of the patient (Fig 3).

DISCUSSION

Recently, we reported (14) the location and distribution of the renal artery origins as noted on transverse CT scans in 200 patients. The conventional wisdom that the right renal artery origin has an anterolateral location and the left renal artery origin has a posterolateral or lateral location was confirmed in that study (14). The best average projection angle (± 1 standard deviation) for depiction of the right renal artery was 24° ± 15 LAO (range, −26° to 70°); for the left renal artery the best average angle was 5° ± 16 LAO (range, −75° to 38°). We were unable to recommend any specific projection or combination of two projections that would result in an adequate number of depictions of the renal artery origins because of the variation in the distribution of renal artery origin locations and because of our lack of knowledge with regard to acceptable projection error.

Our mathematical model of the abdominal aorta and renal artery origins provides insight into the relationship between the incident x-ray beam and the location of the ostium and length of the proximal renal artery that is hidden from view behind the contrast material–filled aorta. With our model, we can assume that a projection error of ±10° is acceptable at attempted profile imaging of the renal artery origin in patients whose abdominal aorta has a diameter, at the level of the renal arteries, of no larger than 3 cm. A projection error of this magnitude will result in a hidden segment that is no more than 0.5 mm in length. If, however, the abdominal aorta is larger than 3 cm in diameter (ie, aneurysmal), a smaller projection error should be accepted. A projection error of ±5° may be more appropriate in those circumstances. As the aortic diameter increases, the length of the hidden segment increases exponentially for a given increment of change in projection angle. The relationship between origin location and the length of hidden renal artery segment becomes close to linear as the aortic diameter decreases, as is the case, for example, in an infant with an aortic diameter of 1 cm.

If the renal artery origin does not seem to be depicted in profile at examination of the angiograms obtained after the initial injection of contrast material, a subsequent projection change of at least 10° may be appropriate because, in the majority of cases, the abdominal aorta is less than 3 cm in diameter. Subsequent injections of contrast material at smaller projection increments (eg, ±5°) will not substantially alter the length of the hidden renal artery segment in those patients and are, therefore, unlikely to result in better visualization of the proximal renal artery segment and origin. Smaller projection increment changes would likely necessitate more subsequent injections of contrast material, which would result in unnecessary contrast material load and radiation exposure to the patient.

A weakness of our assumptions with regard to the allowable projection-angle error and increment changes in projection angle is that they are based on a mathematical model, which is an approximation of reality. We believe, however, that our mathematical model represents a reasonable approximation. Variations in the thickness of the aortic wall and different ratios in the thickness of the contrast material column in the aorta and in the renal artery will affect the visibility through the aortic contrast medium of the proximal renal artery and origin. Optimization of the window levels can often help depict segments of the proximal part of the renal artery and origin that are hidden behind aortic contrast material in images that inadequately profiled these structures.

Conversely, on adequate images, stenoses oriented in the coronal plane in the proximal renal artery and ostium may be difficult to visualize if the angiogram is obtained in the frontal plane. In these instances, compound angulation can be useful (15).

A factor that was thought to have implications with regard to the best projection angles and the best sequence of angles to use was whether one had a specific interest in the left renal artery origin, right renal artery origin, both origins, or either origin. Because the sex of a patient who is to undergo angiography is always known before the start of the procedure, we attempted to analyze our results with this fact in mind. Furthermore, our results are based on the combination of CT findings and our mathematical model. Whether our results are clinically reproducible remains to be proved. The results of early clinical application, at the University of Washington, Seattle, of the recommendations based on the data summarized in Table 2 have shown those recommendations to be quite useful, and our results appear to correlate well with our clinical experience.

The LAO projection has been recommended (16) as the best projection for imaging of both the left and right renal artery origins. Harrington et al (15) used the 15° LAO projection as their initial projection for imaging the renal arteries. With a few refinements, our results are in general accordance with theirs. We found that the 20° LAO view resulted in an approximate yield of 45% of images that adequately profiled the renal artery origins. This was the highest yield attainable with a single projection in a given patient, regardless of sex, when both renal artery origins are of interest.

The question remains, however: Which projection angle should be used next if the 20° LAO projection does not result in adequate depiction? Our results suggest that the recommended second projection angle should be the AP projection, and the third should be the 40° LAO projection. This is, again, true irrespective of the sex of the patient (Table 2). Overall, without regard to sex or the need for evaluation of the right or left artery origin, a combination of the 20° LAO (shallow oblique), AP, and 40° LAO views (in that order) are the most likely to depict the renal arteries.

Specific interest in either the right or left renal artery origin will affect the choice of the initial projection. With regard to the right renal artery origin, LAO projections (20° and 40° LAO, in that order) resulted in the largest number of adequate depictions, compared with the AP projection, which should be considered as a third option. This is true regardless of the sex of the patient. In male patients, the AP projection should be used first if a profile image of the left renal artery is needed, followed by the 20° LAO view. In female patients, the 20° LAO projection should be used first, followed by the AP view. The AP projection combined with a 20° LAO view will likely lead to substantial yields in both male (83% in our study) and female (88% in our study) patients.

An important conclusion is that the RAO projection plays a relatively unimportant role when profile imaging of the left renal artery origin is the specific angiographic goal. This was true regardless of the sex of the patient. The underlying anatomic reason is that only 20% (40 of 200) of the left renal artery origins are in an anterolateral location (14). The RAO view plays virtually no role when imaging the right renal artery origin. The underlying anatomic reason is that only 2% (three of 200) of right renal artery origins are in a posterolateral location (14). Review of angiographic findings of the renal artery origins at our institutions showed that, in most cases, three or more projections were obtained. The three most commonly used projections were the AP, a shallow LAO (15°–20°), and varying degrees of RAO and steep LAO views. The majority of the RAO views were unnecessary and did not aid in depicting the renal artery origins. Occasionally RAO views can be of use when imaging an anterolaterally located left renal artery or when attempting to depict a stenosis in the middle to distal portion of the right renal artery.

In conclusion, therefore, sex, specific site of interest (right or left renal artery origin), and the local diameter of the abdominal aorta are important factors to consider at diagnostic angiography and at therapeutic intervention at the renal artery origins. ■

Acknowledgments: The authors thank Jeroen van der Grond, PhD, for his skilled contribution in generating the graphics and M. Viergever, PhD, and W. A. Grootendorst, PhD, for their assistance in creating the mathematical model of the abdominal aorta and renal artery origins.

References

1. Schwartz CJ, White TA. Stenosis of the renal artery: an unselected necropsy study. Br Med J 1964; 2:1415–1421.
2. McCormack LJ, Dustan HP, Gifford RW, et al. Pathology of renal artery disease. Postgrad Med 1966; 40:348–354.

3. McCormack LJ, Poutasse EF, Meaney TF, et al. A pathologic-arteriographic correlation of renal arterial disease. Am Heart J 1966; 72:188–198.
4. Kaatee R, Beek FJA, Verschuyl EJ, et al. Atherosclerotic renal artery stenosis: ostial or truncal? Radiology 1996; 199:637–640.
5. Weibull H, Bergqvist D, Jonsson K, et al. Long-term results after percutaneous transluminal angioplasty of atherosclerotic renal artery stenosis: the importance of intensive follow-up. Eur J Vasc Surg 1991; 5:291–301.
6. Baert AL. Renal artery stent placement (editorial). Radiology 1994; 191:619–621.
7. Henry M, Amor M, Henry I, et al. Stent placement in the renal artery: three-year experience with the Palmaz stent. JVIR 1996; 7:343–350.
8. van de Ven PJG, Beutler JJ, Kaatee R, et al. Transluminal vascular stent for ostial atherosclerotic renal artery stenosis. Lancet 1995; 346:672–674.
9. Hennequin LM, Joffre FG, Rousseau HP, et al. Renal artery stent placement: long-term results with the Wallstent endoprosthesis. Radiology 1994; 191:713–719.
10. Rees CR, Palmaz JC, Becker GJ, et al. Palmaz stent in atherosclerotic stenoses involving the ostia of the renal arteries: preliminary report of a multicenter study. Radiology 1991; 181:507–514.
11. Rose SC, Gardner JC, Verschuyl EJ, et al. Image magnification in renal and superior mesenteric angiography: CT calculation and assessment of variables. JVIR 1996; 7:573–578.
12. Siegel CL, Ellis JH, Korobkin M, et al. CT-detected renal arterial calcification: correlation with renal artery stenosis on angiography. AJR 1994; 163:867–872.
13. Scott JA, Rabe FE, Becker GJ, et al. Angiographic assessment of renal artery pathology: how reliable? AJR 1983; 141:1299–1303.
14. Verschuyl EJ, Kaatee R, Beek FJA, et al. Renal artery origins: location and distribution in the transverse plane at CT. Radiology 1997; 203:71–75.
15. Harrington DP, Levin DC, Garnic JD, et al. Compound angulation for the angiographic evaluation of renal artery stenosis. Radiology 1983; 146:829–831.
16. Gerlock AJ Jr, Goncharenko V, Sloan OM. Right posterior oblique: the projection of choice in aortography of hypertensive patients. Radiology 1978; 127:45–48.

Robert Kaatee, MD • Frederik J. A. Beek, MD • Eduard E. de Lange, MD • Maarten S. van Leeuwen, MD
Henk F. M. Smits, MD • Peter J. G. van der Ven, MD • Jaap J. Beutler, MD • Willem P. T. M. Mali, MD

Renal Artery Stenosis: Detection and Quantification with Spiral CT Angiography versus Optimized Digital Subtraction Angiography[1]

PURPOSE: **To compare spiral computed tomographic (CT) angiography with optimized digital subtraction angiography (DSA) for accurate detection and quantification of renal artery stenosis.**

MATERIALS AND METHODS: **In 71 consecutive patients with possible renovascular hypertension, spiral CT angiography was performed of the renal arteries before DSA. Optimized DSA (performed with projection angles calculated from axial spiral CT source images) was used as the standard. Two independent observers evaluated spiral CT angiograms for the presence and grade of renal artery stenosis. Sensitivity, specificity, and interobserver variability were calculated.**

RESULTS: **With spiral CT angiography, all 166 renal arteries and accessory arteries were identified correctly by both reviewers. Overall sensitivity and specificity for assessment of stenoses of grade 0 (none), grade 1 (1%–49%), grade 2 (51%–99%), and grade 3 (occlusion) were 97% and 100%, 92% and 98%, 96% and 96%, and 100% and 100%, respectively. Agreement was strong between spiral CT angiographic and DSA findings in assessment of all grades of stenosis (κ coefficient, 0.9 and 0.9, respectively) for the two observers.**

CONCLUSION: **Spiral CT angiography enabled accurate assessment of renal artery stenosis in patients with possible renovascular hypertension and may assist in selecting patients for interventional treatment.**

RENAL artery stenosis resulting from atherosclerosis is the most common cause of secondary hypertension (1). Although secondary hypertension has an estimated prevalence of 3%–5% in the overall population with hypertension, it is important to detect renal artery stenosis because it is potentially curable (2,3). Atherosclerotic renal artery stenosis tends to progress and may lead to atrophy of the poststenotic kidney and progressive renal failure if both kidneys are involved (4). Early identification and treatment of renal artery stenosis can potentially prevent the development of end-stage renal failure (5,6). Currently, conventional x-ray arteriography and digital subtraction angiography (DSA) are the standard modalities for diagnosis of renal artery stenosis. However, considering the relative low prevalence of renal artery stenosis and the invasive nature of these techniques, they are not suitable for screening purposes.

Recently, studies have demonstrated the usefulness of spiral computed tomographic (CT) angiography as a minimally invasive imaging technique for depicting the vascular anatomy of the kidneys and for evaluating pathologic conditions (7–12). Most studies in which spiral CT angiography was evaluated for detection of renal artery stenosis have shown good results, particularly with use of thin collimation and optimized timing of administration of contrast material (7,8). In those studies, conventional arteriography or DSA was used as the standard, and calculations of sensitivity and specificity of spiral CT angiography in evaluation of renal artery stenosis were based on the assumption that arteriography enabled the correct diagnosis. However, several studies have demonstrated that the severity of renal artery stenosis may be overestimated at spiral CT angiography (7–10). It has been suggested that this overestimation may not be real but is in fact the result of underestimation of the stenosis at arteriography or DSA studies that were used as the standard. This underestimation may be caused by inadequate profiling of the proximal segment of the renal artery that usually contains the stenosis (13). An inadequate profile of this segment of the renal artery may lead to incorrect angiographic assessment of stenosis and, consequently, to an inadequate standard.

At standard arteriography or DSA, radiographs are usually obtained in the anteroposterior and shallow (15°–20°) right posterior oblique projections (14). In these projections, however, the proximal segment of the renal artery

Index terms: Computed tomography (CT), angiography, 961.12915, 961.12916 • Computed tomography (CT), comparative studies, 961.12915, 961.12916 • Computed tomography (CT), helical, 961.12915 • Renal angiography, 961.12915, 961.12916 • Renal arteries, stenosis or obstruction, 961.721

Abbreviation: DSA = digital subtraction angiography.

Radiology 1997; 205:121–127

[1] From the Departments of Radiology (R.K., F.J.A.B., M.S.v.L., H.F.M.S., W.P.T.M.M.) and Nephrology (P.J.G.v.d.V., J.J.B.), University Hospital Utrecht, the Netherlands; and the Department of Radiology, University of Virginia Health Sciences Center, Charlottesville (E.E.d.L.). Received November 4, 1996; revision requested January 6, 1997; final revision received June 10; accepted June 16. Supported in part by grant no. C95.1516 from the Dutch Kidney Foundation. **Address reprint requests to** R.K., Department of Radiology, Boven IJ Ziekenhuis, Postbus 37610, 1030 BD Amsterdam, the Netherlands.

may not be visualized optimally relative to the aorta because the two structures may be superimposed. As a result, stenosis involving this segment may be difficult to assess and may be underestimated. Consequently, standard angiography or DSA may be of limited use as the standard when determining the usefulness of spiral CT angiography in assessment of renal artery stenosis.

In an earlier study (13), we showed that there is marked variety in the angles that occur between the proximal portion of the renal artery and the aorta when evaluated in the transverse plane. The origin of the right renal artery tends to be located anterolateral in the aorta and the left posterolateral or lateral, with angles ranging from 75° ventral to 38° dorsal in the transverse plane. Therefore, a high degree of variability in x-ray source and image intensifier angulation is necessary to depict optimally the proximal segment of the renal artery at angiography. Thus, to improve the standard for evaluating spiral CT angiography, it is necessary to obtain radiographs at arteriography or DSA with such projections that the proximal segment of each renal artery is shown fully without superimposition over the aorta.

The purpose of this study was to determine the usefulness of spiral CT angiography for detecting and quantifying renal artery stenosis in patients with hypertension and possible renovascular disease. To avoid potential problems of over- and underestimation of disease, the findings from spiral CT angiography were compared with those from DSA as an "optimized" standard (DSA was performed with projections that ensured depiction of the proximal segment of each renal artery fully).

MATERIALS AND METHODS

Patient Population

The group consisted of 71 consecutive patients in whom renovascular hypertension or ischemic nephropathy was suspected clinically and who underwent spiral CT angiography and DSA for evaluation of the renal arteries for the presence of stenosis. Clinical suspicion of disease was based on the following clinical findings: (*a*) blood pressure greater than 160/90 mm Hg while receiving antihypertensive treatment, (*b*) positive renographic findings after administration of captopril 1 hour before renography, and/or (*c*) increase in the plasma creatinine level greater than 20% after treatment with an angiotensin converting enzyme inhibitor.

The 33 men and 38 women ranged in age from 33 to 79 years (mean, 59 years). In all patients, spiral CT angiography was performed before DSA, with a median interval of 12 days (range, 3–85 days) between the two examinations.

Spiral CT Angiographic Technique

Spiral CT angiography was performed with a commercially available scanner (Tomoscan SR 7000; Philips Medical Systems, Best, the Netherlands). The acquisition was initiated with a localizer scan obtained without contrast material enhancement to determine the level of the renal arteries. Subsequently, a volume acquisition was performed with the following protocol: 140 kV at 250 mA, 30 seconds continuous exposure, 3-mm collimation, and 3 mm/sec table speed. Data were reconstructed with a 180° linear interpolation algorithm; the reconstruction index was 1 mm. Narrower collimation was not used, as this was not available on our CT scanner.

A total of 140 mL of nonionic contrast material (iopromide [300 mg of iodine per milliliter], Ultravist 300; Schering, Weesp, the Netherlands) was injected at a rate of 3 mL/sec. Scanning was performed in descending order over 9 cm beginning at the level of the superior mesenteric artery. The acquisition was performed in a single 30-second breath hold. In the first 35 patients, a fixed scanning delay of 27 seconds was used between the beginning of injection of the contrast agent and the start of the acquisition. In the latter 36 patients, an individual scanning delay was calculated on the basis of the transit time of a preliminary test injection of 15 mL of contrast material, as described elsewhere (7,8).

Spiral CT Angiogram Analysis

The axial source images were postprocessed on a commercially available workstation (Easy Vision CT/MR; Philips Medical Systems) to obtain multiplanar reformations and maximum intensity projections. Multiplanar reformations were generated into a coronal plane in each patient. In cases of a tortuous vessel, a curved planar reformation paralleling the center of the renal artery was also obtained. Before the maximum intensity projections were generated, the spinal column was removed from the volume of interest by reducing the image volume to a 2-cm-thick anteroposterior subvolume or slab through the abdominal portion of the aorta, and a coronal maximum intensity projection was performed on this slab. Since the course of the renal arteries is oblique, generation of multiple slab maximum intensity projections, rotating ± 90° about a craniocaudal axis through the abdominal portion of the aorta with an increment of 5° was necessary to assess the vessels along the entire course. The generated maximum intensity projections were evaluated in a cine mode for interactive image review. The editing procedures for maximum intensity projections were performed by one of the reviewers (R.K.).

The combination of the axial spiral CT angiographic source images, the multiplanar reformation images, and maximum intensity projection images were interpreted by two independent reviewers (R.K., H.F.M.S.) before the DSA studies were performed and without knowledge of any other angiographic studies, if performed previously. Each reviewer determined the severity of renal artery stenosis by visually assessing the width of the narrowest section of the stenotic segment and by comparing that with the width of the uninvolved segment of the renal artery distal to the stenosis. Subsequently, each reviewer classified the results of the vessel assessments into one of the following categories: grade 0 = no stenosis, grade 1 = 1%–49% stenosis, grade 2 = 50%–99% stenosis, and grade 3 = occlusion. In addition, the reviewers indicated whether the stenosis was associated with mural calcification.

The serum creatinine level was measured at two points relative to the spiral CT angiographic examination; the first measurement was obtained the day immediately before spiral CT angiography, and the second measurement was obtained the day before DSA. The median interval between the two measurements was 12 days (range, 3–85 days). Preexisting renal insufficiency was defined as a serum creatinine level greater than 130 μmol/L at entry into the study (15).

DSA Technique and Image Analysis

Intraarterial DSA was performed with a commercially available digital subtraction system (Integris V 3000; Philips Medical Systems). To avoid problems with superimposition of vessels and thus to optimize the DSA studies, the axial spiral CT angiographic source images were evaluated in each case before DSA was performed to measure the angle between the proximal segment of the renal artery and the aorta

Table 1
Grade of Stenosis at Spiral CT Angiography versus That at DSA

Stenosis Grade at DSA	Stenosis Grade at Spiral CT Angiography: 0	1	2	3	Total
Reviewer A					
0	45	0	1	0	46
1	0	23	1	0	24
2	0	5	76	0	81
3	0	0	0	15	15
Total	45	28	78	15	166
Reviewer B					
0	44	0	2	0	46
1	0	21	3	0	24
2	0	2	79	0	81
3	0	0	0	15	15
Total	44	23	84	15	166

Note.—Numbers are the number of arteries. Grades of stenosis: grade 0 = 0%, grade 1 = 1%–49%, grade 2 = 50%–99%, grade 3 = occlusion.

Table 2
Results from the Two Reviewers according to Number of Arteries in Which Stenosis Was Detected with Both Modalities

Grade of Stenosis	No. of Arteries at DSA	Reviewer A: No. of Arteries at CT	Reviewer A: Sensitivity (%)	Reviewer A: Specificity (%)	Reviewer A: PPV (%)	Reviewer A: NPV (%)	Reviewer B: No. of Arteries at CT	Reviewer B: Sensitivity (%)	Reviewer B: Specificity (%)	Reviewer B: PPV (%)	Reviewer B: NPV (%)	Average Results: Sensitivity (%)	Average Results: Specificity (%)
0	46	45	98	100	100	99	44	96	100	100	98	97	100
1	24	28	96	96	82	99	23	88	99	91	98	92	98
2	81	78	94	98	97	94	84	98	94	94	98	96	96
3	15	15	100	100	100	100	15	100	100	100	100	100	100

Note.—NPV = negative predictive value, PPV = positive predictive value.

(renoaortic angle). This measurement was obtained by one of the investigators (R.K.) who did not perform the DSA studies. The measurement was obtained by determining the angle between the longitudinal axis of the proximal portion of the renal artery and the imaginary coronal plane through the longitudinal axis of the aorta. Midstream DSA images were then obtained in left and right anterior oblique views by using projections with angles as determined from the renoaortic measurements. Use of these projections ensured optimal visualization of the proximal segment of the renal artery without superimposition.

After all DSA studies were performed, images were evaluated for renal artery stenosis by two interventional radiologists (F.J.A.B., W.P.T.M.M.) in consensus and without knowledge of the spiral CT angiographic findings. For determination of the severity (grade) of renal artery stenosis, the same classification criteria were used as for spiral CT angiography. The results of the DSA studies were used as the standard of reference for comparison with spiral CT angiography. This way, a total of 166 arteries were visualized at DSA, including 24 accessory arteries. Of the 166 arteries, there were 46 without stenosis (grade 0), 24 with stenoses classified as grade 1, 81 classified as grade 2, and 15 classified as occlusion (grade 3). The stenoses were caused by fibromuscular dysplasia in two patients and by atherosclerosis in the remaining patients.

Statistical Analysis

The sensitivity and specificity in detection of renal artery stenosis were determined for each grade and each reviewer. Interobserver variability between the reviewers was determined by calculating the κ coefficient. This coefficient is a measurement of concordance with a correction for chance agreement, and the results are weighed to distinguish varying degrees of disagreement between two observers or modalities (16,17). The κ value expressed the strength of agreement as follows: 0.20 = poor agreement, 0.21–0.40 = fair agreement, 0.41–0.60 = moderate agreement, 0.61–0.80 = good, and 0.81–1.00 = very good agreement. The variability between the two modalities (spiral CT angiography and DSA) in assessment of all grades of stenoses was also determined for each reviewer by calculating the κ coefficient. Statistical significance of the difference in creatinine levels before and after spiral CT angiography was determined with the Mann-Whitney *U* test.

RESULTS

All 166 renal arteries and all accessory arteries identified at DSA were identified at spiral CT angiography by both reviewers. No additional renal arteries were detected with spiral CT angiography that were not detected with DSA. Reviewer A identified correctly 45 arteries without stenosis, 23 arteries with grade 1 stenosis, 76 arteries with grade 2 stenosis, and all 15 arteries with occlusion (Table 1). Reviewer A overestimated the degree of stenosis in two arteries; in one of these cases, a nonstenotic (grade 0) artery was classified incorrectly as a grade 2 stenosis, and in the other case a grade 1 stenosis was classified incorrectly as grade 2 stenosis. Underestimation occurred in five arteries, and in all of these cases, the reviewer classified grade 2 stenosis as grade 1.

Reviewer B diagnosed correctly 44 arteries without stenosis, 21 with grade 1 stenosis, 79 with grade 2 stenosis, and all 15 with occlusion. Five stenoses were overestimated by this reviewer; in two cases, a nonstenotic artery was classified as grade 2 stenosis, and in three cases, a grade 1 stenosis was classified as grade 2. Underestimation occurred in two grade 2 stenoses, which were both classified as grade 1. Both reviewers indicated that the stenoses were associated with mural calcifications in 28 arteries (16 patients). In three of the five stenoses underestimated by reviewer A and in two stenoses underestimated by reviewer B, calcifications were noted in the arterial wall. Calcifications were not seen in any of the cases of overestimated stenosis.

The independent interpretations made by the two observers showed overall concurrence. The average sensitivity and specificity for assessing stenosis of grade 0 (no stenosis), grade 1 (1%–49% stenosis), grade 2 (51%–99% stenosis), and grade 3 (occlusion) were 97% and 100%, 92% and 98%, 96% and 96%, and 100% and 100%, respectively (Table 2). The variability between the two modalities in assessing all grades combined was low, with κ coefficients of 0.9 and 0.9, respectively, for the two reviewers (95% confidence interval = 0.83, 0.96).

The serum creatinine levels before spiral CT angiography were 54–881 μmol/L (median, 127 μmol/L) in all 71 patients. Of the 71 patients, 35 (49%) had preexisting renal insufficiency (defined as a serum creatinine level greater than 130 μmol/L). At follow-up after spiral CT angiography, the creatinine levels were 64–861 μmol/L (median, 126 μmol/L). In the entire patient population, there was no statistically significant difference between the median creatinine level after spiral CT angiography and the baseline level (before spiral CT angiography) (P = .82). None of the patients showed an increase of more than 20% between creatinine levels obtained before spiral CT angiography and those obtained after. In addition, there was no clinical evidence that any of the patients experienced contrast material–induced nephrotoxicity (ie, consultation of nephrologist, extended hospital stay, and/or hemodialysis).

DISCUSSION

Conventional arteriography or DSA is generally used as the standard modality for evaluation of renal artery stenosis (2). The invasive nature of these procedures poses some risks, however, especially in older patients with moderate to severe atherosclerotic changes. In addition, contrast agent–induced impairment of renal function and cholesterol embolism are of concern (18). To avoid these problems, less invasive modalities have been used as screening procedures for renal artery stenosis. Renal scintigraphy performed with a combination of ^{131}I-Hippuran and diethylenetriaminepentaacetic acid has been used as an initial screening method; however, the reported accuracy is low, with sensitivity of 75% and specificity of 80% (19–22). Scintigraphy after administration of angiotensin converting enzyme inhibitor has been shown to increase both the sensitivity and the specificity; however, this technique is limited in assessment of bilateral disease (1,23).

Some of the early studies in which ultrasonography (US) was used showed promising results in detection of renal artery stenosis (24–26). Later reports, however, demonstrated less favorable results, with relatively low sensitivity and specificity and inadequate visualization of accessory renal arteries (27). An additional limitation of US is that it may be difficult to visualize the proximal renal artery in the presence of overlying gas-filled loops of bowel. More recently, magnetic resonance (MR) angiography has been used to evaluate the renal arteries, but experience with this technique is still limited. Studies in which time-of-flight pulse sequence techniques were used revealed limitations in quantification of renal artery stenosis and detection of accessory renal arteries, with sensitivities of 53%–100% and specificities of 78%–97% (28–32). Accurate detection and quantification of renal artery stenosis with MR angiography performed with bolus enhancement of gadopentetate dimeglumine has yet to be determined (33,34).

Recently, spiral CT angiography has been introduced as a minimally invasive test for evaluation of renal artery stenosis (7–11). As there is no need for arterial catheterization and because the contrast material is administered intravenously, spiral CT angiography may constitute an attractive alternative for evaluating patients in whom renal artery stenosis is suspected.

Vascular surgery and angioplasty have been shown to be beneficial in patients with renal artery stenosis to prevent progression to ischemic nephropathy (35,36). However, these procedures are invasive and may be associated with increased patient morbidity and mortality (36,37). Several studies have indicated that stenoses less than 50% (grade 1 or less) have low risk of progression to occlusion (38,39). Therefore, it is generally considered that no intervention is needed in these patients. Discussion remains as to the degree of stenosis that necessitates intervention. Some studies have shown that when renal artery stenosis is greater than 70%–75%, the risk of occlusion is markedly increased because of substantial reduction of renal plasma flow (38–40). Others found that stenosis of 60% is critical for causing diminished arterial flow and reduction of arterial pressure (41,42).

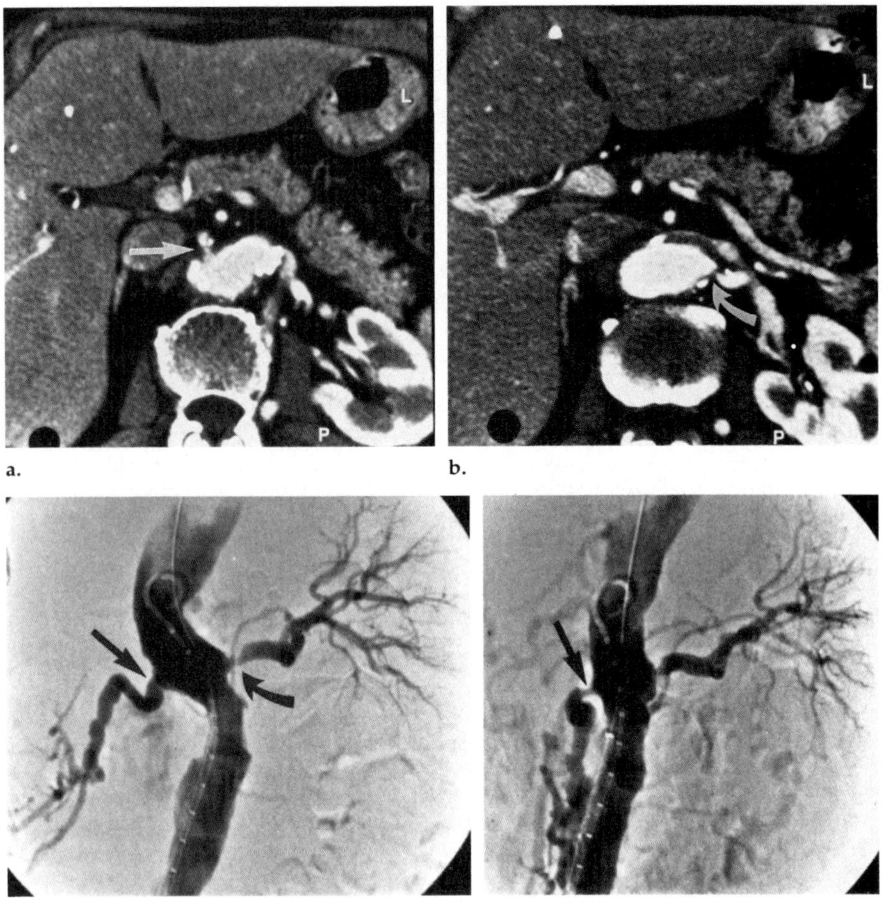

a.

b.

c.

d.

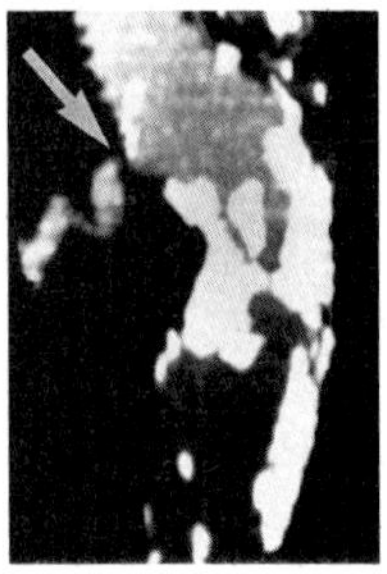
e.

Figure 1. **(a, b)** Axial source CT images show grade 2 stenosis (arrow) in the proximal segment of the **(a)** right and **(b)** left renal arteries. The origin of the right renal artery is located near the anterior aspect of the aorta, with a renoaortic angle of approximately 70°. **(c)** DSA image obtained with standard 15° projection shows no hemodynamically significant stenosis of the proximal segment of the right renal artery (straight arrow). The grade 2 stenosis of the left renal artery (curved arrow) is well demonstrated. **(d)** DSA image obtained with 70° right posterior oblique projection angulation reveals grade 2 stenosis at the origin of the right renal artery (arrow). **(e)** Maximum intensity projection CT angiogram rotated so that the proximal right renal artery is optimally displayed enables visualization of the grade 2 stenosis (arrow).

At our institution, we consider stenosis greater than 50% to be hemodynamically significant. Therefore, we did not consider any other cutoff points in evaluating our patients with renal artery stenosis. Although others have used different grading schemes, most have used 50% stenoses as the threshold for hemodynamically significant stenosis (7,10,11). In cases of complete vessel occlusion (grade 3), there is no need for intervention because of the irreversible changes that usually have occurred to the kidney with the unlikely chance of improvement (43). Thus, accurate identification of patients with grade 2 stenosis is important because these patients represent a group that has a potentially treatable cause of hypertension, and correction of stenosis in these patients helps prevent the development of end-stage renal function (5).

Our results indicate that spiral CT angiography is a highly accurate method for quantifying renal artery stenosis compared with an optimized standard, for which we used DSA. Specifically, the average sensitivities and specificities for assessment of the four grades of renal artery stenosis were high (92%–100%). High concordance (κ coefficient, 0.9) was found between the two reviewers in quantification of

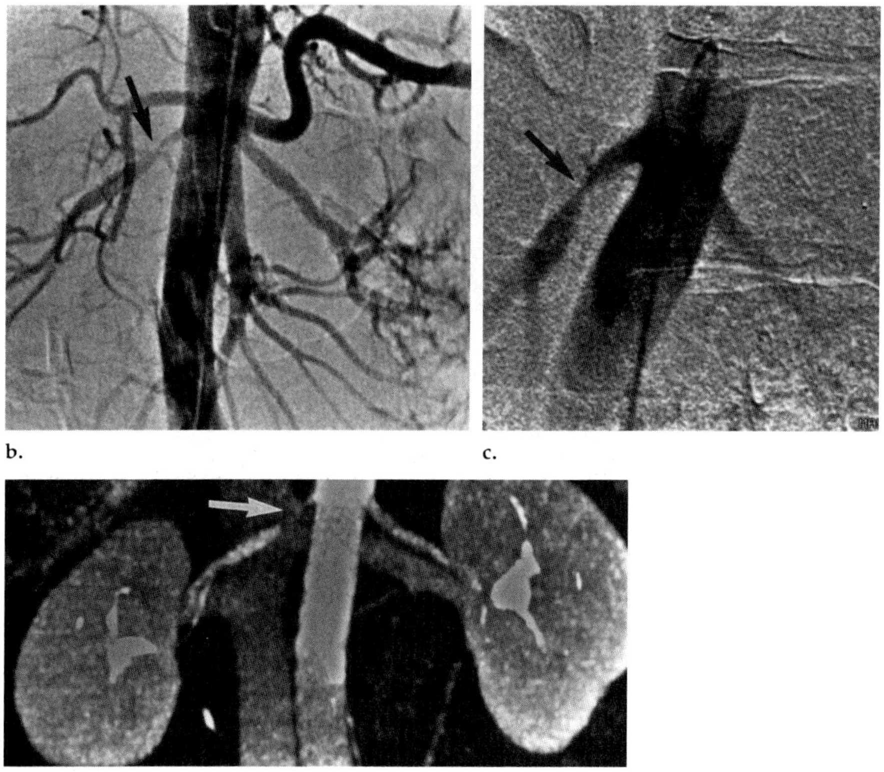

Figure 2. **(a)** Maximum intensity projection CT angiogram shows severe (grade 2) stenosis of the right renal artery (arrow). **(b)** DSA image obtained at standard projection shows that there is a possible mild (grade 1) stenosis (arrow) of the right renal artery. **(c)** DSA image obtained with optimal (48°) right posterior oblique angulation shows that the stenosis (arrow) is more severe (grade 2) than was suggested in **b**, confirming the findings from spiral CT angiography.

the degree of renal artery stenosis with spiral CT angiography. These findings indicate that the reviewers interpreted images consistently, suggesting high reproducibility of spiral CT angiography in assessment of renal artery stenosis. These findings reflect the high accuracy and reliability of the technique in assessment of renal artery stenosis. Of particular importance is the accuracy of spiral CT angiography in depiction of grade 2 stenoses, which are most relevant clinically. We found that these stenoses were identified with an average sensitivity and specificity of 96%. Therefore, spiral CT angiography can be used in selection of patients who need therapeutic intervention for renal artery stenosis.

The results of our study, which to our knowledge involves the largest patient group (71 patients, 166 arteries) reported thus far, compare favorably with those reported by other investigators. However, some investigators evaluated only relatively small numbers of patients, and comparison with those studies is therefore difficult (7,8). When we compared our results with those of other large series of patients, we found higher overall sensitivity and specificity. For instance, Olbricht et al (10) reported overall sensitivity of 95% and specificity of 93% in a series of 62 patients (157 vessels) in which spiral CT angiography was compared with standard DSA. Those investigators noted a relatively high number of false-positive findings (overestimation of the degree of stenosis) in 7% of arteries. The investigators postulated that this overestimation was not real but the result of underestimation of disease from interpretation of standard angiograms that were used as the standard. Overestimation was also involved in our spiral CT angiographic evaluations but to a much lesser extent, occurring only in 2% and 3% of arteries, respectively, for our two observers. Although there is no proof of the true degree of renal artery stenosis in our patients other than the findings from the optimized DSA examinations, it can only be assumed that the reduced overestimation of renal artery stenosis may have been the result of less underestimation of disease on the DSA images we used for our standard (Figs 1, 2).

Another advantage of spiral CT angiography over conventional angiography is that with spiral CT angiography the vessel lumen and the vessel wall with possible calcifications and atherosclerotic plaques are both visualized. As a result, the relationship between stenosis of the renal artery and the wall of the aorta is assessed more accurately, allowing improved distinction between ostial and truncal stenoses as we reported previously (44). This distinction is important for determining the choice of interventional therapy, such as percutaneous angioplasty or stent placement (6,45–48). However, visualization of small intrarenal vessels may be difficult with spiral CT angiography, and accurate assessment of peripheral stenoses beyond the level of the hilum is difficult. Another limitation with spiral CT angiography is that mural calcifications may interfere with evaluation of renal artery stenosis, and in our series calcifications were the major cause of underestimation of disease (7,8,11). In particular, because calcifications are typically positioned eccentric with respect to the vascular lumen, stenoses can go undetected when images are reviewed in only one orientation. Narrowing of the vessel diameter can be, in case of an eccentric calcification at the transition of the aortic wall and the renal artery, in the craniocaudal plane, and luminal patency can be overestimated on the axial images (Fig 3). The extent to which an eccentric calcification causes luminal diameter reduction might be hard to detect on axial images. Therefore, multiplanar reformatting in a second plane is necessary to ensure that craniocaudally oriented stenoses due to mural calcifications will not be missed.

A potential disadvantage of spiral CT angiography is that a relatively large volume of contrast material (120–150 mL) is needed for adequate opacification of the renal arteries. Use of a large volume of contrast material increases the risk of inducing nephrotoxicity. In addition, preexisting renal dysfunction is a risk factor in the development of contrast material–induced nephrotoxicity (49,50). In our study, however, in which there were 35 (49%) patients who had renal insufficiency (creatinine levels >130 μmol/L), we found no evidence of any substantial increase in the serum creatinine level at follow-up. A transient increase in the serum creatinine level may take place within the first 24 hours after a contrast-enhanced body CT examination (18); however, although we did not measure creatinine levels immediately after spiral CT angiography, there was no clinical evidence of nephrotoxicity in any of the patients in the immediate period after spiral CT angiography. It has been reported that in patients with impaired renal function, spiral CT angiography may be unreliable in assessment of renal artery stenosis (10). However, in patients with renal insufficiency, we found no such evidence. Although we did not observe any permanent increase in creatinine levels in our patient population, contrast material–induced renal failure is a conceivable disadvantage to use of spiral CT angiography.

There are several limitations of our study. First, we did not perform a separate analysis for the diagnostic value of the axial source images, multiplanar reformations, and maximum intensity projection reconstructions. Therefore, we cannot determine the usefulness of each of these viewing methods. However, others have addressed this issue and reported that a combination of these viewing modalities may be most suitable for evaluating the renal arteries (7,10,11).

Second, because of the technical limitation of our CT scanner, we used only 3-mm collimation, while use of 2-mm collimation has been suggested by others for optimal image resolution and visualization of the renal arteries (12). Because of this limitation in collimation, we did not increase the pitch, as this would decrease the longitudinal resolution of our images.

Third, with our imaging protocol of 3-mm collimation and a pitch ratio of 1:1, there was the potential that accessory renal arteries would not be included in the image volume, as only 9 cm was covered. However, Boijsen (51) demonstrated that 90% of the accessory renal arteries were within an 87-mm span of the abdominal portion of the aorta, stretching from 17 mm cephalic to 70 mm caudal from the main renal arteries. In our series, we did not encounter any accessory arteries on DSA images that were outside the image volume of the CT scans.

Fourth, the administration of the contrast material bolus for CT was inconsistent in that we used a fixed, 27-second scanning delay in the first half of our patients and variable delays in the remainder. The reason we changed the scanning delay was that with use of the fixed delay, we observed the highest attenuation on images obtained at the end of the acquisition, and we believed that use of variable delays would improve the timing of maximum arterial enhancement (7,8). Although higher injection rates have been suggested for improved visualization of vessels, we did not increase the rate of administration because of increased risk of patient discomfort and extravasation of contrast material at the injection site.

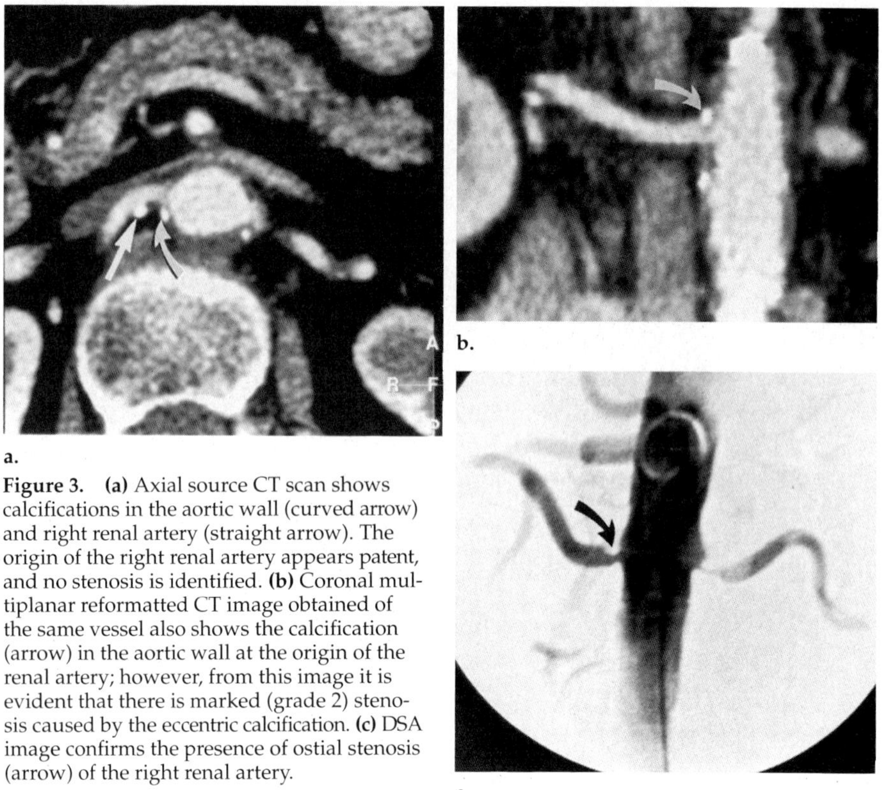

a. b. c.

Figure 3. **(a)** Axial source CT scan shows calcifications in the aortic wall (curved arrow) and right renal artery (straight arrow). The origin of the right renal artery appears patent, and no stenosis is identified. **(b)** Coronal multiplanar reformatted CT image obtained of the same vessel also shows the calcification (arrow) in the aortic wall at the origin of the renal artery; however, from this image it is evident that there is marked (grade 2) stenosis caused by the eccentric calcification. **(c)** DSA image confirms the presence of ostial stenosis (arrow) of the right renal artery.

In our study, we found that spiral CT angiography can be reliable in assessment of renal artery stenosis. The question remains as to what the role of spiral CT angiography is in screening patients with hypertension. In our patient group, the prevalence of renal artery stenosis was high and involved 96 of 166 arteries (grades 2 and 3). This high prevalence is based on the fact that our institution is a tertiary referral center for treatment of renovascular disease. However, in the general population of patients with hypertension, the prevalence of renal artery stenosis is only about 5%, while in patients with a high index of clinical suspicion, the prevalence of renal artery stenosis is approximately 30% (2). If spiral CT angiography is used as a screening test in the latter group and we apply our findings of 96% sensitivity and specificity, we can estimate the diagnostic value of this technique. For instance, in a group of 250 patients with hypertension in whom the prevalence of renal artery stenosis is 30%, spiral CT angiography enables correct identification of 72 of 75 patients with hemodynamically significant (50% or greater) renal artery stenosis and 168 of 175 patients without hemodynamically significant stenosis. Thus, therapy is withheld in three patients, while unnecessary treatment is scheduled in seven patients.

In contrast, if DSA is performed as the only screening procedure, 175 would unnecessarily undergo this invasive and expensive test. Conversely, an advantage of DSA is that treatment such as angioplasty or stent placement can be applied immediately when the diagnosis of renal artery stenosis is made. Clearly, a cost-benefit analysis is needed to assess the role of spiral CT angiography in clinical practice.

In summary, spiral CT angiography is an attractive, minimally invasive procedure for assessment of renal artery stenosis in patients in whom renovascular disease is suspected. In particular, when compared with optimally obtained DSA images, spiral CT angiography allows accurate detection and quantification of renal artery stenosis without substantial risk of contrast material–induced nephrotoxicity. ■

Acknowledgment: We thank Yvonne T. van de Schouw, PhD, for skilled statistical support.

References

1. Pickering TG. Diagnosis and evaluation of renovascular hypertension: indications

for therapy. Circulation 1991; 83(suppl): 147–154.
2. Hillman BJ. Imaging advances in the diagnosis of renovascular hypertension. AJR 1989; 153:5–14.
3. National High Blood Pressure Education Program Working Group. Update of working group reports on chronic renal failure and renovascular hypertension. Arch Intern Med 1996; 156:1938–1947.
4. Schreiber MJ, Pohl A, Novick AC. The natural history of atherosclerotic and fibrous renal artery disease. Urol Clin North Am 1984; 11:383–392.
5. Rimmer JF, Gennari FJ. Atherosclerotic renovascular disease and progressive renal failure. Ann Intern Med 1993; 118:712–719.
6. van der Ven PJG, Beutler JJ, Kaatee R, et al. Transluminal vascular stent for ostial atherosclerotic renal artery stenosis. Lancet 1995; 346:672–674.
7. Galanski M, Prokop M, Chavan A, et al. Renal artery stenoses: spiral CT angiography. Radiology 1993; 189:185–192.
8. Rubin GD, Dake MD, Napel S, et al. Spiral CT of renal artery stenosis: comparison of three-dimensional rendering techniques. Radiology 1994; 190:181–189.
9. Rubin GD, Alfrey EJ, Dake MD, et al. Assessment of living renal donors with spiral CT. Radiology 1995; 195:457–462.
10. Olbricht CJ, Paul K, Prokop M, et al. Minimally invasive diagnosis of renal artery stenosis by spiral computed tomography angiography. Kidney Int 1995; 48:1332–1337.
11. Beregi JP, Elkohen M, Deklunder G, Artaud D, Coullet JM, Wattinne L. Helical CT angiography compared with arteriography in detection of renal artery stenosis. AJR 1996; 167:495–501.
12. Brink JA, Lim JT, Wang G, Heiken JP, Deyoe LA, Vannier MW. Technical optimization of spiral CT for depiction of renal artery stenosis: in vitro analysis. Radiology 1995; 195:157–163.
13. Verschuyl EJ, Kaatee R, Beek FJA, et al. Location of the renal artery origins in the transverse plane. Radiology 1997; 203:71–75.
14. Gerlock AJ Jr, Goncharenko V, Sloan OM. Right posterior oblique: the projection of choice in aortography of hypertensive patients. Radiology 1978; 127:45–48.
15. Runick MR, Goldfarb S, Wexler L, et al. Nephrotoxicity of ionic and nonionic contrast media in 1196 patients: a randomized trial. Kidney Int 1995; 47:254–261.
16. Kramer MS, Feinstein AR. Clinical biostatics: LIV—the biostatics of concordance. Clin Pharmacol Ther 1981; 29:111–113.
17. Dillon EH, Van Leeuwen MS, Fernandez MA, et al. CT angiography: application to the evaluation of carotid artery stenosis. Radiology 1993; 189:211–219.
18. Rudnick MR, Berns JS, Cohen RM, Goldfarb S. Nephrotoxic risk of renal angiography: contrast media associated nephrotoxicity and atheroembolism—a critical review. Am J Kidney Dis 1994; 24:713–727.
19. Chen CC, Hoffer PB, Vahjen G, et al. Patients at high risk for renal artery stenosis: a simple method of renal scintigraphic analysis with Tc-99m DTPA and captopril. Radiology 1980; 176:365–370.
20. Russel CD, Thorstad B, Yester MV, Stutzman M, Baker T, Dubovsky EV. Comparison of technetium-99m MAG_3 with iodine-131 hippuran by simultaneous dual channel technique. J Nucl Med 1988; 29: 1189–1193.
21. Davidson RA, Wilcox CS. Newer tests for diagnosis of renovascular hypertension. Am J Med 1992; 268:3353–3358.
22. King BF Jr. Diagnostic imaging evaluation of renovascular hypertension. Abdom Imaging 1995; 20:395–405.
23. Mann SJ, Pickering TG, Sos TA, et al. Captopril renography in the diagnosis of renal artery stenosis: accuracy and limitations. Am J Med 1991; 90:30–40.
24. Robertson R, Murphy A, Dubbins PA. Renal artery stenosis: the use of duplex ultrasound as a screening technique. Br J Radiol 1988; 61:196–201.
25. Berland LL, Koslin DB, Routh WD, et al. Renal artery stenosis: prospective evaluation of diagnosis with color duplex ultrasound compared with angiography. Radiology 1990; 174:421–423.
26. Hansen KJ, Tribble RW, Reavis SW, et al. Renal duplex sonography: evaluation of clinical utility. J Vasc Surg 1990; 112:227–236.
27. Kliewer MA, Tupler R, Carroll BA, et al. Renal artery stenosis: analysis of Doppler waveform parameters and tardus-parvus pattern. Radiology 1993; 189:779–787.
28. Debatin JF, Spritzer CE, Grist TM, et al. Imaging of the renal arteries: value of MR angiography. AJR 1991; 157:981–990.
29. Yucel KE, Kaufman JA, Prince M, et al. Time of flight renal MR angiography: utility in patients with renal insufficiency. Magn Reson Imaging 1993; 11:925–930.
30. Wladyslaw MWG. Magnetic resonance angiography of renal arteries. Renal Vasc Disease Transplantation 1994; 21:201–214.
31. Hertz SM, Holland A, Baum A, et al. Evaluation of renal artery stenosis by magnetic resonance angiography. Am J Surg 1994; 168:140–143.
32. Servois V, Laissy JP, Feger C, et al. Two-dimensional time-of-flight magnetic resonance angiography of renal arteries without maximum intensity projections: a prospective comparison with angiography in 21 patients screened for renovascular hypertension. Cardiovasc Intervent Radiol 1994; 17:138–142.
33. Holland GA, Dougherty L, Carpenter JP, et al. Breath-hold ultrafast three-dimensional gadolinium-enhanced MR angiography of the aorta and the renal and other visceral abdominal arteries. AJR 1996; 166: 971–981.
34. Snidow JJ, Johnson MS, Harris VJ, et al. Three-dimensional gadolinium-enhanced MR angiography for aortoiliac inflow assessment plus renal artery screening in a single breath-hold. Radiology 1996; 198: 725–732.
35. Jensen G, Zachrisson BF, Delin K, Volkmann R, Aurell M. Treatment of renovascular hypertension: one year results of renal angioplasty. Kidney Int 1995; 48:1936–1945.
36. Novick AC. Options for therapy of ischemic nephropathy: role of angioplasty and surgery. Am J Kidney 1996; 16:53–60.
37. Klinge J, Mali WPTM, Puijlaert CBAJ, Geyskens GG, Becking WB, Feldberg MAM. Percutaneous transluminal renal angioplasty: initial and long-term results. Radiology 1989; 171:501–506.
38. Schreiber MJ, Pohl MA, Novick AC. The natural history of atherosclerotic and fibrous renal artery disease. Urol Clin North Am 1984; 11:383–392.
39. Tollefson DF, Ernst CB. Natural history of atherosclerotic renal artery stenosis associated with aortic disease. J Vasc Surg 1991; 14:327–331.
40. Jacobson HR. Nephrology forum: ischemic renal disease—an overlooked clinical entity? Kidney Int 1988; 34:729–743.
41. May AG, Berg VDL, DeWeese JA, Ros CG. Critical arterial stenosis. Surgery 1963; 54: 250–259.
42. Haimovici H, Zinicola N. Experimental renal artery stenosis: diagnostic significance of arterial hemodynamics. J Cardiovasc Surg 1962; 3:259–263.
43. Geyskens GG, Oei HY, Klinge J, Kooiker CJ, Puylaert CBAJ, Dorhout Mees EJ. Renovascular hypertension: the small kidney updated. J Med 1988; 251:203–217.
44. Kaatee R, Beek FJA, Verschuyl EJ, et al. Atherosclerotic renal artery stenosis: ostial or truncal? Radiology 1996; 199:637–640.
45. Sos TA, Pickering TG, Phil D, et al. Percutaneous transluminal renal angioplasty in renovascular hypertension due to atheroma or fibromuscular dysplasia. N Engl J Med 1983; 309:274–279.
46. Canzanello VJ, Millan VG, Spiegel JE, Ponce SP, Kopelman R, Madias NE. Percutaneous transluminal renal angioplasty in management of atherosclerotic renal vascular hypertension: results in 100 patients. Hypertension 1989; 13:163–172.
47. Weibull H, Bergqvist D, Jonsson K, Hulthen L, Mannheim P, Bergentz SE. Long-term results after percutaneous transluminal angioplasty of atherosclerotic renal artery stenosis: the importance of intensive follow-up. Eur J Vasc Surg 1991; 5:291–301.
48. Rees CR, Palmaz JC, Becker GJ, et al. Palmaz stent in atherosclerotic stenoses involving the ostia of the renal arteries: preliminary report of a multicenter study. Radiology 1991; 181:507–514.
49. Parfrey PS, Griffiths SM, Barreth BJ, et al. Contrast material–induced renal failure in patients with diabetes mellitus, renal insufficiency, or both: a prospective controlled study. N Engl J Med 1989; 320:143–149.
50. Moore RD, Steiberg EP, Powe NR, et al. Nephrotoxicity of high-osmolality versus low-osmolality contrast media: randomized clinical trial. Radiology 1992; 182:649–655.
51. Boijsen E. Angiographic studies of the anatomy of single and multiple renal arteries. Acta Radiol 1959; 183(suppl):1–99.

Martin R. Prince, MD, PhD • Stefan O. Schoenberg, MD[2] • Jennifer S. Ward, BA
Frank J. Londy, RT • Thomas W. Wakefield, MD • James C. Stanley, MD

Hemodynamically Significant Atherosclerotic Renal Artery Stenosis: MR Angiographic Features[1]

PURPOSE: **To identify magnetic resonance (MR) angiographic features of hemodynamically significant renal artery stenosis.**

MATERIALS AND METHODS: **Forty-seven patients underwent MR angiography of the renal arteries, including T1-weighted spin-echo and three-dimensional gadolinium-enhanced spoiled gradient-echo and three-dimensional phase-contrast pulse sequences, followed by renal revascularization. Thirty-five patients (52 arteries) were identified who benefited from renal revascularization, which indicated that they had hemodynamically significant renal artery stenoses. Kidney length, cortical thickness, parenchymal enhancement, and poststenotic dilatation were measured. Arteries were also examined for signal drop-out (dephasing) on phase-contrast angiograms; dephasing was considered severe if the stenotic artery appeared occluded on phase-contrast angiograms.**

RESULTS: **Poststenotic dilatation of greater than 20% was present in 36 (59%) of 52 hemodynamically significant renal artery stenoses, and severe dephasing was present in 45 (87%) of 52. In patients with unilateral hemodynamically significant stenosis or occlusion, mean ischemic kidney length was reduced to 9.3 cm compared with 10.7 cm for the contralateral normal kidney ($P = .009$), mean parenchymal thickness was reduced (1.2 vs 1.7 cm; $P < .001$), and mean parenchymal enhancement was 15% less on the ischemic side ($P = .05$). Severe dephasing on phase-contrast angiograms was present in nine (75%) of 12 unilateral hemodynamically significant stenoses but in only one contralateral normal renal artery ($P < .001$).**

CONCLUSION: **MR angiography depicts features of renal artery stenosis that are markers of hemodynamic significance.**

Several magnetic resonance (MR) imaging and MR angiographic techniques with fundamentally different image contrast mechanisms have been developed for imaging the kidneys and renal arteries (1–22). T1-weighted, spin-echo MR imaging demonstrates the kidney size, parenchymal thickness, corticomedullary differentiation (1), location in the retroperitoneal space, and anatomic variations. Time-of-flight (2–9) and phase-contrast (10–17) MR angiography are flow-sensitive techniques. They produce MR angiograms by depicting the motion of flowing blood. Such flow-sensitive techniques may accurately image the normal renal artery lumen. However, in regions of vascular disease where the normal laminar blood flow is disturbed, the images are often degraded by artifactual signal dropout. One type of artifact, commonly referred to as dephasing, is known to correlate with the severity of stenoses (23,24). Finally, three-dimensional (3D) MR angiography uses an injection of a gadolinium chelate to shorten the T1 of arterial blood (25–31). This latter technique does not depend on the in-flow effect. It provides true anatomic images that are similar to conventional arteriograms. Dynamic imaging during injection of contrast material may also be used to evaluate the symmetry of renal parenchymal enhancement (32) and corticomedullary differentiation (33,34).

In this outcomes study, we tested the hypothesis that a combination of information acquired from T1-weighted spin-echo MR imaging, 3D gadolinium-enhanced MR angiography, and 3D phase-contrast MR angiography enables detection of atherosclerotic renal artery stenoses and accurate prediction of their hemodynamic and functional significance. A renal artery stenosis is considered to be hemodynamically and functionally significant if the patient can have either improved blood pressure control or improved renal function by revascularizing the kidney supplied by that artery.

MATERIALS AND METHODS

Patients

A total of 413 consecutive patients underwent renal artery MR angiography from January 1994 to December 1996 (Table 1). Included were 390 patients initially referred for MR evaluation of the renal arteries or abdominal aorta and 23 additional patients who underwent conventional arteriography of their renal arteries first and consented to undergo subsequent aortorenal MR imaging under a human-use protocol

Index terms: Gadolinium • Magnetic resonance (MR), phase imaging, 961.129412, 961.12942 • Magnetic resonance (MR), three-dimensional, 961.12917, 961.129412, 961.12942 • Magnetic resonance (MR), vascular studies, 961.129412, 961.12942 • Renal arteries, flow dynamics, 961.129412, 961.12942 • Renal arteries, stenosis or obstruction, 961.7213, 961.7214

Abbreviations: VENC = velocity-encoding value, 3D = three-dimensional.

Radiology 1997; 205:128–136

[1] From the Departments of Radiology (M.R.P., S.O.S., J.S.W., F.J.L.) and Surgery (T.W.W., J.C.S.), University of Michigan Medical Center, B2B311G, 1500 E Medical Center Dr, Ann Arbor, MI 48109-0030. Received February 12, 1997; revision requested March 31; revision received June 13; accepted June 18. Supported in part by a grant from the Whitaker Foundation. **Address reprint requests to** M.R.P.

[2] Current address: Department of Radiology, German Cancer Research Center, Heidelberg, Germany.

Table 1
Distribution of 90 Consecutive Patients Undergoing Renal MR Angiography

Clinical Characteristics	No. of Patients
Greater than 75% renal artery stenosis or occlusion	90
Successful anatomic revascularization with balloon angioplasty (n = 16*) or surgery (n = 31)	47
Clinical benefit	35
Group 1: unilateral stenosis	15
Group 2: bilateral stenoses	20
No clinical benefit, group 3	12

* A 17th patient, in whom balloon angioplasty failed, required surgical revascularization.

approved by the Institutional Review Board. Among these 413 patients, MR angiography depicted severe renal artery stenoses in 60, renal artery occlusion in 23, and both in nine. Two of the severe stenoses were due to fibromuscular dysplasia, and these patients were excluded from the current analysis. Renal revascularization was performed in 47 of the remaining 90 patients by means of balloon angioplasty (n = 16), surgery (n = 30), or both (n = 1), the latter due to balloon failure. Among these 47 patients, the mean age was 62 years (age range, 20–84 years) and the mean serum creatinine level was 2.3 mg/dL (200 µmol/L) (23 patients had a serum creatine level >2.0 mg/dL [180 µmol/L]). The 47 patients represent 30% of the 158 patients who underwent renal revascularization at this institution during the study period. One hundred eleven patients underwent revascularization without MR angiography; these patients were younger (mean age, 54 years) and had better renal function (mean serum creatinine level, 1.7 mg/dL [150 µmol/L]). Demographic data on these patients are shown in Table 2. Forty-three patients with renal artery stenosis or occlusion on MR angiograms did not undergo revascularization because of the following: The kidneys were less than 6 cm in length and thus too small to salvage (n = 5), the patient had a short life expectancy (n = 15) or died (n = 2), the patient had a preference for medical management (n = 6) or was lost to follow-up (n = 9), revascularization was pending (n = 4), or the MR angiogram was found to be false-positive when compared with the results of subsequent conventional arteriography (n = 2).

The medical records of the 47 patients who underwent renal revascularization were reviewed retrospectively to determine if the patients benefited from the intervention. For purposes of this study, benefit was defined as a decrease in serum creatinine level greater than or equal to 0.3 mg/dL (30 µmol/L) or a reduction in the number of medications required for blood pressure control. Changes in serum creatinine level were calculated by subtracting an average of three measurements obtained 1 week to 3 months after surgery from an average of three measurements obtained before surgery. The reduction in number of blood pressure medications was determined by counting the number of medications required to control blood pressure at the time of admission and subtracting the number of medications at the time of discharge or at the most recent follow-up visit, which was typically 1–6 months after revascularization. If the medical records were incomplete, patients and referring physicians were interviewed by phone. Of the 26 patients whose improvement was based on reduction in the number of medications, 20 patients (77%) had one or more of their medications eliminated and six patients (23%) received different antihypertensive medications after revascularization but the total number of antihypertensive medications was reduced by two or more.

Imaging Technique

All patients were imaged with a 1.5-T superconducting magnet (Signa; GE Medical Systems, Milwaukee, Wis) with use of the body coil and version 5.3, 5.4, or 5.5 software. Imaging consisted of three pulse sequences. First, a sagittal T1-weighted spin-echo localizer sequence was acquired with the following parameters: 333–385/17–25 (repetition time msec/echo time msec), 16-kHz bandwidth, 8–9-mm section thickness (interleaved with no gap), phase reordering with respiration (respiratory compensation), 256 × 128–256 matrix with frequency encoding superior to inferior, 40–48-cm field of view, and two or four signals acquired. Image acquisition time was 7–9 minutes for 24 sections.

Second, a coronal 3D dynamic gadolinium-enhanced spoiled gradient-echo sequence was acquired. Early in the study, at the 5.3 software level, 22 patients underwent imaging with the following parameters: 24/6.9, 45° flip angle, 28 sections at 2–3-mm section thickness, and 256 × 256 matrix. The total image acquisition time was 3 minutes 20 seconds for one signal acquired. Gadodiamide (Omniscan; Nycomed, Princeton, NJ) or gadopentetate dimeglumine (Magnevist; Berlex Laboratories, Wayne, NJ) was injected beginning at the initiation of imaging and ending 30 seconds before the end of the imaging (26). Later, the software and gradient performance were upgraded. This enabled us to speed up the imaging in the other 25 patients by using the following parameters: 5–14/1.2–2.5, 45° flip angle, 16- or 32-kHz bandwidth, 28–44 sections with 2–3-mm section thickness, 256 × 128–160 matrix, frequency encoding superior to inferior, 28–36-cm field of view, and one signal acquired. No saturation pulses were employed. The total image acquisition time was adjusted from 14 to 58 seconds according to the patient's ability to breath hold and the volume of coverage required. Patients were asked to suspend breathing during this imaging. Gadodiamide or gadopentetate dimeglumine was injected rapidly over 15–20 seconds as an intravenous bolus timed for the maximum arterial gadolinium concentration to occur during the middle of the acquisition when the central lines of k space were acquired (27,30). The same volume of contrast material, 40 mL (two vials; 20 mmol), was used in every patient under 95 kg (210 pounds). Patients weighing more than 95 kg received 60 mL (three vials; 30 mmol) of contrast material. A 20–30-mL saline flush was used to ensure rapid delivery of the entire dose of contrast material and to help flush the contrast material from the veins. An intravenous tubing set (Smart Set; TopSpins, Plymouth, Mich) with an automatic switching mechanism was used to avert any delay between the bolus of contrast material and flush solution.

Third, an axial 3D phase-contrast (35) volume was acquired immediately after the dynamic gadolinium-enhanced acquisition by using the following parameters: 24–25/6.3–8.6, 45° flip angle, 16-kHz bandwidth, 28 sections with 2.5–3.0-mm section thickness, flow compensation, no phase wrap, 256 × 128 matrix, frequency encoding right to left, 28–32-cm field of view, and two signals acquired with velocity encoding in all directions at 20–55 cm/sec. The image acquisition time was 13–14 minutes. Images were reconstructed with the phase difference method, illustrating maximum velocity in all flow directions as well as right-to-left flow to evaluate the retrocaval course of the right renal artery. The velocity-encoding value (VENC) varied from 20 to 55 cm/sec (median, 50 cm/sec). In patients aged 70 years or older, patients with aortic aneurysm, patients with a history of severe cardiac disease (ie, congestive heart failure), and patients with a serum creatinine level greater than 2.0 mg/dL (180 µmol/L), the VENC was set to 20–30 cm/sec. All other patients were imaged with a VENC of 40–55 cm/sec.

Images were reconstructed by a vascular radiologist (M.R.P.) using a computer workstation (GE Medical Systems). Subvolume maximum intensity projection images and single-voxel-thick reformations were made through the origins of each of the major aortic branch vessels. For tortuous renal arteries, individual curved reformations were performed along the course of the vessel identified on the collapsed images.

Image Analysis

Renal artery MR angiograms were evaluated prospectively by a single board-certified radiologist (M.R.P.) specializing in angiography who was blinded to the patients' clinical outcomes and conventional arteriographic results. This evaluation included an assessment of kidney length, number of renal arteries, and a grading of each artery as normal, mildly stenotic (<50%), moderately stenotic (50%–75%), severely stenotic (>75%), or occluded (on 3D gadolinium-enhanced and phase-contrast MR angiograms). This grading was done by subjective impression.

The renal artery MR angiograms subsequently were examined retrospectively with knowledge of the location of stenoses on the basis of either a conventional arteriogram or findings at surgery. The mean time between MR angiography and angioplasty or surgery was 40 days (mean, 0 days to 7 months). Four patients in whom the delay was greater than 2 months had other medical problems that delayed scheduling renal revascularization. One patient with a delay of greater than 2 months elected to delay revascularization for personal reasons, and another patient had scheduling problems due to referral from an outside hospital.

Greater severity of the stenosis on phase-contrast angiograms compared with that on 3D gadolinium-enhanced MR angiograms was assumed to result from signal dephasing that was present on phase-contrast angiograms. If the artery showed a region of complete signal dropout on phase-contrast angiograms before, at, or immediately distal to a renal artery stenosis that gave the appearance of occlusion, this was graded as severe dephasing (Fig 1). Mild dephasing was defined as a signal attenuation on phase-contrast angiograms at the location of a stenosis that appeared more severe than the degree of stenosis on the 3D gadolinium-enhanced MR angiograms. This difference in appearance of stenosis between 3D gadolinium-enhanced MR angiograms and phase-contrast angiograms was also characterized by measuring the length of the stenosis on images from the two sequences. On the phase-contrast angiograms, the measured length of stenosis included the full extent of signal loss. A ratio of apparent stenosis length on the phase-contrast angiogram to actual stenosis length on the 3D gadolinium-enhanced MR angiogram (ie, length ratio) was calculated.

To assess the influence of the VENC on the evaluation of stenosis, the length ratios of the phase-contrast images with a VENC less than 50 cm/sec were compared with the length ratios of those images that were acquired with a VENC of 50 cm/sec or greater. The amount of poststenotic dilatation was determined by measuring the maximum arterial diameter immediately distal to the stenosis and dividing by the more normal renal artery diameter measured 2–3 cm more distally (Fig 2). For comparison with contralateral normal arteries, renal artery diameters were measured at similar sites to those of the stenotic artery.

Thickness of the renal parenchyma was measured at three locations—upper pole, middle pole, and lower pole—on the T1-weighted spin-echo images. These three measurements were averaged to obtain a single value. Corticomedullary differentiation on the T1-weighted spin-echo images was also noted if present. Region-of-interest analysis was used to determine the degree of renal parenchymal enhancement from the 3D spoiled gradient-echo images obtained before and during infusion of contrast material without any change in preimaging parameters.

Table 2
Demographic Information of Patients with and Those without Renal Repair

Patient Characteristic	Renal Artery Stenosis on MR Angiograms: Renal Revascularization: Postoperative Improvement	Renal Artery Stenosis on MR Angiograms: Renal Revascularization: No Postoperative Improvement	Renal Artery Stenosis on MR Angiograms: No Renal Revascularization	Renal Revascularization without MR Angiography
No. of patients	35	12	43	111
Sex				
Female	21	3	16	62
Male	14	9	27	49
Age (y)				
Mean	62	68	66	54
Range	20–84	54–78	54–78	5–89
Serum creatinine level (mg/dL)*				
Mean	2.3	4.5	2.4	1.7
Range	0.9–3.6	1.1–9.0	0.7–9.1	0.4–7.3

* For conversion to SI units, 1 mg/dL = 88.40 μmol/L.

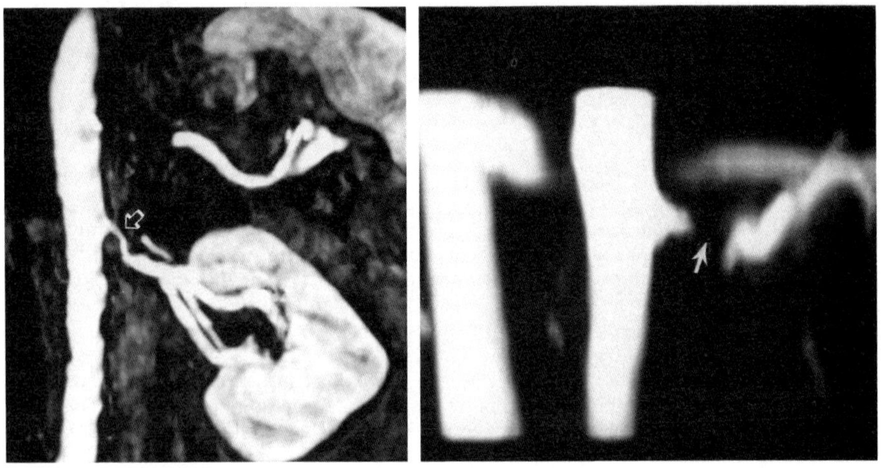

a. b.

Figure 1. **(a)** Coronal oblique maximum intensity projection image from a 3D dynamic gadolinium-enhanced spoiled gradient-echo angiogram (13.8/2.5, 45° flip angle) in a 48-year-old man after a right nephrectomy shows a stenotic left renal artery (arrow). **(b)** Three-dimensional phase-contrast angiogram (23/7.9, 35° flip angle) after injection of contrast material overestimates the severity of the stenosis (arrow) because high-velocity, separated flow with swirling eddy currents just distal to the stenosis causes signal loss from intravoxel dephasing. Dephasing was graded as severe in this patient because the signal dropout simulates occlusion. Left renal artery stenosis was confirmed at surgery (without undergoing angiography), and the patient's blood pressure control and serum creatinine level improved after revascularization.

Statistical Analysis

Differences in kidney length, parenchymal thickness, relative enhancement, and poststenotic dilatation between the normal and ischemic kidneys (where ischemic kidneys are those supplied by an artery with hemodynamically significant stenosis), as well as left and right kidneys, were subjected to statistical analysis by using a paired Student *t* test. Differences between the length ratios of stenoses greater than 50% for different VENCs were analyzed by using an unpaired Student *t* test. Differences in the number of arteries with dephasing on phase-contrast angiograms between ischemic kidneys and kidneys with normal or only mildly stenotic (<50%) renal arteries were subjected to χ^2 statistical analysis. The significance of differences in length ratios between patients who improved and patients who did not improve was tested by using analysis of variance controlling for the variables of age, serum creatinine level, and kidney height. A P value of less than .05 was considered to indicate a statistically significant difference.

RESULTS

The 47 patients who underwent renal revascularization were divided into three groups. Group 1 patients (n = 15) had two kidneys present and benefited from a unilateral renal artery intervention. This group was the most important for testing how well MR features can predict hemodynamic significance of a renal artery stenosis because their improvement was definitive evidence that the treated unilateral stenosis was hemodynamically and functionally significant and that the contralateral renal artery did not have a significant stenosis. Group 2 patients (n = 20) had bilateral renal artery stenoses or a solitary kidney with stenosis and benefited from intervention. This group provided information on features of hemodynamically significant stenoses although

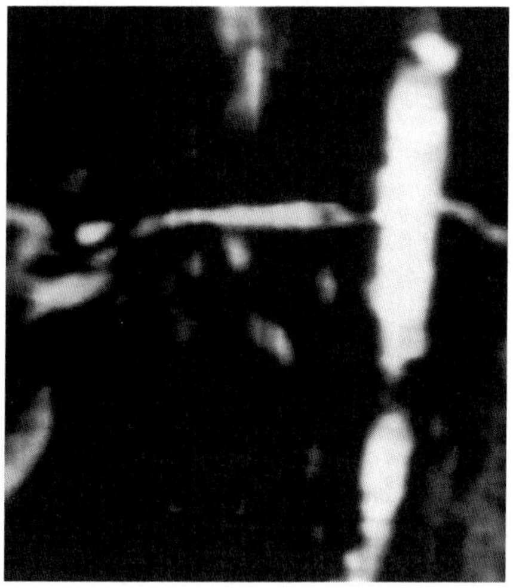

Figure 2. Dynamic 3D gadolinium-enhanced spoiled gradient-echo angiogram (13.5/2.3, 45° flip angle) in a 53-year-old woman with poststenotic dilatation. The vessel is more than 20% greater in diameter immediately distal to the stenosis relative to 2–3 cm downstream.

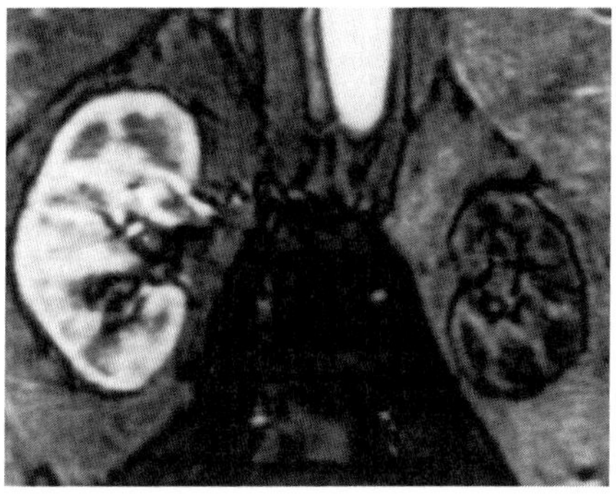

Figure 3. Dynamic 3D gadolinium-enhanced spoiled gradient-echo angiogram (14.1/2.6, 45° flip angle) in a 44-year-old man with unilateral renal artery stenosis. The normal right kidney shows homogeneous cortical enhancement with corticomedullary differentiation, while the smaller left ischemic kidney is not yet enhancing.

there were no contralateral normal arteries for comparison. Group 3 patients ($n = 12$) had unilateral ($n = 7$) or bilateral ($n = 5$) renal artery stenoses but had no reduction in the number of antihypertensive medications or in serum creatinine level after renal revascularization. This group did not benefit from intervention.

Group 1: Unilateral Renal Artery Stenosis

One of these 15 patients had two diseased right renal arteries, one severely stenotic and the other occluded. Thus, 16 renal arteries with hemodynamically significant lesions were identified with MR angiography and correctly graded prospectively as either severely stenotic ($n = 12$) or occluded ($n = 4$). One ischemic kidney (ie, supplied by a significantly stenotic artery) had a small but normal accessory renal artery. The contralateral kidneys known to be free of hemodynamically significant renal artery disease exhibited 16 renal arteries graded as normal ($n = 13$) or mildly stenotic ($n = 3$).

Ischemic kidneys of group 1 patients with unilateral renal artery disease were smaller with a thinner cortex and decreased parenchymal enhancement compared with the contralateral normal kidneys (Fig 3, Table 3). For unilateral renal artery occlusions, these differences were greater compared with unilateral renal artery stenoses (Table 3).

None of the occluded renal arteries were visible on 3D phase-contrast MR angiograms. In nine (75%) of 12 cases, however, hemodynamically significant stenoses exhibited a region of signal dropout encompassing the entire renal artery diameter due to severe dephasing. Mild dephasing was present in two cases. No dephasing was seen in one case. All 16 renal arteries to the contralateral normal kidneys in group 1 patients were visible on phase-contrast angiograms. Three had a dephasing artifact of which only one was severe. This one case of severe dephasing in a normal renal artery occurred at the origin, which is a known pitfall of phase-contrast MR angiography (36) (Fig 4).

Poststenotic dilatation averaged 37% (range, 0%–126%) among the 12 hemodynamically significant renal artery stenoses in the group 1 patients. Postocclusion dilatation was not visible in any of the four occluded renal arteries.

Corticomedullary differentiation on the unenhanced T1-weighted images was observed in only two patients. These were among the youngest patients in the study, ages 20 and 44 years. In one case, the normal kidney had corticomedullary differentiation while the ischemic kidney did not. In the other patient, corticomedullary differentiation was present in both the normal and ischemic kidneys.

Group 2: Bilateral Renal Artery Stenosis or Unilateral Stenosis in a Solitary Kidney

Forty-one renal arteries were present in these 20 patients. Three patients had only one renal artery due to prior nephrectomy and two patients had accessory renal arteries, including one patient with bilateral accessory renal arteries. These 41 renal arteries were prospectively graded as occluded ($n = 1$), severely stenotic ($n = 31$), or moderately stenotic ($n = 9$). No statistically significant asymmetry was seen between the right and left kidney lengths, parenchymal thickness, enhancement, poststenotic dilatation, or signal dephasing (Table 4). Furthermore, these parameters for the patients with bilateral renal artery stenosis were similar to those of patients with ischemic kidneys due to unilateral stenoses in the group 1 patients. Corticomedullary differentiation was not seen in any group 2 patient.

Groups 1 and 2: Further Characterization of Dephasing

Combining the data for groups 1 and 2 showed a statistically significant difference in the presence of dephasing between hemodynamically significant renal artery stenosis and mildly stenotic or normal arteries (Table 5). To further characterize the dephasing on phase-contrast angiograms, a length ratio was measured to compare the apparent stenosis length on each phase-contrast angiogram with the actual stenosis length on the 3D gadolinium-enhanced MR angiogram. For hemodynamically significant stenoses, the length of dephasing on the phase-contrast angiograms was an average of 31% longer than that on the 3D gadolinium-enhanced MR angiograms (length ratio = 1.31 ± 0.62). When separating the length ratios according to the VENC in hemodynamically significant stenoses, the length of dephasing for a VENC of 50 cm/sec or greater was significantly shorter (length ratio = 1.17 ± 0.58) compared with that of a lower VENC less than 50 cm/sec (length ratio = 1.57 ± 0.64, $P = .024$).

Group 3: No Benefit after Revascularization

Twelve patients with severe renal artery stenoses were identified who did not benefit from renal revascularization (Table 6).

Six of these patients underwent balloon angioplasty followed by placement of a renal artery stent. Three patients were undergoing dialysis before the intervention, but in spite of the technical success of angioplasty, the serum creatinine level remained high and dialysis was continued after the stent procedure. Possibly this failure to improve was related to the nephrotoxic insult of the iodinated contrast material, or possibly the deterioration in renal function was too advanced to reverse with revascularization. The fourth patient who did not benefit from balloon angioplasty followed by stent placement had refractory hypertension and a normal serum creatinine level. After stent placement, this patient's serum creatinine level remained normal but he continued to require three medications to control his hypertension. The fifth and sixth patients who did not benefit from intervention had technical failures in deployment of intervascular stents.

The other six patients who did not benefit from revascularization had undergone surgical revascularization (bypass in two patients, endarterectomy in four patients). One of these patients had a reduction in serum creatinine level but died of pneumonia on the 3rd postoperative day. One patient undergoing dialysis before surgery continued with dialysis after surgery. The other four patients had a persistent elevation in serum creatinine level after surgery; one patient required dialysis.

The patients who did not benefit from revascularization demonstrated certain important clinical differences compared with patients who showed improvement after revascularization. The former were significantly older (mean ages, 68 vs 62 years; $P < .01$) and had higher serum creatinine levels (mean levels, 4.5 vs 2.3 mg/dL [400 vs 200 μmol/L]; $P < .01$). All of their stenoses (14 of 14 stenoses) revealed at least mild dephasing on phase-contrast angiograms, with severe dephasing in 12 (86%) of 14 cases. Interestingly, however, the length ratio of these stenoses was significantly shorter ($P = .04$) compared with that of the patients with improvement from revascularization even after controlling for age, serum creatinine level, and kidney height. This indicates that the length of dephasing was less in patients who did not benefit.

Table 3
MR Angiographic Findings in Group 1 Patients with Unilateral Renal Artery Disease (15 Patients, 16 Diseased Arteries)

Finding	Ischemic Kidney	Kidney with Normal Artery	*P* Value
Stenoses and occlusions combined (16 arteries)			
Kidney length (cm)	9.3 ± 1.2	10.7 ± 1.5	.009
Kidney height (VB*)	3.0 ± 0.4	3.4 ± 0.4	.008
Parenchymal thickness (cm)	1.2 ± 0.3	1.7 ± 0.3	<.001
Kidney mass (cm²)†	11.1 ± 3.6	18.1 ± 4.9	<.001
Enhancement	171 ± 102	201 ± 143	.053
Stenoses only (12 arteries)			
Kidney length (cm)	9.7 ± 0.9	10.5 ± 1.4	.05
Kidney height (VB*)	3.1 ± 0.3	3.4 ± 0.4	.043
Parenchymal thickness (cm)	1.3 ± 0.3	1.7 ± 0.3	.0002
Kidney mass (cm²)†	12.2 ± 3.1	17.9 ± 4.7	.0002
Enhancement	149 ± 66	171 ± 88	.135
Dephasing on PC angiograms‡			
Mild or severe	11/12 (92)	3/13 (23)	<.001
Severe only	9/12 (75)	1/13 (8)	<.001
Poststenotic dilatation§	1.42 ± 0.37	1.02 ± 0.37	.026
Occlusions only (four arteries)			
Kidney length (cm)	8.1 ± 1.1	11.2 ± 1.5	.069
Kidney height (VB*)	2.5 ± 0.4	3.5 ± 0.5	.065
Parenchymal thickness (cm)	1.0 ± 0.2	1.7 ± 0.3	.0012
Kidney mass (cm²)†	7.8 ± 2.5	18.7 ± 5.5	.019
Enhancement	240 ± 157	304 ± 224	.163

Note.—Except for dephasing and *P* values, data are presented as the mean ± standard deviation.
* Kidney length measured by number of vertebral bodies to correct for different sizes of patients.
† Kidney length multiplied by parenchymal thickness to give a rough indicator of parenchymal mass.
‡ PC = phase contrast. Data are no. of arteries. Numbers in parentheses are percentages.
§ Ratio of maximum renal artery diameter within 1 cm distal to stenosis divided by the renal artery diameter measured 2–4 cm distal to the stenosis.

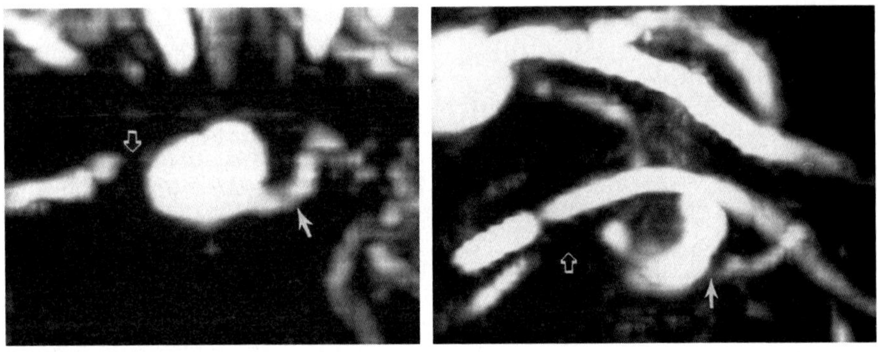

a. b.

Figure 4. **(a)** Dynamic 3D gadolinium-enhanced spoiled gradient-echo angiogram (5.2/1.2, 45° flip angle) in a 77-year-old woman shows severe right renal artery stenosis (open arrow) and normal left renal artery (solid arrow). **(b)** Three-dimensional phase-contrast MR angiogram (25/6.7, 35° flip angle) after injection of contrast material shows false-positive severe dephasing (solid arrow) at the ostium of the normal left renal artery, which is a known pitfall due to turbulent flow. However, the extent of dephasing is less than on the stenotic right side (open arrow).

DISCUSSION

The challenge of reducing the invasiveness of renal artery imaging in patients with renal failure or hypertension has been addressed with numerous imaging techniques (37–39), including ultrasound, nuclear scintigraphy, captopril scintigraphy, intravenous digital subtraction angiography (40), spiral computed tomographic (CT) angiography (41), and MR angiography (1–35). Even conventional arteriography, the reference standard, has important limitations. This is because it is not sufficient to know if a stenosis is present. It is also necessary to determine if the stenosis is hemodynamically significant (ie, causing a pressure drop of functional importance). Data from the current study's 35 patients with hemodynamically significant renal artery lesions, proved by means of a salutary clinical response after renal revascularization, demonstrate the usefulness of MR imaging and MR angiography for identifing physiologic changes that reflect the hemodynamic and functional significance of these stenoses.

Of the MR angiographic parameters studied, the most characteristic sign for hemodynamically significant renal artery stenoses was signal dropout (dephasing) on 3D phase-contrast MR angiograms obtained after administration of contrast material (35). This tendency for a stenotic artery to appear more severely stenotic (mild dephasing) or occluded (severe dephasing) is a well-known phenomenon that has caused flow-sensitive MR angiographic techniques (such as phase-

Table 4
MR Angiographic Findings in Group 2 Patients with Bilateral Renal Artery Stenosis or Occlusion (20 Patients, 41 Arteries)

Finding	Right Kidney	Left Kidney	*P* Value
Kidney length (cm)	9.7 ± 1.8	9.6 ± 1.2	.81
Kidney height (VB*)	3.0 ± 0.6	2.9 ± 0.4	.85
Parenchymal thickness (cm)	1.3 ± 0.4	1.2 ± 0.5	.60
Kidney mass (cm²)†	12.4 ± 5.6	11.3 ± 5.0	.55
Enhancement	180 ± 128	176 ± 115	.93
No. of occlusions	0	1	. . .
No. of stenoses	21	19	. . .
Dephasing on PC angiograms‡			
Mild or severe	21/21 (100)	19/19 (100)	.99
Severe only	18/21 (86)	18/19 (95)	.34
Length ratio§	1.17 ± 0.49	1.44 ± 0.64	.14
Poststenotic dilatation‖	1.3 ± 0.30	1.5 ± 0.15	.20

Note.—Except for no. of occlusions and stenoses, dephasing, and *P* values, data are presented as the mean ± standard deviation.
* Kidney length measured by number of vertebral bodies to correct for different sizes of patients.
† Kidney length multiplied by parenchymal thickness to give a rough indicator of parenchymal mass.
‡ PC = phase contrast. Data are no. of arteries. Numbers in parentheses are percentages.
§ Ratio between length of dephasing on the PC angiograms and length of stenosis measured on the 3D gadolinium-enhanced MR angiograms.
‖ Ratio of maximum renal artery diameter within 1 cm distal to stenosis divided by the renal artery diameter measured 2–4 cm distal to the stenosis.

Table 5
Differences in Dephasing on Phase-Contrast Angiograms of Arteries with Hemodynamically Significant Stenoses versus Normal or Mildly Stenotic Arteries in 35 Patients

Dephasing	Arteries with Significant Stenosis (*n* = 52)	Normal Arteries (*n* = 16)	*P* Value
Mild or severe	51 (98)	3 (19)	<.001
Severe	45 (87)	1 (6)	<.001

Note.—All 35 patients had proved hemodynamically significant stenoses. Numbers in parentheses are percentages.

contrast angiography) to often overestimate the severity of stenoses. This phenomenon is thought to be due to accelerating, swirling, or turbulent flow at or beyond the stenosis that occurs during the dephasing lobe of the readout gradient (23,24,42,43) or during flow encoding. The greater magnitude of dephasing seen at a lower VENC in this study reflects the increased flow-encoding gradient strength required for a lower VENC. Loss of signal may also result from the susceptibility effect of calcific deposits although this effect is likely to be small at the short echo times used in this study. The magnitude of signal loss on phase-contrast angiograms may also be affected by aliasing, which can be reduced by using cardiac gating to adjust the VENC separately for systolic and diastolic flow (44,45). Because dephasing is inherently pulse sequence dependent, its use on equipment from other manufacturers will probably have to be validated.

In this study, the presence of "severe" dephasing was proved, retrospectively, when an artery known to be stenotic on the basis of conventional angiographic or operative correlation appeared occluded on phase-contrast angiograms. Mild dephasing could only be inferred when the artery appeared more stenotic on the phase-contrast angiogram than on the 3D gadolinium-enhanced MR angiogram. The fact that severe dephasing was present in 87% of hemodynamically significant stenoses but in only 6% of normal renal arteries (Table 5) suggests that severe dephasing is a reliable criterion for evaluating the hemodynamic significance of a stenosis. The one false-positive phase-contrast examination with severe dephasing at a normal renal artery origin is a known pitfall of phase-contrast MR angiography (36). Mild dephasing was less useful as an indicator of hemodynamic significance because of its higher false-positive rate.

To identify spin dephasing prospectively, the phase-contrast angiogram can be compared with the 3D gadolinium-enhanced MR angiogram. Regions that show greater stenosis severity on the phase-contrast angiogram compared with the appearance of those regions on the 3D gadolinium-enhanced MR angiogram are assumed to result from dephasing on the phase-contrast angiogram that is not present on the 3D gadolinium-enhanced MR angiogram. The absence of dephasing artifact on the 3D gadolinium-enhanced MR angiogram results from the smaller voxels, shorter echo time, fractional echo (which reduces the size of the dephasing lobe on the read-out gradient), and absence of flow-encoding gradients. For these reasons, the 3D gadolinium-enhanced MR angiograms, when obtained at high resolution with a sufficient dose of contrast material, are believed to accurately reflect the true anatomic features of the renal artery lumen.

Poststenotic dilatation of greater than 20% was also a useful marker of hemodynamic significance. It was present in seven (58%) of 12 hemodynamically significant unilateral stenoses and in 27 (68%) of 40 bilateral stenoses. This is a recognized phenomenon thought to be due to increased force on the vessel wall from deceleration of the jet flow beyond the stenosis. It is, in theory, related to the magnitude of the pressure gradient through the stenosis. In practice, variations in vessel geometry, compliance, and vessel remodeling may be more important in determining the actual extent of poststenotic dilatation.

Dephasing and poststenotic dilatation are obviously not applicable for evaluating the hemodynamic significance of occluded renal arteries. Occlusions, however, were not a problem to evaluate because they are always hemodynamically significant. All unilateral occlusions in the present study were associated with the constellation of markedly decreased kidney length, decreased renal parenchymal thickness, and decreased enhancement, relative to the contralateral normal side. These findings also accompanied hemodynamically significant stenoses but to a lesser degree. The findings of decreased length and decreased parenchymal thickness tended to parallel each other. One might expect variations in patient size to affect the kidney length measurements. However, indexing the kidney length measurement to vertebral body height did not change the statistical significance of size differences.

Hypoperfusion of the kidney due to renal artery stenosis is thought to result in redistribution of blood from the cortex to the medulla, with associated cortical atrophy. Chronic oxygen deficiency causes an adaptive decrease in renal oxygen demand of the kidney, which ultimately decreases renal size (46). These changes are paralleled by an overall decreased and delayed kidney enhancement with loss of the corticomedullary differentiation. Loss of corticomedullary differentiation, however, was not found to be useful in the present study population. This may reflect the advanced age and high frequency of medical renal disease, which are also associated with loss of corticomedullary differentiation.

Some aspects of renal physiology that can be examined with MR imaging but that were not evaluated in this study include excretion of gadolinium contrast material, response to pharmacologic agents, renal parenchymal diffusion coefficient, and renal artery flow profile. Hypoperfusion causes renin-angiotensin–mediated hypertension and hyperconcentration of the urine. Asymmetric, hyperconcentrated gadolinium contrast material in the renal collecting system may be a marker of unilateral renal artery stenosis (47). Asymmetry in the enhancement with gadolinium contrast material produced by captopril may also signify a significant unilateral stenosis (48). Renal artery stenosis may cause a reduction in the renal diffusion coefficient (49) or a change in the flow profile on cine phase-contrast angiograms (50–53). These techniques add additional time to the MR examination.

Table 6

MR Imaging and Clinical Features of Patients Who Benefited from Revascularization versus Those Who Did Not

Feature	Benefit from Revascularization	No Benefit from Revascularization	*P* Value
No. of patients	35	12	...
Mean age (y)	62	68	.043
Mean serum creatinine level (mg/dL)*	2.3	4.5	.0004
No. of patients with renal insufficiency	23 (66)	8 (67)	...
No. of patients receiving dialysis	0	3	...
No. of ischemic kidneys	53	19	...
Kidney length (cm)	9.3	9.0	.18
Kidney height (VB†)	3.0	2.5	.02
Parenchymal thickness (cm)	1.2	1.4	.09
Kidney mass (cm^2)‡	11.7	13.5	.13
Enhancement	176	161	.63
No. of arterial stenoses	52§	14	
No. of arterial occlusions	5	5	
Dephasing on PC angiograms‖			
Mild or severe	51/52 (98)	14/14 (100)	.603
Severe only	45/52 (87)	12/14 (86)	.936
Length ratio#	1.31 ± 0.62	0.92 ± 0.52	.04
Poststenotic dilatation**	1.58	1.36	.12

* For conversion to SI units, 1 mg/dL = 88.40 μmol/L.
† Kidney length measured by number of vertebral bodies to correct for different sizes of patients.
‡ Kidney length multiplied by parenchymal thickness to give a rough indicator of parenchymal mass.
§ Kidneys had stenotic accessory renal arteries.
‖ PC = phase contrast. Data are no. of arteries. Numbers in parentheses are percentages.
\# Ratio between length of dephasing on the PC angiograms and length of stenosis measured on the 3D gadolinium-enhanced MR angiograms. Values are the mean ± standard deviation.
** Ratio of maximum renal artery diameter within 1 cm distal to stenosis divided by the renal artery diameter measured 2–4 cm distal to the stenosis.

This study had a high percentage of patients who did not benefit from renal revascularization. We believe this reflects a bias in the study population resulting from a tendency to order MR angiography for patients with more severe degrees of renal insufficiency and for patients in whom the decision to undertake intervention is difficult to make on the basis of standard tests. The criteria for determining hemodynamic significance of renal artery stenoses defined in the current study may be of greater prognostic value when applied to the entire population of patients suspected of having renal artery stenosis.

Predicting which patient with renal artery stenosis would benefit from revascularization was challenging. Many clinical factors, including age, sex, duration and severity of hypertension, pulmonary hypertension, and serum creatinine levels, are predictive of benefit after intervention (54,55). In this study, the patients who did not improve were significantly older and had higher creatinine levels before revascularization. Patients already undergoing dialysis had a decreased chance of benefiting from revascularization. Of the four patients undergoing dialysis, all continued to undergo dialysis after revascularization. However, discontinuing dialysis is such an enormous benefit that intervention may still be worth pursuing in certain patients. Although severe dephasing was evident for the stenoses in the patients who did not improve, the overall length of dephasing in these cases was significantly less. This may reflect slower renal artery flow in these patients, which causes less turbulence at the stenosis and hence less dephasing. Quantitative renal artery flow measurements might be a better means to identify and accurately evaluate these patients (50–53).

In addition to detecting features of significant renal artery disease, 3D gadolinium-enhanced MR angiography has several important additional advantages over conventional angiography with iodinated contrast material. Gadolinium contrast material is free of nephrotoxicity. It can be used safely at high doses in patients with renal insufficiency (56). It also has a low rate of occurrence of allergic reactions (57–59) and little or no cross-reactivity with iodinated contrast material. Thus, it can be used in patients with known allergy to iodinated contrast material without requiring premedication or other preventative precautions. Gadolinium contrast material only rarely causes nausea or vomiting, even when injected rapidly or immediately after eating. Thus, there is no need for patients to fast before 3D gadolinium-enhanced MR angiography. A final advantage of MR angiography relates to the cross-sectional nature of the imaging data. The 3D cross-sectional data sets allow an infinite variety of projections by computer processing of data acquired from a single bolus injection. Unraveling tortuous arteries and demonstrating renal artery origins in cross section and in perpendicular projections is easily performed at a computer workstation similar to that in CT angiography.

MR angiography has certain limitations and disadvantages. Many patients are not suitable for MR imaging. This includes patients with severe claustrophobia, morbid obesity (too large to fit within the magnet), or patients with implanted electronic devices, orbital metal fragments, certain berry aneurysm clips, and other known MR hazards. The complexity of performing renal artery MR angiography and reconstructing the images as described in this article means that it is available at only a limited number of sites. The best quality studies were obtained on a 1.5-T imaging system with gradient performance sufficient to attain echo times of 2–3 msec and repetition times of 5–10 msec or shorter with 3D gadolinium-enhanced spoiled gradient-echo MR angiography. Technical improvements that decrease the current imaging times (31) and minimize bolus timing errors (60–62) need to be developed and disseminated. Finally, the resolution of current MR angiographic technology, even when performed well, is inferior to conventional arteriography. MR angiography cannot reliably depict intrarenal vascular disease, such as segmental stenoses or the minute aneurysms of vasculitis. It may also fail to depict small collateral vessels that are also helpful for determining the hemodynamic significance of stenoses.

On the basis of these observations, we recommend a simple approach to grading renal artery atherosclerotic disease on MR angiograms. First, assess the renal artery on the 3D gadolinium-enhanced and phase-contrast angiograms to tentatively place the renal artery in one of the following categories: (*a*) normal—renal artery appears normal with both sequences; (*b*) mild stenosis—renal artery appears normal with one sequence but stenotic with the other; (*c*) moderate stenosis—renal artery appears stenotic with both sequences; (*d*) severe stenosis—renal artery appears stenotic on the 3D gadolinium-enhanced MR angiogram but occluded on the phase-contrast angiogram; (*e*) occluded—renal artery appears occluded with both sequences. Then, examine the supporting factors of kidney length, parenchymal thickness, loss of corticomedullary differentiation, asymmetry of enhancement, and poststenotic dilatation and adjust up or down by one grade as necessary. In this scheme, severely stenotic and occluded renal arteries are hemodynamically significant, moderately stenotic arteries are of borderline significance, and normal or mildly stenotic arteries are not significant. It is not yet known if this analysis is suitable for evaluating patients with fibromuscular disease.

In conclusion, MR angiography enables identification of kidney length, parenchymal thickness, symmetry of enhancement, dephasing, and poststenotic dilatation, all of which can be markers of hemodynamically significant renal artery stenosis. ■

Acknowledgments: The authors gratefully acknowledge Thomas L. Chenevert, PhD, Brian H. Hamilton, MD, Qian Dong, MD, Kyung J. Cho, MD, Dasika L. Narasimham, MD, David M. Williams, MD, M. Victoria Marx, MD, Sahira Kazanjian, MD, N. Reed Dunnick, MD, Mel Korobkin, MD, Joel Platt, MD, Isaac Francis, MD, Jim F. M. Meaney, MD, Jeff H. Maki, MD, PhD, Michael V. Knopp, MD, Michael Bock, PhD, and David Stafford-Johnson, MD, for many helpful discussions; all of the MR imaging technologists for performing the studies; Karen E. Travis for assistance with preparation of the manuscript; and Bob Combs for photography.

References

1. Mitchell DG, Tobin M, LeVeen R, et al. Induced renal artery stenosis in rabbits: magnetic resonance imaging, angiography, and radionuclide determination of blood volume and blood flow. Magn Reson Med 1988; 6:113–124.
2. Kim D, Edelman RR, Kent KC, Porter DH, Skillman JJ. Abdominal aorta and renal artery stenosis: evaluation with MR angiography. Radiology 1990; 174:727–731.
3. Lewin JS. Time-of-flight magnetic resonance angiography of the aorta and renal arteries. Invest Radiol 1992; 27:S84–S89.
4. Roditi GH, Smith FW, Redpath TW. Evaluation of tilted, optimized, non-saturating excitation pulses in 3D magnetic resonance angiography of the abdominal aorta and major branches in volunteers. Br J Radiol 1994; 67:11–13.
5. Strotzer M, Fellner CM, Feissler A, et al. Noninvasive assessment of renal artery stenosis: a comparison of MR angiography, color Doppler sonography, and intraarterial angiography. Acta Radiol 1995; 36:243–247.
6. Loubeyre P, Revel D, Garcia P, et al. Screening patient for renal artery stenosis: value of three-dimensional time-of-flight MR angiography. AJR 1994; 162:847–852.
7. Servois V, Laissy JP, Feger C, et al. Two-dimensional time-of-flight magnetic resonance angiography of renal arteries without maximum intensity projection: a prospective comparison with angiography in 21 patients screened for renovascular hypertension. Cardiovasc Intervent Radiol 1994; 17:138–142.
8. Hertz SM, Holland GA, Baum RA, Haskal ZJ, Carpenter JP. Evaluation of renal artery stenosis by magnetic resonance angiography. Am J Surg 1994; 168:140–143.
9. Fellner C, Strotzer M, Geissler A, et al. Renal arteries: evaluation with optimized 2D and 3D time-of-flight MR angiography. Radiology 1995; 196:681–687.
10. Debatin JF, Spritzer CE, Grist TM, et al. Imaging of the renal arteries: value of MR angiography. AJR 1991; 157:981–990.
11. Vock P, Terrier F, Wegmueller H, et al. Magnetic resonance angiography of abdominal vessels: early experience using the three-dimensional phase-contrast technique. Br J Radiol 1991; 64:10–16.
12. Gedroyc WM, Neerhut P, Negus R, et al. Magnetic resonance angiography of renal artery stenosis. Clin Radiol 1995; 50:436–439.
13. Silverman JM, Friedman ML, Van Allan RJ. Detection of main renal artery stenosis using phase-contrast cine MR angiography. AJR 1996; 166:1131–1137.
14. De Cobelli F, Mellone R, Salvioni M, et al. Renal artery stenosis: value of screening with three-dimensional phase-contrast MR angiography with a phased-array multicoil. Radiology 1996; 201:697–703.
15. Duda SH, Schick F, Teufl F, et al. Phase-contrast MR angiography for detection of arteriosclerotic renal artery stenosis. Acta Radiol 1997; 38:287–291.
16. de Haan MW, Kouwenhoven M, Thelissen RP, et al. Renovascular disease in patients with hypertension: detection with systolic and diastolic gating in three-dimensional, phase-contrast MR angiography. Radiology 1996; 198:449–456.
17. Wasser MN, Westenberg J, van der Hulst VP, et al. Hemodynamic significance of renal artery stenosis: digital subtraction angiography versus systolically gated three-dimensional phase-contrast MR angiography. Radiology 1997; 202:333–338.
18. Wielopolski PA, Adamis M, Prasad P, Gaa J, Edelman R. Breath-hold 3D STAR MR angiography of the renal arteries using segmented echo planar imaging. Magn Reson Med 1995; 33:432–438.
19. Li D, Haacke EM, Mugler JP III, Berr S, Brookeman JR, Hutton MC. Three-dimensional time-of-flight MR angiography using selective inversion recover RAGE with fat saturation and ECG-triggering: application to renal arteries. Magn Reson Med 1994; 31:414–422.
20. Borrello JA, Li D, Vesely TM, Vining EP, Brown JJ, Haacke EM. Renal arteries: clinical comparison of three-dimensional time-of-flight MR angiographic sequences and radiographic angiography. Radiology 1995; 197:793–799.
21. Korosec FR, Mistretta CA, Turski PA. ECG-optimized phase contrast line-scanned MR angiography. Magn Reson Med 1992; 24:221–235.
22. Grist TM. Magnetic resonance angiography of renal artery stenosis. Am J Kidney Dis 1994; 24:700–712.
23. Ståhlberg F, Søndergaard L, Thomsen C, Henriksen O. Quantification of complex flow using MR phase imaging: a study of parameters influencing the phase/velocity relation. Magn Reson Imaging 1992; 10:13–23.
24. Evans AJ, Richardson DB, Tien R, et al. Poststenotic signal loss in MR angiography: effects of echo time, flow compensation, and fractional echo. AJNR 1993; 14:721–729.
25. Mustert BR, Dumas MD, Williams DM. In vitro model of arterial stenosis: correlation of MR signal dephasing and transstenotic pressure gradients (abstr). JVIR 1996; 7(suppl):149.
26. Prince MR. Gadolinium-enhanced MR aortography. Radiology 1994; 191:155–164.
27. Prince MR, Narasimham DL, Stanley JC, et al. Breath-hold gadolinium-enhanced MR angiography of the abdominal aorta and its major branches. Radiology 1995; 197:785–792.
28. Kaufman JA, Geller SC, Petersen MJ, Cambria RP, Prince MR, Waltman AC. MR imaging (including MR angiography) of abdominal aortic aneurysms: comparison with conventional arteriography. AJR 1994; 163:203–210.
29. Snidow JJ, Johnson MS, Harris VJ, et al. Three-dimensional gadolinium-enhanced MR angiography for aortoiliac inflow assessment plus renal artery screening in a single breath hold. Radiology 1996; 198: 725–732.
30. Siegelman ES, Gilfeather M, Holland GA, et al. Breath-hold ultrafast three-dimensional gadolinium-enhanced MR angiography of the renovascular system. AJR 1997; 168:1035–1040.
31. Grist TM, Sproat IA, Kennel TW, Korosec FR, Swan JS. MR angiography of the renal arteries during a breath-hold using gadolinium-enhanced 3D TOF with k-space zero-filling and a contrast timing scan (abstr). Proceedings of the Fourth Meeting of the International Society for Magnetic Resonance in Medicine. Berkeley, Calif: International Society for Magnetic Resonance in Medicine, 1996; 63.
32. Mukai J, Kershaw G, Hees PS. Application of magnetic resonance imaging to physiologic and morphologic characterization of renal artery stenosis before and after angioplasty. Am J Physiol Imaging 1992; 7:220–229.
33. Ros PR, Gauger J, Stoupis C, et al. Diagnosis of renal artery stenosis: feasibility of combining MR angiography, MR renography, and gadopentetate-based measurements of glomerular filtration rate. AJR 1995; 165:1447–1451.
34. Vosshenrich R, Kallerhoff M, Grone HJ, et al. Detection of renal ischemic lesions using Gd-DTPA enhanced turbo FLASH MRI:

experimental and clinical results. J Comput Assist Tomogr 1996; 20:236–243.
35. Bass JC, Prince MR, Londy FJ, Chenevert TL. Effect of gadolinium on phase-contrast MR angiography of the renal arteries. AJR 1997; 168:261–266.
36. Loubeyre P, Trolliet P, Cahen R, Grozel F, Labeeuw M, Minh VA. MR angiography of renal artery stenosis: value of the combination of three-dimensional time-of-flight and three-dimensional phase-contrast MR angiography sequences. AJR 1996; 167:489–494.
37. Davidson RA, Wilcox CS. Newer tests for the diagnosis of renovascular disease. JAMA 1992; 268:3353–3358.
38. Wilcox CS. Ischemic nephropathy: noninvasive testing. Semin Nephrol 1996; 16:43–52.
39. Mitty HA, Shapiro RS, Parsons RB, Silberzweig JE. Renovascular hypertension. Radiol Clin North Am 1996; 34:1017–1036.
40. Dunnick NR, Svetkey LP, Cohan RH, et al. Intravenous digital subtraction renal angiography: use in screening for renovascular hypertension. Radiology 1989; 171:219–222.
41. Rubin GD, Dake MD, Napel S, et al. Spiral CT of renal artery stenosis: comparison of three-dimensional rendering techniques. Radiology 1994; 190:181–189.
42. Gatenby JC, McCauley TR, Gore JC. Mechanisms of signal loss in magnetic resonance imaging of stenoses. Med Phys 1993; 20:1049–1057.
43. Schmalbrock P, Yuan C, Chakeres DW, Kohli J, Pelc NJ. Volume MR angiography: methods to achieve very short echo times. Radiology 1990; 175:861–865.
44. Swan JS, Weber DM, Grist TM, Wojtowycz MM, Korosec FR, Mistretta CA. Peripheral MR angiography with variable velocity encoding: work in progress. Radiology 1992; 184:813–817.
45. Saloner D, Selby K, Anderson CM. MRA studies of arterial stenosis: improvements by diastolic acquisition. Magn Reson Med 1994; 31:196–203.
46. Shanley PF. The pathology of chronic renal ischemia. Semin Nephrol 1996; 16:21–32.
47. Walsh P, Rofsky NM, Krinsky GA, Weinreb JC. Asymmetric signal intensity of the renal collecting systems as a sign of unilateral renal artery stenosis following administration of gadopentetate dimeglumine. J Comput Assist Tomogr 1996; 20:812–814.
48. Grenier N, Trillaud H, Combe C, et al. Diagnosis of renovascular hypertension: feasibility of captopril-sensitized dynamic MR imaging and comparison with captopril scintigraphy. AJR 1996; 166:835–843.
49. Müller MF, Prasad PV, Bimmler D, Kaiser A, Edelman RR. Functional imaging of the kidney by means of measurement of the apparent diffusion coefficient. Radiology 1994; 193:711–715.
50. Thomsen C, Cortsen M, Söndergaard L, Henriksen O, Ståhlberg F. A segmented k-space velocity mapping protocol for quantification of renal artery blood flow during breath-holding. JMRI 1995; 5:393–401.
51. Cortsen M, Petersen LJ, Ståhlbert F, et al. MR velocity mapping measurement of renal artery blood flow in patients with impaired kidney function. Acta Radiol 1996; 37:79–84.
52. Schoenberg SO, Knopp MV, Bock M, et al. Renal artery stenosis: grading of hemodynamic changes with CINE phase-contrast MR blood flow measurements. Radiology 1997; 203:45–53.
53. Maier SE, Scheidegger MB, Liu K, Schneider E, Bollinger A, Boesiger P. Renal artery velocity mapping with MR imaging. JMRI 1995; 5:669–676.
54. Barri YM, Davidson RA, Senler S, et al. Prediction of cure of hypertension in atherosclerotic renal artery stenosis. South Med J 1996; 89:679–683.
55. Messina LM, Zelenock GB, Yao KA, Stanley JC. Renal revascularization for recurrent pulmonary edema in patients with poorly controlled hypertension and renal insufficiency: a distinct subgroup of patients with arteriosclerotic renal artery occlusive disease. J Vasc Surg 1992; 15:73–80.
56. Prince MR, Arnoldus C, Frisoli JK. Nephrotoxicity of high-dose gadolinium compared with iodinated contrast. JMRI 1996; 6:162–166.
57. Weiss KL. Severe anaphylactoid reaction after i.v. Gd-DTPA. Magn Reson Imaging 1990; 8:817–818.
58. Jordan RM, Mintz RD. Fatal reaction to gadopentetate dimeglumine. AJR 1995; 164:743–744.
59. Nelson KL, Gifford LM, Lauber-Huber C, Gross CA, Lasser TA. Clinical safety of gadopentetate dimeglumine. Radiology 1995; 196:439–443.
60. Prince MR, Chenevert TL, Foo TK, Londy FJ, Ward JS, Maki JH. Contrast-enhanced abdominal MR angiography: optimization of imaging delay time by automating the detection of contrast material arrival in the aorta. Radiology 1997; 203:109–114.
61. Earls J, Rofsky NM, DeCorato DR, Krinsky GA, Weinreb JC. Hepatic arterial-phase dynamic gadolinium-enhanced MR imaging: optimization with a test examination and a power injector. Radiology 1997; 202:268–273.
62. Prince MR, Grist TM, Debatin JF. 3D contrast MR angiography. New York, NY: Springer Verlag, 1997.

Alan H. Wilman, PhD • Stephen J. Riederer, PhD • Bernard F. King, MD • Josef P. Debbins, MSEE
Phillip J. Rossman, MS • Richard L. Ehman, MD

Fluoroscopically Triggered Contrast-enhanced Three-dimensional MR Angiography with Elliptical Centric View Order: Application to the Renal Arteries[1]

PURPOSE: **To determine the reliability of obtaining arterial-phase, contrast-material–enhanced three-dimensional (3D) magnetic resonance (MR) angiograms of the renal arteries by using a technique that combines two-dimensional real-time MR fluoroscopy and a 3D MR angiographic acquisition with elliptical centric view order.**

MATERIALS AND METHODS: **Twenty-five consecutive patients suspected of having renal artery disease were evaluated with the fluoroscopically triggered technique by using a mean dose of 0.18 mmol/kg gadoteridol. Left renal vein suppression, inferior vena cava suppression, motion artifact, and image quality for depiction of the renal arteries were each evaluated on a five-point scale (1 = best). The findings were compared with those of another 25 consecutive patients who underwent conventional gadolinium-enhanced 3D MR angiography.**

RESULTS: **The fluoroscopically triggered technique produced 4.6 times less left renal vein enhancement than did the conventional method ($P <$ .01). With the fluoroscopically triggered technique, visualization of the renal arteries was adequate for diagnosis in 24 patients (96%) and the overall result (score of 1–3 for all criteria) was of good quality in 22 patients (88%).**

CONCLUSION: **With this fluoroscopically triggered MR angiographic technique, high-quality, arterial phase, relatively motion immune angiograms can be routinely obtained.**

The success of gadolinium-enhanced magnetic resonance (MR) angiography (1,2) is dependent on delivery of the gadolinium chelate through the vascular system to the site of interest. It is well accepted that low-order phase-encoding views dominate image contrast (3); thus, to obtain first-pass arterial-phase images, the central k-space views should ideally be acquired at peak arterial enhancement (4). For two-dimensional (2D) imaging of a single section, this is not difficult to achieve due to the intrinsic high temporal resolution (5–7). However, for three-dimensional (3D) imaging with acquisition times of several tens of seconds, the issue of bolus timing is very important, especially since bolus transit times can vary substantially between patients (8,9). The initial work in 3D gadolinium-enhanced MR angiography used continuous infusion and an imaging time much longer than the variability in transit time, making the timing issue moot (1,10). This approach, however, was susceptible to both respiratory motion and venous contamination, and also suffered from continual dilution of the contrast material due to the lengthened acquisition time. More recent, many 3D studies were performed with use of rapid injection and a rapid acquisition protocol (8,11–14). This approach has the potential to reduce respiratory artifact, venous contamination, and the required dosage of contrast material. With this approach, however, timing the acquisition with the arrival of the bolus of contrast material then becomes extremely important (4,8,11,15).

A number of methods for timing the data acquisition with the arrival of the bolus of contrast material to produce 3D arterial-phase images have already been presented. These include (*a*) estimation of the time of arrival, (*b*) injection of a small amount of contrast material in a test dose to establish timing (16), (*c*) partial k-space updating with increased time resolution (17), and (*d*) line scanning before 3D triggering (18). These methods have all been successful to varying degrees. Nevertheless, each method has a potential drawback as discussed below. For method *a*, the time-to-enhancement variability between patients can be problematic. For method *b*, the test dose causes increased vascular enhancement and causes accumulation of contrast material in the renal pelvis, neither of which is generally desirable. Furthermore this method requires that the cardiac output remain unchanged between the test acquisition and the actual 3D acquisition, which may not always be true. For method *c*, the repetitive sampling of k space ensures an arterial-phase image,

Index terms: Gadolinium, 961.12943 • Magnetic resonance (MR), phase imaging, 961.12942, 961.12943, 961.12949 • Magnetic resonance (MR), technology, 961.12942, 961.12943, 961.12949 • Magnetic resonance (MR), vascular studies, 961.12942 • Renal arteries, MR, 961.12942, 961.12943, 961.12949

Abbreviations: FOV = field of view, FT = Fourier transform, MIP = maximum intensity projection, TR = repetition time, 2D = two-dimensional, 3D = three-dimensional.

Radiology 1997; 205:137–146

[1] From the MR Research Laboratory, Department of Diagnostic Radiology, Mayo Clinic, 200 First St, SW, Rochester, MN 55905. Received April 14, 1997; revision requested May 29; revision received June 23; accepted June 25. Supported by National Institutes of Health grants CA37993 and HL37310, and by GE Medical Systems. A.H.W. supported in part by the Medical Research Council of Canada. **Address reprint requests to** S.J.R.

Figure 1. Schematic diagram of possible contrast-enhanced 3D MR angiographic (*MRA*) acquisitions. In *a*, a typical contrast curve of arterial and venous enhancement is shown. In *b*, the fluoroscopically triggered pulse sequence is shown. This sequence is initiated just before injection of contrast material, and continuous fluoroscopic imaging occurs at an interactively prescribed location. Once the contrast agent is detected, the 3D image with centric phase-encoding order is triggered. For breath-hold studies, breath holding is coached just before triggering. In *c* and *d*, the two possible timings for the conventional sequential phase-encoding order are shown (see text for details). In *e*, the elliptical spiral and sequential view orders are illustrated for an 8 × 8 phase-encoding matrix. During every repetition of a 3DFT acquisition, the signal collected corresponds to one of the points shown, with sampling along an axis corresponding to the frequency direction, k_x, coming out of the plane of the plot. Note that the shaded central views are played out first with the elliptical centric approach. T_{ell} and T_{seq} = time to sample the central views in the elliptical centric method and the sequential method, respectively.

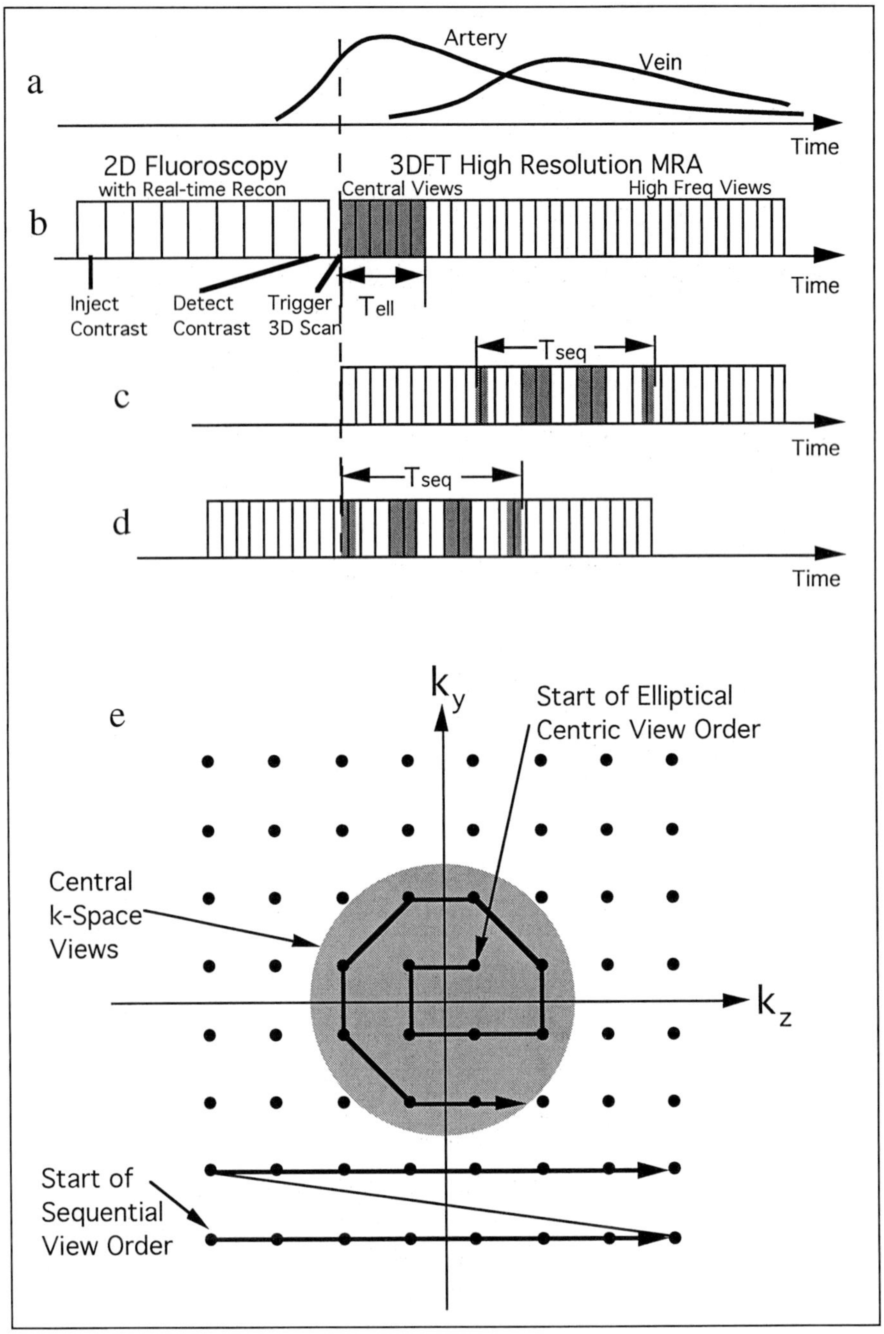

but within a given breath-hold length, the total k-space coverage must be limited to allow for sufficient repetitive view sampling. Finally, although method *d* monitors the bolus arrival in real time, this approach does not give an image-based view of the arrival of contrast material and requires the setting of an automatic threshold level that may not account for variability in the degrees of contrast enhancement between patients.

Thus, we developed a technique for direct monitoring of arrival of the contrast material in a sequence of real-time "MR fluoroscopic" images with means for immediate triggering of a 3D MR angiographic sequence. This technique overcomes all the aforementioned disadvantages by making use of direct monitoring rather than prediction, by maximizing the spatial resolution for a given breath hold, by providing a temporal series of 2D images that illustrates the dynamics of the arrival of contrast material, and by allowing for manual triggering of the 3D acquisition by the operator.

Accurate timing alone is not sufficient to achieve the ideal angiographic result in which the arterial system has high signal intensity and the venous system has no signal. To achieve this, the 3D MR angiographic acquisition is ideally performed in a manner to maximize immunity of the technique to contrast enhancement of the venous vasculature. The question of the determination of the best method for sampling k space has already been raised (8). To this end, we recently developed an "elliptical centric" phase-encoding order for 3D Fourier transform (FT) gradient-echo imaging that has been shown in studies in phantoms and volunteers to provide improved immunity to venous enhancement and to motion compared with many other view orders for 3DFT imaging (19–21).

The purpose of this study was to apply the technique of fluoroscopically triggered contrast material–enhanced 3DFT acquisition in conjunction with the elliptical centric view order in a set of consecutive patients referred for MR imaging evaluation of the renal arteries. We compared the results of this technique with those in a similar set of consecutive patients who underwent conventional contrast-enhanced 3D MR angiographic examination.

MATERIALS AND METHODS

Overview of Fluoroscopic Technique

A timing diagram of contrast-enhanced 3D MR angiography with fluoroscopic triggering and centric view order is shown in Figure 1 parts *a* and *b*. For purposes of discussion, suppose that the origins of the renal arteries are to be imaged by using a 25-second 3DFT MR angiographic acquisition. Before the actual injection of contrast material, all imaging parameters for the 3D sequence are determined and loaded into the pulse sequence controller, and the 3D sequence is thus ready for immediate

Table 1
Evaluation Criteria for Qualitative Evaluation of Contrast-enhanced 3D MR Angiograms

Score	Left Renal Vein Suppression	Inferior Vena Cava Suppression	Motion Artifact	Image Quality for Depiction of Renal Arteries
1	No signal from left renal vein	No signal from inferior vena cava	No visible artifact	Excellent
2	Barely visible signal intensity	Barely visible signal intensity	Minimal artifact	More than adequate for diagnosis
3	Noticeable signal intensity but less than that of the left renal artery	Noticeable signal intensity but less than that of the aorta	Moderate artifact without serious impairment of vessel visualization	Adequate for diagnosis
4	Signal intensity equal to that of the left renal artery	Signal intensity equal to that of the aorta	Moderate artifact with serious impairment of vessel visualization	Less than adequate for diagnosis
5	Signal intensity greater than that of the left renal artery	Signal intensity greater than that of the aorta	Severe artifact, nondiagnostic	No visualization

Table 2
Blood Vessel Signal Intensity Measurements (Normalized to Aortic Noise)

	Conventional 3D MR Angiography		Fluoroscopically Triggered 3D MR Angiography	
Blood Vessel	Before Injection	During Injection	Before Injection	During Injection
Aorta	1.8 ± 1.0	24.5 ± 11.7	2.2 ± 1.4	22.4 ± 10.2
Inferior vena cava	1.6 ± 1.1	6.8 ± 6.0	2.1 ± 1.5	3.2 ± 2.4
Left renal artery	2.1 ± 1.8	19.5 ± 9.1	2.2 ± 1.3	18.2 ± 7.2
Left renal vein	1.8 ± 0.9	14.4 ± 11.1	1.9 ± 0.9	5.2 ± 4.1
Vena cava–to–aorta enhancement ratio	0.26 ± 0.28		0.06 ± 0.05	
Left renal vein–to–artery enhancement ratio	0.88 ± 0.86		0.19 ± 0.18	

execution. Next, a plane is selected to be monitored by the real-time 2DFT fluoroscopic sequence. For the current study, this plane was usually chosen to be a 10-mm-thick sagittal section that contained the thoracic and abdominal aorta as best as possible. With both the 3D and fluoroscopic sequences loaded, execution of the actual contrast-enhanced procedure can commence. As shown in part *b*, just before administration of the contrast agent the fluoroscopic sequence is initiated and applied continuously. While the contrast material is en route to the targeted vasculature, the operator monitors the aorta by viewing the fluoroscopic images, each of which is reconstructed within several hundred milliseconds after acquisition. On seeing the contrast material in the aorta, the operator can optionally direct the patient to hold his or her breath and then immediately trigger the 3DFT MR angiographic sequence. In this way, 3D imaging is initiated while the contrast material is entering the targeted arterial anatomy, at the outset of a breath hold, and with central k-space views acquired during maximal arterial enhancement.

MR Angiographic Sequence: Elliptical Centric View Order

The 3D MR angiographic portion of the technique makes use of the elliptical centric view order (20–22), which, as shown in Figure 1, differs greatly from the conventional sequential view order. In parts *b–d*, the temporal playouts of the two orders are compared. The 3D playout in k space is shown in part *e*, where the two axes shown correspond to the two phase-encoding directions, k_y and k_z. The shaded area represents the "central" views, which correspond to the lowest spatial frequencies and dominate image contrast. For the case of a sequential acquisition of k-space views, the first repetition samples the lowest leftmost point, the next repetition samples the point immediately to the right, and this continues until the lowest row is completely sampled. The next higher row is then sampled similarly, and this process repeats until all desired points are sampled. Conversely, for the elliptical centric view order, the readout during the first repetition of the acquisition starts with one of the k-space points closest to the origin, and in subsequent repetitions points are sampled at progressively larger radii in this k space. In this manner, the central views are sampled earliest in the acquisition, and those points at larger k_y and k_z distances (which sample higher spatial frequencies) are sampled later.

The spacing between the sampled points in the k-space plots of Figure 1 part *e* is dictated by the fields of view (FOVs) along the y and z directions. Here, these FOVs are assumed to be equal, and consequently, the spacings are the same along k_y and k_z. For the general case these FOVs are different, resulting in different spacings along k_y and k_z, which requires a modification of the sampling order to maintain a circular trajectory in k space. Often, the inverse FOV spacing is discounted when plotting k-space indexes, and the points are plotted on a grid with equal spacing. In this case, the circular trajectory of part *e* becomes an elliptical one when the FOVs differ; hence, the name "elliptical centric."

The inherent ability of the elliptical centric view order to provide improved immunity to venous enhancement can perhaps be understood by again considering Figure 1 parts *a–d*. Part *a* demonstrates hypothetic curves that show the behavior over time of contrast enhancement in the arteries followed several seconds later by enhancement in the veins, the specific delay dependent on the vasculature under consideration. Part *b*, after 3D triggering, shows the 3D acquisition corresponding to the elliptical centric view order of part *e*. Each temporal division represents the acquisition of two points of the plot in part *e*. As shown, the 12 points of the central region of part *e* are sampled at the shaded outset of the acquisition in part *b*, here during peak arterial contrast enhancement and before any venous contrast enhancement.

The sequential view order in part *c* differs from the elliptical centric case in part *b* in two important respects. First, the central views are acquired much later during data acquisition, centered halfway through. For the case shown in Figure 1 part *c*, these views would undesirably be sampled well after peak arterial enhancement and during peak venous enhancement. The central views of the sequential acquisition could be matched to peak arterial enhancement as shown in part *d*, but in that case a number of the initial high k-space views would be acquired before the contrast material arrives in the targeted vasculature. A second important difference between sequential and elliptical centric view orders is the time it takes to sample the central views. Ideally, one wishes to sample these views in the shortest time possible at peak arterial enhancement, which will minimize the likelihood of venous enhancement. The elliptical centric method achieves this goal;

however, the sequential approach plays out the central views over a substantially longer time period (compare T_{seq} in part *d* with T_{ell} in part *b*).

To summarize, the elliptical centric view order samples the central views at the outset of the acquisition and acquires the central views in the shortest time possible. The desirability to initiate a 3DFT acquisition with the elliptical view order at the onset of arterial enhancement provides the motivation for a means for accurate triggering.

Table 3
Comparison of Conventional and Fluoroscopically Triggered 3D Contrast-enhanced MR Angiography

Category*	Conventional	Triggered	*P* Value
Left renal vein suppression	2.8 ± 1.2	1.4 ± 0.7	<.0001
IVC suppression distal to renal veins	2.0 ± 0.9	1.2 ± 0.4	<.001
IVC suppression below renal veins	1.3 ± 0.7	1.0 ± 0.0	<.015
Motion artifact	2.0 ± 1.3	1.7 ± 0.8	<.15
Image quality for depiction of renal arteries	2.3 ± 1.2	1.5 ± 0.9	<.02

Note.—Data are presented as the mean ± standard deviation. Images from all 50 patients were evaluated on a five-point scale (1 = best, 5 = worst) as detailed in Table 1.
* IVC = inferior vena cava.

MR Fluoroscopy Sequence

The fluoroscopic portion of the integrated pulse sequence was first used to determine the viewing plane to monitor the arrival of contrast material. This was accomplished in a simple and rapid manner by using a cursor-defined off-isocenter rotation under interactive fluoroscopic control (23). Specifically, beginning with an axial view of the abdomen nominally at the level of the renal artery origins, a cursor was placed on the image at the center of the aorta, and the image plane was then rotated 90° about the cursor into a sagittal view at the prescribed cursor location. If necessary, further small-angle rotations and adjustments in FOV or section thickness were made to improve the length and quality of aortic visualization. Typically, the time for selecting the aortic viewing plane was about 1 minute. Once the viewing plane was established, the patient was coached to hold his or her breath and a test 3D image set was obtained without administration of contrast material to ensure accurate selection of the 3D volume. Next, the sequence as shown in Figure 1 part *b* was performed.

The fluoroscopic image parameters were chosen to produce dynamic 2D images with high spatial resolution under the constraint of keeping the image update rate no slower than about one per second. This temporal resolution was considered marginally sufficient for observing the arrival of contrast material into the abdominal aorta. Thus, the typical fluoroscopic scanning parameters included the following: 13–15/8 (repetition time [TR] msec/echo time msec), 30° flip angle, 10-mm section thickness, 256 (x) × 96 (y) matrix, ±16-kHz receiver bandwidth, and first-order gradient moment nulling in the section-select and frequency directions. The relatively long echo time of 8 msec was necessary to allow for a full echo acquisition at a relatively low bandwidth, for the use of gradient moment nulling, and for oblique imaging with an FOV as small as 200 mm. The use of gradient moment nulling reduced flow dephasing effects; this was particularly valuable in the initial scouting process before the arrival of contrast material. The flip angle was chosen to be large enough to saturate in-plane flow, thus allowing for substantial contrast material enhancement but also to be sufficiently small such that the images obtained before the arrival of contrast material were not completely saturated. As mentioned above, the fluoroscopic imaging rate was approximately one per second (96 views × 13 msec). The 96 views represented three-quarter partial Fourier sampling of 128 views, with the latter quarter zero filled; further symmetric zero filling to 256 points was performed before reconstruction. The reconstruction time was ~500 msec for the 256 × 256 matrix when using a four-coil phased array and a "sum of the squares" reconstruction (24).

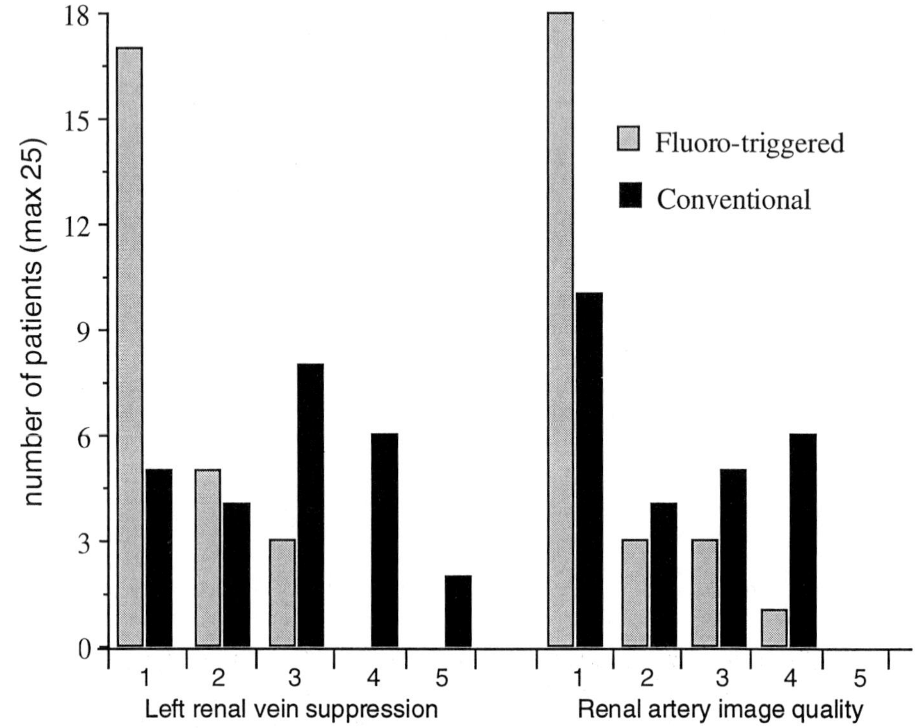

Figure 2. Illustration of the distribution of patients in the evaluation of left renal vein suppression and renal artery image quality. The improvement with the fluoroscopically triggered sequence was statistically significant for both the left renal vein suppression and the renal artery categories. In the latter category, the only grade 4 score in the fluoroscopically triggered acquisitions was due to a verbal communication error.

Instrumentation for Fluoroscopic Triggering

Actual implementation of fluoroscopic triggering of the 3D angiographic sequence requires instrumentation capable of several distinct functions. These include (*a*) the ability to rapidly switch from one pulse sequence to another, (*b*) the ability to reconstruct the 2DFT fluoroscopic images very quickly, and (*c*) the means for allowing the operator to manually trigger the 3DFT sequence. These functions were achieved by making use of an "MR fluoroscopy" apparatus (25), which has recently been described in detail (26). This real-time reconstruction system has been interfaced to a standard whole-body 1.5-T MR imaging unit (Signa; GE Medical Systems, Milwaukee, Wis).

The first function above, sequence switching, is provided by copying both the fluoroscopic and 3D pulse sequences into the pulse controller memory of the MR imaging unit. At the outset of contrast-enhanced imaging, a logic variable is set to "true," and after each 13-msec repetition of the fluoroscopic sequence the variable is evaluated. If "true," the fluoroscopic sequence is repeated; if "false," the sequence controller switches to the 3D sequence. Once triggered, there is an additional 10-msec latency until execution of the 3D se-

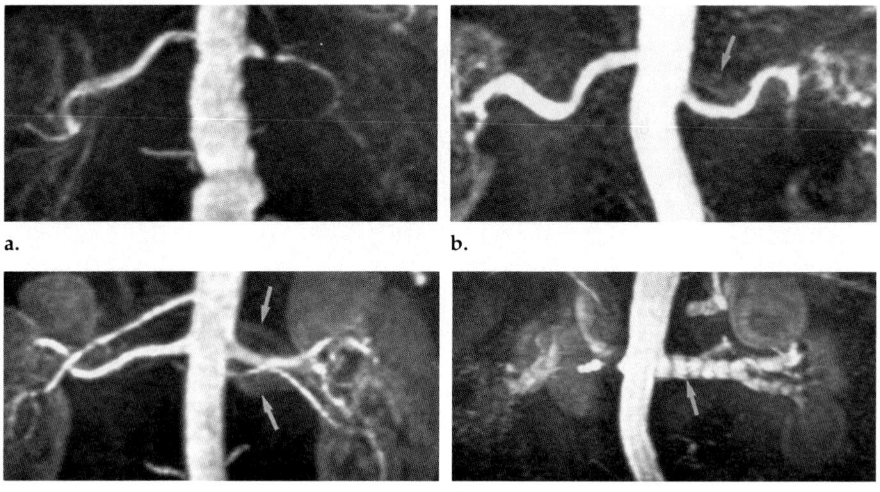

Figure 3. Coronal MIP images from the 3D data sets illustrate varying degrees of left renal vein suppression. **(a)** No renal vein was evident (grade 1). **(b)** Left renal vein (arrow) is barely visible (grade 2). **(c)** Left renal veins (arrows) are noticeable but less so than the renal artery (grade 3). **(d)** Left renal vein signal intensity (arrow) is equal to that of the renal artery (grade 4). The images in **a–c** are from fluoroscopically triggered, elliptical centric phase-encoding order data sets. The image in **d** is from a nontriggered, sequential acquisition data set. In terms of motion artifact, **a** and **b** received a grade of 2 due to minimal artifact, while **c** and **d** had no visible artifact (grade 1).

quence. The second function, high-speed reconstruction, is performed as discussed above with the array processor integral to the instrumentation discussed by Debbins et al (26). The third function, operator intervention, is provided by a direct serial interface from the host computer of the MR fluoroscopy system to the pulse sequence controller. By clicking a mouse corresponding to a "trigger" button on the display screen, the operator causes the logic variable described above to change from true to false. The total delay from acquisition of data for the contrast-filled fluoroscopic image until initiation of the 3DFT MR angiographic sequence is thus 523 msec (500 + 13 + 10) plus the response time of the operator.

Patient Studies

The fluoroscopically triggered breath-hold contrast-enhanced 3D pulse sequence with elliptical centric view order was tested on 25 consecutive patients who had been referred for MR examination of the renal arteries. There were 16 male and nine female patients with a mean age of 64 years ± 17 (age range, 17–78 years) and mean weight of 84 kg ± 21. Their serum creatinine levels ranged from 0.7 to 2.5 mg/dL (60–220 μmol/L) with a mean of 1.5 mg/dL ± 0.7 (130 μmol/L). Each patient received a 30-mL dose (mean dose, 0.18 mmol/kg ± 0.05) of gadoteridol (Prohance; Bracco Diagnostics, Princeton, NJ) by hand injection into a forearm vein with an 18-gauge angiographic catheter at a rate of 3–5 mL/sec. This was followed by a saline flush of 20 mL. The 3D MR angiographic portion of the integrated pulse sequence was prescribed to image the renal arteries and abdominal aorta in the coronal plane. The 3DFT MR angiographic acquisition used radio-frequency spoiling, rewinding of both phase-encoding gradients, 7.2/1.3, 45° flip angle, matrix size of 256 (x) × 128 (y) × 32 (z) with 1.5–2.0-mm section thickness, three-quarter or full FOV in the y direction, ±32-kHz receiver bandwidth, and acquisition time of 24–32 seconds. Either a dual-element "license plate" coil (GE Medical Systems) or a four-element phased-array coil (27) was used. Each patient was instructed to hold his or her breath at end-inspiration immediately before triggering the 3D acquisition.

The results from the fluoroscopically triggered sequence were compared with those in a similar population of 25 consecutive patients (14 men, 11 women; mean age, 64 years ± 11; age range, 35–79 years; mean weight, 78 kg ± 19; serum creatinine level: mean, 1.6 mg/dL ± 0.7 [140 μmol/L]; range, 0.7–3.2 mg/dL [60–280 μmol/L]). The same 30-mL dose (mean dose, 0.20 mmol/kg ± 0.5) and injection scheme were used. These patients had undergone gadolinium-enhanced 3D MR angiography during the 4 months prior to the availability of the fluoroscopically triggered sequence. In these patients, 3D imaging commenced approximately 12–15 seconds after the injection was begun, similar to the technique used by Leung et al (14). This standard 3D technique made use of sequential view order and was typically performed with the following parameters: 45° flip angle, ±32-kHz bandwidth, three-quarter phase FOV, 512 × 128 × 32 matrix with 10.5/1.8 or 512 × 160 × 16 matrix with 12.7/2.4. A dual-element license plate receive coil was used, and the breath-hold length was 20–32 seconds.

Evaluation

The fluoroscopically triggered technique was evaluated in two ways. First, the fluoroscopic portion of the procedure was evaluated by determining if it was possible to trigger the 3D MR angiographic sequence on the basis of visualization of the contrast agent on the fluoroscopic image sequence. Second, the fluoroscopic image sequence for each patient was used to determine the actual time delay from start of injection to arrival of contrast material in the abdominal aorta and the degree of signal enhancement. The latter was defined as the ratio of signal intensity measurements on the fluoroscopic images obtained just before triggering of the 3D image to those obtained just before injection. The signal intensity was the average value from a ~1-cm^2 region of interest within the aorta at the nominal level of the renal arteries.

Qualitative and quantitative evaluations were also performed on the 3D MR angiograms obtained with the fluoroscopically triggered technique with elliptical centric view order and on those obtained with sequential view order with no triggering. Five criteria were chosen for the qualitative evaluation of the 3D MR angiograms by using a five-point scale (Table 1). Evaluations were done on an examination-by-examination basis, with consideration of both hard-copy films and video displays of the maximum intensity projection (MIP) images and individual partitions. Each grade represented the consensus of the three senior authors (A.H.W., S.J.R., B.F.K.). To assess the degree of venous suppression, the signal intensity of the left renal vein relative to that of the left renal artery was graded. Similarly, the degree of contrast enhancement in the inferior vena cava proximal and distal to the confluence with the right renal vein was also evaluated. The degree of apparent motion artifact was also assessed. Finally, the overall quality of each MR angiographic examination in terms of degree of portrayal of the main renal arteries was assessed. For each comparison, the mean and standard deviation of each group were computed, and the Wilcoxon rank-sum test was performed to determine statistical significance ($P < .05$) (28). For the quantitative evaluation, signal intensity measurements were obtained from the 3D MR angiographic source images at the following four locations: the aorta at the level of the renal arteries, the inferior vena cava distal to the confluence with the right renal vein, the main left renal artery, and the main left renal vein. These measurements were normalized to the aortic noise as reported by Prince (2). The venous-to-arterial enhancement ratio, V/A, was computed by taking the differences in signal intensity, SI, between the acquisitions obtained during, SI_d, and those obtained before, SI_b, passage of contrast material and is expressed by the following equation: $V/A = (VSI_d - VSI_b)/(ASI_d - ASI_b)$. Ideally, this enhancement ratio would be 0.

RESULTS

The results from the comparison of the fluoroscopically triggered 3D MR

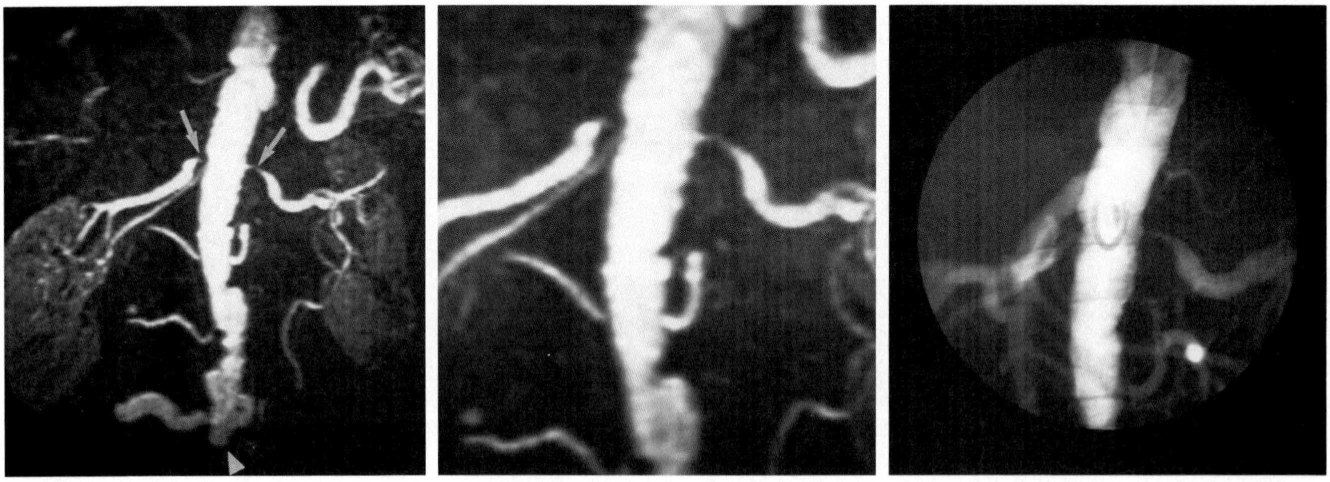

a. b. c.

Figure 4. Angiograms in a patient with bilateral renal artery stenoses and a distal aortic occlusion with collateral flow being supplied by the lumbar arteries. **(a)** Coronal MIP image of 12 sections illustrates the bilateral renal artery stenoses (arrows) and distal aortic occlusion (arrowhead). **(b)** Renal artery portion has been enlarged for comparison with the x-ray angiogram **(c)** for which a pigtail catheter was used. The MR matrix size was 256 (x) × 128 (y) × 32 (z), with 1.5-mm resolution in z. The acquisition time was 34 seconds and the dual-element license plate coil was used.

angiographic sequence with the standard 3D MR angiographic technique are summarized in Tables 2 and 3. The signal intensity measurements of Table 2 show that the fluoroscopically triggered technique produced significantly less venous enhancement for the 3D acquisition during contrast administration. In particular, the venous-to-arterial enhancement ratios differed by a factor of greater than 4 for both the inferior vena cava–to–aorta ratio ($P < .01$) and the left renal vein–to–left renal artery ratio ($P < .001$). The results for the graded evaluation are shown in Table 3, and the corresponding distributions for two individual categories, left renal vein suppression and renal artery image quality, are shown in Figure 2. From Table 3 and Figure 2, it is again clear that the fluoroscopically triggered technique with elliptical centric view order was significantly superior for renal vein suppression. In all of the fluoroscopically triggered cases, the renal vein suppression was sufficiently low such that the main renal arteries could be easily identified on a coronal MIP image of the complete imaging volume. To aid in interpreting the numeric grades presented here, Figure 3 illustrates examples of different grades of left renal vein suppression. These images are coronal MIP images of the renal arteries and veins and represent the first four levels of the left renal vein evaluation scale.

The fluoroscopically triggered method also received a better grading for renal artery quality, and the degree of improvement over the conventional technique was statistically significant (Table 3). In addition, from the distribution in Figure 2, with use of the fluoroscopically triggered sequence, the renal arteries were well visualized in 24 (95%) of the 25 consecutive patients. On the basis of the MR examinations only, it was determined that of the 25 patients in the fluoroscopically triggered group, 15 patients had greater than 60% renal artery stenosis with five of these patients exhibiting bilateral stenoses; one case was indeterminate. The single case of poor visualization (grade 4) was due to improper verbal communication, which led to premature triggering of the 3D image. Of the 25 patients in the conventional technique group, seven patients had greater than 60% stenosis with one having bilateral stenoses, and four cases were indeterminate due to poor quality.

In 18 (72%) of the 25 fluoroscopically triggered cases, the overall result was considered high quality, defined as a score of 1 or 2 for all five evaluation criteria. In 22 (88%) of these 25 cases, the result was considered good quality, defined as a score of 1, 2, or 3 for all criteria. In comparison, for the patients in the conventional method group, the respective frequencies were six (24%) and 14 (56%) of 25 patients.

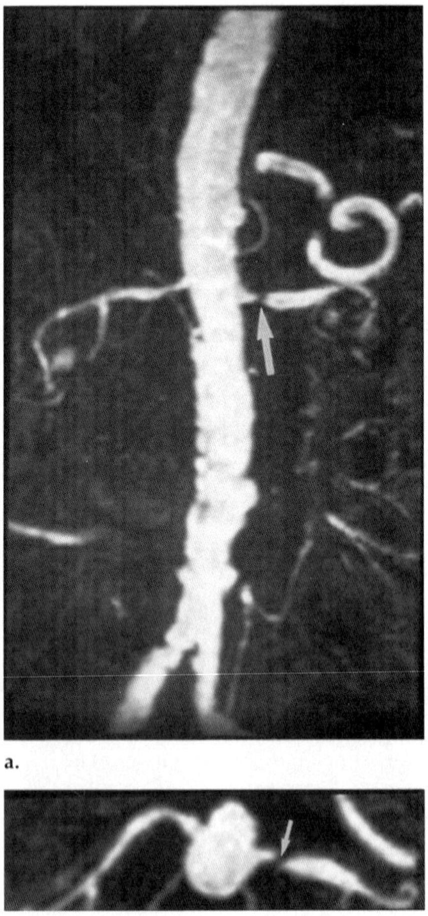

a.

b.

Figure 5. Contrast-enhanced 3D MR angiograms from a fluoroscopically triggered data set with 1.5-mm section-select resolution. By making use of fine resolution in the section-select direction, the vessels may be well visualized from multiple angles. **(a)** Coronal MIP image of the full data set illustrates the left renal artery stenosis (arrow) and moderate atherosclerotic disease of the aorta. **(b)** Selective axial MIP image that includes all of the sections clearly shows the stenosis (arrow) in another orthogonal projection.

The superior image quality of the 3D data sets from the fluoroscopically triggered pulse sequence was particularly helpful in several difficult patients. In Figure 4a, the selective coronal MIP

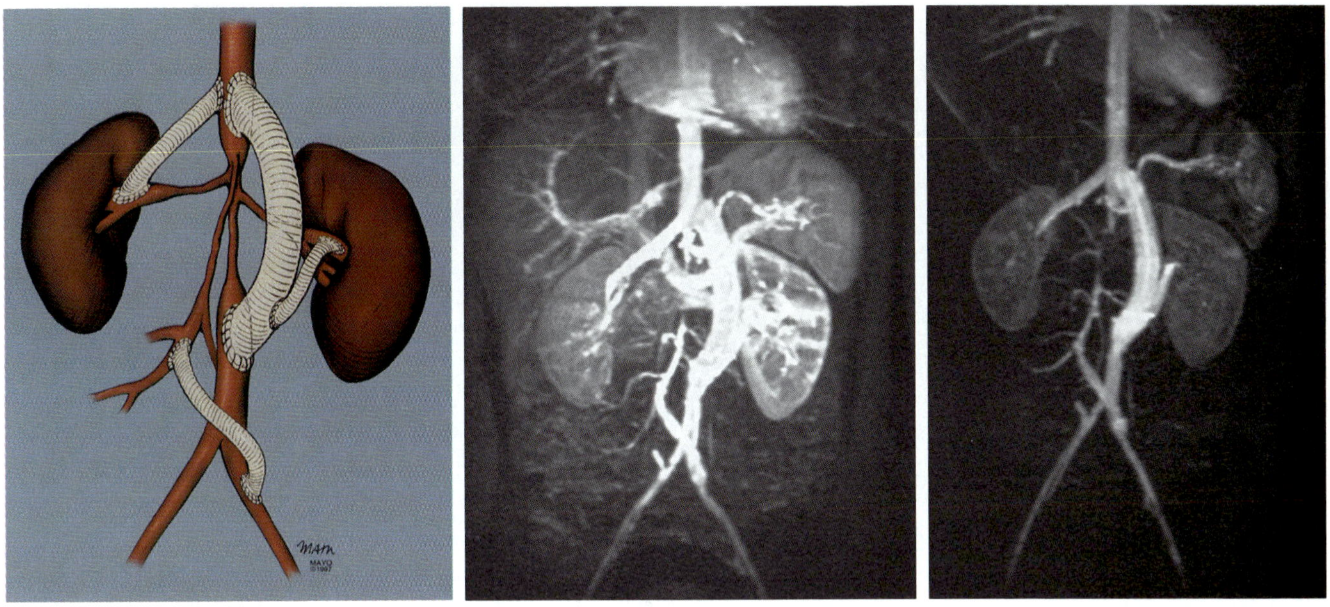

a. b. c.

Figure 6. Takayasu arteritis in a patient with multiple grafts to the aorta. **(a)** Sketch of this patient's specific anatomic features shows the grafts in beige. **(b, c)** Three-dimensional MR angiographic MIP images from this patient's complete data set were obtained by using two different techniques. **(b)** MIP image obtained with the conventional technique that uses sequential phase encoding and estimation of the bolus timing. The 3D acquisition was 32 seconds in duration and was begun 4 seconds after administration of contrast material. The combination of rapid circulation time and sequential phase encoding caused substantial venous enhancement. **(c)** Follow-up MIP image obtained 6 months later with use of the fluoroscopically triggered pulse sequence shows minimal venous signal intensity. The discontinuity in the lumen of the proximal superior mesenteric artery arises from the inflammation and fibrosis of the Takayasu disease. The lumen of the distal superior mesenteric artery is patent with blood supply via a graft from the left iliac artery.

image illustrates a case of bilateral renal artery stenoses and distal aortic occlusion. The accurate bolus timing and lack of venous overlap enabled easy delineation of the aortic and renal abnormalities. The x-ray angiogram of this patient is shown in Figure 4c. In another patient (Fig 5), the 3D nature of the data set, with high z-resolution (1.5 mm in the anteroposterior direction), clearly demonstrated a left renal artery stenosis in both the coronal and axial projections. Finally, Figure 6 illustrates a complex case in which the patient had multiple abdominal vascular grafts as a result of Takayasu arteritis. The initial examination was performed without fluoroscopic triggering, using instead a fixed delay and sequential phase encoding for the 3D sequence. The resultant image in Figure 6b demonstrates extensive venous overlap obscuring the arterial anatomic structures. A follow-up MR angiogram obtained 6 months later with use of fluoroscopic triggering and elliptical centric phase-encoding order clearly shows all grafts, with no venous overlap (Fig 6c).

In all 25 cases, by using the interactive capability of the fluoroscopic system, it was possible to rapidly obtain a sagittal view of the aorta for monitoring the bolus. In 24 of the 25 fluoroscopically triggered cases, it was possible to trigger the 3D MR angiographic sequence on the basis of visualization of arrival of contrast material into this imaging plane. The single failure was that of miscommunication, as mentioned earlier. A typical set of fluoroscopic image frames showing arrival of contrast material into the sagittal imaging plane is shown in Figure 7.

Results from the retrospective quantitative analysis of the fluoroscopic frames are shown in Figure 8. In Figure 8a, the transit times from injection to aortic enhancement are plotted against the enhancement factor (postcontrast maximum intensity divided by precontrast intensity from the fluoroscopic images). For the 24 patients, the average time from injection to enhancement of the aorta at the renal arteries was 15.3 seconds ± 4.0 (mean ± standard deviation) and the range of transit times was 8–25 seconds. In Figure 8b, examples of the complete time course from injection to enhancement are shown. In each case, the 3D MR angiographic sequence was triggered at the last point. A decrease in intensity of the last point was common due to inhalation by the patient. In general, the measured degree of contrast material enhancement in the aorta was far less on the fluoroscopic images than on the 3D images. There are three main reasons for this difference: First, the fluoroscopic images were obtained with use of a lower flip angle and longer TR and thus were subject to increased time-of-flight enhancement; second, the fluoroscopic image sections were typically 10 times thicker than the 3D partitions, and thus the region-of-interest measurements were more influenced by neighboring tissue; and third, the fluoroscopic technique depicted the leading edge of the bolus before maximal enhancement, which ideally would occur by the start of the 3D acquisition a few seconds later.

DISCUSSION

High-quality 3D contrast-enhanced MR angiograms have been demonstrated by many groups without the use of a timing image or direct monitoring. A common approach is to use continuous infusion over the course of the imaging time, with sequential phase-encoding order. The injection is begun such that contrast material will appear in the vessels of interest at the start of imaging. If the timing is accurate, the contrast material will therefore be in the vessels of interest for approximately one-half of the acquisition time before the most central k-space views are acquired. In this time period, the contrast material is likely to migrate into the venous system, and enhancement of the renal vein and vena cava is likely to occur. Reduction of this venous signal intensity can be

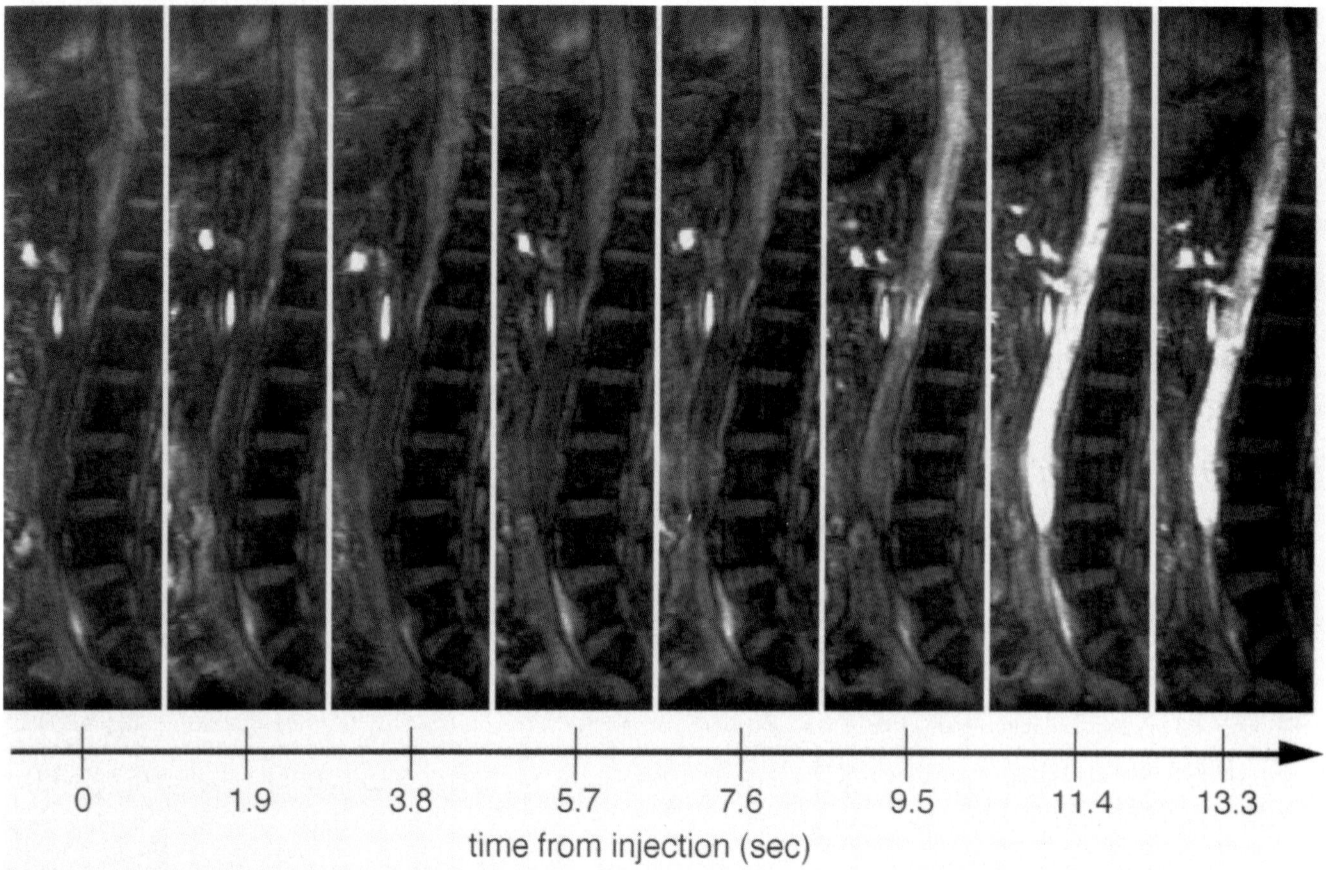

Figure 7. Fluoroscopic images show the arrival of contrast material into the sagittal imaging plane. Only part of each fluoroscopic image is shown, beginning at the time of injection and continuing until when the 3D sequence was triggered. The FOV was 400 mm, and the section thickness was 15 mm. In this case, the TR was 15 msec and a full number of excitations was used, leading to an image update rate of 1.9 seconds.

achieved by using centric ordering; however, the timing of the contrast enhancement then becomes crucial since poor timing can lead to lack of enhancement during the central k-space acquisition. By making use of direct monitoring of the contrast material, consistently accurate timing is possible. When accurate timing is possible, centric encoding may be used and the benefits of improved venous signal suppression and breathing artifact minimization can be reaped.

Recently, venous-suppressed 3D MR angiograms have been obtained by using an initial bolus timing acquisition, followed by a 3D acquisition with sequential order in which the rapid injection is timed such that peak enhancement matches the playout of the central k-space views (16,29). The 3D acquisition is thus similar to Figure 1 part *d*. Although this approach can produce low venous enhancement, it also sacrifices a portion of the high k-space views since many of the initial views are acquired without any contrast material present in the targeted vasculature. The elliptical centric approach also captures the central views at peak arterial enhancement, but these views are captured in a reduced time period as shown in Figure 1. All of the high k-space views are sampled last when the contrast material is still present in the vasculature. Toward the end of the acquisition, venous enhancement will occur, but the effects are minimized since only high k-space views remain to be sampled.

With regard to bolus timing, the test bolus injection has been shown to provide reliable timing. In a study by Earls et al (16), the average additional time for the performance and evaluation of the timing acquisition was 4.5 minutes. With the fluoroscopic approach, the only additional time is that needed for fluoroscopic localization of the monitoring plane, which was less than 1 minute. Since the fluoroscopic method does not use a test dose, no additional kidney or venous enhancement is introduced. Perhaps most important, the fluoroscopic technique monitors the actual arrival of the contrast material for the 3D MR angiographic acquisition. By using direct monitoring of this dose rather than prediction from an acquisition performed a number of minutes earlier, this technique is unaffected by changes in patient heart rate or changes in dose delivery rate (possible with manual injection). Immunity to these variables can only aid in increasing the reliability of the technique.

Direct monitoring of contrast material has already been used in 3D MR angiography (18,30). In that approach, a line image through the aorta was used. While that method can provide accurate timing, it does not provide the scope of information available from a 2D image. The typically sagittal image acquisition used in the present work provides an extended view of the aorta from the heart to the lower abdomen, and because of the high spatial resolution, the origins of the major branching vessels (eg, mesenteric and celiac arteries) are typically well seen. The resultant 2D images allow for retrospective analysis of the dynamics of arrival of contrast material at any point on the image. The fluoroscopic triggering approach also differs from that of Foo et al (18) in that the 3D acquisition is triggered by the operator on the basis of specific enhancement of the vessels of interest, as opposed to an automatic trigger arising from a line of data. An auto-

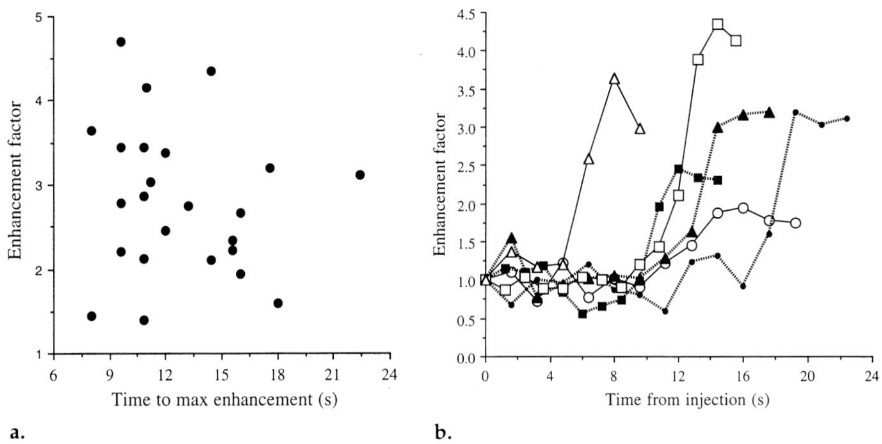

Figure 8. **(a)** Graph of the enhancement factor of the abdominal aorta plotted against the time to maximum enhancement as determined from the fluoroscopic images in 24 patients. The fluoroscopic enhancement factor was defined as the ratio of aortic signal intensity on the 2D image obtained just before 3D triggering to the signal intensity on the image obtained just before injection. One patient was excluded due to premature triggering of the fluoroscopically triggered sequence. **(b)** Specific examples of the time course of arrival of contrast material before 3D triggering are shown for six patients. A decrease in signal intensity of the last point was common due to inhalation by the patient after the breath-hold command.

matic triggering method requires the establishment of a specific trigger threshold of signal enhancement; however, Figure 8a illustrates the varying degrees of enhancement. In addition, manual triggering by an experienced operator eliminates the possibility of false triggering arising from respiratory motion, increased blood inflow, gross patient movement, or unusual enhancement problems (4,8,11,15).

At present, the fluoroscopic imaging approach has a slower updating rate than the line scanning approach, which produces an output point every 400 msec (18). Certainly, the fluoroscopic image update rate could be increased to match this rate by sacrificing spatial resolution, by using a higher bandwidth and shorter TRs, or by using partial k-space updating (3,31). In fact, a 64×64 resolution would probably be sufficient for bolus detection; however, the detailed depiction of vessel anatomic features provided here would be lost. Further research into the ideal trade-off between spatial resolution and image sampling is necessary.

Time-resolved 3D MR angiography (17) can also consistently produce first-pass arterial images. To achieve this, the k-space data from the 3D volume are sampled repetitively during the breath hold. To allow for a high degree of repetitive sampling within a given time, this technique must limit either the FOV coverage or the spatial resolution. The elliptical centric approach presented here maximizes 3D spatial resolution by sampling each k-space point only once and is constrained only by the duration of the breath hold and the length of the bolus.

The elliptical centric encoding scheme has been shown elsewhere to provide superior immunity to breathing artifact (often occurring late in the breath hold) and venous background signal intensity in comparison to many other phase-encoding orders (20,21), including approaches that are based on the centric order used for 2D imaging (32). It is interesting to note, however, that in the present study there was only minor improvement and no statistically significant difference in the degree of motion artifact when using the elliptical centric approach instead of the nontriggered image with sequential phase-encoding order even though the average breath-hold lengths were roughly the same (fluoroscopically triggered, 29 seconds $\pm$ 4; nontriggered, 25 seconds $\pm$ 5). Although initially surprising, we believe that there are two main reasons as to why the superior motion artifact immunity of the elliptical centric approach was not evident in this study. First, the nontriggered, sequential encoding group benefitted from hyperventilation before the start of the 3D acquisition, whereas in the fluoroscopically triggered cases patients breathed quietly until they were told to quickly hold their breath. Second, the fluoroscopic image operator triggered the 3D acquisition immediately after hearing the "hold your breath" command, and it is conceivable that a number of the patients had not fully held their breath at the triggering time. Since the most central views were acquired first, it was important that the patient had stopped moving before triggering the 3D acquisition. Typically, the total time between bolus detection at the thoracic aorta and the 3D triggering was under 5 seconds. During this delay, the bolus progressed distally through the abdominal aorta and into the renal artery tree.

The venous-suppressed MR angiograms shown in this work arise from the combined use of fluoroscopic triggering and an elliptical centric phase-encoding order. Both innovations are important. If one were to perform elliptical centric phase encoding without an accurate bolus timing scheme, it is unlikely that the central views would be acquired at peak arterial enhancement, and this could lead to substantial artifacts (4). Alternatively, if one were to perform fluoroscopic triggering with a sequential phase-encoding order, the bolus would peak long before the central views were acquired (Fig 1 part *c*) resulting in substantial venous enhancement. Hence, the fluoroscopic triggering approach requires the use of a centric phase-encoding order. Our choice of the elliptical centric order was based on the extensive evaluation of centric phase-encoding orders (21). In particular, when the bolus is properly timed, this technique has been shown to limit venous enhancement more effectively than other commonly used 3D centric approaches because the central views are sampled first in the most compact period possible.

The equipment described here for performing the fluoroscopic acquisition and triggering of the 3D acquisition is not presently widely available. Although this equipment was custom developed in our own laboratory, many of the elements are already intrinsic to most commercial MR imaging systems. In fact, the most expensive element of the hardware used here was the array processor, and such a device is already found in virtually all current commercial systems. Implementation of this technique on commercial systems would principally require that the data flow, image reconstruction, and sequence switching be performed faster than is typically done currently.

In addition to cost, another practical aspect of any new technology is the expertise required to operate it. In the initial phases of this project, the equipment was operated by the senior author (A.H.W.). However, as the procedures for fluoroscopic positioning and setup of the 3D MR angiographic acquisition became more standardized, equipment operation for many of the patient studies was done by a technician. We fully expect that MR technologists will be readily capable of operating the fluoroscopic equipment.

In conclusion, fluoroscopic 2D imaging provides a reliable method for timing the arrival of the bolus of contrast material to the specific area of interest. When combined with a 3D MR angiographic acquisition with use of an elliptical centric view order, it is possible to consistently obtain high-quality, high-resolution, arterial-phase, relatively motion immune angiograms. ■

References

1. Prince MR, Yucel EK, Kaufman JA, Harrison DC, Geller SC. Dynamic gadolinium-enhanced 3D abdominal MR arteriography. JMRI 1993; 3:877–881.
2. Prince MR. Gadolinium-enhanced MR aortography. Radiology 1994; 191:155–164.
3. Riederer SJ, Tasciyan T, Farzaneh F, Lee JN, Wright RC, Herfkens RJ. MR fluoroscopy: technical feasibility. Magn Reson Med 1988; 8:1–15.
4. Maki JH, Prince MR, Londy FJ, Chenevert TL. The effects of time varying intravascular signal intensity and k-space acquisition order on three-dimensional MR angiography image quality. JMRI 1996; 6:642–651.
5. Adamis MK, Li W, Wielopolski PA, et al. Dynamic contrast-enhanced subtraction MR angiography of the lower extremities: initial evaluation with a multisection two-dimensional time-of-flight sequence. Radiology 1995; 196:689–695.
6. Wang Y, Johnston DL, Breen JF, et al. Dynamic MR digital subtraction angiography using contrast enhancement, fast data acquisition, and complex subtraction. Magn Reson Med 1996; 36:551–556.
7. Hennig J, Scheffler K, Laubenberger J, Strecker R. Time-resolved projection angiography after bolus injection of contrast agent. Magn Reson Med 1997; 37:341–345.
8. Holland GA, Dougherty L, Carpenter JP, et al. Breath-hold ultrafast three-dimensional gadolinium-enhanced MR angiography of the aorta and the renal and other visceral abdominal arteries. AJR 1996; 166: 971–981.
9. Earls JP, Rofsky NM, DeCorato DR, Krinsky GA, Weinreb JC. Hepatic arterial-phase dynamic gadolinium-enhanced MR imaging: optimization with a test examination and a power injector. Radiology 1997; 202:268–273.
10. Creasy JL, Price RR, Presbrey T, Goins D, Partain CL, Kessler RM. Gadolinium-enhanced MR angiography. Radiology 1990; 175:280–283.
11. Prince MR, Narasimham DL, Stanley JC, et al. Breath-hold gadolinium-enhanced MR angiography of the abdominal aorta and its major branches. Radiology 1995; 197:785–792.
12. Shetty AN, Shirkhoda A, Bis KG, Alcantara A. Contrast-enhanced three dimensional MR angiography in a single breath-hold: a novel technique. AJR 1995; 165:1290–1292.
13. Isoda H, Ushimi T, Masui T, et al. Clinical evaluation of pulmonary 3D time-of-flight MRA with breath holding using contrast media. J Comput Assist Tomogr 1995; 19: 911–919.
14. Leung DL, McKinnon GC, Davis CP, Pfammatter T, Krestin GP, Debatin JF. Breath-hold, contrast-enhanced, three-dimensional MR angiography. Radiology 1996; 201:569–571.
15. Steiner P, McKinnon GC, Romanowski B, Goehde SC, Hany T, Debatin J. Contrast-enhanced, ultrafast 3D pulmonary MR angiography in a single breathhold: initial assessment of imaging performance. JMRI 1997; 7:177–182.
16. Earls JP, Rofsky NM, DeCorato DR, Krinsky GA, Weinreb JC. Breath-hold single-dose gadolinium-enhanced three-dimensional MR aortography: usefulness of a timing examination and MR power injector. Radiology 1996; 201:705–710.
17. Korosec FR, Frayne R, Grist TM, Mistretta CA. Time-resolved contrast-enhanced 3D MR angiography. Magn Reson Med 1996; 36:345–351.
18. Foo TKF, Saranathan M, Prince MR, Chenevert TL. Automated detection of bolus arrival and initiation of data acquisition in fast, three-dimensional, gadolinium-enhanced MR angiography. Radiology 1997; 203:275–280.
19. Wilman AH, Riederer SJ, Breen J, Ehman RL. Elliptical spiral phase encode ordering: a dynamic, field-of-view–dependent scheme for breath-hold contrast-enhanced MR angiography (abstr). Radiology 1996; 201(P):328.
20. Wilman AH, Riederer SJ. An optimal phase encoding order for minimizing motion and maximizing arterial contrast in 3D contrast-enhanced MR angiography (abstr). Proceedings of the Fifth Meeting of the International Society for Magnetic Resonance in Medicine. Berkeley, Calif: International Society for Magnetic Resonance in Medicine, 1997; 252.
21. Wilman AH, Riederer SJ. Performance of an elliptical spiral centric view order for signal enhancement and motion artifact suppression in breathhold three dimensional gradient echo imaging. Magn Reson Med (in press).
22. Wilman AH, Riederer SJ. Improved centric phase encoding orders for three dimensional magnetization prepared MR angiography. Magn Reson Med 1996; 36:384–392.
23. Hangiandreou NJ, Debbins JP, Rossman PJ, Riederer SJ. Interactive selection of optimal section orientations using real-time MRI. Magn Reson Med 1995; 34:114–119.
24. Hayes CE, Hattes N, Roemer PB. Volume imaging with MR phased arrays. Magn Reson Med 1991; 18:309–319.
25. Wright RC, Riederer SJ, Farzaneh F, Rossman PJ, Liu Y. Real-time MR fluoroscopic data acquisition and image reconstruction. Magn Reson Med 1989; 12:407–415.
26. Debbins JP, Riederer SJ, Rossman PJ, et al. Cardiac magnetic resonance fluoroscopy. Magn Reson Med 1996; 36:588–595.
27. Campeau N, Johnson C, Felmlee J, et al. MR imaging of the abdomen with a phased array multicoil: prospective clinical evaluation. Radiology 1995; 195:769–776.
28. Rosner B. Fundamentals of biostatistics. 3rd ed. Boston, Mass: Duxbury, 1990; 304–307.
29. Hany TF, McKinnon GC, Leung DA, Pfammatter T, Debatin JF. Optimization of contrast timing for breath-hold three-dimensional MR angiography. JMRI 1997; 7:551–556.
30. Prince MR, Chenevert TL, Foo TK, Londy FJ, Ward JS, Maki JH. Contrast-enhanced abdominal MR angiography: optimization of imaging delay time by automating the detection of contrast material arrival in the aorta. Radiology 1997; 203:109–114.
31. van Vaals JJ, Brummer ME, Dixon WT, et al. "Keyhole" method for accelerating imaging of contrast agent uptake. JMRI 1993; 3:671–675.
32. Bampton AEH, Riederer SJ, Korin HW. Centric phase encoding order for 3D magnetization-prepared gradient echo sequences: application to abdominal imaging. JMRI 1992; 2:327–334.

Michelle L. Melany, MD • Edward G. Grant, MD • André J. Duerinckx, MD, PhD
Tina M. Watts, RDMS, RVT • Barton S. Levine, MD

Ability of a Phase Shift US Contrast Agent to Improve Imaging of the Main Renal Arteries[1]

PURPOSE: **To evaluate the ability of a phase shift contrast agent to improve Doppler sonographic imaging of the main renal arteries in cases of suspected renal artery stenosis.**

MATERIALS AND METHODS: **In 25 patients in whom renal artery stenosis was suspected, baseline Doppler sonography was performed followed by two studies performed after blinded administration of contrast material or placebo (saline). Each kidney (n = 45) was evaluated for (*a*) visualization of the main renal artery on a scale of 0–4, (*b*) presence of accessory renal arteries, and (*c*) direct Doppler sonographic findings suggestive of renal artery stenosis. Correlative magnetic resonance angiography was performed in 24 patients, and angiograms were obtained in eight kidneys with stenosis at one or both imaging studies.**

RESULTS: **Contrast enhancement was observed in 23 patients. Enhancement was 8–20 minutes. Renal artery visualization scores improved from a mean of 2.56 and 2.71 on baseline and noncontrast scans, respectively, to 3.69 after administration of contrast material. Contrast-enhanced images depicted seven kidneys with accessory renal arteries not seen at other studies. Two of eight cases of stenosis were seen only with contrast-enhanced sonography.**

CONCLUSION: **Use of the phase shift contrast agent appears to enable a reduction in the number of equivocal findings of renal artery stenosis.**

Renal artery stenosis is an uncommon cause (1%–2%) of hypertension; however, it is potentially treatable with angioplasty or surgery. Although angiography remains the diagnostic standard, a widely accepted, noninvasive method of screening has yet to be found. Imaging algorithms vary for evaluating patients suspected of having renovascular hypertension. Some investigators advocate angiography as the initial imaging study for patients in whom there is a high clinical suspicion of renal artery stenosis (1). Angiography, however, is invasive, expensive, and potentially harmful in these patients who may have compromised renal function and may not tolerate iodinated contrast material. Although carbon dioxide angiography eliminates the risks associated with use of iodinated contrast material, a noninvasive method of screening patients is preferable.

In theory, sonography is an ideal technique for screening because it is noninvasive and use of iodinated contrast material is not necessary. Duplex sonography was successful in identification of renal artery stenosis in some series (2–4), but its use as a screening tool for renal artery stenosis remains controversial because other investigators have found Doppler sonography to be of limited value (5,6). Despite the addition of color Doppler sonography, the location of the main renal arteries deep within the abdomen has rendered direct visualization of these vessels difficult. Accessory renal arteries may be present in up to 22% of the population (6). These accessory renal arteries may not be identified with Doppler sonography, yet these vessels may contain stenosis.

Several investigators advocate evaluation of intrarenal Doppler waveforms to determine whether a stenotic lesion is present more proximally in the main renal artery. Earlier observations by Handa et al (7) suggest that systolic upstroke is slowed distal to an area of stenosis, and semiquantitative measurements of prolonged acceleration time and a diminished acceleration index were reported. Martin et al (8) also noted a loss of the early systolic peak distal to a stenosis. Stavros et al (9) suggested that these indirect signs in addition to pattern recognition of the abnormal Doppler waveform are sensitive methods for evaluating renal artery stenosis. Although the "tardus-parvus" phenomenon has proved successful in some series (9–11), other investigators have questioned the usefulness of intrarenal waveform analysis as a screening method (12–14).

During the past several years, there has been renewed interest in the development of sonographic contrast agents. The newest generation of these contrast materials is injected intravenously, crosses into the arterial circulation, and remains active long enough to be clinically useful (15).

Index terms: Ultrasound (US), contrast media • Ultrasound (US), Doppler studies, 961.12983, 961.12988 • Hypertension, renovascular, 961.721, 961.723 • Renal arteries, stenosis or obstruction, 961.721, 961.723

Radiology 1997; 205:147–152

[1] From the Departments of Radiological Sciences (M.L.M., E.G.G., A.J.D.) and Internal Medicine (B.S.L.), University of California Los Angeles; and the Departments of Radiology (M.L.M., E.G.G., A.J.D., T.M.W.) and Internal Medicine (B.S.L.), Veterans Affairs Medical Center West Los Angeles, 11301 Wilshire Blvd, Los Angeles, CA 90073. From the 1996 RSNA scientific assembly. Received November 4, 1996; revision requested December 16; revision received May 9, 1997; accepted June 9. Supported by a grant from Sonus Pharmaceuticals. **Address reprint requests to** M.L.M.

Most contrast agents enhance ultrasound (US) images by producing differences in acoustic impedance between the agent and the surrounding medium; these differences in impedance improve backscattering (echogenicity) of solid tissue and vascular structures. These intravenously administered agents use highly echogenic gaseous microbubbles. The gases are eliminated by means of respiration or may be metabolized.

A contrast agent that substantially improves sonographic depiction of the main renal arteries may provide a relatively noninvasive method of screening patients for renal artery stenosis. We undertook this study to investigate whether perflenapent emulsion (EchoGen; Sonus Pharmaceuticals, Bothell, Wash), a phase shift contrast agent that uses dodecafluoropentane as the enhancing gas, could improve Doppler sonographic evaluation of the main renal arteries for stenosis.

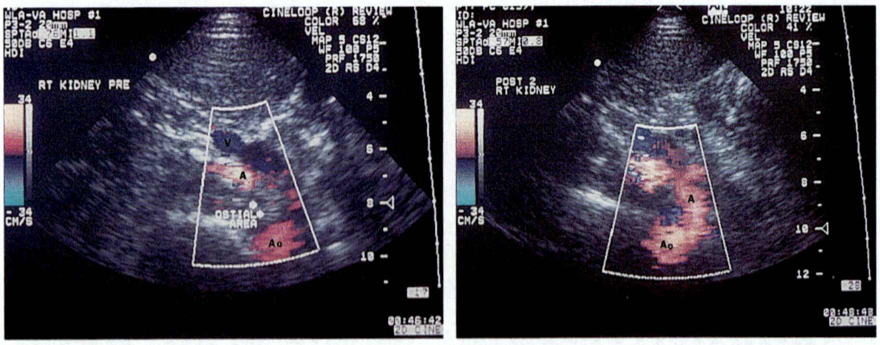

a. b.

Figure 1. Images of a normal right renal artery before and after injection of contrast material. **(a)** US image obtained before injection of contrast material shows that the ostial and retrocaval portions of the right renal artery (*A*) could not be visualized (arrows). **(b)** US image obtained after injection of contrast material demonstrates the entire right renal artery (*A*). *Ao* = aorta, *V* = right renal vein entering inferior vena cava.

MATERIALS AND METHODS

The study was approved by the Institutional Review Board at our hospital. Informed consent was obtained before sonographic examinations and injection of contrast material. Twenty-five male patients, aged 38–68 years (mean, 56 years), were enrolled. The study was performed at a Veterans Administration medical center. There was no attempt to exclude female patients from the study. Patients were referred by clinicians in the Renal Hypertension Clinic. All patients were suspected of having renovascular hypertension on the basis of one or more of the following clinical criteria: hypertension with unexplained deterioration of renal function, severe hypertension that was difficult to control with administration of multiple drugs, hypertension with disparate renal size noted at previous imaging studies, and renal failure induced by angiotensin converting enzyme inhibitors. Routine blood chemistry tests were performed before and after the study, and vital signs were monitored during injection of contrast material and placebo (normal saline) and throughout the sonographic examinations.

The imaging protocol included acquisition of a baseline sonogram followed by two additional studies after injection of contrast material or placebo. The dose of contrast agent administered was 0.05 mL per kilogram body weight of 2% perflenapent emulsion. An equal amount of placebo was administered. Sonography was performed with an HDI Ultramark 9 US machine (Advanced Technology Laboratories, Bothell, Wash). Broadband transducers were used, including a phased-array 2–3-MHz transducer and a curved-array 3–5-MHz transducer. Spectral tracings were obtained from upper- and lower-pole intrarenal arteries. Resistive indexes, acceleration times, and acceleration indexes were calculated (9).

The main renal arteries were evaluated in the sagittal or coronal plane from a flank approach and in the transverse plane through the anterior portion of the abdomen in all patients. Efforts were made to image the main renal artery from the renal hilum to the origin in all studies. Peak systolic and end diastolic velocities were measured at representative sites along the course of each artery. Aortic peak systolic velocities were measured and renal-aortic ratios were calculated.

All scans were obtained by the same technologist who, along with the participating physicians, was blinded with regard to whether the injected material was contrast material or placebo. The blind was removed after all patients were studied and imaging results were dictated. All three scans for each patient were recorded on videotape and reviewed by two experienced sonologists (M.L.M., E.G.G.). Results were determined by consensus. The presence and approximate duration of contrast enhancement were noted for each of the contrast-enhanced examinations.

For each of the scans, the following parameters were evaluated with respect to the intrarenal arteries: acceleration time or time to early systolic peak (normal, <70 msec) and acceleration index or gradient of the early systolic rise (normal, >300 cm/sec^2). The presence of an early systolic peak was also noted (9). For each study, the extrarenal arteries ($n = 45$) were evaluated for (*a*) the ability to visualize the entire main renal artery, (*b*) the number of arteries per kidney, and (*c*) Doppler criteria suggestive of renal artery stenosis (peak systolic velocity >200 cm/sec, renal aortic ratio, >3.5) (4). The ability to visualize the main renal artery was graded on a scale of 0–4: 0 = no visible artery beyond the hilum, 1 = minimal visibility (usually only the distal artery adjacent to the renal hilum), 2 = partial visibility of various segments, 3 = visibility of most of the length of the artery (typically all but the ostial area), and 4 = complete visualization from ostium to renal hilum. A renal artery visualization score was established for each kidney from all scans.

Statistical significance of changes in the number of diagnostic-quality US studies for renal artery visualization before and after administration of contrast material was calculated with a comparison of proportions in paired groups (McNemar test).

A correlative magnetic resonance (MR) angiogram was obtained in 24 of the 25 patients. These images were interpreted by a third radiologist (A.J.D.) who had no knowledge of the sonographic results. The presence of renal artery stenosis and the number of renal arteries that supplied each kidney were noted. The studies were performed with a 1.5-T MR imaging unit (Siemens Medical Systems, Erlangen, Germany). MR angiograms were obtained with two techniques in each patients. The first MR angiographic technique generated two-dimensional images obtained with cardiac-triggered breath-hold MR imaging (12–20–second breath holds) and provided angiographic images of the renal arteries and sections of the abdominal portion of the aorta (section thickness, 7 mm; matrix, 144 × 256; images obtained in mid-diastole; k-space segmented and fat-suppressed turbo fast low-angle shot technique; field of view, 350–400 mm; repetition time, 13 msec; echo time, 8 msec [13/8]).

The second MR angiographic technique was breath-hold, three-dimensional time-of-flight MR angiography performed during the first pass of 20 mL of gadopentetate dimeglumine (Magnevist; Berlex Laboratories, Wayne, NJ) (16). The circulation time of the MR imaging contrast agent was estimated first with a 1-mL injection. Three-dimensional time-of-flight MR angiography was based on a fast imaging with steady state free precession pulse sequence, which necessitated a 29-second breath hold (section thickness, 2.0 mm; slab of 16 or 32 sections; repetition time, 12 or 18 msec; echo time, 5 or 7 msec; flip angle, 40°; field of view, 350–400 mm). A maximum intensity projection algorithm was used to produce three-dimensional time-of-flight MR angiograms.

The results of all imaging studies were reviewed by the participating radiologists and clinicians. If neither sonography nor

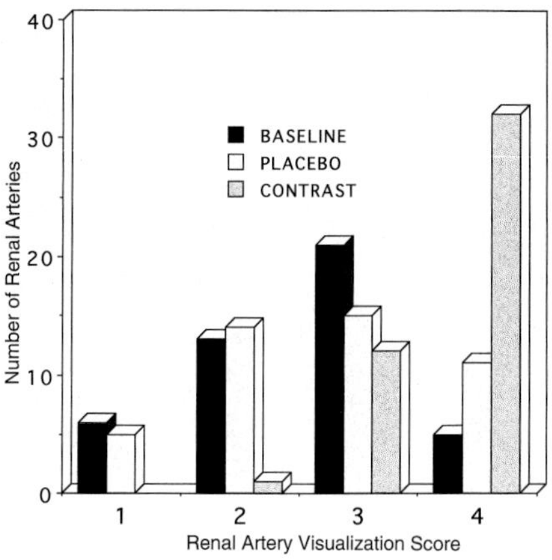

Figure 2. Graph shows renal artery visualization scores for baseline (black bars), placebo (white bars), and contrast-enhanced (gray bars) studies. Renal artery visualization scores are widely scattered for baseline and noncontrast studies. Note improved visualization after administration of contrast material with a preponderance of score = 4 (complete visualization of the main renal artery) after injection of contrast material.

MR angiography showed findings suggestive of renal artery stenosis, no further imaging was considered. In cases in which one or both of the noninvasive tests revealed findings suggestive of renal artery stenosis, correlative arteriography was recommended. In cases with angiographic correlation, this examination was used as the ultimate standard. Lesions that narrowed the renal artery lumen greater than 60% at angiography were considered indicative of renal artery stenosis.

RESULTS

Contrast enhancement was observed in 23 of the 25 patients. The patients in whom we were unable to distinguish between placebo and contrast material were the first two patients studied. In all other patients, varying degrees of increased vessel conspicuity were evident. Lack of contrast enhancement in the two previously described patients may have been due to our inexperience in injecting this type of contrast agent. To administer perflenapent emulsion, the agent must be activated before injection. The activation process necessitates holding the syringe containing the contrast agent in a horizontal position, rapidly pulling back the syringe plunger, and immediately releasing the plunger. This should result in an audible "pop."

Contrast enhancement lasted 8–20 minutes after injection of contrast material (mean, 12.6 minutes ± 3.01). In four patients, contrast enhancement was still present at the end of imaging. Immediately after bolus injection of contrast material, the "color blooming" artifact was identified in most cases. With the blooming phenomenon, gray-scale pixels are displayed as color information in regions where there is actually no flow (17). Manually decreasing the gain was necessary to eliminate the blooming artifact and to maintain adequate image quality.

Among the 25 patients, 45 kidneys were imaged with sonography. Of the five patients in whom only one kidney was examined, two had renal transplants and three had unilateral hypoplastic kidneys. One patient who failed to return for follow-up MR angiography was excluded from the data summarizing multiple renal artery and renal artery stenosis detection. This patient was included in the data outlining differences in main renal artery visualization before and after injection of contrast material because correlative imaging was not necessary for this evaluation.

The scores for imaging of the main renal arteries improved from a mean of 2.56 ± 0.87 and 2.71 ± 0.97 for the baseline and placebo (noncontrast) scans, respectively, to 3.69 ± 0.51 after injection of contrast material (Fig 1). Scores ranged from 1 to 4 for baseline and noncontrast scans and from 2 to 4 for contrast-enhanced scans. In eight kidneys, the main renal artery visualization score did not change between the baseline and contrast-enhanced studies; however, five of these kidneys were visualized completely (score = 4) on the baseline scan. A graphic representation of the changes in renal artery visualization scores is provided in Figure 2.

A single renal artery was identified at US and MR angiography in 29 kidneys. In three kidneys, two renal arteries were found at the baseline study and the contrast-enhanced study, and MR angiography corroborated these findings. Contrast-enhanced scans showed seven additional renal arteries that were not seen on baseline or noncontrast scans. These findings were confirmed at MR angiography (Fig 3). In one case, contrast-enhanced US identified a vessel that was believed to represent a second renal artery not seen at MR angiography. No angiogram was available in this case. In three kidneys, noncontrast and contrast-enhanced US images failed to depict accessory renal arteries that were seen at MR angiography. One patient (with two kidneys) was lost to follow-up and did not undergo a correlative imaging study after sonography. The results of detection of accessory renal arteries before and after administration of contrast material are summarized in Table 1.

No renal artery stenosis was found at duplex sonography or MR angiography in 32 of 43 kidneys in which correlative imaging studies were performed. In only four (12%) of these 32 kidneys was the baseline study able to show the entire main renal artery (score = 4). After injection of contrast material, however, the main renal arteries in 24 (75%) of these 32 kidneys were imaged throughout their course. In this population, the percentage of incompletely visualized main renal arteries was reduced from 88% to 25% after injection of contrast material ($P < .001$).

Renal artery stenosis was diagnosed in the remaining 11 kidneys at Doppler sonographic evaluation. MR angiograms were technically suboptimal in one patient with a renal transplant in whom baseline and contrast-enhanced Doppler sonography showed evidence of renal artery stenosis. This patient refused to undergo follow-up angiography to corroborate the Doppler sonographic finding of stenosis in the transplanted renal artery. Stenoses were confirmed in eight of the remaining 10 kidneys at MR angiography, angiography, or both (Figs 4, 5). Two kidneys had false-positive diagnoses of renal artery stenosis. In one of these kidneys, angiographic and MR angiographic findings were normal, while in the other kidney, MR angiographic findings were negative for renal artery stenosis and angiography could not be performed due to the patient's deteriorating clinical condition (unrelated to renal function). In both of these cases, the suspected renal artery stenosis was reported as being present on baseline and contrast-enhanced US scans.

Of the eight kidneys in which correlative imaging confirmed the diagnosis of renal artery stenosis, in two kidneys the stenotic lesion was not identified at baseline Doppler sonography. In both of these cases, stenosis was seen only after administration of contrast material and renal artery stenosis was confirmed at angiography.

Table 2 demonstrates a summary of these findings. The sensitivity for diagnosis of renal artery stenosis with baseline Doppler sonography was 75% and increased to 100% after administration of contrast material. The specificity was 94% before and after administration of contrast material.

DISCUSSION

The usefulness of Doppler sonography as a screening test for renal artery

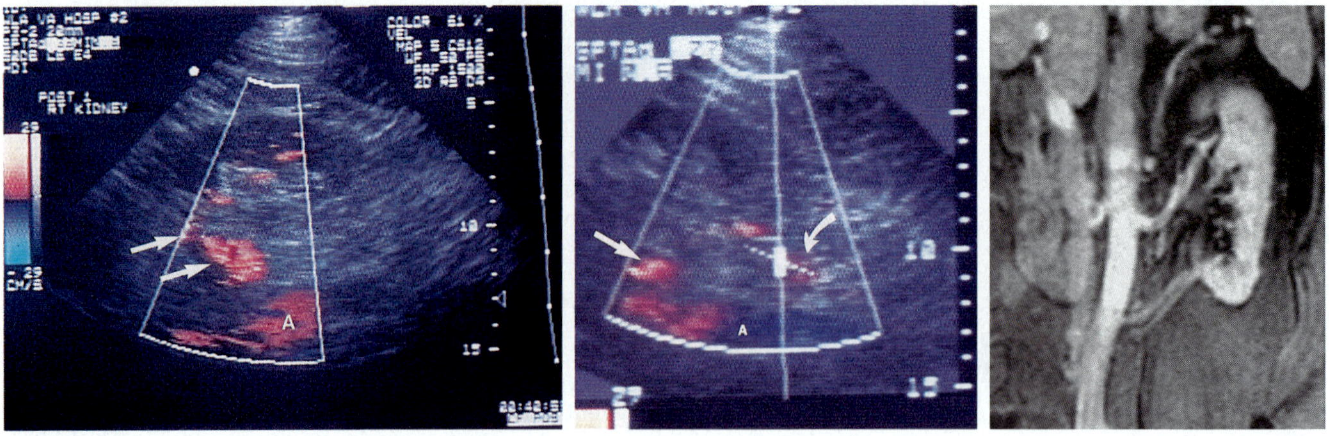

a. b. c.

Figure 3. Images in a patient with two left renal arteries. **(a)** Doppler US image shows the larger, upper-pole renal artery (arrows) is identified before and after injection of contrast material. *A* = aorta. **(b)** US image shows the lower-pole left renal artery (curved arrow), which is visualized only after injection of contrast material. The aorta (*A*) is well visualized, although it is perpendicular to the sound beam and at a depth of 13 cm from the transducer. Visualization of the aorta from the flank approach is often difficult on routine, noncontrast scans. The straight arrow points to upper-pole renal artery. **(c)** MR angiogram (13/8) shows two left renal arteries. An accessory lower-pole renal vein is seen adjacent to the lower-pole renal artery.

stenosis has been evaluated with the focus on detection of increased velocity at the site of stenosis in the main renal artery and/or morphologic changes in the waveform distal to the stenosis. The ability to detect a tardus-parvus waveform and lack of an early systolic peak are believed to be dependent on compliance of the vessel distal to the stenosis, potentially limiting the usefulness of this technique in elderly patients and in patients with atherosclerosis (14).

Direct measurement of peak systolic velocity at the site of a stenosis is hampered by many technical problems including inability to visualize the main renal artery due to patient body habitus or shadowing from adjacent bowel gas. Acquisition of a spectral tracing from the main renal artery can be difficult in patients who are incapable of suspending respiration. Technical difficulties in determining the angle of insonation or in obtaining an angle less than 60° make it impossible to measure the peak systolic velocity accurately in some patients. The presence of multiple renal arteries and the frequent inability to image these often small vessels further limits this technique. At best, evaluation of the main renal arteries necessitates considerable imaging time, is associated with a long learning curve involving a highly motivated operator, and may be influenced further by technical factors described previously.

Use of sonographic contrast agents has been investigated for over 20 years, but these contrast agents have only recently been considered for widespread use. The most widely used agent to date has been human albumin (Albunex; Molecular Biosystems, San Diego, Calif), which has been approved for cardiac imaging by the U.S. Food and Drug Administration. Unfortunately, this agent is destroyed by high pressures in the left ventricle, and use is limited to "one-pass" venous or cardiac applications. Galactose-based compounds (Levovist; Schering, Berlin, Germany) and a number of other agents are also under investigation (18,19).

Table 1

Comparison of Baseline Sonography, Contrast-enhanced Sonography, and MR Angiography in Depiction of Multiple Renal Arteries

No. of Kidneys (*n* = 45)	No. of Renal Arteries Depicted	Renal Arteries Depicted: Baseline Sonography	Contrast-enhanced Sonography	MR Angiography
29	1	Yes	Yes	Yes
3	2	Yes	Yes	Yes
7	2	No	Yes	Yes
1	2	No	Yes	No
3	2	No	No	Yes
2*	...	...	...	...

* Patient was lost to follow-up. No correlative imaging was performed after sonography.

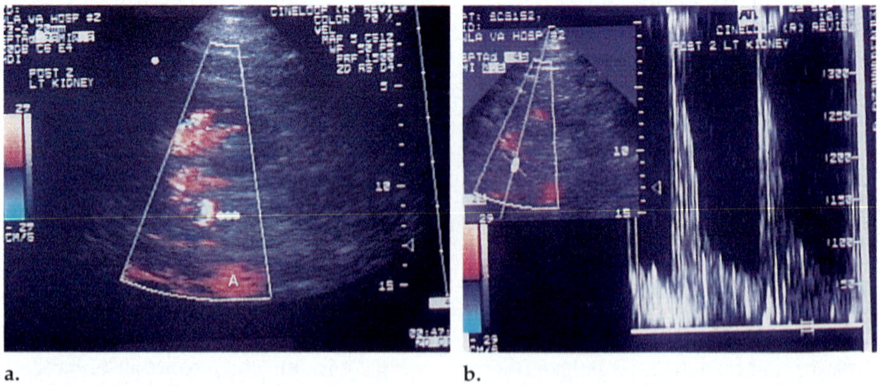

a. b.

Figure 4. **(a)** Doppler US image obtained after injection of contrast material shows the left renal artery is visualized, and a focal area of color aliasing is identified. *A* = aorta. **(b)** US image of spectral analysis in the area of aliasing demonstrates markedly elevated peak systolic velocities (340 cm/sec). Spectral sample was placed over area of color aliasing at real time US. The area of color aliasing is not seen in this spectral image.

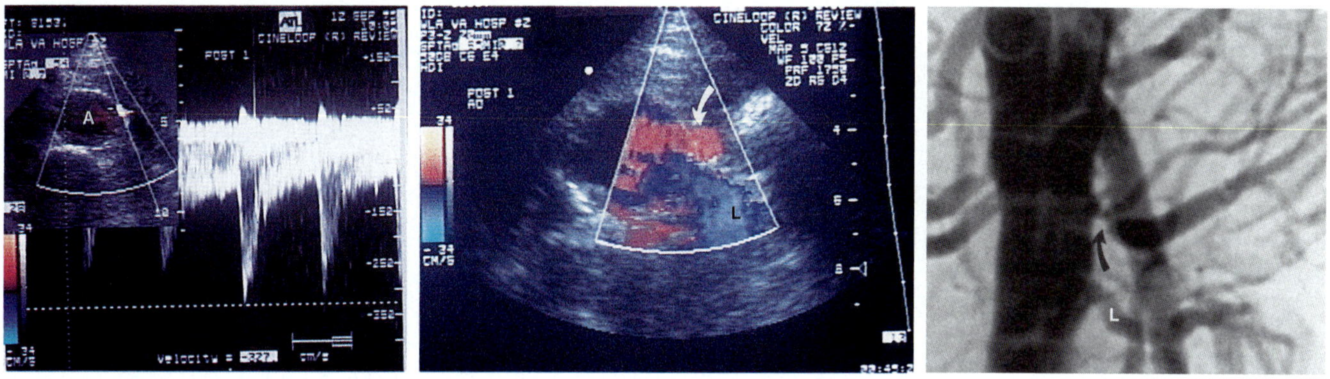

a. b. c.

Figure 5. Renal artery stenosis in a patient with dual renal arteries. **(a)** Transabdominal spectral Doppler US image shows an area of prominent aliasing in a left renal artery originating from the anterolateral aspect of the aorta (*A*). Spectral sampling demonstrated a peak systolic velocity of 327 cm/sec. **(b)** Doppler US image obtained inferiorly shows a second left renal artery (*L*) originating from a more posterior location in the aorta. Spectral analysis revealed normal flow velocities (arrow = left renal vein). **(c)** Conventional angiogram confirms stenosis at the origin of the upper pole of the left renal artery (arrow) and the presence of an additional, lower-pole artery (*L*).

Table 2
Detection of Renal Artery Stenosis with Each Modality

Patient	Angiography	MR Angiography	Baseline US	Contrast-enhanced US
1	NA	Yes	Yes	Yes
2	Yes	Yes	Yes	Yes
3	Yes	Yes	Yes	Yes
4	Yes	Yes	Yes	Yes
5	Yes	Yes	Yes	Yes
6	Yes	No	Yes	Yes
7	Yes	Yes	No	Yes
8	Yes	Yes	No	Yes
9	No	No	Yes	Yes
10	NA	No	Yes	Yes

Note.—NA = no angiogram obtained.

The phase shift contrast agent perflenapent emulsion is unique in that it is a nonechogenic emulsion at room temperature. The boiling point, however, is 28°–30°C; this boiling point allows perflenapent emulsion to convert to a gas, dodecafluoropentane, at body temperature (37°C). Conversion from liquid to gas and a marked decrease in density result in the creation of microbubbles estimated to be approximately 3–5 µm in diameter. These gaseous microbubbles are highly echogenic and are capable of traversing the pulmonary capillary circulation.

Perflenapent emulsion has a calculated concentration of 10^{12} particles per milliliter. These particles persist in solution longer than air microbubbles of the same size owing to the low solubility of this agent in water and slower diffusion in blood. Because dodecafluoropentane is a perfluorocarbon gas, it is not metabolized but rather is eliminated unchanged via the lungs (20). Studies in rats have shown that 82.9% ± 9.4 of the compound is excreted within 5 minutes (21). Perflenapent emulsion, which is not nephrotoxic, appears to be an ideal contrast agent for evaluation of the renal arteries because it passes successfully into the arterial circulation and persists unchanged in the bloodstream for a considerable period. Our study demonstrated contrast enhancement in 23 consecutive patients, and the enhancement persisted for a period that rendered the agent clinically useful.

Perflenapent emulsion improved visualization of the main renal arteries in our patient population. Renal artery visualization scores (as defined in the Materials and Methods section) improved from a mean of 2.56 on the baseline sonogram to 3.69 after injection of the US contrast agent. Postcontrast sonograms enabled improved visualization of the extrarenal portions of the main renal artery and enabled us to better detect the presence of multiple renal arteries. In seven of 10 cases in which multiple renal arteries were identified sonographically, visualization was possible only after administration of the contrast agent.

Our confidence level in exclusion of stenosis in the main renal artery improved with the use of contrast material. At baseline examination of the main renal arteries, findings in 88% of these arteries were deemed equivocal because of lack of visualization of the entire vessel. After injection of contrast material, findings in only 25% of the main renal arteries were equivocal.

In kidneys in which renal artery stenosis was proved, contrast-enhanced scans identified stenoses that were not seen on baseline scans in two of eight cases. Stenosis in both of these cases was confirmed at MR angiography.

Because only a small number of patients had renal artery stenosis ($n = 8$), generalization of our findings of an increase in sensitivity from 75% to 100% with contrast-enhanced duplex sonography to larger population groups may not be valid. In the two kidneys in which Doppler US studies indicated renal artery stenosis and correlative imaging studies revealed normal renal arteries, contrast enhancement did not appear to cause the false-positive diagnosis. In these cases, areas of abnormal flow in the main renal artery suggesting renal artery stenosis were seen on baseline and contrast-enhanced scans. The exact cause of these false-positive diagnoses is not clear. In one of these patients, a small vessel originating from the aorta may have been a mesenteric artery mimicking the origin of the left main renal artery.

In our study, the use of contrast material improved diagnostic confidence by improving our ability to visualize the main renal arteries. However, because of limitations in the study design we cannot comment on the ability of the agent to enable unequivocal exclusion of renal artery stenosis, even in cases in which complete visualization of the main renal arteries was achieved. This inability to completely exclude renal artery stenosis in cases in which the entire main renal artery was seen with contrast-enhanced US is due mainly to the possible existence of small accessory renal arteries that could harbor stenosis yet may not be seen on the contrast-enhanced scans. The ability of contrast material to enable complete visualization of the entire length of all accessory renal arteries was not tested in this investigation. Although the addition of contrast material improved detection of multiple renal arteries, in three cases accessory renal arteries not identified on contrast-enhanced scans were detected with alternate imaging modalities. Identification of the entire length of main and accessory renal arteries, while ideal, may not be essential to improve detection of renal artery stenosis. Renal artery stenosis may be better seen after contrast material is injected, even in incompletely imaged arteries, by virtue of prominent color aliasing at the site of stenosis and flow disturbances distal to stenotic lesions. Future studies in which multiple doses of contrast material are used may improve results by allowing additional scanning time for a more thorough assessment of the renal vasculature in problem cases.

Another limitation of the study is that we did not obtain MR angiograms in all patients. Therefore, with regard to the visualization of multiple renal arteries and stenoses, MR angiography was often used to help refute or corroborate US findings. Recent studies describe MR angiography and digital subtraction angiography as being equally effective in depicting hemodynamically significant stenoses in the main renal arteries (22). In our study population, although angiographic correlation in all patients would have been ideal, it was difficult to justify an invasive procedure and the use of potentially harmful iodinated contrast material in cases in which two noninvasive studies showed no evidence of renal artery stenosis. To determine the usefulness of US contrast agents in the evaluation of renal artery stenosis, larger studies in which results from contrast-enhanced sonography are compared with those from angiography are necessary.

There is debate as to whether contrast material produces increases in detected peak systolic velocity and whether this increase in velocity represents an artifact (17). Alternatively, these agents may not produce artifactually high velocities but may actually allow detection of real, but weak, previously undetected high-velocity signals. Further research is necessary to determine if this phenomenon is found with use of all contrast agents and whether the elevation of velocity is an artifact or real. This elevation of peak systolic velocity could have a great effect on the clinical use of US contrast agents, as the velocity increase would affect disease criteria based on peak velocity measurements such as detection of renal and carotid artery stenosis.

Studies indicate that US contrast agents can provide new information and improve vascular imaging in various ways: Greater lengths of vessels can be seen with contrast enhancement, vessels previously seen as occluded have been found to be patent, vessels not seen without use of contrast material are detected after injection of the agent, improved visualization of stenoses has been reported, and superior identification of runoff vessels has been identified (15). In our study, after injection of contrast material, the number of vessels identified increased and detection of renal artery stenosis improved. Most important, however, is that superior visualization of the main renal arteries after administration of contrast material led to improved diagnostic confidence in our ability to exclude the diagnosis of renal artery stenosis in these vessels. Should this prove true in larger studies and should multiple-dose contrast-enhanced imaging enable improved identification of accessory renal arteries, use of US contrast agents may decrease the need for more invasive, expensive, and potentially harmful imaging tests by providing a definitive method of "ruling out" renal artery stenosis in a well-selected population of patients with hypertension. ■

References

1. Davidson RA, Wilcox CS. Newer tests for the diagnosis of renovascular disease. JAMA 1992; 268:3353–3358.
2. Kohler TR, Zieler E, Martin BS, et al. Noninvasive diagnosis of renal artery stenosis by ultrasonic duplex scanning. J Vasc Surg 1986; 4:450–456.
3. Taylor DC, Kettler MD, Moneta GL, et al. Duplex ultrasound scanning in the diagnosis of renal artery stenosis: a prospective evaluation. J Vasc Surg 1988; 7:363–367.
4. Olin JW, Piedmonte MA, Young JR, DeAnna S, Grubb M, Childs MB. The utility of duplex ultrasound of the renal arteries for diagnosing significant renal artery stenosis. Ann Intern Med 1995; 122:833–838.
5. Desberg AL, Paushter DM, Lammert GK, et al. Renal artery stenosis: evaluation with color Doppler flow imaging. Radiology 1990; 177:749–753.
6. Berland LL, Koslin DB, Routh WD, Keller FS. Renal artery stenosis: prospective evaluation of diagnosis with color Doppler US compared with angiography. Radiology 1990; 174:421–423.
7. Handa N, Fukunaga R, Uehara A, et al. Echo-Doppler velocimeter in the diagnosis of hypertensive patients: the renal artery Doppler technique. Ultrasound Med Biol 1986; 12:945–952.
8. Martin RL, Nanra RS, Wlodarczyk J, Desilva A, Bray AIE. Renal hilar Doppler analysis on the detection of renal artery stenosis. J Vasc Technol 1991; 15:173–180.
9. Stavros AT, Parker SH, Yakes WF, et al. Segmental stenosis of the renal artery: pattern recognition of tardus and parvus abnormalities with duplex sonography. Radiology 1992; 184:487–492.
10. Patriquin HB, Lafortune M, Jequier JC, et al. Stenosis of the renal artery: assessment of slowed systole in the downstream circulation with Doppler sonography. Radiology 1992; 184:479–485.
11. Lafortune M, Patriquin HB, Demeule E, et al. Renal artery stenosis: slowed systole in the downstream circulation—experimental study in dogs. Radiology 1992; 184:475–478.
12. Kliewer MA, Tupler RH, Carroll BA, et al. Renal artery stenosis: analysis of Doppler waveform parameters and tardus-parvus pattern. Radiology 1993; 189:779–787.
13. Kliewer MA, Tupler RH, Hertzberg BS, et al. Doppler evaluation of renal artery stenosis: interobserver agreement in the interpretation of waveform morphology. AJR 1994; 162:1371–1376.
14. Bude RO, Rubin JM, Platt JF, Fechner KP, Adler RS. Pulsus tardus: its cause and potential limitations in detection of arterial stenosis. Radiology 1994; 190:779–784.
15. Needleman L, Forsberg F. Contrast agents in ultrasound. Ultrasound Q 1996; 13:121–138.
16. Prince MR, Narasimham DL, Stanley JC, et al. Breath-hold gadolinium-enhanced MR angiography of the abdominal aorta and its major branches. Radiology 1995; 197:785–792.
17. Forsberg F, Liu J, Burns PN, Merton DA, Rawool NM, Goldberg BB. Artifacts in ultrasonic contrast agent studies. J Ultrasound Med 1994; 13:357–365.
18. Schwarz K, Becher H, Schimpfky C, Vorwerk D, Bogdahn U, Schlief R. Doppler enhancement with SH U 508A in multiple vascular regions. Radiology 1994; 193:195–201.
19. Otis S, Rush M, Boyajian R. Contrast-enhanced transcranial imaging: results of an American phase-two study. Stroke 1995; 26:203–209.
20. Yokayama K, Yamanouchi K, Murashima R. Excretion of perfluorochemicals after intravenous injection of their emulsion. Chem Pharm Bull 1975; 23:1368–1372.
21. Forsberg F, Liu J, Merton DA, Rawool NM, Goldberg BB. Parenchymal enhancement and tumor visualization using a new sonographic contrast agent. J Ultrasound Med 1995; 14:949–957.
22. Wasser MN, Westenberg J, van der Hulst VPM, et al. Hemodynamic significance of renal artery stenosis: digital subtraction angiography versus systolically gated three-dimensional phase-contrast MR angiography. Radiology 1997; 202:333–338.

Pierre Loubeyre, MD, PhD • Emmanuelle Angelie • Florence Grozel, MD
Hassan Abidi, PhD • Van André Tran Minh, MD

Spiral CT Artifact That Simulates Aortic Dissection: Image Reconstruction with Use of 180° and 360° Linear-Interpolation Algorithms[1]

PURPOSE: To evaluate a computed tomographic (CT) artifact that simulates aortic dissection.

MATERIALS AND METHODS: Two groups of 65 patients underwent spiral CT of the chest for reasons other than suspected aortic dissection. In each group, two series of images (10-mm sections) were reconstructed with use of a 180° or 360° linear-interpolation algorithm. Series of images were read by two radiologists, and variance between interpretations was statistically measured.

RESULTS: Among series of images, artifacts were seen on 21–26 (32%–40%) with use of a 180° algorithm and 41 (63%) and 44 (68%) with use of a 360° algorithm. Concordance between reviewers was fair ($\kappa = 0.58$, 0.59) or good ($\kappa = 0.65$) with use of a 180° algorithm and excellent ($\kappa = 0.92$) with use of a 360° algorithm. In one group, with use of a 180° algorithm, two series of reconstructed images were separated by 5 mm; artifact was observed on seven (11%) CT studies (on both series of images) and was located along the left or left anterior side of the aorta.

CONCLUSION: To reduce the frequency of a spiral CT artifact that simulates aortic dissection, two series of segmented images can be reconstructed with a change of image position along the z axis of the aorta and use of a 180° linear-interpolation algorithm.

The appearance of a curvilinear interface in the root of the ascending aorta that simulates aortic dissection is observed on both conventional and spiral computed tomographic (CT) scans (1–5). This artifact is usually limited to images of two or three contiguous sections that are close to the aortic root (5) and is thought to be related to the motion of the aortic wall between end diastole and end systole (1,6). It has been suggested that the artifact can be eliminated by retrospectively reconstructing segmented images from data collected during 0.6 second of a full 1-second scan during conventional axial CT imaging (1). This artifact has not been reported with use of fast (50 msec) CT scanning times, but equipment with fast scanning times is not always readily available. With the widespread acceptance of spiral CT, the presence of such an artifact in the ascending aorta can raise diagnostic problems in a patient who presents with thoracic pain.

Spiral CT necessitates interpolation of the volume data set for the creation of transaxial images (7). The simplest approach is linear interpolation of spiral-projection data sets from adjacent turns (eg, 360° apart). Another possibility, available with most current spiral CT equipment, is to reorder the projection data and perform interpolation with data from views separated by 180° (180° linear interpolation) (8). In this way, fewer averaging artifacts caused by broadening of the section-sensitivity profile are created (8,9). In our initial experience, motion artifacts of the ascending aorta were fewer when a 180° linear-interpolation algorithm was used instead of a 360° linear-interpolation algorithm.

The purpose of this study was to evaluate in a large patient population the frequency and location of this CT artifact that resembles aortic dissection with use of 180° or 360° linear-interpolation algorithms. Modification of this artifact was evaluated with position changes of the reconstructed segmented images with use of the 180° linear-interpolation algorithm. For this evaluation, the 180° linear-interpolation algorithm was chosen because artifacts have been reported to be fewer with use of this algorithm.

MATERIALS AND METHODS

Two groups of 65 patients each underwent consecutive, dynamic, contrast material–enhanced spiral CT examinations of the chest. CT examinations were performed with a Somatom-plus S CT scanner (Siemens Medical Systems, Erlangen, Germany). Patients underwent CT for a variety of unselected clinical indications (eg, lymphoma, lung cancer, mediastinal lymph node disease), excluding suspected aortic dissection or pulmonary embolism. All spiral chest CT examinations were performed during a single breath hold with use of 10 mm/sec table motion, 10-mm collimation, 10-mm contiguous reconstructions from the apex to the diaphragm, 145 mA, and 137 kVp. Contrast enhancement was performed with a monophasic intravenous injection of a 100-mL bolus of ioxi-

Index terms: Aorta, CT, 941.12115, 941.93 • Aorta, dissection, 563.743, 943.743 • Computed tomography (CT), artifact, 941.12115, 941.93 • Computed tomography (CT), image processing, 941.12115, 941.93

Radiology 1997; 205:153–157

[1] From the Departments of Radiology (P.L., F.G., V.A.T.M.) and Epidemiology (H.A.) and Nuclear Imaging and Spectroscopy Research Group (E.A.), Lyon-Sud Hospital, Chemin du Grand Revoyet, 69495 Pierre Benite, France. Received March 7, 1997; revision requested April 11; revision received June 5; accepted June 9. **Address reprint requests to** P.L.

Table 1
CT Series of Images Showing Artifact That Simulates Aortic Dissection

CT Series	No. of CT Series: Reviewer 1	Reviewer 2
SLIM 1*	23 (35)	21 (32)
SLIM 2*	23 (35)	21 (32)
SLIM 3*	26 (40)	23 (35)
WIDE†	41 (63)	44 (68)
SLIM 1* + WIDE†	26 (40)	22 (34)
SLIM 2* + SLIM 3*	13 (20)	8 (12)

Note.—Numbers in parentheses are percentages of 65 series.
* Series obtained with 180° linear-interpolation algorithm.
† Series obtained with 360° linear-interpolation algorithm.

Table 2
CT Images Showing Artifact That Simulates Aortic Dissection

CT Series	No. of CT Images: One	Two	Three	Four	Five	Total No. of Series
SLIM*						
Reviewer 1	38 (53)	19 (26)	10 (14)	3 (4)	2 (3)	72 (100)
Reviewer 2	34 (52)	22 (34)	8 (12)	1 (2)	0 (0)	65 (100)
WIDE†						
Reviewer 1	8 (20)	8 (20)	6 (15)	10 (24)	9 (22)	41 (100)
Reviewer 2	10 (23)	11 (25)	10 (23)	10 (23)	3 (7)	44 (100)

Note.—Numbers are numbers of positive series. Numbers in parentheses are percentages of total number of series. Percentages in WIDE series do not add up to 100 due to rounding.
* All series of images obtained with 180° linear-interpolation algorithm.
† Series obtained with 360° linear-interpolation algorithm.

Table 3
Location of Artifact Simulating Aortic Dissection on CT Series of Images

CT Series	Artifact Location: A	B	C	A + B	A + C	B + C	A + B + C	Total No. of Series
SLIM*								
Reviewer 1	9 (12)	21 (29)	15 (21)	3 (4)	0 (0)	20 (28)	4 (6)	72 (100)
Reviewer 2	0 (0)	23 (35)	21 (32)	2 (3)	0 (0)	18 (28)	1 (2)	65 (100)
WIDE†								
Reviewer 1	4 (10)	3 (7)	4 (10)	2 (5)	3 (7)	5 (12)	20 (49)	41 (100)
Reviewer 2	4 (9)	7 (16)	3 (7)	8 (18)	3 (7)	7 (16)	12 (27)	44 (100)

Note.—Numbers are numbers of CT series. Numbers in parentheses are percentages of total number of series. A = aortic root, B = proximal section of ascending aorta, C = ascending aorta near pulmonary artery.
* All series of images obtained with 180° linear-interpolation algorithm.
† Series obtained with 360° linear-interpolation algorithm.

talamate (Telebrix 35; Guerbet, Aulnay-sous-Bois, France). Injection was performed automatically at a rate of 2 mL/sec through an antecubital vein. Scanning began 25 seconds after injection began. Scanning time varied from 23 to 30 seconds.

In the first group of 65 patients, there were 17 women and 48 men. Patient ages ranged from 25 to 81 years (mean, 60.4 years). For each patient, two series of images were reconstructed; one series (SLIM 1) was reconstructed with a 180° linear-interpolation algorithm, and the other series (WIDE) was reconstructed with a 360° linear-interpolation algorithm.

In the second group of another 65 patients, there were 24 women and 41 men. Patient ages ranged from 18 to 79 years (mean, 59.2). For each patient, two series of images (SLIM 2 and SLIM 3) were reconstructed; in both series, contiguous images were reconstructed with use of a 180° linear-interpolation algorithm. The images of SLIM 3 were reconstructed with an interval position that differed by 5 mm from that of the SLIM 2 images. For example, if the positions of the reconstructed SLIM 2 images were 10, 20, 30, and 40 mm on the topogram, the positions of the reconstructed SLIM 3 images were 15, 25, 35, and 45 mm on the topogram.

For each of the 130 patients, the images of each series (for each patient, there were two series of images; total, 260 series of images) were obtained at window levels appropriate for vascular visualization (level, 50 HU; width, 400 HU). Series of images were retrospectively and independently reviewed by two vascular radiologists (P.L., F.G.). Each reviewer was unaware of the series of images being reviewed.

A series was considered to show the artifact if a curvilinear structure that resembled a double lumen or a dissection flap was seen on at least one image of the series. In this case, the series was considered to be positive and the reviewer noted the following: the number of images in a series on which the artifact was seen and the axial level of the aortic artifact. Three axial levels were selected: (*a*) the aortic root (ie, the area from the aortic valve to the origin of the left coronary artery), (*b*) the proximal section of the ascending aorta (the part of the aorta close to the pulmonary trunk), and (*c*) the part of the ascending aorta close to the right pulmonary artery. The reviewers also noted the location of the artifact along the circumference of the aorta. For this interpretation, the aortic circumference was represented with a clockface. In a simplified analysis, nine possible locations of the artifact were proposed between the following clock positions: 12 and 3, 3 and 6, 6

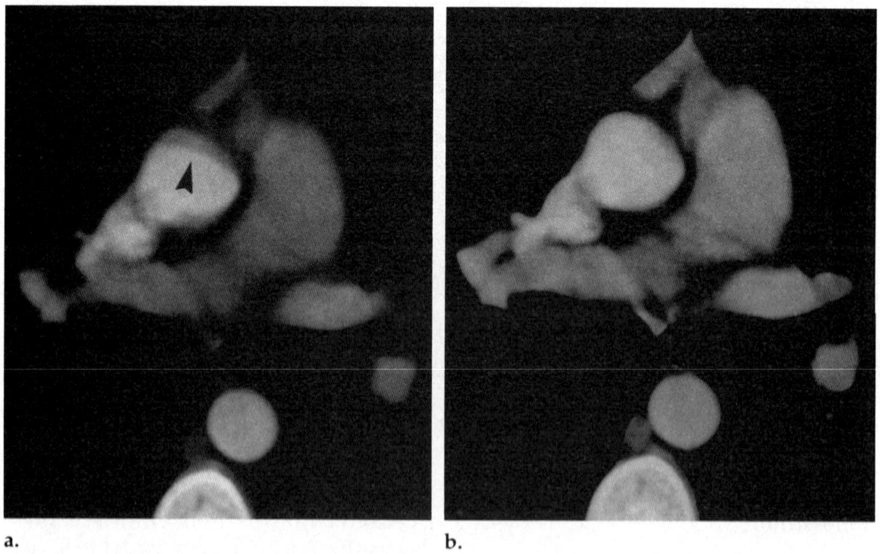

a. b.

Figure 1. Chest CT images in a 30-year-old woman who underwent examination for follow-up of lymphoma. **(a)** With use of a 360° linear-interpolation algorithm, CT image shows an artifact (arrowhead) in the left anterior part of the aorta at the level of the right pulmonary artery that resembles aortic dissection. **(b)** With use of a 180° linear-interpolation algorithm, CT image does not show the artifact.

Table 4
Artifact Location along Aortic Circumference

CT Series	Artifact Location*									Total No. of Images
	12–3	3–6	6–9	9–12	12–6	3–9	6–12	9–3	12–12	
SLIM†										
Reviewer 1	54 (60)	0 (0)	13 (15)	0 (0)	11 (12)	0 (0)	6 (7)	4 (5)	1 (1)	89 (100)
Reviewer 2	44 (60)	1 (1)	5 (7)	6 (8)	12 (16)	1 (1)	4 (5)	0 (0)	0 (0)	73 (100)
WIDE‡										
Reviewer 1	27 (38)	0 (0)	29 (41)	2 (3)	8 (11)	0 (0)	2 (3)	3 (4)	0 (0)	71 (100)
Reviewer 2	19 (29)	0 (0)	22 (33)	2 (3)	13 (20)	0 (0)	4 (6)	2 (3)	4 (6)	66 (100)

Note.—Numbers are number of images that showed the artifact. Numbers in parentheses are percentages of total number of images that showed the artifact. Percentages in SLIM series read by reviewer 2 do not add up to 100 due to rounding.
* Locations along aortic circumference are designated with clock positions.
† All series of images obtained with 180° linear-interpolation algorithm.
‡ Series obtained with 360° linear-interpolation algorithm.

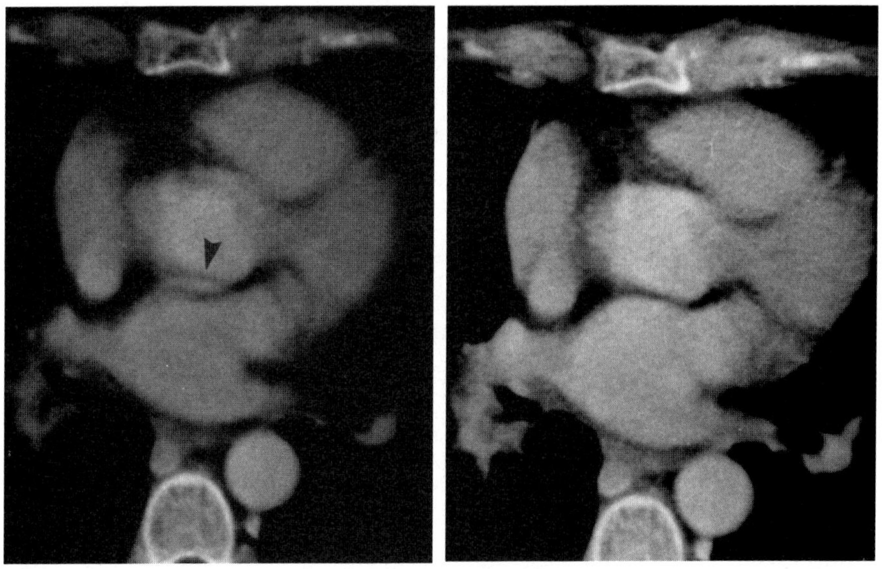

a. b.

Figure 2. Chest CT images in a 52-year-old woman who underwent examination for ovarian carcinoma. **(a)** With use of a 360° linear-interpolation algorithm, CT image shows an artifact (arrowhead) in the aortic root that resembles an intimal flap. **(b)** With use of a 180° linear-interpolation algorithm, CT image does not show this artifact.

and 9, 9 and 12, 12 and 6, 3 and 9, 6 and 12, 9 and 3, or 12 and 12. On the same image, reviewers could choose more than one location of the artifact (eg, between 12- and 3-o'clock positions and between 6- and 9-o'clock positions).

The variance between observers for detecting the artifact was measured with the κ test of concordance. The kappa index (κ) was calculated for each test of concordance.

The variance between observers was measured with a one-way repeated measured analysis of variances, or ANOVA, to detect (*a*) the number of images in a series on which the artifact was observed, (*b*) the axial level of the aortic artifact, and (*c*) the location of the artifact in the aorta. Significant differences were determined when P was less than .05. Concordance between observers was considered fair ($0.5 < \kappa \leq 0.6$), good ($0.6 < \kappa \leq 0.8$), or excellent ($\kappa > 0.8$).

RESULTS

The numbers and percentages of series that showed the artifact for each reviewer are shown in Table 1. For series reconstructed with the 180° linear-interpolation algorithm (series SLIM 1, 2, and 3), the numbers of series that showed the artifact ranged from 21 to 26 (32%–40%). For series reconstructed with the 360° linear-interpolation algorithm (WIDE), the numbers of series that showed the artifact were 41 (63%) and 44 (68%) for reviewers 1 and 2, respectively.

Concordance between reviewers was considered fair for the reading of SLIM 2 ($\kappa = 0.59$) and SLIM 3 ($\kappa = 0.58$) series. Concordance between reviewers was considered good ($\kappa = 0.65$) for the reading of SLIM 1 series and excellent ($\kappa = 0.92$) for the reading of WIDE series.

If a CT study (two series of images) was considered to be positive only when the artifact was seen on both series of reconstructed images, then CT studies in the first group of patients (SLIM 1 + WIDE series) showed the artifact in 26 (40%) cases if read by reviewer 1 and 22 (34%) cases if read by reviewer 2. In the second group of patients (SLIM 2 + SLIM 3 series), CT studies showed the artifact in 13 (20%) cases if read by reviewer 1 and eight (12%) cases if read by reviewer 2 (Table 1). In the second group of patients (SLIM 2 + SLIM 3 series), only seven CT studies (11%) were considered to be positive by both reviewers.

Table 2 shows the number of images on which the artifact was observed in positive series, Table 3 shows the axial levels of the aorta where the artifact was observed, and Table 4 shows the location of the artifact along the aortic circumference. No significant differences were found between reviewers for interpreting these three findings with use of the 180° linear-interpolation algorithm (P = .30, .59, and .31 for the findings, respectively) or the 360° linear-interpolation algorithm (P = .75, .81, and .72 for the findings, respectively).

In seven CT studies (11%) of the second group (SLIM 2 + SLIM 3), the artifacts were observed by both reviewers on both series of images. The findings were as follows: The artifact was observed on one scan (four CT studies) or two scans (three CT studies). The artifact was observed near the right pulmonary artery (four CT studies) or in the proximal section of the ascending aorta (three CT studies). The artifact was noted along the aortic circumference between the 12- and 3-o'clock positions (five CT studies) or the 12- and 6-o'clock positions (two CT studies).

DISCUSSION

During spiral CT, the patient is moved through the gantry while data are acquired simultaneously with multiple 360° acquisitions (8). To compensate for the continuous movement of the patient during the procedure, a planar data set must be calculated from the volume data set so that each image can be reconstructed. With all current spiral CT equipment, two main interpolation algorithms are available for calculating the planar data set from volume scans. For use of a 360° linear-interpolation algorithm, 2 × 360° of coplanar projection data are required to reconstruct a single axial image that is centered at an arbitrary location along the z axis. With the 180° linear-interpolation algorithm, rays from opposing directions are used to reduce the range of data along the z axis (8,10). The 180° linear-interpolation algorithm offers an improved section-sensitivity profile. Broadening of the section-sensitivity profile results in variable degrees of volume-averaging artifacts. Particularly, slight blurring of structures that change along the z axis must be considered (9). In our study, the number of CT series interpreted as showing an artifact that resembled aortic dissection was markedly reduced when a 180° linear-interpolation algorithm was used instead of a 360° linear-interpolation algorithm (Figs 1, 2). As well, the number of images that showed the artifact in each series was markedly reduced with use of a 180° linear-interpolation algorithm.

When reconstructing images with a 180° linear-interpolation algorithm, the artifact in the ascending aorta was still present in a high percentage (from 32% to 40%) of series. When reconstructing images of two series (SLIM 2 and SLIM 3) with use of the same 180° linear-interpolation algorithm but changing the position of the reconstructed images along the z axis in one series, the percentage of series that showed the artifact was not modified (reviewer 1, 23 [35%] of 65 SLIM 2 series and 26 [40%] of 65 SLIM 3 series; reviewer 2, 21 [32%] of 65 SLIM 2 series and 23 [35%] of 65 SLIM 3 series); however, on both the SLIM 2 and SLIM 3 series, the artifact was observed in only 13 (20%) of 65 CT studies by reviewer 1 and eight (12%) of the 65 CT studies by reviewer 2.

Imaging of a structure with a cross section that changes rapidly (eg, the ascending aorta expanding and contracting with the heartbeat) in the direction of travel of the CT table is more likely to result in a volume-averaging artifact than would imaging of a structure that does not change considerably in this direction (7). This observation can explain why the artifacts were noted to disappear or appear when only the position of the reconstructed image along the z axis (SLIM 2 and SLIM 3 CT studies) was changed (Figs 3, 4). Views separated by 180° (with use of a 180° linear-interpolation algorithm) can reveal the same phase of aortic motion if the images are reconstructed at an arbitrary plane; these views can reveal opposing phases of aortic motion if the positions of the reconstructed images are changed along the z axis.

On conventional CT studies, curvilinear motion artifacts that simulate ascending aortic dissection have been frequently observed in the ascending aorta; the position of the artifact has been reported to be predictable and related to the systolic aortic motion from the left anterior to the right posterior positions (5).

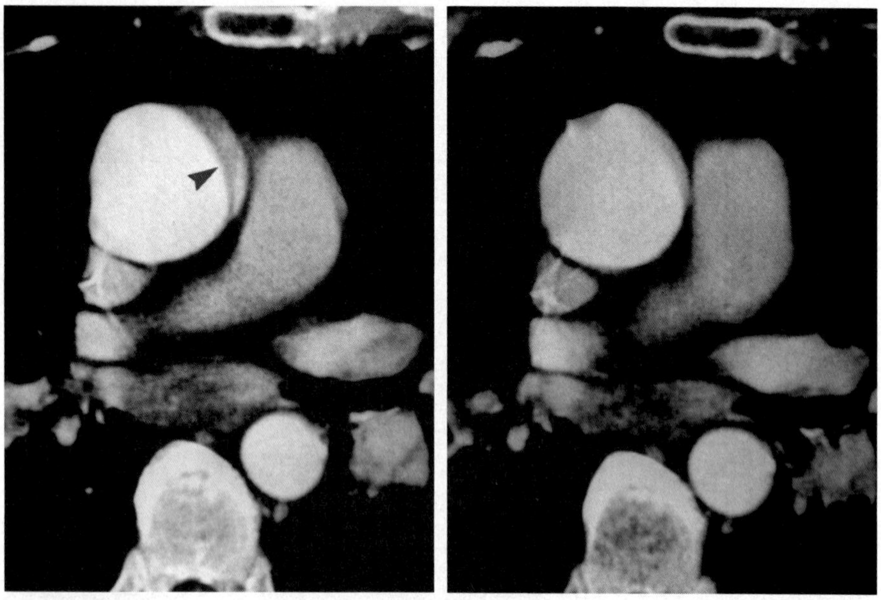

a. b.

Figure 3. Chest CT images in a 69-year-old man who underwent examination for staging of lung cancer. Both images were reconstructed with use of a 180° linear-interpolation algorithm. **(a)** An artifact (arrowhead) along the left anterior circumference of the aorta close to the pulmonary trunk that resembles aortic dissection was noted on images of two contiguous sections. **(b)** CT image with an interval position that differed by 5 mm from that in **a** does not show the artifact.

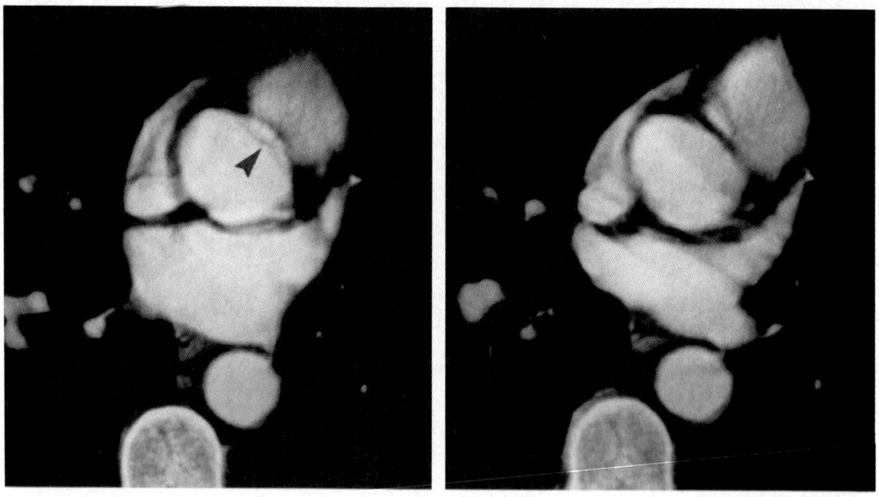

a. b.

Figure 4. Chest CT images in a 60-year-old man who underwent examination for suspected lung cancer. Both images were reconstructed with use of a 180° linear-interpolation algorithm. **(a)** CT image shows an artifact (arrowhead) in the left anterior part (between the 12- and 3-o'clock positions) of the proximal ascending aorta that resembles an intimal flap. **(b)** CT image with an interval position that differed by 5 mm from that in **a** does not show the artifact.

In conclusion, more work is needed to evaluate this imaging artifact. In particular, it would be of interest to assess the value of data from retrospective half-acquisitions that are segmented from the original 1-second scanning data set (11). In our study, however, the artifacts were observed in only 11% of spiral CT studies (on both series of images) when imaging was performed with use of a 180° linear-interpolation algorithm for reconstructing images and the position along the z axis was changed by 5 mm in two series of segmented images. In this case, the artifacts were limited to one or two images and appeared in the proximal section of the ascending aorta or close to the right pulmonary artery in the left or left anterior position along the aortic circumference. ■

References

1. Posniak HV, Olson MC, Demos TC. Aortic motion artifact simulating dissection on CT scans: elimination with reconstructive segmented images. AJR 1993; 161:557–558.
2. Burns MA, Molina PL, Gutierrez FR, Sagel SS. Motion artifact simulating aortic dissection on CT. AJR 1991; 157:465–467.
3. Stanford W. Motion artifact simulating aortic dissection. AJR 1992; 158:1408.
4. Posniak H, Olson M, Demos T. Motion artifact simulating aortic dissection. AJR 1993; 160:420.
5. Duvernoy O, Coulden R, Ytterberg C. Aortic motion: a potential pitfall in CT imaging of dissection in the ascending aorta. J Comput Assist Tomogr 1995; 19:569–572.
6. Set PA, Lomas DJ, Maskell GF, Flower CD, Dixon AK. Artifacts in the ascending aorta on computed tomography: another measure of aortic distensibility? Eur J Radiol 1993; 16:107–111.
7. Kalender WA, Polacin A. Physical performance characteristics of spiral CT scanning. Med Phys 1991; 18:910–915.
8. Kalender WA. Technical foundations of spiral CT. Semin Ultrasound CT MR 1994; 15:81–89.
9. Brink JA, Heiken JP, Balfe DM, Sagel SS, Dicroce J, Vannier MW. Spiral CT: decreased spatial resolution in vivo due to broadening of section-sensitivity profile. Radiology 1992; 185:469–474.
10. Polacin A, Kalender WA, Marchal G. Evaluation of section sensitivity profiles and image noise in spiral CT. Radiology 1992; 185:29–35.
11. Silverman PM, Cooper CJ, Weltman DI, Zeman RK. Helical CT: practical considerations and potential pitfalls. RadioGraphics 1995; 15:25–36.

Book Review

Arthritis in Black and White. 2nd ed.

Anne C. Brower, MD

Philadelphia, Pa: W.B. Saunders & Co, 1996. ISBN 0-7216-5152-6. Cloth, $79.00; pp 442; 561 figures.

Arthritis in Black and White is now in its second edition. The format, with many radiographs of common arthropathies, is similar to that of the first edition. In the second edition, hallmark findings of each of these common arthropathies have been added. This new addition also includes a meager section with a few magnetic resonance (MR) images and brief descriptions of MR imaging characteristics of arthropathies. The second edition also has a new chapter, "The Approach to the Foot."

The text is divided into two major sections. The first section includes six chapters in which changes in specific joints (such as the hand, foot, hip, knee, shoulder, sacroiliac joints, and spine) are demonstrated. In these chapters, there are excellent radiographs that demonstrate the findings of the various arthropathies in each of the joints discussed. There are brief and understandable descriptions of each finding and discussions of the disease process that creates these findings. In the second section, common arthropathies are discussed specifically and radiographic findings of early and late manifestations of the disease processes are demonstrated. Each chapter presents a single arthropathy and begins with a list of its common radiographic characteristics. The affected joints in each arthropathy are discussed individually to provide a direct, simple, and understandable approach.

The textbook is well illustrated with high-quality radiographs. Many of the radiographs included in the first section are shown again in the second section to reemphasize the findings. In the second section, the lists of the common findings of the arthropathies are accurate and concise. The text is also well written and enables a rapid understanding of the key concepts. The textbook offers a good approach to the radiographic diagnosis of common arthropathies.

Other textbooks, such as *Diagnosis of Bone and Joint Disorders*, 3rd ed (six-volume set) by Donald Resnick, MD (Philadelphia, Pa: Saunders, 1995), provide more extensive discussion of arthropathies. However, *Arthritis in Black and White* provides a much more simplified, concise, and understandable approach to the routine identification of common radiographic findings and arthropathies. The textbook is reasonably priced and is a good resource for radiology residents, practicing radiologists, and any clinician who frequently sees patients with articular disorders.

Reviewed by Paul N. Olson, MD

Osamu Matsui, MD • Masumi Kadoya, MD • Jun Yoshikawa, MD • Toshifumi Gabata, MD
Yasuhiro Kawamori, MD • Kazuhiko Ueda, MD • Kouji Nobata, MD
Tsutomu Takashima, MD

Posterior Aspect of Hepatic Segment IV: Patterns of Portal Venule Branching at Helical CT during Arterial Portography[1]

PURPOSE: **To determine the anatomy of the portal venous system in the posterior aspect of segment IV of the liver by using helical computed tomography (CT) during arterial portography (CTAP).**

MATERIALS AND METHODS: **One hundred consecutive patients underwent CTAP. Helical CT during hepatic arteriography was performed in 20 patients. In seven patients with hepatocellular carcinoma in the posterior aspect of segment IV, the feeding arteries were also analyzed.**

RESULTS: **A venule from the intrahepatic portal vein to segment IV was seen in all patients. Other findings included a tiny venule from the distal part of the main left portal vein ($n = 36$), from the proximal left main portal vein ($n = 20$), and from the right portal vein ($n = 18$). Aberrant right gastric venous drainage and/or parabiliary venous drainage directly into the posterior aspect was present in 14 patients. In two patients, a tiny accompanying artery was seen on images from CT during hepatic arteriography. In seven patients with hepatocellular carcinoma, the main feeding artery branched from the right ($n = 2$) or left ($n = 5$) hepatic artery.**

CONCLUSION: **CTAP adequately demonstrates the tiny portal venous and arterial branches from the main right or left portal vein that distribute to the posterior aspect of segment IV. Knowledge of this vascular anatomy is clinically important.**

The posterior aspect of hepatic segment IV presents some challenges as regards determination of vascular anatomy and diagnosis based on imaging findings (1–6). A well-known occasional finding in this region at computed tomography (CT) during arterial portography (CTAP) is a pseudotumor (localized portal venous perfusion defect). Matsui et al (1) found that the major cause of this perfusion defect is aberrant drainage of the right gastric vein directly into the posterior aspect of segment IV, which occurs in approximately 6%–14% of patients. There is a strong correlation between focal sparing in the fatty liver (2), focal fatty changes in the normal liver (3), and focal hyperplastic change in the cirrhotic liver (4) in this region and aberrant right gastric venous drainage into the region (4). In an anatomic study, Couinaud (5) reported that tiny veins flow directly into the posterior aspect of segment IV from the parabiliary venous system and from tiny portal venules that distribute to this region directly from the left portal vein.

Recent advances in helical CT have made possible visualization of the entire tiny vascular system and, as a result, determination of the anatomy of small vessels. The purpose of this study was to determine the portal venous anatomy in the posterior aspect of segment IV by using CTAP and to determine the clinical importance of this anatomy.

MATERIALS AND METHODS

Findings in 100 consecutive patients (64 men, 36 women), aged 41–75 years (mean, 64 years), who underwent CTAP with a helical CT system between April 1994 and February 1996 were included in this study. Findings in 12 patients with advanced hepatocellular carcinoma and/or a tumor that surrounded the hepatic hilus (including the posterior aspect of segment IV) were excluded. Hepatic angiography, including CTAP, was performed in 79 patients with liver cirrhosis who were suspected of having hepatocellular carcinoma and for the detection of liver metastases in 21 patients with colorectal cancer and a normal liver. In addition, helical CT during hepatic arteriography (CTHA) was performed in 20 of the patients.

Both CTAP and CTHA were performed with a commercially available, helical CT scanner (HiSpeed; GE Medical Systems, Milwaukee, Wis). After selective celiac and hepatic arteriography, a 4-F catheter was inserted into the superior mesenteric artery, and the patient was transported to the CT room. For celiac and hepatic arteriography, the patients received approximately 20 mL of iohexol (350 mg of iodine per milliliter) (Omnipaque; Daiichi, Tokyo, Japan); for CTAP, 50–80 mL of iohexol (350 mg of iodine per milliliter) were infused through a catheter in the superior mesenteric artery at a rate of 1.5 mL/sec during CT of the entire liver. Helical CTAP of the entire liver was performed with 7-mm collimation, a table speed of 7 mm/sec, and an overlapping axial reconstruction interval of 3.5 mm. Scanning began 25 seconds after the start of the injection of the contrast medium, and infusion of the contrast medium was

Index terms: Hepatic arteries, CT, 952.12916 • Hepatic veins, CT, 959.12916 • Liver, anatomy, 761.91, 761.929 • Liver, CT, 761.12916 • Liver neoplasms, blood supply, 761.323, 761.332 • Portal vein, anatomy, 957.92 • Portal vein, CT, 957.12916

Abbreviations: CTAP = CT during arterial portography, CTHA = CT during hepatic arteriography.

Radiology 1997; 205:159–162

[1] From the Department of Radiology, Kanazawa University School of Medicine, 13-1 Takara-machi, Kanazawa 920, Japan. Received March 20; revision requested May 8; revision received June 19; accepted June 23. **Address reprint requests to** O.M.

stopped 25 seconds before completion of the scanning.

For the CTHA study, another 4-F catheter was inserted through the ipsilateral femoral artery and into the common hepatic artery, and iohexol was infused at a rate of 1.0–1.5 mL/sec during scanning of the entire liver. In 15 patients, helical CTHA was performed with 7-mm collimation, a table speed of 7 mm/sec, and an axial reconstruction interval of 3.5 mm. In the remaining five patients, helical CTHA was performed with 2-mm collimation, a table speed of 2 mm/sec, and an axial reconstruction interval of 1 mm.

In all patients, findings of the tiny portal venules that branch directly from the main left or right portal vein that distributes to the posterior aspect of segment IV were analyzed. In patients who underwent CTHA, findings of the accompanying tiny arterial branches were analyzed, as well. In all patients, the diameter of the posterior aspect at the axial level of the right hepatic hilus was roughly classified as "small" or "large." When the transverse diameter of the posterior aspect of segment IV was less than half that of the anterior aspect, as shown in Figure 1, it was classified as small; otherwise, it was classified as large. The relationship between the size of the posterior aspect and the number of tiny portal venules depicted on CTAP images was analyzed.

Between April 1994 and February 1996, arteriographic files in seven patients showed a relatively small (diameter < 3 cm) lesion from hypervascular hepatocellular carcinoma in the posterior aspect of segment IV. Hepatocellular carcinoma was diagnosed on the basis of clinical examination findings in five patients and was proved with biopsy results in two patients. In these seven patients, the feeding arteries were analyzed, as well.

The χ^2 statistic was used to test for statistically significant differences.

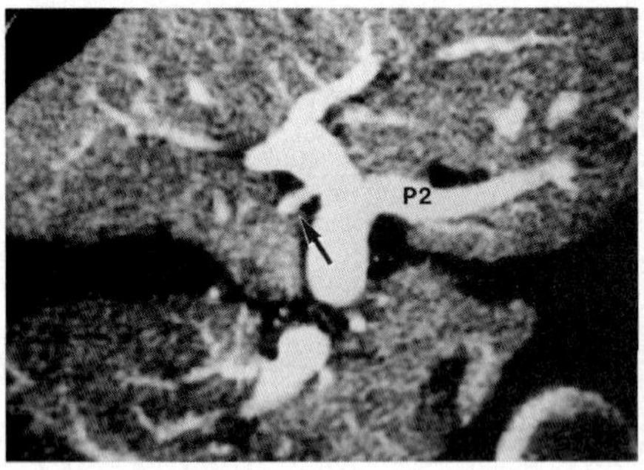

1.

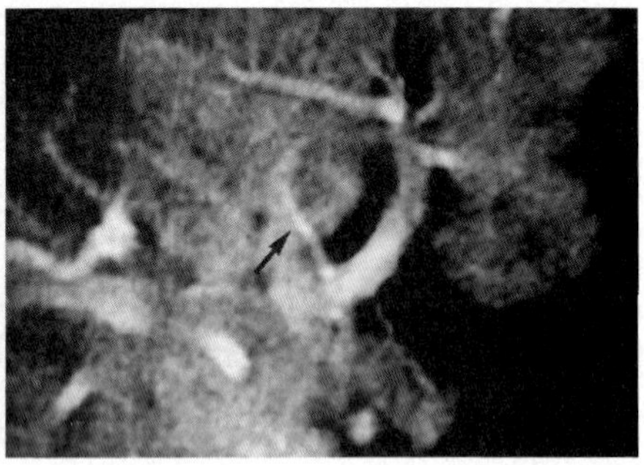

2.

Figures 1, 2. **(1)** CTAP image shows a type 2 tiny portal venule (arrow) distributing to the posterior aspect of segment IV and branching directly from the distal portion (distal to the branching point of the portal venous branch to segment II [*P2*]) of the main left portal vein. **(2)** CTAP image shows a type 3 tiny portal venule (arrow) distributing to the posterior aspect of segment IV and branching directly from the proximal portion of the left main portal vein.

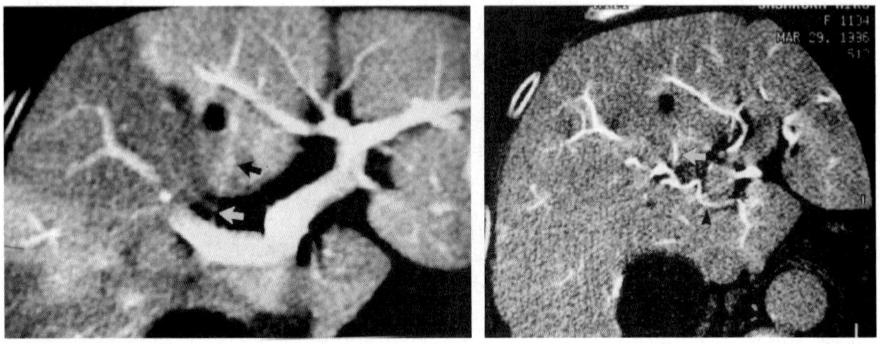

a. b.

Figure 3. Type 4 portal venule. **(a)** CTAP image shows a tiny portal venule (arrows) distributing to the posterior aspect of segment IV and branching directly from the right main portal vein. **(b)** CTHA image shows a tiny artery (arrow) distributing to the posterior aspect of segment IV and branching from the right hepatic artery (arrowhead). The course of this artery was the same as that of the portal venule shown in **a**.

RESULTS

On CTAP images, we observed five types of anatomic patterns of the tiny portal venules that branch directly from the left or right portal vein and distribute to the posterior aspect of segment IV. The type 1 pattern was characterized by portal venules that distribute to the posterior aspect from the intrahepatic portal vein to segment IV. The type 2 pattern was characterized by a tiny portal venule that branched directly from a distal portion (distal to the branching point of the portal vein branch to hepatic segment II) of the main left portal vein (Fig 1). The type 3 pattern was characterized by a tiny portal venule that branched from the proximal portion of the left main portal vein (Fig 2). The type 4 pattern was characterized by a tiny portal vein branch from the right main portal vein or from the proximal end of the anterior superior branch (Fig 3). The type 5 pattern was characterized by a portal perfusion defect (pseudotumor) in the posterior aspect of segment IV, which was probably due to aberrant right gastric venous drainage, drainage from the parabiliary venous system directly into the posterior aspect of segment IV, or both (Fig 4).

Table 1 lists the frequency of these types of branching patterns in the patients in the study group. The type 1 pattern was seen in all patients. Types 2, 3, 4, and 5 were seen in 36 (36%), 20 (20%), 18 (18%), and 14 (14%) patients, respectively.

Table 2 shows the correlation between the distribution of types of these tiny venules demonstrated on CTAP images and the diameter of the posterior aspect of segment IV (large vs small). A small-diameter posterior aspect was noted in 36 of 40 (90%) patients with the type 1 pattern only, in 16 of 33 (48%) patients with the type 1 pattern and another type, in three of 22 (14%) patients with the type 1 pattern and two other types, and in none of five (0%) patients with the type 1 pattern and three other types. The diameter of the posterior aspect was classified as small in 55 (55%) patients; in the remaining 45 (45%) patients, it was classified as large. A small posterior aspect was seen in 46 of 79 patients with liver cirrhosis and in nine of 21 patients without diffuse liver disease. There were no statistically significant differences in the prevalence of a small posterior segment between patients with liver cirrhosis and those without diffuse liver disease (P = .21).

In two of the five patients who underwent CTHA with 2-mm collimation, a tiny artery that branched from the right anterior segmental artery of the liver was accompanied by a type 4 tiny portal vein branch (Fig 3). In the remaining 15 patients who underwent CTHA, the accompanying artery was not visualized.

In two of the seven patients with a relatively small hepatocellular carcinoma in the posterior aspect of segment IV, the main feeding artery branched from the proximal portion of the right anterior artery (Fig 5). The main feed-

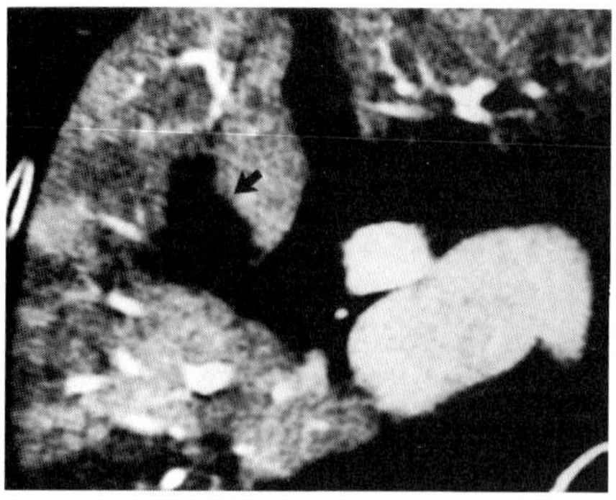

Figure 4. Type 5 portal venule. CTAP image shows a portal venous perfusion defect (pseudotumor) (arrow) in the posterior aspect of segment IV resulting from aberrant right gastric venous drainage (confirmed at arteriography) directly into the posterior aspect of segment IV.

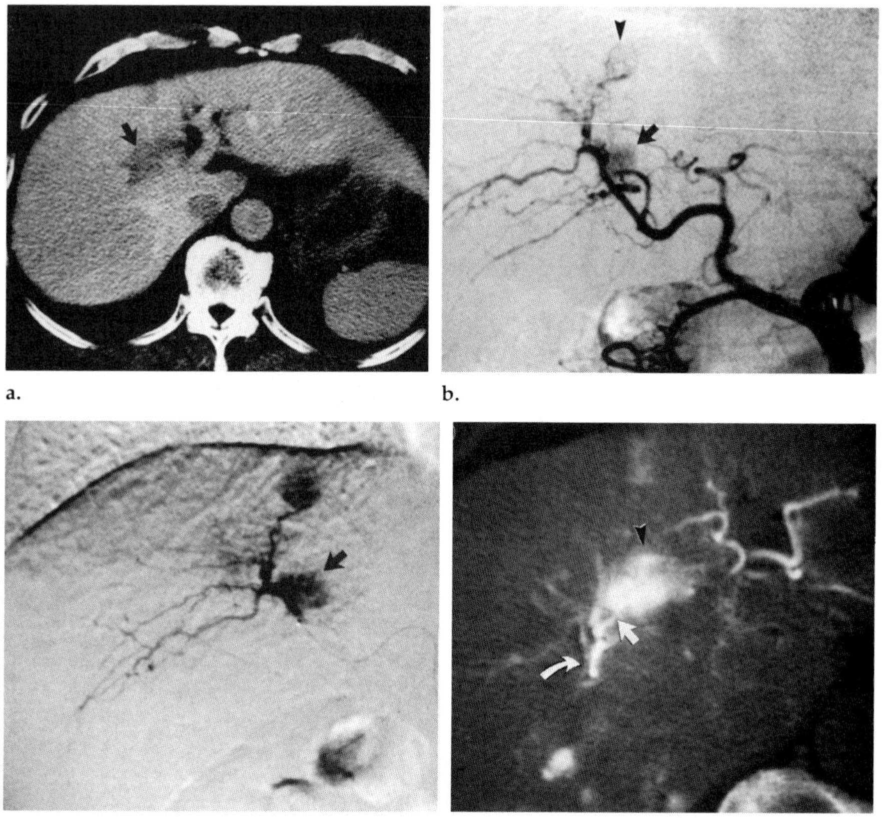

a. b. c. d.

Figure 5. Hepatocellular carcinoma. **(a)** Contrast-enhanced CT scan shows a hypoattenuated mass (arrow) in the posterior aspect of segment IV. **(b)** Celiac arteriogram of the same mass as in **a** shows definite nodular staining (arrow). Another lesion (arrowhead) is also visible. **(c)** Subselective right anterior segmental arteriogram also depicts the same lesion shown in **a** (arrow). The tiny feeding artery branches directly from the proximal end of the right anterior segmental artery. **(d)** CTHA image shows the feeding artery (straight arrow) branching directly from the right hepatic artery (curved arrow) and dense, nodular staining in the posterior aspect of segment IV (arrowhead).

Table 1
Branching Patterns of Portal Venules That Distribute to the Posterior Aspect of Hepatic Segment IV

Branching Pattern	No. of Cases (n = 100)
Type 1	100
Type 2	36
Type 3	20
Type 4	18
Type 5	14

Table 2
Correlation between Branching Pattern and Diameter of Posterior Aspect of Segment IV

	Diameter of Posterior Aspect	
Branching Pattern	Small	Large
Type 1 only (n = 40)	36	4
Type 1 and another type (n = 33)	16	17
Type 1 and two other types (n = 22)	3	19
Type 1 and three other types (n = 5)	0	5

Note.—Data are number of patients.

ing artery was believed to be accompanying a type 4 portal venule. The main feeding artery branched from the left hepatic artery in the other five patients.

DISCUSSION

The intrahepatic vascular anatomy has been thoroughly analyzed in both anatomic and radiologic terms. The main focus, however, has been on the major intrahepatic portal venous and hepatic arterial branches. Owing to advances in modern imaging modalities—especially in helical CT—the tiny intrahepatic vessels can now be visualized (7,8). In our study with helical CTAP, we noted various types of tiny portal venules around the hepatic hilus, especially in the posterior aspect of segment IV. We also noted a particular pattern of vascular supply in tumors located around the hepatic hilus, as well as various kinds of portal venous collateral vessels in patients with portal venous obstruction. Therefore, we analyzed the frequency and branching types of these tiny venules in the posterior aspect on helical CTAP images to evaluate their clinical importance.

In this study, approximately 60% of the patients examined with CTAP had more than one tiny portal venous supply that branched directly from the left or right main portal vein to the posterior aspect, in addition to the branches from the intrahepatic portal vein to segment IV (most frequently from the main left portal vein distal to the branching point of the portal vein branch to segment II).

To our knowledge, there have been no anatomic or radiologic studies, other than those of Couinaud (5,9), in which these venules have been analyzed. Couinaud (9) used injection-cast methods to investigate the tiny portal venules that supply the liver parenchyma around the hepatic hilus and reported that the portal venule that supplies the posterior aspect of segment IV branched directly from the main left portal vein in 30 of 109 patients and from the parabiliary system in 45 of 74 patients. Discrepancies between our data and those of Couinaud may be the result of differing examination techniques, but we consider the results of both analyses to be almost the same. Couinaud, however, did not mention the tiny portal venules that branch from the right and the left portal vein distal to the branching point of the portal vein branch to segment II, probably because of the difficulty of such an analysis with the injection-cast method (9). To our knowledge, therefore, ours is the first report to describe these tiny portal venules that supply the posterior aspect of segment IV.

We did not perform CTHA in every patient. In two of five patients who underwent helical CTHA with 2-mm collimation, however, the tiny artery that accompanied the portal venule branch from the right portal vein was visualized (Fig 3). According to Couinaud (5,9), all of these tiny portal venules are associated with accompanying tiny arteries and biliary ducts. Therefore, we believe the portal venules described here had accompanying arterial branches, most of which were too small to be visualized on CTHA images.

The vascular anatomy determined in this study is similar to that of the caudate lobe (segment I) of the liver. Therefore, the same type of changes in configuration or pseudolesions seen in segment I in patients with diffuse liver disease can be present in the posterior aspect of segment IV. In those patients with a relatively large posterior aspect, a larger number of these tiny portal venules that branch directly from the left or right portal vein were present than in patients with a relatively small posterior aspect (Table 2). In our study, the size of the posterior aspect relative to that of the entire segment IV, however, was not statistically significantly different in patients with cirrhosis compared with those without diffuse liver disease. Therefore, we found no correlation between the deformity of the posterior aspect occasionally seen in cirrhotic livers and the number of these tiny portal venules.

The clinical importance of knowledge of the vascular anatomy of the posterior aspect of segment IV becomes evident in cases of hepatocellular carcinoma (Fig 5). At surgery and transcatheter arterial embolization, it is important to know that hepatic tumors in the posterior aspect can be supplied by the artery that branches from the right hepatic artery or from the proximal portion of the left hepatic artery (10). In addition, these portal venules can be one of the important collateral pathways during intra- and extrahepatic portal venous obstruction. The same type of collateral flow in the biliary system can also be expected. The hypertrophy of liver parenchyma around the hepatic hilus (central hypertrophy) that is occasionally seen in idiopathic portal venous hypertension (thrombosis in the peripheral portal veins) can be well explained in terms of preservation of these tiny portal venules (11,12). The hypertrophy of segment IV seen in patients with Alagille syndrome also may result from this kind of anatomic variation in the biliary system (13).

In conclusion, helical CTAP images in approximately 60% of the patients in this study had one to three tiny portal venules that branched directly from the main right or left portal vein and distributed to the posterior aspect of segment IV. An accompanying tiny artery was also noted on thin-section CTHA scans in some patients. We consider this vascular anatomy to be clinically important. ■

References

1. Matsui O, Takahashi S, Kadoya M, et al. Pseudolesion in segment IV of the liver at CT during arterial portography: correlation with aberrant gastric venous drainage. Radiology 1994; 193:31–35.
2. Matsui O, Kadoya M, Takahashi S, et al. Focal sparing of segment IV in fatty livers shown by sonography and CT: correlation with aberrant gastric venous drainage. AJR 1995; 164:1137–1140.
3. Kawamori Y, Matsui O, Takahashi S, Kadoya M, Takashima T, Miyayama S. Focal hepatic fatty infiltration in the posterior edge of the medial segment associated with aberrant gastric venous drainage: CT, US, MR findings. J Comput Assist Tomogr 1996; 20:356–359.
4. Matsui O, Kadoya M, Yosikawa J, et al. Aberrant gastric venous drainage in cirrhotic livers: imaging findings in focal areas of liver parenchyma. Radiology 1995; 197: 345–349.
5. Couinaud C. The parabiliary venous system. Surg Radiol Anat 1988; 10:311–316.
6. Ito K, Choji T, Fujita T, Matsumoto T, Nakada T, Nakanishi T. Early-enhancing pseudolesion in medial segment of left hepatic lobe detected with multisection dynamic MR. Radiology 1993; 187:695–699.
7. Bluemke DA, Soyer P, Chan BW, Bliss DF, Calhoun PS, Fishman EK. Spiral CT during arterial portography: technique and applications. RadioGraphics 1995; 15:623–637.
8. Soyer P, Bluemke DA, Bliss DF, Woodhouse CE, Fishman EK. Surgical segmental anatomy of the liver: demonstration with spiral CT during arterial portography and multiplanar reconstruction. AJR 1994; 163: 99–103.
9. Couinaud C. Surgical anatomy of the liver revisited. Paris, France: Couinaud, 1989; 98–99.
10. Matsui O, Kadoya M, Yoshikawa J, et al. Small hepatocellular carcinoma: treatment with subsegmental transcatheter arterial embolization. Radiology 1993; 188:79–83.
11. Wanless IR. Micronodular transformation (nodular regenerative hyperplasia) of the liver: a report of 64 cases among 2,500 autopsies and a new classification of benign hepatocellular nodules. Hepatology 1990; 11:187–197.
12. Arai K, Matsui O, Kadoya M, et al. MR imaging in idiopathic portal hypertension. J Comput Assist Tomogr 1991; 15:405–408.
13. Torizuka T, Tamaki N, Fujita T, et al. Focal liver hyperplasia in Alagille syndrome: assessment with hepatoreceptor and hepatobiliary imaging. J Nucl Med 1996; 37:1365–1368.

Neil M. Rofsky, MD • Glyn Johnson, PhD • Mark A. Adelman, MD • Robert J. Rosen, MD
Glenn A. Krinsky, MD • Jeffrey C. Weinreb, MD

Peripheral Vascular Disease Evaluated with Reduced-Dose Gadolinium-enhanced MR Angiography[1]

PURPOSE: **To demonstrate the utility of low-dose gadolinium-enhanced magnetic resonance (MR) angiography of two consecutive anatomic areas for assessment of peripheral vascular disease.**

MATERIALS AND METHODS: **Fifteen patients underwent gadolinium-enhanced MR angiography for evaluation of lower extremity peripheral vascular disease after conventional digital subtraction angiography (DSA). MR angiography was performed with three-dimensional coronal gradient-echo acquisitions before and during administration of gadopentetate dimeglumine. Two separate, contiguous areas were studied with separate doses of 0.075 and 0.1 mmol/kg gadopentetate dimeglumine. MR angiography findings were compared with DSA findings; DSA was the standard of reference. Treatment options were determined first with MR angiograms and then with DSA images.**

RESULTS: **For distinguishing greater than 50% stenosis from 50% or less stenosis, gadolinium-enhanced MR angiography yielded a sensitivity of 97%, a specificity of 96%, and an accuracy of 97%. In 146 (97%) of 150 anatomic segments, there was essential or total agreement on treatments determined with MR angiography and DSA. In two cases (one case of vascular stent placement and one case of surgical anastomosis), extent of disease was overestimated with MR angiography. The MR study of one infrapopliteal area was insufficient for evaluation.**

CONCLUSION: **Accurate gadolinium-enhanced MR angiography of multiple peripheral vascular areas of the lower extremities can be performed in most patients with less than 0.2 mmol/kg contrast material.**

TIME-OF-FLIGHT magnetic resonance (MR) angiography has been used successfully for the evaluation of patients with atherosclerotic occlusive peripheral vascular disease (1–3). MR angiography with use of gadolinium-based contrast material is an alternative to time-of-flight imaging (4–11). With gadolinium-enhanced MR angiography, images can be acquired in the coronal plane. Use of this orientation is much more time efficient than use of the axial orientation that is required with time-of-flight MR angiography. With use of three-dimensional gradient-echo sequences, 45 cm of an anatomic structure can be imaged in 20–50 seconds, depending on the resolution needed; time-of-flight imaging of a similar amount of tissue can take 20 minutes. Furthermore, gadolinium-enhanced MR angiography can provide better images of the iliac artery (9).

The MR contrast material gadopentetate dimeglumine (approved by the U.S. Food and Drug Administration) is associated with a much lower frequency of adverse reactions than iodinated contrast materials (12,13). Gadopentetate dimeglumine has no known nephrotoxicity (14–16) even at high doses (13). Gadolinium-enhanced MR angiography is therefore a safe alternative to conventional angiography for patients with renal insufficiency or other contraindications to iodinated contrast material. Furthermore, gadolinium-enhanced MR angiography is not associated with the arterial complications inherent in catheter-based conventional angiography.

With gadolinium-enhanced MR angiography, a complete peripheral runoff study of two or more anatomic areas can be performed with time-efficient acquisitions. Such a protocol may provide more suitable screening for atherosclerotic occlusive peripheral vascular disease. Most investigators, however, have used at least a double dose (0.2 mmol/kg) (4,9,11) or more (17,18) of gadolinium chelates for imaging of a single anatomic area. For imaging each one of multiple anatomic areas, use of a large dose is undesirable for several reasons: The safety of very large doses has not been tested; the cost of the procedure increases substantially (gadopentetate dimeglumine is approximately $70/20 mL); and, with later acquisitions, the background signal is large, which reduces the contrast between artery and background.

The purpose of this study was to investigate the use of low-dose gadopentetate dimeglumine in MR angiography when imaging two areas of peripheral lower extremity vasculature. We compared results of MR angiography with those of conventional digital subtraction angiography (DSA), which was the standard of reference.

Index terms: Angiography, comparative studies, 92.1211 • Arteries, extremities, 92.12942, 92.12943 • Arteries, stenosis or obstruction, 92.721 • Gadolinium • Magnetic resonance (MR), comparative studies, 92.12942, 92.12943 • Magnetic resonance (MR), vascular studies, 92.12942, 92.12943

Abbreviations: CI = confidence interval, DSA = digital subtraction angiography, MIP = maximum intensity projection.

Radiology 1997; 205:163–169

[1] From the Department of Radiology (N.M.R., G.J., R.J.R., G.A.K., J.C.W.) and Department of Surgery, Division of Vascular Surgery (M.A.A.), New York University Medical Center, 530 First Ave, New York, NY 10016. Received April 4, 1997; revision requested May 7; revision received June 10; accepted June 16. Supported in part by a grant from Berlex Laboratories, Wayne, NJ. **Address reprint requests to** N.M.R.

Table 1
Scoring of Agreement on Treatments Chosen with DSA and MR Angiography

Agreement	Definition
None	Severe disease is seen with one examination only.
Partial	Disease is seen with both examinations, but differences in apparent severity alter treatment chosen.
Essential	Severity of disease seen with the two examinations is not sufficiently different to alter treatment chosen.
Total	The same extent of disease is seen with both examinations.

Table 2
Disease States of Anatomic Segments Studied with DSA and MR Angiography

Disease State	No. of Anatomic Segments (n = 150)
Normal	91
Stenosis, ≤50%	21
Stenosis, >50%	13
Occlusion	25

Table 3
Truth Table for Gadolinium-enhanced MR Angiography of 150 Vascular Segments with DSA as the Standard of Reference

Severity of Disease with MR Angiography	Severity of Disease with DSA	
	High-grade*	Low-grade†
High-grade*	37	4
Low-grade†	1	108

Note.—For MR angiography, sensitivity = 0.97 (95% CI: 0.86, 1.00), specificity = 0.96 (95% CI: 0.91, 0.99), positive predictive value = 0.90 (95% CI: 0.77, 0.97), negative predictive value = 0.99 (95% CI: 0.95, 1.00), and accuracy = 0.97 (95% CI: 0.92, 0.99).
* >50% stenosis and occlusions.
† ≤50% stenosis.

Table 4
Agreement on Treatments Determined with Gadolinium-enhanced MR Angiography and DSA

Agreement	No. of Anatomic Segments	
	All (n = 150)	Diseased Segments Only (n = 59)
Total	140 (93)	49 (83)
Essential	6 (4)	6 (10)
Partial	2 (1)	2 (4)
None	2 (1)	2 (4)
Total and essential	146 (97)	55 (93)
Partial and none	4 (3)	4 (7)

Note.—Numbers in parentheses are percentages.

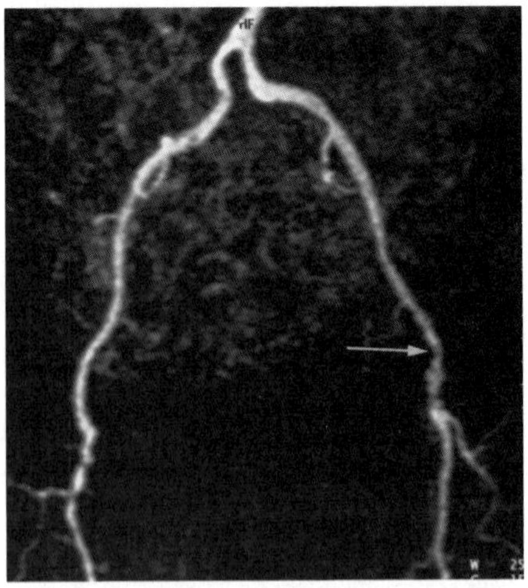

a.

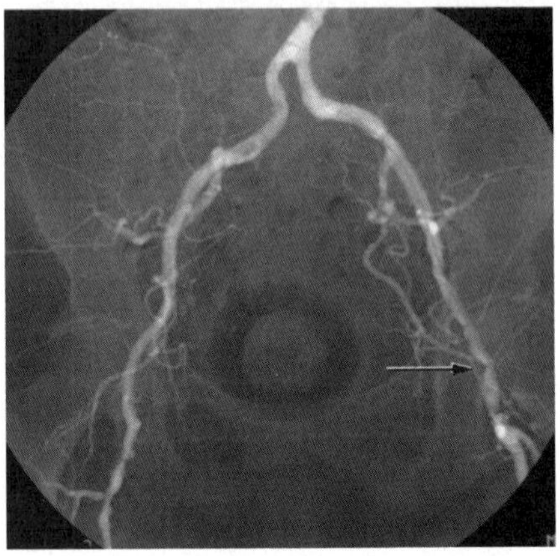

b.

Figure 1. Total and essential agreement between gadolinium-enhanced MR angiography and DSA studies. **(a)** Subtraction MIP MR angiogram (5/2 [repetition time msec/echo time msec], 50° flip angle) of first anatomic area acquired after administration of 0.075 mmol/kg gadopentetate dimeglumine shows multiple stenoses; one focal stenosis (arrow) was judged 50% or less. **(b)** On the DSA image of the same area, the focal stenosis (arrow) that was seen in **a** was judged greater than 50%. Because the patient had experienced symptoms in the other leg, essential agreement was scored. There was otherwise excellent correlation between the two studies and better visualization of smaller branch vessels with DSA.

MATERIALS AND METHODS

Between February 12, 1996, and April 15, 1996, 15 patients underwent conventional DSA and gadolinium-enhanced MR angiography. There were nine men and six women. Patient ages ranged from 49 to 89 years (mean, 66 years). Patients were selected from a group with rest pain, limb-threatening ischemia, or imminent tissue loss who were referred for conventional DSA by vascular surgeons. All patients underwent DSA before MR angiography, and all had atherosclerotic occlusive peripheral vascular disease. Patients were excluded from the study (*a*) because of standard contraindications to MR imaging, (*b*) if the MR study could not be scheduled within 5 days of DSA, or (*c*) if an interventional procedure was performed at the time of DSA. Otherwise, patients were chosen consecutively from the group. The study was approved by the Institutional Board of Research Associates, and informed consent was obtained from all patients before study entry.

DSA

All DSA examinations were performed by experienced angiographers with a Philips Integris 4000 digital angiographic unit (Philips Medical Systems, Shelton, Conn). For imaging of the area from the distal abdominal aorta to the common femoral arteries, a 5-F pigtail catheter was inserted into the abdominal aorta with use of the Seldinger technique. Into the distal aorta, 16 mL of ioxaglate (19.6% sodium, 39.3% meglumine) (Hexabrix; Mallinckrodt, St Louis, Mo) was administered at 8 mL/sec. For all lower extremity evaluations, an average of 60–80 mL of ioxaglate was injected at 4–5 mL/sec through a 5-F dilator into the appropriate external iliac artery. Separate selective injections were performed in the one bilateral evaluation in this series. In all cases, intraarterial digital subtraction images were obtained of separate anatomic areas.

MR Angiography

MR angiography was performed with a circularly polarized volume body coil and a 1.5-T imager (Vision; Siemens, Iselin, NJ) with 25-mT/m gradients and 600-µsec rise times. Gadolinium-enhanced MR examination of two contiguous anatomic areas was performed without knowledge of the DSA results. The areas to be imaged, however, were chosen by the vascular radiologist who performed the DSA; selected areas included at least one area with disease. In 12 patients, the boundaries of the first area were the infrarenal abdominal aorta and the proximal superficial femoral artery and those of the second area were the proximal superficial femoral artery and the midcalf. In three patients, the boundaries of the first area were the lower pelvis and the knee and those of the second area were the knee and the ankle.

Coronal three-dimensional gradient-echo MR images were acquired with the following parameters: repetition time, 5 msec; echo time, 2 msec; and flip angle, 30°–50°. A flip angle of 50° was attempted in all cases. When the specific absorption rate exceeded the recommended level, the flip angle was reduced in 10° decrements until an acceptable specific absorption rate

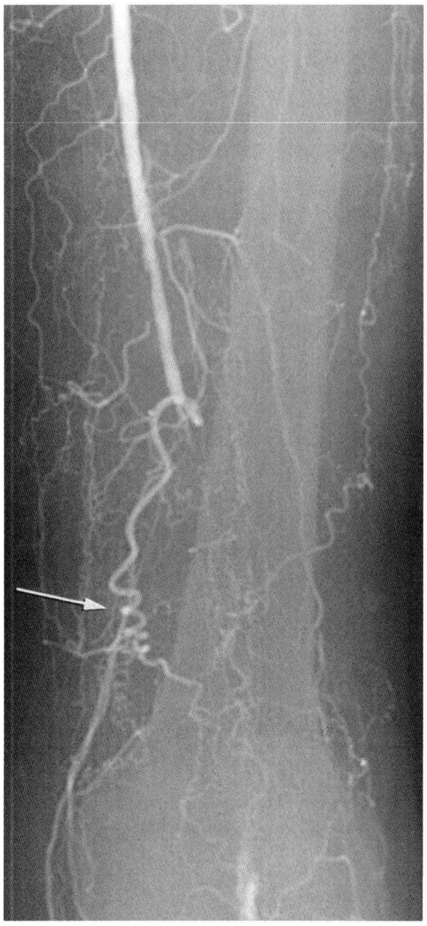

b.

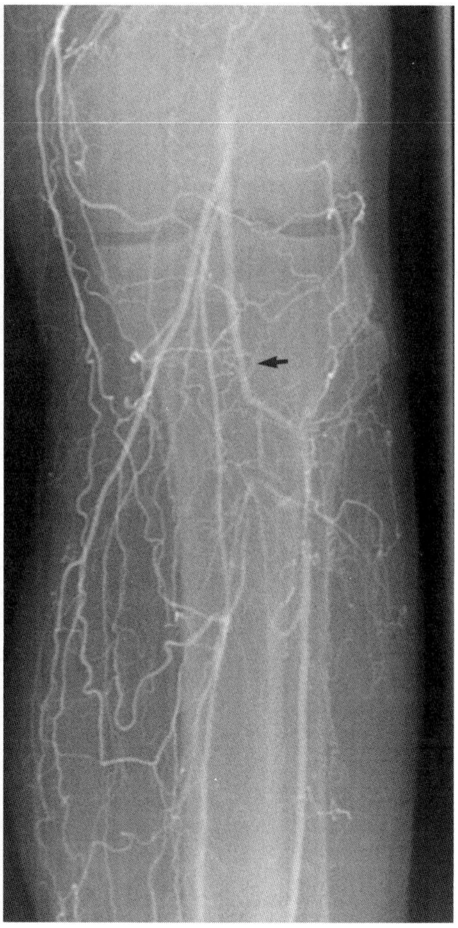

c.

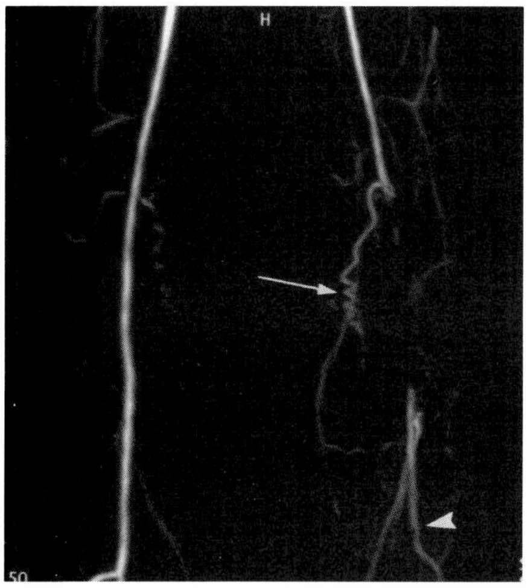

a.

Figure 2. Total and essential agreement between gadolinium-enhanced MR angiography and DSA studies. **(a)** Subtraction MIP MR angiogram (5/2, 50° flip angle) of the second anatomic area acquired after administration of 0.1 mmol/kg gadopentetate dimeglumine shows a long segment of occlusion in the superficial femoral artery and reconstitution of the popliteal artery. A major collateral vessel (arrow) and focal stenosis (arrowhead) in the infrageniculate popliteal artery are also noted. **(b, c)** DSA images of the same area show segmental occlusion of the superficial femoral artery; however, the popliteal stenosis was judged normal in an area with additional overlapping collateral vessels. There was excellent correlation when major collateral vessels (arrow) on DSA and MR angiography images were compared.

was achieved. The field of view was adjusted to cover the anatomic area under study and minimize aliasing. A rectangular field of view was used if possible. In anatomic areas above the knee, the field of view varied from 380 to 480 mm (mean, 410 mm) with a slab thickness between 90 and 120 mm; the data matrix was adjusted so that pixel size was less than 2.8 mm × 1.75 mm (in plane) × 3 mm (section thickness). Below the knee, the field of view varied from 380 to 410 mm (mean, 395 mm) with a slab thickness between 60 and 80 mm; pixel size was less than 2.5 mm × 1.75 mm (in plane) × 2 mm (section thickness). Imaging times were between 30 and 45 seconds. A longer imaging time was required to maintain resolution with a larger field of view.

Images of the first and second anatomic areas were acquired with respective doses of 0.075 and 0.1 mmol/kg gadopentetate dimeglumine (Magnevist; Berlex, Wayne, NJ). The interval between doses was at least 10 minutes and never longer than 15 minutes. Therefore, the cumulative dose of gadopentetate dimeglumine was less than 0.2 mmol/kg. Contrast material was administered through a 22-gauge intravenous catheter in the arm. A bolus was injected manually (at approximately 2 mL/sec) and followed immediately by a 20-mL saline flush.

In each anatomic area, one image before and two images after administration of contrast material were acquired; acquisition parameters in each anatomic area were identical. The second gadolinium-enhanced image, acquired immediately after the first gadolinium-enhanced image, was required to account for individuals with altered cardiovascular dynamics in the absence of a test bolus (19).

In the first anatomic area, image acquisition was begun at the completion of the bolus injection of gadopentetate dimeglumine. This technique has been found to optimize rapid gadolinium-enhanced MR angiography of the aorta. In the second anatomic area, image acquisition was begun 10 seconds after the bolus injection was complete; in the infrapopliteal area, image acquisition was begun 15 seconds after the bolus injection was complete. These delays were estimates derived with the assumption that some additional time is required for contrast material to reach the more distal parts of a given anatomic area.

To minimize background signal intensity, each image acquired before the administration of contrast material was subtracted from the image that showed greater arterial enhancement. The resultant subtraction image was then processed with use of a maximum-intensity-projection (MIP) algorithm, and these processed images were used in the subsequent assessment. The subtraction and MIP software are standard components of the commercially available MR system we used.

The MIP reconstructed images were presented for review in frontal and 30° oblique projections and retrospectively evaluated in a joint review by a vascular surgeon (M.A.A.), a vascular interventional radiologist (R.J.R.), and a radiologist with experience in MR angiography (N.M.R.). The vascular interventional radiologist had performed eight of the 15 DSA studies. The images were reviewed by consensus 3 months after the studies were performed to minimize a bias toward agreement.

Data Analysis

For analysis, the vasculature was divided into 21 segments, which consisted of the infrarenal abdominal aorta and the right and left arteries of the following: common and external iliac arteries; common, superficial, and deep femoral arteries; popliteal arteries; tibioperoneal trunks; anterior and posterior tibial arteries; and peroneal arteries. In each of these segments, the vasculature was scored as follows: normal, 50% or less stenosis, greater than 50% stenosis, or occluded. In cases with multiple sites of disease, only the site with the most severe disease was scored.

Treatment options on the basis of gadolinium-enhanced MR angiography findings alone were discussed before the DSA

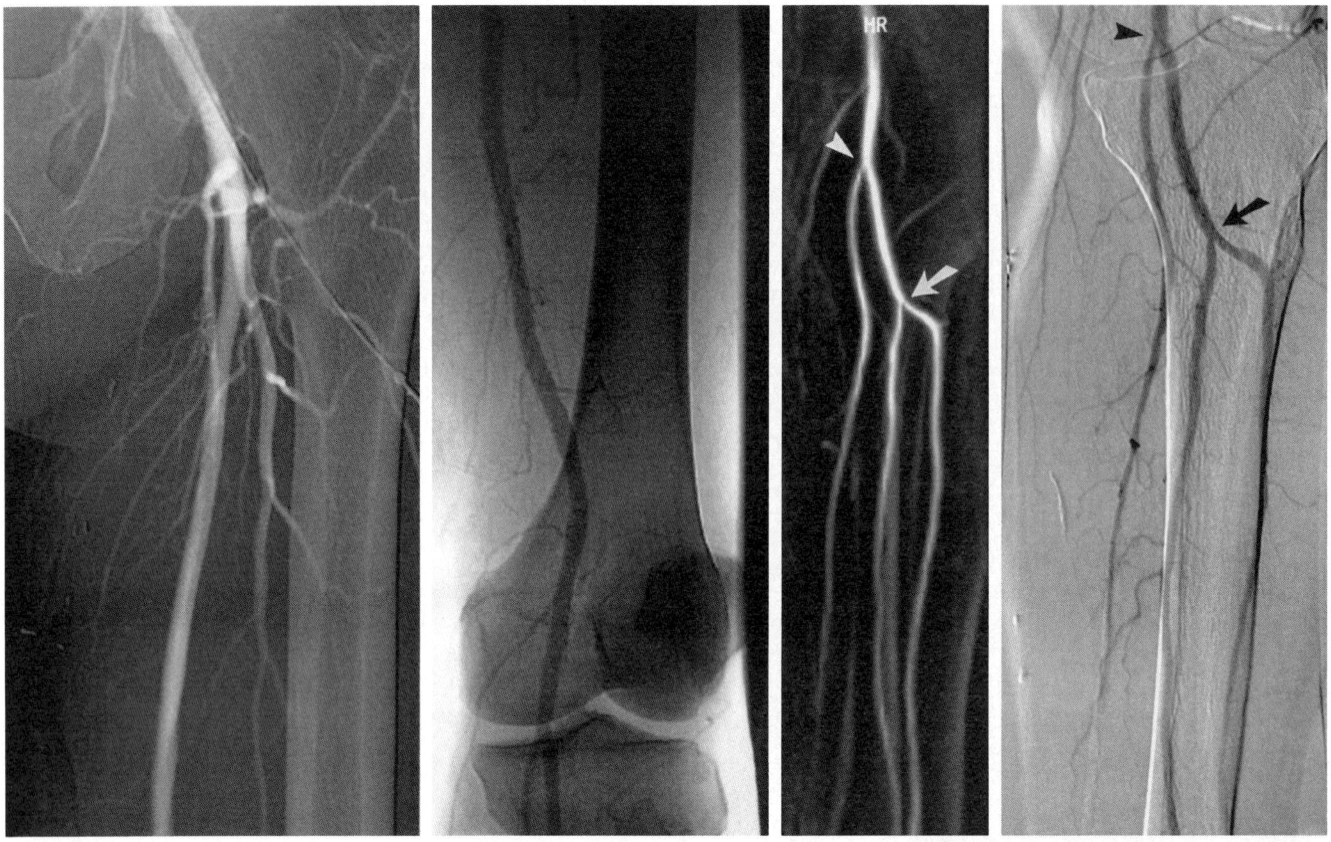

b. c. d. e.

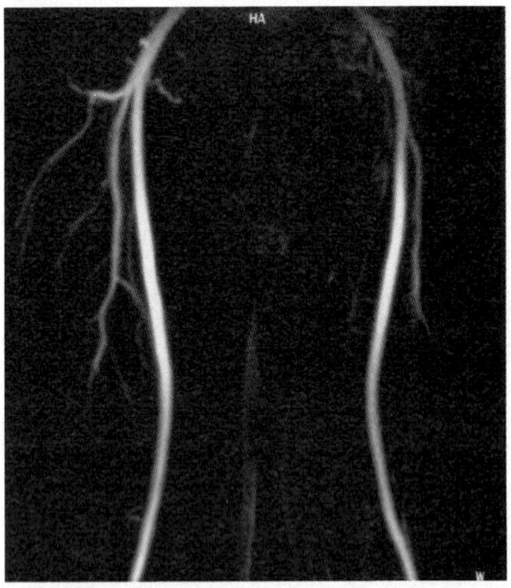

a.

Figure 3. Total agreement between gadolinium-enhanced MR angiography and DSA studies. **(a)** Subtraction MIP MR angiogram (5/2, 50° flip angle) of the first anatomic area after administration of 0.075 mmol/kg of gadopentetate dimeglumine shows no disease. **(b, c)** DSA images of the same area, with use of selective injections of contrast material in the left leg, show no disease in the superficial femoral or popliteal arteries. **(d)** Subtraction MIP MR angiogram of the second (lower) area acquired after administration of 0.1 mmol/kg gadopentetate dimeglumine shows low-grade stenoses (<50%) at the origin of the peroneal artery (arrow) and at the anomalous origin of the posterior tibial artery (arrowhead). There is an occlusion in the mid-posterior tibial artery. **(e)** DSA image shows findings noted in **d**.

images were reviewed. Agreement on treatments chosen with gadolinium-enhanced MR angiography and DSA studies of each anatomic area was then scored on a four-point scale (Table 1): none, partial, essential, and total. In cases of no or partial agreement, the treatment chosen with DSA was different from that selected with MR angiography; however, in cases of essential or total agreement, treatment options were identical.

Statistical Analysis

A truth table was constructed on the basis of the severity and likely clinical significance of disease: positive = greater than 50% stenoses and occlusions, and negative = 50% or less stenoses and normal vessels. DSA results were assumed to provide the true disease state. Sensitivity, specificity, positive predictive value, negative predictive value, and accuracy of gadolinium-enhanced MR angiography were calculated (including the exact confidence interval [CI] for each of these values). The CI was calculated with the assumption of independence of anatomic sites in a patient.

RESULTS

Gadolinium-enhanced MR angiography provided diagnostic results in all 15 patients. In a single anatomic area, however, the MR angiography findings were considered nondiagnostic and the study of this area was excluded from further consideration. In this case, there was insufficient enhancement of the infrapopliteal vessels on MR angiography images to allow confident therapeutic decisions in a patient whose DSA study showed multilevel, severe occlusive disease. Results in the 29 other anatomic areas are summarized in Tables 2–4. In two cases, the second acquisition after gadopentetate dimeglumine administration was used for the MIP reconstructed images. In one of these cases, venous enhancement was prominent but did not impair diagnostic accuracy.

A total of 150 imaged anatomic segments were compared; in 59 (39%) segments, images showed at least some disease (Table 2). Gadolinium-enhanced MR angiography enabled distinction of high-grade from low-grade disease with a sensitivity of 0.97 (95% CI: 0.86, 1.00), a specificity of 0.96 (95% CI: 0.91, 0.99), a positive predictive value of 0.90 (95% CI: 0.77, 0.97), a negative predictive value of 0.99 (95% CI: 0.95, 1.00), and an accuracy of 0.97 (95% CI: 0.92, 0.99) (Table 3).

There was total agreement on treatment determined with DSA and gadolinium-enhanced MR angiography in 140 (93%) of the 150 segments and in 49 (84%) of 59 diseased segments (Table 4). There was total or essential

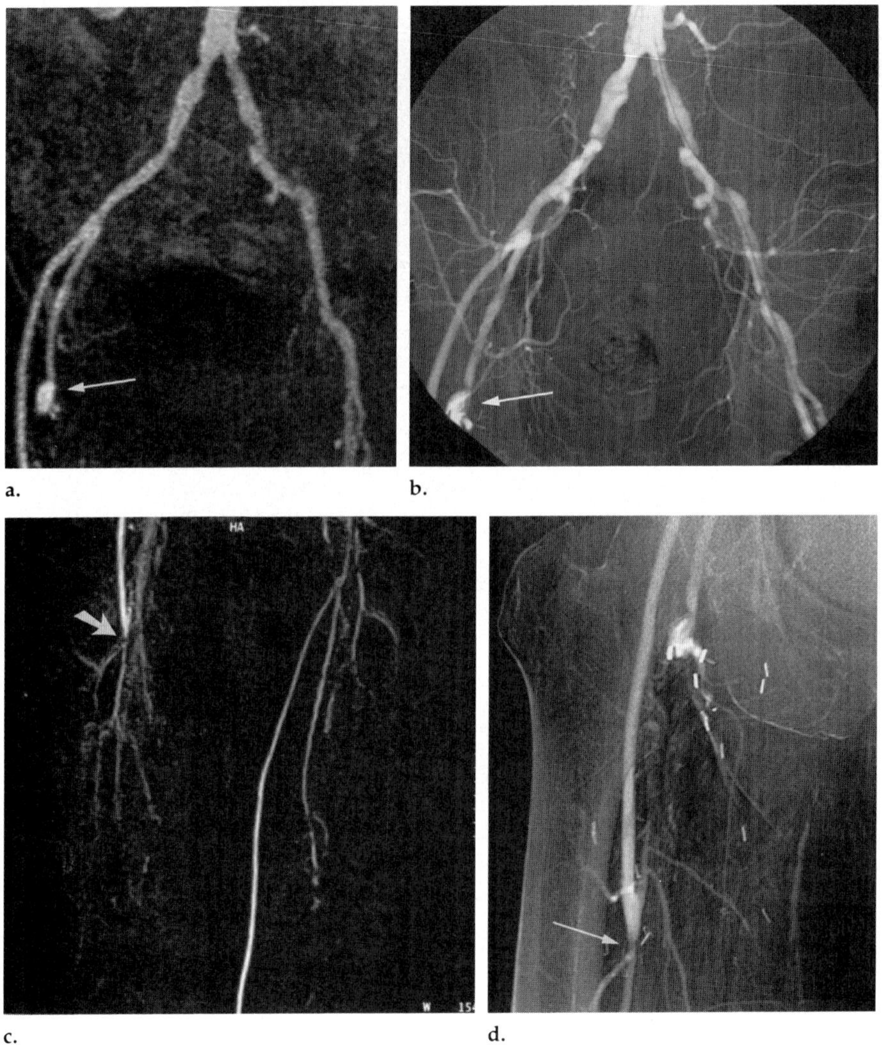

Figure 4. Total and partial agreement between gadolinium-enhanced MR angiography and DSA studies. **(a)** Subtraction MIP MR angiogram (5/2, 50° flip angle) acquired after administration of 0.075 mmol/kg gadopentetate dimeglumine shows multiple atherosclerotic plaques in the first anatomic area. The remnant of a failed graft (arrow) is noted. **(b)** DSA image of the same area shows similar extent of disease and the failed graft remnant (arrow). **(c)** Subtraction MIP MR angiogram (5/2, 50° flip angle) of the second anatomic area acquired after administration of 0.1 mmol/kg gadopentetate dimeglumine shows a high-grade (>50%) stenosis (arrow) at an anastomotic site. **(d)** DSA image of the anastomotic site (arrow) in **c** shows no substantial disease. In the region of the anastomosis, there are multiple surgical clips, which may have resulted in loss of signal intensity on the MR angiogram.

agreement on treatment in 146 (97%) of the 150 segments and in 55 (93%) of 59 diseased segments (Figs 1–3). Agreement on treatment occurred in all segments that were free of disease.

With gadolinium-enhanced MR angiography, severity of disease was overestimated in seven segments and underestimated in three. Among the seven segments in which disease was overestimated, different treatments were selected in four cases. In two of these four cases, diseased vessels had been treated before the study. In one of these segments treated before the study, a critical stenosis that would have prompted surgical exploration was identified at an anastomotic site. In this case, DSA showed much less severe stenosis, which was thought to be clinically inconsequential (Fig 4), and partial agreement was scored. Numerous surgical clips were noted next to the anastomosis. In the other segment treated before the study, a susceptibility artifact from an iliac Palmaz stent (Johnson & Johnson, New Brunswick, NJ) appeared as complete iliac artery occlusion on gadolinium-enhanced MR angiography images; on DSA images, the artery was patent (Fig 5).

DISCUSSION

In this study, the cumulative dose of gadolinium chelate was less than that most investigators currently use for gadolinium-enhanced MR angiography of a single anatomic area. Higher doses have been recommended to reduce the relaxation time of signal from blood to below that of fat and obtain satisfactory contrast between blood and fat on the angiogram (20). The success of our lower doses was largely because we used acquisitions that were more rapid than the 3–4-minute acquisitions originally used by Prince (20). During much of a long acquisition, gadolinium chelates will be distributed nearly uniformly in blood, and therefore, the contrast material will be relatively dilute. Most of our image data were acquired during the first pass of the bolus when concentration of gadopentetate dimeglumine (and hence signal) was much greater. Improved results with rapid acquisitions have been previously reported (7,17,19). Rapid acquisitions, however, necessitate fast imaging sequences and relatively high-performance gradient systems.

A second possible reason for our success with low-dose gadolinium-enhanced MR angiography is the use of subtraction to improve background suppression. Subtraction has been useful in gadolinium-enhanced MR angiography (8,10); use of subtraction is critical when additional anatomic areas are studied with residual contrast material in the veins. When subtraction techniques are employed, there is the possibility that data will be misregistered; misregistration of data is usually caused by physiologic motion or repositioning of the patient between acquisitions before and after administration of contrast material. In this study, the short duration of the acquisitions facilitated reproducibility, and most studies of anatomic areas were not affected by respiratory motion. These factors contributed to the production of high-quality subtraction images.

Korosec et al (18) suggested that all image data should be acquired in the short window between arterial and venous enhancement to avoid venous imaging. Although our acquisitions were somewhat longer than the time between arterial and venous enhancement, we saw minimal signal intensity in veins. Two different factors probably reduced venous signal intensity. First, before venous enhancement, the central k-space lines were acquired, which results in partial suppression of the venous signal. Second, the bolus of gadopentetate dimeglumine is diluted as it passes through the capillary bed; this dilution reduces venous enhancement. We suspect our relatively low doses of gadopentetate dimeglumine contributed to relatively greater dilution.

Doses of gadolinium chelates as high as 0.3 mmol/kg have been used without increased frequency of adverse reactions (13,21–24). Increasing the dose from 0.1 to 0.3 mmol/kg increases contrast between arteries and background; therefore, increased doses may heighten diagnostic accuracy. The relationship between size of dose and diagnostic accuracy, however, has not been established. Despite the apparent safety of high doses of gadolinium chelates, there are several reasons for minimizing the dose. First, more anatomic areas can be studied with use of a dose range that has been proved safe. Although not required in this study, additional doses could be used to repeat acquisitions because initial acquisitions are unsatisfactory (eg, as a result of patient movement). Second, background signal increases as gadolinium chelate moves into the extracellular spaces. Small doses will minimize this effect, and contrast between arteries and background tissue will be improved on subsequent images. Third, as mentioned, low doses may reduce venous signal. Finally, the use of low doses reduces the cost of the examination. The minimum useful dose remains to be determined, and we are investigating the utility of doses that are lower than those used in this study. The optimum and minimum time between consecutive administrations of contrast material also must be determined.

Earls et al (19) used a dose of gadopentetate dimeglumine more efficiently with a timing run. In their study, a small test bolus (1 mL) of gadopentetate dimeglumine was injected mechanically, and the aorta was imaged repeatedly with a rapid two-dimensional sequence. The arrival time of contrast material in the aorta was then determined. With knowledge of the transit time of the contrast material, the time of data acquisition was synchronized with that of the injection, and arterial enhancement was optimized. This approach, however, was not used in our study because our data were acquired before the timing-run method was developed. We were therefore unable to account for the variability in the circulation times and cardiovascular dynamics. We expect to further improve image quality and reliability with the use of a timing run or an automated triggering of the data acquisition (25).

In this study, we used exclusively gadopentetate dimeglumine. Achieving similar results, however, should be possible with any of the other gadolinium chelates that have been approved by the Food and Drug Administration; the relaxivities of the gadolinium chelates in water and citrated human plasma have been shown to be very similar (26).

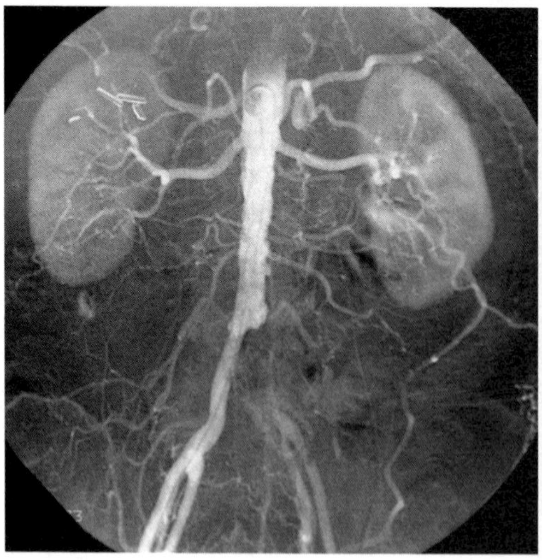

b.

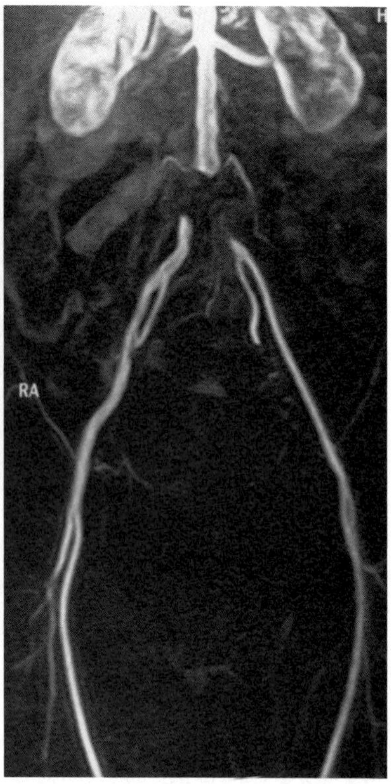

a.

Figure 5. No agreement between MR angiography and DSA studies of a vascular area with a common iliac artery stent. **(a)** Subtraction MIP MR angiogram (5/2, 50° flip angle) acquired after administration of 0.075 mmol/kg gadopentetate dimeglumine shows bilateral occlusions of short segments of the common iliac arteries. **(b)** DSA image of the same area shows a widely patent right common iliac artery; image quality is unaffected by the stent material. There was total agreement with recognition of the short-segment occlusion in the left common iliac artery.

For a complete peripheral runoff study, it is necessary to evaluate more than the two anatomic areas we imaged in this study. In three cases in our study, gadolinium-enhanced MR angiography was used to evaluate the infrapopliteal vessels. In the single nondiagnostic study, we attempted to evaluate severely diseased infrapopliteal vessels. Distal vessels are the most difficult to study with gadolinium-enhanced MR angiography; in these vessels, the concentration of contrast material is reduced and the arrival time of the bolus may be delayed, particularly if proximal vessels are diseased. Delay of contrast material, a problem in catheter-based angiography techniques, may lead to an erroneous diagnosis of vascular occlusive disease (27–29). The use of a timing run, as described, would probably improve gadolinium-enhanced MR angiography of more distal vessels. Nonetheless, there may be advantages with use of time-of-flight MR angiography of these vessels; this technique is dependent only on blood flow in the immediate vicinity of the region imaged (1,2,30,31). The potential time savings, however, that are achievable with coronal or sagittal acquisitions provide motivation for optimizing use of gadolinium-enhanced MR angiography in this anatomic area.

Therapeutic options are best made with the results of a complete evaluation. Severe, diffuse, distal peripheral vascular disease can render a more proximal high-grade stenosis clinically irrelevant. For example, in one case (Fig 2) an essential agreement was scored when the gadolinium-enhanced MR angiogram showed a high-grade (>50%) stenosis in the popliteal artery that was judged to be low grade (≤50%) on the DSA image. Owing to the severity of more distal disease, this discrepancy was not therapeutically relevant. Inclusion of this case diminished the specificity, positive predictive value, and accuracy calculated.

In two cases in which therapeutic disagreement occurred, prior treatment had been administered. In one of these cases, an indwelling vascular stent caused a susceptibility artifact, which resulted in the artifactual appearance of complete occlusion. In this case, the susceptibility artifact was apparent at retrospective review of the source images. In the other case, a therapeutically relevant overestimation of disease at an anastomotic site where multiple surgical clips were present was determined with gadolinium-enhanced MR angiography. Susceptibility artifacts at this site may have contributed to artifactual loss of signal intensity. Therefore, when evaluating the use of gadolinium-enhanced MR angiography, a patient history of intervention must be considered and evaluation of the source images may preclude overestimation of disease caused by artifact. A study of the likelihood of various vascular stents and surgical clips to generate artifact would be useful.

There were several limitations in this study. Selection of anatomic areas with disease introduced potential bias; reviewers knew disease was present in at least one anatomic segment. On the other hand, many anatomic areas included normal and diseased segments, and our results indicated that accurate discrimination of normal and diseased segments is possible. Because only two anatomic areas were evaluated in our study, the therapeutic options were selected with partial information.

Despite these limitations, the results are, nonetheless, encouraging. With a consensus review, we minimized interpretation errors that may result from relative inexperience in interpreting MR angiography or vascular studies. Specialists with expertise in interpreting MR angiography studies may not have a complete knowledge of the intricacies and implications of certain findings when evaluating peripheral vascular disease. Likewise, specialists with expertise in interpreting DSA studies may not be skilled in interpreting MR studies. Nonetheless, a randomized, blinded, prospective comparison of DSA with gadolinium-enhanced MR angiography is needed to confirm our results.

Finally, the use of DSA as a standard of reference and the exclusive use of MIP data in gadolinium-enhanced MR angiography may pose certain limitations. Gadolinium-enhanced MR angiography offers alternative perspectives and cross-sectional data for interpretation; these features were not used fully in this study, and they may provide information that resolves different findings on DSA images. Indeed, gadolinium-enhanced MR angiography may have advantages over DSA. For example, with gadolinium-enhanced MR angiography, the appearance of overlapping vessels that obscures disease sites can be eliminated. In future comparative studies, examination of arterial pressures, intraoperative findings, and use of additional DSA views at sites with discrepant findings may clarify the function of MR angiography.

In conclusion, we demonstrated the potential of gadolinium-enhanced MR angiography with lower doses of contrast material to enable evaluation of peripheral vascular disease. Reduction in examination times may make comprehensive MR angiography of multiple areas of the lower extremity vasculature more feasible. ■

Acknowledgments: We acknowledge the efforts of Douglas R. DeCorato, MD, James P. Earls, MD, Peter Schlossberg, MD, and Jeff Stevenson, BS, and the collaborative assistance of Patrick Lamparello, MD, Thomas S. Riles, MD, and Gary Giangola, MD. We thank Wayne Holyoak, PhD, for statistical assistance.

References

1. Glickerman DJ, Obregon RG, Schmiedl UP, et al. Cardiac gated MR angiography of the entire lower extremity: a prospective comparison with conventional angiography. AJR 1996; 167:445–451.
2. Baum RA, Rutter CM, Sunshine JH, et al. Multicenter trial to evaluate vascular magnetic resonance angiography of the lower extremity. JAMA 1995; 274:875–880.
3. Yucel E, Kaufman J, Geller S, et al. Prospective evaluation of two-dimensional time-of-flight MR angiography in lower extremely atherosclerotic occlusive disease. Radiology 1993; 187:637–641.
4. Prince MR. Gadolinium-enhanced MR angiography. Radiology 1994; 191:155–164.
5. Tartaro A, Severini S, Tonni G, Magarelli N, Carriero A, Bonomo L. Magnetic resonance angiography with gadolinium (Gd-DTPA) versus baseline magnetic resonance angiography in the study of the intracranial circulation. Radiol Med (Torino) 1992; 84:536–543.
6. Prince MR, Narasimham DL, Stanley JC, et al. Gadolinium-enhanced magnetic resonance angiography of abdominal aortic aneurysms. J Vasc Surg 1995; 21:656–669.
7. Prince MR, Narasimham DL, Stanley JC, et al. Breath-hold gadolinium-enhanced MR angiography of the abdominal aorta and its major branches. Radiology 1995; 197:785–792.
8. Adamis MK, Li W, Wielopolski PA, et al. Dynamic contrast-enhanced subtraction MR angiography of the lower extremities: initial evaluation with a multisection two-dimensional time-of-flight sequence. Radiology 1995; 196:689–695.
9. Snidow JJ, Aisen AM, Harris VJ, et al. Iliac artery MR angiography: comparison of three-dimensional gadolinium-enhanced and two-dimensional time-of-flight techniques. Radiology 1995; 196:371–378.
10. Douek PC, Revel D, Chazel S, Falise B, Villard J, Amiel M. Fast MR angiography of the aortoiliac arteries and arteries of the lower extremity: value of bolus-enhanced, whole-volume subtraction technique. AJR 1995; 165:431–437.
11. Krinsky G, Rofsky NM, DeCorato DR, et al. Thoracic aorta: comparison of gadolinium-enhanced three-dimensional MR angiography with conventional MR imaging. Radiology 1997; 202:183–193.
12. Nelson KL, Gifford LM, Lauber-Huber C, Gross CA, Lasser TA. Clinical safety of gadopentetate dimeglumine. Radiology 1995; 196:439–443.
13. Prince MR, Arnoldus C, Frisoli JK. Nephrotoxicity of high dose gadolinium compared with iodinated contrast. JMRI 1996; 6:162–166.
14. Rofsky NM, Weinreb JC, Bosniak MA, Libes RB, Birnbaum BA. Renal lesion characterization with gadolinium-enhanced MR imaging: efficacy and safety in patients with renal insufficiency. Radiology 1991; 180:85–89.
15. Haustein J, Niendorf HP, Krestin G. Renal tolerance of gadolinium-DTPA/dimeglumine in patients with chronic renal failure. Invest Radiol 1992; 27:153.
16. Niendorf HP, Haustein J, Cornelius I, Alhassan A, Clauss W. Safety of gadolinium-DTPA: extended clinical experience. Magn Reson Med 1991; 22:222–228.
17. Holland GA, Dougherty L, Carpenter JP, et al. Breath-hold ultrafast three-dimensional gadolinium-enhanced MR angiography of the aorta and the renal and other visceral abdominal arteries. AJR 1996; 166:971–981.
18. Korosec FR, Frayne R, Grist TM, Mistretta CA. Time-resolved contrast-enhanced 3D MR angiography. Magn Reson Med 1996; 36:345–351.
19. Earls JP, Rofsky NM, DeCorato DA, Krinsky GK, Weinreb JC. Breath-hold single-dose gadolinium-enhanced three-dimensional MR aortography: usefulness of a timing examination and MR power injector. Radiology 1996; 201:705–710.
20. Prince MR. Body MR angiography with gadolinium contrast agents. Magn Reson Imaging Clin N Am 1996; 4:11–24.
21. Nelson KL, Gifford LM, Lauber-Huber C, Gross CA, Lasser TA. Clinical safety of gadopentetate dimeglumine. Radiology 1995; 196:439–443.
22. Yuh WT, Fisher DJ, Runge VM, et al. Phase III multicenter trial of high-dose gadoteridol in MR evaluation of brain metastases. AJNR 1994; 15:1037–1051.
23. Niendorf HP, Haustein J, Louton T, Beck W, Laniado M. Safety and tolerance after intravenous administration of 0.3 mmol/kg Gd-DTPA: results of a randomized, controlled clinical trial. Invest Radiol 1991; 26(suppl 1):221–223; discussion 232–235.
24. Runge VM, Wells JW. Update: safety, new applications, new MR agents. Top Magn Reson Imaging 1995; 7:181–195.
25. Foo TKF, Saranathan M, Prince MR, Chenevert TL. Automated detection of bolus arrival and initiation of data acquisition in fast, three-dimensional, gadolinium-enhanced MR angiography. Radiology 1997; 203:275–280.
26. Tweedle MF. Physiochemical properties of gadoteridol and other magnetic resonance contrast agents. Invest Radiol 1992; 27(suppl):2–6.
27. Dardik H, Miller N, Adler J, et al. Primary and adjunctive intra-arterial digital subtraction arteriography of the lower extremities. J Vasc Surg 1986; 3:599–604.
28. Kahn PC, Boyer DN, Moran JM, et al. Reactive hyperemia in lower extremity arteriography: an evaluation. Radiology 1968; 90:975–980.
29. Oser RF, Picus D, Hicks ME, Darcy MD, Hovsepian DM. Accuracy of DSA in the evaluation of patency of infrapopliteal vessels. JVIR 1995; 6:589–594.
30. Owen RS, Carpenter JP, Baum RA, Perloff LJ, Cope C. Magnetic resonance imaging of angiographically occult runoff vessels in peripheral arterial occlusive disease. N Engl J Med 1992; 326:1577–1581.
31. Cortell ED, Kaufman SC, Cambria RP, Rivitz SM, Waltman AC. MR angiography of the tibial runoff vessels: imaging with the head coil compared with conventional arteriography. AJR 1996; 167:147–151.

Joseph A. Prahlow, MD • Timothy J. O'Bryant, MD • Jeffrey J. Barnard, MD

Cardiac Perforation Due to Wallstent Embolization: A Fatal Complication of the Transjugular Intrahepatic Portosystemic Shunt Procedure[1]

The transjugular intrahepatic portosystemic shunt procedure is an effective intervention for patients with bleeding esophageal varices. Potential complications are numerous but rarely serious. A case of hemopericardium, cardiac tamponade, and death caused by perforation of the right atrium and aorta by a stent after embolization from the liver during stent placement is reported.

Index terms: Esophagus, varices, 71.75 • Esophagus, interventional procedure, 71.1267 • Shunts, portosystemic, 958.453 • Stents and prostheses, 958.1268 • Surgery, complications, 521.458

Radiology 1997; 205:170–172

THE transjugular intrahepatic portosystemic shunt (TIPS) procedure is an effective and relatively safe nonsurgical intervention in patients with bleeding esophageal varices (1–9). When long-term complications such as hepatic encephalopathy and delayed stent stenosis or occlusion are excluded, the overall complication rate associated with TIPS creation is less than 10% (5,9). The mortality rate is less than 2%, with most deaths attributed to intraperitoneal hemorrhage after puncture of the portal vein or the liver capsule (5,6). We report an unexpected technical complication of a TIPS procedure that resulted in death.

CASE REPORT

A 39-year-old man with a history of chronic alcoholism presented at the emergency room with a 12-hour history of hematemesis and melena. At physical examination, scleral icterus and splenomegaly were noted. The patient's laboratory data were as follows: hemoglobin level, 12.4 g/dL (7.7 mmol/L) (mild anemia); platelet count, 133×10^3 cells per cubic millimeter (133×10^9/L); prothrombin time, 14.4 seconds; partial thromboplastin time, 34.2 seconds; albumin level, 3.3 g/dL (33 g/L); total bilirubin level, 1.7 mg/dL (38 μmol/L); aspartate aminotransferase level, 97 U/L; alanine aminotransferase level, 58 U/L, γ-glutamyltransferase level, 1,211 U/L; and alkaline phosphatase level, 248 U/L. At endoscopy, numerous nonbleeding esophageal varices and evidence of actively bleeding portal venous hypertensive gastropathy were seen. The dominant varix was treated with sclerotherapy, and adjunctive intravenous therapy was begun. The patient continued to bleed slowly despite medical and repeated endoscopic therapy, and the interventional radiology department was consulted for consideration of a TIPS procedure. At ultrasonography, patent portal and hepatic veins and splenomegaly were seen.

On the 4th day, the patient underwent an elective TIPS procedure, which was performed in the standard fashion by an experienced operator (T.J.O.) who had performed approximately 60 previous TIPS procedures. The procedure went well at first. Selective catheter placement was performed in the middle hepatic vein, and a 10-F sheath (Cook, Bloomington, Ind) was inserted. A Colopinto needle (Cook) and a long, 21-gauge needle (Cook) were used coaxially to puncture a branch of the right portal vein. A 0.018-inch-diameter wire was passed into the portal vein, and a diagnostic catheter was inserted.

Portal venographic findings confirmed the presence of gastric and esophageal varices (Fig 1). The portal venous anatomy was otherwise normal. Portal vein pressure was 30 mm Hg, and mean right atrial pressure was 8 mm Hg. The tract was dilated with an 8-mm balloon (Ultrathin; Medi-tech/Boston Scientific, Watertown, Mass), and the appropriate stent length was measured by using a guide wire from the right portal vein to the middle hepatic vein near the vena cava. The measurement was approximately 10 cm, and a 12-mm-diameter by 90-mm-long Wallstent (Schneider, Minneapolis, Minn) was deployed from the right portal vein to the vena cava. The stent was constricted at the portal vein wall and initially extended farther superiorly than desired. It was thought that optimal positioning of the upper end would be achieved with dilation, which was performed first with the 8-mm balloon and then with a 12 × 40-mm balloon (Blue Max; Medi-tech/Boston Scientific) (Fig 2).

At this point, fluoroscopic monitoring demonstrated that the stent was in good position. An attempt was made to pass the sheath over the balloon, but despite efforts that included aspiration with a large syringe, reinflation and deflation of the balloon, and pushing of the sheath to the point of buckling, the sheath would not completely cover the balloon. An attempt was then made to remove the partially covered balloon. The balloon was rotated during removal but nonetheless caught on the upper end of the stent, which protruded just into the vena cava, and displaced the stent by approximately 2–3 cm.

It was believed that the procedure could be salvaged by removing the stent and replacing it with another. The balloon was advanced and then withdrawn; however, it caught again and pulled the stent all the way into the right atrium before it slid free. An Amplatz Superstiff guide wire (Medi-tech/Boston Scientific) remained in place through the stent lumen and across the shunt tract, and the balloon and sheath were removed together. A new sheath was inserted to begin the process of stent retrieval, but the patient suddenly had a seizure and became hypotensive and cyanotic. Emergent resuscitation efforts were begun. Intubation was performed and advanced cardiac life-support measures were initiated. The electrocardiogram showed sinus tachycardia, which suggested electromechanical dissociation. At fluoroscopic evaluation of the chest, the endotracheal tube was seen in the midtrachea, and minimal contraction of the right atrium on the stent, which was pinned between the upper aspect of the atrium and the hepatic vein and was held in place by the wire, was noted. The wire was removed to allow the stent to move. A cardiologist attempted pericardiocentesis but obtained only 1–2 mL of fluid during each of three passes. During these efforts, the question was raised as to whether the stent was causing dysrhythmia. The right femoral vein was punctured, and a 25-mm loop snare (Microvena, White Bear Lake, Minn)

[1] From the Southwestern Institute of Forensic Sciences and the Department of Pathology, University of Texas–Southwestern Medical Center, 5230 Medical Center Dr, Dallas, TX 75235 (J.A.P., J.J.B.); and the Department of Radiology, Medical City Hospital, Dallas, Tex (T.J.O.). Received November 8, 1996; revision requested January 3, 1997; revision received May 14; accepted June 16. **Address reprint requests to** J.A.P.

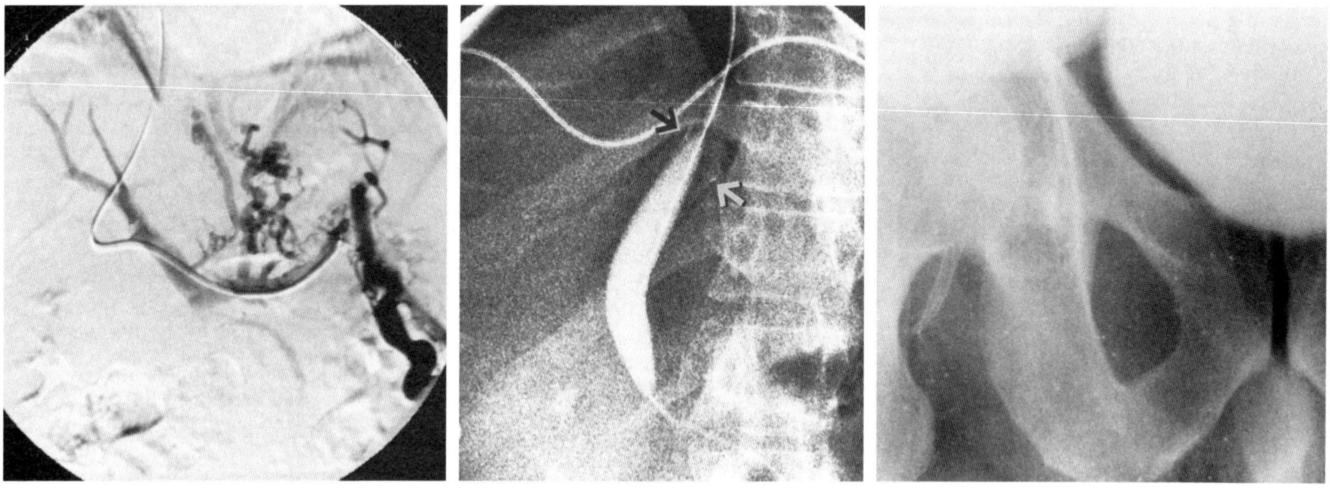

1. 2. 3.

Figures 1–3. **(1)** Digital subtraction image from a portal venogram shows varices, patent splenic and portal veins, and occlusion of the right portal vein beyond the puncture site. **(2)** Fluoroscopic image shows the Wallstent during dilation with a 12-mm-diameter Blue Max balloon. Arrows = superior end of the stent. **(3)** Postmortem radiograph of the right pelvis shows the lower end of the Wallstent crushed by the loop snare used to withdraw it from the heart.

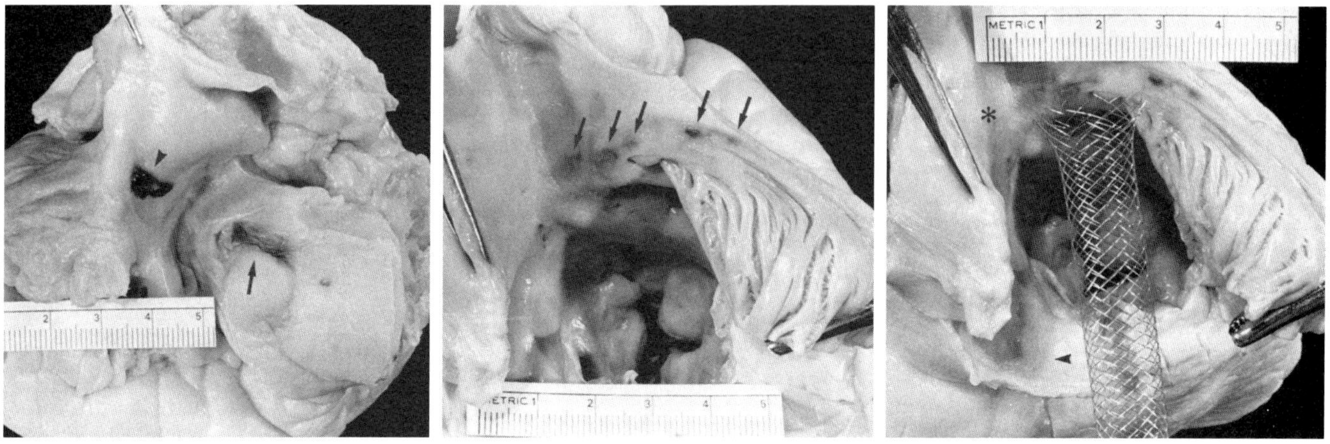

4. 5. 6.

Figures 4–6. **(4)** Cephalocaudal view of the heart at autopsy shows areas of hemorrhage associated with perforations of the right atrium (arrowhead) and aorta (arrow). **(5)** Internal view of the opened right atrium, obtained at autopsy, shows numerous endocardial injuries (arrows). **(6)** Internal view of the opened right atrium shows numerous endocardial injuries adjacent to the proximal end of the Wallstent. Note the inferior vena cava (arrowhead) and superior vena cava (*).

was passed around the lower end of the stent, which was constricted and withdrawn into the iliac vein and left in place. Further efforts at revival were unsuccessful, and the patient died.

Because this death occurred during a medical procedure, it was reported to the medical examiner. An autopsy was performed at the Southwestern Institute of Forensic Sciences in Dallas, Texas, and a postmortem radiograph of the pelvis showed the Wallstent in the right iliofemoral region (Fig 3). At internal examination, advanced cirrhosis, esophageal varices, and massive hemopericardium (600 mL) were seen. No injuries were seen at examination of the apex of the heart; at dissection of the soft tissues of the anterior chest wall, it was noted that the pericardiocentesis punctures did not enter the pericardial sac. A small puncture wound with an adherent epicardial blood clot was seen on the medial aspect of the right atrium just under the auricle (Fig 4). Another puncture wound was noted in the wall of the ascending aorta adjacent to the right atrial wound (Fig 4). Multiple endocardial puncture wounds were seen at internal examination of the right atrium (Fig 5).

Sections of the cirrhotic liver showed an intraparenchymal portosystemic shunt track. The stent was recovered from the right iliofemoral vein. By placing the proximal end of the stent next to the right atrial endocardial injuries, we confirmed that the puncture wounds resulted from the sharp ends of the stent wires (Fig 6).

On the basis of autopsy findings and review of the medical records, the cause of death was determined to be hemopericardium with cardiac tamponade due to perforation of the right atrium and aorta by the Wallstent.

DISCUSSION

The TIPS procedure is an effective and reliable method for decreasing portal venous pressure and controlling variceal bleeding in patients with portal hypertension who fail to respond to endoscopic sclerotherapy (1–9). The TIPS procedure is also beneficial in alleviating ascites (2,4,6) and the hepatorenal syndrome (4) and is useful as a "bridge" to liver transplantation (3,4,6,10).

The stent most commonly used in the United States for creation of a TIPS is the 10-mm-diameter Wallstent. The 12-mm-diameter Wallstent had just been made available for use in the United States at the time this procedure was performed, and it was thought that a larger-diameter shunt might reduce the risk of intrashunt stenosis and thus reduce the need for future intervention. This has since been reported (11) not to be the case. The 12-mm-diameter stent is no longer used for TIPS creation by the author (T.J.O.) or at his institution.

Wallstent migration is unusual because the radial force and the flared ends of the stent contribute to stability (5; manufacturer's recommendation, Schneider). In this case, the stent was protruding just into the vena cava; thus, the fixation mechanism on that end was lacking. The "wings" of the balloon caught on the free end of the stent and dislodged it, but the balloon seemed to pull free as soon as the stent came most of the way out. We believe that when the stent lodged between the upper atrium and the hepatic vein orifice and was held in place by the guide wire, the contraction of the heart on the stent may have caused the perforation. The underlying problem was the inability to cover the balloon with the sheath before removal, despite the use of a 10-F sheath over a balloon on a 7-F shaft. The operator (T.J.O.) strongly believes that had coverage of the balloon with the sheath been accomplished before withdrawal, there would have been no adverse outcome.

Stent dislodgement with subsequent embolization has been reported (2,5,7,8, 10,12) several times and can occur during the procedure or later. Embolization to the right atrium (10,12), the pulmonary artery (2,8), and the internal jugular vein (7) have been reported. Except in one patient with pulmonary artery embolization, who experienced vague, right-sided pulmonary symptoms (2), stent migration has produced no serious sequelae (5,7,8,10,12–16). Stent migration is reportedly (5) less common with the Wallstent because it is longer and exerts self-restraining, radial forces.

This case represents a serious complication of stent migration that, to our knowledge, has been previously unreported. The wire tips at the ends of the Wallstent endoprosthesis are quite sharp, presumably to assist in lodging of the stent in the vessels and tissues during deployment. Unfortunately, exposed wire tips can penetrate vascular walls and cause perforation and subsequent bleeding. In this case, one of the stent wires perforated the right atrium and the ascending aorta, which resulted in hemopericardium and cardiac tamponade. Several other wire tips penetrated, but did not perforate, the right atrial endothelium. The proximity of these injuries to the sinoatrial node suggested that the stent might have induced some sort of arrhythmia; however, the continuous electrocardiographic tracing showed only tachycardia before cardiac arrest occurred.

The TIPS procedure is an effective, reliable, and relatively safe intervention in patients with portal venous hypertension. Several complications can occur, but most are not serious. Previously, stent migration to the right atrium was reported (10,12) to be more of an inconvenience than a potentially life-threatening complication. Perforation of the heart with subsequent bleeding and arrhythmia may result after Wallstent migration. This case alerts the reader to a potentially lethal complication of the TIPS procedure. ■

Acknowledgment: The authors thank Bette Porter for her professional assistance with the photographs in this report.

References

1. Richter GM, Noeldge G, Palmaz JC, et al. Transjugular intrahepatic portacaval stent shunt: preliminary clinical results. Radiology 1990; 174:1027–1030.
2. Zemel G, Katzen BT, Becker GJ, Benenati JF, Sailee DS. Percutaneous transjugular portosystemic shunt. JAMA 1991; 266:390–393.
3. Ring EJ, Lake JR, Roberts JP, et al. Using transjugular intrahepatic portosystemic shunts to control variceal bleeding before liver transplantation. Ann Intern Med 1992; 116:304–309.
4. LaBerge JM, Ring EJ, Gordon RL, et al. Creation of transjugular intrahepatic portosystemic shunts with the Wallstent endoprosthesis: results in 100 patients. Radiology 1993; 187:413–420.
5. Freedman AM, Sanyal AJ, Tisnado J, et al. Complications of transjugular intrahepatic portosystemic shunt: a comprehensive review. RadioGraphics 1993; 13:1185–1210.
6. Miller-Catchpole R. Transjugular intrahepatic portosystemic shunt (TIPS): diagnostic and therapeutic technology assessment (DATTA). JAMA 1995; 273:1824–1830.
7. Rogers CG, Paolini RM, O'Leary JP. Intrahepatic vascular shunting for portal hypertension: early experience with the transjugular intrahepatic porto-systemic shunt. Am Surg 1994; 60:114–117.
8. Rossle M, Haag K, Ochs A, et al. The transjugular intrahepatic portosystemic stent-shunt procedure for variceal bleeding. N Engl J Med 1994; 330:165–171.
9. Rossle M, Haag K, Blum HE. The transjugular intrahepatic portosystemic stent-shunt: a review of the literature and own experience. J Gastroenterol Hepatol 1996; 11:293–298.
10. Freeman RB, FitzMaurice SE, Greenfield AE, Halin N, Haug CE, Rohrer RJ. Is the transjugular intrahepatic portocaval shunt procedure beneficial for liver transplant recipients? Transplantation 1994; 58:297–300.
11. Kuhn-Fulton J, Trerotola SO, Harris VJ, et al. Transjugular intrahepatic portosystemic shunt procedure: efficacy of 10-mm versus 12-mm Wallstents. Radiology 1996; 199:658–664.
12. Valji K, Bookstein JJ, Roberts AC, Oglevie SB, Royster AP, Varney RR. Overdilation of the Wallstent to optimize portal decompression during transjugular intrahepatic portosystemic shunt placement. Radiology 1994; 191:173–176.
13. Cekirge S, Foster RG, Weiss JP, McLean GK. Percutaneous removal of an embolized Wallstent during transjugular intrahepatic portosystemic shunt procedure. JVIR 1993; 4:559–560.
14. Cohen GS, Ball DS. Delayed Wallstent migration after transjugular intrahepatic portosystemic shunt procedure: relocation with a loop snare. JVIR 1993; 4:561–563.
15. Lipton M, Cynamon J, Bakal CW, Sprayregan S. Percutaneous retrieval of two Wallstent endoprostheses from the heart using a single jugular sheath. JVIR 1995; 6:469–472.
16. Hartnell GG, Crenshaw WB, Burger AJ, Hamer AW. Percutaneous removal of a fully expanded Wallstent from the right ventricle with transesophageal echocardiography guidance. JVIR 1996; 7:371–374.

Gwen K. Nazarian, MD • Haraldur Bjarnason, MD • Charles A. Dietz, Jr, MD • Casandra A. Bernadas, BS
Mary C. Foshager, MD • Hector Ferral, MD • David W. Hunter, MD

Refractory Ascites: Midterm Results of Treatment with a Transjugular Intrahepatic Portosystemic Shunt[1]

PURPOSE: **To assess midterm results and examine factors associated with successful treatment of refractory ascites with creation of a transjugular intrahepatic portosystemic shunt (TIPS).**

MATERIALS AND METHODS: **In 50 patients with refractory ascites, TIPS creation was performed. Clinical and ultrasound follow-up were performed. Success was defined as survival with no further therapeutic paracentesis and decreased ascites.**

RESULTS: **Mean follow-up was 11.6 months after the TIPS procedure. Major complications occurred in 16% of patients including intraperitoneal hemorrhage, refractory encephalopathy, and progression of liver and renal failure. Overall mortality was 60% (30 patients). In 23 (62%) of 37 patients not lost to follow-up, ascites was controlled successfully at 1–3 months. A bilirubin level greater than 3.0 mg/dL (52 μmol/L) and creatinine level greater than 1.9 mg/dL (170 μmol/L) were associated with treatment failure (86% treatment failure at 3 months) and early mortality (P = .03). In all 14 patients alive at 1-year follow-up, ascites was controlled successfully.**

CONCLUSION: **TIPS creation is often useful in treatment of severe ascites not controlled with medical therapy. In patients with advanced liver and renal failure, TIPS creation is not associated with a definite benefit and may hasten death.**

A decrease in the volume of ascitic fluid has been noted in patients with hemorrhagic portal hypertension who have undergone nonselective surgical placement of a portosystemic shunt (1–4) or a transjugular intrahepatic portosystemic shunt (TIPS) (5,6). In 1993, we reported our early results from evaluation of the use of TIPS in the treatment of refractory ascites (7). Since that communication, we have performed TIPS procedures in 36 additional patients for the treatment of refractory ascites.

The purpose of this study was to assess midterm results and examine factors that appear to be associated with the success or failure of TIPS creation for the treatment of refractory ascites. In addition, we compared our results with those reported by Crenshaw et al (8) and Ochs et al (9) on the use of TIPS creation for treatment of refractory ascites.

MATERIALS AND METHODS

From September 26, 1991, to November 16, 1995, 50 patients underwent creation of a TIPS for treatment of refractory ascites. The 29 male and 21 female patients ranged in age from 11 to 81 years (mean, 51 years). The causes of liver disease are shown in Table 1. Long-term alcohol abuse (n = 27) and previous viral infection (n = 11) were the most common causes of cirrhosis. Various clinical characteristics are listed in Table 2, including Child-Pugh classification (10). Five patients were treated previously with peritoneovenous shunts that were nonfunctional at examination performed before the TIPS procedure. Twenty-three (46%) patients previously had episodes of encephalopathy, all well controlled medically when the TIPS procedure was performed.

Only patients with severe ascites refractory to standard forms of treatment were included in this nonrandomized prospective trial, which was approved by the Institutional Review Board. Severe ascites that could not be controlled with diuretic therapy, owing to ineffectiveness of the diuretics or the adverse effect of the diuretics on renal function, was considered refractory to medical therapy. The primary care physician and the gastroenterologist at our institution agreed that the ascites could not be managed medically before a patient underwent TIPS creation. All patients entered into the study gave written informed consent to undergo the TIPS procedure. During the study period, all patients with refractory ascites treated at our institution underwent TIPS creation.

Exclusion criteria included electrocardiographic changes compatible with acute myocardial infarction, polycystic liver disease, bacterial peritonitis and positive ascitic fluid cultures, and/or malignant or tuberculous ascites. In addition, patients who refused to accept blood or blood products or were unable to give informed consent were excluded.

Preprocedural Care

A careful clinical history was obtained and physical examination was performed in the Medicine Clinic and at admission to

Index terms: Ascites, 761.77 • Interventional procedures, 761.1267, 95.453 • Liver, cirrhosis, 761.79 • Liver, interventional procedure, 761.1267, 95.453 • Shunts, portosystemic, 761.1267, 95.453

Abbreviation: TIPS = transjugular intrahepatic portosystemic shunt.

Radiology 1997; 205:173–180

[1] From the Department of Radiology, University of Minnesota School of Medicine, 420 Delaware St SE, Box 292 Mayo, Minneapolis, MN 55455-0391 (G.K.N., H.B., C.A.D., C.A.B., M.C.F., D.W.H.); and the Department of Radiology, Louisiana State University Medical Center, New Orleans (H.F.). From the 1996 RSNA scientific assembly. Received March 11, 1997; revision requested April 18; revision received June 9; accepted June 16. **Address reprint requests to** G.K.N.

the hospital. Special emphasis was placed on development of liver disease including a history of bleeding, ascites, and encephalopathy. In all patients, ascites was evaluated and determined refractory to medical management by the attending gastroenterologist. Encephalopathy was graded as follows: grade 1, confused; grade 2, drowsy; grade 3, stuporous; grade 4, coma. Laboratory tests included complete blood cell count, prothrombin time, partial thromboplastin time, bilirubin, albumin, aspartate transaminase, alanine transaminase, alkaline phosphatase, sodium, potassium, chloride, blood urea nitrogen, creatinine, and serum ammonia.

All patients underwent a thorough sonographic evaluation within 24 hours before the TIPS procedure to assess the amount of ascitic fluid, the appearance of the liver parenchyma, and the patency of the portal vein, hepatic veins, hepatic artery, and inferior vena cava. The views used to evaluate fluid volume were carefully standardized to include longitudinal and transverse scans in the right and left lower quadrants and in the right upper quadrant with the patient in the supine position and the transducer position between the anterior and midaxillary lines in the intercostal space. Imaging performed with these patient and transducer positions enabled the best depiction of the Morison pouch. The volume of ascitic fluid was classified as absent (grade 0), mild (grade 1), moderate (grade 2), or massive (grade 3).

Before the procedure, the coagulation status in each patient was corrected, if necessary, with transfusion of fresh frozen plasma or platelets or administration of vitamin K to bring the prothrombin time within the normal range if possible. The patients were also given fluid as indicated to reduce the risk of contrast material–induced nephrotoxicity. No prophylactic antibiotic agents were given. If the patients were extremely uncomfortable or dyspneic, ascitic fluid was drained the evening before or the morning of the procedure.

TIPS Procedure

In some cases, ascitic fluid was removed just before the TIPS procedure in an attempt to facilitate portal venous puncture. Thirteen patients underwent paracentesis during the TIPS procedure in an attempt to increase the angle between the inferior vena cava and the hepatic vein (to facilitate portal venous puncture) or improve their respiratory function. A mean of 3.7 L of ascitic fluid (range, 1.5–7.5 L) was removed.

The TIPS procedure was performed by using the flexible coaxial Rösch-Uchida transjugular access set (Cook, Bloomington, Ind) as described by Rösch et al (11). Wallstents (Schneider, Minneapolis, Minn), 10 or 12 mm in diameter, were used to open the tract. Procedures were performed after administration of local anesthetic (1% lidocaine hydrochloride, Abbott Laboratories, North Chicago, Ill) and intravenous administration of sedatives (fentanyl citrate, Elkins-Sinn, Cherry Hill, NJ; midazolam hydrocholride, Versed, Roche Laboratories, Nutley, NJ; or propofol, Diprivan, Zeneca Pharmaceuticals, Wilmington, Del) in 25 patients or general anesthesia in the other 25 patients. Portal venography and pressure gradient measurements were performed before completion of the procedure to confirm shunt patency and to evaluate the portosystemic gradient after the shunt was created.

The shunts were dilated to 8 mm in diameter with an 8-mm-diameter Blue-Max balloon (Medi-tech/Boston Scientific, Watertown, Mass), and no further dilation was performed unless the portosystemic gradient was 15 mm Hg or greater. If the gradient was 15 mm Hg or greater, the shunt was dilated to 10 mm in diameter. The goal was to keep the shunt diameter as small as possible to relieve portal hypertension while minimizing the risk of encephalopathy. For this reason, the optimal portosystemic gradient was considered slightly higher than the 10–12-mm Hg gradient sought for patients with variceal bleeding.

Postprocedural Care

Immediately after the TIPS procedure, 26 patients were admitted to the regular hospital unit and were discharged from the hospital 1–9 days (mean, 4.2 days) after the procedure. In two patients, extended hospitalization was necessary: in one patient because of liver transplantation, and in the other because of complications of end-stage endometrial carcinoma. Immediately after the procedure, 22 patients were admitted to the intensive care unit and were discharged 3–36 days (mean, 12.7 days) after the procedure. Sonographic evaluation was performed within 24 hours after the TIPS procedure to document shunt function and the volume of ascitic fluid and to assess for any immediate complications. At discharge, a low-protein (40–75 g/d), low-sodium (0.5–2.0 g/d) diet with fluid restriction (1.0–1.5 L/d) was prescribed.

Patients were followed up monthly in the gastroenterology clinic and interventional radiology department. A detailed history was obtained and physical examination was performed. In addition, laboratory tests and sonographic evaluation were performed at 1 month and then at 3-month intervals thereafter. The doses of diuretic agents and lactulose were adjusted by the attending physician. If patients did not return to the clinic as scheduled, contact was established by telephone with the patient or the primary physician in an attempt to ascertain the patient's clinical status. For analysis of shunt function, however, the nonreturning patients were considered lost to follow-up.

Sonographic studies were performed to evaluate changes in blood flow velocity in the shunt, vessel patency, and volume of ascitic fluid. Shunt malfunction was suggested if sonographic evaluation demonstrated (*a*) absence of blood flow within the shunt at color Doppler sonography, (*b*) blood flow less than 60 cm/sec throughout the entire shunt (12) for the first 3 years of the study (the cutoff was then increased to 100 cm/sec after interval review of data from our institution), (*c*) focal velocity elevation at the hepatic vein segment of the shunt 2.5 times or greater than the peak velocity in any other area in the shunt (12), (*d*) gradual or acute decrease in blood flow velocities in the shunt from that of previous ultrasound (US) examinations (typically greater than 80–100 cm/sec throughout the shunt) (13), (*e*) change in direction of intrahepatic portal venous blood flow from hepatofugal to hepatopedal (12,14,15), and/or (*f*) increase in volume of ascitic fluid over that found at previous examinations without a change in medications.

Table 1
Causes of Liver Disease

Cause	No. of Patients*
Long-term alcohol abuse	27
Previous viral infection	11
Toxin exposure	3
Primary biliary cirrhosis	2
Bridging fibrosis	1
Granulomatous liver disease	1
Veno-occlusive disease after bone marrow transplantation	1
Sclerosing cholangitis	1
Biliary atresia	1
Budd-Chiari syndrome	1
Cryptogenic	7

* Five patients had a history of long-term alcohol abuse and viral hepatitis, and one patient had a history of long-term alcohol abuse and toxin exposure.

Angiographic evaluation of the shunt was performed initially at 6-month intervals during the 1st year of the study and when US findings suggested shunt malfunction after the 1st year. Shunt stenoses seen on follow-up angiograms that were associated with a portosystemic gradient of 15 mm Hg or greater were revised by means of balloon angioplasty ($n = 13$), additional stent placement and angioplasty ($n = 2$), or stent placement only ($n = 7$).

Outcome Success and Patency Criteria

Completely successful outcome was defined as complete or near resolution of ascites as seen at subsequent sonographic evaluations. Partial success was defined as no further paracentesis with a decrease in ascites of one grade at US. Treatment was considered a failure when a decrease in ascitic fluid volume could not be demonstrated sonographically or large-volume paracentesis was necessary to relieve severe ascites. In addition, treatment was considered a failure if the patient died during the follow-up interval, even if ascites

Table 2
Clinical Characteristics

Characteristic	No. of Patients
Child-Pugh class	
A	1 (2)
B	28 (56)
C	21 (42)
History of variceal bleeding or portal gastropathy	16 (32)
History of hepatic encephalopathy	23 (46)
Chronic renal insufficiency	15 (30)
Creatinine level (mg/dL)	1.7 ± 1.2 (150 μmol/L ± 110)*
Bilirubin level (mg/dL)	4.7 ± 5.7 (80 μmol/L ± 98)*
Prothrombin time	14.9 ± 3.9
Aspartate transaminase level (U/L)	80.0 ± 51.0

Note.—Numbers in parentheses are percentage of patients with each characteristic. Laboratory values are the means ± standard deviations.
*Values in parentheses are metric conversions.

# Months	0	2	4	6	8	10	12	14	16	18	20	22	24
Total # Patients	48	35	24	21	17	15	14	11	8	8	8	8	7
# No further paracentesis	48	21	17	16	14	12	11	9	7	7	7	7	6

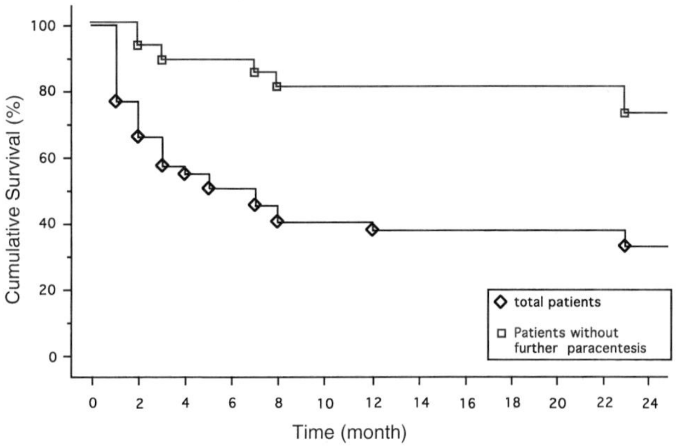

Figure 1. Graph shows cumulative survival rates in all patients and in those who did not undergo further paracentesis.

was controlled. Shunt patency was classified according to the reporting standards of the Society for Vascular Surgery (16) as (*a*) primary patency (ie, an adequately functioning shunt in which additional intervention was not necessary), (*b*) primary assisted patency (ie, an adequately functioning shunt that did not become occluded but some type of intervention was necessary such as balloon angioplasty or additional stent placement to maintain shunt function), and (*c*) secondary patency (ie, restoration of shunt patency after occlusion by means of thrombectomy, thrombolysis, angioplasty, or additional stent placement).

Data Analysis

Life table analysis was used to evaluate shunt patency (16,17). The Student *t* test was used for comparison of means; a *P* value less than .05 indicated statistically significant findings. The predictive value of laboratory results before the TIPS procedure for comparison of success and failure was analyzed with the χ^2 method. A Fisher exact *P* value less than .05 indicated statistically significant findings. Kaplan-Meier analysis was performed to determine cumulative survival rates. A log rank *P* value less than .05 indicated statistically significant predictors of survival.

RESULTS

Technical Success

Creation of the portosystemic shunt was successful in all 50 patients. Shunt formation was achieved with a single stent in 30 patients, two stents in 17 patients, and three stents in three patients. The mean portosystemic gradient was 22 mm Hg ± 6.6 before the TIPS procedure and 11 mm Hg ± 2.8 after the TIPS procedure ($P < .001$).

Clinical Course

Patients were followed up for a mean of 11.6 months (range, 1–59 months) after the TIPS procedure. Thirteen patients died, received liver transplants, or were lost to follow-up before the 4-week follow-up period. Twenty-three (62%) of the remaining 37 patients had decreased ascites and did not undergo further paracentesis at 1–3 months (partial resolution in 10 patients and complete resolution in 13 patients). However, three of these patients died by 3 months; thus, in these three patients, treatment was considered a failure. In 20 (42%) of 48 patients, ascites was controlled and the patients were alive at 3 months; thus, treatment was considered successful in these patients. Among the 27 patients alive and available for follow-up at 3 months after TIPS placement, treatment was considered a failure in seven (26%) and successful in 20 (74%). Total cumulative survival at 3 months was 57%, and for patients who required no further paracentesis, survival was 86% (Fig 1).

At 6-month follow-up, 14 (32%) of 44 patients were alive with controlled ascites, and thus treatment was considered successful. At that time, 20 patients were alive and available for follow-up, 24 patients died, four patients were lost to follow-up, and two patients received liver transplants. Of the 20 patients alive and available for 6-month follow-up, treatment was considered successful in 14 (70%) and a failure in six (30%).

At 1-year follow-up, 14 (33%) of 43 patients were alive with controlled ascites (treatment successful). Twenty-nine patients died, four patients were lost to follow-up, two patients had received transplants, and one patient had not yet been followed up for 1 year. One year after TIPS creation, 14 patients were alive and available for follow-up, and treatment was considered successful in all 14 (100%).

At 36 months, treatment was considered successful in only seven (18%) of 38 patients. At that time, 30 patients died, five patients were lost to follow-up, two patients had undergone liver transplantation, and five patients had not yet been followed up for 36 months. One patient had an occluded shunt. Treatment was considered successful in all seven patients. Treatment was considered successful in the patient whose shunt had occluded because the ascites had not reaccumulated.

Various laboratory values, as shown in Tables 3 and 4, were associated with treatment success or failure. Of the 16 patients with a creatinine level less than 1.9 mg/dL (170 μmol/L) and a bilirubin level less than 3.0 mg/dL (52 μmol/L), 11 (69%) were alive with successfully controlled ascites at 3-month follow-up. Treatment was successful in only one (14%) patient with a creatinine level greater than 1.9 mg/dL (170 μmol/L) and a bilirubin level greater than 3.0 mg/dL (52 μmol/L) at 3 months ($P = .03$). At 6-month follow-up, a creatinine level less than 1.9 mg/dL (170 μmol/L) became a statistically significantly independent predictor of treatment success. By 6 months, all of the patients with a creatinine level greater than 1.9 mg/dL (170 µmol/L) and a bilirubin level greater than 3.0 mg/dL (52 µmol/L) died and, therefore, no treatment successes occurred in that category. The association of various preprocedural laboratory values with patient survival is listed in Tables 5 and 6.

Encephalopathy

Before undergoing TIPS creation, 23 (46%) patients had a history of encephalopathy that was well controlled medically. Among the 23 patients, encephalopathy worsened in six after the TIPS procedure, was stable in eight, and resolved in two. Four of the patients died within 30 days, one underwent transplantation, and two were lost to follow-up.

After the TIPS procedure, 28 (56%) of the 50 patients experienced encephalopathy. In 20 (40%) patients, the encephalopathy was new or worsened. Encephalopathy was new in 14 patients, worsened in six patients, and was stable in eight patients. At some point after the TIPS procedure, 19 (38%) patients were hospitalized for treatment of encephalopathy.

Only two (4%) of the 50 patients had encephalopathy that was refractory to lactulose therapy; in these cases, the shunts were downsized by means of placement of stents of progressively smaller diameter within the shunts. In one patient, two 8-mm-diameter stents were placed within the 10-mm-diameter shunt, increasing the portosystemic gradient from 8 mm Hg to 15 mm Hg. One month later, the shunt was downsized further by placing another 8-mm-diameter stent and a 6-mm-diameter stent within the shunt, increasing the portosystemic gradient to 20 mm Hg. Encephalopathy improved temporarily, but ascites recurred and the patient died 3 months later. In the other patient, an 8-mm-diameter stent was placed within a 10-mm-diameter shunt. Encephalopathy improved temporarily, but the patient died less than 1 month later. Other investigators have used different techniques for downsizing TIPS, such as placement of specially designed hourglass stents within the shunts (18).

Table 3
Laboratory Values as Predictors of Treatment Success 3 Months after the TIPS Procedure

Laboratory Value*	Treatment Outcome: Failure	Treatment Outcome: Success†	*P* Value
Bilirubin >3.0 mg/dL	17	6 (26)	.04
Bilirubin <3.0 mg/dL	11	14 (56)	NS
Creatinine >1.9 mg/dL	11	4 (27)	NS
Creatinine <1.9 mg/dL	16	16 (50)	NS
Creatinine >1.9 mg/dL and bilirubin >3.0 mg/dL	6	1 (14)	.03
Creatinine <1.9 mg/dL and bilirubin <3.0 mg/dL	5	11 (69)	NS

Note.—Numbers in parentheses are percentages. For Tables 3–6, NS = not significant.
* For Tables 3–6, bilirubin, 3.0 mg/dL = 52 µmol/L; creatinine, 1.9 mg/dL = 170 µmol/L.
† Success is defined as survival with controlled ascites.

Table 4
Laboratory Values as Predictors of Treatment Success at 6 Months

Laboratory Value	Treatment Outcome: Failure	Treatment Outcome: Success*	*P* Value
Bilirubin >3.0 mg/dL	17	4 (19)	NS
Bilirubin <3.0 mg/dL	13	10 (44)	NS
Creatinine >1.9 mg/dL	12	1 (7)	.03
Creatinine <1.9 mg/dL	17	13 (43)	NS
Creatinine >1.9 mg/dL and bilirubin >3.0 mg/dL	6	0 (0)	.02
Creatinine <1.9 mg/dL and bilirubin <3.0 mg/dL	6	9 (60)	NS

Note.—Numbers in parentheses are percentages.
* Success is defined as survival with controlled ascites.

Table 5
Laboratory Values as Predictors of Survival at 3 Months

Laboratory Value	Cumulative Survival at 3 Months (%)	No. at Risk	*P* Value
Bilirubin >3.0 mg/dL	34	7	.023
Bilirubin <3.0 mg/dL	72	19	NS
Creatinine >1.9 mg/dL	51	7	NS
Creatinine <1.9 mg/dL	55	19	NS
Creatinine >1.9 mg/dL and bilirubin >3.0 mg/dL	28	1	.001
Creatinine <1.9 mg/dL and bilirubin <3.0 mg/dL	77	12	NS

Other Complications

Complications associated with the TIPS procedure are summarized in Table 7. Two patients had severe bleeding related to the procedure. The first patient developed hypotension during tract dilation for TIPS creation, with substantial hypovolemic shock caused by bleeding from the puncture site into the portal vein. Balloon tamponade controlled bleeding. This complication occurred early in our experience.

In a second patient, hemorrhage was believed to be caused by wedge hepatic venography. Two hours after the procedure, the patient became hypotensive and the hemoglobin decreased 5 g/dL (0.5 g/L). Transfusion of 8 units of packed red blood cells was performed, and the hemoglobin level was stabilized. A computed tomographic scan revealed extravasation from the right lobe of the liver, hemoperitoneum, and a subcapsular hematoma. The patient recovered and was discharged from the hospital 16 days later.

One patient whose shunt occluded within 24 hours was treated with urokinase (Abbokinase; Abbott Laboratories) and angioplasty and received heparin. The patient developed a gastrointestinal hemorrhage caused by portal gastropathy and duodenal ulcers. Heparin was discontinued. The patient developed respiratory compromise and was believed to have fluid overload. Intubation was performed, and aspirate from suctioning revealed blood in the lungs consistent with pulmonary hemorrhage. Four days later, the bleeding resolved and an antiplatelet antibody was diagnosed. The patient was discharged

Table 6
Laboratory Values as Predictors of Survival at 6 Months

Laboratory Value	Cumulative Survival at 6 Months (%)	No. at Risk	*P* Value
Bilirubin >3.0 mg/dL	29	6	.023
Bilirubin <3.0 mg/dL	68	15	NS
Creatinine >1.9 mg/dL	37	4	NS
Creatinine <1.9 mg/dL	52	15	NS
Creatinine >1.9 mg/dL and bilirubin >3.0 mg/dL	0	0	.001
Creatinine <1.9 mg/dL and bilirubin <3.0 mg/dL	71	11	NS

Table 7
Complications Associated with the TIPS Procedure

Complication	No. of Patients	No. with Death as a Result
Major		
Hemoperitoneum	2 (4)	1 (2)
Accelerated liver or renal failure	1 (2)	1 (2)
Progression of renal failure	1 (2)	0 (0)
Refractory encephalopathy	2 (4)	0 (0)
Recurrent gastrointestinal hemorrhage		
Heparin treatment as a cause	1 (2)	0 (0)
Sepsis as a cause	1 (2)	0 (0)
Minor		
Hemolysis	4 (8)	0 (0)
Fever without bacteremia	4 (8)	0 (0)
Fever with bacteremia	3 (6)	0 (0)
Lower-extremity edema	10 (20)	0 (0)

Note.—Numbers in parentheses are percentages.

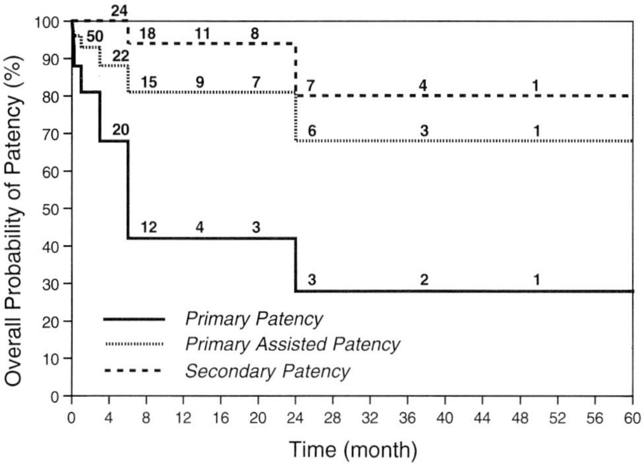

Figure 2. Graph shows rates of overall probability of patency of TIPS.

with a patent shunt and no evidence of further bleeding.

Another patient developed severe acceleration of liver failure with associated renal failure and died of multiorgan failure secondary to candidal sepsis 17 days after the TIPS procedure. An additional patient with a preprocedural creatinine level of 3.2 mg/dL (280 µmol/L) experienced progression of renal failure after the TIPS procedure believed to be related to the contrast material (50 mL) administered during the procedure.

Four patients had evidence of hemolysis. One patient died 2 weeks after the TIPS procedure. Hemolysis resolved in one patient by 2 weeks after the TIPS procedure, in one patient 12 months after TIPS creation, and in one patient by 5 months after TIPS creation (at the time of death). None of the patients required transfusions because of hemolysis. Ten patients developed lower-extremity edema as fluid redistributed shortly after the TIPS procedure. The edema resolved within 3 months in all patients. Four patients developed fever not associated with bacteremia and three patients developed fever associated with bacteremia. One patient developed sepsis and was treated with intravenous antibiotics, with resolution of symptoms several days after the TIPS procedure.

Shunt Patency

Early.—Patency rates are shown in Figure 2. Five shunts were occluded at portography within 24 hours of the TIPS procedure. An 8-mm-diameter shunt occluded during the initial procedure and revision was achieved with a pulse spray of 150,000 U of urokinase into the shunt, then dilation of the shunt to 10 mm and placement of an additional stent. In one patient, the stent recoiled into the tract within 24 hours of placement. Initially, the tract was opened with a 6.8-cm-long, 10.0-mm-diameter stent dilated to 8 mm. US performed at 24 hours showed the portal vein end of the stent lying in the hepatic parenchyma with no blood flow. The shunt was then dilated to 10 mm, and a 4.2-cm-long stent was added and dilated to 10 mm in diameter. In two shunts, 12-mm-diameter stents were placed and dilated only to 8 and 9 mm in diameter, respectively. In another shunt, 10-mm-diameter stents were used and were not dilated after deployment (the tract was dilated to 10 mm in diameter before stent deployment). These three stents were opened with a combination of urokinase, balloon angioplasty, and additional stent placement.

A tight stenosis that involved a 12-mm stent dilated to 10 mm was detected at 24-hour follow-up and was revised by means of balloon angioplasty with a 12-mm-diameter balloon. In one case, the stent recoiled into the tract. Otherwise, there were no cases of shunt occlusion within 24 hours that occurred in the TIPS in which a 10-mm-diameter stent was redilated with an 8-mm-diameter balloon after stent deployment. This lack of occlusion was attributable most likely to the relatively high radial strength of the 10-mm-diameter stent compared with that of the 12-mm-diameter stent (19).

Delayed.—No change in shunt patency occurred between 48 hours and 30 days. In 12 patients, 22 shunt stenoses occurred 30 days or later after shunt placement. Sixteen of these stenoses occurring in 11 patients were associated with recurrent or persistent ascites (Table 8). Eight stenoses occurred in seven patients with massive recurrent or persistent ascites, which was associated with a mean portosystemic gradient of 21 mm Hg (Fig 3). Three stenoses occurred in three patients with moderate persistent or recurrent ascites and a mean portosystemic gradient of 19 mm Hg. Five stenoses occurred in three patients with mild ascites associated with a mean portosystemic gradient of 16.8 mm Hg. Six stenoses occurred in two patients who had no ascites and a mean portosystemic gradient of 18.6 mm Hg. One of these two patients also previously had stenosis that was associated with recurrent ascites.

In nine of 16 stenoses, ascites decreased after shunt revision, usually when ascites was recurrent rather than residual. In one patient, a stenosis with a portosystemic gradient of 17 mm Hg was detected at 5 months after shunt placement. Because of the patient's history of encephalopathy and absence of ascites, the stenosis was observed for 26 months until the shunt was revised eventually due to recurrence of massive ascites associated with a portosystemic gradient of 18 mm Hg.

Four shunt occlusions occurred at 2, 9, 13, and 27 months after TIPS creation. In two of these patients, there was no recurrent ascites and the patients had encephalopathy after the TIPS procedure. As a result, the shunts were not revised. Both patients remain asymptomatic. The other two patients had recurrent massive ascites, and shunt revision was performed. After revision, the ascites resolved in both patients.

Four patients experienced recurrence of bleeding caused by varices or portal gastropathy. Variceal bleeding persisted in two patients with portosystemic gradients less than 12 mm Hg and both patients died after they requested no further therapy. In one patient, bleeding occurred because of shunt malfunction 5 months after the TIPS procedure. In this patient, 2 units of red blood cells were transfused, and bleeding stopped after shunt revision. The other patient had no shunt malfunction, but bleeding occurred 3 months after the TIPS procedure. Stabilization was achieved with two units of red blood cells. However, bleeding occurred again 2 months later and the patient died.

Mortality

Overall, 30 (60%) of the 50 patients died. Within 30 days of the TIPS procedure, 11 (22%) patients died, six of whom had Child-Pugh class C disease and five of whom had Child-Pugh class B disease. At 3 months, 21 (42%) of the 50 patients died, one with Child-Pugh class A disease, 10 with Child-Pugh class B disease, and 10 with Child-Pugh class C disease. At 6 months after the TIPS procedure, 24 (48%) of the 50 patients died, four were lost to follow-up, and two underwent transplantation. Patients died a mean of 3.9 months (range, 1–23 months) after TIPS creation. Fifteen patients had Child-Pugh class C disease, 14 patients had Child-Pugh class B disease, and one patient had Child-Pugh class A disease. Causes of death included liver failure in 11 patients, renal and liver failure in five patients, liver and renal failure combined with sepsis in three patients, and liver failure and sepsis, pneumonia, or variceal bleeding in eight patients. Three patients died of malignancy.

Table 8
Correlation of Shunt Stenosis with Persistent or Recurrent Ascites

Ascites	No. of Stenotic Shunts	Decrease in Ascites after Shunt Revision
Resolved	6	0
Residual mild	3	0
Recurrent mild	2	1
Residual moderate	1	0
Recurrent moderate	2	2
Residual massive	3	2
Recurrent massive	5	4

DISCUSSION

A decrease in the amount of ascites after TIPS creation has been reported by other investigators (5–9,20–22). Crenshaw et al (8) reported a substantial reduction in ascites in 78% of patients with severe ascites, 57% of whom no longer required therapeutic paracentesis. Clearly, the definition of successful treatment is somewhat controversial. We believed that no further need for paracentesis was a clear, objective criterion for success. There most likely were patients in whom treatment was considered a failure, and these patients actually had a reduced need for paracentesis than they would have if TIPS creation was not performed. If the goal is to make patients more comfortable, then a reduced need for paracentesis, although somewhat subjective, is a reasonable definition of success.

Certainly, previously published data showing improved quality of life in and of itself may justify the cost of the TIPS procedure (23). However, if the patient dies within 3–6 months, one may question whether the therapy should be considered successful. The possibility of enhanced patient comfort and decreased need for paracentesis over 3–6 months may not be worth the cost of TIPS creation unless the odds are strongly in favor of success. Our study, as well as the study by Crenshaw et al, showed that patients who survive at least 3–6 months after the TIPS procedure are much more likely to have controlled ascites as a result of the TIPS procedure compared with patients who die within 3–6 months of the procedure.

After reviewing our data and that of Ochs et al (9), which reveal a relatively high mortality in this patient population, we concluded that for the treatment to be considered successful, patients should have an objective improvement in ascites (no further paracentesis) and should survive the follow-up interval. Unfortunately, the 1-year mortality rate of patients with severe ascites who have not undergone TIPS creation has been reported to be approximately 75% (24). It is for this reason we believed it necessary to try to identify factors associated with improved 3–6 month survival and successfully controlled ascites.

Of the 50 patients who underwent TIPS creation in our study, only 42% were alive with controlled ascites at 3 months. Although TIPS creation effectively treated refractory ascites in 62% of patients who survived at least 1 month after the procedure, 8% of these patients died before the 3-month follow-up. Of the patients who were alive at 3 months, treatment was successful in 74%. Treatment success (alive with controlled ascites) was associated with a creatinine level less than 1.9 mg/dL (170 μmol/L) and a bilirubin level less than 3.0 mg/dL (52 μmol/L). Elevated creatinine and bilirubin levels were associated with early mortality and treatment failure. In fact, there was only one 3-month success and no 6-month successes in patients with a creatinine level greater than 1.9 mg/dL (170 μmol/L) and a bilirubin level greater than 3.0 mg/dL (52 μmol/L). Conversely, of patients with a creatinine level less than 1.9 mg/dL (170 μmol/L) and a bilirubin level less than 3.0 mg/dL (52 μmol/L), 69% were successful at 3 months and 60% at 6 months. A bilirubin level less than 3.0 mg/dL (52 μmol/L) was an independent predictor of 3-month success, and the lack of renal insufficiency was a statistically significantly indepen-

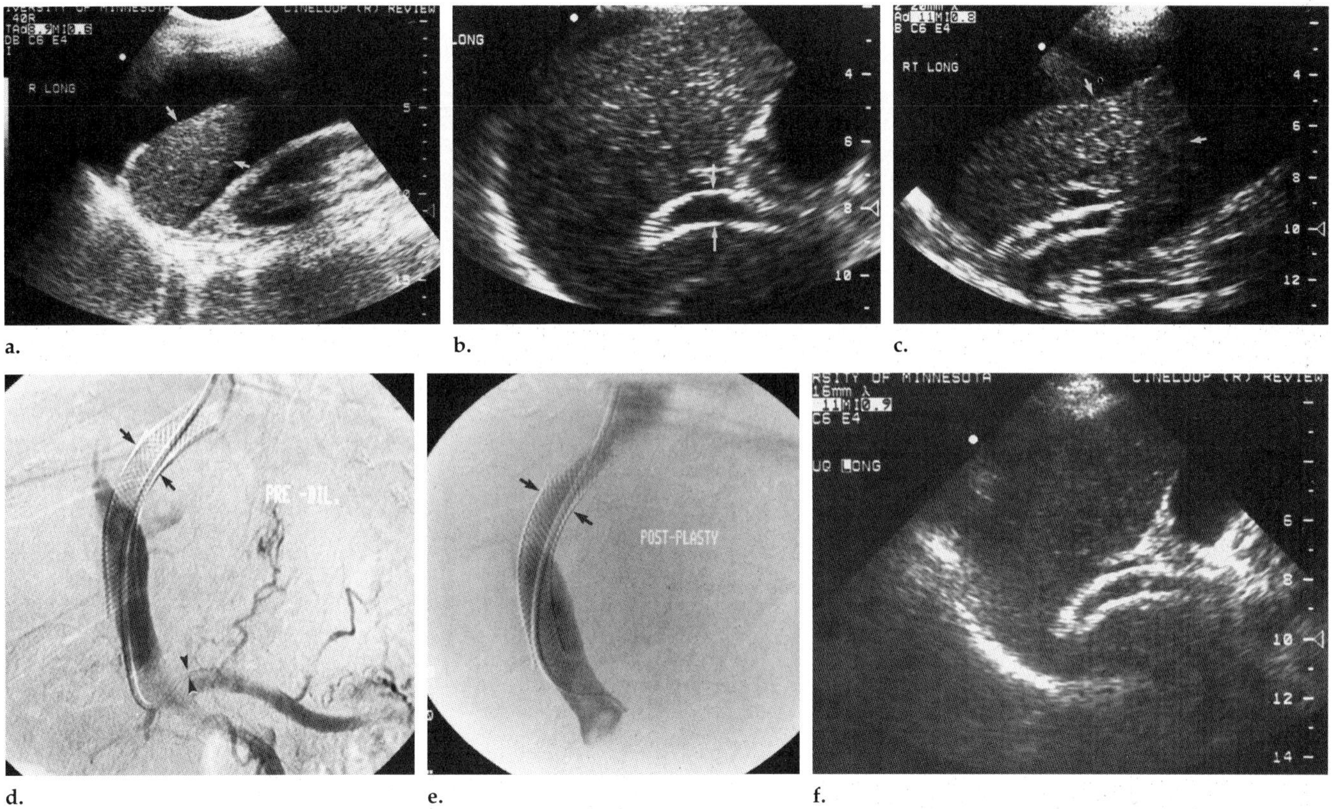

Figure 3. **(a)** Longitudinal US image shows massive ascites surrounding the liver (arrows). **(b)** US image obtained at 2-month follow-up shows the TIPS stent (arrows) with resolution of ascites. **(c)** Follow-up US image obtained 17 months after TIPS creation shows reaccumulation of ascites around the liver (arrows). **(d)** Portogram obtained with the catheter in the main portal vein (arrowheads) shows absence of contrast material within the shunt (arrows) consistent with high-grade stenosis or occlusion. The portosystemic gradient was 22 mm Hg. **(e)** Portogram obtained after dilation of the shunt with a 10-mm-diameter balloon shows the shunt is filled with contrast material (arrows), indicating restoration of shunt patency. The portosystemic gradient was 12 mm Hg after revision. **(f)** US image obtained 1 month after shunt revision shows resolution of ascites around the liver.

dent predictor of 6-month success. No association was shown between treatment failure or early mortality and Child-Pugh class or history of encephalopathy, as suggested previously (7).

Ochs et al (9) defined success as no further need for paracentesis but included patients who may have died during the follow-up interval, showing a 3-month success rate of 82% with a similar complication rate and slightly higher 1-year survival rate of 54%. They also found a low pretreatment bilirubin level (<1.3 mg/dL [22 µmol/L]) and a complete response to treatment to be associated with improved patient survival for at least 1 year. In that study, patients greater than 60 years of age with organic kidney disease had a poor outcome.

Crenshaw et al (8) recently reported their results with TIPS creation for the treatment of severe ascites. The investigators created a TIPS in 50 patients and followed them up a mean of 9 months (range, 1–33 months). The 50 patients we reported were followed up for a similar length of time (mean, 11.6 months; range, 1–59 months). Crenshaw et al defined treatment success somewhat differently (ie, a decrease in frequency of paracentesis). However, our reported rate of successfully controlled ascites of 62% at 1–3 months is similar to their percentage of patients who no longer required paracentesis (57%). The 16% rate of severe complications we reported in our study including hemoperitoneum (4%), renal insufficiency (2%), accelerated liver failure (2%), and refractory encephalopathy (4%) is similar between the two groups. However, Crenshaw et al reported no cases of refractory encephalopathy. They reported a 6% incidence of hemoperitoneum. The mortality rates at 1 month, 6 months, and 1 year, respectively, were nearly identical between the two groups (22% vs 20%, 48% vs 47%, 58% vs 52%). The most common causes of death were liver failure (33% vs 40%) or multiorgan failure (7% vs 6%). We also observed a strong correlation between treatment success and patient survival; thus treatment was likely to be effective if the patient survived 6 months after TIPS creation. Finally, both studies showed that preexisting renal failure adversely affects the probability of treatment success. Treatment success was not shown to be affected statistically significantly by Child-Pugh class in either study.

Our data indicate that the combination of low bilirubin and creatinine levels are associated strongly with treatment success and patient survival, as 69% of such patients were alive with well controlled ascites at 3 months and 60% at 6 months. We also found that revision of shunt stenosis was usually effective in controlling recurrent ascites.

The similarity in results between our study and other studies on separate patient populations provides convincing evidence that TIPS creation is a useful treatment for severe ascites that cannot be controlled with existing medical therapy. In patients without liver and renal failure, ascites can be controlled successfully in most cases after TIPS creation. However, patients with advanced liver and renal failure are unlikely to benefit from TIPS creation. Therefore, careful patient selection and close follow-up is critical to the successful use of TIPS creation for refractory ascites. ■

References

1. Rikkers LF, Sorrell WT, Jin G. Which portosystemic shunt is best? Gastroenterol Clin North Am 1992; 21:179–196.
2. Franco D, Vans C, Traynor O, Smadja C. Should portosystemic shunt be reconsidered in the treatment of intractable ascites in cirrhosis? Arch Surg 1988; 123:987–991.
3. Shear L. Ascites in cirrhosis: a medical or surgical problem? Hepatology 1990; 11:323–325.
4. Rosemurgy AS, McAllister EW, Kearney RE. Prospective study of a prosthetic H-graft portacaval shunt. Am J Surg 1991; 161: 159–164.
5. Zemel G, Katzen B, Becker GJ, Benenati JF, Sallee S. Percutaneous transjugular portosystemic shunt. JAMA 1991; 266:390–393.
6. LaBerge JM, Ring EJ, Gordon RL, et al. Creation of transjugular intrahepatic portosystemic shunts with the Wallstent endoprosthesis: results in 100 patients. Radiology 1993; 187:413–420.
7. Ferral H, Bjarnason H, Wegryn SA, et al. Refractory ascites: early experience in treatment with transjugular intrahepatic portosystemic shunt. Radiology 1993; 189:795–801.
8. Crenshaw WB, Gordon FD, McEniff NJ, et al. Severe ascites: efficacy of the transjugular intrahepatic portosystemic shunt in treatment. Radiology 1996; 200:185–192.
9. Ochs A, Rössle M, Haag K, et al. The transjugular intrahepatic portosystemic stent-shunt procedure for refractory ascites. N Engl J Med 1995; 332:1192–1197.
10. Pugh RNH, Murray-Lyon IM, Dawson JL, Pietroni MC, Williams R. Transection of the oesophagus for oesophageal varices. Br J Surg 1973; 60:646–649.
11. Rösch J, Uchida BT, Barton RE, Keller FS. Coaxial catheter-needle system for transjugular portal vein entrance. JVIR 1993; 4:145–147.
12. Foshager M, Ferral H, Nazarian G, Castaneda-Zuniga W, Letourneau J. Duplex sonography after transjugular intrahepatic portosystemic shunts (TIPS): normal hemodynamic findings and efficacy in predicting shunt patency and stenosis. AJR 1995; 165: 1–7.
13. Dodd G, Zajko A, Orons P, Martin M, Eichner L, Santaguida L. Detection of transjugular intrahepatic portosystemic shunt dysfunction: value of duplex Doppler sonography. AJR 1995; 164:1119–1124.
14. Surratt R, Middleton W, Darcy M, Melson G, Brink J. Morphologic and hemodynamic findings at sonography before and after creation of a transjugular intrahepatic portosystemic shunt. AJR 1993; 160:627–630.
15. Feldstein V, Maitray DP, LaBerge JM. Transjugular intrahepatic portosystemic shunts: accuracy of Doppler US in determination of patency and detection of stenosis. Radiology 1996; 210:141–147.
16. Rutherford RB, Flanigan DP, Gupta SK, et al. Suggested standards for reports dealing with lower extremity ischemia. J Vasc Surg 1986; 4:80–94.
17. Lee ET. Statistical methods for survival data analysis. 2nd ed. New York, NY: Wiley, 1992.
18. Hauenstein KH, Haag K, Ochs A, Langer M, Rössle M. The reducing stent: treatment for transjugular intrahepatic portosystemic shunt-induced refractory hepatic encephalopathy and liver failure. Radiology 1995; 194:175–179.
19. Kuhn-Fulton J, Trerotola SO, Harris VJ, et al. Transjugular intrahepatic portosystemic shunt procedure: efficacy of 10-mm versus 12-mm Wallstents. Radiology 1996; 199:658–664.
20. Quiroga J, Sangro B, Nuñez M, et al. Transjugular intrahepatic portal-systemic shunt in the treatment of refractory ascites: effect on clinical, renal, humoral, and hemodynamic parameters. Hepatology 1995; 21: 986–994.
21. Somberg KA, Lake JR, Tomlanovich SJ, LaBerge JM, Feldstein V, Bass NM. Transjugular intrahepatic portosystemic shunts for refractory ascites: assessment of clinical and hormonal response and renal function. Hepatology 1995; 21:709–716.
22. Wong F, Sniderman K, Liu P, Allidina Y, Sherman M, Blendis L. Transjugular intrahepatic portosystemic stent shunt: effects on hemodynamics and sodium homeostasis in cirrhosis and refractory ascites. Ann Intern Med 1995; 122:816–822.
23. Nazarian GK, Ferral H, Bjarnason H, et al. Effect of transjugular intrahepatic portosystemic shunt on quality of life. AJR 1996; 167:963–969.
24. Bories P, Garcia-Compean D, Michel H, et al. The treatment of refractory ascites by the LeVeen shunt: a multicenter controlled trial (57) patients. J Hepatol 1986; 3:212–218.

Hirohiko Tanihata, MD • Richard R. Saxon, MD • Yasushi Kubota, MD
Dusan Pavcnik, MD, PhD • Barry T. Uchida, BS • Josef Rosch, MD
Frederick S. Keller, MD • Ryusaku Yamada, MD, PhD • Morio Sato, MD, PhD

Transjugular Intrahepatic Portosystemic Shunt with Silicone-covered Wallstents: Results in a Swine Model[1]

PURPOSE: To evaluate the use of impermeable silicone-covered Wallstents for transjugular intrahepatic portosystemic shunt creation.

MATERIALS AND METHODS: A transjugular intrahepatic portosystemic shunt was created in 14 young swine (weight, 20–32 kg) by using impermeable silicone-covered Wallstents. In eight animals, the silicone covering extended from the portal vein to the inferior vena cava. In two swine, the silicone covering ended short of the inferior vena cava, in two it ended short of the portal vein wall, and in two it ended short at each end. Follow-up transhepatic portal venography was performed weekly for 6 weeks or until the shunt was occluded. Animals were then sacrificed for gross and histologic evaluation.

RESULTS: Only two of 14 shunts were patent after 3 weeks; both were stenosed with luminal narrowing of more than 50% in the middle of the shunt. By 6 weeks, all shunts were occluded. At histologic evaluation, a marked foreign-body reaction with superimposed thrombosis was demonstrated.

CONCLUSION: In comparison with uncovered Wallstents, impermeable silicone-covered Wallstents are associated with decreased patency at transjugular intrahepatic portosystemic shunt creation. This is likely due to increased thrombogenicity and a foreign-body reaction.

The use of the transjugular intrahepatic portosystemic shunt (TIPS) has been established as an effective and safe medical procedure to decompress portal venous hypertension and to control acute variceal hemorrhage (1–7). However, there is substantial room for improvement in the long-term primary patency of TIPS. Several authors (4–11) have reported that shunt stenosis and/or occlusion occurs in 25%–85% of patients by 1 year after shunt placement.

The development of a TIPS malfunction appears to be a multifactorial process. TIPS malfunction within the first few weeks after placement is probably a result of acute thrombosis. Stenosis or occlusion of the TIPS 1 month to 1 year after stent placement is probably a result of substantial pseudointimal hyperplasia development in the parenchymal tract (12). Finally, the formation of intimal hyperplasia within the outflow of the hepatic vein (HV) is a cause of late TIPS malfunction that may occur most often 3 months to 1 year after shunt placement (2,9,10).

Transection of an intrahepatic bile duct by means of a TIPS may be a cause of early shunt thrombosis and of the later development of pseudointimal hyperplasia, which causes parenchymal tract stenosis and occlusion. In a recent study (13), substantial biliary injury and biliary epithelial proliferation were absent in patients with a patent shunt and were present in almost all patients with parenchymal tract abnormalities. Therefore, we hypothesized that TIPS patency could be improved by distinguishing flowing blood in the shunt from leaking bile and the exposed surface of the liver parenchyma. In fact, TIPS created with stent-grafts covered with polytetrafluoroethylene (PTFE) that extended from the portal vein (PV) to the inferior vena cava (IVC) substantially improved patency in a swine model (14). Recently, a Wallstent (Schneider, Minneapolis, Minn) with an impermeable silicone covering was developed for use in the tracheobronchial tree. We tested this stent for TIPS creation to determine if this commercially available device could act as an impermeable barrier to transected bile ducts and improve TIPS patency.

MATERIALS AND METHODS

Materials

TIPS were created with silicone-covered Wallstents in 14 young domestic swine, aged 8–10 weeks, that weighed 20–32 kg. All animals had a normal liver and no portal venous hypertension. An impermeable silicone membrane covered most of the stent except 2 cm at the PV end (Fig 1). The visibility of the covered section was enhanced by means of two gold wires braided

Index terms: Liver, interventional procedure, 761.1269, 958.123, 958.1268 • Shunts, portosystemic, 958.453 • Stents and prostheses, 958.1268

Abbreviations: HV = hepatic vein, IVC = inferior vena cava, PTFE = polytetrafluoroethylene, PV = portal vein, TIPS = transjugular intrahepatic portosystemic shunt.

Radiology 1997; 205:181–184

[1] From the Dotter Interventional Institute, Oregon Health Sciences University, Portland (H.T., R.R.S., Y.K., D.P., B.T.U., J.R., F.S.K.); the Department of Radiology, Wakayama Medical College, 27 Banchi, 7 Bancho, Wakayama City 640, Japan (H.T., M.S.); the Department of Radiology, Nara Medical College, Japan (Y.K.); and the Department of Radiology, Osaka City University, Japan (R.Y.). From the 1996 RSNA scientific assembly. Received December 3, 1996; revision requested January 27, 1997; revision received June 12; accepted June 23. **Address reprint requests to** H.T.

Results of TIPS Creation with Silicone-covered Wallstents in 14 Pigs

Pig	No. of Stents	Stent Coverage PV	Stent Coverage IVC	Patency (wk) 0*	Patency (wk) 1	Patency (wk) 3	Patency (wk) 6	Cause of Occlusion	Presence of Bile Duct
1	2	N	Y	Patent	Patent, thrombus	Occluded	NA	Thrombus	N
2	1	Y	Y	Patent	Patent	Patent†	NA	NA	Y
3	1	Y	N	Patent, thrombus	70% stenosis	Occluded	NA	Intimal hyperplasia in HV	Y
4	2	N	Y	Patent	Occluded	NA	NA	Thrombus	N
5	1	Y	Y	Patent, thrombus	Occluded	NA	NA	Thrombus	N
6	1	Y	Y	Patent	Occluded	NA	NA	Thrombus	Y
7	1	Y	Y	Patent, thrombus	Patent, thrombus	Patent, thrombus	Occluded	Intimal hyperplasia in IVC	N
8	2	N	N	Patent	Occluded	NA	NA	Thrombus	Y
9	2	N	N	Patent	70% stenosis	Occluded	NA	Intimal hyperplasia in HV	Y
10	2	Y	N	Patent	Occluded	NA	NA	Thrombus	Y
11	2	Y	Y	Patent	Occluded	NA	NA	Thrombus	Y
12	2	Y	Y	Patent	Occluded	NA	NA	Thrombus	Y
13	2	Y	Y	Patent	Occluded	NA	NA	Thrombus	Y
14	3	Y	Y	Occluded	NA	NA	NA	Thrombus	Y

Note.—N = no, NA = not applicable, Y = yes.
* Indicates immediately after TIPS creation.
† The animal was sacrificed because of failure to thrive.

into the stent. Stent lengths were 4.5, 6.0, or 7.5 cm; all stents had a diameter of 8.0 mm. A rolling membrane delivery system was used to deploy the silicone-covered Wallstents. The membrane was activated by applying contrast material at 5 atm with an inflation device.

Technique

The technique used for TIPS creation has been previously described (7,15). Under sterile conditions, a catheter was placed in the PV by using a right midaxillary transhepatic approach with a 20-gauge needle, a 0.018-inch-diameter Cope-type guide wire, and a 5-F Teflon multi–side-hole catheter that contained a 20-gauge metal cannula. Portal venography was performed through the transhepatic portal catheter with diatrizoate meglumine (Renografin-76; Bracco Diagnostics, Princeton, NJ).

Contrast material was injected into a right ear vein. This allowed visualization and percutaneous catheter placement in the right external jugular vein with an 18-gauge needle by using a ventral approach between the angle of the jaw and the sternum. A 0.035-inch-diameter guide wire (Terumo, Tokyo, Japan) was inserted in the external jugular vein past the right atrium and into the IVC, the subcutaneous tissue was dilated with a 12-F dilator (Cook, Bloomington, Ind), and a coaxial catheter-needle set (RUPS 100; Cook) was used, as previously described (15). After establishing a tract to the PV, 2,000 U of heparin were injected intravenously. An 8-mm-diameter, 6-cm-long angioplasty balloon catheter (Medi-tech/Boston Scientific, Watertown, Mass) was used to dilate the parenchymal tract. One, two, or three silicone-covered Wallstents were used to create a TIPS with the technique that has been previously described (15,16) for TIPS creation in humans. The impermeable silicone covering extended from the PV wall to the IVC in eight animals, from the PV to the HV in two animals, from the parenchymal tract to the IVC (excluding the PV wall) in two animals, and from the parenchymal tract to the HV in two animals.

Follow-up Portal Venography

The animals underwent weekly follow-up with transhepatic portal venography. Animals were sacrificed for the purpose of gross and histologic evaluation when the stents were occluded or at the end of the 6-week study period. One animal was sacrificed at 3 weeks owing to failure to thrive caused by severe encephalopathy. Shunt stenoses were determined by using the narrowest luminal measurement on either the anteroposterior or the lateral view. For the purpose of comparison, luminal narrowing of more than 50% was considered to be relevant.

Histologic Evaluation

Gross evaluation of the shunts removed from the sacrificed animals was performed. The specimens were then placed in 10% formalin for 4 weeks before the shunts and stents were carefully bisected in a longitudinal fashion. Gross and histologic evaluations of the shunts were performed. The silicone-covered stent and bare metal wires were carefully removed to obtain specimens for light microscopy. Approximately six specimens obtained from the PV end, shunt tract, and HV end were embedded in paraffin. The specimens were then sectioned and stained with hematoxylin and eosin.

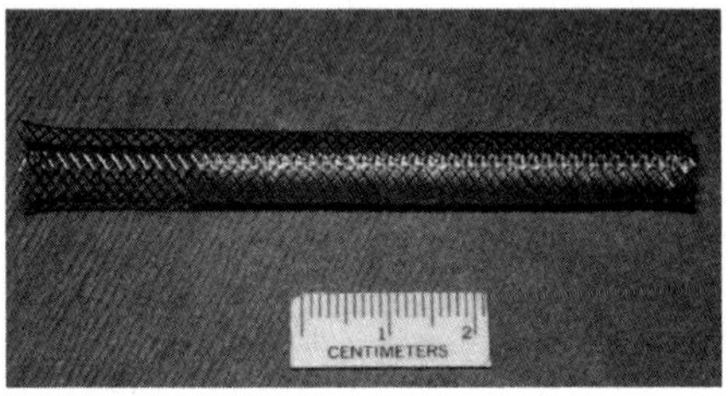

Figure 1. Impermeable silicone-covered Wallstent used for TIPS creation. The membrane covered most of the stent except for 2 cm at the PV end.

RESULTS

Portal Venography

Immediately after TIPS creation, portal venograms showed an occlusion in one animal (Table), and there was evidence of thrombus formation in the covered portion of the TIPS on the ventrodorsal and lateral portal venograms in three animals (Fig 2). Results of follow-up studies obtained at 1–6 weeks showed occlusion or various degrees of shunt narrowing (Table). At the 1-week follow-up, eight (57%) of 14 animals had an occluded shunt, three (21%) animals had a shunt with luminal narrowing of more than 50% in the middle of the graft, and two (14%) animals had a severe (more than 70%) HV stenosis. In four animals (pigs 1, 3, 7, and 9), there was also some evidence of thrombus inside the tract. At the 3-week follow-up, only two animals (pigs 2 and 7) had a patent shunt, but one animal (pig 2) was sacrificed at 3 weeks because of severe encephalopathy. The other animal (pig 7) had a mild HV stenosis (20%), with the presence of a linear defect in the central portion of the parenchymal tract. At the 6-week follow-up, the last shunt was occluded.

In the eight animals with silicone-covered stents that covered the area from the PV wall to the IVC, the shunt was occluded at 0 weeks (immediately after TIPS creation), 1 week, and 6

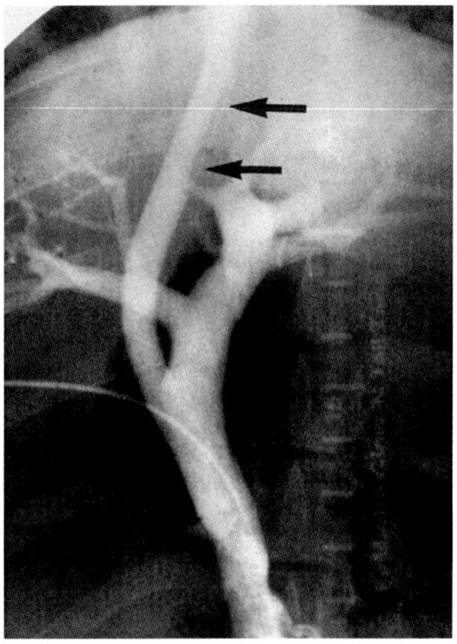

Figure 2. Portal venogram obtained in a swine immediately after TIPS creation shows the presence of thrombus (arrows).

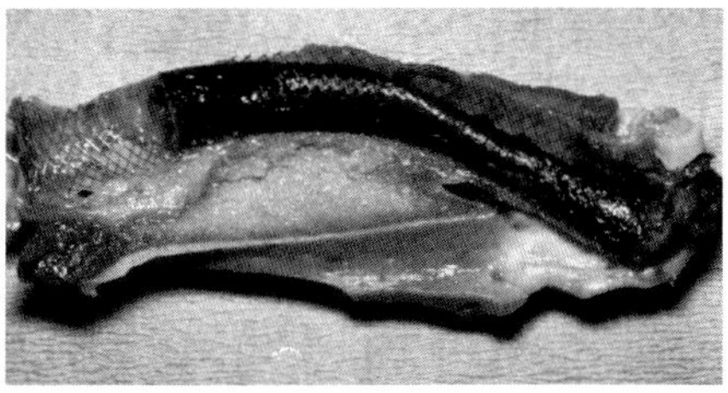

a.

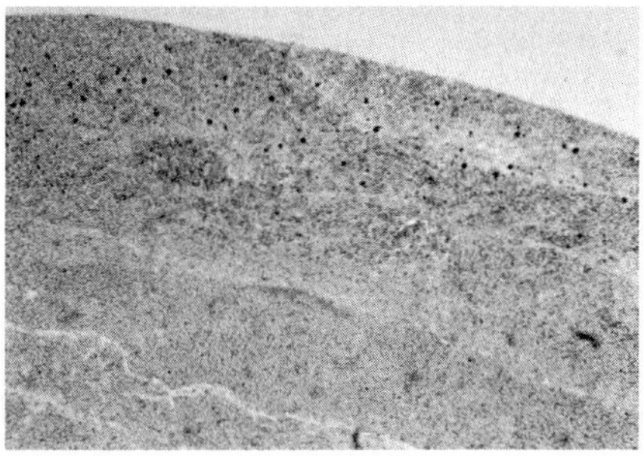

b.

Figure 3. **(a)** Gross specimen of an occluded shunt obtained at 3 weeks shows the TIPS tract filled with thrombus. **(b)** Photomicrograph shows thrombus with clotted blood and no evidence of organization. (Hematoxylin-eosin stain; original magnification, ×4.)

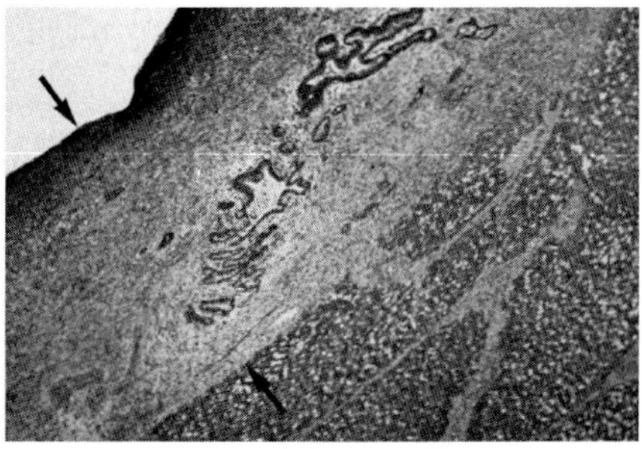

Figure 4. Photomicrograph obtained 1 week after TIPS creation shows hyperplastic granulation tissue and bile ducts within the scar tissue (arrows) that formed between the liver parenchyma and the outside of the silicone cover. (Hematoxylin-eosin stain; original magnification, ×4.)

weeks, with a mean patency of 1.5 weeks. The two shunts with the silicone membrane that covered all but 2 cm of the stent were occluded at 1 and 3 weeks. In the two animals with stents on which the silicone covering ended short of the PV, the shunt was occluded at 1 and 3 weeks; in the two animals with stents on which the silicone covering ended short at each end, the shunt was occluded at 1 and 3 weeks. Because almost all shunts were occluded at 3 weeks, the site where the silicone membrane ended seemed to have little effect on patency.

Gross Pathologic and Histologic Evaluation

At gross examination, occlusive thrombus was noted in the lumen of the TIPS in 12 of the 13 animals (Fig 3a); the exception was the one swine sacrificed because of uncontrollable encephalopathy. At microscopic evaluation, the thrombus was seen to consist only of clotted blood, with no evidence of organization (Fig 3b). Two of the four animals in which the covered stent did not extend into the IVC were sacrificed at 3 weeks because of occlusion; there was narrowing of the HV just beyond the end of the stent. Only one of the 10 animals in which the cover extended into the IVC was sacrificed at 6 weeks because of occlusion; there was intimal hyperplasia in the IVC wall in this animal. At microscopic examination, the narrowing corresponded to intimal hyperplasia, which was due predominantly to proliferation of fibroblasts. There was focal extension of this process along the uncovered ends of the stents (neointima formation); however, the lumen remained free of cellular elements within the covered portion of the stents.

Fibrous tissue reaction in the surrounding hepatic parenchyma, accompanied by occasional smooth muscle cells, was present on the outside of the silicone covering in all 14 animals (Fig 4). Foreign-body–type giant cells were present at the interface of the fibrous tissue and the outer surface of the stent. There was no evidence of the presence of endothelial cells, as expected. Within the fibrous tissue, there were occasional proliferating bile ducts that had irregular lumina and reactive nuclear characteristics in the TIPS of 10 animals. Bile staining was grossly evident in this fibrous tissue in two animals, which was suggestive of damage to the bile ducts at the time of stent placement; however, there was no recognizable bile staining on the inside of the silicone covering. In all animals, there was no evidence of continuity of bile duct proliferation and bile staining with the shunt lumen, which is consistent with the view that the silicone covering prevented the inward migration of biliary epithelial cells or of bile.

DISCUSSION

Development of acute thrombosis, pseudointimal hyperplasia in the TIPS, and/or intimal hyperplasia in the outflow of the HV limits the long-term, primary patency of a TIPS. The theoretic advantage of covered stent-grafts is that the stent-graft can separate flowing blood in the shunt from exposed bile ducts, liver parenchyma, and the injured HV. Results of previous experiments (14) in which PTFE was used as a covering demonstrated improved shunt patency. Unfortunately, a commercially viable PTFE-covered stent-graft is not yet available. We had hoped that the use of an impermeable silicone membrane would yield a similar result; unfortunately, the opposite was true, and patency was worse than with uncovered stents (14).

The use of silicone-covered Wallstents in the vascular system has been previously attempted. Arteriovenous shunts were percutaneously created with silicone-covered Wallstents in an animal model by Trerotola et al (17); however, they demonstrated only a technical feasibility and short-term (2.5–6.5-hour) patency. Therefore, avoidance of the problem of thrombogenesis with impermeable silicone-covered Wallstents has not yet been demonstrated over the long term. In our study, durable patency was not achieved: 13 of 14 shunts were occluded after 6 weeks, and most were occluded by 3 weeks. The early occlusions were not the result of development of pseudointimal or intimal hyperplasia in the HV due to acute thrombosis of the parenchymal tract. Therefore, the thrombogenicity of silicone overwhelmed the potential benefit of a covered stent for TIPS creation.

Silicone is widely used in many applications in veins, including central venous access devices and transvenous pacemaker leads. Thrombosis is one of the most common complications associated with catheters or leads that come in contact with blood. Thrombus related to transvenous pacemaker leads is platelet rich (18). Contact of platelets with surfaces constructed of artificial materials causes platelet activation, adhesion, and aggregation. The resultant degree of thrombosis depends on physiochemical characteristics of the artificial surface (19). The incidence of subclavian vein stenosis when silicone catheters are used for hemodialysis is lower than the incidence of stenosis when PTFE and polyurethane catheters are used (20). In an animal study (21), however, the thrombogenicity of polyurethane leads appeared to be lower than that of silicone leads. Thus far, it has been impossible to avoid complications due to thrombus formation when using silicone-covered devices without the administration of anticoagulation drugs (22,23). This does not seem to be a viable means of improving TIPS patency.

Different lengths of silicone covering were used to evaluate the prevention of intimal hyperplasia development in the outflow of the HV, in the PV wall, or in both. The stents in four animals, including two in which the silicone cover did not cover the PV wall, ended within the HV, short of the IVC. The stents in 10 animals, including another two stents which did not cover the PV wall, covered the entire HV and extended well into the IVC. Histologic findings demonstrated intimal hyperplasia in the outflow of the HV in two of four animals in which the covered stent did not extend into the IVC. However, intimal hyperplasia was also seen in the IVC wall in one of the 10 animals in which the cover extended into the IVC. We did not see this previously with uncovered stents; presumably, the silicone covering stimulated the development of intimal hyperplasia. No intimal hyperplasia occurred in the outflow of the HV in animals with covered stents that extended to the IVC. When stents were placed short of the IVC, intimal hyperplasia was evident after 3 weeks. This finding reiterated a problem associated with covered stent use in TIPS creation: The graft may stimulate intimal hyperplasia in the HV if the covering does not extend to the IVC.

In a previous study (13), a correlation was observed between the presence of biliary epithelium in the neointimal lining of the shunts and thrombotic occlusion of the lumen. It was hypothesized that mucin release from the biliary epithelial cells promoted local thrombus formation and decreased TIPS patency.

In the present study, no biliary epithelium or bile staining were detected inside the impermeable membrane. Interestingly, hyperplastic granulation tissue and a proliferation of bile ducts were detected outside the silicone membrane in 10 animals. Gross evidence of bile staining was also seen outside the covering in two animals but did not leak into the lumen of the shunt. Therefore, the silicone membrane appeared to exclude the effects of biliary injures from the lumen of the shunt. Despite this, thrombosis was present to an even greater extent than has been seen with uncovered shunts.

In conclusion, impermeable silicone-covered Wallstents do not solve the problem of the long-term patency of a TIPS. Thrombogenesis appears to be increased because of the silicone membrane, and a foreign-body reaction was stimulated that resulted in universal early shunt occlusion. ■

References

1. Rossle M, Haag K, Ochs A, et al. The transjugular intrahepatic portosystemic stent-shunt procedure for variceal bleeding. N Engl J Med 1994; 330:165–171.
2. LaBerge JM, Ring EJ, Gorden RL, et al. Transjugular intrahepatic portosystemic shunts with the Wallstent endoprosthesis: results in 100 patients. Radiology 1993; 187: 165–171.
3. Rousseau H, Vinel JP, Bilbao JI, et al. Transjugular intrahepatic portosystemic shunts using the Wallstent prosthesis: a follow-up study. Cardiovasc Intervent Radiol 1994; 17:7–11.
4. Noeldge G, Richter GM, Roessle M, et al. Morphologic and clinical results of the transjugular intrahepatic portosystemic stent-shunt (TIPSS). Cardiovasc Intervent Radiol 1992; 15:342–348.
5. Conn HO. Transjugular intrahepatic portal-systemic shunts: the state of the art. Hepatology 1993; 17:148–158.
6. Helton WS, Belshaw A, Althaus S, Park S, Coldwell D, Johansen K. Critical appraisal of the angiographic portacaval shunt (TIPS). Am J Surg 1993; 165:566–571.
7. Maynar M, Cabrera J, MaPulido-Duque J, et al. Transjugular intrahepatic portosystemic shunt: early experience with a flexible trocar/catheter system. AJR 1993; 161: 301–306.
8. Saxon RR, Barton RE, Petersen BD, Lakin PC, Keller FS, Rosch J. Transjugular intrahepatic portosystemic shunt: middle-term shunt patency (abstr). Radiology 1993; 189(P):227.
9. Haskal ZJ, Pentecost MJ, Soulen MC, Shlansky-Goldberg RD, Baum RA, Cope C. Transjugular intrahepatic portosystemic shunt stenosis and revision: early and middle-term results. AJR 1994; 163:439–444.
10. Hausegger KA, Sternthal HM, Klein GE, Karaic R, Stauber R, Zenker G. Transjugular intrahepatic portosystemic shunt: angiographic follow-up and secondary interventions. Radiology 1994; 191:177–181.
11. LaBerge JM, Ferrell LD, Ring EJ, Gordon RL. Histologic study of stenotic and occluded transjugular intrahepatic portosystemic shunts. JVIR 1993; 4:779–786.
12. LaBerge JM, Somberg KA, Lake JR, et al. Two year outcome following transjugular intrahepatic portosystemic shunt for variceal bleeding: results in 90 patients. Gastroenterology 1995; 108:1143–1151.
13. Saxon RR, Mendel-Hartvig J, Corless CL, et al. Bile duct injury as a major cause of stenosis and occlusion in transjugular intrahepatic portosystemic shunts: comparative histopathologic analysis in humans and swine. JVIR 1996; 7:487–497.
14. Nishimine K, Saxon RR, Kichikawa K, et al. Improved transjugular intrahepatic portosystemic shunt patency with PTFE-covered stent-grafts: experimental results in swine. Radiology 1995; 196:341–347.
15. Rosch J, Uchida BT, Barton RE, Keller FS. Coaxial catheter-needle system for transjugular portal vein entrance. JVIR 1993; 4:145–147.
16. Barton RE, Rosch J, Keller FS, Uchida BT. Transjugular intrahepatic portosystemic shunts. In: Hunter JG, Sackier JM, eds. Minimally invasive surgery. New York, NY: McGraw-Hill, 1993; 269–277.
17. Trerotola SO, Johnson WM, Winkler T, Dreesen RG. Percutaneous creation of arteriovenous hemodialysis graft: work in progress. JVIR 1995; 6:675–681.
18. Davis G, Kaplan K, Kwaan HC. Pulmonary emboli from a platelet-rich thrombus attached to a pacemaker electrode. Pacing Clin Electrophysiol 1983; 6:883–886.
19. Baier RE, Dutton RC. Initial events in interactions of blood with a foreign surface. J Biomed Mater Res 1969; 3:191–206.
20. Beene L, van Leusen R, Deenick B, Bosch FH. The incidence of subclavian vein stenosis using silicone catheters for hemodialysis. Artif Organs 1994; 18:289–292.
21. Palatianos GM, Dewanjee MK, Panoutsopoulos G, Kapadvanjwala M, Novak S, Sfakianakis GN. Comparative thrombogenicity of pacemaker leads. Pacing Clin Electrophysiol 1994; 17:141–145.
22. Freund M, Mantz F, Nicolini P, et al. Experimental thrombosis on collagen coated arterioarterial shunt in rats: a pharmacological model to study antithrombotic agents inhibiting thrombin formation and platelet deposition. Thromb Haemost 1993; 69:515–521.
23. Dollery CM, Sullivan ID, Bull C, Milla PJ. Thrombosis and embolism in long-term central venous access for parenteral nutrition. Lancet 1994; 344:1043–1045.

Andrew J. Fisher, MD • Erik K. Paulson, MD • Douglas H. Sheafor, MD
Constance M. Simmons, RN • Rendon C. Nelson, MD

Small Lymph Nodes of the Abdomen, Pelvis, and Retroperitoneum: Usefulness of Sonographically Guided Biopsy[1]

PURPOSE: **To evaluate the usefulness of sonographically guided percutaneous biopsy of small lymph nodes in the abdomen, retroperitoneum, and pelvis.**

MATERIALS AND METHODS: **From May 1995 through January 1997, 35 sonographically guided lymph node biopsies were performed in 34 patients. All biopsies were performed with a 20- (n = 18) or 22-gauge (n = 10) self-aspirating needle alone or in combination (n = 7). To determine the amount of compression achieved with the transducer, the skin-to-lesion distance on reference computed tomographic (CT) scans was compared with that on sonograms. A biopsy was considered successful if a specific benign or malignant diagnosis was rendered by the pathologist.**

RESULTS: **Of 35 sonographically guided biopsies, 30 (86%) were successful. Diagnoses included 26 (74%) cases of carcinoma, three (9%) cases of benign reactive lymphocytosis confirmed at open biopsy, and one (3%) case of a lymph node with a positive acid-fast bacilli stain. The average lymph node diameter was 2.1 cm (range, 0.9–4.3 cm). With sonography, a mean of 2.5 needle passes (range, 1–5) were made per biopsy. Transducer compression reduced the skin-to-lesion distance from an average of 8.8 cm (at CT) to 4.5 cm.**

CONCLUSION: **Sonographic guidance seems to provide a reasonable alternative to CT in biopsy of small abdominal, pelvic, and retroperitoneal lymph nodes.**

Imaging-guided percutaneous biopsy procedures are a critical component of the diagnosis, staging, and follow-up of suspected or known malignancies. Although European and Asian physicians have routinely used sonographic guidance for biopsies (1–8), radiologists trained in the United States have relied largely on computed tomography (CT) as the modality of choice for biopsy guidance, particularly when targeting lymph nodes in the abdomen and pelvis. Sonography and CT have proved successful and are associated with unique benefits and disadvantages.

Compared with CT, sonographic guidance is less familiar to most American-trained radiologists but has potential advantages over CT guidance. Sonographic guidance with a needle guide is readily mastered and shortens procedure time, facilitates needle tip visualization throughout the entire process, and enables biopsy to be performed during a single breath hold. This technique also ensures that sampling is limited to the lesion. Most, if not all, equipment manufacturers provide needle guides that attach easily to transducers, inside or outside the protective condom, and provide a computer-generated path to the lesion, ensuring accurate needle placement. Other advantages of sonography are mobility of the equipment and no emission of ionizing radiation.

The limitations of sonographic guidance center on the difficulty in visualizing the needle and lesion, particularly when lesions are small or there is overlying bowel gas. In addition, intervening tissues can be difficult to delineate, especially with compression. Many radiologists decline to attempt biopsy of such lesions or perform biopsy with CT guidance. As a result, in some institutions sonography is used primarily for biopsy of large or superficial lesions, as an aid for renal biopsy or paracentesis or thoracentesis, and for biopsy of lesions within the liver.

As experience is gained, radiologists are starting to use sonographic guidance not only for percutaneous biopsy of large or superficial lesions but also for small lesions located deeply or positioned precariously (9). These small lesions include lymph nodes within the abdomen, pelvis, and retroperitoneum. The purpose of this study was to evaluate the usefulness of sonographically guided biopsy of small lymph nodes of the abdomen, pelvis, and retroperitoneum.

MATERIALS AND METHODS

Between May 1995 and January 1997, we performed a total of 35 sonographically guided lymph node biopsies in 34 patients. The average age of the 13 men and 21 women was 59 years (range, 24–88 years). Of these patients, 23 (68%) had a known malignancy, three (9%) had positive results for human immunodeficiency virus, and the remaining eight (24%) had no history of malignancy or condition predisposing

Index terms: Biopsies, technology, 998.1261, 998.12985, 998.12989 • Computed tomography (CT), comparative studies, 998.1261 • Lymphatic system, biopsy, 998.1261 • Ultrasound (US), comparative studies, 998.12985, 998.12989, 998.12911 • Ultrasound (US), guidance, 998.12985, 998.12989

Radiology 1997; 205:185–190

[1] From the Department of Radiology, Duke University Medical Center, Box 3808, Erwin Rd, Durham, NC 27710. Received April 24, 1997; revision requested May 23; revision received June 20; accepted June 25. **Address reprint requests to** E.K.P.

toward lymphadenopathy. Primary tumors in the 23 patients with known malignancy included lymphoma in seven (30%) patients; colon cancer in five (22%); melanoma in two (9%), breast cancer in two (9%), ovarian cancer in two (9%), cervical cancer in two (9%); and pancreatic cancer, ovarian cancer, or cholangiocarcinoma in one patient each (4%). Twenty-two patients were outpatients and 12 were inpatients. Biopsy results were reviewed retrospectively.

The 35 lymph nodes in which biopsy was performed varied widely in location. Eight (23%) were in the porta hepatis or portacaval region, seven (20%) were in an aortocaval or paracaval distribution (six of these seven were inferior to the level of the left renal vein), six (17%) were paraaortic (five of these six lymph nodes were inferior to the left renal vein), four (11%) were in the pelvic area, four (11%) were in the mesenteric region, three (9%) were paraceliac, and three (9%) were adjacent to the superior mesenteric artery.

The mean diameter of the lymph nodes was 2.1 cm. Measurement was based on an average of the transverse and anteroposterior diameters (range, 0.9–4.3) measured sonographically. Of the 35 lymph nodes, 18 (51%) had an average diameter less than 2 cm.

All patients underwent diagnostic CT before biopsy. CT scans were displayed in the interventional radiology suite during the biopsy procedure and were reviewed to choose the optimal site and route for biopsy. A full diagnostic abdominal or pelvic sonogram was not obtained at biopsy; acquisition of preliminary sonograms was limited to identification of an appropriate path to the lymph node in question. Only seven (20%) of the 35 CT scans were obtained at other institutions.

After written informed consent was obtained from each patient, the selected lymph node was identified sonographically and a biopsy path was chosen. To improve visualization of the lymph node, the overlying abdominal wall was compressed with the transducer to displace or minimize intervening bowel loops and fatty tissues. The needle path was interrogated routinely with color Doppler sonography to detect and avoid intervening blood vessels. The route chosen was the shortest possible but also free of intervening critical structures such as large vessels or bile ducts. No particular attempt was made to avoid intervening bowel; in fact, with compression it typically was not possible to differentiate compressed bowel from mesenteric fatty tissue. A path through solid organs was avoided except in cases in which there was no alternative (eg, porta hepatis and portacaval lymph nodes).

All biopsies were performed with a model 128 sonographic unit (Acuson, Mountain View, Calif) except for a single biopsy performed with a Logic 700 unit (GE Medical Systems, Milwaukee, Wis). A 3.25- or 2.5-MHz sector transducer equipped with an attachable needle guide was used. This needle guide directs the needle at a 15° or 30° angle with respect to the orientation of the transducer.

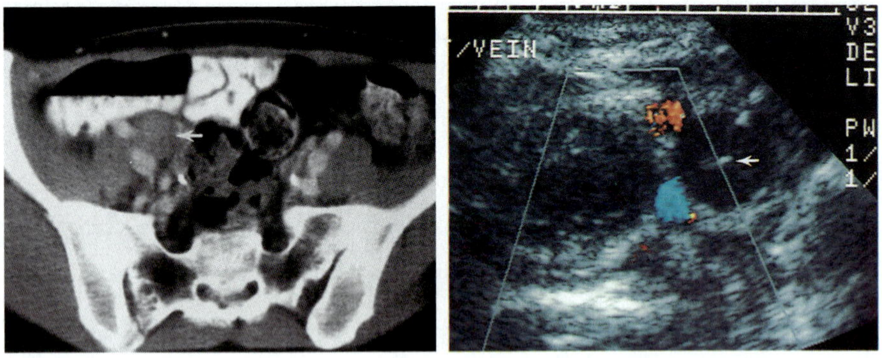

a. b.

Figure 1. Images obtained in a 23-year-old woman in whom non-Hodgkin lymphoma was suspected. **(a)** CT scan shows an enlarged right external iliac lymph node (arrow). **(b)** Sonogram shows the echogenic tip of a 20-gauge needle within the lymph node (arrow). Real-time visualization of the needle tip during the biopsy ensures that the specimen will be obtained exclusively from the lymph node without contamination from adjacent normal tissues or transgression of the adjacent external iliac vein. Non-Hodgkin lymphoma was proved pathologically in this specimen.

Summary of Lymph Node Biopsies according to Site

Location	Success*	Mean Size (cm)†	Mean No. of Needle Passes†
Retroperitoneal (n = 13)			
Paraaortic (n = 6)	5 (83)	1.8 (1.5–2.7)	2.3 (1–4)
Aortocaval (n = 7)	6 (86)	2.1 (0.9–2.8)	2.4 (1–5)
Porta hepatis and portacaval (n = 8)	6 (75)	2.2 (1.5–4.0)	2.5 (1–5)
Pelvic (n = 4)	3 (75)	2.9 (1.9–4.3)	3.0 (2–4)
Mesenteric (n = 4)	4 (100)	2.4 (1.5–3.5)	3.25 (2–4)
Adjacent to the superior mesenteric artery (n = 3)	3 (100)	1.2 (1.2–1.3)	2.3 (1–3)
Paraceliac (n = 3)	3 (100)	1.6 (1.1–2.4)	1.7 (1–2)
Total (n = 35)	30 (86)	2.1	2.5

* Numbers in parentheses are percentages.
† Numbers in parentheses are a range.

After the skin was thoroughly washed with bactericidal soap, the skin site and anterior abdominal wall were infiltrated with 5–10 mL of 1% lidocaine hydrochloride (Xylocaine; Astra, Westborough, Mass) with a 25-gauge needle. Sedation was achieved with intravenous administration of diazepam (Valium; Elkins-Sinn, Cherry Hill, NJ) and/or fentanyl citrate (Sublimaze; Akorn, Decatur, Ill) as necessary.

In all lymph nodes, biopsy was performed with a 20-gauge (n = 18) or 22-gauge (n = 10) self-aspirating Crown needle without suction (Medi-tech/Boston Scientific, Watertown, Mass) alone or in combination (n = 7). In six cases, biopsy was also performed with an 18- or 20-gauge automated spring-loaded cutting needle (Medi-tech/Boston Scientific).

The needle pass technique was as follows: One physician (A.J.F., E.K.P., D.H.S., or R.C.N.) held the transducer while a second manipulated the needle. Initially, the needle pierced the skin and advanced into the subcutaneous fatty tissue. While the patient suspended respiration, the path of the needle guide was aligned with the lymph node and the needle was advanced into it. The stylet was then removed, and, without suction, the needle was passed in and out of the lymph node five to 10 times, with slight rotation. Operators paid careful attention to the needle tip, attempting to avoid sampling adjacent normal structures or blood vessels (Fig 1). The needle was removed (without the stylet), and the patient was instructed to breathe normally.

Biopsies were performed or supervised directly by one of a group of eight attending abdominal radiologists (E.K.P., R.C.N.). A cytopathologist was present during all procedures to determine if adequate tissue was obtained and to provide a preliminary interpretation. The procedure was considered completed once the pathologist determined an adequate sample had been obtained. Patients were monitored in a recovery area for 4–6 hours after the biopsy procedure to monitor vital signs and assess for complications. All outpatients were contacted by a nurse 1 or 2 days after the biopsy procedure to determine complications such as persistent pain, fever, or bleeding at the puncture site. The inpatients were monitored by their clinical team, and the medical records were reviewed for the development of peritonitis, unexplained fever or abdominal pain, abscess, or blood transfusion requirement.

Final pathology reports were reviewed.

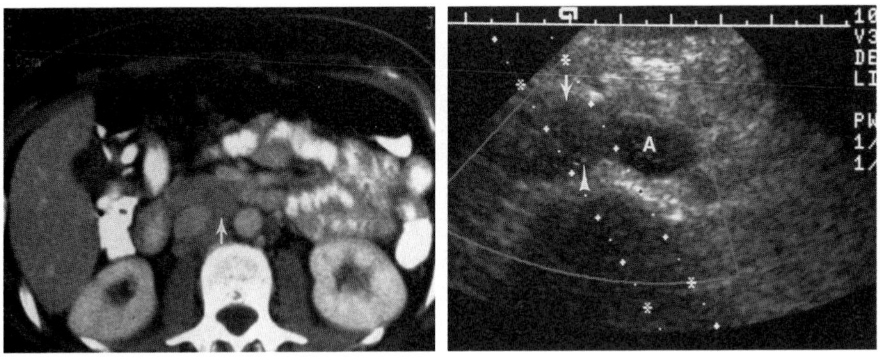

a. b.

Figure 2. Carcinoma of the cervix in a 32-year-old woman. **(a)** CT scan shows an enlarged aortocaval lymph node (arrow). The anteroposterior distance from the skin to the leading edge of the lymph node is 9 cm. **(b)** Sonogram shows that with gradual compression produced with the transducer, the skin-to-lesion distance is reduced to only 3 cm. Displacement and compression of bowel and fatty tissue improve visualization of the lymph node (arrow) and needle tip (arrowhead). *A* = aorta.

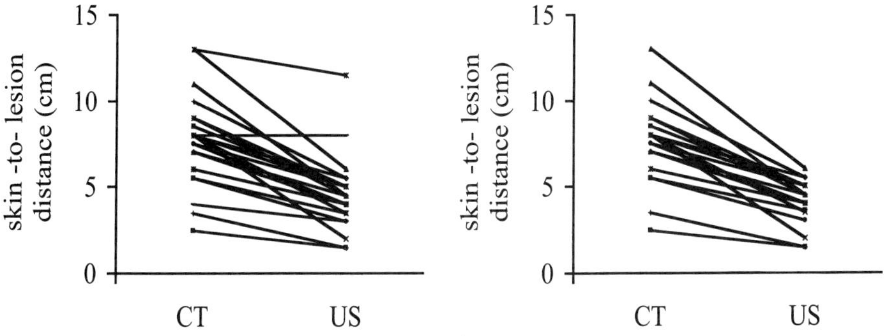

a. b.

Figure 3. **(a, b)** Graphs show comparison of the skin-to-lesion distance measured at CT with that measured at sonographically guided biopsy. **(a)** The lines connect the measurements in all cases in which CT scans and sonograms were available (n = 25). **(b)** The measurements in the seven cases in which liver transgression was necessary were excluded.

The final pathologic diagnosis was based on examination of the cytopathologic specimen in all cases and of the cytopathologic specimen and histopathologic specimen in six cases. A biopsy was considered successful if a specific malignant diagnosis was made or a benign diagnosis was made and confirmed subsequently at open surgical biopsy. A biopsy was considered unsuccessful if the pathology report revealed nonspecific findings such as reactive tissue, suspicious cells, fibrous or fatty tissue, or acute or chronic inflammation. In addition, a specific benign diagnosis not confirmed at open biopsy was deemed unsuccessful even though these biopsy procedures may have resulted in true-negative specimens.

The total room time (n = 35) and procedure time (n = 25) were recorded. Early in our experience, procedure time was not recorded, accounting for the difference in sample size. Room time was defined as the period during which the patient was in the interventional radiology suite, including all preparation (consent, placement of intravenous catheter, patient transfers, etc) and postprocedural monitoring (initial vital signs, hemostasis assessment for pain, dressing of the puncture site, etc) before the patient was transferred to a recovery area. Procedure time was defined as the time from commencement of skin preparation through preliminary cytopathologic interpretation. Differences in the amount of room time necessary for all CT-guided lymph node biopsies (n = 23) performed over a 1-year period were determined with a two-tailed Student t test. For CT-guided biopsies, acquisition of scans was limited to biopsy planning, and a full diagnostic abdominal or pelvic study was not performed. Therefore, although diagnostic scans were available during CT- or sonographically guided biopsies, room time for CT-and sonographically guided biopsies encompassed similar parameters.

Images from the procedure and the diagnostic CT scans, if available, were reviewed retrospectively by two radiologists (A.J.F., E.K.P.) in consensus. As this was a retrospective review, a standard imaging format was not followed for each case. Nevertheless, for each case the sonographic images documented the targeted lymph node and the anticipated needle path as prescribed by the needle guide. To assess the amount of compression of the abdominal wall achieved by applying downward transducer pressure, we measured the shortest distance from the abdominal wall to the leading edge of the lymph node with hand-held calipers. This distance was measured on the CT scans and sonograms. Sonograms and CT scans were available in only 25 cases. The reason for this is that many of the CT scans were from other institutions and had been returned.

RESULTS

Sonographically guided biopsy was successful in 30 (86%) of 35 biopsies. These biopsies yielded new or recurrent metastatic carcinoma in 26 (74%) patients, benign reactive lymphocytes confirmed at subsequent open surgical biopsy in three (9%) patients, and positive findings in a lymph node from acid-fast bacilli stain consistent with *Mycobacterium tuberculosis* in one (3%) patient (Table). The five unsuccessful biopsies yielded nonspecific inflammation, fibrous tissue, or no evidence of malignancy. For analysis purposes, these cases were considered unsuccessful, although no subsequent histopathologic proof of malignant lesions was determined.

The mean lymph node diameter was 2.1 cm (range, 0.9-4.3). Even though these lymph nodes were small, an average of 2.5 needle passes (range, 1–5) were made. Eight procedures were completed successfully in a single pass. A mean of three passes were made in the five unsuccessful biopsies.

Part of the success of sonographic guidance related to the ability to reduce the needle path distance with application of transducer pressure (Fig 2). Under CT guidance, the lymph nodes sampled for biopsy had an average skin-to-lesion distance of 8.8 cm (range, 2.5–13.0 cm). During sonographically guided biopsy, this average distance (shortest measurable path) was only 4.5 cm (range, 1.5–11.5), a reduction of 49% (Fig 3). If the seven cases in which the liver was transgressed are excluded, the difference is more marked. In these biopsies, average skin-to-lesion distance was 9.5 cm on CT scans; this distance was only 4.0 cm with transducer pressure, a reduction of 58%.

Results from the the five unsuccessful biopsies were not substantially different from results from the successful biopsies. Four of the five biopsies yielded primary malignancy. The mean lymph node size was similar (2.2 cm). An average of 3.0 passes were performed compared with 2.4 for successful biopsies. The sonographic depth was comparable (5.0 cm for unsuccessful biopsies vs 4.5 cm for successful biopsies). Clinical or imaging follow-up was performed at our

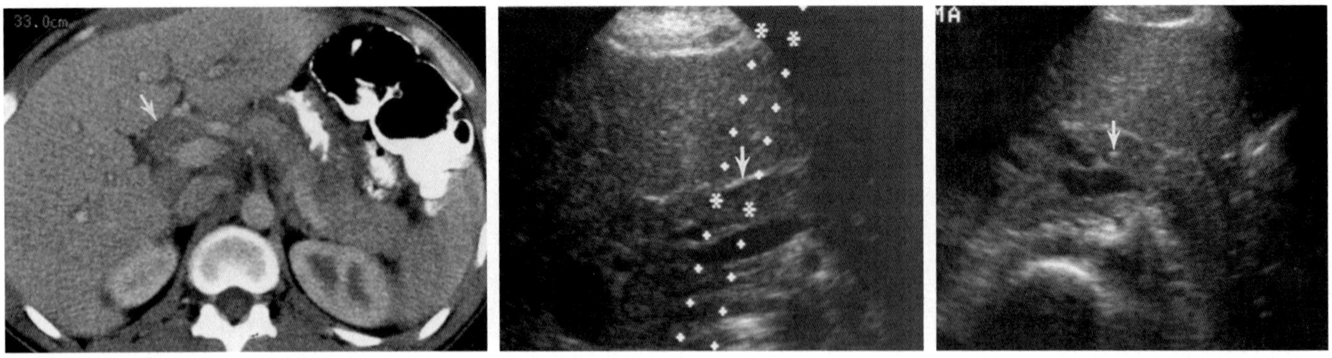

a. b. c.

Figure 4. Images obtained in a 32-year-old man with human immunodeficiency virus. **(a)** CT scan shows an enlarged portocaval lymph node (arrow). Note the proximity of this lymph node to the hepatic artery, portal vein, and common bile duct (not shown). **(b)** Sonogram obtained with needle guidance shows a safe route to the lymph node (arrow), free of intervening critical structures. **(c)** Sonogram shows the needle tip (arrow) within the lymph node, which stained positive for acid-fast bacilli consistent with *M tuberculosis*.

institution in only one of these five cases, and the CT findings showed stable disease at 8 months.

There was a single bleeding complication. In this case, injury to the inferior epigastric artery occurred during needle placement; transcatheter arterial embolization was necessary to obtain hemostasis. All remaining patients tolerated the procedure well; none of the outpatients reported fever, pain, or admission to other hospitals when contacted by our nurse (C.M.S.). None of the inpatients developed peritonitis, unexplained abdominal pain, or abscess or required a blood transfusion after the biopsy procedure. One inpatient had a temperature of 40°C 3 days after biopsy. The patient had no abdominal pain or tenderness, and the fever was attributed to lymphoma. The patient died of respiratory failure 2 weeks later, and an autopsy showed no hematoma, abscess, or injury to bowel.

Although the average room time was 81 minutes for sonographically guided biopsies (range, 45–135 minutes), the average procedure time was 35 minutes (range, 10–85 minutes). The average room time was 95 minutes for CT-guided lymph node biopsies (range, 50–157 minutes). The difference in procedure time between sonographically and CT-guided lymph node biopsies was not statistically significant ($P > .19$).

DISCUSSION

Our results show that sonography is an accurate and safe guidance technique for biopsy of abdominal, pelvic, and retroperitoneal lymph nodes. Our success rate of 86% is on par with results from other institutions, with reported success rates of 75%–91%. Our results confirm the recent study by Memel et al (9), which included 26 patients with abdominal, pelvic, and retroperitoneal lymphadenopathy and yielded tissue adequate for diagnosis in 21 (91%) of 23 sonographically guided procedures. Nagano et al (4) reported a successful procedure in 13 (81%) of 16 pelvic and 21 (81%) of 26 paraaortic lymph node biopsies. Similarly, Al-Mofleh (10) obtained diagnoses in 75% of 37 sonographically guided biopsies. Tikkakoski et al (7) obtained "correct results" in 31 (91%) of 34 abdominal and retroperitoneal lymph node biopsies. Part of the success in European studies probably relates to the increased availability of sonography compared with that of CT. In addition, European cytopathologists may have more familiarity with fine-needle aspiration techniques and analysis than their counterparts in the United States.

Proponents for the use of CT for lymph node biopsy argue that CT provides superior anatomic visualization and detailed delineation of the lesion and adjacent structures. Bowel gas and osseous structures that hinder sonographic localization pose no such problem at CT. In addition, many radiologists prefer the broad field of view provided by CT and the relative ease of needle visualization. However, there are several drawbacks to CT guidance. CT precludes real-time visualization during needle placement and biopsy; in the case of small lymph nodes, lack of visualization during the procedure may result in sampling of adjacent normal tissue. More time is typically necessary to perform a biopsy with CT rather than with sonography. Use of CT in biopsy procedures occupies valuable time on busy CT schedules, which are often already overburdened.

We found that sonographic guidance is useful in biopsy of abdominal, pelvic, and retroperitoneal lymph nodes. With use of a needle guide, the needle can be passed accurately into the lesion during real-time visualization and the procedure may be performed during one or two patient breath holds. Most, if not all, equipment manufacturers provide needle guides, which usually attach to the transducer and provide a computer-generated path to the lesion, ensuring accurate needle placement. Experienced operators may favor the free-hand technique, although we have found the needle guide helpful in efficient and direct placement of the needle into lesions. One drawback of the needle guide is that in some cases it is not possible to follow the prescribed path of the needle due to intervening vital structures. In these cases the free-hand technique is necessary.

Real-time needle tip visualization also helps ensure that sampling will be limited to the lesion; samples are far less likely to be contaminated with extraneous tissue or blood and thus may be easier to interpret by the pathologist. With real-time visualization it is also possible to ensure that the needle excursions are short of adjacent critical structures such as blood vessels or the common bile duct. With sonographic guidance, the length of time that the needle is actually in the patient is often limited to less than 30 seconds.

Another advantage of sonography is its multiplanar capability. The operator can angle and rotate the transducer to avoid adjacent vessels and organs (Fig 4). This type of transducer movement is particularly important for biopsy of portal, pelvic, and retroperitoneal nodes, which are frequently adjacent to large vessels. Biopsies performed outside the axial plane are far more complex when CT is used.

Use of sonography for biopsy of lymph nodes may seem paradoxical because this modality, unlike CT, is not particularly sensitive in the depiction of lymph nodes. Lymph nodes may be difficult to visualize with sonography because of deep location and overlying bowel. Accordingly, it has become our routine always to display previously obtained diagnostic CT scans or magnetic resonance images in the interventional radiology suite to serve as a guide for lymph node identification. We also found that lymph node visualization is improved markedly by applying firm pressure with the transducer to compress and displace overlying fatty tissue and bowel loops, decreasing the necessary depth of sound penetration and the length of needle excursion. Compared with the skin-to-lesion distance on the reference CT scans, the distance from the anterior abdominal wall to the lymph node was reduced by approximately one-half as a result of transducer pressure. Predictably, there was less compression achieved in biopsy of lymph nodes in the porta hepatis because the liver and subcostal region is less compressible than bowel or mesenteric fat.

We made no particular attempt to avoid transgression of intervening small bowel or colon. In fact, with compression it is usually impossible to differentiate bowel from mesenteric or omental fatty tissue. None of our patients received antibiotics and none had complications related to bowel perforation; in selected cases, however, particularly those in which transgression of the colon is anticipated, prophylactic antibiotics may be indicated. Further, in patients with bowel distention or when a 16–18-gauge cutting needle is used, the risk of peritoneal contamination may be increased. In dogs, Petit et al (11) showed no untoward effect from transgressing bowel with needles and catheters.

There was one major complication that resulted from an injury to the inferior epigastric artery and necessitated subsequent embolization, giving our small series a complication rate of 3%. This rate is higher than the reported complication rates associated with percutaneous biopsies of focal lesions within the abdomen. In an extensive review of 11,700 patients undergoing fine-needle abdominal biopsies between 1969 and 1982, Livraghi et al (12) reported a mortality rate of 0.008% with a 0.5% serious and 0.49% minor complication rate. Nolsoe et al (13) reported seven complications (0.2% morbidity) with a mortality rate of 0.028% in a study of 3,500 fine-needle aspiration biopsies between 1969 and 1987. Two cases of portal lymph node biopsies were complicated by bile leaks. Other questionnaire studies with large numbers of patients have yielded mortality rates of 0.006%-0.031% (14–16).

Although careful attention to critical structures may limit complication rates, superficial vessels such as the inferior epigastric artery affected in our one case with complications, or the internal mammary vessels as reported by others (17), can be a source of serious bleeding. Careful attention to superficial vasculature during biopsy planning with color Doppler sonography should limit these cases.

It has been suggested that biopsy of retroperitoneal lymph nodes is performed best with a posterior paraspinal approach. The theoretical advantage of this approach is that should arterial bleeding occur, the result would be a contained retroperitoneal hematoma rather than an intraperitoneal hematoma. In addition, this approach may be less painful than an anterior approach. A disadvantage of sonography compared with CT, however, is that it is often impossible to identify retroperitoneal lymph nodes when a paraspinal window is used. Also, biopsy of pelvic lymph nodes cannot be performed from a posterior approach because of the osseous pelvis. An alternative approach in the pelvis would be an endorectal or endovaginal technique (18).

One limitation of our study is that it is a retrospective review of our experience. It is possible that there were patients who were referred for an imaging-guided lymph node biopsy who were not referred for sonography because it was believed that the node would be inaccessible sonographically. Although we are not aware of such patients, inclusion of these potential cases would bias our results in favor of sonography. Alternatively, it is possible that some lymph nodes were readily amenable to sonographically guided biopsy but not amenable to CT-guided biopsy. This issue could be addressed by a prospective randomized direct comparison of CT versus sonographic guidance. In the 26 consecutive cases reported by Memel et al (9), biopsy with sonographic guidance was successful in 23 (88%) cases; in only three cases was use of a CT scanner necessary. An additional potential limitation of our study is that we used a nonaspiration capillary technique rather than suction generated by attachment of a syringe to the biopsy needle. However, we and others have found that samples obtained with the capillary technique have adequate number of cell clusters and less contamination from blood than samples obtained with the suction technique (19–21).

Although our success rate is high, technical developments in imaging guidance may lead to even higher success and lower complication rates. A number of new techniques and equipment options have already had an effect on sonographic guidance and will most likely improve success and reduce complication rates (22-26).

Sonography is a diagnostically accurate and safe guidance technique for biopsy of abdominal, pelvic, and retroperitoneal lymph nodes. Benefits include continuous needle tip visualization, adjacent vessel identification, scanning in nonaxial planes, and avoidance of ionizing radiation. Sonographic guidance provides a reasonable alternative to CT guidance. ■

References

1. Damgaard-Pedersen K, Von der Maase H. Ultrasound and ultrasound guided biopsy, CT and lymphography in the diagnosis of retroperitoneal metastases in testicular cancer. Scand J Urol Nephrol 1991; 137:139–144.
2. Dodd GD III, Esola CC, Memel DS, et al. Sonography: the undiscovered jewel of interventional radiology. RadioGraphics 1996; 16:1271–1288.
3. Matalon TAS, Silver B. US guidance of interventional procedures. Radiology 1990; 174:43–47.
4. Nagano T, Nakai Y, Taniguchi F, et al. Diagnosis of paraaortic and pelvic lymph node metastasis of gynecologic malignant tumors by ultrasound-guided percutaneous fine-needle aspiration biopsy. Cancer 1991; 68:2571–2574.
5. Nyman RS, Cappelen-Smith J, Brismar J, et al. Yield and complications in ultrasound-guided biopsy of abdominal lesions. Acta Radiol 1995; 36:485–490.
6. Paulson EK. Image guided percutaneous abdominal biopsies. Appl Radiol 1995; 24: 11–15.
7. Tikkakoski T, Siniluoto T, Ollikainen A, et al. Ultrasound-guided aspiration cytology of enlarged lymph nodes. Acta Radiol 1991; 32:53–56.
8. Tikkakoski T, Pairvansalo M, Similuoto T, et al. Percutaneous ultrasound-guided biopsy: fine needle biopsy, cutting needle biopsy, or both? Acta Radiol 1993; 34:30–34.
9. Memel DS, Dodd GD III, Esola CC. Efficacy of sonography as a guidance technique for biopsy of abdominal, pelvic and retroperitoneal lymph nodes. AJR 1996; 167:957–962.
10. Al-Mofleh IA. Ultrasound-guided fine needle aspiration of retroperitoneal, abdominal and pelvic lymph nodes: diagnostic reliability. Acta Cytol 1992; 36:413–415.
11. Petit P, Bret PM, Tough JO, Reinhold C. Risks associated with intestinal perforation during experimental percutaneous drainage. Invest Radiol 1992; 27:1012–1019.

12. Livraghi T, Damascelli B, Lombardi C, Spagnoli I. Risk in fine-needle abdominal biopsy. JCU 1983; 11:77–81.
13. Nolsoe C, Nielsen L, Torp-Pedersen S, Holm HH. Major complications and deaths due to interventional ultrasonography: a review of 8000 cases. JCU 1990; 18: 179–184.
14. Smith EH. The hazards of fine-needle aspiration biopsy. Ultrasound Med Biol 1984; 10:629–634.
15. Smith EH. Complications of percutaneous abdominal fine-needle biopsy. Radiology 1991; 178:253–258.
16. Weiss H, Duntsch U, Weiss A. Risiken der feinnadelpunktion: ergebnisse einer umfrage in der BRD (DEGUM-Umfrage). Ultraschall Med 1988; 9:121–127.
17. Targhetta R, Bourgeois JM, Dauzat M, Marty-Double C, Balmes P. Sonographic guidance in diagnosing anterior mediastinal mass: importance of visualizing internal mammary vessels. JCU 1993; 21:203–206.
18. Zanetta G, Brenna A, Pittelli M, et al. Transvaginal ultrasound-guided fine needle sampling of deep cancer recurrences in the pelvis: usefulness and limitations. Gynecol Oncol 1994; 54:59–63.
19. Mair S, Dunbar F, Becker PJ, DuPlessis N. Fine needle cytology: is aspiration suction necessary? a study of 100 masses in various sites. Acta Cytol 1989; 33:809–813.
20. Fagelman D, Chess P. Non-aspiration fine needle cytology of the liver: a new technique for obtaining diagnostic samples. AJR 1990; 155:1217–1219.
21. Kinney TB, Lee MJ, Ficomena CA, et al. Fine needle biopsy: Prospective comparison of aspiration versus nonaspiration techniques in the abdomen. Radiology 1993; 186:549–552.
22. Bisceglia M, Matalon TAS, Silver B. The pump maneuver: an atraumatic adjunct to enhance US needle tip localization. Radiology 1990; 176:867–868.
23. Winsberg F, Mitty HA, Shapiro RS, Yelt HC. Use of an acoustic transponder for US visualization of biopsy needles. Radiology 1991; 180:877–878.
24. Perella RR, Kimme-Smith C, Tessler FN, Ragavendra N, Grant EG. A new electronically enhanced biopsy system: value in improving needle tip visualization during sonographically guided interventional procedures. AJR 1992; 158:195–198.
25. Hamper UM, Savader BL, Sheth S. Improved needle-tip visualization by color Doppler sonography. AJR 1991; 156:401–402.
26. Feld R, Needleman L, Goldberg BB. Use of a needle vibrating device and color Doppler imaging for sonographically guided invasive procedures. AJR 1997; 168:255–256.

Guenther E. Klein, MD • Dieter H. Szolar, MD • Klaus A. Leber, MD
Radenko Karaic, MD • Klaus A. Hausegger, MD

Basilar Tip Aneurysm: Endovascular Treatment with Guglielmi Detachable Coils—Midterm Results[1]

PURPOSE: To determine the safety and effectiveness of Guglielmi detachable coils in the endovascular treatment of ruptured and nonruptured basilar tip aneurysms.

MATERIALS AND METHODS: A basilar tip aneurysm was occluded with Guglielmi detachable coils in 21 patients. The aneurysmal diameter was small (less than 12 mm) in 15 patients, large (12–25 mm) in four patients, and giant (more than 25 mm) in two patients. Angiographic follow-up ranged from 6 to 48 months (mean, 26 months); clinical follow-up ranged from 1 to 48 months.

RESULTS: Embolization was technically successful in all patients. Complete occlusion was achieved in 14 (67%) patients; 90% occlusion was achieved in seven (33%) patients. There was partial reperfusion of the aneurysm in three patients (14%) after 6 months, which necessitated repeated embolization. The clinical results were excellent in 13 patients, good in six, and fair in one. One patient died 2 months after the embolization due to pulmonary complications. A posterior cerebral artery was occluded in five (24%) patients; one of these patients developed a permanent neurologic deficit, one developed a transient neurologic deficit, and three had no clinical symptoms.

CONCLUSION: Endovascular treatment of a basilar tip aneurysm with Guglielmi detachable coils seems to be a safe and less invasive alternative to surgical clipping.

Because of the deep location of basilar tip aneurysms, surgical treatment is difficult, and there is a high risk of complications (1–7). Hence, the surgical outcome in patients with a basilar tip aneurysm has been shown (7) to be poorer than the outcome in those with an aneurysm in the anterior circulation.

During the past decade, endovascular treatment has gained acceptance as a therapeutic alternative in the care of patients with an intracranial aneurysm that is considered to be inoperable or may be associated with a high surgical risk (8–15). Detachable balloons (8–16) and nondetachable microcoils (17,18) have been widely used. However, these devices are associated with a relatively high complication rate. Higashida et al (13) reported a morbidity rate of 7.4% and a mortality rate of 9.8% associated with the use of balloons. Morbidity and mortality rates associated with the use of nondetachable coils have been reported (17) to be 4.2% and 11.3%, respectively.

With the development of the Guglielmi detachable coil (GDC), the indication for treatment of intracranial aneurysms may have changed. The use of GDCs allows a more controlled and precise placement of these soft platinum microcoils, enabling selective occlusion of saccular aneurysms. The results of preliminary studies (19–25) of the endovascular occlusion of intracranial aneurysms with GDCs have been encouraging.

There have been only a few reports (22,26,27) of the use of GDC for occlusion of basilar tip aneurysms in selected patients. To our knowledge, however, ours is the first report of the use of GDCs in a nonselected study population. Because of the high surgical risk associated with the anatomic location of a basilar tip aneurysm, none of the patients in the present study were considered to be candidates for surgery. We report our results of 4 years of experience with GDC treatment in 21 patients with a ruptured or a nonruptured basilar tip aneurysm.

The purpose of this study was to determine the safety and effectiveness of GDCs in the endovascular treatment of ruptured and nonruptured basilar tip aneurysms in a nonselected population of patients.

MATERIALS AND METHODS

Patients

From December 1992 to December 1996, 21 patients (13 women and eight men) with a basilar tip aneurysm were treated with GDCs. Written informed consent was obtained from all patients, who were physically and mentally able. The patients were aged 31–75 years (mean, 50 years).

At the time of presentation, 16 (76%) patients had a subarachnoid hemorrhage, and two (10%) patients had signs of mass effect (sixth nerve palsy in one patient, headache and vertigo in the other). An aneurysm was found incidentally in three (14%) patients. All 16 patients with a sub-

Index terms: Aneurysm, cerebral, 1753.73 • Aneurysm, therapy, 1753.1264 • Arteries, therapeutic blockade, 1753.1264

Abbreviations: GDC = Guglielmi detachable coil, PCA = posterior cerebral artery.

Radiology 1997; 205:191–196

[1] From the Departments of Radiology (G.E.K., D.H.S., R.K., K.A.H.) and Neurosurgery (K.A.L.), Karl-Franzens Medical School and University Hospital, Auenbruggerplatz 9, 8036 Graz, Austria. From the 1995 RSNA scientific assembly. Received March 11, 1997; revision requested April 11; revision received June 11; accepted June 12. **Address reprint requests to** G.E.K.

Findings in 21 Patients with a Basilar Tip Aneurysm Treated with GDCs

Patient/ Age (y)/Sex	Clinical Finding	Hunt-Hess Grade	Aneurysm Size*	Coil Length (cm)	Occlusion (%)	Complications†	Angiographic Follow-up (mo)‡	Outcome§
1/44/F	Incidental finding	0	Small	26	100	None	45	Excellent
2/49/F	Mass effect	0	Small	24	90	None	26	Excellent
3/57/M	Mass effect	0	Large	65	90	Occlusion of right PCA	26	Fair
4/46/F	Incidental finding	0	Small	18	100	None	18	Excellent
5/75/F	Incidental finding	0	Small	58	100	None	6	Excellent
6/60/M	Subarachnoid hemorrhage	I	Large	110	90	None	18	Excellent
7/42/M	Subarachnoid hemorrhage	I	Small	28	100	None	6	Excellent
8/56/F	Subarachnoid hemorrhage	I	Small	8	100	None	NA	Excellent
9/31/M	Subarachnoid hemorrhage	II	Small	48	100	Occlusion of left PCA	46	Excellent
10/46/F	Subarachnoid hemorrhage	II	Small	8	90	None	25	Excellent
11/50/F	Subarachnoid hemorrhage	II	Small	45	100	Occlusion of left PCA	24	Excellent
12/64/F	Subarachnoid hemorrhage	II	Small	43	100	None	16	Excellent
13/38/F	Subarachnoid hemorrhage	III	Large	84	100	None	48	Excellent
14/34/M	Subarachnoid hemorrhage	III	Small	40	90	None	47	Excellent
15/43/M	Subarachnoid hemorrhage	III	Giant	185	100	Occlusion of PCA	30	Good
16/52/F	Subarachnoid hemorrhage	III	Giant	172	100	None	25	Excellent
17/47/F	Subarachnoid hemorrhage	III	Large	100	100	None	15	Good
18/58/M	Subarachnoid hemorrhage	IV	Small	60	90	None	42	Good
19/67/M	Subarachnoid hemorrhage	IV	Small	20	100	None	6	Good
20/56/F	Subarachnoid hemorrhage	V	Small	70	100	Occlusion of left PCA	NA	Dead
21/47/F	Subarachnoid hemorrhage	V	Small	16	90	None	24	Good

* Small aneurysm had a diameter of less than 12 mm; large aneurysm diameter was 12–25 mm; giant aneurysm was 25 mm in diameter or larger.
† PCA = posterior cerebral artery.
‡ NA = not available.
§ A modified Glasgow scale was used to report outcome: excellent = neurologically intact with no detectable deficit; good = mild deficit; fair = marked hemiparesis, aphasia, or other deficit; poor = comatose.

arachnoid hemorrhage underwent endovascular treatment within 4 days of the onset of symptoms. The Hunt and Hess grading system was used to classify the subarachnoid hemorrhage as grade I in three patients, as grade II in four patients, as grade III in five patients, as grade IV in two patients, and as grade V in two patients.

The aneurysm was small (less than 12 mm in diameter) in 15 patients, large (12–25 mm in diameter) in four patients, and giant (more than 25 mm in diameter) in two patients (Table). The aneurysm in nine patients had a narrow neck (4-mm diameter or smaller); in twelve patients, the aneurysm had a wide neck (larger than 4 mm in diameter). In all patients, the clinical diagnosis of subarachnoid hemorrhage was confirmed with computed tomographic (CT) findings (Fig 2a), and the diagnosis of basilar tip aneurysm was confirmed with findings from four-vessel angiography (Figs 1a, 1b, 2b, 2c, 3b, 3c). Magnetic resonance (MR) images, MR angiograms (Fig 3a), and/or CT angiograms were obtained in all patients who did not have a subarachnoid hemorrhage.

The study protocol included angiographic follow-up at 6 months and 1, 2 (Fig 3f), and 4 years after treatment. The clinical follow-up ranged from 1 month to 4 years. Outcome in patients was classified on the basis of a modified Glasgow scale (23): excellent (neurologically intact), good (mild deficit), fair (marked neurologic deficit), poor (comatose), and dead.

Interventional Procedure

Thirteen procedures were performed with local anesthesia. Sedative and/or analgesic drugs were also administered if deemed necessary. General anesthesia was used in eight patients, who were either in poor medical condition or uncooperative. Heparin (Heparin Immuno; Immuno, Vienna, Austria) (5,000 IU) was administered intravenously for the purpose of systemic anticoagulation.

Initially, intraarterial digital subtraction angiograms of the cerebral vessels were obtained by using a 6-F catheter (Simmons II or Headhunter; Cordis, Miami, Fla) inserted through a transfemoral 6-F introducer sheath. Computer-assisted measurement of the aneurysm was performed to select the appropriate size of GDC. Subsequently, the diagnostic catheter was exchanged for a 6-F guide catheter (Balt, Paris, France) placed in the cervical segment of the dominant vertebral artery. Superselective catheter placement in the aneurysm was accomplished coaxially with a Tracker-18 GDC microcatheter (Target Therapeutics, Fremont, Calif). The coaxial system was continuously flushed with a solution of saline and heparin (1,000 IU heparin per 500 mL normal saline) to prevent thrombus formation between the two catheters. The negotiation of the aneurysm was accomplished with a platinum-tipped 0.016-inch steerable guide wire (Taper; Target Therapeutics). Roadmapping was helpful during this part of the procedure and was used in all cases. Care was taken not to touch the wall of the dome of the aneurysm with the tip of either the guide wire or the microcatheter.

A various number (range, 1–14; mean, 3) of GDCs (Target Therapeutics) of various sizes (2–10 mm in diameter, 8–40 cm in length) were implanted by using a previously described technique (19,22–24). The synthesis and physical properties of GDCs have been described (28) in detail elsewhere. GDC implantation was started with coils that had the largest diameter in relation of the size of the aneurysm. Care was taken to place the first coil in a basket-like configuration in the aneurysm (Fig 1c). Further embolization was performed with smaller coils to fill the remaining cavity (Fig 1d) until control angiograms showed the aneurysm densely packed with GDCs (Figs 1e, 1f, 2d, 2e, 3d, 3e). After placement and before electrolytic detachment of each GDC, a control angiogram was obtained with hand injection of iodixanol (Visipaque; Nycomed, Oslo, Norway) through the guide catheter to confirm the correct site and location of the coil, as well as to demonstrate the patency of the adjacent arteries.

The percentage of occlusion initially achieved was determined on angiograms, with 100% indicative of complete occlusion of the aneurysm. Complete occlusion was defined as occlusion of the aneurysmal sac and neck; 90% occlusion was defined as an occlusion of the aneurysmal sac, with a small, residual open part of the neck.

RESULTS

Superselective catheter placement in the aneurysm with the GDC microcatheter and GDC embolization were technically possible in all 21 (100%) patients. The clinical examination findings, therapeutic results, and complications (if any) are summarized in the Table.

An initial 100% occlusion of the aneurysm was achieved in 14 (67%) patients. Nine of these patients had an aneurysm with a small neck, whereas

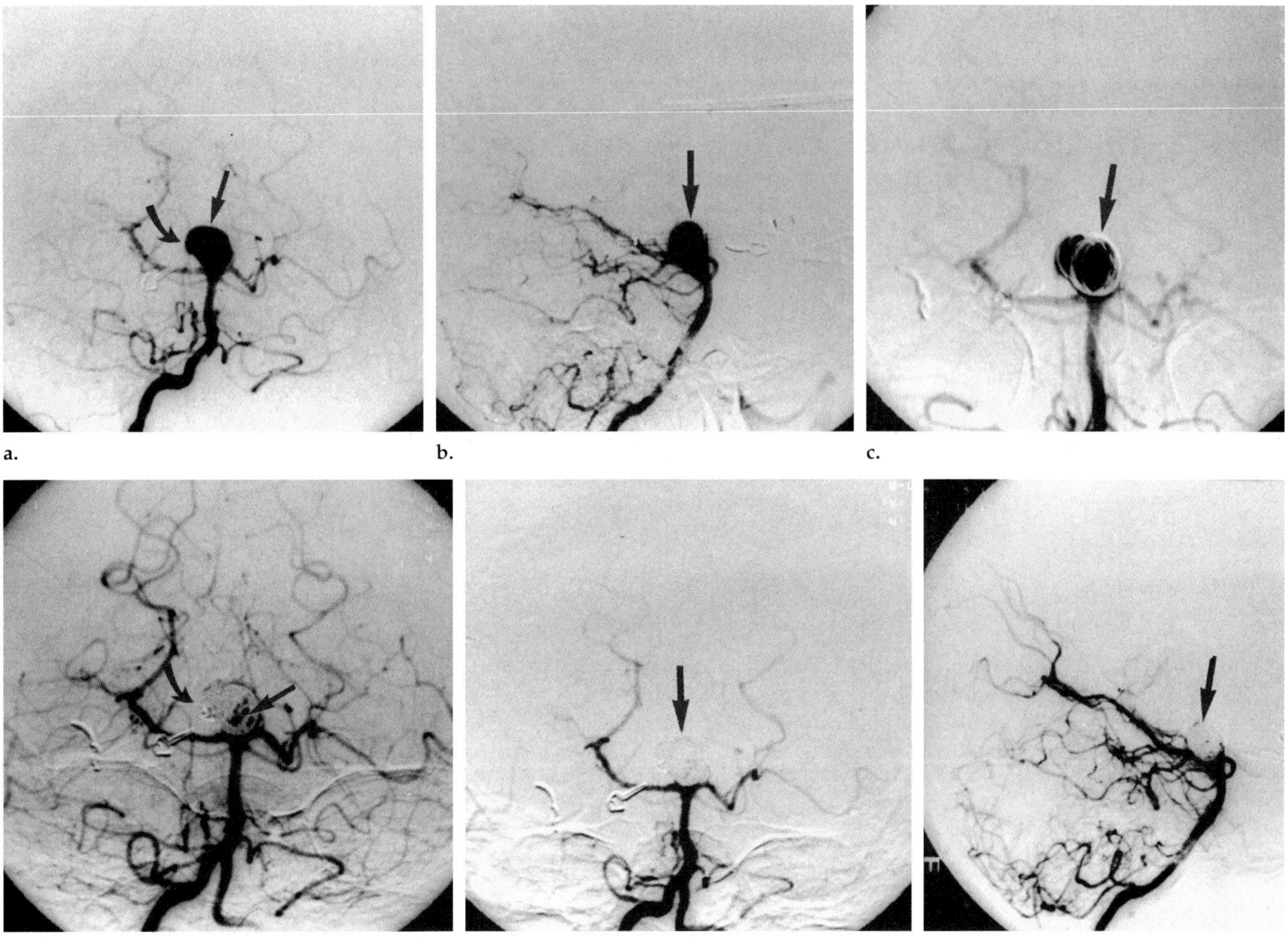

a. b. c. d. e. f.

Figure 1. Vertebral angiograms show the sequence of steps in the use of GDCs to occlude a large basilar tip aneurysm. **(a)** Frontal and **(b)** lateral projections show a large basilar tip aneurysm (straight arrow) with an outpouching of the right dome of the aneurysm (curved arrow in **a**). **(c)** Frontal projection shows the aneurysm (arrow) after delivery of the large-diameter first coil, which acts as a frame for the subsequent smaller-diameter coils. **(d)** Frontal projection shows incomplete occlusion of the aneurysm. The outpouching (curved arrow) is completely occluded at this point, but the central part of the aneurysm (straight arrow) is still perfused. **(e, f)** Postembolization vertebral angiograms obtained in the **(e)** frontal and **(f)** lateral projections show complete occlusion of the aneurysm with GDCs (arrow).

five patients had an aneurysm with a wide neck. In the remaining seven (33%) patients, all of whom had an aneurysm with a wide neck, 90% occlusion of the aneurysm was achieved at initial treatment. In three of these patients, 6-month follow-up angiograms showed that the remnant of the aneurysmal neck had increased in size owing to compaction of the coils. The aneurysm itself remained the same; that is, coil compaction resulted in a recurrence without a change in morphology of the original aneurysm. Repeated treatment was necessary in cases of recurrence. The aneurysm in two of these patients was large; the third patient had a small aneurysm. In the other four patients with a small aneurysm that was 90% occluded after initial treatment, the residual filling was unchanged at follow-up and was considered to be too small for repeated embolization. There was no change in the occlusion at 6-month follow-up angiography in 12 (86%) of the 14 patients with a completely occluded aneurysm after initial treatment. One of the two remaining patients died 2 months after the embolization and the second patient, with an initial 100% occlusion, was treated too recently to have undergone 6-month angiographic follow-up at the time this article was written. In 12 patients, who underwent angiographic follow-up at 24–48 months (mean, 34 months), the occlusion was unchanged. In the patients who underwent repeated treatment, occlusion of the aneurysm remained stable at angiographic follow-up at 18–47 months (mean, 30 months).

In clinical terms, repeated bleeding was prevented in all 16 patients with a ruptured aneurysm. Fourteen of these patients were followed up with angiography at 6–48 months (mean, 25 months). The patient who died 2 months after treatment had no symptoms of repeated bleeding. In the patient who was treated recently, there were no clinical findings of repeated bleeding. The patients with signs of a mass effect ($n = 2$) and those without symptoms ($n = 3$) were followed up at 6–45 months (mean, 24 months); none had signs of hemorrhage at follow-up. In the 11 patients with a Hunt and Hess grade II–IV subarachnoid hemorrhage, the aneurysm showed improvement at the 6-month follow-up. The clinical outcome was excellent in seven patients and good in four patients. Three patients with an initial Hunt and Hess grade I had an excellent clinical outcome at the 6-month follow-up. Of the two patients with a grade V hemorrhage, one had a good outcome at follow-up, and the other died of pulmonary complications 2 months after the embolization. Of the

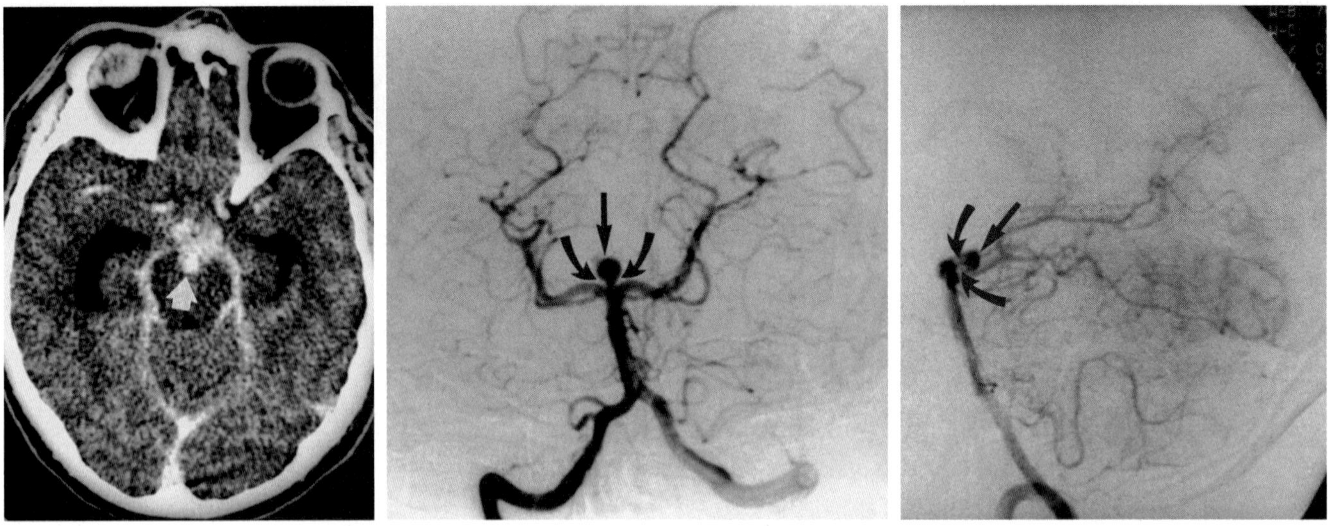

a. b. c.

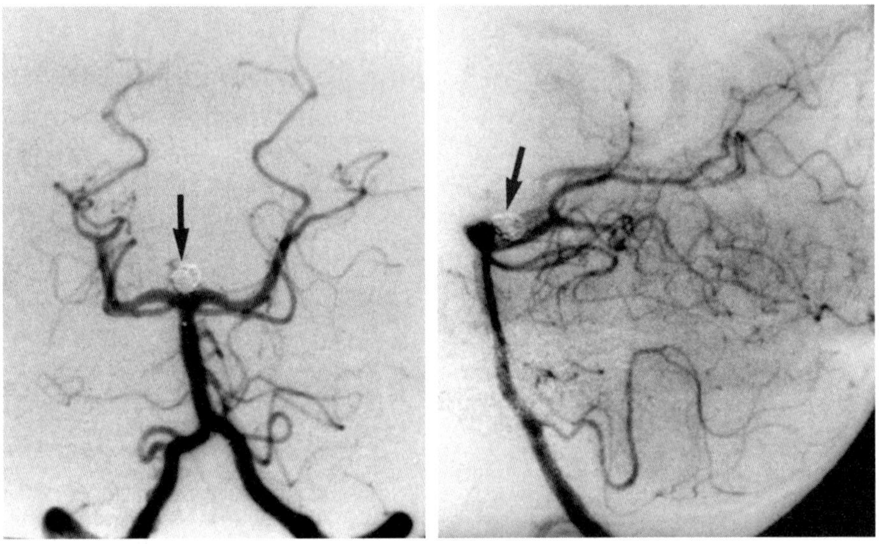

d. e.

Figure 2. Ruptured basilar tip aneurysm. **(a)** Axial CT scan shows subarachnoid hemorrhage and the aneurysm (arrow). **(b, c)** Vertebral angiograms obtained in the **(b)** frontal and **(c)** lateral projections show a small basilar tip aneurysm (straight arrow) with a well-defined neck (curved arrows). **(d, e)** Postembolization vertebral angiograms obtained in the **(d)** frontal and **(e)** lateral projections show complete occlusion of the aneurysm with GDCs (arrow).

two patients with sixth nerve palsy, one had an improved outcome, and the other, who had a large aneurysm accompanied by headache and vertigo, had a worsened outcome with a neurologic deficit. Outcome in the three asymptomatic patients, in whom the aneurysm was detected incidentally, remained unchanged.

There were postoperative and therapy-related complications in five patients, namely, occlusion of one of the PCAs after treatment. In one patient, the PCA was reopened by means of intraarterial fibrinolytic therapy; however, a permanent neurologic deficit resulted. In another patient, a transient neurologic deficit resulted, but the 6-month clinical outcome was good. In a third patient, there was flow reduction in one PCA because the GDCs caused partial compromise of the origin of the PCA. The patient was clinically asymptomatic, and normal perfusion of the formerly compromised PCA was evident at the 6-month follow-up. The other patients were clinically asymptomatic; the PCA had normal perfusion by way of the anterior circulation through the posterior communicating artery. The overall morbidity and mortality rate was 5% (one patient) and 5% (one patient), respectively. There was 0% mortality at 30 days after performance of the procedure.

DISCUSSION

Vertebrobasilar aneurysms account for 5%–15% of all intracranial aneurysms (5). Basilar tip aneurysms are the most common type (51%) of aneurysm in the posterior circulation (29,30). Aneurysms of the posterior circulation, particularly basilar tip aneurysms, are difficult to treat surgically and result in high morbidity and mortality rates (1–7,31). Hence, several endovascular techniques have gained acceptance as an alternative therapy in patients who have this aneurysm. Higashida et al (10–13,15) have reported results in large series of patients who underwent detachable balloon embolization for treatment of intracranial aneurysms. However, such balloons do not adapt to the irregular shape of the aneurysm, thereby causing stress on the aneurysm wall during balloon inflation and resulting in a relatively high risk of aneurysm rupture. Another shortcoming is the possible displacement of the balloon after detachment, which can result in occlusion of parent vessels (13,15). Therefore, only patients with an inoperable basilar tip aneurysm or who were otherwise unable to undergo surgery were selected for endovascular balloon embolization.

With the development of steerable microcatheter guide-wire systems, superselective catheter placement in an aneurysm and delivery of microcoils have become possible. The nontraumatic placement of the tip of the microcatheter in the aneurysm and the implantation of microcoils should eliminate the complications that occur with the use of detachable balloons, such as rupture of the aneurysm.

Casasco et al (17) reported a large series of 71 cases of aneurysm treated with platinum-fiber microcoils. An incomplete occlusion was reported in 11 (15%) of the 71 cases. Two of these patients died because of a repeated hemorrhage. In six patients, there were ischemic complications; in four patients, there was

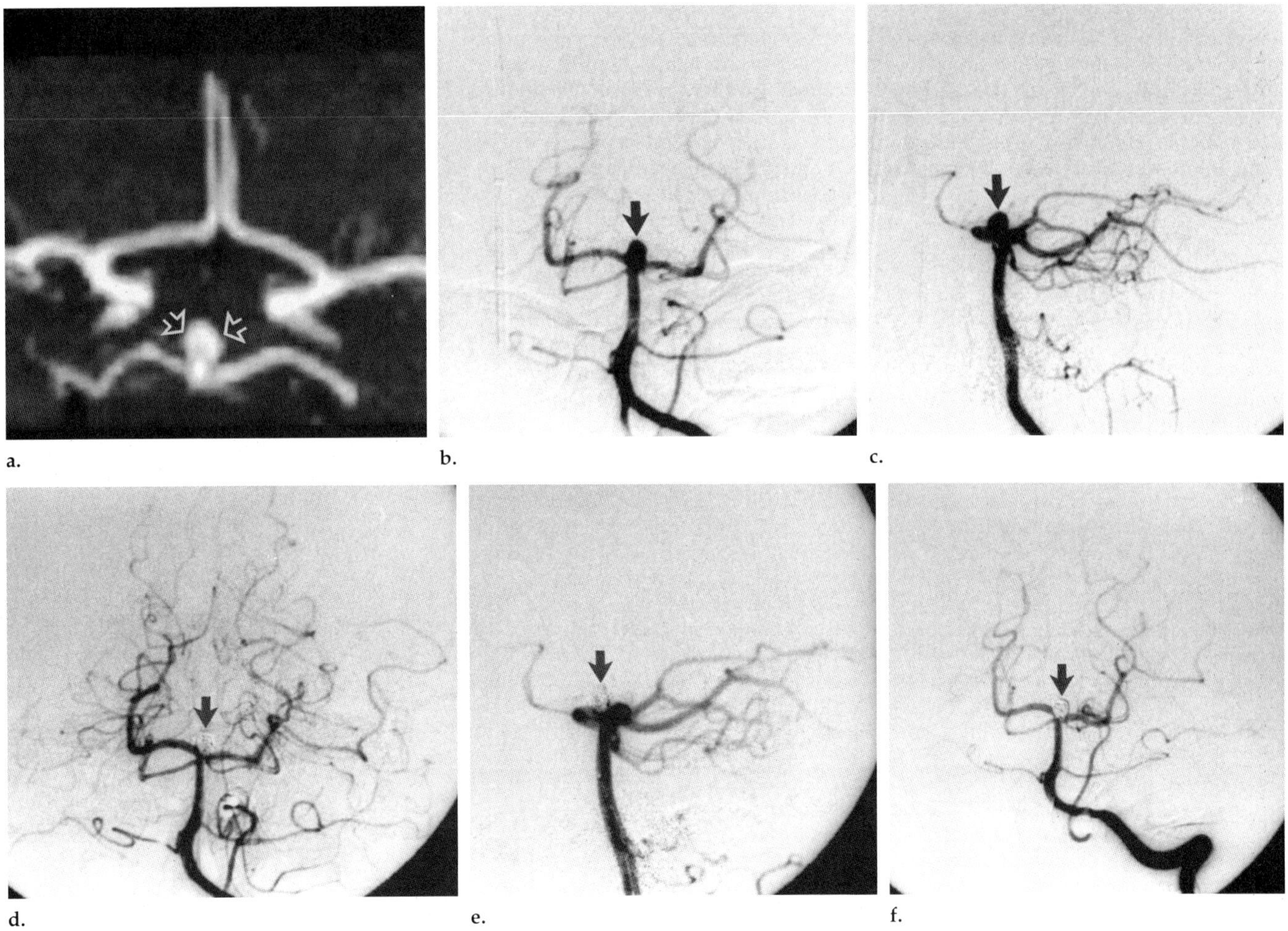

Figure 3. Nonruptured basilar tip aneurysm. **(a)** MR angiogram shows the basilar tip aneurysm (arrows). **(b, c)** Vertebral angiograms obtained in the **(b)** frontal and **(c)** lateral projections show a small, wide-necked basilar tip aneurysm (arrow). **(d, e)** Postembolization vertebral angiograms obtained in the **(d)** frontal and **(e)** lateral projections show complete occlusion of the aneurysm with GDCs (arrow). **(f)** Frontal angiographic projection obtained at 2-year follow-up shows persistent occlusion of the aneurysm (arrow).

occlusion of the parent vessel. These two types of complications were the result of the fact that these microcoils are nondetachable, which seems to cause problems especially in the treatment of a wide-necked aneurysm. When conventional microcoils are used, ischemic complications can result after inadvertent placement of the last coil. Conversely, the attempt to avoid inadvertent placement can result in incomplete occlusion of the aneurysm.

With the development of the GDC, the disadvantages of nondetachable microcoils and detachable balloons can be minimized (32). Controlled delivery is the most important advantage of the GDC: The coil is detached only when the correct position is demonstrated at angiography. In case of inadvertent placement, the GDC can be withdrawn and reinserted. A further advantage is the flexibility and softness of the coils, which enables the filling of outpouchings in the aneurysm and minimizes the risk of rupture. Additionally, during electrolytic detachment of the GDC, electrothrombosis occurs adjacent to the coil, which accelerates the occlusion.

Implantation was started with a GDC with the largest diameter relative to the size of the aneurysm to achieve a basket-like configuration and to bridge the aneurysm neck with a mesh of coils. The remaining cavity was filled with smaller-diameter coils, which were placed in the network of the first coil; this placement prevented bulging into the parent artery.

Problems with GDC implantation can occur because of anatomic features of the aneurysm. Specifically, a wide aneurysmal neck and/or an aneurysm in which the normal branch arteries originate near the neck or are incorporated in the aneurysm can cause difficulties (to the point of impossibility) in the tight packing of the aneurysm. In these circumstances, there is a risk that the coils will bulge into the parent artery or compromise the adjacent origin of the parent artery, and only loose packing and a sometimes incomplete occlusion of the aneurysm can be achieved. Consequently, complete occlusion is possible in a larger percentage of small-necked aneurysms than wide-necked aneurysms (33). A further complication is the development of a remnant aneurysmal neck caused by compaction of the coils due to arterial flow.

Guglielmi et al (22) reported initial 100% occlusion in two cases of a small-necked aneurysm and in one case of a wide-necked aneurysm in their series of 23 cases of basilar bifurcation aneurysm. A 98% occlusion was achieved in two cases of wide-necked aneurysm, and a 95% occlusion was achieved in three cases of a wide-necked aneurysm and in two cases of a small-necked aneurysm. In three cases of a wide-necked aneurysm, more than one embolization was necessary. McDougall et al (27) reported an initial complete occlusion with GDCs in seven of 33 (21%) cases of basilar tip aneurysm. Six patients required repeated treatment because of partial recanalization. In three of these patients, the repeated treatment was successful. Bavinzski et al (26) reported 100% occlusion in seven (33%) of 13 patients. In one case, repeated treatment was performed. All of these previous studies, however, involved a selected group of patients.

Unlike in the studies cited in the preceding paragraph, we performed endovascular treatment in a nonselected population of patients with a basilar tip aneurysm; therefore a comparison of our results with those of surgical series (1–7,31) may be more valid. In our series of 21 patients with a basilar tip aneurysm, an initially complete occlusion was achieved in 14 (67%) patients, and 90% occlusion was achieved in seven (33%) patients. In other studies (22,26, 27,33), the highest percentage of complete occlusions was reported in patients with a small-necked aneurysm. Because of recurrence of partial perfusion of the aneurysmal neck after 6 months, repeated treatment was necessary in three of the patients in our series.

The goal of any treatment for an intracranial aneurysm is to avoid bleeding, to prevent repeated bleeding in a ruptured aneurysm, and to improve neurologic symptoms due to mass effect in a patient with an unruptured aneurysm. In 16 of 21 patients, a basilar tip aneurysm caused subarachnoid hemorrhage before treatment. There was no repeated hemorrhage after treatment, which suggests that an incomplete occlusion (in five patients with a ruptured aneurysm, an initial 90% occlusion was achieved) may protect the aneurysm against repeated rupture (22,23,26,34). Two patients in our series presented with symptoms due to mass effect. Clinical improvement of the symptoms was observed in one of these patients; however, GDC embolization resulted in protection against bleeding in both patients. Three other asymptomatic patients, whose aneurysms were found incidentally, were treated successfully to prevent rupture.

Another disadvantage in treating patients with a wide-necked basilar tip aneurysm is the risk of compromising an adjacent origin of the PCA. The cause for occlusion of the PCA can be either mechanical compression of the origin at an attempted tight packing of the aneurysm or thrombus formation when the intraaneurysmal thrombus shifts to the origin of the parent vessel. The occlusion of one PCA was the most important complication in our series. Occlusion of a PCA occurred in five (24%) patients, and only one of these patients had worsened clinical symptoms intraoperatively; therefore, intraarterial fibrinolytic therapy was started immediately. Despite successful reopening of the artery, the patient developed a permanent neurologic deficit. Guglielmi et al (22) reported one complication (permanent hemianopsia) in a patient with a wide-necked basilar bifurcation aneurysm with bilateral occlusion of the PCAs. In their series of patients with a posterior circulation aneurysm, the morbidity and mortality rates were both 7%. McDougall et al (27) reported one patient with a repeated hemorrhage after treatment and thrombosis of the distal part of the basilar artery and of the P-1 segment of the PCA, which resulted in a permanent neurologic deficit. In one patient, the coil migrated into the P-1 segment of the PCA but did not compromise the parent artery.

In summary, occlusion by means of endovascular coils is a promising alternative therapy in patients with an intracranial aneurysm that should not be treated with surgical clipping because of increased risk to the patient. Surgical clipping of a basilar bifurcation aneurysm is difficult and is associated with high morbidity and mortality rates. Our midterm results indicate that occlusion with GDCs is a less invasive and safe alternative therapeutic method for the treatment of patients with such an aneurysm and that this method should be used preferentially. Moreover, this endovascular approach is not only less invasive than other procedures, but it is also associated with a shorter period of hospitalization. In addition, patients with a poor medical condition can be treated. Long-term follow-up studies, however, are needed before the present results can be confirmed. ■

References

1. Jamieson KG. Aneurysms of the vertebrobasilar system: surgical intervention in 19 cases. J Neurosurg 1964; 21:781–797.
2. Drake CG. Surgical treatment of ruptured aneurysms of the basilar artery: experience with 14 cases. J Neurosurg 1965; 23:457–473.
3. McMurtry JG, Housepian EM, Bowman FO, Matteo RS. Surgical treatment of basilar artery aneurysms: elective circulatory arrest with thoracotomy in 12 cases. J Neurosurg 1974; 40: 486–493.
4. Wilson CB, Hoi Sang U. Surgical treatment for aneurysms of the upper basilar artery. J Neurosurg 1976; 44:537–543.
5. Peerless SJ, Drake CG. Posterior circulation aneurysms. In: Wilkins RH, Rengachary SS, eds. Neurosurgery. Vol 2. New York, NY: McGraw-Hill, 1985; 1422–1437.
6. Yasargil MG, Antic J, Laciga R, et al. Microsurgical pterional approach to aneurysms of the basilar bifurcation. Surg Neurol 1976; 6: 83–91.
7. Kassel NF, Torner JC, Jane JA, et al. The international cooperative study on the timing of aneurysm surgery. II. Surgical results. J Neurosurg 1990; 73:37–47.
8. Romodanov AP, Shcheglov VI. Intravascular occlusion of saccular aneurysms of the cerebral arteries by means of a detachable balloon catheter. In: Krayenbühl H, ed. Advances and technical standards in neurosurgery. Vol 9. New York, NY: Springer-Verlag, 1982; 25–49.
9. Hieshima GB, Higashida RT, Wapewsky J, et al. Balloon embolization of a large distal basilar artery aneurysm: case report. J Neurosurg 1986; 65:413–416.
10. Higashida RT, Hieshima GB, Halbach VV, et al. Intravascular detachable balloon embolization of intracranial aneurysms: indications and techniques. Acta Radiol 1986; 369:594–596.
11. Higashida RT, Halbach VV, Dowd CF, et al. Endovascular detachable balloon embolization therapy of cavernous carotid aneurysms: results in 87 cases. J Neurosurg 1990; 72:857–863.
12. Higashida RT, Halbach VV, Barnwell SL, et al. Treatment of intracranial aneurysms with preservation of the parent vessel: results of percutaneous balloon embolization in 84 patients. AJNR 1990; 11:633–640.
13. Higashida RT, Halbach VV, Dowd CF, Barnwell SL, Hieshima GB. Intracranial aneurysms: interventional neurovascular treatment with detachable balloons—results in 215 cases. Radiology 1991; 178:663–670.
14. Zeumer H, Brückmann H, Adelt D, Hacke W, Ringelstein EB. Balloon embolization in the treatment of basilar aneurysms. Acta Neurochir 1985; 78:136–141.
15. Higashida RT, Halbach VV, Cahan LD, Hieshima GB, Konishi Y. Detachable balloon embolization therapy of posterior circulation intracranial aneurysms. J Neurosurg 1989; 71: 512–519.
16. Guglielmi G. Balloon embolization of a basilar bifurcation aneurysm. AJNR 1990; 11:653–655.
17. Casasco AE, Aymard A, Gobin YP, et al. Selective endovascular treatment of 71 intracranial aneurysms with platinum coils. J Neurosurg 1993; 79:3–10.
18. Numaguchi Y, Pevsner PH, Rigamonti D, Ragheb J. Platinum coil treatment of complex aneurysms of the vertebrobasilar circulation. Neuroradiology 1992; 34:252–255.
19. Guglielmi G, Viñuela F, Dion J, Duckwiler G. Electrothrombosis of saccular aneurysms via endovascular approach. II. Preliminary clinical experience. J Neurosurg 1991; 75:8–14.
20. Bradac GB, Riva A, Bergui M, Stura G, Fontanella M, Bonicalzi V. Endovascular coil embolization of cerebral aneurysms. Riv Neuroradiol 1995; 8:637–644.
21. Scotti G, Righi C, Simionato F, Li MH. Endovascular therapy of intracranial aneurysms with GDC. Riv Neuroradiol 1994; 7:723–733.
22. Guglielmi G, Viñuela F, Duckwiler G, et al. Endovascular treatment of posterior circulation aneurysms by electrothrombosis using electrically detachable coils. J Neurosurg 1992; 77:515–524.
23. Guglielmi G. The GDC system in the treatment of intracranial aneurysms. Riv Neuroradiol 1996; 9:463–470.
24. Massoud TF, Guglielmi G, Viñuela F, Duckwiler G. Endovascular treatment of multiple aneurysms involving the posterior intracranial circulation. AJNR 1996; 17:549–554.
25. Gobin YP, Viñuela F, Gurian JH, et al. Treatment of large and giant fusiform intracranial aneurysms with Guglielmi detachable coils. J Neurosurg 1996; 84:55–62.
26. Bavinzski G, Richling B, Gruber A, Killer M, Levy D. Endosaccular occlusion of basilar artery bifurcation aneurysms using electrically detachable coils. Acta Neurochir 1995; 134:184–189.
27. McDougall CG, Halbach V, Dowd CF, Higashida RT, Larsen DW, Hieshima GB. Endovascular treatment of basilar tip aneurysms using electrolytically detachable coils. J Neurosurg 1996; 84:393–399.
28. Guglielmi G, Viñuela F, Sepetka I, Macellari V. Electrothrombosis of saccular aneurysms via endovascular approach. I. Electrochemical basis, technique, and experimental results. J Neurosurg 1991; 75:1–7.
29. McCormick WF, Nofzinger JD. Saccular intracranial aneurysms: an autopsy study. J Neurosurg 1965; 22:155–159.
30. Bull JW. Contribution of radiology to the study of intracranial aneurysms. Br Med J 1962; 2:1701–1708.
31. Peerless SS, Drake CG. Management of aneurysms of the posterior circulation. In Youmans JR, ed. Philadelphia, Pa: Saunders, 1982; 1764–1806.
32. Halbach V. The "current" status of aneurysm treatment. AJNR 1993; 14:799–800.
33. Zubillaga AF, Guglielmi G, Viñuela F, Duckwiler GR. Endovascular occlusion of intracranial aneurysms with electrically detachable coils: correlation of aneurysm neck size and treatment results. AJNR 1994; 15:815–820.
34. Schievink WI. Intracranial aneurysms. N Engl J Med 1997; 336:28–40.

Norbert G. Campeau, MD • Ronald C. Petersen, MD, PhD • Joel P. Felmlee, PhD
Peter C. O'Brien, PhD • Clifford R. Jack, Jr, MD

Hippocampal Transverse Relaxation Times in Patients with Alzheimer Disease[1]

***PURPOSE:* To determine whether hippocampal relaxation times in magnetic resonance (MR) imaging differ between patients with probable Alzheimer disease and elderly control subjects with normal cognition.**

***MATERIALS AND METHODS:* MR imaging relaxation times were measured in the head and body of the right and left hippocampi in 123 subjects: 62 patients with Alzheimer disease (44 women, 18 men; age range, 65–89 years) and 61 elderly control subjects without cognitive impairment (39 women, 22 men; age range, 65–89 years). Hippocampal relaxation times were correlated with clinical status (patient vs control subject), age, sex, laterality (right vs left), and location within the hippocampus (body vs head). The hippocampal T2 value was correlated with the severity of disease in the patients.**

***RESULTS:* No statistically significant difference in the relaxation times was found between the two clinical groups for the analysis of the right versus left hippocampi and the hippocampal head versus body. In both patients and control subjects, no correlation was found between T2 measurements and age or sex. Twenty-seven patients had a clinical dementia rating (CDR) score of 0.5 (very mild dementia), 21 patients had a CDR score of 1.0 (mild dementia), and eight patients had a CDR score of 2.0 (moderate dementia). The CDR score was not available in six patients. No statistically significant association between T2 values and severity of disease was observed.**

***CONCLUSION:* MR relaxation time measurements in the hippocampus are not useful for the detection of Alzheimer disease.**

The hippocampus and entorhinal cortex are involved early and most severely by the pathologic process of Alzheimer disease (1–4). In addition to neurofibrillary tangles and plaques, gross atrophy and gliosis are characteristic features of Alzheimer disease (5,6). The latter would be expected to prolong the magnetic resonance (MR) imaging tissue relaxation time in patients with Alzheimer disease relative to that in control subjects without dementia.

Increased signal intensity in the hippocampus on T2-weighted MR images has been reported in Alzheimer disease (7). Kirsch and colleagues (8), using a two-point fit, measured the relaxation time in the hippocampus in patients with clinically diagnosed Alzheimer disease and reported that the values exceeded those in age-matched elderly individuals without dementia. They concluded that measurements of hippocampal relaxation time were clinically useful as a marker of both the presence and severity of Alzheimer disease. On the other hand, Laakso and colleagues (9), in a similar but larger study in which the relaxation times of the head and body of the hippocampus were measured in patients with Alzheimer disease, found considerable overlap between the study groups and reported that T2 relaxometry was not a reliable method for diagnosing Alzheimer disease.

To determine whether hippocampal MR imaging relaxation time differs between patients with Alzheimer disease and control subjects, we measured the relaxation times in the head and body of both hippocampi in 123 subjects: 62 patients with Alzheimer disease and 61 elderly control subjects without dementia.

MATERIALS AND METHODS

Patient Selection

Examination of the Mayo Alzheimer's Disease Center and Alzheimer's Disease Patient Registry (10) resulted in identification of 62 patients with Alzheimer disease (44 women, 18 men; mean age, 77.4 years; age range, 65–89 years) who had undergone a protocol MR imaging study of the head that included an eight-echo, coronal Carr-Purcell-Meiboom-Gill (CPMG) pulse sequence through the hippocampi. Sixty-one elderly control subjects (39 women, 22 men; mean age, 80.8 years; age range, 65–89 years) from the same source but without dementia also underwent an identical protocol study. All examinations were performed between September 1994 and April 1996. Alzheimer disease was diagnosed clinically in accordance with the National Institute of Neurological and Communicative Disorders and Stroke–Alzheimer's Disease and Related Disorders Association criteria (11).

Index terms: Dementia, 1341.83 • Hippocampus, 1341.12146, 1341.83 • Magnetic resonance (MR), relaxometry, 1341.12146

Abbreviations: CDR = clinical dementia rating, CPMG = Carr-Purcell-Meiboom-Gill, CSF = cerebrospinal fluid, ROI = region of interest, TE = echo time.

Radiology 1997; 205:197–201

[1] From the Departments of Diagnostic Radiology (N.G.C., J.P.F., C.R.J.), Neurology (R.C.P.), and Health Sciences Research (P.C.O.), Mayo Clinic, East 2 Mayo Building, 200 First St SW, Rochester, MN 55905. Received April 10, 1997; revision requested May 9; revision received June 23; accepted June 25. Supported by National Institutes of Health National Institute of Aging grants AG11378, AG08031, and AG06786; National Institute of Neurological and Communicative Disorders and Stroke grant NS29059; the Dana Foundation; and the Alzheimer's Association. **Address reprint requests to** C.R.J.

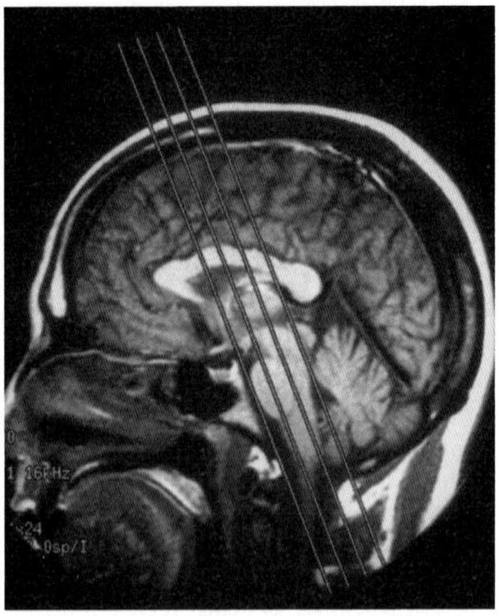

Figure 1. T1-weighted scout image (400/16) demonstrates the prescription of sections for coronal oblique CPMG pulse sequence. Four sections are perpendicular to the left hippocampus, with the most posterior section passing through the posterior commissure.

Table 1
Phantom Study Results

Variable Parameters	Relaxation Time (msec): Mineral Oil Phantom	Relaxation Time (msec): 0.35 mmol/L MnCl Phantom	Relaxation Time (msec): 0.1 mmol/L MnCl Phantom	Constant Parameters
Multisection eight-echo CPMG sequence				
Section thickness (mm)				
3	35.4	38.3	67.5	25-msec echo spacing
5	30.8	41.0	84.0	25-msec echo spacing
10	32.2	34.3	77.0	25-msec echo spacing
Section angle (degrees)				
0	30.8	41.0	84.0	25-msec echo spacing
30	30.9	41.0	85.1	25-msec echo spacing
60	34.8	32.9	72.8	25-msec echo spacing
Echo spacing (msec)				
20	31.3	32.8	71.9	10-mm section thickness
25	31.2	34.3	77.0	10-mm section thickness
30	34.2	36.8	81.0	10-mm section thickness
35	38.6	39.2	83.4	10-mm section thickness
Intersection gap				
4 cm				
Eight separate single-echo acquisitions	32.5	41.8	122.2	25-msec echo spacing, 10-mm section thickness, multisection
Eight-echo CPMG sequence	30.2	33.9	74.6	25-msec echo spacing, 10-mm section thickness, multisection
2 cm				
Eight separate single-echo acquisitions	32.8	41.8	119.3	25-msec echo spacing, 10-mm section thickness, multisection
Eight-echo CPMG sequence	30.4	35.1	73.6	25-msec echo spacing, 10-mm section thickness, multisection
1 cm				
Eight separate single-echo acquisitions	32.7	41.9	121.7	25-msec echo spacing, 10-mm section thickness, multisection
Eight-echo CPMG sequence	29.9	34.1	75.5	25-msec echo spacing, 10-mm section thickness, multisection
Acquisition type				
Eight separate single-echo acquisitions	32.5	42.9	126.1	25–200-msec TEs, 25-msec echo spacing, 10-mm section thickness
Eight-echo CPMG sequence	30.3	33.5	74.4	25–200-msec TEs, 25-msec echo spacing, 10-mm section thickness

Note.—Phantoms built by J.P.F.

Relaxation Time Measurement Technique and Validation

Because no pulse sequence exists for calculating relaxation time on standard 5.X GE software (GE Medical Systems, Milwaukee, Wis), the eight-echo CPMG pulse sequence mentioned above was developed at our institution for this purpose. Phantom (Table 1) and in vivo studies to evaluate the performance of this pulse sequence were performed in healthy young adult volunteers to examine a number of variables that could influence the T2 measurement (12). These included the effects of a multiple-echo acquisition versus multiple single-echo acquisitions, single-section versus multiple-section acquisitions, the section thickness, the section angle, the echo spacing, and the intersection gap.

Imaging Protocol

Each patient and elderly control subject underwent imaging with an eight-echo CPMG pulse sequence on a 1.5-T MR imager (Signa; GE Medical Systems). Sections were acquired in a coronal oblique orientation perpendicular to the hippocampi. Imaging parameters were 3,000/30–240 (repetition time msec/echo time [TE] msec), 30-msec echo spacing, and a 4.0-mm section thickness with an intersection gap of 4.0 mm. The image field of view was 24 cm, and the matrix size was 256 × 192. This pulse sequence produced 32 images from four sections. The coronal oblique sections were prescribed as in Figure 1.

A T1-weighted, three-dimensional, spoiled gradient-recalled-echo pulse sequence (24/9, 124 sections, 1.6-mm thickness) was performed in the same coronal oblique spatial orientation in all subjects as part of the protocol. These T1-weighted images were used for anatomic reference when performing the region of interest (ROI) tracings on the T2 maps.

T2 Map Creation

The T2 maps were calculated from the eight-echo train by using a single exponential decay model on an off-line workstation (Indigo; Silicon Graphics, Mountain View, Calif) with custom software developed at our institution. The CPMG data were postprocessed pixel by pixel to create four coronal oblique T2 maps through the hippocampus. An error-checking algorithm was used to identify pixels in which the data in the successive eight echoes were not monotonically decreasing by assigning a value of zero to these pixels. These pixels therefore appear black on the T2 map and are visually apparent, which allows them to be easily and manually segmented out of the ROI. Motion artifact that occurs in one or more of the eight images would be one cause of nonmonotonically decreasing echoes.

ROI Measurements

The investigators were blinded with respect to the subject's clinical status (patient vs control subject), age, and sex while measuring the relaxation times. Precise ROI tracings of the heads and bodies of the hippocampi were performed by using the ANALYZE software (13). ROIs were drawn to include as much of the hippocampi as possible; partial volume averaging errors were avoided by excluding pixels that bordered white matter and cerebrospinal fluid (CSF) in the hippocampal fissure, choroidal fissure, and temporal horn (Fig 2). Pixels in the T2 map flagged with the error-checking algorithm were manually segmented out of the ROI and therefore did not con-

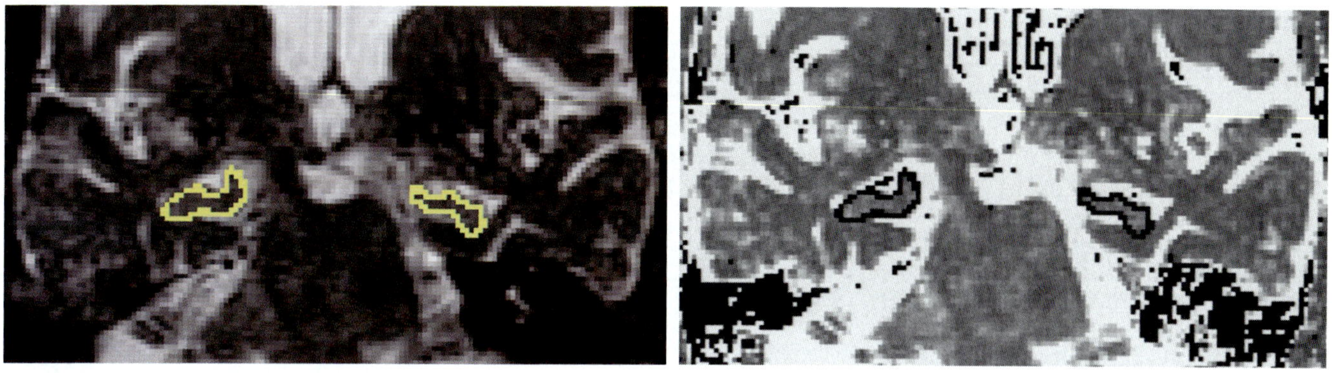

a. b.

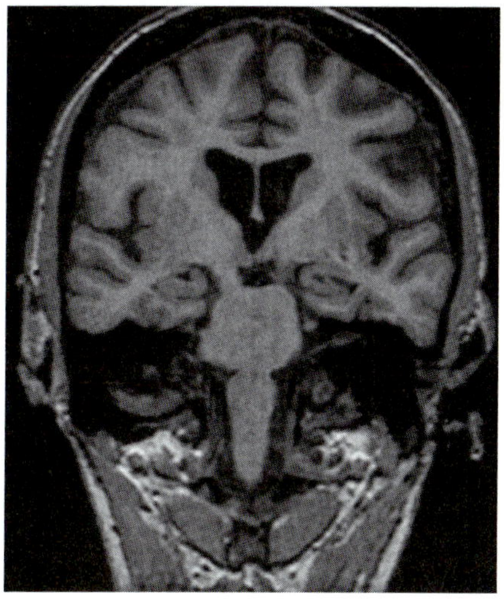

c.

Figure 2. **(a)** T2-weighted CPMG image (1,000/120) through the hippocampal heads. This image of the eight-echo CPMG train was used to draw the ROIs (in yellow) to include as much of the hippocampal parenchyma as possible while excluding border pixels that may cause partial volume artifacts. The ROI shape was not confined to a geometric shape, such as a circle, oval, or rectangle. **(b)** Corresponding T2 map of **a** was constructed off-line pixel by pixel by using data from all eight of the CPMG images. The mean gray-scale value of the pixels in the ROI represents the mean relaxation time (calibrated in milliseconds). Black pixels are those that have been rejected as inaccurate or invalid by an error-checking algorithm of the T2 map–creation routine. **(c)** T1-weighted, three-dimensional, spoiled gradient-recalled-echo image (24/9; 45° flip angle) through the same section of the brain as **a** demonstrates the hippocampal heads. This image was acquired in the same orientation as the T2-weighted images from the CPMG sequence and is used for anatomic reference when drawing the ROIs.

tribute to the calculation of average relaxation time within the ROI. No geometric constraints (ie, circular or rectangular) were placed on ROI shape. The size of the ROI typically was 40–60 pixels (46.9–70.3 mm^2) for the body and 65–90 pixels for the head (50.5–105.45 mm^2). The thin-section, T1-weighted, spoiled gradient-recalled-echo images acquired in corresponding anatomic planes were used in conjunction with the T2 maps to help properly identify the anatomic boundaries of the ROIs.

Reproducibility of the technique for selecting ROIs was validated before data analysis. Repeat ROI measurements performed at separate intervals in five patients demonstrated high reproducibility of the measured T2 values (mean difference, 1.3%).

Data Analysis

Two-sample *t* tests were performed to determine whether the relaxation times of the heads and bodies of the right and left hippocampi varied between the Alzheimer disease group and the nondemented control group. Paired *t* tests were used to assess laterality (right vs left) and position within the hippocampus (body vs head). Stepwise regression was performed to determine whether there was an association of age or sex with relaxation time in control subjects. Two-sample *t* tests were used to determine whether there was any correlation between hippocampal T2 and severity of disease in Alzheimer disease cases as graded with the clinical dementia rating (CDR) score (14).

RESULTS

Relaxation Time Measurement Technique and Validation

The results of the phantom studies are displayed in Table 1. There was little difference in the T2 measurements with changes in section thickness or section orientation (angle) or between single- versus multiple-section acquisitions. The relaxation time is underestimated with the CPMG sequence when compared with a similar measurement calculated by using eight single-echo acquisitions performed at corresponding TEs. This is most likely the result of T1 saturation caused by imperfect 180° spin refocussing at the edges of the imaging section (15). The T2 measurement also decreases with decreasing interecho delay in the CPMG sequence, which also is likely from saturation effects. This effect was more pronounced with longer T1 and T2 values of the phantom material. Several of the healthy, young volunteers underwent imaging with different interecho spacings of 20, 25, 30, and 35 msec. As also observed with the phantoms, measured T2 decreased with decreasing interecho spacing. An interecho spacing of 30 msec was selected for the study, because it was empirically noted in the volunteer data that nearly all the signal decayed at TEs that exceeded 240 msec.

Laterality and Segmental Position within the Hippocampus

The mean relaxation times measured in the head and body of the hippocampus in patients with Alzheimer disease and in elderly control subjects without dementia are summarized in Table 2. No statistically significant difference in the relaxation times between the right and left hippocampi or the head and body of the hippocampus was found between the two clinical groups. To assess the adequacy of sample size to detect a difference, we have computed the 95% confidence intervals for the differences in group means (Table 2). We cannot exclude the possibility that group differences that lie within (or are less than) the computed 95% confidence interval may be present, but group differences greater than the 95% confidence interval would not be consistent with our data.

Age and Sex

No correlation of hippocampal relaxation time with patient age (Table 3) or sex was observed.

Severity of Disease

There were 27 patients with a CDR of 0.5, which indicates very mild dementia; 21 patients with a CDR of 1.0, which indicates mild dementia; and eight patients with a CDR of 2.0, which indicates moderate dementia. The CDR score was not available in six patients. No statistically significant association between T2 values and severity of disease was observed (Table 4) ($P > .10$).

DISCUSSION

Because gliosis is a feature of Alzheimer disease, one might expect T2 measurements in areas of the brain most severely affected (the medial temporal lobe) to differ between patients with Alzheimer disease and control subjects. However, findings of this study demonstrate considerable overlap of the measured relaxation times of the head and body of the hippocampus between the control and Alzheimer disease groups and show that the usefulness of relaxation time in the hippocampus for the detection of Alzheimer disease is limited.

The results from this study are consistent with those of Laakso and colleagues (9) and differ from those of Kirsch and colleagues (8), who reported that prolongation of the MR relaxation time of the hippocampus was useful as a marker of both the presence and the severity of Alzheimer disease. Pitkanen and colleagues (16) reported that the relaxation times of the head and tail of the right hippocampus were slightly prolonged (5–6 msec) relative to the left hippocampal counterparts ($P < .01$) in 55 patients with Alzheimer disease when compared with those in 76 control subjects.

We found no differences between control subjects and patients for T2 measurements of the head versus body and right versus left hippocampus. The standard deviations of the results in this study are also smaller than the standard deviations reported for both of the other studies. In a recent study with MR microscopy at 7 T, the relaxation time of the hippocampus did not correlate with the size of the hippocampus or the numbers of plaques or tangles in Alzheimer disease (17). Because this study was performed in vitro, it is difficult to extrapolate the relevance of these results to clinical imaging results in patients with Alzheimer disease.

The absolute T2 values we measured in our study are lower than those reported in the other studies. This difference is likely due to the pulse sequence parameters used.

Measured relaxation time is substantially reduced when a CPMG pulse sequence is used than when data are acquired with an equivalent number of separate pulse sequences with varying TEs (Table 1). However, this latter approach is impractical for in vivo work owing to time constraints.

Table 2
Relaxation Times of the Hippocampal Head and Body for the Two Clinical Groups

Location	Patient Relaxation Time (msec)	Control Subject Relaxation Time (msec)	95% Confidence Interval
Right hippocampus			
Head	79.370 ± 5.60	79.392 ± 5.67	−2.032, 1.989
Body	78.570 ± 6.63	77.933 ± 6.12	−1.642, 2.916
Left hippocampus			
Head	79.131 ± 6.03	78.345 ± 6.17	−1.391, 2.964
Body	78.445 ± 7.83	77.121 ± 6.12	−1.188, 3.836

Note.—Data are means ± standard deviations.

Table 3
Pearson Correlation between Hippocampal Relaxation Time and Age

Location	Patients: Pearson R	Patients: P Value	Subjects: Pearson R	Subjects: P Value
Right hippocampus				
Head	−.11	NS	−.10	NS
Body	−.16	NS	−.09	NS
Left hipppocampus				
Head	−.15	NS	−.01	NS
Body	−.24	NS	.06	NS

Note.—NS = not significant.

Table 4
Severity of Disease versus Relaxation Times

Location	Mean Relaxation Times (msec) in Patients (N = 56)*: Patients with a CDR of 0.5 (n = 27)	Patients with a CDR of 1.0 (n = 21)	Patients with a CDR of 2.0 (n = 8)
Right hippocampus			
Head	78.739	80.930	79.194
Body	78.893	79.370	76.221
Left hippocampus			
Head	78.894	80.867	77.563
Body	78.204	79.171	79.338

* The CDR score was not available in six patients.

In vivo T2 measurements are influenced by the number of echoes in a CPMG pulse sequence, the echo spacing, and the repetition time (Table 1). Our measurements were performed at 1.5 T, as were the measurements of Laakso and colleagues (9); this is in contrast with those of Kirsch and colleagues (8), which were performed at 0.04 T. Unlike T1 measurements, which are highly dependent on field strength, T2 measurements vary little with field strength over the range used in diagnostic imaging.

Relaxation times obtained from different institutions will vary, depending on the technique used. However, for each given technique, results should be repeatable and consistent. Kirsch and colleagues (8) used two spin-echo acquisitions (1,000/130 and 1,000/200), which were fit to a monoexponential function: $T2 = (TE_2 - TE_1)/\ln(S_1/S_2)$, where S is signal intensity. The technique of Laakso and colleagues (9) was similar to ours, with a 16-echo CPMG sequence and TEs of 22–262 msec; the repetition time was not reported in their article.

We found no difference in the relaxation times with respect to age or sex between the Alzheimer disease group and the nondemented elderly group. The control subjects and patients with Alzheimer Disease in our study were aged 65–89 years. From our study data, it is impossible to comment on how the hippocampal relaxation times might differ from those in healthy, young individuals.

One source of artifact in measuring the T2 values may be due to the effects of partial volume averaging of CSF or adjacent white matter tracts. Because the relaxation time of CSF is much greater than that of the hippocampus, inclusion of only a few CSF volume-averaged pixels can cause a marked increase in the measured T2 value of the ROI. Kirsch and colleagues (8) used ROIs that consisted of three to five pixels, and five to 10 ROIs were defined for each structure. Laakso and colleagues (9) used the largest possible circular ROI, with a minimum of eight but typically 30–50 pixels (40–60 mm^3) within the head, body, and tail of each hippocampus, and avoided boundaries where partial volume effects may occur.

To deal with the complexity of eliminating partial volume effects from the CSF when estimating relaxation times in complex anatomic regions such as the hippocampus, the ROI shapes in this study were precisely drawn by using anatomic images for reference. The shape of the ROI was not confined to a fixed geometric shape, such as a circle or a rectangle. The geometric ROI approach may work reasonably well in the body of the hippocampus but is difficult to apply in the head of the hippocampus while simultaneously attempting to maximize the ROI size.

It is interesting to note that while hippocampal T2 signal intensity is not different between patients with Alzheimer disease and elderly control subjects without dementia, several studies have documented that the hippocampi in patients with Alzheimer disease are statistically significantly atrophic compared with those in control subjects (2,18–25). In contrast, patients with epilepsy due to mesial temporal sclerosis usually have atrophy and elevated T2 signal intensity in one or both hippocampi (16,26,27). This discrepancy between the nature of the MR imaging hippocampal abnormalities between Alzheimer disease and mesial temporal sclerosis probably represents manifestation of fundamentally different pathogenic mechanisms.

In conclusion, the results of this study demonstrate that hippocampal transverse relaxation time measurements are not useful for the detection of Alzheimer disease and do not correlate with the severity of Alzheimer disease. ■

Acknowledgment: The authors acknowledge Ruth Cha, MS, for her assistance with the statistical analysis.

References

1. Tierney MC, Fisher RH, Lewis AJ, et al. The NINCDS-ADRDA Work Group criteria for the clinical diagnosis of probable Alzheimer's disease: a clinicopathologic study of 57 cases. Neurology 1988; 38:359–364.
2. Jack CR, Petersen RC, O'Brien PC, Tangalos EG. MR-based hippocampal volumetry in the diagnosis of Alzheimer's disease. Neurology 1992; 42:183–188.
3. George AE, DeLeon MJ, Stylopoulos LA, et al. CT diagnostic features of Alzheimer's disease: importance of the choroidal/hippocampal fissure complex. AJNR 1990; 11: 101–107.
4. DeLeon MJ, Convit A, DeSanti S, et al. The hippocampus in aging and Alzheimer's disease. Neuroimaging Clin North Am 1995; 5:1–17.
5. Hyman BT, Van Hoesen GW, Damasio AR, Barnes CL. Alzheimer's disease: cell-specific pathology isolates the hippocampal formation. Science 1984; 225:1168–1170.
6. Tomlinson BE, Blessed G, Roth M. Observations on the brains of demented old people. J Neurol Sci 1970; 11:205–242.
7. Fazekas F, Chawlug JB, Alavi A, Hurtig HI, Zimmerman RA. MR signal abnormalities at 1.5 T in Alzheimer's dementia and normal aging. AJR 1987; 149:351–356.
8. Kirsch SJ, Roland WJ, Butcher LL, Beatty J. Prolongation of magnetic resonance T2 time in hippocampus of human patients marks the presence and severity of Alzheimer's disease (letter). Neuroscience 1992; 134:187–190.
9. Laakso MP, Partanen K, Soininen H, et al. MR T2 relaxometry in Alzheimer's disease and age-associated memory impairment. Neurobiol Aging 1996; 17:1–5.
10. Petersen RC, Kokmen E, Tangalos E, Ivnik RJ, Kurland LT. Mayo Clinic Alzheimer's Disease Patient Registry. Aging 1990; 2:408–415.
11. McKhann G, Drachman D, Folstein M, Katzman R, Price D, Stadian EM. Clinical diagnosis of Alzheimer's disease: report of the NINCDS-ADRDA Work Group under the auspices of the Department of Health and Human Services Task Force on Alzheimer's Disease. Neurology 1984; 34:939–944.
12. Grunewald RA, Jackson GD, Connelly A, Duncan JS. MR detection of hippocampal disease in epilepsy: factors influencing T2 relaxation time. AJNR 1994; 15:1149–1156.
13. Robb RA, Hanson DP, Karwoski RA, Larson AG, Workman EL, Stacy MC. ANALYZE: a comprehensive, operator-interactive software package for multidimensional medical image display and analysis. Comput Med Imaging Graph 1989; 13:433–454.
14. Berg L. Mild senile dementia of the Alzheimer type: clinical dementia rating (CDR). Psychopharmacol Bull 1988; 24:637–639.
15. Poon CS, Szumowski J, Plewes DB, Ashby P, Henkelman RM. Fat/water quantitation and differential relaxation time measurement using chemical shift imaging technique. Magn Reson Imaging 1989; 7:369–382.
16. Pitkanen A, Laakso M, Kalviainen R, et al. Severity of hippocampal atrophy correlates with the prolongation of MRI T2 relaxation time in temporal lobe epilepsy but not in Alzheimer's disease. Neurology 1996; 46: 1724–1730.
17. Huesgen CT, Burger PC, Crain BJ, Johnson GA. In vitro MR microscopy of the hippocampus in Alzheimer's disease. Neurology 1993; 43:145–152.
18. Kesslak JP, Nalcioglu O, Cotman CW. Quantification of magnetic resonance scans for hippocampal and parahippocampal atrophy in Alzheimer's disease. Neurology 1991; 41:51–54.
19. Lehericy S, Baulac M, Chiras J, et al. Amygdalohippocampal MR volume measurements in the early stages of Alzheimer's disease. AJNR 1994; 15:927–937.
20. Laakso MP, Soininen H, Partanen K, et al. Volumes of hippocampus, amygdala and frontal lobes in the MRI-based diagnosis of early Alzheimer's disease: correlation with memory functions. J Neural Transm Park Dis Dement Sect 1995; 9:73–86.
21. Soininen HS, Partanen K, Pitkanen A, et al. Volumetric MRI analysis of the amygdala and the hippocampus in subjects with age-associated memory impairment: correlation to visual and verbal memory. Neurology 1994; 44:1660–1668.
22. Pearlson G, Harris GJ, Powers RE, et al. Quantitative changes in mesial temporal volume, regional cerebral blood flow, and cognition in Alzheimer's disease. Arch Gen Psychiatry 1992; 49:402–408.
23. Killany RJ, Moss MB, Albert MS, et al. Temporal lobe regions on magnetic resonance imaging identify patients with early Alzheimer's disease. Arch Neurol 1993; 50:949–954.
24. Convit A, deLeon MJ, Golomb J, et al. Hippocampal atrophy in early Alzheimer's disease: anatomic specificity and validation. Psychiatr Q 1993; 64:371–387.
25. Convit A, deLeon MH, Tarshish C, et al. Hippocampal volume losses in minimally impaired elderly (letter). Lancet 1995; 345: 266.
26. Jack CR Jr, Sharbrough FW, Twomey CK, et al. Temporal lobe seizures: lateralization with MR volume measurements of hippocampal formation. Radiology 1990; 175: 423–429.
27. Jackson GD, Connelly A, Duncan JS, Grunewald RA, Gadian DG. Detection of hippocampal pathology in intractable partial epilepsy: increased sensitivity with quantitative magnetic resonance T2 relaxometry. Neurology 1993; 43:1793–1799.

Wendie A. Berg, MD, PhD • Thorsten L. Krebs, MD • Cristina Campassi, MD
Laurence S. Magder, PhD • Chen-Chih J. Sun, MD

Evaluation of 14- and 11-gauge Directional, Vacuum-assisted Biopsy Probes and 14-gauge Biopsy Guns in a Breast Parenchymal Model[1]

PURPOSE: **To compare commercially available 14-gauge core biopsy guns and 11- and 14-gauge, directional, vacuum-assisted biopsy probes for tissue yield and fragmentation.**

MATERIALS AND METHODS: **One hundred passes were made through fresh turkey breasts by using each of 11 14-gauge, automated biopsy gun–needle combinations and a directional, stereotactic, vacuum-assisted biopsy system equipped with 11- or 14-gauge probes. Specimens were measured for total weight, individual length, diameter, and number of fragments.**

RESULTS: **Among the handheld devices, the Pro-Mag 2.2 gun (Manan Medical Products, Northbrook, Ill) and 14-gauge Biopty-Cut needle (Bard, Covington, Ga) had the greatest yield (17.7 mg per core specimen); this combination also produced the greatest percentage of nonfragmented cores (83%). Directional, vacuum-assisted biopsy specimens were significantly larger ($P < .001$): 36.8 mg per core specimen for the 14-gauge probe and 94.4 mg per core specimen for the 11-gauge probe. Specimens obtained with directional, vacuum-assisted biopsy were more fragmented than those obtained with spring-actuated, two-stage, long-throw, automated biopsy systems.**

CONCLUSION: **Statistically significant differences with various biopsy devices are seen in the breast tissue yield and in fragmentation.**

INCREASED use of nonsurgical, 14-gauge core needle breast biopsy (1–3) has focused increased attention on sources of error (4–6). Errors in targeting are usually the result of operator inexperience (6,7), patient movement, or poor lesion conspicuity. Errors due to incomplete sampling occur most often with lesions that manifest as microcalcifications; overall, an approximately 8%–12% nondiagnostic rate has been observed for such lesions in multiple studies (1,4,8). With sampling, two forms of error exist. The first is the difficulty in histopathologically distinguishing closely related entities in the small amount of material in a core biopsy specimen compared with the material in an excised lesion. The second is the potential for two different histopathologic entities to be interspersed, perhaps both with microcalcifications, but for only one to be sampled (5,7). Increasing the number of specimens obtained (8), the gauge of the needle, or both (9) has been advocated to diminish the underestimation of lesion severity.

In current practice, 14-gauge, automated biopsy guns are most commonly used for stereotactically or ultrasound (US)–guided core needle breast biopsy and have been shown to provide a greater yield of material than do manual guns in animal studies (10). A previous report demonstrated a statistically significantly greater yield of material with a 14-gauge, automated gun than with 16-gauge or 18-gauge devices in cadaveric kidneys (11). A recent report by Nath and colleagues (12) demonstrated statistically significant improvement in the sensitivity for diagnosing breast malignancy ex vivo when larger-gauge Biopty-Cut needles (Bard, Covington, Ga) were used: 100% were diagnosed when a 14-gauge needle was used compared to 92% when a 16-gauge needle and 65% when an 18-gauge needle were used.

While a 14-gauge Biopty-Cut needle (Bard) or a 14-gauge Automatic Cutting needle (Manan Medical Products, Northbrook, Ill) and either a Biopty gun with 23-mm throw (Bard) or a Pro-Mag 2.2 gun with 22-mm throw (Manan Medical Products) have been used in most stereotactically or US-guided core needle biopsy studies described in published reports, findings of a recent study (13) indicate that the Magnum gun (formerly known as the BIP High Speed Multi gun; Bard) and Pro-Mag 2.2 guns yield statistically significantly more material than the Biopty gun and needle in the cadaveric breast. These results were also validated by using fresh turkey breast as a model of breast parenchyma (13).

To address the issues of sampling and underdiagnosis, a directional, vacuum-assisted biopsy system has been developed. This device uses either a 14-gauge or an 11-gauge sampling chamber with a motorized cutting needle and the application of vacuum suction during directional sampling (14). Preliminary results

Index term: Breast, biopsy, 00.1261, 00.1267

Abbreviations: ANOVA = analysis of variance, DCIS = ductal carcinoma in situ.

Radiology 1997; 205:203–208

[1] From the Departments of Diagnostic Radiology (W.A.B., T.L.K., C.C.), Epidemiology and Preventive Medicine (L.S.M.), and Pathology (C.C.J.S.), University of Maryland School of Medicine, 22 S Greene St, Baltimore, MD 21201. Received April 11, 1997; revision requested June 5; revision received June 25; accepted June 27. **Address reprint requests to** W.A.B.

Table 1
Tissue Acquisition with 14-gauge, Spring-actuated, Two-Stage, Long-Throw Automated Biopsy Guns and 14- and 11-gauge Directional, Vacuum-assisted Biopsy Instruments

Device	No. of Core Specimens per 100 Passes	Sample Weight (mg)*	Sample Length (mm)†	No. of Single-Fragment Passes	No. of Two-Fragment Passes	No. of Passes with More than Two Fragments
Pro-Mag 2.2 gun and 14-gauge Biopty-Cut needle	100	17.7 ± 1.5	9.6 ± 1.8	83	12	5
Pro-Mag 2.2 gun and 14-gauge Automatic Cutting needle	97	13.6 ± 1.0	10.1 ± 2.4	58	23	16
Magnum gun and Magnum needle	100	13.6 ± 0.4	9.6 ± 2.2	54	26	20
Monopty gun	100	11.5 ± 0.4	9.2 ± 2.1	51	38	11
Max-Core gun	99	11.4 ± 0.6	7.4 ± 2.1	81	17	1
Channel-Cut gun	100	10.9 ± 0.9	8.9 ± 1.9	27	35	38
Biopty gun and 14-gauge Biopty-Cut needle	100	10.6 ± 0.5	7.6 ± 2.5	61	27	12
Ultra-Cut gun	95	10.4 ± 1.2	7.2 ± 2.2	67	18	10
BioGun	100	9.6 ± 0.4	8.4 ± 2.1	64	26	10
Temno gun	99	8.5 ± 0.4	6.2 ± 2.4	52	27	20
Delta-Cut gun	100	7.0 ± 0.6	6.4 ± 2.2	75	17	8
Directional, vacuum-assisted breast biopsy probe						
14 gauge	100	36.8 ± 1.0	20.7 ± 3.0	32	41	27
11 gauge	100‡	94.4 ± 2.2	26.9 ± 7.1	18	38	44

* Sample weight was calculated by dividing the total weight of material obtained (in grams) by 100. Data are means ± standard errors.
† Data are means ± standard deviations.
‡ After each "round" of six passes, the chamber was examined for residual material. In the course of making 100 passes, an additional eight fragments were obtained from the chamber of the 11-gauge, directional, vacuum-assisted biopsy probe. These were not included in average weight, length, or fragmentation calculations.

have shown improved tissue yields (14) and more accurate diagnosis of lesions that manifest as microcalcifications (15,16). Excision of lesions by using directional, vacuum-assisted biopsy has been demonstrated (14,17).

We performed this study to compare commercially available 14-gauge core biopsy guns and 11- and 14-gauge, directional, vacuum-assisted biopsy probes in terms of tissue yield and fragmentation. To expand on previous results, we evaluated a larger series of currently available 14-gauge core biopsy guns as well as directional, vacuum-assisted biopsy probes with fresh turkey breast as a parenchymal model. We also compared 11-gauge and 14-gauge vacuum-assisted probes. We evaluated the results in the context of yields from a subset of these guns and needles in patient lesions, as assessed with specimen radiography. Implications for diagnostic applications are discussed below.

MATERIALS AND METHODS

Eleven 14-gauge, automated biopsy gun–needle combinations were evaluated: three reusable guns and seven disposable devices; one gun was tested independently with two different needles. The devices tested were the Biopty gun (Bard, Covington, Ga) and Biopty-Cut needle (Bard); the Pro-Mag 2.2 gun (Manan Medical Products, Northbrook, Ill) with the Automatic Cutting needle (Manan Medical Products) or the Biopty-Cut needle; the Magnum gun (Bard) set on 22-mm throw with a 14-gauge Magnum needle (Bard); the Max-Core gun (Bard) and Monopty gun (Bard); the ASAP Channel-Cut (Medi-tech/Boston Scientific, Watertown, Mass) and ASAP Delta-Cut guns (Medi-tech/Boston Scientific); the Ultra-Cut gun (MD Tech, Silver Spring, Md); and two semi-automated devices, the Bio-Gun (E-Z-Em, Westbury, NY) and the Temno gun (Bauer Medical, Clearwater, Fla). A directional, vacuum-assisted biopsy device (Mammotome; Biopsys Medical, Irvine, Calif) equipped with either a 14-gauge or an 11-gauge, vacuum-assisted probe was also evaluated.

Five whole fresh turkey breasts were used at room temperature. Three radiologists (W.A.B., T.L.K., C.C.) experienced in core needle biopsy technique practiced with each gun to perfect the technique before beginning the study. One hundred passes were performed with each gun-needle combination; care was taken not to cross a previous biopsy track. With the directional, vacuum-assisted biopsy probe, one pass was made in each of six directions (the 12 o'clock, 2 o'clock, 4 o'clock, 6 o'clock, 8 o'clock, and 10 o'clock positions) at each probe location. The probe was then repositioned at least 2 cm away for the next series of passes. The "tap tap" maneuver (17), consisting of manually applying the vacuum to the chamber without additional cutting, was performed after each specimen was obtained to ensure that no residual material remained in the chamber.

Specimens were rolled onto filter paper, and the net total specimen was weighed and placed in a petri dish that contained 10% formalin. The cores from each device were measured for length, diameter, and number of fragments by an experienced histopathologist (C.C.J.S.) blinded to the device used.

Groups of specimens from the same gun were pooled together before weighing. The average weight per specimen was calculated by taking the sum of the weights of the pooled specimens and dividing by the total number of specimens that were pooled together. The standard deviation of the weight of individual specimens was estimated on the basis of the variance of the pooled specimens, with adjustment for the number of specimens that were pooled together. The standard error of the mean specimen weights was calculated by dividing the standard deviations by the square root of the number of specimens obtained. When specimens were fragmented, the length of the specimen was calculated as the sum of the lengths of the fragments. Analysis of variance (ANOVA) was used to assess the degree to which differences between guns were statistically significant.

We have reviewed our clinical experience with 66 lesions in 60 patients (age range, 39–81 years), with 100 passes each made with the 11-gauge, directional, vacuum-assisted biopsy probe, the Pro-Mag 2.2 gun–14-gauge Biopty-Cut needle combination for stereotactic biopsy, and the Monopty gun and the Max-Core gun for US-guided biopsy performed in January 1997, after experience had been obtained in more than 400 large-core needle breast biopsies in patients. Biopsy results are presented for 66 cases: 35 masses, 30 clustered microcalcifications, and one focal asymmetric density. Stereotactic sampling was performed on a digital spot-mammographic stereotactic unit (LoRad, Danbury, Conn). A 10-MHz linear transducer (Performa; Acoustic Imaging Technologies, Phoenix, Ariz) was used to provide US guidance. With directional, vacuum-assisted biopsy, sampling was performed as

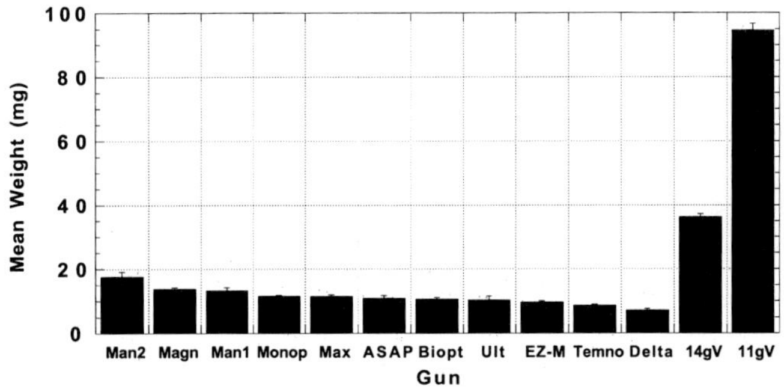

1.

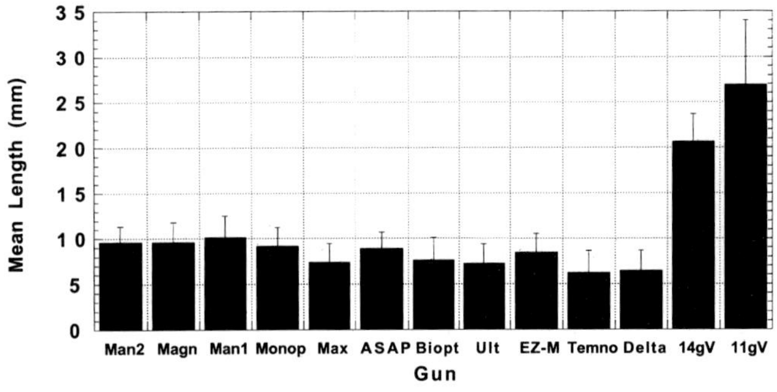

2.

Figures 1, 2. **(1)** Mean weight of turkey breast specimens per pass with a variety of commercially available 14-gauge biopsy gun–needle combinations and 14- and 11-gauge, directional, vacuum-assisted biopsy probes. Error bars show standard errors. **(2)** Mean length of turkey breast specimens obtained with a variety of commercially available 14-gauge biopsy gun–needle combinations and 14- and 11-gauge, directional, vacuum-assisted biopsy probes. Error bars show standard deviation. *ASAP* = ASAP Channel-Cut gun; *Biopt* = Biopty gun–14-gauge Biopty-Cut needle combination; *Delta* = ASAP Delta-Cut gun; *11gV* = 11-gauge, directional, vacuum-assisted biopsy probe; *EZ-M* = Bio-Gun; *14gV* = 14-gauge, directional, vacuum-assisted biopsy probe; *Magn* = Magnum gun and needle; *Man1* = Pro-Mag 2.2 gun–Automatic Cutting needle combination; *Man2* = Pro-Mag 2.2 gun–14-gauge Biopty-Cut needle combination; *Max* = Max-Core gun; *Monop* = Monopty gun; *Temno* = Temno gun; *Ult* = Ultra-Cut gun.

with the turkey breast, with six to 12 specimens obtained per lesion. With 14-gauge biopsy guns, five to nine specimens were obtained per lesion. Prefire and postfire images were obtained for the initial stereotactic pass and for all US passes. Specimens were kept moistened with saline on filter paper. Magnification specimen mammography of all specimens was performed at 22 kVp, 7 mAs. Twenty-three (35%) of the 66 lesions sampled were malignant. A discrete benign process was identified in all other cases (fibroadenoma, focal fibrosis, sclerosing adenosis, apocrine metaplasia, papilloma, fibrocystic changes, lymph node). Microcalcifications were documented in at least three of the passes from each lesion that contained microcalcifications.

RESULTS

Paralleling the results of Burbank and colleagues (14), whose average specimen weight was 31.9 mg with a 14-gauge directional, vacuum-assisted probe and 17.2 mg with the Biopty gun in a series of 345 stereotactic breast biopsies, the yield of breast tissue in our parenchymal model with 14-gauge, directional, vacuum-assisted biopsy was twofold greater than that with the best of the handheld biopsy guns: The average specimen weight was 36.8 mg compared to 17.7 mg with the Pro-Mag 2.2 gun equipped with a 14-gauge Biopty-Cut needle ($P < .001$) (Table 1) (Fig 1). The Pro-Mag 2.2 gun–Biopty-Cut 14-gauge needle combination yielded significantly more material than all the other handheld 14-gauge systems ($P < .001$); the yield of this combination was 2–2½-fold greater than that observed with the Delta-Cut and Temno disposable guns (Fig 1). The Pro-Mag 2.2 gun–Biopty-Cut needle combination yielded fully 67% more material than the more commonly used Biopty gun–Biopty-Cut needle combination and 30% more material than the Magnum gun and needle combination or the Pro-Mag 2.2 gun–Automatic Cutting needle combination, which had previously been shown to be superior (13). A directional, vacuum-assisted biopsy device equipped with an 11-gauge probe yielded an average specimen weight of 94.4 mg, which is 2.6-fold more than the average specimen weight with a 14-gauge probe ($P < .001$) and greater than fivefold the best of the 14-gauge handheld devices ($P < .001$) (Fig 1).

Although the length of the cutting notch varied only from 17 mm to 19 mm across the guns in this series, the lengths of the specimens obtained ranged from 2 mm to 42 mm and the mean lengths of the specimens from 6 mm to 27 mm (Table 1) (Fig 2). Overall, the specimen lengths paralleled the specimen weights; specimens obtained with the directional, vacuum-assisted biopsy probe averaged more than twice as long as those obtained with any of the handheld devices. The average diameter of the specimens ranged from 1.5 mm (14-gauge Bio-Gun) to 1.9 mm (Pro-Mag 2.2 gun with 14-gauge Biopty-Cut needle) across the series of handheld guns; with directional, vacuum-assisted biopsy, the average diameter was 1.9 mm for the 14-gauge probe and 2.6 mm for the 11-gauge probe.

The number of fragments produced in each pass ranged from zero to seven. The least fragmentation was observed with two of the handheld combinations: the Pro-Mag 2.2 gun equipped with the 14-gauge Biopty-Cut needle, with 83 of the passes composed of a single fragment, and the Max-Core single-use gun, with 81 of 99 specimen-containing passes composed of a single fragment (Table 1) (Fig 3). The majority of passes made with either the 14-gauge or the 11-gauge, directional, vacuum-assisted stereotactic biopsy probe had at least two fragments (68% and 82%, respectively).

Similar results have been obtained in patient lesions (Table 2), although we have not tested all gun-needle combinations in clinical practice. In a consecutive series of 100 passes we made in patients with the 11-gauge, directional, vacuum-assisted biopsy probe, we obtained 138 fragments and had five empty passes (in one case, moderate bleeding may have inhibited specimen collection). By contrast, with 100 passes with a Pro-Mag 2.2 gun and a 14-gauge Biopty-Cut needle, 102 fragments were obtained and no passes were empty. With 100 passes of the single-use 14-gauge Monopty gun, 118 fragments were obtained and one pass was empty.

As measured at specimen radiography, with correction for magnification, specimen lengths in patient lesions parallel those in the turkey breast model. The average specimen length we have observed in patient lesions with 11-gauge, directional, vacuum-assisted biopsy has been 19.6 mm (range, 8–31 mm), compared to 13.0 mm with a Pro-Mag 2.2 gun–14-gauge Biopty-Cut needle combination (range, 8–19 mm), 15.0 mm with a 14-gauge Monopty gun (range, 8–24 mm), and 9.2 mm with a Max-Core disposable gun (range, 7–14 mm). We have previously observed greater yields from specimens that include breast parenchyma (13). The improved yield with a Monopty gun over the Pro-Mag 2.2

gun–14-gauge Biopty-Cut needle combination likely reflects preferential use of the Monopty gun in US-guided biopsy performed exclusively through mass lesions versus the yield with the Pro-Mag 2.2 gun–Biopty-Cut needle combination we use in stereotactic biopsy of microcalcifications, for which more of the core specimen is often fat.

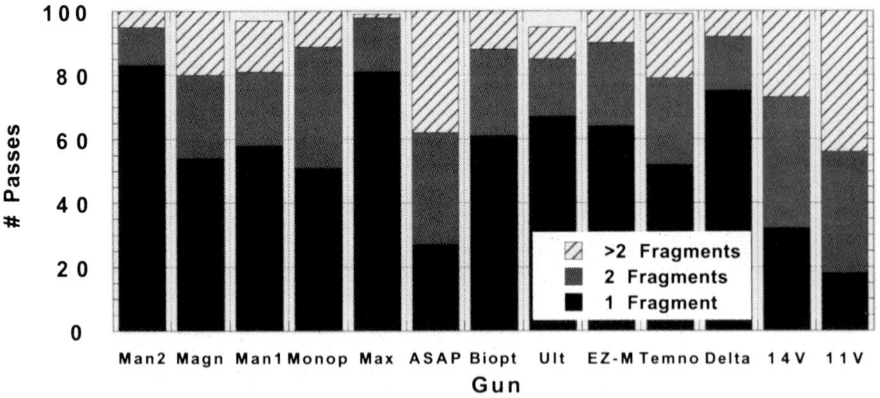

Figure 3. Plot of number of fragments per pass obtained with each gun-needle combination. Unless otherwise specified, 14-gauge needles were used. *ASAP* = ASAP Channel-Cut gun; *Biopt* = Biopty gun–14-gauge Biopty-Cut needle combination; *Delta* = ASAP Delta-Cut gun; *11V* = 11-gauge, directional, vacuum-assisted biopsy probe; *EZ-M* = Bio-Gun; *14V* = 14-gauge, directional, vacuum-assisted biopsy probe; *Magn* = Magnum gun and needle; *Man1* = Pro-Mag 2.2 gun–Automatic Cutting needle combination; *Man2* = Pro-Mag 2.2 gun–14-gauge Biopty-Cut needle combination; *Max* = Max-Core gun; *Monop* = Monopty gun; *Temno* = Temno gun; *Ult* = Ultra-Cut gun.

DISCUSSION

Large-core needle biopsy is generally replacing diagnostic surgical biopsy as the initial procedure of choice to evaluate both palpable and nonpalpable breast lesions. There are certain situations, however, where there is a risk of underdiagnosis of lesion severity when core needle biopsy is used. The first of these is with lesions where both an in situ and an infiltrating carcinoma are present but only one or the other has been sampled. Approximately 20% of lesions diagnosed as ductal carcinoma in situ (DCIS) with 14-gauge, automated core needle biopsy prove to have an infiltrating component at excision (1,15). This may occur more often when DCIS is evident as a mass lesion (Jackman R, unpublished data, 1996). Because axillary lymph node dissection is performed only when an invasive component is known, failure to identify the invasive component initially will in most cases necessitate a second surgical procedure.

If the final diagnosis is DCIS, core needle biopsy has potentially saved a procedure if the lesion is widespread and best managed with mastectomy. An isolated focus of DCIS, usually smaller than 5 cm, would typically be managed by means of needle localization, excisional biopsy (lumpectomy), and radiation therapy. In these cases, diagnostic surgical biopsy may prove to be synonymous with the definitive surgical procedure, and initial core biopsy may have less of a role. Indeed, in patients with lesions that manifested as highly suspicious microcalcifications and that usually proved to be DCIS, initial core needle biopsy spared a surgical procedure only 42% of the time in one series (18); in contrast, with spiculated masses, initial core biopsy spared at least one surgical procedure 77% of the time (19).

Traditionally, for infiltrating carcinomas, axillary lymph node dissection is performed as a second surgical procedure after initial diagnostic biopsy. When the diagnosis has been established at initial core biopsy, axillary lymph node dissection can be performed concurrently with lumpectomy. Furthermore, with initial diagnostic core biopsy, the surgeon can deliberately obtain wider margins at the first surgery when the lesion is known preoperatively to be malignant. Indeed, in one series, the initial surgical procedure resulted in positive margins in 40 (37%) of 107 cancers in which diagnostic surgical biopsy was performed compared with only five (8%) of 62 cancers revealed at initial core biopsy (20). Another 29 (27%) of 107 lesions diagnosed at excisional biopsy showed tumor within one high-power (×40) field of the biopsy margins (20): Reexcision would generally be performed whenever less than 1 cm of uninvolved tissue has been obtained around the tumor.

As has been shown in multiple studies, the diagnosis of atypical ductal hyperplasia at core needle biopsy should prompt excision, because 52%–56% of such lesions prove to be malignant (2,21). This lesion most often manifests as clustered amorphous or pleomorphic microcalcifications (22). Because atypical hyperplasia can be interspersed with carcinoma, such underdiagnosis can result from sampling error. More often, however, we have observed this situation when the lesion is in situ or infiltrating cribriform ductal carcinoma, which closely mimics atypical ductal hyperplasia; this distinction is especially difficult at core biopsy, where only a few ducts are available for review (23). In this situation, carcinoma has been suspected but not diagnosed with core needle biopsy.

Acquisition of larger volumes of material should facilitate accurate diagnosis and preoperative planning. In the largest series that we know of to date, in which 14-gauge core needle biopsy was used, underdiagnosis as discussed above was observed in 12.5% of cases (1). It has been shown that increasing the number of specimens improves the diagnostic yield (8): Whereas the first pass is diagnostic only 70% of the time, diagnosis was achieved in 99% of mass lesions with five passes performed with a Biopty gun and a 14-gauge Biopty-Cut needle. Accurate and complete diagnosis of lesions that manifest as microcalcifications has proved more problematic, with approximately 8% of such lesions missed after acquisition of five (24) to six (8) specimens. Some investigators routinely obtain 10 or more specimens through targeted microcalcifications (25), which has been shown to decrease the frequency of underestimation of disease (15).

Increasing the volume of tissue obtained with each pass may be even more effective than increasing the number of specimens. As has been demonstrated, choice of the most advantageous gun and needle combination can statistically significantly improve tissue yields. Histopathologically, the greater the number of ducts visualized, the greater the certainty of diagnosis. Obtaining a broader specimen, through increasing the diameter of each fragment, further enhances the diagnostic potential.

Visualization of an isolated nest of monomorphic hyperplastic ductal cells could represent a focus of invasive ductal carcinoma (particularly of the cribriform type), DCIS, or atypical ductal hyperplasia. Further, a nest of

Table 2
Tissue Acquisition in Patients

Device	Sample Length (mm) Mean	Range	No. of Fragments	No. of Empty Passes
Pro-Mag 2.2 gun and 14-gauge Biopty-Cut needle	13.0	8–19	102	0
Monopty gun	15.0	8–24	118	1
Max-Core gun	9.2	7–14	100	0
11-gauge, directional, vacuum-assisted breast biopsy probe	19.6	8–31	138	5*

Note.—Specimen radiography was used to analyze the yield from 100 consecutive passes.
* Five passes were empty during biopsy of the same lesion; moderate hemorrhage complicated the procedure.

cells that represent DCIS can be displaced by the core needle biopsy itself, thus mimicking a focus of invasion (26). If many nests of monomorphic hyperplastic ductal cells are present in the stroma, the correct diagnosis of invasion is facilitated. Because standard 14-gauge core needle biopsy results typically show little more than one or two ducts across, such distinctions can be subtle.

Early results with the 14-gauge, directional, vacuum-assisted biopsy probe suggest a decrease in the underdiagnosis rate: Jackman and colleagues (15) reported that, among lesions diagnosed as atypical hyperplasia at core needle biopsy, 26 (48%) of the 54 sampled with 14-gauge, spring-actuated, two-stage, long-throw, automated biopsy guns proved malignant compared to 13 (18%) of the 74 sampled with 14-gauge, directional, vacuum-assisted biopsy probes. In a recent article, Burbank (16) reports that, while eight of 18 lesions diagnosed as atypical ductal hyperplasia with a 14-gauge, automated biopsy gun proved malignant at excision, none of the eight diagnosed as atypical ductal hyperplasia with a 14-gauge, directional, vacuum-assisted biopsy probe proved malignant. Similarly, whereas nine (16%) of 55 lesions diagnosed as DCIS with a 14-gauge, automated biopsy gun proved to have an infiltrating component at excision, all 32 lesions diagnosed as DCIS with a 14-gauge, directional, vacuum-assisted biopsy gun showed only DCIS at excision (16).

To our knowledge, no results have been published on a comparison of 11-gauge and 14-gauge, directional, vacuum-assisted biopsy probes. Given the 70% increase in the diameter of specimens obtained with the 11-gauge probe, it is expected that more of the overall architecture of the lesion is available for review than with any of the 14-gauge options.

Complete removal of lesions is possible with the increased tissue-harvesting capabilities of the directional, vacuum-assisted biopsy probes. Indeed, Burbank and colleagues (14) reported complete "excision" of 48% of lesions in their series, where the average lesion diameter was 9 mm. With a cluster of microcalcifications no larger than 5 mm, 79% of biopsies were excisional. Similarly, Liberman and co-workers (17) reported complete removal of 11 (58%) of 19 lesions 5 mm or smaller.

At present, coaxial clip placement is needed to mark the site for subsequent excision whenever complete removal is suspected at the time of initial core biopsy. At some point in the future, it may prove desirable to excise lesions completely by using directional, vacuum-assisted biopsy, perhaps followed by irradiation. One of the major potential drawbacks of this approach for excision, however, is the difficulty in assessing the margins. This may prove particularly problematic if the degree of fragmentation is great, which would prohibit proper orientation of the specimens with respect to each other. We have observed statistically significantly greater fragmentation with directional, vacuum-assisted biopsy in both the turkey breast model and in patient lesions.

With the four- to fivefold increased cost of directional, vacuum-assisted biopsy probes ($134 for 14 gauge and $200 for 11 gauge) compared to the cost of disposable biopsy guns ($34–$40 each) and the up to 14-fold greater cost compared to the cost of the Biopty-Cut disposable needle ($14), it is important to weigh the potential benefits. Because underestimation or outright miss of a mass lesion at standard 14-gauge core needle biopsy after five passes occurs in only 0.1%–2% of cases (4,24), it may be that the conventional 14-gauge, automated biopsy gun approach is sufficient for masses. Conversely, for lesions that have to be sampled with stereotactic guidance, which include clustered microcalcifications, focal asymmetries, and architectural distortions, the miss rate is higher at 8%–14% (24). In these situations, directional, vacuum-assisted biopsy may be warranted.

Because turkey breast is a relatively homogeneous tissue compared with human breast tissue and breast lesions, actual patient findings may vary. In our own experience, relative comparisons of guns appear to be most valid when similar types of lesions are sampled with each gun. We use the 11-gauge, directional, vacuum-assisted biopsy probe for stereotactic biopsy of microcalcifications and the Pro-Mag 2.2 gun–14-gauge Biopty-Cut needle combination when sampling masses stereotactically. We sample most masses under US guidance by using the Monopty disposable gun.

In conclusion, these results extend previous work (13) and further validate the use of fresh turkey breast as a parenchymal model. Our yields in turkey breast closely parallel those in patient lesions observed by Burbank and colleagues (14). Similarly, with specimen radiography, we have observed similar-length and similar-diameter fragments and a similar degree of fragmentation as that seen in turkey breast with a subset of these guns and needles in patient lesions. As further guns and needle-gun combinations are developed, manufacturers should be encouraged to evaluate the performance in breast parenchymal models before marketing the devices for patient use. These data should serve as a basis for comparison to establish which new guns and needles represent a substantial improvement over existing combinations. ■

Acknowledgments: The authors thank the gun manufacturers for supplying all nonmotorized biopsy guns used in this study at no charge.

References

1. Parker SH, Burbank F, Jackman RJ, et al. Percutaneous large-core breast biopsy: a multi-institutional study. Radiology 1994; 193:359–364.
2. Jackman RJ, Nowels KW, Shepard MJ, Finkelstein SI, Marzoni FA. Stereotaxic large-core needle biopsy of 450 nonpalpable breast lesions with surgical correlation in lesions with cancer or atypical hyperplasia. Radiology 1994; 193:91–95.
3. Rubin E, Dempsey PJ, Pile NS, et al. Needle-localization biopsy of the breast: impact of a selective core needle biopsy program on yield. Radiology 1995; 195: 627–631.
4. Dershaw DD, Morris EA, Liberman L, Abramson AF. Non-diagnostic stereotaxic core breast biopsy: results of rebiopsy. Radiology 1996; 198:323–326.
5. Berg WA. When is core breast biopsy or

fine-needle aspiration not enough? Radiology 1996; 198:313–315.
6. Liberman L, Dershaw DD, Glassman J, et al. Analysis of cancers not diagnosed at stereotaxic core breast biopsy. Radiology 1997; 203:151–157.
7. Berg WA, Hruban RH, Kumar D, Singh HR, Brem RF, Gatewood OMB. Lessons from mammographic-histopathologic correlation of large-core needle breast biopsy. RadioGraphics 1996; 16:1111–1130.
8. Liberman L, Dershaw DD, Rosen PP, Abramson AF, Deutch BM, Hann LE. Stereotaxic 14-gauge breast biopsy: how many core biopsy specimens are needed? Radiology 1994; 192:793–795.
9. Parker SH, Lovin JD, Jobe WE, Burke BJ, Hopper KD, Yakes WF. Nonpalpable breast lesions: stereotactic automated large-core biopsies. Radiology 1991; 180:403–407.
10. Hopper K, Baird D, Reddy V, et al. Efficacy of automated biopsy guns versus conventional biopsy needles in the pygmy pig. Radiology 1990; 176:671–676.
11. Hopper K, Abendroth C, Sturtz K, Matthews Y, Shirk S, Stevens L. Blinded comparison of biopsy needles and automated devices in vitro. II. Biopsy of medical renal disease. AJR 1993; 161:1299–1301.
12. Nath M, Robinson T, Tobon H, Chough D, Sumkin J. Automated large-core needle biopsy of surgically removed breast lesions: comparison of samples obtained with 14-, 16-, and 18-gauge needles. Radiology 1995; 197:739–742.
13. Krebs TL, Berg WA, Severson MJ, et al. Large-core biopsy guns: comparison for yield of breast tissue. Radiology 1996; 200: 365–368.
14. Burbank F, Parker S, Fogarty T. Stereotactic breast biopsy: improved tissue harvesting with the Mammotome. Am Surg 1996; 62:738–744.
15. Jackman R, Burbank F, Parker S, et al. Atypical ductal hyperplasia diagnosed at stereotactic biopsy: improved reliability with 14-gauge, directional, vacuum-assisted biopsy. Radiology 1997; 204:485–488.
16. Burbank F. Stereotactic breast biopsy of atypical ductal hyperplasia and ductal carcinoma in situ lesions: improved accuracy with directional, vacuum-assisted biopsy. Radiology 1997; 202:843–847.
17. Liberman L, Hann LE, Dershaw DD, Morris EA, Abramson AF, Rosen PP. Mammographic findings after stereotactic 14-gauge vacuum biopsy. Radiology 1997; 203:343–347.
18. Liberman L, LaTrenta L, VanZee KJ, Morris E, Abramson A, Dershaw DD. Stereotactic core biopsy of calcifications highly suggestive of malignancy. Radiology 1997; 203: 673–677.
19. Liberman L, Dershaw DD, Rosen PP, Cohen MA, Hann LE, Abramson AF. Stereotaxic core biopsy of impalpable spiculated breast masses. AJR 1995; 165:551–554.
20. Liberman L, LaTrenta L, Dershaw D, et al. Impact of core biopsy on the surgical management of impalpable breast cancer. AJR 1997; 168:495–499.
21. Liberman L, Cohen MA, Dershaw DD, Abramson AF, Hann LE, Rosen PP. Atypical ductal hyperplasia diagnosed at stereotaxic core biopsy of breast lesions: an indication for surgical biopsy. AJR 1995; 164: 1111–1113.
22. Stomper P, Cholewinski S, Penetrante R, Harlos J, Tsangaris T. Atypical hyperplasia: frequency and mammographic and pathologic relationships in excisional biopsies guided with mammography and clinical examination. Radiology 1993; 189:667–671.
23. Ioffe OB, Berg WA, Kumar D. Mammographic-histopathologic correlation of large core needle breast biopsies (abstr). Mod Pathol 1997; 10:20.
24. Brenner RJ, Fajardo L, Fisher PR, et al. Percutaneous core biopsy of the breast: effect of operator experience and number of samples on diagnostic accuracy. AJR 1996; 166:341–346.
25. Parker S, Burbank F. A practical approach to minimally invasive breast biopsy. Radiology 1996; 200:11–20.
26. Youngson BJ, Liberman L, Rosen PP. Displacement of carcinomatous epithelium in surgical breast specimens following stereotaxic core biopsy. Am J Clin Pathol 1995; 103:598–602.

Hanan Sherif, MD • Ahmed-Emad Mahfouz, MD • Hans Oellinger, MD
Jose Hadijuana, MD • Jens-Uwe Blohmer, MD • Matthias Taupitz, MD, PhD
Roland Felix, MD • Bernd Hamm, MD

Peripheral Washout Sign on Contrast-enhanced MR Images of the Breast[1]

PURPOSE: **To assess the value of the peripheral washout sign on delayed contrast material–enhanced magnetic resonance (MR) images in differentiation of benign from malignant breast masses.**

MATERIALS AND METHODS: **In 49 women with 79 breast lesions (55 malignant and 24 benign), dynamic contrast-enhanced MR imaging was performed every 90 seconds during the first 7 minutes and repeated at 10, 20, 30, 40, 50, and 60 minutes after injection of contrast material. Qualitative analysis of the images was performed to evaluate the presence of the peripheral washout sign (a hypointense zone in the periphery of the lesion relative to the center). Quantitative analysis of the images was performed by measuring the signal intensity of the periphery and center of the lesions.**

RESULTS: **The peripheral washout sign was seen in 28 (51%) of the 55 carcinomas on delayed contrast-enhanced MR images (>10 minutes). Quantitative analysis demonstrated different enhancement profiles of the periphery and center of these lesions. The periphery showed early increase and decrease of enhancement, while the center showed gradual increase and persistent enhancement. The peripheral washout sign was not seen in any of the benign lesions. Specificity was 100% and sensitivity was 51% for diagnosis of breast carcinoma.**

CONCLUSION: **Peripheral washout may be a reliable sign of malignancy on delayed contrast-enhanced MR images of the breast.**

Breast cancer is one of the most common malignancies among women (1). Contrast material–enhanced magnetic resonance (MR) imaging of the breast has been used successfully in detection of breast cancer (2–6). With MR imaging, however, it is still difficult to differente benign from malignant lesions because the differentiating signs of these lesions appear similar (4–6). This similarity is evident in that the sensitivity of MR imaging in the diagnosis of malignancy is satisfactory but the specificity has been lower in most studies (4–6). Early enhancement at MR imaging (ie, enhancement within the first 2 minutes after injection of the contrast agent) is considered the hallmark of malignant lesions (2,4,7). Consequently, the morphologic signs suggestive of malignancy, such as irregularity of the border and inhomogeneous or ringlike pattern of enhancement, are seen during this early phase of enhancement (2,4,7–9). However, these signs typically cannot be used alone to differentiate malignant lesions from other rapidly enhancing lesions that are benign, such as fibroadenomas (7).

To our knowledge, no previous study has evaluated possible differentiating signs on delayed contrast-enhanced MR images (obtained more than 10 minutes after injection of contrast material). The purpose of our study was to evaluate the usefulness of the peripheral washout sign on delayed MR images for differentiation of benign from malignant lesions.

MATERIALS AND METHODS

Patients

Initially, this prospective study included 62 women (age range, 23–79 years; mean, 55 years) who underwent MR imaging of the breast for assessment of clinically or mammographically evident masses.

Criteria for inclusion of patients in the image analysis included (*a*) focal enhancing lesions within the first 2 minutes of dynamic contrast-enhanced MR imaging, (*b*) a complete dynamic MR imaging examination according to the protocol described below, and (*c*) histopathologic proof of the diagnosis of focal lesions.

Of the 62 women included in the study initially, 49 patients fulfilled the aforementioned inclusion criteria and were thus included in the image analysis. The remaining 13 women were excluded from the image analysis: Two women were excluded because they could not complete the MR imaging examination; seven women were excluded because they demonstrated early diffuse enhancement of the breast at dynamic MR imaging; and four patients, in whom fibroadenomas were suspected, were excluded because the definite histopathologic diagnosis could not be ascertained.

Lesions

The 49 patients who were included in the image analysis had a total of 79 lesions. Fifty-five lesions were malignant (51 invasive ductal carcinomas, two invasive lobular carcinomas, and two ductal carcinomas in situ with nodular invasive foci). Twenty-four lesions were benign (17 fibroadenomas, three benign phyllodes tumors, three

Index terms: Breast neoplasms, diagnosis, 00.31, 00.32 • Breast neoplasms, MR, 00.121412, 00.12143 • Gadolinium • Magnetic resonance (MR), contrast enhancement, 00.12143

Radiology 1997; 205:209–213

[1] From the Department of Radiology, Rudolf Virchow Hospital, Berlin, Germany (H.S., H.O., J.H., R.F.); the Departments of Radiology (A.E.M., M.T., B.H.) and Gynecology (J.U.B.), Charité Hospital, Humboldt University of Berlin, Schumannstr 20/21, D-10098 Berlin, Germany; and the Department of Radiology, Cairo University Hospital, Cairo, Egypt (A.E.M., H.S.). Received November 8, 1996; revision requested December 26; final revision received June 9, 1997; accepted June 16. **Address reprint requests to** B.H.

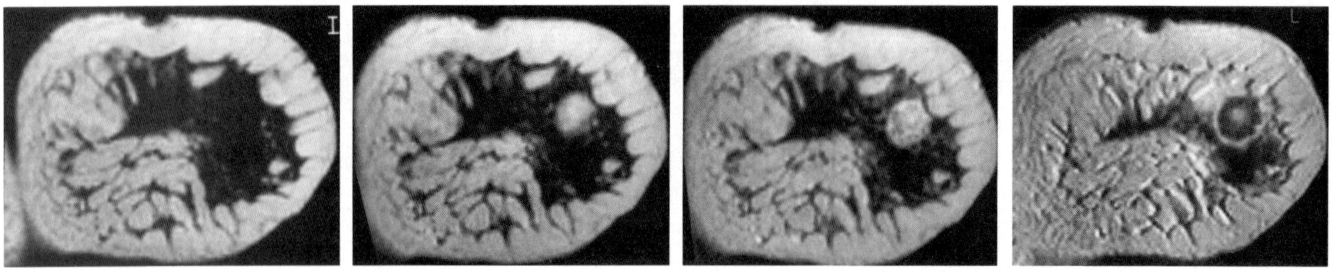

a. b. c. d.

Figure 1. Invasive ductal carcinoma in the upper outer quadrant of the left breast. Coronal, dynamic gadolinium-enhanced, T1-weighted gradient-recalled-echo MR images (11/4.6; flip angle, 25°) obtained **(a)** before, **(b)** 90 seconds after, **(c)** 10 minutes after, and **(d)** 40 minutes after intravenous injection of gadopentetate dimeglumine. **(b)** The entire lesion enhanced rapidly on the 90-second image. The peripheral washout sign is observed on the delayed images and is best seen on the 40-minute image **(d)**. An enhancing perilesional rim is also present and is best seen on the 40-minute image.

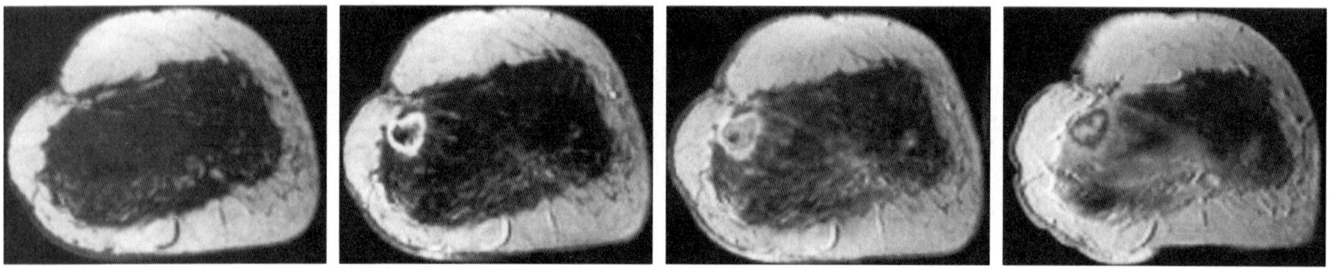

a. b. c. d.

Figure 2. Recurrent invasive ductal carcinoma in the upper outer quadrant of the right breast. Coronal dynamic, gadolinium-enhanced, T1-weighted gradient-recalled-echo MR images (11/4.6; flip angle, 25°) obtained **(a)** before, **(b)** 90 seconds after, **(c)** 10 minutes after, and **(d)** 60 minutes after intravenous injection of contrast material. **(b)** The lesion shows a ringlike pattern of enhancement on the 90-second image. **(c, d)** The peripheral washout sign and the perilesional rim are seen on the delayed images.

cases of nodular proliferative mastopathy, and one case of granulomatous mastitis). On the 90-second contrast-enhanced MR images, the diameter of malignant lesions was 3–36 mm (mean, 16 mm) and the diameter of benign lesions was 7–40 mm (mean, 17 mm). In all lesions, the type was proved histologically.

MR Imaging

MR imaging was performed at 1.5 T (Gyroscan ASC-NT, Philips Medical Systems, Eindhoven, the Netherlands, and Magnetom Vision, Siemens, Erlangen, Germany). Before the examination, an intravenous catheter was placed, usually through an antecubital vein. The intravenous cannula was connected to a mechanical injector by means of a long connecting tube. The patient was then placed in the prone position with both breasts hanging in a double breast coil. A three-dimensional, T1-weighted gradient-recalled-echo sequence was performed with the following parameters: 11/4.6 (repetition time msec/echo time msec); flip angle, 25°; rectangular field of view, 175 × 350 mm; matrix, 128 × 256 (pixel size, 1.37 × 1.37); section thickness, 2.5 mm with no gap; and one signal acquired. A bolus (0.2 mmol/kg) of gadopentetate dimeglumine (Magnevist; Schering, Berlin, Germany) was then injected at a rate of 3 mL/sec followed by 10 mL of saline. Imaging was then repeated with the previously mentioned sequence starting at the following points: 90, 180, 270, and 360 seconds and 10, 20, 30, 40, 50, and 60 minutes. The start of injection was considered the zero point. In 30 of the 49 patients, the entire series of images was obtained with the patient lying in the same position in the magnet throughout the dynamic study. The remaining 19 patients could not lie within the magnet for the entire examination time. In these cases, the patient was removed from the magnet for a short time and then repositioned at the previously mentioned times. This repositioning was performed between the 10- and 20-minute images in two patients, between the 20- and 30-minute images in five patients, between the 30- and 40-minute images in eight patients, and between the 40- and 50-minute images in four patients. Image subtraction was performed on a pixel-by-pixel basis for the first four series of images in the dynamic study.

Image Analysis

Qualitative analysis.—Qualitative analysis was performed independently by three radiologists (H.S., A.E.M., B.H.). The subtracted images were viewed first for identification of the position of the lesions. The corresponding nonsubtracted pre- and postcontrast images at each point of the dynamic study (90 seconds to 60 minutes) were then viewed together to evaluate the presence of the peripheral washout sign. The objective criterion for the presence of this sign is a hypointense zone in the periphery of the lesion relative to its center on delayed contrast-enhanced images. If the peripheral washout sign was noticed, the radiologists were asked to note the point at which it was seen first. Results from the three radiologists were then compared. The peripheral washout sign was considered present when the three radiologists agreed on its presence.

Quantitative analysis.—Quantitative analysis was performed by means of a manually placed region of interest. Two measurements were obtained per lesion: One region of interest was placed in the most enhancing part of the periphery, and another was placed in the center. Placement of these regions of interest was performed initially on the nonsubtracted 90-second image in the dynamic study. The region of interest was then placed in the same positions of the periphery and center on the pre- and postcontrast nonsubtracted images at each point of the study. The area of the region of interest was 0.5–1.5 mm^2 (average area, 1.2 mm^2). The percentage of enhancement was then calculated according to the following equation: enhancement $= (S_{post} - S_{pre}) / S_{pre}$, where enhancement is measured in percent, S_{pre} is the signal intensity before injection of the contrast agent, and S_{post} is the signal intensity after intravenous injection of the contrast agent at each point of the dynamic study. Although images were obtained at all points of the dynamic study in the 19 patients who were removed from the magnet between the imaging series, quantitative analysis was performed in these patients

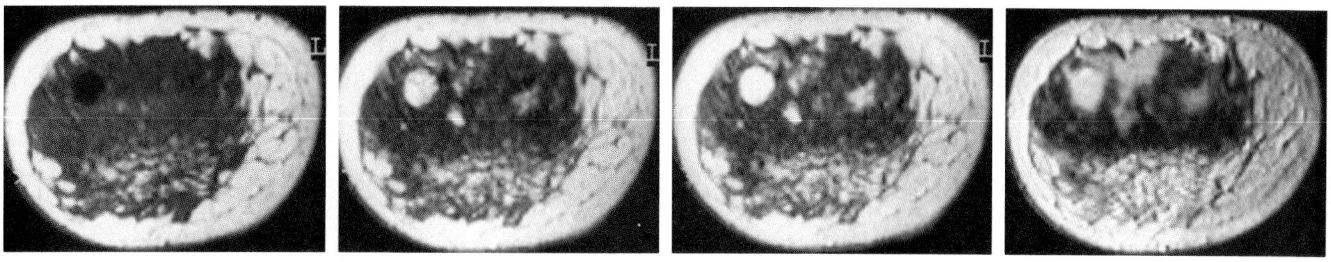
a. b. c. d.

Figure 3. Fibroadenoma in the upper inner quadrant of the left breast. Coronal dynamic, gadolinium-enhanced, T1-weighted gradient-recalled-echo MR images (11/4.6; flip angle, 25°) obtained **(a)** before, **(b)** 90 seconds after, **(c)** 10 minutes after, and **(d)** 60 minutes after intravenous injection of contrast material. **(b)** The entire lesion enhances rapidly on the 90-second image. No peripheral washout is seen on the delayed images up to 60 minutes. Other foci of enhancement caused by mastopathic changes are also present.

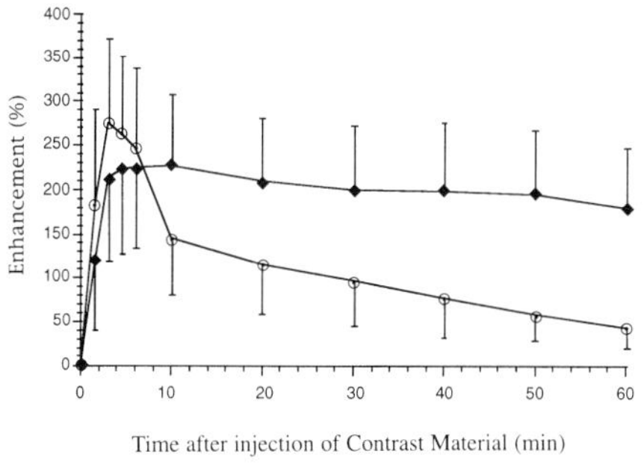

4.

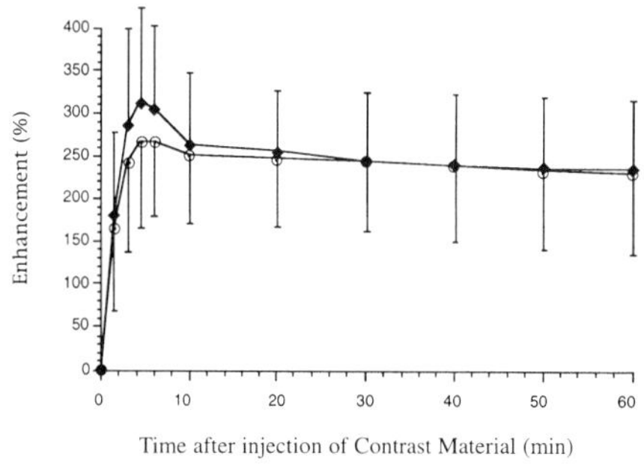

5.

Figures 4, 5. ○ = periphery, ◆ = center. Error bars represent standard deviation. Enhancement-versus-time curves for **(4)** carcinomas that showed the peripheral washout sign ($n = 28$) and **(5)** benign lesions ($n = 24$). **(4)** On the early images obtained after injection of the contrast agent, the periphery enhances more than the center, then the enhancement curve declines steeply. Enhancement of the center increases gradually to reach a plateau. The two curves intersect at 8 minutes. **(5)** Enhancement curves of the periphery and the center follow nearly the same course with an initial increase, the peak of the center slightly higher than that of the periphery, followed by a plateau for both curves.

only up to the point at which they were first removed from the magnet.

Statistical analysis.—Statistical analysis of the qualitative data was performed with the χ^2 test.

RESULTS

Qualitative Analysis

During dynamic contrast-enhanced imaging, the peripheral washout sign was seen (as a decrease of the initially enhancing periphery of the lesion while the center retained initial enhancement) by all three radiologists in 28 (51%) of 55 malignant lesions. The radiologists disagreed as to presence of the sign in six malignant lesions and agreed it was absent in 21 malignant lesions. The time of first appearance of the sign during the dynamic study varied among lesions (range, 3–30 minutes; mean, 14.8 minutes). In all of these 28 lesions, a perilesional rim of enhancement was also seen around the washed-out periphery of the lesion on the delayed images (Figs 1, 2). The peripheral washout sign was seen in none of the benign lesions (Fig 3). No disagreement occurred among the radiologists in the benign lesions. This difference in the occurrence of the peripheral washout sign was statistically significant ($P < .001$). The sensitivity of the peripheral washout sign for indication of malignancy was 51% and the specificity was 100%. All lesions that showed the peripheral washout sign were invasive ductal carcinomas. The lesions that showed the sign were 5–36 mm in diameter (mean, 19 mm), while the lesions that did not show the sign were 3–30 mm in diameter (mean, 12 mm).

Quantitative Analysis

On the basis of the qualitative analysis, three groups of lesions were identified: (*a*) malignant lesions that showed the peripheral washout sign ($n = 28$), (*b*) benign lesions ($n = 24$), and (*c*) malignant lesions that did not show the peripheral washout sign ($n = 27$). The mean enhancement of the periphery and the center were plotted versus time for each of these three groups (Figs 4–6).

For carcinomas that demonstrated the peripheral washout sign, enhancement of the periphery increased rapidly to reach a peak at 180 seconds after injection of the contrast agent followed by a rapid decline, while enhancement of the center increased less rapidly, reaching nearly a plateau at 6 minutes. Curves of the periphery and the center intersected at 8 minutes (Fig 4).

In the benign lesions, enhancement of the periphery and center followed nearly the same course, with an initial increase. The peak enhancement of the center was slightly higher than that of the periphery. The peak was followed by a plateau for both curves (Fig 5).

In cases of carcinomas that did not show the peripheral washout sign, enhancement curves of the periphery and center were identical; however, they differed from those of the benign lesions in that they declined steeply in the delayed portion of the dynamic study (Fig 6).

DISCUSSION

To our knowledge, information about enhancement of breast lesions at dynamic contrast-enhanced MR imaging is available for only the first 7 minutes after injection of contrast material (7). Enhancement patterns that suggest malignancy have been described as appearing within the first 2 minutes after injection of contrast material (2,4,9). However, considerable overlap still exists between enhancement profiles of malignant and those of benign lesions (3,7,8).

In our study, we assessed enhancement every 90 seconds in the first 6 minutes and then every 10 minutes up to 1 hour after injection of contrast material. In these previously unstudied delayed points of the dynamic examination, we noticed the presence of the peripheral washout sign in 51% of the malignant lesions. This proved to be a sign specific for invasive carcinoma (specificity, 100%), as it was not seen in any of the benign lesions. Despite the fact that this sign showed low sensitivity in our series (51%), the absolute specificity still renders it as important as other signs that may be more sensitive but remain, due to some overlap, suggestive rather than pathognomonic signs. Taking into consideration that this sign is not meant to be used alone but in conjunction with other morphologic signs described in other reports (2,8), the low sensitivity of this sign is not a great disadvantage. As the mean point of visual detection of the peripheral washout sign was 14.8 minutes after injection of contrast material, delayed imaging around this time might be recommended in cases of equivocal lesions on early images.

To document and evaluate quantitatively the visually observed peripheral washout sign, we placed a region of interest in the center and a second region of interest in the periphery of the lesion. Almost all previous studies in which quantitative analysis was performed used a single region of interest (8–12). To our knowledge, similar to our work, only one recent study measured the signal intensity in the center as well as the periphery of the lesion (13). However, the time-intensity curves in that study were created from data obtained only during the first 5 minutes after injection of contrast material. The curves obtained during that period were similar to the corresponding parts of our curves before the intersection of the curves of the periphery and center (13).

One of the important results from use of our method of quantitative assessment is that the periphery and the center of some malignant breast lesions show different enhancement characteristics after injection of contrast material at MR imaging. In some malignancies, the periphery enhanced more than the center in the first 2 minutes; the two time-intensity curves intersected at 8 minutes, then the curve of the periphery continued to decline steeply while that of the center remained at a plateau. The use of the time-intensity curves for differentiation of benign from malignant tumors may lead to incorrect results if this difference between the center and the periphery is not considered.

The difference between the curves of malignant lesions that showed the morphologic washout sign and the curves of those that did not show the sign is in the enhancement characteristics of the center, which showed persistent enhancement in the former group and lack of persistent enhancement in the latter group. Conversely, the curve of the periphery showed a steep decline in enhancement for both groups. This steep decline of enhancement may distinguish malignant from benign lesions, in which the peripheral part of the benign lesion also retains enhancement.

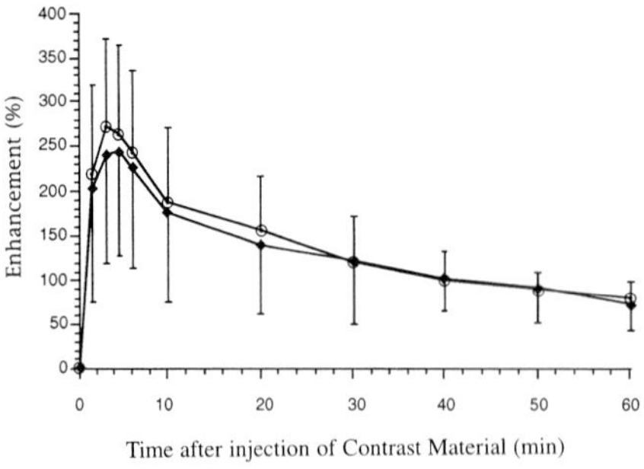

Figure 6. Enhancement-versus-time curve for carcinomas that did not show the peripheral washout sign (n = 27). Enhancement curves of the periphery (○) and center (◆) are identical; however, they differ from those of the benign lesions in that they decline more steeply in the delayed portion of the dynamic study. The error bars represent standard deviation.

All previously reported morphologic signs that suggest malignancy are applied to the distribution phase of the contrast agent (2,4,8). On the basis of our results, we believe that morphologic signs in the elimination phase can be as important as those in the distribution phase. Mussurakis et al (14) used the rates of wash in and washout as criteria for differentiating benign from malignant lesions. However, those investigators did not address the morphologic aspect and, furthermore, did not evaluate the rate of enhancement and washout of the contrast agent in two different regions of the enhancing lesion.

The exact mechanism of the peripheral washout sign is not understood fully. However, because the peripheral washout sign was also reported in malignant liver neoplasms with a specificity of 100% (15), it is probable that the mechanism of peripheral washout is linked to the pathophysiologic mechanisms within malignant tumors regardless of the organ of origin and location.

The amount of gadopentetate dimeglumine within a certain tumor at a certain point in the dynamic MR imaging study depends on the rate of transport of the contrast agent from the intravascular to the interstitial compartment and the opposite rate of transport of the contrast agent from the interstitial to the intravascular compartment (Fig 7). In the distribution phase of the contrast agent, the first rate dominates, resulting in accumulation of the contrast agent in the interstitial space. In the elimination phase of the contrast agent (ie, washout), the reverse occurs.

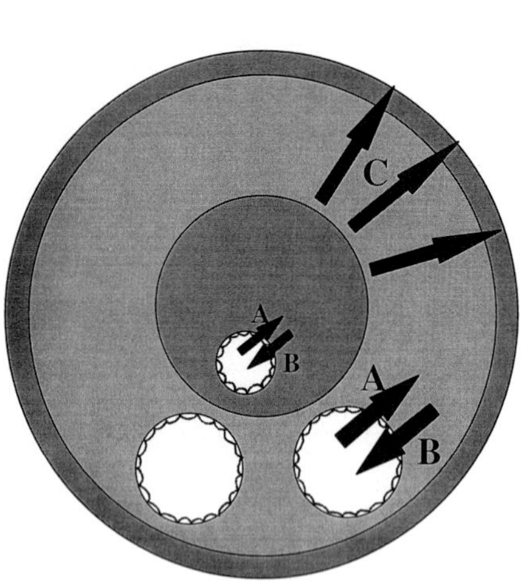

Figure 7. Diagram shows the three rates that possibly determine enhancement and washout of the periphery and center of the tumor. The periphery of the lesion is represented in light gray. The center of the tumor and the perilesional rim of breast parenchyma are represented in dark gray. The capillaries are represented in white. *A* is the transport rate of the contrast agent from the intravascular to the interstitial compartment. *B* is the transport rate of the contrast agent from the interstitial to the intravascular compartment. *C* is the transport rate of the contrast agent within the interstitial space under the force of the interstitial pressure gradient, which drives the interstitial fluid together with the contrast agent from the periphery to the perilesional rim. The turnover of contrast agent is higher in the periphery than in the center (ie, it enhances earlier and is washed out earlier) because (*a*) rates *A* and *B* are probably greater in the periphery than the center due to the larger number and size of capillaries, the greater capillary permeability, and the higher rate of blood flow in the periphery compared with that in the center; and (*b*) rate *C* occurs only in the periphery because there is no pressure gradient in the center.

Among the factors that determine these two rates are the capillary permeability, the size of the capillaries, the number of capillaries within the tissue, and the rate of blood flow. The first three of these factors are linked directly to tumor angiogenesis. Several studies have shown that the vascular growth factor, which is released by the tumor cells, causes an increase in the size and number of capillaries and an increase in the capillary permeability (13,16–19). Recent studies in which immunohistochemical staining of the vessels was used in the periphery and the center of invasive ductal carcinoma demonstrated that the size and number of capillaries and the capillary permeability are higher in the periphery than in the center of malignant neoplasms (13,18,19). It has also been proved that the rate of blood flow is higher in the periphery of malignant tumors than in the center (20,21). The higher blood flow, the larger size and increased number of capillaries, and the higher capillary permeability in the periphery compared with those in the center of the tumor would result in a higher turnover of contrast agent, which is rapidly transported from the intravascular to the interstitial compartment and vice versa. This turnover of contrast material may help explain the greater and faster rise and decline of enhancement in the tumor periphery compared with that in the center in the carcinomas that showed the morphologic peripheral washout sign.

In addition to the transport of contrast material from the intravascular to the interstitial compartment and vice versa, we assume that there is a third mechanism of transport of contrast material within the tumor, transport of contrast material within the interstitial compartment (Fig 7). Such transport occurs under the influence of difference in hydrostatic pressure between the different parts of the interstitial space, the contrast agent being transported from regions of high pressure to regions of lower pressure. This assumption is based on several studies that demonstrated that the interstitial fluid pressure is higher within malignant tumors than in the peritumoral normal tissue (22–26). Moreover, some of these studies demonstrated that the center of the malignant tumor has a uniformly high pressure and the peritumoral normal tissue has a uniformly low pressure. Between these two different pressure zones, the periphery of the tumor represents a zone of radially oriented pressure gradient (24–26). This gradient causes generation of a flux of interstitial fluid. The flux of interstitial fluid propels the contrast agent from the peripheral zone to the outside of the tumor, while the contrast agent in the center of the tumor remains undisturbed owing to the lack of pressure gradient. The perilesional rim of normal breast tissue thus represents the region that continuously receives the contrast agent driven outside the tumor through the interstitial pathway owing to low interstitial pressure. Contrast agent tends to accumulate within this rim (and therefore enhances more than other parts of the normal breast parenchyma).

Because the interstitial pressure is a determinant factor for the delivery of drugs to the tumor (26), the study of the pattern and rate of washout at contrast-enhanced MR imaging of the breast neoplasms may have important consequences in the follow up of breast carcinomas being treated with chemotherapy by offering an approximate simulation of the delivery of drugs to the tumor.

It is not clear why the contrast agent persists in the center of some malignant lesions and is washed out from the periphery (leading to the appearance we describe as the peripheral washout sign) but does not persist in the center of some other malignant lesions. In our study, we admit the lack of a dedicated histopathologic examination of the center and periphery of lesions in these two groups. However, it is highly probable that the difference between the two groups is related to dynamic in vivo factors such as the interstitial pressure rather than the static in vitro histopathologic findings in the resected specimens. We also admit that our description of the rim of enhancement that appears around the washed out periphery of the lesion as "perilesional" has not been based on point-to-point correlation between histopathologic and imaging findings. Such a correlation would be extremely difficult considering the transient in vivo changes in the distribution of contrast material in the periphery of the lesion and the perilesional tissue.

In conclusion, the peripheral washout sign, reported in our study on delayed contrast-enhanced MR images of the breast, is a specific indicator of malignancy. In addition to the value of this sign in differentiation between benign and malignant breast lesions in equivocal cases, it has the potential value of demonstrating the characteristics of the interstitial pressure within malignant tumors. ■

References

1. Kelsey JL. A review of the epidemiology of human breast cancer. Epidemiol Rev 1979; 1:74–109.
2. Heywang-Koebrunner SH, Haustein J, Pohl C, et al. Contrast-enhanced MR imaging of the breast: comparison of two different doses of gadopentetate dimeglumine. Radiology 1994; 191:639–646.
3. Kerslake RW, Fox JN, Carleton PJ, et al. Dynamic contrast-enhanced and fat suppressed magnetic resonance imaging in suspected recurrent carcinoma of the breast: preliminary experience. Br J Radiol 1994; 67:1158–1168.
4. Gilles R, Guinebretiere JM, Lucidarme O, et al. Nonpalpable breast tumors: diagnosis with contrast-enhanced subtraction dynamic MR imaging. Radiology 1994; 191:625–631.
5. Boetes C, Barentsz JO, Mus RD, et al. MR characterization of suspicious breast lesions with a gadolinium-enhanced TurboFLASH subtraction technique. Radiology 1994; 193: 777–781.
6. Harms SE, Flamig DP, Hesley KL, et al. MR imaging of the breast with rotating delivery of excitation off resonance: clinical experience with pathologic correlation. Radiology 1993; 187:1493–1501.
7. Fobben ES, Rubin CZ, Kalisher L, Dembner AG, Seltzer MH, Santoro EJ. Breast MR imaging with commercially available techniques: radiologic-pathologic correlation. Radiology 1995; 196:143–152.
8. Orel SG, Schnall MD, LiVolsi VA, Troupin RH. Suspicious breast lesions: MR imaging with radiologic-pathologic correlation. Radiology 1994; 190:485–493.
9. Gribbestad IS, Nilsen G, Fjosne HE, Kvinnslands S, Haugen OA, Rinck PA. Comparative signal intensity measurements in dynamic gadolinium-enhanced MR. JMRI 1994; 4:477–480.
10. Flickinger FW, Allison JD, Sherry RM, Wright JC. Differentiation of benign from malignant breast masses by time-intensity evaluation of contrast enhanced MRI. Magn Reson Imaging 1993; 11:617–620.
11. Stomper PC, Herman S, Klippenstein DL, et al. Suspect breast lesions: findings at dynamic gadolinium-enhanced MR imaging correlated with mammographic and pathologic features. Radiology 1995; 197:387–395.
12. Tofts PS, Berkowitz B, Schnall MD. Quantitative analysis of dynamic Gd-DTPA enhancement in breast tumors using a permeability model. Magn Reson Med 1995; 33:564–568.
13. Buadu LD, Murakami J, Murayama S, et al. Breast lesions: correlation of contrast medium enhancement patterns in MR images with histopathologic findings and tumor angiogenesis. Radiology 1996; 200:639–649.
14. Mussurakis S, Buckley DL, Bowsley SJ, et al. Dynamic contrast-enhanced magnetic resonance imaging of the breast combined with pharmacokinetic analysis of gadolinium-DTPA uptake in the diagnosis of local recurrence of early stage breast carcinoma. Invest Radiol 1995; 30:650–662.
15. Mahfouz AE, Hamm B, Wolf KJ. Peripheral washout: a sign of malignancy on dynamic gadolinium-enhanced MR images of focal liver lesions. Radiology 1994; 190:49–52.
16. Gilles R, Zafrani B, Guinebretiere JM, et al. Ductal carcinoma in situ: MR imaging–histopathologic correlation. Radiology 1995; 196: 415–419.
17. Hulka CA, Smith BL, Sgroi DC, et al. Benign and malignant breast lesions: differentiation with echo-planar MR imaging. Radiology 1995; 197:33–38.
18. van Dijke CF, Brasch RC, Roberts TP, et al. Mammary carcinoma model: correlation of macromolecular contrast-enhanced MR imaging characterizations of tumor microvasculature and histologic capillary density. Radiology 1996; 198:813–818.
19. Schwickert HC, Stiskal M, Roberts TP, et al. Contrast-enhanced MR imaging assessment of tumor capillary permeability: effect of irradiation on delivery of chemotherapy. Radiology 1996; 198:893–898.
20. Feldmann HJ, Molls M, Hoederath A, Krumpelmann S, Sack H. Blood flow and steady state temperatures in deep-seated tumors and normal tissues. Int J Radiat Oncol Biol Phys 1992; 23:1003–1008.
21. Dewhirst MW, Ong ET, Klitzman B, et al. Perivascular oxygen tensions in a transplantable mammary tumor growing in a dorsal flap window chamber. Radiat Res 1992; 130:171–182.
22. Leunig M, Yuan F, Menger MD, et al. Angiogenesis, microvascular architecture, microhemodynamics, and interstitial fluid pressure during early growth of human adenocarcinoma LS174T in SCID mice. Cancer Res 1992; 52:6553–6560.
23. Less JR, Posner MC, Boucher Y, Borochovitz D, Wolmark N, Jain RK. Interstitial hypertension in human breast and colorectal tumors. Cancer Res 1992; 52:6371–6374.
24. Baxter LT, Jain RK. Transport of fluid and macromolecules in tumors. III. Role of binding and metabolism. Microvasc Res 1991; 41:5–23.
25. Boucher Y, Jain RK. Microvascular pressure is the principal driving force for interstitial hypertension in solid tumors: implications for vascular collapse. Cancer Res 1992; 52:5110–5114.
26. Jain RK. Haemodynamic and transport barriers to the treatment of solid tumours. Int J Radiat Biol 1991; 60:85–100.

Helen M. Fenlon, FRCR • Niall C. Phelan, MSc • Phyllis O'Sullivan, FRCR
Sean Tierney, FRCSI • Thomas Gorey, FRCSI • Joseph T. Ennis, FRCR

Benign versus Malignant Breast Disease: Comparison of Contrast-enhanced MR Imaging and Tc-99m Tetrofosmin Scintimammography[1]

PURPOSE: To compare technetium-99m tetrofosmin scintimammography with contrast material–enhanced magnetic resonance (MR) imaging in the characterization of palpable breast masses.

MATERIALS AND METHODS: Forty-seven patients (mean age, 51 years) with a palpable breast mass were prospectively examined with scintimammography, MR imaging, and conventional mammography 2 weeks before fine-needle aspiration biopsy.

RESULTS: In three patients, MR imaging was aborted. Of the remaining 44 patients, 21 had biopsy-proved cancer and 23 had benign disease. The sensitivity of mammography was 81%; specificity, 82%; positive predictive value (PPV), 85%; and negative predictive value (NPV), 78%. The sensitivity of scintimammography was 95%; specificity, 91%; PPV, 91%; and NPV, 95%. The sensitivity of MR imaging was 90%; specificity, 91%; PPV, 90%; and NPV, 91%. In 11 patients with previous breast cancer, scintimammographic findings were positive in all four with tumor recurrence and negative in all seven with benign disease. Masses were correctly characterized with MR imaging in eight of these 11 patients.

CONCLUSION: Although both techniques accurately differentiate benign from malignant palpable breast masses, scintimammography is more accurate in the posttreatment breast. Because of lower cost, wider availability, and high patient acceptance, scintimammography may provide a valuable alternative to MR imaging for noninvasive characterization of palpable breast disease.

Breast cancer is the leading cause of unpreventable, cancer-related death among women in the Western world. Statistics show that one in nine women will develop breast cancer at some stage during her life (1,2). There is now persuasive evidence that screening with mammography results in earlier cancer detection with improved patient survival (3). Although the high sensitivity of conventional mammography for carcinoma is well documented, interpretative errors may occur in patients with mammographically dense breasts and in patients who have previously undergone breast surgery or radiation therapy (4,5). In addition, the specificity of mammography is limited: As many as two of every three women who are referred for biopsy because of an abnormal mammogram have benign histopathologic results (6–8).

Triple assessment with clinical examination, imaging (mammography and ultrasound [US]), and fine-needle aspiration biopsy, core biopsy, or both is diagnostic in more than 70% of cases (3). US is used to characterize lesions detected at mammography; to evaluate mammographically occult, palpable breast masses; and to guide core biopsy. US, however, cannot be used to confidently exclude cancer, because some malignant lesions, especially noninvasive and diffusely growing carcinomas, may not be visible at US. Furthermore, the sensitivity of US decreases with lesion size. Even with a combination of mammography, US, and fine-needle aspiration biopsy, core biopsy, or both, difficulties may arise in diagnosing cancer in patients with mammographically dense breasts and in patients who have undergone previous breast-conserving surgery or radiation therapy or who have implants.

A variety of adjunctive techniques have been evaluated to improve lesion detection and characterization (9–21). These include color Doppler US, contrast material–enhanced magnetic resonance (MR) imaging, MR spectroscopy, fluorodeoxyglucose positron emission tomography, positron emission tomography of estrogen receptors, and, more recently, nuclear medicine imaging of the breast or scintimammography.

We have recently described the successful use of technetium-99m tetrofosmin as a breast imaging agent (22). The aim of this study was to compare the accuracy of Tc-99m tetrofosmin scintimammography with contrast-enhanced MR imaging in differentiating benign from malignant palpable breast lesions and to correlate results of each technique with findings of conventional mammography and histopathologic outcome.

Index terms: Breast neoplasms, MR, 00.12141, 00.30 • Breast neoplasms, radiography, 00.11, 00.30 • Breast neoplasms, radionuclide studies, 00.1216, 00.30 • Magnetic resonance (MR), comparative studies, 00.12141 • Radionuclide imaging, comparative studies, 00.1216

Abbreviations: FLASH = fast low-angle shot, NPV = negative predictive value, PPV = positive predictive value, SPECT = single photon emission computed tomography.

Radiology 1997; 205:214–220

[1] From the Institute of Radiological Sciences and the Department of Radiology (H.M.F., N.C.P., P.O., J.T.E.), and the Department of Surgery (S.T., T.G.), Mater Misericordiae Hospital, Dublin, Ireland. Received April 4, 1997; revision requested May 9; revision received June 5; accepted June 9. **Address reprint requests to** H.M.F., Department of Radiology, Boston Medical Center, 88 E Newton St, Boston, MA 02118.

MATERIALS AND METHODS

Study Group

Forty-seven consecutive patients who presented to the outpatient department with a palpable breast lump were prospectively examined. All patients had a palpable breast lump suspicious for malignancy that required fine-needle aspiration biopsy. The mean age of the study group was 51 years, and the age range was 28–79 years. Eleven of the 47 patients had a history of breast cancer. Eight of these 11 patients had undergone previous lumpectomy, and three patients had undergone lumpectomy followed by radiation therapy. Patients who had undergone breast biopsy, surgery, or radiation therapy within 12 months of the study were excluded. The study protocol was approved by the institutional review board, and fully informed written consent was obtained in all patients.

Imaging

Imaging was performed before fine-needle aspiration biopsy in all patients. Patients older than 35 years underwent two-view conventional mammography (Mammomat 2; Siemens, Erlangen, Germany). Breast US was performed by using a high-frequency (7.5-MHz) transducer to differentiate solid from cystic lesions (Ultramark 2; Advanced Technology Laboratories, Bothell, Wash). On the same day, all patients underwent Tc-99m tetrofosmin scintimammography and contrast-enhanced MR imaging.

Scintimammography.—Patients were seated parallel to a gamma camera (model ZLC; Siemens) with both arms raised out of the field of view. Patient position was adjusted to obtain a lateral oblique view of the affected breast, including the axilla. A 140-keV energy peak with a 20% window was selected. A high-resolution collimator was used with a 126 × 126 image matrix and a 40-cm field of view without acquisition zoom. The myocardial imaging agent Tc-99m tetrofosmin (Myoview; Amersham International, Buckinghamshire, England; dose, 600 MBq [16 mCi]) was injected intravenously in the arm contralateral to the affected breast; this was followed by a bolus flush of 20 mL of physiologic saline. Planar imaging was performed with the patient seated in an erect position; data acquisition commenced immediately after injection of the radioisotope. A lateral oblique view of the affected breast was acquired immediately over 10 minutes (3–5 million counts). This was followed by acquisition of a 10-minute anterior view of the thorax and of a 10-minute lateral oblique view of the noninvolved breast. External reference markers were not used.

Contrast-enhanced MR imaging.—MR imaging was performed on a 1.5-T superconducting system (Magnetom; Siemens) by using a standard breast coil (Siemens) with a 30-cm field of view. Patients were placed in a slightly oblique prone position to allow optimal visualization of the axillary tail of the involved breast.

A precontrast, T1-weighted, fast low-angle shot (FLASH), three-dimensional localization sequence was performed in the affected breast (600/13 [repetition time msec/echo time msec], 50° flip angle, sagittal orientation, one signal acquired, and 3.75-mm section thickness). These MR images were evaluated to identify the presence and location of an abnormality that corresponded to the palpable lump; a section through the maximum bulk of disease was selected for the dynamic study.

A dynamic profile study was performed by using a T1-weighted, FLASH, two-dimensional, sequential-repeat, single-section sequence through the region of interest (600/13, 50° flip angle, one signal acquired, 3-mm section thickness, sagittal image orientation, and 30 sequence repetitions). Five baseline images were obtained immediately before contrast material administration to ensure the uniformity of signal intensity. Gadopentetate dimeglumine (Magnevist; Schering, Berlin, Germany) was then rapidly intravenously injected at a dose of 0.1 mmol/kg over 20 seconds. The imaging time for each sequence was 12.4 seconds, with a total of 30 sequence repetitions before, during, and after contrast material injection.

A postcontrast, T1-weighted, FLASH, three-dimensional sequence was performed with the same parameters as the precontrast sequence. Digital subtraction with standard software was applied to each set of images, and enhancement profiles were generated for each lesion. The signal intensity of each lesion before, during, and after contrast material injection was calculated in terms of mean pixel values in a computer-drawn region of interest. The region of interest was drawn to encompass the maximum region of enhancement of each lesion as determined on postcontrast images. Mean signal intensity profiles were superimposed on the reference image to indicate the degree and rate of lesion enhancement.

Follow-up.—Patients returned to the outpatient department within 1 week of imaging for fine-needle aspiration biopsy. Patients with suspicious or clearly malignant cytologic findings were referred for surgery irrespective of the findings of scintimammography and MR imaging. Patients with clearly benign cytologic findings who did not undergo surgery were followed up with repeat clinical evaluation and mammography at 1 year to exclude malignancy.

Image interpretation.—Each examination was reported on by two independent observers. MR images were reported on with access to the conventional mammograms but without knowledge of the findings of scintimammography or histopathologic outcome. The scintimammograms were reported on with access to the conventional mammograms but without knowledge of the findings of MR imaging or the histopathologic diagnosis. Before consensus agreement, interobserver variability was evaluated for each modality, with agreement between observers expressed as a κ statistic (23).

By using standard interpretative criteria (24), lesions identified at conventional mammography were classified as either malignant or benign. A scintimammogram was negative when there was bilateral symmetric distribution of radioisotope throughout the breast, with the same intensity as the background soft tissue. A scintimammogram was positive when there was focally increased uptake of radioisotope in either breast on the lateral oblique view (Fig 1). The anterior views were used to help confirm any abnormal findings identified on the lateral oblique views. The MR images were reported as positive for malignancy if a suspicious mass lesion, identified with the precontrast sequence, displayed avid, early, and rapid enhancement to reach a plateaued, steady state of enhancement as assessed with the dynamic profile study (Figs 1, 2). The rate of lesion enhancement was visually assessed. A twofold increase in tumor signal intensity within the first 60 seconds after gadopentetate dimeglumine injection, with a more gradual increase in enhancement over the remaining 4 minutes of imaging, was regarded as highly suspicious for malignancy (12). Absent, delayed, gradually progressive, or diffuse enhancement favored benignity. After fine-needle aspiration biopsy, surgery, or both, the histopathologic diagnoses were correlated with findings of conventional mammography, MR imaging, and scintimammography.

Statistical analysis.—On the basis of the histopathologic findings, the findings of conventional mammography, contrast-enhanced MR imaging, and Tc-99m tetrofosmin scintimammography were classified as true-positive, true-negative, false-positive, or false-negative. The sensitivity, specificity, positive predictive value (PPV), and negative predictive value (NPV) were determined for each imaging modality.

RESULTS

Of the 47 patients, three were excluded from final analysis because of incomplete MR examinations. Two patients were unable to tolerate MR imaging owing to anxiety or claustrophobia, and in one patient the MR images were substantially degraded owing to patient movement. Results of conventional mammography (performed if the patient was older than 35 years), contrast-enhanced MR imaging, and scintimammography were available in the remaining 44 patients, with histopathologic correlation in each case.

Of the 44 patients, 21 had biopsy-proved malignancy while 23 had benign lesions. All 21 patients with malignancy underwent surgery: mastectomy ($n = 8$), segmentectomy ($n = 6$), or lumpectomy ($n = 7$). Of the 21 patients with malignant lesions, 20 had invasive ductal carcinoma and one had mucinous carcinoma. The average tumor size was 1.7 cm (range, 7 mm to

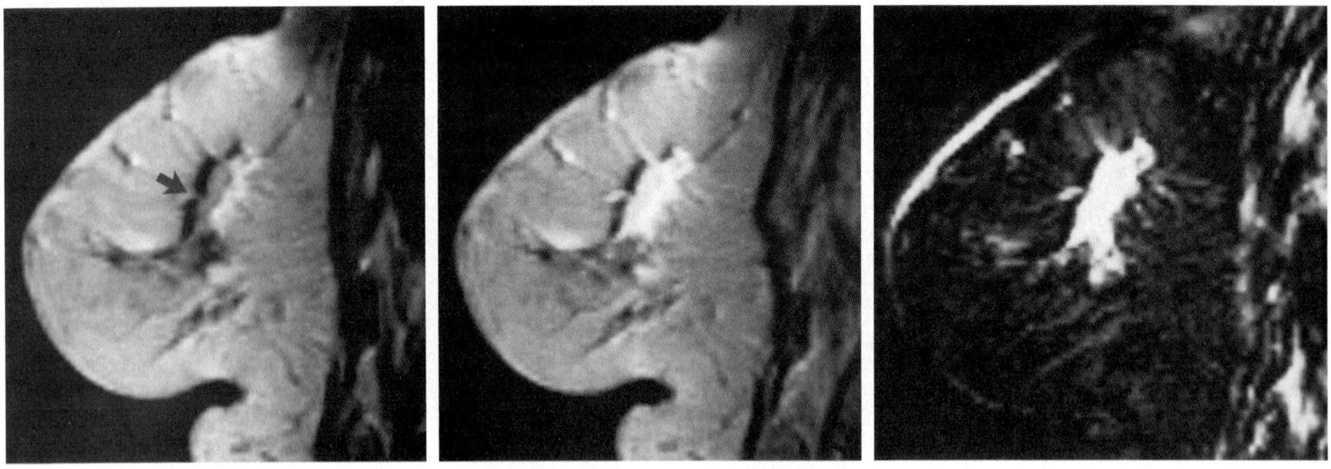

a. b. c.

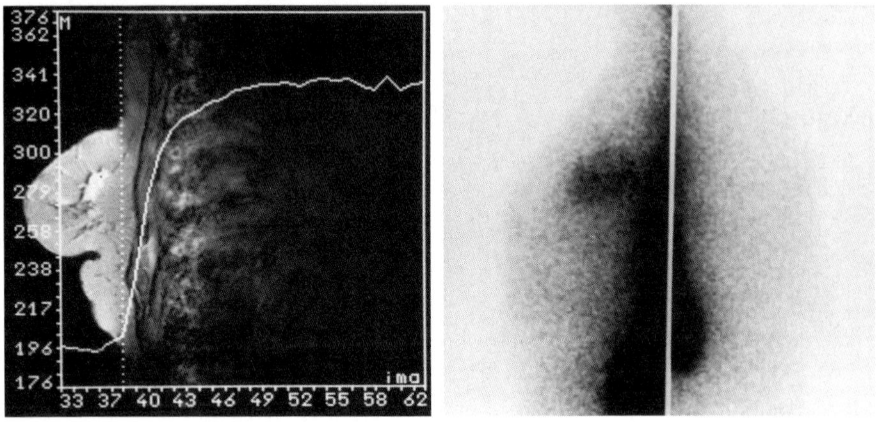

d. e.

Figure 1. Images obtained in a 54-year-old patient. **(a)** Unenhanced, T1-weighted, FLASH, three-dimensional MR image (600/13, 50° flip angle) demonstrates a spiculated mass in the upper outer quadrant of the right breast (arrow). **(b)** Gadolinium-enhanced, T1-weighted, FLASH, two-dimensional MR image (600/13, 50° flip angle) demonstrates marked tumoral enhancement. **(c)** Subtraction MR image illustrates avid enhancement of the mass after contrast material administration. **(d)** Enhancement profile (in arbitrary units of time vs signal intensity) through the lesion demonstrates early and rapid enhancement and attainment of a steady state or plateau consistent with malignancy. **(e)** Lateral oblique Tc-99m tetrofosmin scintimammograms of both breasts demonstrate focal abnormal accumulation of radioisotope in the upper outer quadrant of the right breast. A 2.8-cm invasive ductal carcinoma was subsequently resected.

4.2 cm). Of the 23 patients with fine-needle aspiration biopsy–proved benign lesions, 11 underwent surgical excision; in the remaining 12, clinical and radiologic follow-up findings at 1 year showed no evidence of malignancy. Of the 23 with benign lesions, eight had fibrofatty tissue, six had fibrocystic disease, three had proliferative dysplasia, three had solitary benign cysts, one had a fibroadenoma, one had apocrine metaplasia, and one underwent resection of a radial scar.

Of the 44 patients, 38 underwent two-view mammography (six patients were younger than 35 years). Of these 38 patients, 21 had biopsy-proved malignancy while 17 had benign histopathologic findings (all patients aged 35 years or younger had benign histopathologic findings). In the 21 patients with malignant disease, conventional mammographic findings indicated malignancy in 17 patients and benignity in four patients. Of these four patients with false-negative findings, two patients had mammographically dense breasts and two patients had a history of breast surgery. No mass lesions were visible at conventional mammography in either patient with mammographically dense breasts. In two patients who had previously undergone surgery, focal abnormalities were identified on both standard and compression views. There had been no interval change, however, on serial postoperative mammograms, and these findings were regarded as benign postoperative change rather than recurrent disease (Fig 3). All four mammographically "missed" cancers were invasive ductal carcinomas that measured 1.4, 1.8, 1.9, and 2.2 cm in maximum dimension.

Of the 17 patients with benign disease, 14 patients had mammographic features that indicated benignity and three had mammographic features that indicated malignancy. Of these three patients with false-positive findings, two had fibrofatty change at histopathologic analysis (postoperative change in both patients) while one had a radial scar in a mammographically dense breast. The sensitivity of conventional mammography in our group was 81%, the specificity was 82%, the PPV was 85%, and the NPV was 78%.

Of the 21 patients with biopsy-proved malignancy, 20 had positive Tc-99m tetrofosmin scintimammographic findings. There was one false-negative finding in a patient with severe rheumatoid arthritis in whom positioning was suboptimal because of immobility. Although the study was technically suboptimal, it was considered adequate for interpretation and was included in the final analysis. Focal abnormal radioisotope accumulation was not identified, and the scintimammographic findings were reported as negative. Subsequent excision revealed a 1.9-cm invasive intraductal carcinoma.

Of the 23 patients with benign histopathologic findings, 21 had negative scintimammographic findings. There were two false-positive findings: One in a patient with proliferative dysplasia and another in a patient with a hypercellular (glandular) fibroadenoma. The sensitivity of Tc-99m tetrofosmin scintimammography in this group therefore was 95%, the specificity was 91%, the PPV was 91%, and the NPV was 95%.

Of the 21 patients with biopsy-proved malignancy, 19 had MR findings con-

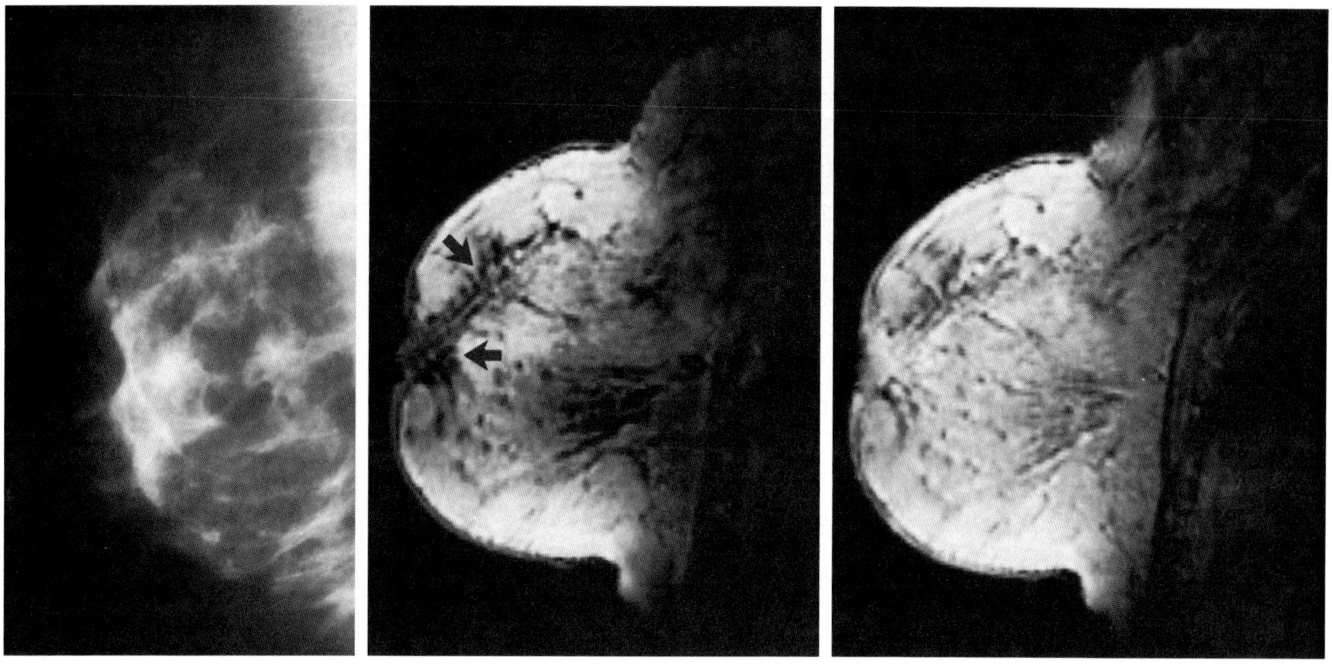

a. b. c.

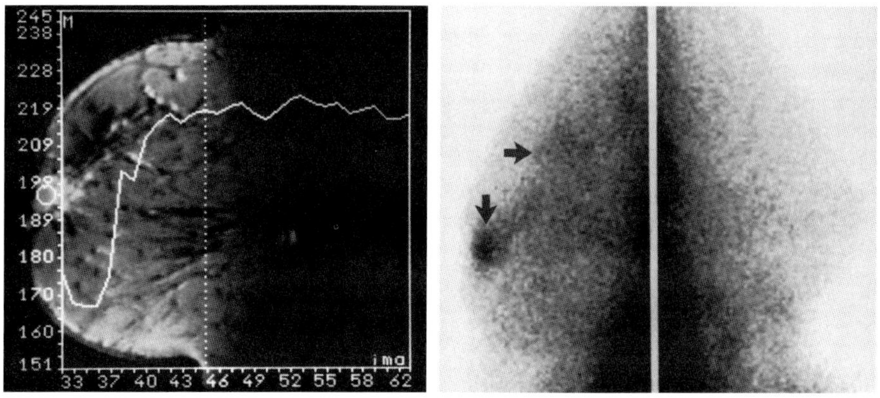

d. e.

Figure 2. Images obtained in a 69-year-old woman 3 years after right-side lumpectomy to treat carcinoma. **(a)** Lateral oblique mammogram demonstrates asymmetric breast density in the retroareolar area and upper outer quadrant of the right breast. These findings had not been present on previous postoperative mammograms and were reported as suspicious for tumor recurrence. **(b)** Unenhanced, T1-weighted, FLASH, three-dimensional MR image (600/13, 50° flip angle) shows a corresponding irregular, hypointense mass (arrows). **(c)** Gadolinium-enhanced T1-weighted, FLASH, two-dimensional MR image (600/13, 50° flip angle) demonstrates diffuse enhancement in the corresponding area. **(d)** Enhancement profile (in arbitrary units of time vs signal intensity) through the retroareolar area demonstrates avid and early enhancement, which indicates suspicion for tumor recurrence. **(e)** Lateral oblique Tc-99m tetrofosmin scintimammograms of both breasts demonstrate multifocal radioisotope accumulation in the right breast (arrows). Multifocal tumor recurrence was confirmed histopathologically after mastectomy.

sistent with malignancy. Two had false-negative MR findings. One false-negative MR finding occurred in a patient with a history of lumpectomy for invasive ductal carcinoma. Although a mass was identified on precontrast MR images, the pattern of enhancement suggested scar or fibrosis rather than tumor recurrence. Conventional mammography in this case was reported to show recurrent disease, and scintimammography clearly demonstrated a focal area of abnormal radioisotope accumulation consistent with recurrent tumor. Tumor recurrence (2.2-cm invasive ductal carcinoma) was confirmed at mastectomy. In the second patient with false-negative findings, a 1.5-cm tumor recurrence (invasive ductal carcinoma) in the axillary tail of the right breast was not adequately imaged with the precontrast localization sequence and was not included in the imaging volume of the dynamic study. No abnormality was identified, and the MR image was incorrectly reported as negative for malignancy.

Of the 23 patients with benign lesions, 21 had negative MR imaging findings. There was one false-positive MR finding in a patient with enhancing focal high-grade proliferative dysplasia and a second false-positive finding in a patient 14 months after lumpectomy, in whom histopathologically proved scar tissue demonstrated avid enhancement. The sensitivity of MR imaging in our group was 90%, the specificity was 91%, the PPV was 90%, and the NPV was 91% (Table).

Interobserver agreement for each modality was high, with a κ statistic of 0.78 for conventional mammography, 0.86 for MR imaging, and 0.90 for scintimammography.

DISCUSSION

Contrast-enhanced MR imaging is increasingly used as an adjunct to conventional mammography and breast US to differentiate benign from malignant breast lesions (11–15,25–34). It provides valuable additional information in mammographically "difficult" cases. Common clinical indications for this noninvasive evaluation are indeterminate mammographic findings, exclusion of malignancy in mammographically dense breasts, and differentiation of scar from recurrent tumor in the postoperative and post–radiation therapy breast; MR imaging is also used as a supplementary evaluation in patients with breast implants and to detect multicentric tumor in patients with cancer who are considering breast-conserving surgery.

Imaging Findings

Modality	Findings: Benign (no. of patients)	Findings: Malignant (no. of patients)	Sensitivity (%)	Specificity (%)	PPV (%)	NPV (%)
Conventional mammography ($n = 38$)	18	20	81 (17 of 21)	82 (14 of 17)	85 (17 of 20)	78 (14 of 18)
MR imaging ($n = 44$)	23	21	90 (19 of 21)	91 (21 of 23)	90 (19 of 21)	91 (21 of 23)
Tc-99m tetrofosmin scintimammography ($n = 44$)	22	22	95 (20 of 21)	91 (21 of 23)	91 (20 of 22)	95 (21 of 22)

Excellent data on the accuracy of MR imaging already exist. Contrast-enhanced MR imaging has a high sensitivity for breast cancer. A normal MR image without evidence of enhancement excludes malignancy with a high degree of confidence (11–15). The figures for specificity, however, are less consistent: 37%–97% (11–15,28–34). Although quantification of enhancement improves discrimination between benign and malignant lesions, diagnostic difficulties arise because benign lesions, such as proliferative dysplasias, inflammatory breast disease, breast abscesses, postoperative scar tissue (less than 6 months after surgery), postradiation fibrosis (less than 18 months after radiation therapy), papillomas, and fibroadenomas, can show avid, early, and rapid enhancement, similar to that of carcinoma (12,29,34). Attention to both lesion morphology and patterns of enhancement helps to diminish the number of false-positive diagnoses of malignancy (35).

Factors that limit the widespread use of contrast-enhanced MR imaging include cost, availability, claustrophobia (in 5%–10% of patients), and patient exclusion because of vascular clips, cochlear implants, or pacemakers. Recent reports suggest that breast scintimammography may be an effective alternative to MR imaging in differentiating benign from malignant breast lesions (16–20,36). A variety of radiopharmaceuticals have been evaluated as breast imaging agents, and a number of imaging protocols have been described.

Waxman and colleagues (16), in a study of thallium-201 scintimammography, reported abnormal accumulation of Tl-201 in 42 of 44 palpable breast cancers. In a study of 30 patients with both mammographically detected and palpable breast lesions, Lee and colleagues (17) reported a sensitivity of 80% and a specificity of 96% with the same radiopharmaceutical. Khalkali and co-workers (18) in an investigation of Tc-99m sestamibi scintimammography reported a sensitivity and specificity of 96% and 87%, respectively, while Palmedo and colleagues (19) reported a sensitivity of 88% and a specificity of 83% for carcinoma with the same technique. In women who underwent routine bone scintigraphy before breast surgery, Piccolo and colleagues (20) described abnormal accumulation of Tc-99m methylene diphosphonate in 158 (92%) of 172 carcinomas and correctly characterized 43 (81%) of 53 lesions for which mammographic findings were indeterminate.

We have recently reported sensitivities and specificities in excess of 90% for carcinoma detection with the use of the lipophilic, cationic, myocardial imaging agent Tc-99m tetrofosmin for breast scintigraphy (22). To expand on our previous work, this study was designed to compare the accuracy of Tc-99m tetrofosmin scintimammography with that of contrast-enhanced MR imaging in clinically suspicious breast lesions, with mammographic and histopathologic correlation in each case. To our knowledge, we are the only group to report the results of Tc-99m tetrofosmin scintimammography and this is the first comparative study of Tc-99m tetrofosmin scintimammography with contrast-enhanced MR imaging.

Both MR imaging and scintimammographic findings were false-positive in a patient with histopathologically proved high-grade proliferative dysplasia with no evidence of malignancy; scintimammographic findings were false-positive in an additional patient with a hypercellular fibroadenoma, while MR imaging findings were suggestive of tumor recurrence in a patient with benign scar tissue 14 months after lumpectomy. Our results reflect those of other investigators who have independently described false-positive scintimammographic and MR imaging findings in cases of high-grade proliferative dysplasia, in patients with hypercellular (glandular or myxoid) fibroadenomas, within 1 year after surgery, and within 18 months of radiation therapy (12,16,29).

In two of three false-negative studies, technical factors, especially poor patient positioning, adversely affected lesion detection and characterization. A false-negative scintimammogram was reported in a patient with advanced rheumatoid arthritis in whom optimal positioning was not achieved because of immobility. A false-negative MR image was obtained in an elderly patient in whom, again owing to suboptimal positioning, the axillary tail of the affected breast was not included in the precontrast sequence and a carcinoma was missed.

With an overall sensitivity of 81% and a specificity of 82%, the results of conventional mammography in our group compare favorably with published data (1–8). Lesion detection at mammography, however, was adversely affected by breast density. Two of four patients with false-negative and two of three patients with false-positive conventional mammographic findings had mammographically dense breasts. In comparison, results of Tc-99m tetrofosmin scintimammography and MR imaging were not affected by breast density. In 13 patients with mammographically dense breasts, all of 13 lesions were correctly characterized with scintimammography, with correct MR diagnoses in 12 of the same 13 patients.

The results of conventional mammography were limited in the postoperative breast. Eleven of our 47 patients had a history of previous surgery, radiation therapy, or both to treat carcinoma; four of the 11 had histopathologic evidence of tumor recurrence. In two of these four patients, recurrent carcinoma was not accurately predicted with conventional mammography (Fig 3); however, mammographic findings suggested tumor recurrence in two of seven patients with postoperative fibrosis alone. Tc-99m tetrofosmin scintimammographic findings were positive in all four patients with recurrent disease (which included one patient with multifocal tumor recurrence [Fig 2]) and negative in all seven patients with benign scar tissue. MR imaging was less accurate in the post-

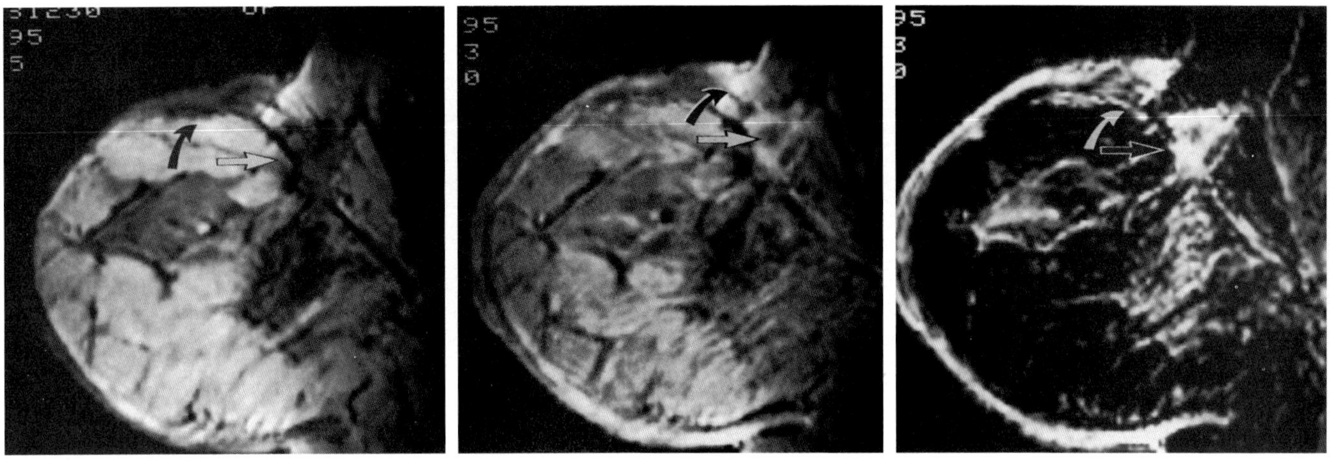

b. c. d.

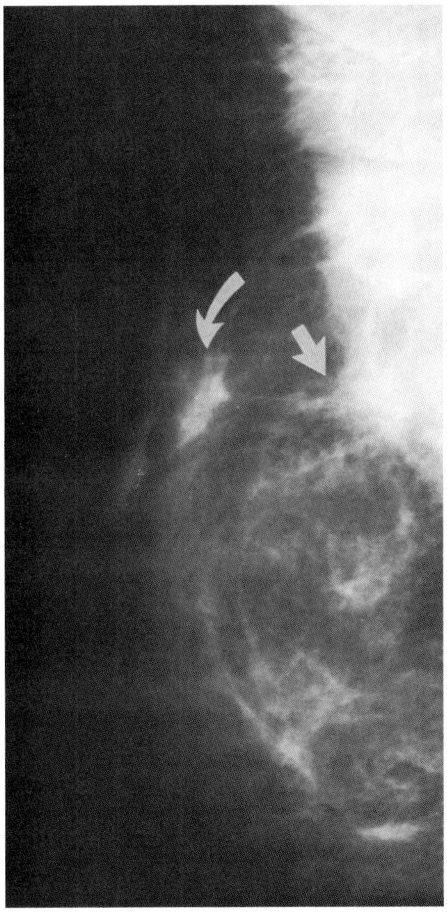

a.

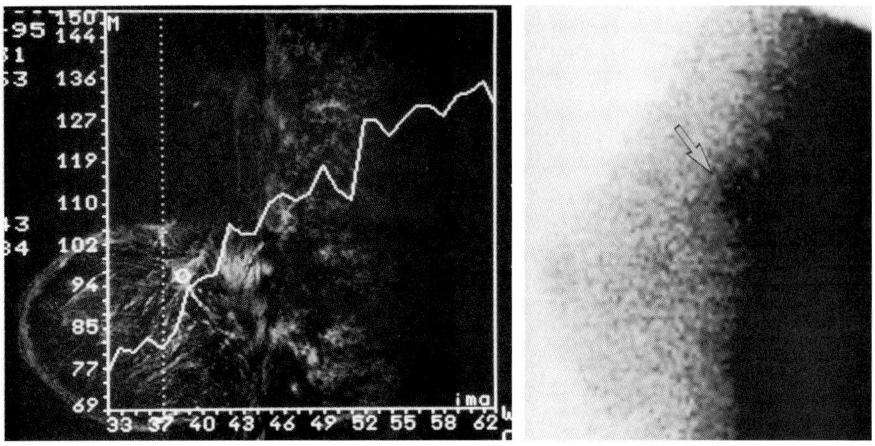

e. f.

Figure 3. Images obtained in a 55-year-old woman with a palpable lump in the upper outer quadrant of the right breast. **(a)** Lateral oblique mammogram obtained 16 months after lumpectomy and radiation therapy for invasive ductal carcinoma shows a spiculated mass in the upper outer quadrant of the right breast (curved arrow) associated with thickening of the overlying skin, with a second spiculated density adjacent to the anterior chest wall (straight arrow). Similar findings had been present on a 6-month follow-up mammogram (not shown) and were reported as posttreatment scar tissue rather than recurrent tumor. **(b)** Unenhanced, T1-weighted, FLASH, three-dimensional MR image (600/13, 50° flip angle) demonstrates a hypointense mass in the posterior part of the right breast (straight arrow) with thickening of the overlying skin (curved arrow). **(c)** Contrast-enhanced, T1-weighted, FLASH, two-dimensional MR image (600/13, 50° flip angle) shows enhancement of both the mass (straight arrow) and the overlying skin (curved arrow). **(d)** Subtraction MR image confirms the extent of enhancement of both the mass (straight arrow) and the overlying skin (curved arrow). **(e)** Enhancement profile (in arbitrary units of time vs signal intensity) through the lesion demonstrates gradual and persistent enhancement of the mass, which is suggestive of postoperative and postradiation fibrosis rather than recurrent tumor. **(f)** Lateral oblique Tc-99m tetrofosmin scintimammogram demonstrates focal abnormal tracer accumulation in the posterior part of the right breast (arrow), which was reported as recurrent tumor. A 2.1-cm recurrent invasive ductal carcinoma was subsequently resected. Histopathologic findings indicated that the more superficial mass seen at conventional mammography associated with thickening of the overlying skin represented benign posttreatment change rather than recurrent tumor.

operative and postradiation breast, with only eight of the 11 lesions correctly characterized, with one false-positive and two false-negative findings.

In the only other comparative study of breast scintigraphy and MR imaging performed to date that we know of, Helbich and colleagues (36) investigated the diagnostic accuracy of planar and single photon emission computed tomographic (SPECT) Tc-99m sestamibi scintimammography and compared the findings of scintigraphy with those of contrast-enhanced MR imaging. These investigators reported sensitivities and specificities for malignancy of 96% and 92%, respectively, for MR imaging, 62% and 88% for planar Tc-99m sestamibi scintimammography, and 83% and 80% for SPECT Tc-99m sestamibi scintimammography. The demographic data in our patient group, including patient age, tumor size, and number of carcinomas studied, are remarkably similar to those of Helbich and co-workers. Although the accuracies of MR imaging reported in their series and ours are similar, the results of planar scintimammography with Tc-99m tetrofosmin in our study surpass those reported by Helbich and colleagues (36) with Tc-99m sestamibi scintigraphy.

Discrepancies between the two studies may relate to the nature of the radioisotope used, the time between radioisotope injection and image acquisition, the manner in which the data were acquired (planar vs SPECT imaging), or the differences in image interpretation. In our experience and that of others, planar imaging had a higher diagnostic accuracy than SPECT, with similar sensitivities for carcinoma and fewer false-positive findings (19). In addition, planar imaging with the patient in an erect position produces scintimammograms that are directly comparable to lateral oblique conventional mammograms, which facilitates lesion detection and localization. Helbich and colleagues (36) commenced image acquisition 15 minutes after the administration of Tc-99m sestamibi. We favor immediate dynamic imaging, because early tumoral accumulation (0–4 minutes) is well recognized, with maximal lesion-to-background differentiation at 10–20 minutes after tracer injection (20).

Both Tc-99m sestamibi and Tc-99m tetrofosmin are lipophilic, cationic imaging agents with a similar mechanism of action. A practical advantage of using Tc-99m tetrofosmin compared with Tc-99m sestamibi for breast imaging is convenience of preparation. Tc-99m sestamibi requires boiling and subsequent cooldown before use. This step is time-consuming and may increase the radiation exposure to medical personnel. Tetrofosmin, on the other hand, is freeze-dried and ready to use and requires no additional preparation.

Issues that require further investigation include the relative accuracy of Tc-99m scintimammography and MR imaging in the detection and characterization of "minimal" tumor and methods for attaining histopathologic diagnosis in patients with nonpalpable lesions detected at scintigraphy alone. We elected to examine only patients with palpable breast abnormalities to compare results of the two techniques under the least demanding of circumstances. Although a 7-mm carcinoma was correctly characterized with both modalities, the favorable results of Tc-99m tetrofosmin scintimammography and MR imaging in our series cannot be extrapolated to include nonpalpable, screening-detected tumors. It is likely that MR imaging will be more accurate than scintimammography in the detection and characterization of subcentimeter lesions; however, further work is required to evaluate this. Although occult, nonpalpable breast lesions detected at MR imaging alone may be localized and biopsy performed under MR guidance, practical difficulties will arise in determining how best to perform biopsy in nonpalpable lesions demonstrated at scintigraphy alone.

Tc-99m tetrofosmin scintimammography and MR imaging exhibit comparable sensitivities and specificities for carcinoma in patients with palpable breast lesions. Both techniques can exclude malignancy with a high degree of confidence, while false-positive results may occur in higher grades of proliferative dysplasia and hypercellular fibroadenomas. Both techniques were useful in the evaluation of the mammographically dense breast, while Tc-99m tetrofosmin scintimammography proved more accurate in the evaluation of the postoperative and postradiation therapy breast.

Because of the lower cost, wider availability, and high patient acceptance, Tc-99m tetrofosmin scintimammography may challenge contrast-enhanced MR imaging as the noninvasive modality of choice to supplement mammography and US in mammographically difficult cases. Dynamic planar imaging with Tc-99m tetrofosmin provides a reliable alternative to MR imaging when MR is not available or poorly tolerated or when findings are equivocal. Further work to compare the results of each technique in nonpalpable, screening-detected lesions is ongoing. ■

References

1. Kopans DB. The positive predictive value of mammography. AJR 1992; 158:521–526.
2. Kelsey JL, Gammon MD. The epidemiology of breast cancer. CA Cancer J Clin 1991; 41:146–165.
3. Tabar L, Fagerberg G, Duffy SW, Day NE, Gad A, Grontoft O. Update of the Swedish Two-County Program of mammographic screening for breast cancer. Radiol Clin North Am 1992; 30:187–210.
4. Jackson VP, Hendrick RE, Feig SA, Kopans DB. Imaging of the radiographically dense breast. Radiology 1993; 188:297–301.
5. Bird RE, Wallace TW, Yankaskas BC. Analysis of cancer missed at screening mammography. Radiology 1992; 184:613–617.
6. Meyer JE, Eberlein TJ, Stomper PC, Sonnenfeld MR. Biopsy of occult breast lesions: analysis of 1261 abnormalities. JAMA 1990; 263:2341–2343.
7. Kopans DB, Swann CA. Observations on mammographic screening and the false-positive mammograms. AJR 1988; 150:785–786.
8. Tabar L, Gad A. Screening for breast cancer: the Swedish trial. Radiology 1981; 138:221–222.
9. Heywang-Kobrunner SH. Nonmammographic breast imaging techniques. Curr Opin Radiol 1992; 4:146–154.
10. McSweeney MB, Murphy CM. Whole breast sonography. Radiol Clin North Am 1985; 23:157–167.
11. Heywang-Kobrunner SH, Fenzl G, Hahn D, et al. MR imaging of the breast: comparion with mammography and ultrasound. J Comput Assist Tomogr 1986; 10:615–620.
12. Stack JP, Redmond RM, Codd MB, Dervan PA, Ennis JT. Breast disease: tissue characterization with Gd-DTPA enhancement profiles. Radiology 1990; 174:491–494.
13. Greenstein OS, Schnall MD, LiVolsi VA, Troupin RH. Suspicious breast lesions: MR imaging with radiologic-pathologic correlation. Radiology 1994; 190:485–493.
14. Turkat TJ, Klein BD, Polan RL, Richman RH. Dynamic MR mammography: a technique for potentially reducing the biopsy rate for benign breast disease. JMRI 1994; 4:563–568.
15. Porter BA, Taylor V, Smith JP, Tsao V. Contrast-enhanced magnetic resonance mammography. Acad Radiol 1994; 1 (suppl):36–46.
16. Waxman AD, Ramanna L, Memsic LD, et al. Thallium scintigraphy in the evaluation of mass abnormalities of the breast. J Nucl Med 1993; 34:18–23.
17. Lee VW, Sax EJ, McAneny DB, et al. A complementary role for thallium-201 scintigraphy with mammography in the diagnosis of breast cancer. J Nucl Med 1993; 34:2095–2100.
18. Khalkali I, Mena I, Jouanne E, et al. Prone scintimammography in patients with suspicion of carcinoma of the breast. J Am Coll Surg 1994; 178:491–497.
19. Palmedo H, Schomburg A, Grunwald F, Mallmann P, Krebs D, Biersack HJ. Technetium-99m-MIBI scintimammography for suspicious breast lesions. J Nucl Med 1996; 37:626–630.
20. Piccolo S, Lastoria S, Mainolfi C, Muto P, Bazzicalupo L, Salvatore M. Technetium-99m-methylene diphosphonate scintimammography to image primary breast cancer. J Nucl Med 1995; 36:718–724.
21. McGuire AH, Dehdashti F, Siegel BA, et al. Positron tomographic assessment of 16 alpha-[^{18}F] fluoro 17-beta-estradiol uptake in metastatic breast cancer. J Nucl Med 1991; 32:1526–1533.
22. Fenlon HM, Phelan NC, Tierney S, Gorey T, Ennis JT. Tc-99m tetrofosmin scintimammography as an adjunct to plain film mammography in palpable breast lesions. Clin Radiol (in press).
23. Fleiss JL. Statistical methods for rates and proportions. New York, NY: Wiley, 1973; 143–147.
24. Sickles WA. Mammographic features of 300 consecutive nonpalpable breast cancers. AJR 1986; 146:661–663.
25. Gilles R, Guinebretiere JM, Shapero LG, et al. Assessment of breast cancer recurrence with contrast-enhanced subtraction MR imaging: preliminary results in 26 patients. Radiology 1993; 188:473–478.
26. Dao TH, Rahmouni A, Campana F, et al. Tumour recurrence versus fibrosis in the irradiated breast: differentiation with dynamic gadolinium-enhanced MR imaging. Radiology 1993; 187:751–755.
27. Hussman K, Renslo R, Phillips JJ, et al. MR mammographic localization: work in progress. Radiology 1993; 189:915–917.
28. Harms SE, Flamig DP, Hesley KL, Evans WP. Magnetic resonance imaging of the breast. Magn Reson Q 1992; 8:139–155.
29. Heywang-Kobrunner SH. Contrast-enhanced MRI of the breast. Basel, Switzerland: Karger, 1990.
30. Harms SE, Flamig DP. MR imaging of the breast. JMRI 1993; 3:277–283.
31. Hickman PF, Moore NR, Shepstone BJ. The indeterminate breast mass: assessment using contrast-enhanced magnetic resonance imaging. Br J Radiol 1994; 67:14–20.
32. Lewis-Jones HG, Whitehouse GH, Leinster SJ. The role of magnetic resonance imaging in the assessment of local recurrent breast carcinoma. Clin Radiol 1991; 34:197–204.
33. Heywang SH, Hilbertz T, Beck R, Bauer WM, Eiermann W, Permanetter W. Gd-DTPA enhanced MR imaging of the breast in patients with postoperative scarring and silicon implants. J Comput Assist Tomogr 1990; 14:348–356.
34. Gribbestad IS, Nilsen G, Fjosne HE, Kvinnsland S, Haugen OA, Rinck PA. Comparative signal intensity measurements in dynamic gadolinium-enhanced MR mammography. JMRI 1994; 4:477–480.
35. Fobben ES, Rubin CZ, Kalisher L, Dembner AG, Seltzer MH, Santoro EJ. Breast MR imaging with commercially available techniques: radiologic-pathologic correlation. Radiology 1995; 196:143–152.
36. Helbich TH, Becherer A, Trattnig S, et al. Differentiation of benign and malignant breast lesions: MR imaging versus Tc-99m sestamibi scintimammography. Radiology 1997; 202:421–429.

Nikos A. Courcoutsakis, MD • Catherine K. Chow, MD • Thomas H. Shawker, MD
J. Aidan Carney, MD, PhD • Constantine A. Stratakis, MD, DSc

Syndrome of Spotty Skin Pigmentation, Myxomas, Endocrine Overactivity, and Schwannomas (Carney Complex): Breast Imaging Findings[1]

PURPOSE: To study the imaging appearances of breast lesions in female patients with Carney complex.

MATERIALS AND METHODS: Seven patients with Carney complex underwent mammography ($n = 5$), ultrasound (US) ($n = 6$), or magnetic resonance (MR) imaging ($n = 6$) in a prospective study. Previous breast images in three patients were reviewed. Mammograms in two additional patients were retrospectively reviewed. Thus, nine patients aged 16–61 were included in this study.

RESULTS: Mammograms showed well-defined, iso- or hypodense masses; most were not calcified. Two lesions contained calcifications; both were biopsy-proved ductal adenomas. US demonstrated solid, hypoechoic, well-circumscribed masses in six patients and complex cystic masses (myxoid fibroadenomas) in one patient. MR imaging with a fat-suppressed, fast spin-echo, T2-weighted sequence demonstrated high-signal-intensity lesions ($n = 5$). Fat-suppressed, spoiled gradient-recalled-echo MR images demonstrated hypointense lesions with variable contrast material enhancement ($n = 5$). Five of seven patients in the prospective review had multiple breast lesions on at least one study. Mammograms and US scans were negative in three patients each. Chest and breast MR images were negative in only one patient.

CONCLUSION: Female patients with Carney complex often have multiple breast masses with variable imaging appearances that probably represent myxoid fibroadenomas or ductal adenomas. MR imaging showed the most lesions. These lesions all demonstrate benign characteristics and should not prompt multiple biopsies.

Carney complex (Mendelian Inheritance in Man catalog no. 160980 [1]) is a familial multiple-neoplasia and lentiginosis syndrome first reported on in 1985 by Carney and colleagues (2). Carney complex is characterized by spotty pigmentation of the skin and mucosae (lentigines and blue nevi); myxomatous tumors of the skin, heart, breast, and other organs; and a variety of endocrine tumors, which include primary pigmented nodular adrenocortical disease, growth hormone–secreting pituitary adenoma, testicular neoplasms (large-cell calcifying Sertoli and Leydig cell tumors), psammomatous melanotic schwannomas, and thyroid follicular tumors (adenoma and papillary and follicular carcinoma) (2–6).

The syndrome is autosomal dominant, and the genetic locus for it has been mapped to the short arm of chromosome 2 (2p16) (7). The disease is familial in approximately half of the patients; in the remaining patients, the syndrome appears sporadically. The complex has many similarities with the familial lentiginoses, for example, Peutz-Jeghers syndrome and the multiple endocrine neoplasias. Accordingly, a variety of tissues derived from mesenchyme or neuroectoderm, which include melanocytes and adrenocortical, thyroid, gonadal, and mammary cells, are affected.

The known breast lesions associated with Carney complex include myxoid fibroadenomas and ductal adenomas (8–10). The former have been found in at least one-fifth of the patients with reported sporadic and familial cases of the complex, while the latter have been described in five patients, which include two in the same family (8–10). The myxomatous lesion is characterized by the accumulation of myxoid material in the stroma that involves single or small groups of nodules (8). Larger aggregates of these lesions result in the formation of a myxoid fibroadenoma. Ductal adenomas are solid tumors with tubular features and are composed of distinct epithelial and myoepithelial cells with a modest amount of fibrous tissue (9,10).

Myxoid tumors and ductal adenomas can be uni- or bilateral and can be present in the same breast. The prevalence has not been prospectively evaluated among affected individuals. Breast lesions were present in 22% of the 51 patients in the largest series published to date that we know of (7).

In the present study, breast imaging was performed in eight patients from four unrelated kindreds and in one

Index terms: Breast neoplasms, diagnosis, 00.30 • Breast neoplasms, MR, 00.121411, 00.121412, 00.121413, 00.121415, 00.12143 • Breast neoplasms, radiography, 00.11 • Breast neoplasms, US, 00.1298 • Carney complex, 00.30 • Gadolinium

Abbreviations: NIH = National Institutes of Health, SPGR = spoiled gradient-recalled echo, STIR = short inversion time inversion recovery.

Radiology 1997; 205:221–227

[1] From the Department of Diagnostic Radiology, Warren Magnuson Clinical Center, National Institutes of Health, Bldg 10, Room 1 C 660, 10 Center Dr, MSC 1182, Bethesda, MD 20892-1182 (N.A.C., C.K.C., T.H.S.); the Department of Laboratory Medicine and Pathology, Mayo Clinic, Rochester, Minn (J.A.C.); the Unit on Genetics of Endocrinology, Section of Pediatric Endocrinology, Developmental Endocrinology Branch, National Institutes of Child Health and Human Development, Bethesda, Md (C.A.S.); and the Department of Pediatrics, Georgetown University Children's Medical Center, Washington, DC (C.A.S.). Received March 14, 1997; revision requested April 25; revision received June 2; accepted June 9. **Address reprint requests to** C.K.C.

sporadic patient with Carney complex (patient with the complex but no family history of the disorder); seven of these individuals were evaluated prospectively to define the prevalence and imaging characteristics of breast involvement. The purpose was to study the mammographic, ultrasound (US), and magnetic resonance (MR) imaging appearance of breast lesions in female patients with Carney complex.

MATERIALS AND METHODS

The institutional review boards of The National Institute of Child Health and Human Development, Bethesda, Md, the National Institutes of Health (NIH), Bethesda, Md, and the Mayo Clinic, Rochester, Minn, approved the contacting of families of patients with Carney complex and the participation of patients and their relatives in the present study after they gave informed consent (National Institutes of Child Health and Human Development protocol 95-CH-0059).

All patients were examined by two of the authors (J.A.C., C.A.S.). Stratakis and colleagues (7) described kindreds CAR.01, CAR.101, and CAR.102 previously. Kindred CAR.110 was reported on elsewhere (11). The medical records, mammographic and other radiologic studies, and tissue specimens obtained in three patients with known breast lesions from unrelated kindreds (CAR.01, CAR.101, and CAR.102) were reviewed retrospectively (Table 1). Tissue slides from available biopsy specimens were reviewed by one of the authors (J.A.C.) for confirmation of the diagnosis. Three patients from kindred CAR.01 and two patients from kindred CAR.102 were then examined prospectively for the presence of breast lesions. In addition, one patient from kindred CAR.110 and one patient without any family history of Carney complex (sporadic case) were enrolled in this protocol (Table 1).

Each patient underwent physical examination and breast imaging. Mammography was performed in five patients, US in six, and MR imaging in six. One patient, a 16-year-old girl, was examined only with US. Four chest MR imaging examinations were performed to evaluate the mediastinum and heart and included both breasts. Four MR examinations were performed with a dedicated breast coil. Two patients underwent both chest and breast MR imaging.

Mammographic examinations (bilateral craniocaudal and mediolateral oblique views) were performed with a Mammomat II unit (Siemens Medical Systems, Iselin, NJ). US was performed by using a 7.5–10.0-MHz linear-array transducer (Acuson, Mountain View, Calif).

Unilateral breast MR imaging was performed with a 1.5-T MR unit (Signa; GE Medical Systems, Milwaukee, Wis) with a commercially available breast coil (model M1085BR; GE Medical Systems). To perform a dynamic examination with a small field of view, we were constrained to performing unilateral, rather than bilateral, examinations. The patient was positioned pronely, and the following imaging protocol was used: (*a*) a sagittal, fat-suppressed, fast spin-echo, T2-weighted sequence (3,933–5,000/98 [repetition time msec/echo time msec], two signals acquired, 256 × 128 matrix, 2- or 3-mm section thickness) and (*b*) a three-dimensional, fat-suppressed, spoiled gradient-recalled-echo (SPGR) sequence (23.9–24/2.5, 30°–60° flip angle, 256 × 128 matrix, 2- or 3-mm section thickness) performed before and after the intravenous administration of gadopentetate dimeglumine (Magnevist; Berlex, Wayne, NJ). Gadopentetate dimeglumine was administered by hand with a bolus injection at a dose of 0.1 mmol per kilogram body weight for 10 seconds.

Contrast material–enhanced images were obtained in three of the four patients who underwent dedicated breast MR imaging. The decision to perform imaging in the left or right breast was based on information from the other imaging modalities that indicated the breast more likely to harbor the larger number of lesions. One patient underwent bilateral breast MR imaging.

Chest MR imaging was performed with a 0.5-T MR unit (Picker, Highland Heights, Ohio) and a body coil. The patient was positioned supinely, and the following imaging protocol was used: (*a*) an axial, motion-artifact–suppressed, spin-echo, T2-weighted sequence (2,050–2,455/30-80, two signals acquired, 128 × 256 matrix, 10-mm section thickness) and (*b*) an axial short-inversion-time inversion-recovery (STIR) sequence (2,455/30/100 [repetition time msec/echo time msec/inversion time msec], four signals acquired, 128 × 256 matrix, 10-mm section thickness).

Table 1
Selected Clinical Findings in Nine Patients with Carney Complex

Patient/ Age (y)	Kindred*	Clinical Findings	Breast Physical Examination
1/35	CAR.110	Lentigines, primary pigmented adrenocortical disease, skin and heart myxomas, thyroid cancer, ovarian tumors	Diffuse nodularity without dominant masses
2/37	CAR.01	Lentigines, primary pigmented adrenocortical disease, thyroid cancer, ovarian cystadenoma	Diffuse nodularity without dominant masses
3/33	CAR.01	Lentigines, primary pigmented adrenocortical disease, thyroid nodules	Diffuse nodularity without dominant masses
4/44	CAR.102	Lentigines, primary pigmented adrenocortical disease, skin and heart myxomas, acromegaly	Diffuse nodularity without dominant masses
5/39	CAR.102	Obligate carrier, lentigines	Diffuse nodularity without dominant masses
6/45	CAR.01	Lentigines, nevi, primary pigmented adrenocortical disease, thyroid nodules, skin myxoma	Diffuse nodularity without dominant masses
7/16	Sporadic case	Lentigines, primary pigmented adrenocortical disease, thyroid nodules	Tanner stage IV
8/61	CAR.102	Lentigines, skin myxoma	Bloody nipple discharge (unilateral)
9/61	CAR.101	Lentigines, skin myxoma	Bloody nipple discharge

* The codes are according to the nomenclature established by Stratakis and colleagues (6).

RESULTS

Pertinent patient data are presented in Table 1. Data from patients 8 and 9 were based on retrospective reviews. Patients 2, 3, 5, and 7 were examined only at the NIH; patients 1, 4, and 6 underwent part of the breast imaging work-up elsewhere, with completion of the work-up at the NIH. Biopsy was performed in lesions diagnosed before the beginning of our protocol; none of the patients examined prospectively underwent biopsy.

In the seven prospectively examined patients, five had multiple breast lesions shown with at least one imaging modality. Only two patients appeared free of breast lesions. One was an obligate carrier of the syndrome, with lentigines as the only manifestation of the syndrome, and the other was an adolescent girl. Six of the seven patients (patients 1–6) had diffuse breast nodularity at physical examination but no dominant masses. One patient (patient 7) was the previously mentioned adolescent girl with Tanner stage IV breast, the breast at the last developmental stage before maturity in which a projection of the areola and papilla form a secondary mound above the level of the breast.

Mammography was performed at our institution in five of the seven patients (patients 1–4 and 6); the obligate carrier and the adolescent girl (patients 5 and 7) were excluded. All of the patients had heterogeneously dense

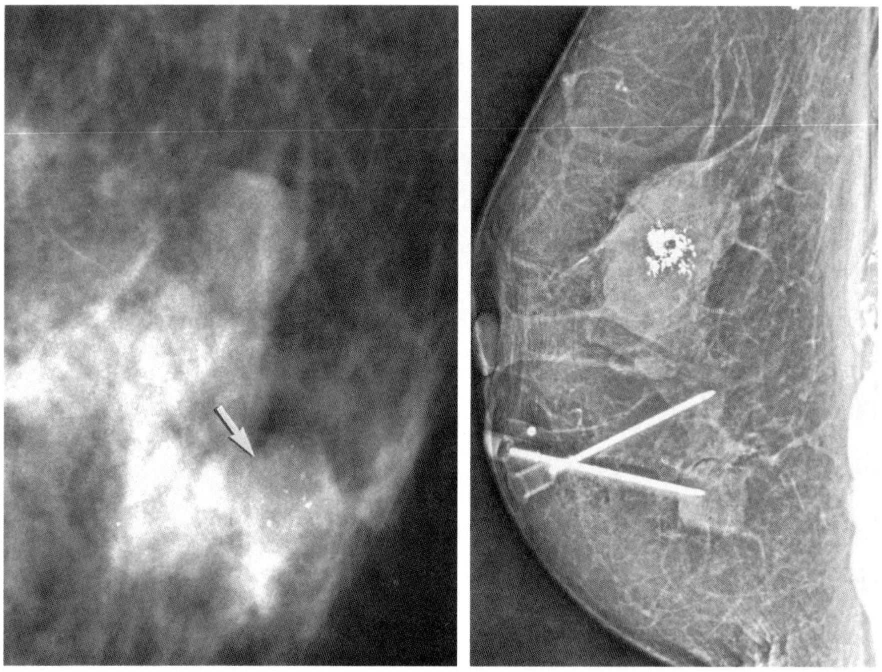

a. b.

Figure 1. Mammographic appearance. **(a)** Mammogram obtained in patient 6 demonstrates two ovoid low-density masses, one without and one with punctate calcification. The latter represents a ductal adenoma (arrow). **(b)** Mammogram obtained in patient 9 demonstrates two low-density masses. The larger mass with clusters of punctate calcifications is a histopathologically proved ductal adenoma. The smaller mass is a fibroadenoma. (Reprinted, with permission, from reference 9.)

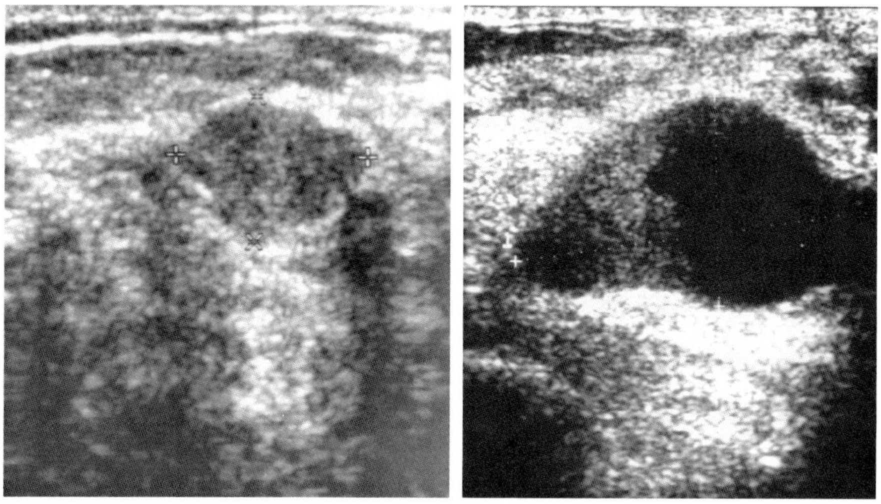

a. b.

Figure 2. US appearance. **(a)** US scan obtained in patient 2 demonstrates one of multiple, well-defined, hypoechoic masses. **(b)** US scan obtained in patient 6 demonstrates one of at least three complex cystic masses. The masses were excised and found to represent myxoid fibroadenomas.

breasts; thus, small masses were not easily appreciated radiologically, and round or ovoid, hypo- or isodense masses were only partially visualized in two patients (patients 4 and 6). Both of these patients were known from previous biopsy results to have had myxoid fibroadenomas or ductal adenomas. Patient 1, who had a "negative" mammogram, had undergone biopsy and confirmation of the presence of at least three myxoid fibroadenomas. Retrospective review of biopsy-proved lesions showed that they were isodense and well defined at mammography. None of the myxoid fibroadenomas was associated with calcifications, while all the biopsy specimens of ductal adenomas contained coarse or punctate calcifications (Fig 1).

US was performed in six patients (patients 1–5, 7). Three patients had one or more solid masses (patients 1, 2, and 4). All lesions appeared homogeneously hypoechoic and well defined (Fig 2a). No cysts were seen. Patient 1 had positive US findings despite negative mammographic findings, as described above. Patient 6 had multiple complex cystic masses at US performed elsewhere (Fig 2b), which were excised and found to represent myxoid fibroadenomas.

Breast MR was performed in four patients (patients 1–4) (Table 2); all of them had multiple lesions documented on the fat-suppressed, fast spin-echo, T2-weighted images. The lesions were small, ovoid, and uniformly hyperintense relative to the surrounding breast parenchyma (Fig 3a, 3b). On the contrast-enhanced, fat-suppressed SPGR images, lesions larger than 10 mm appeared as well-defined hypointense round or oval masses (Fig 3c). Those smaller than 10 mm were difficult to distinguish from the surrounding parenchyma; the presence of contrast material further obscured the smaller lesions that were surrounded by stippled enhancement in the normal breast. Some lesions showed homogeneous enhancement; a few showed septated enhancement (Fig 3d). The number of lesions on the fast spin-echo, T2-weighted images was greater than that on the contrast-enhanced or unenhanced SPGR images (Table 2).

Four patients underwent chest MR imaging (patients 1, 2, 5, and 6); three had multiple lesions with high signal intensity on spin-echo, T2-weighted and on STIR images (Fig 3e), similar to those seen on breast MR images. Only one of the patients examined with MR imaging had no lesions at all. She was the previously mentioned obligate carrier of Carney complex, who had only lentigines as a manifestation of Carney complex.

DISCUSSION

Two different breast tumors have been reported in patients with Carney complex. Myxoid fibroadenomas have been found in 22% of the patients with this disorder (7), while five patients have been reported to have ductal adenoma with tubular features (9,10). These two lesions may coexist in the breast in patients with Carney complex (3,9,10). In the present article, we review the available radiologic and histopathologic findings in two patients with Carney complex who had myxoid fibroadenomas and ductal adenomas and report the findings

Table 2
Imaging Findings

Patient/ Study	Non-NIH Examination Findings: Mammography	Non-NIH Examination Findings: US	Non-NIH Examination Findings: Histologic Analysis	NIH Examination Findings: Mammography	NIH Examination Findings: Bilateral US	NIH Examination Findings: Unilateral or Bilateral MR Imaging
1/R and P	NA	Bilateral, multiple, smoothly marginated, solid masses	At fine-needle aspiration biopsy, three lesions represent myxoid fibroadenomas; fibrocystic changes	Heterogeneously dense breast parenchyma, no masses	In the right breast, four, and in the left breast, two, well-circumscribed, ovoid, solid hypoechoic masses; no cysts on either side	In the right breast, 58 nodular masses (2–18 mm). At fast spin-echo, T2-weighted imaging, high signal intensity. At unenhanced SPGR, discrete lesions of low signal intensity. At contrast-enhanced SPGR, homogeneous lesions, lesions indistinguishable from parenchyma, or septated lesions At chest imaging, multiple nodular lesions. At spin-echo T2-weighted and STIR imaging, high signal intensity
2/P	NA	NA	NA	Heterogeneously dense breast parenchyma, no masses, benign calcifications	In the right breast, no masses; in the left breast, one 15-mm, solid, hypoechoic, ovoid mass; no cysts in either breast	In the left breast, 12 nodular masses (5–15 mm). At fast spin-echo, T2-weighted imaging, high signal intensity. At unenhanced SPGR, discrete lesions of low signal intensity. At contrast-enhanced SPGR, masses indistinguishable from breast parenchyma; the largest mass showed septated contrast material enhancement. At chest imaging, multiple nodular lesions. At spin-echo, T2-weighted and STIR imaging, high signal intensity
3/P	NA	NA	NA	Heterogeneously dense breast parenchyma, no masses	No cysts or solid masses in either breast	In the right breast, seven nodular masses. In the left breast, four nodular masses (3–12 mm). At fast spin-echo, T2-weighted imaging, high signal intensity. At unenhanced SPGR, discrete lesions of low signal intensity. At contrast-enhanced SPGR, masses indistinguishable from breast parenchyma
4/R and P	NA	NA	Bilateral myxomatous lesions	Heterogeneously dense breast parenchyma with bilateral, multiple, round or ovoid, partially obscured, iso- or low-density masses	In the right breast, two solid hypoechoic lesions (14 and 18 mm); in the left breast, one solid hypoechoic lesion (7 mm); no cysts in either breast	In the right breast, 14 nodular masses (3–22 mm). At fast spin-echo, T2-weighted imaging, high signal intensity. At unenhanced SPGR, discrete lesions of low signal intensity

(*Table 2 continues*)

Table 2 (*continued*)
Imaging Findings

Patient/ Study	Non-NIH Examination Findings			NIH Examination Findings		
	Mammography	US	Histologic Analysis	Mammography	Bilateral US	Unilateral or Bilateral MR Imaging
5/P	NA	NA	NA	NA	No cysts or solid masses in either breast	At chest spin-echo, T2-weighted and STIR imaging, no masses
6/R and P	Multiple nodules with fairly smooth margins	Multiple complex cysts (myxoid fibroadenomas) with internal echoes	At fine-needle aspiration biopsy, myxoid fibroadenomas	Heterogeneously dense breast parenchyma, an 8-mm nodule with a cluster of punctate microcalcifications (ductal adenoma), and bilateral, multiple masses (8–14 mm; myxoid fibroadenomas)	NA	At chest imaging, multiple nodular masses. At spin-echo, T2-weighted and STIR imaging, high signal intensity
7/P	NA	NA	NA	NA	Negative	NA
8/R	In the right breast, a poorly defined 10-mm soft-tissue mass with a cluster of rodlike and punctate calcifications (ductal adenoma). In the left breast, a 50-mm soft-tissue mass with a mixed grouping of calcifications of various sizes (ductal adenoma) and a 15-mm mass in the outer lower quadrant without calcification (myxoid fibroadenoma)	NA	Ductal adenomas and a myxoid fibroadenoma	NA	NA	NA
9/R	In the right and left breasts, well-defined masses with coarse calcifications (ductal adenomas) and circumscribed noncalcified lesions (myxoid fibroadenomas)	NA	Ductal adenomas and bilateral myxoid fibroadenoma	NA	NA	NA

Note.—NA = not applicable, P = prospective study, and R = retrospective study.

from seven additional patients from the same or other kindreds.

In our patients, the number of lesions depicted with MR imaging was far greater than the number depicted with US or mammography. Mammography was hampered by the patients' heterogeneously dense parenchyma; US was similarly impeded by the lack of discrimination between the fibroglandular tissue and the presumed myxoid fibroadenomas and ductal adenomas (12–15). Although the MR appearance of these masses was not specific, their multiplicity and uniform appearance suggested a single benign cause. Their enhancement characteristics were not specific, although in one lesion (in patient 2) septated enhancement was found, a pattern that has been reported to be characteristic of fibroadenoma (16,17). A differential diagnosis for the pattern of numerous high-signal-intensity masses on fast spin-echo, T2-weighted images would also include multiple cysts or multiple metastases.

US examination of the six patients ruled out the presence of any cysts, and although patient 6 underwent an outside US examination in which complex cystic lesions were found, histologic diagnosis showed that these were myxoid fibroadenomas. The lack of primary carcinoma or other metastatic lesions in our patients rendered the possibility of metastatic disease very unlikely. Although we have no histopathologic diagnosis for the lesions we visualized, we found little basis for suggesting biopsy to our patients because they were known to have Carney complex and all had a homogeneous population of lesions without malignant characteristics.

Mammographic screening of patients with Carney complex for possible breast cancer is complicated by the presence of multiple masses. In fact, Carney and Toorkey (9) reported on a series of five women with ductal adenomas who were at first misdiagnosed as having infiltrating ductal carcinomas; two of the patients underwent modified radical mastectomy (9). Nevertheless, relying on mammographic signs of malignancy should help to prevent unnecessary intervention. The presence of microcalcifications can be confusing, because they may be difficult to distinguish from carcinoma and are associated with ductal adenomas or fibroadenomas. Although fibroadenomas are known to produce coarse calcifications, most of the lesions (except the ductal adenomas) in our patients were not calcified, possibly because of the younger age.

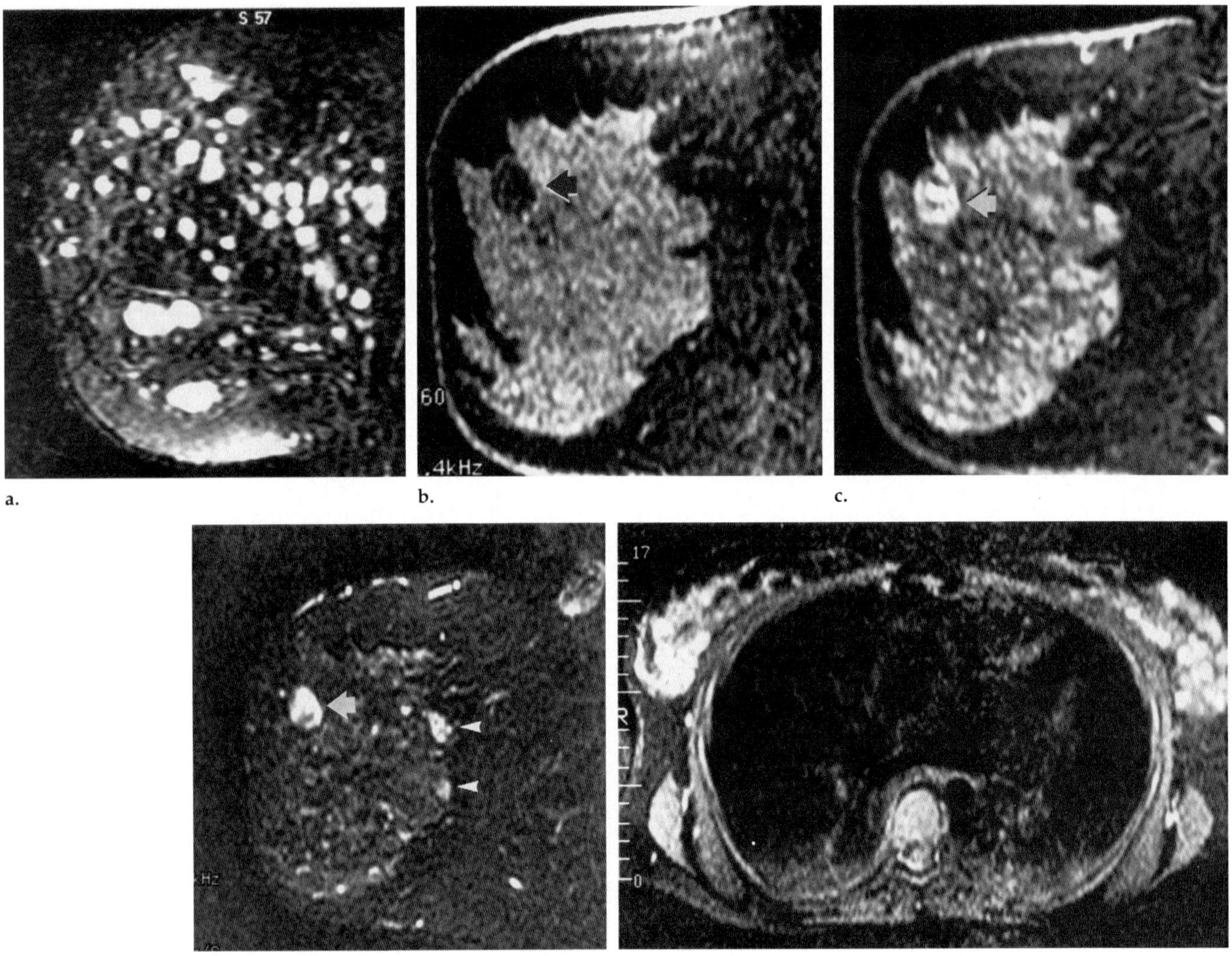

a. b. c. d. e.

Figure 3. MR imaging appearance. **(a)** Sagittal, fat-suppressed, fast spin-echo, T2-weighted MR image (5,000/98) obtained in patient 1 demonstrates numerous hyperintense nodules. **(b, c)** Sagittal, fat-suppressed, SPGR MR images (24/2.5, 30° flip angle) obtained in patient 2 **(b)** before and **(c)** after contrast material administration demonstrate a well-defined hypointense mass (arrow) with septated enhancement. **(d)** Sagittal, fat-suppressed, fast spin-echo, T2-weighted MR image (5,000/98) obtained in patient 2 at the same location demonstrates the hypointense mass (arrow), two additional nodules posteriorly (arrowheads), and an incidental axillary node. **(e)** Chest axial STIR MR image (2,455/30/100) obtained in patient 1 demonstrates numerous nodules in both breasts. The scale is in centimeters.

We have not been able to document an increased rate of breast cancer in our kindreds with Carney complex (7). Although a weak association has been found between the presence of fibroadenomas and breast cancer (18), the presence of myxoid fibroadenomas in the complex reflects a general predisposition toward myxomatous growth that is characteristic of this condition and that, in our experience, does not lead to an increased risk of cancer in patients with the complex. On the other hand, one should not exclude the possibility that malignancy could arise in the context of benign hyperplasia; this appears to be the case in patients with Carney complex who develop thyroid cancer after a long history of benign thyroid tumors (19).

In conclusion, breast masses in Carney complex may represent myxoid fibroadenomas or ductal adenomas. They are benign tumors that can manifest at a young age and are autosomal dominant. We suggest that MR imaging be performed when a solid, benign-appearing mass in a patient with Carney complex is found on a screening mammogram. If additional lesions with similar features exist and no other signs of malignancy are present, the patient can be followed up clinically. Alternatively, stereotactically or US-guided core biopsy of the lesion may be performed. If core biopsy is performed, the pathologist should be apprised of the diagnosis of Carney complex, with the caveat mentioned above. Because ductal adenomas are unusual benign tumors, incidental discovery of such a lesion should prompt one to exclude Carney complex. Clinical work-up for Carney complex includes a search for skin myxomas (eyelid, ear, oral, nasal, vulvar, penile, or other skin site) and exclusion of endocrine hyperactivity (7) so that the potentially lethal components of the syndrome, for example, cardiac myxomas and the occasional malignant tumor, can be identified. ■

References

1. Online Mendelian Inheritance in Man (OMIM). Available at: http://www.ncbi.nlm.nih.gov/Omim/. Accessed February 1997.
2. Carney JA, Gordon H, Carpenter PC, Shenoy V, Go VLW. The complex of myxomas, spotty pigmentation, and endocrine overactivity. Medicine 1985; 64:270–283.
3. Carney JA. The Carney complex (myxomas, spotty pigmentation, endocrine overactivity, and schwannomas). Dermatol Clin North Am 1995; 13:19–26.
4. Carney JA, Young WF. Primary pigmented

adrenocortical disease and its associated conditions. Endocrinologist 1992; 2:6–21.
5. Carney JA. Psammomatous melanotic schwannoma: a distinctive, heritable tumor with special associations, including cardiac myxoma and the Cushing syndrome. Am J Surg Pathol 1990; 14:206–222.
6. Premkumar A, Stratakis CA, Shawker TH, Papanicolaou DA, Chrousos GP. Testicular ultrasound in Carney complex. JCU 1997; 25:211–214.
7. Stratakis CA, Carney JA, Lin JP, et al. Carney complex, a familial multiple neoplasia and lentiginosis syndrome: analysis of 11 kindreds and linkage to the short arm of chromosome 2. J Clin Invest 1996; 97:699–705.
8. Carney JA, Toorkey BC. Myxoid fibroadenoma and allied conditions (myxomatosis) of the breast: a heritable disorder with special associations including cardiac and cutaneous myxomas. Am J Surg Pathol 1991; 15:713–721.
9. Carney JA, Toorkey BC. Ductal adenoma of the breast with tubular features: a probable component of the complex of myxomas, spotty pigmentation, endocrine overactivity, and schwannomas. Am J Surg Pathol 1991; 15:722–731.
10. Carney AJ, Stratakis C. Ductal adenoma of the breast. Am J Surg Pathol 1996; 20: 1154–1155.
11. Gollin SM, Jenkins RB, Swaney WP, Mulvihil JJ, Bartlet D Jr, Nwokoro NA. 10q26: consistent chromosomal breakpoint in two cardiac myxomas from a patient with Carney syndrome (abstr). Am J Hum Genet 1995; 57:A65.
12. Hachiya J, Seki T, Okada M, Nitatori T, Korenaga T, Furuya Y. MR imaging of the breast with Gd-DTPA enhancement: comparison with mammography and ultrasonography. Radiat Med 1991; 9:232–240.
13. Boetes C, Mus RDM, Holland R, et al. Breast tumors: comparative accuracy of MR imaging relative to mammography and US for demonstrating extent. Radiology 1995; 197:743–747.
14. Jackson VP, Rothschild PA, Kreipke DL, Mail JT, Holden RH. The spectrum of sonographic findings of fibroadenoma of the breast. Invest Radiol 1986; 21:34–40.
15. Venta LA, Dudiak CM, Salomon CG, Flisak ME. Sonographic evaluation of the breast. RadioGraphics 1994; 14:29–50.
16. Greenstein Orel S, Schnall MD, LiVolsi VA, Troupin RH. Suspicious breast lesions: MR imaging with radiologic-pathologic correlation. Radiology 1994; 190:485–493.
17. Heywang SH, Wolf A, Pruss E, Hilbertz T, Eiermann W, Permanetter W. MR imaging of the breast with Gd-DTPA: use and limitations. Radiology 1989; 171:95–103.
18. Dupont W, Page DL, Parl FF, et al. Long term risk of breast cancer in women with fibroadenoma. N Engl J Med 1994; 331:10–15.
19. Stratakis CA, Courcoutsakis NA, Doppman JL, Carney JA, Shawker TH. Thyroid gland abnormalities in patients with the "syndrome of spotty skin pigmentation, myxomas, endocrine overactivity and schwannomas (Carney Complex)." J Clin Endocrinol Metab 1997; 82:2037–2043.

Stephen J. Swensen, MD • Gregory L. Aughenbaugh, MD • Jeffrey L. Myers, MD

Diffuse Lung Disease: Diagnostic Accuracy of CT in Patients Undergoing Surgical Biopsy of the Lung[1]

PURPOSE: **To determine if there is a subset of patients undergoing surgical biopsy for diffuse lung disease in whom accurate diagnosis can be made with computed tomography (CT) only.**

MATERIALS AND METHODS: **Two chest radiologists retrospectively reviewed the CT scans of 85 patients in whom surgical biopsy for diffuse lung disease was performed. Thin-section CT images were available in 58 (68%) of the 85 cases. By consensus, the radiologists listed the three most likely diagnoses in order of probability and rated their level of confidence in the first choice.**

RESULTS: **Each of 85 patients with diffuse lung disease had one of 16 diseases. In 79 (93%) cases, the correct diagnosis was one of the three choices. In 54 (64%) cases, the correct diagnosis was the radiologists' first choice. A high level of confidence in the first choice was reached in 20 (24%) cases; all 20 cases were forms of chronic lung disease. In 18 (90%) of these 20 cases, the first choice was correct.**

CONCLUSION: **In a subset of patients with diffuse lung disease who undergo surgical biopsy, accurate diagnosis can be made with CT findings only.**

When introduced in the mid-1980s, thin-section computed tomography (CT) substantially changed the evaluation and treatment of patients who are suspected or known to have diffuse lung disease (1–3). This change has occurred largely because the diagnostic accuracy of thin-section CT is greater than that of chest radiography (4–35). Patients with radiologic findings that are characteristic of specific diffuse lung diseases and compatible clinical findings are frequently treated without lung biopsy. This is particularly true for patients with clinical and radiologic diagnoses of usual interstitial pneumonia, silicosis, sarcoidosis, lymphangitis carcinomatosa, hypersensitivity pneumonitis, asbestosis, eosinophilic granuloma, constrictive bronchiolitis, and lymphangiomyomatosis.

Previous studies of the diagnostic accuracy of CT in diffuse lung disease were well performed and included patients in whom the diagnosis was established with transbronchial or surgical biopsy or on the basis of clinical criteria. In some instances, the diagnosis was known before CT was performed (4–11).

The purpose of this study was to determine if there is a subset of patients who undergo surgical biopsy for diffuse lung disease in whom accurate diagnosis can be made (with a high level of confidence) with CT only. We retrospectively evaluated the CT scans in a consecutive series of patients with diffuse lung disease who underwent lung biopsy by means of thoracotomy or video-assisted thoracoscopic surgery.

MATERIALS AND METHODS

CT scans of all patients with diffuse lung disease who underwent open lung biopsy or video-assisted thoracoscopic surgery between January 7, 1991, and August 3, 1993, were reviewed (36). We defined diffuse as widely distributed throughout both lungs with involvement of all lobes. Eighty-five patients with diffuse infiltrative lung disease were identified. There were 44 male and 41 female patients; patient ages ranged from 9 to 89 years (mean, 48 years). CT scans were obtained with a model 1200SX (Picker International, Highland Heights, Ohio) or a model C-100 (Imatron, South San Francisco, Calif) scanner. Conventional CT was performed with either 10-mm collimation (1200SX) or 6-mm collimation (C-100). All lung-windowed (width, 1,500 HU; level, −600 HU) and mediastinal-windowed (width, 400 HU; level, 20 HU) images were reviewed by a radiologist. Among the 85 patients, 58 (68%) underwent thin-section CT (1-mm collimation at 10-mm intervals with use of a high-spatial-frequency reconstruction algorithm). Two patients underwent a limited thin-section CT study that included only five sections that were spaced evenly throughout the lungs. Three patients underwent thin-section CT with use of 3-mm collimation at 10-mm intervals on the model C-100 scanner. All CT examinations were performed at suspended end inspiration. All CT examinations were performed 2 weeks or less before biopsy.

The CT scans were reviewed retrospectively by two chest radiologists (S.J.S., G.L.A.)

Index terms: Computed tomography (CT), thin section, 60.12118 • Lung, bronchiolitis obliterans, 60.219 • Lung, diseases, 60.2, 60.79 • Lung, fibrosis, 60.792 • Lung, infection, 60.20 • Lung, interstitial disease, 60.79 • Lung, lymphoma/leukemia, 60.34 • Pneumonitis, hypersensitivity, 60.639

Radiology 1997; 205:229–234

[1] From the Departments of Diagnostic Radiology (S.J.S., G.L.A.) and Pathology (J.L.M.), Mayo Clinic, 200 First St SW, Rochester, MN 55905. Received February 26, 1997; revision requested March 24; revision received May 7; accepted May 12. **Address reprint requests to** S.J.S.

who knew the patient's age and sex only. The two reviewers were from the institution where the CT examinations were performed. The reviewers were two of 38 radiologists who originally interpreted the images. In all cases, the time between the original interpretation and the retrospective review was 3–5 years. No information was available regarding the patient's immune status or disease progression. The reviewers were unaware of the specific diseases included in the study, the frequency of specific diagnoses, and the original radiologic interpretations. By consensus, the reviewers listed three diagnostic choices in decreasing order of probability for each patient. The radiologists' confidence in the first choice was recorded with use of a three-level scale: definite, probable, and possible (1).

The patients' histories and pathologic reports were reviewed after the retrospective radiologic predictions were made. The histologic specimens were reexamined by a pathologist (J.L.M.) if (*a*) the radiologists' first choice (made with a high level of confidence) was incorrect ($n = 2$) or (*b*) the correct diagnosis was not included in the radiologists' three choices ($n = 6$).

Table 1
Correct Diagnostic Predictions with CT

Disease	No. of Cases	Diagnostic Predictions: First Choice	Diagnostic Predictions: Top Three Choices
Usual interstitial pneumonia	18	16 (89)	17 (94)
Infection	13	8 (62)	12 (92)
Lymphoproliferative disorder	13	9 (69)	13 (100)
Bronchiolitis obliterans with organizing pneumonia	10	6 (60)	9 (90)
Hypersensitivity pneumonitis	9	7 (78)	9 (100)
Nonspecific interstitial pneumonia with fibrosis	3	0	3
Desquamative interstitial pneumonia	3	0	1
Bronchioloalveolar carcinoma	3	2	3
Diffuse alveolar damage	3	2	2
Chronic bronchiolitis	2	0	2
Eosinophilic granuloma	2	1	2
Drug reaction (chemotherapy)	2	0	2
Congestive heart failure	1	1	1
Lymphangitis carcinomatosa	1	1	1
Hemorrhage	1	0	1
Sarcoidosis	1	1	1
All cases	85	54 (64)	79 (93)

Note.—Numbers in parentheses are percentages of number of cases.

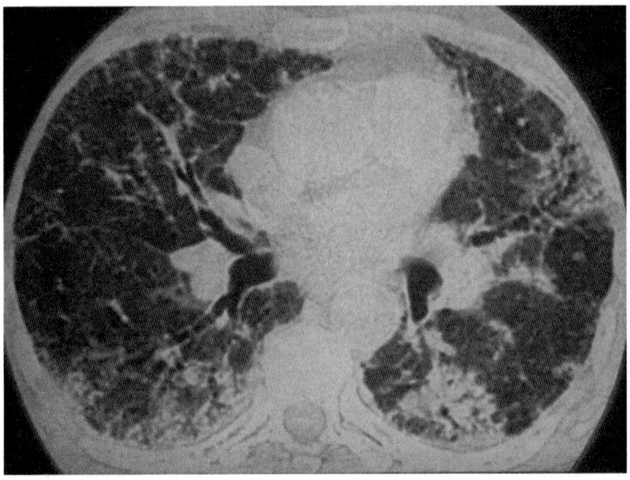

Figure 1. Usual interstitial pneumonia diagnosed in a 68-year-old woman after open lung biopsy. Thin-section CT (1-mm collimation) image shows multifocal regions of consolidation. In some regions, the bronchi are dilated, perhaps from traction. The lung bases (not shown) were relatively spared. The radiologists' three diagnostic choices were bronchiolitis obliterans with organizing pneumonia (first choice made with the lowest level of confidence), chronic eosinophilic pneumonia, and hypersensitivity pneumonitis.

RESULTS

Each of the 85 patients in this study had one of 16 diseases (Table 1). In all cases, a definitive diagnosis was ascertained with pathologic examination of biopsy specimens. Five diseases—usual interstitial pneumonia, infection, lymphoproliferative disorder, bronchiolitis obliterans with organizing pneumonia, and hypersensitivity pneumonitis—accounted for 74% of the total number of diseases. Among the 18 cases of usual interstitial pneumonia, three were associated with scleroderma ($n = 2$) or rheumatoid arthritis ($n = 1$). Infections included pneumocystis pneumonia ($n = 3$), fungal granulomatosis ($n = 6$), cytomegalovirus pneumonia ($n = 2$), cytomegalovirus pneumonia with fungal granulomatosis ($n = 1$), and mycoplasmal pneumonia ($n = 1$). Lymphoproliferative disorders included malignant lymphoma ($n = 10$) and leukemic infiltration ($n = 3$).

In 79 (93%) of the 85 cases, the correct diagnosis was included in the three choices of the radiologists. In 54 (64%) of the 85 cases, the correct diagnosis was the first choice. The correct diagnosis was not included in the three choices in six cases (7%) (Fig 1). These six cases were two cases of desquamative interstitial pneumonia and one case each of usual interstitial pneumonia, pneumocystis pneumonia, bronchiolitis obliterans with organizing pneumonia, and diffuse alveolar damage.

In 20 (24%) of the 85 cases, the first choice was reached with a high level of confidence (Table 2). All of these patients had chronic diffuse lung disease. The first choices reached with a high level of confidence were correct in 18 (90%) of the 20 cases (Figs 2, 3). No cases of infection, bronchiolitis obliterans with organizing pneumonia, bronchioloalveolar carcinoma, diffuse alveolar damage, chronic bronchiolitis, drug reaction, congestive heart failure, or hemorrhage were predicted with a high level of confidence. Usual interstitial pneumonia was predicted most often with the highest level of confidence. Twelve (67%) of the 18 cases of usual interstitial pneumonia were correctly predicted with a high level of confidence. Two cases (one case each of nonspecific interstitial pneumonia with fibrosis and desquamative interstitial pneumonia) were predicted with a high level of confidence as usual interstitial pneumonia (Figs 4, 5). In one of these cases, the pathologic diagnosis at first examination and review was nonspecific interstitial pneumonia with fibrosis and patchy bronchiolitis obliterans with organizing pneumonia. Usual interstitial pneumonia was our pathologist's primary differential diagnosis at review. This patient had polymyositis, was treated with prednisone, and died of pulmonary complications within 6 months of CT. In this case,

Table 2
First Radiologic Choices Made with a High Level of Confidence

Disease	No. of Cases	First Choices	No. Correct
Usual interstitial pneumonia	18	12	12
Infection	13	0	0
Lymphoproliferative disorder	13	1	1
Bronchiolitis obliterans with organizing pneumonia	10	0	0
Hypersensitivity pneumonitis	9	2	2
Nonspecific interstitial pneumonia with fibrosis	3	1	0*
Desquamative interstitial pneumonia	3	1	0*
Bronchioloalveolar carcinoma	3	0	0
Diffuse alveolar damage	3	0	0
Chronic bronchiolitis	2	0	0
Eosinophilic granuloma	2	1	1
Drug reaction (chemotherapy)	2	0	0
Congestive heart failure	1	0	0
Lymphangitis carcinomatosa	1	1	1
Hemorrhage	1	0	0
Sarcoidosis	1	1	1
Total	85	20	18

* Incorrect radiologic diagnosis was usual interstitial pneumonia.

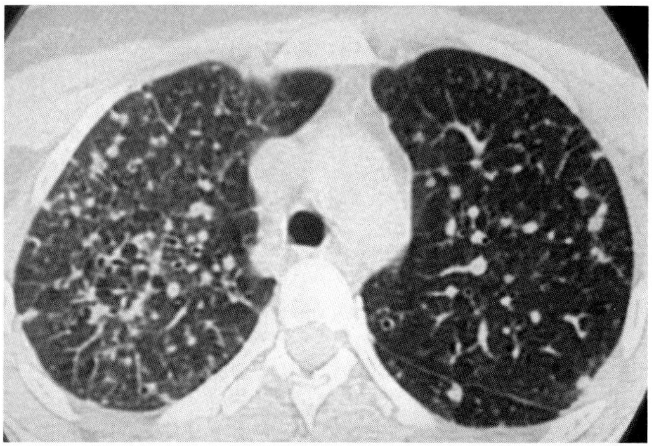

Figure 2. Eosinophilic granuloma diagnosed in a 45-year-old woman after open lung biopsy. Thin-section CT (1-mm collimation) image shows cystic and nodular changes. The lung bases (not shown) were relatively spared. The first radiologic choice (made with a high level of confidence) was eosinophilic granuloma.

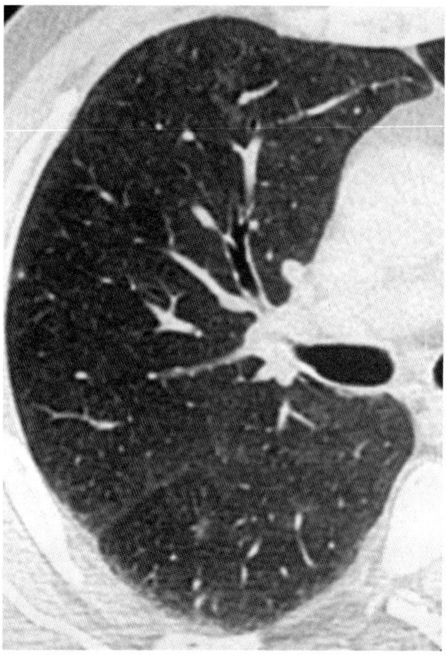

Figure 3. Hypersensitivity pneumonitis diagnosed in a 52-year-old man at pathologic examination. Thin-section CT (1-mm collimation) image shows a faint, diffuse, poorly circumscribed micronodular infiltrative process. The location of micronodules is primarily centrilobular. There are a few scattered focal regions of ground-glass attenuation. The lungs were involved uniformly. The first radiologic choice (made with a high level of confidence) was hypersensitivity pneumonitis.

our first choice (usual interstitial pneumonia) was incorrect; however, our second choice, nonspecific interstitial pneumonia with fibrosis, was correct (Fig 4). In the other case, the pathologic diagnosis at first examination and review was desquamative interstitial pneumonia. Chronic eosinophilic pneumonia was our pathologist's primary differential diagnosis at review. Our choices in this case were as follows: first, usual interstitial pneumonia; second, nonspecific interstitial pneumonia with fibrosis; and third, bronchiolitis obliterans with organizing pneumonia (Fig 5).

DISCUSSION

CT scans provide useful information for the accurate radiologic diagnosis of diffuse lung disease, even in a highly selected subset of patients for whom surgical biopsy is deemed appropriate. A combination of clinical and thin-section CT findings are routinely used to evaluate chronic diffuse lung disease at our institution. The 85 patients who underwent open lung biopsy represent only a small fraction of the approximately 1,000 cases of chronic diffuse infiltrative lung disease seen annually at our institution. In our experience, transbronchial and surgical biopsies of the lung are commonly avoided because diagnoses with use of CT and clinical findings are made with a very high level of confidence. In particular, when a chest radiologist, with use of thin-section CT, confidently diagnoses usual interstitial pneumonia, eosinophilic granuloma, lymphangiomyomatosis, silicosis, sarcoidosis, lymphangitis carcinomatosa, hypersensitivity pneumonitis, asbestosis, or chronic bronchiolitis, and the clinical findings support the diagnosis, surgical biopsy of the lung is performed infrequently. In our series, no cases of lymphangiomyomatosis and only one case of sarcoidosis were diagnosed with examination of surgical biopsy specimens.

We do not recommend that patients undergo biopsy if the clinical and radiologic findings are characteristic of a specific disease; our practice likely resulted in a selection bias in this study. The clinical or radiologic findings in patients who undergo surgical biopsy tend to be atypical or ambiguous (Figs 1, 4, 5). Also, patients are more likely to undergo biopsy if the presumed treatment program involves potential morbidity. Therefore, this subset of patients with diffuse lung disease presents the greatest diagnostic and management difficulties for the physician.

In this study, we included all cases of diffuse lung disease; there was no regard for the acute or chronic nature of the disease or the patient's immune status. We made predictions with a high level of confidence only in cases of chronic diffuse lung disease. To our knowledge, no series has been reported in which a large number of acute or subacute cases were examined and the radiologists were unaware of the clinical features. In our study, if acute or subacute cases had been excluded and the radiologist had known the clinical features (including the patient's immune status), we believe the overall accuracy and number of confident retrospective interpretations would have been higher. For example, no case of infection, diffuse alveolar damage, drug reaction, or hemorrhage was predicted with a high level of confidence.

Only 58 (68%) of 85 patients underwent thin-section CT. Since 1987, we have routinely performed thin-section CT examinations to evaluate diffuse lung disease and bronchiectasis. We have found thin-section CT to be most helpful for evaluating chronic diffuse lung disease. In most cases in which thin-section CT was not performed, pathologic diagnoses of infection, diffuse alveolar damage, drug reaction, and lymphoproliferative disorder were made. The radiologist who supervised the examination knew the clinical features of the case and tailored the study accordingly. In general, our experience indicates that thin-section CT is much less useful in these cases than in most cases of chronic diffuse lung disease.

Others have reported series of chronic lung disease in which radiologists had a high level of confidence in their first-choice diagnoses 49%–63% of the time (4–16). Only 20 (24%) of our 85 first choices were made with a high level of confidence; perhaps this finding resulted from the selection bias. Also, only cases of chronic lung disease were predicted with a high level of confidence. We were correct in 18 (90%) of the 20 cases that we predicted with a high level of confidence (Table 2). This percentage of correct predictions is similar to those of Mathieson et al (4) and Lee et al (6). All 12 of the first-choice predictions of usual interstitial pneumonia made with a high level of confidence were correct. In all of these cases, there were characteristic features on thin-section CT scans of usual interstitial pneumonia, including a predominantly basilar subpleural reticular process with architectural distortion and variable honeycombing.

In less than 10% of our cases (ie, six [7%] of 85 cases), the pathologic diagnosis was not included in our three radiologic predictions (Table 1, Fig 1). In these six cases, the pathologic diagnoses were desquamative interstitial pneumonia ($n = 2$), diffuse alveolar damage, bronchiolitis obliterans with organizing pneumonia, usual interstitial pneumonia, and pneumocystis pneumonia. The level of confidence in our first choice was high in only the one case of desquamative interstitial pneumonia presented (Fig 5). With the exception of the case of usual interstitial pneumonia, all of the incorrect predictions were of diseases that most believe warrant intervention for diagnosis (1–5,7–11). In cases of these diseases, knowledge of clinical history is very helpful for accurately interpreting thin-section CT findings.

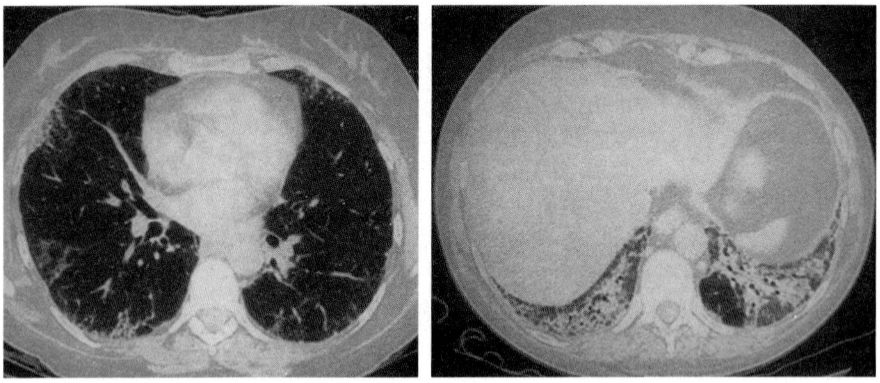

a. b.

Figure 4. Nonspecific interstitial pneumonia with fibrosis and patchy regions of bronchiolitis obliterans with organizing pneumonia diagnosed in a 50-year-old woman at pathologic examination. Thin-section CT (1-mm collimation) images show a diffuse infiltrative process with a basilar and subpleural predominance. **(a)** Image through the upper lungs shows a predominantly subpleural reticular process with some small cysts that are perhaps caused by early honeycombing. **(b)** Image through the lung bases shows a more consolidative process with mild bronchial dilatation that is consistent with traction bronchiectasis. This patient had polymyositis. Our first radiologic choice (made with a high level of confidence) was usual interstitial pneumonia; our second choice was nonspecific interstitial pneumonia with fibrosis.

In our series, there were three cases of nonspecific interstitial pneumonia with fibrosis. In each case, this disease was the second or third choice. In one case of nonspecific interstitial pneumonia with fibrosis (Fig 4), our first choice (made with a high level of confidence) was usual interstitial pneumonia. The thin-section CT scan of this patient showed a diffuse reticular process with a peripheral and basilar predominance. There were small cystic regions consistent with honeycombing. Images of the most basilar areas showed a more consolidative process with mild bronchial dilatation that was consistent with traction bronchiectasis and bronchiolectasis. We thought these findings were more characteristic of usual interstitial pneumonia. The most common pattern on CT images of nonspecific interstitial pneumonia with fibrosis is bilateral patchy areas of ground-glass attenuation with or without consolidated areas or, less commonly, irregular lines (37).

In our study, there were also three cases of desquamative interstitial pneumonia. In one of these cases (Fig 5), our first choice (made with a high level of confidence) was usual interstitial pneumonia. The thin-section CT scan showed bilateral predominantly subpleural regions of ground-glass attenuation in the midlung zones. In the bases, there was a predominantly subpleural reticular process with some ground-glass attenuation and regions of early honeycombing. In desquamative interstitial pneumonia, the reported predominant finding on thin-section CT scans is areas of ground-glass attenuation that involve mainly the lower subpleural lung zones. Irregular lines, cystic changes, and traction bronchiectasis may also be seen, but these findings are usually not prominent (28). On thin-section CT images, the distribution of abnormalities in desquamative interstitial pneumonia may be similar to that seen in usual interstitial pneumonia; however, the greater extent of ground-glass attenuation and the paucity of cystic changes in desquamative interstitial pneumonia should enable the distinction of this condition from usual interstitial pneumonia in most cases (28).

Our accuracy of predicting infection was particularly low (eight [62%] of 13 cases). None of these predictions was made with a high level of confidence. Likely, the clinical history (eg, immunodeficiency, fever, leukocytosis) in these cases would have been very helpful. Clinical history may also have been valuable in the three cases of diffuse alveolar damage.

We believe that thin-section CT is a very helpful and cost-effective examination for evaluating patients sus-

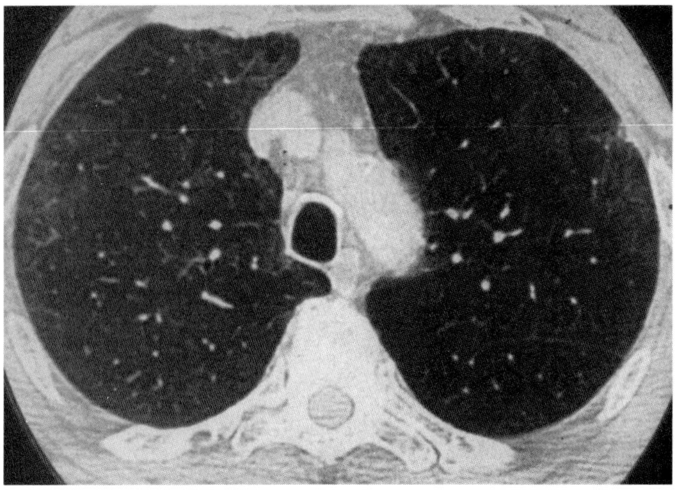

a.

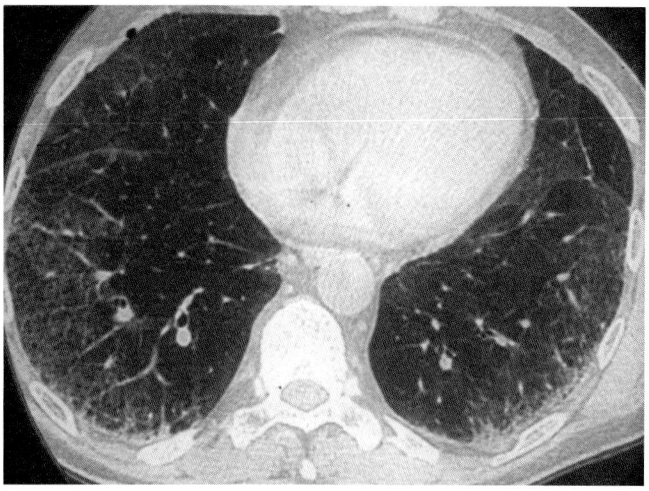

b.

Figure 5. Desquamative interstitial pneumonia diagnosed in a 71-year-old man at pathologic examination. **(a)** Thin-section CT (1-mm collimation) image of the upper lungs shows bilateral, predominantly subpleural ground-glass attenuation. **(b)** Thin-section CT (1-mm collimation) image of the lung bases shows a predominantly subpleural reticular process with regions of ground-glass attenuation. There may be early regions of honeycombing in several regions of the posterior aspects of the lung. Our first radiologic choice (made with a high level of confidence) was usual interstitial pneumonia with a probable reversible component (ie, regions of ground-glass attenuation).

pected or known to have diffuse lung disease whose clinical histories are ambiguous and whose chest radiographs show no findings or nonspecific findings. The use of thin-section CT for examination of diffuse lung disease has positively influenced the treatment of this disease. Today, fewer patients at our institution undergo surgical biopsy of the lung for diagnostic purposes. Now (4–6 years after our study patients were initially evaluated) with thin-section CT, we are more experienced and confident in our evaluation of patients with diffuse lung disease. Furthermore, our colleagues in pulmonary medicine and general thoracic surgery are more confident in the interpretation of thin-section CT studies. Accordingly, more patients with characteristic thin-section CT findings and supportive clinical features are being treated on the basis of these criteria alone and without pathologic confirmation of diagnosis.

In our study, even in cases in which surgical biopsy of the lung was deemed necessary, a confident retrospective diagnosis with CT was made 24% of the time (Figs 2, 3); without clinical information, the radiologists' accuracy was 90%. With better communication between clinical specialists, it is possible that fewer patients will need to undergo surgical biopsy of the lung for a confident, accurate diagnosis of diffuse lung disease.

In conclusion, in a subset of patients who undergo surgical biopsy for evaluation of diffuse lung disease, diagnosis can be made with a high level of confidence with use of CT findings only. ■

References

1. Müller NL, Miller RR. Computed tomography of chronic diffuse infiltrative lung disease: part 1. Am Rev Respir Dis 1990; 142:1206–1215.
2. Müller NL, Miller RR. Computed tomography of chronic diffuse infiltrative lung disease: part 2. Am Rev Respir Dis 1990; 142:1440–1448.
3. Müller NL. Clinical value of high-resolution CT in chronic diffuse lung disease. AJR 1991; 157:1163–1170.
4. Mathieson JR, Mayo JR, Staples CA, Müller NL. Chronic diffuse infiltrative lung disease: comparison of diagnostic accuracy of CT and chest radiography. Radiology 1989; 171:111–116.
5. Leung AN, Staples CA, Müller NL. Chronic diffuse infiltrative lung disease: comparison of diagnostic accuracy of high-resolution and conventional CT. AJR 1991; 157: 693–696.
6. Lee KS, Primack SL, Staples CA, Mayo JR, Aldrich JE, Müller NL. Chronic infiltrative lung disease: comparison of diagnostic accuracies of radiography and low- and conventional-dose thin-section CT. Radiology 1994; 191:669–673.
7. Grenier P, Chevret S, Beigelman C, Brauner MW, Chastang C, Valeyre D. Chronic diffuse infiltrative lung disease: determination of the diagnostic value of clinical data, chest radiography, and CT with Bayesian analysis. Radiology 1994; 191:383–390.
8. Nishimura K, Izumi T, Kitaichi M, Nagai S, Itoh H. The diagnostic accuracy of high-resolution computed tomography in diffuse infiltrative lung diseases. Chest 1993; 104: 1149–1155.
9. Padley SPG, Hansell DM, Flower CDR, et al. Comparative accuracy of high-resolution computed tomography and chest radiography in the diagnosis of chronic diffuse infiltrative lung disease. Clin Radiol 1991; 44:222–226.
10. Grenier P, Valeyre D, Cluzel P, Brauner MW, Lenoir S, Chastang C. Chronic diffuse interstitial lung disease: diagnostic value of chest radiography and high-resolution CT. Radiology 1991; 179:123–132.
11. Remy-Jardin M, Remy J, Deffontaines C, Duhamel A. Assessment of diffuse infiltrative lung disease: comparison of conventional CT and high-resolution CT. Radiology 1991; 181:157–162.
12. Webb WR, Stein MG, Finkbeiner WE, Im JG, Lynch D, Gamsu G. Normal and diseased isolated lungs: high-resolution CT. Radiology 1988; 166:81–87.
13. Swensen SJ, Aughenbaugh GL, Douglas WW, Myers JL. High-resolution CT of the lungs: findings in various pulmonary diseases. AJR 1992; 158:971–979.
14. Bergin CJ, Müller NL. CT in the diagnosis of interstitial lung disease. AJR 1985; 145: 505–510.
15. Murata K, Khan A, Herman PG. Pulmonary parenchymal disease: evaluation with high-resolution CT. Radiology 1989; 170: 629–635.
16. Lynch DA, Newell JD, Logan PM, King TE, Müller NL. Can CT distinguish hypersensitivity pneumonitis from idiopathic pulmonary fibrosis? AJR 1995; 165:807–811.
17. Silver SF, Müller NL, Miller RR, et al. Hypersensitivity pneumonitis: evaluation with CT. Radiology 1989; 173:441–445.
18. Müller NL, Miller RR, Webb WR, et al. Fibrosing alveolitis: CT-pathologic correlation. Radiology 1986; 160:585–588.
19. Aberle DR, Gamsu G, Ray CS, et al. Asbestos-related pleural and parenchymal fibrosis: detection with high-resolution CT. Radiology 1988; 166:729–734.
20. Müller NL. Differential diagnosis of chronic diffuse infiltrative lung disease on high-resolution computed tomography. Semin Roentgenol 1991; 36:132–142.
21. Adler BD, Padley SPG, Müller NL, et al. Chronic hypersensitivity pneumonitis: high-resolution CT and radiographic features in 16 patients. Radiology 1992; 185: 91–95.
22. Müller NL, Kullnig P, Miller RR. The CT findings of pulmonary sarcoidosis: analysis of 25 patients. AJR 1989; 152:1179–1182.
23. Lynch DA, Webb WR, Gamsu G, et al. Computed tomography in pulmonary sarcoidosis. J Comput Assist Tomogr 1989; 13:405–410.
24. Webb WR. High-resolution computed tomography of obstructive lung disease. Radiol Clin North Am 1994; 32:745–757.
25. Templeton PA, McLoud TC, Müller NL, et al. Pulmonary lymphangioleiomyomato-

sis: CT and pathologic findings. J Comput Assist Tomogr 1989; 13:54–57.
26. Moore ADA, Godwin JD, Müller NL, et al. Pulmonary histiocytosis X: comparison of radiographic and CT findings. Radiology 1989; 172:249–254.
27. Brauner MW, Grenier P, Mouelhi MM, et al. Pulmonary histiocytosis X: evaluation with high-resolution CT. Radiology 1989; 172: 255–258.
28. Hartman TE, Primack SL, Swensen SJ, et al. Desquamative interstitial pneumonitis: thin-section CT findings in 22 patients. Radiology 1993; 187:787–790.
29. Murch CR, Carr DH. Computed tomography appearances of pulmonary alveolar proteinosis. Clin Radiol 1989; 40:240–243.
30. Godwin JD, Müller NL, Takasugi JE. Pulmonary alveolar proteinosis: CT findings. Radiology 1988; 169:609–613.
31. Akira M, Yamamoto S, Yokoyama K, et al. Asbestosis: high-resolution CT-pathologic correlation. Radiology 1990; 176:389–394.
32. Mayo JR, Müller NL, Road J, et al. Chronic eosinophilic pneumonia: CT findings in six cases. AJR 1989; 153:727–730.
33. Müller NL, Miller RR. Diseases of the bronchioles: CT and histopathologic findings. Radiology 1995; 196:3–12.
34. Müller NL, Staples CA, Miller RR. Bronchiolitis obliterans organizing pneumonia: CT features in 14 patients. AJR 1990; 154: 983–987.
35. McAdams HP, Rosado-de-Christenson ML, Wehunt WD, Fishback NF. The alphabet soup revisited: the chronic interstitial pneumonias in the 1990s. RadioGraphics 1996; 16:1009–1033.
36. Chadokura M, Colby T, Myers J, et al. Pathologic comparison of video-assisted thoracic surgical with traditional open lung biopsy. J Thorac Cardiovasc Surg 1995; 108: 494–498.
37. Park JS, Lee KS, Kim JS, et al. Nonspecific interstitial pneumonia with fibrosis: radiographic and CT findings in seven patients. Radiology 1995; 195:645–648.

David S. Gierada, MD • Richard M. Slone, MD • Kyongtae T. Bae, MD, PhD • Roger D. Yusen, MD
Stephen S. Lefrak, MD • Joel D. Cooper, MD

Pulmonary Emphysema: Comparison of Preoperative Quantitative CT and Physiologic Index Values with Clinical Outcome after Lung-Volume Reduction Surgery[1]

PURPOSE: **To compare quantitative computed tomographic (CT) and preoperative physiologic values in emphysema with outcome after lung-volume reduction surgery.**

MATERIALS AND METHODS: **In 46 patients, emphysema was quantified by measuring lung attenuation on preoperative CT scans. Quantitative CT and preoperative physiologic values and postoperative outcomes (1-second forced expiratory volume, Pa_{O_2}, and 6-minute walk distance) were compared.**

RESULTS: **Moderately strong correlations were found between several quantitative CT and preoperative physiologic values ($|r| = .29–.58$, $P < .05$) and several quantitative CT and outcome measures ($|r| = .31–.47$, $P < .05$). With stratification, postoperative outcome was better with mean lung attenuation greater than −900 HU; 75% or greater of upper lung below −900 HU (emphysema index); greater than 25% of lung below −960 HU (severe emphysema index); ratio of upper- and lower-lung emphysema indexes 1.5 or greater; volume of normally attenuated lung (−850 to −701 HU) greater than 1 L; and full width at half maximum of attenuation-frequency distribution 80 HU or less. Differences in outcome measures between groups stratified with quantitative CT values were often two- to threefold; patients with greater numbers of favorable quantitative CT values had better outcome. Correlations between preoperative physiologic measures and outcome were few.**

CONCLUSION: **In emphysema, quantitative CT values correlate with outcome. Quantitative assessment of emphysema in candidates for lung-volume reduction surgery is potentially useful.**

With the increasing application of lung-volume reduction surgery during the past several years (1–8), the radiologic assessment of emphysema has gained additional clinical importance. Findings on chest radiographs, computed tomographic (CT) scans, and perfusion scintigraphy studies strongly influence patient selection for lung-volume reduction surgery (9). Features considered favorable for lung-volume reduction surgery include marked thoracic hyperinflation—which indicates a potential for improvement in breathing mechanics with a reduced lung volume—and a heterogeneous, or nonuniform, distribution of emphysema with the presence of severely affected surgical "target areas" amid areas of more mildly emphysematous lung (1–3,9–11). Other favorable radiologic characteristics have been identified by comparing subjective assessments of the severity and distribution of emphysema with the clinical outcome of lung-volume reduction surgery (8–10,12). On preoperative imaging studies, patients with evidence of greater upper-lobe emphysema, greater heterogeneity of severity of emphysema, and a larger percentage of mildly diseased lung have experienced the greatest clinical improvement after lung-volume reduction surgery.

The specific features of the disease can be assessed on CT scans, which depict emphysema with high accuracy (13,14). However, visually estimating the volume and severity of emphysema generally or regionally is difficult, and these estimations are subject to interobserver and intraobserver variations. Visual interpretation may be influenced by several factors, including scanner type and the window and level chosen for filming. Quantitative assessment of emphysema with use of CT virtually eliminates these problems and may allow standardized assessment.

We theorized that, by analyzing pixel-attenuation statistics in different lung-attenuation ranges and lung regions, quantitative CT parameters of emphysema can be defined that are analogous to morphologic features of the disease considered clinically important in the evaluation of patients for lung-volume reduction surgery. The purpose of this study was to define relevant quantitative CT parameters of emphysema and compare them with outcomes of lung-volume reduction surgery. A secondary purpose was to investigate the relationship between quantitative CT and preoperative physiologic values.

MATERIALS AND METHODS

Patients

The study group consisted of a convenience sample of 46 of the first 150 patients

Index terms: Computed tomography (CT), quantitative, 60.12111 • Emphysema, pulmonary, 60.751 • Lung, CT, 60.12111 • Lung, surgery, 60.459

Abbreviations: FEV_1 = forced expiratory volume in 1 second, FVC = forced vital capacity.

Radiology 1997; 205:235–242

[1] From the Mallinckrodt Institute of Radiology (D.S.G., R.M.S., K.T.B.) and the Divisions of General Medical Sciences (R.D.Y.), Pulmonary Medicine (R.D.Y., S.S.L.), and Cardiothoracic Surgery (J.D.C.), Washington University School of Medicine, Barnes-Jewish Hospital North Campus, 216 S Kingshighway Blvd, St Louis, MO 63110. Received February 12, 1997; revision requested April 8; revision received June 9; accepted June 16. D.S.G. is supported in part by the RSNA Research and Education Fund. R.D.Y. is supported in part by the National Heart, Lung, and Blood Institute (National Institutes of Health) grant HL07317 and the Norman P. Knowlton, Jr, MD, Incentive for Excellence Fund of Barnes-Jewish Hospital. **Address reprint requests to** D.S.G.

to undergo bilateral lung-volume reduction surgery at our institution between January 1993 and February 1996. Patients were chosen without knowledge of the results of their preoperative or postoperative pulmonary function tests or radiologic studies. There were 27 women and 19 men; the female preponderance in this group differed from the slight male predominance in the 150 patients. Patient ages of the 46 patients ranged from 36 to 74 years (mean, 58 years ± 9). The pulmonary function of the 46 patients (Table 1) was similar to that of the group of 150 patients (15) from which the 46 patients were chosen. All 46 were former heavy smokers. Three women had α_1-antitrypsin deficiency.

Table 1
Preoperative Values of Quantitative CT and Physiologic Indexes in 46 Patients

Indexes	Mean ± SD*	Range
Quantitative CT		
Mean lung attenuation (HU)	−896 ± 15	−927 to −845
Emphysema index (%)	63 ± 8	45–83
Severe emphysema index (%)	28 ± 10	10–54
Upper-lung index (%)	73 ± 12	32–89
Upper-lung index/lower-lung index	1.6 ± 0.7	0.6–5.5
Volume of normal-attenuation lung (L)	1.1 ± 0.2	0.7–1.9
Full width at half maximum (HU)	86 ± 32	21–178
Physiologic		
Forced expiratory volume in 1 second (FEV_1) (% predicted)	26 ± 7	15–49
Forced vital capacity (FVC) (% predicted)	72 ± 15	42–103
FEV_1/FVC	29 ± 6	20–49
Total lung capacity (% predicted)†	145 ± 19	115–181
Residual volume (% predicted)†	290 ± 63	183–432
Diffusing capacity of lung for carbon monoxide (mL/min per mm Hg)	9 ± 4	3–25
Pa_{O_2} (mm Hg)	61 ± 10	42–80
Pa_{CO_2} (mm Hg)	42 ± 7	28–59
6-minute walk distance (ft)‡	1,100 ± 300	300–1,630

Note.—Emphysema index = percentage of lung volume less than −900 HU, upper-lung index = emphysema index in upper half of lungs, severe emphysema index = percentage of lung volume less than −960 HU, volume of normal-attenuation lung = volume in attenuation range from −850 HU to −701 HU.
* SD = standard deviation.
† Determined with plethysmography; n = 45.
‡ 1 ft = 0.3 m.

CT Technique

CT examinations of the whole lungs were performed at suspended maximum inspiration on a Somatom Plus scanner (Siemens Medical Systems, Iselin, NJ) without intravenously administered contrast material. Technical parameters included the following: 8-mm (n = 8) or 10-mm (n = 38) collimation; 137 (n = 44) or 120 (n = 2) kV; 180 (n = 23), 210 (n = 2), or 255 (n = 21) mAs; and a scan time of 1 second or less. All patients except for one were scanned in incremental mode; one patient was scanned in spiral mode with use of 8-mm collimation and a pitch of 1.5. CT examinations were performed from 1 day to 7 months (median, 2.3 months) before surgery.

CT Image Analysis

All CT images of lung sections were analyzed at a satellite console (Siemens Medical Systems) by a trained technologist with use of Siemens Pulmo CT software. Pulmo CT is a semiautomated image-processing program that enables (*a*) detection and outlining of the lung margins, (*b*) calculation of lung cross-sectional areas and pixel-attenuation statistics of individual imaged sections, (*c*) a graphic display of results, and (*d*) a summarization of results for all imaged sections analyzed (Figure).

Quantitative CT Indexes

The features of emphysema and corresponding quantitative CT indexes were defined as follows:

Indexes of global emphysema severity: (*a*) mean lung attenuation, (*b*) emphysema index (percentage of whole lung with attenuation on CT images below a threshold value of −900 HU) (16–19), and (*c*) severe emphysema index (percentage of whole lung with attenuation on CT images below a threshold value of −960 HU [defined arbitrarily]).

Indexes of regional emphysema severity: (*a*) emphysema indexes in the upper and lower halves of the lungs (instead of being defined with lobar anatomy, upper and lower halves were defined with an equal number of imaged sections of lung) and (*b*) the ratio of the emphysema index of the upper lung to that of the lower lung.

Indexes of emphysema heterogeneity: (*a*) the standard deviation of the mean lung attenuation and (*b*) the full width at half maximum of the attenuation-frequency distribution curve.

Volume of normally attenuated lung: volume of lung with attenuation in the upper normal range (between −850 and −701 HU).

The display of these measurements with use of Pulmo CT is illustrated in the Figure.

Physiologic Indexes and Outcome Measures

Pulmonary function testing was performed according to the standards of the American Thoracic Society (20,21) with use of a Medgraphics System 1085 (Medical Graphics, St Paul, Minn). Spirometry values obtained after administration of aerosolized albuterol were used in all cases. Lung volumes were determined with plethysmography, and the carbon monoxide diffusing capacity was measured with the single-breath technique. Arterial blood samples were obtained with patients at rest breathing room air, and partial pressures of oxygen and carbon dioxide were measured with a model BG3 blood gas analyzer (Instrumentation Laboratory, Lexington, Mass). The 6-minute walk distance was used to measure exercise tolerance (22).

All preoperative physiologic testing was performed (after 6 weeks of pulmonary-exercise rehabilitation) within 1 month before surgery (mean, 3 days ± 6). Six months after lung-volume reduction surgery, the postoperative changes in FEV_1, Pa_{O_2}, and the 6-minute walk distance were used as outcome measures. Data obtained at 3 months were used in three patients, and data obtained at 1 month were used in one patient; in these patients, data at 6 months were not available.

Data Analysis

Comparison of quantitative CT values with preoperative physiologic values and comparison of quantitative CT and preoperative physiologic values with postoperative measures were made with use of Pearson correlation coefficients. Only correlation coefficients with an absolute value of at least .25 were considered clinically potentially significant.

In addition, patients were stratified into groups according to threshold quantitative CT values determined empirically from the data. The threshold values for each quantitative CT index were chosen initially so that there was an approximately equal number of patients in each stratum. After the mean postoperative change in each outcome measure for each stratum was determined, the threshold was varied to follow natural divisions in the grouping of the data. The stratification thresholds that resulted in the greatest mean differences are presented. Differences in mean preoperative physiologic values and mean postoperative measures between groups stratified by using quantitative CT values were compared with use of an unpaired one-tailed Student t test; equal variance was assumed. The same analysis was also performed by stratifying patients on the basis of each preoperative physiologic index and comparing differences in outcome between groups. The Bonferroni correction for multiple tests was applied. Three pa-

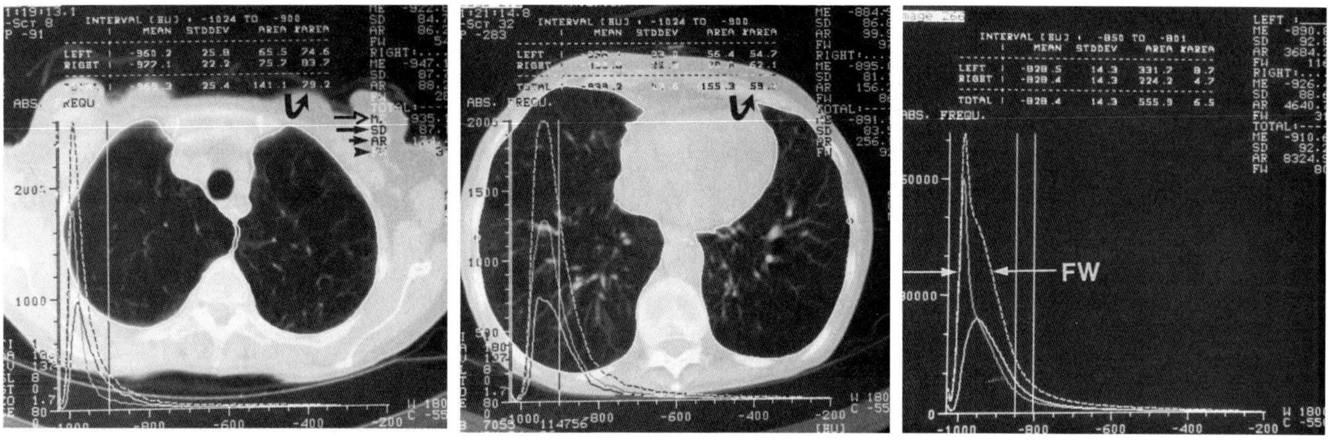

a. b. c.

(a, b) Quantitative data shown on CT images of 10-mm-thick sections through the upper **(a)** and lower **(b)** lungs. The lung margins were automatically outlined, and only attenuation numbers within lung regions were analyzed. The attenuation-frequency distributions are displayed as histograms. The mean lung attenuation (*ME*, open arrow), standard deviation of the mean attenuation (*SD*, long filled arrow), area (*AR*, short arrow), and full width at half maximum (*FW*, arrowhead) are displayed for the total lung section and above that for the left and right lung sections. Statistics for the subrange of attenuation numbers lower than −900 HU, or emphysema index (curved arrow), also are shown. The emphysema index is 79% in **a** and 59% in **b**; there is greater severity of upper-lobe disease. The shapes of the attenuation-frequency histograms also differ between the two scan levels. **(c)** Numerical data and a histogram are displayed for the whole lung with use of summated data from individual imaged sections. Statistics for part of the normal-attenuation subrange (from −850 to −801 HU) are shown. The width of the total-lung histogram at the level of the arrows represents the full width at half maximum (*FW*).

Table 2
Correlation Coeffients Determined by Comparing Values of Preoperative Quantitative CT and Physiologic Indexes with Outcome Measures in 43 Patients

Indexes	Postoperative Change in Physiologic Index: FEV_1	PaO_2	6-minute Walk Distance
Quantitative CT			
Global emphysema severity			
Severe emphysema index	.47 (.001)	.35 (.02)	.32 (.04)
Regional emphysema severity			
Upper-lung index	.37 (.01)	.31 (.04)	NC
Upper-lung index/lower-lung index	.38 (.01)	NC	NC
Heterogeneity			
Full width at half maximum	−.47 (.001)	−.32 (.03)	−.35 (.02)
Standard deviation of mean lung attenuation	.35 (.02)	NC	NC
Volume of normal-attenuation lung	.31 (.04)	NC	NC
Physiologic			
FVC (% predicted)	NC	NC	−.32 (.04)
Total lung capacity (% predicted)	NC	NC	−.25 (.11)
PaO_2	NC	−.34 (.03)	NC
6-minute walk distance	NC	NC	−.34 (.03)

Note.—Numbers are *r* values. Numbers in parentheses are *P* values. NC = no correlation (*r* between −.25 and .25 and $P > .05$).

tients who died in the hospital after surgery were excluded from the analysis of outcome.

RESULTS

Quantitative CT Values versus Outcome Measures

There was fairly wide variability in the values of the quantitative CT and preoperative physiologic indexes of the patients (Table 1). Three patients died of respiratory failure in the early postoperative period and did not undergo postoperative testing. Postoperatively, the mean data of the other 43 patients showed a decrease in total lung capacity of 1.13 L (14%), a decrease in residual volume of 1.77 L (30%), an increase in FEV_1 of 0.36 L (52%), an increase in FVC of 0.54 L (22%), an increase in PaO_2 of 9 mm Hg (15%), and an increase in the 6-minute walk distance of 210 ft (63 m) (19%). All postoperative differences were statistically significant ($P < .0001$, paired *t* test).

The analysis of quantitative CT values was successfully performed in all patients. Many moderately strong correlations were found between values of quantitative CT indexes and improved postoperative outcome measures (Table 2). The correlation coefficients determined by comparing values of global mean lung attenuation and global emphysema indexes with postoperative measures were between −.25 and .25 ($P > .05$).

Significant differences in outcome were found between patient groups stratified by using quantitative CT values (Table 3). A full-width-at-half-maximum value of 80 HU or less was associated with a greater than twofold postoperative improvement in values of FEV_1 and PaO_2 and a greater than threefold improvement in the 6-minute walk distance. A severe emphysema index value greater than 25% and an upper lung emphysema index value 75% or greater were also particularly strongly associated with postoperative improvements. Stratifications by using many other quantitative CT indexes revealed differences in the outcome measures that were of a similar magnitude (Table 3). In each patient, an increasing number of quantitative CT features that were identified as more favorable with stratified comparisons was associated with progressively greater improvement in each outcome measure (Table 4).

Quantitative CT versus Preoperative Physiologic Values

Many moderately strong correlations were found between the values of the preoperative quantitative CT and physiologic indexes (Table 5). The correlations (r values) between all of the values of the quantitative CT indexes and Pa_{O_2} or Pa_{CO_2} were between −.25 and .25 ($P > .05$). Differences in many preoperative physiologic test results were seen between groups stratified by using quantitative CT values (Table 6). The values of mean lung attenuation and volume of normally attenuated lung showed the strongest relationships to many physiologic values in the stratified analysis. The preoperative values of the diffusing capacity of the lung for carbon monoxide were associated with the greatest number of quantitative CT values in the correlation and stratification analyses.

Preoperative Physiologic Values versus Outcome Measures

Few significant correlations were found between the values of the preoperative physiologic indexes and outcome measures (Table 2). The correlation coefficients determined by comparing preoperative values of FEV_1, FEV_1/FVC, residual volume, diffusing capacity of the lung for carbon monoxide, and Pa_{CO_2} with each outcome measure were all between −.25 and .25 ($P > .05$). In the stratified analysis, a preoperative FEV_1 less than 25% of the predicted value, a FVC less than 70% of the predicted value, and total lung capacity less than 150% of the predicted value were each associated with a two to three times greater improvement in the 6-minute walk distance (Table 7). On the basis of stratified preoperative physiologic measures, no obvious trends toward differences in postoperative improvement in FEV_1 or Pa_{O_2} were identified.

Table 3
Outcome Measures of 43 Patients Stratified by Using Preoperative Quantitative CT Values

	Mean Postoperative Increase in Physiologic Index		
Stratification	FEV_1 (L)	Pa_{O_2} (mm Hg)	6-minute Walk Distance (ft)*
Global emphysema severity			
Mean lung attenuation			
>−900 HU (n = 22)	0.31	7	120
≤−900 HU (n = 21)	0.43	12	300
P value	.07	.07	.01
Emphysema index			
<65% (n = 23)	0.33	7	190
≥65% (n = 20)	0.41	12	240
P value	.18	.05	.29
Severe emphysema index			
≤25% (n = 20)	0.28	6	110
>25% (n = 23)	0.44	12	300
P value	.03	.03	.006
Regional emphysema severity			
Upper-lung index			
<75% (n = 22)	0.28	6	160
≥75% (n = 21)	0.46	13	270
P value	.01	.02	.07
Upper-lung index/lower-lung index			
<1.5 (n = 19)	0.26	7	130
≥1.5 (n = 24)	0.45	11	280
P value	.01	.08	.03
Heterogeneity			
Standard deviation of mean lung attenuation			
<95 HU (n = 23)	0.32	9	190
≥90 HU (n = 20)	0.40	10	230
P value	.17	.39	.30
Full width at half maximum			
>80 HU (n = 25)	0.25	6	110
≤80 HU (n = 18)	0.53	14	350
P value	<.001	.008	.001
Volume of normal-attenuation lung			
<1 L (n = 16)	0.26	9	190
≥1 L (n = 27)	0.43	9	230
P value	.03	.42	.31

Note.—By applying the Bonferroni correction, the P value threshold for statistical significance with 24 t tests was .05/24 = .002.
* 1 ft = 0.3 m.

Table 4
Outcome Associated with Number of Favorable Quantitative CT Features

		Mean Postoperative Increase in Physiologic Index		
No. of Quantitative CT Features	No. of Patients	FEV_1 (L)	Pa_{O_2} (mm Hg)	Six-minute Walk Distance (ft)*
≥3	32	0.40	11	250
≥4	26	0.43	11	270
≥5	18	0.51	13	320
≥6	12	0.58	16	400
≥7	9	0.60	18	440

Note.—Favorable quantitative CT features consist of mean lung attenuation −900 HU or less, standard deviation of the mean lung attenuation ≥95 HU, full width at half maximum ≤80 HU, total-lung emphysema index ≥65%, upper-lung emphysema index ≥75%, ratio of upper- to lower-lung indexes ≥1.5, severe emphysema index >25%, and volume of normal-attenuation lung ≥1 L.
* 1 ft = 0.3 m.

DISCUSSION

In candidates for lung-volume reduction surgery, CT is used to identify patients with (a) a heterogeneous distribution of emphysema that is most severe in the upper lobes and (b) a sufficient amount of normal and mildly emphysematous lung to support lung function after resection (9,10). In practice, qualitative evaluation of these features can be difficult, and interobserver variation may be high. For example, we previously found that interobserver agreement (as measured with the mean Pearson correlation coefficient) among four chest radiologists, who graded these features on the conventional preoperative CT scans of 40 patients who had undergone lung-volume reduction surgery, ranged from .5 to .8 for the various features assessed (10). Thus, in many cases, these CT features are likely assessed inconsistently by different observers. Use of quantitative CT indexes to assess emphysema should improve objectivity and consistency and could help standardize the preoperative imaging evaluation of candidates for lung-volume reduction surgery.

Because of the potential advantage, we sought to define quantitative CT parameters that are analogous to pa-

Table 5
Correlation Coefficients Determined by Comparing Values of Quantitative CT and Preoperative Physiologic Indexes in 46 Patients

Quantitative CT Indexes	Preoperative Physiologic Indexes: FEV_1	FVC	FEV_1/FVC	Diffusing Capacity*	6-minute Walk Distance
Global emphysema severity					
Mean lung attenuation	.29 (.05)	NC	.48 (.001)	.58 (<.001)	NC
Emphysema index	NC	NC	−.47 (.001)	−.51 (<.001)	−.29 (.05)
Severe emphysema index	NC	.25 (.09)	NC	−.29 (.05)	−.28 (.06)
Regional emphysema severity					
Upper-lung index	NC	NC	NC	−.30 (.04)	−.32 (.03)
Upper-lung index/lower-lung index	.41 (.005)	NC	.37 (.01)	.43 (.003)	NC
Volume of normal-attenuation lung	.39 (.007)	.35 (.02)	NC	.35 (.02)	NC

Note.— Numbers are *r* values. Numbers in parentheses are *P* values. NC = no correlation (*r* between −.25 and .25 and $P > .05$).
* Diffusing capacity of lung for carbon monoxide.

rameters evaluated qualitatively in the preoperative assessment of patients and determine if quantitative CT provides relevant information for guiding patient selection. Moderately strong correlations were found between the values of quantitative CT indexes and outcome measures, and there were substantial and significant differences in outcome measures between groups of patients stratified by using quantitative CT values of emphysema. Such relationships were not seen between values of preoperative physiologic indexes and outcome measures. These results suggest that quantitative CT analysis provides useful data that cannot be obtained with physiologic testing. Other potential influences on outcome measures—such as general health, cardiac status, comorbid medical conditions, and variations in the volume and location of lung tissue resected among different patients—were not considered.

The determination of emphysema severity by measuring lung attenuation on CT images is a straightforward concept that has been validated by comparing quantitative CT data with pathologic findings (23,24). By definition, emphysema causes the permanent abnormal enlargement of air spaces distal to the terminal bronchiole with destruction of air-space walls (25). On CT images, emphysema appears as a decrease in lung attenuation in the involved areas. The percentage of lung with attenuation below a threshold value is directly related to the amount of macroscopic emphysema. Our study showed that the values of quantitative CT indexes of global and regional emphysema severity were related to outcome measures after lung-volume reduction surgery; this relationship confirms findings discovered by visually grading emphysema severity on imaging studies (8,10).

Unlike the indexes of emphysema severity, there is currently no validated quantitative CT correlate of regional distribution of severity, also referred to as heterogeneity. In clinical practice, heterogeneity is considered an important feature to assess; however, heterogeneity has been defined only loosely in terms of visual analysis. Uniformly severe emphysema throughout the lungs represents low heterogeneity; large bullae superimposed on a background of mostly normal lung represent high heterogeneity. Most patients have a distribution of disease somewhere between these two extremes, and assessment of the extent of heterogeneity can be very subjective. The standard deviation of mean lung attenuation indicates the overall spread of pixel-attenuation values and may serve as a mathematical or statistical index for heterogeneity; however, with the standard deviation of mean lung attenuation, the spatial distribution of the pixel-attenuation values is not considered. There were differences in outcome measures between groups stratified by using the standard deviation, but these differences were smaller than those obtained with other indexes and statistically insignificant. With use of the full width at half maximum, the spatial distribution of emphysema was also not taken into account; however, this index appears more promising as a potential measure of heterogeneity and a predictor of outcome. We found that patients whose attenuation-frequency histograms displayed a narrow, low-attenuation peak showed greater postoperative improvement. Other, more sophisticated mathematical approaches—such as texture analysis (26)—may be better indicators of heterogeneity.

Our results suggest that development of outcome-based quantitative CT selection guidelines for lung-volume reduction surgery may be feasible. Before such guidelines can be determined, several technical issues, which may affect the reliability of quantitative CT data in any individual patient, must be more rigorously studied and the optimal scanning method must be defined. The scanning methods used to quantify emphysema have varied, and no single method has been universally advocated. Some investigations have been performed with use of a conventional section thickness (16,23,27,28). Use of thin-section CT increases the sensitivity of detecting mild emphysema (29,30), and this modality is frequently used. However, use of thin-section CT may be unnecessary to quantify emphysema in candidates for lung-volume reduction surgery because these patients have extensive advanced disease (although use of thin-section CT may improve assessment of less diseased lung regions).

The level of inspiration can affect quantitative CT values (31–33); however, level of inspiration has not been controlled in most quantitative CT studies of emphysema. In one study of 20 patients with emphysema in which lung volume was controlled with use of a spirometer (34), the emphysema index (defined with an attenuation threshold of −910 HU) changed by 33% when lung volume was gated at 10% and 90% of vital capacity. The difference in lung attenuation at different inspiratory levels near total lung capacity may be less because patients with emphysema have a reduced inspiratory capacity. This hypothesis is supported with the finding of no significant difference between the mean emphysema index on ungated inspiratory CT scans and that on expiratory scans in a group of 10 patients before lung-volume reduction surgery (16). However, the inspiratory level could affect the reproducibility of various quantitative CT values in individual patients.

Investigators (23,27,35) have advocated different optimal attenuation thresholds for defining emphysema when pathologic correlation was performed. The purpose of our study was to explore the relationship between quantitative CT values and outcome measures after lung-volume reduction

Table 6
Preoperative Physiologic Test Results in 46 Patients Stratified by Using Quantitative CT Values

	Preoperative Physiologic Indexes						
Stratification	FEV_1 (L)	FVC (L)	FEV_1/FVC	Diffusing Capacity* (mL/min/mm Hg)	Pa_{O_2} (mm Hg)	Pa_{CO_2} (mm Hg)	6-minute Walk Distance (ft)†
Global emphysema severity							
Mean lung attenuation							
≥−900 HU (n = 23)	0.77	2.46	31.7	10.3	62	41	1,220
<−900 HU (n = 23)	0.65	2.47	26.6	7.4	59	42	990
P value	.06	.49	.004	.005	.20	.39	.004
Emphysema index							
<65% (n = 23)	0.76	2.44	31.0	10.2	63	41	1,170
≥65% (n = 23)	0.67	2.48	26.9	7.6	58	42	1,060
P value	.11	.40	.01	.01	.03	.29	.17
Severe emphysema index							
≤25% (n = 20)	0.74	2.50	30.1	10.2	65	42	1,240
>25% (n = 26)	0.69	2.44	28.0	7.9	57	42	1,000
P value	.21	.38	.13	.02	.006	.43	.002
Regional emphysema severity							
Upper-lung index							
<75% (n = 22)	0.72	2.42	29.7	9.5	61	42	1,180
≥75% (n = 24)	0.71	2.50	28.2	8.3	60	41	1,030
P value	.45	.34	.21	.16	.39	.40	.04
Upper-lung index/lower-lung index							
<1.5 (n = 21)	0.65	2.37	27.6	8.7	60	43	1,110
≥1.5 (n = 25)	0.76	2.54	30.0	9.0	61	41	1,100
P value	.05	.18	.09	.39	.44	.19	.43
Volume of normal-attenuation lung							
<1.0 L (n = 17)	0.60	2.20	27.1	7.3	59	44	1,040
≥1.0 L (n = 29)	0.78	2.62	30.0	9.8	62	40	1,140
P value	.003	.01	.06	.02	.19	.05	.15

Note.—By applying the Bonferroni correction, the P value threshold for statistical significance with 42 t tests was .05/42 = .001.
* Diffusing capacity of lung for carbon monoxide.
† One foot = 0.3 m.

surgery; we did not attempt to determine attenuation thresholds that would optimize correlation between quantitative CT data and pathologic findings. Like several other investigators (16–19), we chose a threshold of −900 HU to define the emphysema index for global and regional assessment. Because all patients in our study had severe emphysema, we wanted to see if an even lower threshold would distinguish better the patients that would improve most with lung-volume reduction surgery. Therefore, a severe global emphysema index was defined with the arbitrarily assigned lower threshold of −960 HU. This lower threshold resulted in a stronger correlation of the value of this index with outcome measures than the −900 HU threshold. A different threshold may result in an even stronger correlation. The section thickness can alter the optimal attenuation threshold used for correlation with pathologic findings (23,35); therefore, thresholds that enable the identification of the greatest outcome differences among stratified groups may vary on the basis of section thickness.

Lung-attenuation measurements can be affected considerably by the number and locations of sections analyzed, which have varied widely in previous studies; some investigators have acquired scans at as few as two levels (24,34,36). However, sampling theory indicates that images of many more sections may be needed for adequately precise analysis, depending on the distribution of disease (37). We chose to analyze the whole lung to minimize the possible effects of sampling error. Analysis of fewer imaged sections would be more efficient and may produce equivalent results. Because our studies were not performed with the spiral technique, there was likely some sampling error owing to respiratory variation; however, this is a random event and should not have had a systematic effect on the results.

Like the results of previous studies, our results demonstrate a relationship between quantitative CT attenuation values and pulmonary function in emphysema. The correlations between values of preoperative mean lung attenuation and physiologic indexes in our study are in the range of those correlations determined by others. To our knowledge, correlation coefficients in the literature determined with mean lung attenuation and FEV_1 values range from .15 to .76; correlation coefficients determined with values of mean lung attenuation and those of diffusing capacity of the lung for carbon monoxide (or transfer coefficient) range from .29 to .68 (19,27,34,38,39). Similarly, to our knowledge, the reported correlation coefficients determined with emphysema index and FEV_1 values range from −.15 to −.80, and the correlation coefficients determined with values of the emphysema index and those of the diffusing capacity of the lung for carbon monoxide (or transfer coefficient) range from −.40 to −.73 (19,27,34,38). This fairly wide variation in the correlation coefficients may be related to differences in methodology, patient population, or both. Our correlation coefficient values typically fell in the midrange of reported values.

There were only moderate correlations between values of lung attenuation and preoperative physiologic indexes, but pulmonary function may be affected by factors other than the alveolar destruction that alters lung attenuation in emphysema. For example, expiratory airflow may be impaired to different extents in patients with similar lung densities but different severities of airway disease. Likewise, gas exchange may vary with differences in ventilation-perfusion matching in addition to differences in alveolar destruction. An imperfect correlation is expected because quan-

Table 7
Outcome Meaures of 43 Patients Stratified by Using Preoperative Physiologic Values

Stratification	Mean Postoperative Increase in Physiologic Index: FEV_1 (L)	Pa_{O_2} (mm Hg)	6-minute Walk Distance (ft)*
FVC			
<70% predicted (n = 20)	0.33	10	290
≥70% predicted (n = 23)	0.39	9	140
P value	.24	.40	.03
FEV_1			
<25% predicted (n = 23)	0.37	12	300
≥25% predicted (n = 20)	0.36	7	110
P value	.45	.06	.006
Residual volume†			
<300% predicted (n = 23)	0.32	7	200
≥300% predicted (n = 19)	0.40	11	230
P value	.15	.14	.38
Total lung capacity†			
<150% predicted (n = 25)	0.35	7	280
≥150% predicted (n = 17)	0.36	11	120
P value	.48	.11	.02
Diffusing capacity‡			
≤30% predicted (n = 23)	0.34	11	270
>30% predicted (n = 20)	0.39	7	150
P value	.29	.13	.06
Pa_{O_2}			
<60 mm Hg (n = 20)	0.35	12	230
≥60 mm Hg (n = 23)	0.38	7	200
P value	.36	.09	.37
Pa_{CO_2}			
≤45 mm Hg (n = 29)	0.38	8	180
>45 mm Hg (n = 14)	0.34	12	280
P value	.34	.17	.12
6-minute walk distance*			
<1,200 ft (n = 23)	0.40	11	250
≥1,200 ft (n = 20)	0.34	7	170
P value	.22	.11	.17

Note.—By applying the Bonferroni correction, the P value threshold for statistical significance with 24 t tests was .05/24 = .002.
* 1 ft = 0.3 m.
† Residual volume and total lung capacity of one patient were not available.
‡ Diffusing capacity of lung for carbon monoxide.

titative CT allows assessment of anatomic features and not physiologic features. Assessment of anatomic and physiologic features in candidates for lung-volume reduction surgery is important; these features provide complementary information. Physiologic testing enables the physician to decide if functional impairment is of appropriate severity to warrant the risks of surgery and is important in postoperative assessment. CT (and other radiologic testing) enables the physician to identify the severely impaired patients that are most likely to benefit from surgery.

Most investigators who have compared densitometric and physiologic index values of pulmonary function have focused solely on quantifying the volume of emphysema. We found that the volume of normal lung (defined with an attenuation in the −850 to −701 HU subrange) was also associated with many preoperative physiologic values in the correlation and stratification analyses. The potential physiologic importance of this index also was identified in another study, in which the preoperative volume of normally attenuated lung was highly correlated with FEV_1 after pulmonary resection for lung cancer (40).

In summary, we defined quantitative CT indexes in emphysema that are analogous to features evaluated visually on CT scans of candidates for lung-volume reduction surgery. Many quantitative CT values were correlated with clinical outcome measures, and significant differences were found among groups stratified by using quantitative CT values. The relationships between preoperative physiologic values and outcome measures were much more limited. Standardization of data acquisition and analysis techniques may be needed; however, these data suggest that quantitative CT may aid identification of patients who are candidates for lung-volume reduction surgery and the standardization of the selection process. ■

References

1. Cooper J, Trulock E, Triantafillou A, et al. Bilateral pneumectomy (volume reduction) for chronic obstructive pulmonary disease. J Thorac Cardiovasc Surg 1995; 109:106–119.
2. McKenna RJ Jr, Brenner M, Gelb AF, et al. A randomized, prospective trial of stapled lung reduction versus laser bullectomy for diffuse emphysema. J Thorac Cardiovasc Surg 1996; 111:317–322.
3. Keenan RJ, Landreneau RJ, Sciurba FC, et al. Unilateral thoracoscopic surgical approach for diffuse emphysema. J Thorac Cardiovasc Surg 1996; 111:308–315.
4. Sciurba FC, Rogers RM, Keenan RJ, et al. Improvement in pulmonary function and elastic recoil after lung-reduction surgery for diffuse emphysema. N Engl J Med 1996; 334:1095–1099.
5. Daniel TM, Chan BB, Bhaskar V, et al. Lung volume reduction surgery, case selection, operative technique, and clinical results. Ann Surg 1996; 223:526–531.
6. Brenner M, Yusen R, McKenna RJ Jr, et al. Lung volume reduction surgery for emphysema. Chest 1996; 110:205–218.
7. Kotloff RM, Tino G, Bavaria JE, et al. Bilateral lung volume reduction surgery for advanced emphysema: a comparison of median sternotomy and thoracoscopic approaches. Chest 1996; 110:1399–1406.
8. McKenna RJ Jr, Brenner M, Fischel RJ, Gelb AF. Should lung volume reduction for emphysema be unilateral or bilateral? J Thorac Cardiovasc Surg 1996; 112:1331–1339.
9. Slone RM, Gierada DS. Radiology of pulmonary emphysema and lung volume reduction surgery. Semin Thorac Cardiovasc Surg 1996; 8:61–82.
10. Slone RM, Pilgram TK, Gierada DS, et al. Lung volume reduction surgery: comparison of preoperative radiologic features and clinical outcome. Radiology 1997; 205:685–693.
11. Yusen RD, Lefrak SS. Evaluation of patients with emphysema for lung volume reduction surgery. Semin Thorac Cardiovasc Surg 1996; 8:83–93.
12. Wendt CH, Teel G, Rosenthal B, Dunitz J, Maddaus MA. The increase in FEV-1 in lung reduction surgery correlates to the degree of emphysema in the nonresected lung measured by HRCT (abstr). Am J Respir Crit Care Med 1996; 153:A267.
13. Stern EJ, Frank MS. CT of the lung in patients with pulmonary emphysema: diagnosis, quantification, and correlation with pathologic and physiologic findings. AJR 1994; 162:791–798.
14. Thurlbeck WM, Muller NL. Emphysema: definition, imaging, and quantification. AJR 1994; 163:1017–1025.
15. Cooper JD, Patterson GA, Sundaresan RS, et al. Results of 150 consecutive bilateral lung volume reduction procedures in patients with severe emphysema. J Thorac Cardiovasc Surg 1996; 112:1319–1329.
16. Bae KT, Slone RM, Gierada DS, Yusen RD, Cooper JD. Patients with emphysema: quantitative CT analysis before and after lung volume reduction surgery. Radiology 1997; 203:705–714.
17. Hayhurst MD, Flenley DC, McLean A, et al. Diagnosis of pulmonary emphysema by computerised tomography. Lancet 1984; 2:320–322.
18. Crausman RS, Ferguson G, Irvin CG, Make B, Newell JD. Quantitative chest computed tomography as a means of predicting exercise performance in severe emphysema. Acad Radiol 1995; 2:463–469.
19. Miniati M, Filippi E, Falaschi F, et al. Radiologic evaluation of emphysema in patients with chronic obstructive pulmonary disease: chest radiography versus high

resolution computed tomography. Am J Respir Crit Care Med 1995; 151:1359–1367.
20. American Thoracic Society. Standardization of spirometry: 1987 update. Am Rev Respir Dis 1987; 136:1285–1298.
21. American Thoracic Society. Lung function testing: selection of reference values and interpretive strategies. Am Rev Respir Dis 1991; 144:1202–1218.
22. Butland R, Pang J, Gross E, Woodcock A, Geddes D. Two-, six-, and 12-minute walking tests in respiratory disease. Br Med J 1982; 284:1607–1608.
23. Müller NL, Staples CA, Miller RR, Abboud RT. "Density mask": an objective method to quantitate emphysema using computed tomography. Chest 1988; 94:782–787.
24. Gould GA, MacNee W, McLean A, et al. CT measurements of lung density in life can quantitate distal airspace enlargement: an essential defining feature of human emphysema. Am Rev Respir Dis 1988; 137: 380–392.
25. Snider GL, Kleinerman J, Thurlbeck WM, Bengali ZH. The definition of emphysema: report of a national Heart, Lung, and Blood Institute, Division of Lung Diseases workshop. Am Rev Respir Dis 1985; 132: 182–185.
26. Haralick RM, Shanmugan K, Dinstein I. Textural features for image classification. IEEE Trans SMC 1973; 3:610–621.
27. Gould GA, Redpath AT, Ryan M, et al. Lung CT density correlates with measurements of airflow limitation and the diffusing capacity. Eur Respir J 1991; 4:141–146.
28. Holbert JM, Brown ML, Sciurba FC, et al. Changes in lung volume and volume of emphysema after unilateral lung reduction surgery: analysis with CT lung densitometry. Radiology 1996; 201:793–797.
29. Hruban R, Meziane M, Zerhouni E, et al. High resolution computed tomography of inflation fixed lungs: pathologic-radiologic correlation of centrilobular emphysema. Am Rev Respir Dis 1987; 136:935–940.
30. Miller RR, Müller NL, Vedal S, Morrison NJ, Staples CA. Limitations of computed tomography in the assessment of emphysema. Am Rev Respir Dis 1989; 139:980–983.
31. Rosenblum LJ, Mauceri RA, Wellenstein DE, et al. Density patterns in the normal lung as determined by computed tomography. Radiology 1980; 137:409–416.
32. Kalender WA, Rienmüller R, Seissler W, et al. Measurement of pulmonary parenchymal attenuation: use of spirometric gating with quantitative CT. Radiology 1990; 175: 265–268.
33. Kalender WA, Fichte H, Bautz W, Skalej M. Semiautomatic evaluation procedures for quantitative CT of the lung. J Comput Assist Tomogr 1991; 15:248–255.
34. Lamers RJ, Thelissen GR, Kessels AG, Wouters EF, van Engelshoven JM. Chronic obstructive pulmonary disease: evaluation with spirometrically controlled CT lung densitometry. Radiology 1994; 193: 109–113.
35. Gevenois PA, de Maertelaer V, De Vuyst P, Zanen J, Yernault JC. Comparison of computed density and macroscopic morphometry in pulmonary emphysema. Am J Respir Crit Care Med 1995; 152:653–657.
36. Knudson RJ, Standen JR, Kaltenborn WT, et al. Expiratory computed tomography for assessment of suspected pulmonary emphysema. Chest 1991; 99:1357–1366.
37. Henschke CI. Image selection for computed tomography of the chest: a sampling approach. Invest Radiol 1992; 27:908–911.
38. Kinsella M, Müller NL, Abboud RT, Morrison NJ, DyBuncio A. Quantitation of emphysema by computed tomography using a density mask program and correlation with pulmonary function tests. Chest 1990; 97: 315–321.
39. Heremans A, Verschakelen JA, Van fraeyenhoven L, Demedts M. Measurement of lung density by means of quantitative CT scanning: a study of correlations with pulmonary function tests. Chest 1992; 102:805–811.
40. Wu MT, Chang JM, Chiang AA, et al. Use of quantitative CT to predict postoperative lung function in patients with lung cancer. Radiology 1994; 191:257–262.

Samuel C. Wang, MD • Keith C. Fischer, MD • Richard M. Slone, MD • David S. Gierada, MD
Roger D. Yusen, MD • Stephen S. Lefrak, MD • Thomas K. Pilgram, PhD • Joel D. Cooper, MD

Perfusion Scintigraphy in the Evaluation for Lung Volume Reduction Surgery: Correlation with Clinical Outcome[1]

PURPOSE: **To identify preoperative pulmonary perfusion scintigraphic findings that might be associated with clinical outcome after lung volume reduction surgery.**

MATERIALS AND METHODS: **Preoperative perfusion scintigrams in 103 patients (56 men, 47 women; age range, 41–76 years; mean age, 61 years ± 9) were reviewed and graded for emphysematous heterogeneity (from isolated areas to diffuse distribution), extent of maximally perfused lung, and lobar predominance (upper-lobe vs lower-lobe asymmetry). These findings were correlated with clinical outcome on the basis of pulmonary function, arterial blood gas levels, and exercise test results before and 6 months after surgery.**

RESULTS: **Among the 96 patients who survived surgery, there was an average improvement of 47% in the forced expiratory volume in 1 second (FEV_1), of 20% in arterial oxygen tension, and of 20% in the 6-minute walking distance. Scintigraphic markers correlated best with FEV_1 improvement. The strongest scintigraphic predictor of increase in FEV_1 was upper-lobe predominance (r = .38, $P < .001$), which was followed by heterogeneity (r = .31, P =.002). The seven patients who died had a significantly lower percentage of maximally perfused lung than the survivors (25% vs 34%, P = .004).**

CONCLUSION: **Perfusion scintigraphy can provide modest prognostic information in patients who undergo evaluation for lung volume reduction surgery.**

Chronic obstructive pulmonary disease, including emphysema, is a major cause of death and disability worldwide (1,2). Medical therapy typically includes smoking cessation; drug treatment with bronchodilators, steroids, and antibiotics; supplemental oxygen; pulmonary rehabilitation; and exercise training (3). Emphysema, however, is an irreversible process, and in those patients with advanced disease, there is frequently little functional improvement or symptomatic relief that can be achieved with this standard therapy. Lung transplantation has been effective in treating patients with end-stage emphysema; however, use of this procedure has been limited by the scarcity of donors and by complications associated with long-term immunosuppression and rejection (4,5).

Over the last 4 years, lung volume reduction surgery has emerged as another promising surgical option for select patients with severe debilitating emphysema as a palliative procedure to alleviate symptoms of breathlessness and improve quality of life. Unlike conventional bullectomy, the surgery is not limited to removing individual large bullae, but involves the resection of hyperinflated, nonfunctional areas of lung (6). The rationale for doing this is to (*a*) reduce the total thoracic volume and thus improve chest wall and diaphragmatic respiratory mechanics, (*b*) increase lung elastic recoil and thus decrease airway obstruction, and (*c*) redistribute ventilation to more normal areas of the lung (7–9).

A variety of techniques have been described for lung volume reduction surgery, including bilateral or unilateral stapled resections or laser ablation via sternotomy, thoracotomy, or thoracoscopy (10,11). At our institution, the procedure is performed by means of sternotomy and involves the bilateral, stapled, nonsegmental wedge resection of multiple regions of severely emphysematous lungs (12). Approximately 20%–30% of the volume of the lungs is excised.

Candidates for lung volume reduction surgery undergo extensive preoperative evaluation, which typically includes the performance of ventilation-perfusion scintigraphy (13,14). These scintigrams in conjunction with other radiologic studies serve to provide information about the distribution and overall severity of emphysema. Within the operating room, the scans are used to determine which

Index terms: Emphysema, pulmonary, 60.751 • Lung, perfusion, 60.12171 • Lung, radionuclide studies, 60.12171 • Lung, surgery, 60.459

Abbreviations: ANOVA = analysis of variance, FEV_1 = forced expiratory volume in 1 second, PaO_2 =arterial oxygen tension while breathing room air.

Radiology 1997; 205:243–248

[1] From the Mallinckrodt Institute of Radiology (S.C.W, K.C.F., R.M.S., D.S.G, T.K.P.) and the Divisions of Pulmonary and Critical Care Medicine (R.D.Y., S.S.L.), General Medical Sciences (R.D.Y.), and Cardiothoracic Surgery (J.D.C), Washington University School of Medicine, St Louis, Mo. From the 1996 RSNA scientific assembly. Received April 16, 1997; revision requested May 14; revision received June 24; accepted June 27. R.M.S. supported in part by an RSNA Research and Education Fund seed grant. R.D.Y. supported in part by National Institutes of Health–National Heart, Lung, and Blood Institute grant HL07317 and the Norman P. Knowlton, Jr, MD, Incentive for Excellence Fund of Barnes-Jewish Hospital. **Address reprint requests to** K.C.F., Mallinckrodt Institute of Radiology, Division of Nuclear Medicine, Barnes-Jewish Hospital, 216 S Kingshighway Blvd, St Louis, MO 63110.

lung to operate on first (the most emphysematous lung), and they are also used as a surgical road map for identification of target areas for resection within each lung.

To our knowledge, large, controlled studies that compare the results of lung volume reduction surgery and intensive medical therapy have yet to be done. The preliminary results of lung volume reduction surgery at several centers suggest that substantial improvements in lung function, exercise tolerance, oxygen requirements, quality of life, and perceived dyspnea can be achieved in a majority of carefully selected patients (15–18). However, in this high-risk group of patients with emphysema, poor outcome and death also occur, and considerable uncertainty remains with regard to optimal patient selection, surgical techniques, overall benefit, and duration of response (19). The purpose of this study was to evaluate the preoperative perfusion scans in those patients who underwent lung volume reduction surgery to identify scintigraphic markers that might be associated with good or poor clinical outcome.

MATERIALS AND METHODS

Patients

We retrospectively evaluated findings in a cohort of 103 of the first 110 patients to undergo lung volume reduction surgery at our institution (56 men, 47 women; age range, 41–76 years; mean age, 61 years ± 9). Seven patients were excluded from the study owing to incomplete scintigraphic or clinical follow-up data. General guidelines for patient selection were as outlined in Figure 1. These were not strict guidelines, and not all patients fulfilled each of the criteria.

Imaging Protocol

All patients underwent preoperative ventilation-perfusion scintigraphy by using a large–field-of-view scintillation camera (Siemens Medical Systems, Hoffman Estates, Ill) fitted with a low-energy, medium-resolution, parallel-hole collimator. Ventilation scanning was performed by using either krypton-81m or xenon-133; however, scans were not evaluated in this study.

For perfusion imaging, each patient received 92.5–185.0 MBq (2.5–5.0 mCi) technetium-99m macroaggregated albumin (Mallinckrodt, St Louis, Mo). A reduced number of particles, approximately 200,000, were injected as per our standard protocol in patients with severe lung disease. The posterior view was obtained for 600,000 counts and then anterior, left and right posterior oblique, and left and right lateral projections were acquired for the same time.

Image Interpretation

The perfusion images were independently reviewed and scored by six readers, which included two nuclear medicine physicians (S.C.W., K.C.F.), two chest radiologists (R.M.S., D.S.G.), and two pulmonologists (R.D.Y., S.S.L.). The pulmonologists are members of a dedicated group of specialists involved in the evaluation for emphysema surgery at our institution. They are experienced in the interpretation of ventilation-perfusion scans in this group of patients. The readers were blinded to patient identity and clinical outcome. The images were graded for heterogeneity of disease distribution, for the percentage of lung that was maximally perfused, and for upper- versus lower-lobe predominance of disease.

Heterogeneity was defined as the regional variation in the severity of emphysema throughout the lungs. This was scored from 1 to 10, with high scores indicative of target areas of severely emphysematous lung among areas of mild emphysema and with low scores indicative of diffuse emphysema throughout the lungs, with all regions similarly affected (Fig 2).

The percentage of maximal perfusion was defined as the percentage of the total lung volume perfused at the maximal count density. This was not computer quantified, but was a subjective visual estimate of the extent of disease (Fig 3).

Lobar predominance of disease was graded on a scale of 1 to 5, with a low score representative of predominantly upper-lobe emphysema and a high score representative of predominantly lower-lobe emphysema (Fig 4).

Surgical Method and Clinical Outcome

Bilateral stapled lung volume reduction surgery was performed by means of median sternotomy. Details on surgical technique and postoperative management have previously been described (12,20,21).

All surviving patients included in this study had a minimum postsurgical follow-up of 6 months. Findings on the perfusion scans were correlated with clinical outcome in terms of the difference between preoperative and 6-month postoperative follow-up forced expiratory volume in 1 second (FEV_1), arterial oxygen tension while breathing room air (PaO_2), and distance that the patient could walk in 6 minutes. Postbronchodilator values of FEV_1 were used for data analysis. Arterial blood samples and PaO_2 measurements were obtained while the patients were sitting and breathing room air. The 6-minute walk was performed in a level, premeasured hallway, and the patient was encouraged to walk as far as possible in the allotted time. Supplemental oxygen was given as needed to maintain arterial oxygen saturation of greater than 88%.

- Severe pulmonary emphysema
- Disabling dyspnea despite maximal medical therapy
- Age younger than 75 years
- Ability to participate in pulmonary rehabilitation program
- No coexisting medical problems that would substantially increase surgical risk
- Abstinence from cigarette smoking
- Hyperinflated thorax
- Heterogeneous emphysema distribution
- FEV_1 < 35% predicted
- $PaCO_2$ < 55 mm Hg
- No clinically important pulmonary artery hypertension (mean < 35 mm Hg)

Figure 1. Patient selection guidelines, 1993–1995. *$PaCO_2$* = arterial carbon dioxide tension.

Statistical Analysis

Summary statistics of clinical and scintigraphic data are expressed as mean ± one standard deviation. Reader agreement was examined by calculating Pearson coefficients of correlation for all measurements. The mean response was calculated for all readers for each patient. These average values were compared with clinical outcome by using Pearson correlation coefficients. For each scintigraphic parameter, the patients were also stratified according to score into three subgroups, and the differences in mean outcome values between the subgroups were tested for significance by using the analysis of variance (ANOVA). Stratification was performed by dividing the range of scores by 3. Paired two-tailed Student t tests were performed to determine the significance of outcome improvement within each subgroup. A P value of less than .05 was considered to indicate a statistically significant difference. Multivariate analysis by using backward stepwise regression was performed to find the best model fit between outcome and scintigraphic findings.

RESULTS

Within the 6-month follow-up, seven patients died. Six died of respiratory failure, and one died of cerebrovascular accident. Four died within the first 90 days after surgery. For the 96 surviving patients, the absolute and percentage of improvements in FEV_1, PaO_2, and 6-minute walking distance are presented in Table 1.

The mean interobserver correlation coefficient was .81 for lobar predominance, .56 for heterogeneity, and .41 for percentage of maximal perfusion.

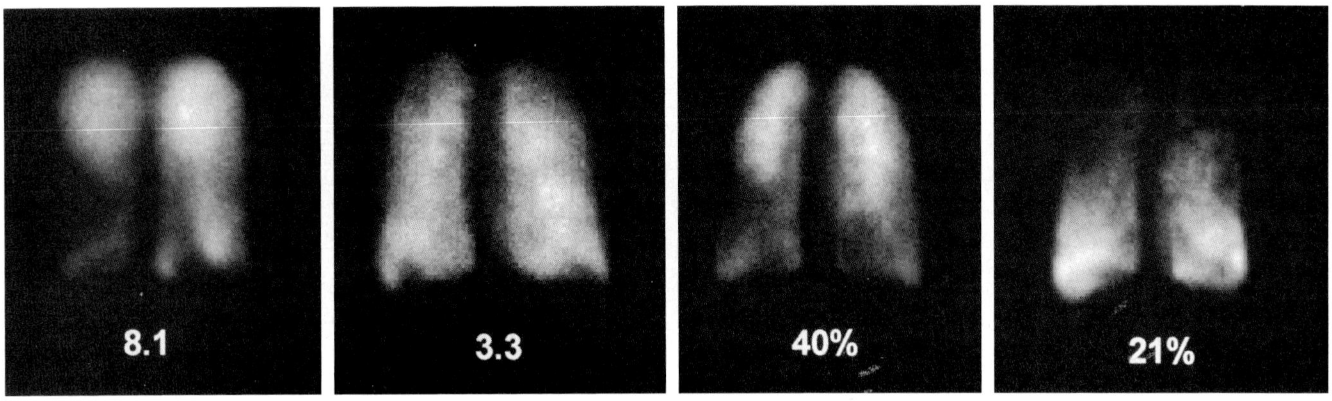

2a. 2b. 3a. 3b.

Figures 2, 3. **(2)** Posterior perfusion images and corresponding mean heterogeneity scores in two patients: **(a)** one with focal areas of severe emphysema and **(b)** one with diffuse areas of emphysema. **(3)** Posterior perfusion images and corresponding mean percentages of maximal perfusion in two patients: **(a)** one with a large portion and **(b)** one with a small portion of lung perfused at the maximal count density.

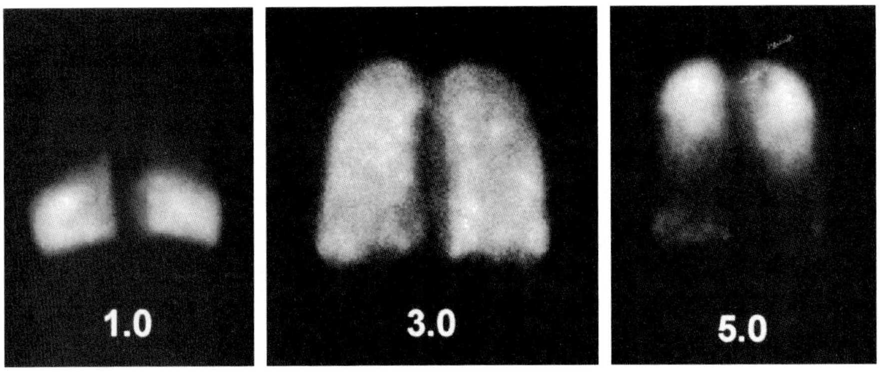

a. b. c.

Figure 4. Posterior perfusion images and corresponding mean lobar predominance scores in three patients: **(a)** one with predominantly upper-lobe emphysema, **(b)** one with evenly distributed emphysema, and **(c)** one with predominantly lower-lobe emphysema.

Table 1
Clinical Results at 6 Months in the 96 Patients

Clinical Parameter	Improvement from Preoperative Value	
	Mean ± Standard Deviation	Range
FEV_1 (L)	0.33 ± 0.29* (47 ± 38)	−0.22 to 1.57
PaO_2 (mm Hg)	9.1 ± 10.2* (20 ± 20)	−11.0 to 54.0
6-minute walking distance (m)	57.0 ± 78.0* (20 ± 34)	−129.5 to 258.2

Note.—Numbers in parentheses are percentages ± standard deviations.
* $P < .001$ (two-tailed Student t test).

There were several correlations between the scintigraphic measures and outcome (Table 2). The outcome measure that most strongly correlated with the scintigraphic measures was FEV_1, followed distantly by PaO_2 and the 6-minute walking distance. The best scintigraphic predictor of increase in FEV_1 was upper-lobe predominance ($r = .38$, $P < .001$) (Fig 5) followed by heterogeneity ($r = .31$, $P = .002$). The percentage of maximal perfusion did not correlate at a significant level with the increase in FEV_1 ($r = .19$, $P = .067$). The best backward stepwise model for predicting the increase in FEV_1 combined lobar predominance and heterogeneity as the independent variables ($r = .52$, $r^2 = .27$).

Table 3 summarizes the patient outcome as stratified by scintigraphic score for lobar predominance, heterogeneity, and maximal perfusion. Patients with upper-lobe emphysema had significantly greater improvement in FEV_1 than did those with evenly distributed or lower-lobe emphysema ($P = .001$). Patients with either upper- or lower-lobe emphysema had significantly greater improvement in the 6-minute walking distance than did those with evenly distributed disease ($P = .016$). Significantly greater improvement in FEV_1 was noted in subgroups with greater heterogeneity ($P = .047$). There was no significant difference in outcome improvement when patients were stratified according to percentage of maximal perfusion. Within each scintigraphic subgroup, patients on the average had statistically significant improvement in FEV_1, PaO_2, and 6-minute walking distance, with the exception of those with evenly distributed emphysema, low heterogeneity scores, or high perfusion scores who did not have statistically significant improvement in the 6-minute walking distance.

Mortality analysis demonstrated a significant difference ($P = .004$) in the percentage of maximal perfusion between the 96 surviving patients (34% ± 8) and the seven who died (25% ± 4) (Table 4). There was also a significant difference in age (60 years ± 9 vs 70 years ± 4, $P = .004$). No statistically significant difference in the heterogeneity and lobar predominance scores was present between the two groups.

DISCUSSION

Appropriate patient selection is an important key to the success of lung volume reduction surgery. Routine diagnostic imaging studies for screening and preoperative evaluation at our institution include posteroanterior and lateral chest radiography during inspiration and expiration, conventional chest computed tomography (CT), and quantitative ventilation-perfusion scintigraphy.

Findings of initial studies (22,23) have indicated that radiologic findings can make an important contribution to predicting the degree of improvement and thereby provide some guidance in developing the criteria for the selection of appropriate patients. Radiographic and CT features found to be suggestive of good outcome include hyperinflation with limited diaphragmatic excursion, predominantly upper-lobe emphysema with heterogeneous distribution, the presence of compressed lung, and some residual normal or mildly emphysematous lung (22,23). Some of these radiologic features are reflected and supported by the scintigraphic features found to be clinically important in this study.

Although there were several statistically significant relationships between the scintigraphic markers studied in this investigation and various measures of clinical outcome, the correlations were often weak, which suggests that factors other than emphysema distribution and relative severity influence outcome. The preoperative patient health profile, surgical technique used, and postoperative management also likely influence the clinical results. The stronger correlation between the scintigraphic markers and FEV_1, as opposed to PaO_2 or the 6-minute walking distance, may reflect the closer relationship between FEV_1 and the prognosis that has been observed in patients with chronic obstructive pulmonary disease (24–26).

The results of this study demonstrate a correlation between measures of clinical outcome (particularly FEV_1) and lobar predominance of disease, as well as the heterogeneity of disease distribution. The greater improvement in FEV_1 seen in patients with predominantly upper-lobe emphysema may have several explanations. It has been observed in several studies that the contribution of the lower lobes to total lung function is greater than that of the upper lobes (27–29). Thus, it is possible that patients with more severe lower-lobe disease will have less reserve for improvement than those with upper-lobe disease.

Alternatively, the difference in FEV_1 outcome may not be directly related to the location of disease, but rather to the underlying histopathologic findings. Panlobular emphysema, which has a basal predominance, may have a different effect on lung function than centrilobular emphysema, which has an upper-lobe predominance. Alpha$_1$-antitrypsin deficiency is a classic example of panlobular emphysema. Smoking is traditionally described as a typical cause of centrilobular emphysema, although panlobular emphysema may also develop (30,31). In centrilobular emphysema, there is distention and destruction of the central part of the acinus formed by the respiratory bronchiole, while the distal alveoli are spared. In panlobular emphysema, there is diffuse enlargement and destruction of the entire acinus. In addition, the small airways in centrilobular emphysema tend to be more inflamed and constricted than those in panlobular emphysema (32).

Given these structural differences, one might expect important mechanical and functional differences. Indeed, findings of the study by Kim and colleagues (30) on centrilobular and panlobular emphysema in smokers indicated that elastic recoil losses were more marked in panlobular than in centrilobular emphysema. Increased elastic recoil is one of the mechanisms shown to be associated with improvement in pulmonary function after lung volume reduction surgery (7). In their analysis of the possible effects of lung volume reduction surgery in emphysematous lungs, Cosio and Majo (32) predicted that, in patients with predominantly centrilobular emphysema, higher elastic recoil pressures could be attained in the volume-reduced lung, with consequent improvement in air flow. In patients with predominantly panlobular emphysema, they predicted that the diffuse involvement of the acinus would prevent a marked increase in elastic recoil and result in little or no improvement after lung volume reduction surgery.

Heterogeneity in the distribution of emphysema has also emerged as an important imaging feature (22,23). This is not surprising, because it is a marker for potential target zones that can be resected without substantially compromising lung function. Resection of these regions of lung, which contribute to volume but not function, increases the ratio of normal to diseased lung. This would not be possible in a lung that was homogeneously diseased.

In this study, upper-lobe emphy-

Table 2
Correlation between Scintigraphic Measures and Clinical Improvement

Scintigraphic Measure	FEV_1 r*	FEV_1 P Value†	PaO_2 r*	PaO_2 P Value†	6-minute Walking Distance r*	6-minute Walking Distance P Value†
Lobar predominance	−.38	<.001	−.24	.021	−.06	.57
Heterogeneity	.31	.002	.02	.83	.26	.010
Percentage of maximal perfusion	.19	.067	−.08	.44	.01	.92

Note.—For lobar predominance, lower scores in this study represented greater upper-lobe emphysema and higher scores represented greater lower-lobe emphysema.
* Pearson correlation coefficient.
† Two-tailed Student t test.

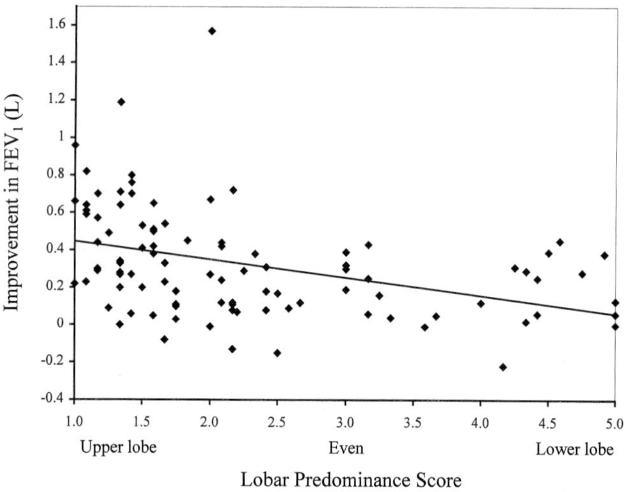

Figure 5. Scatter plot of improvement in FEV_1 as a function of lobar predominance of emphysema. A low score represents predominantly upper-lobe emphysema and a high score represents predominantly lower-lobe emphysema. The best-fit line is illustrated ($r = -.38$).

Table 3
Stratified Comparison of Lobar Predominance, Heterogeneity, and Percentage of Maximal Perfusion with Clinical Improvement

Parameter	Range of Scores	FEV_1 (L)	PaO_2 (mm Hg)	6-minute Walking Distance (m)
Lobar predominance				
Upper ($n = 63$)	1.0–2.3	0.40 ± 0.31*	10.7 ± 11.0*	64.0 ± 77.4*
Evenly distributed emphysema ($n = 19$)	>2.3 to <3.7	0.18 ± 0.15*	6.9 ± 8.8†	14.0 ± 67.7‡
Lower ($n = 14$)	3.7–5.0	0.18 ± 0.19†	5.2 ± 6.8§	87.2 ± 79.2†
P value‖		.001	.122	.016
Heterogeneity				
High ($n = 35$)	7.7–10	0.41 ± 0.35*	7.8 ± 9.4*	78.6 ± 79.2*
Intermediate ($n = 49$)	>5.3 to <7.7	0.29 ± 0.25*	10.4 ± 11.3*	49.7 ± 79.9*
Low ($n = 12$)	0–5.3	0.20 ± 0.13*	8.0 ± 8.4#	23.8 ± 57.6‡
P value‖		.047	.515	.074
Percentage of maximal perfusion				
High ($n = 19$)	42–100	0.42 ± 0.40*	7.9 ± 9.6†	39.3 ± 89.9‡
Intermediate ($n = 53$)	>28 to <42	0.31 ± 0.23*	8.9 ± 10.6*	60.7 ± 71.6*
Low ($n = 24$)	0–28	0.27 ± 0.29*	10.5 ± 10.3*	62.5 ± 85.3†
P value‖		.242	.716	.567

Note.—Data are means ± standard deviations.
* $P < .001$.
† $P < .005$.
‡ Not statistically significant.
§ $P < .05$.
‖ ANOVA.
\# $P < .01$.

Table 4
Mortality Analysis

Scintigraphic Measure	Living Patients ($n = 96$)	Patients Who Died ($n = 7$)	*P* Value*
Lobar predominance	2.3 ± 1.2	2.1 ± 1.0	.738
Heterogeneity	7.0 ± 1.5	7.0 ± 0.6	.882
Percentage of maximal perfusion	34 ± 8	25 ± 4	.004

Note.—Data are mean scores ± standard deviations.
* Unpaired two-tailed Student *t* test.

sema and lower-lobe emphysema were associated with greater improvement in 6-minute walking distance than evenly distributed emphysema. One possible explanation is that many of the patients with evenly distributed emphysema also had low heterogeneity (mean heterogeneity score, 5.2), which was associated with a smaller improvement in the 6-minute walking distance. The large improvement in the patients with lower-lobe emphysema may partly be related to the overall younger age of this group (mean age, 55 years) compared to the ages of the groups with upper-lobe or evenly distributed emphysema (mean age, 60 years or 63 years; $P = .03$, ANOVA). Younger patients may have an increased ability to recover from surgery and regain exercise tolerance than older patients. The difference in age may be related to patients with alpha$_1$-antitrypsin deficiency, who were generally younger and had predominantly basal emphysema.

The results of quantitative CT analyses have previously demonstrated a correlation between the percentage of normal or mildly diseased lung seen on CT scans and measures of clinical improvement (33). In this study, the percentage of maximal perfusion did correlate with an increase in FEV_1, but not at a significant level ($P = .067$). This difference in significance may be explained by the fact that with scintigraphy, the amount of activity that is displayed on an image is based on the relative perfusion. Thus, although regional differences in severity are well demonstrated, the absolute degree of emphysema can be inaccurately estimated. In addition, in this study, the assessment of maximal perfusion was purely subjective. The difficulty with making such an estimate is reflected in the large amount of interobserver variability (mean interobserver correlation coefficient, .41). Preliminary study findings suggest that better correlation may be attained with quantitative methods of lung scan analysis (34).

While the sample size was small, the difference in the percentage of maximal perfusion noted between those patients who survived and those who died points to the potential importance of this variable. The relationship between the percentage of maximally perfused lung and survival suggests that inadequate pulmonary function increases the risk of death. Given an adequate amount of minimally emphysematous lung, however, it seems that other factors are more predictive of the actual degree of improvement.

In this study, only the perfusion images were evaluated. The ventilation images were not analyzed. Several studies have shown that perfusion scintigraphy is at least equivalent if not superior to ventilation scintigraphy in predicting postoperative pulmonary function in patients who undergo lung resection (35–37). Noma and colleagues (38) also found that the sensitivity of single photon emission CT perfusion studies for the detection of mild changes of elastase-induced pulmonary emphysema in pigs was higher than that of ventilation scintigraphy and thin-section CT. Further work needs to be performed to determine whether the additional analysis of ventilation images for factors such as extent of ventilatory defects, severity of retention, and degree of perfusion mismatch would be of use in the prediction of postoperative outcome. ■

Acknowledgment: The authors thank Barry A. Siegel, MD, for his thoughtful review of the manuscript.

References

1. Feinleib M, Rosenberg H, Collins J, et al. Trends in COPD morbidity and mortality in the United States. Am Rev Respir Dis 1989; 140(suppl):S9–S18.
2. Parker SL, Tong T, Bolden S, Wingo PA. Cancer statistics, 1997. CA Cancer J Clin 1997; 47:5–27.
3. Ferguson G, Cherniack R. Management of chronic obstructive pulmonary disease. N Engl J Med 1993; 328:1017–1022.
4. Pohl M, Cooper J. The international status of lung transplantation (abstr). Am J Respir Crit Care Med 1996; 153:829.
5. Low DE, Trulock EP, Kaiser LR, et al. Morbidity, mortality, and early results of single versus bilateral lung transplantation for emphysema. J Thorac Cardiovasc Surg 1992; 103:1119–1126.
6. Snider GL. Reduction pneumoplasty for giant bullous emphysema: implications for surgical treatment of nonbullous emphysema. Chest 1996; 109:540–548.
7. Sciurba FC, Rogers RM, Keenan RJ, et al. Improvement in pulmonary function and elastic recoil after lung-reduction surgery for diffuse emphysema. N Engl J Med 1996; 334:1095–1099.
8. O'Donnell DE, Webb KA, Bertley JC, Chau LK, Conlan AA. Mechanisms of relief of exertional breathlessness following unilat-

eral bullectomy and lung volume reduction surgery in emphysema. Chest 1996; 110: 18–27.

9. Gelb AF, McKenna RJ Jr, Brenner M, Fischel R, Baydur A, Zamel N. Contribution of lung and chest wall mechanics following emphysema resection. Chest 1996; 110: 11–17.
10. Brenner M, Yusen R, McKenna R Jr, et al. Lung volume reduction surgery for emphysema. Chest 1996; 110:205–218.
11. Naunheim KS, Ferguson MK. The current status of lung volume reduction operations for emphysema. Ann Thorac Surg 1996; 62:601–612.
12. Cooper JD, Patterson GA. Lung volume reduction surgery for severe emphysema. Semin Thorac Cardiovasc Surg 1996; 8: 52–60.
13. Yusen RD, Lefrak SS. Evaluation of patients with emphysema for lung volume reduction surgery. Semin Thorac Cardiovasc Surg 1996; 8:83–93.
14. Dennie C, Coblentz CL, LeBlanc P. Evaluation of the emphysematous patient. Chest Surg Clin N Am 1995; 5:635–657.
15. Yusen RD, Trulock EP, Pohl MS, Biggar DG. Results of lung volume reduction surgery in patients with emphysema. Semin Thorac Cardiovasc Surg 1996; 8:99–109.
16. Cooper JD, Trulock EP, Triantafillou AN, et al. Bilateral pneumectomy (volume reduction) for chronic obstructive pulmonary disease. J Thorac Cardiovasc Surg 1995; 109:106–119.
17. Wakabayashi A. Thoracoscopic laser pneumoplasty in the treatment of diffuse bullous emphysema. Ann Thorac Surg 1995; 60:936–942.
18. McKenna RJ Jr, Brenner M, Gelb AF, et al. A randomized prospective trial of stapled lung reduction versus laser bullectomy for diffuse emphysema. J Thorac Cardiovasc Surg 1996; 111:317–322.
19. Tonelli MR, Benditt JO, Albert RK. Clinical experimentation: lessons from lung volume reduction surgery. Chest 1996; 110: 230–238.
20. Cooper JD. Technique to reduce air leaks after resection of emphysematous lung. Ann Thorac Surg 1994; 57:1038–1039.
21. Cooper JD, Patterson GA. Lung-volume reduction surgery for severe emphysema. Chest Surg Clin N Am 1995; 5:815–831.
22. Slone RM, Gierada DS. Radiology of pulmonary emphysema and lung volume reduction surgery. Semin Thorac Cardiovasc Surg 1996; 8:61–82.
23. Slone RM, Pilgram TK, Gierada DS, et al. Comparison of preoperative radiologic features and clinical outcome after lung volume reduction surgery. Radiology 1997; 204:685–693.
24. Anthonisen N, Wright E, Hodgkin J, et al. Prognosis in chronic obstructive pulmonary disease. Am Rev Respir Dis 1986; 133: 14–20.
25. Nocturnal Oxygen Therapy Trial Group. Continuous or nocturnal oxygen therapy in hypoxemic chronic obstructive lung disease: a clinical trial. Ann Intern Med 1980; 93:391–398.
26. Intermittent Positive Pressure Breathing Trial Group. Intermittent positive pressure breathing therapy of chronic obstructive pulmonary disease. Ann Intern Med 1983; 99:612–620.
27. Gurney JW, Jones KK, Robbins RA, et al. Regional distribution of emphysema: correlation of high-resolution CT with pulmonary function tests in unselected smokers. Radiology 1992; 183:457–463.
28. Nairn JR, Prime FJ, Simon G. Association between radiological findings and total and regional function in emphysema. Thorax 1969; 24:218–227.
29. Martelli NA, Hutchison DC, Barter CE. Radiological distribution of pulmonary emphysema: clinical and physiological features of patients with emphysema of upper or lower zones of lungs. Thorax 1974; 29: 81–89.
30. Kim WD, Eidelman DH, Izquierdo JL, et al. Centrilobular and panlobular emphysema in smokers: two distinct morphologic and functional entities. Am Rev Respir Dis 1991; 144:1385–1390.
31. Saetta M, Kim WD, Izquierdo JL, et al. Extent of centrilobular and panacinar emphysema in smokers' lungs: pathological and mechanical implications. Eur Respir J 1994; 7:664–671.
32. Cosio MG, Majo J. Overview of the pathology of emphysema in humans. Chest Surg Clin N Am 1995; 5:603–621.
33. Bae KT, Slone RM, Gierada DS, Yusen RD, Cooper JD. Patients with emphysema: quantitative CT analysis before and after lung volume reduction surgery. Radiology 1997; 203:705–714.
34. Bae KT, Slone RM, Fischer KC, et al. Quantitative analysis of lung scans in patients with emphysema undergoing lung volume reduction surgery (abstr). Radiology 1997; 202(2):57A.
35. Markos J, Mullan BP, Hillman DR, et al. Preoperative assessment as a predictor of mortality and morbidity after lung resection. Am Rev Respir Dis 1989; 139:902–910.
36. Corris PA, Ellis DA, Hawkins T, Gibson GJ. Use of radionuclide scanning in the preoperative estimation of pulmonary function after pneumonectomy. Thorax 1987; 42:285–291.
37. Wemly JA, DeMeester TR, Kirchner PT, Myerowitz PD, Oxford DE, Golomb HM. Clinical value of quantitative ventilation-perfusion lung scans in the surgical management of bronchogenic carcinoma. J Thorac Cardiovasc Surg 1980; 80:535–543.
38. Noma S, Moskowitz GW, Herman PG, Khan A, Rojas KA. Pulmonary scintigraphy in elastase-induced emphysema in pigs: correlation with high-resolution computed tomography and histology. Invest Radiol 1992; 27:429–435.

Karen T. Brown, MD • Lynn A. Brody, MD • George I. Getrajdman, MD • Tracy E. Napp, MD

Outpatient Treatment of Iatrogenic Pneumothorax after Needle Biopsy[1]

PURPOSE: To evaluate prospectively the feasibility of treating iatrogenic pneumothorax after fine-needle aspiration biopsy (FNAB) of the lung with short-term placement of a small-caliber chest tube and to determine whether a 1-hour clamping trial is adequate to identify patients with persistent air leak.

MATERIALS AND METHODS: All patients undergoing FNAB of lung masses over a 28-month period were entered into the study. Patients with symptomatic, enlarging, or greater than 30% pneumothorax were treated with an 8-F chest tube. After 2 hours, the chest tube was clamped, and if the lung remained expanded for an additional hour, the chest tube was removed and the patients were discharged after a brief observation period. Patients were followed up by telephone after 24 hours.

RESULTS: Three hundred fifteen patients underwent FNAB of the lung. Sixty-eight patients (22%) developed a pneumothorax. Chest tubes were placed in 14 patients (4%): Six patients (2%) required admission to the hospital (four for air leaks), and the other eight patients were treated successfully as outpatients, with removal of the chest tube before discharge the day of FNAB.

CONCLUSION: Patients who develop clinically important pneumothorax after FNAB can be safely treated with short-term, small-caliber chest tubes and require hospital admission only if they demonstrate evidence of continued air leak.

Percutaneous fine-needle aspiration biopsy (FNAB) of the lung has been shown to be safe and effective in the diagnosis of pulmonary masses (1–4). Pneumothorax after FNAB is a well-recognized complication. In the past, many patients with iatrogenic pneumothorax after FNAB were admitted to the hospital and treated by surgeons using large-bore chest tubes. Over the past decade, radiologists have taken a more active role in treating this group of patients by using small-caliber percutaneous catheters (5–7). Indeed, some pneumothoraces can be treated with aspiration alone, as recently demonstrated by Yankelevitz et al (8). Although not all patients who develop pneumothorax after FNAB require tube thoracostomy, those treated with chest tubes typically have been admitted to the hospital. Routine hospital admission after chest tube placement adds considerably to the cost of the procedure and is inconvenient for the patient. The purpose of this study was to evaluate the feasibility of short-term treatment with a small-caliber thoracostomy tube to obviate hospital admission.

MATERIALS AND METHODS

Between July 14, 1994, and November 15, 1996, a prospective study was performed that included all patients undergoing lung biopsy performed by one author (K.T.B.). Data collected included patient demographics, size and depth of the lesion undergoing biopsy, number of needle passes made into the lung, presence or absence of pneumothorax on immediate and 2-hour-delayed chest radiographs, requirement for chest tube placement, and the need for hospital admission. All patients were followed up at 24 hours.

Most FNAB procedures of the lung are performed on an outpatient basis at our institution. The patients are monitored after the procedure in our Surgical Day Hospital Post-anesthesia Care Unit (PACU), which is on another floor and in a different building than the interventional radiology area. Patients undergo preprocedure screening, at which time they are instructed to discontinue antiplatelet agents, and preprocedure laboratory studies (complete blood count with platelet count and prothrombin time) are performed. The FNAB procedure is scheduled early in the morning to allow time for treatment should a pneumothorax develop after biopsy. Patients fast the morning of the procedure. After an intravenous catheter is placed, the patient is positioned on the fluoroscopy table (or, less commonly, on the computed tomographic [CT] scanner table); pulse and blood pressure are monitored, and pulse oximetry is initiated. After the lesion is localized, the patient is prepared and draped in a sterile manner and a specimen is obtained, typically with use of a 22-gauge Westcott needle (Becton Dickinson, Franklin Lakes, NJ). A portion of the specimen is reviewed immediately by a cytotechnologist. If the specimen is inadequate, or if material is necessary for special studies or cultures, additional passes are made in an attempt to obtain diagnostic material.

While the patient is still on the table, chest fluoroscopy, (or, if the biopsy was

Index terms: Biopsies, complication, 60.458, 60.732 • Lung, biopsy, 60.126 • Pneumothorax, 60.458, 60.732

Abbreviations: COPD = chronic obstructive pulmonary disease, FNAB = fine-needle aspiration biopsy, PACU = Post-anesthesia Care Unit.

Radiology 1997; 205:249–252

[1] From the Department of Radiology, Vascular/Interventional Section, Memorial Sloan-Kettering Cancer Center, 1275 York Ave, New York, NY 10021. Received December 7, 1996; revision requested January 22, 1997; revision received June 23; accepted June 25. **Address reprint requests to** K.T.B.

performed with CT guidance, axial CT scanning) is performed to assess for pneumothorax, followed by postbiopsy chest radiography. If at any time a large or symptomatic pneumothorax is noted, a chest tube is placed and the chest tube treatment algorithm (Fig 1) is used. We insert an 8-F chest tube (Arrow, Reading, Pa), with use of fluoroscopic guidance and the trocar technique, into the second or third anterior intercostal space. The pleural space is evacuated as completely as possible with a 60-mL syringe. The tube is then attached to a Heimlich chest drain valve (Becton Dickinson, Lincoln Park, NJ), and an immediate postplacement chest radiograph is obtained. Under the assumption that the lung is completely reexpanded, the patients are then given 2 L of oxygen by means of a nasal cannula and observed in the Surgical Day Hospital while their pulse, blood pressure, and oxygen saturation are monitored. A follow-up chest radiograph is obtained after 2 hours of observation, or sooner should the patient become symptomatic. Recurrent pneumothorax is considered evidence that the lung injury resulting from the needle puncture is causing continued air leak that is too large to be handled by a Heimlich valve alone. The chest tube is then placed to a Pleur-Evac (Deknatel, Fall River, Mass) on low wall suction, and the patient is admitted.

In patients whose lungs remain reexpanded, the chest tube is clamped for 1 hour, at which time the chest radiograph is repeated. If the lung remains expanded, the chest tube is removed and a postremoval chest radiograph is obtained. The patient is observed at rest for an additional 30 minutes and then ambulates to the PACU II; there, vital signs are obtained and the patient receives instructions to call or return if notable dyspnea or pleuritic chest pain develops. In patients who do not tolerate a clamping trial, the pneumothorax is reaspirated, the catheter is either reconnected to a Heimlich valve or placed to a Pleur-Evac, and the patient is admitted.

Patients with no pneumothorax, or only a small asymptomatic pneumothorax, on the initial chest radiograph are observed in the Surgical Day Hospital for 2 hours and follow the treatment flow chart outlined in Figure 2. If a small pneumothorax is present, the patient is given 2 L of oxygen by means of a nasal cannula, and some of these patients are positioned with the biopsy site dependent. After the 2-hour observation period, or sooner should the patient become symptomatic, a follow-up chest radiograph is obtained. Patients with no pneumothorax or a small, stable pneumothorax on the 2-hour delayed chest radiograph are discharged within an hour, after spending some time in the PACU II and receiving discharge instructions. These patients are instructed to return, or to be seen at a hospital near their home, if they develop new pleuritic chest pain or shortness of breath.

In patients with a substantial new or enlarging pneumothorax during the observation period, a chest tube is placed if they are symptomatic or the pneumothorax is greater than 30%. If they are not symptomatic and the pneumothorax is less than 30%, a repeat chest radiograph is obtained 1 hour later. Continued evidence of enlargement or the development of serious signs or symptoms at any time is indication for chest tube placement. Once a chest tube is placed, the chest tube treatment algorithm (Fig 1) is followed.

All outpatients are followed-up at 24 hours with a telephone call from one of the nurses in the Surgical Day Hospital. If the patient reports any problems, the nurse contacts the physician who performed the biopsy. Hospitalized patients are visited daily.

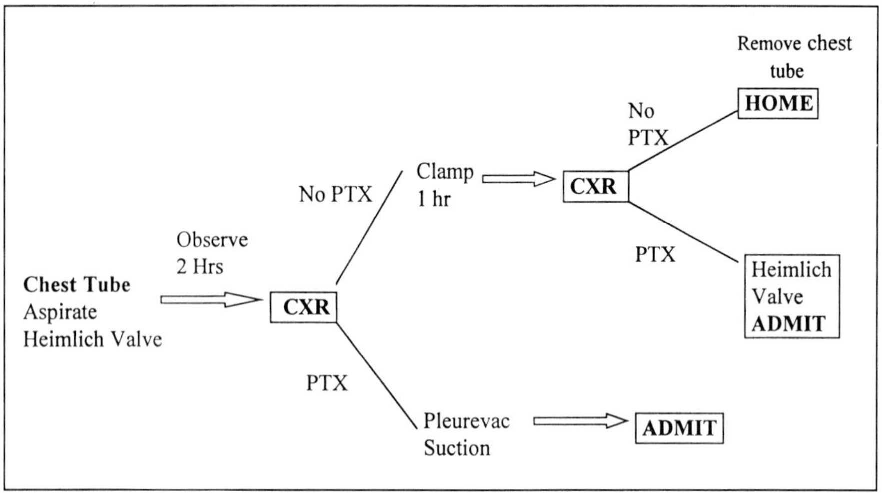

Figure 1. Treatment algorithm for patients who require placement of a chest tube for iatrogenic pneumothorax after FNAB of the lung. *CXR* = chest radiography, *PTX* = pneumothorax.

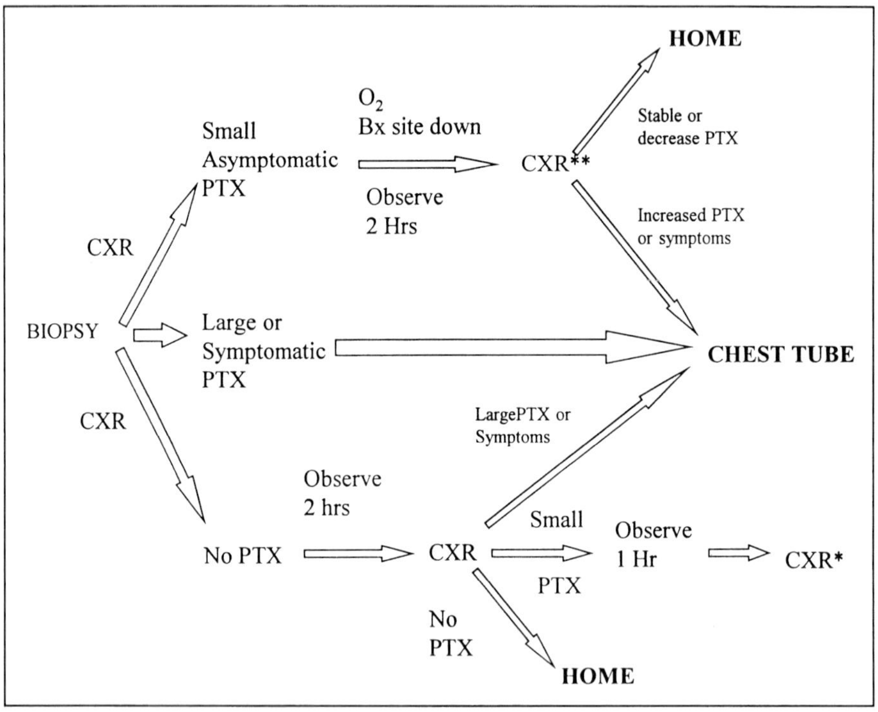

Figure 2. Postbiopsy flow chart used for all patients undergoing FNAB of the lung. *Bx* = biopsy, *CXR* = chest radiography, *PTX* = pneumothorax.

RESULTS

During the study period, 315 patients underwent FNAB of the lung (157 male and 158 female patients; mean age, 63 years; age range, 10–89 years). Overall, 68 patients ([21.5%] 40 men, 28 women; mean age, 64 years; age range, 25–83 years) developed pneumothorax during the period of observation. Fourteen of these 68 patients, or 4.4% of the entire group who underwent biopsy, required tube thoracostomy. In 59 (87%) of the 68 patients with pneumothorax, a diagnosis of malignancy was made with FNAB.

Lesion Characteristics and Number of Passes during FNAB

Category	All Patients (n = 315)	Patients without Pneumothorax (n = 247)	Patients with Pneumothorax (n = 68)	Patients with Treated Pneumothorax (n = 14)
Lesion size (cm)				
Mean	2.5 ± 1.5	2.6 ± 1.6	2.2 ± 1.3*	2.1 ± 0.8*
Range	0.5–10.0	0.5–10.0	0.8–7.0	0.8–3.5
Lesion depth (cm)				
Mean	6.8 ± 2.5	6.5 ± 2.5	8.0 ± 2.4†	9.0 ± 2.7†
Range	1–4	1–4	1–4	1–2
No. of passes				
Mean	1.2 ± 0.5	1.2 ± 0.5	1.3 ± 0.7	1.07 ± 0.3‡
Range	1–4	1–4	1–4	1–2
No. of men§	157 (50)	117 (47)	40 (59)	10 (71)
No. of women§	158 (50)	130 (53)	28 (41)	4 (29)

* Significant difference compared with patients without pneumothorax ($P < .05$).
† Significant difference compared with patients without pneumothorax ($P < .005$).
‡ Significant difference compared with patients with pneumothorax *not* requiring treatment (n = 54) ($P < .05$).
§ Numbers in parentheses are percentages.

In four patients (6%), a specific benign diagnosis (tuberculosis in two, hamartomas in two) was established, and in five patients, nonspecific benign findings were present. The overall diagnostic rate was therefore 93%.

Lesion characteristics and number of passes for each group are listed in the Table. There was a statistically significant difference in lesion depth between the 68 patients who developed a pneumothorax and those who did not. Pneumothorax was more common after biopsy of deeper lesions. There was a significant difference in size as well, with pneumothorax being more common in patients with smaller lesions. There was not, however, a significant difference in the number of passes made between the 68 patients who developed a pneumothorax and those who did not. The only significant difference related to number of needle passes was that patients who developed a pneumothorax that necessitated treatment had significantly fewer passes than those patients with a pneumothorax that did not necessitate treatment.

Of the 14 patients requiring chest tubes, eight patients (2.5% of the total group, 57% of patients with chest tubes placed) were discharged home the day of the FNAB, after removal of the chest tube. Six patients (1.9% of the overall group, 43% of those requiring chest tubes) required hospitalization. Four of the six patients had persistent air leaks when their chest tubes were clamped. All four patients required daily bronchodilator therapy before the biopsy for treatment of severe chronic obstructive pulmonary disease (COPD), with multiple bullae evident on CT scans and forced expiratory volume in 1 second of less than 2 L (35%–40% of predicted). All of these patients required 2–4 days of thoracostomy drainage. The other two patients were not admitted as a result of an air leak. One patient had a small asymptomatic pneumothorax that was treated because of a history of myocardial infarction after an otherwise uneventful bronchoscopy 6 months earlier. Given his fragile cardiac status, we thought it was prudent to treat him with a chest tube and admit him for observation. The other patient had severe COPD and, after the biopsy, which was performed later in the day than usual, had a small asymptomatic pneumothorax that continued to slowly enlarge over a 4-hour observation period. At that time, a chest tube was placed, and because there was not enough time to allow for a safe clamping trial, he was admitted. In these last two patients, the chest tubes were removed within 24 hours and the patients were discharged.

Fifty-four patients with pneumothorax were not treated at the time of FNAB. One of these patients demonstrated enlargement of the pneumothorax by approximately 10% on the 2-hour delayed chest radiograph and was advised to have a chest tube placed, but the patient refused treatment. This patient required chest tube placement at an outside institution the next day. The other 53 patients discharged with a small pneumothorax, as well as the 247 patients discharged with no evidence of pneumothorax, were asymptomatic at 24 hours. In three patients with no evidence of pneumothorax the day of the FNAB, an asymptomatic pneumothorax was discovered incidentally on an imaging study obtained within 3 days of the biopsy; the pneumothorax did not necessitate treatment.

DISCUSSION

Ever since Poe and Kallay (9) demonstrated the safety of performing FNAB of the lung in nonhospitalized patients, the procedure has been moved to the outpatient setting. Gobien et al (10) had already demonstrated the fiscal advantage of needle biopsy of the lung, versus surgical biopsy, in hospitalized patients. Additional cost savings were recognized when the procedure was moved to the outpatient environment. Routine admission of patients treated with chest tubes for iatrogenic pneumothorax after FNAB adds substantially to the cost of caring for these patients, and also disrupts the patient's life. As a result, many techniques have been investigated to diminish the likelihood of patients developing a pneumothorax that necessitates treatment after FNAB. These include limiting the number of pleural surfaces transgressed and the number of punctures made, administering oxygen, and dependent positioning of the biopsy site (11–13). In the best hands, and despite the use of many of these techniques, a certain number of patients will require chest tube placement for treatment of pneumothorax (14), particularly with deeper lesions for which aerated lung must be traversed (15). Patients with severe COPD are known to be at higher risk for pneumothorax than are patients with normal pulmonary function (16,17). It is no surprise then, that despite having had their biopsies performed with a single pass of a 22-gauge needle, all four patients in our study with pneumothorax who required hospitalization for persistent air leak had severe COPD necessitating bronchodilator therapy.

Some authors have demonstrated the feasibility of treating simple pneumothoraces with catheter aspiration alone (8,18), achieving success in 70%–75% of cases in which the pneumothorax was caused by needle puncture. This supports our hypothesis that small pleural injuries resulting from FNAB might be expected to "seal" quickly. In their series of CT-guided biopsies, Yankelevitz et al (8) advocated aspirating the pneumothorax at the time of biopsy. Although this is convenient and does not require preparing and draping a different area, or moving the patient to another room, it is a technique that was demonstrated to be safe in the "immediate" postbiopsy setting in a group of patients the majority of whom were without symptoms. We do not consider patients with limited pulmonary reserve who become symptomatic from a pneumothorax to be good candidates for treatment with aspiration alone. These high-risk patients might get into trouble should their lungs recollapse during the observation period, when a physician might not be immediately available to place a chest tube. Patients who undergo biopsy of contralateral lung lesions after pneumonectomy also fall into this "high-risk" category. In addition, patients who return with delayed evidence of an enlarging pneumothorax are considered to have an air leak that has continued beyond the immediate postbiopsy period. We consider these patients to be at higher risk of having a persistent air leak. In all of these patients, we prefer to place a small catheter anteriorly at the apex of the pleural space that can be used for extended treatment if necessary. We placed eight of the 14 chest tubes immediately, and the other six after a delayed chest radiograph demonstrated a new or considerably enlarged pneumothorax. In all eight patients in whom chest tubes were placed immediately, the lungs were completely reexpanded, but three patients subsequently demonstrated persistent air leaks and required admission to the hospital. Had we treated these eight patients with aspiration alone, sparing five patients the 8-F chest tube would have exposed the other three patients to the risk of developing a complication related to recurrent pneumothorax. Unfortunately, it is difficult to know in advance which of the many higher risk patients (those with COPD, deep lesions, etc) will develop an air leak, and we prefer to err on the side of placing chest tubes in patients for whom aspiration alone might have been sufficient treatment.

We do not have the luxury of being able to observe our post-FNAB patients in our department, or in close proximity. The Surgical Day Hospital PACU is on another floor remote from the special procedures room. If a patient becomes acutely symptomatic from a recurrent pneumothorax during the observation period, or after a clamping trial, it is necessary only to visit them in the Surgical Day Hospital and reaspirate or unclamp the chest tube. This process can be initiated by a nurse at the Surgical Day Hospital if a physician is not immediately available. Our patients tolerated placement of the 8-F chest tube very well, and placement anteriorly and superiorly results in a catheter that is more functional than an intravenous catheter placed at the site of biopsy. This allows for more complete evacuation of the pleural space and can be used for extended treatment if necessary.

Perlmutt et al (19) have demonstrated that most pneumothoraces that occur after FNAB of the lung are detected by 1 hour, with only an additional 2% demonstrated on the 4-hour chest radiograph. In his study, all clinically important pneumothoraces were seen by 1 hour. This led us to believe that recurrent pneumothorax would likely be identified in a similar time period. Indeed, in our study, all four patients with persistent air leaks were identified within 1 hour of chest tube clamping. All eight patients in whom the chest tube was removed after the 1 hour clamping trial did well.

We believe that placing a small chest tube in patients with a symptomatic, large (>30%) or enlarging iatrogenic pneumothorax after FNAB of the lung is safe and effective. Although it may be feasible to treat selected patients with aspiration alone, our study has shown that when a chest tube is necessary, it is feasible to remove the chest tube in many patients a few hours after placement, thus averting hospital admission. The cost of our thoracostomy set is minimal, and there is little patient discomfort experienced during placement. Once the tube is in place, a recurrent pneumothorax can be managed remote from the interventional area. This has been well accepted by our patients. In this small series of 14 patients requiring chest tubes, a 1-hour clamping trial appears to be adequate before removing the chest tube. Further use of this algorithm is warranted in patients with pneumothorax after FNAB in an effort to avert unnecessary hospital admission. ■

References

1. Westcott JL. Percutaneous transthoracic needle biopsy. Radiology 1988; 169:593–601.
2. Conces DJ, Clark SA, Tarver RD, et al. Transthoracic aspiration needle biopsy: value in the diagnosis of pulmonary infections. AJR 1989; 152:31–34.
3. Perlmutt LM, Johnston WW, Dunnick NR. Percutaneous transthoracic needle aspiration: a review. AJR 1989; 152:451–455.
4. Weisbrod GL. Transthoracic percutaneous lung biopsy. Radiol Clin North Am 1990; 28:647–655.
5. Perlmutt LM, Braun SD, Newman GE, et al. Transthoracic needle aspiration: use of a small chest tube to treat pneumothorax. AJR 1987; 148:849–851.
6. Casola G, vanSonnenberg E, Keightley A, et al. Pneumothorax: radiologic treatment with small catheters. Radiology 1988; 166: 89–91.
7. Conces DJ, Tarver RD, Gray WC, et al. Treatment of pneumothoraces utilizing small caliber chest tubes. Chest 1988; 94: 55–57.
8. Yankelevitz DF, Davis SD, Henschke CI. Aspiration of a large pneumothorax resulting from transthoracic needle biopsy. Radiology 1996; 200:695–697.
9. Poe RH, Kallay MC. Transthoracic needle biopsy of lung in nonhospitalized patients. Chest 1987; 92:676–678.
10. Gobien RP, Bouchard EA, Gobien BS, et al. Thin needle aspiration biopsy of thoracic lesions: impact on hospital charges and patterns of patient care. Radiology 1983; 148: 65–67.
11. Cormier Y, Haviolene M, Tardif A. Prevention of pneumothorax in needle lung biopsy by breathing 100% oxygen. Thorax 1980; 141:35–37.
12. Moore EH, Shepard JO, McLoud TC, et al. Positional precautions in needle aspiration lung biopsy. Radiology 1990; 175:733–735.
13. Herman SJ, Weisbrod GL. Usefulness of the blood patch technique after transthoracic needle aspiration biopsy. Radiology 1990; 176:395–397.
14. Li H, Boiselle PM, Shepard JO, et al. Diagnostic accuracy and safety of CT guided percutaneous needle aspiration biopsy of the lung: comparison of small and large pulmonary nodules. AJR 1996; 167:105–109.
15. Harman LB, Austin JM. Complications after CT-guided needle biopsy through aerated verus nonaerated lung. Radiology 1991; 181:778.
16. Fish GD, Stanley JH, Miller KS, et al. Postbiopsy pneumothorax: estimating the risk by chest radiography and pulmonary function tests. AJR 1988; 150:71–74.
17. Kazerooni EA, Lim FT, Mikhad A, et al. Risk of pneumothorax in CT-guided transthoracic needle aspiration biopsy of the lung. Radiology 1996; 198:371–375.
18. Delius RE, Obeid FN, Horst HM, et al. Catheter aspiration for simple pneumothorax: experience with 114 patients. Arch Surg 1989; 124:833–836.
19. Perlmutt LM, Braun SD, Newman GE, et al. Timing of chest film follow-up after transthoracic needle aspiration. AJR 1986; 146: 1049–1050.

Antonio Leone, MD • Alfonso Cerase, MD • Francesco Priolo, MD • Pasquale Marano, MD

Lumbosacral Junction Injury Associated with Unstable Pelvic Fracture: Classification and Diagnosis[1]

PURPOSE: **To determine the types and prevalence of lumbosacral junction injuries associated with an unstable pelvic fracture and to assess the diagnostic value of conventional radiographic and computed tomographic (CT) findings.**

MATERIALS AND METHODS: **Anteroposterior, inlet, and outlet radiographs and CT scans in 97 patients with pelvic disruption were retrospectively reviewed.**

RESULTS: **Unstable pelvic fractures were seen on radiographs in 73 patients, 42 of whom had a sacral fracture. Fourteen of these 42 patients had an associated L5-S1 facet joint injury (three extraarticular, nine articular, and two complex). In three of these 14 patients, the L-5 body was laterally bent by more than 10°, with asymmetric L5-S1 intervertebral space. The diagnosis in nine of the 14 patients with an associated lumbosacral junction injury was rendered on the basis of CT findings only.**

CONCLUSION: **Lumbosacral junction injury must be considered in patients with an unstable pelvic fracture, especially in those with an associated sacral fracture. CT is necessary because these conditions may be overlooked on radiographs, although outlet radiographs are better than CT scans for depicting the possibly associated L5-S1 intervertebral disk lesion.**

Classification systems based on the force vectors of pelvic injuries (1–4), as well as the ubiquity of computed tomography (CT) (5–10), provide a logical approach to the management of pelvic ring disruption and allow early and aggressive treatment, which has dramatically decreased the previously high mortality and complications rates in patients with an unstable pelvic fracture (11–17).

Nevertheless, little progress has been made in decreasing the prevalence of chronic disability due to late complications such as nonunion, malunion, limb-length discrepancy, and low back pain; these complications may result in disability in up to 52% of the patients with a fracture through the sacrum or sacroiliac joint (18,19). In this context, associated lumbosacral junction injuries, which represent a major cause of low back pain (20), can render the reduction of a displaced sacral fracture impossible. In 1990, Isler (20) classified lumbosacral junction injuries. Isler stated that if a sacral fracture passes through or is medial to the S-1 articular process, even a minimal hemipelvic displacement affects the anatomic relationships between the elements of the lumbosacral junction, which results in subsequent posttraumatic degeneration of the L5-S1 facet joints and thus represents an important causative factor for pain in the lumbar or lumbosacral region.

Our purpose was to determine the type and frequency of lumbosacral junction injuries that occur in patients with an unstable pelvic fracture, and to assess the diagnostic value of findings from conventional radiography and CT.

MATERIALS AND METHODS

We reviewed plain radiographs and CT images obtained in 97 consecutive patients with pelvic disruption who were treated, between March 1985 and June 1994, at the Orthopedics and Traumatology Department of the Catholic University of Rome, Policlinico "Agostino Gemelli." Motor vehicle accidents in which the patient was a driver, passenger, or pedestrian were the main cause of injury (88 [91%] patients). Six (6%) of the patients fell from a height, and the remaining three (3%) patients had an occupational injury.

All of the patients underwent preoperative routine radiologic examination because of pelvic trauma; anteroposterior, inlet, and outlet radiographs and pelvic CT images were obtained. In 48 (50%) patients, 45° Judet oblique views were obtained.

The CT study always covered the anatomic region from the L-5 superior end plate to the greater trochanters, including the ischial tuberosities. The scout view was obtained in the anteroposterior view; thus, the axial CT scans were obtained without gantry angulation. In 17 patients, direct coronal oblique CT scans of the sacrum were also obtained after the acquisition of a lateral scout view. A PACE CT scanner (GE Medical Systems, Milwaukee, Wis) was used in 85 (88%) patients; serial 5-mm-thick sections were obtained in these patients, except in the acetabular region, where 3-mm-thick interval sections were obtained. The remaining 12 (12%) patients were examined early in the study period with a 12000 scanner (CGR, Paris, France); 5-mm-thick serial sections were obtained in these patients. A bone algorithm was

Index terms: Pelvis, CT, 33.12111, 44.12111 • Pelvis, fractures, 44.41, 44.422 • Sacrum, fractures, 33.41, 33.42 • Spine, fractures, 331.41, 334.41 • Spine, intervertebral disks, 336.43

Radiology 1997; 205:253–259

[1] From the Institute of Radiology, Università Cattolica del Sacro Cuore, Policlinico Agostino Gemelli, Largo Agostino Gemelli, 8, 00168 Rome, Italy. Received October 17, 1996; revision requested December 16; revision received May 15, 1997; accepted June 2. **Address reprint requests to** A.L.

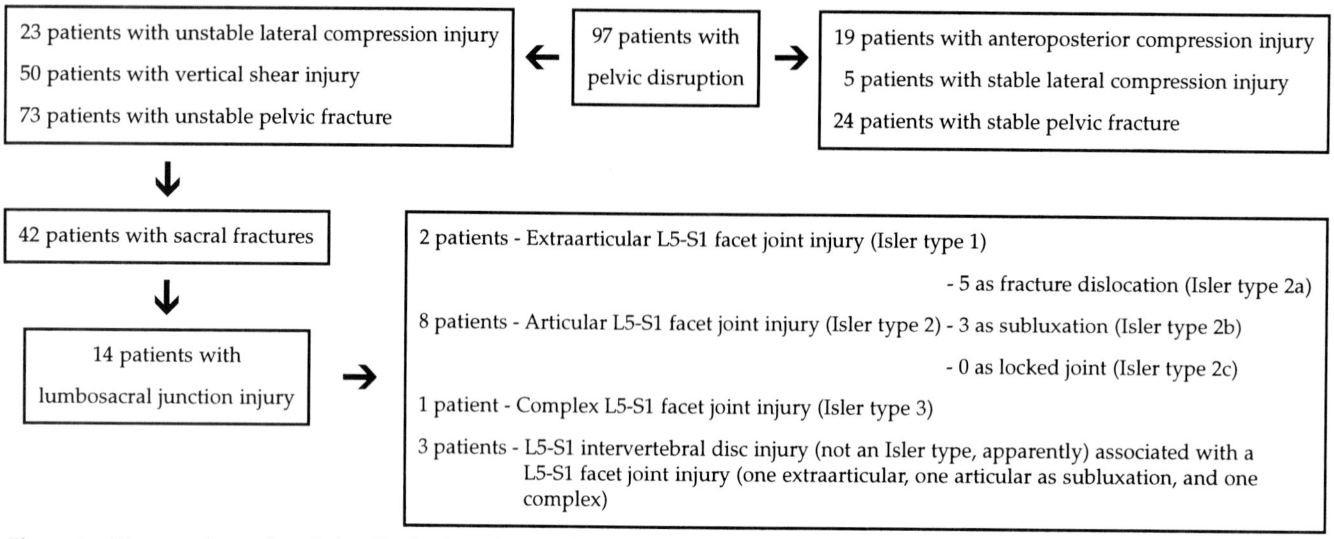

Figure 1. Diagram shows the relative distribution of types of pelvic ring disruption and of associated lumbosacral junction injuries that occurred in patients in our series with an unstable pelvic fracture.

used for reconstruction of the images in 74 (76%) patients. Reformations in the coronal and sagittal planes were obtained in 20 (21%) patients. Total scanning time (exclusive of the time involved in patient transfer and positioning, tube arrangement, time spent on non-imaging–related procedures, etc) was less than 15 minutes; data processing added another 10–15 minutes.

Plain radiographs and CT scans in each patient were retrospectively assessed by two radiologists (A.L., A.C.), who were unaware of clinical findings. To classify each pelvic disruption according to the schema of Pennal et al (2) and Tile (3), the degree of pelvic instability was evaluated on the basis of the evidence of disruption of the posterior tension band of the pelvis (the sacroiliac complex with the addition of iliolumbar, sacrospinous, and sacrotuberous ligaments) (1–3). CT findings were the standard of reference for definition of the fracture pattern. Plain radiographs and CT images were also examined for presence of associated lumbosacral junction injuries (20); other pelvic injuries, including acetabular fractures and proximal femoral injuries, were also noted but were not analyzed in detail. In cases of discrepant interpretations of images, a final conclusion was achieved by means of consensus.

Anteroposterior compression injury was diagnosed in 19 patients; stable lateral compression injury, in five patients; unstable lateral compression injury, in 23 patients; and vertical shear injury, in 50 patients. Only the images in the 73 patients (47 male and 26 female patients; average age, 28.5 years; age range, 13–68 years) with an unstable pelvic fracture were included in the analysis. In 25 patients, follow-up plain radiographs and CT scans were available.

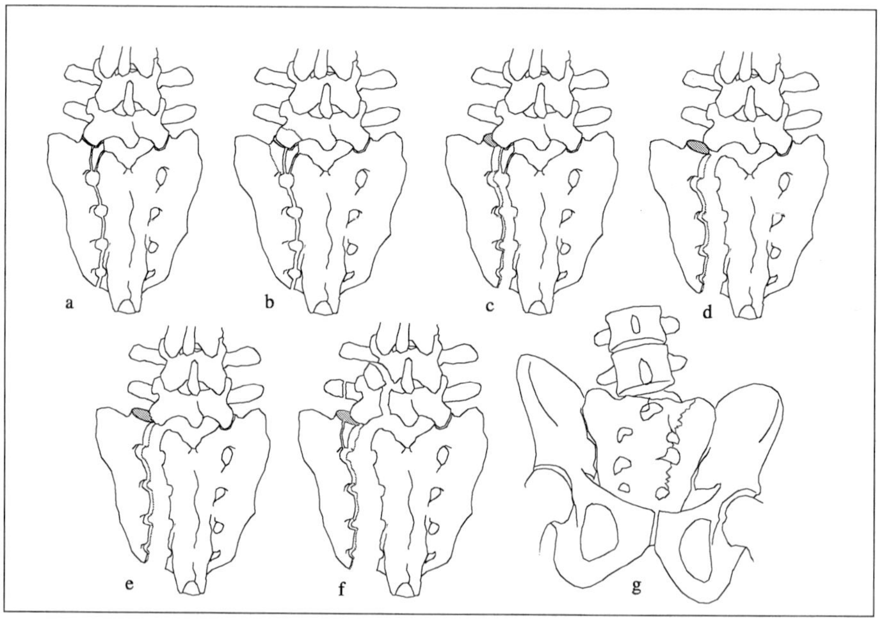

Figure 2. Schematic diagrams of the types of lumbosacral junction injuries associated with unstable pelvic fractures. Posterior view (*a*) shows a vertical sacral fracture passing cranially through or medial to the S-1 articular process, which is a prerequisite for an associated lumbosacral junction injury. Posterior view (*b*) shows an extraarticular L5-S1 facet joint injury. This injury is the result of displacement of the hemipelvis, which causes fracture of the L-5 inferior articular process or the S-1 articular process (Isler type 1). Posterior view (*c*) shows an articular L5-S1 facet joint injury manifesting as a fracture-dislocation. This injury is the result of a sacral fracture that passes cranially through the S-1 articular process and reaches the articular facet surface (Isler type 2a). Posterior view (*d*) shows an articular L5-S1 facet joint injury manifesting as a subluxation. This injury is the result of a sacral fracture that passes medial to the S-1 articular process (Isler type 2b). Posterior view (*e*) shows an articular L5-S1 facet joint injury manifesting as a complete locked facet joint (Isler type 2c). Posterior view (*f*) shows a complex L5-S1 facet joint injury with rotational displacement of the posterior elements, fractures of the interarticular portion and pedicles, and subluxations (Isler type 3). Anterior view (*g*) shows an L5-S1 intervertebral disk injury. Lateral bending of the L-5 body and asymmetry of L5-S1 intervertebral space are depicted. This injury apparently does not have an Isler type classification.

RESULTS

Pelvic Disruption and Associated Lumbosacral Junction Injuries

Of the 73 patients with an unstable pelvic fracture, 23 (32%) had an unstable lateral compression injury, and 50 (68%) had a vertical shear injury. A sacral fracture was noted in 42 (58%) of the 73 patients, including 10 (43%) of the 23 patients with an unstable lateral compression injury and 32 (64%) of the 50 patients with a vertical shear injury. A lumbosacral junction injury associated with a sacral fracture was noted in 14 (19%) of the 73 patients (six male and eight female patients), aged 14–41 years (mean, 25.8 years). A lumbosacral junction injury was present in one (4%) of the 23 pa-

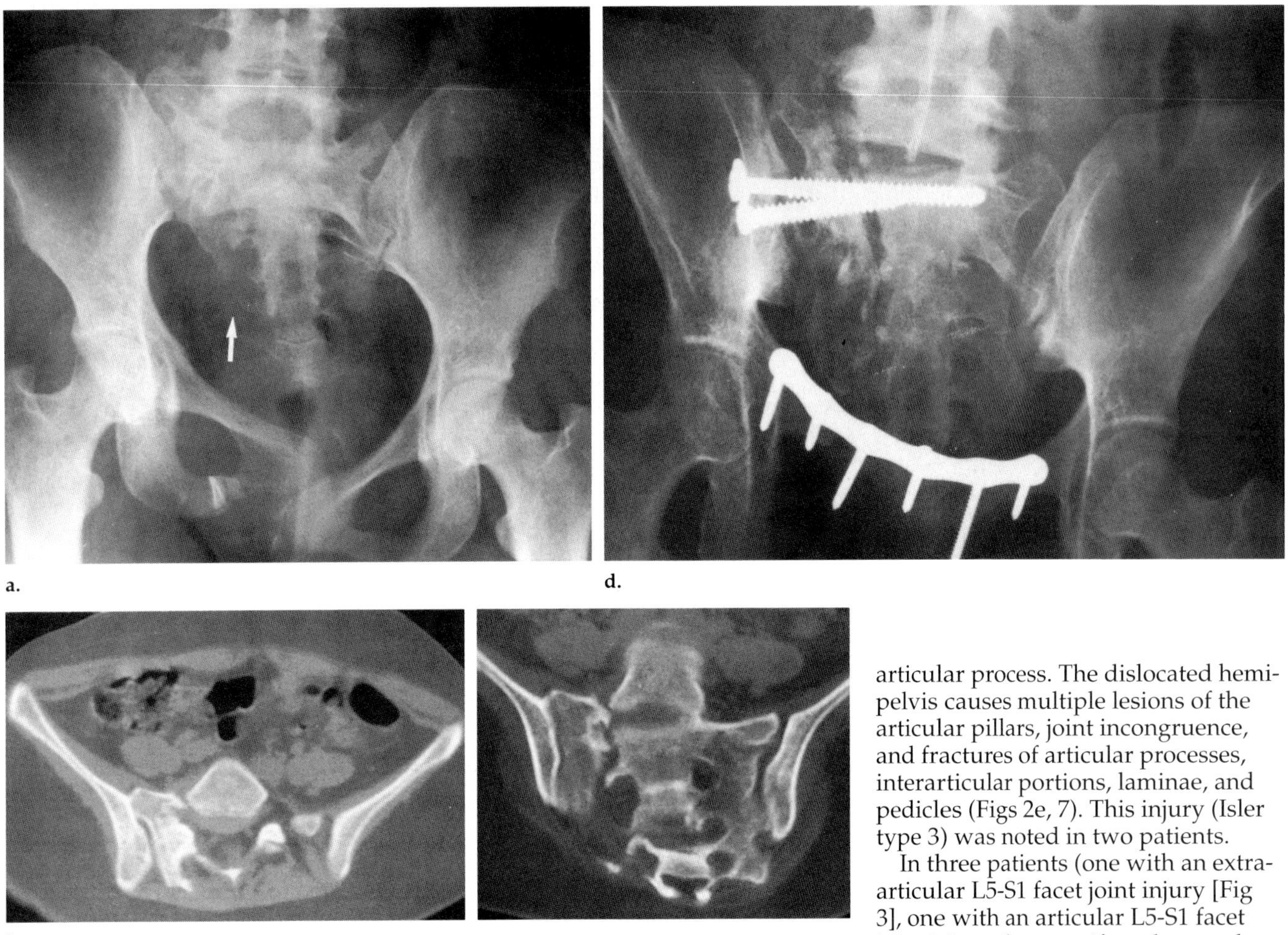

a. d.

b. c.

Figure 3. Extraarticular L5-S1 facet joint injury and L5-S1 intervertebral disk injury associated with a lateral compression pelvic injury in a 15-year-old girl who was involved in a motor vehicle accident. The patient was a passenger in the right front seat. **(a)** Anteroposterior radiograph demonstrates inward rotation and cranial displacement of the right hemipelvis with a locked pubic symphysis. A displaced transforaminal fracture of the right side of the sacrum is also visible (arrow). **(b)** Axial CT scan shows the cranial displacement of the right sacral wing and a bulging L5-S1 disk. **(c)** Coronal CT scan confirms that the vertical transforaminal right sacral fracture passes ipsilaterally through the S-1 articular process and demonstrates lateral bending of the L-5 body, as well as consequent asymmetry of the L5-S1 intervertebral space. **(d)** Outlet radiograph obtained during the immediate postoperative period shows lateral bending of the L-5 body. Despite the persistence of low back pain, the patient refused to undergo revision surgery.

tients with an unstable lateral compression injury and in 13 (26%) of the 50 patients with a vertical shear injury. These results are summarized in Figure 1.

Types of Lumbosacral Junction Injuries

By using the classification scheme of Isler (20), we noted the following types of lumbosacral junction injuries associated with an unstable pelvic fracture (Fig 2):

1. Extraarticular L5-S1 facet joint injury, which is a vertical sacral fracture that passes through or medial to the S-1 articular process. The dislocated hemipelvis causes the fracture of the ipsilateral S-1 articular process or L-5 inferior articular process (Figs 2b, 3). This injury (Isler type 1) was noted in three patients.

2. Articular L5-S1 facet joint injury, which is a vertical sacral fracture that passes through or medial to the S-1 articular process. The dislocated hemipelvis causes a disruption at the level of the L5-S1 facet joint (Isler type 2); the disruption can be a fracture-dislocation (Figs 2c, 4) or a subluxation (Figs 2d, 5, 6). This injury was noted in nine patients: five with a fracture-dislocation (Isler type 2a) and four with a subluxation (Isler type 2b). Complete L5-S1 locked dislocation (Isler type 2c) was never observed in our series.

3. Complex L5-S1 facet joint injury, which is a vertical sacral fracture that passes through or medial to the S-1 articular process. The dislocated hemipelvis causes multiple lesions of the articular pillars, joint incongruence, and fractures of articular processes, interarticular portions, laminae, and pedicles (Figs 2e, 7). This injury (Isler type 3) was noted in two patients.

In three patients (one with an extraarticular L5-S1 facet joint injury [Fig 3], one with an articular L5-S1 facet joint injury that manifested as a subluxation [Fig 5], and one with a complex L5-S1 facet joint injury [Fig 7]), lateral bending of the L-5 body of more than 10°, asymmetry of the L5-S1 intervertebral space, and consequent lateral deformity of the lumbar spine (Fig 2f) were seen. These findings were better demonstrated on the outlet radiographs than on the conventional axial CT scans, even if a careful review of all the CT images indicated that, in one patient, these lesions could also be seen on direct coronal oblique CT scans (Fig 3c); in the same patient, axial CT scans showed a bulging L5-S1 disk (Fig 3b).

Diagnostic Imaging

The diagnosis was determined on the basis of plain radiographic findings in five of the 14 patients with a lumbosacral junction injury, including the three patients with deformity of the lumbar spine. In nine patients, the diagnosis was established only after evaluation of the CT scans. In all 14 patients, the additional anatomic information provided on the CT scans allowed the precise definition of the type of the associated lumbosacral junction injury.

DISCUSSION

Pelvic fractures are a common consequence of high-speed collisions and occupational accidents, because strong external forces are necessary to produce a fracture in a normal pelvis (21, 22). The importance of pelvic fractures lies in the high rate of morbidity and mortality—the latter approaches 30%—mainly because of associated injuries to different organs and systems (cardiovascular, gastrointestinal, respiratory, genitourinary) (11,23,24). Although many reports (11–16,25–27) indicate dramatically decreasing mortality rates associated with rapid diagnosis, multidisciplinary management, early aggressive approach to treatment, and improvement in surgical techniques (eg, preoperative angiography, therapeutic embolization, external fixation, early open reduction with internal fixation), little progress has been made in treating the chronic disability that is a consequence of late complications of pelvic fractures, including nonunion, malunion, leg-length discrepancy, and low back pain. In this context, low back pain, which frequently persists after pelvic ring injuries and represents a major cause of invalidity (17,18,20), may be due to pelvic obliquity, sacroiliac joint instability, or associated lumbosacral junction injury.

Associated lumbosacral junction injuries were described by Isler in 1990 (20) and have been rarely reported (28). This type of injury occurs when a sacral fracture passes cranially through or medial to the S-1 articular process (Fig 2a). In contrast, if a vertical sacral fracture passes lateral to the S-1 articular process, the displacement of the hemipelvis does not cause damage to the lumbosacral junction.

Three different types of associated lumbosacral junction injuries were defined in the Isler (20) classification scheme (Fig 2b–2f): (*a*) extraarticular L5-S1 facet joint injury (type 1); (*b*) articular L5-S1 facet joint injury that manifested as a fracture-dislocation (type 2a), subluxation (type 2b), or complete locked dislocation (type 2c); and (*c*) complex L5-S1 facet joint injury (type 3).

In cases of articular and complex lumbosacral junction injuries, tremendous forces are needed to overcome the sagittal orientation of the facet joints. The injury mechanism for severe hyperflexion, compression, and rotation may account for energy dissipation at the level of the lumbosacral junction (28). The mechanism for forced hyperflexion has been supported by other authors (29).

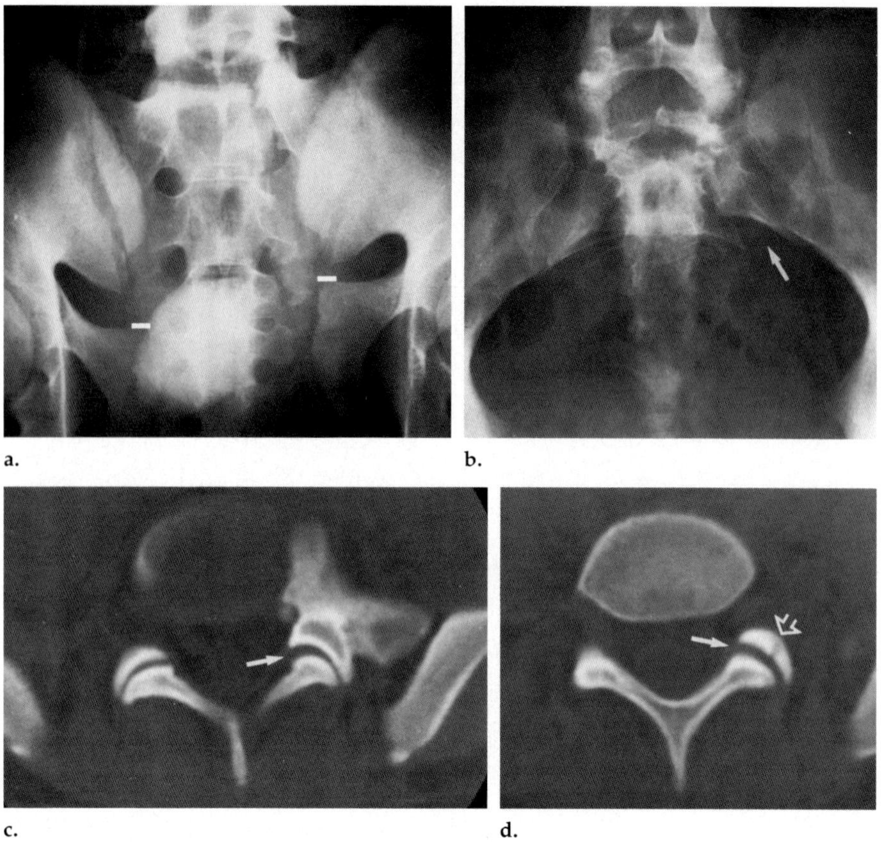

Figure 4. Articular L5-S1 facet joint injury manifesting as a fracture-dislocation in a 16-year-old pedestrian who was involved in a motor vehicle accident. This lumbosacral junction injury was associated with a pelvic ring disruption produced by an anteroposterior force that also contained a shearing element; the injury was thus classified as an unstable vertical shear injury. **(a)** Outlet radiograph shows a left sacral vertical shear fracture extending into the upper two neural foramina and passing through the left S-1 articular process. The white lines indicate anterior upward displacement at the widely disrupted pubic symphysis. **(b)** Inlet radiograph shows severe posterior displacement on the left side (arrow). **(c, d)** Sequential axial CT scans demonstrate the incongruence of the left L5-S1 facet joint (solid arrow) and fracture of the S-1 facet (open arrow).

Isler (20) stated that associated lumbosacral junction injuries are clinically relevant because (*a*) locked dislocation of the L5-S1 joint (a type of injury not observed in our series) can make the reduction of a displaced sacral fracture unfeasible, and (*b*) posttraumatic degeneration of the lumbosacral facet joint may be an important causative factor for lumbosacral pain. Moreover, it is well known that posterior elements are involved in the preservation of motion-segment stability (30). Thus, knowledge of the presence and type of a lumbosacral junction injury, as well as the degree of instability, allows the orthopedic surgeon to choose the adequate treatment (nonsurgical alternatives, open reduction with internal fixation and fusion, or arthrodesis) (28,30).

At a comparison of our data with those of Isler (20) (Tables 1, 2), the overall prevalence of lumbosacral junction injury was clearly higher in our series (19% [14 of 73] vs 6% [12 of 193]). Moreover, there was a higher prevalence, in our series, of this injury associated with an unstable lateral compression injury (4% [one of 23] vs 3% [four of 150]), a vertical shear injury (26% [13 of 50] vs 19% [eight of 43]), and a sacral fracture (33% [14 of 42] vs 9% [12 of 134]). These differences can be explained by the fact that CT scans were obtained in all patients in our series; in the series of Isler, only 27 (24%) of the 113 patients with a sacral fracture associated with an unstable lateral compression injury and 10 (48%) of the 21 patients with a sacral fracture associated with a vertical shear injury underwent CT.

Moreover, ours is the only hospital in central and southern Italy at which open reduction with internal fixation for stabilization of an unstable pelvic ring fracture is performed. Nearly all of our patients were referred from other hospitals, at which only external fixation and conservative treatment is performed. This also accounts for the relative distribution of pelvic disruptions, which differs from that reported elsewhere (1–4,31), with patients with

Table 1
Prevalence of Unstable Pelvic Fracture and Associated Injuries

Type of Injury	Isler (20)	Present Study
All unstable pelvic fractures	193/193 (100)	73/73 (100)
Unstable lateral compression	150/193 (78)	23/73 (32)
Vertical shear	43/193 (22)	50/73 (68)
Sacral fracture	134/193 (69)	42/73 (58)
Unstable lateral compression*	113/150 (75)	10/23 (43)
Vertical shear†	21/43 (49)	32/50 (64)
Lumbosacral junction injury	12/193 (6)	14/73 (19)
Unstable lateral compression	4/150 (3)	1/23 (4)
Vertical shear	8/43 (19)	13/50 (26)
Sacral fracture	12/134 (9)	14/42 (33)

Note.—Numbers in parentheses are percentages.
* Pelvic CT scans were available in 27 (24%) of the 113 patients with unstable lateral compression injury associated with a sacral fracture in the series of Isler (20) and in all of such patients in our series.
† Pelvic CT scans were available in 10 (48%) of the 21 patients with a vertical shear injury associated with a sacral fracture in the series of Isler (20) and in all of such patients in our series.

Table 2
Prevalence of Lumbosacral Junction Injury

Type of Injury	Isler (20)	Present Study
L5-S1 facet joint injury	12	14
Extraarticular	2	3
Articular	6	9
Fracture-dislocation	3	5
Subluxation	2	4
Locked dislocation	1	0
Complex	4	2
L5-S1 intervertebral disk injury	0	3*

Note.—Diagnosis was determined on the basis of CT findings ($n = 37$ in the series of Isler [20], $n = 42$ in our series).
* All injuries were associated with L5-S1 facet joint injuries, including one extraarticular, one articular subluxation, and one complex injury.

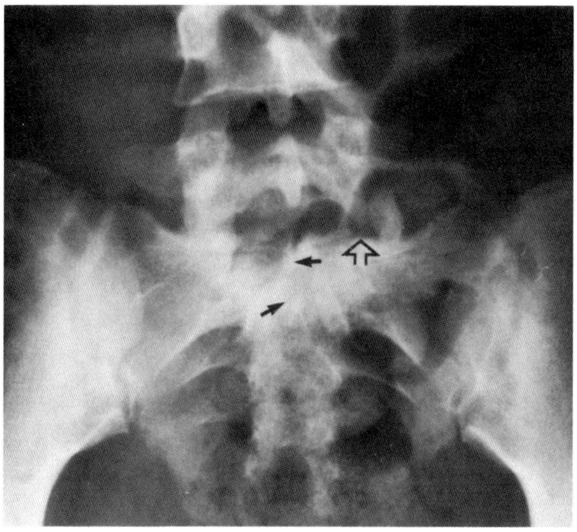

a.

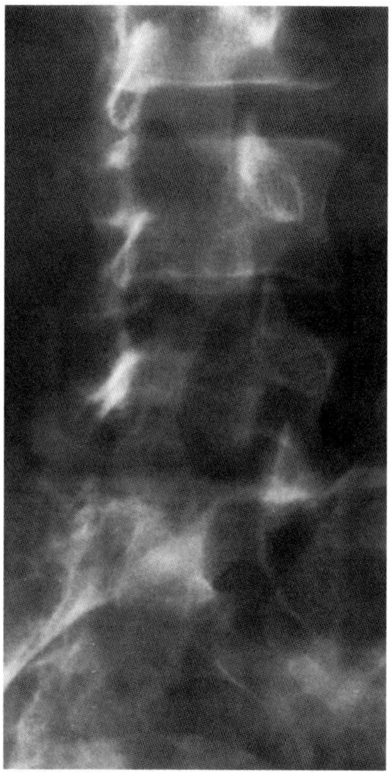

b.

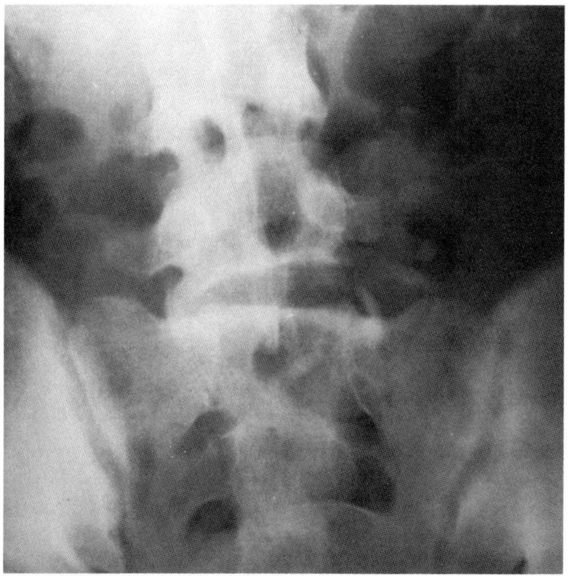

c.

Figure 5. Articular L5-S1 facet joint injury manifesting as a subluxation and L5-S1 intervertebral disk injury associated with a vertical shear injury in a 19-year-old woman involved in a motor vehicle accident. **(a)** Anteroposterior radiograph shows a sacral fracture (solid arrows) and subluxation of the left L5-S1 facet joint (open arrow). **(b)** Oblique radiograph shows the diastasis between left L5-S1 articular facets. **(c)** Outlet radiograph demonstrates lateral bending of the L-5 body and asymmetry of the L5-S1 intervertebral space, which are suggestive of disruption of the L5-S1 intervertebral disk. The fracture of the left L-5 transverse process is also visible.

a vertical shear injury clearly predominant in our series.

There is another important difference between our series and that of Isler: In three patients with a lumbosacral junction injury, the outlet view clearly demonstrated lateral bending of the L-5 body of more than 10°, asymmetry of the L5-S1 intervertebral space, and deformity of the lumbar spine in the coronal plane. These findings were suggestive of disruption of at least part of the L5-S1 fibrous ring (anulus fibrosus) (32,33) and were not visible on conventional axial CT scans because the sections were transverse. In one of these patients, conventional axial CT scans demonstrated a nonspecific bulging of the L5-S1 intervertebral disk (Fig 3).

To our knowledge, the possible association between a sacral fracture and L5-S1 intervertebral disk injuries has been reported (34) in only three pediatric patients; however, no pathologic mechanism was postulated in

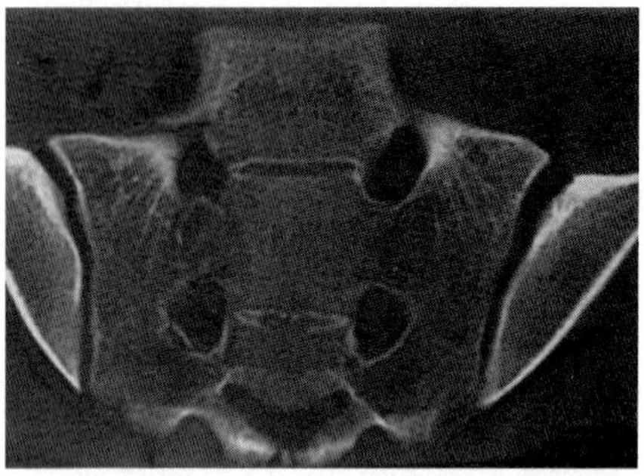

a.

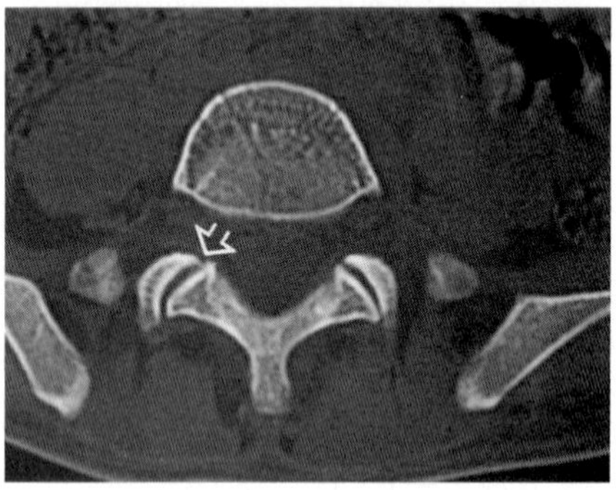

b.

Figure 6. Articular L5-S1 facet joint injury manifesting as a subluxation in a 20-year-old man involved in an occupational accident (fall from a scaffolding). **(a)** Coronal CT scan demonstrates the minimally displaced right vertical sacral fracture. **(b)** Axial CT scan shows incongruence of the right L5-S1 facet joint (arrow).

that report. We think that, in the context of the displacement and proximal migration of the hemipelvis, the S-1 body and articular process cause displacement in the cranial direction of the ipsilateral side of the L5-S1 intervertebral disk and the L-5 body, thereby causing lateral bending of more than 10° of the L-5 body and, thus, the complete failure of the L5-S1 motion segment. The energy of the traumatic incident must be high because it is responsible for bone fractures, as well as disruption of the osteo-disco-ligamentous complex. This lesion causes substantial instability in the coronal plane and, if not reduced, may result in compensatory scoliosis (Fig 7). Thus, we think that the involvement of the L5-S1 intervertebral disk should be considered separately because of the clinical relevance of injuries to this structure.

Diagnostic imaging provides all of the information that the orthopedic surgeon needs to define the pattern of a pelvic injury and to make the correct therapeutic decisions. An accurate restoration of the anatomy of the pelvic ring is essential to the improvement of survival and the reduction of future morbidity. Findings from the anteroposterior, inlet, and outlet views recommended by Pennal et al (2), Tile (3),

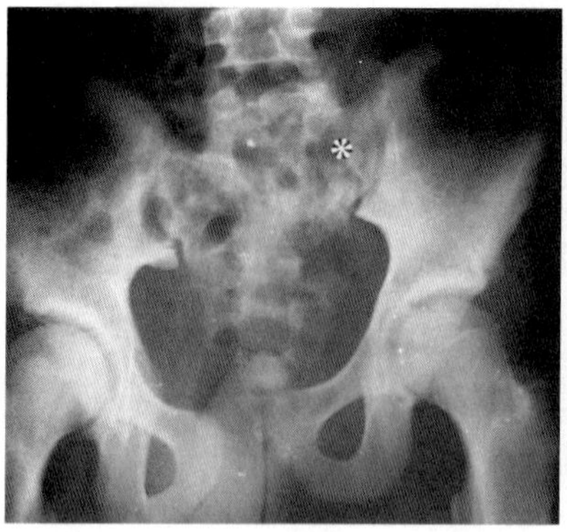

a.

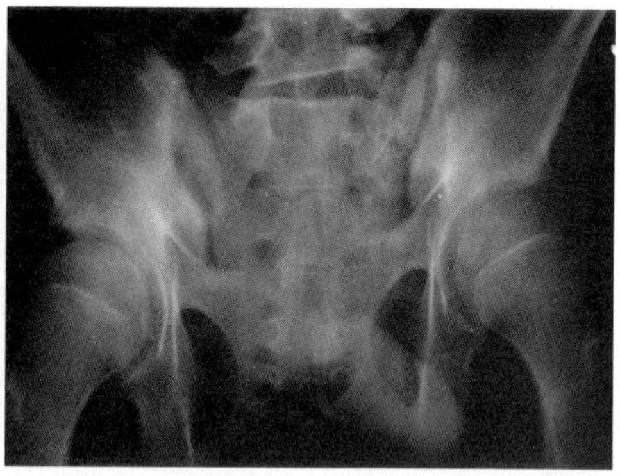

b.

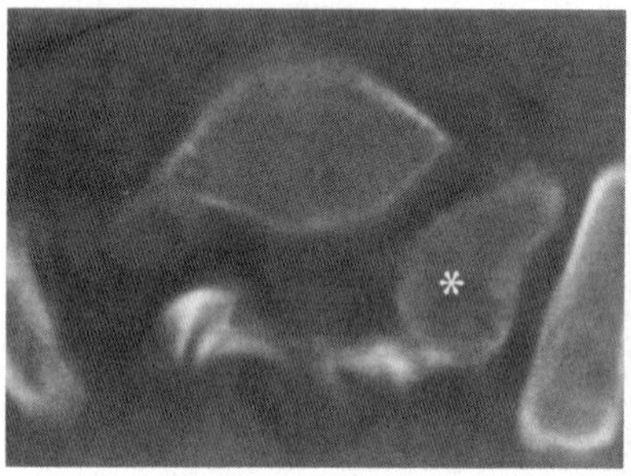

c.

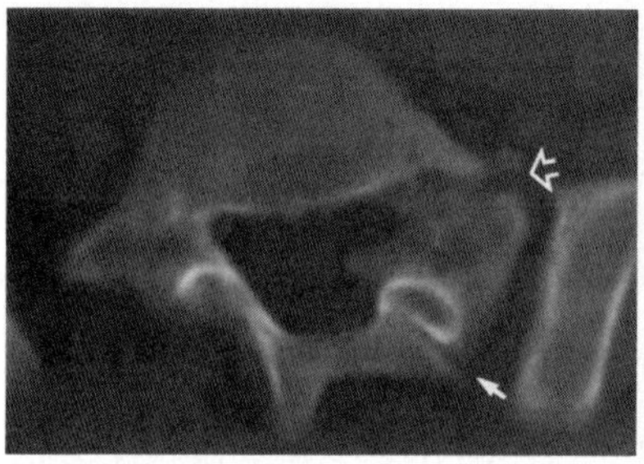

d.

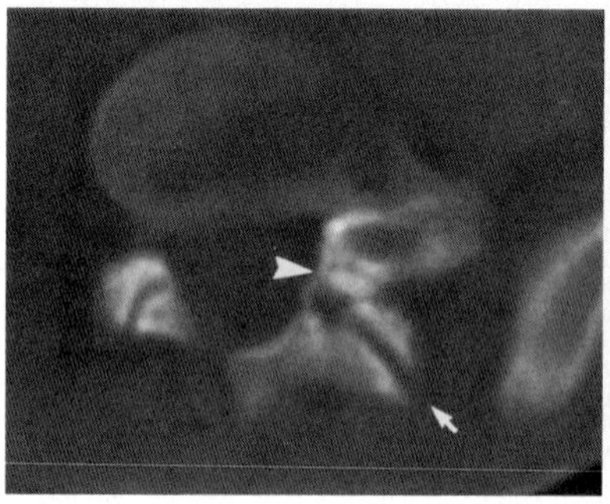

e.

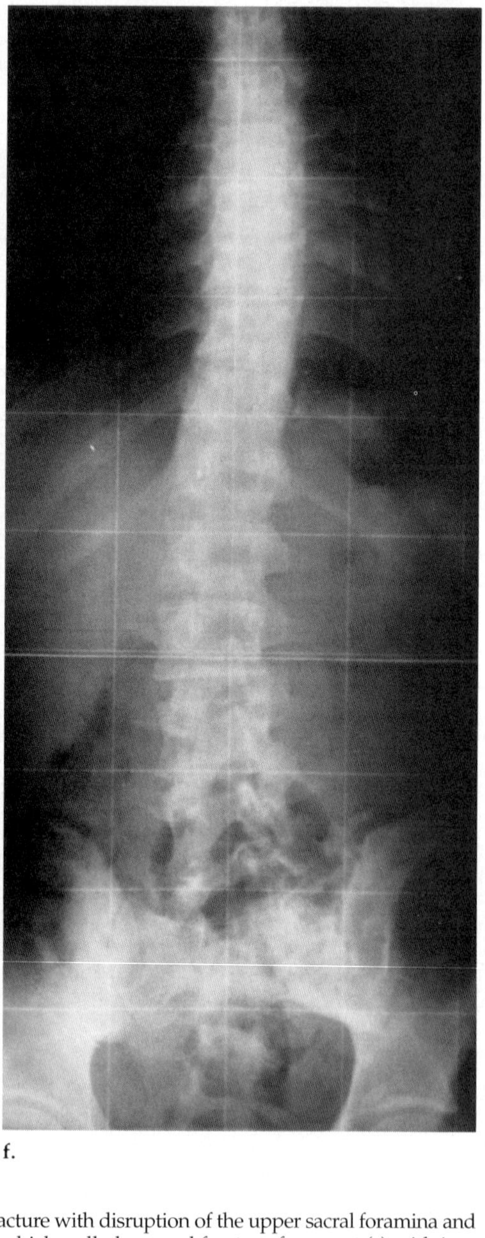

f.

Figure 7. Complex L5-S1 facet joint injury and L5-S1 intervertebral disk injury with a delayed vertical shear injury in a 15-year-old boy involved in a motor vehicle accident. (The poor quality of some CT images is due to faulty operation of laser printer.) **(a)** Anteroposterior radiograph shows a left sacral fracture with disruption of the upper sacral foramina and cranial displacement of the left hemipelvis, which pulled a sacral fracture fragment (*) with it. **(b)** Outlet radiograph clearly demonstrates lateral bending of the L-5 body and asymmetry of L5-S1 intervertebral space, suggestive of a concomitant injury of the L5-S1 intervertebral disk. **(c–e)** Sequential axial CT scans definitely demonstrate the dorsocranial displacement of the left sacral fragment. **(c)** The displaced left sacral fragment (*) is visible at the level of the right L5-S1 facet joint. **(d)** At a higher level than that shown in **c**, the left L5-S1 facet joint (solid arrow) is visible at the level of the L-5 right pedicle, which indicates a marked rotational displacement of the posterior elements of the L-5 body. A fracture of the L-5 left pedicle is also well demonstrated, together with repairing processes (open arrow). **(e)** At a higher level than that shown in **d**, the tip of the L5-S1 facet joint (arrow) is visible at the level of the ipsilateral L4-L5 facet joint (arrowhead). **(f)** Anteroposterior radiograph obtained 5 years later shows compensatory scoliosis of the lumbar spine.

and others (1,35) provide the basis with which pelvic fractures can be detected.

However, it is well known that an optimal evaluation of posterior ring element injuries cannot be accomplished with conventional radiographs alone, especially in cases of sacral fracture, which occurs in 40%–74% of the cases and is often diagnosed late or is even overlooked on radiographs (8,9,36). To our knowledge, only CT demonstrates all sacral and sacroiliac joint fractures, the extent of comminution, the rotation of the hemipelvic fragment, and the status of posterior aspect of the sacroiliac joint, all of which define the residual mechanical stability of the pelvic ring (5–9,36). Thus, it is necessary to obtain CT scans, which are superior to conventional radiographs in the depiction of the force vectors that produce a pelvic injury. For example, if an anteroposterior force also includes a shearing element that renders the hemipelvis unstable, this injury should properly be classified as an unstable vertical shear injury (Fig 4); in such a case, radiographs may be misleading (3,4).

In our study, the diagnosis of lumbosacral junction injury in nine of the 14 patients with this injury was made only on the basis of CT findings. No real estimate of specificity or sensitivity of CT findings for diagnosis of these injuries is possible, however, because of the lack of a reference standard (eg, intraoperative results or long-term follow-up findings) for the evaluation of the diagnostic efficacy of CT.

In conclusion, despite the small number of patients with a lumbosacral junction injury associated with an unstable pelvic fracture ($n = 14$), our results indicate that the prevalence of this injury may often be underestimated or the injury itself overlooked on the basis of radiographic findings, because of poor resolution and the tendency of bowel contents to obscure pelvic anatomic details. Associated lumbosacral junction injuries should be suspected in patients with a concomitant sacral fracture, especially if displacement, even if minimal, is present (Fig 6). Therefore, we recommend that pelvic CT scans that include the region of the lumbosacral junction be obtained in all patients with a severe pelvic ring fracture. It should be kept in mind that residual incongruence between the articular facets has a major effect on the outcome of patients with an unstable pelvic fracture because this incongruence may result in instability, clinically relevant symptoms, or invalidity, even in a patient whose pelvic fracture has been treated with anatomically correct reduction. Furthermore, we draw attention to the possible associated injury of the L5-S1 intervertebral disk. The presence of this injury is likely to indicate important chronic instability and is better evaluated on plain radiographs than on conventional axial CT scans. ■

Acknowledgments: We thank Perla Avegno for her valuable contribution in preparing the manuscript and Roberto Carnassale for his technical assistance in providing the schematic diagrams presented in this article.

References

1. Huittinen VM, Slatis P. Fractures of the pelvis: trauma mechanism, types of injury and principles of treatment. Acta Chir Scand 1972; 138:563–569.
2. Pennal GF, Tile M, Waddell JP, Garside H. Pelvic disruption: assessment and classification. Clin Orthop 1980; 151:12–21.
3. Tile M. Fractures of the pelvis and acetabulum. Baltimore, Md: Williams & Wilkins, 1984; 70–96.
4. Young JWR, Resnik CS. Fractures of the pelvis: current concepts of classification. AJR 1990; 155:1169–1175.
5. Gilula LA, Murphy WA, Tailor CC, Patel RB. Computed tomography of the osseous pelvis. Radiology 1979; 132:107–114.
6. Rafii M, Firooznia H, Golimbu C, Waugh T Jr, Naidich D. The impact of CT in clinical management of pelvic and acetabular fractures. Clin Orthop 1983; 178:228–235.
7. Gill K, Bucholz RW. The role of computerized tomographic scanning in the evaluation of major pelvic fractures. J Bone Joint Surg [Am] 1984; 66:34–39.
8. Dunn EL, Berry PH, Connolly PJ. Computed tomography of the pelvis in patients with multiple injuries. J Trauma 1983; 23: 378–383.
9. Montana MA, Richardson ML, Kilcoyne RF, Harley JD, Shuman WP, Mack LA. CT of sacral injury. Radiology 1986; 161:499–503.
10. Mears DC, Ward AJ, Wright MS. The radiological assessment of pelvic and acetabular fractures using three dimensional computed tomography. Int J Orthop Trauma 1992; 2:196–209.
11. McMurtry R, Walton D, Dickinson D, Kellam J, Tile M. Pelvic disruption in the polytraumatized patient: a management protocol. Clin Orthop 1980; 151:22–30.
12. Ward RE, Clark DG. Management of pelvic fractures. Radiol Clin North Am 1981; 19:167–170.
13. Agnew S. Hemodynamically unstable pelvic fractures. Orthop Clin North Am 1994; 25:715–721.
14. Tile M, Pennal GF. Pelvic disruption: principles of management. Clin Orthop 1980; 151:56–64.
15. Goldstein A, Phillips T, Sclafani SJA, et al. Early open reduction and internal fixation of the disrupted pelvic ring. J Trauma 1986; 26:325–332.
16. Riemer B, Butterfield S, Diamond D, et al. Acute mortality associated with injuries to the pelvic ring: the role of early mobilization and external fixation. J Trauma 1993; 35:671–677.
17. Pohlemann T, Bosch U, Gänsslen A, Tscherne H. The Hannover experience in management of pelvic fractures. Clin Orthop 1994; 305:69–80.
18. Raf L. Double vertical fractures of the pelvis. Acta Chir Scand 1966; 131:298–305.
19. Fell M, Meissner A, Rahmanzadeh R. Langzeitergebnisse nach konservativer behandlung von beckenringverletzungen und konsequenzen fur das heutige management. Zentralbl Chir 1995; 120:899–904.
20. Isler B. Lumbosacral junction injuries associated with pelvic ring injuries. J Orthop Trauma 1990; 4:1–5.
21. Slatis P. Injuries in fatal traffic accidents. Acta Chir Scand 1962; 297(suppl):1–15.
22. Sevitt S. Fatal road accidents: injuries, complications and causes of death. Br J Surg 1968; 55:481–505.
23. Patterson FP, Morton KS. The cause of death in fracture of the pelvis. J Trauma 1973; 13:849–856.
24. Rothenberger DA, Fischer RP, Strare R, et al. The mortality associated with pelvic fractures. Surgery 1978; 84:356–361.
25. Goris RJ, Gimbrère JS, van Nickerk JL, Schoots FJ, Booy LH. Improved survival of multiply injured patients by early internal fixation and prophylactic mechanical ventilation. Injury 1982; 14:39–43.
26. Smith TK, Johnston RM, Bucholz RW, Brommer BB. Symposium: external fixation of pelvic fractures. Contemp Orthop 1983; 7:81–101.
27. Tile M. Pelvic fractures: operative versus non-operative treatment. Orthop Clin North Am 1980; 11:423–464.
28. Connolly PJ, Esses SI, Heggeness MH, Cook SS. Unilateral facet dislocation of the lumbosacral junction. Spine 1992; 17: 1244–1248.
29. Watson-Jones R. Fractures and joint injuries. Baltimore, Md; Williams & Wilkins, 1940; 641.
30. White AA III, Panjabi MM. Clinical biomechanics of the spine. 2nd ed. Philadelphia, Pa; Lippincott, 1990; 342–362.
31. Dalal SA, Burgess AR, Siegel JH, et al. Pelvic fracture in multiple trauma: classification by mechanism is key to pattern of organ injury, resuscitative requirements, and outcome. J Trauma 1989; 29:981–1000.
32. Lumsden RM II, Morris JM. An in vivo study of axial rotation and immobilization at the lumbosacral joint. J Bone Joint Surg [Am] 1968; 50:1591–1602.
33. Nagel DA, Koogle TA, Piziali RL, Perkash I. Stability of the upper lumbar spine following progressive disruptions and the application of individual internal and external fixation devices. J Bone Joint Surg [Am] 1981; 63:62–70.
34. Ehrensperger J. Fractures of the sacrum and disk herniation: rare lesions in the pediatric surgical patient? Eur J Pediatr Surg 1992; 2:173–176.
35. Leone A, Oranski M, Priolo F, Marano P. Le fratture pelviche. Radiol Med 1992; 83: 602–607.
36. Resnik CS, Stackhouse DJ, Shanmuganathan K, Young JW. Diagnosis of pelvic fractures in patients with acute pelvic trauma: efficacy of plain radiographs. AJR 1992; 158:109–112.

Robert R. Brown, MD • Mini N. Pathria, MD • Paul M. Ruggieri, MD • Jon A. Jacobson, MD
Joseph G. Craig, MB, BCh • Donald Resnick, MD

Extensive Intraosseous Gas Associated with Lymphangiomatosis of Bone: Report of Three Cases[1]

Asymptomatic pneumatosis may be found in patients with lymphangiomatosis of bone. The authors report three cases from three institutions in which development of intraosseous gas in association with lymphangiomatosis of bone was found incidentally at imaging. Soft-tissue emphysema also developed in two cases. In all three cases, intraosseous gas developed after biopsy or surgery in the areas involved with lymphangiomatosis.

Index terms: Bone neoplasms, in infants and children, 40.3142, 40.3143 • Lymphangioma, 40.3142, 40.3143, 60.3157 • Lymphangiomatosis, 40.3142, 60.3157 • Lymphatic system, diseases, 40.3142, 40.3143, 60.3157

Radiology 1997; 205:260–262

LYMPHANGIOMATOSIS is a rare disorder, presumably caused by a multifocal congenital malformation of the lymphatic system alone or combined with malformation of the vascular system (1,2). Lymphangiomatosis produces lytic lesions in multiple bones, commonly in association with visceral involvement, particularly of the pleura, lung, and solid abdominal organs (3). We report three cases of disseminated osseous lymphangiomatosis in which extensive intraosseous gas was present in the bone lesions. To our knowledge, this association has not been reported previously.

CASE REPORTS

Case 1.—After an uncomplicated delivery, a male infant was noted to have a right posterior cervical mass diagnosed as a cystic hygroma. At 21 months of age, the patient developed Kasabach-Merritt syndrome (coagulopathy and thrombocytopenia) and was treated with prednisone, aspirin, and dipyridamole. At 3 years of age, disseminated skeletal lesions were discovered on radiographs. Findings from angiography and biopsy of a rib lesion at that time were consistent with hemangiolymphangiomatosis and cystic angiomatosis. At the age of 6 years, the cervical mass increased in size and extended to involve the temporal bone, the base of the skull, and the mediastinum. Histologic examination showed hemangioendothelioma, which was treated with cyclophosphamide and embolization. At the age of 7½ years, a radical neck dissection performed to resect this tumor resulted in Horner syndrome occurring on the right side.

At 8 years of age, the patient developed a large mediastinal mass, bilateral pulmonary infiltrates, and cardiac tamponade. A pericardial window yielded chylous pericardial fluid. Multiple biopsies of the mediastinal mass yielded material that was interpreted as an angiosarcoma at histologic analysis. After surgery, the patient developed massive bilateral chylous pleural effusions. The effusions were treated with thoracic duct ligation and injection of tetracycline into the pleural spaces. At 14 years of age, a retroperitoneal mass developed. Histologically, this mass represented a lymphangioma with chronic inflammation and fibrosis.

At age 15 years, computed tomography (CT), radiography, and magnetic resonance (MR) imaging of the skull base (Fig 1a, 1b) were performed for assessment of headaches. These images demonstrated extensive intraosseous gas in the diploë of the occiput, clivus, petrous bones, and sphenoid wings, as well as subcutaneous emphysema posteriorly. Gas noted at CT was more difficult to appreciate at radiography or MR imaging. One month later, results from biopsies performed of a skull lesion and the C-2 vertebral body revealed benign lymphangiomas. All bone and soft-tissue cultures were negative, and no osteomyelitis or organisms were present at histologic examination. CT performed 1 month after biopsy (Fig 1c) demonstrated progression of gas in the bones of the skull base and upper cervical spine; the gas occupied most of the cancellous bone. No cortical destruction, abnormal mass, or fluid collection was apparent. Soft-tissue emphysema was also noted in the upper portion of the neck. Currently, at the age of 15 years, the patient has an unstable cervical spine, experiences increasing pain, and wears a neck brace.

Case 2.—After this writing, this case was reported in another article (4). Although pneumatization of the cranial bones was mentioned, massive osteolysis of the skull base was emphasized in that report. A 14-year-old girl had cerebrospinal fluid rhinorrhea at initial examination. The patient was the product of a normal pregnancy and had no medical history. At the age of 10 years, the patient developed a Bell palsy that resolved spontaneously. At 13 years of age, the patient reported left-sided hearing loss and occasional headaches. Results of physical examination were normal except for cerebrospinal fluid rhinorrhea that occurred when the patient leaned forward. Radiographs and a CT scan demonstrated a lesion in the first thoracic vertebral body and extensive destruction of the clivus and petrous bones diagnosed as lymphangiomatosis. Biopsy samples obtained from the clivus, sphenoid sinus, and right middle turbinate bone revealed no pathologic changes. No gas was present at that time.

The patient was treated with a right occipital-peritoneal shunt with a high-pressure valve. After the procedure, the patient reported tunnel vision and severe headaches on one side. Minimal left homonymous quadrantanopia was diagnosed. The postoperative course was otherwise unremarkable with no signs of rhinorrhea. The patient was discharged from the hospital 4 days after surgery.

MR images and CT scans obtained 4 and 5 months later, respectively (Fig 2), demonstrated extensive intraosseous gas in the lesions of the skull base and atlas. No other interval change was noted.

Case 3.—A previously healthy 6-year-old boy developed loosening of the right lower molar teeth 9 months after injury to the chin. Several right lower teeth were extracted, and 1 year later more teeth loosened and were removed. During surgery, sulfur granules were detected; the presence of these granules led to suspicion of an actinomycosis infection. The patient was treated with antibiotics. It was subsequently believed that the sulfur granules represented contamination rather than a true infection. At 8 years of age, multiple left upper

[1] From the Department of Radiology 8756, University of California San Diego Medical Center-Veterans Administration Medical Center, 200 W Arbor St, San Diego, CA 92103 (R.R.B., M.N.P., D.R.); the Department of Radiology, Cleveland Clinic Foundation, Ohio (P.M.R.); and the Department of Radiology, Henry Ford Hospital, Detroit, Mich (J.A.J., J.G.C.). Received March 11, 1997; revision requested May 1; revision received May 19; accepted June 2. Supported in part by Veterans Administration grant no. SA-360. **Address reprint requests to** M.N.P.

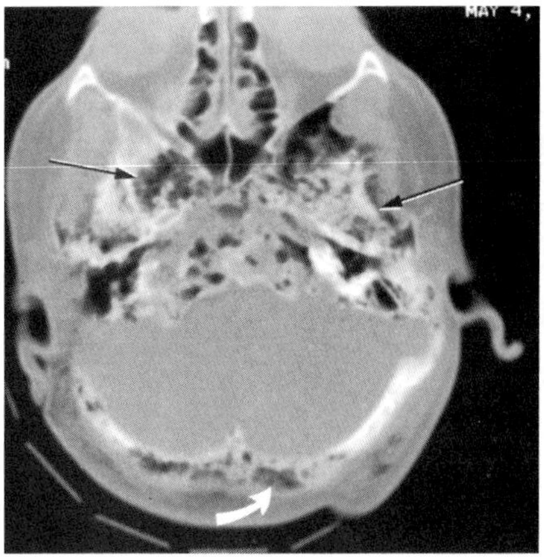

a.

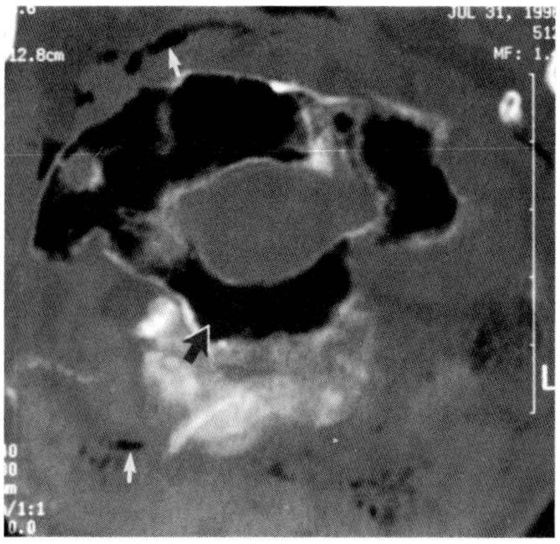

c.

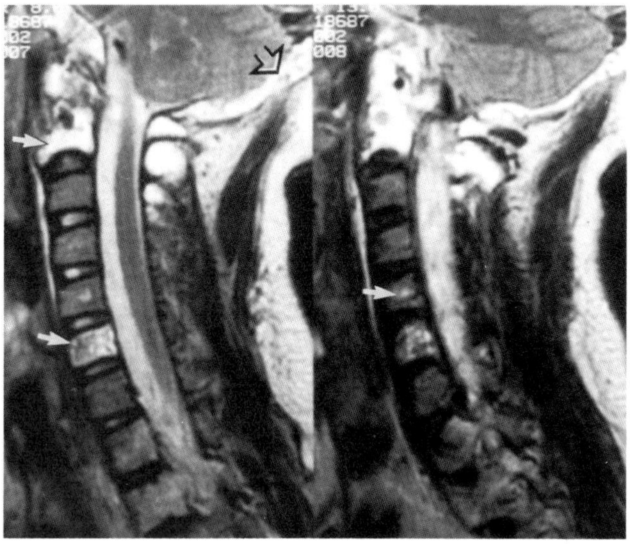

b.

Figure 1. Patient 1. **(a)** CT scan of the skull base demonstrates extensive intraosseous gas in the sphenoid bone (straight arrows) and occipital bone (curved arrow). **(b)** Sagittal MR images (3,000/90 effective [repetition time msec/echo time msec]) of the cervical spine show a mottled appearance to the diploë consistent with pneumatosis (open arrow). Abnormal signal intensity is also seen in the axis and C-5 and C-6 vertebral bodies (solid arrows). **(c)** CT scan of the C-2 vertebral body obtained 3 months later shows complete replacement of the bone marrow cavity with intraosseous gas. The body, posterior elements (large arrow), and transverse processes are involved with lymphangiomatosis. Subcutaneous gas is noted (small arrows).

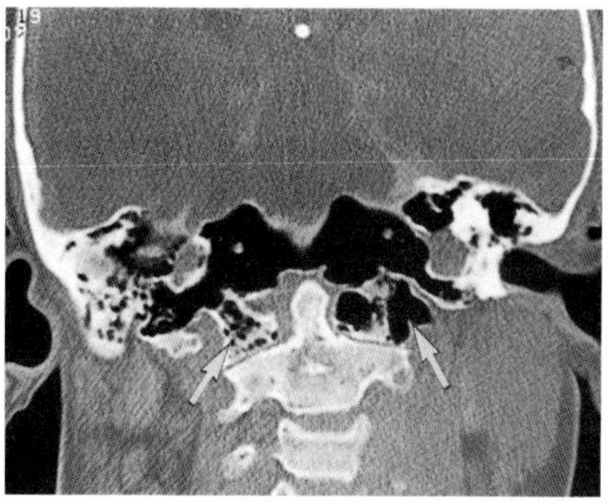

Figure 2. Patient 2. CT scan obtained 5 months after surgery demonstrates extensive pneumatization of the skull base and atlas (arrows).

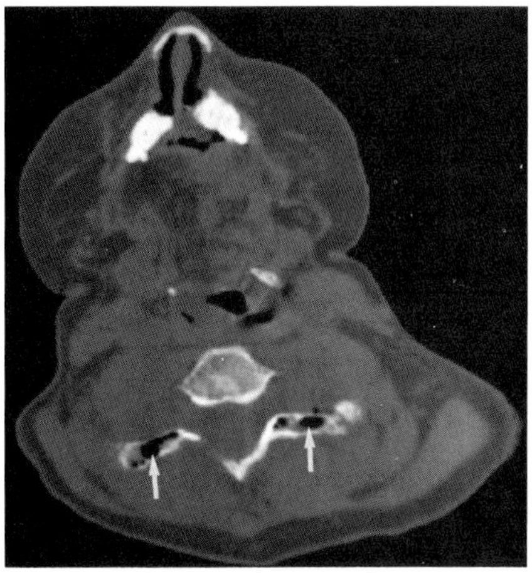

Figure 3. Patient 3. CT scan obtained through the upper thorax confirms intraosseous gas in the transverse processes of T-1 (arrows) that was also seen on radiographs.

teeth loosened, and a defect was noted in the hard palate. Osteolysis was apparent in the right middle cranial fossa and right infratemporal region. Long-term antibiotic therapy and hyperbaric oxygen treatments were administered. Six months later, systemic candidiasis infection developed secondary to placement of a central venous catheter. At 9 years of age, biopsy specimens obtained in the area of osteolysis revealed osteoclasts, and a diagnosis of Gorham disease was made by the pathologist. The patient was treated subsequently with calcitonin.

At 10 years of age, osteolysis was noted to involve the cervical spine, and the diagnosis was changed to generalized angiomatosis. Radiation treatmet and administration of pamidronate disodium, an osteoclast inhibitor, slowed disease progression. Six months later, a feeding tube was placed. At 12 years of age, the cervical spine was fused due to cervical spine impingement and basilar invagination. A large right pleural effusion developed 2 years later; this effusion was not chylous in nature. A chest tube was placed for several weeks and drained 0.5 L/d of fluid from an unknown source. At this time, a bone scan and radiographs demonstrated involvement of the right clavicle and right first rib. Biopsy samples were obtained from the right clavicle, and cultures were negative. The patient subsequently received 14 radiation therapy treatments.

At 15 years of age, radiographs showed gas in the cervical and thoracic spine and right ribs; the presence of gas was confirmed at CT (Fig 3). Gas was also noted in the soft tissues of the right hemithorax and pleural space with the chest tube in place. The patient had no clinical signs of infection.

DISCUSSION

Lymphangiomatosis of bone is an uncommon skeletal disorder. This disease may show a benign course in some patients and cause serious morbidity in others. The histologic, radiologic, and clinical characteristics of lymphangiomatosis overlap those of hemangiomatosis and Gorham massive osteolysis, so that these entities often are grouped together as angiomatous bone lesions. The cause of these disorders is unknown, but most investigators suggest that multifocal angiomatous bone lesions represent a congenital malformation of the vascular or lymphatic system or both (2). At histologic examination, a lymphangioma of bone is a lymph-filled, multilocular cavity with an endothelial lining. If the lymph-filled spaces are replaced by fibrous tissue, definite diagnosis is impossible.

Osseous lymphangiomatosis develops typically during childhood (5). Patients with isolated bone involvement usually are asymptomatic, show slow progression of the osseous disease, and generally have a good prognosis (3,5). Visceral involvement, present in 45% of affected persons, adversely affects the clinical course and the prognosis associated with lymphangiomatosis and results in substantial morbidity (3,5). The most common visceral manifestations of lymphangiomatosis are chylous pleural effusions, pericardial effusion, and soft-tissue lymphedema. Involvement of the lungs, mediastinum, retroperitoneum, abdominal organs, and soft tissues have also been described, with variable frequency. All organ systems may be affected except the central nervous system, which presumably is spared because it lacks a lymphatic system (3).

Lymphangiomas of bone appear as multiloculated radiolucent lesions on radiographs. The most common sites of involvement are the tibia and humerus. Axial involvement, particularly in the skull and flat bones, is also well recognized (5,6). Margination of the lesions may or may not be well defined. Both sclerotic and nonsclerotic borders have been reported. The lesions originate from the medullary portion of bone. Thinning and expansion of the overlying cortex may occur, and rarely, there may be extension of the lesion into adjacent soft tissues and neighboring bones.

CT and MR imaging are both useful in the demonstration of soft-tissue and visceral involvement. However, the CT and MR imaging characteristics of an intraosseous lymphangioma are also nonspecific. Heterogeneous bone marrow with intermediate to high signal intensity is seen on T1- and T2-weighted images. Involved bone may be expanded, and internal septa appear as low-signal-intensity structures. Although the imaging findings are nonspecific, lymphoangiographic demonstration of communication with the lymphatic system establishes the diagnosis (1,5,7,8). Delayed imaging is necessary to allow sufficient time for lymphangiographic contrast material to extend into the lesions. Once the contrast material is located within the intraosseous cavities, it may remain for months after the procedure (8). Although there are numerous descriptions of the imaging features of angiomatous lesions of bone, we have been unable to find any previous reports on the presence of intraosseous gas in these lesions (2,6,9).

Intraosseous pneumatosis has been reported after occurrence of penetrating wounds, after biopsy, and in the presence of compound fractures or osteomyelitis (10,11). Although intraosseous gas has been emphasized as an indicator of osteomyelitis, there are numerous situations in which gas within bone may be present in the absence of open injury or infection. It has been suggested that gas may accumulate anywhere in the body where substantial negative pressure develops and may persist for months (12,13). Intraosseous gas has been described commonly in association with osteonecrosis and typically is seen in a linear fashion within a vertebral body or in the subchondral region at the end of a long bone (14).

In rare cases, intraosseous gas may be identified within an area of neoplastic involvement (14). A gas-fluid level within a sterile, uncomplicated solitary bone cyst has also been described (12). Sterile pneumatocysts of the cervical spine and the iliac bone can be seen, although the presence of gas may be difficult to confirm without CT (13,15,16). On plain radiographs, intraosseous gas is difficult to recognize and its presence may be identified only retrospectively after evaluation with CT (15). MR imaging can demonstrate intraosseous gas as a region of signal void or as a zone of speckled inhomogeneous signal intensity, but the findings are more conspicuous at CT.

In these three patients, the origin of intraosseous gas is not known. Osteomyelitis is an unlikely cause of intraosseous gas in these cases. None of these patients had abnormal laboratory values such as increased sedimentation rate or increased white blood cell count. Two patients underwent biopsy in the area of gas formation, and no organisms grew in culture or were visualized at histologic examination. The third patient did not undergo biopsy after detection of intraosseous gas but had no clinical features of infection, despite months of documented intraosseous pneumatosis. We can only speculate on the origin of the extensive pneumatosis in these lesions. The fluid in these lesions may have resorbed spontaneously, creating negative pressure in the lesions and allowing nitrogen gas from the blood to accumulate in them. It is also possible that the gas may have originated within the lung and entered the abnormal pulmonary lymphatic system, which communicated directly with the abnormal lymphatic system within the bone. The first patient had pulmonary and pleural involvement, demonstrated by evidence of pulmonary infiltrates and previous chylous effusions. The second patient did not have documented pulmonary disease, although chest radiographic findings suggested the presence of mild pulmonary lymphangiomatosis.

Another possible explanation for the pneumatosis is that the intraosseous gas was related to previous surgery. All patients underwent head and neck surgery before pneumatosis was detected. The surgery may have caused abnormal communication between an aerated sinus and the abnormal bone. If surgical exploration disrupted the flow of lymph fluid into these lesions, allowing them to empty, air from a sinus may have entered the endothelial-lined spaces. In the absence of sinus communication, negative pressure within the emptied spaces could allow collection of nitrogen from the blood, leading to intraosseous pneumatosis. Unfortunately, the composition of the gas was not analyzed in these cases, which makes it more difficult to establish the cause of this unusual finding.

In summary, we reported findings in three patients with lymphangiomatosis in whom asymptomatic intraosseous gas was identified after head and neck surgery or after biopsy. To our knowledge, the association of intraosseous pneumatosis and lymphangiomatosis has not been described previously. Although the presence of osseous pneumatosis in lymphangiomatosis must be rare, knowledge of this association may help avert unnecessary biopsy. ■

Acknowledgment: We thank Henry Bone, MD, for assistance.

References

1. Chu JY, Graviss ER, Danis RK, et al. Lymphangiography and bone scan in the study of lymphangiomatosis. Pediatr Radiol 1977; 6:46–48.
2. Latour L, Simeons CJ, Gryspeerdt S, Samson I, Mertens V, Van Damme B. Skeletal cystic angiomatosis. Skeletal Radiol 1996; 25:92–95.
3. Canady AI, Chou SN. Cervical lymphangiomatosis with progressive craniospinal deformity. Neurosurgery 1980; 6:422–425.
4. Frankel DG, Lewin JS, Cohen B. Massive osteolysis of the skull base. Pediatr Radiol 1997; 27:265–267.
5. Nixon GW. Lymphangiomatosis of bone demonstrated by lymphangiography. AJR 1970; 110:582–586.
6. Nazarian GK, Gebarski SS, Niparko JK. Cranial lymphangiomatosis causing CSF otorrhea and recurrent meningitis: CT features. J Comput Assist Tomogr 1990; 14: 121–123.
7. Gafner E, Fuchs WA, Kuffer F. Lymphangiography in lymphangiomatosis of bone. Lymphology 1972; 5:129–131.
8. Winterberger AR. Radiographic diagnosis of lymphangiomatosis of bone. Radiology 1972; 102:321–324.
9. Edwards WH, Thompson RC, Varsa EW. Lymphangiomatosis and massive osteolysis of the cervical spine. Clin Orthop 1983; 177:222–229.
10. Azouz EM, Raymond J. Case report 316: intraosseous gas of the left tibia 24 hours after biopsy. Skeletal Radiol 1985; 13:327–328.
11. Ram PC, Martinez S, Korobkin M, et al. CT detection of intraosseous gas: a new sign of osteomyelitis. AJR 1981; 137:721–723.
12. Hahn PF, Rosenthal DI, Ehrlich MG. Case report 286: gas within a solitary bone cyst of the proximal end of the left humerus. Skeletal Radiol 1984; 12:214–217.
13. Hart BL, Brantly PN, Lubbers PR, Zell BK, Flynn ET Jr. Compression pain in a diver with intraosseous pneumatocysts. Undersea Biomed Res 1986; 13:465–468.
14. Resnick D, Niwayama G, Guerra J, Vint V, Usselman J. Spinal vacuum phenomena: anatomic study and review. Radiology 1981; 139:341–348.
15. Grunshaw MD, Carey BM. Case report: gas within a cervical vertebral body. Clin Radiol 1994; 49:653–654.
16. Ramirez H, Blatt ES, Cable HG, McComb BL, Zornoza J, Hibri NS. Intraosseous pneumatocysts of the ilium. Radiology 1984; 150:503–505.

Martin Kocher, MD • Harald Treuer, PhD • Rolf-Peter Müller, MD

Quantification of Tumor Reoxygenation during Accelerated Radiation Therapy[1]

PURPOSE: **To determine the effect of accelerated fractionated radiation therapy on the reoxygenation of chronic hypoxic tumor cells by means of a three-dimensional Monte Carlo simulation.**

MATERIALS AND METHODS: **Tumor growth (cell cycle time [T_c] of 2 or 5 days), irradiation (α = 0.3 Gy^{-1}, α/β = 10 Gy), oxygen tension (oxygen enhancement ratio of 3.0), capillary network distortion, and shrinkage of a small (10^4-cell) tumor were modeled on a workstation. Conventional (2 Gy delivered five times per week), accelerated (1.6 Gy delivered twice a day for 5 d/wk), and split-course (1.6 Gy delivered twice a day for 5 d/wk with a break in week 3) radiation therapies were simulated with total doses of 50–70 Gy.**

RESULTS: **Tumors grew in cords with a central necrotic area surrounded by hypoxic cells (hypoxic fraction, 25%). If undisturbed tumor shrinkage occurred, complete reoxygenation took 2½ weeks for accelerated, 3–5 weeks for split-course, or 4–6 weeks for conventional radiation therapy. If shrinkage was prevented, the hypoxic fraction rose to 90%–100% at 2–3 weeks. In the shrinking, reoxygenating tumors with a T_c of 2 days, accelerated radiation therapy increased tumor control by 40%–80% over the control with conventional radiation therapy. With split-course therapy, this advantage was lost at doses below 70 Gy. Shrinking tumors with a T_c of 5 days were all controlled with 50 Gy.**

CONCLUSION: **Fast-growing tumors that reoxygenate by shrinking are especially sensitive to acceleration and treatment breaks.**

In recent years, fractionation schedules have been developed to improve the therapeutic ratio for tumors that reside in dose-limiting normal tissue. Interest has been focused on accelerated fractionation in combination with hyperfractionation, which is thought to overcome tumor repopulation and reduce late normal-tissue toxic reactions (1). Although the potentially deleterious effect of split-course irradiation on tumor control has been well recognized, this fractionation scheme has been used to reduce acute toxic reactions (2).

These fractionation schemes do not specifically take into account the relative radioresistance of the hypoxic cell fraction, which may amount to up to 25% in human tumors (3,4). In addition to the processes that increase perfusion in irradiated acutely hypoxic tumors (5), several mechanisms exist that may reoxygenate chronic hypoxic cells during fractionated radiation therapy. A reduced respiration rate in damaged cells and ischemic or mitotic death may contribute to reoxygenation, but the most long-lasting effect is thought to arise from tumor shrinkage, which increases capillary density and brings hypoxic cells closer to the nutrient vessels (6).

In experimental tumors, however, insufficient reoxygenation during accelerated radiation therapy has been observed if the interfraction intervals are too short (7,8). We performed this study to estimate the effect of accelerated radiation therapy on reoxygenation and tumor cell repopulation (9), and thus the effect on tumor control, by means of computer simulation. Unlike other mathematical models of reoxygenation that we know of (10–12), the model provides a three-dimensional spatial representation of the tumor cells, the capillary bed, oxygen tension, and tumor shrinkage (13,14).

MATERIALS AND METHODS

A three-dimensional model was developed with a 33-MHz workstation (model 80486; Intel, Santa Clara, Calif). It consisted of a 75 × 75 × 75 lattice with a 20-μm distance between the lattice positions in all space directions. Monte Carlo simulation techniques were used to generate random numbers that, after adequate transformation, determined individual tumor cell division, radiation-induced cell killing, tumor shrinkage and distortion, and restoration of the capillary network (14).

Capillary Network and Oxygen Supply

The simplified capillary network consisted of capillary cross sections positioned at every seventh lattice position in all space directions, which resulted in a minimum distance between capillaries of 140 μm and a density of about 350 capillaries per cubic millimeter. Cells with a distance in space ([x distance^2 + y distance^2 + z distance^2]$^{1/2}$)

Index terms: Computers, simulation • Dosimetry, **.1299[2] • Neoplasms, blood supply, **.30 • Neoplasms, therapeutic radiology, **.1299, **.30

Abbreviation: T_c = cell cycle time.

Radiology 1997; 205:263–268

[1] From the Departments of Radiotherapy (M.K., R.P.M.) and Stereotactic Neurosurgery (H.T.), University of Cologne, Joseph-Stelzmann-Strasse 9, D-50924 Cologne, Germany. From the 1996 RSNA scientific assembly. Received March 20, 1997; revision requested May 7; revision received June 23; accepted June 25. **Address reprint requests to** M.K.

[2] ** indicates all regions of the body.

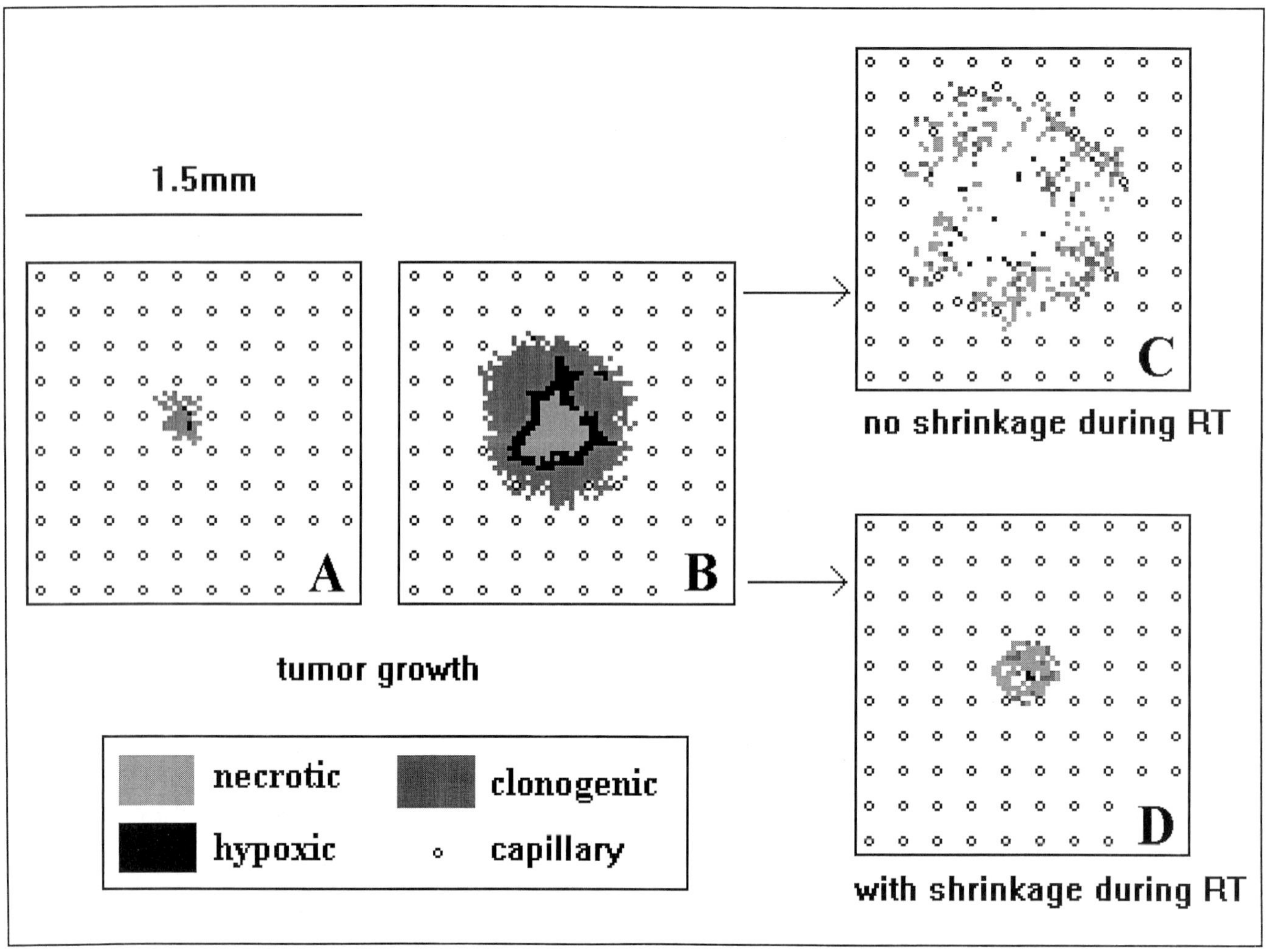

Figure 1. Cross sections of a simulated tumor during growth and radiation therapy. *A,* Early growth phase. *B,* End of growth phase, just before the start of radiation therapy. Tumor cells have grown in cords, the capillary network is deformed, central necrosis has developed, and hypoxic cells reside between the necrotic and the clonogenic cells. *C,* Disturbed shrinkage during radiation therapy (RT) prevents reoxygenation. Capillaries are represented as small circles but occupy only one lattice position in the model. *D,* During radiation therapy. Undisturbed shrinkage of the tumor allows for reoxygenation owing to restoration of the vascular architecture.

of up to 100 μm from the nearest capillary were treated as normoxic, clonogenic tumor cells. Tumor cells with a distance of more than 100 μm up to 140 μm were regarded as hypoxic cells, viable but unable to divide unless reoxygenated. Cells with a distance of more than 140 μm were regarded as necrotic.

Tumor Growth, Shrinkage, and Irradiation

Tumor cells were thought to occupy lattice positions 20 μm apart; no special assumption was made with regard to cell size. The cell cycle time (T_c) of all cells of a tumor was set to either 2 or 5 days. At the beginning of the simulation, a single tumor cell was placed in the center of the capillary network. Cells divided after every interval equal to their T_cs but were desynchronized by randomly adding $(-1 \ldots 1)$ to the time of the next division. At each division, one of the daughter cells stayed in place while the other was randomly placed into one of the 26 ($3^3 - 1$) surrounding lattice positions. If this place was already occupied, all tumor cells and capillaries along the spatial direction of this division were shifted away from the parent cell one lattice distance (20–35 μm) in the direction of the division, thereby leaving a free place for the daughter cell.

The linear-quadratic model was used to simulate the cell kill by irradiation. For oxygenated, clonogenic cells, α was 0.3 Gy^{-1} and α/β was 10 Gy. For the hypoxic tumor cells, an oxygen enhancement ratio of 3.0 was chosen. Oxygen was assumed to be purely dose modifying: $\alpha_{hypoxic} = \alpha_{normal}/(\text{oxygen enhancement ratio})$, and $\beta_{hypoxic} = \beta_{normal}/(\text{oxygen enhancement ratio})^2$. Survival ($S$) was calculated according to the following: $S_{normal} = \exp(-[\alpha_{normal}d + \beta_{normal} \times d^2])$, and $S_{hypoxic} = \exp(-[\alpha_{hypoxic} \times d + \beta_{hypoxic} \times d^2])$.

Irradiation was modeled according to random cell kill, with each cell's probability to survive adjusted to the calculated survival for the selected dose per fraction. For every tumor cell, a random number between 0 and 100 was generated, and the cell survived only if this number fell into the range determined with the equations above. Complete repair between fractions was assumed. During irradiation, clonogenic tumor cells continuously repopulated the tumor without acceleration. Clonogenic cells hit by radiation suffered mitotic death at their next attempt to divide and were resorbed 5 days later. Hypoxic cells were assumed to die after one cell cycle if lethally hit. Reoxygenated tumor cells became clonogenic again at one cell cycle after reoxygenation.

A main property of the model was the simulation of tumor shrinkage. In nonshrinking tumors, passive cell movements were caused only by the cell division procedure. In contrast, in shrinking tumors, elastic tissue forces were assumed that caused cell movements targeted to the center of the tumor and capillary movements directed toward the initial capillary position before distortion due to tumor growth. For this purpose, tumor cells and capillaries underwent random shifts until reaching a position nearer to their target. This process was started at the most inner layers and continued until it reached the most peripheral layers. It was implemented to represent properties of tumor stroma, such as the amount of connective tissue, interstitial pressure, calcifications, and cysts

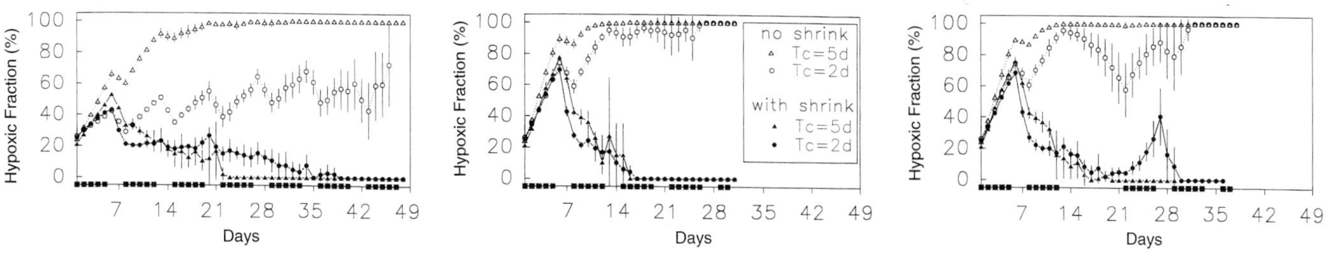

a. b. c.

Figure 2. Time course of the hypoxic cell fraction (means ± standard deviations for five simulation runs) during **(a)** fractionated conventional (2 Gy), **(b)** accelerated (1.6 Gy twice a day), or **(c)** accelerated split-course (1.6 Gy twice a day) irradiation. △ = T_c of 5 days and no shrinkage, ▲ = T_c of 5 days and shrinkage, ○ = T_c of 2 days and no shrinkage, ● = T_c of 2 days and shrinkage, ■ = days of irradiation.

that allow or inhibit tumor shrinkage during irradiation.

Simulation Runs

Irradiation was started at a total tumor cell number of at least 10^4 cells. During irradiation, all cells were counted and the hypoxic cell fraction was calculated according to the following: (number of hypoxic cells)/(number of hypoxic cells + number of clonogenic cells). Three different fractionation schemes were used: conventional (five fractions of 2.0 Gy/wk), accelerated (1.6 Gy delivered twice a day for 5 d/wk, 16 Gy/wk), and accelerated split-course (1.6 Gy delivered twice a day for 5 d/wk, split in week 3) irradiation. Simulation runs were performed for doses of 50, 60, or 70 Gy in tumors with T_cs of 2 or 5 days, with tumor shrinkage allowed or inhibited. After completion of the fractionation schedule, a tumor was regarded as locally controlled if neither a clonogenic nor a hypoxic cell survived after irradiation. Tumor control probability was estimated as (number of controlled tumors)/(number of irradiated tumors). Five tumors were irradiated for each scheme at each dose level.

The Fisher exact test was used to compare tumor control probabilities between the different fractionation schemes and between shrinking and nonshrinking tumors at each dose level. A P value of less than .05 was regarded as indicating a statistically significant difference.

RESULTS

Simulated tumor growth resulted in a spherical tumor nodule. At the end of the growth phase, when tumors contained at least 10,000 cells, the capillary network was deformed, which resulted in a reduced central capillary density. In consequence, a necrotic center developed that was surrounded by a zone of hypoxic cells that made up about 25% of all viable cells (Fig 1).

The time course of reoxygenation was mainly determined by the shrinkage pattern and the fractionation scheme (Fig 2). In the case of undisturbed tumor and stroma shrinkage, the hypoxic fraction increased with the onset of irradiation and started to decrease continuously 5 days after the beginning of irradiation and synchronously with the first removal of necrotic cells. Complete reoxygenation was achieved after 4–6 weeks with conventional, after 2½ weeks with accelerated, and after 3–5 weeks with split-course irradiation. If shrinkage of the tumor stroma was inhibited, tumors soon became completely hypoxic. Minor reoxygenation was caused by ongoing tumor growth that allowed the peripheral tumor cells access to the surrounding capillaries; minor reoxygenation took place during weekend breaks and the split.

Tumor control probability depended on the intrinsic speed of tumor growth, the ability of the tumor to shrink, and the fractionation scheme (Fig 3). Shrinking, slowly growing tumors (T_c of 5 days) were controlled with 50 Gy, regardless of the irradiation schedule. For shrinking tumors with a T_c of 2 days, accelerated fractionation was more likely to control the tumor than the other schedules. At a dose level of 60 Gy, this difference in tumor control was statistically significant ($P < .05$) in a comparison between accelerated fractionation and conventional irradiation. The introduction of the 1-week split was also accompanied by a statistically significant ($P < .05$) loss of tumor control at doses of 60 Gy. For nonshrinking tumors, response curves were shifted to higher doses. A statistically significant ($P < .05$) difference between shrinking and nonshrinking tumors, however, was found only at doses of 50–60 Gy in the slower-growing tumors.

DISCUSSION

Results of the present three-dimensional cellular computer simulation demonstrate that shrinkage of the tumor during fractionated radiation therapy is associated with continuous reoxygenation and an increase in tumor control. Compared with conventional fractionation, accelerated irradiation produced statistically significantly better results in the fast-growing, shrinking tumors. The introduction of a 1-week split into the accelerated scheme led to a pronounced loss of tumor control at a total dose of 50–60 Gy in these tumors. The parameters, patterns and mechanisms of reoxygenation, and data on the processes that determine tumor control were chosen to simulate the behavior of a real tumor.

Choice of Parameters

The basic radiobiologic parameters of the radiosensitivity (15), the α/β ratio (16), and the oxygen enhancement ratio (17) were extracted from textbooks or recently published data on human tumors. Histopathologic (18), immunohistochemical (19), and oxygen partial pressure (20) measurements have shown that sufficient oxygen supply from capillaries by means of diffusion is limited to cells within 100 μm around a capillary and that hypoxic cells reside in the layers at about 100–150 μm. In consequence, capillary lattice distances were chosen to guarantee sufficient oxygenation to at least 99% of all cells as long as no capillary was displaced.

Hypoxic cells were regarded as being clonogenic as soon as becoming reoxygenated but were unable to divide while in the hypoxic state. This assumption was based on the measurements of tumor cell kinetics in tumor cords by Moore and colleagues (21). The highest mitotic index was found in the immediate vicinity of the subtending vessel but fell to almost zero at a distance of more than 80 mm from the vessel. The percentage of clonogenic cells (75%; 25% were hypoxic, nondividing cells) at the end of the growth phase is close to the growth fraction of 0.78–0.83 calculated for human tumor cords by Moore and colleagues. The potential tumor doubling time was about $1.2T_c$ (2.4 or 6 days), which is also close to the value in human carcinomas (22), according to $T_c \cdot \ln(2)/\ln(1 + \text{growth fraction})$.

For the dependence of tumor growth and radiosensitivity on oxygen tension, the two-compartment model as described by Tannock (23), with well-oxygenated and hypoxic cells rather than a graded radiosensitivity, was used. No clearly defined values were found in the literature for the time it takes to resorb necrotic tumor cells, a process that is thought to take some days (24). To not introduce too many variables into the model, a value of 5 days was arbitrarily chosen. The graphic representation of a model tumor cross section (Fig 1) resembles that of a histopathologic section of a partly hypoxic and necrotic tumor as described by Thomlinson and Gray (18), which suggests that the pattern of tumor growth and the calculation of oxygen supply were adequately modeled.

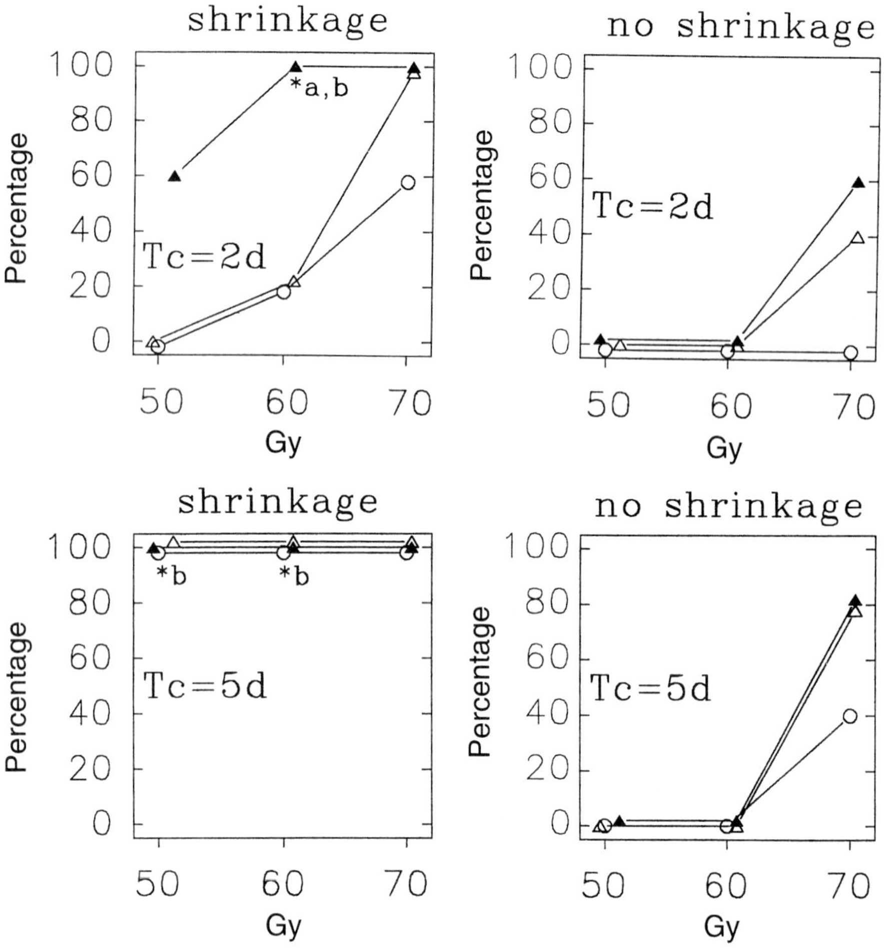

Figure 3. Tumor control rates (elimination of all clonogenic and hypoxic tumor cells in five simulation runs at each dose level) after fractionated irradiation. Accelerated irradiation increased the control rates the most in fast-growing, shrinking, reoxygenating tumors. The Fisher exact test was used to compare different fractionation schemes and to compare shrinking and nonshrinking tumors at each dose level. ○ = conventional irradiation (2 Gy), △ = split-course irradiation (1.6 Gy delivered twice), ▲ = accelerated irradiation (1.6 Gy delivered twice), *a = $P < .05$ in a comparison between conventional and split-course irradiation, *b = $P < .05$ in a comparison between shrinking tumors and nonshrinking tumors.

Patterns and Mechanisms of Reoxygenation

In the available experimental studies, different patterns of reoxygenation during or after fractionated irradiation were found. Howes and colleagues (25) observed marked tumor shrinkage associated with almost complete reoxygenation of mammary carcinoma cells treated with 3 Gy five times in 9 days. In contrast, hypoxic fractions never decreased enough to be substantially below pretreatment values in nonshrinking squamous cell carcinomas (26) or human melanoma xenografts (27). Teicher and colleagues (28) even found hypoxic fractions of up to 70%–85% 24–48 hours after 3 Gy had been delivered five times in rat mammary carcinomas.

Data on the time course of hypoxic tumor cell fractions for overall treatment times of more than 10 days are even more limited and rely on methods such as oxygen electrodes that may not be directly comparable to the paired survival curve assay (29). Koh and colleagues (30) determined the fractional hypoxic tumor volume with fluorine-18 misonidazole positron emission tomography in seven patients with non–small-cell lung cancer. It changed from 20%–84% at the beginning to 3%–65% at the end of a course of conventionally fractionated radiation therapy. In contrast to carcinomas, which often regress rapidly, macroscopic sarcomas rarely shrink during the first weeks of fractionated therapy (31). In experimental sarcomas treated with 60 Gy in 4 weeks, an increase of up to 38% in week 4 was measured (32). Brizel and colleagues (33) measured the oxygen partial pressure in patients with sarcoma. After 10–16 Gy were given in daily 2-Gy fractions, the tumor median oxygen partial pressure decreased, that is, reoxygenation was not observed.

Insufficient tumor shrinkage may result from increased interstitial pressure (34), invasion of inflammatory cells (24), or the presence of large necrotic regions (35). It is interesting that findings of recent investigations suggest that tumor reoxygenation can be enhanced with paclitaxel, probably by means of extensive apoptotic cell death followed by the removal of killed cells and tumor shrinkage 2–3 days later (36). In summary, the computer model is in good agreement with experimental and clinical data that suggest that tumor shrinkage has a main influence on the reoxygenation of hypoxic tumor cells, which may disappear, persist, or increase during fractionated irradiation.

Tumor Control

Experimental (37) and clinical (2) evidence exists that accelerated radiation therapy increases local control only in tumors with short doubling times. Findings of European Organization for Research and Treatment of Cancer trial 22851 (2) demonstrated that patients with tumors with a potential tumor doubling time of at most 4 days had a substantially higher local control rate when treated with 1.6 Gy three times per day than those with a potential tumor doubling time of more than 4 days. The simulation results fit these data such that the increase in tumor control owing to accelerated therapy was absent (shrinking tumors) or reduced (nonshrinking tumors) in tumors with a T_c of 5 days (potential tumor doubling time around 6 days) when compared with that in tumors with a T_c of 2 days (potential tumor doubling time around 2.4 days).

The Continuous Hyperfractionated Accelerated Radiation Therapy, or CHART, protocol (1.5 Gy delivered three times per day with no weekend break) increased local tumor control by 15% in patients with head and neck tumors and a T_c of 3–4 days and increased survival in patients with non–small-cell lung cancer by 10% (1), although all of the late side effects due to this aggressive treatment remain to be evaluated. The results of the Continuous Hyperfractionated Accelerated Radiation Therapy regime can be related to the simulation results if one assumes a patient population to have 50% shrinking and 50% nonshrinking tumors, with each 50% of the tumors having a T_c of 2 or 5 days. An overall increase in tumor control of 20% at 60 Gy would result from 1.6 Gy delivered twice per day compared to 2 Gy delivered once per day, which is close to the clinical figures.

Split-course irradiation has been used in accelerated fractionation for head and neck tumors to keep acute toxic reactions low. Wang and colleagues (38) demonstrated the loss of local control when patients with carcinomas of the oropharynx and larynx had a midcourse break of more than 2 weeks. In agreement with this finding, the simulation results suggest that fast-growing tumors that become reoxygenated during treatment are especially sensitive to treatment breaks.

In conclusion, the results of the computer simulation support the view that reoxygenation induced by tumor shrinkage during fractionated radiation therapy has a major effect on local control. Under the assumption of continuous tumor cell repopulation, accelerated fractionation schemes increase local control rates the most in fast-growing tumors that shrink easily owing to the absence of necrosis, inflammatory cells, calcifications or fibrosis of the tumor stroma. This kind of tumor also seems to be especially sensitive to treatment breaks.

The present simulation was designed in an attempt to integrate the known processes that determine tumor control in radiation therapy. Owing to the limited size of the lattice, larger tumors that induce neoangiogenesis and often have several hypoxic regions could not be modeled. Also, apoptosis was not considered but may be introduced by changing α and β values. Implementation on a more powerful computer will allow an increase in size that approaches that of real macroscopic tumors. These extensions probably will allow the fitting of the simulation parameters to clinical and radiologic data. In individual patients, the presence or absence of badly perfused, hypoxic regions could be determined and the speed of tumor regression could be measured in repetitive contrast material–enhanced computed tomographic examinations; in addition, the dose distribution and fractionation could be adapted according to the prediction of the model. Complex therapies such as the combination of brachytherapy and external beam therapy might be tested and optimized in virtual tumors before being applied to the patient. ■

References

1. Saunders MI, Dische S, Barett A, Parmar MKB, Harvey A, Gibson D. Randomized multicentre trials of CHART vs conventional radiotherapy in head and neck and non-small-cell lung cancer: an interim report. Br J Cancer 1996; 73:1455–1462.
2. Begg AC, Hofland I, Van Glabekke M, Bartelink H, Horiot JC. Predictive value of potential doubling time for radiotherapy of head and neck tumor patients: results from the EORTC cooperative trial 22851. Semin Radiat Oncol 1992; 2:22–25.
3. Gatenby RA, Kessler HB, Rosenblum JS, et al. Oxygen distribution in squamous cell carcinoma metastases and its relationship in outcome of radiation therapy. Int J Radiat Oncol Biol Phys 1988; 14:831–838.
4. Urtasun RC, Koch CJ, Franko AJ, Raleigh JA, Chapman JD. A novel technique for measuring human tissue Po_2 at the cellular level. Br J Cancer 1986; 54:453–457.
5. Dewhirst MW, Oliver R, Tso CY, Gustafson C, Secomb T, Gross JF. Heterogeneity in tumor microvascular response to radiation. Int J Radiat Oncol Biol Phys 1990; 18:559–568.
6. Hall EJ. The oxygen effect and reoxygenation. In: Hall EJ, ed. Radiobiology for the radiologist. Philadelphia, Pa: Lippincott, 1994; 133–152.
7. Kitakabu Y, Shibamoto Y, Sasei K, Ono K, Abe M. Variations of the hypoxic fraction in the SCC VII tumors after single dose and during fractionated radiation therapy: assessment without anesthesia or physical restraint of mice. Int J Radiat Oncol Biol Phys 1991; 20:709–714.
8. Grau C, Khalil AA, Nordsmark M, Horsman MR, Overgaard J. The relationship between carbon monoxide breathing, tumor oxygenation and local tumor control in the CH3 mammary carcinoma in vivo. Br J Cancer 1994; 69:50–57.
9. Urano M, Nishimura Y, Yaes R. The relative significance of repopulation and hypoxic clonogens in the fractionated radiotherapy of a mouse tumor. Radiat Res 1995; 142:204–211.
10. Brown JM, Koong A. Therapeutic advantage of hypoxic cells in tumors: a theoretical study. J Natl Cancer Inst 1991; 83:178–185.
11. Denekamp J, Joiner MC. The potential benefit from a perfect radiosensitizer and its dependence on reoxygenation. Br J Radiol 1982; 55:657–663.
12. Scott OCA. Mathematical models of repopulation and reoxygenation in radiotherapy. Br J Radiol 1990; 63:821–823.
13. Duechting W, Vogelsaenger T. Aspects of modelling and simulating tumor growth and treatment. J Cancer Res Clin Oncol 1983; 105:1–12.
14. Kocher M, Treuer H. Reoxygenation of hypoxic cells by tumor shrinkage during irradiation: a computer simulation. Strahlenther Onkol 1995; 4:219–230.
15. Okunieff P, Hoeckel M, Dunphy EP, Schlenger K, Knoop C, Vaupel P. Oxygen tension distributions are sufficient to explain the local response of human breast tumors treated with radiation alone. Int J Radiat Oncol Biol Phys 1993; 26:631–636.
16. Joiner MC. The linear-quadratic approach to fractionation. In: Steel GG, ed. Basic clinical radiobiology. London, England: Edward Arnold, 1993; 55–64.
17. Palcic B, Skarsgard LD. Reduced oxygen enhancement ratio at low doses of ionizing irradiation. Radiat Res 1984; 100:328–339.
18. Thomlinson RH, Gray LH. The histological structure of some human lung cancers and the possible implications for radiotherapy. Br J Cancer 1955; 9:539–549.
19. Cline JM, Thrall DE, Page RL, Franko AJ, Raleigh JA. Immunohistochemical detection of a hypoxia marker in spontaneous canine tumors. Br J Cancer 1990; 62:925–931.
20. Dewhirst MW, Secomb TW, Ong ET, Hsu R, Gross JF. Determination of local oxygen consumption in tumors. Cancer Res 1994; 54:3333–3336.
21. Moore JV, Hasleton PS, Buckley CH. Tumor cords in 52 human bronchial and cervical squamous cell carcinomas: inferences for their cellular kinetics and radiobiology. Br J Cancer 1985; 51:407–413.
22. Begg AC. Cell proliferation in tumors. In: Steel GG, ed. Basic clinical radiobiology. London, England: Edward Arnold, 1993; 14–22.
23. Tannock IF. Oxygen diffusion and the distribution of cellular radiosensitivity in tumours. Br J Radiol 1972; 45:515–524.
24. Brammer I, Jung H. Cell loss in irradiated tumours. In: Beck-Bornholdt HP, ed. Current topics in clinical radiobiology of tumors. Berlin, Germany: Springer Verlag, 1993; 129–145.
25. Howes AE, Page A, Fowler JF. The effect of single and fractionated doses of x rays on the effective proportion of hypoxic cells in C_3H mouse mammary tumors. Br J Radiol 1972; 45:250–256.
26. Kitakabu Y, Shibamoto Y, Sasai K, Ono K, Abe M. Variations of the hypoxic fraction in the SCC VII tumors after single dose and during fractionated radiation therapy: assessment without anesthesia or physical restraint of mice. Int J Radiat Oncol Biol Phys 1991; 20:709–714.
27. Rofstad EK. Hypoxia and reoxygenation in human melanoma xenografts. Int J Radiat Oncol Biol Phys 1989; 17:81–89.
28. Teicher BA, Sotomayor, EA, Dupuis NP, Kusumoto T, Menon K. Reduced oxygenation in a rat mammary carcinoma after chemo- or radiation therapy and reoxygenation with perflubron emulsion/carbogen breathing. J Cancer Res Clin Oncol 1994; 120:593–598.
29. Fenton BM, Kiani MF, Siemann DW. Should direct measurements of tumor oxygenation relate to the radiobiological hypoxic fraction of a tumor? Int J Radiat Oncol Biol Phys 1995; 33:365–373.

30. Koh WJ, Bergmann KS, Rasey JS, et al. Evaluation of oxygenation status during fractionated radiotherapy in human non-small cell lung cancers using [F-18]fluoromisonidazole positron emission tomography. Int J Radiat Oncol Biol Phys 1995; 33: 391–398.
31. Denekamp J. Physiological hypoxia and its influence on radiotherapy. In: Steel GG, Adams GE, Horwich A, eds. The biological basis of radiotherapy. Amsterdam, The Netherlands: Elsevier, 1989; 115–134.
32. Zywietz F, Reeker W, Kochs E. Tumor oxygenation in a transplanted rat rhabdomyosarkoma during fractionated irradiation. Int J Radiat Oncol Biol Phys 1995; 32: 1391–1400.
33. Brizel DM, Scully SP, Harrelson JM, et al. Radiation therapy and hyperthermia improve the oxygenation of human soft tissue sarcomas. Cancer Res 1996; 56:5347–5350.
34. Znati CA, Rosenstein M, Boucher Y, Epperly MW, Bloomer WD, Jain RK. Effect of radiation on interstitial fluid pressure and oxygenation in a human tumor xenograft. Cancer Res 1996; 56:964–968.
35. Murata R, Shibamoto Y, Sasai K, et al. Reoxygenation after single irradiation in rodent tumors of different types and sizes. Int J Radiat Oncol Biol Phys 1996; 34:859–864.
36. Milas L, Hunter NR, Mason KA, Milross CC, Saito Y, Peters LJ. Role of reoxygenation in induction of enhancement of tumor radioresponse by paclitaxel. Cancer Res 1995; 55:3564–3568.
37. Sarkaria JN, Fowler JF, Lindstrom MJ, Jordan VC, Mulcahy RT. The decreased influence of overall treatment time on the response of human breast tumor xenografts following prolongation of the potential doubling time (Tpot). Int J Radiat Oncol Biol Phys 1995; 31:833–840.
38. Wang CC, Efird J, Nakfoor B, Martins P. Local control of T3 carcinomas after accelerated fractionation: a look at the gap. Int J Radiat Oncol Biol Phys 1996; 35:439–441.

Thoracic Spiral CT: Delivery of Contrast Material Pushed with Injectable Saline Solution in a Power Injector[1]

Kenneth D. Hopper, MD
Timothy J. Mosher, MD
Claudia J. Kasales, MD
Thomas R. TenHave, PhD
Danielle A. Tully, MA
Jill S. Weaver, BSRT

A method of power injection of contrast material pushed with injectable saline solution during thoracic computed tomography (CT) was evaluated in 75 patients to help decrease the amount of contrast material necessary. Patients received 50–125 mL of 60% nonionic contrast material alone or pushed with 50 mL of saline. A volume of 75 mL of contrast material pushed with saline provided enhancement of the thoracic vasculature equal to that provided by a 125-mL volume of contrast material administered alone ($P < .001$) and caused significantly less beam-hardening artifact ($P < .01$).

Index terms: Computed tomography (CT), contrast media, 56.12112, 94.12912 • Computed tomography (CT), helical, 56.12112, 56.12115, 94.12912, 94.12915 • Contrast media, experimental studies, 56.12112, 94.12912 • Thorax, CT, 56.12112, 56.12115, 94.12912, 94.12915

Radiology 1997; 205:269–271

THE past several years have witnessed an explosion in new computed tomography (CT) technology. The widespread introduction of spiral (helical) CT has led to a dramatic increase in scanning speed, optimization of contrast, and available image-processing options. Spiral CT has opened the door to dynamic scanning.

As these new capabilities have increased, however, the demand for intravenous delivery of contrast material in these patients has increased. Injection rates of 2.5–5.0 mL/sec are usually necessary, and the use of a power injector has become essential. Spiral CT performed with rapid injection not only optimizes contrast enhancement but also allows a reduction in the amount of intravenous contrast material necessary for high-quality body imaging.

Because of the need to use power injectors and rapid injection rates with spiral CT, many radiologists have begun to use only nonionic contrast material for these types of procedures. Use of fast injection rates with ionic contrast material leads to increased nausea and vomiting for the patient; and large extravasations of ionic contrast material cause more serious complications than those caused by nonionic media. The American College of Radiology has recently included the use of a power injector with a high injection rate as a criterion for the selective use of nonionic contrast material because of the seriousness of extravasation of ionic contrast material. Pressure is increasing for all physicians to continually reduce costs, however, and the expense of nonionic contrast material is a sensitive item on the budget.

At our institution, we use the strengths of spiral CT plus contrast material pushed with saline to obtain high-quality contrast material–enhanced CT scans in the chest with 75 mL of 60% nonionic contrast material. Herein we explain this technique and provide data to support its routine clinical use.

Materials and Methods

Technique.—In this method of delivering contrast material pushed with saline, the saline solution costs 75 cents for a 50-mL bottle at our institution. Intravenous contrast material and saline are both clear and immersible. Nonionic contrast material is three times osmolar, however, whereas saline is isoosmolar. For that reason, they are not easily mixed.

The first step in loading the contrast material and saline is for the technologist to turn the injector nozzle straight up so that it is vertical. At this point, 75 mL of 60% nonionic contrast material is drawn into the syringe. Because it is heavier than the saline, the contrast material must be drawn into the syringe first when the injector is in a vertical position.

The technologist then carefully loads 50 mL of saline into the syringe. With most injectors, the saline may be loaded automatically by pressing the automatic-load switch on the injector. Some newer injectors load at a faster rate, however, which causes undue mixing of the saline and contrast material. When this type of injector is used, the contrast material should be loaded manually by counterrotating the injector dial. The additional time needed for the technologist to open and load the saline is 1 minute.

Figure 1. Radiograph of an upright syringe obtained after the saline was loaded on top of the contrast material shows an obvious fluid-fluid level between the radiolucent saline and the radiopaque contrast material with virtually no mixing.

Now the saline lies on top of the more dense nonionic contrast material with virtually no mixing of the two liquids (Fig 1). Even though both liquids are clear, the denser contrast material visibly layers in the dependent portion of the syringe. All air is then evacuated from the syringe, and the intravenous catheter and connecting tubing is attached and filled with saline. With a continuous steady slow motion, the technologist then inverts the injector so that its nozzle is pointed directly down at the floor. During this inversion, the saline flows over the top of the contrast material (Fig 2), and their positions in the syringe are reversed. At this point, three layers of liquid are visible (Fig 3). The two largest layers are the unmixed saline and contrast material. Between these two layers is a third layer that contains mostly saline with some admixed contrast material.

The goal of this method is to use the unmixed layer of saline to clear the sy-

[1] From the Department of Radiology (K.D.H., T.J.M., C.J.K., J.S.W.) and the Center for Biostatistics and Epidemiology (T.R.T., D.A.T.), Penn State University, 500 University Dr, Box 850, Hershey, PA 17033. Received April 21, 1997; revision requested May 29; revision received June 16; accepted June 19. **Address reprint requests to** K.D.H.

ringe and intravenous catheter and connecting tubing and to clear the contrast material from the patient's arm. Despite the inversion process, the intravenous catheter and connecting tubing remains filled with saline. Our experience is that extravasation, when it occurs, usually happens at the beginning of the power injection. By filling the intravenous catheter and connecting tubing with saline, the first few milliliters of liquid injected into the patient is saline, not contrast material. If extravasation occurs, this initial injection of saline offers an added safety margin while the technologist observes the insertion site of the intravenous catheter during contrast material injection. There is little additional mixing of the saline and contrast material during the next 30 minutes after the injector has been inverted. Once the contrast material has been injected, the heparin lock is filled with saline, and additional flushing is not necessary.

Early in our experience, we attempted to load the contrast material first, with the injector in its normal position, followed by the saline. Because contrast material is much denser than saline, however, we experienced unacceptable mixing.

Patients.—Seventy-five patients undergoing medically indicated contrast-enhanced thoracic CT were recruited to participate in this study from March through May 1996. This study was approved by and performed under the auspices of our institutional review board. Once entered into the study, the patients were assigned randomly and equally into one of six categories: (*a*) injection of 50 mL of contrast material pushed with 50 mL of saline (five patients), (*b*) injection of 75 mL of contrast material pushed with 50 mL of saline (15 patients), (*c*) injection of 75 mL of contrast material alone (15 patients), (*d*) injection of 100 mL of contrast material pushed with 50 mL of saline (15 patients), (*e*) injection of 100 mL of contrast material alone (15 patients), and (*f*) injection of 125 mL of contrast material alone (10 patients).

CT scanning.—All CT examinations were performed in the same manner. With scanning started 20 seconds after initiation of the injection of contrast material, consecutive 8-mm-thick sections were obtained with a commercially available unit (PQ5000 spiral scanner; Picker International, Highland Heights, Ohio) (300 mA; 120 kV; pitch, 1.5).The entire chest was scanned during one breath hold. In all patients, 60% nonionic contrast material was injected at a rate of 2.5 mL/sec. In the middle ascending aorta and main pulmonary artery, three region-of-interest measurements were obtained with their standard deviations and averaged. In addition, the artifact on each thoracic image was evaluated to determine any effect caused by the contrast material. The artifact on each image was graded by a single experienced radiologist (T.J.M.) who reviewed the scans in a randomized order and was blinded to the volume of contrast material and the method of delivery used. The following 5-point scale was used: 1 = very sharp vessel edges, no artifact; 2 = sharp vessel edges, minimal artifact involves 25% or less of the wall or extends 3 mm or less into the image; 3 = sharp vessel edges, mild artifact involves 50% or less of the wall or extends 6 mm or less into the image; 4 = sharp vessel edges, moderate artifact involves more than 75% of the wall or extends 10 mm or less into the image; 5 = blurred vessel edges, extensive artifact involves more than 75% of the wall or extends more than 10 mm into the image.

Figure 2. Radiograph of the same syringe after it was slowly rotated horizontally shows the saline flowing over the top of the contrast material.

Statistical analysis.—Analysis of variance was performed by means of Dunnetts test to adjust the *P* values for multiple comparisons of all variables except the image artifact. The presence of image artifact was analyzed by means of logistic regression analysis.

Results

The use of 50 mL of 60% nonionic contrast material pushed with 50 mL of saline provided inadequate opacification of the aorta and pulmonary artery (Table). Use of 75 mL of 60% nonionic contrast material pushed with saline provided opacification of the pulmonary artery and the middle ascending aorta that was equivalent to that achieved with administration of either 100 or 125 mL of contrast material alone. The use of 75 mL of contrast material alone provided inadequate opacification of the main pulmonary artery ($P < .001$). In addition, the use of 75 mL of contrast material pushed with saline caused significantly less artifact ($P < .01$) than did the use of 125 mL of contrast material alone (mean scores, 2.1 and 3.6, respectively). The amount of artifact produced when 75 mL of contrast material was used, however, was the same alone and pushed with saline (mean scores, 1.9 and 2.1, respectively). When 75 mL of contrast material was pushed with saline, opacification of the aorta was increased (254.8 HU with saline vs 238.1 HU alone), but this difference was not statistically significant. Use of saline tended to produce better opacification of the pulmonary artery with 100 mL compared with 75 mL of contrast material (292.6 HU vs 243.1 HU, respectively). This difference was not statistically significant, however, and use of a larger volume of contrast material caused a large increase in artifact (mean scores, 3.6 vs 2.1, respectively).

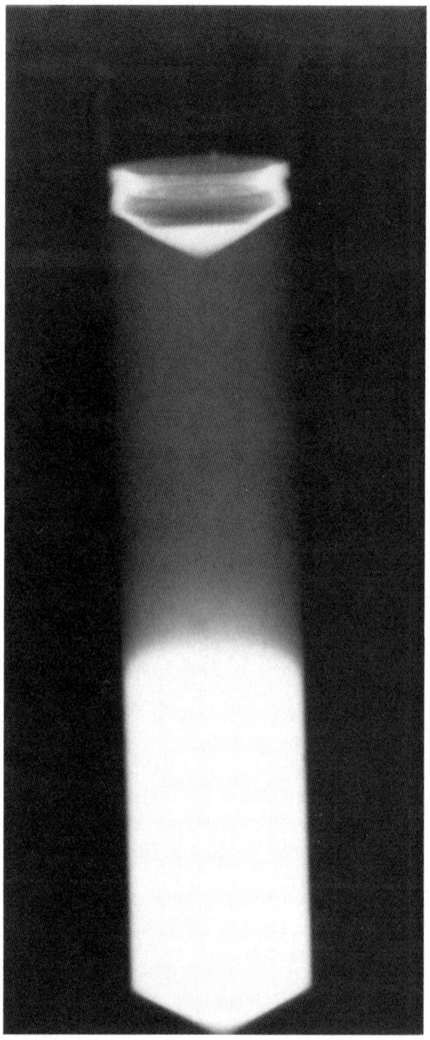

Figure 3. Radiograph of the same syringe after inversion shows three layers of fluid, with the more radiolucent saline in the upper half of the syringe and the radiopaque contrast material in the dependent portion. There is relative nonmixing of the contrast material and the saline.

Summary of Results with Push of Saline

Volume of 60% Nonionic Contrast Material (mL)	Main Ascending Thoracic Aorta				Main Pulmonary Artery				Artifact *	
	Without Saline		With Saline		Without Saline		With Saline			
	n	Mean Attenuation (HU)	*n*	Mean Attenuation (HU)	*n*	Mean Attenuation (HU)	*n*	Mean Attenuation (HU)	Without Saline	With Saline
50	0	. . .	5	151.6 (38.6)	0	. . .	5	120.8 (53.7)†	. . .	. . .
75	15	238.1 (67.8)	15	254.8 (83.7)	15	148.4 (43.1)‡	15	243.1 (98.5)	1.9‡	2.1
100	15	268.5 (74.1)	15	263.8 (77.8)	15	258.0 (90.8)	15	292.6 (79.1)	2.7	3.6
125	10	225.2 (100.7)	0	. . .	10	272.4 (37.8)	0	. . .	3.6	. . .

Note.—Standard deviation is given in parentheses.
* Score: 1 = best (no artifact), 5 = worst (extensive artifact).
† $P < .01$ versus 125 mL without saline.
‡ $P < .001$ versus 125 mL without saline

Discussion

The results of this study show that use of a power injector and reduced volumes of 60% nonionic contrast material pushed with saline allows contrast-enhanced thoracic CT scans to be obtained with consistent high-quality vascular and hepatic opacification. When this technique is used, attenuation values in the main pulmonary artery for the chest and in the liver for the abdomen consistently show a minimum increase of 60–70 HU. The cost savings per patient of use of a smaller volume of nonionic contrast material are also a benefit.

We have used the contrast material push with saline in more than 3,000 patients undergoing thoracic or abdominal CT. This technique consistently produces high-quality contrast-enhanced CT images with an average savings in contrast material of 50 mL per patient. In addition, we have found that artifact from dense contrast material in central veins is reduced when pushed with saline.

The use of uniphasic injections of contrast material at a rate of at least 2.0–2.5 mL/sec, combined with spiral CT, allows good parenchymal and vascular enhancement with a reduced amount of contrast material (1–4). Although the use of injections of a bolus of contrast material during spiral CT can increase lesion detection (5), at least one article (6) has recently reported that attempts to reduce the volume of contrast material potentially may decrease detection of focal hypovascular hepatic lesions. Freeny et al (6) did not address contrast material requirements for examinations other than hepatic CT. If a chest CT examination is to be performed with 150 mL of contrast material alone to optimally evaluate the liver for metastases, we believe use of 100 mL of contrast material pushed with saline could be substituted and could provide equivalent hepatic opacification. We are currently evaluating this technique for abdominal and pelvic CT.

The product inserts for nonionic contrast media state that the contrast material is not to be mixed. The technique of contrast material pushed with saline relies on the relative nonmixing of the two liquids. Indeed, the minimal mixing that does occur is about the same as that experienced when saline is used to clear an intravenous catheter and tubing after hand injection of nonionic contrast material. Given the increased osmolality of saline compared with nonionic contrast media, this technique would perform at least as well with ionic contrast materials.

In conclusion, the results of our study indicate that high-quality contrast-enhanced thoracic CT scans can be obtained with use of only 75 mL of contrast material when pushed with saline. Opacification of the pulmonary arteries was poor with the use of 75 mL of contrast material alone. The vascular opacification afforded with 75 mL of contrast material pushed with saline was equivalent to that provided with 125 mL of contrast material alone. Beam-hardening artifact caused by the presence of dense contrast material in the innominate veins and superior vena cava was significantly less ($P < .001$) with 75 mL of contrast material pushed with saline than with larger volumes of contrast material alone or pushed with saline. ■

References

1. Silverman PM, Brown B, Wray H, et al. Optimal contrast enhancement of the liver using helical (spiral) CT: value of SmartPrep. AJR 1995; 164:1169–1171.
2. Birnbaum BA, Jacobs JE, Yin D. Hepatic enhancement during helical CT: a comparison of moderate rate uniphasic and biphasic contrast injection protocols. AJR 1995; 165:853–858.
3. Brink JA, Heiken JP, Forman HP, Sagel SS, Molina PL, Brown PC. Hepatic spiral CT: reduction of dose of intravenous contrast material. Radiology 1995; 197:83–88.
4. Herts BR, Paushter DM, Einstein DM, Zepp R, Friedman RA, Obuchowski N. Use of contrast material for spiral CT of the abdomen: comparison of hepatic enhancement and vascular attenuation for three different contrast media at two different delay times. AJR 1995; 164:327–331.
5. Hollett MD, Jeffrey RB Jr, Nino-Murcia M, Jorgensen MJ, Harris DP. Dual-phase helical CT of the liver: value of arterial phase scans in the detection of small (1.5 cm) malignant hepatic neoplasms. AJR 1995; 164:879–884.
6. Freeny PC, Gardner JC, vonIngersleben G, Heyano S, Nghiem HV, Winter TC. Hepatic helical CT: effect of reduction of iodine dose of intravenous contrast material on hepatic contrast enhancement. Radiology 1995; 197:89–93.

Virtual Cystoscopy: Early Clinical Experience[1]

Helen M. Fenlon, FRCR
Timoth V. Bell, MD
Heideh K. Ahari, MD
Sarwat Hussain, MD

Virtual cystoscopy was performed in 13 patients with hematuria and abnormal findings at conventional cystoscopy. Perspective volume-rendering algorithms were applied to helical computed tomographic data to generate interactive, intraluminal views of the bladder mucosa after insufflation of room air. At conventional cystoscopy, 29 masses appeared to arise from the bladder mucosa and two were hypertrophied median lobes of the prostate. At virtual cystoscopy, 30 masses arose from the bladder (one prostate mass was misinterpreted as an intrinsic bladder mass). Results at virtual cystoscopy were comparable to those at conventional cystoscopy but were obtained without the associated risks.

Index terms: Bladder, CT, 83.12115, 83.12119 • Computed tomography (CT), comparative studies, 83.12115, 83.12119 • Computers, diagnostic aid, 83.12119. Virtual reality imaging, 83.12115, 83.12119

Radiology 1997; 205:272–275

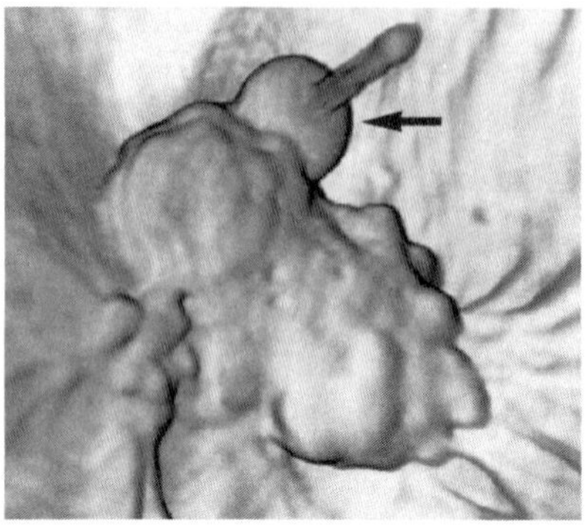

1.

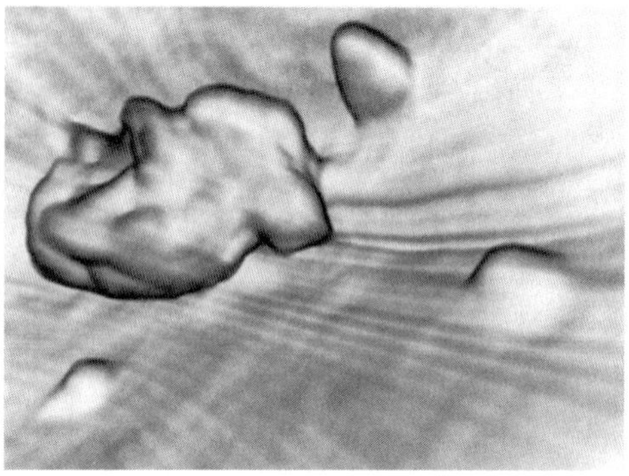

2.

Figures 1, 2. **(1)** Bladder carcinoma. An 8-cm (maximum dimension) sessile mass arising at the bladder neck is shown at virtual cystoscopy. A 12-F Foley catheter is present adjacent to the mass (arrow). **(2)** Bladder carcinoma. A 4-cm sessile mass and three adjacent polyps smaller than 1 cm are shown at virtual cystoscopy.

In the clinical setting of hematuria, conventional radiology is used to evaluate the upper urinary tract before cystoscopy (1). Once a diagnosis of bladder carcinoma has been established, cross-sectional imaging may be performed for tumor staging and follow-up (2–5). Conventional cystoscopy, however, remains the mainstay for diagnosis, management, and follow-up of bladder carcinoma. Repeat surveillance cystoscopy examinations are also necessary at frequent intervals to assess disease control.

Recent advances in computer-assisted virtual-reality data-postprocessing techniques have led to the development of a variety of novel computed tomography (CT) techniques including virtual colonoscopy and virtual bronchoscopy (6–8). Virtual-reality imaging involves postprocessing of volumetric CT data to create a "virtual environment." Immersion in this virtual environment permits interactive navigation through any hollow, air-distended viscus and thus simulates conventional endoscopy.

The aim of this study was to investigate the value of virtual cystoscopy in the identification of mucosal abnormalities of the urinary bladder in patients with hematuria and abnormal findings at conventional cystoscopy.

Materials and Methods

Patients.—Thirteen consecutive patients (nine men and four women aged 61–83 years [mean, 69 years]) with macroscopic hematuria and abnormal findings at conventional cystoscopy were studied prospectively between November 1996 and February 1997. All patients underwent virtual cystoscopy within 24 hours of conventional cystoscopy. The study protocol was approved by our institutional review board, and informed, written consent was obtained from each patient.

Technique.—A 12-F Foley catheter was used to drain the urinary bladder of residual urine and to distend it with 300–550 mL of room air, according to patient tolerance. An anteroposterior scout view of the pelvis was obtained to plan the helical CT scan. A single-breath-hold helical CT scan (PQ 5000 helical scanner; Picker International, Cleveland, Ohio) was obtained of the air-distended bladder with use of the following scanning parameters: collimation (section thickness) of 3 mm, table speed of 3 mm per 360° rotation, smallest field of view to fit, 120 mA, 110 kVp, and a 512 × 512 matrix. Images were reconstructed at 1-mm intervals (reformatting index of 1) with a 2-mm section overlap. Patients were then moved into a prone or prone-oblique position, and helical CT was repeated with the same parameters.

CT data from the two acquisitions were downloaded to an independent workstation (Voxel Q; Picker International). Commercially available, perspective volume-rendering algorithms (Voyager 1 and epi-Scope 3.4 software; Picker International) were used to compute the helical CT data to generate intraluminal views of the bladder mucosa with interactive capabilities. These views simulated those of conventional cystoscopy. The interactive data sets were viewed directly at the workstation for interpretation.

Image interpretation.—Images in the 13 virtual cystoscopy examinations were interpreted by two staff radiologists (H.M.F., S.H.) who were unaware of the findings at conventional cystoscopy. Differences in interpretation between the two observers were resolved by consensus.

The number, size, morphology, and exact location of masses observed at virtual cystoscopy were recorded. Note was made of whether a mass appeared to be intrinsic to the bladder or arose from the prostate. Masses were described as sessile or pedunculated. Sessile masses were defined as those lesions that were broader at their base than they were high (Figs 1, 2). In a trabeculated bladder, masses were reported if a focal contour abnormality was identified that was out of propor-

[1] From the Department of Radiology, Boston Medical Center, Boston University School of Medicine, 88 E Newton St, Boston, MA 02118.
Received March 24, 1997; revision requested May 19; revision received June 16; accepted June 19. **Address reprint requests to** H.M.F.

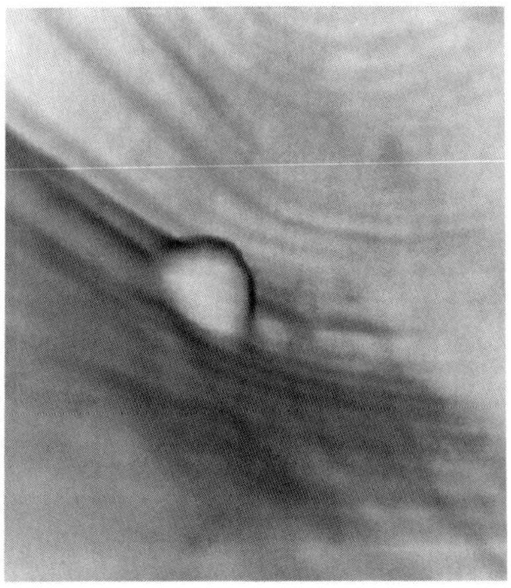

3.

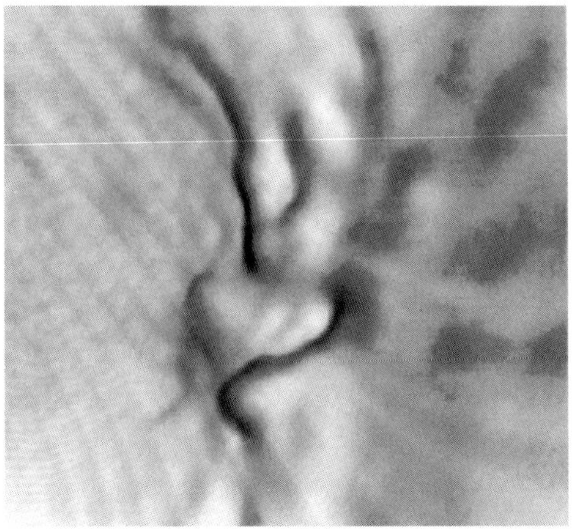

4.

Figures 3, 4. **(3)** Recurrent bladder carcinoma. A 3-mm (maximum dimension) bladder mass, the smallest found in our study, is shown at virtual cystoscopy. **(4)** Chronic mucosal ulceration. A magnified view of a virtual cystoscopy image shows focal mucosal nodularity. At conventional cystoscopy, a corresponding area of subtle mucosal granularity was identified that was a result of long-term bladder catheterization.

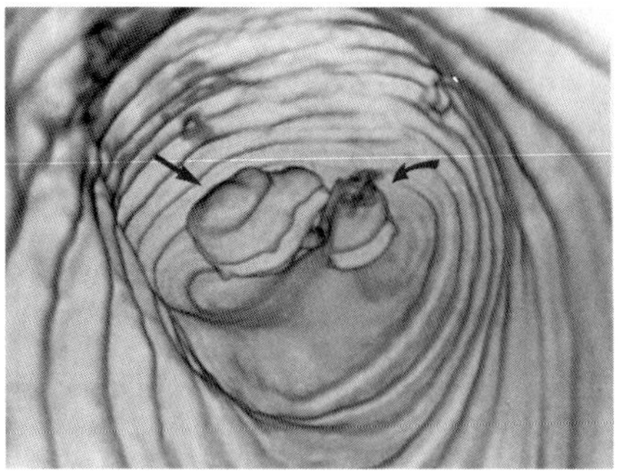

Figure 5. Motion artifact. This virtual cystoscopy image is degraded by ring artifact secondary to patient motion in a patient with a prominent median lobe of the prostate (straight arrow) that was misinterpreted as an intrinsic bladder tumor. Note artifactual distortion of the adjacent Foley catheter balloon (curved arrow).

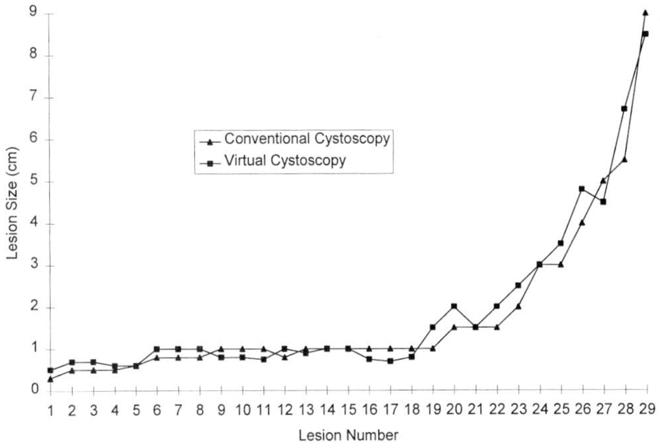

Figure 6. Comparison of lesion maximum dimension estimated from conventional and virtual cystoscopy images.

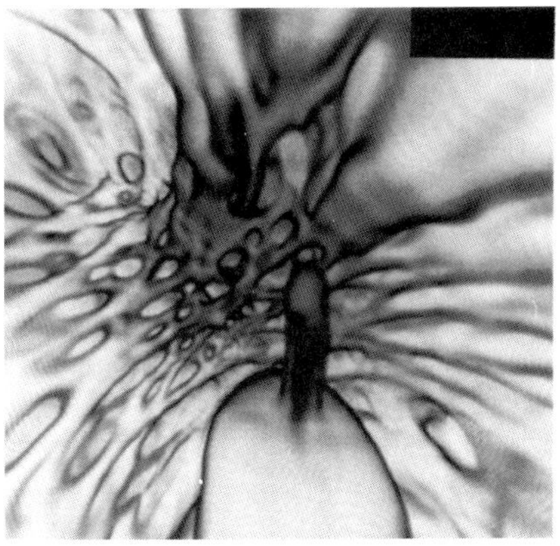

Figure 7. Bladder trabeculation. Virtual cystoscopy image shows a heavily trabeculated bladder in a patient with bladder outflow obstruction. A Foley catheter is shown in the foreground.

tion to the degree of adjacent trabeculation. The location of bladder lesions identified at virtual cystoscopy was described with conventional cystoscopic terminology for a patient in a supine position. The degree of bladder trabeculation (on a scale of 0–3; 0 = none, 3 = severe) and the presence of bladder diverticula were noted. The degree of bladder distention, adequacy of drainage of urine, and presence of imaging artifacts were also recorded.

Results

All 31 of the lesions detected at conventional cystoscopy were visualized at virtual cystoscopy. At conventional cystoscopy, 29 of the 31 masses were found to arise from the bladder, and two were found to represent hypertrophied median lobes of prostate. The prostatic origin of these two masses was subsequently confirmed by means of transrectal ultrasound. Intrinsic bladder masses seen at conventional cystoscopy (n = 29) ranged in maximum dimension from 0.3 to 9.0 cm (mean, 1.8 cm). Nineteen masses measured 1 cm or less (Fig 3). Seven masses were pedunculated and 22 were sessile. Nine masses had an irregular ulcerated surface, and 20 were smooth with intact bladder mucosa. Nineteen of the 29 bladder masses were transitional cell carcinomas, nine were masses with varying degrees of dysplasia, and one mass was a focal area of mucosal nodularity and ulceration secondary to long-term bladder catheterization (Fig 4).

Virtual cystoscopy showed 30 masses arising from the bladder and one arising from the prostate; a median lobe of prostate was misdiagnosed as a bladder mass in one patient (Fig 5). Virtual cystoscopy allowed accurate assessment of size (including 19 masses that were 1 cm or smaller in maximum dimension), location, and morphology (pedunculated or sessile) for all 29 bladder masses. The size of masses determined at virtual cystoscopy was within 1.2 cm of the size estimated at conventional cystoscopy for all masses larger than 5 cm and within 5 mm of the estimated size for lesions smaller than 5 cm (Fig 6). Seven masses were reported to have an irregular surface and 22 masses were found to be smooth at virtual cystoscopy, compared with nine and 20 lesions, respectively, at conventional cystoscopy.

At virtual cystoscopy, the degree of bladder trabeculation was judged to be mild in five patients, moderate in four, and severe in two (Fig 7). Prominent bladder trabeculation was documented in five conventional cystoscopy examinations. Bladder diverticula were seen in four patients at virtual cystoscopy; this finding was confirmed in all four patients at conventional cystoscopy. The mean bladder capacity was 410 mL (range, 280–550 mL). In no patient did residual urine or lack of adequate bladder distention interfere with correct diagnosis.

The average duration of the CT cystoscopy examination was 23 minutes (range, 18–33 minutes). This period included the time necessary to obtain patient consent, perform catheterization, acquire data, and remove the catheter. Data acquisition necessitated an average scanning time of 15–20 seconds and an average reconstruction time (to complete virtual cystoscopic navigations) of 15 minutes. The procedure was well tolerated by all patients, and no complications were reported.

Discussion

Although conventional cystoscopy is the main method of investigating bladder abnormalities, it has some limitations. This technique, which is used routinely to examine patients with hematuria, is invasive, time-consuming, and expensive. Sedation is frequently necessary, and iatrogenic injury to the urethra and bladder may occur. Urinary sepsis develops in 5%–10% of patients, and the mucosa at the bladder neck and within bladder diverticula is not accessible for easy scrutiny. Bladder tumors can be detected with intravenous pyelography, contrast material–enhanced cystography, sonography, contrast-enhanced CT, and magnetic resonance imaging. To our knowledge, however, no reliable radiologic technique exists for the detection and follow-up of bladder disease (1,9). The development of a safe noninvasive reliable method has obvious appeal.

A variety of CT techniques have recently been proposed as alternatives to conventional cystoscopy for detection and characterization of bladder tumors. Vining et al (10) described three-dimensional renderings of the air-distended urinary bladder at CT cystoscopy in one healthy volunteer and two patients with known bladder tumors. These investigators successfully used software to achieve image segmentation and used volume rendering to gain an intraluminal perspective of the bladder mucosa. More recently, Narumi et al (11) reported the results of three-dimensional surface-shaded displays of helical CT data sets of the air-distended bladder in a nonblinded evaluation of bladder tumors. Their results with surface-shaded three-dimensional reconstructions were encouraging in tumors larger than 1 cm in maximum dimension. Only 79% of lesions smaller than 1 cm were identified, however, and only 39% of those detected were correctly characterized as either sessile or pedunculated.

Vining et al (10) and Narumi et al (11) used two different rendering algorithms for virtual-reality data processing: volume rendering and surface-shaded display. In our experience at CT endoscopy of the colon and tracheobronchial tree, use of volume-rendering algorithms provides a more accurate representation of lesion morphology and tissue composition than surface-shaded display. Volume-rendered images are "data rich"; they use 100% of the available CT data for three-dimensional reconstruction and have a fluoroscopic appearance rather than the flat opaque appearance of images created with surface-shaded display. In addition to showing greater anatomic detail, volume-rendered images contain fewer smoothing and blurring artifacts. A sense of depth, distance, and motion can be achieved by also using a perspective algorithm (perspective volume rendering). This algorithm is a computer-graphics technique that causes the object to grow larger as the observer approaches. When combined with real-time viewing (5–30 frames per second), use of this technique conveys the effect of traveling through the bladder lumen in vivo.

Volume-rendering algorithms generate a tissue volume by assigning varying degrees of opacity on the basis of the CT attenuation coefficient of each voxel. The percentage-classifier algorithm, used in volume rendering, determines the relative components of each voxel and accounts for volume averaging of different tissue types within a single voxel. Voxels are classified according to the density of their tissue constituents; this system enables a prediction of the probability that a voxel belongs to a specific tissue type (12). Computer processing in surface-shaded display involves manipulation of CT data by means of a marching-cubes algorithm to create a "wire frame" model, the surface of which is filled in. Depending on the CT attenuation threshold selected, tissues of different densities can be either included or removed. The net effect is the display of a tissue interface that simulates a flat opaque anatomic specimen. Light and shade from a simulated light source are used to achieve a three-dimensional perspective. Although surface-shaded display allows rapid three-dimensional reconstruction and is less demanding computationally than volume rendering, surface-shaded displays use only 10% of the available helical CT data and, compared with volume-rendered images, lack depth and detail (12).

Unlike the initial study by Vining et al (10), in which prototype, site-specific segmentation software was used, our virtual cystoscopy study was performed with commercially available, scanner-based software. Use of volume rendering allowed us to achieve a substantial improvement in detection of lesions smaller than 1 cm in maximum dimension compared with Narumi et al (11), who used surface-shaded display. When virtual cystoscopy was used, all 31 lesions were successfully identified, including 19 masses that measured 1 cm or less (the smallest being a 3-mm sessile polyp) and an area of subtle mucosal nodularity at the bladder dome.

Diagnostic benefits of virtual cystoscopy compared with conventional cystoscopy include its ability to accurately record tumor maximum dimension and volume without magnification or distortion. The ability to evaluate tumor dimensions objectively is valuable in the follow-up of treatment, especially in trials that compare different therapeutic regimens. In addition, a lesion within the bladder can be precisely localized at virtual cystoscopy by referencing external landmarks that may be useful for tumor mapping before transurethral resection. Certain areas of the bladder mucosa are recognized as potential blind spots at conventional cystoscopy. Because of the limited flexibility of both rigid and fiberoptic cystoscopes, the mucosa at the bladder neck can be difficult to visualize. Similar difficulties occur in the examination of patients with prominent bladder trabeculation and of the mucosa within bladder diverticula. By means of the interactive capabilities of virtual cystoscopy, these limitations can be overcome. The viewpoint of the observer can be manipulated through 360° in any axis, and thus the bladder mucosa can be examined from any perspective. Virtual cystoscopy also allows the mucosa of small bladder diverticula to be easily examined. Although uncommon, diverticular carcinoma is difficult to detect at conventional cystoscopy and has a poorer prognosis than neoplasm that originates within the main bladder lumen owing to earlier transmural invasion (13).

Display of CT data as virtual cystoscopy images affords a number of advantages compared with interpretation of axial CT scans alone. Virtual cystoscopy allows data from more than 100 CT images to be compressed into one interactive data set. The data set can be easily manipulated, and tumor measurements can be recorded in any dimension. At virtual cystoscopy, masses are seen "en face"; in comparison, axial CT images depict the bladder wall in profile. Abnormalities can be examined from any perspective, which facilitates lesion characterization and evaluation of surface morphology.

Although bladder catheterization can be performed by using catheters of a variety of sizes, we routinely use a small catheter to reduce the potential risk of urethral trauma. Bladder catheterization is easier to perform and less traumatic than fiberoptic cystoscopy, especially in patients with urethral strictures and prostatic hypertrophy. We are currently investigating the use of an anterior urethral catheter position, without formal bladder catheterization, for air distention of the bladder. This technique theoretically should minimize urethral trauma and reduce the risk of urinary sepsis. We have used anterior urethral catheterization successfully for virtual cystoscopy in a limited number of patients (unpublished data), but further work is needed to confirm our initial results.

Image artifacts and certain interpretive pitfalls were encountered in our study. Stair-step artifact, which appears as a series of concentric rings, was most obvious at the bladder dome. This artifact, which is a function of the scanning parameters selected, can be minimized by reformatting the data with a minimal 50% overlap between sections. Partial-volume effects may render the bladder wall relatively translucent and result in "shine through" from adjacent, gas-distended loops of small and large bowel. The presence of residual intravesical urine may obscure lesions in the dependent bladder, although this problem is easily overcome with use of both supine and prone or prone-oblique patient positioning during acquisitions.

Data acquisition should be performed in the helical mode with a single breath hold to eliminate breathing artifact and reduce section-to-section misregistration. Although acquisition times are short (approximately 15 seconds), motion artifacts can occur and can degrade image quality. In one of our patients in whom a median lobe of prostate was misinterpreted as an intrinsic bladder lesion, considerable ring artifact occurred due to patient movement (tremor secondary to Parkinson disease) and resulted in substantial image degradation (Fig 5). The radiation dose for virtual cystoscopy is less than half that needed for conventional helical CT in the pelvis. Because subject contrast is high (air-tissue interface) during virtual cystoscopy, the radiation dose to the patient can be reduced to 70 mA without a perceptible loss in image quality (8).

A major limitation of virtual cystoscopy compared with conventional cystoscopy is its inability to depict subtle alterations in mucosal texture. Although many of these subtle changes are benign, important entities such as "velvety patches" of dysplastic mucosa and "sandy patches" of urinary schistosomiasis may be difficult to identify on reconstructed images. Work is ongoing to develop automated computer algorithms for virtual colonoscopy that will assign varying degrees of color and opacity depending on colonic wall thickness. The application of such algorithms in the evaluation of the bladder at virtual cystoscopy may help increase conspicuity and detection of subtle mucosal lesions.

Virtual-reality imaging is still in its infancy. Software manufacturers promise faster parallel processing with decreased computation time, improved navigation techniques, more accurate spatial localization, increased spatial resolution, and more precise measurement techniques. Even with the limitations of existing commercially available software, virtual cystoscopy represents an exciting and novel approach to the diagnosis of bladder disease. In this study, virtual cystoscopy yielded results comparable to those obtained with conventional cystoscopy in patients with documented bladder disease. There were, however, fewer potential complications and a reduction in patient inconvenience, time, and discomfort. Further work is ongoing to prospectively evaluate the accuracy of virtual cystoscopy in a larger group of patients with hematuria but without documented bladder disease. ■

References

1. Webb JAW. Imaging in hematuria. Clin Radiol 1997; 52:167–171.
2. Kim B, Semelka RC, Ascher SM, Chalpin DB, Carroll PR, Hricak H. Bladder tumor staging: comparison of contrast-enhanced CT, T1- and T2-weighted MR imaging, dynamic gadolinium-enhanced imaging, and late gadolinium-enhanced imaging. Radiology 1994; 193:239–245.
3. Tanimoto A, Yuasa Y, Imai Y, et al. Bladder tumor staging: comparison of conventional and gadolinium-enhanced dynamic MR imaging and CT. Radiology 1992; 185:741–747.
4. Husband JE. Staging bladder cancer. Clin Radiol 1992; 46:153–159.
5. Havard AC. Technical report: the post-micturition CT scan as an aid to staging bladder cancer. Clin Radiol 1992; 45:201–202.
6. Kauczor HU, Wolcke B, Fischer B, Mildenberger P, Lorenz J, Thelen M. Three-dimensional helical CT of the tracheobronchial tree: evaluation of imaging protocols and assessment of suspected stenoses with bronchoscopic correlation. AJR 1996; 167:419–424.
7. Vining DJ. Virtual endoscopy: is it reality (editorial)? Radiology 1996; 200:30–31.
8. Hara AK, Johnson CD, Reed JE, Ehman RL, Ilstrup DM. Colorectal polyp detection with CT colography: two- versus three-dimensional techniques (work in progress). Radiology 1996; 200:49–54.
9. Stonelake PS, Wallace DMA. Investigation of adults with hematuria. Br Med J 1990; 301:1396–1397.
10. Vining DJ, Zagoria RJ, Liu K, Stelts D. CT cystoscopy: an innovation in bladder imaging. AJR 1996; 166:409–410.
11. Narumi Y, Kumatani T, Sawai Y, et al. The bladder and bladder tumors: imaging with three-dimensional display of helical CT data. AJR 1996; 167:1134–1135.
12. Johnson PT, Heath DG, Bliss DF, Cabral B, Fishman EK. Three-dimensional CT: real-time interactive volume rendering. AJR 1996; 167:581–583.
13. Donaldski M, White EM, Ghahremani GG, Patel SK. Carcinoma arising in urinary bladder diverticula: imaging findings in six patients. AJR 1993; 161:817–820.

Transrectal US-guided Seminal Vesiculography[1]

Thomas R. Jones, MD
Ronald J. Zagoria, MD
Jonathan P. Jarow, MD[2]

Transrectal ultrasound (US)–guided seminal vesiculography is a technique that couples US with radiography to evaluate male-factor infertility. Seminal vesiculography was performed in 12 patients after needle puncture of the seminal vesicle to inject contrast material for radiography. Seminal vesiculography helped imaging of the distal male reproductive tract (vas deferens, seminal vesicles, ejaculatory ducts). This method is an improvement over standard vasography for evaluation of infertility in men with suspected ejaculatory-duct obstruction.

Index terms: Seminal vesicle, 845.1287, 856.12985 • Sterility • Ultrasound (US), guidance, 845.1287, 845.12985

Radiology 1997; 205:276–278

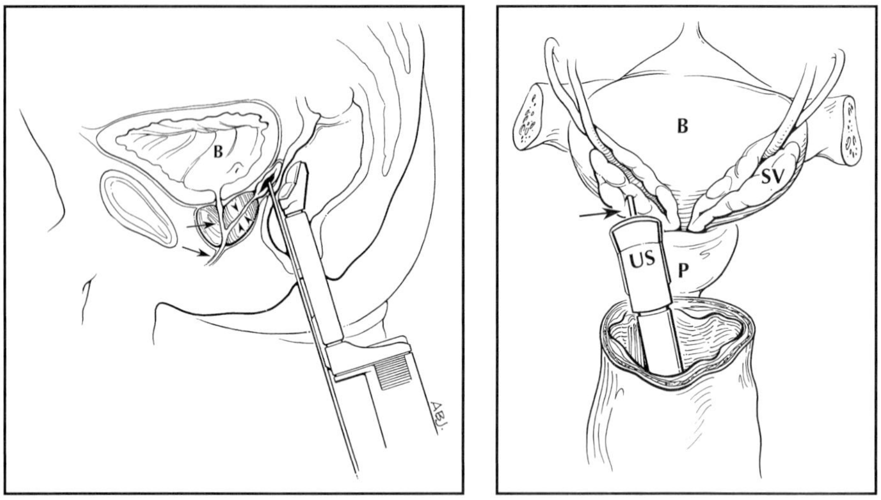

a. b.

Figure 1. Diagram of transrectal puncture of the seminal vesicle for vesiculography. **(a)** Sagittal view illustrates use of transrectal US to guide needle puncture of the seminal vesicle for injection of contrast material. Bladder (*B*), urethra (arrows), and ejaculatory duct (arrowheads) are indicated. **(b)** Coronal view from behind the bladder illustrates the sonography probe (*US*) in the rectum used to guide needle (arrow) puncture of one of the seminal vesicles. Also shown are the contralateral seminal vesicle (*SV*), bladder (*B*), and prostate gland (*P*).

Approximately 20% of couples in the United States have difficulty conceiving, and a male factor is present in approximately one-half of these couples. Obstruction of the ejaculatory duct is an uncommon cause of male infertility but is important because it is potentially curable. The typical semen-related findings in patients with complete ejaculatory-duct obstruction include low ejaculate volume, no fructose, and azoospermia (1). In contrast, patients with partial ejaculatory-duct obstruction may have normal to low ejaculate volume, normal or reduced sperm count, or abnormal sperm motility (1–3). Patients with ejaculatory-duct obstruction may also demonstrate hemospermia or perineal pain.

Vasography via either a puncture or partial-thickness vasotomy of the scrotal vas deferens has been the traditional radiologic imaging modality used to examine patients with suspected ejaculatory-duct obstruction (1). Vasography is an invasive test that often necessitates the use of anesthesia and carries an uncalculated risk of vasal stricture formation (4). The alternative approach of retrograde transurethral cannulation of the ejaculatory ducts is not used because it is technically very difficult. More recently, transrectal ultrasonography (US) has been proposed as an imaging method to help diagnose ejaculatory-duct obstruction (2,5,6). There are no generally accepted criteria, however, for diagnosis of this disorder with transrectal US, and the accuracy of such a diagnosis is still unknown (6).

Herein we describe an alternative, minimally invasive approach for imaging the distal male reproductive tract by combining transrectal US with conventional radiography to perform seminal vesiculography. Seminal vesiculography can be performed on an outpatient basis without the use of anesthesia. It also is less invasive and technically easier than vasography, and it avoids the risk of vasal injury. Seminal vesiculography is performed by means of direct needle puncture of the seminal vesicle with transrectal US guidance and subsequent opacification of the seminal vesicle and distal male reproductive tract with water-soluble contrast material (7). Needle puncture of the seminal vesicles can be performed through the rectal wall by using the needle guide of the US transducer or by using an US-guided free-hand technique through the perineum. Seminal vesiculography provides excellent visualization of the pelvic vas deferens, seminal vesicles, and ejaculatory ducts and can be used to rule out obstruction or abnormalities in any of these organs.

Materials and Methods

Seminal vesiculography was performed in 12 patients with suspected ejaculatory-duct obstruction on the basis of clinical and laboratory findings. All patients underwent bowel and antibiotic preparation consisting of a single cleansing enema the morning of the procedure and fluoroquinolone administered orally for 24 hours starting the night before the procedure.

Transrectal US was performed with the patient in the lithotomy position. A commercially available US unit (EUB 450; Hitachi, Tokyo, Japan) with a 6.5-MHz biplanar transducer was used. With real-time US guidance, each seminal vesicle was identified in the sagittal plane and was punctured with a 17-gauge, 30-cm-long needle (Figs 1, 2). Seminal vesicle fluid was routinely aspirated and examined microscopically for sperm (8). Use of a 17-gauge or

[1] From the Departments of Radiology (T.R.J., R.J.Z.) and Urology (J.P.J.), Bowman Gray School of Medicine, Wake Forest University, Medical Center Blvd, Winston-Salem, NC 27157. From the 1996 RSNA scientific assembly. Received March 11, 1997; revision requested April 23; revision received June 10; accepted June 16. **Address reprint requests to** R.J.Z.
[2] Current address: Department of Urology, Johns Hopkins Medical School, Baltimore, Md.

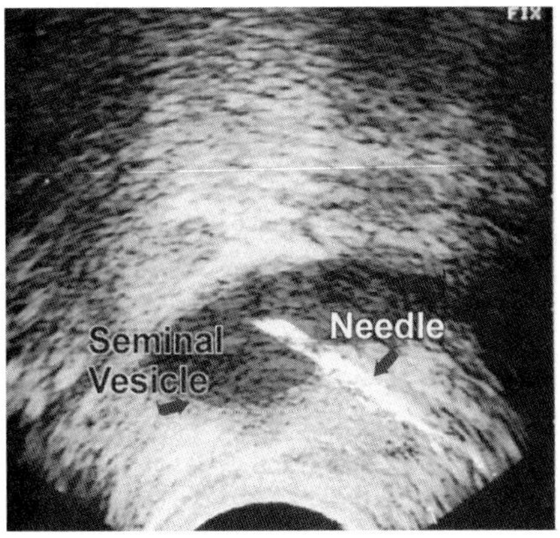

Figure 2. Transrectal US image of seminal-vesicle puncture. Transverse sonogram obtained during transrectal needle puncture for seminal vesiculography shows a dilated seminal vesicle, a finding suggestive of ejaculatory-duct obstruction.

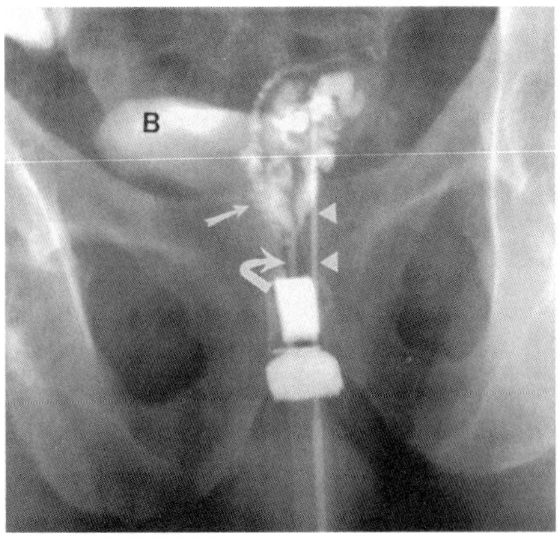

Figure 3. Normal transrectal seminal vesiculogram. Contrast material has been injected through the needle (arrowheads) to opacify the left seminal vesicle, the ampulla of the vas deferens (straight arrow), and the ejaculatory duct (curved arrow). Contrast material is shown in the bladder (*B*), a finding that indicates patency of the ejaculatory duct.

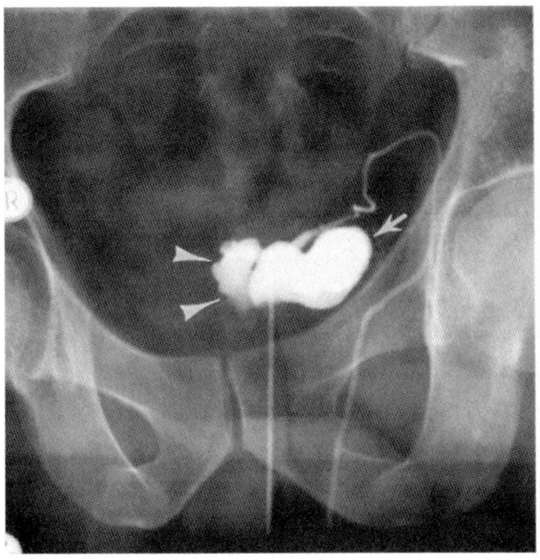

Figure 4. Seminal vesiculogram indicates ejaculatory-duct obstruction. The left seminal vesicle (arrow) and the ampulla of the vas deferens (arrowheads) are very dilated. Retrograde filling of the vas deferens, a common finding with this technique, is also shown. Opacification of the ejaculatory duct, urethra, or bladder is not shown.

larger needle is necessary for successful aspiration from the seminal vesicle.

A total of 5–20 mL of dilute, nonionic, water-soluble contrast material was then instilled with fluoroscopic monitoring. Patency of the ipsilateral ejaculatory duct was demonstrated when the contrast material opacified the seminal vesicle, the ampulla of the vas deferens, and the ejaculatory duct, with free spillage of contrast material into the prostatic urethra and bladder (Figs 3, 4). Retrograde flow of contrast material into the inguinal and scrotal vas deferens is common, and the procedure should be closely monitored to avoid reflux of the contrast agent into the epididymis.

The procedure was then repeated with puncture of the contralateral seminal vesicle.

Results

Seminal vesiculography was technically successful in all 12 patients. All radiographic images were of diagnostic quality, and patient discomfort was minimal. Use of anesthetics was not necessary, and general anesthesia was used only when seminal vesiculography was coupled with ejaculatory-duct recanalization procedures. There were no immediate complications. One patient developed left epididymitis after seminal vesiculography owing to reflux of contrast material to the epididymis. The epididymitis resolved after treatment with a combination of oral antibiotics and nonsteroidal antiinflammatory agents.

Discussion

Obstruction of the ejaculatory duct is suggested clinically by symptoms of painful ejaculation, perineal pain, hemospermia, and infertility (1). This disorder may be congenital or acquired. Congenital causes of ejaculatory-duct obstruction include atresia or stenosis of the ejaculatory duct; ectopic ureter; and utricular, mullerian, or wolffian duct cysts that may extrinsically compress the ejaculatory ducts (1). Acquired obstruction may be caused by urethral instrumentation with catheters or endoscopes, infection or inflammation, and obstructing calculi. Most cases, however, are idiopathic. Although ejaculatory-duct obstruction is an infrequent cause of male infertility, its correct identification is important, as it represents a potentially curable cause of infertility. Ejaculatory-duct obstruction can be treated with transurethral resection or with newer recanalization techniques (9). When seminal vesiculography is used, ejaculatory-duct obstruction is shown by the presence of enlarged seminal vesicles and the absence of opacification with contrast material of the prostatic urethra and bladder (Fig 4).

Much like hysterosalpingography in women, this technique does not provide a means to diagnose partial obstruction. Seminal vesiculography in patients with partial ejaculatory-duct obstruction will also show flow of contrast material into the urethra and bladder. We do not yet have a radiologic modality that can help accurately establish the diagnosis of partial ejaculatory-duct obstruction.

Seminal vesiculography performed with transrectal US guidance represents a useful technique in the evaluation of obstructive causes of male-factor infertility. This technique differs from earlier descriptions of seminal-vesicle puncture in which this procedure was performed either blindly across the rectal wall (10) or, if US guidance was involved, by using a transperineal approach (11,12). Transrectal US-guided seminal vesiculography avoids the potential complications associated with traditional vasography and thus represents a safer means of imaging the distal male reproductive tract (13). Variations of this technique may be used to guide puncture and aspiration of prostatic and periprostatic cysts, as well as to perform recanalization and balloon dilation of obstructed ejaculatory ducts with catheter and guide-wire techniques (9). ■

References

1. Pryor JP, Hendry WF. Ejaculatory duct obstruction in subfertile males: analysis of 87 patients. Fertil Ster 1991; 56:725–730.
2. Hellerstein DK, Meacham RB, Lipshultz LI. Transrectal ultrasound and partial ejaculatory duct obstruction in male infertility. Urology 1992; 39:449–452.
3. Meacham RB, Hellerstein DK, Lipshultz LI. Evaluation and treatment of ejaculatory duct obstruction in the infertile male. Fertil Ster 1993; 59:393–397.
4. Poore RE, Schneider A, DeFranzo AJ, Humphries ST, Woodruff RD, Jarow JP. Comparison of puncture versus vasotomy techniques of vasography in an animal model. J Urol (in press).
5. Belker AM, Steinbock GS. Transrectal prostate ultrasonography as a diagnostic and therapeutic aid for ejaculatory duct obstruction. J Urol 1990; 144:356–358.
6. Jarow JP. Transrectal ultrasonography of infertile men. Fertil Ster 1993; 60:1035–1039.
7. Riedenklau E, Buch JP, Jarow JP. Diagnosis of vasal obstruction with seminal vesiculography: an alternative to vasography in select patients. Fertil Ster 1995; 64:1224–1227.
8. Jarow JP. Seminal vesicle aspiration in the management of patients with ejaculatory

duct obstruction. J Urol 1994; 152:899–901.
9. Jarow JP, Zagoria RJ. Antegrade ejaculatory duct recanalization and dilation. Urology 1995; 46:743–746.
10. Meyer JJ, Hartig PR, Koos GW, McKinley CR. Transrectal seminal vesiculography. J Urol 1979; 121:129–130.
11. Abe M, Watanabe H, Kojima M, Saitoh M, Ohe H. Puncture of the seminal vesicles guided by a transrectal real-time linear scanner. J Clin Ultrasound 1989; 17:173–178.
12. Asch MR, Toi A. Seminal vesicles: imaging and intervention using transrectal ultrasound. J Ultrasound Med 1991; 10:19–23.
13. Goldstein M. Vasography and technique of testis biopsy. In: Rajfer J, ed. Common problems in infertility and impotence. Chicago, Ill: Year Book Medical, 1990.

Pathologic Conditions in the Small Bowel: Findings at Fat-suppressed Gadolinium-enhanced MR Imaging with an Optimized Suspension of Oral Magnetic Particles[1]

Sonja C. Faber, Dipl Phys
Michael K. Stehling, MD, PhD
Nicolaus Holzknecht, MD
Jörg Gauger, MD
Thomas Helmberger, MD
Maximilian Reiser, MD

Depiction of small-bowel pathologic conditions was optimized with use of a negative luminal contrast agent, spectral fat suppression, and gadolinium enhancement in an excised gut phantom. The method was applied in nine patients in conjunction with standard enteroclysis examinations. Bulk susceptibility effects of oral magnetic particles were canceled with use of a diamagnetic methylcellulose suspension. In the ileum, fat suppression and contrast between bowel wall and lumen was judged good or excellent in eight and nine patients, respectively. In eight of nine patients, additional mesenteric findings were depicted.

Index terms: Contrast media, experimental studies • Gastrointestinal tract, MR, 70.12143 • Iron • Magnetic resonance (MR), contrast enhancement, 70.12143

Radiology 1997; 205:278–282

The primary diagnostic modality for examinations in the small bowel is enteroclysis. Enteroclysis gives only indirect information about the bowel wall and extraluminal processes, however, and exposes the patients (who are often young) to large doses of ionizing radiation (average dose per small-bowel examination in Germany, 16 mSv) (1).

In the past, magnetic resonance (MR) imaging in the gastrointestinal tract was limited by the presence of artifacts due to peristaltic and respiratory motion (2,3) as a result of long data acquisition times and by the lack of a suitable luminal contrast agent. Recent improvements in MR technology, however, now allow sufficiently fast imaging in the gut to obtain good image quality (4). Also, a number of suitable positive (5–8) and negative (3,9–12) bowel contrast agents have become available. We have used oral magnetic particles, which provide negative luminal contrast (3,13–17). In previous studies of oral magnetic particles, excellent image quality was achieved with T2-weighted spin-echo (SE) sequences but susceptibility artifacts were observed with gradient-echo sequences (15–17). Gradient-echo sequences, however, are the most suitable and widely used for multisection T1-weighted breath-hold imaging.

To our knowledge, the scope of previous studies on MR imaging in the small bowel was limited to the visualization and delineation of the bowel wall and lumen. In none of the previous studies was use of a negative oral contrast agent combined with fat-suppressed gradient-echo imaging and gadolinium enhancement to highlight the bowel wall and its pathologic condition against the black background and lumen.

Oral magnetic particles cancel signal from water protons that diffuse in the local gradients caused by the particles, but unfortunately they also have a paramagnetic bulk susceptibility that causes macroscopic field distortions and hampers spectral fat suppression.

This study had three purposes: (*a*) To find a way to use oral magnetic particles to provide a black lumen on T1-weighted, T2-weighted, and short inversion time inversion-recovery (STIR) images without susceptibility problems at the lumen-tissue interface (on the basis of an idea reported by Liebig et al [18] and Briggs et al [19]). (*b*) To use fat saturation, with STIR and spectral fat saturation, respectively. (*c*) To administer gadopentetate dimeglumine (Magnevist; Schering, Berlin, Germany) intravenously as a positive contrast agent to highlight inflammatory and neoplastic processes on T1-weighted fat-saturated images.

Materials and Methods

Contrast agent.—Oral magnetic particles, the main component of the negative oral contrast agent (Abdoscan; Nycomed, Oslo, Norway), consist of superparamagnetic iron oxide crystals less than 50 nm in diameter that are precipitated on a resin carrier particle. The complete particle contains approximately 25% iron oxide by weight with a diameter of 3.5 µm (12,15). The effect of superparamagnetism has been described previously in detail (20,21). In the presence of an external magnetic field, superparamagnetic particles produce microscopic magnetic-field gradients that increase the spin dephasing of water protons that diffuse through them, resulting in a shortening of the transverse relaxation time T2. Additionally, the gradient fields cause a shift, $\Delta\omega$, of the resonance frequency. If this bulk susceptibility effect is strong enough, $\Delta\omega$ will make spectral fat suppression impossible. This effect occurs especially at the bowel wall–fat interface.

The combination of the paramagnetic ($\chi_{mag} > 0$) oral magnetic particles (OMP), where χ_{mag} is the magnetic susceptibility, with a diamagnetic substance (DS) ($\chi_{mag} < 0$) in appropriate quantities should result in a cancellation of the bulk susceptibility effect. This can be described with the following equation: $c_1\, \chi_{mag}(\text{OMP}) + c_2$

[1] From the Department of Diagnostic Radiology, Klinikum Grosshadern, University of Munich, Marchioninistr 15, D-81377 Munich, Germany. Received April 18, 1997; revision requested May 15; revision received June 12; accepted June 19. **Address reprint requests to** S.C.F.

χ_{mag}(DS) = χ_{mag}(bowel wall–fat), where c_1 and c_2 are constants (18,19,22). To our knowledge, the only suitable diamagnetic substances for use in patients are water ($\chi_{mag} = 12.9 \times 10^{-6}$ in centimeter-gram-second [cgs] units) and $BaSO_4$ ($\chi_{mag} = 71.3 \times 10^{-6}$ in cgs units). To increase the viscosity of water, methylcellulose was added. Both the methylcellulose and $BaSO_4$ suspensions are standard contrast agents used in bowel examinations (23,24).

MR imaging.—All measurements were performed on a 1.5-T MR imager (Magnetom Vision; Siemens, Erlangen, Germany) with a circular polarized body array coil.

In vitro studies were performed to find the ratio at which bulk susceptibility equals that of fat. We have prepared a dilution series of oral magnetic particles (Abdoscan) with $BaSO_4$ suspension and with methylcellulose suspension. A plastic container filled with vegetable oil (to simulate fat) was used to hold 12 test tubes (diameter = 3 cm) that were filled with the different mixtures of oral magnetic particles with methylcellulose and $BaSO_4$ suspensions. A water load was added to ensure correct frequency adjustment of the radio-frequency coil.

To visualize the susceptibility effects of the oral-magnetic-particles mixtures, a field mapping sequence was used (25,26). The optimal mixing ratio that zeros the bulk susceptibility effects was identified on the basis of the homogeneous field distribution around the test tubes filled with this mixture. To ensure that this mixing ratio provided sufficient signal attenuation, the signal intensities of the mixtures were measured on images obtained with different pulse sequences.

To assess the amount of sedimentation of oral magnetic particles (OMP) in the methylcellulose suspension (MCS), the concentration gradient $\partial[OMP/(MCS + OMP)]/\partial s$ (where s is distance) was determined as follows. Before image acquisition, the test tubes were shaken to guarantee optimal distribution of oral magnetic particles and then allowed to rest for 4 hours. The signal intensities of one section at the top of the test tube and one near the bottom were measured and related to the OMP/(MCS + OMP) concentration by means of a calibration curve, respectively. $\partial[OMP(MCS + OMP)]/\partial s$ was obtained by dividing the difference in the OMP/(MCS + OMP) concentrations of the two sections by the distance s of the two sections.

To test the contrast agent mixture ex vivo, fresh bovine intestine was filled with the optimized oral-magnetic-particles–methylcellulose-suspension mixture, the optimized oral-magnetic-particles–$BaSO_4$-suspension mixture, and the unmodified oral magnetic particles, respectively, and placed in the oil-filled plastic container. Spectral fat suppression and a short inversion time inversion-recovery (STIR) sequence were applied on this phantom. The following pulse sequences were used: T1-weighted SE (repetition time msec/echo time msec = 300/12; flip angle, 90°; section thickness, 3 mm; field of view, 200 × 200 mm; matrix, 256 × 256; acquisition time, 61 seconds; one signal acquired; intersection gap, 1.5 mm) with spectral fat suppression, T2-weighted turbo SE (4,000/90; flip angle, 180°; section thickness, 3 mm; field of view, 200 × 200 mm; matrix, 256 × 256; acquisition time, 140 seconds; one signal acquired; intersection gap, 1.5 mm) with spectral fat suppression, T1-weighted fast low-angle shot (FLASH) (124/4.8; flip angle, 75°; section thickness, 3 mm; field of view, 225 × 300 mm; matrix, 144 × 256; acquisition time, 18 seconds; one signal acquired; intersection gap, 1.5 mm) with spectral fat suppression, and fast STIR (2,000/30; flip angle, 180°; section thickness, 3 mm; field of view, 200 × 200 mm; matrix, 256 × 256; acquisition time, 75 seconds; one signal acquired; intersection gap, 1.5 mm).

In volunteer and patient studies, 800 mL of the optimized oral-magnetic-particles–methylcellulose-suspension and oral-magnetic-particles–$BaSO_4$-suspension mixtures were orally administered to one and two male volunteers, respectively, to test tolerance and to design the sequence protocol for MR imaging examination. Tolerance was subjectively rated by the volunteers. Pulse sequences were chosen from our routine abdominal protocol. The criteria for pulse-sequence selection were multisection option and an acquisition time short enough to allow imaging in one breath hold.

We examined nine patients (four male, five female, aged 16–64 years) with known small-bowel diseases (seven with Crohn disease, one with small-bowel metastasis of malignant melanoma, and one with backwash ileitis in ulcerative colitis) directly after they underwent enteroclysis. The latter was performed with the method described by Sellink (27) and Herlinger (28) modified by the addition of oral magnetic particles to the methylcellulose suspension. Oral magnetic particles did not noticeably alter the x-ray absorption. Prior to MR imaging, endoscopy was performed in eight of the nine patients and a double-contrast-enema examination of the colon with barium in three. All patients and volunteers gave their informed consent prior to examination.

Immediately after enteroclysis, 20 mg of a spasmolyticum hyoscine butylbromide (Buscopan; Boehringer Ingelheim, Ingelheim, Germany) was administered intravenously to paralyze peristaltic activity. At the MR unit, 600–800 mL of the optimized oral-magnetic-particles–methylcellulose suspension was administered rectally. Gadopentetate dimeglumine was injected intravenously in a dose of 0.1 mmol per kilogram of body weight during the MR examination. The following pulse sequences were used just before and after injection of gadopentetate dimeglumine: T1-weighted spoiled gradient echo (FLASH) (140/4.1; flip angle, 75°; section thickness, 8 mm; field of view, 240 × 320 mm; matrix, 144 × 256; acquisition time, 20 seconds; one signal acquired; intersection gap, 1.6 mm; 17 sections) without spectral fat suppression, T1-weighted FLASH (124/4.8; flip angle, 75°; section thickness, 8 mm; field of view, 240 × 320 mm; matrix, 144 × 256; acquisition time, 18 seconds; one signal acquired; intersection gap, 1.6 mm; four sections) with spectral fat suppression, and T2-weighted half-Fourier single-shot turbo SE (4.3/60; flip angle, 140°; section thickness, 8 mm; field of view, 240 × 320 mm; matrix, 144 × 256; acquisition time, 19 seconds; one signal acquired; intersection gap, 1.6 mm; 17 sections). The patients were asked to hold their breath during image acquisition.

In image reading and assessment, images were read and scored by two radiologists (N.H., J.G.) independently. Signal attenuation in the bowel lumen and the resulting contrast between bowel wall and lumen was scored as (*a*) no darkening effect, no contrast; (*b*) slightly darker than bowel wall, low contrast; (*c*) darker than bowel wall, intermediate contrast; (*d*) much darker than bowel wall, good contrast; or (*e*) total luminal signal void, excellent contrast. Fat saturation and susceptibility effects were graded as (*a*) very strong susceptibility effects, more than 80% of bowel wall effaced, fat saturation not possible; (*b*) strong susceptibility effects, 50%–80% of bowel wall effaced, fat saturation insufficient; (*c*) intermediate susceptibility effects, 20%–50% of bowel wall effaced, fat saturation moderate; (*d*) weak susceptibility effects, less than 20% of bowel wall effaced, fat saturation good; or (*e*) no susceptibility effects, less than 5% of bowel wall effaced, fat saturation excellent.

Results

In vitro studies.—The viscosity of a 2.0% (weight) methylcellulose suspension was sufficient to avoid sedimentation of the oral magnetic particles over several hours. Four hours after preparation, the mean difference in oral-magnetic-particles content between two sections separated by 1 cm was less than 7%. Sedimentation of oral magnetic particles was thus judged to be negligible during the average duration of the MR examination even when peristaltic mixing was stopped with pharmacologic paralysis.

The respective amounts of $BaSO_4$ or methylcellulose suspensions to cancel the bulk susceptibility effect of oral magnetic particles was determined from the images of magnetic-field distribution as 1.75 parts (volume) of $BaSO_4$ suspension to one part (volume) of oral magnetic particles, or four parts (volume) of methylcellulose suspension to one part (volume) of oral magnetic particles, respectively.

Use of these optimized concentrations of diluted oral magnetic particles resulted in sufficient signal attenuation. Signal attenuation was better with T2- than with T1-weighted pulse sequences.

Filled into the bovine gut, neither oral-magnetic-particles–methylcellulose or $-BaSO_4$ suspensions caused any noticeable bulk susceptibility effects and both allowed spectral suppression of the oil directly abutting the gut. With both lumen and surroundings black, the intestinal wall stood out bright against the background, even before gadopentetate dimeglumine was injected. The bulk susceptibility of unmodified oral magnetic particles prevented fat suppression near the bowel wall, which hampered the delineation of the latter (Fig 1). Nonspectral fat suppression with a STIR sequence also provided good images of the intestinal wall, independent of bulk susceptibility. Simultaneous gadolinium enhancement, however, is impossible with STIR sequences, since fat and gadolinium-enhanced tissue have similar T1 relaxation times.

Volunteer and patient studies.—The heavier oral-magnetic-particles–$BaSO_4$-suspension mixture was tolerated less well (slight constipation and gastric malaise) than the oral-magnetic-particles–methylcellulose-suspension mixture. Consequently, the latter was used for the subsequent patient examinations.

The signal intensity of the bowel lumen was reported as much darker than the bowel wall or as a total signal void with good or excellent contrast in the jejunum in four (N.H.) or three (J.G.) of the nine patients, in the ileum in nine (N.H.) or seven (J.G.), and in the colon in nine. Fat saturation was judged as good or excellent and susceptibility effects as weak or nonexistent in the jejunum in six (N.H.) or seven (J.G.) and in the ileum and colon in nine.

In all patients, the inflammation-altered parts (Fig 2) and extraluminal compression and stenosed segments (Fig 3) of the bowel seen at small-bowel enteroclysis, double-contrast-enema examination of the colon with barium, or endoscopy were depicted at MR imaging. Also depicted at MR imaging were mesenteric lymphadenopathy in six of the nine patients (Fig 2), involvement of the right ureter in one, and a sinus tract between the ileum and sigmoid colon in one.

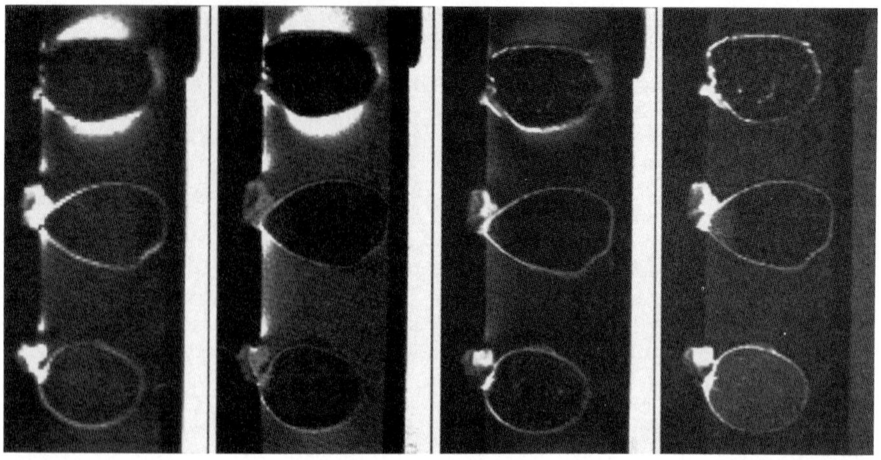

Figure 1. Pieces of bovine small bowel filled with (top) unmodified oral magnetic particles, (middle) oral-magnetic-particles–$BaSO_4$-suspension mixture (1:1.75, volume), and (bottom) oral-magnetic-particles–methylcellulose-suspension mixture (1:4, volume). From left to right the images were acquired with T1-weighted FLASH, T1-weighted SE, T2-weighted fast SE, and fast STIR. In the FLASH and SE sequences, spectral fat suppression was applied; in the STIR sequence, inversion time of 150 msec was used to suppress the signal from fat. Unmodified oral magnetic particles prevented spectral fat suppression along the magnetic-field lines near the bowel wall–oil interface and resulted in a partial suppression of water signal in the bowel wall. The modified oral-magnetic-particle mixtures allowed spectral fat suppression, which resulted in excellent delineation of the intestinal wall against the lumen and surrounding oil.

Discussion

The combination of fat saturation and gadolinium enhancement proved useful for detecting various pathologic conditions in the abdomen (29–31) by decreasing the bright signal from fat and highlighting the contrast-enhanced lesions. Semelka et al (32) and Anderson et al (33) conclude that the optimal assessment of inflammatory bowel disease with MR imaging necessitates the administration of an oral contrast agent in addition to gadopentetate dimeglumine.

To our knowledge, however, there are no prior reports about the use of a combination of an intraluminal contrast agent, gadolinium enhancement, and fat suppression in the small bowel.

Findings in our in vitro studies have shown that the appropriate mixture of oral magnetic particles with $BaSO_4$ or methylcellulose suspensions yields an artifact-free, negative gastrointestinal contrast agent that allows spectral fat suppression. We have confirmed these findings in patients and shown that the simultaneous, intravenous administration of gadopentetate dimeglumine results in the expected highlighting of inflammatory and neoplastic diseases of the bowel against a black background, thus optimizing the sensitivity of MR imaging to such disease processes.

One disadvantage remains: The oral-magnetic-particles–methylcellulose-suspension mixture was applied transduodenally via a probe that bypassed the stomach, rendering the procedure invasive and time-consuming and necessitating fluoroscopy for probe placement. Oral administration of the contrast agent may alter its consistency and result in the presence of a fragmented volume of contrast material in the small bowel. This needs to be investigated in future studies. The concentration of the contrast agent as it moves down from the jejunum to the colon, however, did not seem to alter strongly as fat suppression in the colon was still excellent. Slightly inferior intraluminal contrast in the jejunum was thought to be caused by the delay between small-bowel enteroclysis and MR imaging, which was typically 20 minutes. If MR imaging supported with the oral-magnetic-particles–methylcellulose-suspension mixture proves to be a sufficient replacement for enteroclysis, the contrast material should be administered in the MR unit to optimize the delay between administration and imaging.

Larger correlated studies are needed to compare findings at enteroclysis with those at MR imaging. We believe such studies will prove MR imaging to

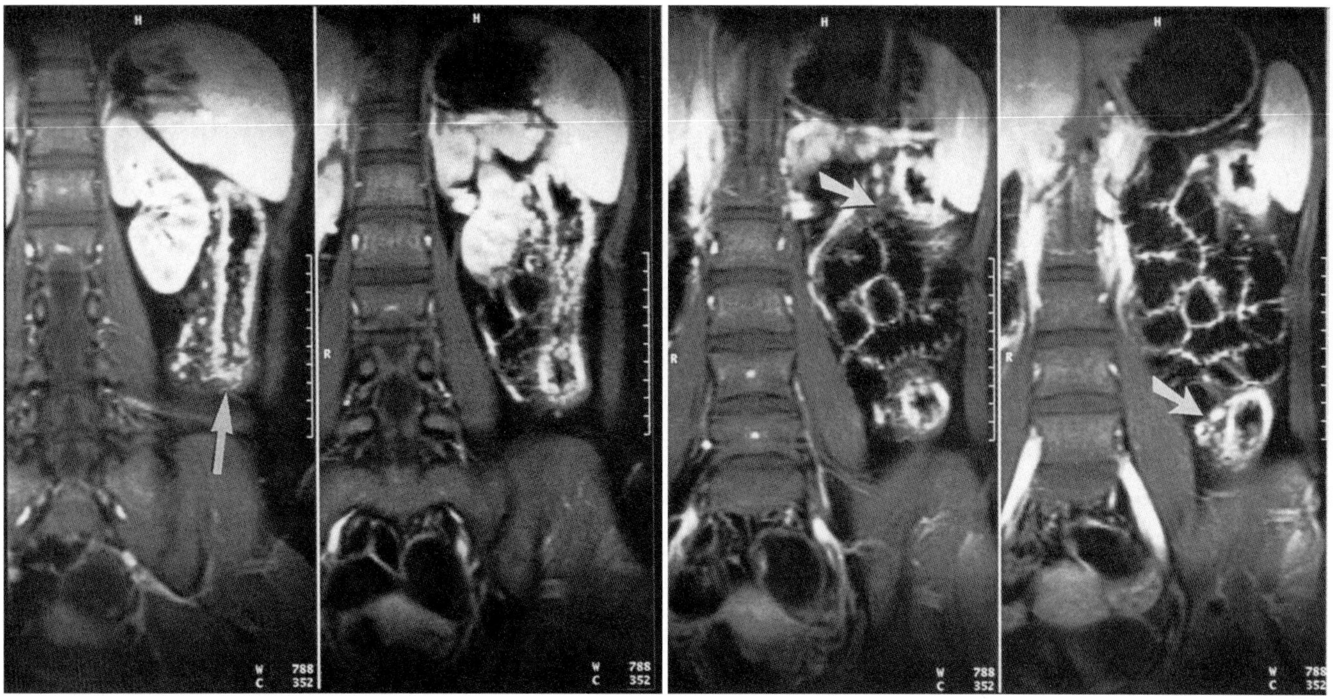

Figure 2. Images obtained in a 54-year-old man with an 11-year history of ulcerative colitis. Four consecutive coronal gadolinium-enhanced, fat-suppressed, T1-weighted, gradient-echo images obtained after transduodenal and rectal administration of oral-magnetic-particles–methylcellulose-suspension mixture show sufficient distention of the stomach and small bowel; most of the small-bowel folds are visualized clearly. The left colonic flexure and the descending colon show bowel-wall thickening up to 10 mm (arrow on left) and mesenteric lymphadenopathy (arrows on right).

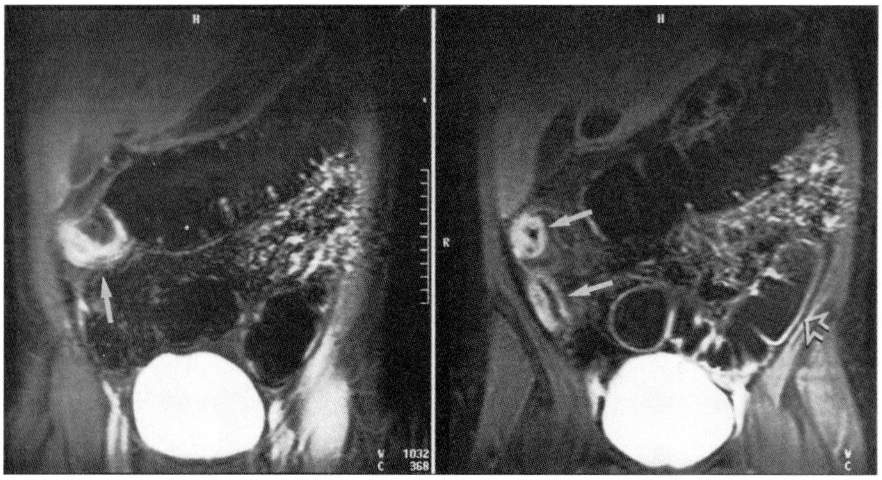

Figure 3. Images obtained in a 38-year-old woman with an 8-year history of Crohn disease and previous resection of the terminal ileum and caecum owing to stenosis. The patient was seen with symptoms of recurrent stenosis. Coronal gadolinium-enhanced, T1-weighted, fat-suppressed, gradient-echo images highlight a recurrent 10-cm-long stenosis at the ileocolonic anastomosis (solid arrows). Note the marked enhancement of the wall of the stenosis, the descending colon (open arrow), and sigmoid colon that correlated with inflammatory changes at endoscopy.

be a more sensitive and perhaps specific method for the detection, characterization, staging, and assessment of activity of small-bowel disease.

Acknowledgment: This article is part of a PhD thesis of the University of Munich, Germany. We thank Joerg Reinhardt, MD, from Nycomed for his observations and for providing the contrast agent for the in vitro studies.

References

1. Kaul A, Bauer B, Bernhardt J, Nosske D, Veit R. Effective doses to members of the public from the diagnostic application of ionizing radiation in Germany. Eur Radiol (in press).
2. Wood ML, Henkelman RM. MR image artifacts from periodic motion. Med Phys 1985; 12:143–151.
3. Bach-Gansmo T, Dupas B, Gayet-Delacroix M, Lambrechts M. Abdominal MRI using a negative contrast agent. Br J Radiol 1993; 66:420–425.
4. Riederer SJ. Recent technical advances in MR imaging of the abdomen. JMRI 1996; 6:822–832.
5. Vlahos L, Gouliamos A, Athanasopoulou A, et al. A comparative study between Gd-DTPA and oral magnetic particles (OMP) as gastrointestinal (GI) contrast agents for MRI of the abdomen. Magn Reson Imaging 1994; 12:719–726.
6. Bernardino ME, Weinreb JC, Mitchell DG, Small WC, Morris M. Safety and optimum concentration of a manganese chloride–based oral MR contrast agent. JMRI 1994; 4:872–876.
7. Hiraishi K, Narabayashi I, Fujita O, et al. Blueberry juice: preliminary evaluation as oral contrast agent in gastrointestinal MR imaging. Radiology 1995; 194:119–123.
8. Hirohashi S, Uchida H, Yoshikawa K, et al. Large scale clinical evaluation of bowel contrast agent containing ferric ammonium citrate in MRI. Magn Reson Imaging 1994; 12:837–846.
9. Ros PR, Steinman RM, Torres GM, et al. The value of barium as a gastrointestinal contrast agent in MR imaging: a comparison study in normal volunteers. AJR 1991; 157:761–767.
10. Li KCP, Tart RP, Fitzsimmons JR, Storm BL, Mao J, Rolfes RJ. Barium sulfate suspension as a negative oral MRI contrast agent: in vitro and human optimization studies. Magn Reson Imaging 1991; 9:141–150.
11. Brown JJ, Duncan JR, Heiken JP, et al. Perfluoroctylbromide as a gastrointestinal contrast agent for MR imaging: use with and without glucagon. Radiology 1991; 181:455–460.
12. Mattrey RF, Trambert MA, Brown JJ, et al. Perflubron as an oral contrast agent for MR

imaging: results of a phase III clinical trial. Radiology 1994; 191:841–848.
13. Lonnemark M, Hemmingson A, Ericson A, Gundersen HG, Bach-Gansmo T. Oral superparamagnetic particles for magnetic resonance imaging. Acta Radiol 1990; 31: 303–307.
14. Lonnemark M, Hemmingson A, Bach-Gansmo T, et al. Effect of superparamagnetic particles as oral contrast medium at magnetic resonance imaging. Acta Radiol 1989; 30:193–196.
15. MacVicar D, Jacobsen TF, Guy R, Husband JE. Phase III trial of oral magnetic particles in MRI of abdomen and pelvis. Clin Radiol 1993; 47:183–188.
16. Øksendal AD, Jacobsen TF, Gundersen HG, Rinck PA, Rummeny E. Superparamagnetic particles as an oral contrast agent in abdominal magnetic resonance imaging. Invest Radiol 1991; 26:67–70.
17. Rinck PA, Smevik O, Nilsen G, et al. Oral magnetic particles in MR imaging of the abdomen and pelvis. Radiology 1991; 178:775–779.
18. Liebig T, Stoupis C, Ros PR, Ballinger JR, Briggs RW. A potentially artifact free oral contrast agent for gastrointestinal MRI. Magn Reson Med 1993; 30:646–649.
19. Briggs RW, Wu Z, Mladinich CRJ, et al. In vivo animal tests for an artifact-free contrast agent for gastrointestinal MRI. Magn Reson Imaging (in press).
20. Bean CP, Livingston JD. Superparamagnetism. J Appl Phys 1959; 30:120–129.
21. Bach-Gansmo T. Ferrimagnetic susceptibility contrast agents. Acta Radiol Suppl 1993; 387:9–30.
22. Chauvel B, Cathelineau G, Balac S, Lecerf J, de Certaines JD. Cancellation of metal-induced MRI artifacts with dual component paramagnetic and diamagnetic material: mathematical modelization and experimental verification. JMRI 1996; 6:936–938.
23. Antes G, Lissner J. Double contrast technique of the small bowel with barium and methylcellulose. ROFO 1981; 134:10–15.
24. Antes G, Kruis W. Whipple's disease demonstrated by double contrast small bowel enema with barium and methylcellulose. Eur J Radiol 1982; 2:238–241.
25. Romeo F, Hoult DI. Magnetic field profiling: analysis and correcting coil design. Magn Reson Med 1984; 1:44–65.
26. Boesch C, Gruetter R, Martin E. Temporal and spatial analysis of fields generated by eddy currents in superconducting magnets: optimization of corrections and quantitative characterization of magnet/gradient systems. Magn Reson Med 1991; 20:268–284.
27. Sellink JL. X-ray differential diagnosis in small bowel disease: a practical approach. Dordrecht, The Netherlands: Kluwer, 1988.
28. Herlinger H. A modified technique for double contrast small bowel enema. Gastrointest Radiol 1978; 3:201–207.
29. Semelka RC, Shoenut JP, Kroeker MA, MacMahon RG, Greenberg HM. Renal lesions: controlled comparison between CT and 1.5-T MR imaging with nonenhanced and gadolinium-enhanced fat-suppressed spin-echo and breath-hold FLASH techniques. Radiology 1992; 182:425–430.
30. Semelka RC, Lawrence PH, Shoenut JP, Heywood M, Kroeker MA, Lotocki R. Primary ovarian cancer: prospective comparison of contrast-enhanced CT and pre- and postcontrast fat-suppressed MR imaging with histologic correlation. JMRI 1993; 3:99–106.
31. Okizuka H, Sugimura K, Yoshzako T, Yasushi K, Wada A. Rectal carcinoma: prospective comparison of conventional and gadopentetate dimeglumine enhanced fat-suppressed MR imaging. JMRI 1996; 6:465–471.
32. Semelka RC, John G, Kelekis NL, Burdeny DA, Ascher SM. Small bowel neoplastic disease: demonstration by MRI. JMRI 1996; 6:855–860.
33. Anderson CM, Brown JJ, Balfe DM, et al. MR imaging of Crohn disease: use of perflubron as gastrointestinal contrast agent. JMRI 1994; 4:491–496.

Letters to the Editor

■ Differentiation between Benign and Malignant Breast Lesions with MR Imaging and Scintimammography

From:
Fabienne Servais, MD, Didier C. Blocklet, MD, Alain E. Seret, PhD, Andre Lenaers, MD, PhD, and Andre C. Schoutens, MD
Department of Nuclear Medicine, Hôpital Universitaire Erasme, Université Libre de Bruxelles
Route de Lennik 808, B-1070 Brussels, Belgium

Editor:
We read with interest the article by Helbich and colleagues, "Differentiation of Benign and Malignant Breast Lesions: MR Imaging versus Tc-99m Sestamibi Scintimammography," in the February 1997 issue of *Radiology* (1). A specificity of 30%–70% had been reported for the differentiation of benign from malignant breast lesions with magnetic resonance (MR) imaging (2,3). The improved specificity of nuclear MR reported in the article by Helbich and colleagues is probably due to the use of the latest refinements of nuclear MR and the use of better diagnostic criteria.

On the basis of our own experience with technetium-99m sestamibi scintimammography for the detection of malignant breast lesions, we highlight the following points: (*a*) The prone position is essential to achieve better separation of the deep breast structures from the high-activity myocardium and liver. (*b*) A preset count of 500 kilocounts with an all-purpose collimator provides breast images with inadequate data; thus, one may be unable to correctly distinguish some lesions from background activity. We routinely accumulate 3,000–8,000 kilocounts in 10 minutes (counts from the breasts represent less than 3% of the total counts). (*c*) Published study findings show that single photon emission computed tomography (SPECT) does not improve the diagnostic accuracy over that of planar scintimammography and even degrades specificity (4–8).

We no longer practice SPECT. We obtain information in about 20–30 minutes with Tc-99m sestamibi scintimammography. This compares favorably with the MR imaging time (about 30 minutes [1]).

Let us also propose that planar images in scintimammography be improved with the triple-energy window acquisition and scatter-correction method (9). The method offers better delineation of breast tumors, especially deep ones.

References

1. Helbich TH, Becherer A, Trattnig S, et al. Differentiation of benign and malignant breast lesions: MR imaging versus Tc-99m sestamibi scintimammography. Radiology 1997; 202:421–429.
2. Palmedo H, Grünwald F, Bender H, et al. Scintimammography with technetium-99m methoxyisobutylisonitrile: comparison with mammography and magnetic resonance imaging. Eur J Nucl Med 1996; 23:940–946.
3. Tiling R, Sommer H, Pechmann M, et al. Comparison of technetium-99m-sestamibi scintimammography with contrast-enhanced MRI for diagnosis of breast lesions. J Nucl Med 1997; 38:58–62.
4. Nagaraj N, Waxman A, Ashok G, et al. Comparison of SPECT and planar Tc-99m sestamibi (MIBI) imaging in patients with carcinoma of the breast (abstr). J Nucl Med 1994; 35:229P.
5. Palmedo H, Schomburg A, Grünwald F, Mallmann P, Krebs D, Biersack HJ. Technetium-99m-MIBI scintimammography for suspicious breast lesions. J Nucl Med 1996; 37:626–630.
6. Palmedo H, Schomburg A, Grünwald F, Bender H, Mallmann P, Biersack HJ. Mammoscintigraphy with Tc-99m MIBI: planar and SPECT imaging techniques in patients with suspicious breast nodules (abstr). J Nucl Med 1995; 35:51P.
7. Diggles L, Khalkhali I. SPECT prone dependent-breast scintimammography (SMM) (abstr). Eur J Nucl Med 1994; 21:S28.
8. Khalkhali I, Cutrone JA, Mena IG, et al. Scintimammography: the complementary role of Tc-99m sestamibi prone breast imaging for the diagnosis of breast carcinoma. Radiology 1995; 196: 421–426.
9. Ichihara T, Ogawa K, Motomura N, Kubo A, Hashimoto S. Compton scatter compensation using the triple-energy window method for single- and dual-isotope SPECT. J Nucl Med 1993; 34:2216–2221.

From:
E. S. Delpassand, MD, and Edward F. Jackson, PhD
Division of Diagnostic Imaging, M. D. Anderson Cancer Center
1515 Holcombe Boulevard, Box 083, Houston, TX 77030

Editor:
In the article by Dr Helbich and colleagues (1), the sensitivities of MR imaging and planar scintimammography are reported as 96% and 62%, respectively. A high sensitivity of MR imaging has been reported by several investigators in the literature. The reported average sensitivity of planar imaging for both palpable and nonpalpable breast lesions is between 80% and 89% (2,3). However, the authors used planar imaging with patients in the supine position, which can limit the sensitivity of this modality. The value of imaging with patients in the prone position has been well established in the literature (4). Also, of a total of 26 malignant lesions, seven were smaller than 1 cm in greatest dimension. Scintimammography is generally not recommended in these cases.

The authors of this article report specificities of 82% and 88% for MR imaging and planar scintimammography, respectively. The specificity for MR imaging reported in this article is probably the highest reported in the literature. I believe this is partly due to the bias in the analysis of MR images by the investigators. In describing the method for reviewing MR images, the authors state that if there was no agreement between the two investigators who analyzed the MR images, the final decision was made by consensus. Initially, both radiologists were blinded to the patient's history; the findings of mammography, ultrasound (US), and scintimammography; and the histopathologic diagnosis. However, in cases in which the two observers disagreed, both observers were provided with the clinical history and copies of the mammograms and US scans. With MR images and this additional information, the observers decided whether a lesion was present.

The authors' approach was completely different for the scintimammographic studies. In the case of the nuclear studies, all images were read independently by two experienced observers. In four cases, the original two observers were not in agreement and the final diagnosis was made by a third observer who was also blinded to the clinical history and imaging findings. Therefore, all the scintigraphic studies were interpreted without the benefit of other imaging modalities. It is also not clear how many MR images were interpreted with the benefit of other pertinent clinical and diagnostic study findings. The reported specificity of MR imaging for breast cancer in the literature is 31%–59% (5,6).

The three-dimensional, fast, T1-weighted imaging techniques used in this study, while not necessarily providing optimal temporal resolution, do provide reasonable anatomic coverage. Given the promising sensitivity and specificity, one does wonder whether improved temporal resolution, and a more sophisticated analysis of the contrast agent uptake rates, might further improve the specificity of the dynamic MR imaging data. The use of empirical or pharmacokinetic models, when fit to contrast agent uptake data with improved temporal resolution, may well improve the already promising results of this study with a simplistic analysis of the uptake data. Two-dimensional, fast gradient-echo acquisition techniques on modern imagers allow around 15 sections to be acquired in approximately 20 seconds with 128 × 256 acquisition matrices and a 220-mm field of view. It would be interesting to compare the results of this study with the results of a study in which the anatomic coverage and spatial resolution were slightly more limited than in this study but with substantially improved temporal resolution.

References

1. Helbich TH, Becherer A, Trattnig S, et al. Differentiation of benign and malignant breast lesions: MR imaging versus Tc-99m sestamibi scintimammography. Radiology 1997; 202:421–429.
2. Waxman A, Nagaraj N, Ashok G, et al. Sensitivity and specificity of Tc-99m methoxyisobutylisonitrile (MIBI) in the evaluation of primary carcinoma of the breast: comparison of palpable and nonpalpable lesions with mammography (abstr). J Nucl Med 1994; 35:22P.
3. Waxman AD. The role of Tc-99m methoxyisobutylisonitrile in imaging breast cancer. Semin Nucl Med 1997; 27:40–54.
4. Khalkhali I, Mena I, Diggles L. Review of imaging techniques for the diagnosis of breast cancer: a new role of prone scintimammography using technetium-99m sestamibi. Eur J Nucl Med 1994; 21:357–362.
5. Harms SE, Flamig DP, Hesley K, et al. Fat-suppressed three-dimensional MR imaging of the breast. RadioGraphics 1993; 13: 247–267.
6. Nguyen K, Waxman A, Gupta P, et al. Comparison of Tc-99m methoxyisobutylisonitrile (MIBI) and MRI in breast malignancy: the significance of concordant and discordant findings (abstr). J Nucl Med 1996; 37:35P.

From:

Iraj Khalkhali, MD
Department of Radiology, Harbor–University of California Los Angeles Medical Center
Harbor–University of California Los Angeles Professional Building, 21840 South Normandie Avenue, Suite 500, Torrance, CA 90502

Editor:

We enthusiastically read the article by Helbich and colleagues (1). We congratulate the authors on the data collection and statistical analysis used in their study.

They reported on 66 women with 75 breast lesions. The findings of MR imaging of the breast during the intravenous administration of gadopentetate dimeglumine were compared with those of planar and SPECT scintimammography after the intravenous injection of 740-MBq Tc-99m sestamibi. Histopathologic proof was available in 63 lesions; the remaining 12 lesions were clinically followed up.

The authors concluded that the sensitivities and specificities for breast malignancy were, respectively, 96% and 82% for MR imaging, 62% and 88% for planar scintimammography, and 83% and 80% for SPECT scintimammography (1).

MR imaging of the breast in this cohort was performed with patients in the prone position, whereas planar and SPECT scintimammography were performed with patients in the supine position. In our experience, prone scintimammography is superior to supine breast imaging. When we initiated the use of scintimammography at Harbor–University of California Los Angeles Medical Center, we performed imaging in 20–30 patients in the supine position with a technique similar to that used by Helbich and colleagues (1).

We found that prone scintimammography is the technique of choice for nuclear medicine breast imaging. This has resulted in improvement in the sensitivity for the diagnosis of breast carcinoma (2). This observation has been confirmed by several other investigators (3–5). Preliminary findings of a combined multicenter clinical trial at 42 institutions in the United States and Canada in 673 patients with palpable (286 patients) or nonpalpable (387 patients) breast abnormalities who underwent scintimammography in the prone position demonstrated a higher sensitivity (85%)(6) than that reported by Helbich and colleagues.

Helbich and co-workers stated that the reason for not using the prone position was that they lacked a commercially available special table for prone imaging. We have noted in several publications (3,5,7) that even without the use of a special table, prone imaging can be performed and a sensitivity higher than that reported by Helbich and colleagues can be achieved.

In prone studies, many investigators have effectively used thick foam with the side cut out instead of a special table. Incidentally, at the time of our publication, as noted in Materials and Methods, the table was commercially available (2).

Recently, Tiling and colleagues (7), from the University of Munich, Munich, Germany, reported on a similar study in which breast MR imaging was compared with prone planar and Tc-99m sestamibi SPECT scintimammography in which a foam pad was used. In 56 patients with breast abnormalities, they demonstrated superior specificity of Tc-99m sestamibi SPECT breast imaging compared with that of MR imaging of the breast. They found that overall planar prone breast imaging with Tc-99m sestamibi had a sensitivity of 88% and a specificity of 83%. Breast MR imaging demonstrated a sensitivity and specificity of 91% and 52%, respectively (7).

Furthermore, Helbich and colleagues reported on 10 breast lesions that had false-negative Tc-99m sestamibi scintimammographic findings. It should be noted that four of these patients were women with stage T1b and 1.0–1.5-cm carcinoma. There were four additional patients who had T1c carcinomas larger than 1 cm but smaller than 2 cm in diameter. It should be emphasized that the current nuclear medicine cameras do not allow us to detect breast carcinomas that are 1.2 cm in diameter or smaller (2). This also relates to the location of the tumor. We have observed that carcinomas in the medial part of the breast are more likely to be missed with this technique, because, at the present time, we are able to obtain only lateral images of the breast with the patient in a prone position (2). Because of the inherent limitation of current nuclear medicine detectors, we do not recommend scintimammography in women with lesions smaller than 1.2 cm in diameter detected at mammography or physical examination.

References

1. Helbich TH, Becherer A, Trattnig S, et al. Differentiation of benign and malignant breast lesions: MR imaging versus Tc-99m sestamibi scintimammography. Radiology 1997; 202:421–429.
2. Khalkhali I, Cutrone JA, Mena IG, et al. Scintimammography: the complementary role of Tc-99m sestamibi prone breast imaging for the diagnosis of breast carcinoma. Radiology 1995; 196: 421–426.
3. Taillefer R, Robidoux A, Lambert R, et al. Tc-99m sestamibi prone scintimammography to detect primary and axillary lymph node involvement. J Nucl Med 1995; 36:1758–1765.
4. Villanueva-Meyer J, Leonard MH, Briscoe E, et al. Mammoscintigraphy with technetium-99m-sestamibi in suspected breast cancer. J Nucl Med 1996; 37:926–930.
5. Palmedo H, Brunwald F, Bender H, et al. Scintimammography with technetium-99m-methoxyisobutylisonitrile: comparison with mammography and magnetic resonance imaging. Eur J Nucl Med 1996; 23:940–946.
6. Khalkhali I, Villanueva-Meyer J, Edell S, et al. Diagnostic accuracy of Tc99m sestamibi breast imaging in breast cancer detection (abstr). J Nucl Med 1996; 37:74P.
7. Tiling R, Sommer H, Pechmann M, et al. Comparison of techne-

tium-99m-sestamibi scintimammography with contrast-enhanced MRI for diagnosis of breast lesions. J Nucl Med 1997; 38:58–62.

Dr Helbich and colleagues respond:

We thank all correspondents for their interest in our article (1). They have raised important points that deserve further attention.

We agree with all correspondents that planar sestamibi scintimammography with patients in the prone position might have some advantages over imaging with patients in the supine position owing to the excellent separation of deep breast structures from the myocardium and liver. Although the advantages of prone imaging over supine imaging in scintimammography have never been proved in a comparative study to our knowledge, they have been recognized as valid (2–4).

It is undisputed that prone, planar scintimammography with a specially developed scintimammographic table was mentioned by Dr Khalkhali, a pioneer in this field, in one of his first articles (5). However, it is also obvious that the data collection of our study (1) had been finalized before this was confirmed by other groups (2–4,6). Nonetheless, Scopinaro and colleagues (7) and, more recently, Moretti and co-workers (8) reported good results of planar scintimammography performed in the supine position. As stated in our article, the special table for prone scintimammography is not available in our country. The less expensive technique in which the patient undergoes imaging in the prone position on foam cushions was described as our study was in the process of data collection (2).

In our study, four of 10 carcinomas could not be detected with planar imaging in the supine position but were demonstrated with SPECT (1). If we consider the patient position as a possible disadvantage in our study and if we assume that all four carcinomas with positive tracer uptake at SPECT would have been demonstrated with planar imaging performed in the prone position, we would have obtained a sensitivity of 83% and a specificity of 80% (1). Similar results are reported in the literature for prone planar imaging (2–6). However, three of these four carcinomas were smaller than 2 cm in diameter (T1c tumors). To solve the problem of the lower sensitivity in small breast lesions, Dr Khalkhali does not recommend scintimammography in lesions smaller than 1.2 cm. This recommendation is based on the assumption that the detection of a lesion is a function of size in scintimammography. However, scintimammography is a technique in which the most important parameter is tracer uptake in the lesion compared with that in the surrounding tissue, not size. The exclusion of lesions smaller than 1.2 cm is an enormous limitation. Thus, MR imaging of the breast has a definite advantage, because there is a low rate of false-negative cases in such small lesions (9).

Dr Khalkhali mentioned the divergent results in the specificity of MR imaging of the breast in our study (82%) compared to that (52%) in a study by Tiling and colleagues (10). It is well known that the results of MR imaging of the breast show a great variability for various reasons (eg, choice of pulse sequence, sequence parameters, and interpretation guidelines for breast lesions) (9). However, the low specificity reported by Tiling and colleagues might be explained by their subjective criteria in comparing the enhancement of a lesion with that of fatty tissue, without consideration of quantitative parameters (10).

We agree with Servais and colleagues that the 500 kilocounts we acquired in our study was rather low. We are now using a protocol with a zoom over the breast to exclude the liver and a time limitation of 10 minutes per frame instead of a count limitation.

We do not share the opinion of Servais and colleagues that SPECT scintimammography has been adequately analyzed in the literature (4,11,12). Of these studies, only one has been published as a peer-reviewed article to our knowledge (4). Thus, a comparison, especially of the technical parameters, is not possible. It seems that SPECT scintimammography attains high sensitivity at the cost of lower specificity in comparison with planar scintimammography, because of improved spatial resolution and an increased target-to-background ratio (4,11,12). However, a single carcinoma missed at planar scintimammography more than overbalances the problems of a few false-positive SPECT scintimammographic findings. Thus, it is questionable to renounce SPECT in this early state of scintimammography.

The patient position in SPECT imaging seems to be less important, as demonstrated in our study, in which SPECT in the supine position yielded a high sensitivity and specificity (1). Similar results were confirmed by other groups with SPECT performed in the prone position (4).

The group of Dr Servais obtains valuable information with planar scintimammography in 20–30 minutes. Other groups report that they start 5–10 minutes after sestamibi application with an acquisition time of 10 minutes for each position (both right and left lateral views and one anterior view), which results in a procedure time of 35–40 minutes (4,10). Moreover, Dr Khalkhali recommends additional imaging after 60 minutes (5,6). In contrast, routine MR imaging of the breast takes about 15–30 minutes (9).

Dr Servais' disregard for SPECT is inconsistent with his proposal to use a triple-energy window for scatter correction (13). Furthermore, scatter correction can be a major problem, especially in SPECT combined with quantitative evaluation. Thus, scatter correction may not improve the results of planar as well as SPECT scintimammography.

We do not share the opinion of Drs Delpassand and Jackson that the specificity of 82% for MR imaging of the breast in our study is the highest reported in the literature (1). Furthermore, it should be emphasized that in the current literature the specificity for MR imaging of the breast is 31%–100% (9).

It seems to be a misunderstanding of Drs Delpassand and Jackson that the specificity in our study (1) might be biased by our analysis. As described in Materials and Methods, consensus with regard to the presence of a lesion was obtained only in cases of disagreement. On the basis of this information, further quantitative analyses of the lesions were performed to attain the final diagnosis. Thus, both radiologists were not provided with additional information from other imaging modalities, such as mammography or US, for the final diagnosis. Therefore, the approach to MR imaging of the breast is not totally different from the approach to scintimammography. On the other hand, in most of the scintimammographic studies, the readers are provided information about the side and the exact localization of the suspicious lesion with an anatomic marker (1–3,5–8).

We agree with Drs Delpassand and Jackson that improved temporal resolution seems to be a valuable tool for MR imaging of the breast. There are two studies that confirm their idea (14,15). Both Boetes and colleagues (14) and Hulka and co-workers (15) report a sensitivity of 95% and 86% and a specificity of 86% and 93% by using a temporal resolution of 11.5 seconds and 6 seconds, respectively. Although pharmacokinetic models seem to be promising, Müller-Schimpfle and co-workers (16) recently reported that a pharmacokinetic model of time-intensity curves is not beneficial compared with standard analysis of breast MR imaging data.

Finally, it is hoped that all of the correspondents agree that both methods will serve as valuable adjuncts in the differentiation of benign and malignant lesions but that further studies are necessary to evaluate standard protocols for both modalities.

References

1. Helbich TH, Becherer A, Trattnig S, et al. Differentiation of benign and malignant breast lesions: MR imaging versus Tc-99m sestamibi scintimammography. Radiology 1997; 202:421–429.
2. Taillefer R, Robidoux A, Lambert R, et al. Tc-99m sestamibi prone scintimammography to detect primary and axillary lymph node involvement. J Nucl Med 1995; 36:1758–1765.
3. Villanueva-Meyer J, Leonard MH, Briscoe E, et al. Mammo-

scintigraphy with technetium-99m-sestamibi in suspected breast cancer. J Nucl Med 1996; 37:926–930.
4. Palmedo H, Schomburg A, Grünwald F, Mallmann P, Krebs D, Biersack HJ. Technetium-99m-MIBI scintimammography for suspicious breast lesions. J Nucl Med 1996; 37:626–630.
5. Khalkhali I, Mena I, Jouanne E, et al. Prone scintimammography in patients with suspicion of carcinoma of the breast. J Am Coll Surg 1994; 178:491–497.
6. Khalkhali I, Cutrone JA, Mena IG, et al. Scintimammography: the complementary role of Tc-99m sestamibi prone breast imaging for the diagnosis of breast carcinoma. Radiology 1995; 196:421–426.
7. Scopinaro F, Schillaci O, Scarpini M, et al. Technetium-99m sestamibi: an indicator of breast cancer invasiveness. Eur J Nucl Med 1994; 21:984–987.
8. Moretti JL, Azaloux H, Boisseron D, Kouyoumdjian JC, Vilcoq J. Primary breast cancer imaging with technetium-99m-sestamibi and its relation with p-glycoprotein overexpression. Eur J Nucl Med 1996; 23:980–986.
9. Heywang-Köbrunner SH, Beck R. Contrast-enhanced MR imaging of the breast. 2nd ed. Berlin, Germany: Springer, 1995.
10. Tiling R, Sommer H, Pechmann M, et al. Comparison of technetium-99m-sestamibi scintimammography with contrast-enhanced MRI for diagnosis of breast lesions. J Nucl Med 1997; 38:58–62.
11. Nagaraj N, Waxman A, Ashok G, et al. Comparison of SPECT and planar Tc-99m-sestamibi (MIBI) imaging in patients with carcinoma of the breast (abstr). J Nucl Med 1994; 35:229P.
12. Diggles L, Khalkhali I. SPECT prone dependent-breast scintimammography (SMM) (abstr). Eur J Nucl Med 1994; 21:S28.
13. Ichihara T, Ogawa K, Motomura N, Kubo A, Hashimoto S. Compton scatter compensation using the triple-energy window method for single- and dual-isotope SPECT. J Nucl Med 1993; 34:2216–2221.
14. Boetes C, Barentsz JO, Mus RD, et al. MR characterization of suspicious breast lesions with a gadolinium-enhanced TurboFLASH subtraction technique. Radiology 1994; 193:777–781.
15. Hulka CA, Smith BL, Sgroi DC, et al. Benign and malignant breast lesions: differentiation with echo-planar MR imaging. Radiology 1995; 197:33–38.
16. Müller-Schimpfle M, Ohmenhäuser K, Sand J, Stoll P, Claussen CD. Dynamic 3D-MR mammography: is there a benefit of sophisticated evaluation of enhancement curves for clinical routine? JMRI 1997; 7:236–240.

Thomas H. Helbich, MD,*[,1] Alexander Becherer, MD,[†] Thomas Leitha, MD,[†] and Gerhard H. Mostbeck, MD*
Departments of Radiology* and Nuclear Medicine[†], University of Vienna, Vienna, Austria

■ Popliteal Vascular Disease: MR Imaging and MR Angiography

From:
Mathias Goyen, MD
Department of Radiology, University Hospital Bochum
In der Schornau 23, 44892 Bochum, Germany
e-mail: *mathias.goyen@ruhr-uni-bochum.de*

Editor:
I read with great interest the excellent article "Popliteal Vascular Disease: Evaluation with Spiral CT Angiography" by Beregi and colleagues (1) in the May 1997 issue of *Radiology*.

When discussing several imaging options for assessing popliteal vascular disease, magnetic resonance (MR) imaging and MR angiography also deserve to be mentioned. Several recently published study findings show that MR imaging and MR angiography offer some advantages for morphologic examination in patients with popliteal vascular diseases.

With regard to suspected popliteal artery aneurysms, MR imaging and MR angiography proved to be excellent techniques for defining the morphology of the popliteal fossa (2,3). Recent reports have indicated the use of MR angiography in the diagnosis of popliteal artery entrapment syndrome (4–6) and cystic adventitial disease (7–9).

In conclusion, there are multiple imaging options for investigating suspected popliteal vascular disease, amongst them the use of spiral CT angiography, which Beregi and co-workers showed to be efficient. However, the radiologist chooses the modality on the basis of the patient, available equipment, and expertise.

[1] Current address: Department of Radiology, Contrast Media Laboratory, University of California, San Francisco, 505 Parnassus Avenue, Room S-372, San Francisco, CA 94143-0628

References

1. Beregi JP, Djabbari M, Desmoucelle F, Willoteaux S, Wattinne L, Louvegny S. Popliteal vascular disease: evaluation with spiral CT angiography. Radiology 1997; 203:477–483.
2. Kolb M, Guhl L, Arlart IP. Magnetic resonance tomography and magnetic resonance angiography in diagnosis of complicated popliteal artery aneurysm. Radiologe 1997; 37:145–151.
3. Butler MG, Fuchigami KD, Chako A. MRI of posterior knee masses. Skeletal Radiol 1996; 25:309–317.
4. Forster BB, Houston JG, Machan LS, Doyle L. Comparison of two-dimensional time-of-flight dynamic magnetic resonance angiography with digital subtraction angiography in popliteal artery entrapment syndrome. Can Assoc Radiol J 1997; 48:11–18.
5. Gorres G, Guckel C, Steinbrich W. Diagnostic possibilities of magnetic resonance tomography (MRT) and magnetic resonance angiography (MRA) in popliteal artery entrapment syndrome (PAES). Aktuelle Radiol 1995; 5:31–35.
6. Di Cesare E, Simonetti C, Morettini G, Spartera C. Popliteal artery entrapment: MR findings. J Comput Assist Tomogr 1992; 16:295–297.
7. Decleir P, de Foer B, de Schepper A, Sijs J, Michielsen J. MR imaging of cystic adventitial disease of the popliteal artery: 2 cases. Rofo Fortschr Geb Rontgenstr Neuen Bildgeb Verfahr 1997; 166:167–169.
8. Berger MF, Weber EE. MR imaging of recurrent cystic adventitial disease of the popliteal artery. JVIR 1993; 4:695–697.
9. Crolla RM, Steyling JF, Hennipmann A, Slootweg PJ, Taams A. A case of cystic adventitial disease of the popliteal artery demonstrated by magnetic resonance imaging. J Vasc Surg 1993; 18: 1052–1055.

■ Postmyelographic Headaches

From:
Charles E. Seibert, MD
Department of Radiology, Radiology Imaging Associates, Columbia-Swedish Medical Center
501 East Hampden Avenue, Englewood, CO 80110

Editor:
Thirty-five years of experience with thousands of myelographic and diagnostic lumbar punctures prompts me to agree with the statement made Dr Susan B. Peterman in the September 1996 issue of *Radiology* (1) that "the smaller the gauge of the spinal needle the lower the PDPH [post–dural puncture headache] rate." Since the advent of low-osmolality, nonionic contrast material, my partners and I have used a 26-gauge needle, currently the 26-gauge, 3.5-cm Quincke point needle (Becton Dickinson, Franklin Lakes, NJ), for either diagnostic lumbar puncture or injection of nonionic contrast material. The needle is easily placed within a few minutes in a standard fluoroscopy suite by using an oblique, paramidline, sublaminar approach. The needle is steered by pointing the bevel, with knowledge that the needle tip moves slightly in the direction opposite the stylette needle notch. The subarachnoid position is confirmed by means of the return of cerebrospinal fluid with gentle suction with a 3-mL syringe and the 20-inch plastic connector tube that comes in the myelographic tray (Baxter Healthcare, Round Lake, Ill). A midline approach is not used because the thick interspinous ligament often causes the small needle to veer off course.

In addition, I disagree with the statement from Dr Christine C. Hoeffel that "it is not feasible to use a very small needle to inject iodinated contrast media" (2). The simple addition of a 10-mL luer-lock control syringe (Luer-Lok; Becton Dickinson) that has a thumbhole plunger so that extra pressure can be created easily and of a luer-lock small connector tube, such as the Plexufix Brachial Plexus Anesthesia Set (Braun Medical, Bethlehem, Pa), allows predictable delivery of the viscous contrast material easily and quickly. A frequent frustration is the loss of the expensive contrast material as it sprays on the patient's back if non–luer-lock tubing pops off of a non–luer-lock syringe. These technical modifications make a small needle not only feasible but easy to use.

References

1. Peterman SB. Postmyelography headache rates with Whitacre versus Quincke 22-gauge spinal needles. Radiology 1996; 200: 771–778.
2. Hoeffel CC. Post–dural puncture headache (letter). Radiology 1996; 203:579–580.

Barium Sulfate versus Water-Soluble, Low-Osmolarity Contrast Medium in Esophageal Examinations

From:
Abida Z. Ginai, MD, PhD
Department of Radiology, University Hospital Dijkzigt and Erasmus University Rotterdam
Dr Molewaterplein 40, 3015 GD Rotterdam, The Netherlands

Editor:
The article by Gollub and Bains (1) in the February 1997 issue of *Radiology* came as a surprise. The article is a review of esophageal leaks examined with dilute barium sulfate in 12 patients.

Since 1983, we at the Department of Radiology of the University Hospital, Rotterdam, The Netherlands, have performed more than 2,500 examinations with water-soluble, low-osmolarity contrast media (ioxaglate sodium and ioxaglate meglumine [Hexabrix; Mallinckrodt Medical, St Louis, Mo]), with no pulmonary edema at aspiration and no clinically important leakage missed.

Gollub and Bains (1) include only eight references for this extremely important topic, and all the references are dated 1952–1975. In the first paragraph, the authors point out that "barium within the peritoneal cavity has been shown to cause chemical peritonitis," with reference to a Zheutlin and colleagues article from 1952. Then the authors state "extrapolation of these data to the mediastinum has lead to the accepted clinical practice of use of water-soluble contrast material in possible leaks of the esophagus." Extrapolation is actually not necessary, because actual animal experimental studies, which include studies of the effects on the lungs and mediastinum, have been performed more recently (2,3). Clinical use of lower-osmolarity contrast medium in the esophagus also appears to be safe (4).

One needs to be aware of the dangers (which include mortality) of barium aspiration in children and in debilitated older individuals, especially postoperatively.

The authors, at the end of their article, recommend the use of diatrizoate meglumine and diatrizoate sodium, which is sold under the trade name of Gastroview (Mallinckrodt Medical) or Gastrografin (Schering, Berlin, Germany) and has an osmolarity of 1,900 mOsm/kg water, which is more than six times that of plasma. Use of such a highly osmolal contrast medium may be dangerous because of an increased chance of aspiration and possible pulmonary edema.

Low-osmolality, water-soluble contrast media such as ionic dimers (eg, ioxaglate sodium and ioxaglate meglumine) and nonionic monomers (eg, iohexol [Omnipaque; Nycomed, Princeton, NJ] and iopamidol [Iopamiro; Bracco, Milan, Italy]), with osmolalities of ±600 mOsm/kg water at 300 mg of iodine per milliliter), are therefore safer for oral use.

In light of the available data, it appears that the postoperative esophageal examination should be performed initially with one of the newer lower-osmolarity contrast media.

If the correct technique of examination is used, especially if combined with rapid imaging or video recording, demonstration of even small leaks would almost be adequate.

References

1. Gollub MJ, Bains MS. Barium sulfate: a new (old) contrast agent for diagnosis of postoperative esophageal leaks. Radiology 1997; 202:360–362.
2. Ginai AZ, Ten Kate FJW, Ten Berg RGM, Hoornstra K. Experimental evaluation of various available contrast agents for use in the gastrointestinal tract in case of suspected leakage: effects on lungs. Br J Radiol 1984; 57:895–901.
3. Ginai AZ, Ten Kate FJW, Ten Berg RGM, Hoornstra K. Experimental evaluation of various available contrast agents for use in the gastrointestinal tract in case of suspected leakage: effects on mediastinum. Br J Radiol 1985; 58:585–592.
4. Ginai AZ. Clinical use of Hexabrix for radiological evaluation of leakage from the upper gastrointestinal tract based on experimental study. Br J Radiol 1987; 60:343–346.

Drs Gollub and Bains respond:

We thank Dr Ginai for her comments on our article on the use of barium sulfate in esophageal leaks (1). Dr Ginai makes several points that we believe can be summarized as follows. (*a*) No references after 1975 are cited. (*b*) Extrapolation of peritoneal data to the mediastinum is not necessary. (*c*) Aspiration of barium in children and debilitated older individuals is dangerous. (*d*) Diatrizoate meglumine and diatrizoate sodium in other clinical scenarios is best not used owing to the risk of pulmonary edema from high-osmolarity contrast media compared with the risk from ioxaglate sodium and ioxaglate meglumine, iohexol, or iopamidol; thus, postoperative esophagography should begin with a low-osmolarity or iso-osmolar contrast medium.

Dr Ginai and colleagues have vast experience in esophagography with water-soluble, low-osmolarity media; several published articles describe their experience (2–4). Unfortunately, our initial computer literature search overlooked these articles from the *British Journal of Radiology*.

It is true that one need not extrapolate data from barium studies performed in the peritoneum to the mediastinum. We quoted a reference that discussed barium injections in the mediastinum (5), in which 10 rats, despite granuloma formation, were clinically well at the 90-day follow-up examination.

Dr Ginai's statement that aspiration of barium in children and debilitated adults is dangerous is not supported by a reference. In fact, barium in the bronchial tree is generally innocuous and used to be used for bronchography. Large volumes may produce transient reduction in pulmonary function, but most of it is cleared by bronchociliary action or phagocytosis in the peripheral airways. The remainder is expelled back into the airways and cleared by means of coughing and bronchociliary action (6).

We agree that under ideal circumstances a lower-osmolar, water-soluble contrast medium is preferable to diatrizoate meglumine and diatrizoate sodium; however, a comparison of relative costs (Hexabrix, $1.22/mL; Omnipaque, $0.38/mL; Gastroview, $0.08/mL) reveals that it becomes less practical (in the setting of health care cost containment) when performing many studies. We use iohexol for esophagography in our pediatric patients with similar clinical risk factors.

References

1. Gollub MJ, Bains MS. Barium sulfate: a new (old) contrast agent for diagnosis of postoperative esophageal leaks. Radiology 1997; 202:360–362.
2. Ginai AZ, Ten Kate FJW, Ten Berg RGM, Hoornstra K. Experimental evaluation of various available contrast agents for use in the gastrointestinal tract in case of suspected leakage: effects on lungs. Br J Radiol 1984; 57:895–901.
3. Ginai AZ, Ten Kate FJW, Ten Berg RGM, Hoornstra K. Experimental evaluation of various available contrast agents for use in the gastrointestinal tract in case of suspected leakage: effects on

mediastinum. Br J Radiol 1985; 58:585–592.
4. Ginai AZ. Clinical use of Hexabrix for radiological evaluation of leakage from the upper gastrointestinal tract based on experimental study. Br J Radiol 1987; 60:343–346.
5. James AE, Montaki RJ, Chaffee V, Strecker EP, Vessal K. Barium or gastrografin: which contrast media for diagnosis of esophageal tears? Gastroenterology 1975; 68:1103–1113.
6. Huston J Jr, Wallace DO, Cunningham GJ. Pulmonary reaction to barium sulfate in rats. Arch Pathol 1952; 53:430–438.

Marc J. Gollub, MD,* and Manjit S. Bains, MD†
Departments of Radiology* and Thoracic Surgery†, Memorial Sloan-Kettering Cancer Center
1275 York Avenue, New York, NY 10021

Errata

"Optimization of Thoracic Spiral CT: Effects of Iodinated Contrast Medium Concentration." Radiology 1996; 201:785–791.
Page 785, the affiliation for Paul Stark, MD, should read as follows: "Department of Radiology, Stanford University School of Medicine **and VA Palo Alto Health Care System, Calif.**"

Sum & Substance: "Renal Vein Occlusion: A Review." Radiology 1997; 204:78.
Page 78, in the first column, last paragraph, third sentence, the following bold-faced words should have been deleted: "Renal **magnetic resonance (MR)** images obtained with technetium-99m diethylenetriaminepentaacetic acid, or DTPA, also show persistent intensity in an enlarged kidney."

In Memoriam

Michael J. Feinberg, MD
1947–1996

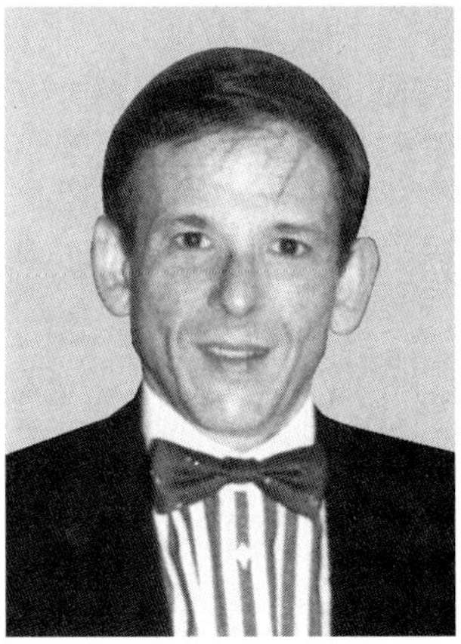

Dr Michael J. Feinberg died unexpectedly in his sleep of cardiovascular disease on December 18, 1996. Michael was born on July 21, 1947, in Brooklyn, NY. His family moved to Asbury Park, NJ, where he grew up. He graduated from Rutgers University in 1969 and received his MD degree from Hahnemann University, Philadelphia, Pa, in 1973. Having decided on a career in radiology, he was accepted for a residency position at the Albert Einstein Medical Center, Philadelphia. After serving as attending radiologist at St Charles General Hospital, New Orleans, La, and Sacred Heart Hospital, Norristown, Pa, Michael returned to the Albert Einstein Medical Center in 1983. From 1983 to 1991, he also held a position at the Philadelphia Geriatric Center. During this time, he was a clinical instructor of diagnostic radiology at the Temple University School of Medicine, Philadelphia. Between 1991 and 1993, he served at the Buffalo General Hospital, Buffalo, NY. In 1993, he moved to North Shore University Hospital, Manhasset, NY. He was appointed assistant professor of radiology at Cornell University Medical Center and later at the New York University School of Medicine. Michael was physician-in-charge of gastrointestinal radiology until his untimely death.

Michael developed an interest in dysphagia in the elderly and began to study swallowing in great detail. His most important contribution to medicine became a better understanding of the normal effects of aging on swallowing and how to distinguish these effects from disease-related dysphagia in the elderly. He also made important contributions to our understanding of bolus transportation. Michael was a careful researcher, but he also devoted his time to education and showed great didactic skills. During the years, he won several awards for his presentations.

Dr Feinberg was a member of the American College of Radiology, the Radiological Society of North America, the American Institute of Ultrasound in Medicine, the Society of Gastrointestinal Radiology, and the Dysphagia Research Society. He was the recipient of many awards for his research in swallowing disorders.

Michael was a wonderful friend and colleague, and his unexpected and untimely death has left all of us with a great emptiness. He is survived by his loving and devoted wife Imelda and their son Samuel.

—Olle Ekberg, MD

Fazlur R. Khan, MD
1936–1996

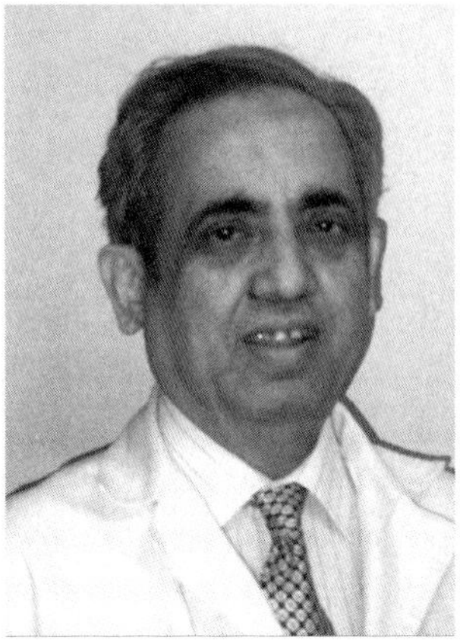

Dr Fazlur R. Khan died on September 21, 1996, after a sudden and brief illness. He was born in Bhopal, India, on May 6, 1936. He completed his medical education at the Laiquit Medical College, Karachi, Pakistan, in 1961. He was senior house officer at the Wimbledon Hospital, London, England, and thereafter at Western Infirmary, Glasgow, Scotland, in the radiation therapy department from 1961 to 1963. He came to the United States in 1963 and worked as chief resident and Beltratron fellow at the Memorial Hospital and Sloan Kettering Institute, New York, NY, from 1963 to 1965. During the latter part of 1965, he joined Michael Reese Hospital, Chicago, Ill, as senior fellow in radiation therapy and thereafter was associate attending until 1970. In 1971, he accepted the position of director of the Department of Radiation Therapy at Weiss Memorial Hospital, Chicago, where he continued until 1978.

In 1979, Dr Khan became the chief of radiation oncology at Northwest Community Hospital, Arlington Heights, Ill. During his stewardship, he was instrumental in building a superb radiation oncology department, integrating cutting-edge technology and sophisticated equipment for the management of cancer.

In the academic sphere, Dr Khan had one passion, and that was teaching. He was an excellent teacher, having students all around the country. He was extremely committed to new ideas and pursuing research. He had over 50 papers presented at or published in various national and international conferences and journals. Dr Khan will be remembered for his many professional accomplishments, personal warmth, enthusiasm, and vision.

He is survived by his wife, two children, and two grandchildren.

—Bhogaraju S. Devi, MD

Robert E. L. Stuart, Jr, MD
1927–1996

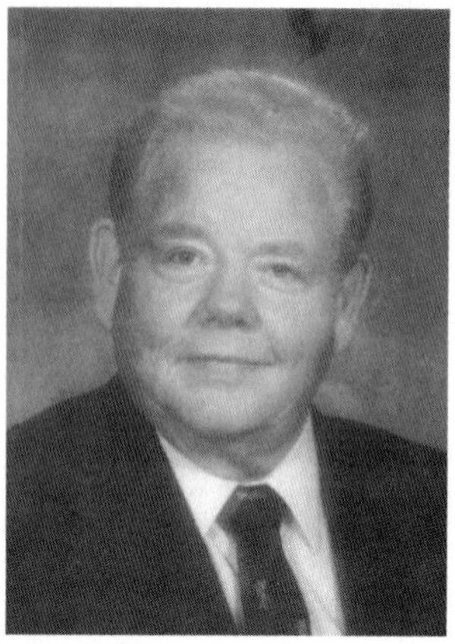

Dr Robert E. Lee "Red" Stuart, Jr, our colleague and friend, died of heart failure, on August 30, 1996, at age 69 years, at his home in Kentwood, La. Dr Stuart was born on July 20, 1927, in Long Beach, Miss, and grew up in Gulfport, Miss. He received his BS degree from the University of Mississippi and his MD degree from the University of Tennessee in 1951. After completing an internship at Baptist Memorial Hospital, Memphis, Tenn, he returned to Gulfport and practiced general medicine until completing his radiology training in 1962 at Ochsner Foundation Hospital, New Orleans, La. American Board of Radiology certification followed in 1964.

In 1963, Dr Stuart became the first radiologist to practice in Hammond, La. He served his patients at Seventh Ward General Hospital (now North Oaks Medical Center), and for many years, he traveled to neighboring towns providing radiology services to patients in small communities. He introduced radiation therapy to the Hammond area, was the first radiologist in Louisiana to institute separate billing, and founded the North Oaks School of Radiologic Technology. Dr Stuart was active in multiple state and national medical societies and in 1978 served as president of the Radiologic Society of Louisiana, a component chapter of the American College of Radiology. The honor of fellow of the American College of Radiology was granted to him in 1978, and upon cessation of practice in 1996, Dr Stuart received the status of fellow emeritus.

His interests outside of medicine were broad, including a love of reading, raising horses and ostriches, music, deep sea fishing, and his grandchildren. Dr Stuart will be missed by his many colleagues and friends.

He is survived by his wife, Caroline; two sons, Lee and Jerome; one daughter, Sandy Miller; and six grandchildren.

—John P. Miller, MD

Karl H. Ueberschar, MD
1924–1995

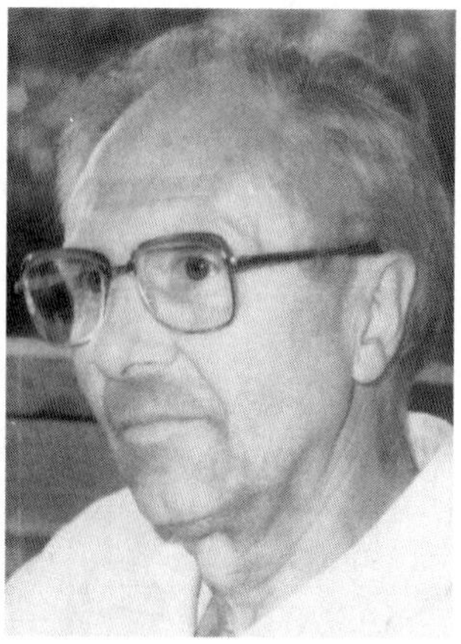

Dr Karl Heinz Ueberschar died on June 4, 1995, at age 70 years. He was born on September 30, 1924, in Eisleben, Germany. In 1949, he graduated from the Medical School in Muenster, Germany. He completed his internship and residency at the University Hospital (Charité) of the Humboldt University, Berlin, Germany. It was there that he received his MD degree and certificate in diagnostic radiology and radiation therapy. In May 1959, he immigrated to Canada and moved to Regina, the capital of the province of Saskatchewan. He completed another internship and 1 year of residency in diagnostic radiology at the Regina Grey Nuns' Hospital (now Pasqua Hospital). In 1961, he passed the Canadian medical licensing examination and received his certificate in diagnostic radiology. He then joined the group of diagnostic radiologists at Pasqua Hospital, which also operated an office in the Regina Medical and Dental Building, and he worked at the Plains Health Center as well as several smaller offices in and around Regina.

In 1965, he obtained his Canadian citizenship and in 1972 his fellowship in the Royal College of Physicians and Surgeons of Canada. In the same year, he became the director of the radiology department of Pasqua Hospital, a position he held until 1978. He was appointed clinical assistant professor of radiology at the University of Saskatchewan in 1975 and was promoted to clinical associate professor in 1979. From 1978 until his retirement in 1989, he was the managing director of the Radiology Associates of Regina.

Throughout his career, he showed much enthusiasm for his work and enjoyed conferring with his clinical colleagues. He also thoroughly enjoyed teaching medical students and residents.

Dr Ueberschar always liked to travel—in Europe, North America, and Japan. He organized and went on many ski trips to the Alps and Rocky Mountains as well as numerous fishing and canoe trips on the Churchill and Nahanni rivers in northern Canada.

He is survived by his wife, Hanna; his daughter, Elisabeth Logothetis; his son-in-law, Christopher Logothetis; and two grandchildren, Richard and Irene.

—Karl H. Ficke, MD

Abstracts of Current Literature

Abdomen and Gastrointestinal System

Major Bile Duct Injuries during Laparoscopic Cholecystectomy Follow-up after Combined Surgical and Radiologic Management. Keith D. Lillemoe, Scot A. Martin, John L. Cameron, et al. *Ann Surg* 1997; 225:459–471. (K.D.L., The Johns Hopkins Hospital, 600 N Wolfe St, Blalock 603, Baltimore, MD 21287)

Objective: The authors provide the results of follow-up evaluation after combined surgical and radiologic management of 89 patients with major bile duct injuries during laparoscopic cholecystectomy. *Summary Background Data:* The incidence and mechanism of injury of major bile duct injuries during laparoscope cholecystectomy has been clearly defined. Furthermore, a number of series have described the management of these injuries by means of surgical, endoscopic, and radiologic techniques with excellent short-term results. Long-term follow-up data, however, are lacking. *Methods:* Data were collected prospectively in 89 patients with major bile duct injuries after laparoscopic cholecystectomy, treated at a single institution between July 1, 1990, and July 1, 1996. Patients referred with injuries underwent early percutaneous transhepatic cholangiography and biliary drainage. Based on the cholangiographic appearance and clinical situation, management consisted of either percutaneous balloon dilation or surgical reconstruction with a Roux-en-Y hepaticojejunostomy with transanastomotic stenting. Follow-up was obtained by personal interview during October 1996. *Results:* Two patients died without an attempt at definitive therapy. Both deaths were caused by sepsis and multisystem organ failure present at the time of transfer to the authors' institution. The remaining 87 patients were managed initially by means of either balloon dilation ($n = 28$) or surgical reconstruction ($n = 59$). Ten patients have not completed treatment and still have biliary stents in place. Evaluation of 25 patients completing treatment after balloon dilation (mean follow-up, 27.8 months) showed a success rate of 64%. Evaluation of 52 patients completing treatment after surgical reconstruction (mean follow-up, 33.4 months) showed a success rate of 92%. All failures were managed successfully with either surgical reconstruction or balloon dilation. *Conclusion:* Major bile duct injuries can be managed successfully with combined surgical and radiologic techniques. This series provides, for the first time, significant follow-up data on a large number of patients, with overall success rates of 64% after balloon dilation and 92% after surgical reconstruction. The combination of surgery and balloon dilation resulted in a successful outcome in 100% of patients treated.
AUTHORS' ABSTRACT

Laparoscopic Adrenalectomy: A New Standard of Care. J. Kenneth Jacobs, Richard E. Goldstein, Richard J. Geer. *Ann Surg* 1997; 225:495–502. (J.K.J., St Thomas Hospital, 4230 Harding Rd, Nashville, TN 37205)

Objective: The authors review their experience with laparoscopic adrenalectomy in patients with benign adrenal neoplasms. Efficacy, safety, and cost-effectiveness of the procedure are examined. *Background:* Laparoscopic adrenalectomy is replacing open adrenalectomy in some medical centers as the standard surgical approach for uncomplicated tumors. However, laparoscopic adrenalectomy often is considered more difficult and more expensive than traditional "open" surgery. *Methods:* Perioperative and postoperative records as well as hospital charges from the first 19 patients undergoing laparoscopic unilateral adrenalectomies at the authors' medical institutions were examined and compared with records in 19 patients who underwent open unilateral adrenalectomies. *Results:* None of the 19 patients undergoing unilateral laparoscopic adrenalectomy required conversion to open adrenalectomy. Mean operative times as well as total hospital charges were similar in those patients undergoing either laparoscopic or open adrenalectomy. However, the morbidity and postoperative length of hospital stay were significantly less in those patients undergoing laparoscopic adrenalectomy. *Conclusion:* Laparoscopic adrenalectomy can be performed safely and with the benefits associated with minimally invasive surgery. In addition, the procedure is cost-effective. These factors suggest that laparoscopic adrenalectomy should be the preferential surgical technique for benign adrenal disease.
AUTHORS' ABSTRACT

The Prognostic Significance of Intratumoral Natural Killer Cells in Patients with Colorectal Carcinoma. Santiago Coca, Javier Perez-Piqueras, David Martinez, et al. *Cancer* 1997; 79:2320–2328. (S.C., Departamento de Anatomía Patológica, Hospital del Aire, Arturo Soria 82, 28027 Madrid, Spain)

Background: Natural killer (NK) cells have a spontaneous cytotoxic capacity against tumor cells. These cells represent a small proportion of human colon carcinoma-infiltrating lymphocytes. Their prognostic significance in these tumors has yet to be determined. *Methods:* One hundred fifty-seven patients who each had a colectomy for large bowel adenocarcinoma were studied. No patient received adjuvant therapy. Immunohistochemical stains were performed for NK cells using the monoclonal antibody CD57. The number of NK cells was counted with a MICRON image analyzer. The total area studied for each tumor was 1 cm^2. In this area, 50 intratumoral fields of 0.173 mm^2 were selected. The degree of NK infiltration was classified as little (<50 NK cells), moderate (50–150 NK cells), or extensive (>150 NK cells). The Kaplan-Meier method was used to obtain survival figures. Multivariate analyses were performed by using the Cox regression model. *Results:* At 5 years, patients with little or moderate NK infiltration showed significantly shorter survival rates (overall and disease-free survival) than those with extensive infiltration ($P < .01$). Three significant factors affecting survival were selected in a stepwise fashion in increasing order as follows: TNM stage, NK infiltration, and lymphocytic infiltration. Patients with TNM stage III disease and extensive NK infiltration showed significantly longer survival rates than those with little or moderate infiltration ($P < .001$). In these patients, multivariate analysis with the Cox regression model identified two significant variables: number of involved lymph nodes and NK cell infiltration. *Conclusion:* In patients with colorectal carcinoma, an extensive intratumoral infiltration of NK cells is associated with a favorable tumor outcome. Intratumoral infiltration of NK cells can be used as a variable wide prognostic value, especially in patients with TNM stage III disease.
AUTHORS' ABSTRACT

The Clinical Significance of Focal Active Colitis. Joel K. Greenson, Robert A. Stern, Steven L. Carpenter, et al. *Hum Pathol* 1997; 28:729–733. (J.K.G., Rm 2G332, Box 0054, Department of Pathology, University of Michigan Hospitals, 1500 E Medical Center Dr, Ann Arbor, MI 48109-0054)

Focal crypt injury by neutrophils (cryptitis/crypt abscesses), or focal active colitis (FAC), is a common isolated finding in endoscopic colorectal biopsies. FAC is often thought of as a feature of Crohn disease but may also be seen in ischemia, infections, partially treated ulcerative colitis, and as an isolated finding in patients undergoing endoscopy to exclude neoplasia. Clinical, endoscopic, and pathologic data were retrospectively reviewed from 49 patients with FAC, who had no other diagnostic findings at colorectal biopsy and no history of chronic inflammatory bowel disease. The histologic findings were correlated with clinical diagnoses. Follow-up information was available for 42 of 49 patients with FAC. None developed inflammatory bowel disease; however, 19 patients had an acute self-limited colitislike diarrheal illness, 11 had incidental FAC (patients without diarrhea who underwent endoscopy to exclude colonic neoplasia and were found to have asymptomatic FAC), six had irritable bowel syndrome, four had antibiotic-associated colitis, and two had ischemic colitis. Twenty patients were immunosuppressed, and 19 were taking nonsteroidal antiinflammatory drugs. No histologic features predicted final diagnoses. FAC did not predict the development of chronic colitis, even when mild crypt distortion or slight basal plasmacytosis was present. The preponderance of acute self-limited colitis and antibiotic-associated colitis among the patients with FAC, along with the high number of

immumosuppressed patients, support the conclusion that most FAC cases are infectious. The incidental detection of FAC in patients undergoing endoscopy to exclude colonic neoplasia was not clinically significant. The role of nonsteroidal antiinflammatory drugs in FAC deserves further study.
AUTHORS' ABSTRACT

Thorax

Nodular Histiocytic/Mesothelial Hyperplasia: A Lesion Potentially Mistaken for a Neoplasm in Transbronchial Biopsy. John K. C. Chan, K. T. Loo, Bryan K. C. Yau, et al. *Am J Surg Pathol* 1997; (J.K.C.C., Department of Pathology, Queen Elizabeth Hospital, Wylie Road, Kowloon, Hong Kong)

This report describes two examples of nodular histiocytic/mesothelial hyperplasia seen at transbronchial biopsy that initially led to serious consideration of neuroendocrine neoplasm or meningioma. The biopsies showed nodular collections of cohesive polygonal or round cells with ovoid or deeply grooved nuclei and a moderate amount of finely granular cytoplasm. Nuclear pleomorphism was mild. Immunohistochemical studies showed few cells staining for cytokeratin and the mesothelial marker HBME-1, whereas most cells were decorated by the histiocytic marker PG-M1 (CD68). This lesion appears to be identical to nodular mesothelial hyperplasia as described in hernia sacs and mesothelial/monocytic incidental cardiac excrescences, and the authors propose modifying the designation to "nodular histiocytic/mesothelial hyperplasia" to take into account the marked predominance of histiocytes over mesothelial cells. The clues to recognition of the true nature of the lesion are clinicopathologic correlation and identification of strips of low cuboidal (mesothelial) cells in the vicinity, and the diagnosis can be further confirmed by immunohistochemical staining. Nodular histiocytic/mesothelial hyperplasia probably results from irritation to the mesothelial lining by various causes leading to focal aggregation of histiocytes within retraction pockets or crevices of the serosal cavity.
AUTHORS' ABSTRACT

The Histological Spectrum of Chronic Necrotizing Forms of Pulmonary Aspergillosis. Samuel A. Yousem. *Hum Pathol* 1997; 28:650–656. (S.A.Y., Department of Pathology, Rm NW 625, UPMC Montefiore, 200 Lothrop St, Pittsburgh, PA 15213-2582)

Chronic necrotizing pulmonary aspergillosis is a rare, locally destructive form of chronic aspergillosis that is recognized as a clinical syndrome but has been poorly defined histologically. In this study, 10 cases were evaluated from a morphologic perspective. Three distinct forms emerged. One form ($n = 4$) resembled a necrotizing, granulomatous pneumonia centered around a central zone of infarctlike necrosis of parenchyma resulting from angioinvasive aspergillus. The second pattern ($n = 4$) was that of a granulomatous bronchiectatic cavity with a central fungus ball and subtle tongues of necrosis and inflammation extending into and through the fibrous wall of the cavity. A final form ($n = 2$) had a bronchocentric granulomatosislike appearance with a necrotizing granulomatous bronchitis/bronchiolitis associated with luminal necrotic debris and replacement of mucosa by a palisaded histiocytic reaction. Despite the varied histomorphology, all patients survived the aspergillus infection after antifungal therapy and surgical resection. The different forms of pulmonary aspergillosis are briefly discussed, and the differential diagnosis, with particular regard to mycetomas and allergic forms of bronchocentric granulomatosis, is highlighted.
AUTHOR'S ABSTRACT

Pleuropulmonary Blastoma: A Clinicopathologic Study of 50 Cases. John R. Priest, Michael B. McDermott, Smita Bhatia, et al. *Cancer* 1997; 80:147–161. (Louis P. Dehner, Division of Surgical Pathology, Barnes-Jewish Hospital [South Campus], 1 Barnes Hospital Plaza, St Louis, MO 63110)

Background: Pleuropulmonary blastoma (PPB) is a unique dysontogenetic neoplasm of childhood that appears as a pulmonary and/or pleural-based mass and is characterized histologically by a primitive, variably mixed blastematous and sarcomatous appearance. *Methods:* Histologic material from all cases was reviewed and the tumors subclassified as type I (purely cystic), type II (cystic and solid), or type III (purely solid). Data regarding presenting symptoms, family history, operative findings, pathologic subtypes, therapeutic interventions, and outcome were correlated with survival by standard statistical methods. *Results:* The series comprised 24 male and 26 female patients. Respiratory difficulty with or without fever was the most common clinical symptom reported. Cyst formation in the affected lung was identified radiographically in 19 children (38%) at or before the definitive pathologic diagnosis. The ages at presentation of the seven type I, 24 type II, and 19 type III PPBs were significantly different: 10, 34, and 44 months, respectively ($P < .001$). Local recurrence developed in one of seven type I PPBs (14%) and in 18 of 43 type II and III PPBs (46%); distant metastasis occurred in 13 patients, chiefly to the brain/spinal cord or bone, and was observed only in those with type II or type III PPB. Patients with pleural or mediastinal involvement fared significantly worse than those without such involvement. Five-year survival was 83% for type I and 42% for types II and III. Survival differences on the basis of pathologic subtype did not reach statistical significance. *Conclusion:* PPB is an aggressive, intrathoracic neoplasm of early childhood with an unfavorable outcome. Although survival differences among patients with different histologic subtypes of disease did not reach statistical significance, the apparently better outcome for patients with purely cystic type I tumors may be borne out in a large series. These observations support the premise that types I and III PPB are bridged morphologically by type II PPB with its combined cystic and solid features. The PPB should be regarded as the pulmonary dysontogenetic analogue to Wilms tumor in the kidney, neuroblastoma in the adrenal gland, and hepatoblastoma in the liver. Molecular genetic investigations, especially in constitutional PPB, should be revealing. In view of the poor outcomes for patients with type II or III PPB, new and aggressive therapies must be developed.
AUTHORS' ABSTRACT

Breast

A Comparative Study of Pure Tubular and Tubulolobular Carcinoma of the Breast. I. Green, B. McCormick, M. Cranor, et al. *Am J Surg Pathol* 1997; 21:653–657. (Paul P. Rosen, Department of Pathology, Memorial Sloan-Kettering Cancer Center, 1275 York Ave, New York, NY 10021)

Tubular carcinoma is a distinctive subtype of invasive, well-differentiated, mammary ductal carcinoma that has a good prognosis when treated with modified radical mastectomy. Little is known about tubulolobular carcinoma (TLC). The purpose of this study was to compare the frequency of prognostic factors in pure tubular carcinoma (PTC) and TLC. The authors studied 90 cases of pure PTC and 17 cases of TLC. The following results were found for PTC: size, 0.5–1.8 cm (mean, 1.2 cm); multifocality, 18 of 90 cases (20%); axillary lymph-node dissection, 51 patients; positive axillary lymph nodes, six of 51 cases (12%); recurrence, one of 90 cases (1%) (local). The following results were found for TLC: size, 0.6–2 cm (mean, 1.3 cm); multifocality, five of 17 cases (29%); axillary lymph-node dissection, 14 patients; positive axillary lymph nodes, six of 14 cases (43%); recurrences, two of 17 cases (12%) (one local and one systemic, each after mastectomy). The relationship between multifocality and positive axillary lymph nodes was as follows: in PTC, the percentage of positive axillary lymph nodes was 33% in multifocal cases and 7% in nonmultifocal cases; in TLC, that percentage was 60% in multifocal cases and 33% in nonmultifocal cases. In conclusion, multifocality and positive axillary lymph nodes were more frequent in TLC than in PTC. Multifocality appeared to predispose to positive lymph nodes in both PTC and TLC. The distribution of prognostic factors suggest that TLC is a higher-grade lesion than PTC. Long-term follow-up is needed to correlate multifocality with recurrence after breast-conserving therapy.
AUTHORS' ABSTRACT

Breast Involvement by Extranodal Rosai-Dorfman Disease: Report of Seven Cases. I. Green, R. F. Dorfman, Juan Rosai. *Am J Surg Pathol* 1997; 21:664–668. (J.R., Department of Pathology, Memorial Sloan-Kettering Cancer Center, 1275 York Ave, New York, NY 10021)

Seven cases of breast involvement by

extranodal Rosai-Dorfman disease are presented. The patients were female, and their ages ranged from 15 to 84 years. Three patients had disease confined to the breast; one had involvement of the breast and ipsilateral axillary lymph nodes, and two had bilateral breast involvement as well as disseminated systemic disease. In all cases the clinical and radiographic presentation of the breast lesion raised the possibility of a malignant tumor. All but one of the lesions were treated with excisional biopsy. Microscopically, the lesions were relatively circumscribed, often multinodular masses, located in the breast stroma, with or without associated involvement of the subcutaneous tissue and dermis. They were composed of sheets of S-100 protein-positive large histiocytes displaying lymphocytophagocytosis, scattered in a polymorphous background of mature lymphocytes and plasma cells. The microscopic differential diagnosis includes idiopathic granulomatous mastitis, infective granulomas, Langerhans cell histiocytosis, Erdheim-Chester disease, fibrous histiocytoma, and malignant melanoma.
AUTHORS' ABSTRACT

Genitourinary System

Papillary (Chromophil) Renal Cell Carcinoma: Histomorphologic Characteristics and Evaluation of Conventional Pathologic Prognostic Parameters in 62 Cases. Mahul B. Amin, Christopher L. Corless, Andrew A. Renshaw, et al. *Am J Surg Pathol* 1997; 21:621–635. (M.B.A., Department of Pathology, Henry Ford Hospital, 2799 W Grand Blvd, Detroit, MI 48202)

For more than 2 decades, papillary renal cell carcinoma has been recognized as a possible distinct clinicopathologic subtype of renal cell carcinoma (RCC). However, the histologic criteria for its diagnosis and the clinical outcome are still debated. In an attempt to clarify the diagnostic criteria and resolve issues pertaining to biologic potential, the authors have evaluated the histologic spectrum of 62 papillary RCCs and assessed the significance of conventional pathologic prognostic parameters (Fuhrman nuclear grade [NG], pathologic stage [Robson and TNM], tumor size, multifocality, necrosis, and foam cells) and correlated these with outcome. The mean age of patients was 61.8 years (range, 22–83 years), and men were more commonly affected (1.8:1). Grossly, most tumors were well circumscribed, averaged 6.7 cm in size (range, 1.8–18 cm), and were predominantly localized to the renal poles (polar vs midrenal, 3:1). Multifocality was a prominent feature (24 cases), and in three cases tumors were bilateral. Microscopically, papillary RCCs were predominantly papillary or tubulopapillary, often with a thick fibrous capsule, foam cells, necrosis, hemorrhage, and multifocality. Thirty-five percent of these tumors were low grade (NG I or II) and 65% high grade (NG III or IV). Sixteen tumors presented in a higher stage (stages III and IV), and the overall stage correlated with NG (χ^2, P = .009). Tumors were further distinguished by cytoplasmic features: eosinophilic (42%), basophilic (34%), and mixed (24%). Eosinophilic tumors were predominantly high grade, and basophilic tumors low grade (χ^2, P = .000). A mean follow-up of 57 months showed progression (metastasis, recurrence, or death due to disease) in 21%, whereas 63% were free of disease. Eleven percent died of unrelated causes, and 5% were lost to follow-up. Kaplan-Meier survival analysis showed that both high NG and stage were strongly associated with decreased survival (P = .0000 each), as were decreased foam cells (P = .0025) and vascular invasion (P = .0002). Comparison of 196 reported cases of papillary RCC, including the current series, with reported large series of conventional RCC indicates that papillary RCC usually presents at an early stage, and stage I (Robson) papillary RCC has better 5-year survival rates (87%–100%) than does RCC of the same stage (65%–75%). The overall 5-year survival rate for papillary carcinoma (82%–90%) was also higher than that of conventional RCC (44%–54%). In a Cox proportional hazard regression model, TNM stage appeared to be the only significant variable (P = .0000; hazard ratio, 10.1) in predicting outcome among papillary RCCs. Based on this experience, the authors conclude that (*a*) papillary RCC is a malignant tumor, with a tendency to present at a lower stage, but with a distinct potential for progression and aggressive behavior; (*b*) stratification of these tumors according to cell type, amount of foam cells, presence or absence of vascular invasion, nuclear grade, and pathologic stage provides useful prognostic information; and (*c*) the better 5-year survival rate of papillary RCC (overall and for stage I tumors) compared with that of conventional RCC suggests that it is a tumor with lower malignant potential. Thus, histologic subcategorization of a renal carcinoma as papillary RCC appears to have prognostic implications.
AUTHORS' ABSTRACT

Laparoscopic Pelvic Lymph Node Dissection Following Definitive Radiotherapy for Carcinoma of the Prostate. Greg O. Lund, Howard N. Winfield, James F. Donovan, et al. *J Urol* 1997; 157:548–551. (From the Department of Urology, University of Iowa College of Medicine, Iowa City)

Purpose: Laparoscopic pelvic lymph node dissection is an effective and minimally invasive approach to the clinical staging of adenocarcinoma of the prostate. The authors report their experience with this technique in patients in whom full-course pelvic radiation therapy had failed and who were being considered for salvage local therapy. *Materials and Methods:* In 14 patients disease was staged by means of transperitoneal laparoscopic pelvic lymph node dissection performed for persistent adenocarcinoma of the prostate at least 20 months (average, 49.5) following external-beam radiation therapy and/or brachytherapy. All patients were healthy, had no evidence of metastatic disease, and were considered to be candidates for salvage therapy. *Results:* A total of 13 patients underwent successful laparoscopic pelvic lymph node dissection, while one sustained an enterotomy requiring conversion to open surgery. The normal surgical planes were more difficult to dissect, with the obturator lymph node packets appearing smaller and more fibrotic than in nonirradiated patients, yielding an average of 7.1 total nodes. The average operative time was 167 minutes, and postoperative hospitalization was comparable to that in reported series of nonirradiated patients. Four patients (28%) with metastatic pelvic lymph nodes underwent subsequent orchiectomy. Nine patients with negative lymph nodes underwent ultrasound-guided transperineal placement of radioactive gold or palladium seeds. One patient underwent salvage radical retropubic prostatectomy. *Conclusion:* Laparoscopic pelvic lymph node dissection following full-course pelvic irradiation is technically feasible, albeit more difficult than in nonirradiated patients. This approach appears to be an excellent minimally invasive technique for the clinical restaging of persistent adenocarcinoma of the prostate in patients being considered for salvage therapy.
AUTHORS' ABSTRACT

Outcome for Surgically Staged Localized Prostate Cancer Treated with External Beam Radiation Therapy. Curt R. Powell, Thomas K. Huisman, Robert H. Riffenburgh, et al. *J Urol* 1997; 157:1754–1759. (C.R.P., Clinical Investigation Department, Naval Medical Center, 34800 Bob Wilson Dr, San Diego, CA 92134-5000)

Purpose: A retrospective analysis was performed in patients with surgically staged localized prostate cancer treated with external-beam radiation therapy; it examined 10-year overall, cause-specific, and disease-free survivals based on lack of clinical recurrence and two separate prostate-specific antigen criteria for cure. *Materials and Methods:* The authors analyzed 145 patients who received external-beam radiation therapy after negative results of staging pelvic lymphadenectomy for prostate cancer. Follow-up data were available for 129 patients (90%). Disease was stage A in 29 patients (22.5%), stage B in 64 (49.6%), stage B2/C in two (17%), and stage C in 14 (10.9%). The average potential follow-up from date of diagnosis was 11.5 years (minimum, 7.2 years). Eighty-seven patients potentially can be followed up for longer than 10 years. Disease-free survival status was based on normal digital rectal examination findings, lack of symptoms suggesting metastasis, and application of two separate prostate-specific antigen criteria of 4 ng/mL or less (group 1) or 1.5 ng/mL or less (group 2). Survival was analyzed with the Kaplan-Meier actuarial method. *Results:* Actuarial overall survival rates at 10 and 15 years were 63.7% and 49.6%, respectively, and cause-specific survival was 84.2% and 80%, respectively. Disease-free survival rates were 54.5% and 32.4%, respectively,

for group 1, and 42.3% and 9.6%, respectively, for group 2. *Conclusion:* The improved patient selection inherent in surgical staging before definitive external-beam radiation therapy provides for improved overall and cause-specific survival over that of patients without surgical staging. Biochemical disease-free survival also appears to be improved.
AUTHORS' ABSTRACT

A Multicenter Clinical Trial Investigating the Use of a Fluoroscopically Controlled Cutting Balloon Catheter for the Management of Ureteral and Ureteropelvic Junction Obstruction. Glenn M. Preminger, Ralph V. Clayman, Stephen Y. Nakada, et al. *J Urol* 1997; 157:1625–1629. (S.Y.N., Department of Surgery—Division of Urology, University of Wisconsin Medical School, G5/343 Clinical Science Center, 600 Highland Ave, Madison, WI 53792)

Purpose: The authors assessed the efficacy of a fluoroscopically controlled cutting balloon catheter for the treatment of ureteropelvic junction and ureteral strictures. *Materials and Methods:* A multicenter trial was performed that included 66 endopyelotomies and 49 endoureterotomies. To the authors' knowledge this study represents the largest number of patients with ureteropelvic junction obstruction and ureteral strictures tested with this device to date. *Results:* With a mean follow-up of 7.8 months (range, 1–17.9 months) the patency rate was 77% for endopyelotomy, with 72% of the primary and 100% of the secondary ureteropelvic junction obstructions remaining patent. The patients undergoing endoureterotomy were followed up for an average of 8.7 months (range, 1.2–17.0 months), with a patency rate of 55%. *Conclusion:* A cutting balloon endoscopic incision is effective in the majority of cases, with patency rates for endopyelotomies and endoureterotomies that mirror those of current endourologic reports on other, albeit more time-intensive and more invasive, incisional techniques.
AUTHORS' ABSTRACT

Long-term Followup of a Bladder Carcinoma Cohort: Questionable Value of Radical Radiotherapy. Sten Holmäng, Hans Hedelin, Göran Borghede, et al. *J Urol* 1997; 157:1642–1646. (S.H., Department of Urology, Sahlgrenska University Hospital, Göteborg, Sweden)

Purpose: The authors studied the outcome of radical radiation therapy for bladder carcinoma in all patients from a well-defined region. *Materials and Methods:* All 701 cases of new bladder carcinoma between 1987 and 1988 in western Sweden were prospectively documented and followed until 1994. Between 1987 and 1994, 74 of the 701 patients (mean age, 73 years; range, 54–88 years) were treated with external-beam radiation therapy (≥70 Gy). *Results:* At least 84% of the patients had persistent tumor, a local recurrence, or a symptomatic contracted bladder after external-beam radiation therapy. Seven patients (9.5%) died of early or late treatment-related complications. Of only eight long-term survivors, six had undergone radical transurethral resection before external-beam radiation therapy. *Conclusion:* Full-dose external-beam radiation therapy in patients with bladder carcinoma was associated with high local recurrence and serious complication rates. It must be questioned whether elderly patients actually benefit from full-dose radiation therapy.
AUTHORS' ABSTRACT

Cardiovascular System

Spontaneous Closure of Selected Iatrogenic Pseudoaneurysms and Arteriovenous Fistulae. Boulos Toursarkissian, Brent T. Allen, Drazen Petrinec, et al. *J Vasc Surg* 1997; 25:803–809. (B.T.A., 1 Barnes Plaza, Ste 5103 QT, St Louis, MO 63110)

Purpose: The authors report their approach to the management of postcatheterization femoral artery pseudoaneurysms and arteriovenous fistulas in an attempt to determine the frequency of spontaneous resolution of selected lesions. *Methods:* The authors studied 196 pseudoaneurysms, 81 arteriovenous fistulas, and nine combined lesions that were identified by means of duplex scanning. Indications for immediate surgical repair included pseudoaneurysm larger than 3 cm, enlarging hematoma, pain, groin infection, nerve compression, limb ischemia, concomitant surgical procedure, and patient refusal or inability to comply with follow-up. All other lesions were observed. *Results:* One hundred thirty-nine patients underwent prompt surgical repair, and 147 patients were initially managed without operation. There were no limb-threatening complications associated with nonoperative management in this subset of patients. Eighty-six percent of the lesions being observed resolved spontaneously within a mean of 23 days, whereas 14% required surgical closure for a variety of reasons (at a mean of 111 days after the initial diagnosis). There was no statistically significant difference in the rate of spontaneous pseudoaneurysm closure (89%) as opposed to fistulas (81%) (P = .17). By life-table analysis, 90% of selected pseudoaneurysms had resolved by 2 months. Patients selected for observation underwent an average of 2.6 duplex scans per patient, versus 1.4 scans per patient for those treated with immediate surgery (P < .01). *Conclusion:* The natural history of stable pseudoaneurysms and arteriovenous fistulas is benign and frequently results in spontaneous resolution, which allows properly selected patients to be managed without operation.
AUTHORS' ABSTRACT

Percutaneous Transluminal Angioplasty and Primary Stenting of the Iliac Arteries in 288 Patients. Timothy M. Sullivan, Mary Beth Childs, J. Michael Bacharach, et al. *J Vasc Surg* 1997; 25:829–839. (T.M.S., Department of Vascular Surgery, S-61, The Cleveland Clinic Foundation, 9500 Euclid Ave, Cleveland, OH 44195)

Purpose: This study reports the initial and late results of percutaneous transluminal angioplasty (PTA) and intravascular stenting for atherosclerotic occlusive disease of the iliac arteries. *Methods:* The preprocedural and postprocedural clinical records, arteriograms, segmental limb pressure measurements (ankle-brachial index [ABI] and thigh-brachial index [TBI]), and pulse volume recordings of 288 patients who underwent PTA and primary stenting of the common iliac (n = 354 [69.4%]) and external iliac (n = 156 [30.6%]) arteries were reviewed. Initial and late clinical, hemodynamic, and angiographic success were assessed according to objective criteria. Data on patients who underwent unsuccessful attempts at iliac stent placement are unavailable; results are not reported on an intent-to-treat basis. *Results:* Clinical follow-up data (mean, 11.9 months) are available for 268 of 288 patients (93.1%) and for 394 of 424 limbs (92.9%). The initial success rates, as defined by TBI, ABI, and clinical limb status, were 90.2%, 87.8%, and 74.6%, respectively. The Kaplan-Meier estimates of angiographic patency (101 arteries) were 96%, 81%, and 73% at 6, 12, and 24 months. Cumulative patency rates were 84%, 76%, and 57% on the basis of TBI, ABI, and clinical limb status at 24 months. Factors associated with initial success included the need for multiple stents (P = .0001), greater initial stenosis (P = .0001), less severe baseline ischemia (P = .007), younger age (P = .0015), and the preprocedural patency of the ipsilateral superficial femoral artery (P = .002). A higher degree of initial stenosis (P < .001) and superficial femoral artery patency (P = .004) were also associated with late success. *Conclusion:* PTA and stenting of the iliac arteries is associated with reasonable angiographic, hemodynamic, and clinical success. The outcome is favorably affected by greater initial stenosis and extent of disease, less severe baseline ischemia, younger age, and patency of the ipsilateral superficial femoral artery.
AUTHORS' ABSTRACT

Musculoskeletal

Lesions of the Bones of the Hands and Feet. Mary L. Ostrowski, Harlan J. Spjut. *Am J Surg Pathol* 1997; 21:676–690. (M.L.O., Department of Pathology, MS-205, Methodist Hospital, 6565 Fannin, Houston, TX 77030)

Neoplasms and their simulators in the bones of the hands and feet include the majority of those found in other skeletal sites, and a disproportionate number of some. The authors examined the clinical, radiologic, and pathologic features of 240 lesions of the hand and foot bones. Benign tumors and lesions including reactive and reparative conditions comprised 203 cases. The largest single category of neoplasms was that with cartilaginous differentiation, with

enchondromas (29 cases) and chondrosarcomas (15 cases) the most common. Noncartilaginous malignant tumors were infrequent and displayed typical radiologic and pathologic features. Florid reactive periostitis, bizarre parosteal osteochondromatous proliferations, and giant cell reparative granulomas made up a larger percentage of lesions in these locations than in other skeletal sites. Lesions of the bones of the hands and feet may frequently be sampled for biopsy or treated at hospitals without large orthopedic tumor services. Thus, it is important for the surgical pathologist to be aware of the frequency and characteristics of lesions that may present in these sites.
AUTHORS' ABSTRACT

Stress Fracture of the Tibia after Arthrodesis of the Ankle or the Hindfoot. Cobi Lidor, Linda R. Ferris, Reginald Hall, et al. *J Bone Joint Surg [Am]* 1997; 79:558–564. (C.L., Department of Surgery, Division of Orthopedic Surgery, Duke University Medical Center, Durham, NC 27710)

The authors studied 12 patients who had a stress fracture of the tibia and one patient who had a stress fracture of the fibula after arthrodesis of the ankle or the foot. A second stress fracture subsequently developed in two patients. All but two patients were managed nonoperatively, and the fractures healed uneventfully. One patient who was managed operatively had a below-the-knee amputation to treat a painful nonunion of a tibial fracture, and the other had interlocking intramedullary nailing for a displaced fracture. All but one of the arthrodesis sites had fused before the stress fracture occurred. All of the stress fractures that occurred after arthrodesis of the ankle were in the middle and distal aspects or the distal aspect of the tibia, while those that occurred after triple arthrodesis were in the distal aspect of the fibula or the medial malleolus. Although six of the 13 patients still had uncorrected alignment and deformity after the arthrodesis, optimum alignment after the arthrodesis did not preclude the occurrence of a stress fracture. The authors conclude that stress fracture must be considered in the differential diagnosis of pain months or even years after solid fusion at the site of an ankle or triple arthrodesis.
AUTHORS' ABSTRACT

Pediatrics

Diagnostic Testing for Acute Head Injury in Children: When are Head Computed Tomography and Skull Radiographs Indicated? Kimberly S. Quayle, David M. Jaffe, Nathan Kuppermann, et al. *Pediatrics* 1997; 99:e11, *http://www.pediatrics.org*. (K.S.Q., Department of Pediatrics, Division of Emergency Medicine, Washington University School of Medicine, 1 Children's Pl, St Louis, MO 63110-1077)

Brain injury is the leading cause of death and disability in pediatric trauma victims. Head injuries in children account for 260,000 hospital admissions each year, and nearly 5 million children present to hospital emergency departments for evaluation and care of head injuries. Morbidity and mortality associated with significant intracranial injury may be ameliorated by early diagnosis and treatment. Diagnostic strategies differ among individuals and institutions. Skull radiographs have been used in evaluation of children with head trauma but their value is controversial. Head computed tomography (CT) is the diagnostic method of choice for diagnosis of intracranial disorders in patients with head trauma. A defined set of clinical screening criteria for the evaluation of head injury does not exist for children but would be valuable in decision making.

The purpose of this study was to evaluate clinical features that are associated with head injuries and that affect the decision to obtain imaging studies. Prospective data collection and predetermined selection criteria were used. A prospective cohort of children with mild, moderate, and severe nonpenetrating head injuries received standardized evaluation to collect clinical information in the form of patient history, physical examination, and imaging studies. Patients younger than 18 years who presented to the emergency department with histories or physical findings of nontrivial head injury were eligible for the study. Nontrivial head injuries were defined as those causing headache, amnesia, vomiting, drowsiness, loss of consciousness, seizure, dizziness, or significant physical findings, including altered mental status, neurologic deficit, and altered head surface anatomy.

A total of 1,201 children with head injuries were seen, 410 with nontrivial injuries. Data were collected in 321 patients. The ages of the study patients ranged from 2 weeks to 17¾ years, with 42% of the study patients younger than 2 years. A fall was the mechanism of injury in more than half of the patients. Seventy-four percent of the patients were discharged home from the emergency department. Nineteen percent were admitted to general care, and 7% were admitted to intensive care. One child died as a result of severe pulmonary injury after being struck by a motor vehicle. Head CT was performed in 98% of all study children, and skull radiography in 89%. Discrepancies between skull radiography and head CT in identifying the presence of a linear skull fracture occurred in 10 cases. In eight children skull radiography demonstrated linear fractures, whereas CT did not. In two children, head CT showed linear skull fractures, whereas skull radiography did not. In two cases there were discrepancies regarding whether a fracture was depressed. Twenty-seven intracranial injuries (8%) were identified, and 50 skull fractures were diagnosed (16%).

The data suggest stratified clinical approaches to pediatric patients. Because altered mental status, focal neurologic deficit, signs of basilar skull fracture, and seizure are independent predictors of intracranial injury, patients with these findings should undergo head CT and/or neurosurgical consultation. Intracranial injuries did occur in patients without the clinical features listed above, and 15 patients would not have received head CT if any of the independent predictors had been used as the only criteria for imaging studies. Only one of these 15 underwent surgery. Clinicians must determine when to obtain head CT in children who have vomiting, amnesia, headache, drowsiness, or history of a loss of consciousness but who have none of the independent predictors that were identified. Careful observation may be chosen rather than head CT, with the realization that intracranial injuries may be missed. The majority of these injuries will not require surgery.

Based on these data and a review of the literature, guidelines have been developed for practice. Head CT is recommended for head-injured children with altered mental status, focal necrologic deficits, signs of a basilar skull fracture, seizure, or a palpable depression of the skull. Because intracranial injuries occur in the absence of these findings, head CT should be considered for neurologically normal children with histories of loss of consciousness, vomiting, headache, drowsiness, or amnesia. Careful observation of these children at home or in the hospital may be an alternative approach depending on the availability of head CT, hospital beds, and reliable caregivers. Children without the symptoms or signs listed above may be carefully observed at home by reliable adults. Neurologically normal children who have normal head CT results may also be safely observed at home when reliable caregivers are available.
BEVERLY P. WOOD, MD
Childrens Hospital, Los Angeles, Calif

Childhood Poisoning Involving Transdermal Nicotine Patches. Alan Woolf, Keith Burkhart, Thomas Caraccio, et al. *Pediatrics* 1997; 99:e4, *http://www.pediatrics.org*. (A.W., Massachusetts Poison Control System, 300 Longwood Ave, Boston, MA 02115)

Transdermal nicotine patches (TNPs) are established systems of drug delivery that have demonstrated efficacy in helping adults to curtail cigarette smoking. Four brands of TNP delivery up to 22 mg in a 24-hour period; however, 27%–74% of the total nicotine may remain in a TNP after use. As much as 83 mg of residual nicotine may remain in a used TNP, the equivalent to the nicotine content of four to seven cigarettes. Therapeutic use of TNPs in adults has been associated with a variety of adverse effects, including rashes, allergic skin reactions, nausea and vomiting, sleep disturbances, headaches, and chest pain. Manifestations of nicotine poisoning in children have been seen after the ingestion of cigarettes or nicotine containing gum. There has been concern that children might be seriously poisoned from inadvertent exposure to a TNP. Thirty-four U.S. Poison Centers were recruited to monitor incoming poisoning calls for instances of an unintentional exposure to TNPs among children. Information about the date and time of the poisoning, circumstances of exposure, type and lot number of the TNPs, clinical symptoms and signs, clinical course, complications, management and

outcomes were recorded. Thirty-three cases of pediatric poisoning by exposure to a TNP were reported. Three additional cases had been reported to the manufacturer before the time of study onset. The mean age of the children was 3 years. In most cases the child had discovered a new or discarded TNP or a TNP had accidentally become affixed the child's skin. Five children became symptomatic after oral exposure to a TNP and had transient and local signs of toxicity, gagging, or a burning sensation of the mouth or tongue. Children with dermal exposures more often had systemic complaints of nausea and vomiting. Most of the children were exposed to a TNP that released approximately 0.9 mg nicotine per hour. A previously used TNP was less likely than a newly opened TNP to produce symptoms. Irrespective of the route, the duration of exposure to the TNP patch was roughly correlated with symptoms of toxicity. Almost all of the 18 oral exposures were less than 10 minutes in duration, and only five of the children developed any symptoms. Of the 18 dermal TNP exposures, seven of eight children exposed for 20 minutes or longer developed toxicity, as opposed to two of 10 children exposed for less than 20 minutes. Because TNPs are now available without prescription, children and adolescents are likely to have greater access to them. Clinicians should be aware of the toxic effects of pediatric TNP exposures.
Beverly P. Wood, MD
Childrens Hospital, Los Angeles, Calif

Magnesium Sulfate in Labor and Risk of Neonatal Brain Lesions and Cerebral Palsy in Low Birth Weight Infants. Nigel Paneth, James Jetton, Jennifer Pinto-Martin, et al. *Pediatrics* 1997; 99:e1, *http://www-.pediatrics.org*. (N.P., Program in Epidemiology, College of Human Medicine, Michigan State University, A 206 East Fee Hall, East Lansing, MI 48824)

Magnesium sulfate is widely used in obstetric practice to treat preeclampsia and eclampsia and to attempt to arrest the progress of premature labor. A recent case-control study in infants weighing less than 1,500 g at birth demonstrated a substantial reduction in cerebral palsy in children whose mothers received magnesium sulfate in labor. This observation matches the multiple catalytic roles of magnesium in cellular enzyme systems and neuronal functioning, particularly with evidence that magnesium can block the *N*-methyl-D-aspartate receptor and thus prevent excitatory amino acids, commonly released during episodes of hypoxia and ischemia, from producing neuronal damage. Low-birth-weight infants were assessed with cranial ultrasound (US) in the neonatal period, at 4 hours, 24 hours, and 7 days, and were examined at 2 years of age for the presence or absence of cerebral palsy. Neonatal outcomes included death in the first 28 days, sonographic diagnosis of germinal matrix or intraventricular hemorrhage, and sonographic diagnosis of parenchymal lesions and ventricular enlargement. Three hundred sixty-two infants were exposed to magnesium sulfate and 280 infants had US-diagnosed neonatal brain lesions; of these, 113 children received the diagnosis of either disabling or nondisabling cerebral palsy. In a small subset of infants, those with onset of parenchymal lesions at 7 days of age or later, magnesium exposure was associated with a significantly reduced risk of disabling cerebral palsy. The hypothesis that magnesium sulfate use reduces the risk of neonatal brain lesions or cerebral palsy in low-birth-weight infants was not statistically supported in this study, although a modest reduction in risk of disabling cerebral palsy cannot be excluded. The data suggest that magnesium exposure may be associated with reduction in the risk of cerebral palsy in low-birth-weight infants who have late-onset brain lesions, but this unpredicted observation requires confirmation in another data set.
Beverly P. Wood, MD
Childrens Hospital, Los Angeles, Calif

Number and Activation of Circulating Polymorphonuclear Leukocytes and Platelets Are Associated with Neonatal Respiratory Distress Syndrome Severity. Frank Brua, Willem van Oeveren, Albert Okken, et al. *Pediatrics* 1997; 99:672–680. (F.B., Division of Neonatology, Beatrix Children's Hospital, University Hospital Groningen, Hanzeplein 1, 9713 EZ Groningen, The Netherlands)

In preterm newborn infants with respiratory distress syndrome (RDS), an exaggerated pulmonary inflammatory response occurs in the first days of life and is considered an important determinant of bronchopulmonary dysplasia (BPD). Characteristic of this inflammatory response is an increase of activated polymorphonuclear leukocytes (PMNs) and alveolar macrophages in the pulmonary interstitium and small airways. Activated PMNs can cause lung tissue injury by release of toxic oxygen radicals, arachidonic acid metabolites, and proteolytic enzymes. Activity of the proteolytic enzyme elastase with reduced levels of α-1 proteinase inhibitor has been associated with lung connective tissue destruction and the development of BPD. Activated alveolar macrophages release leukotriene B_4, complement B_4, complement C5–derived anaphylatoxin C5a, and cytokines, which are found in pulmonary effluent fluid of preterm ventilated newborn infants at risk for BPD. These agents aggravate lung dysfunction by stimulating chemotaxis and endothelial adherence of activated PMNs with subsequent breakdown of the alveolar-capillary membrane structures. A decrease of circulating leukocytes has been found in preform infants with severe RDS. The total leukocyte count was lower in a severe RDS group than in a mild to moderate RDS group, significant on days 2 and 3. The mean PMN counts of both study groups differed significantly, and this study has indicated that a decreased number of circulating PMNs in infants with severe RDS is accompanied by increased activation of these cells represented by systemic release of elastase. The numbers of circulating total leukocytes, PMNs, and platelets decrease in preterm infants with severe RDS. Simultaneously, elastase and thromboxane release increase in these infants. The decreased number and increased activation of circulating PMNs and platelets correlates with hypoxia and acidosis at birth and also with high-pressure ventilation and hyperoxia throughout the study period. Decreased numbers and increased activation of circulating PMNs and platelets are correlated with decreased values for continuous measures of RDS severity, and it is speculated that activated PMNs and platelets sequester in the lungs and induce increased alveolar capillary permeability and lung tissue injury, contributing to RDS severity.
Beverly P. Wood, MD
Childrens Hospital, Los Angeles, Calif

Miscellaneous

Spindle Cell Carcinoma of the Larynx: Review of 26 Cases Including DNA Content and Immunohistochemistry. Jean E. Lewis, Kerry D. Olsen, Thomas J. Sebo. *Hum Pathol* 1997; 28:664–673. (J.E.L., Mayo Clinic, 200 First St SW, Rochester, MN 55905)

Spindle cell carcinoma is uncommon, with a predilection for the upper aerodigestive tract. Its histogenesis has not been resolved, although most authors support the sarcomatoid carcinoma concept. Ploidy analysis and proliferation indexes have not been reported for laryngeal spindle cell carcinoma. The authors examined the pathologic and clinical features of 26 patients (25 men, one woman; mean age, 64 years) with laryngeal spindle cell carcinoma treated at the Mayo Clinic from 1960 to 1990. Twenty-three tumors were examined with digital image analysis for DNA content of the spindle cell population (13 tumors had a sufficient squamous component to be analyzed separately). The glottis was involved most frequently (19 patients); 21 tumors were grossly polypoid. Twenty-three tumors were biphasic, and three were monophasic. Overall, 17 tumors (65%) showed keratin positivity in the spindle cell component. Polyclonal antikeratin (15 positive cases), 34βE12 (15 positive), and AEI/AE3 (12 positive) were the most sensitive markers. Spindle cells were diploid in five tumors (22%) and nondiploid in 18 (78%); conventional squamous cell carcinoma was diploid in four cases and nondiploid in nine. DNA ploidy results were concordant between the two populations in 11 of 13 tumors (85%). The mean percentage of MIB-1 staining was 31% in the sarcomatoid component and 45% in the squamous component. In the primary treatment group of 22 patients (median follow-up, 6.4 years), four (18%) had local recurrence, three (14%) had distant metastasis, and four (18%) died of disease. The presence of a nondiploid spindle cell population in 78% of cases of laryngeal spindle cell carcinoma is interpreted as evidence of a neoplastic rather than reactive process. Keratin positivity in nearly two-thirds of tumors supports the theory of epithelial origin of these tumors (sarcomatoid carcinoma).
Authors' Abstract

William P. Shuman, MD

CT of Blunt Abdominal Trauma in Adults[1]

THIS article reviews the current state of the art for use of computed tomography (CT) in adult patients with blunt abdominal trauma, with emphasis on helical CT. It reviews the optimal helical CT technique in these patients and discusses the clinical presentation and CT findings of traumatic injury to organs of the peritoneal and retroperitoneal spaces. Throughout the article, references are made to alternative diagnostic techniques. The concluding section discusses the use of ultrasound (US) and the relative roles of helical CT and US in acutely traumatized patients.

Parameters for Helical CT of Abdominal Trauma

Category	Parameters
Contrast material	
Oral	Concentration, 2%–5%; total dose, 500–750 mL; administer 5–40 minutes before scanning
Intravenous	Concentration, 60%–75%; total dose, 130–180 mL; administer 70–90 seconds before scanning
Section	5–8-mm-thick, 5–8-mm reconstruction, pitch of 1–2
Extent of scanning	Inferior lungs to inferior edge of ischia

HELICAL CT TECHNIQUE

Helical CT has been a major advancement in the evaluation of trauma patients because scanning can be accomplished more quickly, with more intense bolus contrast material enhancement. In addition to faster scanning and image reconstruction times, automated trauma protocols and rapid patient handling procedures have reduced patient turnaround time for abdominal trauma CT to the 6–10-minute range. Helical CT can rapidly accomplish combined studies of the chest, abdomen, pelvis, head, and extremities as required.

CT technique in patients with abdominal trauma requires water-soluble oral contrast material, usually 500 mL administered through the nasogastric tube in the emergency department and an additional 250 mL administered in the CT room (Table). Dilute (2%–5%) water-soluble oral contrast material can be administered during 20–40 minutes if the patient's condition permits; if not, oral contrast material can be administered through a nasogastric tube from a hanging bag during resuscitation and transport to the CT room. Although previously controversial, complications from the use of oral contrast material in trauma patients more recently have been shown to be very rare and not consequential (1,2). Oral contrast material provides much better CT evaluation of injury to the stomach, duodenum, bowel, and pancreas and better evaluation for hemoperitoneum, especially in thin patients (2). Nonionic intravenous contrast material is often employed to reduce the risk of vomiting since many trauma patients present with a full stomach and also have head trauma, both of which increase the frequency of vomiting. Trauma patients often are immobilized in a neck collar on the CT table, which predisposes to aspiration. If necessary, the frequency of vomiting in trauma patients can be reduced through the use of intravenous metoclopramide (10–20 mg) given at the time oral contrast material is administered (3). Selective use of rectal contrast material may help distinguish colon from other organs or hemoperitoneum in thin patients who have little intraabdominal fat; additionally, rectal contrast material can be valuable for identifying colonic injury, particularly in pelvic trauma.

Intravenous contrast material is usually administered at 2–4 mL/sec for a total volume of 150–180 mL beginning 70–90 seconds before initiation of helical CT. Timing scanning during the peak of organ enhancement is important since early scanning can produce artifacts that may simulate injury (especially in the spleen and kidneys) and late scanning can decrease sensitivity to injuries that are present (4). Radiologists at several centers have had success with the use of a computer-assisted contrast material bolus tracking technique to determine the time to begin scanning. After beginning the intravenous injection, this program periodically (every 2 seconds) samples attenuation in user-selected regions of interest in target organs (such as

Index terms: Abdomen, CT, 78.12115 • Abdomen, injuries, 78.41 • Abdomen, US, 78.12981, 78.12989 • Computed tomography (CT), helical, 78.12115 • State-of-art reviews • Trauma, 78.41

Radiology 1997; 205:297–306

[1] From the Department of Diagnostic Imaging, Evergreen Hospital Medical Center, 12040 NE 128th St, Kirkland, WA 98034; and the Department of Radiology, University of Washington, Seattle. Received June 3, 1997; revision requested June 27; revision received July 15; accepted July 21. **Address reprint requests to** the author.

liver) with low-dose scanning until the organ attenuation reaches a predetermined threshold. The program then automatically begins the diagnostic portion of the study. The use of biphasic helical CT with scanning in the arterial enhancement phase and later organ enhancement phase may have value in select cases, but this issue has not yet been investigated.

Breath holding may not be possible in trauma patients; scanning during respiration creates less artifact with helical CT than with nonhelical CT. Scanning should include the inferior lung fields to the inferior aspect of the ischia with 5–8-mm-thick sections and a pitch of 1–2. Images are rapidly available since up to 100 sections can be acquired in 75 seconds, and image reconstruction is performed in 1–3 seconds per section. These images should be immediately reviewed by a radiologist experienced in trauma CT (5). Review of all CT images at multiple window settings (lung, bone, standard soft tissue, narrow) is important to detect lung contusion, pneumothorax, pneumoperitoneum, bone injury, and subtle abdominal organ injury (6). Multiple-window review is most easily and quickly accomplished at the CT console by using the rapid paging mode. Results are best communicated directly to emergency department personnel and attending trauma surgeons within minutes of the completion of the CT examination. If appropriate, the patient may proceed directly from helical CT to the operating room.

Such rapidly available CT information may enable "focused trauma surgery": Surgeons can go directly to sites of CT-identified active hemorrhage or other focal injury rather than needing to explore the entire abdomen and retroperitoneum to find all acute abnormalities (7). For this reason, in some centers with helical CT in or near the emergency department, scanning marginally unstable trauma patients may be undertaken on the assumption that time spent in the helical CT scanner saves time in the operating room or enables arteriographic catheter embolization of active hemorrhage. Alternatively, stable, minimally injured patients with normal findings at helical CT may be safely discharged to home and may not require a period of in-hospital observation as would be needed if a less specific imaging modality, such as US, were used (8,9). This early safe discharge to home after a negative CT study for some patients may result in substantial economic savings compared with admitting all patients for observation after a negative, but less specific, US study (10).

CT OF HEMOPERITONEUM

Very small volumes of hemoperitoneum are accurately detected with CT. This should prompt a thorough search for organ injury since hemoperitoneum may be the most obvious initial clue (11–13). Hemoperitoneum starts near the site of injury and spreads along traditional pathways. From the liver, in the supine position, blood collects in the Morison pouch or adjacent to the right lobe but then passes down the right paracolic gutter to the pelvis. From the spleen, blood passes via the phrenocolic ligament to the left paracolic gutter and the pelvis. Large amounts of blood may collect in the dependent pelvis without much hemoperitoneum evident in the upper abdomen. This emphasizes the importance of including the pelvis in every trauma CT examination. The "sentinel clot sign" describes adjacent, focal, higher attenuation clotted blood as a marker for the organ that is the major source of hemorrhage, should multiple organs be injured (14). Quantification of the volume of intraperitoneal blood with CT has been attempted in the past, but this information now has less value since stable patients with very large volumes of hemoperitoneum often are treated without surgery (15,16).

The attenuation of intraperitoneal blood varies widely. Active hemorrhage during intravenous administration of contrast material may measure 180 HU or higher. Clotted blood typically measures 60–100 HU (17), fresh unclotted blood measures 30–45 HU, and serum (after clotting) or anterior blood in a supine patient (after the hematocrit effect) can measure as low as 0 HU and often is less than 20 HU (18). These attenuation numbers for hemoperitoneum can be affected by the patients intravascular hematocrit and by dilutional effect from intraperitoneal fluid, such as ascites, urine, or succus from ruptured bowel. Other causes of low-attenuation intraperitoneal fluid might include bile, urine, or lavage fluid from diagnostic peritoneal lavage. Very high attenuation fluid usually represents extravasated intravascular contrast material, indicating active bleeding adjacent to an injured organ. Occasionally such high attenuation can be difficult to differentiate from extravasated oral contrast material, but adjacent injured gut or free intraperitoneal location of contrast material can be helpful clues that indicate leakage of oral contrast material. Repeat scanning after an appropriate time delay and without intravenous contrast material can help differentiate these two possibilities.

CT OF SPLENIC TRAUMA

The spleen is the most frequently injured abdominal organ during blunt abdominal trauma (19–21). While several CT grading systems for splenic injury have been published, no CT grading scheme enables prediction of the need for splenic surgery (22–26). Such prediction has become less important with the increasing popularity of nonsurgical management of splenic injury. Up to 91% of stable patients with splenic injury can be treated conservatively with observation, especially in young patients (15,19,27). The spleen has shown impressive capacity to heal, even after fragmentation, which supports the trend toward nonsurgical management. Such a nonsurgical approach may require delayed repeat CT examinations but only if the subsequent clinical course suggests a developing complication (28–30). If CT depicts a large nonperfused portion of spleen, active hemorrhage, contrast blush (ie, hyperattenuating collection of contrast material [32]) in the splenic parenchyma, or pseudoaneurysm (Fig 1), surgery may be indicated (31,32). Active hemorrhage detected with CT (Fig 1) also can be controlled by means of arteriography plus transcatheter embolization of the splenic artery, which lowers splenic perfusion pressure but does not devascularize the spleen because of its rich collaterals (33). This approach has the advantage of retaining the spleen and thus averting the up to 50 times greater risk of sepsis that occurs in patients in whom the spleen has been removed (33). Delayed rupture of the spleen up to 10 days later does occur; it is most frequently associated with subtle, low-grade splenic injury (Fig 2) and subcapsular hematoma (34,35). Since these types of injuries do not have associated hemoperitoneum, they often are missed at both diagnostic peritoneal lavage and limited US when

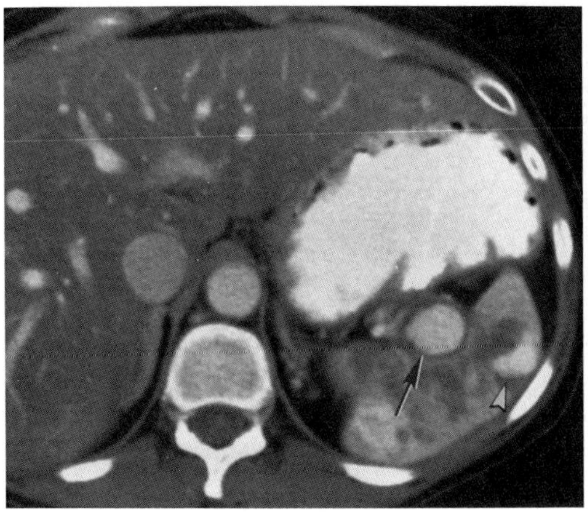
1.

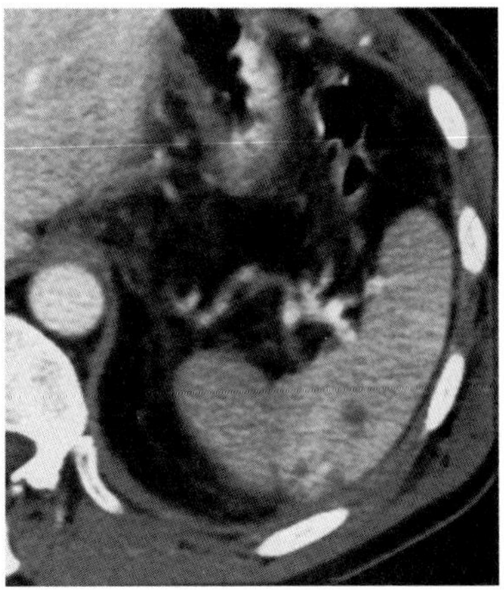
2.

Figures 1, 2. **(1)** Helical CT scan shows a shattered spleen with a pseudoaneurysm (arrow) and active hemorrhage (arrowhead). Note variable perfusion of different splenic segments. **(2)** Helical CT scan shows an isolated small splenic contusion. This limited injury had no associated hemoperitoneum. Delayed rupture of this spleen occurred 2 days later.

used to screen for hemoperitoneum.

CT is about 95% sensitive to the presence of splenic injury and accurately depicts the extent (21). Of note, 40% of patients with splenic injury have associated left-sided rib fractures (36). Rapid infusion of an intravenous bolus of contrast material is important because splenic parenchymal injury may be missed on unenhanced scans and a slow infusion may actually obscure injury (11). Intravenous contrast material also helps in evaluation of splenic perfusion and detection of active hemorrhage (37).

CT findings of splenic injury are varied. On enhanced scans, a subcapsular hematoma appears as a crescentic region of low attenuation that compresses normal parenchyma, usually lateral in location. The intrasplenic hematoma is round and low in attenuation (early), may be inhomogeneous, and may later contain high-attenuation clot. Occasionally a splenic contusion may present as only mottled parenchymal enhancement (Fig 2), sometimes with associated hemoperitoneum, adjacent clot, or thickening of the lateroconal fascia (13). A splenic laceration connects opposed visceral surfaces and, when multiple, defines a shattered spleen. All patients with splenic lacerations will have perisplenic fluid. Of note, the size of the spleen can change substantially from scans obtained soon after trauma to those obtained at later follow-up (38). This change is attributed to initial adrenergic contraction in response to volume loss or parenchymal injury.

CT pitfalls include scanning too early (20–50 seconds) during the inhomogeneous "red pulp" (ie, sinusoidal) stage of enhancement, an appearance that may also be produced by marked hypotension. Later phase scans (70–100 seconds) will clarify this early inhomogeneity. Normal splenic clefts may be misinterpreted as lacerations, but they will not have associated intraperitoneal fluid, are smooth in contour, and are usually medially located in the spleen. Elongation of the contiguous left lobe of the liver may simulate a linear laceration in the spleen (13). Motion, beam-hardening, volume-averaging, or streak artifacts can usually be recognized by employing multiple window settings and checking for similar artifacts in other organs.

CT OF LIVER TRAUMA

The liver is the second most frequently injured (20%) intraabdominal viscus, in part due to its relatively fixed position, large size, and friability (4). Liver laceration is half as frequent as splenic laceration but results in greater morbidity; 45% of patients with liver injury also have splenic injury (11). With extensive injury that includes the thin liver capsule, intraperitoneal hemorrhage may be marked due to the dual blood supply of the liver and inability of liver veins to contract to foster hemostasis (4). If the liver capsule remains intact, injuries may be less consequential due to containment of hemorrhage (36). The liver has the remarkable ability to heal after even complex and severe injury and does not appear to be prone to delayed rupture, such as occurs after splenic injury (13). CT evidence of healing typically may take 1–6 months but may take up to 15 months with a more severe injury (39).

On CT scans, the most frequent site of injury is the posterior segment of the right lobe of the liver, in part because it is large but also because it is near the ribs and spine. While injuries to the left lobe of the liver are less common than those to the right lobe, left lobe injuries are more often associated with damage to the retroperitoneum (duodenum and pancreas) and to the transverse colon (6). The most common liver lacerations are perivascular, paralleling the right and middle hepatic arteries and posterior branches of the right portal vein. Hepatic vein damage occurs in approximately 13% of liver injuries, often as a result of avulsion of the right hepatic vein from the inferior vena cava. Such vein damage may be suggested on CT scans by multiple lacerations around the inferior vena cava or porta hepatis (4). Advanced notice of possible hepatic vein avulsion may prepare surgeons for massive hemorrhage that can occur when the liver is lifted off the inferior vena cava. Laceration that extends only to the bare area of the liver may not have associated peritoneal signs, is often associated with CT findings of retroperitoneal blood, and will be missed with diagnostic peritoneal lavage or US used to screen for hemoperitoneum (40).

Periportal low attenuation (tracking) is found at CT in up to 22% of patients with blunt abdominal trauma. The cause is controversial and may be either blood tracking adjacent to portal branches or may be dilated periportal lymphatics (13,41, 42). Diffuse periportal low attenuation may be due to dilated interlobar lymphatics from elevated central venous pressure after vigorous intravenous fluid resuscitation or injury to the lymphatic system of the liver. Focal periportal low attenuation may be due to localized dissecting hemorrhage or bile. Focal periportal tracking is associated with a high occurrence of hepatic injury and should stimulate a careful search of CT scans (43). Neither diffuse nor focal periportal tracking preclude nonsurgical management of liver injury (44).

CT is the most sensitive test for detecting and characterizing traumatic injury to the liver (12). Helical CT scans of the liver obtained entirely during the period of peak enhancement provide excellent delineation of liver parenchyma and the porta hepatis. Liver lacerations appear on CT scans as nonenhancing irregular, linear, round, or branching regions of low attenuation. Lacerations may extend to the visceral surface to produce isolated parenchymal fragments or complex parallel lines of a "bear-claw" appearance (4). Focal hepatic devascularization may appear as wedges of low attenuation that extend to the liver surface. Liver intraparenchymal hematomas are masslike, well-defined regions of decreased attenuation compared with enhanced parenchyma (Fig 3), while contusions are less well defined. Subcapsular hematomas appear as crescentic lenticular fluid collections that cause compression of underlying parenchyma and are often associated with rib fractures (11). Intrahepatic or subcapsular gas may be detected, usually 1–3 days after injury. Such gas is usually due to necrosis, not infection (45). Active, ongoing hemorrhage on enhanced CT scans appears as focal, irregular areas of high attenuation (80–350 HU), sometimes with adjacent sentinel clot. Several CT grading criteria have been proposed for liver injury, but, as with the spleen, none correlates well with the need for surgical intervention or subsequent complication (46,47).

Focal fatty infiltration can be a pitfall in CT of liver trauma because it can simulate a hematoma. Diffuse fatty infiltration can create a pitfall by making low-attenuation hematoma harder to identify. These problems can be solved by using narrow window settings to identify fat. Other pitfalls include an unusually elongated left lobe of the liver, which may appear separated from the right lobe; a prominent cleft in the undersurface of the liver; and streak or beam-hardening artifact from air-fluid levels in the stomach or from ribs.

Surgical series have shown that up to 80% of liver injuries in adults and up to 97% in children can be treated without surgery, especially in the absence of associated injuries to other organs that would require surgery and in the absence of marked hemodynamic instability (15,16,48–53). This nonsurgical approach largely has been made possible by the increased diagnostic confidence produced with CT (6). Active hemorrhage detected with CT may be treated with angiography and selective embolization with considerable

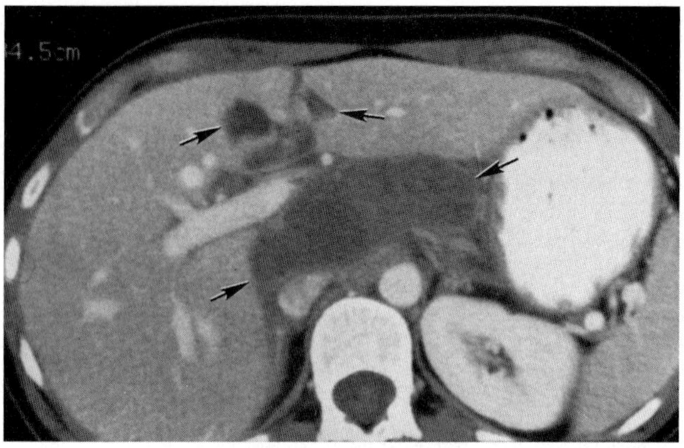

Figure 4. Helical CT ▶ scan shows multiple intrahepatic and porta hepatis bilomas (arrows) detected 4 days after trauma. These required only a single percutaneous drain.

success (54). Delayed complications occur in about 20% of liver injuries due to portal triad injury or devitalized liver tissue. These complications include recurrent bleeding, arterioportal fistula, pseudoaneurysm, biloma (Fig 4), and obstructive jaundice from mass effect of bilomas or hematoma. Bile in a liver hematoma results in delayed healing rates and biloma in some cases. Delayed CT before discharge may be more important after liver injury than after splenic injury due to the greater number of potential delayed complications (55,56). On such delayed CT scans, arterioportal fistulas appear as early and intense contrast enhancement of the portal vein, whereas pseudoaneurysms appear as rounded focal areas of intense enhancement adjacent to arterial structures. Bilomas are round or crescentic, well-defined, low-attenuation regions either within the liver parenchyma or adjacent to the liver. The mass effect of a biloma can press on branch or main hepatic bile ducts, resulting in biliary dilatation.

CT OF GALLBLADDER AND BILIARY TRAUMA

The gallbladder is rarely injured during abdominal trauma due to its well-protected recessed location. Only 2% of abdominal injuries for which laparotomy is performed include the gallbladder; many have associated injuries of the liver or duodenum (4,57). Unfortunately, alcohol causes distention of the gallbladder by increasing bile flow while causing contraction of the sphincter of Oddi (58), presumably making the gallbladder more prone to injury at the same time the alcohol makes trauma more likely. Delay in diagnosis of gallbladder rupture can lead to major complications, so early detec-

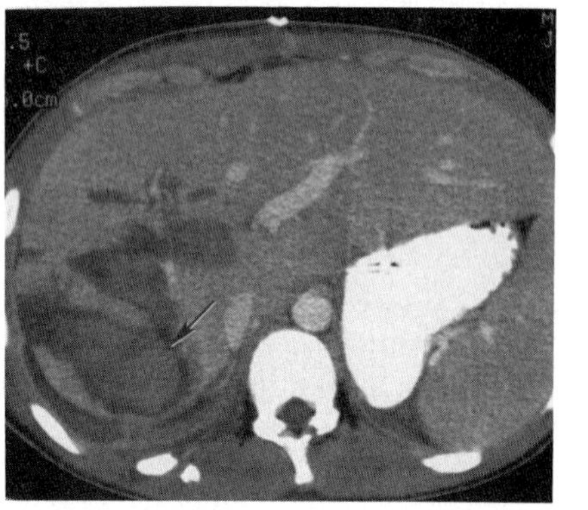

Figure 3. Helical CT scan shows extensive liver laceration and hyperattenuating intraparenchymal hematoma (arrow). Note adjacent lower attenuation fluid. This patient was successfully treated without surgery.

tion and surgical intervention are important (59).

The spectrum of traumatic gallbladder injuries ranges from wall contusion and laceration to traumatic perforation or cholecystectomy with avulsion of the cystic duct and artery (4). Cystic artery avulsion may result in major blood loss leading to hemodynamic instability (58). Uninfected bile in the peritoneal space may produce little or no symptoms for long periods of time. Alternatively, since the gallbladder is extraperitoneal, bile leak from a ruptured gallbladder may be contained in the extraperitoneal gallbladder fossa. For these reasons, neither clinical signs and symptoms nor bile obtained at diagnostic peritoneal lavage is a reliable indicator of gallbladder injury. The diagnosis is frequently not made before laparotomy.

CT findings of gallbladder injury are varied and include pericholecystic fluid (most common), blurring of the contour of the gallbladder, focal thickening or discontinuity of the gallbladder wall (Fig 5), or an enhancing mucosal flap seen within the

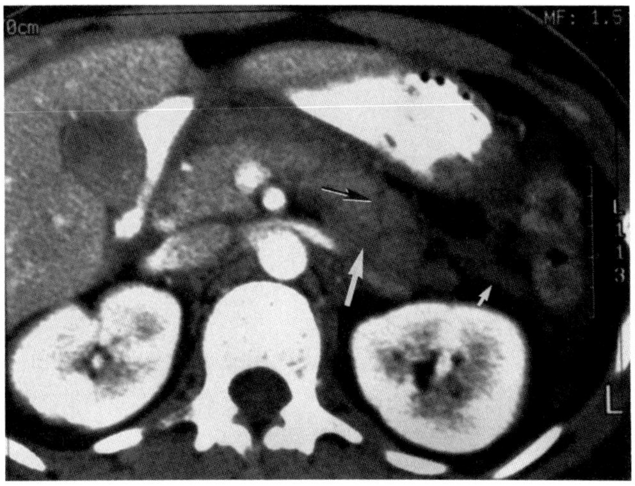

Figure 6. Helical CT scan shows fracture of the tail of the pancreas. Note the vertical line across the pancreas (black arrow), fluid posterior to the tail of the pancreas (large arrow), and thickening of the left anterior pararenal fascia (small arrow).

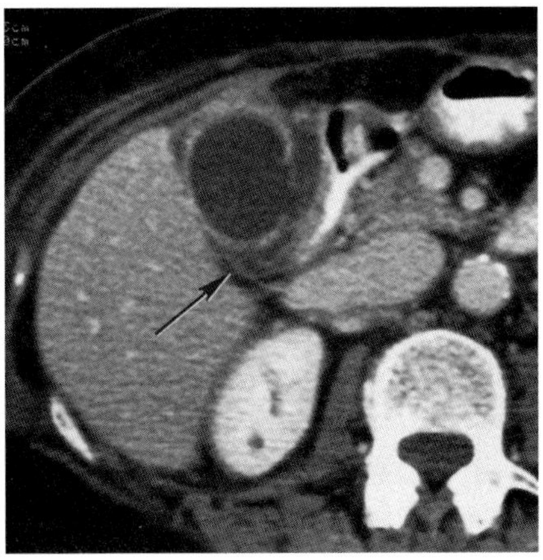

Figure 5. Helical CT scan shows gallbladder rupture. Note discontinuity of the gallbladder wall, mass effect on the duodenum, and free bile (arrow).

lumen (4,59). Additionally, blood (high attenuation) may be found in the gallbladder lumen along with mass effect on the adjacent duodenum (Fig 5)(59). A ruptured gallbladder may be collapsed or be associated with focal periportal tracking in the liver near the porta hepatis. Adjacent liver lacerations or duodenal injury is common, as is intraperitoneal free fluid, which may be of high attenuation (blood) or low attenuation (bile). US-guided paracentesis may be a useful technique to determine the nature of the fluid. Alternatively, hepatobiliary radionuclide imaging may depict bile leak from the gallbladder; delayed images (4 hours) are important. US findings of gallbladder injury include focal hypoechoic thickening of the gallbladder wall, pericholecystic fluid, echogenic mass in the gallbladder, and free intraperitoneal fluid (60). The CT diagnosis of gallbladder injury is challenging since some of the signs are nonspecific, including pericholecystic fluid and intraluminal hemorrhage (59). Blood in the gallbladder may come from liver injury, may by itself cause cholecystitis, or may obstruct the cystic duct with clot. Further, the gallbladder probably can reseal after traumatic microperforation, creating the impression of false-positive CT findings. Delayed CT or US of the gallbladder region at 1–3 weeks may be useful for detection of complications and confirmation of healing if a cholecystectomy is not performed (59).

Of all injuries to the extrahepatic biliary tract, 80% are to the gallbladder and only 20% are to the bile ducts (61,62). Bile duct laceration may be partial or complete; either is associated with a 20% mortality (62). Laceration is most commonly located either where the hepatic duct exits the liver or where the bile duct enters the head of the pancreas, sites of relative fixation (61). Associated injuries of the portal vein or hepatic artery are very rare because these structures are more elastic than the bile duct. Clinical diagnosis of bile duct injury is difficult since free uninfected intraperitoneal bile may produce no symptoms or bile may be contained in an extraperitoneal location; diagnosis before surgery is rare and may be delayed in patients not undergoing surgery (61). CT findings of bile duct injury include edema in the hepatoduodenal ligament area, free intraperitoneal fluid, and associated liver or duodenal injuries.

CT OF PANCREATIC TRAUMA

Pancreatic injury is encountered in only about 3% of abdominal trauma cases that require surgery (12). The mechanism of injury is midline compression against the vertebral column and shear across the neck of the pancreas. Trauma from a steering wheel, seat belt, bicycle handlebar, or football helmet are frequent causes (63). Pancreatic injury is more common in young adults, possibly because of less retroperitoneal fat to act as a protective buffer (11). Pancreatic injury is almost always associated with other organ injury, especially of the liver and duodenum (63). Immediate laparotomy with repair or resection of the pancreas proximal to the fracture is curative. Delay in diagnosis results in recurrent pancreatitis, pseudocyst, fistula, or abscess formation with attendant mortality of 20% (12,64,65). Leukocytosis and hyperamylasemia are uncommon early on and are nonspecific findings that can result from bowel injury (36,64). The retroperitoneal location of the pancreas may delay the manifestation of clinical signs and symptoms (63).

CT is the most effective imaging modality for diagnosing pancreatic injury, but a high index of suspicion is required (65–67). The spectrum of CT findings includes subtle edema or fluid in the peripancreatic fat, focal or diffuse pancreatic enlargement, irregularity of the pancreatic contour, or a fracture line with separation across the long axis of the pancreas in the body or neck (Fig 6)(68). More remote signs include fluid around the superior mesenteric artery, fluid in the transverse mesocolon or lesser sac, fluid between the pancreas and the splenic vein, and thickening of the left anterior pararenal fascia (Fig 6)(11,65,68–70). The presence of retroperitoneal fluid collections suggests pancreatic duct disruption, which may require emergent endoscopic retrograde cholangiopancreatography or magnetic resonance pancreatography for diagnosis (71). While CT sensitivity has been high in reported small series, CT findings may be minimal even with pancreatic transection, since the elastic pancreatic parenchyma may resume its normal contour (65,66). Rarely, major pancreatic duct injury may be present without changes on initial early CT scans (66,67,72). Delayed CT 24–48 hours after injury may often uncover findings not present on earlier scans.

CT pitfalls result from volume-averaging, beam-hardening, and streak artifacts and poor bowel opacification. The duodenum and jejunum can produce a "pseudofracture" appearance against the adjacent pancreas. The use of helical CT may improve the detection of pancreatic injury

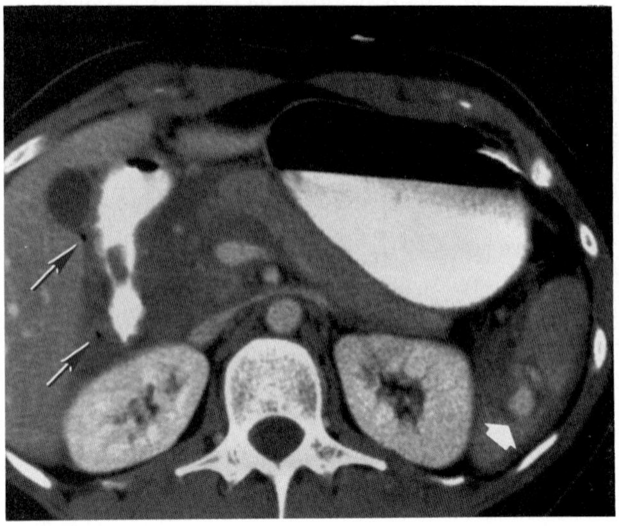

7.

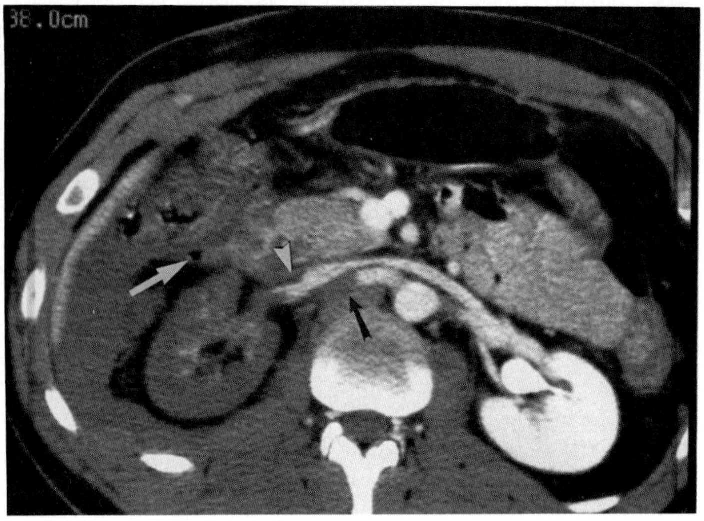

8.

Figures 7, 8. **(7)** Helical CT scan shows duodenal perforation with thickening of the wall, extraluminal gas (arrows), and adjacent fluid. Note active splenic hemorrhage. **(8)** Helical CT scan shows evidence of renal vascular trauma. Note absence of perfusion of the right kidney, thrombus in the right renal artery (black arrow), and thrombus in the right renal vein (arrowhead). Fluid in the anterior pararenal space is contiguous with a perforated duodenum, which shows wall thickening and extraluminal gas (white arrow).

through better parenchymal enhancement with arterial phase imaging, better blood vessel identification, and decreased partial-volume effect by using breath holding, thin collimation, and overlapped reconstructions (65).

US is suitable for diagnosing focal or diffuse pancreatitis or pseudocyst, but US generally does not depict pancreatic fracture (65,73). Because of the retroperitoneal location of the pancreas, fluid aspirated at diagnostic peritoneal lavage may be negative and may not show increased amylase (11).

CT OF BOWEL AND MESENTERIC TRAUMA

About 5% of patients undergoing surgery after trauma have bowel or mesenteric injury, often associated with other organ injuries (74). Again, clinical signs and symptoms may be absent, minimal, or delayed beyond 24 hours. However, delay in surgical therapy markedly increases morbidity, especially rupture of the retroperitoneal duodenum (second and third portions) for which mortality reaches 65% if the diagnosis is not made soon after injury (75). Whereas duodenal perforation or transection necessitates rapid surgery, duodenal hematoma does not. CT findings of focal wall thickening in the duodenum can be seen in either case; however, extraluminal gas or contrast material are seen at CT only with perforation (Figs 7, 8)(76). CT findings may be subtle with only tiny extraluminal gas bubbles or minimal duodenal fold thickening. Abnormality in the right anterior pararenal space can be a particular hint of duodenal injury, as can injury to the adjacent head of the pancreas.

Small-bowel injury generally occurs at points of fixation such as the ligament of Treitz or at the ileocecal valve. Direct injury occurs on the mesenteric side, whereas blow-out injury from increased intraluminal pressure occurs along the antimesenteric border (77). At CT, intramural hematoma appears as focal bowel wall thickening of greater than 3 mm; if the hematoma is large, obstruction can result (36). Free intraperitoneal air is seen at CT in only 32% of bowel ruptures, and extravasation of oral contrast material is not common; therefore, these are specific but not sensitive findings (11). Care should be taken to search CT scans with both broad window (for gas) and narrow window (for subtle extraluminal contrast material or intramural hematoma) settings (78). Focal discontinuity of bowel wall and the sentinel clot sign adjacent to bowel are additional suggestive CT findings (79). Streaky CT attenuation in the mesentery correlates with small-intestine rupture and may be due to both direct mesenteric injury and chemical irritation of the mesentery from spilled intestinal contents (77). The CT finding of intraperitoneal fluid in the absence of organ injury, particularly triangular areas of low-attenuation fluid between bowel loops, should prompt a careful search of bowel with judicious use of additional oral contrast material (Fig 9)(18,78). These patients may be treated conservatively and may not require surgery.

Overall, the sensitivity of CT to traumatic bowel injury varies between 88% and 92% with an accuracy of 94% despite the subtle nature of CT findings (79–81). These high accuracy numbers for CT are particularly relevant to the nonsurgical management of solid-organ injuries, since such an approach should only be undertaken if bowel perforation is ruled out with certainty. Here, the inability of US to facilitate diagnosis of the subtle signs of bowel perforation suggests that US lacks the sensitivity needed to enable safe nonsurgical therapy of abdominal trauma (81).

Three additional points regarding bowel injury should be mentioned. First, diffuse thickening of small-bowel wall with increased CT contrast enhancement plus luminal fluid dilatation are signs of hypotensive "shock bowel" and not perforation. Shock bowel is usually associated with a slitlike inferior vena cava, a normal colon, and recovery of normal bowel function after resuscitation (82). Additional CT findings associated with shock-related hypotension may include a small aorta from reactive arterial constriction, decreased enhancement of the spleen, and marked enhancement of the ad-

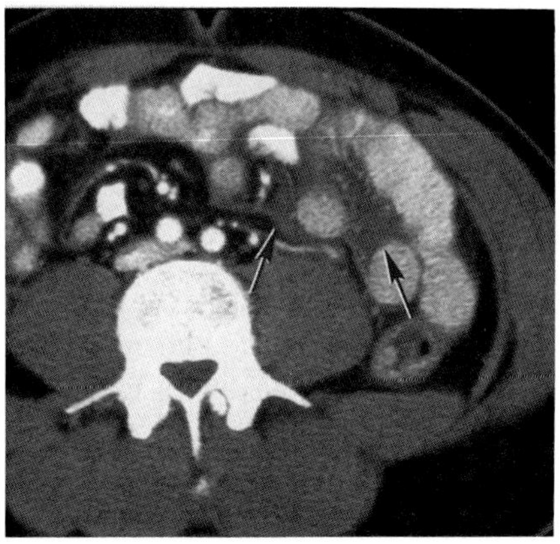

Figure 9. Helical CT scan shows a triangular area of intraperitoneal fluid (arrows) between small-bowel loops associated with occult perforation. Finding of such collections should stimulate a thorough search for bowel injury. Note excellent opacification of the small bowel with oral contrast material.

renal glands. Particularly in children and young adults, blood pressure may be normal despite considerable volume loss and evidence of that volume depletion on CT scans.

Second, free intraperitoneal air can often be present on CT scans in trauma patients in the absence of hollow-viscus injury (83,84). This air may be due to sealed-off microperforations after barotrauma, pneumothorax (via the diaphragm), or subcutaneous dissection from the chest, especially if a chest tube is present. Air may also enter through the female genital tract. While such air detected with CT has no clinical consequence, it should prompt a careful search for other CT signs of organ injury and close clinical observation of the patient to rule out perforation necessitating surgery.

Third, rarely mesenteric injury may be isolated and not associated with other bowel or organ injury. Such injuries may consist of mesenteric hematoma or avulsion of a portion of the mesentery from bowel, which may result in considerable blood loss or focal bowel wall ischemia (85). Given the rarity of this injury, the sensitivity of CT has not been reported. CT findings might consist of a focal mesenteric hematoma of varying attenuation or streaky mesenteric attenuation.

CT OF URINARY TRACT TRAUMA

Injury to the kidneys is very common in blunt abdominal trauma, but parenchymal contusions and minor superficial lacerations that do not necessitate surgery account for 95% of cases (86). Patients with hematuria of less than 35 red blood cells per high-power field, with no history of hypotension and with no pelvic fracture, probably need no imaging of their urinary tract (87). Occasionally, trauma to the renal pedicle or traumatic renal vein thrombosis may have no associated hematuria; this presents a diagnostic dilemma that requires correlation with mechanism and severity of trauma. In patients with gross hematuria or any hematuria plus a pelvic fracture or diastasis of the symphysis, CT is needed to evaluate the kidneys, ureters, and other abdominal structures since there is a strong correlation between renal injury and injury to other organs (88). Delayed CT images are important to check for urine leak, which is typically treated with placement of a ureteral stent. Delayed CT is also useful to separate extravasated urine (which accumulates) from extravasated arterial contrast material (which dilutes after the bolus is stopped). CT provides better information than intravenous pyelography regarding the extent of renal parenchymal injury and hematoma, the status of the collecting system, and the presence of renal vascular injury (Fig 8)(11). Even major renal lacerations with urine leak in stable patients may be treated nonsurgically, with observation and placement of a stent in the ureter. However, injuries with persistent large urine leak, ureteropelvic junction avulsion, enlarging central or subcapsular hematoma, or extensively devitalized parenchyma (particularly in an immunocompromised patient) need surgical intervention (89,90). Treatment of the devascularized kidney is controversial, but surgeons at some centers do not attempt salvage if the contralateral kidney is intact.

Helical CT in the arterial phase (20–30 seconds) is useful to help delineate renal arterial injury (Fig 8). Helical CT in the early cortical phase (40–70 seconds) of the renal parenchyma may not depict injury. Later imaging in the nephrogram phase (80 seconds or later) for detection of renal parenchymal and venous injury and delayed images (2–10 minutes) for detection of extravasation of urine or blood are important to complete the evaluation.

Contusions appear on CT scans as focal patchy areas of decreased enhancement or as a striated nephrogram similar to that seen with pyelonephritis. Renal lacerations are irregular, linear low-attenuation areas in the parenchyma. Lacerations that connect two cortical surfaces through the hilum are termed fractures. Multiple separated renal fragments, which may be perfused or nonperfused, are termed shattered kidney. The subcapsular hematoma appears on CT scans as a superficial, crescentic, low-attenuation area that compresses the adjacent renal parenchyma. Helical CT may depict nonocclusive intimal injury of the main renal artery or show wedge-shaped decreased parenchymal perfusion due to segmental arterial injury. The cortical rim sign of a devascularized kidney often is not present in the acute setting, during which only diffuse nonperfusion is demonstrated. Renal vein thrombosis appears as a persistent nephrogram on delayed scans; the thrombus may be directly visualized in the renal vein at CT (Fig 8)(11). With US, quantifying complex renal injuries, identifying urine leak, and evaluating vascular damage is time consuming and challenging, if not impossible, in the acutely traumatized patient (91). Further, US is notorious for not depicting even a large retroperitoneal hematoma (92).

Bladder injuries are rare; about 70% are associated with pelvic fractures (11). In patients with hematuria, bladder trauma can be evaluated by adding a CT cystogram to the routine CT examination of the abdomen. Before a cystogram is obtained, the urethra should be evaluated for injury, particularly in patients with pelvic fracture. Blood at the urethral meatus, a "floating" prostate, inability to pass a Foley catheter, or symphysis diastasis all suggest urethral injury and should be evaluated with a urethrogram (93). If the urethra is not injured, CT cystography is performed with 350 mL of 5% contrast material instilled into the bladder through a Foley catheter (94). Routine trauma CT scans are then obtained, including scans through the bladder and low pelvic region.

On CT cystograms, contusions appear as focal thickening of the bladder wall of variable attenuation. Bladder ruptures appear as extravasated contrast material and can be extraperitoneal (usually associated with a pelvic fracture) or intraperitoneal (usually rupture of the dome from a blow to a full bladder). In extraperitoneal rupture, contrast material is seen in the perivesicular fat and prevesical space, the anterior abdominal wall and thigh, and the penis and scrotum; it is usually treated with suprapubic drainage. In intraperitoneal rupture, contrast material is seen in the pericolic gutters, around loops of bowel, or in the pouch of Douglas; it is usually treated with surgery (20,95).

WHAT ABOUT TRAUMA US?

A review of the literature advocating the use of US in patients with blunt abdominal trauma between 1989 and 1997 shows three distinct roles proposed for this modality. The first proposed role for US is to confirm the presence of hemoperitoneum in a hemodynamically unstable patient just before taking the patient to the operating room (96,97). In this role, US is advocated as a quicker, less invasive replacement for diagnostic peritoneal lavage, although it carries a false-negative rate of about 18%. Most authors report the sensitivity of US for detection of hemoperitoneum is about 82%; a few report a somewhat higher sensitivity (96–103). Most also report that US can be performed quickly when limited to evaluation for hemoperitoneum, usually in less than 3 minutes (101,104).

The second proposed role for US is to search for hemoperitoneum in stable patients with blunt trauma on the assumption that patients with positive US findings (hemoperitoneum) can be worked up with subsequent CT and patients with negative US examinations can be admitted for observation (100–105). Since at many trauma centers intraabdominal injury is found in only 10%–20% of patients, this approach might considerably decrease the use of CT. It is argued that surgeons and emergency room physicians can learn to do such limited focused US examinations after 8 hours of lectures and a few clinical cases for experience (103). Others, however, document with data that it can take up to 3 years of experience at performing abdominal US in a busy trauma center before the false-positive rate becomes acceptably low (100,106). Most authors who advocate US for detection of hemoperitoneum state that the decision of whether to perform US in each patient was at the discretion of the trauma attending physician, a major potential source of bias in selecting cases that may make trauma US appear safer and more sensitive than would a series of unselected cases. Some such published series also exclude patients with hematuria or "suspected retroperitoneal injury" (101,105). None of the studies accounted for the cost of admitting and observing all patients, necessitated by the relatively low sensitivity of US to hemoperitoneum (about 82%) and the inexact correlation between the presence of hemoperitoneum and the presence of injury necessitating observation or surgery. Embedded within these published series is a consistent rate of important missed intraabdominal abnormalities, such as small-bowel perforation, duodenal perforation, pancreatic fracture, and subcapsular splenic hematoma with subsequent delayed rupture (98,100, 102,103,105,107). These are the exact types of injuries that carry increased morbidity if diagnosis is delayed. These are also the types of injuries that must be detected accurately if a nonsurgical approach is taken with solid-organ trauma. Regardless, it is this limited role for US (ie, detection of hemoperitoneum in stable patients) that has been advocated most recently in the trauma literature.

The final proposed role for US is searching for both hemoperitoneum and organ plus viscus injury in the peritoneum and retroperitoneum in stable trauma patients. In this role, the training and experience of the US examiner become paramount. Many trauma radiologists with considerable experience in US are not comfortable relying on US alone for detecting organ injury or bowel perforation. Virtually all radiologists would advise against its use to detect injury in the retroperitoneum. Reported sensitivities of US for detection of organ injury in the trauma literature vary between 41% and 93% but tend toward the lower portion of this range (108–110). Predictably, this approach, which was much in vogue in the early 1990s, has been less evident more recently.

CONCLUSION

Hemodynamically unstable patients who are brought to the emergency department with blunt abdominal trauma may need to go directly to the operating room. Alternatively, a rapid US examination performed by well-trained and experienced personnel (preferably readily available radiologists) may give useful information about the presence of hemoperitoneum. Diagnostic peritoneal lavage is very sensitive in the detection of intraperitoneal hemorrhage; however, it does not enable identification of the source of hemoperitoneum, detection of retroperitoneal injuries, or separation of inconsequential from clinically important bleeding. It is worth noting that in those fortunate institutions that have helical CT in the emergency department (or nearby), a helical CT examination can produce more definitive diagnostic information in about the same time as it takes to perform a complete US examination (evaluating for organ injury plus hemoperitoneum) or diagnostic peritoneal lavage. For this reason, rapid-process helical CT may change the treatment of some marginally unstable trauma patients by providing information that enables precise localization of injury or active hemorrhage before surgery. Additionally, angiography with embolization of active hemorrhage detected with helical CT has shown great promise for stopping bleeding while preserving function, particularly in the spleen and in the pelvis.

Hemodynamically stable patients who are brought to the emergency department after blunt abdominal trauma or patients who stabilize after initial resuscitation are candidates for rapid work-up with helical CT. In these patients, the following two decisions need to be made: (*a*) Is urgent surgery needed? and (*b*) if surgery is not needed, is a period of observation necessary or can the patient be safely discharged to home? The answers to both of these questions depend on accurately finding and quantifying all organ plus viscus injuries or active bleeding, best accomplished with helical CT. Patients with severe multiple-organ injury or active bleeding may need surgery even if they are hemodynamically stable. Conversely, stable patients with organ injury may not need surgery (or may need only angiography plus embolization) even if they have a large amount of hemoperitoneum. In this setting, the limitations with US include inability to evaluate the retroperitoneum (kidneys, duodenum, and pancreas), inability to detect bowel injuriy or active bleeding, relatively decreased sensitivity to hemoperitoneum and to solid-organ injury, and inability to distinguish intraperitoneal fluid such as ascites or urine from blood. Regardless of the imaging modality employed, the availability of an experienced radiologist to provide immediate interpretation is critical for the best patient care. ■

References

1. Clancy TV, Ragozzino MW, Ramshaw D, et al. Oral contrast is not necessary in

the evaluation of blunt abdominal trauma by computed tomography. Am J Surg 1993; 166:680–685.
2. Federle MP, Peitzman A, Krugh J. Use of oral contrast material in abdominal trauma CT scans: is it dangerous? J Trauma 1995; 38:51–53.
3. Page B, Dallara J. Metoclopramide in trauma CT scanning: preventing emesis of oral radiographic contrast. Am J Emerg Med 1996; 14:373–376.
4. Shanmuganathan K, Mirvis SE. CT evaluation of the liver with acute blunt trauma. Crit Rev Diagn Imaging 1995; 36:73–113.
5. Wechsler RJ, Spettell CM, Kurtz AB, et al. Effects of training and experience in interpretation of emergency body CT. Radiology 1996; 199:717–720.
6. Jeffrey RB, Olcott EW. Imaging of blunt hepatic trauma. Radiol Clin North Am 1991; 29:1299–1310.
7. DiGiacomo JC, McGonigal MD, Haskal ZJ, et al. Arterial bleeding diagnosed by CT in hemodynamically stable victims of blunt trauma. J Trauma 1996; 40:249–252.
8. Fried AM, Humphries R, Schofield CN. Abdominal CT scans in patients with blunt trauma: low yield in the absence of clinical findings. J Comput Assist Tomogr 1992; 16:717–721.
9. Brasel KJ, Borgstrom DC, Kolewe KA, Weigelt JA. Abdominal computed tomography scan as a screening tool in blunt trauma. Surgery 1996; 120:780–784.
10. McKenney KL, McKenney MG, Nunez DB, Martin L. Cost reduction using ultrasound in blunt abdominal trauma. Emerg Radiol 1997; 4:3–6.
11. Roberts JL. CT of abdominal and pelvic trauma. Semin Ultrasound CT MR 1996; 17:142–169.
12. Raptopoulos V. Abdominal trauma: emphasis on computed tomography. Radiol Clin Norh Am 1994; 32:969–987.
13. Wolfman NT, Bechtold RE, Scharling ES, Meredith JH. Blunt upper abdominal trauma: evaluation by CT. AJR 1992; 158: 493–501.
14. Orwig D, Federle MP. Localized clotted blood as evidence of visceral trauma on CT: the sentinel clot sign. AJR 1989; 153: 747–749.
15. Pachter HL, Knudson MM, Esrig B, et al. Status of nonoperative management of blunt hepatic injuries in 1995: a multicenter experience with 404 patients. J Trauma 1996; 40:31–38.
16. Croce MA, Fabian TC, Menke PG, et al. Nonoperative management of blunt hepatic trauma is the treatment of choice for hemodynamically stable patients. Ann Surg 1995; 221:744–755.
17. Federle MP, Jeffrey RB. Hemoperitoneum studied by CT. Radiology 1983; 148:187–192.
18. Levine CD, Patel UJ, Silverman PM, Wachsberg RH. Low attenuation of acute traumatic hemoperitoneum on CT scans. AJR 1996; 166:1089–1093.
19. Haller JA, Papa P, Drugas G, Colombani P. Nonoperative management of solid organ injuries in children: is it safe? Ann Surg 1994; 219:625–631.
20. Gay SB, Sistrom CL. Computed tomographic evaluation of blunt abdominal trauma. Radiol Clin North Am 1992; 30: 367–387.
21. Federle MP. Computed tomography of blunt abdominal trauma. Radiol Clin North Am 1983; 21:461–474.
22. Becker CD, Spring P, Glattli A, Schweitzer W. Blunt splenic trauma in adults: can CT findings be used to determine the need for surgery? AJR 1994; 162:343–347.
23. Kohn JS, Clark DE, Isler RJ, Pope CF. Is computed tomographic grading of splenic injury useful in the nonsurgical management of blunt trauma? J Trauma 1994; 36:385–389.
24. Mirvis SE, Whitley NO, Gens DR. Blunt splenic trauma in adults: CT-based classification and correlation with prognosis and treatment. Radiology 1989; 171:33–39.
25. Smith JS, Wengrovitz MA, DeLong BS. Prospective validation of criteria, including age, for safe, nonsurgical management of the ruptured spleen. J Trauma 1992; 33:368–369.
26. Umlas SL, Cronan JJ. Splenic trauma: can CT grading systems enable prediction of successful nonsurgical treatment? Radiology 1991; 178:481–487.
27. Garber BG, Yelle JD, Smith RF, Lorimer JW, Carson C. Management of splenic injuries in a Canadian trauma center. Can J Surg 1996; 39:474–480.
28. Allins A. Limited value of routine followup CT scans in nonoperative management of blunt liver and splenic injuries. Am Surg 1996; 62:883–886.
29. Lawson DE, Jacobson JA, Spizarny DL, Pranikoff T. Splenic trauma: value of follow-up CT. Radiology 1995; 194:97–100.
30. Ciraulo DL, Nikkanen HE, Palter M, et al. Clinical analysis of the utility of repeated computed tomographic scan before discharge in blunt hepatic trauma. J Trauma 1996; 41:821–824.
31. Gavant ML, Schurr M, Flick PA, et al. Predicting clinical outcome of nonsurgical management of blunt splenic injury: using CT to reveal abnormalities of splenic vasculature. AJR 1997; 168:207–212.
32. Schurr MJ, Fabian TC, Gavant M, et al. Management of blunt splenic trauma: computed tomographic contrast blush predicts failure of non-operative management. J Trauma 1995; 39:507–513.
33. Sclafani SJ, Weisberg A, Scalea TM, Phillips TF, Duncan AO. Blunt splenic injuries: nonsurgical treatment with CT, arteriography, and transcatheter arterial embolization of the splenic artery. Radiology 1991; 181:189–196.
34. Kluger Y, Paul DB, Raves JJ, et al. Delayed rupture of the spleen: myths, facts, and their importance—case reports and a literature review. J Trauma 1994; 36:568–571.
35. Farhat GA, Abdu RA, Vanek VW. Delayed splenic rupture: real or imaginary. Am Surg 1992; 58:340–345.
36. Roberts JL, Dalen K, Bosanko CM, Jafir SZ. CT in abdominal and pelvic trauma. RadioGraphics 1993; 13:735–752.
37. Shammuganathan K, Mirvis SE, Sover ER. Value of contrast enhanced CT in detecting active hemorrhage in patients with blunt abdominal trauma or pelvic trauma. AJR 1993; 161:65–69.
38. Goodman LR, Aprahamian C. Changes in splenic size after abdominal trauma. Radiology 1990; 176:629–632.
39. Bulas DI, Eichelberger MR, Sivit CJ, et al. Hepatic injury from blunt trauma in children: follow-up evaluation with CT. AJR 1993; 160:347–351.
40. Patten RM, Spear RP, Vincent LM, Hesla RB, Jurkovich GJ. Traumatic laceration of the liver limited to the bare area: CT findings in 25 patients. AJR 1993; 160:1019–1022.
41. Patrick LE, Ball TI, Atkinson GO, Winn KJ. Pediatric blunt abdominal trauma: periportal tracking at CT. Radiology 1992; 183:689–691.
42. Shammuganathan K, Mirvis SE, Amoroso M. Periportal low density on CT in patients with blunt trauma: association with elevated venous pressure. AJR 1993; 160: 279–283.
43. Yokota J, Sugimoto T. Clinical significance of periportal tracking on computed tomographic scan in patients with blunt liver trauma. Am J Surg 1994; 168:247–250.
44. Davis KA, Brody JM, Cioffi WG. Computed tomography in blunt hepatic trauma. Arch Surg 1996; 131:255–260.
45. Abramson SJ, Berdon WE, Kaufman RA, et al. Hepatic parenchymal and subcapsular gas after hepatic laceration caused by blunt abdominal trauma. AJR 1989; 153:1031–1032.
46. Mirvis SE, Whitley NO, Vainwright JR, Gens DR. Blunt hepatic trauma in adults: CT-based classification and correlation with prognosis and treatment. Radiology 1989; 171:27–32.
47. Becker CD, Gal I, Baer HU, Vock P. Blunt hepatic trauma in adults: correlation of CT injury grading with outcome. Radiology 1996; 201:215–220.
48. Meredith JW, Young JS, Bowling J, Roboussin D. Nonoperative management of blunt hepatic trauma: the exception or the rule? J Trauma 1994; 36:529–536.
49. Boone DC, Federle M, Billiar TR, Udekwu AO, Pietzman AB. Evolution of management of major hepatic trauma: identification of patterns of injury. J Trauma 1995; 39:344–350.
50. Sherman HF, Savage BA, Jones LM, et al. Nonoperative management of blunt hepatic injuries: safe at any grade? J Trauma 1994; 37:616–621.
51. Goff CD, Gilbert CM. Nonoperative management of blunt hepatic trauma. Am Surg 1995; 61:66–68.
52. Croce MA, Fabian TC, Kudsk KA, et al. AAST organ injury scale: correlation of CT-graded liver injuries and operative findings. J Trauma 1991; 31:806–812.
53. Bond SJ, Eichelberger MR, Gotschall CS, Sivit CJ, Randolph JG. Nonoperative management of blunt hepatic and splenic injury in children. Ann Surg 1996; 223:286–289.
54. De Toma G, Mingoli A, Modini C, Cavallaro A, Stipa S. The value of angiography and selective hepatic artery embolization for continuous bleeding after surgery in liver trauma: case reports. J Trauma 1994; 37:508-511.
55. Knudson MM, Lim RC, Oakes DD, Jeffrey RB. Nonoperative management of blunt liver injuries in adults: the need for continued surveillance. J Trauma 1990; 30:1494–1500.
56. Bynoe RP, Bell RM, Miles WS, et al. Complications of nonoperative management of blunt hepatic injuries. J Trauma 1992; 32:308–315.
57. Sharma O. Blunt gallbladder injuries: presentation of twenty-two cases with review of the literature. J Trauma 1995; 39: 576–580.
58. Jeffrey RB, Federle MF, Laing FC, Wing VW. Computed tomography of blunt trauma to the gallbladder. J Comput Assist Tomogr 1986; 10:756–758.
59. Erb RE, Mirvis SE, Shanmuganathan K. Gallbladder injury secondary to blunt trauma: CT findings. J Comput Assist Tomogr 1994; 18:778–784.
60. Gembala RB, Flynn DE, Radecki PD, Friedman AC, Caroline DF. Sonographic diagnosis of traumatic gallbladder avul-

sion. J Ultrasound Med 1993; 5:299–301.
61. Parks RW, Diamond T. Non-surgical trauma to the extrahepatic biliary tract. Br J Surg 1995; 82:1303–1310.
62. Jurkovich GJ, Hoyt DB, Moore FA, et al. Portal triad injuries. J Trauma 1995; 39:426–434.
63. Smith DR, Stanley RJ, Rue LW. Delayed diagnosis of pancreatic transection after blunt abdominal trauma. J Trauma 1996; 40:1009–1013.
64. Emmick RH, Petersen SR. Evaluation of pancreatic injury after blunt abdominal trauma. Ann Emerg Med 1996; 27:658–661.
65. Lane MJ, Mindelzun RE, Jeffrey RB. Diagnosis of pancreatic injury after blunt abdominal trauma. Semin Ultrasound CT MR 1996; 17:177–182.
66. Wong YC, Wang LJ, Lin BC, et al. CT grading of pancreatic injuries: prediction of ductal disruption and surgical correlation. J Comput Assist Tomogr 1997; 21:246–250.
67. Nelson MG, Jones DR, Vasilakis A, Timberlake GA. Computed tomographic diagnosis of acute blunt pancreatic transection. W Va Med J 1994; 90:274–278.
68. Sivit CJ, Eichelberger MR, Taylor GA, et al. Blunt pancreatic trauma in children: CT diagnosis. AJR 1992; 158:1097–1100.
69. Lane MJ, Mindelzun RE, Sandhu JS, McCormick VD, Jeffrey JB. CT diagnosis of blunt pancreatic trauma: importance of detecting fluid between the pancreas and the splenic vein. AJR 1994; 163:833–835.
70. Sivit CJ, Eichelberger MR. CT diagnosis of pancreatic injury in children: significance of fluid separating the splenic vein and pancreas. AJR 1995; 165:921–924.
71. Clements RH, Reisser JR. Urgent endoscopic retrograde pancreatography in the stable trauma patient. Am Surg 1996; 62:446–448.
72. Dodds WJ, Taylor AJ, Erickson SJ, Lawson TL. Traumatic fracture of the pancreas. J Comput Assist Tomogr 1990; 14:375–378.
73. Jeffrey RB, Laing FC, Wing VW. Ultrasound in acute pancreatic trauma. Gastrointest Radiol 1986; 11:44–46.
74. Nghiem HV, Jeffrey RB, Mindelzun RE. CT of blunt trauma to the bowel and mesentery. Semin Ultrasound CT MR 1995; 16:82–90.
75. Motateanu M, Mirescu D, Schwieger AF, Laverriere C. Computed tomography of retroperitoneal duodenal rupture in blunt abdominal trauma. Eur J Radiol 1992; 15:163–165.
76. Kunin JR, Korobkin M, Ellis JH, et al. Duodenal injuries caused by blunt abdominal trauma: value of CT in differentiating perforation from hematoma. AJR 1993; 160:1221–1223.
77. Hagiwara A, Yukioka T, Satou M, et al. Early diagnosis of small intestine rupture from blunt abdominal trauma using computed tomography: significance of the streaky density within the mesentery. J Trauma 1995; 38:630–633.
78. Levine CD, Patel UJ, Wachsberg RH, et al. CT in patients with blunt abdominal trauma: clinical significance of intraperitoneal fluid detected on a scan with otherwise normal findings. AJR 1995; 164: 1381–1385.
79. Rizzo MJ, Federle MP, Griffiths BG. Bowel and mesenteric injury following blunt abdominal trauma: evaluation with CT. Radiology 1989; 173:143–148.
80. Mirvis SE, Gens DR, Shanmuganathan K. Rupture of bowel after blunt abdominal trauma: diagnosis with CT. AJR 1992; 159: 1217–1221.
81. Sherck JM, Shatney C, Sensaki K, Selivanov V. The accuracy of computed tomography in the diagnosis of blunt small-bowel perforation. Am J Surg 1994; 168:670–675.
82. Mirvis SE, Shanmuganathan K, Erb R. Diffuse small bowel ischemia after blunt abdominal trauma (shock bowel): CT findings and clinical significance. AJR 1994; 163:1375–1379.
83. Hamilton P, Rizoli S, McLellan B, Murphy J. Significance of intra-abdominal extraluminal air detected by CT scan in blunt abdominal trauma. J Trauma 1995; 39:331–333.
84. Kane NM, Francis IR, Burney RE, et al. Traumatic pneumoperitoneum: implications of computed tomography diagnosis. Invest Radiol 1991; 26:574–578.
85. Nolan BW, Gabram SG, Schwartz RJ, Jacobs LM. Mesenteric injury from blunt abdominal trauma. Am Surg 1995; 61:501–506.
86. Matthews LA, Spirnak JP. The nonoperative approach to major blunt renal trauma. Semin Urol 1995; 13:77–82.
87. Eastham JAS, Wilson TG, Ahlering TE. Radiographic evaluation of patients with blunt renal trauma. J Urol 1992; 148:266–267.
88. Kristjansson A, Pedersen J. Management of blunt renal trauma. Br J Urol 1993; 72:692–696.
89. Thall EH, Stone NN, Cheng DL, et al. Conservative management of penetrating and blunt type III renal injuries. Br J Urol 1996; 77:512–517.
90. Husmann DA, Gilling PJ, Perry MO, et al. Major renal lacerations with devitalized fragment following blunt abdominal trauma. J Urol 1993; 150:1774–1777.
91. Pollack HM, Wein AJ. Imaging of renal trauma. Radiology 1989; 172:297–308.
92. Shuman WP, Hastrup W, Kohler TR, et al. Suspected leaking abdominal aortic aneurysm: use of sonography in the emergency room. Radiology 1988; 168:117–119.
93. Fuhrman GM, Simmons GT, Davidson BS, Buerk CA. The single indication for cystography in blunt trauma. Am Surg 1993; 59:335–337.
94. Lis LE, Cohen AJ. CT cystography in the evaluation of bladder trauma. J Comput Assist Tomogr 1990; 14:386–389.
95. Sivit CJ, Cutting JP, Eichelberger MR. CT diagnosis and localization of rupture of the bladder in children with blunt abdominal trauma: significance of contrast material extravasation in the pelvis. AJR 1995; 164:1243–1246.
96. Lentz KA, McKenney MG, Nunez DB, Martin L. Evaluating blunt abdominal trauma: role for ultrasonography. J Ultrasound Med 1996; 15:447–451.
97. Wherett LJ, Boulanger BR, McLellan BA, et al. Hypotension after blunt abdominal trauma: the role of emergent abdominal sonography in surgical triage. J Trauma 1996; 41:815–820.
98. Jehle D, Guarino J, Karamanoukian H. Emergency department ultrasound in the evaluation of blunt abdominal trauma. Am J Emerg Med 1993; 11:342–346.
99. Ma OJ, Mateer JR, Ogata M, et al. Prospective analysis of a rapid trauma ultrasound examination performed by emergency physicians. J Trauma 1995; 38:879–885.
100. Rozycki GS, Ochsner MG, Schjmidt JA, et al. A prospective study of surgeon performed ultrasound as the primary adjuvant modality for injured patient assessment. J Trauma 1995; 39:492–500.
101. Boulanger BR, Brenneman FD, McLellan BA, et al. A prospective study of emergent abdominal sonography after blunt trauma. J Trauma 1995; 39:325–330.
102. Boulanger BR, McLellan BA, Brenneman FD, et al. Emergent abdominal ultrasound as a screening test in a new diagnostic algorithm for blunt trauma. J Trauma 1996; 40:867–874.
103. Thomas B, Falcone RE, Vasquez D, et al. Ultrasound evaluation of blunt abdominal trauma: program implementation, initial experience, and learning curve. J Trauma 1997; 42:384–390.
104. Huang MS, Liu M, Wu JK, et al. Ultrasonography for the evaluation of hemoperitoneum during resuscitation: a simple scoring system. J Trauma 1994; 36:173–177.
105. Mckenney MG, Martin L, Lentz K, et al. 1000 consecutive ultrasounds for blunt abdominal trauma. J Trauma 1996; 40:607–612.
106. Forster R, Pillasch J, Zielke A, Malewski U, Rothmund M. Ultrasonography in blunt abdominal trauma: influence of the investigators' experience. J Trauma 1992; 34:264–269.
107. Healey MA, Simons RK, Winchell RJ, et al. A prospective evaluation of abdominal ultrasound in blunt trauma: is is useful? J Trauma 1996; 40:875–885.
108. Bode PJ, Niezen RA, Van Vugt AB, Schipper J. Abdominal ultrasound as a reliable indicator for conclusive laparotomy in blunt abdominal trauma. J Trauma 1993; 34:27–31.
109. Rothlin MA, Remo N, Amgwerd M, et al. Ultrasound in blunt abdominal and thoracic trauma. J Trauma 1993; 34:488–495.
110. Tso P, Rodriguez A, Cooper C, et al. Sonography in blunt abdominal trauma: a preliminary progress report. J Trauma 1992; 33:39–44.

Andrew H. Cragg, MD • Michael D. Dake, MD

Treatment of Peripheral Vascular Disease with Stent-Grafts[1]

Expandable metallic stents are now commonly used to treat peripheral vascular disease. Endoluminal stents have demonstrated utility in preventing recoil after angioplasty and in reducing restenosis in certain vascular beds. Just as stent placement represented an evolutionary step up from the interventional technology of balloon angioplasty, stent-grafts now are bridging the fields of vascular surgery and interventional radiology. The use of metallic expandable stents to anchor traditional surgical bypass grafts in an endoluminal location has created an opportunity to treat both vascular occlusive disease and aneurysmal disease in a less invasive, interventional fashion. This article outlines the progress made in the development and implementation of endovascular stent-grafts for the treatment of peripheral vascular disease.

RATIONALE FOR USE

The rationale for using stent-grafts in occlusive disease follows the surgical tenet of bypassing the obstructed vessel with a prosthetic conduit. Rather than an extraanatomic bypass, however, the endoluminal stent-graft acts as an endovascular bypass. In so doing, it is hoped that patency after treatment of long lesions (more than 10 cm) or smaller-caliber vessels (less than 6 mm) may be superior to that after conventional balloon angioplasty. Treatment of these lesions with balloon angioplasty is associated with a relatively high recurrence rate. Since the endoluminal bypass lines the diseased vessel with prosthetic material, the vessel may be less susceptible to neointimal ingrowth, which is associated with angioplasty failure.

The rationale for treating peripheral aneurysmal disease with stent-grafts is to isolate the diseased portion of the vessel with an endovascular lining. The expandable portion of the endovascular graft creates a friction seal in the more normal portion of the treated vessel proximal and distal to the aneurysmal lesion. Isolation of the aneurysmal segment in this fashion should result in effective obliteration of the aneurysm and reduce the risk of rupture or distal embolization.

HISTORY OF ENDOLUMINAL GRAFT DEVELOPMENT

In 1969, Charles Dotter proposed the placement of tightly wound steel coils to act as endoluminal stents (1). This concept laid the groundwork for subsequent efforts by a number of investigators to refine this concept for treating both occlusive and aneurysmal disease. During the 1980s most investigators concentrated on the development of open-framework, expandable metallic stents for treating occlusive disease. Some investigators began developing the concept of treating aneurysmal disease with prototype endoluminal stent-grafts (2–4). Experimental work at that time centered around the development of tube grafts of various designs. These included closely wound metallic coils, expandable stents with thin-walled urethane covering, and bulkier designs with conventional graft fabric covering (Fig 1). In 1984, we found that a closely wound metallic tube graft successfully excluded an artificially created aneurysm in a dog (3). Early clinical application of this technique was described by Volodos et al (5). They described the treatment of an iliac aneurysm with use of an expandable Dacron-covered stent. Subsequently, in 1991, Parodi et al described the application of endoluminal stent-graft technology to the treatment of aortic aneurysms (6,7). Since that time there has been widespread interest in this technology for treatment of aortic aneurysms and peripheral occlusive and aneurysmal disease.

GRAFT DESIGNS

Most endoluminal graft designs for peripheral vascular uses have been of a tube-graft–type construction. Aortic stent-grafts are also constructed in a bifurcated fashion. Peripheral stent-grafts are distinguished in two principal ways: by (*a*) the type of stent framework used and (*b*) the type of graft fabric used. Most designs use conventional stents mated to standard bypass graft material. The general characteristics of the known commercial stent-grafts are described in the Table.

Conventional Graft Materials

In most designs to date, conventional graft materials such as polytetrafluoroethylene (PTFE) and polyester (Dacron) have been used. PTFE

Index terms: Aneurysm, iliac, 98.73 • Aneurysm, peripheral, 92.73 • Arteries, grafts and prostheses, 92.1268, 98.1268 • Arteries, stenosis or obstruction, 92.411, 98.411 • Arteries, transluminal angioplasty, 92.1286, 98.1286 • State-of-art reviews

Radiology 1997; 205:307–314

[1] From the Fairview-University Medical Center, 2450 Riverside Ave, Minneapolis, MN 55454 (A.H.C.) and the Department of Radiology, Stanford University Medical Center, Stanford, Calif (M.D.D.). Received April 7, 1997; revision requested April 30; revision received July 10; accepted July 11. **Address reprint requests to** A.H.C.

Abbreviations: AVF = arteriovenous fistula, PTFE = polytetrafluoroethylene, TIPS = transjugular intrahepatic portosystemic shunt.

Commerical Peripheral Stent-Grafts

Name	Vendor	Stent/Graft Material	Stent Location	Diameter (mm)	Length (cm)	Introducer Size (F)	Clinical Status*
Wallgraft	Schneider	Steel alloy/polyester	Inside graft	6–10	3–9	9–11	Active IDE
Hemobahn	Prograft	Nitinol/PTFE	Outside graft	5–12	5–15	8–12	Active IDE
Corvita graft	Schneider	Steel alloy/polycarbonate urethane	Integrated	6–12	Variable	9–10	Active IDE
Passager	Boston Scientific	Nitinol/polyester	Inside graft	5–12	3–10	8–10	Active IDE

* IDE = investigational device exemption.

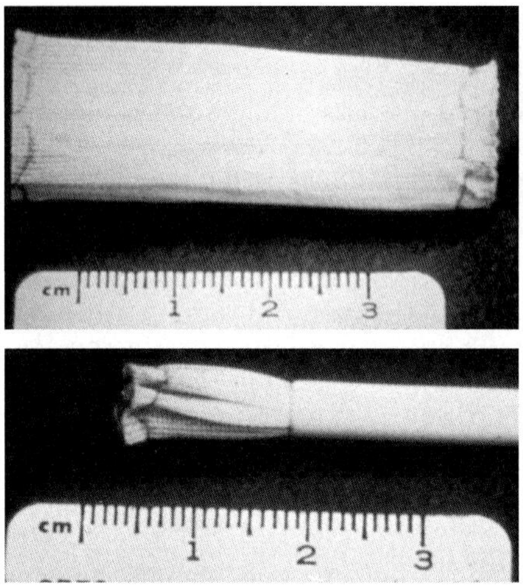
1.

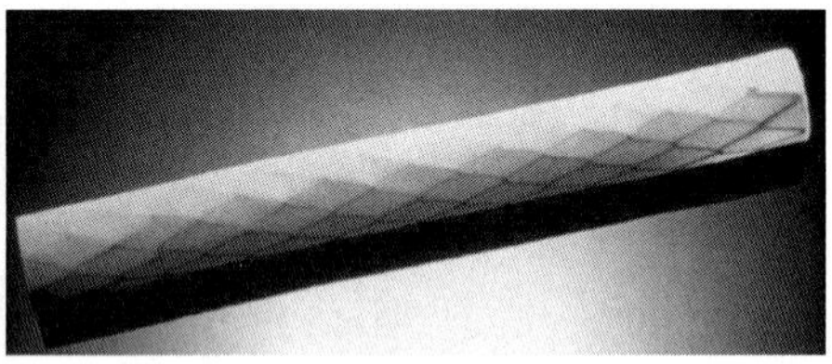
2.

Figures 1, 2. **(1)** Early prototype of endovascular graft. The basic design of expandable stent grafts is demonstrated in this device, which consists of an expandable metallic stent framework covered by conventional polyester graft material. **(2)** Newer graft design. Clinical use of stent-grafts has been facilitated by development of flexible stent frames and thin-walled graft materials. This design uses a nitinol stent that fully supports a polyester graft less than 0.1 mm thick.

has the advantage of being dilatable over a fairly wide range of sizes. In this fashion, a smaller-diameter graft can be introduced through a sheath and then enlarged with an angioplasty balloon to three or four times its nominal diameter. PTFE has a recoil after angioplasty of about 30%, however, which makes overdilation necessary. This phenomenon is a disadvantage when dilation is performed in situ. Polyester graft material has the advantage of a known implant history and compatibility. The graft material is not elastic, however, and is somewhat more bulky than PTFE. For this reason, most grafts have been constructed with ultrathin woven polyester graft material.

Graft thickness ranges from 0.1 to 0.3 mm. Because the polyester is not elastic, it is not dilatable in situ. For this reason, a graft of precise diameter is necessary for a specific application.

Alternative Graft Materials

Most stent-graft designs to date have used approved graft materials. As mentioned, the primary graft materials have been PTFE and polyester. Other polymers may be more suitable for stent-graft use because of their elastomeric nature and lower profile. It may be possible to make thin, strong materials that could be more suitably attached to a stent framework and that would have a lower introduction profile than the rather bulky conventional graft materials used today. Alternative graft materials will have to meet the same standards as conventional graft materials in terms of biocompatibility, porosity, and durability. As such, use of these materials will depend on the results of longer-term implant studies.

Unsupported Stent-Grafts

A common prototype design for peripheral implantation is an expandable stent placed at the end of a conventional segment of graft material. The stent can be either balloon expandable or self-expanding and is generally placed on the inside of the graft. It is sewn onto the graft with conventional surgical suture. The advantage of this type of graft is that long segments can be easily constructed by using longer graft segments. The profile of the graft is also lower because one does not have a long segment of intervening stent in the graft. Since the grafts cannot be pushed in the standard fashion through delivery sheaths without risk of longitudinal collapse, specialized delivery mechanisms are needed to deploy the grafts in proper position. Either the stents can be crimped onto balloon delivery catheters or the leading edge of the stent-graft must be tethered in some fashion as the graft is pushed through the delivery sheath. A potential disadvantage of this design is that the unsupported segment of the graft may be prone to radial compression by the surrounding blood vessel and plaque. In most designs to date, conventional graft materials such as PTFE or polyester have been used.

Fully Supported Stent-Grafts

In some stent-graft designs, a contiguous stent supports the entire length of the graft (Fig 2). The advantage of this design is that the graft is less prone to kinking and external compression. Since the metallic endoskeleton extends along the length of the graft, it can be used to push the graft into position. This procedure requires a less complicated delivery mechanism. A potential disadvantage is that the stent-graft has a substantial amount of metal in the flow surface, since the stent courses along the length of the entire graft.

Some stent-graft designs use stents coursing along the inside of the graft material, and others support the graft with use of an external stent framework. Potential advantages of an endoskeleton include simplified manufacturing and more secure fixation of the graft to the stent. In cases where vessel sealing between graft and vessel wall is critical, the smooth outer covering of the graft material may be advantageous. When the stent is placed on the outside of the graft, a potential advantage is a smoother flow surface, since none of the stent material is in the flow lumen.

PHYSIOLOGIC RESPONSE AND HEALING

Limited basic research has been conducted to evaluate the tissue response to endovascular graft placement. Important issues include the healing response of endoluminal versus extraanatomic graft material, as well at the effect of porosity on the potential ingrowth of intimal hyperplasia. Among important issues that have not been addressed is the durability of thin-walled fabrics used for endoluminal stent-grafts compared with their thicker counterparts used for surgical extraanatomic bypass. This issue is particularly important in the treatment of aneurysms in which prevention of rupture may depend on the long-term integrity of the graft material.

The tissue response to endovascular graft material has been most commonly studied with use of PTFE material. Clowes et al (8) studied the effect of porosity on graft healing. Healing in surgically placed PTFE grafts occurred from the anastomotic region toward the center of the graft. In grafts 7–9 cm long, healing was 60% complete at 12 months. Golden et al (9) showed that porosity also affects the healing rate and mechanism. These investigators found that pore sizes between 60 and 90 µm were optimal to promote graft healing. As pore size increases, both polyester and PTFE graft material can heal by means of transmural migration of endothelial cells (10).

Palmaz et al (11) studied the effect of overdilation on the physical properties of PTFE graft material (11). In that study, grafts were dilated to three to five times the nominal diameter. Elastic recoil was approximately 23%. Porosity was only minimally affected by dilation of the graft material; however, longitudinal and radial tensile strength, as well as suture strength, were decreased, suggesting that overdilation of PTFE graft material associated with stent placement may weaken the material and predispose it to localized disruption.

Dolmatch et al (12) studied the tissue response to PTFE-covered Palmaz stents with the graft covering either inside or outside of the stent. Bare Palmaz stents were used as a control. In this model, there was little transgraft tissue penetration, and neointimal formation appeared to proceed from the ends of the stent-graft toward the center. Intimal thickness was greater and patency was less when the graft material was on the inside of the stent rather than the outside.

Marin et al (13) studied the development of intimal hyperplasia and healing of grafts in humans. In this study, a total of seven grafts were explanted between 2 weeks and 7 months after placement. Histopathologic analysis was performed. At 3 weeks, organized thrombus was seen on the grafts. At 6 weeks, a perianastamotic endothelium was seen. Endothelium was found 1–3 cm from the ends of the stent-grafts at 3 months and 8 cm from the ends at 5 months. There was little evidence of hyperplasia external to the graft within the excluded plaque. There was little tissue ingrowth through the graft as well. In a separate study, Marin et al (14) examined angiograms of patients with iliac artery stent-grafts to determine the effect of the covering on the development of intimal hyperplasia. At 4–6-month follow-up, they found that lumen diameter was larger on the covered portion of an implanted Palmaz stent than on the uncovered portion. They suggested that the low-porosity covering of PTFE graft material may inhibit stent-related restenosis.

Chuter and Green (15) described near-complete healing of a polyester graft material in a canine model at 18 months. PTFE and polyester grafts have both demonstrated healing in experimental models. The healing of graft materials is known to be less complete in humans. The effect of endoluminal placement on graft healing with these two graft materials is still uncertain.

An interesting reaction to endovascular placement of polyester grafts has been described: A local inflammatory reaction may occur in the immediate postimplantation period. Blum et al (16) noted a "postimplantation syndrome" in 87 of 154 patients (56%) treated with an endoluminal polyester-covered aortic graft (16). Patients developed a fever associated with leukocytosis and elevation of C-reactive protein level. Fever lasted 4–10 days without evidence of infection or bacteremia. Link et al (17) described a local perivascular inflammatory response after endovascular stent-graft placement. This response, which has been associated with perivascular thickening seen at magnetic resonance imaging, appears to be transient, resolving over a period of 4–6 weeks. In animals, Link et al (18) demonstrated a perivascular inflammatory reaction after carotid implantation that was thought to be due to the polyester graft material. The cause of this phenomenon is unknown. The response is curious given the long implant history of polyester (Dacron) grafts. To our knowledge, this reaction has not been described with PTFE graft material.

CLINICAL APPLICATIONS

Clinical applications of stent-grafts are expanding as grafts become available for use. In the United States, clinical use has been limited largely to custom devices and limited trials sponsored by the Food and Drug Administration. Outside the United States, thousands of implants have been placed to treat a wide spectrum of peripheral vascular diseases. A summary of some of these applications is included in this section.

Aneurysms

Results of short-term follow-up of relatively small groups of patients treated with endoluminal stent-grafts are now being published. In the largest series to our knowledge, Marin et al (19) described the treatment of 11 patients with iliac aneurysms. Fourteen aneurysms were treated successfully, with a mean follow-up of 11 months; 100% patency was established. Complications in this group included transient colonic ischemia, a groin lymphocele, and distal embolization.

Razavi et al (20) described the treatment of eight patients with iliac aneurysms with use of a combination of prototype stent-grafts. Implantation and aneurysm exclusion were accomplished in every case, with a mean follow-up of 5 months. All grafts remained patent during the follow-up period.

Successful treatment of peripheral aneurysms follows the same principles as aortic aneurysm exclusion. Nonaneurysmal segments of the treated artery that are proximal and distal to the aneurysm are necessary to allow effective sealing of the endoluminal graft (Fig 3). A "cuff" of normal-caliber vessel at least 1 cm long is preferred. As such, vessel caliber and condition are important determinants of success.

In some situations, tapered grafts may be necessary (20). In other situ-

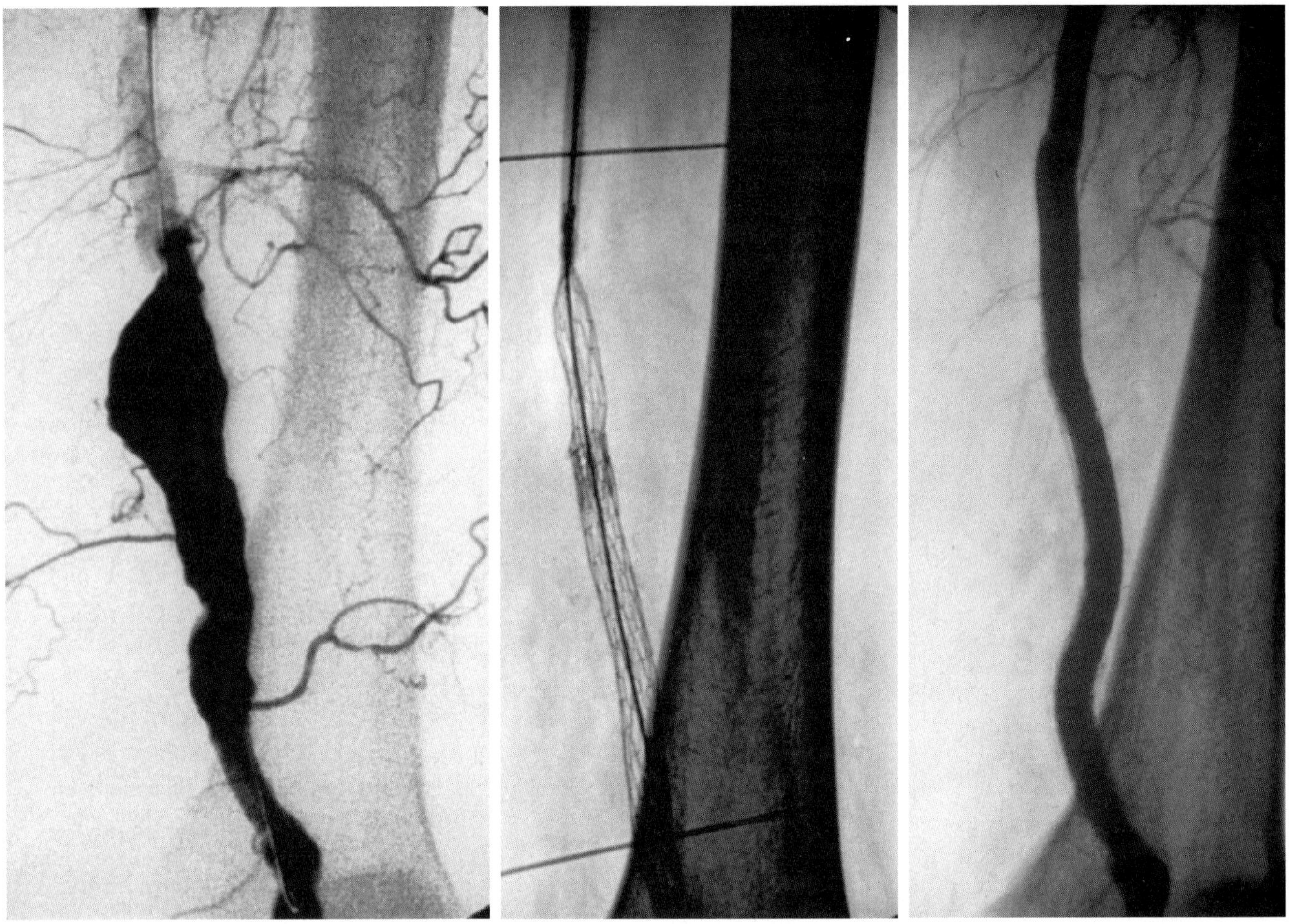

a. b. c.

Figure 3. Peripheral aneurysm. **(a)** A large atherosclerotic aneurysm is demonstrated in the distal left superficial femoral artery. **(b)** The metallic portion of a fully supported stent-graft (Endopro, MinTec) is seen at fluoroscopy during deployment across the aneurysmal segment. Two separate 8-mm-diameter stent-grafts were placed. At the stent junction, a stent strut is angled. This angulation was corrected with balloon expansion of the stent-graft. **(c)** Angiogram obtained at 1-year follow-up shows that the aneurysm is excluded and the graft is widely patent. (Case courtesy of U. Albrechtsson, MD, Lund University, Lund, Sweden.)

ations, coil embolization of feeding vessels may be necessary to isolate the aneurysm for successful graft placement (21).

As has been described with aortic aneurysms (22), delayed rupture of iliac aneurysms is possible if complete exclusion is not obtained. Follow-up of treated aneurysms can generally be accomplished with computed tomographic (CT) angiography or conventional angiography. As such, it is relatively straightforward to follow up these patients by minimally invasive means. We prefer follow-up with CT angiography or duplex ultrasonography at 1 and 6 months to document aneurysm exclusion.

Anecdotal experience with less common peripheral aneurysms has also been reported. Henry et al (23) described the treatment of six femoropopliteal aneurysms with placement of an expandable polyester-covered stent-graft. In these patients, exclusion was possible with good patency. Rousseau et al (24) described similar success in eight patients with iliac, popliteal, and subclavian aneurysms. A determination of the fatigue resistance of the stent or stent-graft components will be necessary over a longer follow-up period if these devices are to be placed across bending joints.

There have been anecdotal reports about stent-graft treatment of aneurysms in other vascular beds. Successful treatment of a renal artery aneurysm (25), a traumatic subclavian pseudoaneurysm (26), and carotid false aneurysm (7) has been described. In general, favorable results can be expected in the treatment of pseudoaneurysms if the vessel caliber is large enough and if there are good segments of vessel both proximal and distal to the pseudoaneurysm to accommodate graft sealing.

Trauma and Arteriovenous Fistula

Treatment of arteriovenous fistulas (AVFs) would also appear to be a good application of stent-graft technology (Fig 4). Symptomatic AVFs, which tend to occur in larger vessels, are well suited to stent-graft placement because they may be normal both proximal and distal to the fistula and have relatively high flow. Parodi (7) described successful treatment of five traumatic AVFs with a balloon-expandable stent-graft. In that series, successfully treated lesions included two AVFs of the subclavian artery, a fistula between the common iliac artery and inferior vena cava occurring after surgery, an aortocaval fistula occurring after a gunshot wound, and a fistula between the superficial femoral artery and vein occurring after a gunshot wound. Others have reported similar anecdotal results for treatment of

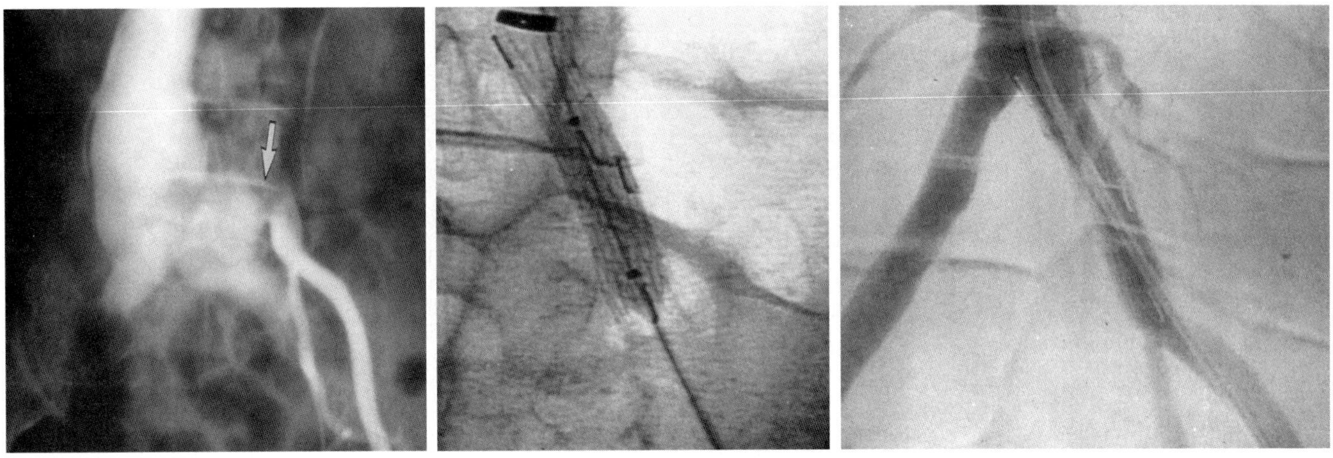

a. b. c.

Figure 4. AVF. **(a)** A high-flow connection (arrow) between the left common iliac artery and vein is demonstrated during injection of contrast medium into the left common iliac artery. **(b)** A balloon is used to model a stent-graft after deployment across the fistula. **(c)** Angiogram obtained immediately after the procedure demonstrates obliteration of the fistula. (Case courtesy of Manuel Maynar, MD, Nuestra Señora del Pino Hospital, Las Palmas, Canary Islands, Spain.)

central AVFs of the common iliac artery (27,28) and subclavian artery (29). Spark et al (30) reported treatment of a peroneal artery fistula with an expandable Dacron graft. Eighteen-month follow-up showed patency of the 5-mm-diameter graft. This finding is notable because patency of small-caliber grafts would be expected to be poor.

Use with Transjugular Intrahepatic Portosystemic Shunts

Stent-grafts have also been used to manage complications related to transjugular intrahepatic portosystemic shunts (TIPS). Cohen et al (31) reported successful treatment of a hepatobiliary fistula with use of a prototype balloon-expandable stent-graft. In this case, the stent-graft was expanded inside a Wallstent (Schneider/Pfizer, Minneapolis, Minn) to seal a leak into a left intrahepatic duct. Experimental studies evaluating the use of stent-grafts for creation of TIPS are also being reported (32). Stent-grafts may limit the ingrowth of cellular elements along the TIPS track that can cause restenosis in shunts created with standard noncovered stents.

Occlusive Disease

The use of stent-grafts for treatment of occlusive disease is of particular interest to both surgeons and interventionalists. For interventionalists, stent-grafts have the potential to expand the range of angioplasty to include longer lesions, which presently are associated with high rates of restenosis when treated with simple angioplasty. For surgeons, stent-grafts offer an alternative to conventional surgical bypass. In both situations, stent-grafts act as an endoluminal lining that isolates the native plaque-filled lumen from the circulation (Fig 5). Theoretically, a low-porosity graft should limit the ingrowth of cellular elements and reduce the frequency of restenosis along the length of the treated vascular segment. Numerous reports are now available on the use of this technique for treatment of occlusive disease (33–35).

Stent-graft systems that use both PTFE and polyester graft material have been used for this application. In addition to differences in graft material, however, the primary difference between various systems is whether or not the graft is inserted with a fully supported stent structure or in an unsupported fashion with stents acting as anastomotic mechanisms only at the ends of the graft. As mentioned previously, the advantage of the latter system is that the graft is flexible, tends to have a lower profile, and may be easier to introduce in longer lengths. A disadvantage is the tendency of plaque elements to recoil and cause compression of the graft. Anecdotal experience with intravascular US with this approach demonstrates substantial compression of unsupported endoluminal grafts.

Fully supported stent-grafts have the advantage of resisting elastic recoil due to the nature of their expandable framework. A disadvantage is the relatively large amount of metal on the flow surface of a longer graft. Newer designs now incorporate stents on the outside of the graft so that blood-to-stent contact is minimized. All of the stent-graft systems under testing appear to have the same limitations as surgical bypass grafts. In general, grafts of smaller caliber (less than 6 mm) have relatively high restenosis rates. In our experience, patency of 5-mm-diameter femoral stent-grafts is uncommon after 2 years. Early reocclusion occurs due to thrombosis; late reocclusion, 3–6 months after placement, is usually due to intimal hyperplasia at the margins of the graft (Fig 6).

In 1993, we described our initial experience with femoropopliteal endovascular graft placement (33). Using a variety of techniques and both supported and unsupported stent-grafts, we were able to recanalize and successfully place grafts in long-segment femoropopliteal occlusions. While the initial technical success was high, virtually all of these stent-grafts occluded within 2 years. This occlusion was usually due to intimal hyperplasia at the ends of the graft. In some situations, however, rigid balloon-expandable stents were used to deploy the grafts. Compression of these stents with activity resulted in graft occlusion. Anecdotal experience with a new stent-graft configuration in which graft material is present on the inside of an expandable stent shows promise for patency in femoropopliteal occlusions. In our small series, stent-grafts in four of five patients remained patent up to 4 years.

Marin et al have published extensively on the use of stent-grafts for the treatment of occlusive disease.

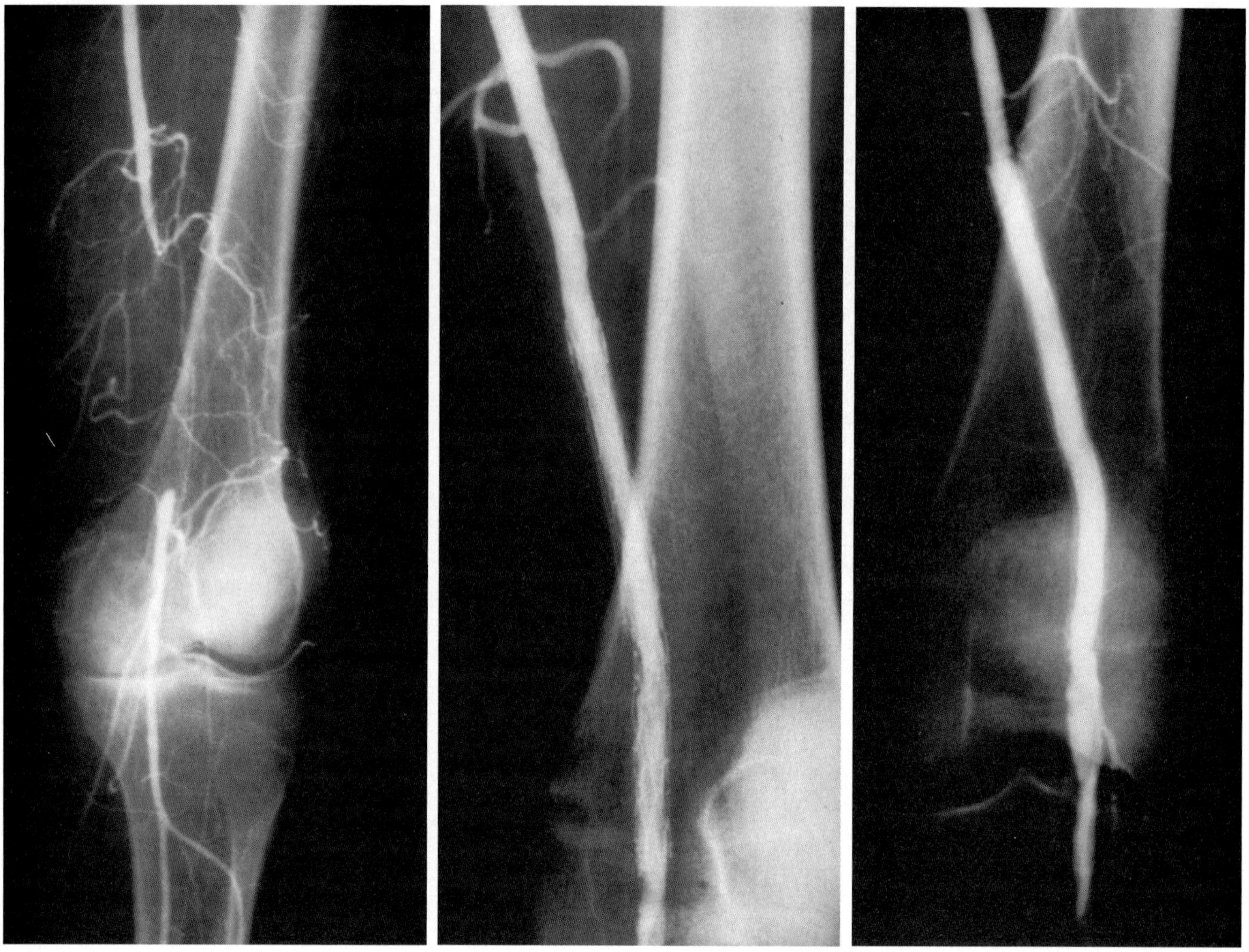

a. b. c.

Figure 5. Popliteal occlusion. **(a)** A 10-cm occlusion of the left popliteal artery did not respond to thrombolysis or angioplasty. **(b)** A stent-graft was placed with an excellent initial result. **(c)** At 1-year follow-up the graft was widely patent. The patient remains asymptomatic at 4 years.

They described their experience with 96 procedures in 92 patients (34), including 48 with iliac or femoral occlusive disease. Initial technical success was achieved in 91% of patients. At follow-up of 13 months, primary patency for aortoiliac reconstructions was 77%, and secondary patency was 95%. There was a 98% limb salvage rate and a 10% rate of major complications. The 30-day mortality rate was 6%. This group has placed stent-grafts by using a variety of innovative, combined surgical and interventional techniques often involving a proximal stent-graft "anastomosis" with a distal surgical anastomosis.

Henry et al (23) has described a large series of patients with peripheral occlusive and aneurysmal disease treated with a commercial expandable polyester stent-graft (Endopro System 1; MinTec, LaCiotat, France). In their series, the rate of patency of treated iliac occlusion was 98% at a mean follow-up of 18 months. The primary patency rate for treatment of femoropopliteal occlusions was much lower, 57%, also at a mean follow-up of 18 months. The secondary patency rate was 80%. Pernes et al (35) reported on their experience with the same stent-graft for the treatment of iliac occlusions. In 10 patients with 12 lesions at mean follow-up of 7 months, the primary patency was 80%.

These early studies have demonstrated the feasibility of endovascular stent-graft placement for treatment of occlusive disease. It has also demonstrated the limitations of these grafts, particularly in smaller-caliber vessels. Further modifications of stent-graft design may improve the patency of these grafts, but it is likely that widespread use for treatment of long-segment occlusive disease will be limited until pharmacologic or physiologic mechanisms for restenosis are defined.

FUTURE DIRECTIONS

Initial studies appear to demonstrate the effectiveness of stent-grafts for treatment of isolated peripheral aneurysms and AVFs. Stent-graft technology is being refined rapidly by commercial vendors, and it is likely that in the next several years, effective stent-graft systems will be available for these indications.

The use of stent-grafts for the treatment of occlusive disease is still of uncertain benefit. At present, primary patency rates for smaller-caliber grafts (less than 6 mm in diameter), in the infrainguinal location in particular, are similar to the those of balloon angioplasty: around 50% at 2 years (23). To be clinically competitive, endoluminal grafts must have

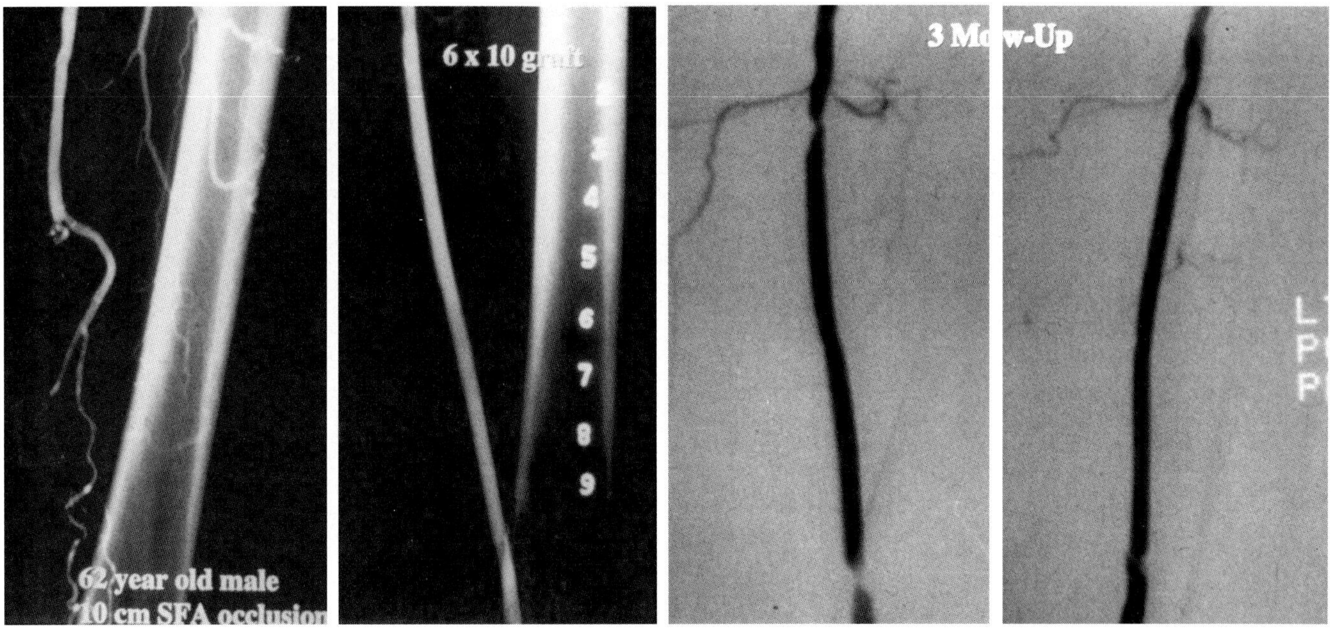

a. b. c. d.

Figure 6. Femoral occlusion. **(a)** A 10-cm occlusion of the left superficial femoral artery. **(b)** Occlusion was treated with a fully supported stent-graft, with an excellent initial result. **(c)** At 3 months, the patient returned with focal stenoses at both the proximal and distal ends of the graft. This result is usually due to intimal hyperplasia at the stent-graft margins. **(d)** Angioplasty was used to assist patency.

patency rates approaching those of prosthetic surgical extraanatomic bypass. Some important issues that need to be addressed are graft introduction profile, graft compression, and anastomotic intimal hyperplasia.

Future areas of research in peripheral stent-grafts should include the development of composite stent and graft configurations that combine the advantages of a flexible biocompatible graft material and a strong expandable stent framework into a single unit. This type of design may provide a more secure relationship between the stent and graft material and a lower introduction profile.

Many of the larger stent-grafts in use today require relatively large sheaths for deployment (12–14 F for graft diameters of 10–12 mm); therefore, a reduction in the stent-graft deployment profile would be an important development. Second-generation stent-graft designs should incorporate this type of design feature. For peripheral use, the stent-graft introduction profile should be less than 9 F.

For occlusive disease, stent-grafts function by excluding the occlusive plaque from the flow lumen and blocking the development of intimal hyperplasia after angioplasty or a related intervention. They do not, however, limit the response to injury at the ends of the graft, a common site for restenosis. Modification of stent-grafts to address these problems may be possible. Potential graft modifications include the attachment of a pharmacologic agent to the ends of the graft to limit smooth muscle hyperplasia; the use of radiation in conjunction with the stent-graft, delivered either to the surface of the stent-graft or locally to the blood vessel; or further mechanical modification to the stent-graft itself to provide a smooth anastomotic zone after implantation.

Stent-grafts, which have been used to a notable degree clinically for only the past 2–3 years, have already had a large effect on the treatment of peripheral vascular disease. It seems likely that their role will continue to expand as we develop and refine the techniques of minimally invasive therapy. ■

References

1. Dotter CT. Transluminally-placed coil-spring endarterial tube grafts: long term patency in canine popliteal artery. Invest Radiol 1969; 4:329–332.
2. Cragg A, Lund G, Rysavy J, Castaneda F, Castaneda-Zuniga W, Amplatz K. Nonsurgical placement of arterial endoprostheses: a new technique using nitinol wire. Radiology 1983; 147:261–263.
3. Cragg A, Lund G, Rysavy J, Salomonowitz E, Castaneda-Zuniga W, Amplatz K. Percutaneous arterial grafting. Radiology 1984; 150:45–49.
4. Mirich D, Wright KC, Wallace S, et al. Percutaneously placed endovascular grafts for aortic aneurysms: feasibility study. Radiology 1989; 170:1033–1037.
5. Volodos NL, Karpovich IP, Troyan VI, et al. Clinical experience of the use of self-fixing synthetic prostheses for remote endoprosthetics of the thoracic and the abdominal aorta and iliac arteries through the femoral artery and as intraoperative endoprosthesis for aorta reconstruction. Vasa 1991; 33(suppl):93–95.
6. Parodi JC, Palmaz JC, Barone HD. Transfemoral intraluminal graft implantation for abdominal aortic aneurysms. Ann Vasc Surg 1991; 5:494–499.
7. Parodi JC. Endovascular repair of abdominal aortic aneurysms and other arterial lesions. J Vasc Surg 1995; 21:549–557.
8. Clowes AW, Kirkman TR, Clowes MM. Mechanisms of arterial graft failure. II. Chronic endothelial and smooth muscle cell proliferation in healing polytetrafluoroethylene prostheses. J Vasc Surg 1986; 3:877–884.
9. Golden MA, Hanson SR, Kirkman TR, Schneider PA, Clowes AW. Healing of polytetrafluoroethylene arterial grafts is influenced by graft porosity. J Vasc Surg 1990; 11:838–845.
10. Florey HW, Greer SJ, Kiser J, Poole JCF, Telander R, Werthessen NT. The development of the pseudointima lining fabric grafts of the aorta. Br J Exp Pathol 1962; 43:655–660.
11. Palmaz F, Sprague E, Palmaz JC. Physical properties of polytetrafluoroethylene bypass material after balloon dilation. JVIR 1996; 7:657–663.
12. Dolmatch BL, Tio FO, Li XD, Dong YH. Patency and tissue response related to two types of polytetrafluoroethylene-covered stents in the dog. JVIR 1996; 7:641–649.
13. Marin J, Veith F, Cynamon J, et al. Human transluminally placed endovascular stented grafts: preliminary histopathologic analysis of healing grafts in aortoiliac and femoral artery occlusive disease. J Vasc Surg 1995; 21:595–604.
14. Marin J, Veith F, Cynamon J, et al. Effect of polytetrafluoroethylene covering of Palmaz stents on the development of intimal hyperplasia in human iliac arteries. JVIR 1996; 7:651–656.

15. Chuter TAM, Green RM. Experimental study of endovascular grafting for aortic aneurysm. In: Yao JST, Pearce WH, eds. Aneurysms: new findings and treatments. Norwalk, Conn: Appleton & Lange, 1993; 325–333.
16. Blum U, Voshage G, Lammer J, et al. Endoluminal stent-grafts for infrarenal abdominal aortic aneurysms. N Engl J Med 1997; 336:13–20.
17. Link J, Muller-Hulsbeck S, Brossmann J, Steffens J, Heller M. Perivascular inflammatory reaction after percutaneous placement of covered stents. Cardiovasc Intervent Radiol 1996; 19:345–347.
18. Link J, Feyerabend B, Grabener M, et al. Dacron-covered stent-grafts for the percutaneous treatment of carotid aneurysms: effectiveness and biocompatibility—experimental study in swine. Radiology 1996; 200:397–401.
19. Marin M, Veith F, Lyon R, Cynamon J, Sanchez L. Transfemoral endovascular repair of iliac artery aneurysms. Am J Surg 1995; 170:179–182.
20. Razavi M, Dake M, Semba C, Nyman U, Liddell R. Percutaneous endoluminal placement of stent-grafts for the treatment of isolated iliac artery aneurysms. Radiology 1995; 197:801–804.
21. Cynamon J, Marin M, Veith F, et al. Endovascular repair of an internal iliac artery aneurysm with use of a stented graft and embolization coils. JVIR 1995; 6:509–512.
22. Lumsden A, Allen R, Chaikof E, et al. Delayed rupture of aortic aneurysms following endovascular stent grafting. Am J Surg 1995; 170:174–178.
23. Henry M, Amor M, Cragg A, et al. Occlusive and aneurysmal peripheral arterial disease: assessment of a stent-graft system. Radiology 1996; 201:717–724.
24. Rousseau H, Gieskes L, Joffre F, et al. Percutaneous treatment of peripheral aneurysms with Cragg Endopro system. JVIR 1996; 7:35–39.
25. Bui B, Oliva V, Leclerc G, et al. Renal artery aneurysm: treatment with percutaneous placement of a stent-graft. Radiology 1995; 195:181–182.
26. Pastores S, Marin M, Veith F, Bakal C, Kvetan V. Endovascular stented graft repair of a pseudoaneurysm of the subclavian artery caused by percutaneous internal jugular vein cannulation: case report. Am J Crit Care 1995; 4:472–475.
27. Marin ML, Veith FJ. Endovascular stents and stented grafts for the treatment of aneurysms and other arterial lesions. Adv Surg 1996; 29:93–109.
28. Zajko A, Little A, Steed D, Curtiss E. Endovascular stent-graft repair of common iliac artery–to–inferior vena cava fistula. JVIR 1995; 6:803–806.
29. Gomez-Jorge J, Guerra J, Scagnelli T, Mendez K, Yrizarry J. Endovascular management of a traumatic subclavian arteriovenous fistula. JVIR 1996; 7:599–602.
30. Spark J, Blanshard K, Scott J. Endovascular graft placement for a symptomatic iatrogenic peroneal arteriovenous fistula. Eur J Vasc Endovasc Surg 1996; 11:496–498.
31. Cohen G, Young H, Ball D. Stent-graft as treatment for TIPS-biliary fistula. JVIR 1996; 7:665–668.
32. Nishimine K, Saxon RR, Kichikawa K, et al. Improved transjugular intrahepatic portosystemic shunt patency with PTFE covered stent-grafts: experimental results in swine. Radiology 1996; 196:341–347.
33. Cragg AH, Dake MD. Percutaneous femoropopliteal graft placement. JVIR 1993; 4:455–463.
34. Marin M, Veith F, Cynamon J, et al. Initial experience with transluminally placed endovascular grafts for the treatment of complex vascular lesions. Ann Surg 1995; 222:449–469.
35. Pernes JM, Auguste M, Hovasse D, Gignier P, Lasry B, Lasry JL. Long iliac stenosis: initial clinical experience with the Cragg endoluminal graft. Intervent Radiol 1995; 196:67–71.

Eric J. Russell, MD

Diagnosis of Hyperacute Ischemic Infarct with CT: Key to Improved Clinical Outcome after Intravenous Thrombolysis?[1]

PUBLIC awareness of stroke as a treatable condition is improving because of efforts promoting the concept of "brain attack" and the availability of a host of therapies currently under investigation or proved to be effective at reducing morbidity.

Early ischemic stroke is a dynamic event with a therapeutic window measured in hours (1). This short interval provides opportunity, which has led to a series of therapeutic clinical trials evaluating the efficacy and safety of, among other strategies, intravenous and intraarterial administration of thrombolytic medications. It is hoped that thrombolytics will result in rapid restoration of perfusion, resulting in reversal of ischemia and improved neurologic outcome with a low risk of serious intracranial bleeding (2). This strategy has been used in a recent clinical trial in the United States with intravenously administered recombinant tissue plasminogen activator (rt-PA) conducted by the National Institute of Neurological Disorders and Stroke (3) in which patients treated within 3 hours of stroke onset were 30% more likely to have minimal or no disability 3 months after treatment than were placebo-treated control patients.

Unfortunately, there is a price to pay for attempted recanalization: increased risk of symptom-producing hemorrhage. In that study (3), mortality in the treated group was often related to hemorrhage (17% at 3 months in the rt-PA–treated group, 21% in the placebo-treated group). In some studies (4), the risks outweighed the benefits because of hemorrhage.

The European Cooperative Acute Stroke Study (ECASS) trials, upon which the current article (5) and another recent article (6) by von Kummer et al are based, is an interesting case in point. The ECASS study, a double-blind, placebo-controlled trial with eligibility based on symptoms and CT findings, was conducted in Europe between late 1992 and early 1994 at 75 centers in 14 European countries. By study design, patients with hemorrhage on CT scans or with major early CT signs of infarct (eg, diffuse swelling or parenchymal hypoattenuation of more than 33% of the territory of the middle cerebral artery [MCA]), were to be excluded. All centers received a booklet with examples of the CT exclusion criteria.

Initial review of ECASS data (7) showed no benefit in patients who received rt-PA when compared with those who received a placebo, due primarily to the high morbidity associated with delayed hemorrhage. However, at detailed review of study data, serious violations of the protocol were found with regard to 17.4% of patients; most often, these violations were related to the presence of early CT findings of stroke, which were overlooked by local investigators but were later detected by a panel of six experts in neuroradiology. Patients with subtle CT evidence of ischemia of more than 33% of the MCA territory should have been excluded from the study but were instead included and treated. A number of these patients experienced excess morbidity and mortality, which skewed study results. Had the local readers been better able to detect the early CT signs of ischemia, overall study results would have been dramatically improved.

As eloquently stated by the ECASS investigators in a recent publication (8), "Intravenous thrombolysis in acute ischemic stroke is effective...in a defined subgroup of stroke patients...without extended infarct signs on the initial CT scan. However, the identification of this subgroup is difficult and depends on recognition of early major CT signs of early infarction."

For this reason, von Kummer et al (5) analyzed the ECASS data by categorizing the study population on the basis of the results of the expert panel review of CT findings. From this, they found that a subpopulation of study patients benefitted from therapy, with lower risk, and that this population could be distinguished on the basis of CT findings. The CT finding predictive of therapeutic benefit (and improved neurologic outcome at 90 days) was the presence of parenchymal hypoattenuation of 33% or less of the MCA territory. No benefit and an increased risk of hemorrhage (relative to the placebo-treated group) were found for rt-PA–treated patients without any detectable hypoattenuation and for those with hypoattenuation that involved more than 33% of the MCA territory. The ischemic zone therefore must be not too small or too big, but "just the right size" for intravenous rt-PA therapy to result in benefit without excess morbidity.

The clinical importance of hypoattenuation in hyperacute stroke has been previously reported. In a study of thrombolytic therapy by Okada et al (9), four of 10 patients had early CT signs within 3 hours of the onset of symptoms, none had recanalization after thrombolysis, and only one experienced clinical improvement, whereas four of six with negative CT findings had an excellent or good outcome. These data suggest that negative CT findings are predictive of improved outcome, contrary to the results of von Kummer et al.

Positive CT findings of ischemia were predictive of hemorrhagic transformation in a study by Boazzo et al (10). In 36 patients with supratentorial ischemia in whom CT was performed within 4 hours of ictus, hemorrhagic infarct was present in 18 (50%) patients on follow-up CT scans obtained 7 days later. In 25 of 36 patients with early CT findings of hypoattenuation, the lentiform nucleus alone was affected in 14, the lentiform nucleus and cortex were affected in five, and the cortex only was affected in six. Furthermore, 18 of these 25 (72%) patients in whom hypoattenuation was seen had hemorrhagic transformation. Hemorrhagic transformation did not occur in any of the 11 patients in whom early hypoattenua-

Index terms: Brain, CT, 10.12111 • Brain, infarction, 13.781,13.782 • Brain, ischemia, 13.7691, 13.781 • Cerebral blood vessels, thrombosis, 174.7691, 174.781 • Editorials • Thrombolysis, 174.1265

Radiology 1997; 205:315–318

[1] From the Department of Radiology, Northwestern University Medical School, Northwestern Memorial Hospital, Olson Pavilion, Ste 3426, 710 N Fairbanks Ct, Chicago, IL 60611. Received August 28, 1997; accepted September 2. **Address reprint requests to** the author.

See also the article by von Kummer et al (pp 327–333) in this issue.

tion was not seen, despite the fact that five of these patients had angiographically documented occlusion of the MCA. Also, there is a direct correlation between the size of an ischemic area and the probability of hemorrhagic transformation (11). These data are in agreement with the findings of von Kummer et al. It should be stressed that many patients with hemorrhagic transformation experienced no clinical deterioration as a result of the hemorrhage (12–14) and that hemorrhagic transformation and parenchymal hematoma are quite different in importance (15).

CT scans are clearly better at depicting subtle shifts of brain water and for detecting early ischemia than was once supposed (16). Seven years ago, Truwit et al (17) reported a series of patients with acute infarct evaluated with CT in which parenchymal areas of hypoattenuation were seen in eight of 10 patients within 2 hours, and in 18 of 21 patients within 4 hours. Tomura et al (18) obtained CT scans within 6 hours of stroke onset in 25 patients with embolic infarct of the MCA or the internal carotid artery distribution. Scans were analyzed for obscured outline of the lentiform nucleus, slight decrease in tissue attenuation, and sulcal effacement; one or more of these findings were present in 23 of 25 (92%) patients. Lentiform nucleus obscuration was the most frequent (92%) and earliest finding (appearance within 1 hour, in some cases).

In an earlier article, von Kummer et al (16) reviewed data in 53 patients with MCA occlusion in whom CT scans were prospectively obtained 46–292 minutes after symptom onset, before rt-PA treatment. Early CT scans in 43 of 53 (81%) patients showed hypoattenuation. The authors concluded that "extended" hypoattenuation or local swelling on CT scans was predictive of fatal outcome and failure of thrombolysis. Of note, von Kummer et al admitted that "volumetry of very subtle findings is difficult at best," although they visually classified the lesions as absent, small, large, or total. Early low attenuation in more than 50% of the territory of the MCA was predictive of mortality as high as 85% and of poor outcome in survivors. In a commentary about the article by von Kummer et al, Tomsick (19) referred to his own previous research (20) and likewise drew the conclusion that early CT signs exist that are predictive of poor outcome but that interobserver variability might cloud the issue.

The results reported in two recent articles by Toni et al (21,22) support another study finding. It appears to be better to withhold intravenously administered rt-PA from patients in whom CT scans obtained during the hyperacute phase of stroke depict no hypoattenuation. In support of this contention is their finding that, in a series of 152 patients with a first stroke who underwent CT within 5 hours of symptom onset, a negative CT scan was an independent predictor of early spontaneous clinical improvement and a good clinical outcome.

The findings of von Kummer et al (5) are important for many reasons. If these findings are reproducible, we are now clearly obliged to ensure that those who interpret emergency CT studies in patients with acute stroke are aware of these findings and skilled enough to detect and accurately report the findings in a timely fashion. The results of this study point to the value of high-quality image interpretation in decision making: Experience and talent help. The expert panel of six academic neuroradiologists disagreed with the results of more than 50 interpretations by the local radiologists, which were made at the time of decision by readers who had already had the benefit of a training manual. Herein lies the problem. If in the heat of the moment, when stroke decisions are often made, local readers in a project of this quality cannot reliably use study criteria, these criteria must be quite subtle.

In a related article (23), von Kummer et al suggested that neuroradiologists can assess subtle CT signs of cerebral infarct within the first 6 hours of symptom onset with moderate to substantial interobserver agreement. However, with regard to the prediction of the percentage of MCA territory affected (crucial to the decision as to whether a patient should be treated or not), complete, pairwise agreement between the predictions of readers as to the percentage of arterial territory affected was rather low (23% and 26% for right and left hemisphere, respectively). In other words, although the chance-adjusted agreement of six expert neuroradiologists was substantial, the percentage agreement in the same volume category was low. Because the authors distinguished percentages of affected tissue in 20% increments, they concluded that larger percentages (33%–50%) would be more reliable predictors, which led to the current report. This uncertainty and the substantial problems experienced at the local study sites in detection of these changes brings into question the reliability of this technique. The carrot is real, however: Meticulous application of these guidelines in the hands of expert CT scan readers may well save lives when deciding who should undergo intravenous thrombolysis.

What can we do? Do we have a sufficient number of capable readers in the community? Should we develop vast teleradiology networks of experienced neuroradiologists who are "up all night" to look for subtle cortical lucency and the insular ribbon sign on uncompressed, transmitted images? If expert radiologists will not be there or are not available to read the studies, should we train emergency room physicians and neurologists with little experience with the subtleties of CT scans to interpret images and make these decisions? This ties into a key imaging issue of the 1990s: the interpretation of images in real time, when it matters for patient care. We must be there to make a difference and to add value.

Certain imaging strategies must be routinely used to optimize detection of subtle early ischemia on CT scans. We all occasionally see images that are poorly recorded at inappropriate window and level settings. Even standard settings will not be equally effective in all cases. Although not discussed in the article by von Kummer et al (5), I would guess that the changes sought for on these CT scans would have been more easily detected if electronic soft copy (not hard copy) images had been used for interpretation. Subtle differences between gray and white become much more easily detectable when a reader can sit at the CT console or independent review console and continuously manipulate and narrow window settings.

Technical factors also play a key role in generating sufficient contrast resolution for the detection of subtle soft-tissue changes. Whereas newer helical CT scanners are fast and efficient for the acquisition of a whole brain study in the setting of acute stroke, the technique typically used for spiral acquisition (1-second scanning) is suboptimal for subtle contrast resolution. A nonspiral study with high dose (3-second scanning, high milliampere setting) should optimize detection of these changes and should be used routinely for such crucial decisions.

The difficulty in estimating the percentage of the territory of the MCA affected is another key issue. It is difficult to locate the ischemic zone, and estimation of the extent is even more of a challenge. Ischemic zone borders may be too poorly defined to result in accurate estimates of volume. Also, there is sufficient evidence in the literature (24–28) to suggest that this territory varies from patient to patient. In other studies (29) with results that suggest accuracy, older, more visible infarcts were classified, and the results do not necessarily apply to cases of more acute subtle stroke. One might find it difficult to make life-or-death decisions on the basis of an estimation of a strict one-third volume limit determined from barely visible findings, not to mention the risk of medicolegal reviews of such judgements when therapeutic complications arise. As Hachinski (7) has written,"seldom has the balance between deliverance and disaster been so finely poised."

Although CT scanning after administration of a bolus of contrast material can now be applied when the newer helical CT scanners are used to produce information about cerebral perfusion that may compare favorably with perfusion magnetic resonance (MR) imaging data (30,31), the future will tell whether the combination of CT signs of hypoattenuation and helical CT perfusion data will rival diffusion/perfusion MR imaging. It is clear, however, that MR imaging is the competition, and the competition is gaining. von Kummer et al are indirectly telling us that we need to use a more accurate tool to rapidly assess the presence of acute ischemia, one that could also more reliably (with less chance of interobserver disagreement) be used for acute stroke trials.

Standard MR imaging pulse sequences are not enough, because T1 and T2 signal intensity do not reliably change in the majority of cases within 8 hours after ictus (32). Optimized standard MR imaging can demonstrate increased signal intensity in gray matter on proton-density images obtained within 3 hours of embolic infarct (33). Local swelling without change in signal intensity, loss of intravascular flow voids, and intravascular and early parenchymal enhancement may also provide clues to the presence of hyperacute infarct (34). Still, we need more.

The better tool is fast (echo-planar) diffusion-weighted MR imaging (35–40). Diffusion-weighted MR imaging is sensitive to the random motion of water. Sensitization is accomplished by adding two rapidly switched gradient pulses to standard or echo-planar MR imaging sequences. As regional cerebral perfusion drops, calcium and sodium accumulate in cells and water is drawn in, which results in restricted (slow) diffusion. Diffusion-weighted MR images can readily depict this hyperacute cytotoxic edema as a change in signal intensity because of the redistribution of water from the extracellular to the more restrictive intracellular space. With adequate gradient coil strength, a complete survey of the brain for restricted water diffusion can be acquired in less than 1 minute. The contrast afforded by this technique is spectacular: a bright white ischemic zone, hard to miss even in the middle of the night. Acute ischemia becomes visible within minutes of the ictus (36). Should one argue that CT is still necessary for detection of hemorrhage, T2*-weighted echo-planar MR imaging permits detection of early parenchymal hemorrhage owing to the sensitivity to magnetic susceptibility (41), although detection of subarachnoid hemorrhage is still somewhat suspect.

The real problem is availability. High-quality imaging requires modern MR equipment with improved gradient coils and appropriate software. Whereas we have been lucky enough to use this technique for more than 2 years, with excellent results, some MR imager manufacturers have only recently provided such capability, and others still lag behind.

Both CT and MR imaging solutions are currently imperfect. The real challenge, outlined several years ago by Bryan and colleagues (42,43), is "where is the dead tissue that cannot be treated, and where is the tissue at risk of dying that might be treated?" With MR imaging, we can focus on the dynamic pathophysiologic processes seen with acute ischemia, not just on anatomy. Magnetic susceptibility–sensitive contrast-enhanced echo-planar imaging can generate transit-time data and provide a quantitative measurement of cerebral blood flow (44–46). Perfusion images can be used to evaluate flow in cerebral microvasculature and can reveal regions of perfusion deficit that correspond to major vascular territories. With it, we can produce functional perfusion maps of "at-risk" ischemic areas, which can then be compared with diffusion maps of dying tissue to estimate the presence of salvageable brain (36,45). The potential to identify in real time the "ischemic penumbra" of reversibly ischemic brain tissue is close.

MR spectroscopy may add another dimension to the "complete" MR imaging evaluation of acute stroke. In cases of acute ischemia, hypoxia and hypoglycemia result in loss of cellular energy homeostasis due to lack of a substrate for oxidative phosphorylation, which leads to decreased high-energy metabolites and the accumulation of lactate. In vivo spectroscopy is now practical. In one recent MR spectroscopic study (47), abnormal metabolite distributions could be detected in all ischemic lesions larger than 1 cm in diameter. In the center of infarcts larger than the section thickness (2 cm), the *N*-acetyl-aspartate level decreased to 20% as early as 1 day, the choline level decreased to 67%, and the creatine level decreased to 51%. Large amounts of lactate were detected in all acute infarcts, although no cases were studied within 1 day of symptom onset (47).

Studies are needed to investigate the utility of MR spectroscopy in the setting of hyperacute stroke. Phosphorus-31 and proton MR spectroscopy may also be used to differentiate ischemic penumbra from irreversible injury by using metabolic criteria. As Baker et al (48) have suggested, there may be phosphocreatinine–inorganic phosphate or lactate–*N*-acetyl-aspartate ratios above which injury is irreversible. Spectroscopy may also be potentially useful for the evaluation of tissue responses to neuroprotective agents—calcium or sodium-calcium channel blockers in acute ischemia (49,50).

Another advantage of MR techniques in patients with acute stroke is the flexibility of MR angiography. By considering the lack of efficacy of intravenous thrombolysis in treating large-vessel occlusion, it would be useful to distinguish between emboli in distal branches of the MCA, occlusion of the main MCA, and occlusion of the intracranial internal carotid artery bifurcation before deciding on the route of thrombolytic delivery. With the CT pattern of ischemia, there is no distinction between carotid arterial and MCA occlusion (10). Results of a study by Wolpert et al (51) confirmed that intravenous rt-PA is not effective at lysing thrombi in the proximal part of a large vessel: Only one third of the treated MCA occlusions recanalized partially. Also, severe branch stenosis associated with thrombosis can be detected at MR angiography (52) and can be treated with angioplasty (53). Although time-of-flight, phase-contrast, and spin-labeling techniques are available and are reasonably accurate (54,55), newer contrast-enhanced subtraction MR angiographic techniques offer extensive coverage with quickly obtained, complete screening studies (56,57). By using an ultrafast three-dimensional gradient-echo time-of-flight sequence with a timed bolus administration of gadolinium and a phased-array head and neck coil, it is possible to complete a survey from the aortic arch to the circle of Willis in under 10 seconds of scanning time, which permits a reduction in motion artifact.

Perhaps with rapid identification of large-vessel occlusion on MR angiograms, intraarterial thrombolysis could be used when intravenous thrombolysis is unsuccessful. CT angiography could certainly be added to a screening nonenhanced CT study to address some of these issues; however, serious difficulties exist, including the relatively intensive reconstruction time and the contrast material load needed for imaging. The absence of the more sensitive baseline MR imaging examination is perhaps the key point. I refer the reader to excellent discussions in the literature (58–60) of both sides of this issue.

MR imaging will likely win in the end. For the time being, we radiologists must become more expert at reading CT scans in cases of acute stroke—and more available—if we are to provide the needed decision making. We must also consider incorporation of MR imaging into forthcoming clinical stroke trials. ■

References

1. Baron JC, von Kummer R, Del Zoppo GJ. Treatment of acute ischemic stroke: challenging the concept of a rigid and universal time window. Stroke 1995; 26:2219–2221.
2. Pessin MS, Del Zoppo GJ, Estol CJ. Thrombolytic agents in the treatment of stroke. Clin Neuropharmacol 1990; 13:271–289.
3. The National Institute of Neurological Disorders and Stroke rt-PA Stroke Study Group. Tissue plasminogen activator for acute ischemic stroke. N Engl J Med 1995; 333:1581–1587.
4. Foulkes MA, Wolf PA, Price TR, et al. The stroke data bank: design, methods and baseline characteristics. Stroke 1988; 19: 547–554.
5. von Kummer R, Allen KL, Holle R, et al. Acute stroke: usefulness of early CT findings before thrombolytic therapy. Radiology 1997; 205:327–333.
6. von Kummer R, Nolte PN, Schnittger H, et al. Detectability of cerebral hemisphere ischaemic infarcts by CT within 6 hours of stroke. Neuroradiol 1996; 38:31–33.
7. Hachinski V. Thrombolysis in stroke: between the promise and the peril (editorial). JAMA 1996; 276:995–996.
8. Hacke W, Kaste M, Fieschi C, et al. Intravenous thrombolysis with recombinant tissue plasminogen activator for acute hemispheric stroke: the European Cooperative Acute Stroke Study (ECASS). JAMA 1995; 274:1017–1025.
9. Okada Y, Sadoshima S, Nakane H, et al. Early computed tomographic findings for thrombolytic therapy in patients with acute brain embolism. Stroke 1992; 23:20–23.
10. Boazzo L, Angeloni U, Bastianello S, et al. Early angiographic and CT findings in patients with hemorrhagic infarction in the distribution of the middle cerebral artery. AJNR 1991; 12:1115–1121.
11. Ott BR, Zamani A, Kleefield J, Funkenstein HH. The clinical spectrum of hemorrhagic infarction. Stroke 1986; 17:179–185.
12. Yamaguchi T, Minematsu K, Choki J, et al. Clinical and neuroradiological analysis of thrombotic and embolic cerebral infarction. Jpn Circ J 1984; 48:50–58.
13. Hornig CR, Dorndorf W, Agnoli AL. Hemorrhagic infarction: a prospective study. Stroke 1986; 17:179–185.
14. Pessin MS, Teal PA, Caplan LR. Hemorrhagic infarction: guilt by association? AJNR 1991; 12:1123–1126.
15. Lodder J. CT-detected hemorrhagic infarction: relation with the size of the infarct and the presence of midline shift. Acta Neurol Scand 1984; 70:329–335.
16. von Kummer R, Meyding-Lamade U, Forsting M, et al. Sensitivity and prognostic value of early CT in occlusion of the middle cerebral artery trunk. AJNR 1994; 15:9–15.
17. Truwit CL, Barkovich AJ, Gean-Marton A, et al. Loss of the insular ribbon: another early CT sign of acute middle cerebral artery infarction. Radiology 1990; 176:801–806.
18. Tomura N, Uemura K, Inugami A, et al. Early CT finding in cerebral infarction: obscuration of the lentiform nucleus. Radiology 1988; 168:463–467.
19. Tomsick TA. Sensitivity and prognostic value of early CT in occlusion of the middle cerebral artery. AJNR 1994; 15:16–18.
20. Tomsick T, Brott T, Barsan W, et al. Thrombus localization with emergency cerebral CT. AJNR 1992; 13:257–263.
21. Toni D, Fiorelli M, Bastinello S, et al. Hemorrhagic transformation of brain infarct: predictability in the first 5 hours after stroke onset and influence on clinical outcome. Neurology 1996; 46:341–345.
22. Toni D, Fiorelli M, Bastinello S, et al. Acute ischemic stroke improving during the first 48 hours of onset: predictability, outcome and possible mechanisms—a comparison of early deteriorating strokes. Stroke 1997; 28:10–14.
23. von Kummer R, Holle R, Grzyska U, et al. Interobserver agreement in assessing early CT signs of middle cerebral artery infarction. AJNR 1996; 17:1743–1748.
24. van der Zwan A, Hillen B. Review of the variability of the territories of the major cerebral arteries. Stroke 1991; 22:1078–1084.
25. Brott T, Marler JR, Olinger CP, et al. Measurements of acute cerebral infarction: lesion size by computed tomography. Stroke 1989; 20:871–875.
26. Damasio H. A computed tomographic guide to the identification of cerebral vascular territories. Arch Neurol 1983; 40:138–142.
27. Berman SA, Hayman LA, Hinck VC. Correlation of CT cerebral vascular territories with function. III. Middle cerebral artery. AJNR 1984; 5:161–166.
28. Takahashi S, Suzuki M, Matsumoto K, et al. Extent and location of cerebral infarcts on multiplanar MR images: correlation with distribution of perforating arteries on cerebral angiograms and on cadaveric microangiograms. AJR 1994; 163:1215–1222.
29. Wardlaw JM, Sellar R. A simple practical classification of cerebral infarcts on CT and its interobserver reliability. AJNR 1994; 15:1933–1939.
30. Hamberg LM, Hunter GJ, Halpern EF, et al. Quantitative high-resolution measurement of cerebrovascular physiology with slip-ring CT. AJNR 1996; 17:639–650.
31. Shih TTF, Huang KM. Acute stroke: detection of changes in cerebral perfusion with dynamic CT scanning. Radiology 1988; 169:469–474.
32. Mohr JP, Biller J, Hilal SK, et al. Magnetic resonance versus computerized tomographic imaging in acute stroke. Stroke 1995; 26:807–812.
33. Shimosegawa E, Inugami A, Okudera T, et al. Embolic cerebral infarction: MR findings in the first 3 hours after onset. AJR 1993; 160:1077–1082.
34. Yuh WTC, Crain MR, Loes DJ, et al. MR imaging of cerebral ischemia: Findings in the first 24 hours. AJNR 1991; 12:621–629.
35. Warach S, Gaa J, Siewart B, et al. Acute human stroke studied by whole brain echo planar diffusion weighted magnetic resonance imaging. Ann Neurol 1995; 37:231–241.
36. Sorensen AG, Buonanno FS, Gonzalez RG, et al. Hyperacute stroke: evaluation with combined multisection diffusion-weighted and hemodynamically weighted echo-planar MR imaging. Radiology 1996; 199:391–401.
37. Warach S, Chien D, Ronthal M, Edelman RR. Fast magnetic resonance diffusion-weighted imaging of acute human stroke. Neurology 1992; 42:1717–1723.
38. Fisher M, Sotak CH. Diffusion-weighted MR imaging and ischemic stroke. AJNR 1992; 13:1103–1105.
39. Le Bihan D. Diffusion/perfusion MR imaging of the brain: from structure to function (editorial). Radiology 1990; 177:328–329.
40. Le Bihan D, Turner R, Douek P, Patronas N. Diffusion MR imaging: clinical applications. AJR 1992; 159:591–599.
41. Ebisu T, Tanaka C, Umeda M, et al. Hemorrhagic and nonhemorrhagic stroke: diagnosis with diffusion-weighted and T2-weighted echo-planar MR imaging. Radiology 1997; 203:823–828.
42. Bryan RN. Imaging of acute stroke (editorial). Radiology 1990; 177:615–616.
43. Bryan RN, Levy LM, Whitlow WD, Killian JM, Preziosi TJ, Rosario JA. Diagnosis of acute cerebral infarction: comparison of CT and MR imaging. AJNR 1991; 12:611–620.
44. Edelman RR, Mattle HP, Atkinson DJ, et al. Cerebral blood flow: assessment with dynamic contrast-enhanced T2*-weighted MR imaging at 1.5 T. Radiology 1990; 176:211–220.
45. Warach S, Wei L, Ronthal M, Edelman RR. Acute cerebral ischemia: evaluation with dynamic contrast-enhanced MR imaging and MR angiography. Radiology 1992; 182:41–47.
46. Rosen BR, Belliveau JW, Chien D. Perfusion imaging by nuclear magnetic resonance. Magn Reson Q 1989; 5:263–281.
47. Lanfermann H, Kugel H, Heindel W, et al. Metabolic changes in acute and subacute cerebral infarctions: findings at proton MR spectroscopic imaging. Radiology 1995; 196:203–210.
48. Baker LL, Kucharczyk J, Sevick RJ, et al. Recent advances in MR imaging/spectroscopy of cerebral ischemia. AJR 1991; 156:1133–1143.
49. Kucharczyk J, Chew W, Derugin N, et al. Nicardipine reduces ischemic brain injury: magnetic resonance imaging/spectroscopy study in cats. Stroke 1989; 20:268–274.
50. Mathews VP, Barker PB, Blackband SJ, et al. Cerebral metabolites in patients with acute and subacute strokes: concentrations determined by quantitative proton MR spectroscopy. AJR 1995; 165:633–638.
51. Wolpert SM, Bruckmann H, Greenlee R, et al. Neuroradiologic evaluation of patients with acute stroke treated with recombinant tissue plasminogen activator. AJNR 1993; 14:3–13.
52. Johnson BA, Heiserman JE, Drayer BP, Keller PJ. Intracranial MR angiography: its role in the integrated approach to brain infarction. AJNR 1994; 15:901–908.
53. Tsai FY, Berberian B, Matovich V, et al. Percutaneous transluminal angioplasty adjunct to thrombolysis for acute middle cerebral artery rethrombosis. AJNR 1994; 15:1823–1829.
54. Furst G, Hofer M, Steinmetz H, et al. Intracranial stenoocclusive disease: MR angiography with magnetization transfer and variable flip angle. AJNR 1996; 17:1749–1757.
55. Korogi Y, Takahashi M, Nakagawa T, et al. Intracranial vascular stenosis and occlusion: MR angiographic findings. AJNR 1997; 18:135–143.
56. Prince MA. Body MR angiography with gadolinium contrast agents. Magn Reson Imaging Clin N Am 1996; 4:11–24.
57. Levy RA, Prince MR. Arterial-phase three-dimensional contrast-enhanced MR angiography of the carotid arteries. AJR 1996; 167:211–215.
58. Brant-Zawadzki M. CT angiography in acute ischemic stroke: the right tool for the job? AJNR 1997; 18:1021–1023.
59. Knauth M, von Kummer R, Jansen O, et al. Potential of CT angiography in acute ischemic stroke. AJNR 1997; 18:1001–1010.
60. Shrier DA, Tanaka H, Numaguchi Y, et al. CT angiography in the evaluation of acute stroke. AJNR 1997; 18:1011–1020.

Michael Laniado, MD • Andreas F. Kopp, MD

Liver-Specific Contrast Media: A Magic Bullet or a Weapon for Dedicated Targets?[1]

In an editorial on hepatic contrast material enhancement in magnetic resonance (MR) imaging published in 1993, Mitchell (1) asked the question, Is hepatobiliary contrast material a magic bullet for sensitivity and specificity? Superparamagnetic iron oxides (SPIOs), another type of liver-specific MR contrast medium that selectively accumulates in the reticuloendothelial system (RES) in the liver and spleen, were the subject of an editorial in 1994 in which Weissleder (2) discussed the attractive possibility of a one-step diagnosis (detection and characterization) provided by using SPIOs. Since then, more articles have been published that deal with clinical and experimental studies of liver-specific contrast media for both computed tomography (CT) (3–6) and MR imaging (7).

In this issue of *Radiology*, Schmitz et al (8) report that gadolinium ethoxybenzyl diethylenetriaminepentaacetic acid (EOB-DTPA) and ytterbium EOB-DTPA were used as hepatobiliary contrast media for CT in dogs at dose levels of 0.5 mmol/kg (ie, approximately 10 times the dose that is tested in clinical trials with Gd-EOB-DTPA for MR imaging of the liver [9,10]). Because of the uptake of the EOB-DTPA ligand into the hepatocytes and the favorable x-ray absorbing properties of the lanthanides gadolinium and ytterbium, liver enhancement is about 32 HU (8). This compares favorably with the degree of enhancement measured 80 minutes after infusion of 0.5 mmol/kg Gd-EOB-DTPA in five patients (6). In that study, liver-to-tumor attenuation difference increased from 24 HU ± 8 before administration of contrast material to 54 HU ± 12 after administration of contrast material (6).

The history of liver-specific contrast agents for MR imaging dates back to the mid-1980s (11), and the CT history of such agents is even older (12). However, only the RES agent ferumoxides (AMI-25, Feridex IV, Advanced Magnetics, Cambridge, Mass, or Endorem, Laboratoire Guerbet, Aulnay-sous-Bois, France) is on the market, and the hepatobiliary contrast medium mangafodipir trisodium injection (Teslascan; Nycomed Imaging, Oslo, Norway) has recently received new drug approval. Therefore, it is worthwhile to ask where we are and where we need to go with liver-specific contrast material.

Today, it takes about 10 years from the design of a contrast medium to sale of the first vial. Within approximately the past 10 years, technical advances in CT that effect liver imaging have included helical scanning, bolus tracking, and dedicated power injectors. Using modern CT technology, Kuszyk et al (13) reported a high sensitivity of 91% for portal phase contrast material–enhanced helical scanning of malignant hepatic tumors larger than 1 cm. As for MR imaging of the liver, technical advances were breath-hold scanning, fast spin-echo sequences, fat-suppression techniques, and phased-array body coils, among others, that were developed since 1987. With the MR technology of today (ie, gradient switching capability of 25 mT/m, rise time of 600 µsec, circularly polarized body array coil, half-Fourier rapid acquisition with relaxation enhancement [RARE]), eight contiguous sections free of respiratory artifacts can be obtained in 16 seconds (14). This plain T2-weighted imaging technique has a high accuracy for detection and characterization of focal liver lesions (14). Thus, the question is whether the shorter life cycle of technologic innovations, along with the availability of the safe extracellular contrast media, will make liver-specific contrast material for CT and/or MR imaging superfluous.

One approach to the question if and when liver-specific contrast media are required for lesion detection and characterization is to compare the potential of CT and MR imaging with and without the use of liver-specific contrast media. With regard to lesion detection with CT, imaging results with two liver-specific compounds—perfluorooctylbromide, or PFOB (15), and ethiodized oil emulsion, or EOE-13 (16)—were excellent, but safety issues precluded these materials from further clinical testing. Of the newly developed CT agents, only Gd-EOB-DTPA underwent clinical trials, but data are too limited to draw conclusions on imaging results and safety. Also, in MR imaging with liver-specific contrast media, side effects in early clinical trials with AMI-25 (17) and mangafodipir trisodium (18) raised safety concerns. After a reformulation of the initial preparation (AMI-25) and a change in the dosing regime (AMI-25 and mangafodipir trisodium), further studies revealed a favorable safety profile for both contrast media (2,19). Meanwhile, a number of recent clinical articles have indicated that hepatobiliary and RES-directed contrast media in MR imaging increase sensitivity compared with that of unenhanced and gadolinium-enhanced MR imaging, without decreasing specificity (10,20–23). To the best of our knowledge, no study has so far included a comparison of contrast-enhanced helical CT and MR imaging with a liver-specific contrast medium. However, CT during arterial portography (CTAP) with (24) and without (25) helical scanning was performed in two trials with SPIO-enhanced MR imaging. On the basis of a segmental analysis, the combination of a T2-weighted spin-echo sequence and a moderately T1-weighted gradient-echo sequence after infusion of SPIOs was more sensitive than nonhelical CTAP (25). With helical scanning, but with only a T1-weighted gradient-echo sequence after administration of contrast material, CTAP was more sensitive but less specific than MR imaging with SPIOs in identifying involved liver segments (24).

Index terms: Contrast media • Editorials • Liver, CT, 761.12112 • Liver, MR, 761.12143

Radiology 1997; 205:319–322

[1] From the Department of Diagnostic Radiology, Eberhard-Karls-Universität Tübingen, Hoppe-Seyler-Strasse 3, 72076 Tübingen, Germany. Received August 28, 1997; accepted September 2. **Address reprint requests to** M.L.

See also the article by Schmitz et al (pp 361–366) in this issue.

Abbreviations: CTAP = CT during arterial portography, EOB-DTPA = ethoxybenzyl diethylenetriaminepentaacetic acid, RARE = rapid acquisition with relaxation enhancement, RES = reticuloendothelial system, SPIO = superparamagnetic iron oxide.

From the brief literature review, there is good evidence that MR imaging with liver-specific contrast material is the most sensitive noninvasive method for the detection of focal lesions that may even challenge CTAP. What questions the value of the numerous studies is that only very few were performed with the rapidly evolving MR or CT equipment of today. On the other hand, one potential role of liver-specific contrast material may be to compensate for limitations in technology. For example, Deckers et al (26) prospectively compared postcontrast MR imaging in 20 patients at 0.2 and 1.5 T. At both field strengths, the detection rate for liver lesions after infusion of SPIOs was not statistically significantly different. Another weak point of most trials is the lack of correlation with intraoperative ultrasound and palpation. Hagspiel et al (27) have shown that these methods are more sensitive than MR imaging with liver-specific contrast material, especially in lesions smaller than 10 mm.

Characterization of focal lesions is another important issue in liver imaging. For this purpose, dynamic MR studies with a gadolinium chelate bolus injection have become a valuable addition to heavily T2-weighted sequences (28,29). But will the radiologist use extracellular gadolinium contrast media for lesion characterization and liver-specific contrast media for detection? More likely, "one-stop shopping" for detection and characterization is the future approach (1,2), and liver-specific contrast media will have to fulfill this requirement to challenge the established methods. Indeed, the limited data dealing with the potential of liver-specific contrast media in the differential diagnosis of focal liver lesions are promising (30). Because the hepatobiliary contrast media, Gd-EOB-DTPA, and the RES agent, Resovist ([ferrixan] Schering, Berlin, Germany), can be injected as a bolus (10,21), the early time course of enhancement in lesions closely resembles the pattern that is well known from dynamic studies with extracellular gadolinium agents (31,32). Delayed images can further narrow differential diagnosis in that tumors with residual hepatobiliary function or Kupffer cells show enhancement and vice versa (30). If only delayed images are obtained, lesion characterization may be inferior to that of gadolinium bolus studies (33). Thus, the hepatobiliary and RES-directed contrast media that were initially designed to improve lesion detection also have the potential to replace extracellular gadolinium contrast media for lesion characterization.

Another approach to the question if and when liver-specific contrast media are required is to consider the clinical needs in imaging of focal liver lesions. To a large extent, these needs depend on the individual situation. In a patient without cancer and a liver lesion detected but not characterized at routine sonography, the need is to exclude malignancy. MR imaging with T2-weighted sequences and dynamic imaging after bolus injection of an extracellular gadolinium contrast medium is the method of choice for this purpose, and there is no need to use liver-specific contrast media. The scenario is different if the lesion is detected during staging sonography in a patient with newly diagnosed cancer or if the patient presents with symptoms of liver cirrhosis. In both cases, not only is lesion characterization essential to rule out metastases or hepatocellular carcinoma but so is screening for additional lesions. Unlike the first case, MR imaging with a liver-specific rather than an extracellular gadolinium contrast medium is recommended for both characterization and detection of additional metastases or foci of hepatocellular carcinoma. Although CTAP may be even more sensitive, it is not an alternative to MR imaging in this clinical setting because of its limitations in lesion characterization. A third scenario is a patient with a potentially resectable liver metastasis from colorectal cancer seen at follow-up sonography. Because the detection of additional lesions has an effect on the therapeutic approach, again, MR imaging with a liver-specific contrast medium has to be considered as the most sensitive noninvasive method. However, on the basis of individual experience, at many institutions, CTAP is still the preferred procedure before liver surgery (34).

The challenge of detecting a second metastasis depends on the primary tumor. An unequivocal benefit of liver resection has been documented for metastases of colorectal cancer (35). When dealing with other primary tumors, the role of liver surgery and, thus, the potential role of liver-specific contrast media are different. In a postmortem study, investigators compared the number of small (< 10 mm) liver metastases in patients with at least one metastasis larger than 1 cm. In colorectal cancer, the ratio was 1.6:1 compared with 4.5:1 in a variety of other malignant tumors (36). Consequently, resection of liver metastases can be a curative approach in colorectal cancer, and the use of liver-specific contrast material is justified before surgery. However, the limited role of surgery in liver metastases of other primary tumors questions the need for liver-specific contrast media.

The issue of lesions smaller than 10 mm has to be looked at in more detail when discussing where we are and where we need to go with liver-specific contrast media. The improvement in sensitivity provided by these agents is greatest for lesions in this range (21). However, the results of a study that used biphasic helical CT in patients with colorectal cancer showed that 78% of subcentimeter foci are not metastatic (37). How important and how reliable is characterization of such a lesion at the time of its detection rather than relying on follow-up studies? Again, the clinical scenario determines the challenge. Is a 5-mm lesion in the left lobe of the liver that is detected only on MR images with SPIOs but that cannot be characterized, enough reason to cancel right hemihepatectomy in a patient with colorectal cancer who has three metastases in the right lobe? Likewise, will a woman with a T2N0 breast cancer receive chemotherapy in addition to surgery and adjuvant radiation therapy if MR imaging with a liver-specific contrast medium shows a subcentimeter liver lesion that may or may not be a metastasis? Does it make a difference to detect a 5-mm lesion compared with its detection at a size of 20 mm 6 months later without a liver-specific contrast medium when characterization as a metastasis can be reliably performed with unenhanced T2-weighted sequences and gadolinium-enhanced dynamic MR imaging? At least, in colorectal cancer metastatic to liver, size is a prognostic factor (38), and the application of liver-specific contrast media to lower the detection threshold will contribute to an improved patient outcome. The potential problem of increasing the number of false-positive metastases can best be avoided when baseline and follow-up studies are always performed with a liver-specific contrast medium. Then any new lesion, even in the subcentimeter range, represents a metastasis that can be appropriately treated.

A third approach to the question if and when liver-specific contrast media are required may consider the cost-sensitive environment of today. If liver-specific contrast media are inexpensive relative to the imaging study itself and/or the extracellular contrast medium, the willingness to use them will be great and vice versa. As an example, oral contrast media in CT are inexpensive enough to be given to almost every patient scheduled for an abdominal study, although, in retrospect, bowel opacification might not have always been needed. The price per dose of Endorem, the only RES contrast medium for MR imaging available in Germany, presently is approximately 100% higher compared with the extracellular gadolinium compounds. It is difficult to predict the price level when other agents from different providers will enter the market. However, from the recent history of the extracellular gadolinium agents, one may infer that prices will not decline substantially with a second or third competitor in this field. But will marketing strategies for extracellular contrast media apply to liver-specific agents? For example, it took a surprisingly short period of time to convince even the toughest skeptics that extracellular gadolinium contrast media add important information in many applications of MR imaging. In the field of liver-specific contrast media, the scenario is less straightforward, with different concepts (positive vs negative enhancement) (23), different sequences (spin echo vs gradient echo), different administration regimes (infusion vs bolus injection) (21), different concepts of delivery of contrast media to the hepatocyte (intact molecule vs cleavage of an ion) (19) and, most important, conflicting results (improved vs unchanged detection rate) (34). Will this force the pharmaceutical companies to lower the price level? Or will the financial investment that may be comparable to that of developing an extracellular agent, with only a fraction of expected sales figures for a liver-specific contrast medium, force the companies to keep prices high?

If liver-specific contrast media remain relatively costly, when are they worth their price and when do they help to save money? Semelka et al (39) calculated the procedural cost of CTAP and MR imaging with an extracellular gadolinium compound. The cost savings resulting from substituting MR imaging for CTAP was $2,225 per patient (39). If it would be MR imaging with the more costly liver-specific contrast medium, the cost savings per patient would still be considerable. One patient population that needs CTAP is a colorectal cancer subgroup. It has been calculated that in the United States, approximately 7,000 of these patients per year are candidates for resection of hepatic metastases (40). Thus, the potential for cost savings in the United States is about $14,000,000 per year. However, if all new cases of colorectal cancer (150,000 per year in the United States) would be imaged with liver-specific contrast medium for staging and follow-up, hoping that more patients will be candidates for curative liver surgery, the added cost would be considerable. For example, in Germany, MR imaging of the liver is not part of the routine imaging workup for patients with colorectal cancer, and it is more expensive than sonography and CT. The expenses to save or to prolong the life of an additional patient in whom liver metastasis was diagnosed early enough to allow curative metastatectomy would then be determined by the money that is spent on such a screening program.

Where are we with liver-specific contrast media in 1997? There is one agent for MR imaging on the market, there is one with new drug approval, and others are in clinical trials (7). The status of CT agents is less advanced, but clinical trials have already been initiated (3–5,8). The consensus is that these agents provide improved lesion detection. The greatest benefit is in surgical candidates for liver resection in whom CTAP might be replaced by MR imaging with use of liver-specific contrast media. MR studies also suggest that lesion characterization is possible with liver-specific contrast media (19,23,32), but data are too limited to draw final conclusions. Although the development of liver-specific contrast media started many years ago, these agents are not in routine clinical use today. There are different potential reasons for this delay, including the relatively short time that the first compound has been on the market, the lack of a "quantum step" forward in sensitivity provided by these agents compared with the sensitivity of competing imaging modalities, and the price of liver-specific contrast media.

More challenging than a statement about where we are is to answer the question, Where do we need to go? There is presently no agent for CT or MR imaging in preclinical testing that promises to be substantially better than the clinically available hepatobiliary and RES-directed contrast media. It will be interesting to compare the potential of CT and MR imaging enhanced with liver-specific contrast media to the potential of state-of-the-art imaging strategies (eg, dual-phase, contrast-enhanced helical CT). On the other hand, the new techniques (eg, RARE) should be combined with the use of liver-specific contrast media (eg, SPIOs) to see if the detection of small lesions can be further improved. However, when lesions in the 5-mm range can be detected, characterization may become a problem.

CT is less costly than MR imaging and is better suited to screen the abdomen and pelvis for extrahepatic disease. Therefore, cost-effective strategies have to be developed to image the liver with a hepatobiliary contrast medium and the abdomen and pelvis with an extracellular contrast medium. Also, the need to acquire unenhanced images with both CT and MR imaging has to be reevaluated when liver-specific contrast media are used. Clearly, cost effectiveness could be further improved if the liver-specific contrast media would be available at the same price as the extracellular agent, but this is a marketing and not a scientific issue. Finally, it will be our duty to define patient populations who will benefit most from the use of state-of-the-art technology and liver-specific contrast media. Today, surgical candidates with liver metastases from colorectal cancer represent one of the few patient groups in which liver-specific contast media may be routinely used. Even if prices for liver-specific contrast media will decrease and even with cost-effective imaging strategies, it will be important to perform outcome studies to ascertain the clinical setting in which detection of additional and/or small lesions and their characterization have an effect on therapy and prognosis and in which liver-specific contrast media are affordable. At present, liver-specific contrast media are more a weapon for dedicated targets than a bullet for all purposes. ■

References

1. Mitchell DG. Hepatobiliary contrast material: a magic bullet for sensitivity and specificity? Radiology 1993; 188:21–22.
2. Weissleder R. Liver MR imaging with iron oxides: toward consensus and clinical practice. Radiology 1994; 193:593–595.
3. Lee FT, Chosy SG, Naidu SG, et al. CT depiction of experimental liver tumors: contrast enhancement with hepatocyte-selective iodinated triglyceride versus conventional techniques. Radiology 1997; 203:465–470.
4. Seltzer SE, Blau M, Herman LW, et al. Contrast material–carrying liposomes: biodistribution, clearance, and imaging characteristics. Radiology 1995; 194:775–781.
5. Weichert JP, Longino MA, Spigarelli MG, Lee FT, Schwendner SW, Counsell RE. Computed tomography scanning of Morris hepatomas with liver-specific polyiodinated triglycerides. Acad Radiol 1996; 3:412–417.
6. Schmitz SA, Häberle JH, Balzer T, Shamsi K, Boese Landgraf J, Wolf KJ. Detection of focal liver lesions: CT of the hepatobiliary system with gadoxetic acid disodium, or Gd-EOB-DTPA. Radiology 1997; 202:399–405.
7. Van Beers BE, Gallez B, Pringot J. Contrast-enhanced MR imaging of the liver. Radiology 1997; 203:297–306.
8. Schmitz SA, Wagner S, Schuhmann-Giampieri G, Krause W, Bollow M, Wolf KJ. Gd-EOB-DTPA and Yb-EOB-DTPA: two prototypic contrast media for CT detection of liver lesions in dogs. Radiology 1997; 205:361–366.
9. Hamm B, Staks T, Muhler A, et al. Phase I clinical evaluation of Gd-EOB-DTPA as a hepatobiliary MR contrast agent: safety, pharmacokinetics, and MR imaging. Radiology 1995; 195:785–792.
10. Reimer P, Rummeny EJ, Shamsi K, et al. Phase II clinical evaluation of Gd-EOB-DTPA: dose, safety aspects, and pulse sequence. Radiology 1996; 199:177–183.
11. Lauffer RB, Greif WL, Stark DD, et al. Iron-EHPG as an hepatobiliary MR contrast agent: initial imaging and biodistribution studies. J Comput Assist Tomogr 1985; 9:431–438.
12. Fisher HW. Improvement in radiographic

contrast media through the development of colloidal or particulate media: an analysis. J Theor Biol 1977; 67:653–670.
13. Kuszyk BS, Bluemke DA, Urban BA, et al. Portal-phase contrast-enhanced helical CT for the detection of malignant hepatic tumors: sensitivity based on comparison with intraoperative and pathologic findings. AJR 1996; 166:91–95.
14. Van HL, Bosmans H, Aerts P, et al. Focal liver lesions: fast T2-weighted MR imaging with half-Fourier rapid acquisition with relaxation enhancement. Radiology 1996; 201:817–823.
15. Bruneton JN, Falewee MN, Francois E, et al. Liver, spleen, and vessels: preliminary clinical results of CT with perfluorooctylbromide. Radiology 1989; 170:179–183.
16. Miller DL, Vermess M, Doppman JL, et al. CT of the liver and spleen with EOE-13: review of 225 examinations. AJR 1984; 143:235–243.
17. Stark DD, Weissleder R, Elizondo G, et al. Superparamagnetic iron oxide: clinical application as a contrast agent for MR imaging of the liver. Radiology 1988; 168:297–301.
18. Kopp AF, Laniado M, Aicher KP, Gronewäller EF, Claussen CD. Mangan-DPDP als kontrastmittel für die MR-tomographie fokaler Leberläsionen. Fortschr Röntgenstr 1992; 157:539–547.
19. Torres CG, Lundby B, Tufte Sterud A, McGill S, Gordon PB, Strand Bjerknes H. MnDPDP for MR imaging of the liver: results of an independent image evaluation of the European phase III studies. Acta Radiol 1997; 38:631–637.
20. Blakeborough A, Ward J, Wilson D, et al. Hepatic lesion detection at MR imaging: a comparative study with four sequences. Radiology 1997; 203:759–765.
21. Kopp AF, Laniado M, Dammann F, et al. MR imaging of the liver with Resovist: safety, efficacy, and pharmacodynamic properties. Radiology 1997; 204:749–756.
22. Caudana R, Morana G, Pirovano GP, et al. Focal malignant hepatic lesions: MR imaging enhanced with gadolinium benzylpropionictetra-acetat (BOPTA)—preliminary results of phase II clinical application. Radiology 1996; 199:513–520.
23. Bernardino ME, Young SW, Lee JK, Weinreb JC. Hepatic MR imaging with Mn-DPDP: safety, image quality, and sensitivity. Radiology 1992; 183:53–58.
24. Oudkerk M, Van den Heuvel AG, Wielopolski PA, Schmitz PIM, Borel Rinkes IHM, Wiggers T. Hepatic lesions: detection with ferumoxide-enhanced T1-weighted MR imaging. Radiology 1997; 203:449–456.
25. Seneterre E, Taourel P, Bouvier Y, et al. Detection of hepatic metastases: ferumoxides-enhanced MR imaging versus unenhanced MR imaging and CTAP. Radiology 1996; 200:785–792.
26. Deckers F, Corthouts E, Nackaerts Y, Ozsarlak O, Parizel PM, De Schepper AM. The influence of MR field strength on the detection of focal liver lesions with superparamagnetic iron oxide. Eur Radiol 1997; 7:1–6.
27. Hagspiel KD, Neidl KF, Eichenberger AC, Weder W, Marincek B. Detection of liver metastases: comparison of superparamagnetic iron oxide–enhanced and unenhanced MR imaging at 1.5 T with dynamic CT, intraoperative US, and percutaneous US. Radiology 1995; 196:471–478.
28. Hamm B, Thoeni RF, Gould RG, et al. Focal liver lesions: characterization with nonenhanced and dynamic contrast material–enhanced MR imaging. Radiology 1994; 190:417–423.
29. Schima W, Saini S, Echeverri JA, Hahn PF, Harisinghani M, Mueller PR. Focal liver lesions: characterization with conventional spin-echo versus fast spin-echo T2-weighted MR imaging. Radiology 1997; 202:389–393.
30. Denys A, Arrive L, Servois V. Hepatic tumors: detection and characterization at 1-T MR imaging enhanced with AMI-25. Radiology 1994; 193:665–669.
31. Vogl TJ, Kummel S, Hammerstingl R, et al. Liver tumors: comparison of MR imaging with Gd-EOB-DTPA and Gd-DTPA. Radiology 1996; 200:59–67.
32. Reimer P, Rummeny E, Marx C, et al. Characterization of focal liver lesions with Resovist as a new SPIO: clinical value of dynamic enhancement with T1- and T2-weighted MRI (abstr). Eur Radiol 7:S293.
33. Kettritz U, Schlund JF, Wilbur K, Eisenberg LB, Semelka RC. Comparison of gadolinium chelates with manganese-DPDP for liver lesion detection and characterization: preliminary results. Magn Reson Imaging 1996; 14:1185–1190.
34. Soyer P. Will ferumoxides-enhanced MR imaging replace CT during arterial portography in the detection of hepatic metastases? prologue to a promising future. Radiology 1997; 201:610–611.
35. Fong Y, Cohen AM, Fortner JG, et al. Liver resection for colorectal metastases. J Clin Oncol 1997; 15:938–946.
36. Schulz W, Borchard F. Größe der lebermetastasen bei geringer metastasenzahl: eine quantitative studie an postmortalen lebern. Fortschr Röntgenstr 1992; 156:320–324.
37. Redvanly RD, Jones MT, Chezmar JL. Prevalence and significance of <10 mm liver lesions on spiral CT in patients with clorectal cancer. Presented at the 97th Annual Meeting of the American Roentgen Ray Society, Boston, Mass, May 4–9, 1997.
38. Seifert JK, Junginger T. Resektion von lebermetastasen kolorektaler Tumoren: eine uni- und multivariate analyse von prognosefaktoren. Langenbecks Arch Chir 1996; 381:187–200.
39. Semelka RC, Schlund JF, Molina PL, et al. Malignant liver lesions: comparison of spiral CT arterial portography and MR imaging for diagnostic accuracy, cost, and effect on patient management. JMRI 1996; 6:39–43.
40. Ferrucci JT. Liver tumor imaging: current concepts. AJR 1990; 155:473–484.

Harry J. Cloft, MD, PhD • David F. Kallmes, MD • Jacques E. Dion, MD, FRCPC

A Second Look at the Second-Look Angiogram in Cases of Subarachnoid Hemorrhage[1]

The article by Dr du Mesnil de Rochemont et al (1) in the March 1997 issue of *Radiology* was an interesting case series, but we do not agree with the authors' conclusion. We believe that the statistics they used do not logically lead to their conclusion. The following are statistics used by the authors to reach their conclusion: (*a*) The risk of permanent neurologic deficit associated with angiography is 0.1%–0.5%, (*b*) the risk of a transient neurologic deficit associated with angiography is 0.5%–2.2%, (*c*) the risk of rebleeding in patients with an untreated ruptured aneurysm is 50% within 6 months, and (*d*) the rate of false-negative angiograms in patients with a ruptured aneurysm is approximately 2%.

If approximately 2% of ruptured aneurysms were overlooked at initial angiography (false-negative studies), then given the 50% rate of rehemorrhage at 6 months, 1% of patients with a negative angiogram would be expected to experience rehemorrhage within 6 months. This rate of rehemorrhage may actually be higher than 1%, given that the authors also state that, on the basis of a review of the literature, the risk of rehemorrhage after a negative angiogram is 1%–12%. The rate of false-negative angiograms would have to fall below 1% (which would result in a risk of rehemorrhage of 0.5%) to compare favorably with the highest risk of permanent neurologic deficit associated with angiography (ie, 0.5%).

Additionally, patients in whom the aneurysm reruptures have an 80% mortality rate (2) or a higher morbidity rate than those who have ischemic complications due to angiography. In that case, the false-negative rate of angiograms would have to be even less than 1% to justify the decision not to perform angiography a second time.

We also take issue with some of the statistics used above. du Mesnil de Rochemont et al (1) state that the rate of false-negative findings on angiograms is "less than 2%,", yet they report false-negative results in three of 66 (5%) patients. Reasons were given for why the aneurysms were overlooked, yet retrospective reevaluation in a study such as this does not change a false-negative angiogram into a true-positive one. Perhaps, however, a conclusion of their study should be that, in the setting of subarachnoid hemorrhage, all negative angiograms should be reevaluated, perhaps by a radiologist other than the initial reader.

It would also be interesting to know the outcome in patients in whom a negative angiogram was obtained who do not undergo angiography a second time. Did any of these patients experience a rehemorrhage that would add to the false-negative rate of the initial angiograms?

The risk associated with angiography in patients with subarachnoid hemorrhage may also have been overstated, because the complications reported in two large, prospective trials (3,4) occurred largely in patients evaluated for transient ischemic attack and ischemic stroke.

The rate of false-negative angiograms in patients with a nonaneurysmal perimesencephalic pattern of subarachnoid hemorrhage may be much lower than the rate in patients without this pattern. The initial angiogram in patients with the nonaneurysmal perimesencephalic pattern of subarachnoid hemorrhage depicts an aneurysm in up to 9% of patients (5,6). There are insufficient data to determine the rate of aneurysm detection when a second angiogram is obtained in patients with the pattern of hemorrhage defined for nonaneurysmal perimesencephalic subarachnoid hemorrhage. In this particular group of patients, the rate of aneurysm detection achieved by obtaining a second angiogram may, in fact, be too low to warrant acquisition of a second angiogram. Yet, because a posterior fossa aneurysm can rupture and cause a nonaneurysmal perimesencephalic subarachnoid hemorrhage pattern (5,6), one cannot conclusively state that acquisition of a second angiogram is unreasonable in patients with this pattern of hemorrhage.

Some patterns of subarachnoid hemorrhage other than the nonaneurysmal perimesencephalic subarachnoid hemorrhage pattern should raise a high level of concern for aneurysm, even if the negative first angiogram is technically good. For example, if a patient had interhemispheric subarachnoid hemorrhage and an inferior medial frontal lobe hematoma, we would be extremely concerned about an aneurysm of the anterior communicating artery or of the pericallosal artery and would insist on a second angiogram if the first angiogram was negative.

An important issue not raised by the authors is what constitutes an adequate angiogram. If one were to assume that a single, technically excellent angiogram is always adequate, as du Mesnil de Rochemont et al (1) contend, one would have to define what constitutes an adequate angiogram. Because angiography may be as much an art as a science, the acquisition of oblique projections used to show more clearly an area of suspicion (because the pattern of subarachnoid hemorrhage was noted on computed tomographic scans or on initial anteroposterior and lateral angiographic projections) depends to a large degree on the experience of the angiographer.

This is a difficult area to explore, which may be why the authors chose

Index terms: Aneurysm, cerebral, 17.73 • Angiography, complications, 17.44 • Arachnoid, hemorrhage, 10.2521 • Carotid arteries, angiography, 17.1248 • Cerebral angiography, 10.124 • Devil's Advocate

Radiology 1997; 205:323–325

[1] From the Department of Radiology, University of Virginia Health Sciences Center, Box 170, Charlottesville, VA 22908. Received April 14, 1997; accepted May 8. **Address reprint requests to** H.J.C.

not to do so. Yet, other technical issues are less ambiguous. If no aneurysm is visualized, the external carotid arteries must always be evaluated (either separately or with common carotid artery injections) to exclude a dural arteriovenous fistula as the cause of subarachnoid hemorrhage. It is not clear from the article by du Mesnil de Rochemont et al (1) whether or not the external carotid arteries were consistently evaluated. Arteriovenous fistulas in the dura mater or pia mater of the cervicomedullary region have been reported (7) to be a cause of subarachnoid hemorrhage and may not be identified unless both vertebral arteries are evaluated. The authors did not discuss the possibility of a dural arteriovenous fistula as a possible cause of subarachnoid hemorrhage, which could have been overlooked for such technical reasons.

On the basis of the available data in the literature, we believe that a second angiographic examination is still generally indicated in patients with subarachnoid hemorrhage in whom the initial angiogram was negative, especially if the pattern is not that described for nonaneurysmal perimesencephalic subarachnoid hemorrhage. We continue to obtain a second angiogram in patients with the nonaneurysmal perimesencephalic subarachnoid hemorrhage pattern, because this pattern can be associated with an aneurysmal subarachnoid hemorrhage (5,6), and we believe that it remains to be proved that the risk associated with angiography outweighs the risk of rupture of an undiscovered aneurysm in these patients.

References

1. du Mesnil de Rochemont R, Heindel W, Wesselmann C, et al. Nontraumatic subarachnoid hemorrhage: value of repeat angiography. Radiology 1997; 202:798–800.
2. Rosenorn J, Eskesen V, Schmidt K, Ronde F. The risk of rebleeding from ruptured intracranial aneurysms. J Neurosurg 1987; 67:329–332.
3. Heiserman JE, Dean BL, Hodak JA, et al. Neurologic complications of cerebral angiography. AJNR 1994; 15:1408–1411.
4. Dion JE, Gates PC, Fox AJ, Barnett HJM, Blom RJ. Clinical events following neuroangiography: a prospective study. Stroke 1987; 18:997–1004.
5. Schwartz TH, Solomon RA. Perimesencephalic nonaneurysmal subarachnoid hemorrhage: review of the literature. Neurosurgery 1996; 39:433–440.
6. Kallmes DF, Clark HP, Dix JE, et al. Ruptured vertebrobasilar aneurysms: frequency of the nonaneurysmal perimesencephalic pattern of hemorrhage on CT scans. Radiology 1996; 201:657–660.
7. Deveikis JP, Allen RB, Dickenson LD, Ross DA, Chandler WF. Cervico-medullary arteriovenous fistulae: a frequently unrecognized etiology of subarachnoid hemorrhage. Presented at the 34th Annual Meeting of the American Society of Neuroradiology, Seattle, Wash, June 23–27, 1996.

Richard du Mesnil de Rochemont, MD • Walter Heindel, MD

Reply[2]

The comments by Dr Cloft et al stimulate discussion about the value of repeat angiography in patients with nontraumatic subarachnoid hemorrhage of unknown origin. We thank Dr Cloft and colleagues for their comments, and we shall state the reasons for our different point of view.

Cloft et al point out that the risk and benefit of repeat angiography in patients with subarachnoid hemorrhage critically depends on (*a*) the precise risk of angiography, (*b*) the rate of rebleeding, and (*c*) the rate of false-negative initial angiograms. Cloft et al use statistics derived from the literature and mentioned in our article (1); these statistics are quite uncertain and do not reflect our experience.

Cloft et al assert that the risk associated with angiography in patients with subarachnoid hemorrhage may be overstated, because the complications reported in two large prospective trials (2,3) occurred largely in patients evaluated because of transient ischemic attack and ischemic stroke. On the other hand, angiography performed because of subarachnoid hemorrhage may be associated with an increased risk because of technical reasons. In patients with subarachnoid hemorrhage of unknown origin, selective placement of catheters in the internal and external carotid arteries and in one or both vertebral arteries is necessary, whereas most patients with ischemic attack only need undergo angiography of the common carotid artery.

In patients with subarachnoid hemorrhage, more angiograms are usually obtained, so that the catheter is left in place for a longer period. This may increase the risk of ischemic events. To our knowledge, no prospective study has yet been performed that examines the specific risk associated with angiography in patients with subarachnoid hemorrhage.

The rate of rehemorrhage of thrombosed or small aneurysms that may be overlooked at initial angiography is unknown. The numbers reported in the literature refer to patients with a proved aneurysm who did not undergo surgery for one reason or another. Many circumstances may influence the risk of rebleeding. For example, in the series of Rosenorn et al (4), the risk of rebleeding was substantially dependent on the clinical Hunt and Hess grade in the patient. Other factors related to rebleeding include patient sex and age; shape, size, and direction of the aneurysm; and variation in blood pressure (5).

In our retrospective investigation (1), no aneurysm was depicted on the second study that was also not visible on the initial study. In the patients in whom a negative initial angiogram was obtained, no documented rehemorrhage was observed. All three false-negative angiograms were the result of observer error or of technical problems. We concluded, therefore, that if one can avoid such mistakes, the risk associated with repeat angiography will outweigh the risk of rupture of an undetected aneurysm.

One way to minimize observer error is to submit all negative angiograms for reevaluation by a radiologist other than the initial reader, as Cloft et al suggest. Of course, we cannot dismiss the objection by Cloft et al that a re-

[2] From the Department of Diagnostic Radiology, University of Cologne, Joseph-Stelzmann Strasse 9, D-50924 Cologne, Lindenthal, Germany. Received and accepted July 10, 1997. **Address reprint requests to** R.d.M.d.R.

evaluation does not change a false-negative angiogram into a true-positive one. This remains an inevitable problem of a retrospective study, which can be solved only by means of further prospective studies.

Cloft et al are critical of the fact that we do not raise the issue of what constitutes an adequate angiogram. In our article (1), we provided some criteria to define what we believe to be an adequate angiogram: (*a*) visualization of all vascular territories, (*b*) use of compression at angiography to visualize the anterior and posterior communicating arteries (if these vessels are not visualized spontaneously), (*c*) acquisition of at least four projections (anteroposterior, lateral, two oblique) of the vascular territory of the internal carotid artery, and (*d*) evaluation of the external carotid artery (if no aneurysms are visualized). We agree that further projections depend largely on the experience of the angiographer.

In conclusion, the diagnostic approach has changed at our institution. In patients with subarachnoid hemorrhage, only one adequate angiogram is obtained because we believe that the risk associated with performance of angiography a second time outweighs the benefit. The data from our retrospective study should stimulate prospective—eventually multicenter—trials to answer the remaining questions. ■

References

1. du Mesnil de Rochemont R, Heindel W, Wesselmann C, et al. Nontraumatic subarachnoid hemorrhage: value of repeat angiography. Radiology 1997; 202:798–800.
2. Heiserman JE, Dean BL, Hodak JA, et al. Neurologic complications of cerebral angiography. AJNR 1994; 15:1408–1411.
3. Dion JE, Gates PC, Fox AJ, Barnett HJM, Blom RJ. Clinical events following neuroangiography: a prospective study. Stroke 1987; 18:997–1004.
4. Rosenorn J, Eskesen V, Schmidt K, Ronde F. The risk of rebleeding from ruptured intracranial aneurysm. J Neurosurg 1987; 67:329–332.
5. Mayberg MR, Batjer H, Dacey R, et al. Guidelines for the management of aneurysmal subarachnoid hemorrhage: a statement for health care professionals from a special writing group of the Stroke Council, American Heart Association. Stroke 1994; 25:2315–2328.

Book Review

Intramedullary Spinal Cord Tumors

Georges Fischer, MD, and Jacques Brotchi, MD, PhD

New York, NY: Thieme Medical, 1996. ISBN 0-86577-593-1. Cloth, $109.00; pp 127; 198 figures; tables.

In the preface, the authors indicate that they wish to report their experience with intramedullary spinal cord tumors. Their series of 171 cases represents considerable experience with over five cases per year during the 30 years since publication of the previous monographs on the subject. Not even physicians at busy neurosurgical centers see these lesions more often; this fact indicates the utility of the book for neurosurgeons.

There are 127 pages and 198 figures in the book. It is divided into three sections, and each section has three or four chapters. The first section gives an overview of the subject. The 20 pages on neuroradiologic topics are located in the second chapter, on diagnosis. The second section, on treatment, contains four chapters in which glial tumors, malignant nonglial tumors, benign nonglial tumors, and diseases that mimic tumors are discussed. The third section is a review of results. In the third chapter, there is a three-page summary of postoperative imaging findings.

The sections on imaging are concise, and the pictures are good. The legends add explanation to the text. However, the discussion is limited to magnetic resonance (MR) imaging. Basic MR imaging findings are discussed; there is no discussion of imaging sequences, MR spectroscopy, or intraoperative ultrasound. In fairness to the authors, however, this book represents their experience, and the monograph was never meant to be encyclopedic.

The intraoperative photographs are spectacular. For a neuroradiologist, it is exciting to correlate these photographs with MR and computed tomographic images of spinal tumors. The section on postoperative neuroradiologic follow-up gives precise, cogent, and useful guidance for the radiologist.

In summary, for a neuroradiologist, this book has some unique advantages and enables a deeper understanding of the needs of the neurosurgeon. Because intramedullary spinal cord tumors occur relatively infrequently and most of their diagnostic features and differential diagnoses are covered in general neuroradiologic textbooks, neuroradiologists in very specialized centers may benefit most from this monograph.

Reviewed by David S. Martin, MD

Rüdiger von Kummer, MD • Kathryn L. Allen, PhD • Rolf Holle, PhD • Luigi Bozzao, MD
Stefano Bastianello, MD • Claude Manelfe, MD • Erich Bluhmki, PhD • Peter Ringleb, MD
Dieter H. Meier, MD • Werner Hacke, MD

Acute Stroke: Usefulness of Early CT Findings before Thrombolytic Therapy[1]

PURPOSE: **To determine whether the extent of subtle parenchymal hypoattenuation detected on computed tomographic (CT) scans obtained within 6 hours of ischemic stroke is a factor in predicting patients' response to thrombolytic treatment.**

MATERIALS AND METHODS: **The baseline CT scans of 620 patients, who received either recombinant tissue plasminogen activator (rt-PA) or a placebo, in a double-blind, randomized multicenter trial were prospectively evaluated and assigned to one of three categories according to the extent of parenchymal hypoattenuation: none, 33% or less (small), or more than 33% (large) of the middle cerebral artery territory. The association between the extent of hypoattenuation on the baseline CT scans and the clinical outcome in the placebo-treated and the rt-PA–treated groups after 3 months was analyzed.**

RESULTS: **In 215 patients with a small hypoattenuating area, treatment increased the chance of good outcome. In 336 patients with a normal CT scan and in 52 patients with a large hypoattenuating area, rt-PA had no beneficial effect but increased the risk for fatal brain hemorrhage.**

CONCLUSION: **The response to rt-PA in patients with ischemic stroke can be predicted on the basis of initial CT findings of the extent of parenchymal hypoattenuation in the territory of the middle cerebral artery.**

Stroke is a syndrome characterized by a sudden central neurologic deficit caused by intracranial hemorrhage or ischemia. After confirmation of cerebral ischemia at imaging, patients with similar clinical symptoms may differ in terms of the nature of the vascular disturbance and the extent of the initial ischemic damage. Thus, the cerebral pathophysiologic characteristics may vary in time and space among individuals. This makes the care of individual patients and the design of stroke studies extremely difficult, because it is unlikely that any specific treatment will be of similar benefit to all stroke patients, irrespective of the time interval from stroke onset.

With this in mind, two recent major studies of thrombolysis by the European Cooperative Acute Stroke Study (ECASS) (1) and the National Institute of Neurological Disorders and Stroke (NINDS) (2) included only patients examined within 3 and 6 hours of stroke onset. Investigators in both studies used computed tomographic (CT) findings to exclude patients with a primary hemorrhage; other patients were excluded on the basis of neurologic scores and clinical symptoms. Symptoms that were resolving before the randomization process were considered indications of a transient ischemic attack rather than of a stroke. In contrast to the NINDS trial, the ECASS protocol was intended to exclude patients with major ischemic strokes already visible on the baseline CT scan.

Careful selection of patients for a specific treatment such as thrombolytic therapy for stroke may result in improved safety and efficacy, but patients who might have benefitted can be excluded, as well. Recently, Baron et al (3) challenged the concept of an identical therapeutic time "window" in all stroke patients. Although used in the ECASS stroke trials, the relevance of inclusion and exclusion criteria based on CT findings has not yet been shown prospectively. These criteria were based solely on the speculation that hypoattenuation indicates ischemic edema, and thus irreversibly damaged tissue, that will not benefit from reperfusion and may have an increased risk of bleeding after treatment with the thrombolytic agent. Limited clinical observations (4) have suggested that this is the case.

Index terms: Brain, CT, 10.12111 • Brain, edema, 10.861 • Brain, infarction, 10.781 • Brain, ischemia, 10.7691, 10.781 • Cerebral blood vessels, thrombosis, 174.7691, 174.781 • Thrombolysis, 174.1265

Abbreviations: ECASS = European Cooperative Acute Stroke Study, NINDS = National Institute of Neurological Disorders and Stroke, rt-PA = recombinant tissue plasminogen activator.

Radiology 1997; 205:327–333

[1] From the Department of Neuroradiology, Technische Universität, Fetscherstrasse 74, D-01307 Dresden, Germany (R.v.K.); the Department of Neurochemistry, Institute of Neurology, London, England (K.L.A.); the GSF–National Research Center for Environment and Health, Institute for Medical Informatics and Health Services Research, Neuherberg, Germany (R.H.); the Department of Neuroradiology, Università degli Studi di Roma La Sapienza, Rome, Italy (L.B., S.B.); the Department of Diagnostic and Interventional Neuroradiology and MRI Unit, Hôpital Purpan, Toulouse, France (C.M.); Boehringer Ingelheim, Germany (E.B., D.H.M.); and the Department of Neurology, University of Heidelberg, Germany (P.R., W.H.). Received May 9, 1997; revision requested June 9; revision received June 23; accepted June 25. Supported by Boehringer Ingelheim, Germany, and Karl Thomae, Biberach, Germany. **Address reprint requests to** R.v.K.

E.B. and D.H.M. are employed by Boehringer Ingelheim, which is seeking approval for the use of recombinant tissue plasminogen activator in the treatment of ischemic stroke.

See also the editorial by Russell (pp 315–318) in this issue.

By analyzing the ECASS data, we aimed to determine whether there is justification for exclusion of patients from treatment with intravenous recombinant tissue plasminogen activator (rt-PA) if signs of extensive ischemic edema are already visible on baseline CT scans. The results of such an analysis may help to define more precisely those patients who are candidates for thrombolysis, as well as provide information about the value of CT in patients with acute stroke.

MATERIALS AND METHODS

Seventy-five centers in 14 European countries recruited 620 patients with the clinical diagnosis of hemispheric stroke and who were admitted to a hospital between December 1992 and March 1994. The patients were randomly assigned to receive treatment with a placebo ($n = 307$) or with intravenous administration of 1.1 mg per kilogram body weight of rt-PA (Alteplase; Boehringer Ingelheim, Germany) ($n = 313$). The trial was conducted in a double-blind fashion. Five patients were randomly assigned to the groups but were not treated; therefore, 305 patients received a placebo, and 310 patients received rt-PA. A baseline CT scan was obtained in all patients; the scans were judged to be technically acceptable for the local investigators. The design of this study and the main results were recently published (1).

In addition to inclusion criteria based on clinical data, the study protocol provided inclusion criteria based on CT findings, with the intention of excluding from the analysis findings in patients with areas of parenchymal hypoattenuation that exceeded one-third of the territory of the middle cerebral artery or if diffuse swelling of the hemisphere was present. Parenchymal hypoattenuation was defined as a region of abnormally decreased attenuation of brain structures (relative to attenuation of other parts of the same structures or of the contralateral counterparts) that could be visually recognized and was consistent with recent hypoperfusion of an arterial territory. We hypothesized that even subtle degrees of hypoattenuation indicated net uptake of tissue water caused by severe focal ischemia. Focal brain swelling was defined as any focal narrowing of the cerebrospinal fluid space (eg, effacement of cortical sulci or ventricular compression).

All investigators received a booklet of CT scans that showed early ischemic tissue changes of varying extent. In anticipation that the local investigators would not always detect subtle parenchymal hypoattenuation (in fact, a 10% rate of false inclusions was anticipated, and the study population was enlarged accordingly) three independent neuroradiologists (R.v.K., L.B., C.M.) from different countries (Germany, Italy, and France) were asked to assess additionally brain pathologic conditions prospectively on all CT scans obtained at 0 (baseline), 1, and 7 days after symptom onset. The neuroradiologists performed their assessments simultaneously and independently.

The independent assessors were blinded to any clinical information, although blinding to follow-up scans was not guaranteed in each case. They evaluated each scan for pathologic parenchymal hypoattenuation, tissue swelling, and scan quality. A scan was defined as "not readable" when gray and white matter attenuation could not be differentiated. A scan was defined as "poor" when gray and white matter of the brain could be differentiated with difficulty because the CT window was too large or because of the presence of motion artifacts. CT scans with some motion or beam-hardening artifacts but with good contrast between gray and white matter attenuation were considered to be of "moderate" quality. All remaining scans were defined as "good."

The size of the area with decreased attenuation was estimated as a percentage of the middle cerebral arterial territory by using three categories: "none," "33% or less," and "more than 33%." In the following text we refer to hypoattenuation of 33% or less of the middle cerebral arterial territory as "small" and to greater degrees of hypoattenuation as "large."

Parenchymal hypoattenuation of the anterior and posterior cerebral arterial territories was assessed separately. Four patients had an isolated posterior cerebral arterial infarct, and five patients had an isolated anterior cerebral arterial infarct. These nine patients were included in the group with no middle cerebral arterial infarct. In three patients, the anterior cerebral arterial infarct contributed to a large middle cerebral arterial infarct, and the findings in these patients were analyzed accordingly. The panel of three neuroradiologists functioned as final arbiter with regard to CT findings. When the panelists disagreed, a common reading session was used to render a final judgment.

Clinical neurologists, blinded with regard to treatment and the judgment of the CT scan reading panel, assessed the severity of neurologic symptoms with the Scandinavian stroke scale (5) at patient admission; disability was assessed 90 days after stroke onset by using the modified Rankin scale (6). The clinical outcome of patients was considered to be "good" if the Rankin score was 0 or 1 (patient was cured with no functional deficit 90 days after the stroke); outcome was considered to be "poor" if the Rankin score was 4–6. Cause of death was individually assessed without knowledge of clinical information, findings from the last CT scan, and autopsy reports, in selected cases.

We used the individual readings, the agreement rates, and the κ statistic to determine interobserver reliability. The association of neuroradiologic characteristics and clinical outcome events was tested with the Kruskal-Wallis test, the χ^2 test with the Yates correction, or, if indicated, the Fisher exact test. We calculated the 95% confidence interval for proportions. The response to rt-PA in different subgroups of patients was assessed with odds ratios and 95% confidence intervals for different outcome events (7).

RESULTS

According to the judgment of the CT reading panel, good quality CT scans were obtained in 166 (27%) of 620 patients, moderate quality scans were obtained in 314 (51%) patients, poor quality scans were obtained in 123 (20%) patients, and unreadable scans were obtained in eight (1%) patients. CT scans in nine (1%) patients were not available for assessment by the CT reading panel, including the scans in the five patients who were not treated.

In 314 (52%) of 603 cases, all three neuroradiologists were in agreement with regard to whether an abnormal area of parenchymal attenuation indicative of recent focal ischemia was visible ($\kappa = 0.34$). Pairwise agreement was 63%–72% (κ range, 0.30–0.45). Agreement was reached in 86% of cases ($\kappa = 0.36$) with regard to whether the extent of the area of hypoattenuation of the middle cerebral arterial territory (33% or less, more than 33%), with pairwise agreement of 90%–91% (κ range, 0.23–0.51). Interobserver agreement was 68% ($\kappa = 0.34$) with regard to focal brain swelling, with pairwise agreement of 77%–80% (κ range, 0.30–0.37). Examples of different types of parenchymal hypoattenuation and focal brain swelling are shown in Figure 1.

Table 1 presents the assessment of the extent of ischemic edema by the CT reading panel. The earliest CT scan that showed parenchymal hypoattenuation of any degree was obtained 35 minutes after the onset of symptoms. Scans obtained during the 1st hour after stroke in five (20%) of 25 patients showed focal parenchymal hypoattenuation, as did scans obtained during the 2nd hour in 53 (42%) of 127 patients. There was no clear association between the time of the CT examination and the percentage of patients with small or large areas of parenchymal hypoattenuation during the first 6 hours after the onset of symptoms ($P = .10$) (Fig 2).

Focal brain swelling was seen on scans in 129 (21%) of 603 patients. Brain swelling was visible on scans in only six (2%) of 336 patients without associated parenchymal hypoattenuation, in 75 (35%) of 215 patients with a small area of hypoattenuation, and in 48 (92%) of 52 patients with a large area of hypoattenuation ($P < .0001$).

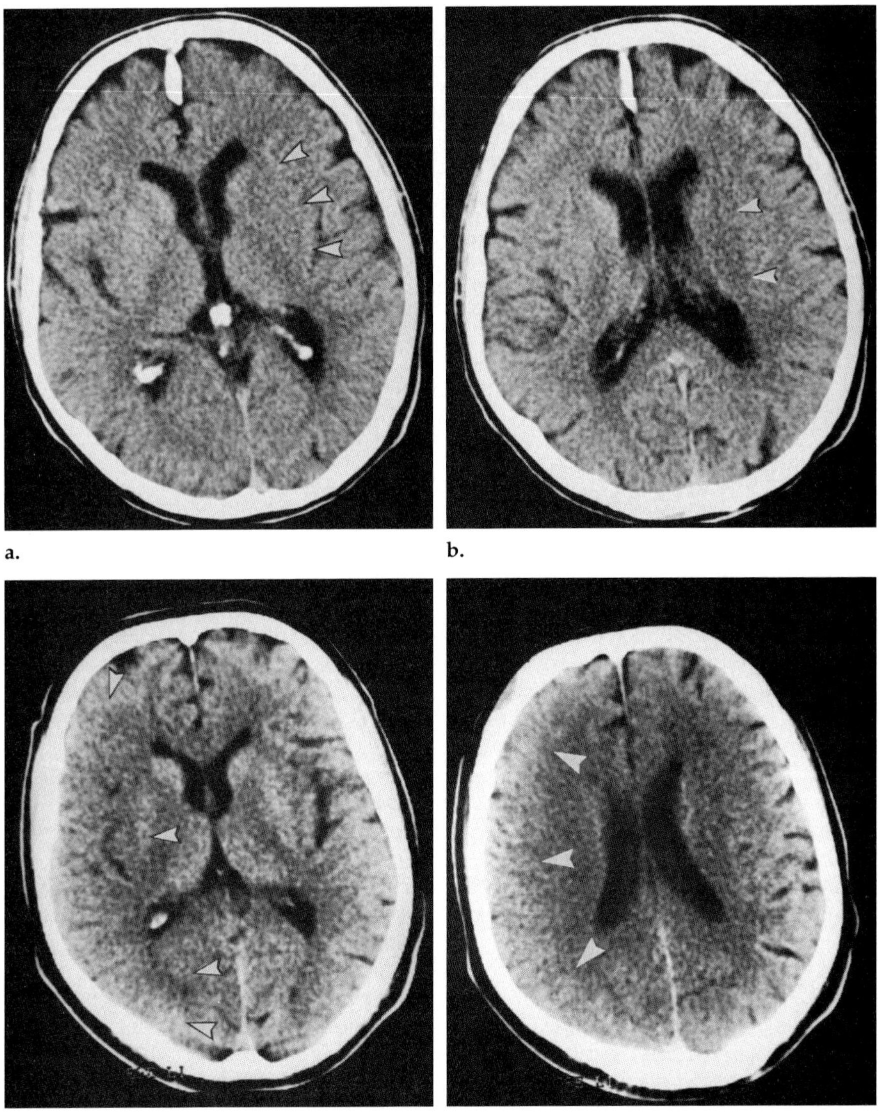

Figure 1. Early CT findings after ischemic stroke. **(a, b)** Unenhanced CT sections obtained 3 hours after the onset of left-sided hemiparesis in a 62-year-old man. The area of diminished attenuation is restricted to the left lentiform nucleus (arrowheads), and the extent is less than 33% of the territory of the middle cerebral artery. This patient was randomly assigned to the placebo group. He was moderately disabled (Rankin score, 3) 3 months after the stroke. **(c, d)** Unenhanced CT scans obtained 2 hours after symptom onset in a 71-year-old man. The lower section (c) shows slight parenchymal hypoattenuation (arrowheads) of the lateral frontal lobe, the insular cortex, the lentiform nucleus, and the temporal lobe. On both sections, brain swelling with effacement of sulci is obvious. The parenchymal hypoattenuation clearly exceeds 33% of the medial cerebral arterial territory. This patient was randomly assigned to the placebo group and died of midbrain incarceration 2 days after the stroke.

Patients with no, small, or large parenchymal hypoattenuation did not differ with regard to age, sex, assignment to treatment group, or time between symptom onset and initiation of treatment (Table 2). The Scandinavian stroke score determined at admission decreased (indicative of more severe stroke) as the extent of estimated parenchymal hypoattenuation increased ($P < .0001$).

In the placebo group, severe disability and mortality (modified Rankin score, 4–6) at 90 days after the stroke were statistically significantly associated with the extent of parenchymal hypoattenuation as shown on the initial CT scan ($P < .0001$). Sixteen (76%; 95% confidence interval = 55%, 89%) of 21 patients with a large hypoattenuating area had a poor clinical outcome (modified Rankin score, 4–6), 65 (59%; 95% confidence interval = 49%, 68%) of 110 patients with a small hypoattenuating area had a poor outcome, and 57 (34%; 95% confidence interval = 27%, 41%) of 169 patients with no hypoattenuating area had a poor outcome. Cause of death was extensive brain edema in five (24%) of 21 patients with a large hypoattenuating area, in nine (8%) of 110 patients with a small hypoattenuating area, and in one (1%) of 169 patients with no hypoattenuating area. No patients with a large area of hypoattenuation on the baseline CT scan died as a result of brain hemorrhage. However, in the placebo group, five (5%) of 110 patients with a small hypoattenuating area and two (1%) of 169 patients with no hypoattenuating area died of a cerebral hemorrhage.

Figure 3 shows the disability at 90 days in patients in both treatment arms according to the extent of parenchymal hypoattenuation on the initial CT scan. Table 3 presents the odds ratio (which is derived by dividing the odds of an outcome in the group that received rt-PA by the odds of the same outcome in the group that received the placebo) for the 90-day outcome of no disability, overall mortality, fatal brain edema, and fatal brain hemorrhage.

In patients with no parenchymal hypoattenuation on the baseline CT scan, no statistically significant effect on the odds ratio for no disability at 90 days was found. In this subgroup, however, nine (5%) of 167 rt-PA–treated patients died of cerebral hemorrhage versus two (1%) of 169 placebo-treated patients ($P = .0338$). In patients with a small area of parenchymal hypoattenuation, rt-PA increased the cure rate from 10% (11 of 110) to 28% (29 of 105) ($P = .0014$), although the risks were not statistically significantly affected. Two (6%) of 31 patients with a large area of parenchymal hypoattenuation were cured after treatment with rt-PA versus three (14%) of 21 patients in the placebo group ($P = .3826$). In this subgroup, five (16%) of 31 patients treated with rt-PA died of cerebral hemorrhage compared with none of the 21 patients treated with the placebo ($P = .0732$).

CT scans in nine (10%) of 87 patients treated within 3 hours of stroke onset showed an ischemic edema with an extent that exceeded 33% of the middle cerebral arterial territory. Of these, four of five patients in the placebo-treated group and three of four patients in the rt-PA–treated group had a poor clinical outcome.

DISCUSSION

The ECASS was designed to be a study of the efficacy and safety of rt-PA administered intravenously in carefully selected stroke patients treated within 6 hours of symptom onset. By applying clinical and CT exclusion criteria, the ECASS protocol was an attempt to exclude patients with slight or severe clinical symptoms and with CT signs of large edema already visible within the first 6 hours of stroke onset. The stroke population discussed here, therefore, is clearly not representative of stroke patients in general. Because the individual exclusion criteria were not recorded, we can only presume that the proportion of patients with mild symptoms or with large ischemic lesions would be larger in an unselected population of patients with stroke. Stratification of the study population into three groups with no, a small, or a large area of hypoattenuation (indicative of ischemic edema) on the baseline CT scan became possible because the central CT scan reading panel of ECASS investigators distinguished 52 patients with large ischemic edema that had been overlooked by local investigators, with the result that these patients were wrongly enrolled in the study (8).

The designers of the ECASS protocol anticipated that the overall awareness for early CT signs of infarct would be low because these signs can be subtle and were not well acknowledged in the radiologic literature when the study was started. The protocol therefore specified that a panel of three independent neuroradiologists should assess all CT scans independently and simultaneously. These radiologists were blinded to all clinical information, and had to assess signs of recent cerebral ischemia on CT scans of heterogeneous quality from different European countries.

The quality of the CT scans was rated as poor in 20% of the available and readable scans. This may explain, in part, the low interobserver agreement ($\kappa = 0.34$) in detecting ischemic lesions, which was lower than that in a recent test (9) of six observers, who achieved a κ of 0.58 for detection of parenchymal areas of hypoattenuation on CT scans obtained within 6 hours of stroke onset. The subtlety of the hypoattenuation caused by ischemic water uptake during the first 2 hours after focal ischemia seems, however, to be the major factor contributing to a low interobserver agreement. We speculate that the use of imaging modalities with which ischemic edema can be more clearly demonstrated, such as diffusion-weighted magnetic resonance imaging, will result in a higher interobserver agreement with regard to the extent of the ischemic lesion during the 1st hours after symptom onset.

With regard to the exclusion criterion of "parenchymal hypoattenuation that exceeds one-third of the middle cerebral arterial territory," the 86% interobserver agreement was high, but the chance-adjusted agreement rate was surprisingly low ($\kappa = 0.36$). The paradox of high agreement but a low κ can be partly explained in terms of the low prevalence of patients with a large area of parenchymal hypoattenuation, because most such patients were excluded from the study before assignment to a treatment group. Feinstein and Cicchetti (10) showed that κ is affected by prevalence and cannot be used as an index of reliability when observer variability is tested without an analysis of how proportionate changes in the marginal total values affect the calculation of κ. In the test (9) of six observers mentioned earlier, the κ for the ordinal rating of the extent of hypoattenuation in cases of acute stroke was 0.65 for the right hemisphere and 0.57 for the left hemisphere. Although a κ of 0.40–0.80 is indicative of moderate to good interobserver agreement, we appreciate that even extensive ischemic edema can be overlooked owing to low technical quality of the scanner or insufficient training of the observer.

We cannot exclude the possibility that the members of the CT scan reading panel were biased because of knowledge of the follow-up scans at the evaluation of the baseline scans. For example, a normal follow-up scan will increase the willingness of an observer who is in doubt about a finding to read the baseline scan as normal, whereas a large edema on a follow-up scan will stimulate the observer to search for early signs of large edema. Thus, the setting of the ECASS CT scan reading panel does not reflect the real world, which was better represented by the practices of the local investigators. On the other hand, we do not doubt that these three experienced neuroradiologists independently detected real pathologic findings that may become apparent to others after training in CT scan reading has increased their awareness. One of the panelists (R.v.K.) and colleagues (11) have recently shown that recognition of ischemic hypoattenuation is possible within 6 hours of stroke onset even when readers are blinded to the results of follow-up CT and clinical data. Clinical information about the site of cerebral ischemia may also improve the observer's awareness. We therefore believe that the estimation of the brain edema apparent on CT scans obtained within 6 hours of symptom onset can be used to differentiate the patient population in future stroke trials. This hypothesis is now being tested in the ongoing second ECASS trial (ECASS II).

Table 1
Extent of Ischemic Edema on CT Scans

CT Finding	Treatment rt-PA	Treatment Placebo
Parenchymal hypoattenuation*		
None ($n = 336$)	167	169
33% or less ($n = 215$)	105	110
More than 33% ($n = 52$)	31	21
Brain swelling		
Present ($n = 474$)	238	236
Absent ($n = 129$)	65	64
CT scan not available ($n = 17$)	10	7

* Extent of parenchymal hypoattenuation was estimated as a percentage of the territory of the middle cerebral artery.

Brain edema plays a major role in the pathophysiology of ischemic stroke. Brain edema causes progressive microcirculatory compression and thereby aggravates the primary ischemic insult (12). If focal cerebral blood flow is reduced below the critical level of 10–15 $mL \cdot 100\ g^{-1} \cdot min^{-1}$ by means of experimental permanent occlusion of the middle cerebral artery, cortical water content increases immediately and steadily from 80.7% to 83.0% wet weight within 4 hours (13). This 2.3% net uptake of water is accompanied by an increase in tissue sodium concentration, a decrease in tissue potassium concentration, a shift of water from the extra- to the intracellular compartment, and a linear increase in brain volume within 4 hours of middle cerebral arterial occlusion (13).

The early water uptake without marked permeability changes of the blood-brain barrier is named "cytotoxic" or "cellular" edema and is caused by osmotic and ionic gradients between blood and ischemic brain tissue and by pinocytosis of water in the presence of remaining blood flow (incomplete ischemia) (14). Brain edema under such conditions does not resolve if the tissue is reperfused after 1 hour of ischemia. Moreover, reperfusion can further enhance edema in areas of dense ischemia (14). Above the critical flow level of 10–15 $mL \cdot 100\ g^{-1} \cdot min^{-1}$, brain edema does not develop (13,15).

The gray scale on CT scans reflects different x-ray attenuation in tissue,

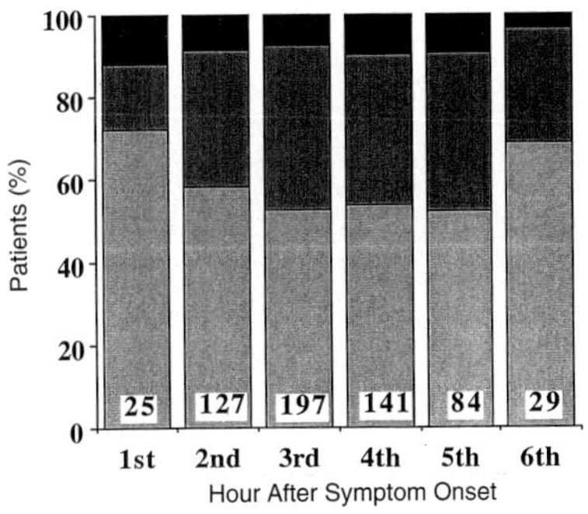

2.

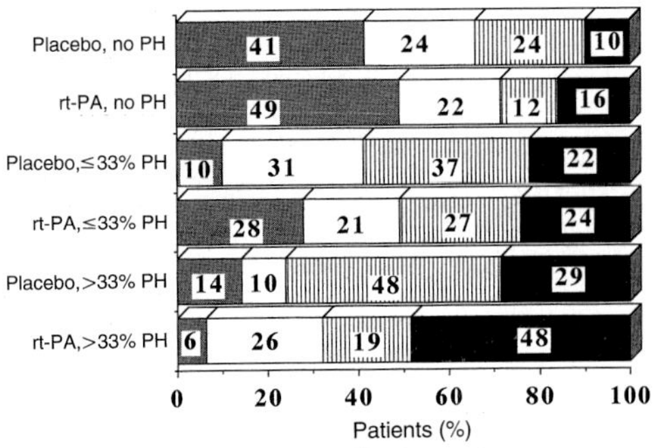

3.

Figures 2, 3. **(2)** Graph shows the percentage of patients with no (light gray bars), a small (33% or less of the middle cerebral arterial territory) (dark gray bars), or a large (more than 33% of the middle cerebral arterial territory) (black bars) area of hypoattenuation (indicative of ischemic edema) depicted on CT scans at different time points after stroke onset. The absolute numbers of patients are printed in the bars. **(3)** Graph shows clinical outcome at 3 months scored with the modified Rankin scale in three placebo and three rt-PA treatment groups of patients stratified according the extent of ischemic edema on baseline CT scans. The numbers in the bars are the number of patients. *PH* = parenchymal hypoattenuation, gray bars = Rankin score of 0–1, white bars = Rankin score of 2–3, striped bars = Rankin score of 4–5, black bars = dead.

Table 2
Baseline Characteristics of Patients and Extent of Early Ischemic Edema

	Parenchymal Hypoattenuation*			
Characteristic	None (n = 336)	33% or Less (n = 215)	More than 33% (n = 52)	P Value
Age (y)†	66 ± 11	65 ± 12	65 ± 11	.45
Women (%)	36	39	38	.76
Scandinavian Stroke score†	31 ± 11	26 ± 9	21 ± 9	<.0001
Received rt-PA (%)	50	49	60	.36
Time to treatment (h)†	4.4 ± 1.1	4.4 ± 1.0	4.3 ± 1.1	.88

* Extent of parenchymal hypoattenuation was estimated as a percentage of the territory of the middle cerebral artery.
† Data are means ± 1 standard deviation.

which is linearly proportional to the electron density or water content of tissue (16,17). A 1% increase in tissue water content causes a 2–3 HU decrease in x-ray attenuation (18). Under the conditions of acute focal cerebral ischemia, x-ray attenuation may also be affected because of changes in focal cerebral blood volume.

We interpret the rare observation of focal brain swelling without concomitant parenchymal hypoattenuation to be an effect of compensatory vasodilation in regions of low perfusion pressure. Thus, CT findings may reflect a mixture of effects that both increase and decrease x-ray attenuation during the early course of ischemic edema.

In the case of middle cerebral arterial trunk occlusion, which causes severe focal ischemia mainly in the basal ganglia, parenchymal hypoattenuation is regularly visible within the first 6 hours after the onset of symptoms (4,19–21). It has been observed (4,22,23) that such parenchymal hypoattenuation can, at an early stage, delineate a volume of tissue that will subsequently become necrotic and—if the hypoattenuating area exceeds 50% of the middle cerebral arterial territory—is associated with a mortality rate of 85%. It seems logical to assume, therefore, that even subtle abnormal parenchymal hypoattenuation on CT scans in patients with a stroke syndrome is indicative of edema caused by focal hypoperfusion. We have observed that ischemic brain edema can appear on CT scans within 1 hour of stroke onset.

We presume that visibility of cerebral ischemia at CT is primarily determined by the degree and extent of ischemia. If hypoperfusion is profound, with values below 10–15 $mL \cdot 100\ g^{-1} \cdot min^{-1}$, ischemic edema will occur early (15). Conversely, a normal CT scan in a patient with stroke indicates a lesser degree of hypoperfusion and indicates potential reversibility of the functional disturbance. The ECASS now provides data to study the importance of these early CT findings.

Our results support the clinical and prognostic relevance of ischemic edema as assessed on CT scans obtained within 6 hours of the onset of symptoms: The extent of ischemic edema was clearly associated with the patient's neurologic score as regards state of disability at admission. Moreover, large ischemic edema was statistically significantly associated with poor clinical outcome at 90 days after stroke. Almost one half of the patients in the placebo group with large edema became severely disabled, and 29% died; most of them died of space-occupying edema, but, interestingly, none died of cerebral hemorrhage.

The clinical response to rt-PA was clearly different in patients with no, small, or large ischemic edema. The chance of cure due to treatment with rt-PA was not statistically significantly increased in patients with no edema relative to the already beneficial course in placebo-treated patients. The cure rate was statistically significantly improved after rt-PA treatment only in patients with a small edema. We think that small areas of hypoattenuation—often situated in the basal ganglia—represent the "tip of an iceberg" of a large hypoperfused tissue volume. Thrombolytic treatment may "rescue" this ischemic, but as yet not irreversibly damaged, tissue if the collateral blood supply does not fail until arterial recanalization is achieved. We recently observed (24) that patients with middle cerebral arterial trunk occlusion experienced a good clinical outcome after arterial recanalization that occurred not earlier than 8 hours after symptom onset.

In patients with a large edema, the proportion of cured patients was lower (0.41) in the rt-PA–treated group compared with the placebo-treated group. The small number of patients with a large edema (n = 52) and the associated large 95% confidence interval of the odds ratio (0.06, 2.70) indicate that this reduction of the odds ratio does not reach a level of statistical significance. This means that rt-PA may be ineffective in patients with a large ischemic edema; the possibility that rt-PA is actually detrimental could not be proved because of the small number of patients. In the group with no visible edema on the baseline CT scan, nine rt-PA–treated and two placebo-treated patients died of cerebral hematoma. This statistically significant difference must be substantiated with further studies. It could mean that—given the risks—treatment with rt-PA is inappropriate in patients with a normal CT scan,

Table 3
Response to rt-PA Treatment as a Function of Degree of Parenchymal Hypoattenuation

	No Hypoattenuated Area (n = 336)				Small Hypoattenuated Area (n = 215)				Large Hypoattenuated Area (n = 52)			
90-day Outcome	rt-PA Odds	Placebo Odds	Odds Ratio*	95% CI	rt-PA Odds	Placebo Odds	Odds Ratio*	95% CI	rt-PA Odds	Placebo Odds	Odds Ratio*	95% CI
No disability	79/88	70/99	1.27	0.82, 1.95	29/76	11/99	3.43†	1.61, 7.33	2/29	3/18	0.41	0.06, 2.70
Death	26/141	17/152	1.65	0.86, 3.17	25/80	24/86	1.12	0.59, 2.12	15/16	6/15	2.34	0.72, 7.63
Fatal edema	2/165	1/168	2.04	0.18, 22.67	11/94	9/101	1.31	0.52, 3.31	8/23	5/16	1.11	0.31, 4.02
Fatal hemorrhage	9/158	2/167	4.76‡	1.01, 22.35	4/101	5/105	0.83	0.22, 3.19	5/26	0/21	NA§	NA§

Note.—CI = confidence interval.
* The odds ratio is used to demonstrate response to rt-PA treatment. The odds ratio is determined by dividing the odds of a given outcome in the rt-PA treatment group (numerator) by the odds of the same outcome in the placebo treatment group (denominator). An odds ratio of 1.00 would indicate that rt-PA treatment did not affect the prevalence of the given outcome event. If the 95% CI does not include 1.00, the likelihood of the given outcome is substantially improved or diminished because of rt-PA treatment. For example, a patient with a small hypoattenuated area who receives rt-PA is more than 3 times as likely to have no disability compared with a patient who receives the placebo (odds ratio = 3.43). Although the likelihood of the no disability outcome after rt-PA treatment was diminished, relative to treatment with the placebo, in patients with a large hypoattenuated area, this reduction was not statistically significant.
† P = .0014.
‡ P = .0338.
§ The odds ratio and 95% CI could not be calculated because no patient had a fatal hemorrhage in the placebo group (P = .0732). NA = not applicable.

which indicates a beneficial natural course, obtained within the first 6 hours after stroke onset.

In summary, our observations, although limited by the attempt to exclude patients with mild symptoms or with a large ischemic edema and by the artificial setting of the CT evaluation, support the hypothesis that the assessment of ischemic edema within the first 6 hours of symptom onset by using CT may help predict different responses to intravenous thrombolytic treatment. Because we studied the vast majority (86%) of our population beyond the 3rd hour after symptom onset, this statement may not be valid for CT studies obtained less than 2 hours after onset, when the increase in tissue water is still too small to cause a visible decrease in x-ray attenuation.

It appears that the beneficial effect of rt-PA treatment is most pronounced in patients with a small ischemic edema visible on CT scans, whereas rt-PA treatment in patients in whom normal CT scans are obtained is not superior to the beneficial natural course but may increase the risk of fatal hemorrhage. Our findings strongly suggest that a parenchymal area of hypoattenuation in excess of one third of the middle cerebral arterial territory is indicative of both poor clinical outcome and ineffectiveness of treatment with intravenously administered rt-PA. Moreover, these observations suggest that intravenous rt-PA may be detrimental in patients with a large early edema. Observations by others support these findings: In the Multicenter Acute Stroke Trial–Europe study (25), treatment with intravenous streptokinase resulted in an increase in mortality, mainly because of hemorrhagic transformation of cerebral infarcts in severely ill patients. In 187 (64%) of 291 patients in this study population, baseline CT scans showed edema. (The extent of the area of parenchymal hypoattenuation was not reported.) In the NINDS trial (2), four (9%) of 45 patients with intracranial hemorrhage had baseline CT evidence of cerebral edema, compared with 4% of the study population as a whole. (The NINDS study did not differentiate between small and large edema.)

We conclude that it is important to assess the extent of ischemic edema on CT scans before thrombolytic treatment of ischemic stroke, as long as no better tools for the differentiation of reversible from irreversible ischemic damage are widely available. The association between the extent of initial ischemic damage and the response to thrombolytic treatment must be substantiated in further trials. On the basis of our results, however, it seems clear that patients with a large brain edema should not undergo rt-PA treatment. Consequently, strenuous efforts should be made to increase the awareness in physicians who care for patients with stroke of the subtle CT findings that indicate early ischemic brain edema. ■

Acknowledgments: We gratefully acknowledge the help of the following ECASS local investigators and committees. J. Klingelhöfer, MD (Munich, Germany); P. Krauseneck, MD (Bamberg, Germany); D. Schneider, MD (Leipzig, Germany); O. Hielscher, MD (Gelsenkirchen, Germany); T. Büttner, MD (Bochum, Germany); G. Hennen, MD (Wuppertal, Germany); P. Marx, MD (Berlin, Germany); C. H. Lücking, MD (Freiburg, Germany); K. Felgenhauer, MD (Göttingen, Germany); W. Hacke, MD (Heidelberg, Germany); W. Müllges, MD (Würzburg, Germany); G. Krieter, MD (Regensburg, Germany); A. Schwartz, MD (Mannheim, Germany); G. Krämer, MD (Mainz, Germany); H. C. Diener, MD (Essen, Germany); O. Busse, MD (Minden, Germany); M. Wiersbitzky, MD (Greifswald, Germany); A. Ferbert, MD (Kassel, Germany); K. F. Druschky, MD (Karlsruhe, Germany); H. Lechner, MD (Graz, Austria); G. Ladurner, MD (Salzburg, Austria); W. Schmutzhard, MD (Innsbruck, Austria); J. Bogousslavsky, MD (Lausanne, Switzerland); A. Vignolo, MD (Brescia, Italy); G. Regesta, MD (Genoa, Italy); G. Re, MD (Bologna, Italy); L. Pecorari, MD (Moncalieri, Italy); A. Lagi, MD (Florence, Italy); C. Argentino, MD (Rome, Italy); G. Ferrari, MD (Verona, Italy); A. Mamoli, MD (Bergamo, Italy); F. Mironi, MD (Mantua, Italy); Markku Kaste, MD (Helsinki, Finland); T. Erilä, MD (Tampere, Finland); I. Sivenius, MD (Kuopio, Finland); K. Murros, MD (Jyväskylä, Finland); H. Liukkonen, MD (Mikkeli, Finland); C. Hedman, MD (Lahti, Finland); A. Muuronen, MD (Kotka, Finland); K. Sotaniemi, MD (Oulu, Finland); L. Thomassen, MD (Bergen, Norway); O. Rosjo, MD (Nordbyhagen, Norway); N. Brautaset, MD (Tonsberg, Norway); B. Indredavik, MD (Trondheim, Norway); P. M. Sandset, MD (Oslo, Norway); J. Petersson, MD (Malmö, Sweden); H. Radberg, MD (Linköping, Sweden); A. Térent, MD (Söderhamn, Sweden); C. Carlström, MD (Stockholm, Sweden); Lena Kjällman, MD (Göteborg, Sweden); K. Overgaard, MD, O. Munck, MD (Copenhagen, Denmark); G. Boysen, MD (Hvidovre, Denmark); E. Enevoldsen, MD (Odense, Denmark); T. St Jensen, MD (Aarhus, Denmark); M. Campbell, MD (Bristol, England); S. A. Hawkins, MD (Belfast, Northern Ireland); C. L. Franke, MD (Heerlen, The Netherlands); J. Vos, MD (Amsterdam, The Netherlands); C. W. G. M. Frenken, MD (Nijmegen, The Netherlands); A. A. W. Op de Coul, MD (Tilburg, The Netherlands); W. Verslegers, MD (Merksem, Belgium); P. Cras, MD (Edegem, Belgium); P. Laloux, MD (Godinne, Belgium); D. Blecic, MD (Brussels, Belgium); M. Marchau, MD (Brugge, Belgium); J. R. Fève, MD (Nantes, France); G. Rancurel, MD (Paris, France); M. Weber, MD (Nancy, France); M. H. Mahagne, MD (Nice, France); V. Larrue, MD, G. Chollet, MD (Toulouse, France); P. Trouillas, MD (Lyon, France); J. M. Blard, MD (Montpellier, France); P. Caussanel, MD (Auch, France); J. M. Orgogozo, MD (Bordeaux, France); F. Arnoud, MD (Perpignan, France); L. Cunha, MD (Coimbra, Portugal); J. Castillo, MD (Santiago de Compostela, Spain); D. Tejedor, MD (Madrid, Spain); A. Chomorro, MD (Barcelona,

Spain); H. Sancho, MD (Valencia, Spain); A. Dávalos, MD (Gerona, Spain).

Steering Committee: Werner Hacke, MD, Chairman (Heidelberg, Germany); Cesare Fieschi (Rome, Italy); Markku Kaste (Helsinki, Finland).

Advisors to the Steering Committee: Marc Verstraete, Emmanuel Lesaffre (Leuven, Belgium); Werner Feuerer (Biberach, Germany).

Regional Coordinators: for Scandinavia, Gudrun Boysen (Hvidovre, Denmark); for the Benelux countries and England, Albert H. J. Hijdra (Amsterdam, Netherlands); for France and Spain, André Bes (Toulouse, France); for Italy, Danilo Toni (Rome, Italy); for Germany, Switzerland, and Austria, Michael Hennerici (Mannheim, Germany).

Ethical and safety monitoring committee: Klaus Poeck, Chairman (Aachen, Germany); Gregory del Zoppo (La Jolla, Calif); Hermann Zeumer (Hamburg, Germany); Gian-Luigi Lenzi (Rome, Italy); Jochen Mau (Düsseldorf, Germany).

Data management was provided by Innovex, Freiburg, Germany. Materials used in this study were supplied by Boehringer Ingelheim.

References

1. Hacke W, Kaste M, Fieschi C, et al. Safety and efficacy of intravenous thrombolysis with a recombinant tissue plasminogen activator in the treatment of acute hemispheric stroke. JAMA 1995; 274:1017–1025.
2. The National Institute of Neurological Disorders and Stroke rt-PA Stroke Study Group. Tissue plasminogen activator for acute ischemic stroke. N Engl J Med 1995; 333:1581–1587.
3. Baron JC, von Kummer R, del Zoppo GJ. Treatment of acute stroke: challenging the concept of a rigid and universal time window. Stroke 1995; 26:2219–2221.
4. von Kummer R, Meyding-Lamade U, Forsting M, et al. Sensitivity and prognostic value of early computed tomography in middle cerebral artery trunk occlusion. AJNR 1994; 15:9–15.
5. The Scandinavian Stroke Study Group. Multicenter trial of hemodilution in ischemic stroke: background and study protocol. Stroke 1985; 16:885–890.
6. van Swieten JC, Koudstaal PJ, Visser MC, Schouten HJA, van Gijn J. Interobserver agreement for the assessment of handicap in stroke patients. Stroke 1988; 19:604–607.
7. Altman D. Practical statistics for medical research. London, England: Chapman & Hall, 1991; 268–269.
8. von Kummer R, Bozzao L. Thrombolysis for acute stroke (letter). JAMA 1996; 275: 984–985.
9. von Kummer R, Holle R, Grzyska U, et al. Interobserver agreement in assessing early CT signs of middle cerebral artery infarction. AJNR 1996; 17:1743–1748.
10. Feinstein AR, Cicchetti DV. High agreement but low kappa. I. The problems of two paradoxes. J Clin Epidemiol 1990; 43: 543–549.
11. von Kummer R, Nolte PN, Schnittger H, Thron A, Ringelstein EB. Detectability of hemispheric ischemic infarction by computed tomography within 6 hours after stroke. Neuroradiology 1996; 38:31–33.
12. Hossmann KA, Schuir FJ. Experimental brain infarcts in cats. I. Pathophysiological observations. Stroke 1980; 11:583–592.
13. Schuir FJ, Hossmann KA. Experimental brain infarcts in cats. II. Ischemic brain edema. Stroke 1980; 11:593–601.
14. Ianotti F, Hoff J. Ischemic brain edema with and without reperfusion: an experimental study in gerbils. Stroke 1983; 14: 562–567.
15. Hossmann KA. Viability thresholds and the penumbra of focal ischemia. Ann Neurol 1994; 36:557–565.
16. Rieth KG, Fujiwara K, Di Chiro G, et al. Serial measurements of CT attenuation and specific gravity in experimental cerebral edema. Radiology 1980; 135:343–348.
17. Torack RM, Alcala H, Gado M, Burton R. Correlative assay of computerized cranial tomography (CCT), water content and specific gravity in normal and pathological postmortem brain. J Neuropathol Exp Neurol 1976; 35:385–392.
18. Unger E, Littlefild J, Gado M. Water content and water structure in CT and MR signal changes: possible influence in detection of early stroke. AJNR 1988; 9:687–691.
19. Tomura N, Uemura K, Inugami A, Fujita H, Higano S, Shishido F. Early CT finding in cerebral infarction. Radiology 1988; 168: 463–467.
20. Truwit CL, Barkovich AJ, Gean-Marton A, Hibri N, Norman D. Loss of the insular ribbon: another early CT sign of acute middle cerebral artery infarction. Radiology 1990; 176:801–806.
21. Horowitz SH, Zito JL, Donnarumma R, Patel M, Alvir J. Computed tomographic–angiographic findings within the first five hours of cerebral infarction. Stroke 1991; 22:1245–1253.
22. Hacke W, Schwab S, Horn M, Spranger M, De Georgia M, von Kummer R. "Malignant" middle cerebral artery territory infarction: clinical course and prognostic signs. Arch Neurol 1996; 53:309–315.
23. Skriver EB, Olsen TS. Contrast enhancement of cerebral infarcts: incidence and clinical value in different states of cerebral infarction. Neuroradiology 1982; 23:259–265.
24. von Kummer R, Holle R, Rosin L, Forsting M, Hacke W. Does arterial recanalization improve outcome in carotid territory stroke? Stroke 1995; 26:581–587.
25. The Multicenter Acute Stroke Trial–Europe Study Group. Thrombolytic therapy with streptokinase in acute ischemic stroke. N Engl J Med 1996; 335:145–150.

Saga of a Driver, a Snake, and a Fish

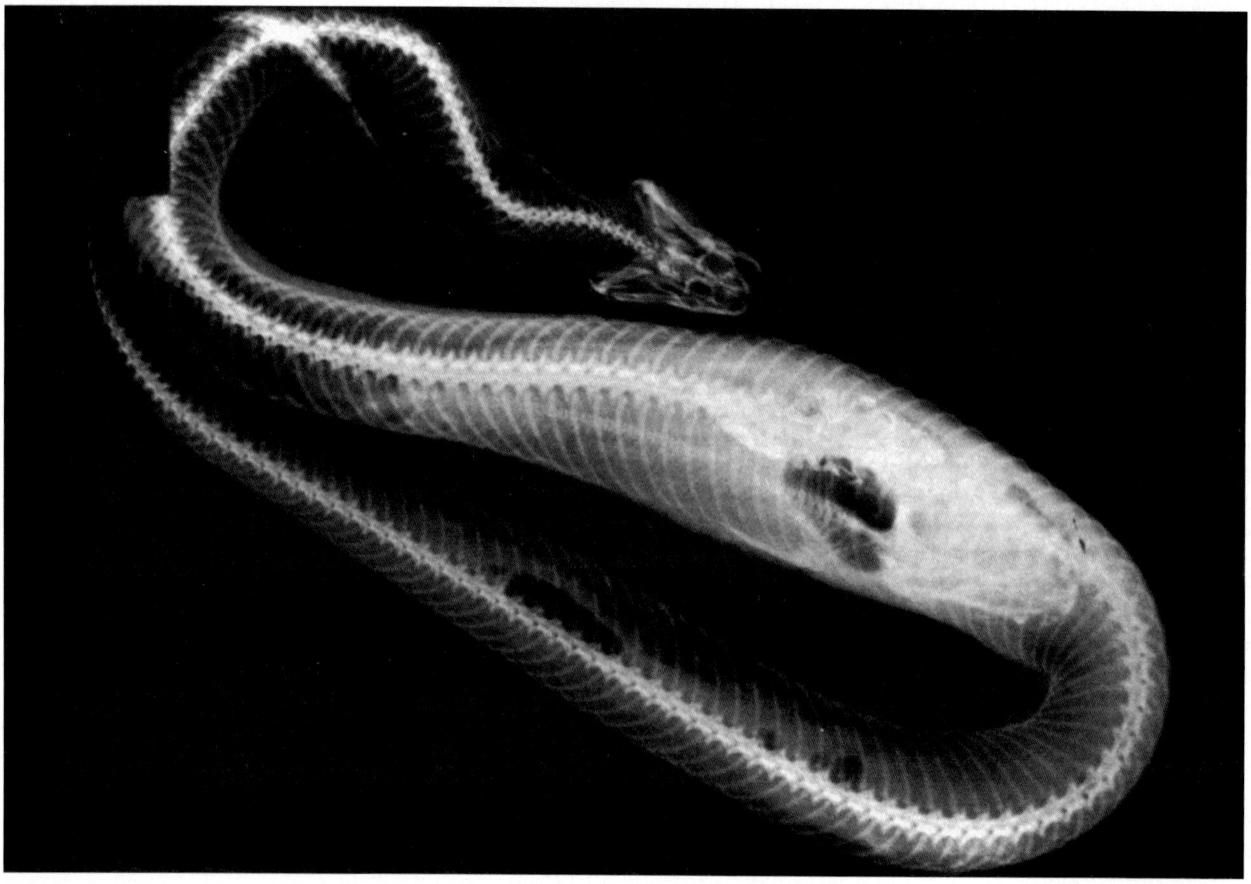

While changing a tire on the shoulder of a rural county road in north central Florida, a car driver was bitten by a snake. The snake was then beaten severely, which resulted in multiple fractures of the skull and, subsequently, death. Both the driver and the snake were transported to the emergency room of a university hospital. The driver was treated and fully recovered. The snake was radiographed, which revealed, in addition to the extent of the head trauma, a fish in its stomach.

Courtesy of Volker Wenzel, MD, Ulm, Germany

Colin P. Derdeyn, MD • Christopher J. Moran, MD • DeWitte T. Cross III, MD
Eric W. Sherburn, MD • Ralph G. Dacey, Jr, MD

Intracranial Aneurysm: Anatomic Factors That Predict the Usefulness of Intraoperative Angiography[1]

PURPOSE: **To correlate the size and location of intracranial aneurysm with the need to reposition the aneurysm clip after intraoperative angiography.**

MATERIALS AND METHODS: **In 199 consecutive patients with 234 clipped intracranial aneurysms, 273 intraoperative angiographic studies were retrospectively reviewed. Aneurysm size and location, determined with preoperative angiographic and surgical reports, were correlated with the frequency of clip repositioning because of parent- or branch-vessel compromise or unexpected residual aneurysm.**

RESULTS: **Findings from intraoperative angiograms resulted in clip repositioning in 46 of 273 (16.8%) studies. Clip repositioning was statistically significantly less frequent with aneurysms of the posterior communicating (three of 52 [5.7%] studies) and anterior choroidal (none of 12 studies) arteries. High rates of clip repositioning were found in aneurysms of the superior hypophyseal artery (seven of 18 [38.9%] studies), superior cerebellar artery (three of five [60.0%] studies), and bifurcation of the internal carotid artery (three of nine [33.3%] aneurysms). In 98 conventional follow-up angiographic studies, seven (7%) false-negative cases with unsuspected aneurysm neck remnant were found.**

CONCLUSION: **The rate of clip repositioning in aneurysms of the posterior communicating or anterior choroidal arteries was less than that at other locations ($P < .05$). Intraoperative angiography may not be necessary when aneurysms are at these two locations.**

INTRAOPERATIVE angiography after clipping of intracranial aneurysms is an established, useful procedure (1–4). The advantages of intraoperative angiography, compared with those of conventional postoperative studies, are all related to timing. Despite limitations inherent in intraoperative angiography, information gained with this technique can lead to modifications at initial surgery that prevent complications or obviate the need for a second operation. Modifications may involve the adjustment of an aneurysm clip because of parent- or branch-vessel compromise or filling of residual aneurysm.

The yield (ie, relative frequency of abnormal studies that lead to changes in the surgical approach) of intraoperative angiography, however, is relatively low. In a recent report (4) of the largest series of which we are aware (100 intraoperative angiographic studies after aneurysm clipping), a 12% frequency of clip repositioning or other changes in therapy due to angiographic findings was reported. This rate of revision is similar to that reported in other series (1–3). The yield of intraoperative angiography could be improved if the technique were performed only in patients in whom an abnormal study was likely to be obtained.

The purpose of this study was to determine if such a group of patients could be identified preoperatively on the basis of aneurysm size and location.

MATERIALS AND METHODS

After the clipping of 234 aneurysms in 199 patients between January 1994 and December 1996, 273 consecutive intraoperative angiograms were obtained. Two factors account for the difference between the number of aneurysms and the number of angiographic studies. First, repeated angiographic studies after clip repositioning were considered separately from the initial angiographic results during the same surgical procedure. Second, in patients with multiple clipped aneurysms, each angiographic examination of a treated aneurysm was considered a separate study.

This series of patients did not include those who were treated for a dissecting aneurysm ($n = 4$) or those who underwent emergent intraoperative angiography in the operating room before craniotomy ($n = 4$). Also not included in this series were patients whose aneurysms were treated with surgical techniques (eg, trapping or proximal ligation) other than clipping of the aneurysm neck. One patient underwent surgical exploration without clipping. During the 3-year study period, six patients underwent craniotomy and surgical clipping without follow-up intraoperative angiography.

A 5-F femoral sheath was placed during preoperative diagnostic angiography or while the patient was in the operating room (usually after the administration of anesthesia and before surgery). While not in use, the sheath was continuously flushed with heparinized saline at arterial pressure. A radiolucent operating table (Skytron, Grand Rapids, Mich) and carbon-fiber head holder (Mayfield radiolucent skull clamp; Ohio Medical, Cincinnati) were used in all patients. The femoral

Index terms: Aneurysm, intracranial, 17.73 • Angiography, intraoperative, 17.73

Radiology 1997; 205:335–339

[1] From the Section of Neuroradiology, Mallinckrodt Institute of Radiology (C.P.D., C.J.M., D.T.C.); and the Department of Neurology and Neurosurgery (Neurological Surgery) (E.W.S., R.G.D.), Washington University School of Medicine, 510 S Kingshighway Blvd, St Louis, MO 63110 ;. Received April 23, 1997; revision requested June 13; revision received June 24; accepted July 8. **Address reprint requests to** C.P.D. C.P.D. supported by a grant from the RSNA/Siemens Medical Systems Research and Education Fund.

sheath was draped to allow access during angiography. Care was taken to avoid placement of radiopaque materials over the patient's head, neck, and chest. The operating room table was positioned to allow space for the bedside angiographic unit.

Selective catheter placement of the desired vessel was performed in standard fashion with the 5-F arterial sheath immediately before angiography. Manual injections were performed. Three views of each lesion were routinely obtained, including anterior, lateral, and oblique projections, and attempts were made to duplicate useful preoperative views. In many patients, the neurosurgical head-holding device prevented precise duplication of standard views.

A bedside digital subtraction unit (OEC Diasonics, Salt Lake City, Utah) that consisted of a C-arm fluoroscope, a digital image processor and storage unit, and a video monitor was used in all cases. This unit allows performance of routine fluoroscopy and real-time digital subtraction angiography. The recorded images could be reviewed at different speeds and frame-by-frame. Permanent hard-copy images were made for the radiologic file with a photographic unit. The preoperative diagnostic studies were available in the operating room for comparison in all cases. All studies were interpreted by the attending neuroradiologist (C.P.D., C.J.M., D.T.C.), and results were discussed with the neurosurgeon (R.G.D.). The femoral sheath was removed in either the recovery room or the intensive care unit, which allowed routine observation by the nursing staff of the puncture site and lower extremity.

The medical records, including surgical and radiographic reports, were reviewed in all patients. Information gathered included (*a*) information about the intraoperative or postoperative complications possibly attributable to angiography or surgery, (*b*) the recorded findings of the intraoperative studies, and (*c*) the surgeon's notes about intraoperative decisions made on the basis of the angiographic results. Preoperative and intraoperative angiograms and surgical reports were reviewed to determine aneurysm size and location. Measured diameters of aneurysms of the anterior circulation were corrected for magnification with the method described by Zubillaga and coworkers (5). With this method, the actual diameter of the internal carotid artery proximal to the bifurcation is assumed to be 3.4 mm. A proximal basilar artery diameter of 3.3 mm was used in cases of aneurysm of the posterior circulation (5). Aneurysm size was graded as follows: small (diameter < 10 mm), large (diameter, 10–25 mm), and giant (diameter > 25 mm). Statistical analysis was performed with the χ^2 test, with statistically significant differences inferred at the $P < .05$ level. Aneurysm location was categorized by using established conventions. Internal carotid artery aneurysms were named for the nearest branch vessel of origin (eg, superior hypophyseal artery aneurysms) even if the vessel was not visible on angiograms.

At our institution, postoperative angiography is generally reserved for patients who do not respond to medical treatment for vasospasm and who are candidates for endovascular treatment. These postoperative studies were reviewed, and findings were correlated with those from the intraoperative study to assess accuracy with intraoperative angiograms.

Table 1
Revision of Clip Placement according to Aneurysm Location

Arterial Location	No. of Studies	No. of Revisions	Frequency of Revisions (%)*	No. of Aneurysms	No. of Revisions	Frequency of Revisions (%)*
All sites	273	46	16.8 (±4.5)	234	30	12.8 (±4.2)
Middle cerebral	60	14	23.3 (±10.6)	49	8	16.3 (±10.3)
Anterior communicating	52	8	15.4 (±9.8)	45	5	11.1 (±9.2)
Posterior communicating	52	3	5.7 (±6.3)†	50	3	6.0 (±6.6)
Ophthalmic	23	3	13.0 (±13.7)	20	2	10.0 (±13.1)
Superior hypophyseal	18	7	38.9 (±22.8)†	11	3	27.3 (±26.5)†
Pericallosal	14	3	21.4 (±22.8)	11	2	18.2 (±22.8)
Basilar tip	14	1	7.7 (±13.4)	13	1	7.7 (±14.5)
Anterior choroidal	12	0	0.0 (±25.0)	12	0	0.0 (±27.3)
Bifurcation of internal carotid artery	12	3	25.0 (±24.5)	9	3	33.3 (±30.7)†
Superior cerebellar	5	3	60.0 (±42.9)	3	2	66.6 (±53.3)†
Posterior inferior cerebellar	4	0	0.0 (±75.0)	4	0	0.0 (±75.0)
Posterior cerebral	3	1	33.3 (±53.3)	3	1	33.3 (±53.3)
Anterior cerebral (A1 segment)	2	0	0.0	2	0	0.0 (±0.0)
Vertebrobasilar junction	1	0	0.0	1	0	0.0 (±0.0)
Anterior inferior cerebellar	1	0	0.0	1	0	0.0 (±0.0)

* Numbers in parentheses are 95% confidence level.
† Rate of revision was statically significantly different than the overall rate ($P < .05$).

RESULTS

Aneurysm clips were repositioned on the basis of intraoperative angiographic findings from 46 of 273 (16.8% ± 4.5 [mean ± 95% confidence level]) studies of 234 aneurysms (Table 1). The repositioning rate per aneurysm was lower (30 of 234 [12.8% ± 4.2] aneurysms) than the 16.8% rate per angiographic study. The 46 intraoperative angiograms with findings that led to revision of clip placement were performed in 30 cases of aneurysm. Two or more revisions were necessary in 10 of these 30 aneurysms. Findings from an initial study that led to clip repositioning were, therefore, associated with a statistically significantly higher rate of subsequent revision of clip placement (10 of 30 [33.3% ± 16.9] aneurysms).

The frequency of clip repositioning was statistically significantly higher than average for aneurysms in the superior hypophyseal and superior cerebellar arteries. The frequency of clip repositioning was statistically significantly higher for aneurysms at the bifurcation of the internal carotid artery compared with the frequency for all clipped aneurysms, but not when the number of studies performed was considered. High rates of clip repositioning that did not reach statistical significance were also seen for aneurysms in the middle cerebral artery and pericallosal artery. The rate of clip repositioning was also statistically significantly more frequent for large aneurysms (Table 2).

The rate of clip repositioning was statistically significantly lower than average for aneurysms in the posterior communicating artery and in the anterior choroidal artery. If these two similar and adjacent locations along the posterior wall of the supraclinoid internal carotid artery proximal to the bifurcation are considered together, the revision rate was even smaller (three of 64 [4.7% ± 5.1%] angiograms and three of 60 [4.8% ± 5.3%] aneurysms) and achieved statistical significance for all aneurysms, as well as for total studies.

The reasons for clip repositioning could be grouped into two categories: (*a*) parent- or branch-vessel compromise and (*b*) residual aneurysm. The category of residual aneurysm encompassed three situations: persistent filling of the sac, filling of a neck remnant, or filling of an unclipped adjacent lobe or of a second aneurysm. The relative frequency of these two findings

Table 2
Revision of Clip Placement according to Aneurysm Size

Size	No. of Studies	No. of Revisions	Frequency of Revisions (%)*	No. of Aneurysms	No. of Revisions	Frequency of Revisions (%)*
All sizes	273	46	16.8 (±4.5)	234	30	12.8 (±4.2)
Small	240	37	15.4 (±4.6)	215	24	11.2 (±4.2)
Large	22	8	36.4 (±20.1)†	19	5	26.3 (±19.8)†
Giant	6	1	16.7 (±29.8)	5	1	20.0 (±35.1)

* Numbers in parentheses are 95% confidence level.
† Rate of revision was statistically significantly different than the overall rate ($P < .05$).

Table 3
Reasons for Revision of Clip Placement according to Aneurysm Location

Arterial Location	No. of Studies	Vessel Compromise (%)	Residual Aneurysm (%)	No. of Aneurysms	Vessel Compromise (%)	Residual Aneurysm (%)
All sites	273	17	29	234	11	19
Middle cerebral	60	11	3	49	6	2
Anterior communicating	52	0	8	45	0	5
Posterior communicating	52	0	3	50	0	3
Ophthalmic	23	0	3	20	0	2
Superior hypophyseal	18	0	7	11	0	3
Pericallosal	14	3	0	11	2	0
Superior cerebellar	5	0	3	5	0	2
Basilar tip	14	1	0	13	1	0
Bifurcation of the internal carotid	12	2	1	9	2	1
Posterior cerebral	3	0	1	3	0	1

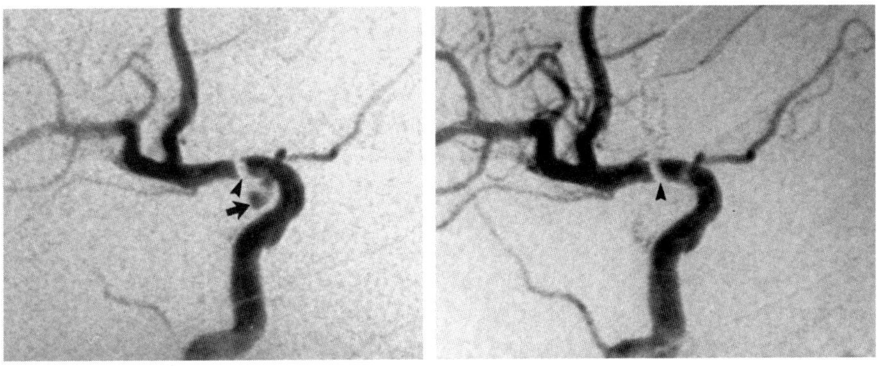

a. b.

Figure 1. Unexpected filling of residual aneurysm at the superior hypophyseal artery after initial clip placement. **(a)** Oblique lateral intraoperative angiogram demonstrates residual filling of the aneurysm sac (arrow). On the basis of this information, the jaws of the aneurysm clip were opened, and the clip was extended anteriorly. A subtraction artifact (arrowhead) of the fenestrated aneurysm clip overlies the supraclinoid carotid artery. **(b)** Same view from the repeated intraoperative angiogram demonstrates no filling of the aneurysm and no compromise of internal carotid artery flow. Arrowhead = subtraction artifact due to the presence of the clip.

for each aneurysm location is shown in Table 3. For internal carotid artery aneurysms above the dural ring but proximal to the bifurcation, all repositionings were undertaken because of residual aneurysm. At the superior hypophyseal location, three of 11 aneurysms continued to fill after initial clipping (Fig 1). In two of these three aneurysms, multiple surgical adjustments were needed to exclude the aneurysm from the circulation. All anterior communicating artery aneurysms that needed clip revision were for residual aneurysm, as well. At the trifurcation of the middle cerebral artery, most revisions were necessary to improve parent-or branch-vessel flow (abnormal findings from 11 of 14 intraoperative angiograms led to repositioning) (Fig 2).

Conventional angiography was performed in 98 of the 234 cases of clipped aneurysms. Unexpected residual aneurysm was noted in seven (7% false-negative rate) cases. One of the seven false-negative studies is shown in Figure 3. No unexpected parent- or branch-vessel compromise was seen. No complications were observed after intraoperative angiography.

DISCUSSION

The goal of surgery in cases of aneurysm is to exclude the aneurysm from the circulatory system without compromising flow through parent or branch vessels. The frequency of incomplete aneurysm obliteration is not known. Feuerberg et al (6) found residual aneurysm in one of 27 (4%) treated intracranial aneurysms. Clipped aneurysms with small (1–2 mm in length) neck remnants have been shown to enlarge and bleed (6–8). Branch-vessel occlusion caused by an aneurysm clip may also complicate surgery. After the clipping of 78 consecutive aneurysms, MacDonald et al (9) reported nine unexpected major-vessel occlusions on postoperative angiograms obtained urgently or routinely. Six of these occlusions resulted in disability due to infarct. In addition, residual aneurysm was seen in six patients. Three of these six patients with residual aneurysm underwent repeated surgery. The frequency of these undesired events was 19.2% (15 of 78 aneurysms)and was similar to the rate of clip repositioning observed in our large series and to that reported by other investigators (1–4).

The data from our investigation suggest that certain aneurysm locations and sizes are associated with particular rates of clip replacement after intraoperative angiography. A low rate of clip repositioning after intraoperative angiography was observed with aneurysms at the relatively easily exposed and well-visualized supraclinoid segment of the internal carotid artery. A change in clip placement was not necessary in any of the 12 aneurysms of the anterior choroidal artery. Revision of clip placement was necessary in only three of the 50 aneurysms of the posterior communicating artery. These findings contrast with those of Alexander et al (4). In their study of 100 craniotomies, clip repositioning was necessary in five of 27 aneurysms of the posterior communicating artery. Not all patients in their series, however, underwent intraoperative angiography; among patients who did not undergo intraoperative angiography were six patients with aneurysms of the posterior communicating artery.

High frequencies of unexpected residual aneurysm that necessitated clip manipulation were observed at the superior hypophyseal artery, at the bifurcation of the internal carotid artery, and at the superior cerebellar artery. Aneurysms arising from the superior hypophyseal artery can be difficult to visualize; these aneurysms are close to the cavernous sinus and the relatively fixed position of the internal carotid artery at the dural ring, which makes exposure of the aneurysm neck challenging. All revisions of clip placement in aneurysms of the superior hypophyseal artery were performed for residual filling of the aneurysm sac (Fig 1). Adequate exposure of aneurysms of the superior cerebellar artery and of the bifurcation of the internal carotid artery may also be difficult. Parent- or branch-vessel compromise was a frequent finding after clipping of aneurysms of the middle cerebral artery. Aneurysms at this location often involve origins of branch vessels, and complete obliteration of the aneurysm may be difficult without compromising parent- or branch-vessel flow.

Large aneurysms were associated with higher rates of clip repositioning. This finding is not surprising because visualization of parent and branch vessels can be more difficult with larger aneurysms. Giant aneurysms were not associated with high rates of revision, but only six of these lesions were included in this series. Alexander et al (4) found a statistically significantly higher frequency of clip repositioning in the 11 giant aneurysms they studied.

No complications attributable to intraoperative angiography were encountered in this retrospective review. Derdeyn et al (3) noted one possible embolic complication in 87 transfemoral catheter placements at intraoperative angiography. Alexander et al (4) reported one possible embolic complication in 100 transfemoral studies. The working conditions in the operating room are different from those in the angiography suite, and the apparent improvement in the complication rate of Alexander et al may reflect the benefit of experience.

The resolution on intraoperative angiograms is not as high as that on conventional angiograms. Small vessels such as the anterior choroidal artery and perforating vessels often are not visualized on intraoperative angiograms. In addition, the head holder can limit the angles at which angiographic projections are obtained. Conventional angiography in a dedicated angiography suite offers biplane capability, which doubles the number of views obtained with each injection and provides higher resolution and greater flexibility with regard to projections. Despite the limitations of intraoperative angiography, however, diagnostic information regarding parent- and branch-vessel patency and the status of the clipped aneurysm is usually obtained. The radiologist performing these studies must be thoroughly familiar with the preoperative cerebral angiogram to ensure that intraoperative images will optimally provide clinically relevant information.

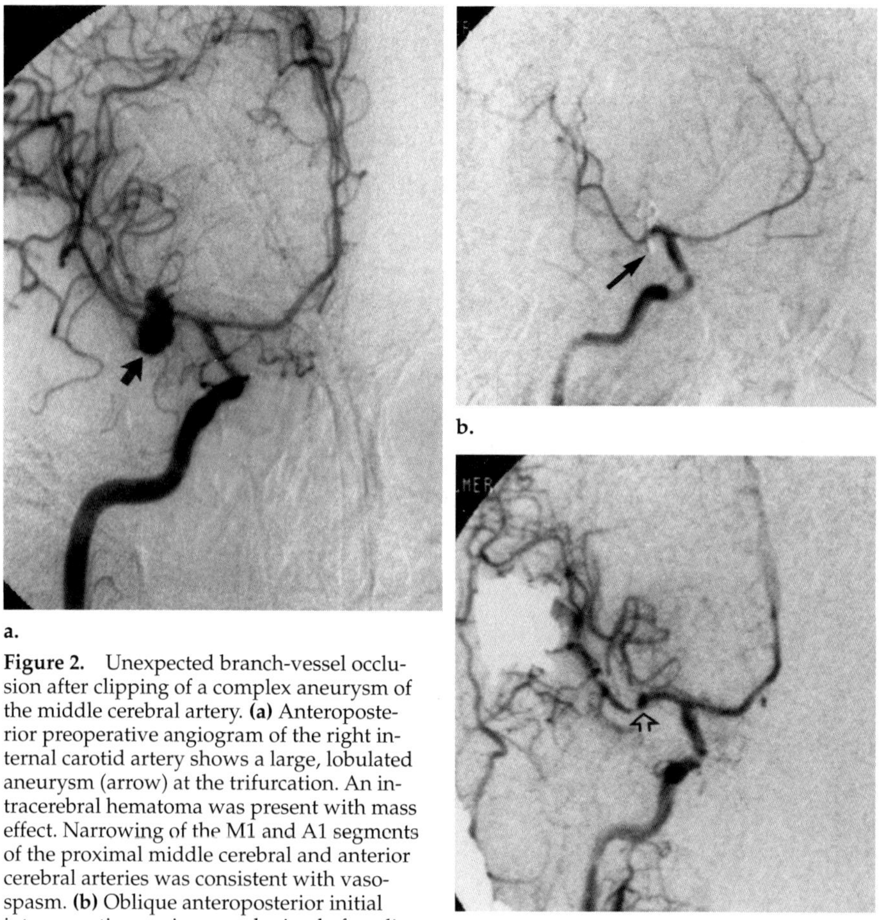

a. b. c.

Figure 2. Unexpected branch-vessel occlusion after clipping of a complex aneurysm of the middle cerebral artery. **(a)** Anteroposterior preoperative angiogram of the right internal carotid artery shows a large, lobulated aneurysm (arrow) at the trifurcation. An intracerebral hematoma was present with mass effect. Narrowing of the M1 and A1 segments of the proximal middle cerebral and anterior cerebral arteries was consistent with vasospasm. **(b)** Oblique anteroposterior initial intraoperative angiogram obtained after clipping demonstrates no filling of the aneurysm or of the previously visualized branches of the middle cerebral artery. Arrow = subtraction artifact due to the presence of the aneurysm clip. **(c)** Angiogram acquired after the clip was repositioned shows restoration of flow to the branch. Of necessity, the residual aneurysm (arrow) was left in place.

An unexpected residual aneurysm neck was identified on seven of the 98 (7%) postoperative angiograms in this series; note that no vessel occlusions were found. In general, the false-negative results obtained in cases of small neck remnants were often attributable to limited resolution and limited availability of angiographic projections with the current intraoperative angiographic equipment (Fig 3). The actual rate of false-negative findings from intraoperative angiography in cases of an unsuspected residual aneurysm cannot be determined from our data because only those patients suspected of having vasospasm underwent conventional angiography after surgery. Our 7% rate is similar to that found in other studies of this technique. Martin et al (1) noted three false-negative intraoperative studies in their series with angiographic follow-up in 62 patients. Two residual aneurysm sacs were overlooked, and a small residual nidus of an arteriovenous malformation was overlooked in a third case. In the series of Barrow et al (2), one residual aneurysm sac was noted in 17 postoperative studies after aneurysm clipping. With subsequent angiography, Derdeyn et al (3) observed two unexpected, small residual aneurysms (false-negative studies) on 25 studies of aneurysms.

While intraoperative angiography clearly offers several advantages in

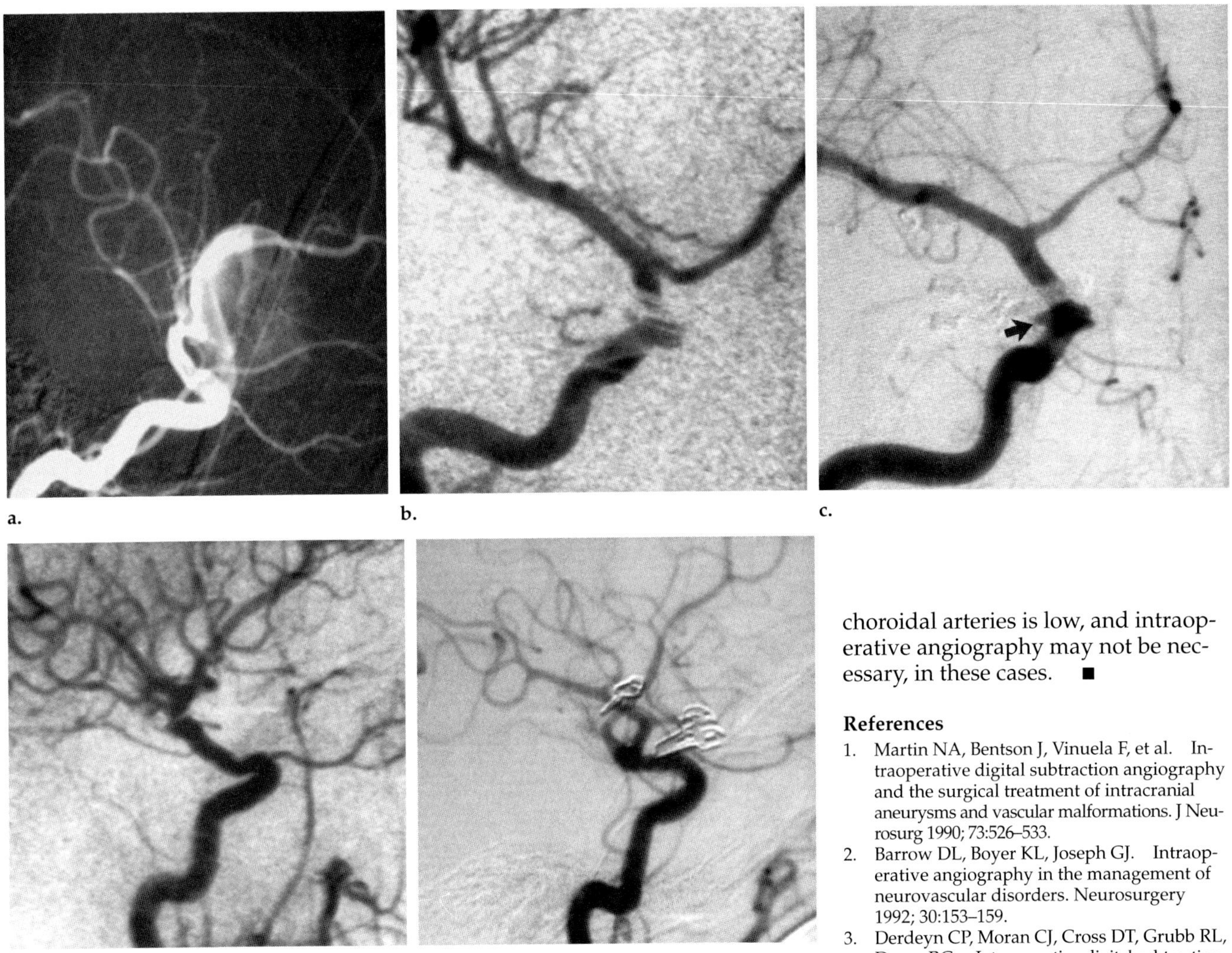

a. b. c.

d. e.

Figure 3. False-negative intraoperative angiogram. **(a)** Preoperative angiogram shows a large internal carotid artery aneurysm at the ophthalmic level. **(b)** On the anteroposterior intraoperative angiogram, no definite residual aneurysm filling is depicted, and the study was considered to be normal. **(c)** A similar view from the postoperative angiogram shows definite residual lateral filling (arrow) of the aneurysm beneath the clips. **(d)** Findings on the lateral intraoperative angiogram are unremarkable and are similar those on **(e)** the postoperative lateral angiogram.

the surgical treatment of aneurysms, this procedure also has some limitations. First, intraoperative angiography necessitates more operating-room time (average of 45 minutes [3]) and consequently increases cost. Second, intraoperative angiography is associated with a small risk of angiographic complications. Third, intraoperative angiographic equipment does not provide the resolution available with equipment in modern angiography suites. The magnitude of the rate of false-negative intraoperative angiograms in cases of aneurysm neck remnant and the subsequent effect of this rate on outcome are unknown. Finally, the information gained with intraoperative angiography may not result in improved outcome. For example, despite identification of an abnormality such as branch-vessel occlusion and rapid surgical correction, an infarct may still occur (3).

The data from this study demonstrate that different aneurysm diameters and locations are associated with different rates of clip repositioning after intraoperative angiography. The yield of intraoperative angiography is high in cases of large aneurysms and of aneurysms of the superior hypophyseal artery, superior cerebellar artery, and bifurcation of the internal carotid artery. The need for intraoperative angiography should be anticipated in these situations. The rate of clip repositioning in aneurysms of the posterior communicating and anterior choroidal arteries is low, and intraoperative angiography may not be necessary, in these cases. ■

References

1. Martin NA, Bentson J, Vinuela F, et al. Intraoperative digital subtraction angiography and the surgical treatment of intracranial aneurysms and vascular malformations. J Neurosurg 1990; 73:526–533.
2. Barrow DL, Boyer KL, Joseph GJ. Intraoperative angiography in the management of neurovascular disorders. Neurosurgery 1992; 30:153–159.
3. Derdeyn CP, Moran CJ, Cross DT, Grubb RL, Dacey RG. Intraoperative digital subtraction angiography: a review of 112 consecutive examinations. AJNR 1995; 16:307–308.
4. Alexander TD, Macdonald RL, Weir B, Kowalczuk A. Intraoperative angiography in aneurysm surgery: a prospective study of 100 craniotomies. Neurosurgery 1996; 39: 10–18.
5. Zubillaga AF, Guglielmi G, Vinuela F, Duckwiler GR. Endovascular occlusion of intracranial aneurysms with electrically detachable coils: correlation of aneurysm neck size and treatment results. AJNR 1994; 15:815–820.
6. Feuerberg I, Lindquist C, Lindqvist M, Steiner L. Natural history of postoperative aneurysm rests. J Neurosurg 1987; 66:30–34.
7. Drake CG, Vanderlinden RG. The late consequences of incomplete surgical treatment of cerebral aneurysms. J Neurosurg 1967; 27:226–238.
8. Lin T, Fox AJ, Drake CG. Regrowth of aneurysm sacs from residual neck following aneurysm clipping. J Neurosurg 1989; 70: 556–560.
9. MacDonald R, Wallace M, Kestle J. Role of angiography following aneurysm surgery. J Neurosurg 1993; 79:826–832.

Book Review

3D Contrast MR Angiography

Martin R. Prince, MD, PhD, Thomas M. Grist, MD, and Jorg F. Debatin, MD

Brooklyn, NY: Springer-Verlag New York, 1997. ISBN 3-540-62577-1. Paperback, $32.00; pp 177; 44 figures.

3D Contrast MR Angiography is a short and very readable introduction to a complex and often confusing subject. Many of the liabilities of traditional magnetic resonance (MR) angiographic methods can be eliminated with use of three-dimensional, contrast material–enhanced MR angiography. With this technique, bolus injection of paramagnetic contrast material and use of high-performance gradient systems allow acquisition of large-field-of-view, high-resolution volumes of data in a single breath hold. Image contrast is based on the considerable T1 shortening of signal in blood induced by the paramagnetic contrast material, rather than on flow-dependent phenomena. Data sets can be acquired in a fraction of the time needed with more traditional techniques; therefore, motion artifacts can be reduced drastically, and patient tolerance is often much improved.

The authors'stated goal is to "familiarize the reader with the basic principles of 3D contrast MRA. All relevant technical aspects are addressed, imaging protocols are provided, and tailored imaging strategies are described for different vascular regions." The authors have succeeded admirably. This book is well worth the investment for anyone interested in learning to apply these techniques.

The introductory chapter is the strongest and well worth the price of the book. This chapter is organized into a series of questions and answers about fundamental concepts of contrast-enhanced MR angiography. There are excellent discussions of dosages and injection rates of contrast material. The importance of timing the injection and image acquisition so that arrival of the bolus of contrast material coincides with sampling of the center of k space is repeatedly emphasized. Strategies to achieve this goal are outlined. The authors strongly recommend use of a test bolus, and this technique is explained. Subtraction techniques are discussed. Optimization of various imaging parameters and strategies to reduce imaging time are reviewed briefly. For the nonexpert radiologist, these matters are not always easy to understand or even read about; however, the presentation in this book is lucid and painless.

The book is divided into nine chapters. The first chapter introduces the basic concepts of contrast-enhanced MR angiography and occupies almost one-third of the book. The other chapters are organized by anatomic region. There are basic, brief descriptions of the pathologic entities encountered frequently, and these entities are probably well known to the practicing radiologist. A paragraph is devoted to answering the question, Why use 3D contrast MR angiography? and the technique and imaging strategies are discussed subsequently. A useful feature in each of these chapters is a paragraph in which the additional sequences needed for a complete examination are outlined.

An extensive and up-to-date bibliography is provided for the ambitious reader. A glossary of technical terms can also be found.

My criticisms are relatively minor. The discussions of technique for individual vascular regions are variable: Some chapters provide extensive information about recommended repetition times, echo times, matrix sizes, and acquisition planes; in other chapters, information is considerably less extensive. Future editions might be improved with tables that provide detailed recommendations for imaging parameters in each of the regions discussed. The authors, who are leaders in the field, are strong advocates of the technique. Some of their statements may be overly optimistic regarding contrast-enhanced MR angiography and overly dismissive regarding other techniques: For example, "3D Contrast MRA is likely to become the standard method for diagnosing pulmonary embolus in the near future."

These few quibbles aside, *3D Contrast MR Angiography* is an excellent book. It is short, readable, and affordable and provides a good introduction to an exciting and evolving field.

Reviewed by Jim Glockner, MD, PhD

Siegfried A. Thurnher, MD • Roland Dorffner, MD • Majda M. Thurnher, MD
Friedrich W. Winkelbauer, MD • Georg Kretschmer, MD • Peter Polterauer, MD
Johannes Lammer, MD

Evaluation of Abdominal Aortic Aneurysm for Stent-Graft Placement: Comparison of Gadolinium-enhanced MR Angiography versus Helical CT Angiography and Digital Subtraction Angiography[1]

PURPOSE: **To determine whether magnetic resonance (MR) angiography can be used alone to evaluate abdominal aortic aneurysms (AAAs) for endovascular placement of stent grafts.**

MATERIALS AND METHODS: **Sixty-one patients with AAAs underwent gadolinium-enhanced MR angiography of the abdominal aorta and pelvic arteries. Measurements of the size and extent of the AAAs were compared with helical computed tomographic (CT) and digital subtraction angiographic measurements; 95% confidence intervals for the differences in the means were determined.**

RESULTS: **Because of the larger field of view, MR angiography was superior to CT angiography in assessing visceral iliac artery disease. Both modalities were equal in evaluating the proximal extent of the AAA (mean difference, −0.16 mm; 95% CI, −0.31, 0.64) and in measuring all aortic dimensions (eg, mean difference in the proximal neck diameter, −0.74 mm; 95% CI, −0.98, −0.49). MR angiography was inferior to CT angiography in depicting accessory renal arteries (seven of 12) and in grading renal artery stenoses (sensitivity, 100% [95% CI, 0.90, 1.00]; specificity, 84% [95% CI, 0.74, 0.91]).**

CONCLUSION: **Gadolinium-enhanced MR angiography is a fast, reliable means of providing all the information relevant to the preoperative assessment of endovascular aortic stent-graft placement.**

Considerable progress has been made over the past 2 decades in the diagnosis and evaluation of abdominal aortic aneurysms (AAAs) before surgical repair. However, the limitations of angiography, ultrasound (US), conventional computed tomography (CT), and magnetic resonance (MR) imaging as imaging modalities used alone in the evaluation of AAAs have been well described (1–11). Aortography is invasive, time-consuming, costly, and may result in underestimation of aneurysm size. Noninvasive means, such as US, conventional CT, and MR imaging cannot reliably be used to grade stenosis of visceral vessels. In practical terms, no contemporary single imaging technique adequately provides all of the necessary anatomic detail required for planning aortic reconstruction in patients with AAA. Thus, more than one imaging study is commonly performed in most institutions.

Recently, helical CT angiography and contrast agent–enhanced MR angiography have been introduced as noninvasive techniques for the evaluation of AAAs that combine the advantages of conventional CT or MR imaging and aortography (12–19). With the introduction of covered endovascular stent grafts to treat aneurysms, the precise determination of the diameter and length of the aorta and iliac arteries and the anatomy and dimension of the aneurysm has become fundamental to successful stent-graft placement (20–22). Major problems with stent grafts include lumbar artery refilling, securing of the anastomoses, and difficulties in the insertion of bifurcated grafts. CT enables proper preoperative and postoperative assessment of aneurysm repair (23–25). To our knowledge, no prospective study has been performed to compare CT angiographic and contrast agent–enhanced MR angiographic techniques.

The purpose of this study was to determine whether MR angiography can be used alone to provide all the information necessary for endovascular placement of stent grafts in patients with AAAs. We compared the findings of contrast-enhanced MR angiography with those of helical CT and digital subtraction angiography (DSA). Particular attention was given to the dimensions of the aorta and aneurysm and the depiction of renal and iliac arteries, because disease in these vessels can affect surgical or interventional planning.

MATERIALS AND METHODS

Patients

From January 1995 to November 1996, 97 patients who were referred for non-

Index terms: Aneurysm, aortic, 981.731 • Aorta, CT, 981.12915, 981.12916 • Aorta, grafts and prostheses, 981.1268 • Aorta, MR, 981.12942 • Computed tomography (CT), comparative studies, 981.12916 • Gadolinium • Magnetic resonance (MR), comparative studies, 981.12942 • Magnetic resonance (MR), vascular studies, 981.12942

Abbreviations: AAA = abdominal aortic aneurysm, CI = confidence interval, DSA = digital subtraction angiography, MIP = maximum intensity projection.

Radiology 1997; 205:341–352

[1] From the Departments of Radiology (S.A.T., R.D., M.M.T., F.W.W., J.L.) and Vascular Surgery (G.K., P.P.), University Hospital, Währinger Gürtel 18-20, A-1090 Vienna, Austria. Received January 17, 1997; revision requested March 10; revision received May 29; accepted June 16. **Address reprint requests to** S.A.T.

mergent, preoperative evaluation of AAA underwent intraarterial DSA and CT angiography. Of these patients, 36 were excluded from the study because the clinical demand for the MR imaging suite precluded scheduling of research MR angiography or because the patients had contraindications for CT or MR angiography, such as contrast agent allergies, pacemakers, and intracranial aneurysm clips.

The 61 patients enrolled in the study underwent contrast-enhanced MR angiography of the abdominal aorta and pelvic arteries. The study group consisted of 53 men and eight women with a mean age of 71.3 years (age range, 43–89 years). Informed consent was obtained from all patients. All imaging studies were performed within 2 weeks in every patient. Any patient who was eligible for surgical treatment of infrarenal AAA was considered for stent-graft placement. Basically, patient exclusion criteria for the insertion of stent grafts included a proximal aortic neck less than 15 mm long, more than 25 mm in diameter, or both; a distal aortic neck (cuff) less than 15 mm long, more than 25 mm in diameter (exclusion criteria for tube graft placement), or both; a distal neck of the common iliac artery more than 12 mm in diameter (exclusion criteria for bifurcated graft placement); severe stenosis of the superior mesenteric artery or dominant inferior mesenteric artery (with arc of Riolan); and involvement of both hypogastric arteries in the aneurysm (20).

MR Technique

MR angiography was performed with a superconducting MR imager at 1.0 T (NT 10; Philips Medical Systems, Eindhoven, The Netherlands) with use of a whole-body coil. Three sequences were performed.

Initially, two-dimensional, multiplanar (multistack) turbo-field-echo localizer images were obtained in the axial, sagittal, and coronal planes; the images were centered at the iliac crest with a repetition time of 11 msec and an echo time of 4.6 msec (11/4.6) with a flip angle of 50°. Other parameters were a 45-cm field of view, a 10-mm section thickness, a 128 × 256 matrix, one signal acquired, and a total acquisition time of 12 seconds.

Next, axial, T2-weighted, short–acquisition time, turbo spin-echo images were obtained through the abdominal aorta and iliac arteries. Imaging parameters were 1,800/120 (effective), a 90° flip angle, an echo train length of 28, a 35–38-cm field of view, a 10-mm section thickness, a 192 × 256 matrix, 21 sections, a 10% intersection gap, respiratory gating, superior and inferior presaturation, no phase wrap, four signals acquired, and a total acquisition time of 1 minute 53 seconds.

Finally, three-dimensional, turbo-field-echo, contrast-enhanced, time-of-flight MR angiography was performed in a single breath hold. Patients hyperventilated for at least 30 seconds before the start of the sequence. The multistack localizer and axial T2-weighted images served as scout images to ensure the proper placement of the imaging volume and the selection of imaging parameters. The coronal volume was positioned with the top edge at the diaphragm and the caudal end at the level of the femoral heads to image the aorta and pelvic arteries from the celiac trunk to the common femoral arteries. The front margin of the volume was anterior to the origin of the superior mesenteric artery, anterior to the wall of the aneurysm, and just anterior to the common femoral vessels. Posteriorly, the volume covered the renal hilus.

We developed this last sequence by modifying the protocol of Prince and colleagues (16,17,19). Initially (in 13 patients), we used the following parameters: 18.5/4.6, a 40° flip angle, a 35 × 19-cm rectangular field of view, a 2.5-mm section thickness, a 128 × 256 matrix, 30–38 coronal sections, first-order gradient moment nulling (flow compensation), two signals acquired, caudal presaturation slab, and a 48–53-second acquisition time (shallow breathing). To avoid aliasing in the right-to-left direction, a foldover suppression technique was applied. After May 1995, we modified the protocol to reduce the imaging time, maximize the arterial signal intensity by injecting the same amount of contrast agent in a shorter time, and eliminate respiratory artifacts by means of breath holding (48 patients). The following were the changed parameters: 8.5/2.8, a 40° flip angle, a 2.0-mm section thickness, 40–50 coronal sections, no presaturation slab, and a delayed reconstruction algorithm. This technique required a total acquisition time of 28–34 seconds.

Gadopentetate dimeglumine (Magnevist; Schering, Berlin, Germany) was injected during the acquisition through a 20-gauge intravenous catheter. All patients received 40 mL of gadopentetate dimeglumine within 30–45 seconds (1.0–1.5 mL of gadopentetate dimeglumine per second) regardless of patient weight. Injections were performed by hand and in all cases by the same radiologist (S.A.T.) to ensure uniformity of the injection technique. The circulation time from the injection site to the abdominal and pelvic arteries was estimated on the basis of age and hemodynamic state. The imaging delay between the start of the injection and the start of the MR sequence was 15–45 seconds.

In addition, in one patient, axial, T1-weighted, spin-echo MR images (500/20, 90° flip angle) with a 10-mm section thickness (Fig 1) were obtained after the contrast-enhanced MR angiographic sequence was performed.

Images were reconstructed by experienced radiologic technologists by using a computer workstation (Philips Medical Systems). Both single-voxel, thick, coronal reformations and maximum intensity projections (MIPs) in coronal and sagittal views (15° increments) were obtained. In addition, axial reconstructions of the three-dimensional data set were performed by using a 5-mm section thickness.

Total imaging time (including positioning of the patient on the table) was about 10 minutes. Postprocessing (MIP, axial reconstructions) was performed within 5 minutes. Thus, a complete imaging study was achieved within 15 minutes.

CT Technique

CT angiograms were obtained with a Somatom Plus-S scanner (Siemens Medical Systems, Erlangen, Germany). Thirty nonhelical sections were obtained, with contiguous 10-mm collimation before administration of the contrast agent, to determine the range of coverage for helical scanning. Patients hyperventilated for at least 30 seconds before the start of scanning. Contrast-enhanced breath-hold helical CT scans were obtained in the craniocaudal direction by using the following parameters: 3-mm collimation width, 6-mm table speed, 2:1 pitch ratio, 210 mA, 192-mm coverage, and 32-second exposure time. All patients received 120 mL of nonionic contrast agent (Jopamiro 300 [jopamidol]; Bracco, Milan, Italy) through a 20-gauge catheter positioned in an antecubital vein by using a power injector (Liebel-Flarsheim, Cincinnati, Ohio) with an injection rate of 4 mL/sec and a scan delay of 25 seconds. CT scanning covered the area from the origin of the superior mesenteric artery to the iliac bifurcation.

Linear interpolation (180°) of the helical data was always used before image reconstruction. Axial images were reconstructed at 1-mm increments and were subsequently edited by an experienced radiologic technologist to exclude unwanted parenchymal organs, bones, and venous structures by means of manual, two-dimensional, region-of-interest drawing. Three-dimensional renderings were generated as MIP images and shadow surface displays. The MIP images were calculated at 15° increments in the z and x axes. The threshold value (110–170 HU) was chosen to maximize contrast in vascular structures.

DSA Technique

Angiographic examinations were performed with a DSA unit (Multistar or Angiostar; Siemens Medical Systems) according to the Seldinger technique with transfemoral insertion of a 5-F calibrated pigtail catheter with 1-cm increments (Cook, Queensland, Australia). With the catheter tip placed in the abdominal aorta at a point proximal to the ostium of the renal arteries, iopromide (Ultravist 300; Schering; n = 14) or ioversol (Optiray 320; Mallinckrodt Medical, St Louis, Mo; n = 47) was injected at a rate of 12 mL/sec for 3 seconds. The catheter was then repositioned just above the aortic bifurcation for pelvic angiography performed with the injection of contrast agent at 10 mL/sec for 2 seconds. Anteroposterior and lateral projections of the abdominal aorta and anteroposterior and oblique projections of the iliac arteries were obtained in each patient. Because a calibrated catheter was used, no corrections for magnification were per-

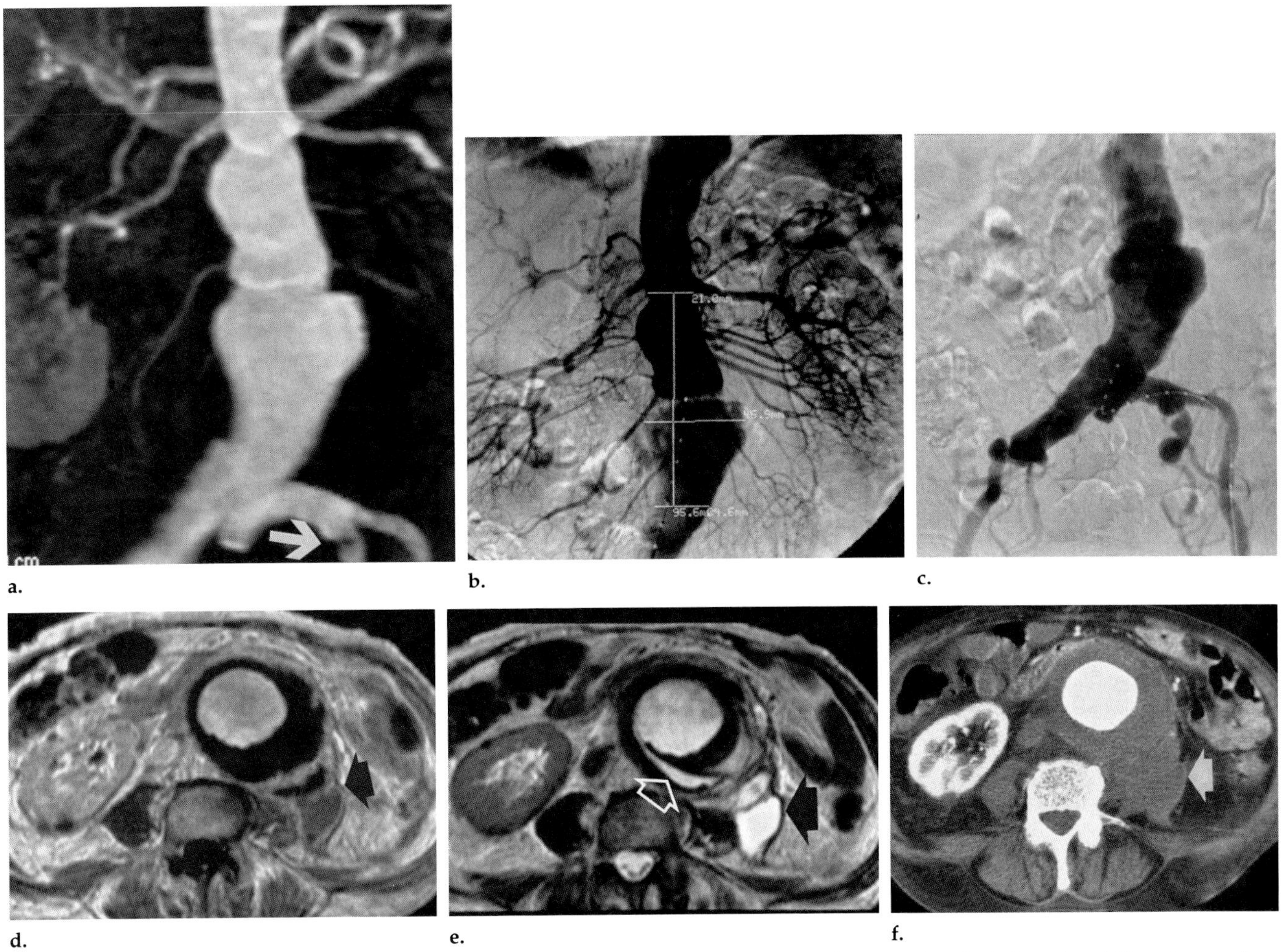

Figure 1. Images obtained in an 81-year-old man with a type VI juxtarenal aortic aneurysm that extends to both iliac artery bifurcations and with a contained aortic rupture. The short proximal neck and the extension into both iliac artery bifurcations preclude stent-graft placement. **(a)** MIP, three-dimensional, time-of-flight MR angiogram (8.5/2.8, 40° flip angle) shows patent renal arteries, a juxtarenal AAA, and severe kinking of the left common iliac artery. Note the 90° stenosis of the left hypogastric artery (arrow). **(b, c)** DSA images show the **(b)** aorta and **(c)** iliac arteries and confirm the juxtarenal extension of the AAA and the aneurysmal involvement of both common iliac arteries. **(d)** Axial, T1-weighted, spin-echo MR image (500/20), **(e)** axial T2-weighted, turbo spin-echo MR image (1,800/120 [effective], 90° flip angle), and **(f)** axial CT angiogram reveal retroperitoneal hemorrhage (solid arrow). The inhomogeneous, high-signal-intensity mural thrombus includes the site of aortic rupture (open arrow in **e**) and is best appreciated in **e.**

formed when measurements were made on DSA images.

Image Analysis

CT scans and MR images were individually interpreted by two experienced radiologists (S.A.T., R.D.), who reviewed by means of consensus. The individual axial CT scans and MR images, coronal unprocessed two-dimensional "source" MR angiograms, and MIP images from the CT and MR examinations were analyzed. The DSA images were independently analyzed by another experienced radiologist (J.L.). Findings of helical CT or MR angiography were then correlated with those of DSA.

Aneurysms were classified as suprarenal (dilatation of the infrarenal aorta up to or above the level of the renal artery ostium), juxtarenal (origin of aneurysm less than 15 mm below the renal arteries), or infrarenal (aneurysm extends cranially more than 15 mm below the renal arteries). The distal extent of the aneurysm was defined as the first part of the aneurysm that had a nearly normal caliber. The aneurysm was considered to extend into the iliac arteries if there was no nonaneurysmal segment proximal to the aortic bifurcation and if the outer diameter of the common iliac arteries exceeded 12 mm. The course of the abdominal aorta and the iliac arteries, kinking or tortuosity in particular, and thrombus formation were evaluated. Additional findings such as horseshoe kidneys and retro- or circumaortic renal veins were noted.

In an attempt to define the AAA type for the appropriate choice of the stent graft or surgical procedure, we performed a modified classification of the aneurysms according to Richter and colleagues (21) (Table 1).

Measurements were performed electronically on an EasyVision workstation (Philips Medical Systems) and on a Sienet workstation (Siemens Medical Systems) for CT and DSA images. The following measurements were obtained: minimal diameter of the aorta at the level of and 1½ cm below the renal arteries, maximum outer diameter of the aneurysm, maximum diameter of the common and external (on MR angiograms and DSA images) iliac arteries, craniocaudal dimensions of the aneurysm and the infrarenal aorta, distance from the renal artery ostium to the proximal extent of the aneurysm (proximal neck), distance from the distal extent of the aneurysm to the aortic bifurcation (distal cuff), and degree of kinking of the infrarenal aorta (Fig 2). The diameter of regions of the aorta determined to be tortuous was defined as the diameter perpendicular to the direction of tortuosity. This was because aortic tortuosity can result in oblique CT sections and, hence, in overestimation of the aortic diameter. The celiac arteries, proximal segments of the superior and inferior mesenteric arteries, and the main renal arteries were graded as normal (grade 0), mildly stenotic (<50%, grade 1), moderately stenotic (50%–75%, grade 2), severely stenotic (76%–99%, grade 3), and occluded or not visualized (grade 4). Accessory renal arteries were recorded individually. Renal arteries were not evaluated for stenoses beyond the proximal 4 cm of the vessel,

Table 1
Classification of AAA with Regard to Stent-Graft Placement

	Proximal Aortic Neck		Distal Aortic Neck		Common Iliac Artery		
AAA Type	Diameter (mm)	Length (mm)	Diameter (mm)	Length (mm)	Diameter (mm)	Extension (mm)	Suggested Stent Graft
I	≤25	≥15	≤25	≥15	≤12	. . .	Tube
II	≤25	≥15	≥25	≤15	≤12	Aortic bifurcation	Bifurcated
III	≤25	≥15	≥25	≤15	≥12	Common iliac artery	Bifurcated
IV	≤25	≥15	≥25	≤15	≥12	Bifurcation of one common iliac artery	Bifurcated and embo HA*
V	≤25	≥15	≥25	≤15	≥12	Bifurcation of two common iliac arteries	Open repair†
VI	≥25	≤15	≥25	≤15	≥12	Common iliac artery	Open repair†

* embo HA = preoperative embolization of ipsilateral hypogastric artery and extension of iliac stent-graft limb into ipsilateral external iliac artery.
† In selected cases, placement of a bifurcated stent graft, preoperative embolization of an ipsilateral hypogastric artery, extension of iliac stent-graft limbs into both external iliac arteries, an additional bypass graft from the contralateral hypogastric artery to the distal external iliac artery, or a combination of these may be performed.

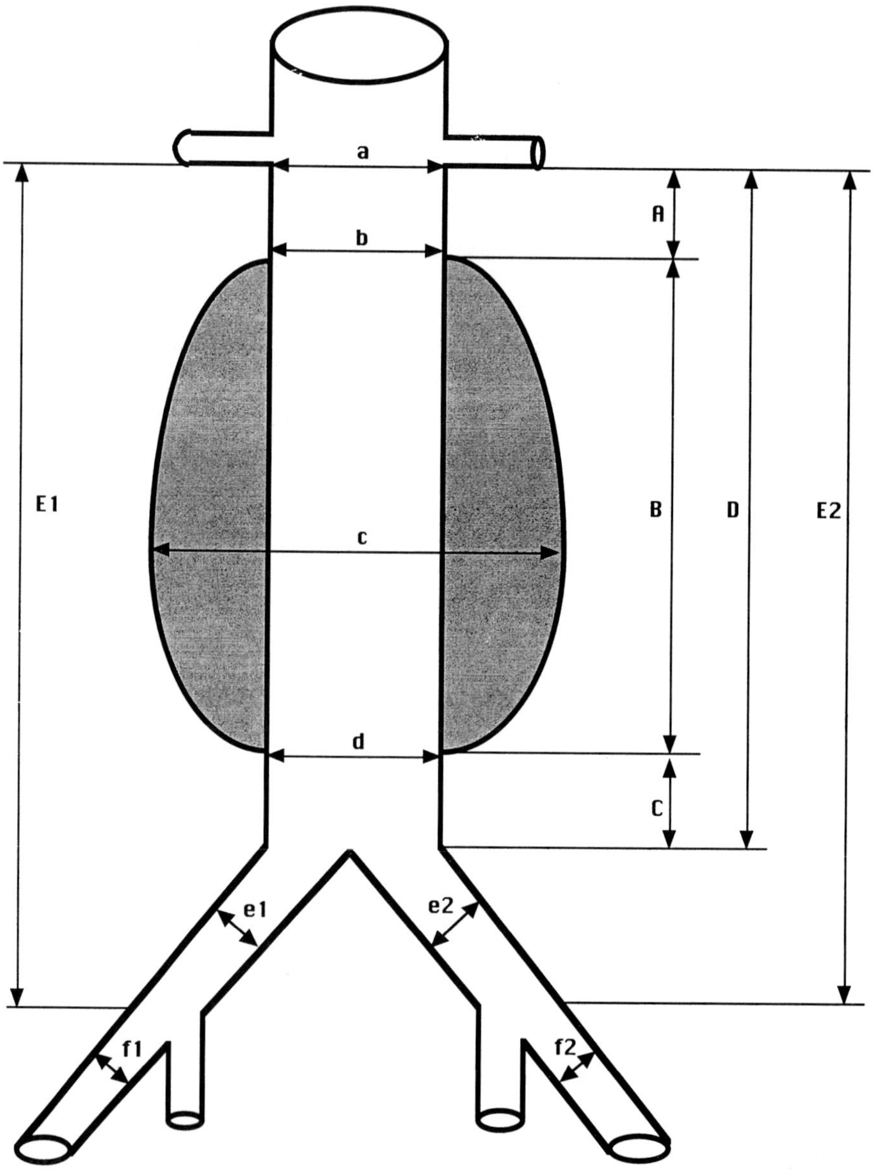

Figure 2. Measurement of the infrarenal aorta, iliac arteries, and AAAs for stent-graft placement. *A* = length of proximal neck, *B* = length of AAA, *C* = length of distal neck (cuff), *D* = length of infrarenal aorta, *E1* = distance from renal artery ostium to right iliac bifurcation, *E2* = distance from renal artery ostium to left iliac bifurcation, *a* = diameter of the aorta at the renal arteries, *b* = diameter of the aorta at 1½ cm below the renal arteries, *c* = maximum diameter of the AAA, *d* = diameter of the aorta at 1½ cm above the bifurcation, *e1* = maximum diameter of the right common iliac artery, *e2* = maximum diameter of the left common iliac artery, *f1* = maximum diameter of the right external iliac artery, and *f2* = maximum diameter of the left external iliac artery.

because the distal portions of the arteries were not consistently depicted.

The stent grafts that were evaluated, Stentor and Miahle-Stentor (Mintec, Great Bahama, Bahamas) and Vanguard (Boston Scientific, Watertown, Mass), are described in detail elsewhere (20). In brief, the devices are available in standard diameter (range, 20–26 mm) and length (range, 80–100 mm [tube graft] and 140–165 mm [bifurcated graft]) or can be custom-made.

For data analysis, DSA was used as the standard of reference to determine the number of main and accessory renal arteries and to demonstrate and grade the celiac artery, superior and inferior mesenteric artery, and common and external iliac artery stenoses. CT scans, which included three-dimensional reformations, were used as the standard of reference to determine the proximal and distal extents of the aneurysm and to measure the dimensions of the abdominal aorta and proximal common iliac arteries.

Statistical methods included calculation of the mean difference between MR angiographic and CT angiographic measurements with two-sided 95% confidence intervals (CIs) (Table 2). The two-tailed Student *t* test for the mean differences was considered to indicate a statistically significant difference at a *P* value of .05. Sensitivity for the degree of renal artery stenoses was calculated as TP/(TP + FN), where *TP* represents true-positive and *FN* represents false-negative findings. Specificity was calculated as TN/(TN + FP), where *TN* represents true-negative and *FP* represents false-positive findings. Ninety-five percent CIs for sensitivity and specificity were calculated by using the standard method of Clopper and Pearson (26). Different analyses for the degree of stenosis (>50% and >75%) were performed.

RESULTS

MR angiography provided high-quality images that resembled CT an-

Table 2
Mean Vascular Measurements and Mean Differences between MR Angiography and Helical CT Angiography

Measurement/Label on Fig 2	MR Angiography	CT Angiography	Mean Difference	Standard Deviation	95% CI
Minimal diameter of aorta at renal artery ostium (mm)/a	26 ± 6	26 ± 6	−0.16	1.31	−0.50, 0.17
Minimal diameter of aorta 1½ cm below renal arteries (mm)/b	29 ± 10	30 ± 10	−0.74	0.96	−0.98, −0.49
Maximum outer diameter of AAA (mm)/c	57 ± 15	59 ± 16	−0.21	4.84	−1.45, 1.03
Diameter of aorta 1½ cm above bifurcation (mm)/d	31 ± 8	30 ± 9	−0.55	1.04	−1.35, 0.74
Maximum diameter of right common iliac artery (mm)/e1	18 ± 10	19 ± 10	−0.52	2.05	−1.05, 0.002
Maximum diameter of left common iliac artery (mm)/e2	16 ± 11	17 ± 11	−0.20	1.27	−0.53, 0.13
Maximum diameter of right external iliac artery (mm)/f1	9 ± 4	8 ± 5	−0.31	1.04	−0.58, 0.17
Maximum diameter of left external iliac artery (mm)/f2	8 ± 3	8 ± 4	−0.02	0.87	−0.24, 0.21
Length of proximal neck (mm)/A	22 ± 20	22 ± 20	0.16	1.86	−0.31, 0.64
Length of AAA (mm)/B	94 ± 36	98 ± 33	−3.46	3.38	−4.32, −2.59
Length of distal neck (cuff) (mm)/C	6 ± 17	7 ± 15	−0.38	2.27	−0.96, 0.20
Length of infrarenal aorta (mm)/D	118 ± 21	122 ± 18	−3.82	2.46	−4.45, −3.19
Distance from renal artery ostium to right iliac bifurcation (mm)/E1	147 ± 24	NA	NA	NA	NA
Distance from renal artery ostium to left iliac bifurcation (mm)/E2	141 ± 21	NA	NA	NA	NA

Note.—MR and CT measurements are means ± standard deviations. NA = not available.

Table 3
Number of Main and Accessory Renal Arteries Detected at MR Angiography, Helical CT Angiography, and DSA

Renal Arteries	MR Angiography	CT Angiography	DSA
Main	118	121	121
Accessory	7	12	12
Total	125	133	133

Note.—DSA was the standard of reference.

giograms in many aspects. The MR angiograms were unacceptable for diagnosis (suboptimal arterial enhancement owing to prolonged circulation time) in two patients. In these patients, MR angiography was successfully repeated within 3 days. In all 61 patients, the abdominal aorta, common iliac arteries, and origins of the celiac artery, superior and inferior mesenteric arteries, and renal arteries were visualized on MR angiograms. In two patients with extremely tortuous iliac vessels, a short posterior segment of the common iliac artery was not included in the three-dimensional volume, which resulted in pseudo-occlusion of this vessel at MR angiography. At helical CT angiography, the range of coverage of the abdominal aorta and pelvic arteries was limited in all patients because of the technique chosen. Thus, the celiac, superior mesenteric, external iliac, and common femoral arteries could not be assessed by using CT.

The gadolinium-based contrast agent was well tolerated in all patients.

Proximal Extent of the Aneurysm

Of the 61 patients, four patients had a suprarenal origin of the aortic aneurysm as defined at CT. In two of these patients, the abdominal aneurysm was an extension of a thoracic aneurysm. Eleven patients had juxtarenal AAAs (type VI) with a neck less than 15 mm from the origin of the renal arteries. Forty-six patients had an infrarenal aortic aneurysm (types I–V). MR findings of the level of the aneurysm neck correlated with CT and angiographic findings in all patients. The mean proximal neck length (± the standard deviation) was 22 mm ± 20 for both MR and CT angiography (mean difference, 0.16 mm; standard deviation of the difference, 1.86; 95% CI, −0.31, 0.64) (Table 2). The mean aortic diameters at the level of and 1½ cm below the renal artery ostium were 26 mm ± 6 and 29 mm ± 10, respectively, for MR angiography and 26 mm ± 6 and 30 mm ± 10, respectively, for CT angiography.

Distal Extent of the Aneurysm

Choice of a stent graft (tube vs bifurcated) depends on the distal extent of the AAA. Only 17 patients had a normal-appearing distal cuff of at most 25 mm in diameter and at least 15 mm in length at CT and MR angiography. In three of these 17 patients, additional aneurysms of the common iliac artery were found. Thus, a total of 14 patients were eligible for tube stent-graft placement (however, in one of these 14 patients, the proximal neck was too short for stent-graft fixation). Another 26 patients had an AAA that reached the aortic bifurcation (type II aneurysm). MR and CT angiographic findings were equal in this respect to angiographic findings (mean difference, −0.38 mm; standard deviation, 2.27; 95% CI, −0.96, 0.20). Distal extension of the AAA to one or both common iliac arteries was found in 18 patients with type III–V aneurysms: 11 had aneurysms limited to the common iliac artery (type III aneurysm), four had an aneurysm that extended to one iliac artery bifurcation (type IV aneurysm), and three had aneurysms that extended to both iliac artery bifurcations (type V aneurysm). The diameter of aneurysms of the common iliac arteries was 16–55 mm. MR measurements correlated with CT angiographic and DSA measurements.

Measurements of the Aneurysm

The mean AAA diameter was 57 mm ± 15 (range, 31–90 mm) with MR angiography and 59 mm ± 16 with CT angiography (Table 2). The mean AAA length was 94 mm ± 36 with MR angiography and 98 mm ± 33 with CT angiography (mean difference, −3.46 mm; standard deviation, 3.38; 95% CI, −4.32, −2.59). The mean length of the infrarenal aorta was 118 mm ± 21 with MR angiography and 122 mm ± 18 with CT angiography (mean difference, –3.82 mm; standard deviation, 2.46; 95% CI, −4.45, −3.19). In nine patients, severe kinking of the infrarenal aorta (at the beginning of the aneurysm) of more than 60° was demonstrated with all modalities, which precluded stent-graft placement.

Renal Artery and Accessory Renal Artery Evaluation

In the 61 patients, DSA showed a total of 133 renal arteries (61 patients had 122 main arteries, eight patients had one accessory renal artery, two patients had two accessory renal arter-

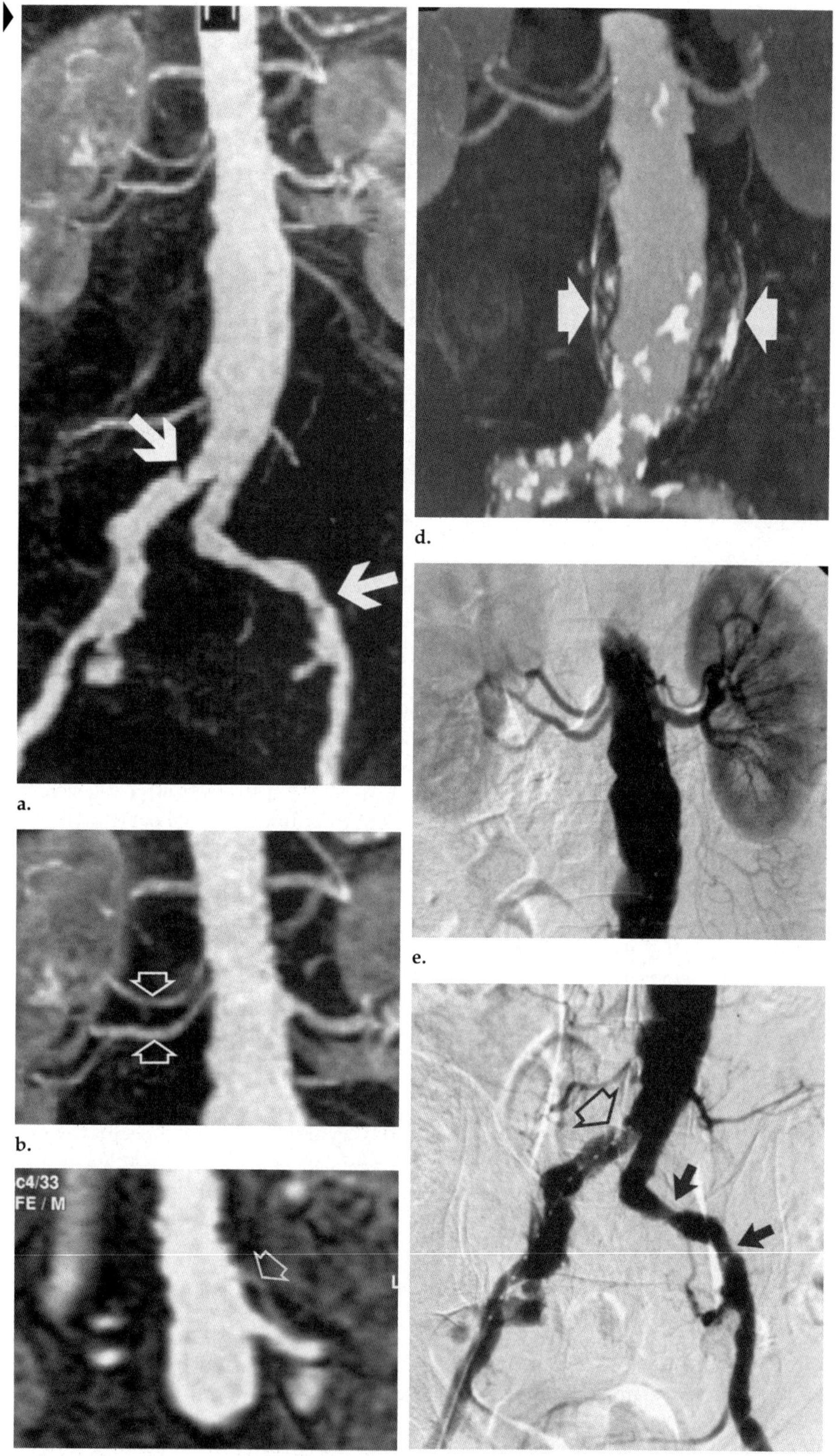

Figure 3. Images obtained in a 69-year-old man with a type IV infrarenal aortic aneurysm, two accessory renal arteries, right and left common iliac artery stenoses, and a right common iliac artery aneurysm that extends to the iliac bifurcation. The imaging findings indicate eligibility for bifurcated stent-graft placement (after balloon angioplasty of both iliac arteries and catheter embolization of the right hypogastric artery). **(a)** Gadolinium-enhanced, MIP, three-dimensional, time-of-flight MR angiogram (8.5/2.8, 40° flip angle) demonstrates an AAA that is limited to the infrarenal aorta, right and left common iliac artery stenoses (arrows), and moderate kinking of the left common iliac artery. **(b)** Focused MIP MR angiogram (8.5/2.8, 40° flip angle) shows two right renal arteries (arrows). **(c)** Source MR angiogram (8.5/2.8, 40° flip angle) reveals an additional left accessory renal artery (arrow). **(d)** MIP CT angiogram shows an infrarenal AAA with a calcified mural thrombus (arrows) and four renal arteries. Note the calcified plaques that obscure the common iliac artery stenosis. **(e)** DSA image shows the abdominal aorta and confirms the diagnosis of four renal arteries and mural irregularity of the AAA. **(f)** DSA image shows the pelvic arteries with eccentric stenosis of the right common iliac artery (open arrow) and two stenoses of the left common iliac artery (solid arrows) *(Fig 3 continues)*.

ies, and one patient had an occlusion of one main renal artery). MR angiography showed 125 renal arteries (94.0%) and did not show three main and five accessory renal arteries (Table 3, Fig 3). CT angiography showed all renal arteries. Three of the five accessory renal arteries missed at MR angiography were smaller than 2 mm in diameter. Two main and two accessory renal arteries were not demonstrated at MR angiography by using the initial non–breath-hold imaging protocol. In one patient, a patent main renal artery was misinterpreted as occluded at MR angiography owing to metallic artifacts from a previously placed Palmaz stent (Fig 4). Two of the accessory renal arteries were obscured on a full-volume MIP image but were correctly diagnosed on restricted-volume MIP or reformatted MR images (Fig 3).

At DSA, 17 (13.9%) of 122 main renal arteries demonstrated a hemodynamically significant stenosis (50% or greater; $n = 16$) or proximal occlusion ($n = 1$). Interpretation of MR angiograms matched that of DSA images in 82 renal arteries (Table 3). For the threshold of 50% stenosis, the specificity was 83.9% (73 of 87; 95% CI, 0.74, 0.91) and the sensitivity was 100% (35 of 35; 95% CI, 0.90, 1.00). For the threshold of 75% stenosis, the specificity was 76.5% (88 of 115; 95% CI, 0.68, 0.84) and the sensitivity was 100% (seven of seven; 95% CI, 0.59, 1.00). Overestimation of stenosis with MR angiography by one or two grades was found in 29 (23.7%) or 11 (9.0%) renal arteries, respectively (Table 4). In contrast, interpretation of CT angiograms matched that of DSA images in 115 renal arteries (94.3%). In seven main renal arteries (5.7%), the degree of stenosis was overestimated by one grade on CT angiograms.

Visceral Artery Evaluation

MR angiography correctly demonstrated all 59 normal celiac arteries and two celiac arteries with 50% stenosis

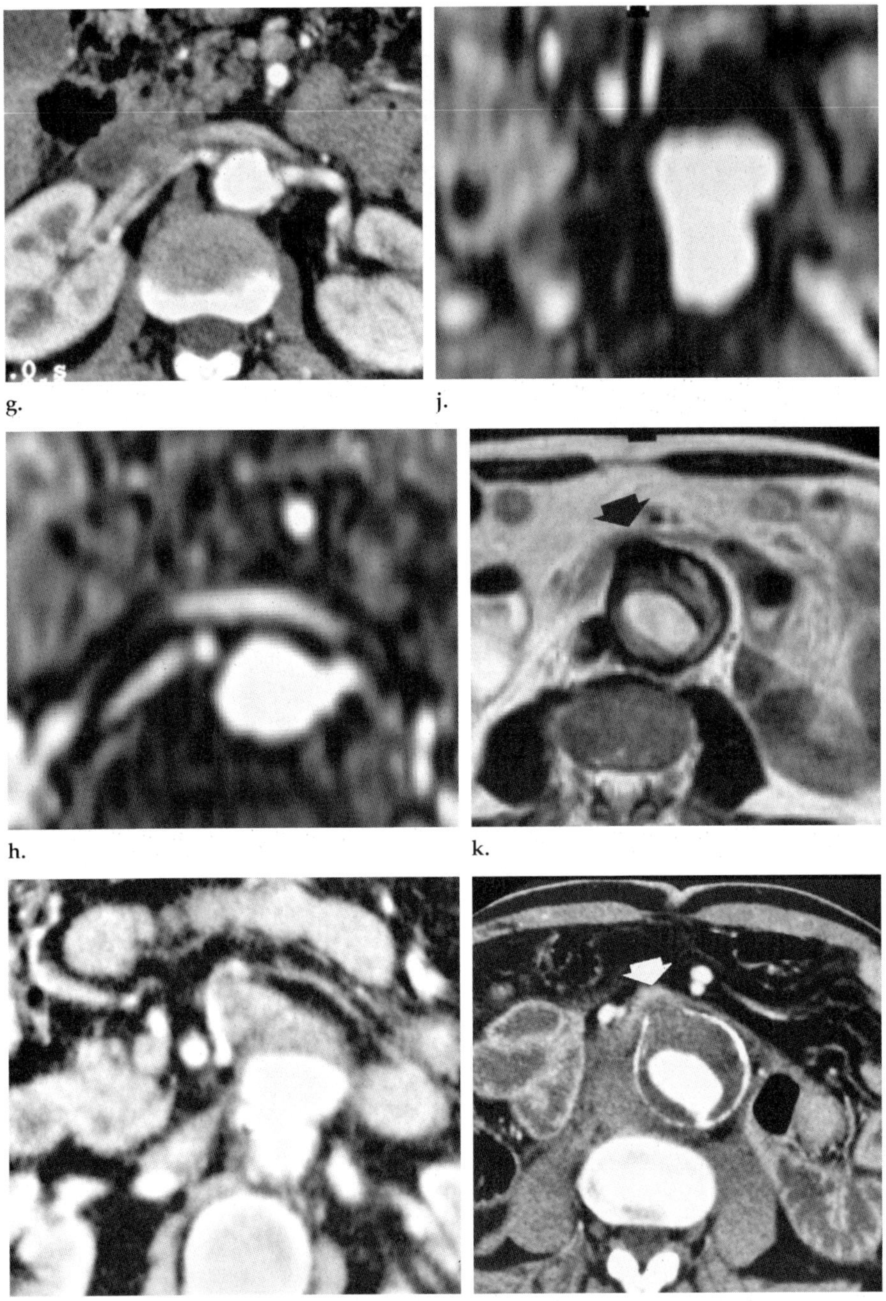

Figure 3 (*continued*). **(g, i)** Axial CT angiograms and **(h, j)** axial reformations from the three-dimensional MR angiographic data set obtained **(g, h)** at the level of and **(i, j)** 1½ cm below the lower renal artery ostium are identical with respect to the dimension of the aortic lumen. **(k)** Axial, T2-weighted, turbo spin-echo MR image (1,800/120 [effective], 90° flip angle) and **(l)** CT angiogram obtained at the level of the maximum diameter of the AAA. **k** shows inhomogeneous thrombus formation (arrow), whereas **l** shows a focal area of discontinuity of mural calcification and bulging of the thrombus (arrow).

(Table 4). Of the 61 superior mesenteric arteries that were imaged, one had a stenosis of 50% identified at DSA and MR angiography. The inferior mesenteric artery was occluded in 38 patients (62.3%), stenotic in 13 patients (21.3%), and patent in 10 patients (16.4%). MR angiography and CT angiography correctly demonstrated all inferior mesenteric artery occlusions and stenoses.

Iliac Artery Evaluation

Both MR and CT angiography showed aneurysmal dilatation (>15 mm) of the common iliac arteries in 12 patients (21 arteries). The dimensions of iliac artery aneurysms were shown correctly with both MR angiography and CT angiography but were underestimated with DSA owing to mural thrombus formation. Twenty common iliac artery stenoses (right side, 12 stenoses; left side, eight stenoses) and two occlusions (right) were correctly demonstrated and graded with MR angiography (Figs 4, 5). In addition, in five patients aneurysms of the hypogastric arteries were found at MR angiography. In three patients, stenoses greater than 50% were demonstrated in the external iliac artery with both MR angiography and DSA. Severe kinking of the common iliac arteries, external iliac arteries, or both was demonstrated in 27 arteries; arteriotomy of the external iliac artery was necessary in three patients and appropriate selection of a common femoral artery for insertion of the 18-F sheath in 24 patients. Assessment of distal common iliac, external iliac, and hypogastric arteries was not possible with CT angiography in our study because of the limited range of coverage.

Thrombus Formation

Both CT angiography and MR angiography were similarly well suited for the depiction of mural thrombus formation in the infrarenal aortic segment. However, characterization of calcified plaque was possible only at CT angiography (Fig 3).

Inflammatory Reaction and Rupture of AAA

Inflammatory periaortic reactions, contrast-enhancing periaortic reactions, or both were demonstrated in four patients at both MR angiography and CT angiography. In one of them, bilateral hydronephrosis was found.

In one patient, signs of a previous, contained rupture of the AAA with a large adjacent retroperitoneal hematoma was demonstrated at both MR imaging and CT (Fig 1).

Anatomic Variations

Both MR imaging and CT provided additional anatomic information not shown with DSA (Table 5). Renal cystic disease was demonstrated with both modalities in 18 patients. Variant venous anatomy was correctly identified on axial MR angiograms and axial CT angiograms (retroaortic left renal veins, two patients). All imaging modalities revealed a horseshoe kidney, with a third middle renal artery, in one patient.

Choice of Stent-Graft Procedure

Basically, 46 of 61 patients had an infrarenal AAA with a proximal neck sufficient for stent-graft placement according to imaging findings. Of 61 patients, 17 had a normal-appearing distal aortic cuff. In three of these 17 patients, additional aneurysms of the common iliac artery precluded tube stent–graft placement. In another patient, the proximal neck was too short for stent-graft fixation. Thus, only 13 of these 17 patients were eligible for tube stent–graft placement. Twenty-nine patients fulfilled the anatomic requirements for bifurcated stent-graft placement. Appropriate selection of the stent graft and dimensions was achieved by using MR angiography in all patients. Severe kinking of the common iliac arteries, external iliac arteries, or both was demonstrated in 27 arteries (in 22 patients) at MR angiography and DSA, which precluded insertion of the 18-F sheath in these vessels. In addition, in three patients, severe stenoses of the external iliac arteries that necessitated balloon angioplasty were detected at MR angiography and confirmed with DSA. CT angiography as a sole imaging modality was inadequate in 23 patients owing to the limited range of coverage with exclusion of the distal portion of the common iliac arteries.

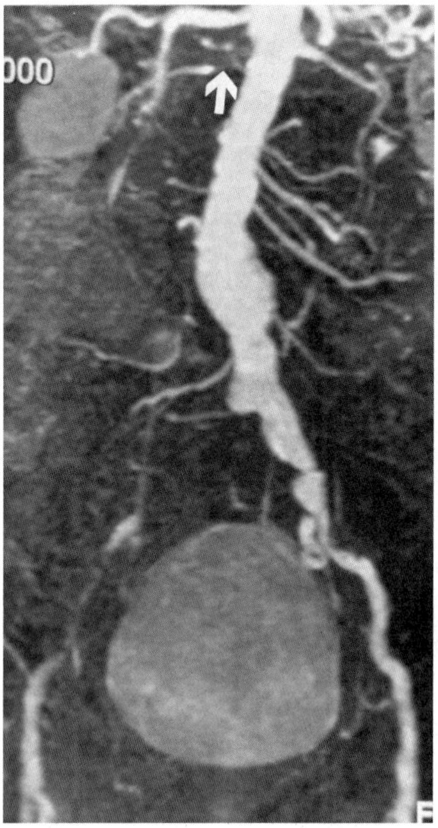

a.

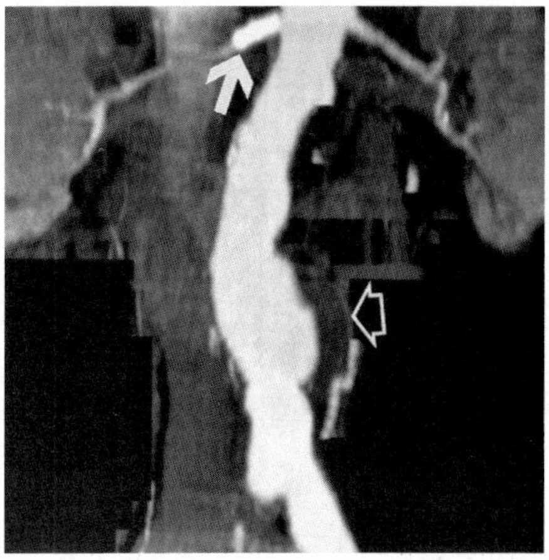

b.

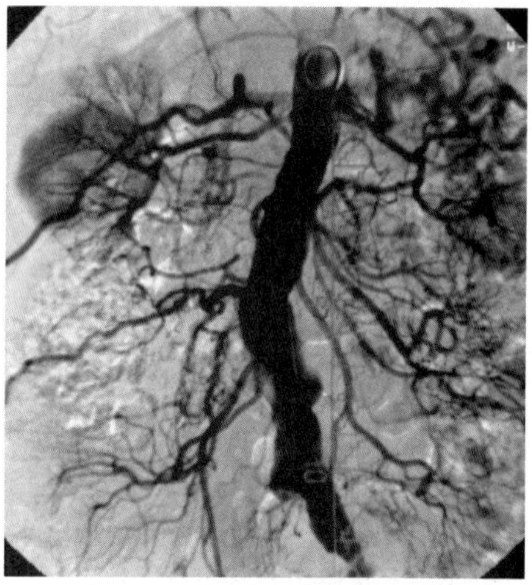

c.

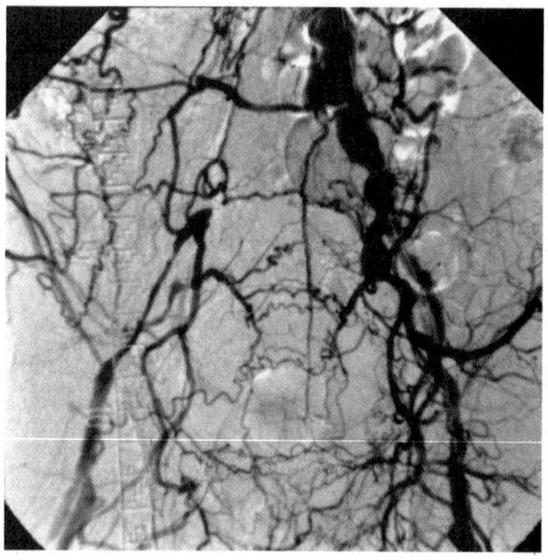

d.

Figure 4. Images obtained in a 71-year-old man with a type I infrarenal aortic aneurysm, a Palmaz stent in the right renal artery, right common iliac artery occlusion, severe right external iliac artery stenosis, and multiple left external iliac artery stenoses. After balloon angioplasty of the left external iliac artery, this patient was eligible for aortic tube stent grafting. **(a)** MIP, three-dimensional, time-of-flight MR angiogram (8.5/2.8, 40° flip angle) reveals a pseudo-occlusion of the right renal artery (arrow) due to metallic artifacts from a previous Palmaz stent. Right common iliac artery occlusion and stenoses in both external iliac arteries are clearly visible, whereas the infrarenal AAA with a long proximal neck is hard to detect. **(b)** MIP CT angiogram shows the stent in the right renal artery (solid arrow) and a small infrarenal AAA with a mural thrombus (open arrow). The limited range of coverage precludes evaluation of the status of the iliac arteries. **(c, d)** DSA images show the **(c)** aorta and **(d)** pelvic arteries and confirm the MR angiographic findings.

DISCUSSION

Recently, endovascular placement of aortic stent grafts has been developed for the treatment of AAAs (20–22). Compared with open surgical repair, this evolving alternative method is less invasive because of the insertion of the stent-graft device from a remote arteriotomy site. However, a variety of additional screening tests are needed to obtain the necessary information for successful stent-graft placement.

The true proximal extent of the AAA is the most crucial preoperative data for the interventional radiologist and surgeon (11). For secure anchoring of the stent graft, a sufficient segment of nonaneurysmal aorta proximal and distal to the aneurysm without relevant vascular branches must be present (20,21). For the device used in our study, a 15-mm distance from the renal artery ostium to the aneurysm is currently believed to be adequate for fixation (20). Of the 61 patients in our study, 46 met this requirement, as confirmed at both MR and CT angiography.

For safe anchoring of the stent graft and treatment of the aneurysm, the device has to be oversized by at least 1 mm in diameter (25). Inaccurate preoperative measurement of aortic dimensions and subsequent choice of an undersized stent-graft device may result in fatal stent-graft migration, leakage, or occlusion of the aortoiliac bifurcation. Our data showed agreement between MR angiographic and CT angiographic measurements of the diameter of the abdominal aorta at the level of the renal artery ostium (26 mm ± 6 [both MR angiography and CT angiography]) and 1½ cm below the renal artery ostium (29 mm ± 10 [MR angiography] vs 30 mm ± 10 [CT angiography]), even in regions of the aorta determined to be tortuous.

For tube graft placement, a distal nonaneurysmal aortic segment of at least 15 mm in length is mandatory (20). Both MR and CT angiography showed a normal distal cuff in 17 patients. Three of these patients had additional aneurysms of the common iliac arteries. Thus, only 13 patients met this criterion for tube stent–graft placement.

Table 4
Grading of Visceral Artery Stenosis with MR Angiography and Helical CT Angiography

Artery	Correctly Assessed		Overestimation of Stenosis: By One Grade		Overestimation of Stenosis: By Two Grades	
	MR Angiography	CT Angiography	MR Angiography	CT Angiography	MR Angiography	CT Angiography
Celiac trunk (n = 61)	61	NA	0	NA	0	NA
Superior mesenteric (n = 61)	61	61	0	NA	0	NA
Renal (n = 122)*	82	115	29	7	11	0
Inferior mesenteric (n = 61)	61	61	0	0	0	0

Note.—NA = not available. DSA was the standard of reference. Data are numbers of vessels.
* There were no underestimations of stenosis. For the threshold of 50% renal artery stenosis, the specificity of MR angiography was 83.9% (95% CI, 0.74, 0.91) and the sensitivity was 100% (95% CI, 0.90, 1.00). For the threshold of 75% renal artery stenosis, the specificity was 76.5% (95% CI, 0.68, 0.84), and the sensitivity was 100% (95% CI, 0.59, 1.00).

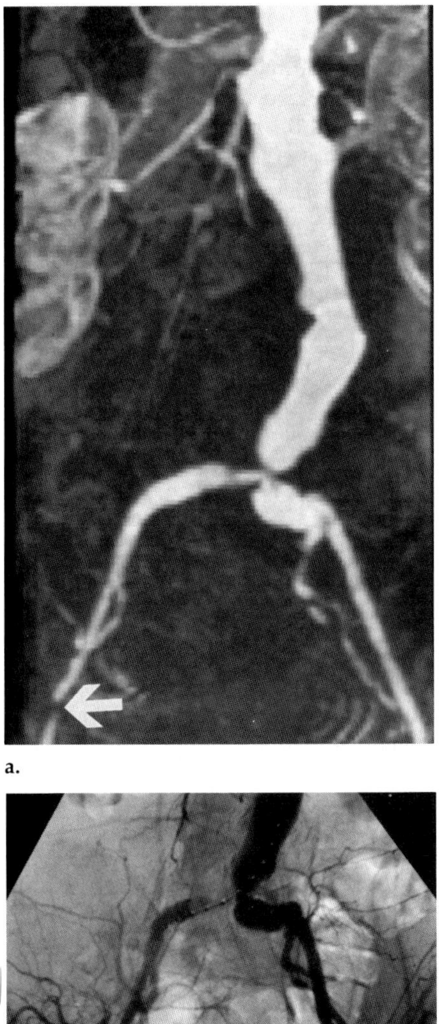

a.

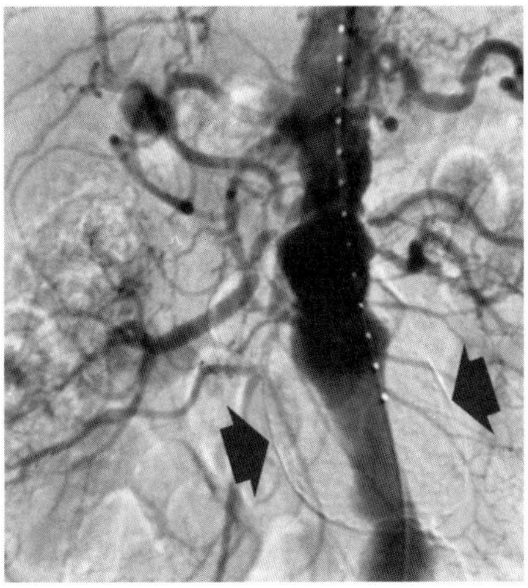

b.

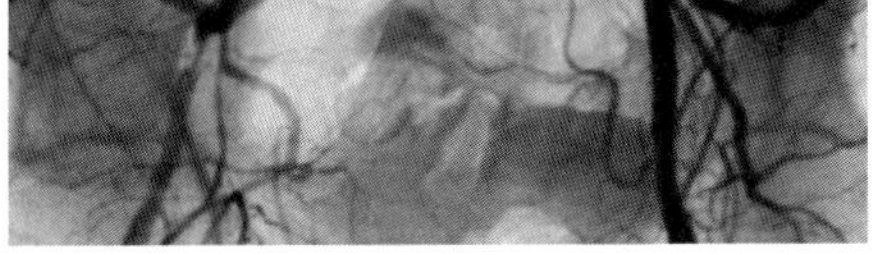

c.

Figure 5. Images obtained in a 68-year-old woman with a type VI juxtarenal aortic aneurysm, right and left common iliac artery stenoses, and a left common iliac artery aneurysm that extends to the iliac bifurcation. The short proximal neck precludes stent-graft placement. **(a)** MIP, three-dimensional, time-of-flight MR angiogram (8.5/2.8, 40° flip angle) demonstrates a large AAA that extends cranially to the renal arteries and distally to the aortic bifurcation. Both renal artery stenoses were incorrectly classified as severe. Angiogram shows 90° stenoses at the aortic bifurcation, which extend into both common iliac arteries, and at the right external iliac artery (arrow). **(b, c)** DSA images of **(b)** the abdominal aorta and **(c)** the iliac arteries confirm the diagnosis of AAA and pelvic artery stenoses. The rim of calcification (arrows in **b**) permits estimation of the true dimensions of the aneurysm.

Accurate measurement of true AAA diameter and changes in diameter are crucial for timing endovascular or surgical repair. The current surgical recommendation is to treat aneurysms that are at least 5 cm in diameter (1). Recently, findings of a random multicenter study in which the intraobserver and interobserver variability in CT measurements of AAA diameters was assessed showed a variable degree of precision because of differences in measurement techniques and imaging modalities (27). However, calipers and a magnifying glass were used for CT measurements in that study.

In contrast, we measured AAA dimensions with electronic calipers provided by a workstation. Thus, we found a high degree of agreement in measurements of maximum aneurysm diameter between MR angiography (57 mm ± 15) and CT angiography (59 mm ± 16; mean difference, −0.21 mm; standard deviation, 4.84; 95% CI, −1.45, 1.03). MR angiographic and CT angiographic measurements of tortuous AAAs are problematic, but tortuosity in the widest region of the aneurysm was rare in our series. Measurements of the length of the aneurysm and infrarenal aorta correlated less well between MR angiography and CT angiography; however, the difference was not statistically significant. In our study, aortic and AAA lengths were generally shorter with MR angiography than with CT angiography (118 mm ± 21 vs 122 mm ± 18 and 94 mm ± 36 vs 98 mm ± 33). We believe that differences in our study resulted from uncertainty of the reader as to where the aneurysm began and as to the exact measurements along the long axis of a tortuous aorta.

Recently, findings of a study in which helical CT and MR angiography were compared in the measurement of phantom tortuous AAA length for intraluminal graft placement showed 97.8% and 96% accuracy (r = .999) for CT angiography and MR angiography, respectively (28). The accuracy was not affected by angulation between the phantom and imaging sections of less than 30° in that study. We found that even though measurements were performed carefully with electronic calipers and a defined protocol, variability in measurements of AAA dimensions at CT and MR angiography is not uncommon. These variations in the measurement of aortic length must be taken into account in the selection of exact stent-graft dimensions. Efforts to reduce variation in measurement are warranted.

The high sensitivity (100% [35 of 35]) but relatively low specificity (83.9% [73 of 87] for a threshold of 50% stenosis; 76.5% [88 of 115] for a threshold of 75% stenosis) of MR angiography for correctly grading main renal artery stenoses in the present study were unexpected. Previous reports by others have noted a sensitivity for these lesions of 71%–100% and a specificity of up to 98% (7,9). However, some investigators (7–9) graded stenoses as not hemodynamically significant (<50%), hemodynamically significant (50%–99%), or occluded. By using our grading system, arterial occlusive disease will, in fact, occasionally be overestimated by at least one grade with MR angiography. Although still used as the standard of reference for comparison purposes, angiography of renal arteries may have inherent inaccuracies as well, particularly owing to eccentric plaques and overlying vessels (1). With regard to this critical subgroup, the information required and the plans for stent-graft placement were equal with both DSA and MR angiography.

The detection of small accessory renal arteries has been notoriously poor with MR angiography, with sensitivities of 28%–92%. Previous articles on gadolinium-enhanced, three-dimensional MR angiography without breath holding reported an increased sensitivity in identifying accessory renal arteries of up to 100% (7,17). The importance of breath-hold MR angiography for the elimination of respiratory artifact is emphasized by the fact that four (two main and two accessory renal arteries) of eight renal arteries missed in our study were imaged without the breath-hold technique. The remaining three accessory renal arteries that were not visualized in our study were smaller than 2 mm in diameter.

In general, 12% of patients with AAAs are noted to have substantial accessory renal vasculature (2). Because vessels greater than 2 mm in diameter may be end arteries that supply substantial renal parenchyma, it is often necessary to revascularize them. In our series, in two patients in whom accessory renal artery ostia were occluded by means of endovascular treatment of AAA, follow-up studies have shown unexpected persistent perfusion of the renal parenchyma (24).

Patency of celiac and superior mesenteric arteries is important for mesenteric circulation after stent-graft placement. Our data showed good correlation between MR angiography and DSA in depicting hemodynamically significant stenosis of the proximal part of these vessels (Table 4). In a total of three patients, stenoses of the celiac and superior mesenteric arteries were correctly graded by means of MR angiography.

The evaluation of iliac arteries is crucial, because occlusive disease of the iliac arteries, extreme tortuosity of the iliac arteries, or both may be an obstacle to stent-graft introduction. The 18-F introducer sheath used in our study requires a minimum vessel luminal diameter of 6 mm. Furthermore, aneurysms of the common iliac artery that extend to the iliac bifurcation may necessitate preoperative embolization of the ipsilateral hypogastric artery to avoid retrograde filling of the aneurysm after stent-graft insertion. Previous studies in which conventional MR angiography has been performed without contrast agent enhancement have shown limited success in the evaluation of iliac arteries owing to in-plane saturation. In our study, the dimensions and tortuosity of the iliac arteries and aneurysms or stenoses were best shown by means of dynamic contrast-enhanced MR angiography, because the injection of gadopentetate dimeglumine minimized the saturation effects. The CT angiographic protocol precluded display of the distal common and external iliac arteries. DSA was considered the standard of reference for iliac artery stenosis; however, the true size of iliac aneurysms was consistently underestimated owing to mural thrombus formation.

Thrombotic material attached to the walls results in underestimation of aortic diameter and misinterpretation of the proximal extent of the AAA at aortography. In our study, both MR angiography and CT angiography were well suited for the depiction of mural thrombus formation and, hence, the measurement of the true axial diameter of the abdominal aorta.

Other findings of our study likely to be detected at MR angiography and CT angiography and not at DSA include inflammatory changes of the aneurysm and anatomic variations in the abdomen, such as retroaortic veins (Table 5).

This article describes a combination of MR imaging and angiographic sequences, performed in less than 15 minutes, that can consistently provide the anatomic data needed to plan surgical interventions in patients with AAAs. Gadolinium-enhanced, three-dimensional MR angiography can overcome many limitations encountered with standard time-of-flight and phase-contrast MR angiographic techniques. Gadopentetate dimeglumine rarely has shown clinically important side effects, is nonnephrotoxic, and thus is safe for patients with renal insufficiency.

In our study, we have shown that for evaluation of AAA a minimum of two MR sequences is necessary: first, an axial T2-weighted sequence for the definition of an aortic aneurysm, the maximum diameter of it, perianeurysmal inflammatory changes, the presence of thrombus, the distal extent of the aneurysm, signs of aortic rupture, and additional anatomic variations; second, a dynamic, breath-hold, gadolinium-enhanced, three-dimensional, time-of-flight MR angiographic sequence with coronal and axial reconstructions and MIPs to produce images similar to those in biplane angiography. MR angiograms are best for evaluating the patency and location of aortic branches, kinking of the aorta, and stenotic or aneurysmatic lesions and tortuosity of the iliac arteries.

Although we considerably decreased imaging times in the second protocol,

Table 5
Additional Findings of MR Angiography and Helical CT Angiography

Finding	MR Angiography	CT Angiography
Thoracic aortic aneurysm	2	2
Kinking of AAA (>60°)	9	9
Inflammatory periaortic reaction	4	4
Rupture of AAA	1	1
Hydronephrosis	2	2
Horseshoe kidney	1	1
Renal cystic disease	18	18
Retro- or circumaortic renal vein	2	2
Kinking of iliac artery (>90°)	27	NA
Hypogastric artery aneurysm	5	NA

Note.—NA = not available. Data are numbers of patients.

we left the dose of gadopentetate dimeglumine unchanged from that used initially. A double dose of gadopentetate dimeglumine (40 mL) was generally required to produce high signal intensity within the vessels for MIP reconstructions, in part because of our failure to accurately and reliably determine circulation times. It has been suggested that an additional test dose of contrast agent be administered to enable a more accurate assessment of circulation times (18,29). However, such measurement would result in parenchymal enhancement and a reduced contrast-to-noise ratio on subsequent MR angiograms.

Contrast-enhanced MR angiographic depiction of small vessels was still inferior to DSA; however, in some respects, MR angiography has proved to be advantageous. Aneurysms and iliac arteries are demonstrated with high signal intensity in their entirety on a single large–field-of-view image. MR angiography provides cross-sectional images in any plane, which allows accurate measurement of aneurysm size, and allows depiction of the origins of the aortic branch vessels, which may not be possible with biplanar DSA when arteries overlap with the aneurysm. Reformatted MIP images are particularly useful for evaluating the relationship of the renal arteries to the AAA neck in complex cases. Parietal thrombus formation is readily identified at MR angiography. This information is important for planning endoluminal stent-graft placement.

Although gadolinium-enhanced MR angiography is conceptually similar to helical CT, it has the advantage of avoiding iodinated contrast agents or ionizing radiation and requires less critical timing for contrast agent injection. The images are acquired in the plane of the aorta, which allows MR angiography to cover a much greater length of the aorta and iliac vessels with great detail in a single injection. Postprocessing was far faster with MR angiography than with CT angiography. In our series, the postprocessing of MR angiographic data, including axial image and MIP reconstructions, lasted less than 5 minutes, whereas CT angiography required up to 1½ hours. The cost of gadolinium-based contrast agents is comparable to the cost of nonionic contrast agents used for helical CT. For these reasons, gadolinium-enhanced MR angiography may become the primary imaging modality for the preoperative evaluation of AAA at our institution.

Certain limitations of gadolinium-enhanced MR angiography must be considered. Open surgery is the standard for accurate determination of the proximal extent of the AAA. Because surgical proof was not possible in our study, we had to use CT as the standard of reference, which may result in failure to correctly estimate the proximal extent of the aneurysm (11). The CT angiographic technique used in our study was hampered by a limited scan time of 32 seconds. Current helical CT systems with longer scan times would adequately image both the aorta and iliac arteries.

Inaccuracy in the estimation of circulation time may result in incomplete opacification of the aorta, pelvic arteries, or both on contrast-enhanced MR angiograms. Recently, the combined use of a power injector and a timing examination with a test bolus during axial, turbo, fast low-angle shot imaging has been shown to improve the aortic signal-to-noise ratio statistically significantly (29).

MR angiography cannot be offered to patients with contraindications to MR angiography, such as implanted pacemakers. Although MR angiography was able to depict most stenoses, the severity of renal artery lesions was overestimated in some patients, and evaluation of the hemodynamic and functional importance is impossible. In addition, the inaccuracy of MR angiography for accessory renal arteries is still a major limitation of this imaging modality. Nevertheless, it is desirable to tailor invasive DSA to answer specific questions in a limited number of patients. Furthermore, MR angiography may be of limited value in postoperative follow-up studies after successful stent-graft placement, because metallic artifacts from a stent will hamper exact evaluation of complications, such as perigraft channels.

Gadolinium-enhanced MR angiography is still in the early phase of development, and technologic advances are occurring at a rapid pace. Improvements will include higher field strength, better field uniformity, faster gradients, specialized coils, and new imaging sequences. Outstanding results have been shown by the MR angiography group of the University of Wisconsin—Madison (30). They used a new technique called time-resolved imaging of contrast kinetics, or TRICKS, to perform either unenhanced or non–time-resolved contrast-enhanced MR angiography with digital subtraction.

In conclusion, gadolinium-enhanced MR angiography is a new and evolving technology that can provide exact anatomic information for the planning of endovascular aortic stent-graft placement. MR angiography displays all the information necessary for the diagnosis and staging of aneurysmal disease without the use of ionizing radiation in a short time. DSA can be reserved for select cases when specific questions are not adequately resolved with MR angiography. It is our contention that because it is noninvasive, fast, and accurate, the increasing use of MR angiography as a sole preoperative imaging technique is warranted in the majority of patients. ■

References

1. Ernst CB. Abdominal aortic aneurysms. N Engl J Med 1993; 328:1167–1172.
2. Bell DD, Gaspar MR. Routine aortography before abdominal aortic aneurysmectomy. Am J Surg 1992; 144:191–193.
3. Todd GC, Nowygrod R, Benvenisty A, et al. The accuracy of CT scanning in the diagnosis of abdominal and thoracoabdominal aortic aneurysms. J Vasc Surg 1991; 13:302–310.
4. Siegel CL, Cohan RH. CT of abdominal aortic aneurysms. AJR 1994; 163:17–29.
5. Cohan RH, Siegel CL, Korobkin M, et al. Abdominal aortic aneurysm: CT evaluation of renal artery involvement. Radiology 1995; 194:751–756.
6. Sivananthan UM, Rees MR, Ridgway J, Ward J, Bann K. Fast MRI with turbo-FLASH sequences in aortoiliac disease. Lancet 1991; 338:1090–1091.
7. Peterson MJ, Cambria RP, Kaufman JA, et al. Magnetic resonance angiography in the preoperative evaluation of abdominal aortic aneurysms. J Vasc Surg 1995; 21:891–899.
8. Ecklund K, Hartnell GG, Hughes LA, Stokes KR, Finn JP. MR angiography as the sole method in evaluating abdominal aortic aneurysms: correlation with conventional techniques and surgery. Radiology 1994; 192:345–350.
9. Kaufman JA, Geller SC, Petersen MJ, Cambria RP, Prince MR, Waltman AC. MR imaging (including MR angiography) of abdominal aortic aneurysms: comparison with conventional angiography. AJR 1994; 163:203–210.
10. Gomes MN, Davros WJ, Zeman RK. Preoperative assessment of abdominal aortic aneurysm: the value of helical and three-dimensional computed tomography. J Vasc Surg 1994; 20:367–376.
11. Van Hoe L, Baert AL, Gryspeerdt S, et al. Supra- and juxtarenal aneurysms of the abdominal aorta: preoperative assessment with thin-section spiral CT. Radiology 1996; 198:443–448.
12. Zeman RK, Silverman PM, Vieco PT, Costello P. CT angiography. AJR 1995; 165: 1079–1088.
13. Costello P, Gaa J. Spiral CT angiography of abdominal aortic aneurysms. RadioGraphics 1995; 15:397–406.
14. Rubin GD, Walker PJ, Dake MD, et al. Three-dimensional spiral computed angiography: an alternative imaging modality for the abdominal aorta and its branches. J Vasc Surg 1993; 18:656–665.
15. Creasy JL, Prince RR, Presbrey T, Goins D, Partain CL, Kessler RM. Gadolinium-enhanced MR angiography. Radiology 1990; 175:280–283.
16. Prince MR, Yucel EK, Kaufman JA, Harrison DC, Geller SC. Dynamic gadolinium-

enhanced 3DFT abdominal MR arteriography. JMRI 1993; 3:877–881.
17. Prince MR. Gadolinium-enhanced MR aortography. Radiology 1994; 191:155–164.
18. Holland GA, Dougherty L, Carpenter JP, et al. Breath-hold ultrafast three-dimensional gadolinium-enhanced MR angiography of the aorta and the renal and other visceral abdominal arteries. AJR 1996; 166: 971–981.
19. Prince MR, Narasimham DL, Stanley JC, et al. Breath-hold gadolinium-enhanced MR angiography of the abdominal aorta and its major branches. Radiology 1995; 197:785–792.
20. Blum U, Langer M, Spillner G, et al. Abdominal aortic aneurysms: preliminary technical and clinical results with transfemoral placement of endovascular self-expanding stent-grafts. Radiology 1996; 198:25–31.
21. Richter GM, Palmaz JC, Allenberg JR, Kauffmann GW. Percutaneous stent grafts for aortic aneurysms: preliminary experience with a new procedure. Radiologe 1994; 34:511–518.
22. Murphy KD, Richter GM, Henry M, Encarnacion CE, Le VA, Palmaz JC. Aortoiliac aneurysms: management with endovascular stent-graft placement. Radiology 1996; 198:473–480.
23. Rozenblit A, Marin ML, Veith FJ, Cynamon J, Wahl SI, Bakal CW. Endovascular repair of abdominal aortic aneurysm: value of postoperative follow-up with helical CT. AJR 1995; 165:1473–1479.
24. Dorffner R, Thurnher S, Youssefzadeh S, et al. Spiral CT-angiography in the assessment of abdominal aortic aneurysms after stent grafting: value of maximum intensity projections. J Comput Assist Tomogr 1997; 21:472–477.
25. Moritz JD, Rotermund S, Keating DP, Oestmann JW. Infrarenal abdominal aortic aneurysms: implications of CT evaluation of size and configuration for placement of endovascular aortic grafts. Radiology 1996; 198:463–466.
26. Hartung J. Statistik. Munich, Germany: Oldenbourg, 1982; 204.
27. Lederle FA, Wilson SE, Johnson GR, et al. Variability in measurement of abdominal aortic aneurysms. J Vasc Surg 1995; 21:945–952.
28. Liu Y, Sampson C, Dorros G, Blechinger J, Wann LS. Measurement of phantom tortuous abdominal aortic aneurysm length for intraluminal graft placement: CT angiography or MR angiography? (abstr). Radiology 1996; 201(P):329.
29. Earls JP, Rofsky NM, DeCorato DR, Krinsky GA, Weinreb JC. Breath-hold single-dose gadolinium-enhanced three-dimensional MR aortography: usefulness of a timing examination and MR power injector. Radiology 1996; 201:705–710.
30. Korosec FR, Frayne R, Grist TM, Mistretta CA. Time-resolved, contrast-enhanced 3D MR angiography (abstr). Radiology 1996; 201(P):328.

Hans Peter Weskott, MD • Kerstin Holsing, MD

US-based Evaluation of Hemodynamic Parameters in the Common Carotid Artery: A Nomogram Trial[1]

PURPOSE: **To evaluate hemodynamic data of the common carotid artery (CCA) with an ultrasound (US)-based technique in an age- and sex-matched healthy population.**

MATERIALS AND METHODS: **Measurements from a color M-mode tracing of each CCA in 205 healthy subjects (age range, 20–87 years) were performed with a time domain processing system. Lumen change of the color M-mode tracing, flow velocity, volume flow rate, and diastolic volume index (DVI) were calculated five times. Blood pressure was measured after the US examination. Fifteen subjects were excluded from the nomogram trial because of hypertension, and 12 and four subjects were excluded because of an asymptomatic carotid artery stenosis or atrial fibrillation, respectively.**

RESULTS: **Mean volume flow rate in the CCA of the remaining 174 healthy volunteers was 415.0 mL/min ± 87.0 (men [*n* = 84], 441.0 mL/min ± 95.5; women [*n* = 90], 390.2 mL/min ± 70.5). The following statistically significant associations were noted: between vessel lumen and sex and blood pressure; between peak systolic velocity and sex and age; between volume flow rate and sex, age, and systolic blood pressure; and between DVI and age, heart rate, and systolic and diastolic blood pressure.**

CONCLUSION: **Time domain processing is an intrasessionally well-reproducible US method for measuring velocities and volume flow in the CCA.**

Ultrasound (US) has become the first choice for imaging and detecting cardiac and vascular diseases. Our knowledge of hemodynamics and its regulation mechanisms has expanded greatly since blood flow velocity and its indexes can be calculated by using the pulsed-wave Doppler (frequency domain) technique. The systolic peak velocity ratio and the ratio of the velocity of the internal carotid artery to the velocity of the common carotid artery (CCA) are considered to be the most important Doppler-based hemodynamic parameters in assessing the degree of an arterial stenosis (1–3).

Because there are abundant clinical reasons to ascertain the volume of blood delivered to a tissue bed, many attempts have been made to estimate the volumetric flow rate in different vessels. The most common US-based technique uses a calculation that includes the mean velocities over a cardiac cycle and the vessel diameter. Although US-based velocity calculation has become a reliable and reproducible parameter, the estimation of blood volume flow potentially has many errors (4–6).

Since 1991, the calculation of velocities and the estimation of volume flow rates can be achieved by using a time domain processing US technique (Color Velocity Imaging, CVI, and Color Velocity Imaging–Quantification, CVI-Q; Philips Medical Systems, Irvine, Calif) (7–9). For volume flow estimation, a time averaging of the Doppler power spectrum is applied. To quantify volume flow, this US technique integrates the time-varying flow profile in a vessel with the cross-sectional measurements derived from M-mode sampling across the vessel lumen. The advantages of time domain processing are high spatial and temporal resolution compared with that of color Doppler systems. In previous studies, this technique has been shown to have an excellent accuracy and a good reproducibility under in vitro and in vivo conditions (10–12). The correlation coefficients between CVI-Q and a flow pump with a pulsatile or continuous volume flow setting in a 4- and 8-mm tube ranged between R^2 = .994 and R^2 = .998; in vivo comparison of flow velocities calculated by using CVI and pulsed-wave Doppler demonstrated an R^2 of .995 (13). Validation studies showed an error of under 8% for flows above 200 mL/min in a flow phantom, an interoperator repeatability of 15.30% in vivo, and an intraoperator repeatability ranging between 9.92% and 13.74% (14).

In this study, the velocity and the volumetric blood flow calculations in the CCA in a healthy age- and sex-matched population were performed by using the time domain processing method. Most of the previously published studies either were not age- and sex-matched or did not take blood pressure into account (Table 1) (15–22).

Index terms: Carotid arteries, flow dynamics, 904.91, 904.92 • Carotid arteries, US, 904.12983, 904.12989 • Ultrasound (US), Doppler, 904.12983 • Ultrasound (US), technology, 904.12989

Abbreviations: CCA = common carotid artery, DVI = diastolic volume index.

Radiology 1997; 205:353–359

[1] From the Department of Internal Medicine II, Städtisches Krankenhaus Siloah, Hannover 30449, Germany. From the 1996 RSNA scientific assembly. Received December 3, 1996; revision requested January 27, 1997; revision received June 13; accepted June 25. **Address reprint requests to** H.P.W.

Table 1
Published Results of US-based Volume Flow in the CCA

Study	Year	Method	Volume Flow* (mL/min) All Subjects	Men	Women	Age (y) Mean/Range	Dependent on Age	Sex	Blood Pressure
Payen et al (15)	1982	TAV	387 ± 183 (*n* = 11)	NM	NM	39/20–56	NM	NM	NM
Uematsu et al (16)	1983	Flow meter	456 ± 66 (*n* = 120)	480 ± 90	402 ± 29	NM	Yes	Yes	NM
Uematsu and Folstein (17)	1985	Flow meter	486 ± 78 (*n* = 27)	NM	NM	NM/5–60	Yes	Yes	NM
Bouthier et al (18)	1985	TAV	396 ± 19 (*n* = 38)	NM	NM	NM	Yes	NM	Yes
Benetos et al (19)	1986	TAV	429 ± 21 (*n* = 21)	NM	NM	NM	NM	NM	Yes
Meyd et al (20)	1992	QFM	513 ± 92 (*n* = 40)	NM	NM	62/32–80	NM	NM	NM
Hamada et al (21)	1993	TAV	564 ± 60 (*n* = 28)	NM	NM	71.4 ± 7.2*	NM	NM	NM
Schöning et al (22)	1994	TAV	470 ± 120 (*n* = 48)	NM	NM	35 ± 12*/20–63	Yes†	No	NM
Eicke and Tegeler (12)	1995	TDP	352 ± 65 (*n* = 125)	375 ± 70	330 ± 60	NM	No	Yes	No

Note.—NM = not mentioned, QFM = quantitative carotid blood flow technique, TAV = time averaged velocity, TDP = time domain processing.
* Data are presented as the mean ± standard deviation.
† In this study, an age-related increase of volume flow of the CCA was reported.

Measuring and interpreting volumetric flow rate in a human vessel is a major challenge, considering the physiologic hemodynamic changes and the varying demands for blood supply of the end organ (23). An increase in vessel diameter depending on age and a difference in vessel diameter for the different sexes has been described by Hansen et al (24).

The volume flow through the conduit arteries is modulated by a large number of factors, among which cardiac output and heart rate are the most important. Apart from the physiologic modulation, numerous conditions are known to increase cardiac output (25).

The cardiac output decreases with age and may be reduced by up to 20% in the elderly (26). To maintain a constant blood flow in the most important organs, a decrease of cardiac output leads to a redistribution of blood, with the brain, small intestine, and heart receiving a higher proportion (27,28).

To assess the physiologic hemodynamic changes in the CCA, a nomogram trial of a healthy, age- and sex-matched population was performed. Volunteers in whom hypertension was first diagnosed at the time of the study were evaluated separately.

Table 2
Physiologic Characteristics of the Nomogram Population

Sex	Age (y)	Body Mass Index (kg/m²)	Heart Rate (bpm)	Blood Pressure (mm Hg) Systolic	Diastolic
Female (*n* = 90)	45 ± 16	26.3	74 ± 12	116 ± 12	75 ± 7.1
Male (*n* = 84)	47 ± 16	23.2	70 ± 11	121 ± 11	76 ± 7.7
All (*n* = 174)	46 ± 16	24.7	72 ± 12	119 ± 12	75 ± 7.4

Note.—Except for body mass index, data are presented as the mean ± standard deviation. Fifty-three of the patients were smokers.

Table 3
Distribution of the 174 Volunteers by Age, Sex, and Smoking Habit

Age (y)	Women (*n* = 90) Nonsmokers	Smokers	Men (*n* = 84) Nonsmokers	Smokers	All
20–29	9	8	12	3	32
30–39	10	6	8	7	31
40–49	12	5	8	7	32
50–59	11	4	10	5	30
60–69	13	3	14	2	32
>70	9	0	5	3	17
All	64	26	57	27	174

MATERIALS AND METHODS

Volunteers

Two hundred five volunteers without a history of acute or chronic organ disease and not currently taking medication were included in the study. The volunteers' age, sex, weight, height, heart rate, body mass, and smoking history were recorded. For the evaluation of marked arteriosclerosis of the CCA or the extracranial internal carotid artery, gray-scale US, CVI, and pulsed-wave Doppler US evaluations were performed on each volunteer before the examination. Afterward, the blood pressure was measured in both arms and considered normal if it did not exceed 140/90 mm Hg.

Fifteen of the 205 volunteers were excluded from the nomogram trial owing to an elevated blood pressure that exceeded 140/90 mm Hg at rest. Twelve of the 205 volunteers had a greater than 50% stenosis of the CCA or internal carotid artery and were therefore excluded from the study. Four of the 205 volunteers were excluded because of an asymptomatic atrial fibrillation.

The clinical data of the 174 volunteers included in the study are listed in Table 2. Table 3 shows the age, sex, and smoking habit distribution of the volunteers.

US Technique

All carotid examinations were performed with a 7.5-MHz linear-array transducer, in CVI and CVI-Q technique (Philips Medical Systems). The readings of all velocities and volume flow numbers were based on the color M-mode tracing time domain processing calculation.

The CCA was insonated from the neck lateral to the sternocleidomastoid muscle, with the operator maintaining the recommended scanning guidelines (Fig 1). The scan line for the M-mode was placed in the midportion of the CCA where the CCA is relatively straight and not too close to the bifurcation. The angle correction was performed on a color-suppressed, magnified image. The mean angle of insonation was 59.3° ± 3.8.

Measurement after a rest period of 10 minutes

Measurement in supine position

Long-axis scan plane in the center of the vessel (greatest vessel diameter)

Angle of insonation between 40° and 70°

Color threshold just below noise

Smallest scale without aliasing

Figure 1. Scanning guidelines for volume flow measurements.

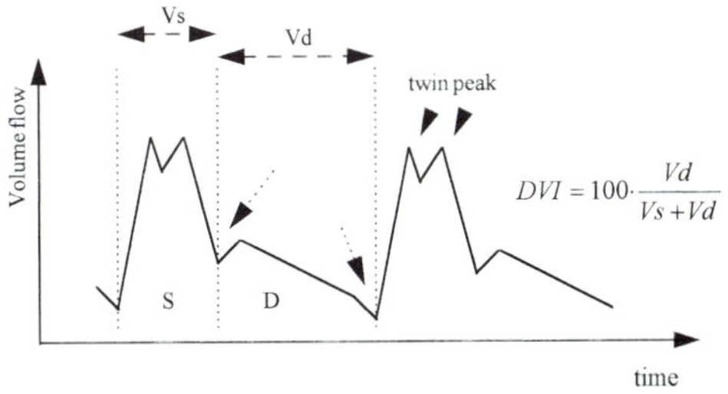

a.

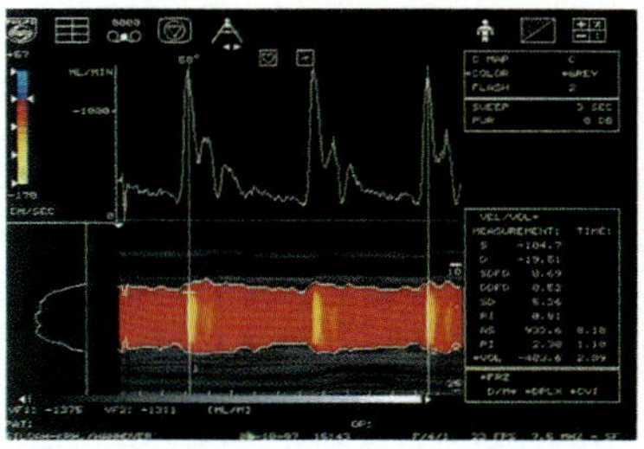

b.

Figure 2. **(a)** Calculations from the velocity and volume flow curve. The dotted arrows indicate the systolic onset and the aortic valve closure. Two arrowheads mark the first systolic peaks. D = diastole, S = systole, V_d and V_s = time interval in which volume flow during diastole or systole, respectively, is measured. **(b)** Color M-mode tracing of the CCA. Volume flow is calculated during the time interval between the two cursors. When switching to the velocity curve, a third cursor indicates the end-diastolic velocity.

Table 4
Correlation between DVI and Heart Rate in the 174 Healthy Volunteers

Volunteers	Regression	R^2 Value	P Value
Smokers	$y = -0.22 \times 57.16$	.154	<.0001
Non-smokers	$y = -0.31 \times 64.79$	.344	<.0001

All US measurements were performed five times from the color M-mode tracing of the midportion of the right and left CCAs, respectively: The functional systolic lumen was defined as the greatest width of the color M-mode tracing and the functional diastolic lumen as the smallest bandwidth just before systolic onset.

After an automatic tracing of the color M-mode band, a velocity or volume flow curve is displayed (Fig 2). The display can be switched between the velocity curve with three cursors and the volume flow curve with two cursors. The cursors indicate the systolic and end-diastolic velocities and the time interval over which the volume flow was calculated automatically or after adjustment. The aortic valve closure can be identified easily by a well-defined, sharp notch at the end of the end-systolic deceleration.

The total volume flow was calculated from all displayed cardiac cycles at a sweep time of 3 seconds. The cursor position was realigned if the automatic positioning was incorrect.

A volume flow–related index (diastolic volume index [DVI]), which is based on a US measurement of the fractional volumetric blood flow during one single cardiac action, is introduced. The diastolic portion of the total volume flow was measured as the diastolic percentage of flow in relation to the total volume flow rate (Fig 2). The duration of diastole was defined as the time interval between the end-diastolic velocity and the notch at end systole. Instead of relating two velocities from the velocity curve to each other (resistive or Pourcelot index), the DVI expresses the proportion of the diastolic flow to the total volume flow and is theoretically angle independent. The calculation of DVI is as follows: $DVI = 100[V_d/(V_s + V_d)]$, where V_d = volume flow during diastole, and V_s = volume flow during systole.

The duration of diastole depends on the heart rate, and so will the DVI. A frequency corrected DVI, DVI_C, can be calculated if we know the mean heart rate, HR_{mean}, and the relation between the DVI and the heart rate (slope of the regression curve, S_r) in a healthy population: $DVI_C = DVI + (HR - HR_{mean}) \times S_r$; when substituting the known values, $DVI_C = DVI + (HR - 72) \times 0.286$. This relation can be described by the regression of the correlation curve (Table 4).

The color M-mode tracing of the velocity-volume flow curve has a characteristic envelope, which is characterized by a central notch leading to a "twin peak" sign during systole (Fig 2).

Statistical Analysis

The data were expressed and statistically analyzed by using the SPSS-PC package (SPSS for Windows; SPSS, Chicago, Ill). Continuous variables are expressed as means (± 1 standard deviation). We used analysis of variance for the comparison of continuous variables. The difference between two specific groups was calculated with the Scheffe post hoc test. Correlation between two continuous variables was examined by means of regression analysis with the mean least squares estimate based on a linear model. A P value of less than .05 was considered to indicate statistical significance in all analyses. To characterize the intrasessional reproducibility of the five measurements in the two carotid arteries in the male or female group, the standard deviation of the mean values was expressed as a percentage of the mean value.

RESULTS

The average duration of the US examination was 25 minutes, but an additional time of 5 minutes per patient was needed for the computer-based calculations.

Functional Lumen

The width of the systolic and diastolic color band expresses the perfused vessel lumen and depends on the sensitivity of the US device for detection of slow flow. This changing color tracing width represents the functional lumen. The average functional CCA lumen during systole and diastole of all volunteers regardless of sex was 6.7 mm ± 0.5 and 5.3 mm ± 0.5, respectively (Table 5). The standard deviation as a percentage of mean value of the five measurements for the systolic lumen was 4.0% for the male volunteers and 4.4% for the female volunteers and for the diastolic lumen was 5.1% and 4.8%, respectively. Both lumina showed a highly significant association with sex (P = .0001, Fig 3) and with age in the elderly. The change in systolic and diastolic lumina differed significantly between both sexes (P = .0001).

The volunteers with unsuspected hypertension (n = 15) had a systolic lumen of 6.95 mm ± 0.29 and a diastolic lumen of 4.67 mm ± 0.38. Compared with an age-related group of healthy volunteers, the difference of 2.28 mm in lumen change during a cardiac cycle was highly significant (P = .0001).

Velocity Measurements

Peak systolic velocity was related highly significantly to age and sex (P = .0001). The standard error was 1.76 for the male volunteers and 1.41 for the female volunteers. The standard deviation as a percentage of mean value of the five measurements for the peak systolic velocity was 5.4% for the male volunteers and 6.8% for the female volunteers. The decline of the peak systolic velocity began in the 3rd decade of life for both sexes. The standard deviation as a percentage of

Table 5
US Measurements of the CCA by Age and Sex

Age (y)	Functional Lumen (mm)				Peak Systolic Velocity (cm/sec)		End-diastolic Velocity* (cm/sec)	Volume Flow (mL/min)		
	Systolic		Diastolic							
	Male	Female	Male	Female	Male	Female		Male	Female	DVI*
20–29	7.00 ± 0.49	6.58 ± 0.52	5.52 ± 0.48	5.30 ± 0.43	119.8 ± 17.4	106.0 ± 11.6	21.9 ± 4.2	487.6 ± 116.7	429.3 ± 69.2	44.5 ± 5.5
30–39	7.15 ± 0.54	6.24 ± 0.28	5.50 ± 0.46	4.87 ± 0.32	114.5 ± 14.7	100.8 ± 17.4	20.7 ± 4.0	466.6 ± 84.2	384.1 ± 57.2	41.3 ± 4.7
40–49	6.85 ± 0.46	6.43 ± 0.32	5.31 ± 0.52	5.09 ± 0.39	105.8 ± 16.0	88.4 ± 12.1	21.3 ± 4.0	434.6 ± 67.4	401.6 ± 66.0	41.7 ± 5.1
50–59	6.85 ± 0.34	6.35 ± 0.39	5.53 ± 0.45	5.23 ± 0.43	84.7 ± 13.1	80.5 ± 13.4	22.2 ± 5.0	445.1 ± 90.7	375.8 ± 77.6	42.8 ± 4.5
60–69	7.03 ± 0.74	6.69 ± 0.53	5.47 ± 0.66	5.34 ± 0.54	81.3 ± 15.7	67.0 ± 9.0	18.0 ± 3.0	408.2 ± 86.1	371.2 ± 62.2	41.0 ± 6.4
>70	7.17 ± 0.69	6.65 ± 0.41	5.13 ± 1.11	5.03 ± 0.54	74.6 ± 17.7	73.3 ± 10.9	15.0 ± 4.0	375.5 ± 94.7	363.4 ± 78.7	32.4 ± 6.1
All	6.99 ± 0.55	6.48 ± 0.45	5.43 ± 0.61	5.15 ± 0.46	98.5 ± 22.8	87.4 ± 19.0	20.2 ± 4.6	440.1 ± 96.3	390.2 ± 70.6	41.3 ± 6.2

Note.—Data are presented as the mean ± standard deviation.
* End-diastolic velocity and DVI were not statistically significantly associated with sex.

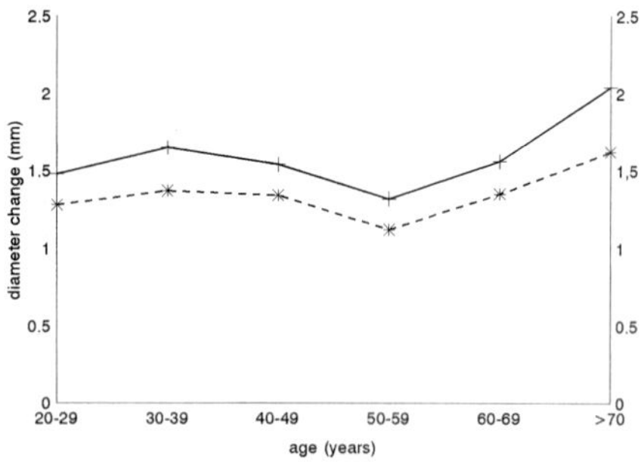

Figure 3. Change in functional lumen (systolic minus diastolic lumen) related to age and sex. Solid line = male subjects, dotted line = female subjects.

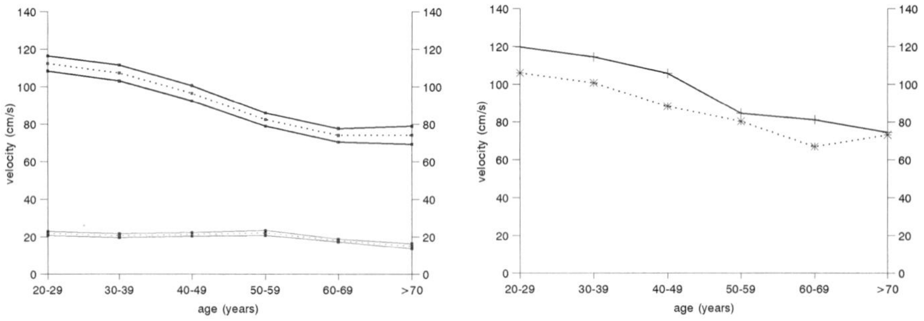

a. b.

Figure 4. **(a)** Graph of the 95% confidence intervals of the peak systolic (lines in upper part of graph) and the end-diastolic (lines in lower part of graph) velocities related to age in the 174 subjects. Dotted lines = mean velocities. **(b)** Graph of mean peak velocities related to age in the 84 men (solid line) and 90 women (dotted line).

mean value of the five measurements for the diastolic velocity was 10.5% for the male volunteers and 10.8% for the female volunteers. Figure 4a demonstrates the 95% confidence interval for the peak systolic and the end-diastolic velocities and Figure 4b the mean peak velocities for both sexes. The end-diastolic velocity at the instant before the systolic velocity upstroke showed a significant association with age ($P = .0001$) but not with sex or vessel side.

Volume Flow Rate

No significant difference in volume flow was found when comparing left and right CCAs. The male subgroup had a significantly higher flow (440.1 mL/min ± 96.3 per CCA; standard error of the mean = 7.52; $P = .0001$) than that of the female subgroup (390.2 mL/min ± 70.6 per CCA; standard error of the mean = 5.35) (Table 5).

The mean standard deviation of the five measurements (five for each side) was 25.8 mL/min ± 12.5 in the female group and 25.7 mL/min ± 11.6 in the male group. The standard deviation as a percentage of mean value of the five measurements for the volume flow in the male and female groups was 5.7% and 6.5%, respectively. The high standard deviation was not only a reflection of the interindividual range in flow calculation but also was significantly associated with age and sex ($P = .0001$). Figure 5a demonstrates the 95% confidence interval for the volume flow and Figure 5b the mean volume flow rates for both sexes. The volume flow rates in the healthy volunteers did not correlate with systolic blood pressure ($r^2 = .001$), body surface ($r^2 = .07$), height ($r^2 = .10$), or weight ($r^2 = .04$). With an increasing heart rate, the total volume flow remained constant.

DVI Measurements

The fractional diastolic volume flow, the DVI, depended on age but—unlike vessel lumen, velocities, and total volume flow—not on sex (Fig 6, Table 5). Figure 6 demonstrates the 95% confidence interval for the DVI. The mean DVI was 41.3 ± 6.2. The standard deviation as a percentage of mean value of the five measurements for the DVI was 5.0% for the male volunteers and 5.2% for the female volunteers. The DVI was influenced significantly by age only in the elderly ($P = .0001$) but not by sex (female, 40.9 ± 6.0; male, 41.9 ± 6.3; $P = .16$).

The DVI decreased with increasing heart rate or age ($P = .0001$). The DVI correlated with smoking ($P = .001$) and heart rate. In comparison with nonsmokers, the smokers had an increased heart rate, but the frequency corrected DVI (DVI_C) did not correlate with smoking. Heart rate and DVI were closely linked. As smokers had a higher heart rate and subsequently a shorter duration of diastole, the DVI had to be corrected by heart rate (Table 4). With all investigated measurements, we found no statistically significant differences between sides; this finding is similar to that of other reports.

Subjects with Hypertension

At the end of the examination, blood pressure was measured after a rest period of at least 25 minutes. Fifteen of the 205 volunteers were found to have an asymptomatic hypertension. Two of the measured parameters showed a highly significant difference compared with those in the healthy volunteers: change in vessel lumen

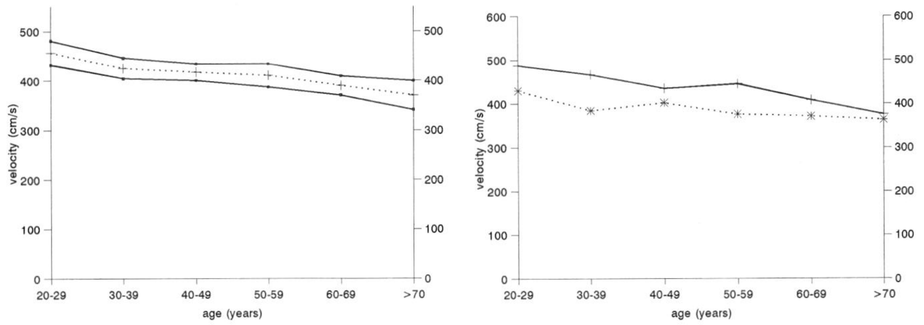

a. b.

Figure 5. **(a)** Graph of the 95% confidence interval of the volume flow rate related to age in the 174 subjects. Dotted line = mean volume flow rate. **(b)** Graph of the mean volume flow rate related to age in the 84 men (solid line) and 90 women (dotted line).

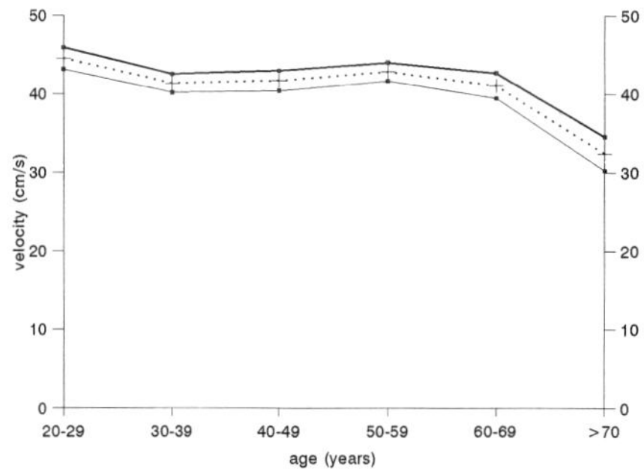

Figure 6. Graph of the 95% confidence interval of the DVI related to age in the 174 subjects. Dotted line = mean DVI.

Table 6
Hemodynamic Parameters in the CCA of Hypertensive Subjects versus That in the Healthy Volunteers

Subjects	Age (y)	Sex Ratio*	Peak Systolic Velocity (cm/sec)	Volume Flow (mL/min)	DVI	Blood Pressure (mm Hg) Systolic	Blood Pressure (mm Hg) Diastolic
Hypertensive (n = 15)	56 ± 13	1.4	78.3 ± 16.5	369 ± 110	31.6 ± 6.1	163 ± 19	96 ± 11
Normotensive (n = 171)	46 ± 16	1.5	92.8 ± 21.5	415 ± 87	41.3 ± 6.2	119 ± 12	75 ± 7

Note.—Except for sex ratio, data are presented as the mean ± standard deviation.
* The sex ratio was calculated by the number of men (digit 1) and women (digit 2) divided by the *sum* of all subjects.

Table 7
Association between Blood Pressure and Functional Lumen, Volume Flow Rate, and DVI in the 30 Volunteers Aged 50–59 Years versus That in the 15 Hypertensive Subjects

Blood Pressure	Peak Systolic Velocity	Functional Lumen Systolic	Functional Lumen Diastolic	Functional Lumen Systolic Minus Diastolic	Volume Flow	DVI
Systolic	<.08	<.029	<.0003	<.01	<.01	<.0001
Diastolic	<.04	<.15	<.0045	<.046	<.046	<.0035

Note.—Data are presented as P values.

and DVI. All other hemodynamic parameters, such as volume flow and peak systolic and end-diastolic velocity, did not reach statistical significance. In the group of hypertensive subjects, the lumen change during a cardiac cycle was significantly higher compared with that of the normotensive subjects (Table 6).

The DVI in the hypertensive subjects was significantly lower than that in an age-matched healthy control group (Table 7).

DISCUSSION

The major hemodynamic factors that determine blood pressure and volume flow are cardiac output and total peripheral resistance. Many humoral and neural regulation mechanisms try to keep volume flow within a certain range at rest. US detection of local vessel wall changes (24), the hemodynamics in arterial stenosis (21), and the effect of cerebral diseases on the flow of the extracranial vessels (17,21) have been described. To our knowledge, only little attention has been paid so far to physiologic changes in cardiac output, heart rate, or blood pressure on the hemodynamics in the CCA as they change. With time domain processing, several hemodynamic data were obtained from a color M-mode tracing of the CCA in an age- and sex-matched healthy population.

The automatically calculated width of a color M-mode tracing changes during the cardiac cycle and depends on the sensitivity for slow flow at a setting that is capable of imaging the high systolic velocities without aliasing. Thus, these so-called functional lumina cannot be compared with the two-dimensional lumen measurements usually performed to register changes of the compliance of the arterial wall. A sex-dependent difference in the vessel lumen has been described previously (24). In our study, the functional lumen was significantly smaller in the female group. Therefore, the difference between the systolic and diastolic lumina was higher in the male group as well. In hypertensive subjects, the change between systolic and diastolic bandwidth was significantly higher than in the control group of the same age and was independent of the age or sex. This finding is not surprising as older hypertensive patients have a high blood pressure amplitude as well. This group of volunteers was unaware of the arterial hypertension (and were asymptomatic) and at the time of this study did not have any vascular or cardiac disease; the vessel wall compliance could be higher than in symptomatic hypertensive patients.

DVI was calculated in addition to lumen calculations, velocity measurements, and estimation of volume flow rates. All velocities were calculated from the color M-mode tracing that was based on a time domain processing technique. It could be proved that all velocity and volume flow rate calculations had a good intraindividual reproducibility during one examination session.

The peak systolic velocity was the most sensitive parameter of all recorded hemodynamic data, indicating the aging of the volunteers. Its decline started in the 3rd decade, long before the volume flow or DVI decreased. This finding is described by Uematsu et al (16), who used an ultrasonic volume flow meter. The peak systolic velocity was highly significantly associated with age as well as sex. The end-diastolic velocity was quite constant over the years and dropped only in the elderly.

The volume flow decreased significantly with aging ($P = .0001$). Subjects in the 3rd decade had a volume flow rate of 456 mL/min; this rate decreased to 370 mL/min in volunteers older than 70 years. Uematsu et al (16) described a decline in volume flow rate from 479 mL/min between the 3rd and 4th decades to 402 mL/min in subjects older than 61 years, measured with an ultrasonic volume flow meter. The lower volumetric flow may be due to the high prevalence of diastolic dysfunction in old age (29). Another characteristic hemodynamic feature in the elderly is the reduced vascular compliance and the concomitant rise in systemic arterial pressures for a given increase in cardiac output (29). It was therefore interesting to see that the fractional volume flow during diastole, the DVI, decreased highly significantly as well. Therefore, all these US-based hemodynamic parameters are helpful in the understanding of changes that come with aging.

Another finding was that the peak systolic velocity, volume flow rate, and functional vessel lumen correlated strongly with sex ($P = .0001$), while end-diastolic velocity and DVI correlated significantly only in the elderly. The lower volume flow in women can be explained with the significantly smaller CCA lumen; as the flow velocities are also lower in the female group, a general sex-dependent difference in hemodynamics may be present. A sex-dependent difference in portal venous and hepatic arterial flow was described previously (30).

Among nine published studies (Table 1) in which volume flow in the CCA was estimated, five studies were based on calculation of the time average velocity and the vessel cross-sectional area (15,18,19,21,22); in one study, a time domain processing technique was applied (12). The reported volume flow rate ranged between 352 mL/min (12) and 564 mL/min (21). Seven of these studies (15,17,18–22) included less than 50 subjects (n = 11–48). Of the nine studies, three (12,16,17) (n = 125, 120, and 27, respectively) found a sex dependence, and four (16–18,22) found an age relation in volume flow. Although in two recent studies (21,22) (n = 28 and 48, respectively), a relation of volume flow between men and women could not be proved, a 12% and 17% lower volume flow in women was found in two other studies (12,17). In the current study, we found a marked difference in volume flow between the men and women, with an 11% lower flow volume recorded for the women.

Studies about the volume measurement by means of other imaging modalities, such as magnetic resonance imaging, are rare and report on only very small numbers of examined healthy subjects (31): In two healthy subjects, the volume flow rate in the CCA was estimated to be 250 and 580 mL/min, respectively.

The reason for the large range of assumed normal volume flow rates evaluated with US techniques are numerous: Inter- and intraobserver variability, a variability in velocity and volume numbers between different US devices, different angles of insonation, and attenuation of the sound waves by the tissue are some explanations with regard to the operator and to technical and scanning conditions. Blood velocity and volume flow are being influenced by many physiologic parameters and by cardiovascular medication. For a nomogram trial, therefore, selection of only healthy subjects is most important; the health of the subjects should be proved by measuring the basic hemodynamic parameters at the time of examination.

In addition to sex and age, heart rate also influences these US hemodynamic parameters. As heart rate rises, a shortening of diastole will influence the diastolic volume flow. As expected, a statistically significant difference in DVI was found between smokers and nonsmokers. It is well known that smokers have a higher heart rate compared with that of nonsmokers (32). The higher heart rate of smokers was statistically significantly linked to a lower DVI.

Cerebral blood flow is also influenced by blood pressure. Systolic and diastolic velocities, volume flow rate, and the DVI in the group of hypertensive volunteers differed significantly from the numbers found in the age-related group of the nomogram trial. These findings can be explained by an age-related increase in the total peripheral resistance (29) and a decline in left ventricular diastolic function that is well known even in healthy subjects without evidence of altered left ventricular systolic function at rest (33). A decrease of volume flow was also described in other vessel regions. A reduction of blood flow in the forearm in hypertensive subjects was reported by Panza et al (34), and myocardial ischemia during a hypertensive crisis (without coronary heart disease) may also be explained by a decrease in volume flow within the coronary vascular bed (35).

Noninvasive methods to monitor end-organ effects of elevated blood pressure concentrated so far on the intima proliferation, the detection of early arteriosclerosis, and the change in vessel lumen. Another approach to detection of early hemodynamic changes in hypertensive patients is the evaluation of changes in the peak velocity, the total volume flow, and especially the fractional diastolic volume flow rates that may also be helpful in monitoring drug therapy. The data from this trial may especially help to evaluate intraindividual hemodynamic changes in cerebrovascular and cardiac diseases. Furthermore, these parameters may be helpful to better understand and monitor the treatment of patients receiving cardiovascular medication. ■

References

1. Scoutt LM, Zawin ML, Taylor KJW. Doppler US. II. Clinical applications. Radiology 1990; 174:309–319.
2. Hunink MGM, Polak JF, Barlan MM, et al. Detection and quantification of carotid artery stenosis: efficiacy of various Doppler velocity parameters. AJR 1993; 160:619–625.
3. Derdeyn CP, Powers WJ, Moran CJ, Cross DT, Allen BT. Role of Doppler US in screening for carotid atherosclerotic disease. Radiology 1995; 197:635–643.
4. Gill RW. Measurement of blood flow by ultrasound: accuracy and sources of error. Ultrasound Med Biol 1985; 11:625–641.
5. Burns PN. Measuring volume flow with Doppler ultrasound: an old nut. Ultrasound Obstet Gynecol 1992; 2:130–131.
6. Ranke C, Hendrickx P, Roth U, Brassel F, Creuzig A, Alexander K. Color and conventional image-directed Doppler ultrasonography: accuracy and sources of error in quantitative blood flow measurements. JCU 1992; 20:187–193.
7. Bonnefous O, Pesque P. Time domain formulation of pulse Doppler ultrasound and blood velocity estimation by cross correlation. Ultrason Imaging 1986; 8:73–85.
8. Embree PM, O'Brian WD Jr. Volumetric blood flow via time-domain correlation: experimental verification. IEEE Trans Ultrason Ferroelec Freq Contr 1990; 37:176–189.
9. Picot PA, Embree PM. Quantitative volume flow estimation using velocity profiles. IEEE Trans Ultrason Ferroelec Freq Contr 1994; 41:340–345.
10. Rickey DW, Rankin R, Fenster A. A velocity evaluation phantom for colour and

pulsed Doppler instruments. Ultrasound Med Biol 1992; 18:479–494.
11. Forsberg F, Liu JB, Russel KM, Guthrie SL, Goldberg BB. Volume flow estimation using time domain correlation and ultrasonic flowmetry. Ultrasound Med Biol 1995; 21:1037–1045.
12. Eicke BM, Tegeler CH. Ultrasonic quantitative flow volume. In: Tegler CH, Babikian VL, Gomez CR, eds. Neurosonology. St Louis, Mo: Mosby–Year Book, 1995; 101–110.
13. Lee W, Bendick P, Best AM, Koslowski N, Kirk JS, Comstock CH. Time domain ultrasonography during pregnancy. J Ultrasound Med 1994; 13:457–463.
14. Harrington K, Deane C, Campbell S. Measurement of volume flow with time domain and M-mode imaging: in vitro and in vivo validation studies. J Ultrasound Med 1996; 15:715–720.
15. Payen DM, Levy BI, Menegalli DJ, Lajat YI, Levenson JA, Nicolas FM. Evaluation of human hemispheric blood flow based on noninvasive carotid blood flow measurements using the range-gated Doppler technique. Stroke 1982; 13:392–398.
16. Uematsu S, Yang A, Preziosi TJ, Kouba R, Toung TJ. Measurement of carotid blood flow in man and its clinical application. Stroke 1983; 14:256–266.
17. Uematsu S, Folstein MS. Carotid blood flow measured by an ultrasonic volume flowmeter in carotid stenosis and patients with dementia. J Neurol Neurosurg Psychiatr 1985; 48:1230–1233.
18. Bouthier J, Benetos A, Simon A, Levenson J, Safar M. Pulsed Doppler evaluation of diameter, blood velocity and blood flow of common carotid artery in sustained essential hypertonus. J Cardiovasc Pharmacol 1985; 7:99–104.
19. Benetos A, Safar ME, Laurent S, et al. Common carotid blood flow in patients with hypertension and stenosis of the internal carotid artery. J Clin Hyperten 1986; 1:44–45.
20. Meyd CJ, Abu-Shakra S, Bleeker ML. Carotid high flow ratio most accurately predicts significant stenosis. Arch Neurol 1992; 49:864–869.
21. Hamada T, Takita M, Kawano H, Noh-tomi A, Okayama M. Difference in blood flow volume of the common carotid artery between vascular and nonvascular dementia detected by colour duplex sonography. J Neurol 1993; 240:191–194.
22. Schöning M, Walter J, Scheel P. Estimation of cerebral blood flow through color duplex sonography of the carotid and vertebral arteries in healthy adults. Stroke 1994; 25: 17–22.
23. O'Rourke M. Systolic blood pressure: arterial compliance and early wave reflection, and their modification by antihypertensive therapy. J Hum Hypertens 1989; 3:47–52.
24. Hansen F, Mangell P, Sonesson B, Länne T. Diameter and compliance in the human common carotid artery: variations with age and sex. Ultrasound Med Biol 1995; 21:1–9.
25. Braunwald W. Heart disease: a textbook of cardiovascular medicine. Philadelphia, Pa: Saunders, 1984.
26. Buchwalski R. Einschwemmkatheter: technik, auswertung und praktische konsequenzen. Erlangen, Germany: Perimed Spitta Medizinische Verlagsgesellschaft, 1992.
27. Saxena PR, Schoemaker RG. Organ blood flow protection in hypertension and congestive heart failure. Am J Med 1993; 94(suppl 4a):S4–S12.
28. Matsumoto M, Sekimoto H, Goriya Y, et al. Simultaneous cardio-cerebral ultrasonic measurement technique for assessing the interrelationship between cardiac circulations in elderly subjects: a preliminary study. Ultrasound Med Biol 1992; 18:45–49.
29. Epstein FH. Age in the cardiovascular system. N Engl J Med 1992; 327:1735–1739.
30. Leen E, Goldberg JA, Robertson J, et al. Detection of hepatic metastasis using duplex/color Doppler sonography. Ann Surg 1991; 214:599–604.
31. Bendel P, Buonocore E, Bockisch A, Besozzi MC. Blood flow in the carotid arteries: quantification by using phase-sensitive MR imaging. AJR 1989; 152:1307–1310.
32. Czernin J, Sun K, Brunken R, Böttcher M, Phelps M, Schelbert H. Effect of acute and long term smoking on myocardial blood flow and coronary flow reserve. Circulation 1995; 91:2891–2897.
33. Bonow RO, Vitale DF, Bacharach SL, Maron BJ, Green MV. Effects of aging on asynchronous left ventricular regional function and global ventricular filling in normal human subjects. J Am Coll Cardiol 1988; 11: 50–58.
34. Panza JA, Casino PR, Kilcoyne CM, Quyyumi AA. Role of endothelium-derived nitric oxide in the abnormal endothelium: dependent vascular relaxation of patients with essential hypertension. Circulation 1993; 87:1468–1474.
35. Elliott PM, Kaski JC. Coronary blood flow in hypertension. Editorials Cardiol 1995; 1:27–31.

Book Review

Imaging in Obstetrics and Gynecology

Patricia Lipford Abbitt, MD

Baltimore, Md: Williams & Wilkins, 1997. ISBN 0-683-18212-9. Cloth, $89.00; pp 360; 280 figures; tables.

The author, a radiologist, uses a teaching-file format in this textbook to present 289 clinical histories and images as unknowns, which are followed with differential diagnoses and discussions. There are five chapters, which cover early pregnancy, the fetus, difficulties during pregnancy, pelvic masses, and hysterosalpingography. The largest number of cases, 129, are of pelvic masses; the smallest, 27, concern hysterosalpingography. Each chapter has a short introduction, and the format in each is the same: clinical history, images, imaging findings, differential diagnoses, correct diagnosis, and a short discussion. Each case is listed in the table of contents. There is a detailed index, and at the conclusion of each chapter, there is a list of selected reading.

This is a fairly large book, measuring 9 × 11 inches (23 × 28 cm) and containing 360 pages. The backing is sturdy with easily read print and good-quality images. Although the vast majority of images are ultrasound images (except for those in the chapter on hysterosalpingography, of course) there are a few computed tomographic and magnetic resonance images. There are no line drawings or graphs. In this single-authored textbook, the style of writing is consistent without intended redundancy. The case selection is broad and has been drawn from teaching files at major medical centers. Because labeling of images is sparse, there are some cases in which the discussed feature might be less obvious to some observers; however, for the most part, the findings are well demonstrated.

This book is not intended to replace major textbooks of obstetric and gynecologic imaging but is informative and deals with everyday topics with an engaging writing style. The price is reasonable. I believe most radiologists—especially those outside large teaching centers—would enjoy this book.

Reviewed by James G. Hazel, Jr, MD

Stephan A. Schmitz, MD • Susanne Wagner, DVM • Gabriele Schuhmann-Giampieri, PhD
Werner Krause, PhD • Matthias Bollow, MD • Karl-Jürgen Wolf, MD

Gd-EOB-DTPA and Yb-EOB-DTPA: Two Prototypic Contrast Media for CT Detection of Liver Lesions in Dogs[1]

PURPOSE: To characterize computed tomographic (CT) attenuation of iodine, gadolinium, and ytterbium in vitro and to study CT liver enhancement after administration of two prototypic hepatocyte-directed contrast media in dogs.

MATERIALS AND METHODS: Samples with increasing concentrations of iodine, gadolinium, and ytterbium were measured for CT attenuation in a water phantom at tube voltages of 80, 120, and 137 kV. Three groups of five adult beagle dogs each received a 0.5 mmol/kg dose of either gadoxetic acid disodium (gadolinium ethoxybenzyl diethylenetriaminepentaacetic acid [EOB-DTPA]) or Yb-EOB-DTPA as intravenous infusions or Yb-EOB-DTPA as an intravenous bolus injection.

RESULTS: At 120 kV, in vitro CT attenuation of gadolinium and ytterbium exceeded that of iodine by 41% and 45%, respectively, when measured at equal mass concentrations (in milligrams per milliliter of saline). In dogs, CT liver enhancement values above the precontrast liver attenuation were 32.6 HU ± 2.3, 31.4 HU ± 1.1, and 33.4 HU ± 5.2 after 0.5 mmol/kg Gd-EOB-DTPA or Yb-EOB-DTPA infusion or Yb-EOB-DTPA bolus, respectively. The values were not significantly different ($P > .05$)

CONCLUSION: Both Gd-EOB-DTPA and Yb-EOB-DTPA provide excellent CT liver enhancement in dogs. CT liver enhancement is not significantly altered by either the absorbing element (gadolinium vs ytterbium) or the mode of application (infusion vs bolus).

Several contrast media with liver-specific uptake have been designed to improve the detection and possibly the tissue characterization of liver lesions. These substances have pharmacokinetic properties that allow them to accumulate in either hepatocytes or cells of the reticuloendothelial system ([RES] or Kupffer cells) and thus demonstrate focal lesions, which do not take up the contrast media. A number of such contrast media have been studied in clinical investigations (1–3) and applied in practice (4) for magnetic resonance (MR) imaging. Gadoxetic acid disodium (gadolinium ethoxybenzyl diethylenetriaminepentaacetic acid [Gd-EOB-DTPA]) is one example of a hepatobiliary contrast medium with selective uptake into the hepatocyte followed by biliary excretion. Good evidence exists for the potential of Gd-EOB-DTPA as a liver-specific contrast medium in MR imaging (5,6).

In principle, liver-specific contrast media could also improve focal lesion detection with computed tomography (CT). However, we questioned whether the concentration of Gd-EOB-DTPA in liver would be high enough for sufficient enhancement because CT generally requires administration of a higher dose of contrast medium than that of MR imaging. This question arises especially because from both animal and human studies it is known that a considerable fraction of the dose is also distributed in the extracellular space and cleared via the kidneys and that the fraction of biliary excretion in rats decreases from 80% to 53% to 33% with increasing doses of 0.05, 0.5, and 1.5 mmol Gd/kg Gd-EOB-DTPA (2). But excellent CT liver enhancement of 33 HU ± 6 and 34 HU ± 8 has been achieved after intravenous infusion of 0.5 mmol Gd/kg Gd-EOB-DTPA in dogs and humans, respectively (7,8). This is explained not only by the pharmacokinetic properties of the EOB-DTPA carrier molecule that allow it to accumulate in the hepatocytes but also by the efficacy of the x ray–absorbing element. At equal mass concentrations, lanthanide elements are known to absorb x rays better than iodine, about 40% better in the case of gadolinium (9). Other lanthanide elements, such as dysprosium ($Z = 66$) or ytterbium ($Z = 70$) may have even higher x-ray absorption than gadolinium ($Z = 64$) owing to their higher atomic number.

After a preclinical study examining the pharmacokinetic and tolerance data of several metal complexes with the EOB-DTPA ligand and different

Index terms: Computed tomography (CT), contrast media, 761.12114 • Contrast media, comparative studies, 761.12114 • Contrast media, experimental studies, 761.12114 • Gadolinium • Liver neoplasms, diagnosis, 761.12114 • Ytterbium

Abbreviations: EOB-DTPA = ethoxybenzyl diethylenetriaminepentaacetic acid, EOE = ethiodized oil emulsion, LD50 = median lethal dose, RES = reticuloendothelial system, ROI = region of interest.

Radiology 1997; 205:361–366

[1] From the Department of Radiology, University Hospital Benjamin Franklin, Free University of Berlin, Hindenburgdamm 30, 12200 Berlin, Germany (S.A.S., S.W., K.J.W.); Research Laboratories, Diagnostic Research, Schering, Berlin, Germany (G.S.G., W.K.); and the Department of Radiology, Charité Hospital, Humboldt-University Berlin, Germany (M.B.). Received November 4, 1996; revision requested December 12; final revision received May 15, 1997; accepted May 19. **Address reprint requests to** S.A.S.

See also the editorial by Laniado and Kopp (pp 319–322) in this issue.

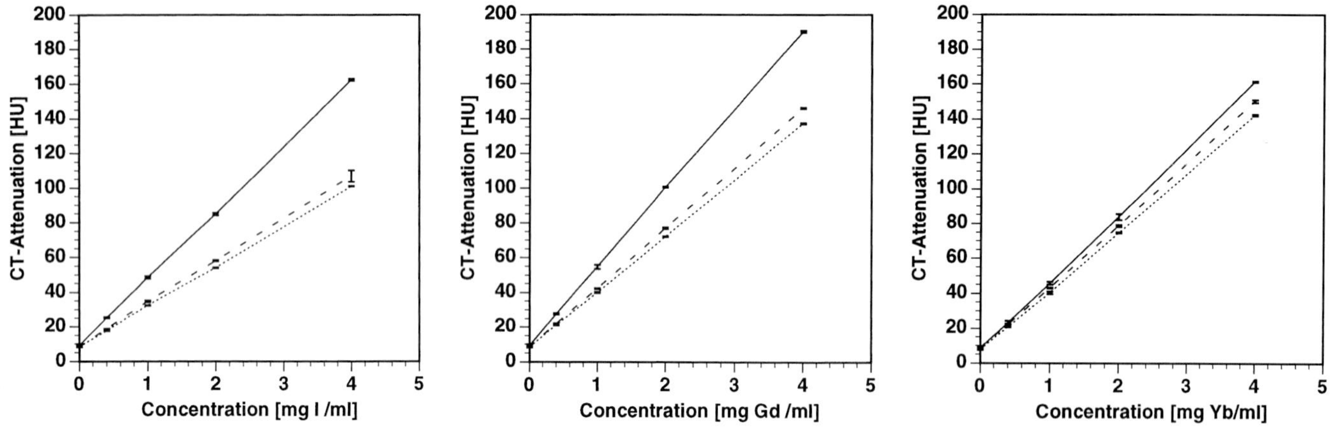

a. b. c.

Figure 1. Three plots of CT attenuation for samples of different mass concentrations of **(a)** iodine, **(b)** gadolinium, and **(c)** ytterbium. The measurements were performed at tube voltages of 80 (solid line), 120 (broken line), and 137 (dotted line) kV. Values represent the means of five measurements with the standard deviation as error bars. (Error bars were plotted with vertical lines. Because the errors are very small, the error bars may not be visible but only their endings indicated by small horizontal lines.)

lanthanides (eg, lanthanum, cerium, praseodymium, gadolinium, dysprosium, ytterbium, and lutetium), as well as nonlanthanides (eg, lead and bismuth), it was concluded that especially Gd-EOB-DTPA and Yb-EOB-DTPA seem to be useful as liver-specific contrast media for CT (10). In that series, in vitro complex stability, cardiovascular tolerance, and acute toxicity (median lethal dose [LD50]) were similar for Gd-EOB-DTPA and Yb-EOB-DTPA.

On the basis of the pharmacokinetic and tolerance data as well as the physical properties of ytterbium, we conducted experiments to determine whether Yb-EOB-DTPA is as favorable as or even more suited than Gd-EOB-DTPA for hepatic CT. In addition, two modes of application, infusion versus bolus injection, were tested with equal doses of Yb-EOB-DTPA. In vitro, CT attenuation of iopromide as well as Gd-EOB-DTPA and Yb-EOB-DTPA samples was related to the chemical iodine, gadolinium, and ytterbium concentrations to characterize the attenuation properties of these elements.

MATERIALS AND METHODS

Contrast Media

Iopromide (Ultravist; Schering, Berlin, Germany) was used as a solution of 300 mg of iodine per milliliter. The investigative drugs Gd-EOB-DTPA and Yb-EOB-DTPA were supplied as sterile aqueous solutions by Schering, at concentrations of 0.25 mol Gd/L and 0.25 mol Yb/L, respectively.

In Vitro Measurements

Ten-milliliter dilution series of iopromide, Gd-EOB-DTPA, and Yb-EOB-DTPA each with 0.0, 0.4, 1.0, 2.0, and 4.0 mg of iodine, gadolinium, or ytterbium per milliliter, respectively, were prepared with 0.9% saline in 2-cm polyethylene tubes. The tubes were centered in a water-filled acrylic cylinder 20 cm in diameter. A commercially available scanner (Somatom Plus S; Siemens, Erlangen, Germany) was used. The CT attenuation (in Hounsfield units) of each sample was measured five times at 80, 120, and 137 kV (450–500 mA, 4–6 seconds, 8-mm section thickness) by placing a 1-cm region of interest (ROI) at the center of each polyethylene tube. The phantom was not moved between scanning, and the ROIs were kept at the identical positions by using a memory function of the standard evaluation software of the CT scanner. The mean and the standard deviation of the five measurements was calculated on a personal computer.

For 80, 120, and 137 kV, the mean of the five measured CT attenuation values, y, was related to the iodine, gadolinium, or ytterbium concentration, x (in milligrams of iodine, gadolinium, or ytterbium per milliliter), by using linear regression analysis: $y = a \cdot x + b$, where a represents the slope of the line and b the attenuation related to the saline in the polyethylene tube. The slope values are expressed as Hounsfield units per milligram per milliliter, where Hounsfield unit is the attenuation value measured in the ROI and milligram denotes the mass of the absorbing element (eg, iodine) in 1 mL of 0.9% sodium chloride water. Confidence levels of 95% were calculated in the regression analysis. Similarly, slope values (expressed as Hounsfield units per micromole per milliliter) were calculated for molar iodine, gadolinium, and ytterbium concentrations. For each tube voltage, the slope of the regression line for gadolinium and ytterbium was compared with that for iodine, and the difference was determined.

Animal Experiments

To provide reliable results, maintenance and care of the experimental animals were performed in accordance with the guidelines described in the German Tierschutzgesetz (Animal Protection Act). Fifteen female adult beagle dogs (9.7–13.2 kg) were included in the study. Before imaging, the animals were anesthetized by intravenous injections of 15 mg/kg ketamine-HCL (Ketanest-50; Parke-Davis, Freiburg, Germany), 2 mg/kg xylazine (Rompun-2%; Bayer, Leverkusen, Germany), and 0.05 mg/kg lormetazepam (Noctamid; Schering). To avoid motion artifacts, suxamethonium chloride (Pantolax-2%; Curamed, Karlsruhe, Germany) was administered for muscle relaxation at a dose of 2 mg/kg. Respiration was controlled by a mechanical pump (Schuler Animal Respirator; Braun-Melsungen, Melsungen, Germany). Imaging was performed at breath hold.

There were three study groups of five animals each. The animals received a dose of 0.5 mmol Gd/kg or 0.5 mmol Yb/kg. The volume was 19.4–26.4 mL. The contrast medium was introduced into a vein on the extensor surface of a foreleg. In two groups, Gd-EOB-DTPA or Yb-EOB-DTPA was infused during 10 minutes by means of a mechanical pump (Infusomat; Braun-Melsungen). In the third group, Yb-EOB-DTPA was manually injected as a bolus during approximately 10 seconds. After the imaging experiments, the animals were observed with regard to their general appearance, their food and water consumption, and their production of urine and stool for 24 hours.

Imaging was carried out before as well as 10, 30, 45, and 90 minutes after the administration of contrast medium; we used a commercially available CT scanner (Somatom Plus S; Siemens). Axial breath-hold images of identical liver sections were acquired (8-mm section thickness, 3 seconds, 120 kV, 495 mAs).

Quantitative Image Analysis

Operator-defined ROIs 1.5 cm in diameter were placed in selected liver regions with a high uptake of contrast medium.

Table 1
Attenuation Concentration Characteristics of Iodine, Gadolinium, and Ytterbium on CT Scans Obtained at Different Tube Voltages

Tube Voltage (kV)	Attenuation per Mass Concentration (HU/mg/mL)			Attenuation per Molar Concentration (HU/μmol/mL)		
	Iodine	Gadolinium	Ytterbium	Iodine	Gadolinium	Ytterbium
	Absolute					
80	38.1 (37.1, 39.0)	45.2 (44.7, 45.9)	38.3 (37.7, 38.8)	4.83 (4.71, 4.95)	7.11 (7.03, 7.22)	6.63 (6.52, 6.71)
120	24.4 (23.7, 25.1)	34.4 (33.8, 34.9)	35.4 (34.9, 36.0)	3.10 (3.01, 3.19)	5.41 (5.32, 5.49)	6.12 (6.04, 6.23)
137	22.9 (22.1, 23.7)	32.1 (31.5, 32.6)	33.6 (33.2, 34.1)	2.91 (2.80, 3.01)	5.05 (4.95, 5.13)	5.81 (5.74, 5.90)
	In Percentage of Iodine					
80	100	119	101	100	147	137
120	100	141	145	100	175	198
137	100	140	147	100	174	200

Note.—Data represent the mean of five CT attenuation measurements determined at 80-, 120-, and 137-kV tube voltage in a sample containing 1 mg or 1 μmol of iodine in iopromide, gadolinium in Gd-EOB-DTPA, or ytterbium in Yb-EOB-DTPA in 1 mL of saline water. The values in parentheses are the lower and upper limit of the 95% confidence interval.

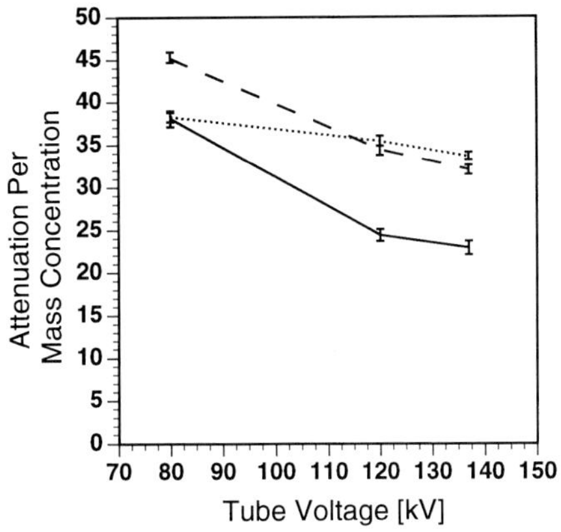

a.

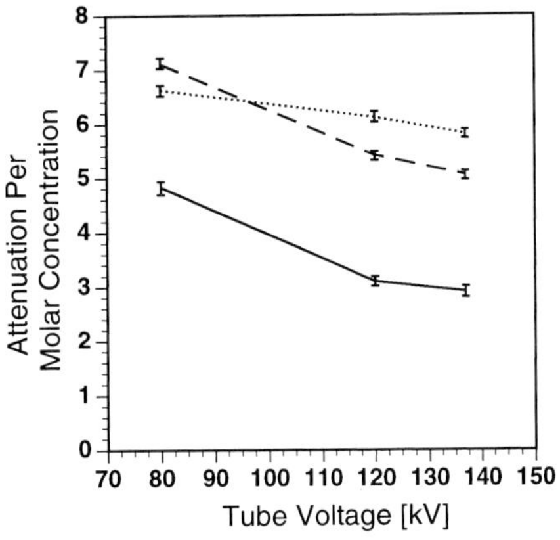

b.

Figure 2. Two plots with slope values for iodine (solid line), gadolinium (broken line), and ytterbium (dotted line) derived by means of regression analysis (Fig 1). Each data point represents a slope value as a function of tube voltage. The slope values are plotted as attenuation per **(a)** mass concentration (in Hounsfield units per milligram per milliliter) or **(b)** molar concentration (in Hounsfield units per micromole per milliliter) .

Liver vessels and bile ducts were excluded from the measurement. CT enhancement, defined as the net increase of liver CT attenuation, was calculated as the difference between the unenhanced and contrast material–enhanced measurements. A statistical analysis was performed to compare the 45- and 90-minute postcontrast liver enhancement between the groups by using the Student *t* test for unpaired samples. A *P* value less than .05 was considered to indicate a statistically significant difference. To describe enhancement over time, the point of maximum enhancement was determined. A ratio of the mean enhancement at 45 minutes was calculated in relation to the maximum enhancement value of each group. The ratio is expressed as a percentage.

RESULTS

In Vitro Measurements

Regression analysis demonstrated a linear relationship between the CT attenuation and the concentration of iodine, gadolinium, or ytterbium (Fig 1). The slope lines crossed the CT attenuation axis between 7 and 10 HU. This intercept was determined by the sodium chloride contained in the samples that did not influence the slope values. In this experiment, slope values express attenuation as a function of the mass concentrations. For all elements studied, attenuation decreased when measured at increasing tube voltages of 80, 120, or 137 kV.

At equal mass concentrations and 80 kV, there were only slight differences between the three elements, with gadolinium being 19% and 18% more effective than iodine and ytterbium, respectively (Table 1). However, the absolute attenuation of mass concentration values decreased at 120 kV from those at 80 kV for all elements, but less markedly for ytterbium than for iodine and gadolinium. Gadolinium and ytterbium were 41% and 45% more effective than iodine at 120 kV and similarly 40% and 47% more effective at 137 HU (Fig 2a).

To further compare the absorbing elements, slope values of their molar concentrations were also calculated, since the amount of absorbing metal transported by a particular carrier relates to its molar rather than its mass concentration (Table 1). At equal molar concentrations and 80 kV, both gadolinium and ytterbium absorbed x rays 47% and 37% more effectively than iodine. A 75% and 74% higher efficacy was found with gadolinium at 120 and 137 kV and 98% and 100% with ytterbium (Fig 2b).

Animal Experiments

All animals completed the imaging experiment. No adverse reactions were observed during the 24-hour period. The mean liver CT enhancement values 90 minutes after the Gd-EOB-DTPA and Yb-EOB-DTPA infusions and the Yb-EOB-DTPA bolus were 32.6 HU ± 2.3, 31.4 HU ± 1.1, and 33.4 HU ± 5.2 (mean ± standard deviation), respectively. There was no statistically significant difference between the groups at 45 and 90 minutes. After 45 minutes, the mean CT liver enhancement values after the Gd-EOB-DTPA and Yb-EOB-DTPA infusions and the Yb-EOB-DTPA bolus were 87.1%, 89.2%, and 88.6% of the maximum enhancement of each group. The mean and standard deviation of liver enhancement values for the three groups are presented in Table 2. Figure 3 shows a dog liver before and 90 minutes after bolus injection of 0.5 mmol Yb/kg Yb-EOB-DTPA.

DISCUSSION

The major findings of this study are that an infusion of 0.5 mmol/kg Yb-EOB-DTPA provides good CT liver enhancement of 31.4 HU ± 1.4 in dogs and is comparable to Gd-EOB-DTPA in this respect. These results compare favorably with two other liver-specific techniques, RES-directed ethiodized oil emulsion (EOE-13) and hepatocyte-directed delayed CT, which enhanced the liver by 32.5 HU (11) and 20 HU (12), respectively, and allowed detection of focal liver lesions as sensitively as CT during arterial portography (12). The latter is currently regarded as the most sensitive technique for focal lesion detection (13).

However, it is not justifiable to conclude on the basis of simple liver enhancement values that Gd-EOB-DTPA would be as effective as EOE-13, since RES-directed contrast media are more effectively deposited in the liver (79% of the dose in the case of EOE-13) than is Gd-EOB-DTPA. In the present study, the contrast medium fractions that cleared either via the bile or the kidney were not quantified, but approximately 50% of a 0.5 mmol Gd/kg Gd-EOB-DTPA dose in rats is cleared via the kidneys, since there is a larger fraction distributed in the extracellular space (2).

In addition, it was shown in a clinical study of Gd-EOB-DTPA infusions that there is also statistically significant CT enhancement of liver metastatic lesions (8). In that study, tumor attenuation after infusion of 0.5 mmol Gd/kg Gd-EOB-DTPA was 38 HU ± 7.4, 45 HU ± 7, and 42 HU ± 8 before and at 30 and 150 minutes after administration of contrast material, respectively. This enhancement of 7 and 4 HU after 30 and 150 minutes, respectively, reflects the distribution of Gd-EOB-DTPA in the extracellular space of the metastatic lesion. At 150 minutes after administration of contrast material, the 4-HU tumor enhancement was very low compared with the 34-HU liver enhancement that was optimal at this point, composing only 7.4% of the 54-HU ± 12 difference in tumor-liver attenuation. Since enhancement of the metastatic lesion is negligible compared with that of liver, comparison of Gd-EOB-DTPA data with EOE-13 data still seems reasonable because the net effect is an increase of about a 30-HU difference in tumor-liver attenuation.

In all groups in our study, approximately 90% of the maximum enhancement was reached as early as 45 minutes after administration of contrast medium. The shape of the enhancement time curve indicates saturation of liver uptake. However, there was still 10% liver uptake of the contrast medium even after 45 minutes.

Table 2
CT Enhancement above Precontrast Liver Attenuation after Intravenous Administration of Gd-EOB-DTPA and Yb-EOB-DTPA in Adult Dogs

Time (min) after Administration of Contrast Material	Gd-EOB-DTPA Infusion	Yb-EOB-DTPA Infusion	Yb-EOB-DTPA Bolus
Before administration	0.0 ± 0.0	0.0 ± 0.0	0.0 ± 0.0
10	18.4 ± 3.4	15.6 ± 2.7	17.2 ± 3.6
30	24.2 ± 2.3	25.4 ± 2.3	26.8 ± 5.1
45	28.4 ± 3.6	28.0 ± 3.2	29.6 ± 4.3
90	32.6 ± 2.3	31.4 ± 1.1	33.4 ± 5.2

Note.—The bolus injection was given manually over approximately 10 seconds. The infusion was performed in 10 minutes with use of a pump. The start of the infusion is the zero point of the postcontrast period. Data are presented as the mean ± standard deviation of five liver enhancement measurements for each time point.

The mode of application, infusion versus bolus injection, of Yb-EOB-DTPA neither influenced maximum liver enhancement (31.4 HU ± 1.1 and 33.4 HU ± 5.2 90 minutes after administration) nor the speed of liver enhancement, which was exemplified by single measurements at 45 minutes (28.0 HU ± 3.2 and 29.6 HU ± 4.3). We expected infusions to maintain high blood concentration levels over a longer period, thus allowing more contrast medium to enter the liver, but the data from the present study do not support this hypothesis.

Doses higher than 0.5 mmol Gd/kg Gd-EOB-DTPA, however, may saturate contrast medium uptake as shown by Schuhmann-Giampieri et al (2). This may increase the contrast medium concentration in the extracellular space without changing the intracellular concentration of contrast medium, thus decreasing the difference in liver-tumor attenuation.

Besides insufficient liver enhancement or undesirable enhancement of metastatic lesions due to distribution of the contrast medium in the extracellular space, tumors originating from the hepatocytes, such as adenomas, focal nodular hyperplasias, and hepatocellular carcinomas, may also take up the contrast medium and thus remain undetected. Depending on its reproducibility, uptake of contrast material may very well be a criterion for tissue differentiation. In a clinical study, liver lesions were seen as hypoattenuating defects in the liver so that they may remain undetected due to their similar appearance to vessels (8).

The strong CT liver-enhancing potential of Gd-EOB-DTPA, which was originally developed for MR imaging, is quite surprising since it contains only one absorbing metal atom with each EOB-DTPA carrier molecule, whereas current extracellular contrast media, such as iopromide, have three. The CT liver enhancement is explained to some extent by the high x ray–absorbing efficacy of the lanthanide elements. This phenomenon is well known and has been the subject of several studies on both extracellular (14,15) and intracellular (16,17) contrast media for CT. As in those studies, our phantom measurements showed a marked decrease in attenuation with increasing tube voltage from 80 to 137 kV for all elements studied: gadolinium, ytterbium, and iodine. However, at clinically applied tube currents of 120 and 137 kV, the attenuation changed only slightly with equal mass concentrations of gadolinium and ytterbium but was still 41% and 45% (120 kV) and 40% and 47% (137 kV) higher than with iodine.

At equimolar concentrations, which are of particular interest since as mentioned the EOB-DTPA molecule carries one metal molecule, the attenuation of gadolinium and ytterbium was 75% and 98% (120 kV) and 74% and 100% (137 kV) higher than that of iodine. These data are based on slope values of in vitro sample measurements at 80, 120, and 137 kV of iodine (38.1, 24.4, and 22.9 HU/mg/mL), gadolinium (45.2, 34.4, and 32.1 HU/mg/mL) and ytterbium (38.3, 35.4, and 33.6 HU/mg/mL). The slope values at 120 kV found by other groups are very similar for iodine (iohexol, 27.3 HU/mg/mL), gadolinium (gadodiamide, 37.4 HU/mg/mL; Gd-DTPA, 39.7 HU/mg/mL)(18), and ytterbium (Yb-DTPA, 36.1 HU/mg/mL)(15). Attenuation generally increases with higher atomic numbers: iodine ($Z = 53$), gadolinium ($Z = 64$) and ytterbium ($Z = 70$). However, some additional attenuation results from charac-

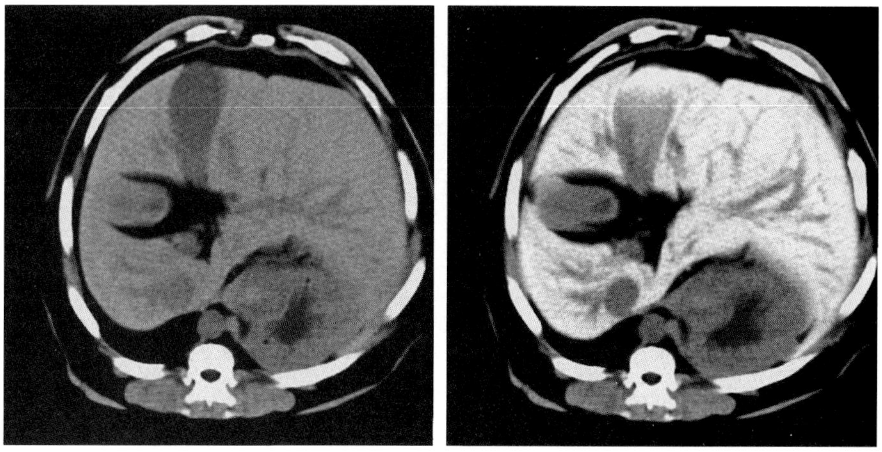

a. b.

Figure 3. Two axial CT scans (window width, 150 HU; center, 50 HU) obtained in a dog **(a)** before and **(b)** 90 minutes after an intravenous bolus injection of 0.5 mmol ytterbium per kilogram Yb-EOB-DTPA. The enhancement of the liver was 37 HU. Improved delineation of the vasculature is clearly evident.

teristic absorption due to the k-edge if covered by the polyenergetic spectrum of the CT scanner. The k-edge for iodine, gadolinium, and ytterbium is at 33.16, 50.23, and 61.31 KeV, respectively (19). K-edge interactions explain to some extent the fact that, at 80 kV, gadolinium has a higher attenuation than ytterbium despite its smaller atomic number. Pilot experiments demonstrated that in vitro measurements are very sensitive to the surrounding material. We chose an anthropomorphic water phantom to reduce possible misregistration, since placement of the samples in air might lead to beam hardening, edge artifacts, or edge enhancement of image-reconstruction algorithms.

Contrary to RES-directed contrast media, such as EOE-13 and perfluorooctylbromide, further development of which was limited by tolerance problems (13,20), only minor side effects were observed in volunteers who received doses of up to 0.1 mmol Gd/kg Gd-EOB-DTPA (21). In a clinical study (phase IIa) with doses of 0.2, 0.35, and 0.5 mmol Gd/kg, adverse events were observed in four of 15 patients (8). Two of these four patients noted mild burning either at the site of the infusion cannula or retrosternally during infusion. Both adverse events ceased immediately after reducing the infusion flow. One patient reported mild nausea accompanied by an epigastric pressure sensation, and another reported moderate upper right abdominal undulating pain that was previously observed on several occasions. These events began after 4–5 hours and lasted 4–8 hours. In three patients, aspartate aminotransferase (formerly serum glutamic oxaloacetic transaminase) levels increased by about 12–26 U/L and alanine aminotransferase (formerly serum glutamic pyruvic transaminase) levels increased by 21–48 U/L from normal or moderately elevated baseline levels. It was concluded at the end of the study that patient tolerance of Gd-EOB-DTPA in doses of up to 0.5 mmol Gd/kg is acceptable and justifies further scientific evaluation.

The tolerance of several metal complexes with EOB-DTPA as a ligand was tested in rats for lanthanum, cerium, praseodymium, gadolinium, dysprosium, ytterbium, and lutetium, as well as for lead and bismuth (10). It was found that gadolinium and ytterbium were among the metals with the highest complex stability ($\leq$10% binding to bone meal). The acute toxicity (LD50) in mice was approximately 10 mmol/kg for both Gd-EOB-DTPA and Yb-EOB-DTPA. The neural tolerance (LD50) was 416 µmol for Yb-EOB-DTPA and 283 µmol for Gd-EOB-DTPA after intracisternal injection in rats. No physiologically relevant cardiovascular changes were observed for either drug. The bone concentration of gadolinium and ytterbium in rats was less than 10 nmol/g of bone 6 hours after administration of 0.5 mmol/kg Gd-EOB-DTPA and Yb-EOB-DTPA, indicating a high stability and clearance of these contrast media from the body. It was concluded that both Gd-EOB-DTPA and Yb-EOB-DTPA were well suited for further scientific evaluation.

In a clinical study, more liver lesions were detected on CT scans after administration of Gd-EOB-DTPA than on unenhanced CT scans (8). It was concluded that CT with Gd-EOB-DTPA enhancement may be potentially useful for the detection of liver lesions. To find an even more effective contrast medium, Yb-EOB-DTPA was tested in the present study. Although there was no statistically significant difference in maximum liver enhancement between Yb-EOB-DTPA and Gd-EOB-DTPA in the present dog study, ytterbium attenuation was 13% better than gadolinium in vitro at equal molar concentrations and 120 kV, which justifies further evaluation of Yb-EOB-DTPA.

On the basis of the costs of current gadolinium-containing MR imaging contrast media, the potential cost of Gd-EOB-DTPA may be prohibitively high for use in CT as compared with MR imaging and CT during arterial portography. CT may necessitate administration of Gd-EOB-DTPA at doses three to five times higher than the current clinical dose of gadopentetate dimeglumine in MR imaging. At this stage of development, we cannot estimate how much a CT dose of Yb-EOB-DTPA would cost.

In conclusion, both Gd-EOB-DTPA and Yb-EOB-DTPA are promising liver-specific hepatocyte-directed CT contrast media. Both Gd-EOB-DTPA and Yb-EOB-DTPA provide excellent CT liver enhancement in dogs. Although at equimolar concentrations ytterbium has better attenuation properties than gadolinium, CT liver enhancement was not statistically significantly altered by the absorbing element (gadolinium vs ytterbium). Similarly, the mode of application (infusion vs bolus) did not change liver enhancement after 90 minutes. Clinical studies are necessary to collect more safety data and to determine the diagnostic benefit provided by the detection of focal liver lesions and the possible tissue characterization. ■

References

1. Hamm B, Vogl TJ, Branding G, et al. Focal liver lesions: MR imaging with Mn-DPDP—initial clinical results in 40 patients. Radiology 1992; 182:167–174.
2. Schuhmann-Giampieri G, Schmitt-Willich H, Press WR, Negishi C, Weinmann HJ, Speck U. Preclinical evaluation of Gd-EOB-DTPA as a contrast agent in MR imaging of the hepatobiliary system. Radiology 1992; 183:59–64.
3. Reimer P, Rummeny EJ, Daldrup HE, et al. Clinical results with Resovist: a phase 2 clinical trial. Radiology 1995; 195:489–496.
4. Weissleder R. Liver MR imaging with iron oxides: toward consensus and clinical practice. Radiology 1994; 193:593–595.
5. Mühler A, Clément O, Vexler V, Berthezéne Y, Rosenau W, Brasch RC. Gadolinium-ethoxybenzyl-DTPA hepatobiliary enhancement: comparison of spin echo and STIR imaging for detection of experimental liver metastases. Radiology 1992; 184:207–213.
6. Schmitz SA, Mühler A, Wagner S, Wolf KJ. Functional hepatobiliary imaging with Gd-

EOB-DTPA: a comparison of MR imaging and ^{153}Gd-EOB-DTPA scintigraphy in rats. Invest Radiol 1996; 31:154–160.

7. Schmitz SA, Wagner S, Schuhmann-Giampieri G, Krause W, Wolf KJ. A prototype liver-specific contrast medium for CT: preclinical evaluation of gadoxetic acid disodium, or Gd-EOB-DTPA. Radiology 1997; 202:407–412.
8. Schmitz SA, Häberle HJ, Balzer T, Shamsi K, Boese-Landgraf J, Wolf KJ. Detection of focal liver lesions: CT of the hepatobiliary system with gadoxetic acid disodium, or Gd-EOB-DTPA. Radiology 1997; 202:399–405.
9. Schmitz SA, Wagner S, Schuhmann-Giampieri G, Wolf KJ. Evaluation of gadobutrol in a rabbit model as a new lanthanide contrast agent for computed tomography. Invest Radiol 1995; 30:644–649.
10. Krause W, Schuhmann-Giampieri G, Bauer M, Press WR, Muschick P. Ytterbium- and dysprosium-EOB-DTPA: a new prototype of liver-specific contrast agents for computed tomography. Invest Radiol 1996, 31: 502–511.
11. Miller DL, Vermess M, Doppman JL, et al. CT of the liver and spleen with EOE-13: review of 225 examinations. AJR 1984; 143: 235–243.
12. Perkerson RB, Erwin BC, Baumgartner BR, et al. CT densities in delayed iodine hepatic scanning. Radiology 1985; 155:445–446.
13. Miller DL, Simmons JT, Chang R, et al. Hepatic metastases detection: comparison of three CT contrast enhancement methods. Radiology 1987; 165:785–790.
14. Unger E, Gutierrez F. Ytterbium-DTPA: a potential intravascular contrast agent. Invest Radiol 1986; 21:802–807.
15. Zwicker C, Langer M, Langer R, Keske U. Comparison of iodinated and noniodinated contrast media in computed tomography. Invest Radiol 1991; 26:162–164.
16. Havron A, Davis M, Seltzer S, Paskin-Hurlburt A, Hessel S. Heavy metal particulate contrast materials for computed tomography of the liver. J Comput Assist Tomogr 1980; 4:642–648.
17. Seltzer S, Douglass F, Davis M, et al. Hepatic contrast agents for computed tomography: high atomic number particulate materials. J Comput Assist Tomogr 1981; 5: 370–374.
18. Engelbrech V, Koch JA, Rassek M, Mödder U. Gadolinium-DTPA and gadodiamide as an alternative contrast medium for CT. ROFO 1996; 165:24–28.
19. Weast RC, Selby SM, eds. Handbook of chemistry and physics: a ready-reference book of chemical and physical data. Cleveland, Ohio: Chemical Rubber, 1981.
20. Bruneton JN, Falewée MN, François E, et al. Liver, spleen, and vessels: preliminary clinical results of CT with perfluorooctylbromide. Radiology 1989; 170:179–183.
21. Hamm B, Staks T, Mühler A, et al. Phase I clinical evaluation of Gd-EOB-DTPA as a hepatobiliary MR contrast agent: safety, pharmacokinetics, and MR imaging. Radiology 1995; 195:785–792.

Luigi Solbiati, MD • S. Nahum Goldberg, MD • Tiziana Ierace, MD • Tito Livraghi, MD
Franca Meloni, MD • Marina Dellanoce, MD • Sandro Sironi, MD • G. Scott Gazelle, MD, MPH

Hepatic Metastases: Percutaneous Radio-Frequency Ablation with Cooled-Tip Electrodes[1]

PURPOSE: **To assess the feasibility and safety of using cooled-tip electrodes to increase the volume of coagulation necrosis obtained or reduce the number of treatment sessions necessary with percutaneous tumor radio-frequency (RF) ablation.**

MATERIALS AND METHODS: **Twenty-nine patients with 44 hepatic metastases (1.3–5.1 cm diameter) from colorectal ($n = 22$), gastric ($n = 5$), pancreatic ($n = 1$), or breast ($n = 1$) carcinoma were treated with RF ablation using cooled-tip, 18-gauge electrodes with 2–3 cm tip exposure. Each tumor was treated in one or two treatment sessions.**

RESULTS: **Technical success, ablation of all visualized tumor, was achieved in 40 (91%) metastases. Findings at computed tomography (CT) and magnetic resonance (MR) imaging performed 3–6 months after treatment confirmed complete necrosis of the entire metastasis in 66%. Disease-free survival was 50% at 12 months and 33% at 18 months, with localized progression of disease in 34% of treated lesions. Overall survival was 100%, 94%, and 89% at 6, 12, and 18 months, respectively. Only one complication, self-limited hemorrhage, was seen.**

CONCLUSION: **Use of cooled-tip electrodes was a safe and feasible adjunct for tumor RF ablation therapy that produced larger volumes of coagulation necrosis with fewer electrode insertions than is produced with other RF ablation techniques.**

Index terms: Liver neoplasms, secondary, 761.33 • Liver neoplasms, therapy, 761.1269 • Radio-frequency (RF) ablation, 761.33

Abbreviation: RF = radio-frequency.

Radiology 1997; 205:367–373

METHODS for imaging-guided percutaneous tumor ablation, such as radio-frequency (RF)–induced tissue coagulation, have been used in early clinical trials for the treatment of hepatocellular carcinoma (1), hepatic (2,3) and cerebral (4) metastases, and osteoid osteomas (5). With ultrasound (US) or computed tomographic (CT) guidance, an electrode is placed percutaneously directly into the tumor. When attached to the appropriate generator, RF energy is emitted from the exposed, noninsulated portion of the electrode. This energy translates into ion agitation that is converted into heat, which induces cellular death as a result of coagulation necrosis. With use of conventional monopolar RF ablation techniques, the diameter of tissue coagulation achievable with a single electrode insertion is limited to 1.6 cm as a result of tissue charring and the associated elevation of impedance (6,7). Because of this, performance of multiple electrode insertions is necessary to treat all but the smallest tumors.

We and others have recently described a modified cooled-tip RF electrode that can coagulate up to a 5-cm-diameter area of normal muscle or a 2.3-cm-diameter area of normal liver in vivo (8,9). The cooled-tip electrode is a thin conventional RF electrode welded into a dual-lumen 18-gauge insulated cannula. These chambers communicate at the tip of the electrode, which allows internal cooling of the probe tip with chilled saline perfusate. As a result, heating of the tissues nearest the RF electrode is reduced, which allows greater energy deposition. This permits increased tissue heating and coagulation further from the electrode without tissue charring. Use of this electrode, therefore, could potentially reduce the technical complexity and the time necessary to achieve adequate coagulation necrosis for a given tumor size, by decreasing the number of probe insertions necessary to treat lesions larger than approximately 1 cm in diameter. This clinical study was conducted to study the effectiveness of cooled-tip RF ablation as a treatment for patients with small hepatic metastases.

MATERIALS AND METHODS

The study was carried out with the approval of the Ethics Committee of the Ospedale Generale, Busto Arsizio, Italy. Informed consent was obtained from all patients at the time of enrollment.

Twenty-nine patients with 44 metachronous liver metastases from documented primary malignancies were treated with percutaneous application of RF ablation from July 1, 1995, to September 1, 1996. Primary tumors were colorectal ($n = 22$), gastric ($n = 5$), pancreatic ($n = 1$), or breast ($n = 1$) adenocarcinomas. All patients had undergone surgical resection of the pri-

[1] From the Department of Radiology, Ospedale Generale, Piazzale Solaro, 3, 21052 Busto Arsizio (VA), Italy (L.S., T.I., M.D.); the Department of Radiology, Massachusetts General Hospital, Harvard Medical School, Boston, Mass (S.N.G., G.S.G.); the Department of Radiology, Ospedale Civile, Vimercate, Italy (T.L., F.M.); and the Department of Radiology, Ospedale San Raffaele, Milan, Italy (S.S.).
Received April 9, 1997; revision requested May 7; revision received July 9; accepted July 11. Supported in part by a grant from Radionics, Burlington, Mass. **Address reprint requests to** L.S.

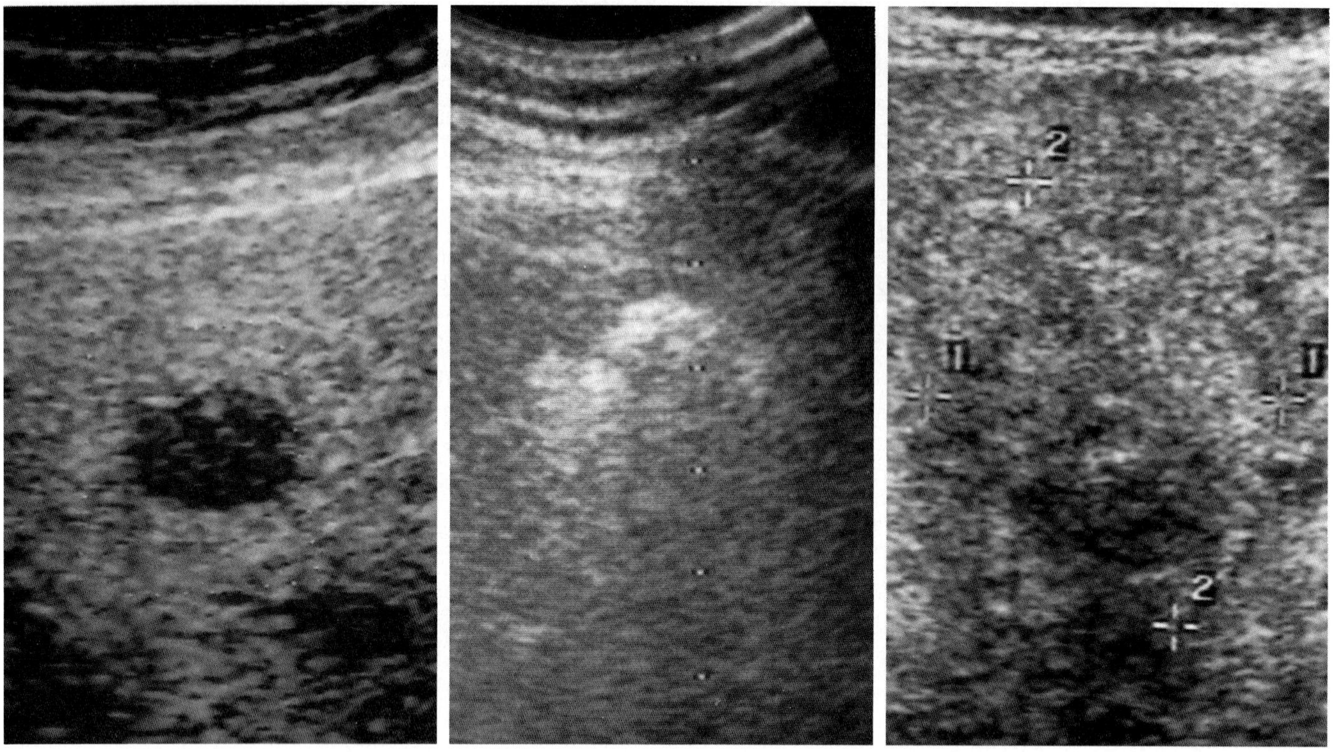

a. b. c.

Figure 1. Sonographic findings in a 63-year-old man. **(a)** US scan depicts a 2.4-cm-diameter hypoechoic colorectal metastasis. **(b)** US scan obtained during RF ablation depicts a wide hyperechoic area surrounding and enveloping the tumor, which is no longer visible. **(c)** Seven-day follow-up US scan shows a 3.9 × 3.4-cm inhomogeneous, hypo- and hyperechoic area (calipers) that replaces the tumor and represents coagulative necrosis.

mary tumor 6–30 months prior to RF ablation. At initial surgery, two (7%) patients underwent additional resection of one and five synchronous liver metastases, respectively. Pathologic proof of malignancy of at least one metastasis was obtained in all patients with US-guided fine-needle aspiration biopsy. Twenty patients had solitary metastases, and nine patients had multiple (two to four) metastases, so a total of 44 lesions were treated with RF ablation. Among the nine patients with multiple metastases, five had two metastases, two had three metastases, and two had four metastases each. Metastases ranged in diameter from 1.3 to 5.1 cm and were further classified by size. Twelve (27%) metastases were less than 2 cm in diameter, and 20 (45%) were between 2 and 3 cm in diameter. All metastases were at least 1 cm away from the hepatic hilum, gallbladder, or bowel wall, with 16 (36%) located in Couinaud segments VII and VIII.

Disease in patients was staged according to the system of Gayowski et al (10). In this system, solitary lesions less than 2.0 cm in diameter are stage mT1, and a lesion 2 cm or greater in diameter is mT2. Multiple unilobar metastases less than 2 cm in diameter are also stage mT2, and such lesions that are 2 cm or greater in diameter are stage mT3. Tumor involving both lobes of the liver or exhibiting invasion of a major portal vessel are stage mT4. In our population, disease in four (14%) patients was stage mT1, in 17 (59%) was stage mT2, in three (10%) was stage mT3, and in five (17%) was stage mT4. No concurrent chemotherapy or other medical treatments were administered to these patients during the entire study.

Pretreatment imaging evaluation of the metastases with US, contrast material–enhanced CT, and magnetic resonance (MR) imaging was performed in all cases. CT (Xpress; Toshiba Medical Systems, Tokyo, Japan) was performed with helical technique (5-mm-thick sections, 7-mm collimation, 1:1 pitch, 120 or 140 kV, 280–300 mA). Unenhanced images were acquired, as well as dual-phase contrast-enhanced images during power injection of 200 mL of 60% iopamidol (Iopamiro; Bracco, Milan, Italy) at a rate of 3 mL/sec. At MR imaging (1.5-T Advanced Signa; GE Medical Systems, Milwaukee, Wis), unenhanced images were acquired with two pulse sequences (spin-echo T1-weighted [repetition time msec/echo time msec = 600/17, with 256 × 192 matrix and two signals acquired] or fat-suppressed fast spin-echo T2-weighted [5,000/120, with 256 × 256 matrix and four signals acquired]). Subsequently, a bolus of gadopentetate dimeglumine (Magnevist; Schering, Berlin, Germany) was injected at standard dose (0.1 mmol per kilogram of body weight), and fast multiplanar spoiled gradient-recalled echo imaging (125/4.2, with 90° flip angle, 256 × 192 matrix, and one signal acquired) was performed at three consecutive 30-second intervals. This triphasic approach allowed evaluation of the liver during the hepatic arterial, portal venous, and parenchymal phases. Finally, gadolinium-enhanced T1-weighted spin-echo and fat-suppressed T1-weighted spin-echo imaging was performed.

Technique

All patients were treated with conscious sedation (neuroleptanalgesia). An anesthetic cream containing prilocaine and xylocaine (EMLA; Astra Tech, Moeindal, Sweden) was applied to the skin surface 1 hour before treatment. Subsequently, both a neuroleptic (droperidol [Sintodian; Farmitalia, Milan, Italy], 1.25–2.5 mg) and an analgesic (fentanyl [Fentanest; Farmitalia], 50–250 μg) were intravenously administered by an anesthesiologist, with continuous cardiovascular and respiratory monitoring.

Cooled-tip RF electrodes with 2–3 cm of exposed metallic tip (Radionics, Burlington, Mass) were used to deliver the RF energy to the tissues. In each treatment session, a single electrode was placed within the tumor with US guidance. With the aid of a needle-guide attachment, the tip of the electrode was positioned at the liver-tumor interface. Electrodes were easily visualized with US, and only one pass was usually necessary for accurate placement.

Grounding was achieved by attaching a large grounding pad with more than 400 cm^2 surface area to the patient's thigh. The electrode was then attached to a 500-kHz monopolar RF generator (model 3-D; Radionics) capable of producing 100 W of

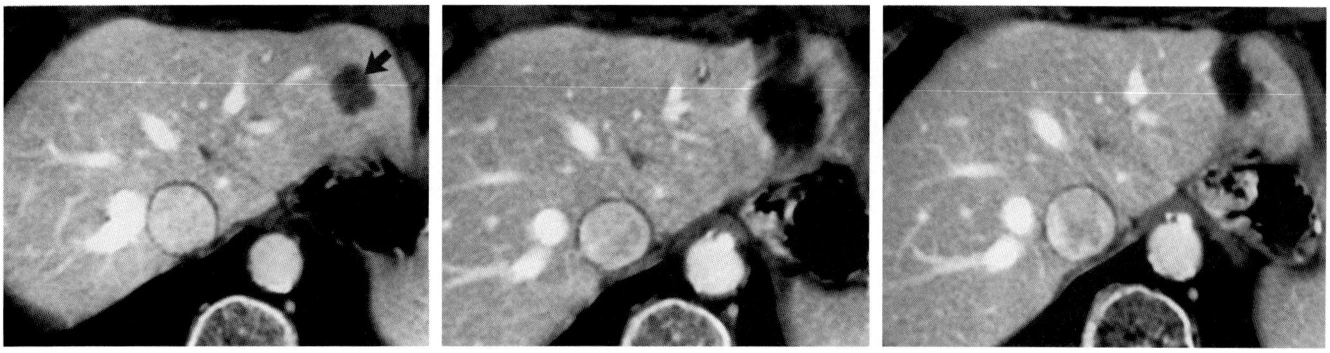

a. b. c.

Figure 2. CT findings in a 70-year-old woman. **(a)** CT scan obtained before RF ablation depicts a 2.0-cm-diameter liver metastasis (arrow) from gastric carcinoma. **(b)** Fifteen-day follow-up CT scan reveals a 4.2 × 2.6-cm focus of hypoattenuation enveloping the tumor. **(c)** Twelve-month follow-up CT scan shows marked regression of the hypoattenuating treatment area to 3.0 × 1.8 cm.

power. During lesion ablation, a thermocouple (embedded within the electrode tip) continuously measured the local temperature. Tissue impedance was monitored continuously by means of circuitry incorporated within the generator. A peristaltic pump (Watson-Marlow, Medford, Mass) was used to infuse 0°C normal saline solution into the cooling lumen of the RF electrode at a rate sufficient to maintain a tip temperature of 20°–25°C. Use of more than 2 L of saline was not necessary in any procedure.

RF energy was delivered in the following manner. Initially, after baseline tissue impedance was measured, generator output was slowly increased to 950–1,100 mA. If an increase in impedance equal to or greater than 10 Ω above baseline was observed, the current was reduced in 50-mA intervals until stable impedance was observed. This reduction in generator output was necessary to prevent tissue boiling, which then leads to increased impedance and limited energy deposition (11). RF application lasted 12–25 minutes, as findings in previous studies demonstrated maximal coagulation at this duration in normal swine liver (8). As indirect measures of tissue heat deposition, the maximum tip temperature at the conclusion of each treatment session was recorded, as well as the time for the tip temperature to decline to 60°C.

Assessment of Treatment Efficacy

CT and MR imaging were performed 7–14 days after the procedure with the same parameters. US was not used to help measure treatment efficacy as we have previously demonstrated that acute US changes cannot help predict the ultimate extent of induced coagulation necrosis (2). Treatment efficacy at this time was assessed on the basis of results at diagnostic imaging, as findings in previous studies have documented close correlation of imaging findings with pathologically proved coagulation necrosis (1–3,8). At CT, areas of hypoattenuation that did not enhance after administration of contrast material were considered to represent necrotic tissue; at MR imaging, hypointense areas on unenhanced T1- and T2-weighted images were considered to represent necrosis. Technical success was defined as a lack of unablated residual tumor at CT or MR imaging at 7–14 days after RF ablation. In cases in which residual tumor was identified, a second RF ablation treatment was performed.

Interval change in tumor size was also studied with follow-up CT and MR imaging at 3–18 months, at 3–4-month intervals. Follow-up findings were classified into two groups: size decreased or unchanged (which implied total necrosis) or size enlarged (which implied incomplete treatment). With these results, the percentage of successfully treated lesions and the disease-free survival rates per patient were calculated.

RESULTS

A total of 51 RF ablation sessions were performed. Thirty-seven (84%) of the 44 metastases in 22 patients were treated in a single session, whereas the remaining seven tumors (in seven patients) necessitated a second RF ablation session. Technical success—defined as a lack of residual unablated tumor at follow-up CT or MR imaging 7–14 days after completion of treatment—was possible in 40 (91%) of 44 tumors. Of the four patients with the remaining four (9%) tumors, three refused further treatment and one underwent hepatic metastasectomy.

Duration of RF application ranged from 12 to 25 minutes for each electrode insertion. Mean total procedure time was 45 minutes per session, including the time necessary for tumor localization, treatment, electrode removal, and immediate postprocedure US. No technical problems were encountered. In 40 (78%) treatment sessions, stable impedance (75–95 Ω) was observed for the duration of the procedure with 950–1,100 mA of current. In the remaining 11 (22%) sessions, current had to be decreased to 800–900 mA owing to rising tissue impedance. For all treatments, tip temperature increased from 20°–25°C (owing to tip cooling) to higher than 80°C immediately after the cessation of cooling. Tip temperature remained above 60°C for a minimum of 2 minutes in all cases.

Imaging

A hyperechoic area that initially surrounded the electrode tip and subsequently enveloped the tumor was observed with US during 50 of the 51 RF ablation sessions (Fig 1). This region was of variable diameter (2.5–5.0 cm) and grossly corresponded to the actual extent of coagulation. Follow-up US 2–4 hours and 1–7 days after the procedure demonstrated a decrease in the echogenicity of the foci, with a partly hyperechoic and partly iso- or hypoechoic echo pattern that could hardly be differentiated from that of the background liver (Fig 1c). Also, the partial obscuration of the characteristic peritumor halo observed in treated metastases precluded accurate assessment of induced coagulation. Similarly, findings at US, with or without the aid of color-flow and power Doppler, did not help precise assessment of coagulation size 1–4 weeks after the procedure.

Initial follow-up contrast-enhanced CT images were obtained 7–10 days after the procedure in every case and depicted foci of hypoattenuation that were devoid of characteristic parenchymal enhancement (Fig 2). T1- and T2-weighted gadolinium-enhanced MR images obtained at the same time revealed hypointense and unenhancing foci (Fig 3). These findings were similar to those previously reported by Solbiati et al (2). With both CT and MR imaging, the treatment area for a single electrode insertion was 2.8 cm ±

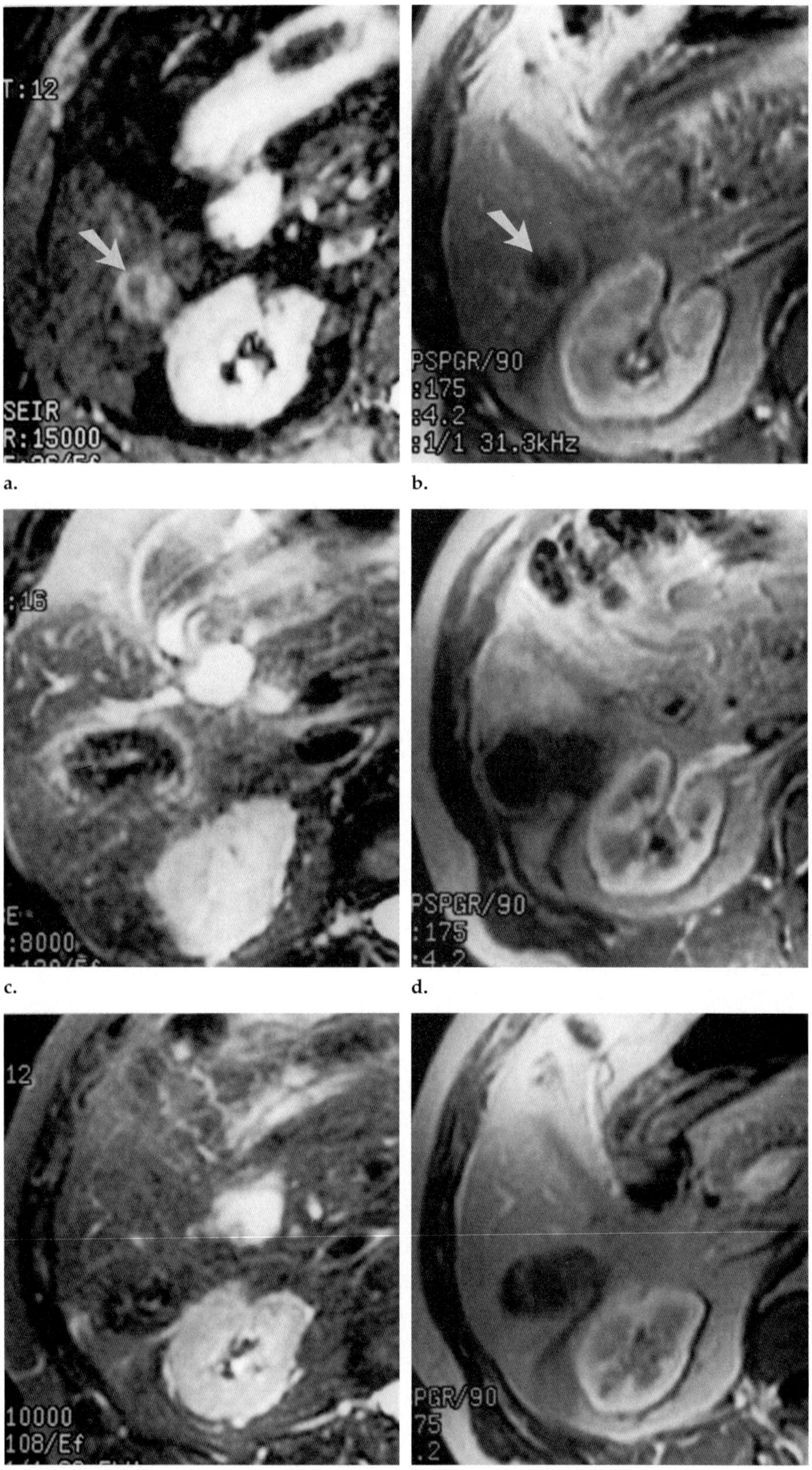

a. b. c. d. e. f.

Figure 3. MR imaging findings in a 71-year-old man. Before RF ablation, **(a)** T2-weighted and **(b)** gadolinium-enhanced T1-weighted MR images depict a 1.9-cm-diameter colorectal metastasis (arrow). Fifteen-day follow-up **(c)** T2-weighted and **(d)** gadolinium-enhanced T1-weighted MR images reveal a 4.3 × 2.4-cm hypointense unenhancing area. Six-month follow-up **(e)** T2-weighted and **(f)** gadolinium-enhanced T1-weighted MR images reveal a reduction in the size of the homogeneously hypointense treatment area without evidence of peripheral tumor regrowth.

0.3 (mean ± standard deviation) in diameter (range, 2.5–3.1 cm) and 3.4 cm ± 0.3 long.

Long-term Follow-up

Imaging and clinical follow-up at 3–4 months and longer (range, 3–18 months; mean, 10.3 months) was possible in 42 of 44 patients. Two patients could not be followed up beyond 3 months as one patient underwent metastasectomy at 60 days and the second was lost to follow-up after the 3-month evaluation. Twenty-one patients with 30 metastases were followed up for at least 6 months. One patient died during the study period of diffuse hepatic metastases 7 months after RF ablation.

Fifteen (34%) of the 44 treated metastases showed evidence of local tumor recurrence (primarily peripheral regrowth) at 6 months. Pathologic confirmation was obtained in one of these patients, who then underwent metastasectomy. No additional evidence for local recurrence was observed in the 21 patients in whom imaging follow-up was performed beyond 6 months. Treated metastases ($n = 33$) in these patients, however, showed either a marked reduction in the region of nonenhancing hypoattenuation ($n = 13$) (Fig 2c) or were unchanged in appearance from the initial 7–14-day follow-up imaging examination ($n = 20$).

Smaller tumors were more likely ($P < .05$) to undergo complete treatment than larger tumors. None of the 12 tumors less than 2 cm in diameter developed recurrent local or distant disease during follow-up. Fourteen (70%) of 20 tumors that were 2–3 cm in diameter, and seven (58%) of 12 metastases more than 3 cm in diameter showed no evidence of regrowth. Thus for 11 (25%) of 44 lesions, follow-up CT or MR imaging performed 7–14 days after RF ablation did not depict residual unablated peripheral tumor.

In four metastases, local tumor regrowth was circumferential (Fig 4). Most of these lesions were therefore believed to be untreatable due to unfavorable geometry. In the remaining seven tumors that demonstrated local regrowth, unablated tumor was observed in only one margin of the metastasis. In four of seven cases, the area of tumor regrowth was adjacent to a large blood vessel (Fig 5). Six of the seven patients with focal tumor regrowth consented to undergo repeat treatment of the tumor with RF ablation. Repeat treatment was performed 3–6 months after the initial treatment and resulted in coagulation of the residual tumor in two (33%) of the six cases.

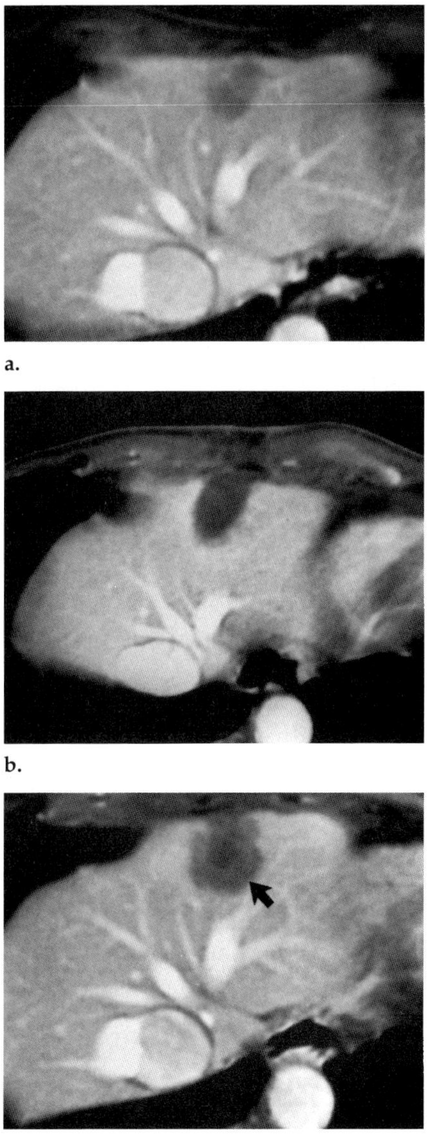

a.

b.

c.

Figure 4. CT findings of inadequate treatment of tumor margins in a 72-year-old woman. **(a)** Pretreatment CT scan depicts a 2.6-cm-diameter solitary colorectal metastasis. **(b)** Fifteen-day follow-up CT scan depicts apparently complete treatment, with no rim of unablated tumor. The size of the coagulation area, however, is not larger than the original metastasis. **(c)** Three-month follow-up CT scan depicts peripheral tumor regrowth (arrow).

Disease-free survival at 6 months was achieved in 16 (76%) of 21 patients. Adequate treatment of the initial lesion was achieved in two of the remaining five patients, but these patients developed additional hepatic or distant metastases. At 12 months, disease-free survival was achieved in nine (50%) of 18 patients. Three (33%) of nine patients followed up for 18 months were disease free. Overall survival ($n = 29$) was much greater than disease-free survival: 100% at 6 months, 94% at 12 months, and 89% at 18 months. Among the 18 patients with disease recurrence after adequate local treatment, four (22%) had new hepatic metastases and two (11%) had distant (pulmonary or lymph node) metastases.

Complications

All procedures were performed with conscious sedation (neuroleptanalgesia). In five (10%) of the 51 sessions, mild pain or discomfort was noted by the patient. All of these lesions were located peripherally, adjacent to the Glisson capsule. A second dose of 50–100 μg of fentanyl alleviated the pain in all cases.

One patient in whom a metastasis located in the dome of the liver was treated reported abdominal pain 3–4 hours after the procedure. Orthostatic hypotension was noted and CT depicted a small intraperitoneal hemorrhage. This patient was admitted to the hospital for observation but did not require transfusion as the hematocrit stabilized at 0.362 g/L (a 0.045 g/L decrease) over 72 hours. In the remaining 28 patients, no complications were observed during 2–4 hours of postprocedure observation, and all were discharged uneventfully on the day of the procedure. No late complications were encountered.

DISCUSSION

There has recently been increased interest in imaging-guided minimally invasive percutaneous therapy to treat hepatic malignancies. Injection of coagulative agents such as ethanol has been demonstrated as an effective treatment for hepatocellular carcinoma (12) but not for metastatic disease (13). Thermal methods such as RF (1–3), laser (14, 15), and microwave (16, 17) are now being explored for the treatment of secondary malignancies. Herein, we report our experience with tumor RF ablation with cooled-tip electrodes. Use of these electrodes increases coagulative necrosis by allowing deposition of more energy without tissue charring .

With use of conventional monopolar RF techniques, the diameter of tissue coagulation from a single electrode insertion is limited to 1.6 cm because of tissue charring and the associated elevation in impedance (6,7). Thus, performance of multiple electrode insertions is necessary to ensure adequate treatment of all lesions more than 1 cm in diameter. Goldberg et al (18) demonstrated that RF can be applied simultaneously to multiprobe arrays, which increases the volume of coagulation necrosis that can be obtained in a single treatment session. In clinical practice, however, this technique is both technically challenging and time-consuming (2). Other strategies for increasing the extent of coagulation necrosis with RF include injection of saline during RF application (3) and the use of bipolar technology (19). Livraghi et al (3) induced coagulation necrosis up to 4 cm in diameter with a single RF application by injecting saline, but they noted limited reproducibility and irregularly shaped regions of coagulation with this technique. McGahan et al (19) used bipolar RF ablation techniques by inserting two electrodes. Although this method resulted in increased coagulation compared with conventional monopolar techniques, the volume of induced necrosis was not only less than that produced with multiprobe arrays but was also irregularly shaped without conformation to the spheric geometry of most hepatic neoplasms (19).

Goldberg et al (8) and Lorentzen (9) recently reported modification of the RF electrode to enable tip cooling during RF application. Use of internal cannulas allows continuous perfusion of the electrode tip with 0°C saline. Although this reduces heat deposition in the tissues nearest the electrode, cooling of the electrode tip allows greater RF energy deposition by preventing overheating of tissues nearest the electrode tip. This overheating can result in charring and lead to elevated tissue impedance, which prevents further delivery of RF energy. Tip cooling, therefore, permits tissues farther from the electrode to be heated sufficiently to induce coagulation and thereby produces a larger volume of coagulation. With use of this cooled-tip method and a single probe insertion in animal experiments, Goldberg et al (8) obtained coagulation necrosis more than 5 cm in diameter in muscle tissue in vivo, more than 4 cm in diameter in liver tissue ex vivo, and 2.4 cm in diameter in normal liver tissue in vivo. This extent of coagulation is larger than that reported for a single application of microwave (16, 17) or single-fiber laser (14, 15) therapy.

Our results suggest that this technique can be performed readily and is associated with minimal complications. More importantly, no more than two sessions with one or two 20–25-minute insertions with the cooled-tip system were necessary for the treatment of tumors up to 3.5 cm in diameter. Compared with our previous findings (2,20) and those of Rossi et al

(1), this represents a remarkable reduction in both the time for any individual treatment session and the overall number of treatment sessions necessary for a given tumor size.

Results obtained with cooled-tip RF application compare favorably with those previously reported with other RF ablation techniques. In our study, overall survival was 94% at 12 months and 89% at 18 months. Disease-free survival was 50% at 1 year, with a majority of the treatment failures due to the presence of new intra- and extrahepatic metastases. Rossi et al (1) treated 11 patients with 13 hepatic metastases with multiple insertions of conventional monopolar and bipolar RF electrodes in multiple treatment sessions. Although all but one of the tumors were less than 3.5 cm in diameter, only one patient was alive without evidence of tumor at 1 year, and local recurrence was evident at CT or pathologic examination in 55% of patients. In this same group, results were better in 39 patients with hepatocellular carcinoma, with median survival of 44 months and local recurrence in less than 10% in a mean follow-up of 22.6 months.

Solbiati et al (2) treated 31 tumors in 16 patients with metastatic gastrointestinal carcinomas 1.5–7.5 cm in diameter with conventional monopolar RF techniques alone and with multiprobe arrays. Complete treatment without evidence of local tumor growth was achieved in 66.6%, and all of these tumors were less than 3 cm in diameter. Disease-free survival was achieved in 50% of patients, with a mean 16.6-month follow-up. Overall survival in these patients is reported as 100% at 1 year and 61.5% at 2 years (20). Livraghi et al (3) treated 14 patients with 24 hepatic metastases 1.2–4.5 cm in diameter and one patient with cholangiocarcinoma with conventional RF electrodes and simultaneous infusion of saline. Complete necrosis at 6 months was achieved in 52% of the tumors, all of which were less than 3.5 cm in diameter.

Imaging findings after RF ablation in this study are similar to those previously published (1–3). Although US was useful for treatment guidance, gray-scale sonographic findings during the RF ablation procedure did not help predict the extent of coagulation necrosis. In most cases, a hyperechoic focus that increased in size during the procedure was seen surrounding the distal portion of the electrode. This region was of variable size and often of irregular shape and contour. Follow-up imaging 1–4 hours after the procedure often demonstrated complete resolution of this hyperechoic area, which we believe represents microbubbles of gas that form in the heated tissue. The findings in this study further confirm our earlier findings of the limited value of US in long-term follow-up (2).

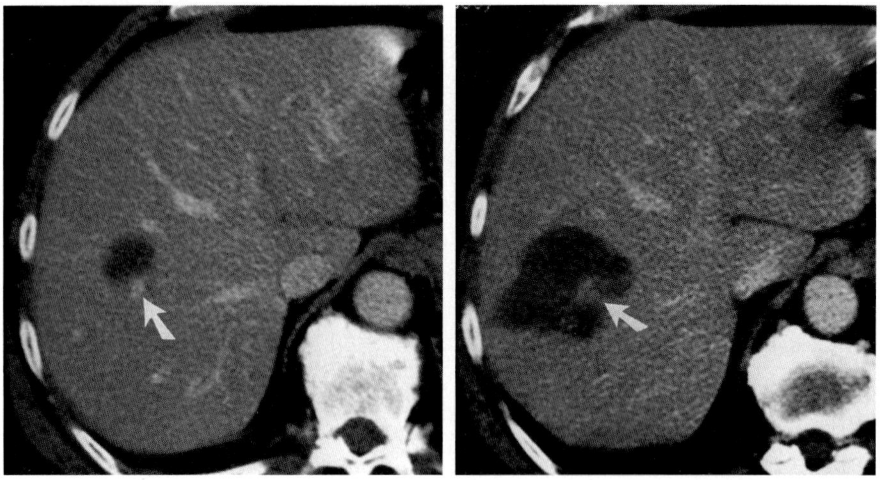

a. b.

Figure 5. CT findings of inadequate coagulation adjacent to large vessels in a 65-year-old man. **(a)** Pretreatment CT scan reveals a 2.3-cm-diameter colorectal metastasis adjacent to an intrahepatic vessel (arrow). **(b)** Six-month follow-up CT scan demonstrates a 3.7-cm-diameter area of coagulation that should have adequately treated the tumor, but persistent perivascular tumor growth extends to one edge of the treatment focus (arrow).

Follow-up contrast-enhanced spiral CT performed 7–14 days after RF ablation demonstrated regions of hypoattenuation devoid of parenchymal enhancement. The region of coagulation was differentiated from hypoattenuating tumor on delayed images, on which persistent hypoattenuation was noted in coagulated tissues but not in unablated tumor. T1- and T2-weighted MR images characteristically reveal hypointense areas devoid of gadolinium enhancement. All cases of local tumor regrowth were detected at follow-up axial CT and MR imaging within 3–6 months. Completely treated tumors demonstrated either variable reduction or unchanged size of the region of induced coagulation necrosis at follow-up imaging at 6 months or later. Increased conspicuity of residual tumor at 3–6-month follow-up was most often a result of continued tumor growth. Occasionally, this differentiation was difficult on initial follow-up CT scans, as only a thin rim of tumor was present.

Although our results with the cooled-tip RF ablation technique are encouraging, they must be interpreted in view of several important limitations. The 18-month follow-up period in this study is too short to allow detection of meaningful differences in survival compared with other treatment strategies. Full evaluation of this technique will necessitate performance of larger studies with longer follow-up. In addition, although the average volume of induced coagulation was increased compared with other techniques, the coagulation necrosis mean diameter of 2.8 cm in this study limits the practical efficacy of this ablative strategy to smaller lesions. Thus, better results were achieved for metastases less than 2 cm in diameter (100% success) compared with those more than 3 cm in diameter (58% success).

In conclusion, our results in 29 patients with 44 hepatic metastases suggest that percutaneous RF ablation with cooled-tip electrodes is feasible and safe. Use of the cooled-tip technology simplifies the RF ablation procedure, increases the extent of induced coagulation necrosis, and reduces the number of electrode insertions or treatment sessions necessary to treat a given metastasis. ■

References

1. Rossi S, Di Stasi M, Buscarini E, et al. Percutaneous RF interstitial thermal ablation in the treatment of hepatic cancer. AJR 1996; 167:759–768.
2. Solbiati L, Ierace T, Goldberg SN, et al. Percutaneous US-guided RF tissue ablation of liver metastases: long-term follow-up. Radiology 1997; 202:195–203.
3. Livraghi T, Goldberg SN, Monti F, et al. Saline-enhanced radio-frequency tissue ablation in the treatment of liver metastases. Radiology 1997; 202:205–210.
4. Anzai Y, Lufkin R, DeSalles A, Hamilton DR, Farahani K, Black KL. Preliminary experience with MR-guided thermal ablation of brain tumors. AJNR 1995; 16:39–48.
5. Rosenthal DI, Springfield DS, Gebhart MC, Rosenberg AE, Mankin HJ. Osteoid osteoma: percutaneous radio-frequency ablation. Radiology 1995; 197:451–454.

6. Goldberg SN, Gazelle GS, Dawson SL, Rittman WJ, Mueller PR, Rosenthal DI. Tissue ablation with radio frequency: effect of probe size, gauge, duration, and temperature on lesion volume. Acad Radiol 1995; 2:399–404.
7. McGahan JP, Brock JN, Tessluk H, Wei-Zhong G, Schneider P, Browning PD. Hepatic ablation with use of radio-frequency electrocautery in the animal model. JVIR 1992; 3:291–297.
8. Goldberg SN, Gazelle GS, Solbiati L, Rittman WJ, Mueller PR. Radio-frequency tissue ablation: increased lesion diameter with a perfusion electrode. Acad Radiol 1996; 3:636–644.
9. Lorentzen T. A cooled needle electrode for radio-frequency tissue ablation: thermodynamic aspects of improved performance compared with conventional needle design. Acad Radiol 1996; 3:556–563.
10. Gayowski TJ, Iwatsuki S, Madariaga JR, et al. Experience in hepatic resection for metastatic colorectal cancer: analysis of clinical and pathologic risk factors. Surgery 1994; 116:703–711.
11. Goldberg SN, Gazelle GS, Halpern EF, Rittman WJ, Mueller PR, Rosenthal DI. Radio-frequency tissue ablation: importance of local temperature along the electrode tip exposure in determining lesion shape and size. Acad Radiol 1996; 3:212–218.
12. Livraghi T, Giorgio A, Giuseppe M, et al. Hepatocellular carcinoma and cirrhosis in 746 patients: long-term results of percutaneous ethanol injection. Radiology 1995; 197:101–108.
13. Mueller PR, Charboneau JW, Chezmar JL, Unger EC, Botet JF, Kane RA. North American experience with percutaneous alcohol ablation in 141 patients: complications and overview (abstr). Radiology 1995; 197(P):200.
14. Amin Z, Donald JJ, Masters A, et al. Hepatic metastases: interstitial laser photocoagulation with real-time US monitoring and dynamic CT evaluation of treatment. Radiology 1993; 187:339–347.
15. Vogl TJ, Muller PK, Hammerstingl R, et al. Malignant liver tumors treated with MR imaging–guided laser-induced thermotherapy: technique and prospective results. Radiology 1995; 196:257–265.
16. Murakami R, Yoshimatsu S, Yamashita Y, Matsukawa T, Takahashi M, Sagara K. Treatment of hepatocellular carcinoma: value of percutaneous microwave coagulation. AJR 1995; 164:1159–1164.
17. Seki T, Wakabayashi M, Nakagawa T, et al. Ultrasonically guided percutaneous microwave coagulation therapy for small hepatocellular carcinoma. Cancer 1994; 74:817–825.
18. Goldberg SN, Gazelle GS, Dawson SL, Mueller PR, Rittman W, Rosenthal DI. Radio-frequency tissue ablation using multiprobe arrays: greater tissue destruction than multiple probes operating alone. Acad Radiol 1995; 2:670–674.
19. McGahan JP, Wei-Zhong G, Brock JM, Tesluk H, Jones CD. Hepatic ablation using bipolar radio-frequency electrocautery. Acad Radiol 1996; 3:418–422.
20. Solbiati L, Goldberg SN, Ierace T, Livraghi T, Sironi S, Gazelle GS. Follow-up of liver metastases treated with percutaneous radio-frequency ablation: clinical outcome and survival rates (abstr). Radiology 1996; 201(P):268.

Book Review

MRI of the Knee. 2nd ed.

Edited by Peter L. Munk, MD, CM, FRCPC, and Clyde A. Helms, MD
Philadelphia, Pa: Lippincott-Raven, 1996. ISBN 0-397-51642-8. Cloth, $130.00; pp 364; 408 figures; tables.

This is the second edition of a much admired book. Although we were unable to locate the first edition for comparison, the preface reveals that chapters on the pediatric knee and postoperative knee have been added and the chapter on technique has been revised. Additionally, the bibliography has been updated, and many new illustrations have been added.

The first chapter, on technique, is very readable. In this chapter, excellent images demonstrate the various sequences, and some suggested protocols for magnetic resonance (MR) imaging of the knee are discussed. The next chapter, on the cruciate ligaments, is well laid out. In this chapter, the value of coronal and sagittal views is stressed. In the following chapter, the extensor mechanism and patellofemoral joint are discussed. Once again, this chapter is well written and covers such topics as patellar instability, peripatellar bursitis, synovial folds, and cartilaginous abnormalities.

The fourth chapter, on the menisci, is also very well laid out and illustrated. The following chapter, on the collateral ligaments and related structures, includes a nice discussion of the posterolateral complex of the knee with some useful diagrams. In chapter 6, the various internal structures of the knee and the associated pitfalls of imaging are reviewed. Chapter 7, on traumatic osteochondral disease of the knee, provides high-resolution MR images and a nice discussion on spontaneous osteonecrosis. Osteochondritis dissecans and occult fractures are also covered in this chapter.

The next chapter covers arthritis and inflammatory diseases of the knee. In the following chapter, tumors of the knee are discussed. Both chapters are helpful and well illustrated. The chapter on tumors also contains a discussion of cysts associated with the knee joint; however, Baker cysts are covered in only about 200 words and with three figures. This chapter is also the longest and appears to be a mini-textbook on bone and soft-tissue tumors. This chapter is very interesting, well written, and useful.

The final two chapters are new: "The Pediatric Knee" covers topics (some of which have been covered elsewhere) such as discoid menisci, soft-tissue lesions, arthritis, and infections. Chapter 11 is well illustrated and covers the complex subject of the postoperative knee in a succinct and useful fashion.

Overall, I believe this is an excellent and worthwhile book. I urge all radiologists who are performing MR imaging of the knee to purchase this book. It would also be most useful for radiology residents who are preparing for the board examinations.

Reviewed by Harry J. Griffiths, MD

Ernst-Peter K. Strecker, MD • Irene B. L. Boos, DVM • Dieter Göttmann, MD

Femoropopliteal Artery Stent Placement: Evaluation of Long-term Success[1]

PURPOSE: To evaluate the long-term success of femoropopliteal artery stent placement after technical failure of balloon angioplasty and to determine potential factors predictive of stent failure.

MATERIALS AND METHODS: In 80 patients, flexible tantalum stents were implanted for treatment of residual stenosis greater than 30% after balloon angioplasty of femoropopliteal artery stenoses (n = 33) or occlusions (n = 47). Follow-up examinations were performed at 1–72 months to evaluate early and late stent failure according to risk factors such as lesion type, anatomic location, stent length, runoff quality, and restenosis after balloon angioplasty.

RESULTS: Early stent thrombosis occurred within 10 days after stent placement in four (5%) patients; the frequency was higher ($P < .01$) in stents longer than 4 cm (14%) versus that in stents 4 cm or shorter (2%). For all stents, the 2-year primary patency rate was 51% and the 3-year rate was 48%. The 2-year primary patency rate was significantly better ($P < .05$) for shorter stents (59%) versus that for longer stents (30%) and for treated stenoses (73%) versus treated occlusions (33%). Multivariate analysis revealed that lesion type and lesion length were the most reliable factors predictive of stent failure.

CONCLUSION: Successful stent therapy does not seem to depend on the type of stent used but rather on lesion type, lesion length, and other predisposing factors.

Of the interventional methods introduced for treatment of occlusive vessel disease, balloon dilation is the percutaneous treatment of choice for therapy of peripheral arterial occlusive disease occurring in the femoral and popliteal arteries. Stents proved to be a valuable adjunct to percutaneous transluminal angioplasty (PTA), however, when PTA was unsuccessful because of elastic recoil of the vessel wall, stenosing vessel wall dissection, or occluding intimal flap. With the development of the stent technique, successful treatment is possible in cases of complex lesions and arterial occlusions that cannot be treated with PTA alone. The long-term success of stent therapy and PTA is impaired by restenosis caused by intimal hyperplasia, especially in small-diameter arteries such as the coronary and femoropopliteal arteries.

The purpose of this study was to evaluate the long-term success of placement of flexible tantalum stents in femoropopliteal arteries after unsuccessful PTA and to determine factors predictive of stent failure.

MATERIALS AND METHODS

Between April 1988 and July 1996, balloon dilation of femoropopliteal arterial lesions was performed in 970 patients. Eighty of these patients (22 women, 58 men; mean age, 63.9 years; range, 37–90 years) were entered into the single-center prospective study on femoropopliteal artery stent implantation. Secondary stent implantation was indicated when biplanar angiography performed after PTA revealed residual stenosis of at least 30% as measured with a caliper from the angiogram. Residual stenoses were caused by vessel wall dissection in 35 (44%) patients or elastic recoil in 43 (54%) patients. Stent implantation was indicated in two (2%) patients because of occlusion of the arterial lumen by an intimal flap.

Exclusion criteria for stent implantation were missing consent to the procedure or noncompliance with the following medication regimen. Residual lesions exceeding 15 cm in length were considered not suitable for stent therapy.

Before angioplasty, lesions were determined to be caused by arterial stenosis in 33 patients and occlusion in 47 patients. In eight patients, the treated lesion was localized in the common femoral artery, in 53 patients in the superficial femoral artery, and in 19 patients in the popliteal artery (Table). In addition, data were included from two of these patients who had occlusion of a synthetic femoral bypass graft and underwent placement of a stent into the proximal graft anastomosis. Data were excluded from statistical analysis in one patient with a long occlusion of the popliteal artery who had undergone a ring stripper procedure. Fourteen patients had a secondary lesion that had developed after angioplasty; the other 66 patients had de novo lesions.

The overall mean lesion length was 6 cm, as measured before recanalization or angioplasty. Stenoses had a mean length of 2.9 cm (range, 1–11 cm), and occlusions

Index terms: Arteries, extremities, 921.721, 922.721, 924.721 • Arteries, grafts and prostheses, 921.1268, 922.1268, 924.1268 • Arteries, stenosis or obstruction, 921.721, 922.721, 924.721 • Arteries, transluminal angioplasty, 921.1286, 922.1286, 924.1286

Abbreviation: PTA = percutaneous transluminal angioplasty.

Radiology 1997; 205:375–383

[1] From the Department of Radiology, Diakonissen Hospital, Diakonissenstr 28, Karlsruhe, Germany. Received September 30, 1996; revision requested November 19; final revision received June 25, 1997; accepted June 27. **Address reprint requests to** E.P.K.S.

E.P.K.S. receives royalties from Medi-tech/Boston Scientific.

had a mean length of 8.2 cm (range, 1–30 cm). Occlusions were significantly longer than stenoses (Student *t* test, $P < .01$); 32 (68%) of the occlusions were longer than 4 cm.

Stents were placed only in the portion of the vessel in which residual stenosis was present after PTA was performed; therefore, the stent length did not necessarily correspond to the length of the original lesion. Long stents, including those that traversed two or more anatomic sites, were determined according to the area in which the largest portion of the stent was placed.

Risk factors associated with vascular disease were cigarette smoking (54 [67%] patients), arterial hypertension (31 [39%] patients), elevated serum cholesterol level (41 [51%] patients), and diabetes mellitus (20 [25%] patients). In 54 (67%) patients, more than one of these risk factors were present.

Clinical symptoms were determined on the basis of a classification by Fontaine (1). Four (5%) patients had mild claudication (stage IIa, painless walking distance >250 m), 63 (79%) patients had severe claudication (stage IIb, painless walking distance <250 m), four (5%) patients had pain while resting (stage III), and nine (11%) patients had tissue loss or gangrene (stage IV). At Doppler sonography performed before the procedure, the mean ankle-brachial index was 0.52 (range, 0.00–0.95).

Conventional balloon angioplasty was performed before stent implantation in all patients. In 16 of 47 patients with an arterial occlusion, initial recanalization was performed by means of local fibrinolysis; in six patients with chronic occlusions present for more than 6 months, slow-rotation angioplasty was performed for recanalization. Initially, balloon dilation was performed over a period of 20 seconds. In cases of residual stenosis, repeat balloon dilation was necessary; the balloon was inflated for a period of up to 5 minutes. Dilation of lesions was performed with a balloon that had a diameter equal to that of the artery as measured with a ruler from the conventional angiogram or the digital subtraction angiogram (x-ray magnification was disregarded).

Runoff status was rated as good in 50 patients and poor in 30 patients. Good runoff status was defined as patency or stenosis less than 50% of the femoropopliteal arteries distal to the area with the stent combined with patency or stenosis less than 50% of at least two crural arteries. Poor runoff status was defined as occlusion or stenosis greater than 50% of the femoropopliteal arteries distal to the area with the stent and occlusion or stenosis greater than 50% of more than one crural artery.

Inflow status was good in all patients, with no occlusion or stenosis greater than 50% in the iliac arteries or in the femoral artery proximal to the lesion in which the stent was placed.

The study protocol was approved by the government presidency (Regierungspräsidium). Written informed consent was obtained from all patients before stent implantation.

Lesion Location and Characteristics

Anatomic Location of Lesion	No. of Patients	Lesion Type		Length of Stent Placed	
		Stenosis	Occlusion	≤4 cm	>4 cm
Common femoral artery	8	4	4	5	3
Proximal and middle third of the superficial femoral artery	25	11	14 (including 2 graft anastomoses)	20	5
Distal third of the superficial femoral artery	28	11	17	19	9
Popliteal artery	19	7	12	15	4
Total	80	33	47	59	21

Stent Type

The technical properties of the balloon-expandable tantalum stent (Strecker stent; Medi-tech/Boston Scientific, Natick, Mass) and the delivery technique used have been described in detail previously (2,3). Briefly, the stent is balloon-expandable, is inserted through an introducer sheath (PVB Medizintechnik, Kirchseeon, Germany, or Terumo, Frankfurt, Germany), and consists of a cylindric, electropolished tantalum filament knit with a wire diameter of 0.1 mm. Within certain limits, this prosthesis is flexible and elastic in both expanded and nonexpanded states. The loosely connected wire loops enable inherent flexibility of the stent, allowing introduction of the catheter-stent assembly through curved arteries and implantation into arteries that lie over the hip joint.

Correct positioning of the stent in the area to be treated is facilitated because shortening of the stent during dilation is compensated for by the design of the stent. With this design, longitudinal compression of the overlapping loops occurs in the nonexpanded state. In addition, the stent is clearly visible at fluoroscopy due to the radiopacity of tantalum. The stent is fixed to the expansion site of the PTA balloon with silicone sleeves, which overlap the stent ends. During balloon inflation, the sleeves roll backward from the balloon shoulders, leaving the expanded stent free for implantation. Until the end of 1995 (55 patients had been treated with stents), introducer sheaths with a length of 8 cm and a diameter of 7.5–9.0 F were used. The improved catheter-stent assembly used since that time has a thin-walled high-pressure balloon, which allows reduction of the introducer sheath to 7 F for stents with an expanded diameter of 5–8 mm. Available stents have a length of 2, 4, or 8 cm.

Stent Placement Procedure

After PTA was performed unsuccessfully, an introducer sheath corresponding to the size of the catheter-stent assembly as described previously was exchanged and the catheter-stent assembly was introduced over the guide wire in place. With the old catheter-stent assembly, the balloon that expanded the stent was 1 mm larger in diameter than the previously used PTA balloon. With the improved catheter-stent assembly with a high-pressure balloon, the balloon that expanded the stent had the same diameter as the previously used PTA balloon. The stent chosen was long enough to cover the area of residual stenosis completely. In cases of long lesions, two stents were implanted consecutively from distal to proximal with the ends overlapping at least 10 mm (tandem fashion). The lesion was localized with the road mapping procedure. The nondilated stents were positioned according to the markers on the PTA catheter and then dilated until expanded completely, and the balloon catheter of the improved stent design tolerated a pressure of 12 bar.

In nine patients, six with common femoral artery lesions and three with lesions in the utmost proximal portion of the superficial femoral artery, PTA and stent implantation were performed via the contralateral femoral artery by using the crossover method (Fig 1). With this method, the catheter-stent assembly was introduced over the guide wire leading over the aortic bifurcation (Fig 1). When this technique is used it is not necessary to place a sheath over the aortic bifurcation.

In six patients, all treated before 1993, ipsilateral popliteal puncture was performed without sonographic guidance, and the catheter-stent assembly was introduced with this popliteal approach. This approach was used in two patients who had calcified occlusions of the common femoral artery that could not be crossed with a guide wire or a catheter from the contralateral femoral artery and in three patients with occlusion of the superficial femoral artery in whom proximal-to-distal guide wire passage was not technically feasible. In one patient, the popliteal approach was necessary because femoral access was contraindicated owing to the presence of an aortobifemoral bypass graft.

Owing to the high complication rate associated with the popliteal access technique, the pull-through method is preferred in cases of failed proximal-to-distal guide wire passage of an occlusion in the superficial femoral artery. For the pull-through method, the popliteal artery was punctured previously with only a cannula (Surflo intravenous catheter; Terumo) to cross the lesion with a single hydrophilic

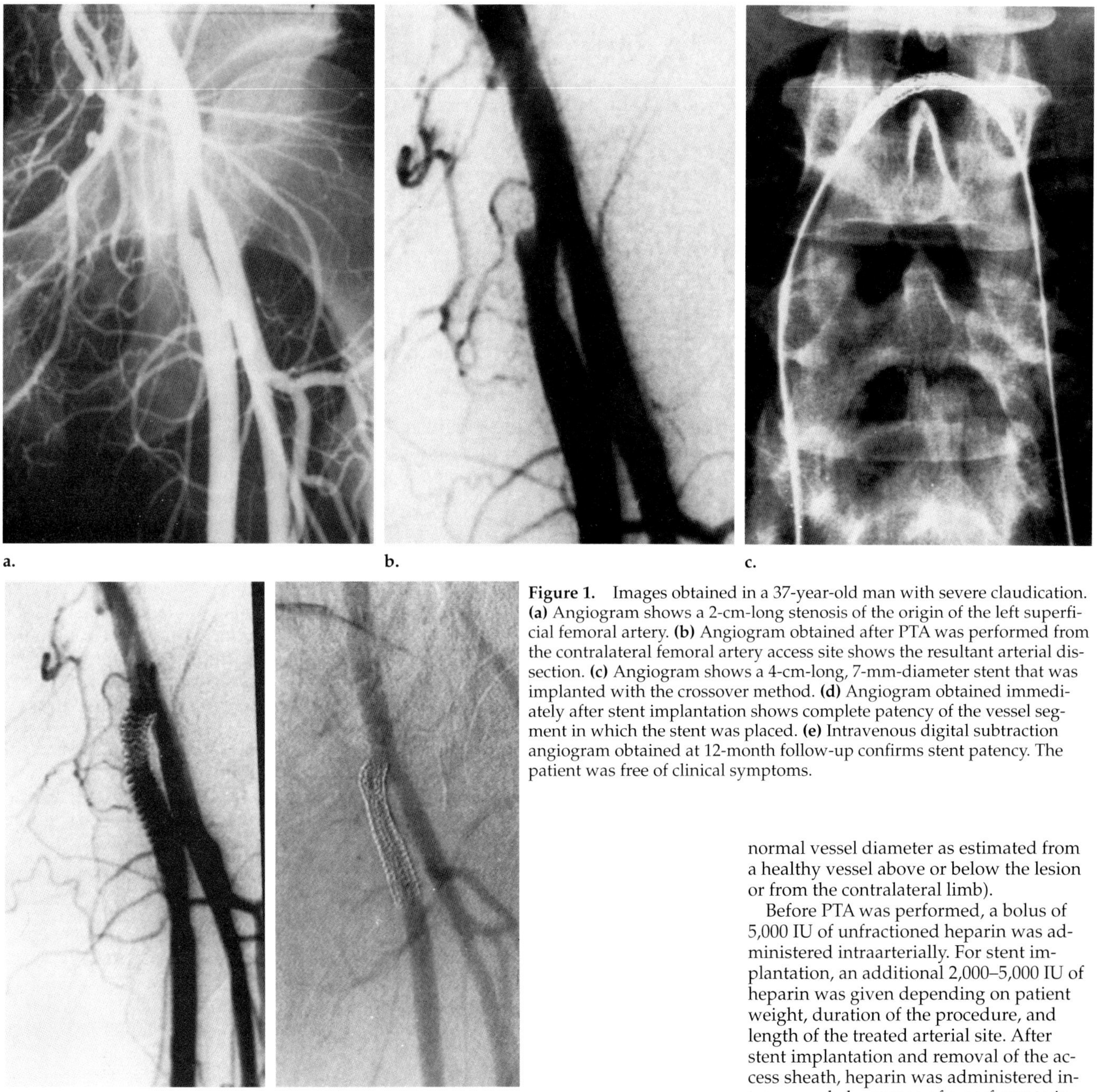

Figure 1. Images obtained in a 37-year-old man with severe claudication. **(a)** Angiogram shows a 2-cm-long stenosis of the origin of the left superficial femoral artery. **(b)** Angiogram obtained after PTA was performed from the contralateral femoral artery access site shows the resultant arterial dissection. **(c)** Angiogram shows a 4-cm-long, 7-mm-diameter stent that was implanted with the crossover method. **(d)** Angiogram obtained immediately after stent implantation shows complete patency of the vessel segment in which the stent was placed. **(e)** Intravenous digital subtraction angiogram obtained at 12-month follow-up confirms stent patency. The patient was free of clinical symptoms.

guide wire (lubricious guide wire M; Terumo) from the distal to proximal direction and to pass the guide wire through a femoral introducer sheath and then outside the patient's body. Thus, use of a popliteal introducer sheath can be avoided. All further procedures such as balloon dilation or stent implantation can then be performed from the femoral access site.

In 11 patients, two stents were implanted in a tandem fashion. In three patients who were treated earlier in the study, the extrinsic forces from the vessel wall were too strong to allow the stent to open completely when the balloon pressure recommended by the manufacturer was used; thus, the balloon catheter was withdrawn carefully and dilation was completed with a PTA balloon that accepted higher pressures (Blue-Max; Meditech/Boston Scientific). When a stent collapsed partially after balloon deflation (collapse occurred in five patients with severly calcified lesions), repeat dilation was performed with inflation over 1 minute or with a balloon with a diameter 1 mm larger than the balloon used previously. With the improved catheter-stent assembly design, repeat dilation was not necessary. After stent implantation, angiograms were obtained that included the peripheral arteries down to the level of the arterial trifurcation in the ankle to exclude any iatrogenic distal embolization. Stent placement was considered technically successful when biplanar control angiography revealed a lumen diameter of at least 80% of the reference vessel diameter (eg, the normal vessel diameter as estimated from a healthy vessel above or below the lesion or from the contralateral limb).

Before PTA was performed, a bolus of 5,000 IU of unfractioned heparin was administered intraarterially. For stent implantation, an additional 2,000–5,000 IU of heparin was given depending on patient weight, duration of the procedure, and length of the treated arterial site. After stent implantation and removal of the access sheath, heparin was administered intravenously by means of a perfusor to increase the partial thromboplastin time to two or three times normal (ie, the partial thromboplastin time measured in each patient before heparin treatment). Heparin treatment was administered for 3–5 days; patients with a presumably higher risk of thrombosis (ie, stents placed in long lesions, occlusions, or popliteal arteries) received intravenous anticoagulation therapy for the entire 5-day period. In addition, aspirin (100 mg) was administered orally every day to prevent platelet aggregation, thus initiating lifelong daily use of aspirin by the patient. The two patients in whom stents were placed in bypass graft anastomoses received coumadin for anticoagulation during the first 6 months after stent placement. The clinical follow-up period was 1–72 months.

Clinical symptoms before and after treatment were determined with the classification by Fontaine for painless walking distance. Clinical success was defined according to the guidelines of the Society of Cardiovascular and Interventional Radiology (4,5): relief or substantial improvement of symptoms (increase in painless walking distance of one Fontaine stage or more [eg, from stage IIb to IIa or from stage III to IIb]), increase in the ankle-brachial index of at least 0.15, and/or normalization of segmental pulse quality. The pulse quality and Doppler sonographic ankle-brachial index were determined before treatment; at 3 days and 3, 6, and 12 months after implantation; and finally at annual intervals. Follow-up digital subtraction angiography was performed when clinical symptoms deteriorated substantially (eg, from Fontaine stage I to IIa or from IIa to IIb or within one Fontaine stage from a painless walking distance of 2,000 m to 500 m), and/or the ankle-brachial index decreased more than 0.15 during the follow-up period. An occluded stent or a stenosis with more than 50% lumen obstruction were considered stent restenosis. When the ankle-brachial index, clinical symptoms, and pulse status did not change during follow-up compared with data obtained after intervention, the stent was considered patent.

Statistical Analysis

Risk factors analyzed were the type of lesion treated with a stent (primary diagnosis of stenosis vs occlusion), length of the underlying original lesion (≤4 cm vs >4 cm), length of the stent used to treat residual stenosis after PTA (≤4 cm vs >4 cm), runoff status (good vs poor femoral runoff), anatomic localization of the lesion with the stent (common femoral artery and the proximal and middle third of the superficial femoral artery vs distal femoral and popliteal arteries), and restenosis after previous PTA (secondary vs de novo lesion).

The frequency of acute stent thrombosis was determined for each risk group, and comparison between the groups was performed with the χ^2 test (6).

Long-term results were analyzed with the Kaplan-Meier method (7) to determine cumulative patency rates. Patency rates were expressed as the percentage ± standard deviation and were determined for the different risk groups. Statistical comparison was performed with the log rank test (8).

Multivariate analysis was performed by means of log-linear analysis to determine the predictive value of several risk factors for initial clinical results and long-term success or failure (9) in simultaneous consideration of the interactions between the single risk factors.

RESULTS

Technical Results

Stents were implanted successfully in all patients. The length of the lesion in which a stent was placed was 4 cm or less in 59 patients and greater than 4 cm in 21 patients.

Incomplete stent expansion due to a rigid vessel wall was observed in two patients; however, residual stenosis was 10% in these patients. These stenoses were not considered hemodynamically significant, however, because the patients showed clinical improvement indicative of a successful procedure.

No cases of stent collapse and/or compression were observed during the follow-up period in any of the patients.

Primary Clinical Results

In three patients, the postprocedural ankle-brachial index could not be measured exactly because of medial sclerosis, and in five patients the ankle-brachial index was not measured because of ongoing local treatment of peripheral ulcers. In the 72 patients in whom the ankle-brachial index was measured, the mean ankle-brachial index improved by more than 0.15, from 0.51 before the procedure (range, 0.00–0.95) to 0.85 after the procedure (range, 0.52–1.03) ($P < .05$).

Postprocedural improvement in clinical symptoms (increase in painless walking distance of at least one Fontaine stage) was noted in 70 (88%) patients. In nine (11%) patients, the Fontaine stage remained unchanged, including four patients with early stent thrombosis and five patients with peripheral ulcers for which local treatment was still necessary. These patients also showed an increase in painless walking distance immediately after intervention, however, but remained categorized in Fontaine stage IV as long as peripheral ulcers were still present (Fig 2). After stent implantation, 56 (70%) patients had an unlimited painless walking distance (stage I), 10 (12%) patients were classified as stage IIa, and six (8%) patients were classified as stage IIb. Five (6%) patients were classified as stage III and three (4%) patients remained at stage IV (Fig 3).

With stratification of the initial clinical results to the risk factors (lesion type, stent length, anatomic location, runoff status, de novo or secondary lesion), multivariate analysis revealed that only stent length was a suitable factor predictive of successful treatment (partial association, $P = .02$). Of 59 patients with short stents (≤4 cm), 46 (78%) achieved stage I painless walking distance, but only 10 (48%) of the 21 patients with stents longer than 4 cm achieved stage I painless walking distance.

Clinical Complications

Complications at the puncture site occurred in four (5%) patients. Treatment was necessary in three (4%) patients.

In two patients, a pseudoaneurysm developed at the femoral puncture site. One of these patients underwent surgery. In the other patient, compression performed with color Doppler sonographic guidance was unsuccessful, and percutaneous coil embolization was then performed successfully.

In two patients in whom puncture of the popliteal artery was performed without sonographic guidance, an arteriovenous fistula developed. One of these patients underwent surgery. In the other patient, the fistula was tiny and clinically inapparent; therefore, no therapy was administered. During 60 months of follow-up, the fistula did not change size or occlude spontaneously.

Distal embolization of thrombus or plaque material was found in eight (10%) patients; this complication occurred only in patients with long occlusions. In five of these eight patients, recanalization of the occluded lesion was achieved with local fibrinolysis; in three patients, only PTA was performed for recanalization. Successful treatment of distal embolization included local fibrinolysis ($n = 4$), aspiration thrombectomy ($n = 1$), local fibrinolysis combined with aspiration thrombectomy ($n = 1$), surgical thrombectomy ($n = 1$), and no therapy ($n = 1$).

The overall percentage of procedure-related complications necessitating surgery was 4% (three of 80 patients). The overall percentage of complications for which any therapy was necessary was 12% (10 of 80 patients).

Thrombotic stent occlusion occurred within the first 10 days after stent placement in four (5%) patients. The occlusion was treated by means of local fibrinolysis in three patients. In one of these patients, stent thrombosis occurred 1 hour after stent implantation while the patient was still in the radiology suite undergoing PTA of a lesion in the contralateral limb. In this patient, thrombosis was caused by incomplete coverage of the lesion, with an intimal dissection present distal to the stent; therefore, implantation of a second stent was necessary after fibrinolysis. Another patient later underwent surgical thrombectomy for treatment of a repeated reocclusion. In the fourth patient, percutaneous stent retrieval was performed after repeated stent thrombosis because of arterial spasm.

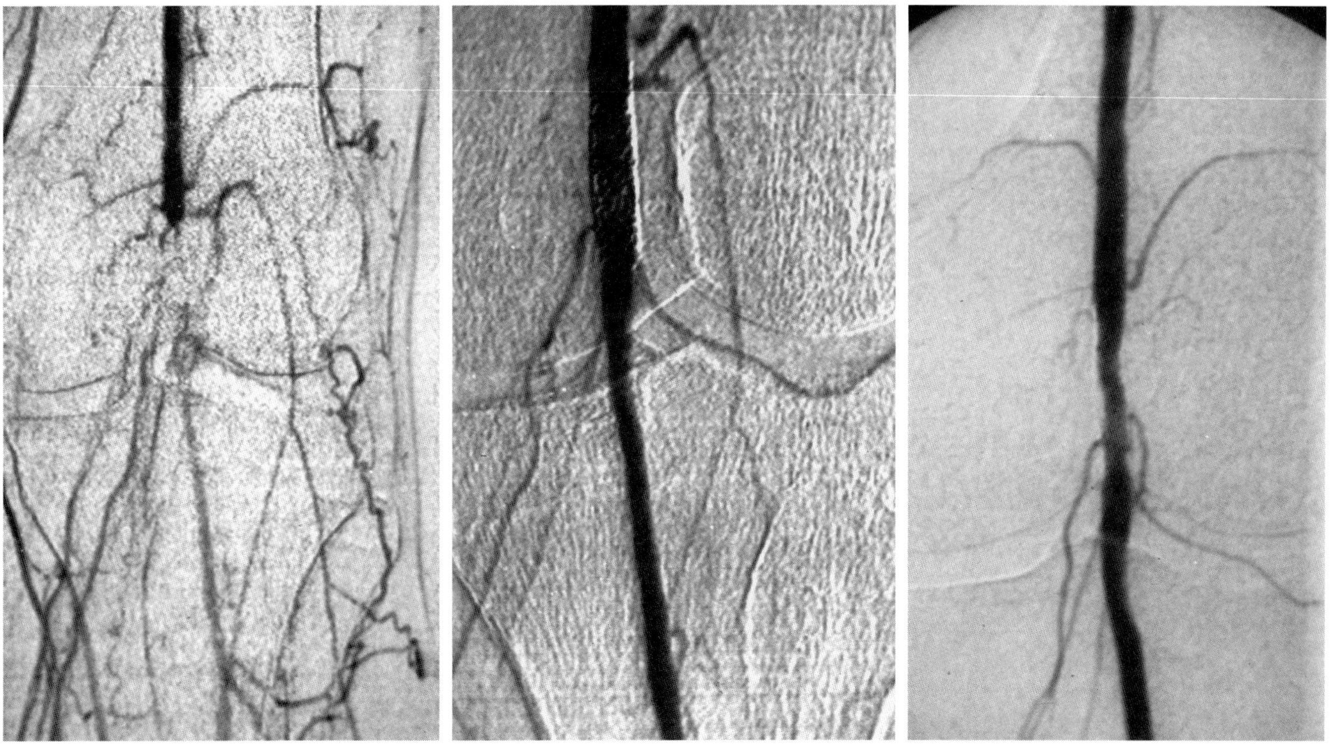

a. b. c.

Figure 2. Images obtained in a 65-year-old man with severe claudication and necrosis of the second toe. **(a)** Angiogram shows a 7-cm-long occlusion of the left popliteal artery. **(b)** Repeated balloon dilations failed and resulted in a 1.5-cm-long residual stenosis. A 2-cm-long, 5-mm-diameter stent was implanted. Angiogram obtained immediately after the procedure demonstrates a widely patent vessel. **(c)** The second toe was amputated 2 days after stent implantation, the surgical wound healed without problems, and the patient achieved an unlimited painless walking distance. Intravenous digital subtraction angiogram obtained at 48-month follow-up shows stent patency with mild neointimal hyperplasia. The patient was free of clinical symptoms.

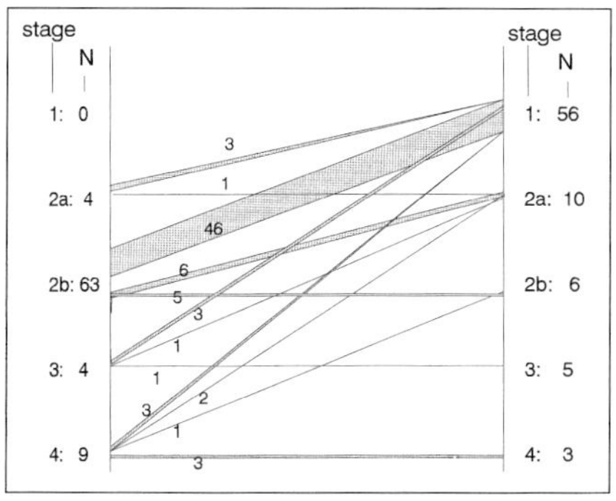

Figure 3. Diagram shows the clinical symptoms according to the classification by Fontaine in all patients before (left) and after (right) stent therapy. N = number of patients.

The frequency of early stent thrombosis was statistically significantly higher in areas longer than 4 cm in which stents were placed (three [14%] of 21 patients) versus areas with stents 4 cm or shorter (one (2%) of 59 patients [χ^2 test, $P < .05$]). Stent thrombosis was also observed more frequently in patients with previous arterial occlusion (three [6%] of 47 patients) than in patients with previous arterial stenosis (one [3%] of 33 patients); however, this difference was not statistically significant. Because most of the long lesions were arterial occlusions and the frequency of stent thrombosis was low and statistical subgroups were small, it could not be proved in our study which of the two risk factors (lesion type or lesion length) was more predictive of stent failure.

Follow-up and Long-term Results

Follow-up examinations were performed in 68 (85%) patients up to the time of this writing. The longest follow-up period after stent implantation was 72 months (mean, 12 months). All 68 patients underwent clinical follow-up; in 21 patients stent patency was monitored with duplex sonography. Angiographic follow-up was performed in 40 of the 68 patients (arteriography in 33 patients and intravenous digital subtraction angiography in seven patients). In 30 of the 40 patients, angiographic follow-up was indicated because of deterioration of clinical symptoms and the ankle-brachial index in the treated limb. The other 10 patients reported clinical symptoms in the untreated contralateral limb and therefore underwent angiography. At that time, the treated limb was also followed up angiographically. Stent restenosis (>50% lumen obstruction) or reocclusion proved at angiography occurred in 25 patients 2–72 months after implantation. This number included the two patients in whom stents were placed in bypass anastomoses, which reoccluded at 13 and 25 months after stent implantation, respectively. Five patients with clinical deterioration in the limb in which stents were placed had newly developed lesions located more proximal or distal to the stent. Six patients died during the follow-up period; none of the deaths were attributable to procedure-related early or late complications.

Figure 4 shows results of life-table analysis performed with the Kaplan-Meier method to determine patency rates. According to the standards proposed by Rutherford and Becker (4), patients with early clinical failure such as acute thrombotic stent occlusions were included in the estimation of patency rates.

For the total cohort of patients, the 1-year primary patency rate was 76% ± 5.5, the 2-year primary patency rate was 51% ± 8.3, and the 3-year primary patency rate was 48% ± 10.6 (Fig 4a).

The 2-year primary patency rate

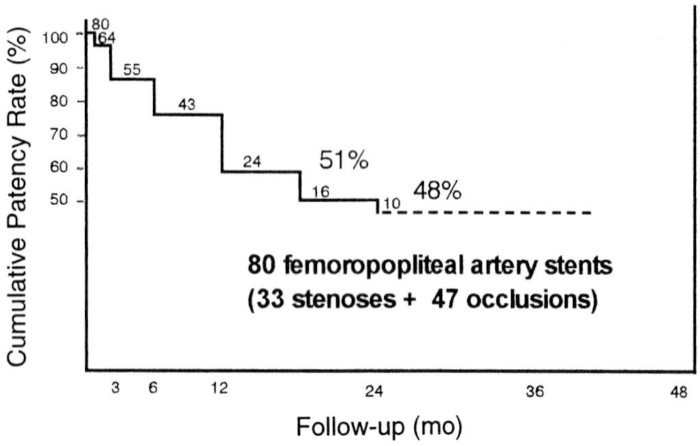

a.

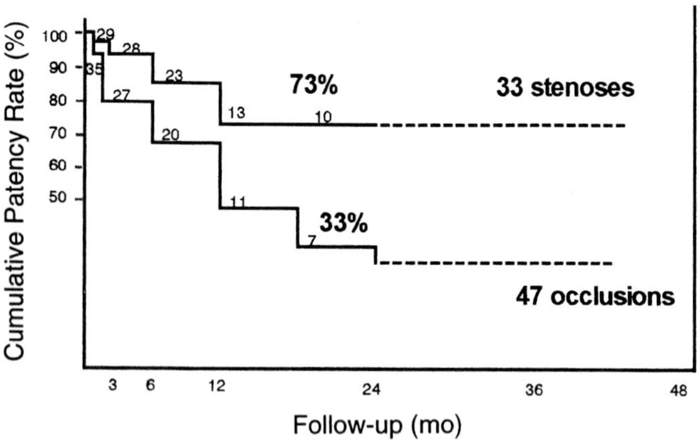

b.

Figure 4. Graphs show primary cumulative patency rates for **(a)** 80 femoropopliteal arteries in which stents were placed, **(b)** 33 treated stenoses and 47 treated occlusions, and **(c)** 59 stents 4 cm or shorter and 21 stents longer than 4 cm. Patency rates were determined with Kaplan-Meier life-table analysis and are reported as the percentage ± standard error. Solid lines indicate estimated patency rates with a standard error less than 10%, and dotted lines indicate patency rates with a standard error greater than 10%. Numbers at each interval indicate the number of patients examined in that interval.

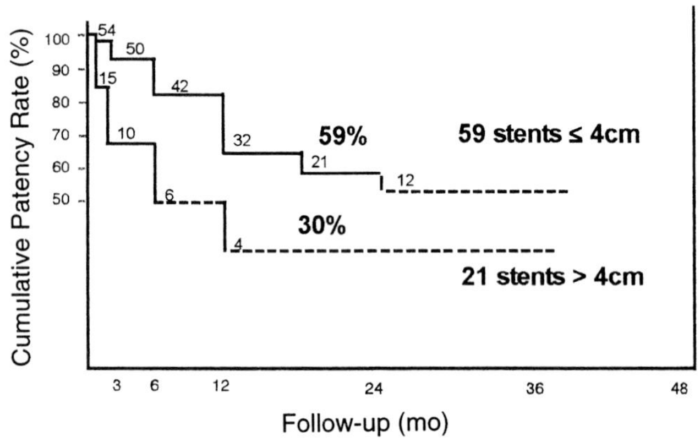

c.

was better for treated stenoses (73% ± 11.2) than that for treated occlusions (33% ± 9.9); this difference was statistically significant (log rank test, $P < .01$) (Fig 4b).

The 2-year primary patency rate was also statistically significantly better in stents 4 cm or shorter (59% ± 8.3) versus that for stents longer than 4 cm (30% ± 18.2; log rank test, $P < .05$) (Fig 4c).

For de novo lesions, the 2-year primary patency rate was 59% ± 8.6 versus 29% ± 12.1 for secondary lesions; however, this difference was not statistically significant.

With regard to length of the underlying lesion, the 2-year primary patency rate was 61% ± 10.6 for lesions 4 cm or shorter and 39% ± 12.6 for lesions longer than 4 cm; this difference was not statistically significant. In addition, there was no statistically significant difference between patency rates according to runoff and anatomic localization. The 2-year primary patency rate was 55% ± 11.1 for patients with good runoff status 45% ± 12.8 for patients with poor runoff status. In the group of patients with a stent placed in the common femoral artery or the proximal or middle third of the superficial femoral artery, the 2-year primary patency rate was 57% ± 12.5; for patients with stents located in the distal third of the superficial femoral artery or the popliteal artery, the 2-year primary patency rate was 45% ± 11.0.

Primary patency of stents of the older design and that of stents of the new design did not differ statistically significantly.

The restenosis rate was determined for stents located in the common femoral or the popliteal artery. These stents were subjected to possible bending movement because they were placed over articular joints. Restenosis occurred in three (38%) of eight stents placed in the common femoral artery (two of four occlusions and one of four stenoses) and five (26%) of 19 popliteal artery stents (five of 12 occlusions and zero of seven stenoses). Conversely, restenosis occurred in 21 (40%) of 53 stents located in other superficial femoral arteries not situated near articular joints. At statistical evaluation, restenosis rates were not different from each other.

The restenosis rate was also determined in 14 patients in whom restenosis after previous PTA was the indication for stent placement. Stent restenosis occurred in eight (57%) of 14 patients. Compared with the restenosis rate of lesions treated for the first time (17 of 66 patients, 26%), this difference was statistically significant (χ^2 test, $P < .05$).

On the basis of multivariate analysis in which the interactions between the risk factors was considered, the restenosis rate was influenced not only by the type of lesion (stenotic vs occluded lesion and de novo lesion vs restenotic lesion after previous PTA) but also by stent length and the quality of runoff, the latter two risk factors showing a strong correlation (partial association, $P = .041$). In lesions with longer stents, the frequency of restenosis was not dependent on the type of lesion, whereas in short stents the risk of restenosis was lower in segments with stenosis than in segments with occlusion. Considering the interaction between risk factors, stent length greater than 4 cm proved to be the most predictive factor for restenosis within the first 12 months after stent implantation (partial association: $P = .005$ [6 months] and $P = .015$ [12 months], respectively). For the long term, the type of lesion proved to be of major importance; totally occluded segments demonstrated the higher risk for stent restenosis (partial association, $P = .05$ [24 months] and $P = .045$ [36 months], respectively).

DISCUSSION

PTA was the first and is the most accepted interventional method for the treatment of femoropopliteal lesions, and extensive long-term studies were performed to determine several risk factors associated with restenosis after PTA. For PTA of femoropopliteal stenoses and occlusions, Matsi et al (10) reported a 3-year primary patency rate of 42% overall and of 63% in a group of selected patients. Johnston et al (11) reported a 2-year primary patency rate of 53% for all dilated femoropopliteal arteries and a 3-year rate of about 50%. In low-risk lesions, the 3-year patency rate can reach 78% (12); in high-risk lesions this patency rate can even decrease to less than 30% (13,14). The higher frequency of restenosis after PTA was found to be associated with treated occlusions, long lesions, small-diameter vessels, and poor runoff status (10–14). These factors were also found to increase the risk of stent failure. This was proved in our study and in previous studies, as well as in studies in which different stent designs were used (15–17). Because most of the long lesions were arterial occlusions and the frequency of stent thrombosis was low and statistical subgroups were small, it could not be proved in our study which of the two risk factors (lesion type or lesion length) was more predictive of stent failure.

The results of our study compare well with those of studies in which other types of stents were used. In our study, the 2-year primary patency rate was 73% for stents placed for treatment of stenosis. Liermann et al (17) reported a primary patency rate of 82% after 18 months with implantation of tantalum stents in femoropopliteal stenoses. In a study in which the Wallstent (Schneider Europe, Zürich, Switzerland) was used in a group of patients with mainly short lesions and stenoses, the 1–2-year primary patency rate was 76% (18). Henry et al (15) reported a 4-year primary patency rate of 80% in femoral artery stenoses treated with the Palmaz stent (Johnson & Johnson Interventional Systems, Warren, NJ).

Comparison of results from different studies is limited owing to different patient cohorts and criteria for assessment of stent patency. However, impaired mid- and long-term stent patency in high-risk lesions seems to be a common phenomenon. Success rates are less favorable for femoropopliteal occlusions, long lesions, small-diameter vessels, and secondary lesions. In our study, 2-year stent patency decreased to 32% in occlusions and was 31% in lesions in which longer stents were placed. Liermann et al (17) reported a 19-month primary patency rate of 60% for occlusions and a lower patency rate for stents placed in the distal portion of the superficial femoral artery and the popliteal artery than that for stents placed in the proximal portion of the superficial femoral artery. In a study in which the Wallstent was used (19), the 1-year primary patency rate was 49% in a small series of patients, most of whom had occlusions. In another small series in which the Wallstent was used, Zollikofer et al (20) reported a high rate of early thrombosis and a restenosis rate of 77% in patients with long lesions and occlusions. In the study of Henry et al (15) in which the Palmaz stent was used, the 4-year patency rate was only 39% for treated occlusions and 44% for small-diameter vessels such as the lower portion of the superficial femoral artery and the popliteal artery.

Because the success rate in treated occlusions is less favorable, Henry et al (15) proposed that total occlusions should be covered more completely with stents to decrease primary restenosis rates. In contrast, we proved in our study that stent patency decreases with the length of the segment with a stent. The prognostic value of the length of the underlying lesion did not appear to be particularly important, since the difference in patency rates between short and long lesions was less pronounced. Our recommendation, therefore, is to introduce as little stent material as possible, meaning that a stent should be placed only in the length of the residual stenosis after PTA. As a consequence, implantation of stents in the femoral artery should be recommended as a secondary treatment, although our own unpublished experience with implantation of stents in the iliac artery suggests that primary stent implantation may be justified in complex and ulcerative lesions to avoid peripheral embolization of plaque or thrombus material. A further indication for placement of stents in the femoropopliteal area as a primary treatment might be secondary lesions caused by restenosis after previous PTA. According to our observations and to those of other investigators (17), the risk of restenosis is higher in those lesions.

The response-to-injury theory states that the more stress applied to the vessel wall, the higher the proliferative response will be and reaction of the vascular wall could possibly be diminished after stent placement as a primary treatment. This theory is supported by experimental data of Cwikiel et al (21) and by early results of a clinical study comparing primary stent implantation and PTA in short de novo lesions (22).

Among different stent designs, each type of stent has been reported to have certain advantages and disadvantages, compared with other stents. A stent made of stainless steel or tantalum may undergo external plastic deformation, whereas a nitinol stent is more elastic. A balloon-expandable stent may cause less sustained stress to the vessel wall after adjusted initial placement than a self-expandable stent that exerts continuous pressure on the vessel wall until it reaches the preset maximum diameter; however, this observation is speculative (23). A rigid stent may have a higher radial force than a flexible stent. Conversely, contradictory results have been published with regard to occurrence of medial atrophy with use of rigid and flexible stents in animal experiments (24,25), and no difference was found between rigid and flexible stents with regard to occurrence of neointimal hyperplasia (25).

The flexible tantalum stent used in our study revealed some valuable advantages. Since this stent is made of tantalum, it is well depicted with fluoroscopy and does not interfere with magnetic resonance imaging, which might be necessary in some patients. The radiopacity of the tantalum stent enables easy imaging-guided placement; ease of placement is supported by the fact that only minimal shortening occurs during stent expansion. With the various stent lengths available (2, 4, or 8 cm), the amount of stent material to be implanted can be adjusted to the length of the lesion, thus reducing the number of overlapping stents in long lesions.

The flexibility of the knitted tantalum stent used in our study enables introduction of even a long stent through a contralateral artery (used in the crossover method); this method has been necessary in some patients. The flexibility of the stent also enabled placement in arteries leading over articular joints (eg, common femoral and popliteal arteries), although this type of placement is not usually recommended because of possible compression during joint flexion, inducing arterial elongation and kinking. However, stent compression was not observed in our study. With the small number of patients in whom stents were placed in the common femoral or popliteal arteries, the rates of early stent thrombosis or of restenosis were not different from those at other anatomic sites. In contrast, some patients have experienced good long-term patency in this anatomic region thus far.

In general, the frequency of restenosis due to intimal hyperplasia remains a major problem after stent implantation. In a further attempt to overcome these limitations, a polyester-covered nitinol stent (Cragg Endopro; Meditech/Boston Scientific) was developed with the purpose of preventing proliferation of smooth muscle cells through the stent mesh into the arterial lumen. Late restenosis caused by intimal hyperplasia could not be avoided and occurred especially at the stent ends (26–28). This phenomenon had also been observed previously in experimental studies in which covered stent-grafts were used (29). In femoropopliteal occlusions treated with the polyester-covered nitinol stent, reocclusion rates of 30%–43% were reported for the first 12–18 months after implantation (26,27, 30,31).

In the peri- and early postprocedural periods, the rate of acute stent failure due to early stent thrombosis can be decreased by a thoroughly administered anticoagulation regimen combined with antiplatelet treatment; 1–3 days of intravenous heparin administration and orally administered aspirin are standard therapy in many institutions thus far. Warfarin may be suitable to help decrease the occurrence of thrombotic stent occlusion (16); however, according to our unpublished experience, the risk of hemorrhagic complications must be considered. Clinical studies of new antiplatelet drugs such as ticlopidine hydrochloride have shown progress in the area of medical treatment (32,33); however, clinical side effects restrict the duration of therapy. In another ongoing study, a 3-week regimen of anticoagulation with use of reviparin sodium, a low-molecular-weight heparin, has been performed to prevent early thrombotic stent occlusion; the first clinical results are promising (34). Whether use of reviparin sodium can also influence the rate of late restenosis due to intimal hyperplasia must be determined.

Local therapy of the arterial site in which a stent was placed may be another method of prevention of stent restenosis. Local irradiation of femoropopliteal arteries with the afterloading technique has been described (35) with encouraging results. Another type of local therapy involves use of drug-releasing stents, which are being developed and tested with promising results (36).

Our long-term results of stent therapy in the femoropopliteal area suggest that this technique remains a valuable treatment to overcome the limitations of PTA. In arterial stenoses, long-term success of stent therapy is favorable compared with the results of PTA alone. In cases of arterial occlusions, long lesions, and restenotic lesions, long-term success is impaired by a high rate of restenosis. Therefore, in cases of high-risk lesions, the decision to perform stent placement and the technique used should be considered carefully. Conversely, stent therapy remains a possible primary treatment that does not adversely affect secondary or tertiary treatment if necessary (eg, repeat PTA in cases of restenosis, thrombolysis, or surgical procedures) and is a valuable alternative for patients in whom surgery is not recommended.

In conclusion, the success of stent therapy in general does not seem to depend on the stent design used, although one design may be more advantageous in a certain lesion than another design. In contrast, the characteristics of the underlying lesion to be treated and the state of atherosclerotic disease (characterized by lesion type, lesion length, and runoff status) and other predisposing factors seem to play a major role in long-term success of stent therapy. Stent therapy should therefore be accompanied by complex medical treatment. To eventually decrease further systemic progression of atherosclerotic disease, risk factors for vascular disease such as smoking, arterial hypertension, hypercholesterolemia, diabetes, and hypercoagulability should be minimized. ■

References

1. Alexander K, Brunner U, Ehringer H. Krankheiten der gefässe. In: Siegenthaler W, Kaufmann W, Hornbostel H, Waller HD, eds. Lehrbuch der inneren medizin. Stuttgart, Germany: Verlag, 1992; 184–185.
2. Strecker EP, Liermann D, Barth KH, et al. Expandable tubular stents for the treatment of arterial occlusive diseases: experimental and clinical results—work in progress. Radiology 1990; 175:97–102.
3. Strecker EP, Kuhn FP, Liermann D, et al. Strecker flexible tantalum stent. In: Kim D, Orron DE, eds. Peripheral vascular imaging and intervention. St Louis, Mo: Mosby–Year Book, 1992; 541–552.
4. Rutherford RB, Becker GJ. Standards for evaluating and reporting the results of surgical and percutaneous therapy for peripheral artery disease. JVIR 1991; 2:169–174.
5. Standards of Practice Committee of the Society of Cardiovascular and Interventional Radiology. Guidelines for percutaneous transluminal angioplasty. Radiology 1990; 177:619–626.
6. Sachs L. Angewandte statistik. Berlin, Germany: Springer-Verlag, 1992; 269.
7. Kaplan EL, Meier P. Nonparametric estimation from incomplete observations. J Am Stat Assoc 1958; 53:457–481.
8. Peto R, Peto J. Asymptotically efficient rank invariant procedures. J R Stat Soc 1972; 135:185–207.
9. Bishop YMM, Fienberg SE, Holland PW. Discrete multivariate analysis. Cambridge, Mass: MIT Press, 1975.
10. Matsi PJ, Manninen HI, Vanninen RL, et al. Femoropopliteal angioplasty in patients with claudication: primary and secondary patency in 140 limbs with 1–3-year follow-up. Radiology 1994; 191:727–733.
11. Johnston KW, Rae M, Hogg-Johnston SA, et al. Five-year results of a prospective study of percutaneous transluminal angioplasty. Ann Surg 1987; 206:403–412.
12. Jeans WD, Armstrong S, Cole SEA, Horrocks M, Baird RN. Fate of patients undergoing transluminal angioplasty for lower-limb ischemia. Radiology 1990; 177: 559–564.
13. Johnston KW. Femoral and popliteal arteries: reanalysis of results of balloon angioplasty. Radiology 1992; 183:767–771.
14. Strunk H, Clouse M, Stokes K, Thelen M. Früh-und spätergebnisse der perkutanen transluminalen angioplastie (PTA) beim diabetiker. ROFO 1991; 154:315–320.
15. Henry M, Amor M, Ethevenot G, et al. Palmaz stent placement in iliac and femoropopliteal arteries: primary and secondary patency in 310 patients with 2–4-year follow-up. Radiology 1995; 1967:167–174.
16. Thornton M, Grüntzig A, Hollman J. Coumadin and aspirin in the prevention of recurrence rate after successful coronary angioplasty. Circulation 1984; 69:721–727.
17. Liermann D, Strecker EP, Peters J. The Strecker stent: indications and results in iliac and femoropopliteal arteries. Cardiovasc Intervent Radiol 1992; 15:298–305.
18. Rousseau H, Raillat C, Joffre F, et al. Treatment of femoropopliteal stenoses by means of self-expandable endoprostheses: midterm results. Radiology 1989; 172:961–964.
19. Sapoval MR, Long AL, Raynaud AC, Beyssen BM, Fiessinger JN, Gaux JC. Femoropopliteal stent placement: long-term results. Radiology 1992; 184:833–839.
20. Zollikofer CL, Antonucci F, Pfyffer M, et al. Arterial stent placement with use of the Wallstent: midterm results of clinical experience. Radiology 1991; 179:449–456.
21. Cwikiel W, Harnek J, Zoucas E, Stenram U. Comparison of effects of the self-expandable nitinol Strecker stent vs angioplasty on the normal artery: an experimental study in pigs. Cardiovasc Intervent Radiol 1995; 18(suppl):90.
22. Richter GM, Roeren TK, Simon C. First report on long-term results of the randomized European femoral stent versus angioplasty trial (abstr). JVIR 1996; 7:196.
23. Shapiro MJ, Levin DC. Percutaneous femoropopliteal graft placement: is this the next step? Radiology 1993; 187:618–619.
24. Barth KH, Virmani R, Froelich J, et al. Paired comparison of vascular wall reactions to Palmaz stents, Strecker tantalum stents, and Wallstents in canine iliac and femoral arteries. Circulation 1996; 93:2161–2169.
25. Schürmann K, Vorwerk D, Kulisch A, et al. Neointimal hyperplasia in low-profile nitinol stents, Palmaz stents, and Wallstents: a comparative experimental study. Cardiovasc Intervent Radiol 1996; 19:248–254.
26. Blum U, Flügel P, Ebert S, et al. Stent-grafting for stenotic/occlusive lesions of femoropopliteal arteries. Presented at the 38th Annual World Congress of the International College of Angiology, Cologne, Germany, 1996.

27. Link J, Müller-Hülsbeck S, Brossmann J, Schwarzenberg H, Steffens JC, Heller M. Ummantelte stents bei oberschenkelarterienverschlüssen: ein erfahrungsbericht nach 2-jähriger anwendung (abstr). ROFO 1996; 164:107.
28. Henry M, Amor M, Cragg A, et al. Occlusive and aneurysmal peripheral arterial disease: assessment of a stent-graft system. Radiology 1996; 201:717–724.
29. Strecker EP, Gabelmann A. Coated stents for the prevention of intimal hyperplasia after stent implantation (abstr). Cardiovasc Intervent Radiol 1996; 19(suppl):81.
30. Zeitler E. Experience with the Cragg Endopro stent in the superficial femoral artery (abstr). Cardiovasc Intervent Radiol 1994; 17(suppl):558.
31. Henry M. Les endoprothèses au niveau des artères fémorales et poplitées. Actual Vasc Int 1996; 36:6–14.
32. Schömig A, Neumann FJ, Kastrati A, et al. A randomized comparison of antiplatelet and anticoagulant therapy after the placement of coronary-artery stents. N Engl J Med 1996; 334:1084–1089.
33. Karrillon GJ, Morice MC, Benveniste E, et al. Intracoronary stent implantation without ultrasound guidance and with replacement of conventional anticoagulation by antiplatelet therapy: 30-day clinical outcome of the French multicenter registry. Circulation 1996; 94:1519–1527.
34. Strecker EP, Göttmann D, Vetter S, Boos I. Low molecular weight heparin (reviparin) for the prevention of restenosis after femoropopliteal stent implantation (abstr). Cardiovasc Intervent Radiol 1996; 19(suppl):107.
35. Liermann D, Herrmann G, Schopohl B, et al. Endovascular afterloading with 192 iridium HDR in the treatment of recurrent intimal hyperplasia in stented peripheral arteries. In: Liermann D, ed. Stents: state of the art and future developments. Morin Heights, Quebec, Canada: Polyscience, 1995; 299–314.
36. Strecker EP, Gabelmann A. Prevention of intimal hyperplasia after stent implantation by drug releasing stents: an experimental study (abstr). Cardiovasc Intervent Radiol 1995; 18(suppl):103.

Ray's Days

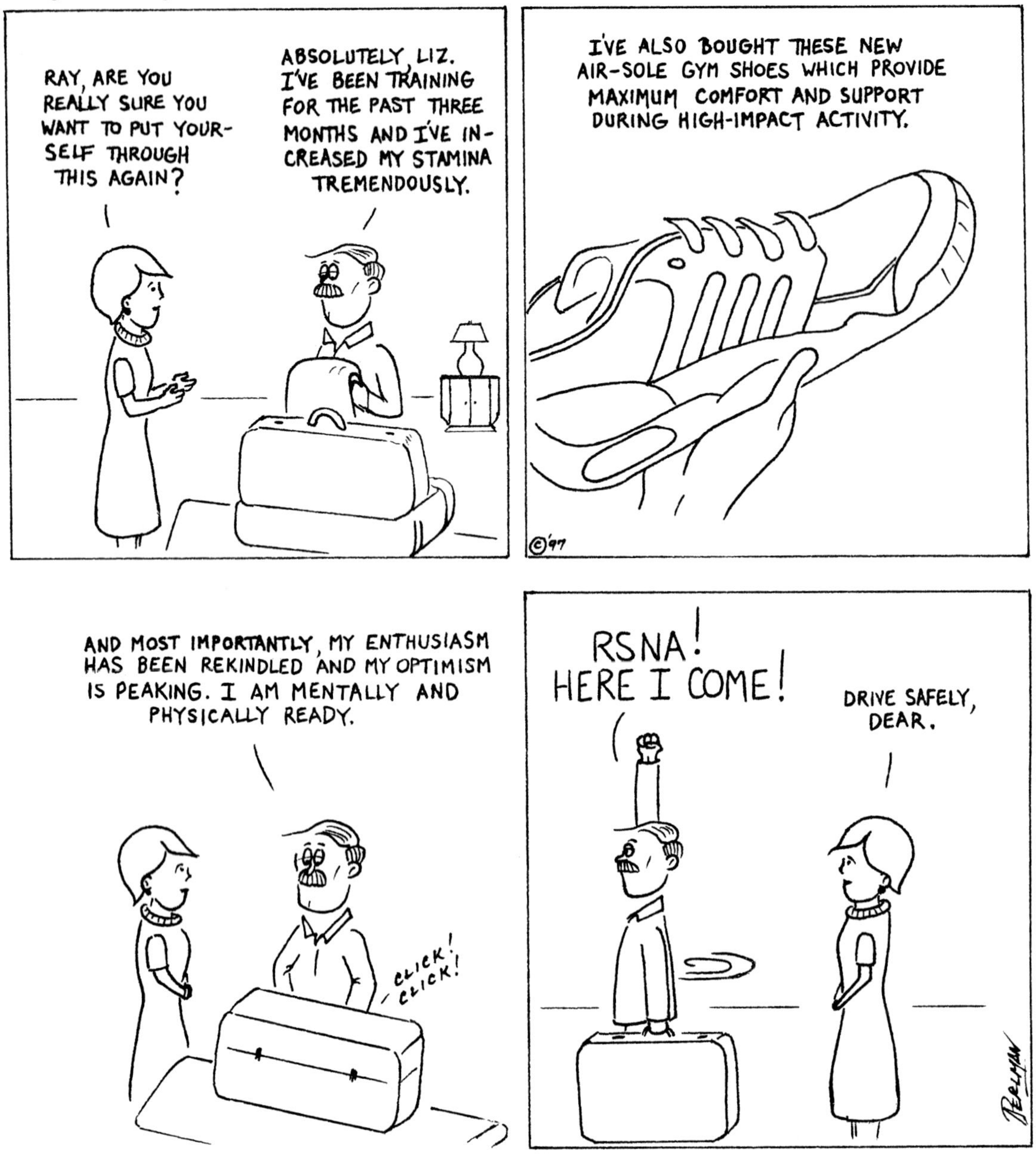

Steven J. Perlman, MD, Cincinnati, Ohio

Rafael Ruiz-Cruces, MD, PhD • Manuel Pérez-Martínez, PhD • Alberto Martín-Palanca, MD
Alberto Flores, MD • Javier Cristófol, MD • Manuel Martínez-Morillo, MD, PhD
Antonio Díez de los Ríos, PhD

Patient Dose in Radiologically Guided Interventional Vascular Procedures: Conventional versus Digital Systems[1]

PURPOSE: **To calculate the difference in the patient radiation dose in radiologically guided interventional vascular procedures between conventional and digital systems and to estimate the effective dose and the energy imparted with the digital system.**

MATERIALS AND METHODS: **A total of 318 procedures (in 318 patients) in 15 different examination groups were analyzed. The dose-area product was determined by using a transmission chamber fitted to an x-ray–tube light-beam diaphragm; the effective dose was determined by using software.**

RESULTS: **Urinary and biliary tract procedures showed small differences in the average dose-area product between conventional and digital systems. The dose-area products in the vascular procedures were higher with the digital than with the conventional system. The average effective dose and energy imparted were 0.88 mSv and 129 mJ, respectively, in the subcutaneous placement of a reservoir for analgesic administration and as much as 25.7 mSv and 829 mJ, respectively, in spermatic vein embolization.**

CONCLUSION: **The dose-area product was higher with the digital system than with the conventional system in 13 of the 15 groups. To reduce the patient dose in vascular interventional radiology procedures, the training of personnel and the frequent use of conventional fluoroscopy and low-dose imaging are required.**

Radiologically guided interventional vascular procedures and diagnostic vascular radiologic examinations have increased in number substantially during the past few years. These minimally invasive diagnostic and therapeutic procedures have experienced increased utilization because of the combination of diagnostic and therapeutic benefits. This has reduced the number of complicated surgical interventions but has increased the use of ionizing radiation (1).

In the past few years, interventional vascular procedures have been performed with conventional fluoroscopy and radiography. The equipment used has improved the quality of the images and has reduced the tube current owing to the incorporation of image intensifiers and TV monitors.

In contrast, radiography in the guidance of interventional vascular procedures has substantially progressed with digital imaging. In Europe, new digital imaging equipment coexists with traditional equipment (analog radiography). In the future, traditional equipment will be replaced by digital equipment, because traditional equipment requires a long exposure time, a high dependence on the grade of black-white contrast, and selection of the images after processing, whereas digital radiography has advantages such as easy storage, the ability to modify the images, rapid acquisition of the images, and rapid access to information (1).

Evaluation of the patient radiation dose in radiologically guided interventional vascular procedures in Spain requires measurement of the dose-area product and the surface dose in the most irradiated region by using thermoluminescence dosimeters. Some studies have evaluated the patient dose in interventional vascular procedures performed with both conventional and digital imaging (2,3). It is thought that digital procedures decrease the patient dose-area product. Plunkett and co-workers (3) observed that the total integral patient dose in patients who underwent cerebral digital subtraction angiography was one-third of that in patients who underwent conventional angiography owing to the reduction in fluoroscopy time. A later article (4) presented the patient dose in conventional angiography. In general, these doses (4) are lower than those in other digital subtraction angiographic studies (5).

Interventional vascular procedures and, above all, radiologic examinations are subject to quality assurance programs to evaluate the patient dose. This is a legal requirement in countries of Health Care Level I (6,7). Thus, the purpose of this research has been to evaluate the patient dose in inter-

Index terms: Dosimetry, 9*.126[2] • Radiations, exposure to patients and personnel, 9*.126 • Radiations, measurement, 9*.126

Radiology 1997; 205:385–393

[1] From the Department of Radiology and Medical Physics (R.R.C., M.P.M., M.M.M., A.D.d.l.R.) and the Radioprotection and Medical Physics Research Group (R.R.C., M.P.M., A.F., J.C., A.D.d.l.R.), School of Medicine, University of Málaga, Campus de Teatinos, s/n, 29071 Málaga, Spain; and the Department of Vascular and Interventional Radiology, Nuestra Señora Virgen de la Victoria University Hospital of Málaga, Málaga, Spain (A.M.P). Received February 28, 1997; revision requested April 3; revision received May 28; accepted June 30. Supported in part by project 94-1346 of the Sanitary Investigations Fund of the Ministerio de Sanidad of Spain and project 1030 of the Consolidated Groups of Research in Andalusia Autonomic Community. **Address reprint requests to** R.R.C.

[2] 9* indicates vascular system, location unspecified.

ventional vascular procedures at Nuestra Señora Virgen de la Victoria University Hospital of Málaga, Málaga, Spain. Our work was divided into two parts: first, to determine the difference in the dose-area product between patients who undergo conventional procedures and patients who undergo digital subtraction angiographic procedures and, second, to evaluate the organ dose, effective dose, energy imparted, and risk of fatal cancer in procedures performed with digital systems.

MATERIALS AND METHODS

In the interventional vascular radiology service of the Nuestra Señora Virgen de la Victoria University Hospital of Málaga, 7,643 examinations were performed in 7,643 patients from January 1991 to July 1996. An average of 1,273 patients per year underwent these examinations. Fifty percent of the examinations involved arteriography, usually arteriography of the lower limbs. The rest were interventional procedures, such as vascular endoprosthesis placement, angioplasty, nephrostomy, ureteral dilation, percutaneous cholangiography with biliary drainage, biliary drainage, and embolization of the spermatic vein.

Dosimetric Method

The dose-area product was determined by using a Diamentor M2 transmission chamber (PTW, Freiburg, Germany) fitted to an x-ray–tube light-beam diaphragm. The transmission chamber is a combination of a large-area ionization chamber and a control unit that integrates the air kerma over the entire area of the x-ray beam. This equipment was calibrated by the PTW service group before this research task was started. The radiation dose calculated from the exposure measured with a radiation-output evaluator (NERO [Noninvasive Evaluator of Radiation Output] 6000M; Victoreen, Cleveland, Ohio) was in concordance with the dose calculated with the transmission-chamber dose-area product. The energy response of this chamber was flat within ±5% for applied tube potentials between 50 and 100 kVp.

To calculate the organ dose (8), 248 thermoluminescence dosimeters (TLD-100; Harshaw-Bicron, Wermelskirchen, Germany) made of lithium fluoride, magnesium, and titanium were used; these were placed on the surface of the skin. This part of the research was conducted only with the digital system. For "complex" examinations (those with fluoroscopy and radiography), we used nine thermoluminescence dosimeters in each woman and six thermoluminescence dosimeters in each man, as proposed by Padovani and co-workers (8); dosimeters were located in the following areas: one in the thyroid zone; two in the pectoral zone (on the breasts in women); two in the scapular zone; two on the iliac fossa (in women); two in the lumbar zone over the ovaries (in women); and one on a testicle (in men). The method of Padovani and co-workers allows only approximate estimation of the organ dose in five organs: thyroid, breast, lung, ovary, and testis. This method is not valid for calculating the dose in other organs (the organ dose was calculated in a total of 29 organs with the EFF-DOSE software [version 1.02; National Board of Health, National Institute of Radiation Hygiene, Bronshoj, Denmark]). The method of Padovani and co-workers is not valid for estimating the entrance surface dose in complex examinations.

For interventional vascular procedures, which involve considerably long fluoroscopic examinations and variations in beam direction and field size, the entrance surface dose cannot be conveniently measured with thermoluminescence dosimeters. The organ dose calculated with the thermoluminescence dosimeters in the five organs was compared with the organ dose calculated with EFF-DOSE, which allowed us to estimate the effective dose with the weighting factors proposed in a 1994 United Kingdom National Radiological Protection Board report (9) and as suggested in a 1991 International Commission on Radiological Protection publication (10). In addition, EFF-DOSE was used to calculate the effective equivalent dose as per the method in a 1977 International Commission on Radiological Protection publication (11). The EFF-DOSE program is based on four parameters: kilovoltage, the total beam filtration of the x ray, the dose-area product, and the projections used.

The thermoluminescence dosimeters were read with a microprocessor-based thermoluminescence dosimeter reader (model 2800MI; Victoreen) in an atmosphere of inert nitrogen with a pureness of 99.9995%. The thermoluminescence dosimeters were annealed in a Theldo oven (PTW) before and after the reading; at the second annealing, the energy absorbed was released so that the dosimeter reading returned to its original state. The set of thermoluminescence dosimeters was calibrated by the Institute of Energy Techniques of the Polytechnic University of Barcelona, Barcelona, Spain. This is a center authorized by the European Community (Brussels, Belgium) to ensure the quality of radiographic examinations per the International Standards Organizations. After one standard irradiation, the thermoluminescence dosimeters were read and the readings were averaged. Thus, a correction factor for each dosimeter was assigned.

The energy imparted to the patient with the digital system can be calculated from the transmission-chamber reading (in gray · square centimeters) by using the factors given by Shrimpton and co-workers (12,13). In peripheral arteriography of the lower limbs, where the beam does not totally intercept the patient's body, we have considered 75% of the results given by the transmission chamber (14).

Finally, we calculated the risk of fatal cancer with the coefficient proposed in a 1991 International Commission on Radiological Protection report (10). The fatal cancer risk is 5×10^{-2} Sv^{-1} instead of the older value of 1.25×10^{-2} Sv^{-1} (11). The risk estimate has been averaged for all ages and sexes; consequently, the risk is overestimated in older patients.

Interventional Vascular Radiology Equipment

Conventional and digital radiology equipment for interventional vascular procedures.— An angiographic, radiographic, and fluoroscopic 45–100-kV imager (Angioskop-33; Siemens Medical Systems, Erlangen, Germany) with a high-frequency generator was used in conventional interventional vascular procedures. The target angle of the x-ray tube was 15°. The total beam filtration for the x-ray tube was 3.0-mm aluminum; the transmission chamber that we used added filtration of 0.5-mm aluminum. The total filtration was therefore equivalent to 3.5-mm aluminum. This equipment presents a 2.4–3.7 mm half-value layer for 60–100 kV.

The operating console (Polimat 100; Siemens Medical Systems) indicated the kilovoltage and milliamperage used in every procedure. These were 40–110 kV and 0.5–5.0 mA for fluoroscopy and 40–110 kV and 60–500 mA for radiography.

An image intensifier (on the Angioskop-33) was used. The 33-cm-diameter metallic intensifier has a titanium screen input surface that contained three circular fields of 33, 27, or 17 cm in diameter. This intensifier has a Sircam camera (Siemens Medical Systems). The radiologic images were obtained by using an indirect x ray with an image intensifier and 10 × 10-cm film. In the conventional system, the maximum dose per image was 75 μR (1.93×10^{-5} mC/kg), with a maximum of three images per second.

In 1995, a digital subtraction system (Digitron-3; Siemens Medical Systems) was added to the conventional angiographic, radiographic, and fluoroscopic equipment. With this equipment, the digital image is formed by using an analog-digital converter of 10 bits per pixel. The images were 256 × 256 pixels and 512 × 512 pixels.

The image intensifier used with the digital equipment was the same as that used with the conventional equipment; however, an additional digital television system (TV Videomed N system; Siemens Medical System) also was used. With the digital system, the image acquisition is not continuous but pulsed.

Table 1 shows the technical data for the digital system. With the digital system, several selectable doses or image-acquisition modes (low mode 1, low mode 2, high mode 1, high mode 2) are available and can be selected with the microprocessor. Digital subtraction angiographic systems can be used to perform fluoroscopy and radiography. The exposure can be produced with either fluoroscopy or radiogra-

Table 1
Technical Data for the Digital System

Parameters	Image-Acquisition Modes: Low Mode 1	Low Mode 2	High Mode 1	High Mode 2
Matrix	256 × 256	256 × 256	512 × 512	512 × 512
Maximum radiation time (sec)	50	50	25	25
Tube rating (kW)	9	9	11	11
Dose rate*				
Fluoroscopy (μR/sec)†				
Standard	20 (5.16)	20 (5.16)	20 (5.16)	20 (5.16)
High dose	40 (10.32)	40 (10.32)	40 (10.32)	40 (10.32)
Digital subtraction angiography (microroentgen per frame)‡	100 (25.8)	200 (51.6)	500 (129)	1,000 (258)
Pulsed radiography (microroentgen per frame)‡				
Two frames per second maximum pulse rate	34 (8.8)	68 (18)	170 (44)	340 (88)
Four frames per second maximum pulse rate	18 (4.6)	36 (9.3)	90 (23)	180 (46)
Six frames per second maximum pulse rate	7 (1.8)	14 (3.6)	35 (9.0)	70 (18)
Eight frames per second maximum pulse rate	5 (1.3)	10 (2.6)	25 (6.4)	50 (13)
Twelve frames per second maximum pulse rate	4 (1.0)	8 (2.1)	20 (5.2)	40 (10)
Twenty-five frames per second maximum pulse rate	1.8 (0.46)	3.6 (0.93)	9 (2.3)	18 (4.6)
Fifty frames per second maximum pulse rate	0.8 (0.21)	1.6 (0.41)	4 (1.0)	8 (2.1)

Note.—In conventional systems, the maximum dose per image was 75 μR (19 nC/kg), with a maximum of three images per second.
* The dose rate was measured at the image intensifier without the antiscatter grid.
† 20 μR/sec = 0.8 μR dose per video frame; 40 μR/sec = 1.6 μR per video frame. The numbers in parentheses are the dose rates in nanocoulombs per kilogram per second.
‡ The numbers in parentheses are the dose rates in nanocoulombs per kilogram per frame.

phy. The radiographic parameters of kilovoltage and milliamperage for digital system operation are set automatically by the control system (Digimatic Z115; Siemens Medical Systems) in the generator.

Conventional (standard) and digital (high-dose) fluoroscopic examinations were performed. No pulsed fluoroscopy was performed with this equipment.

Calibration of equipment.—The service group of Siemens Medical Systems calibrated the equipment monthly. In addition, the equipment was checked daily at each session by the radiologic protection service of the Nuestra Señora Virgen de la Victoria University Hospital by using the radiation-output evaluator. The National Institute of Standards and Technology (Gaithersburg, Md) had previously calibrated the radiation-output evaluator before this study.

Procedures

Each of 15 vascular and interventional procedures were performed in at least nine cases with conventional and with digital equipment (Table 2) for a total of 318 procedures. In each case, the following data were obtained: patient data, the dose-area product (in gray · square centimeter) measured in the transmission chamber, the technical parameters used in fluoroscopy and radiography, the thickness of the examined region, and the average source-to-skin distance. In addition, we read the thermoluminescence dosimeters used with the digital system, initially and subsequently, with the thermoluminescence dosimeter reader.

The same personnel of the interventional vascular radiology service of the university hospital performed all the procedures with both conventional and digital systems. The staff of this service consists of two interventional vascular radiologists, three nurses, and one nursing assistant.

Cerebral arteriography.—In each case in which it was performed, cerebral arteriography was thoroughly successful and depicted the area irrigated by the anterior, middle, and posterior cerebral arteries. The most frequent diagnosis was of a vascular intracranial abnormality (aneurysm, arteriovenous malformation, or tumoral vascularization). All procedures selected were performed via an artery for comparison of the dose from the conventional system with that from the digital system.

To calculate the organ dose (with factors from a 1991 International Commission on Radiological Protection report [11]) and the effective dose with EFF-DOSE, the dose-area product in the posteroanterior head projection and the dose-area product in the right lateral head projection were determined separately. The total effective dose was estimated by adding the two values.

Abdominal arteriography.—Different arteriographic examinations have been included in this group: celiac-mesenteric trunk angiography, hepatic arteriography, and renal arteriography, for which the irradiated regions were the same. There were differences from one patient to another in the radiologic techniques used, the duration of fluoroscopy, and the number of images obtained.

The posteroanterior abdominal projection was selected to evaluate the effective dose with EFF-DOSE, because the patient remains in the supine position on the radiologic table for this projection.

Lower-limb arteriography.—Arteriography of the lower limbs was the most common procedure in this work. It was performed in 30 patients. Conventional and digital methods were used in the femoral artery. Both methods radiate an area from the pelvis (distal aorta) to the distal third of the leg.

In interventional radiology, procedures such as angioplasty are frequently performed in the lower limbs, and it is possible to find differences in the radiologic technique, field, fluoroscopy time, and number of images obtained. In this research, all treatment procedures were performed with arteriography of the lower limbs to avoid distortion of the results.

To calculate the effective dose with EFF-DOSE in these procedures, the pelvis or anteroposterior colon was selected; the dose rate and the radiation beam (that intercepts the lower-limb zone) that is influenced in this zone were taken into account (14).

Biliary tract procedures.—Three procedures were analyzed: percutaneous cholangiography with biliary drainage, the extraction of biliary stones, and the placement of a prosthesis in the biliary route. The zone irradiated in these procedures was always the renal-hepatic zone. To calculate the effective dose with EFF-DOSE in the digital procedures, the posteroanterior kidney projection was selected with consideration of the common zone of irradiation (9, fig 6).

Urinary tract procedures.—The urinary tract was irradiated in four procedures: nephrostomy (the most common), renal catheterization, ureteral catheterization, and ureteral dilation. Fluoroscopy was centered on the kidney and the ureter. These procedures are the only ones in which an anteroposterior projection was used, owing to the prone position of the patient.

To calculate the organ dose and the effective dose with EFF-DOSE, the following projections were selected: the posteroanterior renal projection in nephrostomy and the anteroposterior abdominal projection in the rest of the procedures.

Spermatic vein embolization.—Embolization of the spermatic vein was performed in young patients with clinically diagnosed varicocele. The irradiated area was the left anteroposterior pelvic zone, because in all cases it was the left spermatic vein that was embolized. Therefore, we selected the anteroposterior pelvic projection to evaluate the organ dose and the effective dose with EFF-DOSE.

Subcutaneous reservoir placement.—It was possible to study 21 cases (11 conventional and 10 digital) of subcutaneous reservoir

Table 2
Parameters for the Radiologic Examinations and Procedures

Procedure	No. of Patients	Mean Patient Age (y)	Fluoroscopy Kilovoltage	Fluoroscopy Milliamperage	Radiography Kilovoltage	Radiography Milliampere Seconds	Radiography No. of Images
Cerebral arteriography							
Conventional system	9	51.3	84.0	4.6	67.3	15.03	172.3
Digital system	9	47.9	85.2	3.5	73.2	19.60	80.7
Celiac arteriography							
Conventional system	9	69.8	87.5	4.7	81.0	40.51	112.4
Digital system	10	64.4	92.8	4.5	82.0	42.61	42.8
Hepatic arteriography							
Conventional system	9	63.9	85.6	4.8	81.5	40.17	90.9
Digital system	9	67.0	90.5	4.2	82.1	40.50	24.8
Renal arteriography							
Conventional system	9	57.0	83.9	4.5	79.1	42.21	92.1
Digital system	10	55.3	82.7	4.6	80.1	45.47	33.5
Lower-limb arteriography							
Conventional system	18	61.7	81.5	3.6	66.9	36.91	92.1
Digital system	12	63.2	83.5	3.2	70.5	45.19	42.8
Lower-limb angioplasty							
Conventional system	9	69.0	80.6	3.7	64.8	43.81	119.5
Digital system	10	63.4	82.0	3.4	71.0	45.10	82.6
Percutaneous cholangiography with biliary drainage							
Conventional system	16	62.0	81.5	4.5	79.7	46.44	8.5
Digital system	14	64.8	93.1	3.5	83.1	44.86	3.8
Biliary stone extraction							
Conventional system	9	55.4	84.9	4.6	81.9	50.53	23.0
Digital system	9	56.6	86.4	4.3	81.8	51.32	1.2
Biliary Wallstent prosthesis placement							
Conventional system	9	60.1	81.6	4.4	79.5	45.49	19.6
Digital system	9	63.5	85.6	4.4	81.3	43.38	1.6
Ureteral catheterization							
Conventional system	10	51.4	82.2	4.7	75.9	28.62	20.6
Digital system	10	58.8	88.9	3.8	81.0	40.92	1.3
Nephrostomy							
Conventional system	11	57.1	83.5	4.2	75.8	49.75	8.5
Digital system	14	60.8	91.8	3.5	80.5	44.09	2.4
Renal catheterization							
Conventional system	10	59.7	83.2	4.2	75.0	45.21	2.0
Digital system	13	63.3	84.7	4.2	77.5	42.30	1.2
Ureteral dilation							
Conventional system	10	58.0	85.5	4.3	80.6	46.24	10.4
Digital system	10	57.7	87.3	4.4	82.3	42.70	1.3
Spermatic vein embolization							
Conventional system	10	25.6	79.1	4.5	73.6	41.74	37.8
Digital system	10	23.9	79.9	4.3	80.7	42.50	2.2
Subcutaneous reservoir placement							
Conventional system	11	56.8	80.7	4.5	76.3	43.13	1.6
Digital system	10	44.8	80.9	4.5	78.0	46.25	1.3

placement in the shoulder or pectoral zone in patients who were distressed during the treatment of tumoral pain. We have chosen the anteroposterior shoulder projection (EFF-DOSE software V1.02 User's Manual; National Board of Health, National Institute of Radiation Hygiene, 1995) to estimate the organ dose and the effective dose.

RESULTS

In the calibration of the Siemens Medical Systems equipment throughout the two periods of this research, the maximum coefficients of variation obtained in the parameters of reproducibility, linearity, and efficiency were less than 4.5%. Recurrently, the dose estimated from the exposure measured with the radiation-output evaluator was compared with the dose calculated from the transmission-chamber dose-area product. The maximum coefficient of error was 5.1% (minimum coefficient of error, 3.4%). Correction factors were applied when necessary.

The maximum percentage of variation in the calibration of the thermoluminescence dosimeters was 3.9%. Each thermoluminescence dosimeter was assigned an identity number of 1–248; the correction factor was related to the average value.

Table 2 summarizes the total number of patients in whom procedures were performed, the average age of the patients, the radiologic techniques used, and the total number of images obtained with conventional and with digital systems.

Lower-limb arteriography and percutaneous cholangiography with biliary drainage were the most frequent studies; they composed almost 19% of the studies performed.

The average age of the patients who underwent embolization of the spermatic vein was 25.6 years for conventional methods or 23.9 years for digital methods. The average age of the patients who underwent other procedures ranged from 44.8 years in those who underwent subcutaneous reservoir placement with the digital system to 69.8 years in those who underwent arteriography of the celiac-mesenteric trunk with the conventional system.

In fluoroscopy, the average kilovoltage was higher than that in procedures performed with the digital system,

Table 3
Dose-Area Product and Procedure Time

Procedure	Coefficient of Variation (%)	Dose-Area Product (Gy · cm^2) Total*	Maximum	Minimum	Median	Third Quartile	Total Time (sec)*
Cerebral arteriography							
Conventional system	39	50.53 ± 19.57	79.52	21.23	53.61	64.20	930 ± 556
Digital system	46	82.83 ± 38.14	131.86	39.16	74.82	118.01	1,059 ± 551
Celiac arteriography							
Conventional system	31	78.25 ± 23.89	121.76	47.46	70.82	90.73	818 ± 263
Digital system	25	109.59 ± 27.47	165.71	86.35	96.11	114.87	614 ± 216
Hepatic arteriography							
Conventional system	24	73.63 ± 17.67	97.89	47.46	70.83	87.69	912 ± 307
Digital system	20	88.30 ± 17.30	109.80	51.23	93.80	98.36	588 ± 321
Renal arteriography							
Conventional system	19	81.57 ± 15.51	107.89	61.76	78.07	89.78	630 ± 178
Digital system	34	74.55 ± 25.27	105.67	31.20	81.03	92.19	394 ± 246
Lower-limb arteriography							
Conventional system	75	27.99 ± 21.09	81.08	10.91	16.07	32.04	324 ± 197
Digital system	31	58.17 ± 18.30	90.31	39.05	51.84	71.14	335 ± 94
Lower-limb angioplasty							
Conventional system	89	79.59 ± 70.48	234.25	23.83	65.49	67.71	1,779 ± 1,002
Digital system	67	81.41 ± 54.52	160.56	14.84	92.96	120.49	912 ± 479
Percutaneous cholangiography with biliary drainage							
Conventional system	78	64.07 ± 50.54	199.43	13.71	47.57	85.41	856 ± 670
Digital system	57	43.02 ± 24.54	90.39	11.39	38.93	63.23	662 ± 351
Biliary stone extraction							
Conventional system	36	64.27 ± 22.85	100.28	39.76	58.82	78.97	940 ± 451
Digital system	52	75.07 ± 39.18	155.63	21.36	72.42	89.07	1,202 ± 521
Biliary Wallstent prosthesis placement							
Conventional system	34	84.16 ± 28.19	128.99	44.31	78.54	105.67	1,004 ± 412
Digital system	44	86.67 ± 38.02	154.90	36.36	83.63	106.70	960 ± 379
Ureteral catheterization							
Conventional system	42	40.32 ± 16.85	65.79	10.77	40.21	49.07	588 ± 132
Digital system	32	41.14 ± 13.04	58.90	25.68	41.01	50.97	801 ± 234
Nephrostomy							
Conventional system	51	21.49 ± 10.86	45.21	7.89	19.06	26.70	334 ± 119
Digital system	59	22.73 ± 13.31	51.36	7.05	21.12	32.64	595 ± 219
Renal catheterization							
Conventional system	52	17.04 ± 8.79	29.49	7.27	16.73	20.43	240 ± 72
Digital system	42	20.51 ± 8.70	34.80	7.80	22.00	25.41	272 ± 95
Ureteral dilation							
Conventional system	48	62.56 ± 30.17	128.44	28.44	56.56	74.90	907 ± 348
Digital system	38	62.72 ± 23.72	105.46	35.13	54.35	75.39	1,044 ± 139
Spermatic vein embolization							
Conventional system	44	80.35 ± 34.97	134.58	37.33	79.06	102.91	1,186 ± 438
Digital system	40	106.32 ± 42.41	180.37	43.16	101.80	134.89	1,821 ± 855
Subcutaneous reservoir placement							
Conventional system	23	8.60 ± 1.97	11.10	4.01	8.90	9.88	417 ± 108
Digital system	69	18.50 ± 12.76	40.13	6.18	11.70	29.97	465 ± 236

* Mean ± standard deviation.

with the exception of the kilovoltage in renal arteriography. However, in renal arteriography, the milliamperage was higher than that in procedures performed with the conventional system. In the rest of the digital procedures, the average milliamperage was equal to or lower than that reported in the conventional procedures, with the exception of that in ureteral dilation.

In radiography, the average kilovoltage selected was higher in the radiographic procedures performed with the digital system, with the exception of the kilovoltage in the extraction of biliary stones. Similarly, the average milliampere second was higher in the procedures performed with the digital system, with the exception of percutaneous cholangiography with biliary drainage, placement of a biliary prosthesis, nephrostomy, renal catheterization, and ureteral dilation.

Moreover, the average number of images in digital procedures was lower than that in conventional procedures. The mean percentage of reduction in the number of images was 60%. The range was from 19% in subcutaneous reservoir placements to 95% in biliary stone procedures. The cause of this decrease in the number of images with the digital system was multifactorial: (*a*) Diagnosis was difficult with the small images (10 × 10 cm) produced with the conventional system; (*b*) in the vascular procedures, there were more repetitions of series with the conventional system than with the digital system (ie, in one case in which cerebral arteriography was performed, a total of 300 images were obtained with the conventional system, while a maximum of 110 images were obtained with the digital system); and (*c*) the training, by means of experience and daily practice, of the interventional vascular radiology service staff members improved.

Table 3 presents the average, maximum, minimum, median, and third quartile dose-area products and the coefficients of variation for conventional and digital procedures. In addition, it presents mean values of the procedure times.

For the procedures performed with digital methods, the average third quartiles of the dose-area product were higher than those estimated for the conventional system, with the exception of those for percutaneous cholangiography with biliary drainage.

The average dose-area product in the urinary and biliary tract procedures showed smaller differences between conventional and digital systems. However, these differences were more evident in the vascular procedures. Perhaps this is evidence that these procedures require acquisition of more images than do nonvascular examinations.

Table 4 shows the average source-to-skin distance, the thickness (diameter) of the irradiated section (in centimeters), and the estimated average irradiated area and average entrance surface dose. The estimated surface dose was higher for the digital vascular procedures than for the conventional procedures, with the exception of those in renal arteriography. In the rest of the procedures, this trend was not seen.

Table 5 shows the average organ dose from the digital procedures in the thyroid, breasts, lungs, ovaries, and testicles as measured with thermoluminescence dosimeters on the skin surface as per Padovani and coworkers (8). Similarly, the effective dose (10) and the effective dose equivalent (11) are shown; they were calculated from the average dose-area product by using EFF-DOSE according to the projections recommended by the National Radiological Protection Board (9).

Finally, Table 6 summarizes the average dose-area product, the effective dose, the energy imparted, and the risk of fatal cancer in digital interventional vascular radiology. The range of the average effective dose for digital procedures was 0.88 mSv in subcutaneous reservoir placement to 25.70 mSv in spermatic vein embolization. The range of the energy imparted was 129 mJ in subcutaneous reservoir placement to 829 mJ in spermatic vein embolization. The range of the fatal cancer risk was 44 cases per 1 million procedures in subcutaneous reservoir placement to 1,285 cases per 1 million procedures in spermatic vein embolization. Celiac arteriography had the most energy imparted at 854 mJ.

Table 4
Average Source-to-Skin Distance, Thickness and Area of Irradiated Section, and Surface Dose

Procedure	Source-to-Skin Distance (cm)*	Thickness of Irradiated Section (cm)	Mean Area of Irradiated Section (cm^2)	Surface Dose (mGy)*
Cerebral arteriography				
Conventional system	69.78 ± 1.09	20.11	317.62	159.1 ± 61.6
Digital system	67.56 ± 2.51	20.33	324.61	255.2 ± 117.5
Celiac arteriography				
Conventional system	66.67 ± 1.32	26.89	567.90	137.8 ± 42.1
Digital system	68.70 ± 1.64	27.50	593.96	184.5 ± 46.2
Hepatic arteriography				
Conventional system	67.11 ± 2.03	26.44	549.05	134.1 ± 32.2
Digital system	68.56 ± 1.13	26.78	563.26	156.8 ± 3.07
Renal arteriography				
Conventional system	68.13 ± 2.23	25.13	495.99	164.5 ± 31.3
Digital system	68.10 ± 2.28	24.50	471.44	158.1 ± 53.6
Lower-limb arteriography				
Conventional system	67.67 ± 2.68	19.52†	299.26	93.5 ± 70.5
Digital system	65.25 ± 0.45	19.71†	305.11	190.6 ± 60.0
Lower-limb angioplasty				
Conventional system	66.11 ± 1.36	19.78†	307.29	259.0 ± 229.4
Digital system	65.50 ± 0.85	19.60†	301.72	269.8 ± 180.7
Percutaneous cholangiography with biliary drainage				
Conventional system	67.63 ± 1.63	27.75	604.81	105.9 ± 83.6
Digital system	67.86 ± 1.88	26.43	548.64	78.4 ± 44.7
Biliary stone extraction				
Conventional system	67.11 ± 1.69	27.00	572.56	112.3 ± 39.9
Digital system	69.00 ± 1.73	26.67	558.64	134.4 ± 70.1
Biliary Wallstent prosthesis placement				
Conventional system	67.67 ± 1.22	26.56	554.05	151.9 ± 50.9
Digital system	68.56 ± 1.13	26.11	535.43	162.0 ± 71.0
Ureteral catheterization				
Conventional system	66.20 ± 1.62	26.10	535.02	75.3 ± 31.5
Digital system	67.40 ± 2.41	26.90	568.32	72.4 ± 22.9
Nephrostomy				
Conventional system	66.09 ± 3.27	25.27	501.53	42.8 ± 21.7
Digital system	68.57 ± 1.70	26.64	557.39	40.8 ± 23.9
Renal catheterization				
Conventional system	66.50 ± 3.14	26.30	543.25	31.4 ± 16.2
Digital system	68.85 ± 1.86	26.92	569.17	36.0 ± 15.3
Ureteral dilation				
Conventional system	68.00 ± 2.36	26.40	547.39	114.3 ± 55.1
Digital system	67.10 ± 1.73	24.90	486.95	128.8 ± 48.7
Spermatic vein embolization				
Conventional system	66.70 ± 2.11	22.40	394.08	203.9 ± 88.7
Digital system	67.40 ± 0.97	22.50	397.61	267.4 ± 106.7
Subcutaneous reservoir placement				
Conventional system	68.18 ± 1.94	25.36	505.11	17.0 ± 3.9
Digital system	68.20 ± 1.87	25.30	502.73	36.8 ± 25.4

* Mean ± standard deviation.
† Mean thickness for pelvis, thigh, and leg.

DISCUSSION

It is easy to calculate the patient dose with the dose-area product. This permits comparison of the results of both conventional and digital systems; however, information about radiologic risk cannot be deduced directly from the dose, because radiologic risk depends on the body area irradiated.

The working document of the European Evaluation Program of Risks in Interventional and Vascular Radiology under the auspices of the European Commission (7) proposes classification of the related procedures to avoid distortion of the dose-area product. However, in this way, the coefficient of variation is increased owing to the different methods, different zones and organs irradiated, and different procedure times.

We think that the procedures must be studied in terms of the methods instead of in terms of physics concepts. We have considered a minimum of nine performances of each conventional and digital procedure, with the evaluation of 15 different procedures.

We wanted to complete the findings reported in other articles that have compared patient doses in conventional and digital studies (3,15). In patients with atherosclerotic cerebrovascular disease, Plunkett and coworkers (3) calculated an average

Table 5
Average Organ Dose and Effective Dose in Digital Systems

Procedure	Projection	Thyroid (mGy)	Breast (mGy)	Lung (mGy)	Ovary (mGy)	Testicle (mGy)	Effective Dose* (mSv)	Effective Dose Equivalent* (mSv)	Ratio of Effective Dose to Effective Dose Equivalent
Cerebral arteriography	Posteroanterior and right lateral head								
Thermoluminescence dosimeter		6.67	1.46	3.98	0.28	0.05	NC	NC	NC
EFF-DOSE		5.72	0.04	0.22	0.00	0.00	2.50	4.47	0.56
Celiac arteriography	Posteroanterior abdominal								
Thermoluminescence dosimeter		0.94	2.53	16.17	11.73	0.26	NC	NC	NC
EFF-DOSE		0.00	0.24	1.32	28.15	2.83	15.36	20.34	0.75
Hepatic arteriography	Posteroanterior abdominal								
Thermoluminescence dosimeter		1.18	2.65	15.53	23.64	0.18	NC	NC	NC
EFF-DOSE		0.00	0.19	1.06	22.68	2.28	12.38	16.39	0.75
Renal arteriography	Posteroanterior abdominal								
Thermoluminescence dosimeter		0.45	0.68	4.67	2.23	0.45	NC	NC	NC
EFF-DOSE		0.00	0.16	0.88	18.79	1.87	10.29	13.64	0.75
Lower-limb arteriography	Posteroanterior pelvic								
Thermoluminescence dosimeter		0.23	0.14	2.43	23.74	7.89	NC	NC	NC
EFF-DOSE†		0.00	0.04	0.04	11.31	41.65	8.99	12.07	0.74
Lower-limb angioplasty	Posteroanterior pelvic								
Thermoluminescence dosimeter		0.29	0.24	3.42	33.06	9.29	NC	NC	NC
EFF-DOSE†		0.00	0.05	0.05	15.83	58.29	12.58	16.89	0.74
Percutaneous cholangiography with biliary drainage	Posteroanterior kidney								
Thermoluminescence dosimeter		0.43	1.47	5.01	6.75	0.08	NC	NC	NC
EFF-DOSE		0.03	0.41	2.73	1.51	0.02	6.57	14.82	0.44
Biliary stone extraction	Posteroanterior kidney								
Thermoluminescence dosimeter		0.68	2.20	9.02	7.16	0.34	NC	NC	NC
EFF-DOSE		0.05	0.63	4.44	2.36	0.04	10.85	24.82	0.44
Biliary Wallstent prosthesis placement	Posteroanterior kidney								
Thermoluminescence dosimeter		0.32	0.92	7.24	7.49	1.04	NC	NC	NC
EFF-DOSE		0.06	0.73	5.13	2.73	0.04	12.53	28.66	0.44
Ureteral catheterization	Anteroposterior abdominal								
Thermoluminescence dosimeter		0.09	0.32	0.62	4.27	2.21	NC	NC	NC
EFF-DOSE		0.00	0.12	0.30	8.18	1.54	5.11	5.28	0.75
Nephrostomy	Anteroposterior kidney								
Thermoluminescence dosimeter		0.16	0.24	0.45	1.68	0.43	NC	NC	NC
EFF-DOSE		0.02	0.44	1.36	0.85	0.02	5.49	5.62	0.97
Renal catheterization	Anteroposterior abdominal								
Thermoluminescence dosimeter		0.23	0.25	0.52	1.18	0.28	NC	NC	NC
EFF-DOSE		0.01	0.11	0.27	7.38	1.39	4.61	4.77	0.97
Ureteral dilation	Anteroposterior abdominal								
Thermoluminescence dosimeter		0.07	0.27	0.37	4.54	2.15	NC	NC	NC
EFF-DOSE		0.00	0.34	0.82	22.50	4.20	14.09	14.58	0.97
Spermatic vein embolization	Posteroanterior pelvic								
Thermoluminescence dosimeter		0.07	...	11.47	...	14.83	NC	NC	NC
EFF-DOSE		0.00	...	0.10	...	114.27	25.70	34.49	0.74
Subcutaneous reservoir placement	Anteroposterior shoulder								
Thermoluminescence dosimeter		0.92	0.32	20.21	0.19	0.02	NC	NC	NC
EFF-DOSE		1.24	0.52	4.07	0.00	0.00	0.88	0.94	0.94

Note.—NC = not calculatable.
* Calculated with EFF-DOSE.
† In lower-limb arteriography and lower-limb angioplasty, organ doses and effective doses have been calculated with 75% of the dose-area product.

dose-area product of 27.79 Gy · cm^2 with the conventional system and of 15.91 Gy · cm^2 with the digital system. This means a decrease of 42% with the digital system (intravenous injection of contrast material). Similarly, Pavlicek and co-workers (16) were able to decrease the organ dose (to the bone marrow, the lens of the eye, and the thyroid) by using a digital subtraction system. They attributed this decrease to the use of small fields and less fluoroscopy.

In contrast, our determinations of the dose-area product in cerebral arteriography (Table 3) are higher with the digital system (82.83 Gy · cm^2) than with the conventional system (50.53 Gy · cm^2). This supposes an increase of 64% with the digital system (arterial injection of contrast material). The increase is due to the use of higher technical parameters (kilovoltage and milliampere seconds) with digital imaging than with conventional imaging.

The staff members of the interventional vascular radiology service were the same throughout the study. This allows us to eliminate discussion about the consistency of the methods used in all the procedures, as well as about changes in the professional training of the staff. However, the image-acquisition modes deserve special attention (Table 1). In general, radiologists use high modes 1 and 2 instead of low modes 1 and 2. As is logical, they seek a better image for diagnosing disease (a priority of the radiologist); thus, in theory, a greater radiation dose is delivered to the patient and more radiation disperses toward the staff. Also, the use of conventional, pulsed, or digital (high-dose) fluoroscopy influences the patient dose (recommendation of reference 1, p 42).

The dose-area product attained with the digital system and reported here was compared with the dose-area products attained by other authors. Vañó and co-workers (17) performed arteriography of the lower limbs in 40 cases, cerebral arteriography in 13 cases, renal arteriography in 14 cases, and percutaneous cholangiography with biliary drainage in 10 cases and established average dose-area products of 66.63, 68.16, 92.92, and 68.87 Gy · cm², respectively. Steele and Temperton (5) had average dose-area products of 27.38, 42.91, 136.67, and 94.98 Gy · cm² in carotid, femoral, hepatic, and renal arteriography, respectively. Thwaites and co-workers (14) presented an average dose-area product of 26.26 Gy · cm² for lower-limb arteriography.

The dose-area product estimated in the embolization of the spermatic vein was high. Furthermore, the patients were young people who received a high dose in the testicular zone.

However, it is difficult to estimate the organ dose. Our work presents the organ dose for the five organs selected by Padovani and co-workers (8); it was calculated by using thermoluminescence dosimeters and was compared with the dose estimated with EFF-DOSE, with the selection of simple projections. These values do not present a proportional relationship. Perhaps the solution is to introduce dosimeters into phantoms (Random-Phantoms; Alderson Research Laboratories, Stanford, Conn) and to simulate the digital interventional vascular radiology procedures, the radiologic parameters (eg, kilovoltage and milliampere seconds), and the procedure times. Actually, a 1994 memorandum of the National Radiological Protection Board (9) presents the method that most closely simulates reality and provides approximate values for simple and complex examinations.

Retrospectively, we are not confident that a reasonable organ dose can be obtained with this small number of dosimeters and locations sampled under actual clinical conditions. We have compared only the results derived from the thermoluminescence dosimeters with those derived from the dose-area products according to a 1994 National Radiological Protection Board memorandum (9).

The dose-area product is experimental and allows us to calculate such other interesting measurements in the radiologic examinations as the surface dose (by dividing the dose-area product by the area irradiated), the energy imparted, and the effective dose. The effective dose was estimated by using EFF-DOSE and by adjusting the irradiated fields in digital interventional vascular procedures to match those used in simple exploration projections. In addition, the effective dose can be estimated by using conversion coefficients selected by Hart and co-workers (9, p 36). However, the effective dose estimated with EFF-DOSE is more realistic, because it uses more parameters such as kilovoltage and total equivalent filtration in millimeters of aluminum.

Table 6
Average Dose-Area Product, Effective Dose, Energy Imparted, and Risk of Fatal Cancer in Digital Procedures

Procedure	Dose-Area Product (Gy · cm²)	Effective Dose (mSv)	Energy Imparted (mJ)	Risk of Fatal Cancer (Cases per Million)
Cerebral arteriography	82.83	2.50	579.81	125
Celiac arteriography	109.59	15.36	854.80	768
Hepatic arteriography	88.30	12.38	688.74	619
Renal arteriography	74.55	10.29	581.49	514
Lower-limb arteriography	58.17	8.99	305.39	449
Lower-limb angioplasty	81.41	12.58	427.40	629
Percutaneous cholangiography with biliary drainage	43.02	6.57	344.16	328
Biliary stone extraction	75.07	10.85	600.56	542
Biliary Wallstent prosthesis placement	86.67	12.53	693.36	626
Ureteral catheterization	41.14	5.11	320.89	255
Nephrostomy	22.73	5.49	170.48	274
Renal catheterization	20.51	4.61	159.98	230
Ureteral dilation	62.72	14.09	489.22	704
Spermatic vein embolization	106.32	25.70	829.30	1,285
Subcutaneous reservoir placement	18.50	0.88	129.50	44

The average effective dose attained by Feygelman and co-workers (18) was 10.6 mSv (range, 2.7–23.4 mSv) in cerebral arteriography. Approximately 67% of the total dose (10.6 mSv) was due to fluoroscopy (18). However, these values were calculated with old factors from 1977 recommendations of the International Commission on Radiological Protection (11) and are higher than those in Table 5. The effective dose attained by Berthelsen and Cererblad (19) during the embolization of intracerebral arteriovenous malformations was estimated as 6–43 mSv. Naturally, these values are higher than those attained in diagnostic arteriography. However, Bergeron and co-workers (20) estimated, in eight neurovascular interventional procedures, a surface dose range of 129–1,335 mGy (with thermoluminescence dosimeters) and an average effective dose of 1.67 mSv (range, 0.44–3.44 mSv). Our determinations of the effective dose and the surface dose in cerebral arteriography are within the range of values presented by Bergeron and co-workers (20).

Geterud and co-workers (21) estimated the patient dose during 11 percutaneous kidney stone extractions. According to factors in the 1977 recommendations of the International Commission on Radiological Protection (11), the average effective dose equivalent was 4.2 mSv and the average energy imparted was 285 mJ. In addition, these doses are similar to those estimated by us in the interventional renal procedures, ureteral catheterization, nephrostomy, and renal catheterization.

Finally, Steele and Temperton (5) showed average measurements of energy imparted of 308, 257, 1,636, and 1,085 mJ and estimated average fatal cancer risks of 200, 200, 1,150, and 800 cases per million in carotid, femoral, hepatic, and renal arteriography, respectively.

Achieving a patient dose "as low as reasonably achievable" in interventional vascular procedures depends on the basic principles of dose limitation, exploration time, source-to-skin distance, and shielding. The actual use of these principles will depend on how effectively this information is communicated to staff members and on their education, training, and expertise in performing low-dose fluoroscopy.

In our case, it was recommended that we use low modes 1 and 2 instead of high modes 1 and 2 for image acquisition. More conventional (standard) than digital (high-dose) fluoroscopy should be performed.

Our study included a small sample of cases to evaluate the estimated risk of interventional vascular procedures, but we believe that our findings can be compared with findings of other studies. ■

Acknowledgments: The authors thank the staff of the radiology service of Nuestra Señora Virgen de la Victoria University Hospital of Málaga, Málaga, Spain, and especially the head of the service, Luis Angel Arribas de Rodrigo, MD, for his support during this research.

References

1. Balter S, Shope TB. Syllabus: a categorical course in physics—physical and technical aspects of angiography and interventional radiology. Oak Brook, Ill: Radiological Society of North America, 1995; 1–258.
2. Jeans WD. The development and use of digital subtraction angiography. Br J Radiol 1990; 63:161–168.
3. Plunkett M, Gray J, Kispert D. Radiation exposure from conventional and digital subtraction angiography of cerebral vessels. AJNR 1986; 7:665–668.
4. Díaz-Romero F, Hernandez-Armas J. Dose and detriment to patients from vascular and interventional radiology (D-18). In: Sources and effects of ionizing radiation. New York, NY: United Nations Scientific Committee on the Effects of Atomic Radiation, 1993; 232–233.
5. Steele HR, Temperton DH. Patient dose received during digital subtraction angiography. Br J Radiol 1993; 66:452–456.
6. Royal decree 2071/1995: quality control in radiodiagnostics. Official bulletin of Spain. Madrid, Spain: Boletin Oficial Español, 1996; 20.
7. European Commission. Council directive 84/466/EURATOM of September 3rd 1984 establishing fundamental measures concerning radiation protection of persons undergoing medical examinations and treatments. Off J Eur Community 1984; 1:265.
8. Padovani R, Contento G, Fabretto M, Malisan MR, Barbina V, Gozzi G. Patients' doses and risks from diagnostic radiology in northeast Italy. Br J Radiol 1987; 60:155–156.
9. Hart D, Jones DG, Wall BF. Estimation of effective dose in diagnostic radiology from entrance surface dose and dose-area product measurements. National Radiological Protection Board publication no. R262. Chilton, England: National Radiological Protection Board, 1994; 1–57.
10. Recommendations of the International Commission on Radiological Protection: publication 60. Ann ICRP 1991; 21:1–201.
11. Recommendations of the International Commission on Radiological Protection: publication 26. Ann ICRP 1977; 1:1–53.
12. Shrimpton PC, Wall BF, Jones DG, et al. A National survey of doses to patients undergoing a selection of routine x-ray examinations in English Hospitals. National Radiological Protection Board publication no. R200. Chilton, England: National Radiological Protection Board, 1986; 1–186.
13. Shrimpton PC, Wall BF, Jones DG, et al. Doses to patients from routine diagnostic x-ray examinations in England. Br J Radiol 1986; 59:749–758.
14. Thwaites JH, Rafferty MW, Gray N, Black J, Stock B. A patient dose survey for femoral arteriogram diagnostic radiographic examinations using a dose-area product meter. Phys Med Biol 1996; 41:899–907.
15. Nitatori T. Radiation in digital subtraction angiography. J Kyorin Med Soc 1987; 18: 527–533.
16. Pavlicek W, Weinstein MA, Modic MT, Buonocore E, Duchesneau PM. Patient doses during digital subtraction angiography of the carotid arteries: comparison with conventional angiography. Radiology 1982; 145:683–685.
17. Vañó E, Gonzalez L, Fernandez JM, Guibelalde E. Patient dose values in interventional radiology. Br J Radiol 1995; 68:1215–1220.
18. Feygelman VM, Huda W, Peters K. Effective dose equivalent to patients undergoing cerebral angiography. AJNR 1992; 13:845–849.
19. Berthelsen B, Cererblad A. Radiation doses to patients and personnel involved in embolization of intracerebral arteriovenous malformations. Acta Radiol 1991; 32:492–497.
20. Bergeron P, Carrier R, Roy D, Blais N, Raymond J. Radiation doses to patients in neurointerventional procedures. AJNR 1994; 15:1809–1812.
21. Geterud K, Larsson A, Mattson S. Radiation doses to patients and personnel during fluoroscopy at percutaneous renal stone extraction. Acta Radiol 1989; 30:201–205.

Book Review

Diagnostic Breast Imaging

Sylvia H. Heywang-Köbrunner, MD, Ingrid Schreer, MD, and D. David Dershaw, MD
New York, NY: Thieme Medical, 1996. ISBN 0-86577-636-9 (TMP), 3-13-102891-2 (GTV).
Cloth, $98.00; pp 415, 674 figures; tables.

The authors, who are from Germany and the United States, review in this textbook the current status of breast imaging techniques. The textbook is comprehensive and encompasses all aspects of breast evaluation—including history, physical examination and clinical findings, anatomic structures, pathologic processes, mammography, sonography, magnetic resonance (MR) imaging, localization techniques, and percutaneous biopsy. In addition, a discussion of screening mammography and current controversies surrounding this topic is included.

The text is systematically structured and divided into three main areas: methods of breast examination, appearance of breast disease, and diagnostic imaging of the breast. In each area, multiple chapters are divided into sections and subsections. This division can be particularly helpful if one wishes to go directly to a section on a particular area, such as the indications for sonography of fibroadenoma. However, this division also results in a less smoothly flowing text. There are excellent summaries, highlighted in blue for easy reference, at the end of each section.

The quality of the figures and tables is excellent. The pathologic findings on mammograms, sonograms, and MR images are seen easily. The diagrams and tables have been well thought out and are presented clearly. Rarely, arrows or figures described in the text are absent.

A few modifications would have been helpful. The section on the pathologic nature of invasive carcinoma might be expanded. In this section, the various types of invasive carcinoma have been arranged in decreasing order of frequency. This arrangement means lobular carcinoma precedes medullary and mucinous carcinomas and may imply, to the inexperienced reader, that medullary and mucinous carcinomas are types of lobular, not ductal, carcinomas. In addition, the value of MR imaging is stressed heavily, and the importance of sonography is deemphasized as a result. Perhaps, the emphasis on MR imaging is a reflection of practice in Europe, or the authors have found this modality to be of greater value; however, I doubt that most physicians at breast imaging centers in the United States emphasize MR imaging as the authors do. An expansion of the role of sonography would be useful.

In summary, this is an excellent textbook that encompasses the entire spectrum of breast imaging. This book should appeal to the novice and experienced mammographer. I can recommend this book without hesitation to anyone interested in diagnostic breast imaging.

Reviewed by Joseph H. Tashjian, MD

Kwan H. Ng, PhD[2] • Robert J. Aus, MS • Larry A. DeWerd, PhD • John R. Vetter, PhD

Entrance Skin Exposure and Mean Glandular Dose: Effect of Scatter and Field Gradient at Mammography[1]

PURPOSE: **To investigate the effect of scatter and x-ray field gradient on entrance skin exposure and mean glandular dose by using the measurement protocol of the American College of Radiology.**

MATERIALS AND METHODS: **The exposure difference between the off-axis geometry of the American College of Radiology protocol and the central-axis geometry was measured by using eight common ionization chambers and two mammographic units (Senographe DMR; GE Medical Systems, Milwaukee, Wis; and Mam-CP II; Transcontinental X-ray, Charlotte, NC) at 25, 28, and 30 kVp. The field gradient was also measured on film with a scanning densitometer.**

RESULTS: **The central-axis exposure was 2.0%–3.6% higher than the off-axis exposure for the Senographe DMR unit and 3.1%–8.0% higher for the Mam-CP II unit. The maximum phantom scatter was 0.7% (Senographe DMR) and 1.3% (Mam-CP II).**

CONCLUSION: **Entrance skin exposure varies, depending on the type of ionization chamber and the characteristics of the mammographic unit. Determination of mean glandular dose with the American College of Radiology protocol may lead to underestimates of the actual measured dose by 4%–8% for the x-ray machines used in this study.**

Mammography is generally regarded as the most accurate and reliable technique for the detection of minimal, nonpalpable breast cancer. However, the carcinogenic risk associated with the absorbed dose to the breast has been a concern to many people, and the radiation absorbed dose associated with mammography has been the subject of considerable research (1–3) in recent years.

Breast cancer almost always arises in glandular breast tissue. The average radiation absorbed dose to glandular breast tissue is the most useful measure of radiation risk at mammography and is the currently accepted descriptor of dose to the breast (2). Average radiation absorbed dose to glandular breast tissue represents a "true" mean dose to the most vulnerable tissue of the breast and most appropriately characterizes the radiation risk of carcinogenesis due to mammography.

The mean glandular dose D_g is determined by the relation $D_g = D_{gN} \cdot X_{ESE}$, where D_{gN} is the normalized average glandular dose (ie, average glandular dose per unit entrance skin exposure [ESE]), and X_{ESE} is the ESE associated with each exposure. D_{gN} is a function of the incident x-ray spectrum, the thickness of the compressed breast, and the composition of the breast (4,5). Factors that contribute to the error in the calculation of mean glandular dose are the uncertainty in the exposure measurement (6) and in the values of D_{gN}. In addition, by measuring the exposure in an off-axis position, a systematic bias discrepancy with regard to the measurement at the central axis can be introduced.

The method to determine mean glandular dose that is recommended by the American College of Radiology (ACR) protocol uses the data of Wu et al (4), which necessitates that the ESE be measured free in air. For convenience, the ACR has chosen to use the exposure measured off-axis with the phantom in the beam as an estimate of the central-axis ESE free in air. The procedure for measuring breast entrance exposure is to position the ionization chamber in the x-ray field beside the mammographic phantom, 4 cm from the chest-wall edge of the image receptor, and with the center of the chamber level with the top surface of the phantom (7). The accuracy of the ACR method depends on how well the off-axis measurement approximates the central-axis ESE free in air. There may be other conflicting effects arising from scatter, namely, side scatter from the phantom and back scatter from the image receptor (8,9). The dose table in the ACR's mammography quality control manual, physicists section (7), was derived from the data of Wu et al (4), whose calculation was based on the ESE measured free in air at the central axis of the beam. In Europe and in England, the mean glandular dose is calculated by using the method based on the work of Dance (10), which is in

Index terms: Breast radiography, radiation dose, 00.11 • Dosimetry • Radiations, measurement

Abbreviations: ACR = American College of Radiology, ESE = entrance skin exposure, TLD = thermoluminescent dosimeter.

Radiology 1997; 205:395–398

[1] From the Radiation Calibration Laboratory, Department of Medical Physics, University of Wisconsin–Madison, 1300 University Ave, Madison, WI 53706. From the 1996 RSNA scientific assembly. Received December 4, 1996; revision requested January 22, 1997; revision received July 21; accepted July 23. **Address reprint requests to** L.A.D.
[2] Current address: Department of Radiology, University of Malaya, Kuala Lumpur, Malaysia.

report 59 of the Institute of Physical Sciences in Medicine (11). This method is based on Monte Carlo simulation of air-kerma measurements at the central axis.

The authors of American Association of Physicists in Medicine report number 31 (12) also recommended placement of the ionization chamber to one side of the phantom for measurement of the dose at mammography. In this report, it was stated that "since this measurement is necessarily not made on the central axis, care should be taken to verify that no large exposure gradient exists between the measurement position and the central axis." However, the authors of the report do not suggest how to overcome this problem, nor do they state what care is needed. In the mammography quality control manual (7), it is mentioned that mammographic imaging systems have a substantial x-ray intensity gradient in the anode-cathode direction, but there is no mention of the transverse-axis gradient. It is emphasized that maintenance of a constant chamber position during measurements is crucial.

The objective of the present study was to investigate the effect of scatter and the transverse x-ray field gradient on ESE and mean glandular dose at mammography by using a measurement performed with the ionization chamber positioned beside the mammographic phantom. The entrance surface dose was measured at the central axis for comparison.

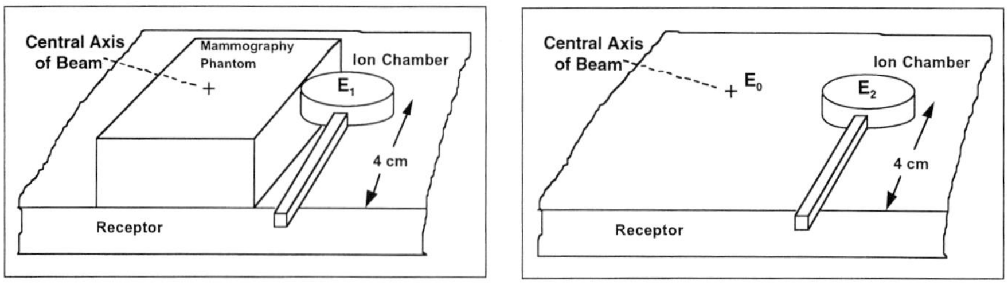

a. b.

Figure 1. Ionization (*Ion*) chamber setup geometry for ESE measurement. E_0 = exposure at the beam center, E_1 = off-axis exposure at the side of the phantom, E_2 = off-axis exposure without the phantom. **(a)** Diagram shows the setup geometry based on the ACR protocol. The ionization chamber is positioned beside the phantom. **(b)** Diagram shows the setup geometry with the ionization chamber and no phantom.

Table 1
Physical Characteristics of Ionization Chambers

Chamber Model	Geometry	Active Volume (cm^3)	Outer Diameter (cm)	Window Material	Window Thickness (mm)
10x5-6 (Radcal)	Cylindric	6.0	2.46	Polycarbonate	0.33000
MC-1 (Precision Radiation Measurement, Nashville, Tenn)	Parallel plate	1.0	2.90	Beryllium	0.25000
PS-033 (Capintec, Ramsey, NJ)	Parallel plate	0.5	3.18	Aluminized polyester film	0.00360
303 (CNMC, Nashville, Tenn)	Parallel plate	3.0	4.12	Polycarbonate	0.25000
10x5-6M (Radcal)	Parallel plate	6.0	4.40	Metalized polyester	0.00635
A11 (Exradin, Lisle, Ill)	Parallel plate	0.6	4.46	Kapton film	1.00000
315 (CNMC)	Parallel plate	15.0	6.35	Polycarbonate	0.25000
96035 (Keithly Instruments, Cleveland, Ohio)	Parallel plate	15.0	6.40	Graphite-coated polycarbonate	0.25000

MATERIALS AND METHODS

This study was performed with two clinical mammographic units, both fitted with a molybdenum anode and a molybdenum filter (Senographe DMR; GE Medical Systems, Milwaukee, Wis; and Mam-CP II; Transcontinental X-ray, Charlotte, NC). Three kilovolt-peak settings (25, 28, and 30 kVp) were used.

The ACR-accredited program phantom (Model 156; Radiation Measurements, Middleton, Wis) was used in this study. This phantom approximates a 4.2-cm thickness of compressed breast tissue composed of 50% adipose and 50% glandular tissue. The phantom has a total thickness of 4.5 cm and consists of an image-quality insert constructed of dental wax in a depression in a polymethylmethacrylate block.

The procedure used was as follows: First, an exposure was performed with the automatic exposure control system in automatic mode, with the phantom present, and the milliampere-second setting was recorded. Subsequent exposures based on this milliampere-second setting were performed in the manual mode. The ionization chamber setup geometry is illustrated in Figure 1. The first exposure, E_1, which is performed according to the ACR protocol, is termed the off-axis exposure and is performed at the side of the phantom. The phantom was then removed, and a second off-axis exposure, E_2, was performed. A final exposure, E_0, was performed at the center of the x-ray beam without the phantom.

Three terms were derived from the measurements obtained with these procedures. Exposure deviation was calculated with $(E_0 - E_1)/E_0$, field gradient was calculated with $(E_0 - E_2)/E_0$, and phantom scatter was calculated with $(E_1 - E_2)/E_0$. These three exposures were repeated with eight types of ionization chambers, all of which are commonly used in mammographic exposure measurements. All chambers were plane-parallel plate chambers, except the Radcal 10x5-6 (Radcal, Monrovia, Calif), which is a cylindric chamber that has been used in the past. The physical characteristics of these chambers are listed in Table 1. All of the ionization chambers have calibration factors that were constant within ±3% for molybdenum-molybdenum beams with a half-value layer of 0.2–0.5 mm aluminum and that were traceable to the National Institute of Standards and Technology, Washington, DC. The chambers operate with voltage saturation and have an acceptably low current leakage (less than 10^{-14} A).

Phantom scatter was also measured with thermoluminescent dosimeters (TLDs) composed of lithium fluorine with magnesium and titanium impurities (Harshaw TLD-100; Bicron, Solon, Ohio). Ten TLDs were arranged horizontally, and four were fixed vertically to the side of the phantom adjacent to the ionization chamber. These TLDs received only scatter radiation from the phantom because the primary radiation was absorbed by a strip of lead 2 mm thick placed on the edge of the phantom. The accuracy of these TLD measurements at the 95% confidence level is 10% (13).

In addition, an exposure was obtained with Kodak TMG film (Eastman Kodak, Rochester, NY), without a screen. Film digitization and densitometry were performed by using a 12-bit gray-scale scanner with an optical density range of 0.15–2.90 and a spatial resolution of 0.35 mm (V-scan 4 TT6012; Oxberry–Vision Ten, Carlspadt, NJ) and SSGI software (SSGI, Chico, Calif). The beam-intensity profile was measured along the transverse axis at the position 4 cm from the chest wall.

RESULTS

The exposure deviations ranged from 2.0% to 3.6% with the Senographe DMR unit and from 3.1% to 8.0%

Table 2
Comparison of Field Gradient, Exposure Deviation, and Phantom Scatter at 28 kVp in Two Mammography Units

	GE Senographe DMR			Transcontinental Mam-CP II		
Chamber Model	Field Gradient without Phantom (%)	Exposure Deviation with Phantom (%)	Phantom Scatter (%)	Field Gradient without Phantom (%)	Exposure Deviation with Phantom (%)	Phantom Scatter (%)
10x5-6 (Radcal)	2.7	2.6	0.1	4.1	4.8	−0.7
MC-1 (Precision Radiation Measurement)	2.6	2.1	0.5	4.5	3.4	1.1
PS-033 (Capintec)	2.4	2.2	0.2	5.7	5.6	0.1
303 (CNMC)	3.3	3.0	0.3	4.8	3.9	0.9
10x5-6M (Radcal)	3.2	2.7	0.5	5.8	5.6	0.2
A11 (Exradin)	2.7	2.6	0.1	5.1	4.7	0.4
315 (CNMC)	3.7	3.6	0.1	5.9	5.5	0.4
96035 (Keithly Instruments)	2.9	3.1	−0.2	8.0	7.9	0.1

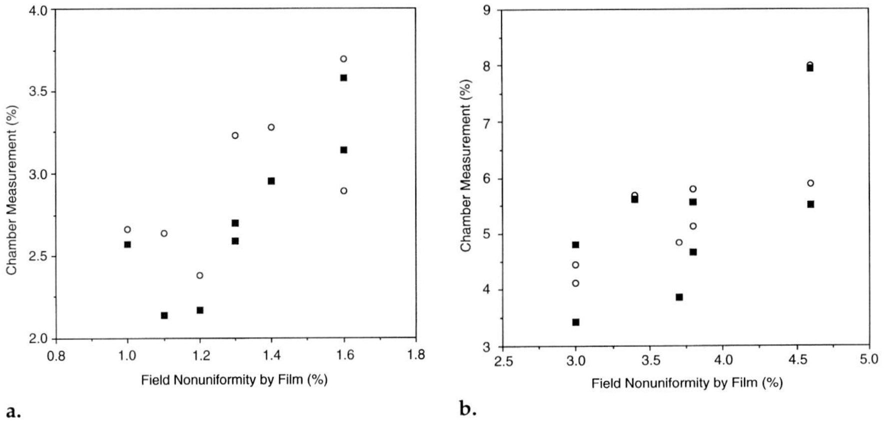

Figure 2. Scatter plots show the percentage field gradient (○) and the percentage exposure deviation (■) based on ionization chamber measurements with the increase of field nonuniformity measured with film and the **(a)** Senographe DMR and **(b)** Mam-CP II mammographic units.

with the Mam-CP II unit. The field gradients ranged from 2.1% to 3.7% with the Senographe DMR unit and from 3.6% to 8.0% with the Mam-CP II unit. Phantom scatter contributed up to 0.7% with the Senographe DMR unit and up to 1.3% with the Mam-CP II unit. Great care was taken to ensure reproducibility of the setup geometry to within 1 mm. The maximum overall uncertainties in the measurements, which take into account chamber characteristics, x-ray generator output, and variations in chamber placement, were 0.41%, 0.45%, and 0.48% for exposure deviation, field gradient, and phantom scatter, respectively. At least three readings were obtained for each setting, and the uncertainties were added in quadrature and are expressed as a percentage of the central axis measurement. Phantom scatter measured with TLDs was 1.1%–4.7% with the Senographe DMR unit and 1.5%–3.1% with the Mam-CP II unit. The standard deviation for the TLD measurements was 0.9%.

Table 2 lists field gradient and exposure deviation measurements for both mammographic units at 28 kVp. (Because measurements obtained at 25 and 30 kVp were similar to the 28-kVp measurements, only the latter are listed in Table 2.)

By using the beam-intensity profile obtained with films, the center of the field was determined to be 0.5%–2.5% and 2.0%–4.6% higher than the off-axis position with the Senographe DMR and Mam-CP II units, respectively. Figure 2 shows the scatter plots of the percentage field gradient and percentage exposure deviation (based on ionization chamber measurements) versus the field nonuniformity measured with film for both clinical mammographic units at 28 kVp. The film measurements for these figures were obtained at points that corresponded to the central- and off-axis chamber positions.

DISCUSSION

The exposure deviation was lower than the field gradient for most chambers due to the contribution of phantom scatter. Phantom scatter was small (less than 1%) in all cases. The negative phantom scatter values shown in Table 2 are probably the result of the presence of the phantom causing a reduction in the backscatter contribution from the image receptor. This reduction affected the Radcal 10x5-6 the most because it is a cylindric chamber, so it is sensitive to radiation from all directions. The back wall of most chambers is thick enough that the backscatter contribution is low. In the case of the Keithley 96035 chamber, the value in Table 2 falls within the uncertainties of the measurement; thus, it is difficult to attribute the negative phantom scatter value to this cause.

The anode-cathode field gradient (heel effect) at mammography was measured by Wu et al (4), who used relative ESEs measured at different distances from the chest wall. The ESE varies by 7% for an 8-cm chest wall–to-nipple distance with a Mam-CP unit at 30 kVp and a 54-cm source-to-chamber–plane distance. To our knowledge, however, there are no reported data about the relative ESEs across the image receptor (transverse to the anode-cathode axis). Our data indicate that there is a difference of up to 3.6% (Senographe DMR) and 8.0% (Mam-CP II), expressed in terms of exposure deviation, between the off-axis position of the ACR protocol measurement and the central-axis measurement. This is due largely to the field gradient effect (the radiation intensity falloff in the transverse direction to the anode-cathode axis). This difference between the off-axis and central-axis measurements is substantial even when one considers the uncertainty of 5.3% for all values of mean glandular dose listed in tables 2–6 in the article by Wu et al (4).

Part of the field gradient across the transverse direction can be attributed to the increased source-to-chamber distance because of the off-axis chamber placement. For the chamber with the maximum diameter, this would cause the off-axis measurement to be 2% lower (1% for the smallest diameter) than the central-axis measurement. Therefore, the inverse square dependence does not completely account for the field gradient. Because the two mammographic units have source-to-film distances within 0.5 cm, the differences in the exposure deviations and field gradients between the units are not due to a difference in the inverse square factor.

Figure 2 shows that both the field gradient and the exposure deviation increase generally with increases in field nonuniformity. Field nonuniformity is a major contributor to the results for the field gradient and exposure deviation measured with the chamber. The results of linear regression analysis indicate a weak linear correlation: For the Senographe DMR field gradient and exposure deviation, $r^2 = .46$ and .72, respectively; for the Mam-CP II field gradient and exposure deviation, $r^2 = .66$ and .47, respectively. These correlations indicate that other factors, such as the design and configuration of the ionization chamber, introduce uncertainties in the measurement of the exposure deviation and field gradient.

The chambers listed in Table 2 are presented in the order of increasing chamber diameter. Generally, exposure deviation and field gradient tend to increase with an increase in chamber diameter. This is because as the diameter of the chamber increases, the chamber is positioned further from the center of the beam (because of the presence of the phantom) and thus is exposed to a higher field gradient. This demonstrates that the measurements are highly dependent on ionization chamber used. Because mean glandular dose is determined by applying multiplicative factors to ESE, mean glandular dose could be *underestimated* by up to 3.6% (Senographe DMR) and 8.0% (Mam-CP II) when compared with ionization chamber measurements obtained at the center of the field.

In conclusion, the designers of the ACR dosimetry protocol chose to use the exposure measured off-axis with the phantom in the beam as an estimate of the central-axis ESE free in air. The accuracy of the ACR method depends on how well this off-axis measurement approximates the central-axis ESE free in air. As our results show, there is variation in values that depends on the chamber and the mammographic x-ray units used. Thus, the mean glandular dose determined on the basis of the ACR protocol could underestimate the actual measured dose by 4%–8% for the x-ray machines used for this report. Our work shows that this difference depends on the mammographic unit, the type of chamber, and the kilovolt-peak setting. Due consideration should thus be given to the above-mentioned factors and to the "best" method of measuring ESE to better perform breast dosimetry. A method that could be used is to determine a correction factor that converts the off-axis measurement to a central-axis measurement. As demonstrated, this correction factor would need to be specific to a given mammographic unit, ionization chamber, and kilovolt-peak setting. Implementation of this correction factor would eliminate the underestimation of ESE caused by the off-axis measurement and, to a lesser extent, phantom scatter, but would still allow the ESE to be measured in the same manner as it is presently determined. ■

Acknowledgments: The authors acknowledge the helpful discussion with John LeHeron, PhD, of the National Radiation Laboratory, Christchurch, New Zealand. The authors also thank Todd R. McNutt, PhD, and Eric Hendee, MS, of the Department of Medical Physics, University of Wisconsin–Madison, for their help in film densitometry.

References

1. Rosenstein M, Andersen L, Warner G. Handbook of glandular tissue doses in mammography. HHS publication (FDA) no. 85-8239. Washington, DC: U.S. Department of Health and Human Services, 1985.
2. National Council on Radiation Protection and Measurements. Mammography: a user's guide. NCRP report no. 85. Washington, DC: Government Printing Office, 1986; 40–56.
3. Dodd GD. American Cancer Society guidelines from the past to the present. Cancer 1993; 72(suppl 4):1429–1432.
4. Wu X, Barnes GT, Tucker DM. Spectral dependence of glandular tissue dose in screen-film mammography. Radiology 1991; 179:143–148.
5. Wu X, Gingold EL, Barnes GT, Tucker DM. Normalized average glandular dose in molybdenum target–rhodium filter and rhodium target–rhodium filter mammography. Radiology 1994; 193:83–89.
6. Gentry JR, DeWerd LA. TLD measurements of in vivo mammographic exposures and the calculated mean glandular dose across the United States. Med Phys 1996; 23:899–903.
7. American College of Radiology. ACR mammography accreditation program: physicist's manual. Reston, Va: American College of Radiology, 1992.
8. Barnes GT, Brezovich IA. The intensity of scattered radiation in mammography. Radiology 1978; 126:243–247.
9. Ng KH, Aus RJ, DeWerd LA, Pearson DW. Dependence of backscatter factors on atomic number for a molybdenum anode with molybdenum filter for the 25 kVp to 35 kVp range. Presented at the Annual Meeting of the American Association of Physicists in Medicine, Philadelphia, Pa, 1996.
10. Dance DR. Monte Carlo calculation of conversion factors for the estimation of mean glandular breast dose. Phys Med Biol 1990; 35:1211–1219.
11. Law J, Dance DR, Faulkner K, Fitzgerald MC, Ramsdale ML, Robinson A. The commissioning and routine testing of mammographic x-ray systems. Report 59, 2nd ed. York, England: Institute of Physical Sciences in Medicine, 1994; 67–74.
12. Standardized methods for measuring diagnostic x-ray exposures. AAPM report no. 31. New York, NY: American Institute of Physics, 1991; 12.
13. DeWerd LA, Chiu NB. The determination of radiation dose by mail for diagnostic radiological examinations with thermoluminescent dosemeters. Radiat Protect Dosim 1993; 47:509–512.

Loren T. Niklason, PhD • Bradley T. Christian, PhD • Laura E. Niklason, MD, PhD • Daniel B. Kopans, MD
Donald E. Castleberry, PhD • Beale H. Opsahl-Ong, PhD • Cynthia E. Landberg, PhD
Priscilla J. Slanetz, MD • Angela A. Giardino, MD • Richard Moore, BS • Douglas Albagli, PhD
Michael C. DeJule, MS • Paul F. Fitzgerald, AAS • David F. Fobare, MS • Brian W. Giambattista, PhD
Robert F. Kwasnick, PhD • Jianqiang Liu, PhD • Stanley J. Lubowski, AAS • George E. Possin, PhD
James F. Richotte, AAS • Ching-Yeu Wei, PhD • Reinhold F. Wirth, MS

Digital Tomosynthesis in Breast Imaging[1]

PURPOSE: To describe and evaluate a method of tomosynthesis breast imaging with a full-field digital mammographic system.

MATERIALS AND METHODS: In this tomosynthesis method, low-radiation-dose images were acquired as the x-ray source was moved in an arc above the stationary breast and digital detector. A step-and-expose method of imaging was used. Breast tomosynthesis and conventional images of two imaging phantoms and four mastectomy specimens were obtained. Three experienced readers scored the relative lesion visibility, lesion margin visibility, and confidence in the classification of six lesions.

RESULTS: Tomosynthesis image-reconstruction algorithms allow tomographic imaging of the entire breast from a single arc of the x-ray source and at a radiation dose comparable with that in single-view mammography. Except for images of a large mass in a fatty breast, the tomosynthesis images were superior to the conventional images.

CONCLUSION: Digital mammographic systems make breast tomosynthesis possible. Tomosynthesis may improve the specificity of mammography with improved lesion margin visibility and may improve early breast cancer detection, especially in women with radiographically dense breasts.

The best method of detecting early stage breast cancer is mammography (1). It has been shown that finding breast cancer in its early stages saves lives (2). Even with the recent advances in mammographic imaging, 10%–30% of breast cancers may be missed, and other cancers are not detected early enough to make a cure possible (3–7). The main reason that breast cancers are missed is that the cancer is often obscured by radiographically dense, fibroglandular breast tissue (8–14). Holland and colleagues (8) found that 76% of missed cancers were in dense breasts.

This article describes a tomosynthesis method that allows the radiologist to see through the "structured noise" of normal breast tissue to improve the detection and characterization of early breast cancer. In conventional screen-film tomography, the x-ray source and the screen-film detector move in opposite directions, so that only features in one plane of the image remain in sharp focus. In tomography, one exposure is necessary for each imaged plane. One of two tomographic methods is typically used: the Twinning method (Fig 1) or the Grossman method (Fig 2). In the tomosynthesis method proposed here (Fig 3), multiple images are acquired as the x-ray tube is moved in an arc above the stationary breast and detector. The radiation dose is low for the acquisition of images at each angle, and the total radiation dose for the acquisition of all of the images is equivalent to or slightly higher than the dose in standard single-view mammography. By shifting and adding the digital images, it is possible to reconstruct any plane in the breast that is parallel to the detector. This technique can provide a series of images of the entire breast, with each image displaying only one plane of the breast in sharp focus.

Several authors (15–17) have demonstrated tomosynthesis with film as a detector by using the methods derived by Ziedses des Plantes (18). Miller and colleagues (15) concluded that, in general, images must be obtained from at least eight angles to produce a high-quality tomosynthesis image. Although these authors demonstrated that it was possible to use film as a detector, the system was too complicated for routine clinical use.

Electronic image acquisition has been performed by using an image intensifier as a detector and an analog-to-digital converter to obtain digital images from multiple angles in numerous applications of tomosyn-

Index terms: Breast neoplasms, radiography, 00.30, 00.121 • Breast radiography, radiation dose, 00.121 • Breast radiography, technology, 00.121 • Radiography, digital, 00.121 • Radiography, technology, 00.121

Abbreviation: ACR = American College of Radiology.

Radiology 1997; 205:399–406

[1] From the Department of Radiological Sciences, Massachusetts General Hospital, Harvard Medical School, Edwards 517, 50 Blossom St, Boston, MA 02114 (L.T.N., L.E.N., D.B.K., P.J.S., A.A.G., R.M.); the Department of Nuclear Medicine, Kettering Memorial Hospital, Kettering, Ohio (B.T.C.); and General Electric Corporate Research and Development, Schenectady, NY (D.E.C., B.O.O., C.E.L., D.A., M.C.D., P.F.F., D.F.F., B.W.G., R.F.K., J.L., S.J.L., G.E.P., J.F.R., C.Y.W., R.F.W.). From the 1996 RSNA scientific assembly. Received March 31, 1997; revision requested May 28; revision received and accepted July 8. **Address reprint requests to** L.T.N.

Patent applied for by Massachusetts General Hospital, Boston.

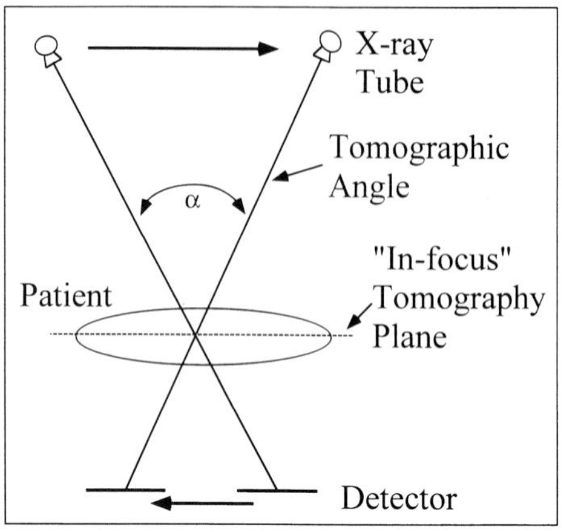

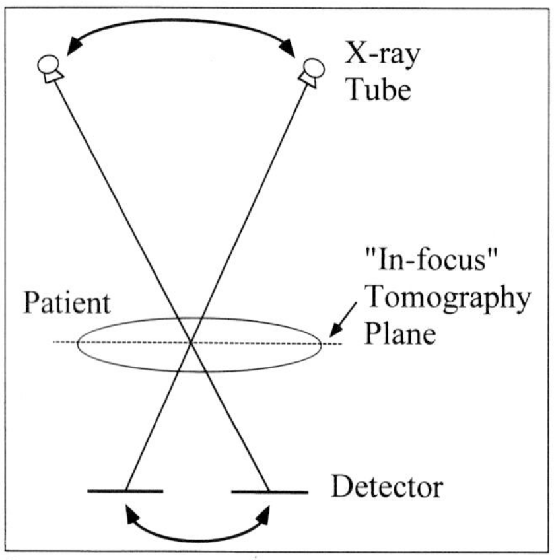

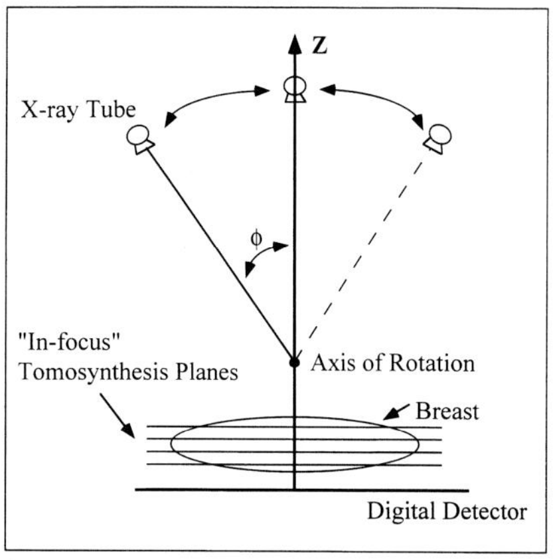

1. 2. 3.

Figures 1–3. **(1)** Twinning geometry for tomographic imaging. The x-ray source and detector move parallel to the in-focus tomographic plane. α = tomographic angle. **(2)** Grossman geometry for tomographic imaging. The x-ray source and detector move in an arc. **(3)** Proposed geometry for breast tomosynthesis. The x-ray source is stationary during each x-ray exposure and is then moved along an arc above the breast to the next position. The number of positions is variable. The breast and digital detector remain stationary. Z = distance above the digital detector, ϕ = x-ray–source angle.

thesis outside of mammography (19–27). Both linear and circular x-ray–tube motions have been investigated. The feasibility of tomosynthesis has been demonstrated in angiography (20–22,24,26). Tomosynthesis has also been investigated in tomography of the lung (20) and the ear (27) and in knee arthrography (20). Images superior to conventional tomograms have been obtained by reducing the streak artifacts by means of one-dimensional filtering of the linear tomosynthesis images (19,27–29). Chakraborty and colleagues (27) have suggested a one-dimensional, unsharp masking technique called self-masking tomosynthesis. Additional methods to reduce the contribution of out-of-focus structures to the in-focus plane have been explored (30–32). Unfortunately, the use of an image intensifier with a curved detector surface has limited the success of these previous attempts at digital tomosynthesis.

Despite numerous studies that have explored the use of tomosynthesis, successful clinical application has been delayed by the lack of a full-field, flat, digital detector with rapid readout. Digital imaging technology has now been introduced that makes tomosynthesis imaging of the breast practical in a clinical setting. The full-field, digital mammographic system undergoing clinical evaluation at our institution is ideally suited for the clinical application of tomosynthesis because of the following properties: low noise; large, flat surface area with minimal image distortion; and rapid image readout.

The proposed method of tomosynthesis was developed at our institution and represents an extension of the technology described in earlier reports. The main differences between this and previous studies are primarily the use of a stationary detector and of existing mechanical arm systems that translate the x-ray tube in an arc above the detector. We have derived reconstruction methods to allow tomosynthesis image reconstruction for this geometry. We believe that tomosynthesis has the potential to improve current mammographic imaging by increasing the sensitivity and specificity in the detection of breast carcinoma. Thus, we performed this study to describe and evaluate a method of tomosynthesis breast imaging with a full-field digital mammographic system.

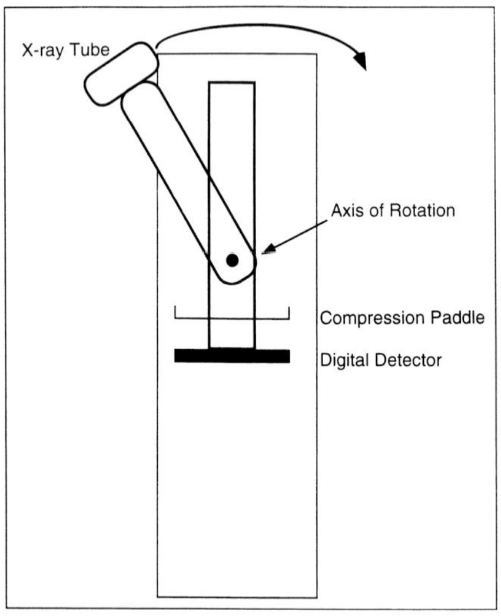

Figure 4. Mammographic system used for tomosynthesis. The x-ray tube is on a rigid mechanical arm that pivots about a point above the breast.

MATERIALS AND METHODS

A schematic of the mammographic system used for digital breast tomosynthesis is shown in Figure 4. The basic system is a mammographic system (model DMR; GE Medical Systems, Milwaukee, Wis) with a full-field digital image receptor. The system has been modified to allow imaging at any angle up to ±27° from the perpendicular to the detector. As shown in Figure 4, the x-ray source pivots about a point above the detector. The x-ray source is stationary during the exposure and then is manually moved to the next position before the next image is obtained.

The digital detector is composed of cesium iodide phosphor on an amorphous silicon transistor-photodiode array. This detector was developed by General Electric Corporate Research and Development (Schenectady, NY). The pixel pitch is 100 μm and the image readout time is 300 msec. The tomosynthesis images were obtained without an antiscatter grid to avoid grid cutoff for the angled projections. The x-ray–source angle (ϕ in Fig 3) was determined with a precision inclinometer (model 02538-01; Lucas Control System Products, Hampton, Va) with a range of ±20° and an accuracy of ±0.1° for 0°–10° and of ±1% for 10°–20°.

The tomosynthesis projection images were obtained at discrete x-ray–source positions as the tube was moved above the breast, as shown in Figure 5. For simplicity, only four x-ray–source positions are shown in Figure 5; however, the number of x-ray–source positions is variable. The tomosynthesis images in any plane in the breast may be reconstructed by using the method shown. The projection images from x-ray–source positions 1–4 were transformed, as described in the Appendix, to simulate images obtained from x-ray–source positions 1a–4a (Fig 5). After transformation of the images, the geometry is similar to Twinning geometry, except that the detector does not move. De-

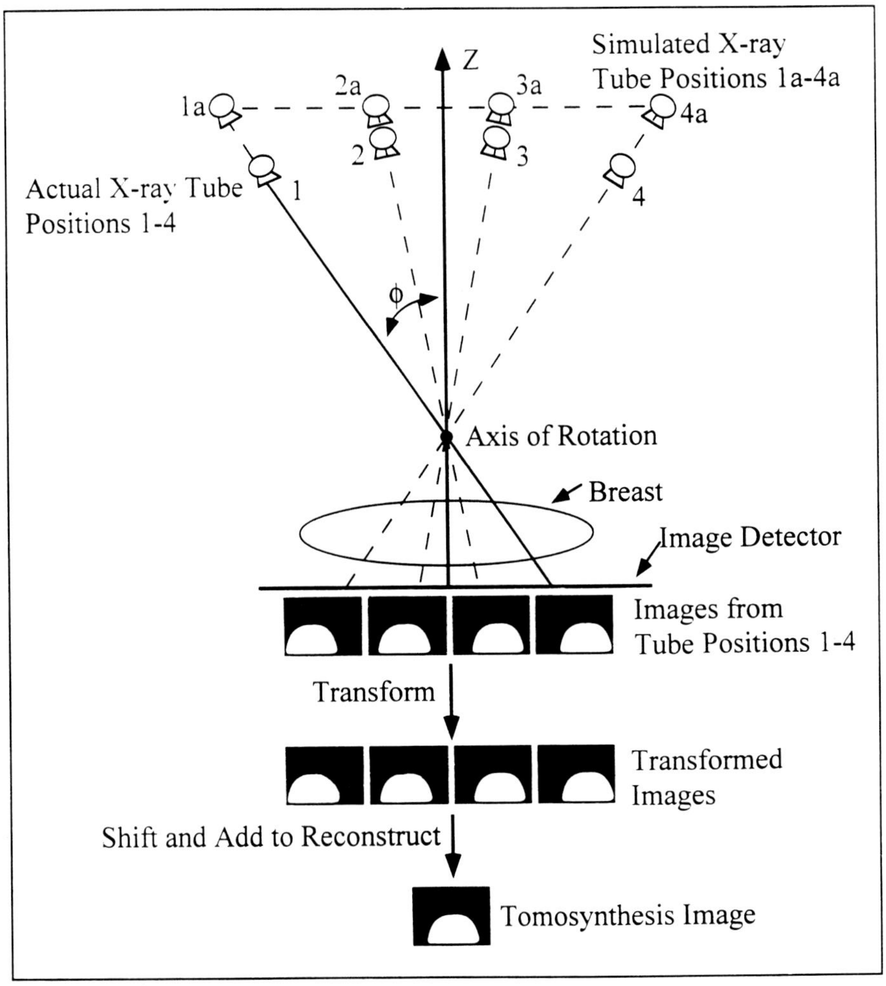

Figure 5. Tomosynthesis reconstruction method with four x-ray–tube positions shown. Images are obtained from positions 1–4 and are transformed, by using the algorithms described in the Appendix, to construct images that would be obtained from source positions 1a–4a. These images simulate tomographic images obtained by using Twinning geometry and may be shifted and combined to create a tomosynthesis image at any level in the breast. Z = distance above the digital detector, ϕ = x-ray–source angle.

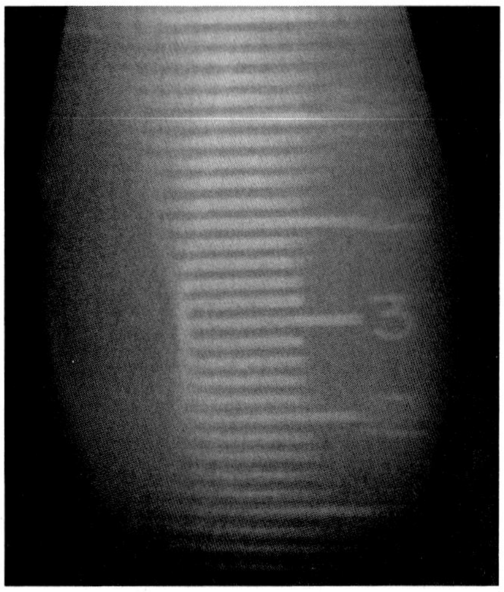

Figure 6. Tomosynthesis image of a Picker tomographic phantom reconstructed at 3 cm above the detector platform demonstrates the thickness of the in-focus plane for the tube motion.

tector motion is simulated by shifting the images in the computer. The transformation and shifting algorithms may be repeated to reconstruct the tomographic planes at any height above the detector. The mathematic reconstruction algorithms are derived in the Appendix.

Images were obtained in one of two tomographic phantoms (one made by Picker International, Cleveland, Ohio, and the other the accreditation phantom of the American College of Radiology [ACR], Reston, Va). The tomosynthesis images of both phantoms were obtained with the following parameters: 26 kVp, molybdenum filter, molybdenum target, 20 mAs per view, and nine views at −20°, −15°, −10°, −5°, 0°, 5°, 10°, 15°, and 20° from the detector perpendicular. A conventional screen-film image of the ACR phantom was obtained at 26 kVp and 126 mAs with a molybdenum target and a molybdenum filter. The total mean glandular radiation dose for the tomosynthesis images was 1.4 times that for the conventional screen-film images. A conventional digital image of the ACR phantom also was obtained by using the same technique as in screen-film imaging, except that 120 mAs was used. Radiation dose estimates for the tomosynthesis projection images, compared to those for the conventional images, take into account differences in the source-to-object distance and in the x-ray–path length through the object.

Images of four unfixed mastectomy specimens were obtained. The specimens were placed in a polymerized methyl methacrylate box and compressed by using a movable top plate. Tomosynthesis specimen images were obtained at seven to nine projections and with a total tomographic angle of 30°–40°. The total radiation dose was varied 0.89–1.74 times that in conventional mammography in the same specimen. Tomosynthesis images of the specimens were reconstructed on a workstation (Sparc 20; Sun Microsystems, Mountain View, Calif). After the initial images were acquired for each angle, we reconstructed tomographic images at 1.5–3.0-mm spacing to display in-focus tomosynthesis images of the entire breast.

Conventional screen-film mammograms were obtained with film (MR5II; Agfa, Ridgefield Park, NJ) and screens (MR detail; Agfa) by using extended processing. These images were obtained with automatic exposure control by using a conventional screen-film system. The kilovolt peak, focal spot sizes, radiation output, and half-value layers of this unit were all closely matched to those of the digital unit.

The two units were installed in the same room, and adjustments were made to match the above parameters during installation. A molybdenum target and a molybdenum filter were used to obtain all of the specimen images, which included the digital, tomosynthesis, and screen-film images.

A preliminary reader study was performed to compare tomosynthesis images with screen-film images of all lesions in the specimens. The conventional screen-film image was shown next to the tomographic image that best demonstrated the mass or calcification in each specimen on a standard, high-intensity, mammographic view box. The digital tomosynthesis images were printed by using a laser imager (40 µm pixel size; Agfa).

Three board-certified radiologists (D.B.K., P.J.S., A.A.G.) with special expertise in mammography were asked to compare the visibility of a mass or a cluster of calcifications in each specimen. Before reading, the location of the lesion was identified by an expert reader (D.B.K.) and marked with an arrow. The readers scored the lesion visibility, lesion margin visibility, and confidence in the classification of benign versus malignant lesions. Scoring was based on a five-point scale: (*a*) conventional images were diagnostically superior, (*b*) conventional images were superior, (*c*) conventional and tomosynthesis images were equal, (*d*) tomosynthesis images were superior, and (*e*) tomosynthesis images were diagnostically superior.

RESULTS

Figure 6 is a tomosynthesis image obtained in a tomography phantom

a.

b.

Figure 7. Images of the ACR phantom. (a) Digital tomosynthesis image. (b) Conventional digital image. (c) Screen-film image.

c.

reconstructed to have an in-focus plane at 3 cm above the detector platform. This figure demonstrates the thickness of the in-focus plane. This image was obtained at a total tomosynthesis angle (2 × ϕ in Fig 3) of 40°. This 40° tomosynthesis angle is equivalent to a tomographic angle of 29.4° (α in Fig 1) in conventional linear tomography for an in-focus plane at 3 cm above the detector platform. The in-focus plane thickness would be expected to be 2.5 mm for this tomographic angle according to conventional geometry (33). This calculated in-focus plane thickness agrees well with that in the tomosynthesis image (Fig 6).

Images of an ACR phantom obtained by using tomosynthesis, conventional screen-film imaging, and conventional digital imaging are shown in Figure 7. The tomosynthesis image of the ACR phantom was reconstructed at the level of the targets. The masses and fibers are seen as well with tomosynthesis as with conventional digital imaging. The fourth calcification group is seen with tomosynthesis, but not as clearly as with conventional imaging. The borders of the calcifications are not as sharp on the tomosynthesis image as they are on the conventional images, because the tomosynthesis image is the summation of nine different projections. Nonetheless, the image quality of the tomosynthesis image is sufficient to pass the ACR criteria for phantom images (34).

The preliminary reader scores are shown in the Table. Except for the tomosynthesis images of a 3-cm mass in a fatty breast, the tomosynthesis images were judged to be superior in lesion visibility, margin visibility, and confidence in classification. In the three subtle lesions, which were in regions of radiographically dense tissue, tomosynthesis images were judged to be diagnostically superior by at least two of the three radiologists for the three parameters. Images of two of the specimens are shown in Figures 8 and 9.

Figure 8 shows tomosynthesis and standard screen-film images of mastectomy specimen 1 (Table), which contained a mass with associated calcifications distributed over a 3-cm^2 area. The tomosynthesis images were reconstructed from seven projections obtained from −15° to +15° in increments of 5°. The total mean glandular radiation dose for acquisition of all of the tomosynthesis images was 1.06 times the radiation dose for acquisition of a single-view, screen-film mammogram. As indicated in the Table, the mass is difficult to detect on the conventional image (Fig 8a). However, the mass is clearly demonstrated

Preliminary Reader Study: Tomosynthesis versus Conventional Imaging of Mastectomy Specimens

Specimen Number	Lesion Description	X-ray–Source Arc	Tomographic Dose/ Conventional Dose*	Parameter	Conventional Imaging Diagnostically Superior	Conventional Imaging Superior	Conventional and Tomo-synthesis Imaging Equal	Tomo-synthesis Imaging Superior	Tomosynthesis Imaging Diagnostically Superior
1	Subtle irregular mass	30°	1.06	Lesion visibility	–	–	–	+	++
				Lesion margin visibility	–	–	–	–	+++
				Confidence in lesion classification	–	–	–	+	++
2	Subtle calcification cluster	40°	1.05	Lesion visibility	–	–	–	+	++
				Lesion margin visibility	–	–	–	+	+
				Confidence in lesion classification	–	–	–	+	++
3	Subtle rounded mass	40°	0.89	Lesion visibility	–	–	–	+	++
				Lesion margin visibility	–	–	–	–	+++
				Confidence in lesion classification	–	–	–	+	++
	Rounded mass	40°	0.89	Lesion visibility	–	–	+	++	–
				Lesion margin visibility	–	–	–	+	++
				Confidence in lesion classification	–	–	–	+	++
	Architectural distortion	40°	0.89	Lesion visibility	–	–	–	–	+++
				Lesion margin visibility	–	–	–	–	+++
				Confidence in lesion classification	–	–	–	–	+++
4	3-cm mass with irregular margins	30°	1.74	Lesion visibility	–	–	+++	–	–
				Lesion margin visibility	–	+	+	+	–
				Confidence in lesion classification	–	–	+++	–	–

Note.—Scores are for three readers; each individual score is marked by a "+." A "–" indicates that there is no score. One reader did not score the margin visibility of the calcification cluster.

* The ratio of the mean glandular radiation dose for tomosynthesis (sum of the doses from all projections) to that for conventional imaging.

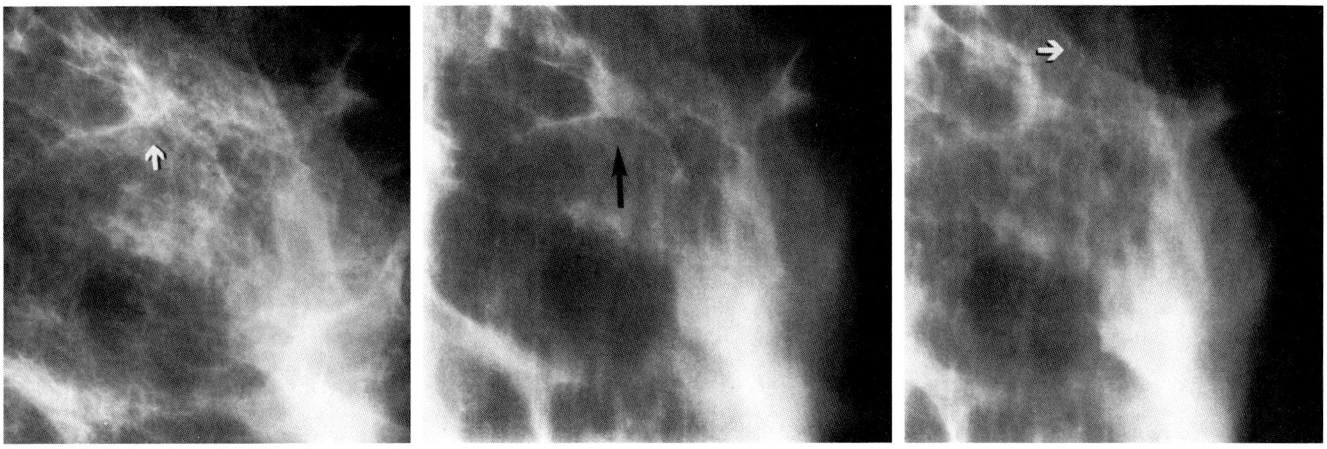

a. b. c.

Figure 8. Images of a mastectomy specimen that contains a subtle mass and associated calcifications. **(a)** Screen-film image obtained at 26 kVp and 197 mAs faintly shows the mass (arrow). **(b)** Tomosynthesis image reconstructed at 7.1 cm above the detector demonstrates the mass (arrow), which was difficult to detect on **a.** Tomosynthesis images were obtained at 5° intervals over a 30° arc. Each image was obtained at 26 kVp and 30 mAs. The total mean glandular radiation dose for acquisition of the tomosynthesis images was approximately equal to the radiation dose for acquisition of one screen-film image in the same specimen. **(c)** Tomosynthesis image reconstructed with the in-focus plane at 6.4 cm above the detector shows a group of microcalcifications (arrow) at this level.

on the tomosynthesis image reconstructed at 7.1 cm above the detector (Fig 8b). The tomosynthesis image reconstructed at 6.4 cm above the detector demonstrates several calcifications at this level (Fig 8c). Figure 8c demonstrates the ability to maintain the contrast and sharpness of small objects in the reconstructed plane wth the algorithms. Figure 8 also demonstrates the ability to determine whether calcifications are associated with a mass and the three-dimensional relationships between masses and calcifications.

Figure 9 shows tomosynthesis images and standard projection digital images of mastectomy specimen 3

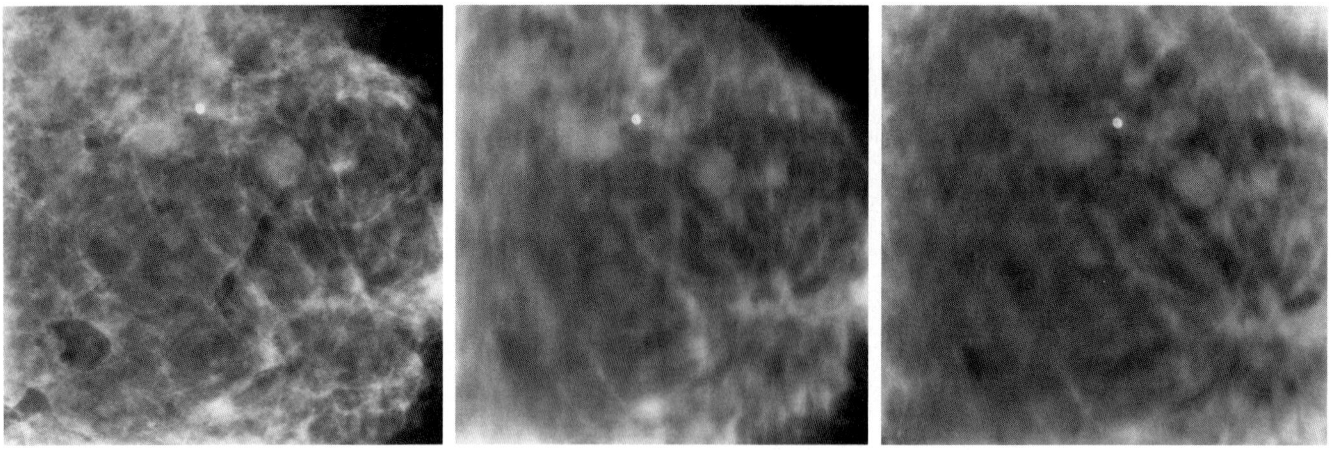

a. b. c.

Figure 9. Images of a mastectomy specimen that contains two masses in the upper central regions of the images and an area of architectural distortion in the lower right. **(a)** Conventional digital image obtained at 25 kVp and 100 mAs. **(b)** Tomosynthesis image with the in-focus plane at 4.45 cm above the detector demonstrates two masses and an area of architectural distortion. One of the masses and the area of architectural distortion are better depicted on **b** than on **a.** The tomosynthesis images were obtained at nine positions at −20° to +20° from the detector perpendicular at 5° intervals. Each image was obtained at 25 kVp and 10 mAs. The total mean glandular radiation dose for acquisition of the tomosynthesis images was 0.89 times that for acquisition of the conventional images in the same specimen. **(c)** Same tomosynthesis image as **b** but with self-masking with a kernel that corresponds to 200 pixels (2 cm).

(Table), which contained two masses and an area of architectural distortion. The digital image (Fig 9a) was obtained with conventional imaging geometry by using the same technical parameters as in screen-film imaging. One mass is clearly visible on the conventional digital image; however, the margins are better depicted on the tomosynthesis image (Fig 9b) reconstructed at 4.45 cm above the detector. Another mass slightly above and to the left of the first mass is seen on the tomosynthesis image but not on the conventional image. In addition, a lower-right area of architectural distortion is displayed well on tomosynthesis images but poorly on the conventional image (Fig 9). The total mean glandular dose for tomosynthesis imaging was 0.89 times the dose for conventional imaging. Thus, even at a radiation dose less than the dose for acquisition of a single mammogram, the tomosynthesis images provide improved lesion visibility compared with the lesion visibility on conventional images.

Figure 9c is a self-masking tomosynthesis image obtained at the same level as Figure 9b, at 4.45 cm above the detector, by using a method similar to that of Chakraborty and colleagues (27). In the self-masking tomosynthesis method, a one-dimensional, unsharp mask is used to reduce streaking artifacts. This image demonstrates a reduction in low-frequency noise.

DISCUSSION

For the last 2 decades, efforts to bring tomosynthesis into the clinical environment have been unsuccessful (19–27). These efforts have been hampered by the lack of a digital, flat-panel detector with rapid image readout. Recent advances in detector development have now made clinical application of tomosynthesis possible. Our results indicate that breast tomosynthesis is capable of producing high-quality breast images that may contain information that is currently not visible with conventional imaging.

Phantom studies demonstrate the ability to attain in-focus planes and the ability to depict small microcalcifications. Tomosynthesis images of the ACR phantom, which has no structured noise, demonstrate an image quality comparable with that of conventional images at 1.4 times the radiation dose.

The value of tomosynthesis imaging is evident in images with substantial structured noise from radiographically dense tissue, as demonstrated in the reader study. Although the number of specimens is small, tomosynthesis images of mastectomy specimens demonstrate an improvement in the depiction of lesions. In three of the four specimens, lesions were seen with tomosynthesis that were either not seen or poorly seen with conventional imaging.

The method proposed for tomosynthesis in this study is different from most previous implementations because the images are obtained at discrete tube positions rather than continuously as the tube moves. Consequently, the blurring of structures is not the smooth blurring typical of continuous image acquisition. For example, if nine images are used in the tomosynthesis data set, objects above or below the in-focus plane will be displayed as nine separate objects on the reconstructed image. Each object will have approximately one-ninth the contrast of the original object. For high-contrast objects such as a large calcification, nine images of the calcification may be visible. Although we use the term "blurring," the images of structures outside the in-focus plane are essentially repeated in the direction of x-ray–source motion. High-frequency information is retained, although the contrast of out-of-plane structures is greatly reduced.

Self-masking tomosynthesis (Fig 9c) reduces low-frequency information in the direction of the x-ray–source motion (27). Because of discrete sampling for the proposed method, other image-processing methods may be better suited to reducing the contribution of out-of-focus structures from planes above or below the in-focus plane. A method similar to that of Kolitsi and colleagues (30) will be tested in the future. This method identifies the plane of an out-of-focus structure such as a dense calcification and computes its contribution to all other planes. The image of the structure may then be removed from all planes except for the plane that contains the structure in focus.

There are several potential uses of tomosynthesis for breast imaging. Tomosynthesis may prove to be a valuable screening tool in women with radiographically dense breasts. The ability to see into the middle of the breast by blurring the superimposed structures may

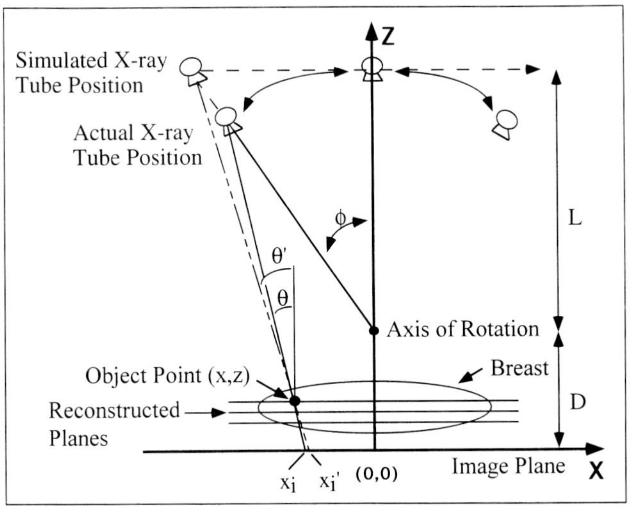

Figure A1. Geometry for tomosynthesis image reconstruction. Diagram defines the angles, distances, and coordinate system used for the reconstruction algorithms. Z = distance above the digital detector.

allow important improvements in the sensitivity of mammographic screening in the early detection of breast cancer. Tomosynthesis may depict cancers in dense breasts or multifocal cancers at a small fraction of the cost of magnetic resonance imaging, which has recently been proposed as another method for detecting these cancers (35).

Tomosynthesis may also be used for problem solving or diagnostic breast imaging. Current mammographic techniques have poor specificity, as 70%–90% of all breast biopsy results are negative (36–38). Tomosynthesis may provide the radiologist with an improved image of a potential lesion. The results shown in the Table indicate that improved depiction of lesion margins may allow the radiologist to have greater confidence in lesion classification and decrease the number of biopsies with benign results. It may also be possible to perform the entire diagnostic evaluation of a lesion with tomosynthesis. Compared with current diagnostic examinations, in which it is necessary to obtain a large number of mammograms, tomosynthesis may save time and reduce patient radiation exposure.

Tomosynthesis will provide three-dimensional information on the dimensions of a lesion, on whether microcalcifications are associated with a mass, and on how they are distributed. The three-dimensional distribution of calcifications is thought to be a useful indicator in discriminating between benign and malignant lesions and thus may also have a positive effect on clinical management (39).

The tomosynthesis method is readily adaptable to current mammographic systems with minor modifications. This geometry has several advantages: (*a*) there are no moving parts near the breast or abdomen; (*b*) existing mammographic machines may be easily altered to allow this type of motion, because many already provide the ability for the tube to move in an arc above the breast; and (*c*) a unit modified for tomosynthesis imaging will still be completely usable for routine breast imaging, which eliminates the need for a dedicated tomosynthesis system. The development of motorized motion of the x-ray tube should allow the acquisition of all of the tomosynthesis images in approximately 3–5 seconds. This is sufficiently rapid to make the system clinically applicable, because these exposure times are similar to exposure times in the acquisition of magnification views with current systems.

In summary, these early results demonstrate that tomosynthesis imaging may be a valuable clinical tool for the early detection of breast cancer and the characterization of benign and malignant lesions.

APPENDIX

The proposed system for breast tomosynthesis imaging is shown in Figure 10. This system requires a different image reconstruction algorithm. As shown in Figure A1, the tomographic angle ϕ is given by the angle of the x rays intersecting the perpendicular to the image plane at the axis of rotation of the x-ray tube. For any given point in the object (x,z), we may define an angle θ as the angle of the x rays intersecting that point relative to the perpendicular to the image plane. The angle θ is a function of ϕ, x, and z, and is given by $\theta(\phi,x,z) = \arctan (L\sin\phi + x)/(L\cos\phi + D - z)$, where L is the distance between the axis of rotation and the x-ray–tube position and D is the distance between the axis of rotation and the image plane (as defined in Fig A1). From this angle, we may derive point x_i, which is the projection of the object point (x,z) onto the image plane:

$$x_i(\phi, x, z) = z(L \sin \phi + x) / (L \cos \phi + D - z). \quad \text{(A1)}$$

$x_i(\phi,x,z)$ is the image point formed by x rays emitted from an x-ray tube that is rotated about the axis. The magnification (M) of points in the object is a function not only of the position z, but also of the angle ϕ: $M(\phi,z) = (L\cos\phi + D)/(L\cos\phi + D - z)$.

Because magnification varies with ϕ and z, it is not possible to reconstruct a tomographic plane by simply shifting and adding the digital images. To facilitate the reconstruction, it is helpful to construct the images that would be produced if the x-ray tube were moved according to the Twinning principle (Fig 1). Thus, if the x-ray tube were rotated by a tomographic angle ϕ, but was constrained to remain in the horizontal plane at a distance of $L + D$ from the image, then the angle of the x rays intersecting an object point would be given as follows:

$$\theta'(\phi, x, z) = \arctan (L\tan \phi + x) / (L + D - z). \quad \text{(A2)}$$

From Equation (A2), it follows that the image point x_i', which is the projection of the object point (x,z) onto the new image plane, is given as follows:

$$x_i'(\phi, x, z) = x + z (L \tan \phi + x) / (L + D - z). \quad \text{(A3)}$$

The proposed x-ray gantry for digital tomosynthesis produces images with image points as defined by Equation (A1). For every x_i in the image, we may use the known value of ϕ and a selected z to determine an object point x with Equation (A1). The values of ϕ, x, and z may then be applied to Equation (A3) to determine a value for x_i' in the new image. The set of new images thus produced may then be used to reconstruct a tomographic plane at z by means of a simple linear shifting process that is analogous to the Twinning method. An example of the method is shown schematically in Figure 5 with projections from tube positions 1–4.

The technique for construction of a new set of images for each desired tomographic plane results in a small distortion of image information for structures outside the plane. This is because the x-ray paths through the object that occur with rotation of the focal spot about an axis are slightly different from those that occur with movement of the focal spot within a horizontal plane. The magnitude of the distortion increases with the distance from the reconstructed plane and also increases with the distance from the central axis of the image (ie, $x = 0$). The distortion for all points that lie exactly on the reconstructed plane is zero. This off-plane distortion is small compared with the blurring caused by tomography. Because it is our intention to blur the structures above or below the in-focus plane, we do not expect that distortion produced by this technique will have any important effects on the tomographic image quality. The method will allow exact reconstruction of all of the objects in the in-focus plane. ■

Acknowledgments: The team from Massachusetts General Hospital, Boston, acknowledges the help of Maria Hanley, RT(M), and thanks Donald Plewes, PhD, for helpful discussions on the removal of the out-of-plane structures from the images. The team from General Electric Corporate Research and Development, Schenectady, NY, acknowledges the invaluable assistance of many present and former colleagues, both at General Electric Corporate Research and Development and GE Medical Systems. In particular, Jack Kingsley, PhD, Henri Rougeot, PhD, and Gene Hilton, PhD, played key roles in the early development of the digital detector technology and associated imaging systems.

References

1. Baker LH. Breast cancer detection demonstration project: five-year summary report. CA Cancer J Clin 1982; 32:194–225.
2. Tabar L, Duffy SW, Krusemo UB. Detection method, tumor size and node metastases in breast cancers diagnosed during a trial of breast cancer screening. Eur J Cancer Clin Oncol 1987; 23:959–962.
3. Hilman BJ, Fajardo LL, Hunter TB, et al. Mammogram interpretation by physician assistants. AJR 1987; 149:907–911.
4. Kalisher L. Factors influencing false negative rates in xeromammography. Radiology 1979; 133:297–301.
5. Bassett LW, Bunnell DH, Jahanshahi R, Gold RH, Arndt RD, Linsman J. Breast cancer detection: one versus two views. Radiology 1987; 165:95–97.
6. Baines CJ, Miller AB, Wall C, et al. Sensitivity and specificity of first screen mammography in the Canadian national breast screening study: a preliminary report from five centers. Radiology 1986; 160:295–298.
7. Haug PJ, Tocino IM, Clayton PD, Bair TL. Automated management of screening and diagnostic mammography. Radiology 1987; 164:747–752.
8. Holland R, Mravunac M, Hendriks JHCL, Bekker BV. So-called interval cancers of the breast. Cancer 1982; 49:2527–2533.
9. Martin J, Moskowitz M, Milbrath JR. Breast cancers missed by mammography. AJR 1979; 132:737–739.
10. Holland R, Hendriks JHCL, Mravunac M. Mammographically occult breast cancer: a pathologic and radiologic study. Cancer 1983; 52:1810–1819.
11. Feig S, Shaber G, Patchefsky A, et al. Analysis of clinically occult and mammographically occult breast tumors. AJR 1977; 128:403–408.
12. Ma L, Fishell E, Wright B, Hanna W, Allan S, Boyd NF. Case-control study of factors associated with failure to detect breast cancer by mammography. J Natl Cancer Inst 1992; 84:781–785.
13. Jackson VP, Hendrick RE, Feig SA, Kopans DB. Imaging of the radiographically dense breast. Radiology 1993; 188:297–301.
14. Bird R, Wallace T, Yankaskas B. Analysis of cancers missed at screening mammography. Radiology 1992; 184:613–617.
15. Miller ER, McCurry EM, Hruka B. An infinite number of laminagrams from a finite number of radiographs. Radiology 1971; 98:249–255.
16. Garrison JB, Grant DG, Guier WH, Johns RJ. Three dimensional roentgenography. AJR 1969; 105:903–908.
17. Richards AG. Variable depth laminography. Biomed Sci Instrum 1969; 6:194–199.
18. Ziedses des Plantes BG. Eine neue methode zur diffenzierung in der rontgenographie (planigraphie). Acta Radiol 1932; 13: 182–192. [German]
19. Sone S, Kasuga T, Sakai F, et al. Chest imaging with dual-energy subtraction digital tomosynthesis. Acta Radiol 1993; 34:346–349.
20. Sone S, Kasuga T, Sakai F, et al. Development of a high-resolution digital tomosynthesis system and its clinical application. RadioGraphics 1991; 11:807–822.
21. Kruger RA, Sedaghati M, Roy DG, et al. Tomosynthesis applied to digital subtraction angiography. Radiology 1984; 152:805–808.
22. deVries N, Miller FJ, Wojtowycz MM, et al. Tomographic digital subtraction angiography: initial clinical studies using tomosynthesis. Radiology 1985; 157:239–241.
23. Baily NA, Lasser EC, Crepeau RL. Electrofluoroplanigraphy. Radiology 1973; 107: 669–671.
24. Baily NA, Crepeau RL, Lasser EC. Fluoroscopic tomography. Invest Radiol 1981; 16: 126–132.
25. Maravilla KR, Murry RC, Horner S. Digital tomosynthesis: technique for electronic reconstructive tomography. AJR 1983; 141: 497–502.
26. Maravilla KR, Murry RC, Diehl J, et al. Digital tomosynthesis: technique modification and clinical application for neurovascular anatomy. Radiology 1984; 152:719–724.
27. Chakraborty DP, Yester MV, Barnes GT, Lakshminarayanan AV. Self-masking subtraction tomosynthesis. Radiology 1984; 150:225–229.
28. Edholm PR, Quiding L. Reduction of linear blurring in tomography. Radiology 1969; 92:1115–1118.
29. Edholm P, Quiding L. Elimination of blur in linear tomography. Acta Radiol 1970; 10:441–447.
30. Kolitsi Z, Panayiotakis G, Pallikarakis N. A method for selective removal of out-of-plane structures in digital tomosynthesis. Med Phys 1993; 20:47–50.
31. Ghosh Roy DN, Kruger RA, Yih B, Del Rio P. Selective plane removal in limited angle tomographic imaging. Med Phys 1985; 12:65–70.
32. Ruttiman UE, Qi XL, Webber RL. An optimal synthetic aperture for circular tomosynthesis. Med Phys 1989; 16:398–405.
33. Littleton JT, Winter FS. Linear laminography: simple geometric interpretation of its clinical limitations. Am J Roentgenol Radiat Ther Nucl Med 1965; 95:981–991.
34. Committee on Quality Assurance in Mammography. Mammography quality control manual. Reston, Va: American College of Radiology, 1994.
35. Harms SE, Flamig DP, Hesley KL, et al. MR imaging of the breast with rotating delivery of excitation off resonance: clinical experience with pathologic correlation. Radiology 1993; 187:493–501.
36. Kopans DB. The positive predictive value of mammography. AJR 1992; 158:521–526.
37. Hall FM, Storella JM, Silverstone DZ, Wyshak G. Nonpalpable breast lesions: recommendation for biopsy based on suspicion of carcinoma at mammography. Radiology 1988; 167:353–358.
38. Sickles EA. Mammographic features of 300 consecutive nonpalpable breast cancers. AJR 1986; 146:661–663.
39. Ng KH, Looi LM, Bradley DA. Microcalcification clustering parameters in breast disease: a morphometric analysis of radiographs of excision specimens. Br J Radiol 1996; 69:326–334.

Fred Burbank, MD • Nancy Forcier, MD

Tissue Marking Clip for Stereotactic Breast Biopsy: Initial Placement Accuracy, Long-term Stability, and Usefulness as a Guide for Wire Localization[1]

PURPOSE: To determine initial placement accuracy, long-term stability, and usefulness as a guide for wire localization for metallic marker clips placed percutaneously after stereotactic breast biopsy.

MATERIALS AND METHODS: One hundred forty-nine marker clips were placed percutaneously with a straight-needle or through-probe method, and clip positions were measured. The locations of 31 marker clips were followed up from deployment to first follow-up mammography. Thirty-six biopsy sites with marker clips were excised surgically and examined; 18 of these marker clips were targets for wire localization. The locations of 22 benign lesions were measured over time to calibrate the measurement system.

RESULTS: Baseline variability was 8 mm. Initial marker clip deployment averaged 5 mm above baseline from the center of the target lesion ($P \leq .01$). Compared with baseline variability, marker clips remained in place from initial deployment to first imaging follow-up (mean, 8.6 months). Potentially clinically meaningful misplacement rates (deployment > 24 mm from target lesion center) were 7% for the through-probe method and 11% for the straight-needle method (not significantly different; $P = .33$).

CONCLUSION: The marker clips appear to be useful targets for wire localization when the entire target lesion is removed at directional, vacuum-assisted breast biopsy. Upright, two-view mammography is recommended after deployment of the marker clip to document location.

When percutaneous breast biopsy was first performed with fine-needle aspiration to establish a cytologic diagnosis for a mammographically identified lesion, the concern that fine-needle aspiration would remove the entire target lesion was not addressed, to our knowledge. Conversely, insufficient acquisition of tissue has become the "Achilles' heel" of fine-needle aspiration breast biopsy (1). After the introduction of automated core needle breast biopsy by Parker et al (2) in 1990, concern that a small target lesion might be removed entirely with use of this technique led Dershaw (3) and Sullivan (4) to recommend that automated core needle breast biopsies be performed only on lesions greater than 5 mm in diameter.

Dronkers (5) reported that in six (8.6%) of 70 18-gauge automated core needle breast biopsies (Crown-Core-Cut Needle; Biomed Instrumente Produkte, Turkenfeld, Germany), "... the lesion disappeared after the stereotactic biopsy". Similarly, Mikhail and colleagues (6) reported that in 60 lesions in which breast biopsy was performed with a 14-gauge automated core needle (Biopty-Cut Needle; Bard Gynecology and Radiology, Covington, Ga), three (5%) lesions were malignant and "... were so small that the ... needle biopsy completely removed the focus of malignant cells ... ".

An even higher frequency of total excision of all visible target lesion landmarks has been reported after directional, vacuum-assisted breast biopsy. In a study in which 14-gauge directional, vacuum-assisted probes (Mammotome; Biopsys Medical, Irvine, Calif) were used (these probes remove 35–45 mg of tissue per specimen), Burbank reported that 50% of the target lesions could not be identified mammographically immediately after stereotactic breast biopsy and that 48% of the lesions could not be identified at the first imaging follow-up months after the stereotactic biopsy (7,8). Excisional breast biopsies that demonstrate histologically clear margins of atypical ductal hyperplasia, ductal carcinoma in situ, and infiltrating breast cancer for lesions 5 mm in diameter and smaller have been reported in 30% of the 14-gauge directional, vacuum-assisted breast biopsies (9).

Furthermore, directional, vacuum-assisted breast biopsies are now being performed percutaneously with 11-gauge probes. The 11-gauge probe removes approximately 90–100 mg of tissue per specimen (10). At this level of percutaneous removal of breast tissue, all visible signs of the target lesion may be removed at an even higher frequency than reported previously.

When total removal of the target lesion occurs during a diagnostic percutaneous stereotactic breast biopsy and the target lesion proves to be

Index terms: Biopsies, technology, 00.1261, 00.1267 • Breast, biopsy, 00.1261, 00.1267 • Breast neoplasms, diagnosis, 00.31, 00.32 • Stereotaxis, 00.1267

Radiology 1997; 205:407–415

[1] From the Mission Breast Care Center, Mission Medical Tower, 26732 Crown Valley Pkwy, Ste 170, Mission Viejo, CA 92691 (F.B.); and the Woman's Choice Health Pavilion, Irvine Medical Center, Irvine, Calif (N.F.). Received April 21, 1997; revision requested June 16; revision received July 7; accepted July 8. **Address reprint requests to** F.B.

F.B. and N.F. are shareholders in Biopsys Medical.

See also the article by Liberman et al (pp 417–422) in this issue.

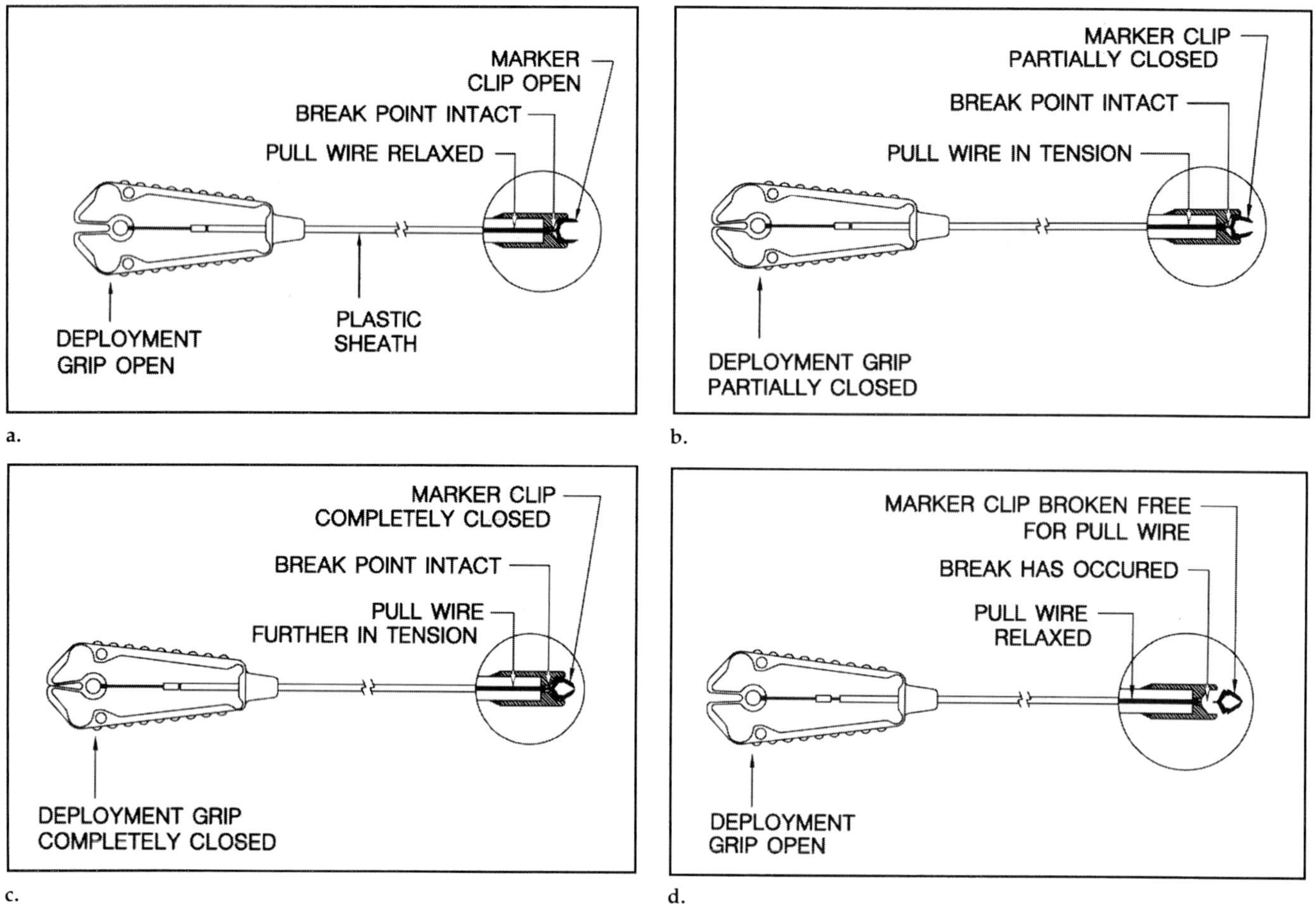

Figure 1. Diagram shows the closure sequence of the marker clip.

atypical ductal hyperplasia, ductal carcinoma in situ, or infiltrating breast cancer, the question remains as to how the biopsy site can be identified accurately for presurgical wire localization. Another question remains as to how the biopsy site can be identified unambiguously during 3 or more years of imaging follow-up when the target lesion proves to be benign.

To address the problem of total removal of a target lesion during directional, vacuum-assisted stereotactic breast biopsy, a 15-gauge, 2 × 2-mm, percutaneous metallic marker clip was developed (MicroMark; Biopsys Medical) and approved by the US Food and Drug Administration on March 15, 1995 for placement in soft tissues. The marker clip and deployment system adds a cost of $75 and approximately 1–2 minutes to the stereotactic breast biopsy procedure.

The purpose of this study was to determine (*a*) the initial accuracy of placement of a marker clip immediately after directional, vacuum-assisted breast biopsies; (*b*) stability of the marker clip after placement from time of insertion to the first follow-up mammographic study; and (*c*) the usefulness of the marker clip as a mammographic guide during wire localization before therapeutic breast surgery.

MATERIALS AND METHODS

A total of 171 patients were studied; 22 patients (average age, 46.8 years; range, 38–85 years) contributed benign control lesions for calibration of the measurement system. In 149 patients (average age, 53.5 years; range, 32–86 years), biopsy was performed with a 14- or 11-gauge directional, vacuum-assisted probe (Biopsys Medical) and marker clips were placed. Between December 8, 1995, and January 28, 1997, 49 (33%) directional, vacuum-assisted biopsies were performed with 14-gauge directional, vacuum-assisted probes and 100 (67%) biopsies were performed with 11-gauge probes. Two radiologists (F.B., N.F.) performed all marker clip placements. The details of performing a directional, vacuum-assisted breast biopsy have been published previously, including complication rates (10,11). Each patient gave informed consent before undergoing biopsy and receiving a marker clip.

Aggregate specimen weights were measured and reported by the attending pathologist at Mission Hospital Regional Medical Center as part of the gross pathologic description for each directional, vacuum-assisted breast biopsy sample. Directional, vacuum-assisted biopsies were categorized as excisional or incisional by examining two ×8 magnified stereotactic digital mammograms and two upright, craniocaudal and mediolateral oblique mammograms obtained after biopsy and marker clip placement. If no residual signs of the target lesion were seen on either of these two sets of mammograms, the biopsy was categorized as excisional. If residual signs of the target lesion were present, the biopsy was categorized as incisional.

Figure 1 shows the percutaneous 2 × 2-mm marker clip and marker clip assembly. The marker clip has two shapes, depending on whether it is open or closed. When open, the marker clip resembles a tiny horseshoe. When closed, the two limbs of the horseshoe are pinched together, forming a diamond shape. The marker clip assembly consists of a deployment grip, a pull wire attached to the deployment grip at one end and attached to the marker clip at the other end, and a plastic sheath that separates the deployment grip from the marker clip. As tension is applied to the pull wire by squeezing the deployment grip, the marker clip changes from the open shape to the closed shape. When breast tissue is trapped between the limbs of the marker clip, the marker clip is then attached or "clipped" to that tissue similar to the action of a surgical vascular clip. As progressively more tension is applied, the marker clip breaks free from the pull wire. At deployment, the marker clip is free from the deployment assembly and is attached to breast tissue at or near the directional, vacuum-assisted breast biopsy site. For purposes of description, the marker clip deployment sequence is shown as four separate steps. In practice, the process occurs almost instantaneously (one rapid motion).

Two marker clip deployment methods were used in this study. The first marker clip deployment method is referred to as the "straight-needle" method. The second deployment method is referred to as the "through-probe" method.

For the straight-needle deployment method, six steps were necessary: (*a*) a directional, vacuum-assisted biopsy was performed with a 14-gauge probe (43 deployments) (11); (*b*) the directional, vacuum-assisted probe and motorized probe driver were removed from the stereotactic breast biopsy table and set aside; (*c*) a purpose-built needle holder was placed on the stereotactic breast biopsy table (this needle holder was secured to a straight 13-gauge needle with a pointed, bevel-tipped trocar); (*d*) a new set of coordinates was generated by the computer to position the tip of the straight needle at the biopsy site; (*e*) the straight needle with a central trocar was advanced to the biopsy site; and (*f*) the trocar was removed and the percutaneous marker clip assembly was advanced down the shaft of the straight needle, and the marker clip was attached to the wall of the biopsy cavity as shown in Figure 1.

The through-probe deployment method consisted of two steps: (*a*) directional, vacuum-assisted biopsy was performed with a 14-gauge probe (six deployments) or an 11-gauge probe (100 deployments); and (*b*) the marker clip assembly was advanced through the directional, vacuum-assisted probe, and the marker clip was attached to the wall of the biopsy cavity as shown in Figure 1.

To evaluate accuracy of marker clip placement and placement stability over time, a measurement system was needed to describe accurately the location of the marker clip and the target lesion within the breast. The American College of Radiology Breast Imaging and Reporting System contains a breast lesion location system (12). Although this method is suitable for generally defining the location of a lesion within the breast, it is not suitable for describing small differences in the position of two objects that may be close to one another within the breast. Consequently, we developed and tested a new measurement system, the "mask measurement system."

The mask measurement system transfers information from two mammograms to one sheet of clear x-ray film referred to as the "mask." After information is hand-traced from the two mammograms to the mask, the mask contains information from both mammograms. The first mammogram defines the shape of the breast and the location of an object of interest on the mask. The second mammogram is fitted to the mask, and the object of interest on the second mammogram is drawn on the mask. The objects of interest, whose locations are compared on the masks, can be a target lesion and a marker clip (first context, described later), a marker clip at two points in time (second context), or a target lesion at two points in time (third context).

If the position of an object within the breast was identical on two mammograms and if the breast projected to the same location on each mammogram, then two tracings of the objects on the mask would superimpose exactly. In this idealized example, the tracings of the superimposed objects on the mask could be described as exactly "on target." However, a breast never projects as exactly the same shape on any two mammograms. Furthermore, when a marker clip is placed in the breast, it may or may not embed in the desired location. Finally, even if the marker clip is deployed accurately, it may move from one location to another over time. When the tracing of an object is not in the ideal position on the mask, the object is described as "off target." The distance (in millimeters) that an object is off target is measured directly on a mask with a ruler.

The craniocaudal mask describes the distance off target in one projection; the mediolateral oblique mask describes the distance off target in another projection. To combine the information from the craniocaudal and mediolateral oblique mammogram masks, a single, continuous, dependent variable was defined and referred to as the "average distance off target." The average distance off target has three meanings, depending on three contexts.

Initial Accuracy of Marker Clip Deployment

In the first context, the average distance off target of the marker clip with respect to the target lesion immediately after stereotactic directional, vacuum-assisted breast biopsy and deployment of the marker clip was measured by creating a mask of the craniocaudal and mediolateral oblique mammograms obtained before biopsy. The mask for each projection was created by stapling a clear sheet of x-ray film on top of the craniocaudal and mediolateral oblique mammograms obtained before biopsy (Fig 2a). With use of a bright light, the skin line, the nipple, and an outline of the lesion were traced by hand onto the mask with an indelible film marker (Fig 2b). For mass lesions, the lesion borders were traced; for clustered microcalcification lesions, the outermost edges of the cluster were traced. The center of each lesion was marked with a dot.

After directional, vacuum-assisted biopsy was performed, the marker clip was delivered percutaneously at or near the biopsy site by means of the straight-needle (43 deployments) or through-probe (106 deployments) deployment method. Craniocaudal and mediolateral oblique mammograms were obtained immediately after biopsy and marker clip deployment to define the locations of the marker clip within the breast in the craniocaudal and mediolateral oblique projections (Fig 2c). The target lesion was commonly removed entirely, distorted, or obscured as a result of the directional vacuum-assisted biopsy. Consequently, the target lesion was often no longer visible or identifiable on the mammograms obtained after biopsy and marker clip placement. The marker clip, however, was always clearly visible.

Finally, the craniocaudal mask was placed on top of the craniocaudal mammogram obtained after biopsy and marker clip placement, and the mediolateral oblique mask was placed on top of the mediolateral oblique mammogram obtained after biopsy and marker clip placement. The skin outlines from each corresponding mask and mammogram obtained after biopsy were fitted together with use of a bright light and the position of the nipple as the fulcrum to achieve the best overall "fit." Once the fit was optimal, the position of the marker clip was drawn as a diamond on the craniocaudal and mediolateral oblique masks with an indelible marker (Fig 2d).

The craniocaudal and mediolateral oblique masks then contained the locations of the two objects of interest: the target lesion and the marker clip. The distance from the center of the target lesion to the center of the marker clip was measured (in millimeters) on the masks in the craniocaudal and mediolateral oblique projections (Fig 2d). The distances between the target lesion and the marker clip in the craniocaudal and mediolateral oblique projections were averaged: average distance = [(craniocaudal distance + mediolateral oblique distance)/2], creating the average distance off target for the initial deployment of the marker clip. The average distance off target in this context is a measurement of the marker clip distance from the target lesion center. Since two deployment methods were used in this study, the average distance off target was analyzed according to deployment method.

Stability of Marker Clip Placement Over Time

In the second context, the stability of marker clip placement over time was measured by comparing the position of the marker clip on the craniocaudal and mediolateral oblique masks immediately after biopsy and marker clip deployment to the position of the marker clip on craniocaudal and mediolateral oblique mammograms obtained at first imaging follow-up. As before, the skin outlines from the mammograms obtained at first imaging follow-up were fitted to the craniocaudal and mediolateral oblique masks by using the nipple as the fulcrum to create the best fit between each follow-up mammogram first imaging follow-up mammogram and the corresponding mask.

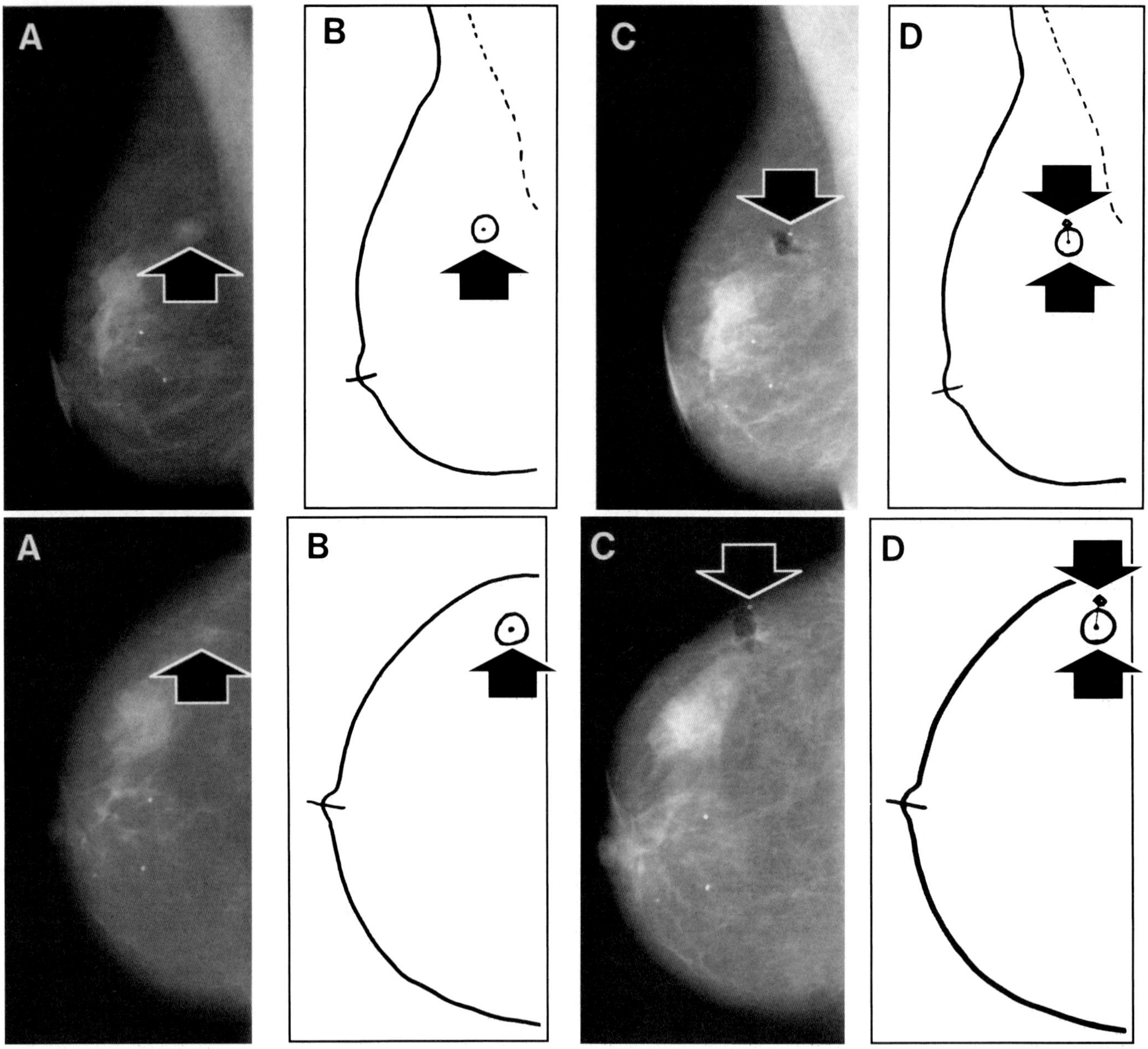

Figure 2. Measurement steps for the placement of a marker clip with respect to a target lesion in the left breast. (*A*) Craniocaudal (bottom) and mediolateral oblique (top) mammograms obtained before biopsy show a 12 × 14-mm nodule (arrow). (*B*) Corresponding masks define the skin outline, the nipple along the skin outline, the margins of the lesion (arrow), and the center of the lesion (dot) in both projections. (*C*) Craniocaudal (bottom) and mediolateral (top) mammograms obtained immediately after directional, vacuum-assisted breast biopsy show that most of the lesion was removed at biopsy. An air-filled cavity is seen at the lesion site. The marker clip (arrow) is attached to the wall of the air-filled cavity. (*D*) Corresponding masks have been fitted to the mammogram. The position of the marker clip is drawn on the mask (arrows). A line was drawn between the center of the lesion and the center of the marker clip in each view. In the craniocaudal projection (bottom), the line is 10 mm; in the mediolateral oblique projection (top), the line is 8 mm. The average distance off target is 9 mm ([10 + 8]/2). The target lesion was an infiltrating lobular carcinoma.

The marker clip distance off target over time was then measured on the craniocaudal and mediolateral oblique masks as the distance from the center of the marker clip immediately after deployment to the center of the marker clip during the first imaging follow-up. The craniocaudal and mediolateral oblique distances were averaged: average distance = [(craniocaudal distance + mediolateral oblique distance)/2], creating the average distance off target of the marker clip over time. The average distance off target in this context is a measurement of how far the marker clip did or did not move from the immediate position after biopsy to the position at the first imaging follow-up. Thirty-one marker clips were followed up from deployment to the first follow-up mammographic study.

Mask Measurement System Calibration

In the third context, the average distance off target of the mask measurement system was evaluated by comparing the position of the center of a well-defined benign breast lesion in craniocaudal and mediolateral oblique projections at two points. It was assumed that the center of a benign lesion would not move within the breast over time and that any apparent movement of the benign lesion would reflect variability in the measurement system rather than movement.

In the biopsy database (Breast Center Manager; Biopsys Medical) at the Mission Breast Care Center, 56 lesions proved benign histologically at previous automated core needle breast biopsy and at 3-year imaging follow-up were identified and reviewed. The details of performing an automated core needle breast biopsy have been published previously (2,11). All lesions were greater than 10 mm in length and width. From these 56 lesions, 22 lesions were selected as the benign control lesions because they were particularly well depicted in the craniocaudal and mediolateral oblique views and on the mammograms obtained before biopsy and at first imaging follow-up. The average time to first follow-up mammography was 8.6 months after automated core needle biopsy for these 22 benign control lesions.

To calibrate the measurement system, craniocaudal and mediolateral oblique "control" masks were created before biopsy for the 22 well-defined benign control lesions. As before, the craniocaudal and mediolateral oblique masks created before biopsy defined the location of the skin, the nipple, and the benign control lesion at the first point. The first follow-up mammograms were placed under the masks and "fitted" as before. The position of the benign control lesion at a second point was then drawn on the mask.

The distance off target over time for the benign control lesions was measured on the masks in the craniocaudal and mediolateral oblique projections as the distance from the center of the benign control lesion at one point to the center of the benign control lesion at a second point. The craniocaudal and mediolateral oblique distances were averaged: average distance = [(craniocaudal distance + mediolateral oblique distance)/2], creating the average distance off target for the benign control lesions.

Because the average distance off target of the benign control lesions is a direct measurement of the variability of the measurement system, this average distance off target was used as the measurement system baseline. For the initial marker clip deployment average distance off target to be statistically meaningful according to the straight-needle deployment method or the through-probe deployment method, the average distance off target for the deployment method must be statistically significantly greater than the average distance off target for the controls. Similarly, for the marker clip average distance off target over time to be statistically meaningful, the average distance off target over time for the marker clip must be statistically significantly greater than the average distance off target for the controls.

The comparison of the average distances off target for the benign control measurements, for the straight-needle and the through-probe deployment methods, and for the marker clip stability measurements over time was performed with an analysis of variance. Pair-wise comparisons of average distance off target measurements were performed with the Student *t* test.

The usefulness of the marker clip as a guide for wire localization was evaluated by examining the clinical records of all patients with atypical ductal hyperplasia, ductal carcinoma in situ, or infiltrating breast cancer who had completed surgical therapy. Thirty-six biopsy sites with marker clips were excised surgically and examined. The process of using the marker clip as the target at wire localization is shown in Figure 3.

All biopsies were performed at Mission Breast Care Center with a prone stereotactic breast biopsy table (Mammotest; Fisher Imaging, Denver, Colo). Clinical data were entered at Mission Breast Care Center into the clinical database program. Data were exported from the clinical database program and analyzed with a statistical program (StatView; Abacus Concepts, Berkeley, Calif).

RESULTS

Table 1 shows the average aggregate specimen weights, the average of the number of specimens obtained, the average of the individual weights per specimen, the average of the mean lesion diameters ([maximum length + maximum width]/2), and the percentage of excisional biopsies according to probe size. In 108 (72%) of the 149 biopsies, no visible sign of the target lesion remained after stereotactic directional, vacuum-assisted breast biopsy. These biopsies were categorized as excisional biopsies. More 11-gauge biopsies (79, 79%) were excisional than 14-gauge biopsies (29, 59%) ($P \leq .03$, χ^2 test.) Of the 149 lesions, 88 (59%) were characterized as clustered microcalcification lesions and 61 (41%) were characterized as masses.

Tables 2 and 3 and Figure 4 show the results of analysis of variance for comparison of the average distance off target for measurements obtained in the 22 benign control lesions, the 43 measurements obtained with the straight-needle deployment method, the 106 measurements obtained with the through-probe deployment method, and the 31 measurements obtained at first imaging follow-up. The average distance off target counts, means, standard deviations, and standard errors for these four independent variables are shown in Table 2. As shown in Table 3, the average distance off target for the control measurements, the two deployment method measurements, and the first imaging follow-up measurements were significantly different ($P \leq .01$).

The source of this statistically significant difference is shown in Figure 4, an interaction bar plot that depicts the data contained in Table 2. The mask measurement system has approximately 8 mm of inherent variability in accuracy. That is, the measurement system generated an average distance off target of 8 mm in the mediolateral oblique and craniocaudal projections for the 22 benign control lesions. This "apparent" motion of 8 mm is the baseline against which marker clip placement accuracy and stability are compared.

The average distance off target was 12.6 mm for both the straight-needle marker clip deployment method and the through-probe deployment method. However, as shown by the error bars in Figure 2 and demonstrated in Table 2, the standard error of the straight-needle deployment method was 2.7 times the standard error of the through-probe deployment method (1.9 vs 0.7). When the average distance off target data for the two deployment methods were combined, the average distance off target mean of 12.6 was significantly different than the control average distance off target mean of 7.7 mm ($P \leq .01$, Student *t* test). On average, the marker clips were placed about 5 mm away from the centers of the target lesions (12.6 mm − 7.7 mm = 4.9 mm). The average distance off target did not correlate with the weight of tissue or the number of specimens removed (r = 0.003 and 0.04, respectively; not statistically significant [$P \leq .1$]).

Finally, the measurements obtained at first imaging follow-up in the 31 marker clip placements demonstrated that the average distance off target (8.7 mm) for the first imaging follow-up measurements are not significantly different than the average distance off target measurements (7.7 mm) for the benign control lesions ($P > .4$, Student *t* test). Once the marker clips were placed, no measurable movement was found to occur over time.

Although the mean of the average distance off target for the two clip deployment methods was only 5 mm greater than the average distance off target for the controls, potential clinically meaningful misplacements of the marker clip were observed. An average distance off target of 24 mm was arbitrarily defined as a potential clinically meaningful deployment error. The average distance off target frequency distribution according to initial deployment method are shown in Figures 5 and 6. In these two frequency distributions, the bar graph intervals for the average distance off target were set at 8 mm to correspond to the baseline variability seen in the mask measurement system. Five (11%) of the 43 straight needle deployments showed an average distance off target of 24 mm or greater (black areas in Figure 5). Similarly, seven (7%) of the 106 through-probe deployments generated average distance off target measurements of 24 mm or greater, corresponding to the black areas in Figure 6. The difference in misplacement rates (11% vs 7%) for the two deployment methods was not statistically significant ($P = .33$, Fisher exact test).

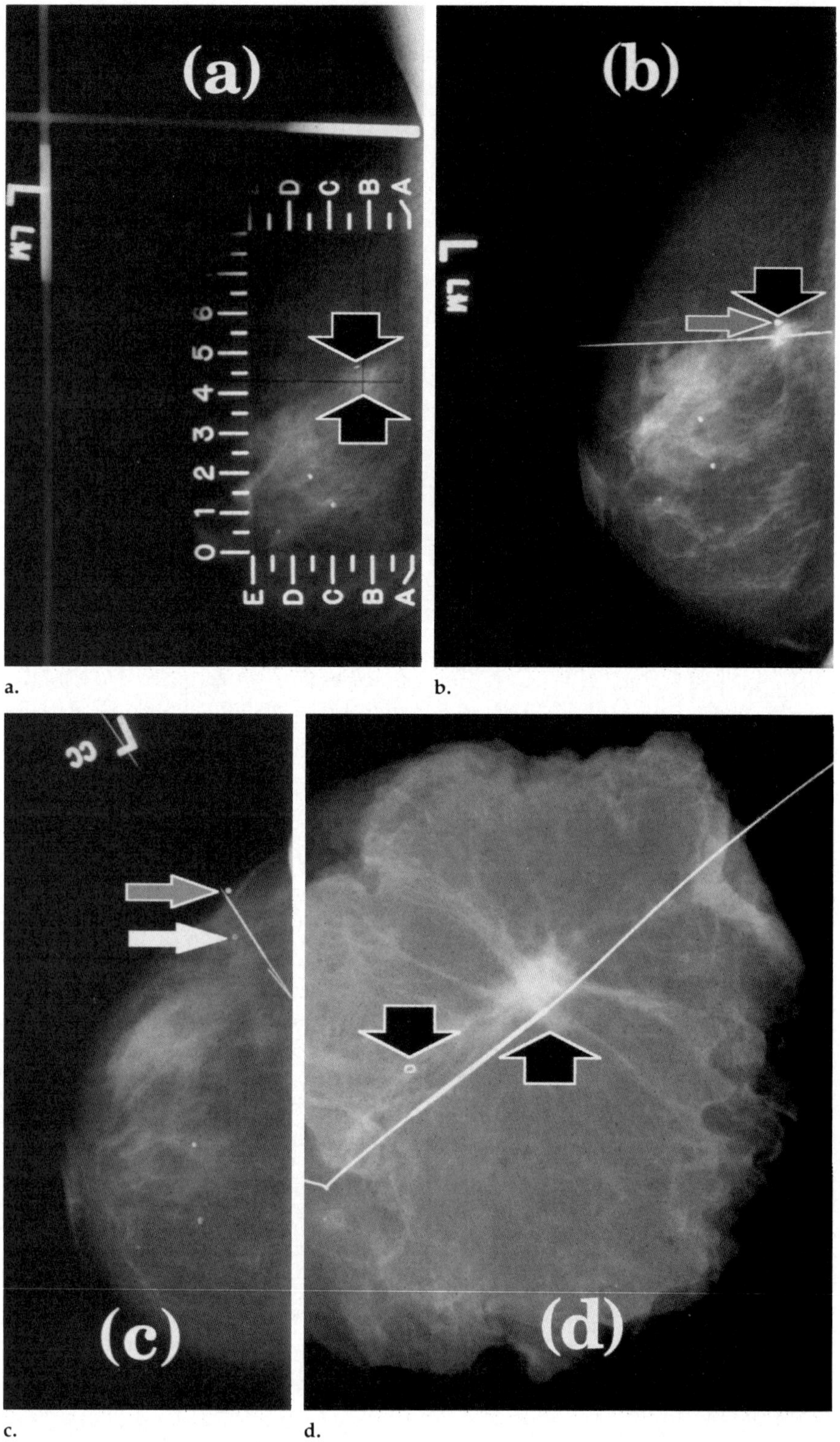

Figure 3. Photographs of mammograms show the steps necessary to use a marker clip as a target for wire localization before surgery. Wire localization was performed in the same lesion shown in Figure 2. **(a)** Lateromedial mammogram obtained with an alphanumeric grid placed over the left breast in the lateromedial projection. Wax pencil lines have been drawn on the lateromedial mammogram grid over the region of residual target lesion (upward-pointing arrow) just adjacent to the marker clip (downward-pointing arrow). A stiffened localization wire (Kopans Spring Hookwire; Cook, Bloomington, Ind) was then placed where the wax pencil lines cross in the lateromedial projection. **(b)** Lateromedial mammogram helps verify the position of the localization wire. The black arrow highlights the marker clip; the gray arrow highlights a "BeBe" (Beekley Spots with Pik-Up; Beekley Corporation, Bristol, Conn), which has been placed at the skin entry site of the wire. **(c)** Craniocaudal mammogram shows the position of the localization wire, the marker clip (white arrow), and the skin BeBe (gray arrow). **(d)** Magnified (×2) radiograph of the surgical specimen cut and compressed in a plastic transportation and compression container (TranSpec; E-Z-Em, Westbury, NY) shows the residual target lesion (upward-pointing arrow), the marker clip (downward-pointing arrow), and the localization wire. The marker clip has been moved away from the target lesion with surgical transection of the specimen and pressure from the plastic compression container.

Of 149 marker clips placed, 36 (24%) patients subsequently underwent surgical therapy. At stereotactic biopsy, infiltrating breast cancer was diagnosed in 20 (56%) of the 36 lesions, ductal carcinoma in situ in 13 (36%) lesions, and atypical ductal hyperplasia in three (8%) lesions. The type of surgery performed, whether the marker clip was used as a guide for wire localization, whether a radiograph was obtained of the surgical specimen, and the distribution of histologic diagnoses are summarized in Table 4.

In eight (22%) of the 36 lesions, no preoperative wire localization was performed. Seven of the eight surgeries were mastectomies and the other surgery was breast-conserving surgery directed by palpation of a hematoma presumed by the surgeon to be at the directional, vacuum-assisted breast biopsy site. In 10 (28%) of the 36 lesions, the marker clip was used as the target for wire localization. However, no radiograph was obtained of the specimen because the biopsy site was readily visible during surgery and radiography was deemed redundant by the surgeon. In 18 (50%) of the 36 lesions, the marker clip was used as the target for wire localization and a radiograph was obtained of the specimen. On all 18 (100%) of these radiographs, the marker clip and the previous biopsy site were identified positively in the specimen.

In 29 (81%) of the 36 lesions, the biopsy site and residual tumor were identified positively at histopathologic examination. In the remaining seven (19%) lesions, the biopsy site was also identified positively, and the pathologist concluded that the target lesion had been excised with clear margins at directional, vacuum-assisted breast biopsy before wire localization and surgical therapy. No evidence of tumor seeding or epithelial displacement was identified in any of the 36 surgical specimens (13).

DISCUSSION

With use of 14-gauge and 11-gauge directional, vacuum-assisted breast

Table 1
Comparison of 14- and 11-gauge Directional, Vacuum-assisted Probes according to Specimen Weight, Specimen Number, Lesion Diameter, and Percentage of Excisional Biopsies

Probe Size	No. of Biopsies	Average Aggregate Weight (mg)*	Average No. of Specimens Obtained†	Average of Individual Weights per Specimen (mg)‡	Average of Mean Lesion Diameters (mm)§	Excisional Biopsies (%)‖
14	49	1,171	27	44	9.1	59
11	100	1,949	19	105	7.8	79

* Weights were determined in the pathology department. $P \le .0001$ (unpaired t test).
† $P \le .0001$ (unpaired t test).
‡ $P \le .0001$ (unpaired t test).
§ $P \ge .13$ (unpaired t test); no statistically significant difference in measurements.
‖ $P \le .03$ (unpaired t test).

Table 2
Analysis of Variance of Average Distance off Target according to Count, Mean, Standard Deviation, and Standard Error

Independent Variables	Count	Mean	Standard Deviation	Standard Error
Benign control lesions	22	7.7	3.8	0.8
Deployment method				
13-gauge straight needle	43	12.6	12.3	1.9
11-gauge through probe	106	12.6	7.2	0.7
First imaging follow-up	31	8.7	4.4	0.8

Table 3
Overall Results of Analysis of Variance

	df	Sum of Squares	Mean Square	F Value	*P* Value
Independent variables ($n = 4$)	3	744	248	3.9	≤.01
Residual	198	12,616	64	. . .	. . .

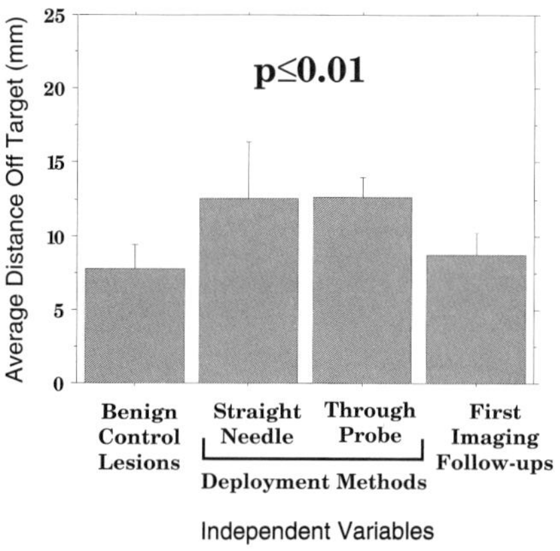

Figure 4. Bar graph shows the plotted average distance off target for each of the four independent variables. Thin bars define the 95% confidence intervals.

biopsies, it is the clinical goal to perform a diagnostic percutaneous breast biopsy as completely and accurately as imaging-guided wire localization and open surgical breast biopsy. With the current directional, vacuum-assisted probes, the goal is not to perform therapeutic breast surgery percutaneously. However, to perform a complete diagnostic breast biopsy, "enough" breast tissue must be obtained percutaneously in all breast lesions. "Enough" tissue may be more tissue than many radiologists are accustomed to removing.

We believe that when stereotactic targeting is nearly perfect, the volume of tissue described in Table 1 for 14-gauge probes is just sufficient to consistently perform a complete and accurate diagnostic breast biopsy. Furthermore, we believe that the volume of tissue obtained with the 11-gauge probe (Table 1) may be sufficient to compensate for small stereotactic targeting errors that occur occasionally. Consequently, we now perform only 11-gauge directional, vacuum-assisted breast biopsies.

Data are available in the literature for atypical ductal hyperplasia and ductal carcinoma in situ lesions that clearly support our first belief. When the diagnosis of atypical ductal hyperplasia is ascertained at percutaneous breast biopsy and surgery is performed subsequently and ductal carcinoma in situ or infiltrating breast cancer is identified at the biopsy site within the surgical specimen, the degree of disease in the breast has been underestimated at percutaneous biopsy (14). Similarly, if ductal carcinoma in situ is identified at percutaneous breast biopsy and infiltrating breast cancer is later identified at surgery, the degree of disease in the breast has been underestimated at percutaneous biopsy (14). When 14-gauge, automated core needle breast biopsies are performed, with acquisition of five to eight specimens per lesion, rates of underestimation of atypical ductal hyperplasia and ductal carcinoma in situ are high, approximately 50% and 20%, respectively (15–17). Even when 17 to 19 specimens are obtained with 14-gauge, automated core needle biopsy, the rate of underestimation of atypical ductal hyperplasia decreases only to 44% and that of ductal carcinoma in situ decreases only to 16% (14).

When 16 or 17 specimens are obtained with 14-gauge, directional vacuum-assisted biopsy, the rate of underestimation of atypical ductal hyperplasia decreases to 18% and the rate of underestimation of ductal carcinoma in situ decreases to 9% (18), (unpublished data). Although these rates are improved compared with rates of underestimation associated with 14-gauge automated core needle biopsies, underestimation of disease at the biopsy site still exists.

To eliminate underestimation of atypical ductal hyperplasia and ductal carcinoma in situ, approximately 30 specimens must be obtained from each lesion with 14-gauge directional, vacuum-assisted biopsy (14). At this level of percutaneous tissue acquisition, over 1 g of tissue is obtained (Table 1). Furthermore, when we use the 11-gauge directional, vacuum-assisted probes, nearly 2 g of tissue are removed at the biopsy site (Table 1).

When over 1 g of tissue is removed from lesions in which the average diameter is 1 cm or less, all mammographic signs of the lesion may be removed as well. If fact, for small lesions (5 mm in diameter or less), we expect to remove all visible signs of the lesion during the directional, vacuum-assisted breast biopsy. The marker clip was developed to ensure that a target would still be present for subsequent wire localization and therapeutic surgery.

Our study demonstrates that on average, the marker clip was deployed about 5 mm from the center of the target lesion (12.6 mm − 7.7 mm = 4.9 mm). Since the average lesion diameter for the 149 marker clip placements was approximately 10 mm, the overall accuracy of deployment was good. On average, the marker clips were placed just outside the margin of each lesion. Although no clinical problems were encountered from any of the marker clip deployments in our study, there were potential clinically meaningful exceptions to this general rule. In 11% of the straight-needle deployments and 7% of the through-probe deployments, the average distance off target was 24 mm or more. An average distance off target of 24 mm or more could potentially lead to a clinical problem at wire localization and therapeutic surgery. We could not predict from the manipulation of the marker clip deployment system when an off-target deployment had occurred. We were aware of off-target placements only as we examined the two-view mammograms obtained immediately after biopsy.

If the position of the marker clip with respect to the target lesion is known immediately after placement of the marker clip, a deployment error of 24 mm or more would not necessarily lead to a clinical problem. If the position of the marker clip with respect to the target lesion is known, then any error in deployment of the marker clip can be taken into account at wire localization and surgery. However, if the position of the marker clip with respect to the target lesion is not known and the average distance off target is large, then a clinical problem might occur. This clinical problem may occur particularly if the patient underwent stereotactic biopsy and marker clip placement at one site and wire localization and surgery were performed at another. At the second site, it might be assumed incorrectly that the marker clip was exactly on target. Consequently, we believe it is important to document the position of the marker clip after each deployment with a standard two-view, upright mammogram. This two-view upright mammogram should then become a part of the patient record and be available for review before wire localization is performed.

We do not believe it is sufficient to repeat stereotactic mammography while the patient is still on the biopsy table and to use the stereotactic mammogram to measure deployment accuracy. It is possible to calculate the x, y, and z coordinates of the marker clip from a repeat stereotactic mammogram. However, the coordinates calculated may give the operator a false sense of security, since in compression the coordinates of the marker clip are almost always close to the coordinates of the center of the target lesion. Because of the accordion-like character of the breast with bands of tough fibrous tissue alternating with bands of softer, fatty tissue, this method of documenting marker clip position is not reliable. The marker clip may attach to a band of fibrous tissue that in compression is close to the center of the target lesion but when the clip is out of compression it is at some distance from the center of the lesion. To avoid this pitfall, the stereotactic mammograms should be used only to document that the marker clip was deployed. To determine where the marker clip was deployed, upright standard mammography is necessary.

Our study also demonstrates that the marker clip did not change position over the follow-up period of the study (mean, 8.6 months). The average distance off target for marker clip measurements at first imaging follow-up were not statistically significantly different from the average distance off target measurements for the benign control lesions. Therefore, once the location of the marker clip is documented with upright mammography after deployment, it can be safely assumed that the marker clip will remain where deployed for at least 8.6 months. Stability over longer periods has not been documented, to our knowledge.

Marker clip misplacements (average off target distance > 24 mm) were more frequent when the straight-needle deployment method was used than when the through-probe deployment method was used (11% vs 7%, not statistically significant). Furthermore, the straight-needle deployment method necessitated more deployment steps than were necessary for

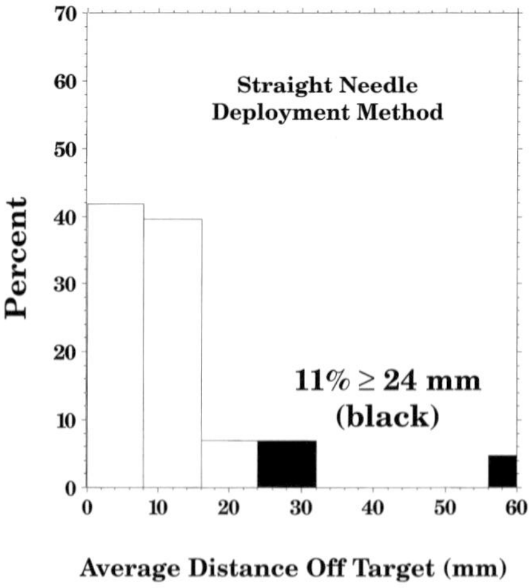

5.

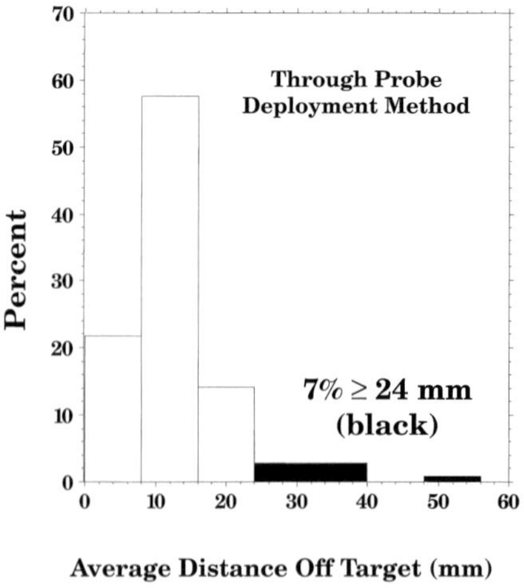

6.

Figures 5, 6. Graphs show the percentage distribution of the average distance off target for the **(5)** straight-needle deployment method and the **(6)** through-probe method. The white bars represent an average distance off target of less than 24 mm; the black bars represent an average distance off target of 24 mm or greater. For the straight-needle deployment method, 11% of the average distance off target measurements were 24 mm or greater, and for the through-probe method, 7% of the average distance off target measurements were 24 mm or greater.

Table 4
Type of Surgery Performed and Histologic Diagnosis in 36 Lesions

Surgery Performed	Metallic Clip Used for Localization	Radiograph Obtained of Surgical Specimen	Histologic Diagnosis: Infiltrating Breast Cancer	Ductal Carcinoma In Situ	Atypical Ductal Hyperplasia	Total*
Mastectomy	No	No	4	3	0	7 (19)
Breast conserving	No	No	1	0	0	1 (3)
Breast conserving	Yes	No	6	3	1	10 (28)
Breast conserving	Yes	Yes	9	7	2	18 (50)

* Numbers in parentheses are percentages.

the through-probe method, more time was necessary to perform the straight-needle method because of the greater number of steps, and the straight needle is no longer available from the manufacturer. Consequently, we currently perform only through-probe deployments.

The marker clip was a successful guide for wire localization before surgery. In all 18 cases in which the marker clip was used as a surrogate for the target lesion for wire localization before surgery, the marker clip and the biopsy cavity were identified in each of the 18 surgical specimens.

The mask measurement system for defining the position of the lesion and the marker clip on one image was developed specifically for this study. However, we soon observed that other radiologists who performed wire localization at our center were pulling the masks from the research files at wire localization to analyze the masks before placement of a localization wire. The masks contain all the information necessary to use the marker clip as a reference point at wire localization regardless of whether the marker clip is exactly on target. Consequently, we continue to create a set of masks for each marker clip deployed from mammograms obtained before and after biopsy and marker deployment.

The most common question asked by patients before signing consent for placement of a marker clip was in regard to the size of the clip being placed in the breast. We initially used a small air gap between our thumb and index finger to show marker clip size and informed the patients that the clip was 2 mm. However, this communication method was not very effective, as most patients did not think in terms of millimeters and the space between index finger and thumb was a crude approximation of clip size. To overcome this communication gap, we attached an actual marker clip to an exposed (black) sheet of x-ray film. Against this black background, the marker clip is clearly visible. Once the size of the marker clip was seen, the patients generally expressed no further concern about having the marker clip placed permanently in the breast. We keep the marker clip sample pinned to the wall in the stereotactic breast biopsy room and find it a useful communication aid to obtain informed consent.

Before we used the marker clip, we were able to perform wire localization successfully in all lesions in which stereotactically guided biopsy was performed and surgery was necessary. In small lesions, however, we had a degree of concern with regard to the time between stereotactic biopsy and wire localization. We were particularly concerned when a patient was to be transferred to another facility for wire localization and definitive breast cancer surgery. In the hope that residual blood or air might remain at the biopsy site to identify the biopsy site if the target lesion were removed entirely at stereotactic biopsy, we attempted to minimize the time from stereotactic biopsy to wire localization. This source of concern has now been eliminated. Because of the marker clip, we are now confident that wire localization can be performed successfully at any time after stereotactic breast biopsy whether residual blood or air from the biopsy are present at wire localization.

Finally, with the availability of the marker clip, it is not necessary to place lower size limits on lesions that can undergo stereotactic biopsy. For small lesions (< 5 mm in diameter), we anticipate that in a high percentage of cases all visible signs of the target lesion will be removed. However, because a marker clip is placed after each stereotactic biopsy of these smaller lesions, we are confident that the biopsy site can be reached accurately at wire localization with the marker clip as the surrogate target. Furthermore, even when a marker clip is off target, knowledge of the direction and magnitude of the deployment error allows the marker clip to be used as a clear-cut point of reference for wire localization. ■

References

1. Pisano ED, Tsimikas J, Fajardo L, et al. RDOG5: stereotactic fine needle aspiration (FNA) and core needle biopsy (CNB) in the work-up of lesions detected by mammography—insufficiency sample rate across multiple centers in a nationwide trial. Presented at the 27th National Conference on Breast Cancer, Dallas, Tex, 1996.
2. Parker SH, Lovin JD, Jobe WE, et al. Stereotactic breast biopsy with a biopsy gun. Radiology 1990; 176:741–747.
3. Dershaw DD. Needle core biopsy of mammographic lesions (letter). AJR 1995; 164:260.
4. Sullivan DC. Needle core biopsy of mammographic lesions (letter). AJR 1994; 162: 601–608.
5. Dronkers DJ. Stereotaxic core biopsy of breast lesions. Radiology 1992; 183:631–634.
6. Mikhail RA, Nathan RC, Weiss M, et al. Stereotactic core needle biopsy of mammographic breast lesions as a viable alternative to surgical biopsy. Ann Surg Oncol 1994; 1:363–367.
7. Burbank F, Parker SH, Fogarty TJ. Stereotactic breast biopsy: improved tissue harvesting with the Mammotome. Am Surg 1996; 62:128–150.
8. Burbank F. Mammographic findings after 14-gauge automated needle and 14-gauge directional vacuum-assisted stereotactic breast biopsy. Radiology 1997; 204:153–156.
9. Burbank F. Frequency of excisional breast biopsy with clear margins with the Biopsys Mammotome (abstr). Mini Invasive Ther Allied Technol 1996; 5(suppl):39.
10. Burbank F. Stereotactic breast biopsy: comparison of 14- and 11-gauge Mammotome probe performance and complication rates. Am Surg 1997 (in press).
11. Burbank F. Stereotactic breast biopsy: its history, its present, and its future. Am Surg 1996; 62:128–150.
12. American College of Radiology (ACR). Breast Imaging Reporting and Data System (BI-RADS). 2nd ed. Reston, Va: American College of Radiology, 1995.
13. Youngson BJ, Cranor M, Rosen PP. Epithelial displacement in surgical breast specimens following needling procedures. Am J Surg Pathol 1994; 18:896–903.
14. Burbank F. Stereotactic breast biopsy of atypical ductal hyperplasia and ductal carcinoma in situ lesions: improved accuracy with a directional, vacuum-assisted biopsy instrument. Radiology 1997; 202:843–847.
15. Jackman RJ, Nowels KW, Shepard MJ, Finkelstein SI, Marzoni FA. Stereotaxic large-core needle biopsy of 450 nonpalpable breast lesions with surgical correlation in lesions with cancer or atypical hyperplasia. Radiology 1994; 193:91–95.
16. Liberman L, Cohen MA, Dershaw DD, Abramson AF, Hann LE, Rosen PP. Atypical ductal hyperplasia diagnosed at stereotaxic core biopsy of breast lesions: an indication for surgical biopsy. AJR 1995; 164: 1111–1113.
17. Liberman L, Dershaw DD, Rosen PP, et al. Stereotaxic core biopsy of breast carcinoma: accuracy at predicting invasion. Radiology 1995; 194:379–381.
18. Jackman RJ, Burbank F, Parker SH, et al. Atypical ductal hyperplasia diagnosed with stereotactic biopsy: improved reliability with 14-gauge, directional vacuum-assisted breast biopsy. Radiology 1997; 204: 485–488.

Laura Liberman, MD • D. David Dershaw, MD • Elizabeth A. Morris, MD
Andrea F. Abramson, MD • Cynthia M. Thornton, RT(R)(M) • Paul Peter Rosen, MD

Clip Placement after Stereotactic Vacuum-assisted Breast Biopsy[1]

PURPOSE: To assess accuracy and usefulness of placement of a localizing clip after stereotactic, vacuum-assisted breast biopsy.

MATERIALS AND METHODS: Retrospective review was performed of 57 lesions that underwent placement of a localizing clip after stereotactic vacuum-assisted biopsy with an 11-gauge (n = 42) or 14-gauge (n = 15) probe. The clip was placed when images obtained after stereotactic biopsy suggested that the lesion seen at mammography was removed. Coordinates of the clip on stereotactic images obtained after placement were compared with lesion coordinates determined before biopsy. Surgery was performed in 25 cases. Mammographic and histopathologic findings were reviewed.

RESULTS: The distance from clip to lesion site was less than 1 cm in 40 (95%) of 42 lesions that underwent clip placement with the 11-gauge probe versus 11 (73%) of 15 lesions that underwent clip placement after 14-gauge biopsy ($P < .04$). The biopsy site was identified in the surgical specimen in 19 (100%) lesions with clips after 11-gauge biopsy and five (83%) of six lesions with clips after 14-gauge biopsy. No complications occurred.

CONCLUSION: A localizing clip can be placed in proximity to the stereotactic biopsy site through an 11-gauge probe. Clip placement can enable accurate localization for surgical excision.

A radiopaque localizing clip has been approved by the U.S. Food and Drug Administration for placement after directional, vacuum-assisted breast biopsy (1–3). The goal of clip placement is to enable subsequent surgical excision of the biopsy site, even if the mammographic findings associated with the original lesion were removed completely. To date, there is little published experience with regard to use of the clip, to our knowledge (1–3). This study was undertaken to assess the accuracy and usefulness of placement of a localizing clip after stereotactic, vacuum-assisted breast biopsy to enable subsequent surgical excision of the biopsy site.

MATERIALS AND METHODS

From May 1, 1996, to April 24, 1997, stereotactic, vacuum-assisted biopsy was offered as an alternative to surgical biopsy for mammographically evident lesions in which surgery would otherwise have been performed unless (*a*) the patient had a bleeding diathesis, (*b*) the patient was unable to tolerate the procedure, or (*c*) the thickness of compressed breast parenchyma was inadequate to accommodate the tip and bowl of the biopsy probe (22 mm for the 14-gauge probe and 27 mm for the 11-gauge probe). No lesions were excluded because of small size. A 2 × 2-mm radiopaque localizing clip (MicroMark; Biopsys Medical, Irvine, Calif) was placed after vacuum-assisted biopsy when stereotactic images obtained after tissue acquisition suggested that the mammographic findings associated with the original lesion were or may have been removed completely. Clips used before February 5, 1997, were constructed of titanium; clips used after that time were constructed of stainless steel.

Biopsies with 11-gauge Probes

Retrospective review was performed of mammograms of 96 consecutive lesions that underwent stereotactic biopsy with an 11-gauge directional, vacuum-assisted biopsy instrument (Mammotome; Biopsys Medical) from October 31, 1996, to April 24, 1997. In 44 (46%) lesions, the radiopaque localizing clip was placed through the 11-gauge probe after biopsy. Two lesions were excluded because the stereotactic images obtained after clip placement were not available. The remaining 42 lesions in 39 patients (age range, 43–81 years; median, 58 years) were included in the study. Mammographic findings in these 42 lesions were calcifications in 26, uncalcified mass in 14, and mass and calcifications in two. The median lesion size was 7 mm (mean, 7 mm; range, 2–15 mm).

Biopsies were performed with patients prone on a dedicated table (StereoGuide DSM; LoRad, Danbury, Conn). The 11-gauge probe was placed to a depth 2 mm proximal to the calculated depth of the center of the lesion to acquire tissue. A median of 13 specimens (mean, 14; range, 8–34) were obtained per lesion. The protocol was to obtain a minimum of eight specimens per lesion by rotating the aperture of the bowl around the face of the clock in 1.5-hour increments (1–5). Additional specimens were obtained to sample a larger area of breast tissue at the discretion of the radiologist performing the biopsy.

Index terms: Biopsies, technology, 00.1261 • Breast, biopsy, 00.1261 • Breast neoplasms, diagnosis, 00.31, 00.32 • Stereotaxis, 00.1261

Radiology 1997; 205:417–422

[1] From the Departments of Radiology, Breast Imaging Section (L.L., D.D.D., E.A.M., A.F.A., C.M.T.), and Pathology (P.P.R.), Memorial Sloan-Kettering Cancer Center, 1275 York Ave, New York, NY 10021. Received May 6, 1997; revision requested June 5; revision received July 21; accepted July 23. **Address reprint requests to** L.L.

See also the article by Burbank and Forcier (pp 407–415) in this issue.

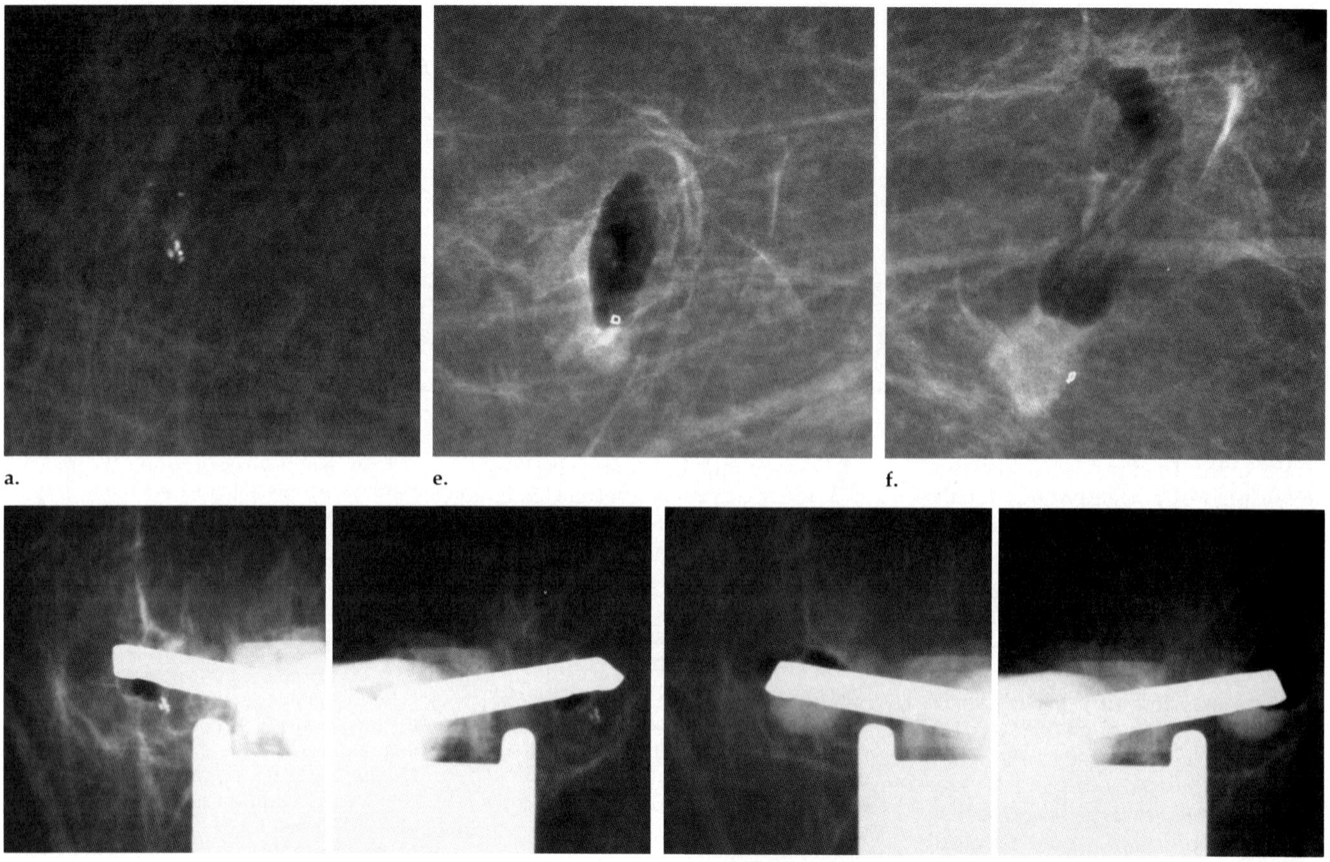

a. e. f.

b. c.

Figure 1. Clip placement through the 11-gauge probe in a 63-year-old woman. **(a)** Collimated craniocaudal mammogram demonstrates a cluster of pleomorphic calcifications measuring 1.0 cm in the longest dimension. **(b)** Stereotactic images obtained after acquisition of the first specimen reveal the probe in proximity to the remaining calcifications. **(c)** Stereotactic images obtained after tissue acquisition show air and hematoma at the biopsy site. No residual calcifications are identified. **(d)** Stereotactic images obtained after suctioning and clip placement show air at the biopsy site. The clip is attached to a side wall of the biopsy cavity. Collimated **(e)** craniocaudal mammogram and **(f)** mediolateral oblique mammogram obtained after clip placement demonstrate the biopsy cavity and accurate positioning of the clip. Histopathologic analysis revealed benign breast tissue with adenosis and microcalcifications.

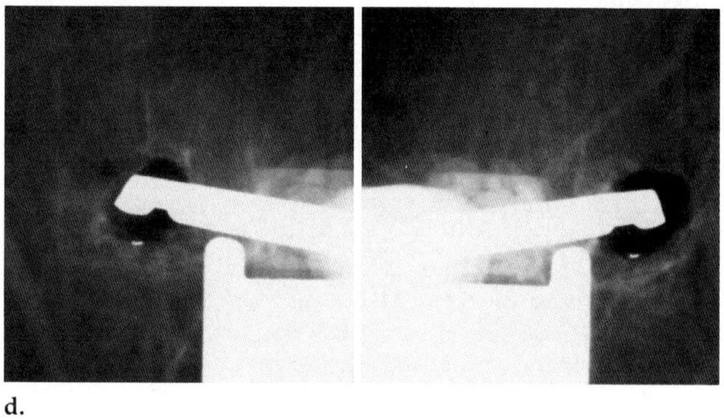

d.

The decision to obtain additional specimens was based on results of radiography of the specimens in lesions evident as calcifications, visual inspection of the tissue specimens, and assessment of stereotactic images. In lesions containing calcifications, radiography of the specimens was performed with ×1.8 magnification at 22 kVp and 4 mAs (3).

After tissue acquisition was complete, the biopsy cavity was suctioned by pulling the cutter all the way back, turning off the vacuum, pinching off the back vacuum tubing, pressing the "VAC" button to apply continuous vacuum to the bowl, and rotating the open bowl 360° twice (Burbank F, oral communication, May 1996). Stereotactic images were obtained after biopsy to ascertain if the mammographic findings associated with the original lesion had been removed.

Clip placement through the 11-gauge probe is illustrated in Figure 1. Before clip placement, the "tap tap" maneuver was used (3). To perform this maneuver, the cutter was pulled back, the vacuum was shut off, and the front vacuum tube was pinched off. The cutter was then brought forward to the precut stop position so that the tip of the cutter was at the proximal end of the bowl. The operator toggled the vacuum and manipulated the cutter manually from the proximal to distal end of the bowl and back many times by turning the dial on the probe driver. Additional short bursts of vacuum were applied while the cutter was pulled back. This maneuver allowed tissue fragments in the bowl or shaft of the probe to be pulled into the cutter lumen, collected, and cleared from the system.

The probe was then withdrawn an additional 5 mm in the depth (z) direction, to a location 7 mm proximal to the initial calculated z coordinate. The direction of clip placement around the face of the clock was chosen on the basis of (*a*) the location of the probe with respect to the lesion on pre- and postfire stereotactic images and (*b*) images obtained after tissue acquisition. If the probe was "low" with respect to the lesion, for example, the clip was placed in the 12-o'clock position; if the probe was "high," the clip was placed in the 6-o'clock position. The radiologist set the direction of clip placement by turning the aperture of the bowl of the probe and the opening of the clip introducer to the desired axis.

The clip was introduced to the first of two black marks on the clip introducer, and vacuum was applied selectively to the bowl (collecting chamber) of the probe by pinching off the vacuum tubing in the back. The clip was then advanced from the first to the second black mark on the introducer, the clip was deployed by pressing the squeeze handles, and vacuum was released. The clip introducer was withdrawn by pulling the squeeze handles; during withdrawal, forward pressure was maintained on the hub of the clip introducer

Table 1
Location of the Clip Relative to Lesion Site

Distance on Stereotactic Images (mm)	Biopsy Method	
	11-gauge (*n* = 42)	14-gauge (*n* = 15)
Total		
Median	5.6	6.7
Mean	5.5	7.9
Range	2.3–12.0	1.5–26.8
<5 mm	18 (43)*	4 (27)*
5–9 mm	22 (52)*	7 (47)*
≥10 mm	2 (5)*	4 (27)*
X		
Median	1.0	0.9
Mean	1.2	1.4
Range	0.0–3.6	0.2–3.8
Y		
Median	3.1	1.5
Mean	3.0	2.3
Range	0.2–5.9	0.7–6.1
Z		
Median	3.8	5.6
Mean	3.8	6.9
Range	0.3–11.9	0.2–26.6
Z error†		
Deep	23 (55)*	11 (73)*
Superficial	19 (45)*	4 (27)*

* Refers to the number of lesions. Numbers in parentheses are percentages.
† Refers to the depth of the clip relative to the lesion site.

until both black marks emerged from the hub. After the clip introducer was withdrawn completely, the bowl of the aperture was rotated 180° and closed, and the probe was removed. Stereotactic images were obtained after clip placement to confirm clip deployment.

The stereotactic images were reviewed. The coordinates of the clip were obtained by "targeting" on the clip and were compared with coordinates of the lesion determined before biopsy. The distance from clip to lesion site on stereotactic images in any direction (x, y, or z) was calculated as the absolute value of the difference between the coordinate of the clip and the lesion in that direction. The total distance from clip to lesion site on stereotactic images was calculated as the square root of the sum of the squares of the x, y, and z distances, per the Pythagorean theorem (6).

A mammogram was obtained after biopsy that consisted of craniocaudal and mediolateral oblique views of the breast in which biopsy was performed to ascertain the location of the clip relative to the biopsy site on standard projections. Hematoma was observed on mammograms obtained after biopsy in 29 (69%) of 42 lesions. Mammograms obtained after biopsy suggested that the original mammographic lesion was removed in 30 (71%) of 42 lesions, obscured in 10 (24%), and diminished in two (5%).

Surgery was subsequently performed on 19 lesions. Surgical procedures after clip placement included mastectomy in seven lesions in five patients and excision after

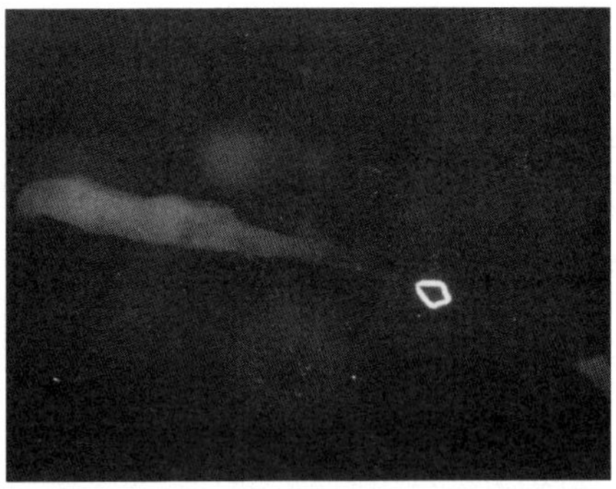

Figure 2. Radiograph of a tissue fragment retrieved from the probe in a case in which the clip failed to deploy in the breast. The clip attached to this fragment. This case illustrates the importance of thorough cleaning of the probe before placing the clip.

preoperative needle localization in 12 lesions in 12 patients. Needle localization images in 11 lesions were reviewed. The median interval from stereotactic biopsy to needle localization was 21 days (mean, 30 days; range, 10–92 days). In all 19 lesions in which surgery was performed, surgical histopathologic findings were reviewed.

Biopsies with 14-gauge Probes

A retrospective review was performed of mammograms of 85 consecutive lesions in which stereotactic vacuum-assisted biopsy was performed with a 14-gauge probe (Mammotome; Biopsys Medical) from May 1, 1996, to October 30, 1996, according to the protocol described previously (3). A localizing clip was placed in 20 (24%) lesions. Five lesions were excluded because stereotactic images after clip placement were not obtained; the remaining 15 lesions were included in the study. These 15 lesions occurred in 15 patients (age range, 43–80 years; median, 56 years). A median of 16 specimens (mean, 17; range, 8–39) were obtained per lesion. Mammographic findings in these 15 lesions were calcifications in 11, uncalcified mass in two, and mass and calcifications in two. The median lesion size was 4 mm (range, 3–10 mm).

Clip placement after 14-gauge vacuum-assisted biopsy differed from clip placement through the 11-gauge probe. Because the clip cannot be placed through the 14-gauge probe, the probe was withdrawn after the biopsy cavity was suctioned. Stereotactic images were obtained and a side wall of the biopsy cavity was targeted. The side wall was targeted because it was necessary for the clip to attach to tissue to deploy in the breast. It was believed preferable for the clip to attach to a side wall of the biopsy cavity rather than to a near or far wall owing to potential error in the depth (z) direction in the compressed breast. Targeting the side wall for clip placement after 11-gauge biopsy was not necessary because clip placement through the 11-gauge probe is accomplished with the use of vacuum to pull tissue into the bowl of the probe.

After the side wall was targeted, a 13-gauge calibrated trocar-style biopsy needle (Manan Medical Products, Northbrook, Ill) was placed, stereotactic images were obtained to confirm accurate positioning, and the clip was deployed. Stereotactic images were obtained to confirm deployment of the clip. Coordinates of the clip on the stereotactic images were compared with lesion coordinates before biopsy. Mammograms obtained immediately after stereotactic biopsy and clip placement in these 15 lesions showed a hematoma in 11 (73%). Mammograms obtained after biopsy suggested that the original mammographic lesion was completely removed in nine (60%) of 15 lesions, obscured in one (7%), and diminished in five (33%).

Six lesions underwent needle localization a median of 15 days (mean, 21 days; range, 11–51 days) after stereotactic 14-gauge vacuum-assisted biopsy. Needle localization images and surgical histopathologic findings were reviewed. Data were analyzed with a computerized statistics program (Epi-Info; Centers for Disease Control, Atlanta, Ga). Statistical significance of results was determined with the χ^2 and Fisher exact tests.

RESULTS

Table 1 shows the distance from the clip to the lesion site on stereotactic images obtained after biopsy. The distance from the clip to the lesion site was less than 1 cm in 40 (95%) of 42 lesions in which clips were placed through the 11-gauge probe versus 11 (73%) of 15 lesions in which clips were placed after 14-gauge vacuum-assisted biopsy ($P < .04$). The largest errors were in the depth or z axis. No complications or untoward reactions to the clip were encountered.

In two additional lesions in which stereotactic 11-gauge vacuum-assisted biopsy was performed during this period, the clip attached to fragments in the bowl of the probe and failed to deploy in the breast (Fig 2). One of these was the first case in which clip placement was attempted through the 11-gauge probe; the other occurred in the 2nd month of our experience with this clip.

Needle localization images in 11 patients who had undergone clip placement after 11-gauge stereotactic vacuum-assisted biopsy revealed hematoma at the biopsy site in four (36%) patients. These hematomas were 0.6–2.4 cm (median, 1.5 cm; mean, 1.5 cm). Needle localization images in six patients who had undergone clip placement after 14-gauge stereotactic vacuum-assisted biopsy showed no evidence of hematoma. No air was identified on images obtained during needle localization.

In all 19 lesions in which surgery was performed after clip placement through the 11-gauge probe, the biopsy site was identified at histopathologic analysis of the surgical specimen (Fig 3). Correlation of stereotactic 11-gauge vacuum biopsy findings and surgical histopathologic findings is shown in Table 2. There were no atypical ductal hyperplasia or ductal carcinoma in situ "underestimates" (2). In three ductal carcinoma in situ and two atypical ductal hyperplasia lesions, surgical histopathologic analysis demonstrated no residual carcinoma or atypical ductal hyperplasia, respectively, although the biopsy sites were identified.

Of six lesions that underwent surgery after 14-gauge stereotactic vacuum-assisted biopsy and clip placement, the biopsy site was identified at histopathologic analysis in five (83%) lesions (Table 3). In one patient in whom ductal carcinoma in situ was diagnosed at 14-gauge vacuum-assisted biopsy, the clip was 3 mm distant from the biopsy site on stereotactic images obtained after biopsy. Needle localization of the clip was performed, but neither the clip nor the carcinoma were removed at surgery. Subsequent reexcision yielded the clip and revealed ductal carcinoma in situ.

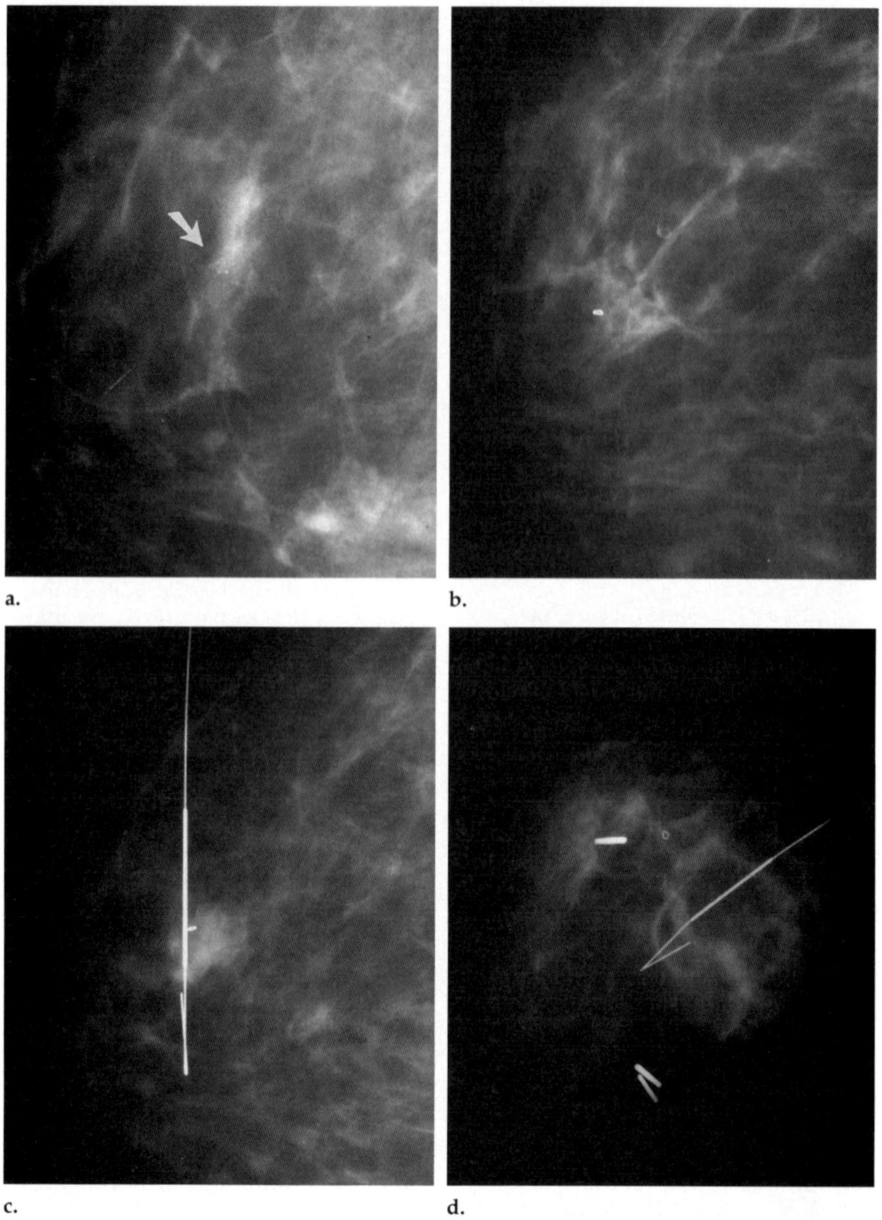

Figure 3. **(a)** Collimated mediolateral oblique mammogram in a 45-year-old woman demonstrates a cluster of pleomorphic calcifications (arrow) measuring 0.5 cm in the longest dimension. **(b)** Collimated mediolateral oblique mammogram obtained after stereotactic 11-gauge vacuum-assisted biopsy and clip placement demonstrates no residual calcifications. The clip is located within the biopsy cavity. Histopathologic analysis revealed ductal carcinoma in situ. **(c)** Collimated mediolateral oblique mammogram obtained during needle localization demonstrates the wire localizing the clip. **(d)** Radiograph of the specimen shows the clip. Surgical histopathologic analysis revealed ductal carcinoma in situ.

DISCUSSION

A directional, vacuum-assisted biopsy instrument is available for performing percutaneous breast biopsy (1–5,7,8). Larger volumes of tissue are obtained with this equipment than with an automated gun for two reasons. First, the vacuum instrument enables acquisition of larger tissue specimens, with mean specimen weights of 17 mg for the automated gun and needle (5), 34 mg for the 14-gauge vacuum-assisted instrument (5), and 100 mg for the 11-gauge vacuum-assisted biopsy instrument (Burbank F, oral communication, April 1997). Second, the ability of the vacuum instrument to obtain multiple samples with a single insertion and to suction blood from the biopsy site facilitates acquisition of a larger number of tissue specimens than was feasible previously (5).

Because of the large volumes of tissue that may be removed with the vacuum device, the mammographic findings associated with the original lesion may be removed completely at vacuum-assisted biopsy. In two previously published series of 14-gauge vacuum-assisted biopsy, Burbank et al (5) and Liberman et al (3) reported complete removal of the mammographic findings in 48% and 13%, respectively, of all lesions, and in 79% and 58%, respectively, of lesions 5 mm in diameter or less. Complete removal of the mammographic lesion does not ensure complete excision of the histologic process (3). Mammographic findings after stereotactic vacuum-assisted biopsy are transient and cannot be relied on to localize the biopsy site for subsequent surgical excision (3). Safe use of the vacuum biopsy instrument, therefore, necessitates the ability to place a localizing marker in proximity to the biopsy site to enable subsequent surgical excision if necessary.

Our findings show that after placement of the localizing clip through an 11-gauge probe, the biopsy site was identified successfully in 100% of lesions in which surgical excision was performed. After clip placement, needle localization can be performed successfully, even if the mammographic findings associated with the original lesion have been removed completely. For patients who undergo mastectomy after clip placement, a radio-

Table 2
Correlation of Stereotactic 11-gauge Vacuum-assisted Biopsy and Surgical Findings

Stereotactic Biopsy Findings	Surgical Findings: Benign	Atypical Ductal Hyperplasia	Ductal Carcinoma In Situ	Invasive Carcinoma
Benign	4*	0	0	0
Atypical ductal hyperplasia	2	0	0	0
Ductal carcinoma in situ	2†	1	4	0
Invasive carcinoma	0	0	0	6

* Includes one lesion yielding fibroepithelial tumor (fibroadenoma vs phyllodes tumor) at stereotactic biopsy that was proved to be a fibroadenoma at surgery, one lesion yielding lobular carcinoma in situ at stereotactic biopsy and surgery, and two lesions yielding benign ductal hyperplasia at stereotactic biopsy and benign findings at surgery. The latter two lesions were excised during mastectomy for carcinoma at a separate site in one patient and during breast-conserving therapy for carcinoma at a separate site in the other patient.

† Both were clusters of calcifications that were 0.9 and 1.0 cm, respectively, in the longest dimension. The biopsy cavities were identified at surgery but no residual ductal carcinoma in situ was found.

Table 3
Correlation of Stereotactic 14-gauge Vacuum-assisted Biopsy and Surgical Findings

Stereotactic Biopsy Findings	Surgical Findings: Benign	Ductal Carcinoma In Situ	Invasive Carcinoma
Atypical ductal hyperplasia	0	1	0
Ductal carcinoma in situ	1*	2	1
Invasive carcinoma	0	0	1

* Findings from subsequent surgical excision yielded ductal carcinoma in situ.

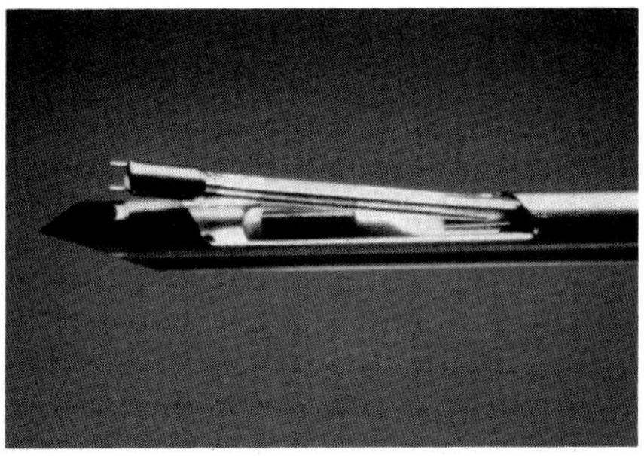

Figure 4. Photograph shows the localizing clip and introducer inside the 11-gauge probe. Note that the clip emerges from the introducer in a sloped or "ramped" configuration so that the vector of force is not entirely along the direction of compression. (Image courtesy of Biopsys Medical.)

graph can be obtained of the mastectomy specimen to assist the pathologist in identification of the biopsy site.

Clip placement is more accurate through the 11-gauge probe than through the introducer needle used after 14-gauge vacuum-assisted biopsy. First, placement of the clip after 14-gauge biopsy necessitates removing the probe from the breast and positioning a new needle. This repositioning allows the possibility of patient or lesion movement, which can diminish accuracy. Second, when placing the clip through the introducer needle after 14-gauge biopsy, the vector of force is entirely along the direction of compression of the breast. This vector of force maximizes the likelihood of error in the depth or z axis. Z-axis errors are potentially of serious consequence. In the compressed breast, as in an accordion, structures that are distant in the z axis are brought close together; when compression is released, structures that were close together move farther apart. Therefore, small errors in the z axis in compression could translate into larger errors when compression is released. The clip placed through the 11-gauge probe is introduced in an angled or "ramped" configuration, such that the vector of force is not entirely in the direction of compression (Fig 4). Furthermore, the operator uses vacuum to pull tissue into the bowl of the probe rather than merely pushing the clip out into the tissue.

Our initial experience with the clip has taught us several lessons. First, it is helpful to suction the blood out of the biopsy cavity and obtain stereotactic images after tissue acquisition is complete to ascertain whether the mammographic findings associated with the original lesion have been removed. If so, clip placement is appropriate (9). Second, the probe must be free of tissue fragments before clip placement, as illustrated by the two cases in which the clip failed to deploy. Clearing of tissue fragments can usually be accomplished by performing the tap tap maneuver (3); occasionally, if clogging of the probe has been a substantial problem during tissue acquisition, we remove the probe from the breast and flush it, as is done at the outset of the procedure, before clip placement. Third, stereotactic images should be obtained after clip placement and probe removal to ensure that the clip has deployed before releasing compression. Finally, it is prudent to obtain a mammogram of the breast that underwent biopsy and clip placement. Observed distances between the clip and lesion site on stereotactic images may underestimate the true distances, particularly in the depth or z axis, owing to the "accordion effect" of compression. By allowing an assessment of the location of the clip relative to the biopsy site on standard projections, the mammogram obtained after biopsy serves as a useful guide for subsequent needle localization.

There are other potential applications of a localizing clip that were not addressed in our study. There have been reports of preliminary experience with magnetic resonance (MR) imaging–guided biopsy and needle localization of breast lesions (10–17). One limitation of MR imaging–guided needle localization procedures is the inability to document lesion retrieval, because contrast enhancement, which is often essential for lesion detection at MR imaging, is not observed in the resected specimen. If a clip could be placed at MR imaging–guided biopsy or localization, radiography of the surgical specimen could confirm retrieval of the clip, supporting successful retrieval of the lesion. The clip described in our study is compatible with a magnet of field strength 1.5 T or less; the probe is not MR imaging–compatible, but clip placement could occur outside the magnet after placement of an MR imaging–compatible introducer (15,16). Edeiken-Monroe et al (18) reported preliminary experience with sonographically guided implantation of metallic markers to permanently localize the tumor bed in patients with breast cancer receiving preoperative chemotherapy. In eight (42%) of 19 cases, the metallic marker was the only remaining evidence of the site of the tumor bed. A localizing clip could therefore be useful to mark the tumor site in these women with locally advanced breast cancer. Mumtaz et al (19) described percutaneous treatment of breast cancers with interstitial laser photocoagulation. The role of percutaneous ablative procedures in the treatment of breast cancer has not been established, but placement of a localizing marker at the tumor site could play a role in this evolving technique. It may be necessary to improve on the accuracy of marker placement over that reported in our study for use in guiding therapy.

In summary, our data demonstrate that a localizing clip can be placed in proximity to the biopsy site after stereotactic vacuum-assisted biopsy. Clip placement is more accurate through the 11-gauge probe than after 14-gauge biopsy. After clip placement, the biopsy site can be identified for subsequent surgical excision, even if the mammographic findings associated with the original lesion have been removed completely. ■

Acknowledgments: We thank Lynda T. Zingaro, RT(R)(M), and Youngduk Paik, RT(R)(M), for expert technical support and David C. Perlman, MD, for invaluable assistance.

References

1. Parker SH, Burbank F. A practical approach to minimally invasive breast biopsy. Radiology 1996; 200:11–20.
2. Burbank F. Stereotactic breast biopsy of atypical ductal hyperplasia and ductal carcinoma in situ lesions: improved accuracy with directional, vacuum-assisted breast biopsy. Radiology 1997; 202:843–847.
3. Liberman L, Hann LE, Dershaw DD, Morris EA, Abramson AF, Rosen PP. Mammographic findings after stereotactic 14-gauge vacuum biopsy. Radiology 1997; 203:343–347.
4. Parker SH, Stavros AT, Dennis MA. Needle biopsy techniques. Radiol Clin North Am 1995; 33:1171–1186.
5. Burbank F, Parker SH, Fogarty TJ. Stereotactic breast biopsy: improved tissue harvesting with the Mammotome. Am Surg 1996; 62:738–744.
6. Kane JW, Sternheim MM. Plane geometry and trigonometric functions. In: Physics. New York, NY: Wiley, 1978; 627.
7. Jackman RJ, Burbank F, Parker SH, et al. Atypical ductal hyperplasia diagnosed at stereotactic breast biopsy: improved reliability with 14-gauge, directional, vacuum-assisted biopsy. Radiology 1997; 204:485–488.
8. Meyer JE, Smith DN, DiPiro PJ, et al. Stereotactic breast biopsy of clustered microcalcifications with a directional, vacuum-assisted device. Radiology 1997; 204:575–576.
9. Burbank F. Mammographic findings after 14-gauge automated needle and 14-gauge directional, vacuum-assisted stereotactic breast biopsies. Radiology 1997; 204:153–156.
10. Heywang-Kobrunner SH, Beck R, Hilbertz T, et al. Needle localization of breast lesions detected with MR imaging. Radiology 1990; 177:190–191.
11. Fischer U, Vosshenrich R, Keating D, et al. MR-guided biopsy of suspect breast lesions with a simple stereotaxic add-on device for surface coils. Radiology 1994; 192:272–273.
12. Orel SG, Schnall MD, Newman RW, Powell CM, Torosian MH, Rosato EF. MR imaging-guided localization and biopsy of breast lesions: initial experience. Radiology 1994; 193:97–102.
13. Orel SG, Schnall MD, Powell CM, et al. Staging of suspected breast cancer: effect of MR imaging and MR-guided biopsy. Radiology 1995; 196:115–122.
14. Brenner RJ, Shellock FG, Rothman BJ, Giuliano A. Magnetic resonance imaging-guided preoperative breast localization using freehand technique. Br J Radiol 1995; 68:1095–1098.
15. Heinig A, Heywang-Kobrunner SH, Viehweg P, Schaumloffel U, Heske N. Ein neues nadelsystem zur MR-gestuzten lokalisation und transkutanen biopsie von suspekten defunden in der brust: in-vitro-untersuchungen bei 1.0 Tesla. ROFO 1997; 166:342–345.
16. Heywang-Kobrunner SH, Kolem H, Heinig A, Viehweg P. A new design for a breast biopsy device suitable for MR application (abstr). Eur Radiol 1997; 7(suppl):243.
17. Kuhl CK, Elevelt A, Leutner CC, Gieseke J, Pakos E, Schild HH. Interventional breast MR imaging: clinical use of a stereotactic localization and biopsy device. Radiology 1997; 204:667–675.
18. Edeiken-Monroe BS, Fornage BD, Holmes FA. A preliminary report of sonographically guided implantation of metallic markers to permanently localize the tumor bed in patients with breast cancer receiving preoperative chemotherapy (abstr). AJR 1997; 168(suppl):98.
19. Mumtaz H, Hall-Craggs MA, Wotherspoon A, et al. Laser therapy for breast cancer: MR imaging and histopathologic correlation. Radiology 1996; 200:651–658.

Liane E. Philpotts, MD • Carol H. Lee, MD • Laura J. Horvath, MD • Irena Tocino, MD

Canceled Stereotactic Core-Needle Biopsy of the Breast: Analysis of 89 Cases[1]

PURPOSE: To determine reasons for cancellation of stereotactic core-needle breast biopsy and outcome in canceled cases.

MATERIALS AND METHODS: Among 572 scheduled stereotactic core-needle biopsies, 89 cases (16%) in 88 patients were canceled. In canceled cases, mammogram origin, mammographic abnormality, reason for cancellation, and outcome were determined.

RESULTS: In canceled cases, 50 (57%) of 88 patients were referred from another facility. Mammographic abnormality in most cases (72 [81%] of 89 canceled biopsies) was a mass(es); calcifications occurred in 14 cases (16%). Reasons for cancellation included (*a*) lesion was not recognized (26 cases [29%]), (*b*) lesion was reassessed as benign (17 cases [19%]), (*c*) cysts were diagnosed with ultrasound (US) (12 cases [13%]) or aspiration (11 cases [12%]), (*d*) lesion location was suboptimal (12 cases [13%]), (*e*) patient was intolerant of procedure (seven cases [8%]), and (*f*) other (four cases [4%]). Numbers of canceled biopsies from another facility and those from the authors' institution differed in cases in which lesions were reassessed as benign (12 and five cases, respectively) or cysts were diagnosed with US (10 and two cases, respectively). Lesions that could not be targeted included many pseudolesions and three cancers.

CONCLUSION: Complete work-up, including US examination, of breast lesions is necessary before stereotactic core-needle biopsy is scheduled. Inability to recognize a suspected lesion on stereotactic images should not preclude biopsy with another method.

Stereotactic core-needle biopsy has been used commonly to diagnose impalpable breast abnormalities on mammograms. Lesions appearing as masses or calcifications can be sampled successfully with the technique (1–7). Increased use of this procedure at many institutions over the past few years has led to a reduced number of open surgical biopsies that necessitate preoperative needle localization and has shifted the spectrum of procedures performed daily by breast radiologists.

Many lesions found with mammography are accessible with stereotactic core-needle biopsy; however, cases scheduled are frequently canceled. Cancellation can cause anxiety and inconvenience for the patient, including time lost from work or other activities and possible delay of diagnosis of a suspected abnormality. In the breast-imaging department, there can be loss of the technologist's or radiologist's time, suboptimal use of equipment and rooms, waste of supplies, and loss of time available for other patients.

To improve the efficiency of daily breast imaging procedures and provision of services and to understand the limitations of stereotactic core-needle biopsy, we performed a retrospective review of cases in which scheduled stereotactic core-needle biopsy was canceled. The origin of the mammogram, mammographic finding, reason for cancellation, and outcome were assessed.

MATERIALS AND METHODS

From July 1992 to December 1995, 572 patients were scheduled to undergo stereotactic core-needle biopsy of the breast. At our institution, it is policy to offer stereotactic core-needle biopsy to all patients who must undergo biopsy because of a mammographic abnormality and in whom the procedure is believed to be technically feasible. The indications for stereotactic core-needle biopsy were the same as those for excisional biopsy. Lesions appearing as masses, architectural distortion, or calcifications were considered. Cases were not excluded on the basis of lesion size. Most biopsies were scheduled after the patient consulted with a breast surgeon. During the entire study, it was not our policy for a breast radiologist to review all mammograms before scheduling the biopsy. Patient requirements of the procedure were (*a*) a compressed breast thickness of at least 3 cm, (*b*) the ability to tolerate and cooperate in the prone position, (*c*) no bleeding diathesis or use of anticoagulant agents, and (*d*) weight less than 300 lb (135 kg). Features that were considered not feasible were (*a*) lesions in very posterior or superficial locations and (*b*) very faint calcifications (like those noted on magnified images only). At our institution during the study period, ultrasound (US)-guided core biopsy was not performed commonly, and thus stereotactic core-needle biopsy represented the primary nonsurgical means of diagnosing impalpable breast lesions.

All stereotactic core-needle biopsies were performed with a dedicated table (Lorad, Danbury, Conn) with patients in the prone position. A 14-gauge core-biopsy needle (Bard Urological, Covington, Ga) and an automatic long-throw gun (Biopty

Index terms: Breast, abnormalities, 00.31, 00.32, 00.81 • Breast, biopsy, 00.1267 • Breast radiography, 00.119

Radiology 1997; 205:423–428

[1] From the Department of Diagnostic Radiology, Yale University School of Medicine, 333 Cedar St, New Haven, CT 06520. From the 1996 RSNA scientific assembly. Received May 19, 1997; revision requested June 13; revision received July 22; accepted July 23. **Address reprint requests to** L.E.P.

gun; Bard Urological) were used; a short-throw gun was used when breast thickness was not sufficient to accommodate the long throw. Digital imaging was used in the vast majority of cases. Screen-film imaging was available but used infrequently. The technique of targeting lesions has been described (8). There was no standard procedure; however, on the day of the scheduled biopsy, patients—especially those referred from other facilities—may have undergone mammography or US examination before stereotactic core-needle biopsy at the discretion of the radiologist. Imaging was also more likely to be performed if a period of time had elapsed from the date of the mammogram that resulted in the recommendation of biopsy.

A review of the records of the breast-imaging department revealed that 89 (16%) (in 88 patients) of 572 stereotactic core-needle biopsies were canceled on the day of the scheduled procedure. The origin of the patient's mammogram (another facility or our institution) was documented. Patients with mammograms from other facilities were referred specifically for core biopsy of a reported abnormality. The mammographic abnormality for which biopsy was recommended was categorized as (*a*) a mass or asymmetric density, (*b*) calcifications, or (*c*) an unknown abnormality (no record available). The following reasons for cancellation of the stereotactic core-needle biopsy were recorded: (*a*) the lesion could not be recognized, (*b*) the lesion was reassessed as benign, (*c*) a cyst(s) was diagnosed, (*d*) the lesion was not in an optimal location, (*e*) the patient could not tolerate the procedure, and (*f*) other. Those cases in which a lesion was not recognized consisted of those in which the lesion was not seen well enough on scout ("straight") or stereotactic images for confident targeting. Those cases in which lesions were reassessed as benign were those in which mammograms acquired on the day of scheduled biopsy did not show a lesion that necessitated biopsy. These patients were never placed on the stereotactic table. The lesion was not in an optimal location if the lesion was in the far posterior portion of the breast (outside the image field) or in a very superficial location or if the compressed breast was so thin that the sample notch would not traverse the lesion and/or the needle would strike the image receptor. The patient could not tolerate the procedure if the patient's weight or discomfort precluded the procedure or the patient could not maintain a motionless, prone position. The reason for cancellation was correlated with the mammographic abnormality and the place of origin of the mammogram.

The outcome of patients after cancellation of the stereotactic core-needle biopsy was assessed. The number of patients who underwent biopsy with other methods was determined. In those patients for whom mammographic surveillance was recommended, the follow-up protocol involved unilateral mammography at 6 months and bilateral mammography at 12 months and annually thereafter. Follow-up information was available in 35 (80%) of 44 patients; duration of follow-up was 4–52 months (mean, 25 months). Clinical follow-up only (absence of clinically evident breast cancer) was available in three of the 35 patients.

RESULTS

In 50 (57%) of the 88 patients, findings on mammograms from other facilities resulted in the recommendation of biopsy. The mammograms of 38 patients (43%) were acquired at our institution. Of the 483 scheduled stereotactic core-needle biopsies that were performed successfully, 189 cases (39%) were referred from another facility and 294 (61%) were from our institution. Therefore, the cancellation rate of cases referred from another facility was 21% (50 of 239 scheduled biopsies) and that from our institution was 11% (39 of 333 scheduled biopsies). The mammographic finding in most (72 [81%] of 89) canceled cases was a mass or asymmetric density. Calcifications were the finding in only 14 cases (16%). The mammographic abnormality was classified unknown in three cases (3%).

The reasons for cancellation of stereotactic core-needle biopsy as they relate to the mammographic finding or place of origin of the patient's mammogram are shown in Table 1. The most common reason for cancellation was the lesion could not be recognized (26 [29%] of 89 canceled biopsies). In most of these cases, masses or asymmetric densities (22 [85%] of 26 cases) were identified. In only four cases (15%) were calcifications too faint to target accurately with stereotactic biopsy.

Mammographic images acquired on the day of the scheduled procedure resulted in reassessment of the reported abnormality as benign in 17 cases (19%); the four cases of calcifications consisted of benign processes such as milk of calcium (n = 1), rim calcifications (n = 1), and diffuse calcifications (n = 2). Additional imaging in 13 cases of suspected mass or asymmetric density revealed that parenchyma was normal (n = 9) or the lesion was smaller or had resolved (n = 4).

Diagnosis of a cyst(s) with US or aspiration—occurring in 12 (13%) and 11 (12%) cases, respectively—was another common reason for cancellation of stereotactic core-needle biopsy. In all of these cases, masses were the mammographic finding.

Only 12 (13%) of the 89 biopsies were canceled because of suboptimal lesion location. A very posterior or superficial location of the lesion precluded stereotactic core-needle biopsy in eight cases (9%), and breasts were too thin when compressed in four cases (4%). In seven cases (8%), the patient could not tolerate the procedure; in most of these cases, the patient could not maintain a motionless, prone position.

When numbers of canceled cases from another facility were compared with those from our institution, the main differences were found in cases in which the lesion was reassessed as benign or cysts were diagnosed with US. Twelve (71%) of 17 cases in which the lesion was reassessed as benign were from another facility. Ten (83%) of 12 cases in which masses proved to be simple cysts with US at scheduled biopsy were from another facility. By contrast, more cases of cysts necessitating aspiration for diagnosis (7 [64%] of 11 cases) were from our institution.

In 19 (21%) of the 89 canceled cases, the appearance of lesions warranted biopsy with use of another method. Needle localization and excisional biopsy were performed in 16 cases (18%), fine-needle aspiration (with stereotactic or mammographic guidance) in two (2%), and US-guided core-needle biopsy in one (1%). The reasons for cancellation of the stereotactic core-needle biopsy in these 19 cases were the lesion could not be recognized (n = 6), lesion reassessed as benign (n = 2) (biopsy was performed at the patient's request), suboptimal location of lesion (n = 9), and patient unable to tolerate the procedure (n = 2). Among these cases, cancer was found at pathologic examination in three cases (all were masses). In two of these cases, stereotactic core-needle biopsy was canceled because the lesion could not be recognized; in one case, the patient could not tolerate the procedure. All cancers were invasive ductal carcinoma, although one was a tubular subtype.

Excluding the 19 cases in which immediate biopsy was performed with alternative methods and the 23 cases in which cysts were diagnosed, follow-up information was available in 38 of the other 47 cases. In three cases, a change in the mammographic findings prompted recommendation for repeat biopsy. In two of the three cases (in which stereotactic core-needle biopsy was canceled because the lesion could not be recognized), biopsy specimens obtained at 6 and 24 months (of a mass and calcifications, respectively) showed benign findings. In the third case, a follow-up mammogram obtained 2 years after stereotactic core-

Reasons for Cancellation of Stereotactic Core-Needle Biopsy on the Basis of Mammographic Findings or Origin of Mammogram

Reason for Cancellation	Mammographic Finding: Mass(es) (n = 72)	Mammographic Finding: Calcifications (n = 14)	Mammographic Finding: Unknown (n = 3)	Origin of Mammogram: Another Facility (n = 50)	Origin of Mammogram: Yale (n = 39)	Total (n = 89)
Lesion not recognized on stereotactic images	22 (85)	4 (15)*	0 (0)	11 (42)	15 (58)	26 (29)
Lesion on mammogram reassessed as benign	13 (76)	4 (24)	0 (0)	12 (71)	5 (29)	17 (19)
Cyst						
Diagnosed with US	12 (100)	0 (0)	0 (0)	10 (83)	2 (17)	12 (13)
Diagnosed with aspiration	11 (100)	0 (0)	0 (0)	4 (36)	7 (64)	11 (12)
Lesion location posterior or superficial	6 (75)	2 (25)	0 (0)	3 (38)	5 (62)	8 (9)
Breasts too small	2 (50)	2 (50)	0 (0)	3 (75)	1 (25)	4 (4)
Patient unable to tolerate biopsy	3 (43)	2 (29)	2 (29)	3 (43)	4 (57)	7 (8)
Other	3 (75)	0 (0)	1 (25)	4 (100)	0 (0)	4 (4)†

Note.—Numbers are numbers of canceled biopsies. Numbers in parentheses are percentages of totals. Percentages that do not add up to 100 are due to rounding.

* Calcifications were too faint to target.

† Cases included one case each of an intrammammary lymph node (diagnosed with US), a dilated duct (diagnosed with US), and a palpable lesion. In the fourth case, the reason for cancellation was not known.

needle biopsy was canceled (because the lesion could not be recognized) demonstrated a change; pathologic examination of an excisional biopsy specimen revealed invasive ductal carcinoma (Fig 1). Although this case was problematic because the originally identified lesion could not be targeted, follow-up mammography (with spot-compression views) at 6 and 12 months did not demonstrate a lesion. In another 32 cases, the following information with follow-up mammography was available: Lesions appeared stable (n = 11) or smaller (n = 12) or had resolved (n = 9). In the other three cases, there was no clinical evidence of disease. In nine cases, no follow-up information was available.

DISCUSSION

Stereotactic core-needle biopsy of many lesions seen on mammograms is replacing surgical excisional biopsy. Stereotactic core-needle biopsy is performed ideally with a dedicated table and digital imaging, but the procedure can be performed with upright add-on units and screen-film systems. When the procedure is performed on a dedicated table, certain restrictions apply. Patients can weigh no more than 300 lb (135 kg) with use of the Lorad or Fischer units because the table may be damaged or malfunction with more weight. The patient must be able to cooperate with use of this equipment; if the patient cannot tolerate the motionless, prone position, the biopsy may not be possible. With use of an automatic sampling gun, the breast must be thick enough (usually a minimum of 3 cm) to accommodate the throw of the needle. Lesion position in the breast is also important; very superficial or posterior targets may be impossible to sample with the technique.

A new vacuum-suction device, the Mammotome (Biopsys Medical, Irvine, Calif), enables stereotactic sampling of lesions without the need to fire the needle and facilitates biopsy of very superficial or posterior lesions or lesions in small breasts. Also, this device may allow sampling of calcifications with greater ease. An "air-gap" technique, with use of a second fenestrated paddle on the side of the breast next to the image receptor, increases the thickness of the compressed breast. Use of this new equipment and technique will likely enable the sampling of more lesions in small breasts with stereotactic core-needle biopsy.

Upright add-on stereotactic units—although probably less desirable for patient comfort and sampling accuracy than dedicated tables—provide potentially better access to lesions in the posterior and axillary portions of the breast. In the upright position, the changing of positioning allows a greater amount of breast tissue to be placed on the fenestrated compression plate. Also, patients unable to tolerate the prone position may be able to undergo successfully a stereotactic core-needle biopsy on the upright unit. Knowledge of the limitations of available equipment allows (*a*) exclusion of certain cases before scheduling a biopsy and (*b*) recommendation of alternative biopsy options.

A thorough work-up of suspected lesions before scheduling stereotactic core-needle biopsy is necessary. Because our institution is a referral center, we see many patients who have undergone mammography at another facility and come for stereotactic core-needle biopsy. Often, adequate work-up with spot-compression and magnification views and high-quality US examination has not been performed before recommendation of biopsy. Performance of such studies often results in the lesion being reassessed as benign, and thus the biopsy is canceled. The cancellation rate (21%) of cases from another facility was almost twice that (11%) of cases at our institution. Seventy-one percent of cases canceled because the lesion was reassessed as benign were from another facility. Mass lesions for which stereotactic core-needle biopsy is recommended should be identified on at least two mammographic projections (required for needle localization). Although with stereotactic biopsy, an area is targeted from one direction, reliance on this feature should not preclude a thorough work-up. High-quality US examination of most masses should be performed before stereotactic core-needle biopsy is recommended. Findings on sonograms may obviate biopsy of simple cysts and lesions with benign features. The higher number of cases from another facility in which simple cysts were demonstrated with US indicates the insufficient evaluation of these masses before recommendation of biopsy. Conversely, at our institution, there were more cases of cysts that necessitated aspiration for diagnosis (because US criteria for simple cysts were not met). Aspiration is a procedure; however, it was not the originally scheduled, tissue-sampling procedure and often necessitates a change of equipment, location, and technologic support.

Despite exclusion of ineligible patients and a thorough work-up of cases before scheduling of stereotactic core-needle biopsy, our results show there will be many cases in which lesions cannot be sampled. In our series, lesions that could not be targeted with stereotactic biopsy represented the most common reason for cancellation (29%). Many of these cases, in retrospect, represented pseudolesions (superimposed normal parenchyma); however, there were a small number of cancers that could not be targeted. The technique of targeting with stereotactic biopsy necessitates that a mass be seen adequately on two angled images, acquired generally at 15° from the scout image. A density that appears prominent on one projection may appear less distinct with this imaging method (Fig 2). Successful targeting of lesions with stereotactic core-needle biopsy depends on radiographic conspicuity, which depends on factors such as lesion shape, margins, and density with regard to the surrounding tissue. The results of our study indicate that one cannot always predict that a lesion will not be recognized on stereotactic images. A "target-on-scout" technique is available with some equipment (Mammotest; Fischer Imaging, Denver, Colo) and allows targeting to be performed with the scout view and one of the two stereotactic images. This technique permits use of the best images and may improve targeting of ill-defined densities.

In cases in which a lesion cannot be targeted with stereotactic biopsy, differentiation of a true lesion from a pseudolesion is necessary and can be difficult. This differentiation depends on imaging expertise and thus is best performed by or under the supervision of an experienced breast imaging radiologist. The differentiation of a true lesion from a pseudolesion often necessitates reevaluation of the current and past mammograms and the procurement of additional images. Evaluation with US and magnetic resonance (MR) imaging may aid this differentiation. While there is minimal literature on this subject, we have frequently performed these additional imaging studies to aid our evaluation of an area. Normal findings on sonograms and MR images support a recommendation of follow-up (9). An abnormality detected on these images may indicate the need for biopsy with a method other than stereotactic core-needle biopsy.

In those patients who do not undergo stereotactic core-needle biopsy or biopsy with use of another method (particularly those patients with a mass that is reassessed as benign or pseudolesions that cannot be targeted), adherence to a follow-up protocol is important and should be emphasized to these patients. A suspected change in an abnormality on follow-up mammograms would prompt a new recommendation of biopsy. In three cases (3%) in our series, mammograms showed interval change that prompted biopsy at a later date. Failure to follow up these cases with mammography could result in a delay of diagnosis of a suspected lesion.

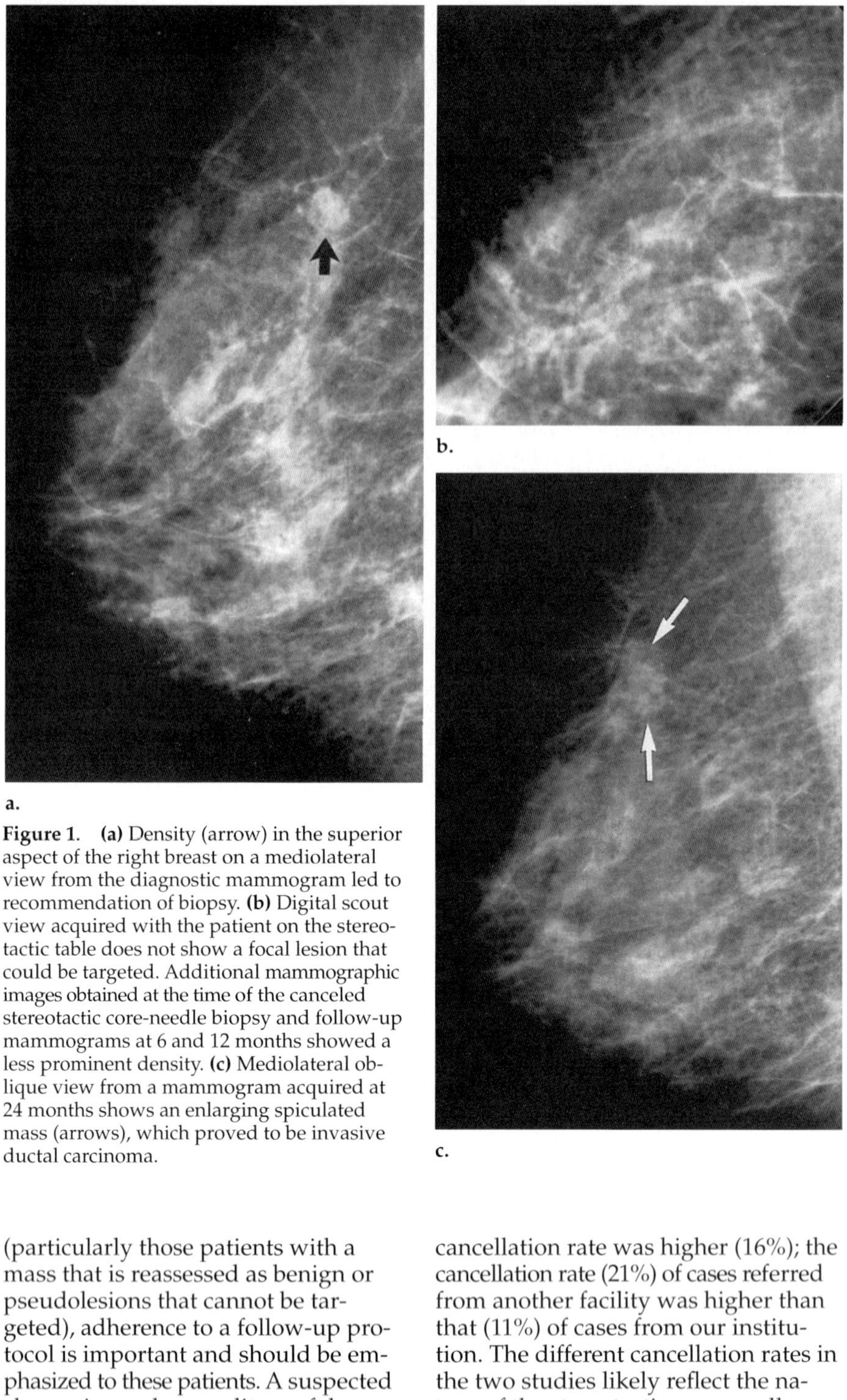

a. b. c.

Figure 1. **(a)** Density (arrow) in the superior aspect of the right breast on a mediolateral view from the diagnostic mammogram led to recommendation of biopsy. **(b)** Digital scout view acquired with the patient on the stereotactic table does not show a focal lesion that could be targeted. Additional mammographic images obtained at the time of the canceled stereotactic core-needle biopsy and follow-up mammograms at 6 and 12 months showed a less prominent density. **(c)** Mediolateral oblique view from a mammogram acquired at 24 months shows an enlarging spiculated mass (arrows), which proved to be invasive ductal carcinoma.

In a study of canceled cases that were scheduled for needle localization before surgical biopsy, Meyer et al (10) found a cancellation rate of 8.8%; all canceled cases were referred from another facility. In our study of stereotactic core-needle biopsy, the overall cancellation rate was higher (16%); the cancellation rate (21%) of cases referred from another facility was higher than that (11%) of cases from our institution. The different cancellation rates in the two studies likely reflect the nature of the stereotactic core-needle biopsy compared with that of needle localization. In both procedures, cancellations are common because lesions are reassessed as benign; however, the requirements of stereotactic core-needle biopsy are unique, and consequently, the number of canceled cases may be increased.

Lesions containing calcifications constituted only a small percentage (16%) of our canceled cases. At our institution during the study period, calcified lesions constituted 37% of cases in which stereotactic core-needle biopsy was recommended (11). The

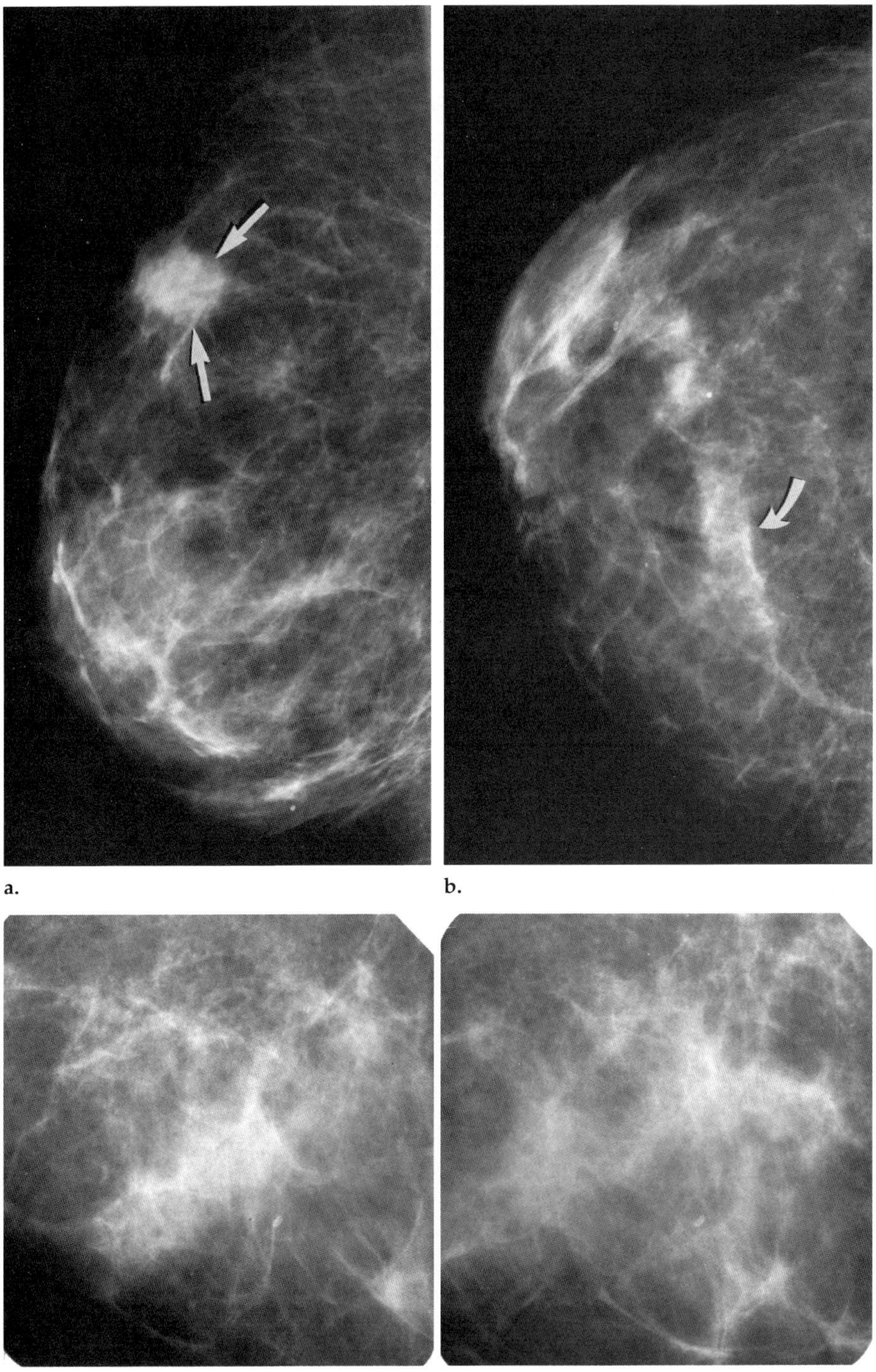

a. b. c.

Figure 2. **(a)** Mediolateral view from a mammogram of the right breast shows a density (arrows) in the superior portion. **(b)** Craniocaudal projection from the same mammogram shows the abnormality (arrow) less conspicuously. **(c)** Mediolateral stereotactic images do not demonstrate a targetable lesion, and the abnormality was thought to represent normal parenchyma. The appearance of the area on follow-up mammograms had not changed for 2 years.

cancellation rate (6%) in these cases was significantly less than that (18%) in cases of masses ($P < .01$). With currently available digital-imaging systems, the visualization of microcalcifications is excellent (12). While targeting of microcalcifications depends primarily on adequate image resolution, targeting of masses depends on radiographic conspicuity; masses must be identifiable on two stereotactic views.

Potentially avoidable situations (ie, lesions reassessed as benign, cysts diagnosed, and features of three "other" cases) that led to cancellation occurred in 48% of all cancellations. Unavoidable situations that led to cancellation illustrate the true limitations of the technique. These cases represented 51% of the all cancellations, and reasons included the lesion could not be recognized, lesion location, and patient factors. (In 1% of cases, the reason for cancellation was not known.) If cases in which cancellation was potentially avoidable were excluded, the overall percentage of canceled cases would have been reduced by approximately half.

New methods of percutaneous biopsy of breast lesions—such as that used with the Mammotome and the air-gap and target-on-scout techniques—should allow more lesions to be diagnosed with stereotactic core-needle biopsy (13). The recently introduced ABBI (Advanced Breast Biopsy Instrumentation; US Surgical, Norwalk, Conn) system is a stereotactic-guided method used to remove large cores of tissue and is an alternative method to open surgical biopsy. Because similar equipment and targeting are used with stereotactic core-needle biopsy, comparable or more restricted requirements regarding patients and lesions will need to be met. Open surgical procedures will still likely be performed in those cases in which stereotactic core-needle biopsy cannot be performed.

To decrease the number of canceled stereotactic core-needle biopsies, it is now our policy to require review by a breast radiologist of all cases referred from another facility before the biopsy is scheduled. Cases in which additional work-up, including US examination, is needed can be identified before biopsy. Any referral center in which stereotactic core-needle biopsy is performed would probably benefit from a such a policy. A ideal schedule would be one that can accommodate canceled stereotactic core-needle biopsies and unscheduled cases in which immediate biopsy is needed after work-up. This schedule may necessitate assignment of an initial level of suspicion to a lesion on a screening study so that time or equipment can be allotted appropriately. In all facilities, a "double reading" (especially by individuals experienced with mammography and aware of limitations of the technique) in cases in which stereotactic core-needle biopsy is recommended could decrease the number of inappropriate recommendations of biopsy and thus cancellations. In addition, measuring compressed breast thickness at diagnostic mammography identifies those patients with inadequate breast thickness, and alternative methods of biopsy can be recommended. Questioning patients about anticoagulant use, a bleeding diathesis, or weight is also recommended to avoid cancellations for such reasons.

The results of our study demonstrate the reasons for cancellation of stereotactic core-needle biopsy of the breast at a referral center. The findings indicate that complete work-up, including high-quality US examination, of lesions is necessary before biopsy is scheduled so that unnecessary or canceled biopsies are minimized. Consideration of biopsy requirements, including breast thickness and lesion characteristics (ie, lesion position in the breast) with respect to available equipment enables exclusion of cases that are inappropriate for stereotactic core-needle biopsy. Newer techniques of percutaneous biopsy should allow more lesions to be sampled with stereotactic core-needle biopsy and thus result in fewer cancellations. The inability to recognize a density on stereotactic images should not preclude biopsy with an alternative method if a lesion is suspected. Differentiating a lesion from a pseudolesion can be difficult, and sonography and MR imaging may provide additional information. Mammographic follow-up of suspected pseudolesions is strongly recommended to assess for interval change and the need for prompt repeat biopsy. ■

Acknowledgments: We thank M. Christina Cates, RTRM, for dedicated technical support and J. Grant Thomson, MD, for invaluable assistance.

References

1. Parker SH, Lovin JD, Jobe WE, Burke BJ, Hopper KD, Yakes WF. Nonpalpable breast lesions: stereotactic automated large-core biopsies. Radiology 1991; 180:403–407.
2. Dronkers DJ. Stereotaxic core biopsy of breast lesions. Radiology 1992; 183:631–634.
3. Elvecrog EL, Lechner MC, Nelson MT. Nonpalpable breast lesions: correlation of stereotaxic large-core needle biopsy and surgical biopsy results. Radiology 1993; 188:453–455.
4. Gisvold JJ, Goellner JR, Grant CS, et al. Breast biopsy: a comparative study of stereotaxically guided core and excisional techniques. AJR 1994: 162:815–820.
5. Parker SH, Burbank F, Jackman RJ, et al. Percutaneous large-core breast biopsy: a multi-institutional study. Radiology 1994; 193:359–364.
6. Liberman L, Dershaw D, Rosen PP, Cohen MA, Hann LE, Abramson AF. Stereotactic core biopsy of impalpable spiculated breast masses. AJR 1995; 165:551–554.
7. Mainiero MB, Philpotts LE, Lee CH, Lange RC, Carter D, Tocino I. Stereotaxic core needle biopsy of breast microcalcifications: correlation of target accuracy and diagnosis with lesion size. Radiology 1996; 198:665–669.
8. Liberman L, Dershaw DD, Rosen PP, Abramson AF, Deutch BM, Hann LE. Stereotaxic 14-gauge breast biopsy: how many core biopsy specimens are needed? Radiology 1994; 192:793–795.
9. Muller-Schimpfle M, Stoll P, Stern W, Kurz S, Dammann F, Claussen CD. Do mammography, sonography, and MR mammography have a diagnostic benefit compared with mammography and sonography? AJR 1997; 168:1323–1329.
10. Meyer JE, Sonnenfeld MR, Greenes RA, Stomper PC. Cancellation of preoperative breast localization procedures: analysis of 53 cases. Radiology 1988; 169:629–630.
11. Lee CH, Egglin TK, Philpotts LE, Mainiero MB, Tocino I. Cost-effectiveness of stereotactic core needle biopsy: analysis by means of mammographic findings. Radiology 1997; 202:849–854.
12. Parker SH, Stavros AT, Dennis MA. Needle biopsy techniques. Radiol Clin North Am 1995; 33:1171–1186.
13. Parker SH, Burbank F. A practical approach to minimally invasive breast biopsy. Radiology 1996; 200:11–20.

Susan G. Orel, MD • Carol Reynolds, MD • Mitchell D. Schnall, MD
Lawrence J. Solin, MD • Douglas L. Fraker, MD • Daniel C. Sullivan, MD

Breast Carcinoma: MR Imaging before Re-excisional Biopsy[1]

PURPOSE: To investigate the role of magnetic resonance (MR) imaging in the examination of patients after excisional biopsy of breast carcinoma before re-excision.

MATERIALS AND METHODS: Forty-seven patients underwent contrast material–enhanced MR imaging after initial excisional biopsy of breast carcinoma before further surgery.

RESULTS: The positive predictive value of MR imaging for predicting residual disease was 82%; the negative predictive value was 61%. Fourteen patients had multifocal ($n = 6$) or diffuse ($n = 8$) carcinoma. The extent of tumor was correctly identified with MR imaging alone in nine of the 14 patients, with both mammography and MR imaging in three patients, with mammography alone in one patient, and with no imaging modality in one patient. In four of the 14 patients, management was altered from re-excision to mastectomy ($n = 3$) or from breast-conservation therapy to mastectomy ($n = 1$).

CONCLUSION: MR imaging has a high positive predictive value for predicting residual tumor after excisional biopsy. The identification of mammographically and clinically unsuspected multifocal or extensive residual tumor may lend support for mastectomy rather than re-excision. However, false-negative findings due to postsurgical changes and false-positive findings due to enhancement of granulation tissue and benign breast tissue remain limitations.

When used as a diagnostic imaging tool in patients with an abnormal mammogram or palpable mass, magnetic resonance (MR) imaging has been shown to be highly sensitive in the identification of invasive breast carcinoma, with reported sensitivities of 86%–100% (1–4). Reported sensitivities of MR imaging in the identification of ductal carcinoma in situ (DCIS) have been more variable, at 40%–100% (1,5–8). In addition to depicting mammographically and clinically detected carcinoma, MR imaging can depict mammographically and clinically occult carcinoma, according to several investigators (1,4,9). On the basis of the results of these studies, it has been suggested that MR imaging could be used as an adjunctive imaging technique to identify the extent of breast carcinoma and to thereby guide treatment planning (1,9). The MR imaging detection of unsuspected multifocal carcinoma has changed treatment recommendations in some cases (9).

Reports of MR imaging–detected multifocal carcinoma have led to an increase in the requests to perform MR imaging in women after excisional biopsy of newly diagnosed breast carcinoma. In particular, this has applied to women who have not undergone MR imaging preoperatively to identify unsuspected multifocal disease. The purpose of this study was to investigate the role of MR imaging in the examination of women after excisional biopsy for breast carcinoma before further surgical intervention.

MATERIALS AND METHODS

Between June 1993 and August 1996, 47 women (age range, 29–81 years; mean age, 49 years) underwent MR imaging after excisional biopsy for breast carcinoma. All patients had positive or close surgical margins and were undergoing evaluation for possible breast-conservation therapy. Five of the 47 patients, three with DCIS at re-excision and two with false-positive MR imaging findings, have been previously reported on (8,10). Findings at presentation and mammographic findings are summarized in Tables 1 and 2. The histopathologic findings of the initial excisional biopsy specimen are summarized in Table 3. The time from excision to MR imaging was 6–40 days (mean, 18 days), and the time from MR imaging to re-excision or mastectomy was 0–28 days (mean, 8 days).

The initial excisional biopsy was performed at an outside institution in 29 patients and at the University of Pennsylvania Medical Center, Philadelphia, in 18 patients. At our institution, when a lesion is suspected to be malignant, a 1–2-cm margin of excision within the breast tissue is planned if possible. The breast tissue is generally not approximated because this will tend to distort the overlying fat and

Index terms: Breast neoplasms, diagnosis, 00.30 • Breast neoplasms, MR, 00.121412, 00.121415, 00.12143 • Breast neoplasms, postoperative, 00.30, 00.45 • Gadolinium

Abbreviations: A_z = area under the receiver operating characteristic curve, DCIS = ductal carcinoma in situ, NPV = negative predictive value, PPV = positive predictive value, ROC = receiver operating characteristic, SPGR = spoiled gradient-recalled echo.

Radiology 1997; 205:429–436

[1] From the Departments of Radiology (S.G.O., M.D.S., D.C.S.), Pathology (C.R.), Radiation Oncology (L.J.S.), and Surgery (D.L.F.), University of Pennsylvania Medical Center, 3400 Spruce St, Philadelphia, PA 19104. Received May 14, 1997; revision requested June 27; revision received July 18; accepted July 21. Supported in part by American Cancer Society grant EDT-108 and National Institutes of Health grant 1-RO1-A60190-01. **Address reprint requests to** S.G.O.

skin. This practice will leave a variably sized seroma in most cases. Clips that mark the initial surgical site or the re-excision cavity are placed at the discretion of the surgeon.

MR imaging was performed with a 1.5-T system (Signa; GE Medical Systems, Milwaukee, Wis) equipped with a prototype high-performance gradient system. All patients underwent imaging in the prone position with a specially designed compression array (11). Sagittal, T1-weighted, spin-echo (500–600/17 [repetition time msec/echo time msec]) and sagittal, fat-suppressed, T2-weighted, fast spin-echo (4,000/120 [effective]) sequences were performed with a 12–16-cm field of view, a 3-mm section thickness, a 1-mm gap, and a 256 × 256 matrix. The entire breast was then imaged before and after the bolus administration of 20 mL of gadopentetate dimeglumine (Magnevist; Schering, Berlin, Germany) with a sagittal, three-dimensional volume, fat-suppressed fast spoiled gradient-recalled-echo (SPGR) sequence (minimal repetition time/minimal echo time, 18-cm field of view, 2-mm section thickness, no gap, and a 256 × 512 matrix). Each patient received 20 mL of gadopentetate dimeglumine regardless of body weight. The gadopentetate dimeglumine was injected as a bolus followed by 20 mL of physiologic saline. Imaging was initiated during the saline injection. The three-dimensional volume, fast SPGR sequence changed with time, and the imaging time for each three-dimensional volume decreased from 3 minutes 30 seconds to 90 seconds. For the 90-second sequence, the entire breast volume was imaged four times (total of 6 minutes). Eight patients underwent MR imaging–guided wire localization. The details of this procedure have been previously described (12).

At our institution, postbiopsy mammography is recommended in patients with mammographically detected carcinomas that contain microcalcifications. Postbiopsy mammograms were obtained in 15 of the 17 patients with calcium-containing lesions. These mammograms were read by one of three dedicated mammographers (including S.G.O. and D.C.S.). Magnification images were obtained when requested by the interpreting radiologist.

The MR images were read prospectively and jointly by two radiologists (S.G.O., M.D.S.), who had knowledge of the mammographic findings, before re-excisional biopsy. The radiologist did not know whether the margins of the initial excisional biopsy specimen had been positive or close and did not know which margins were positive. The studies were reported as (*a*) positive for residual tumor, (*b*) equivocal (residual tumor vs postsurgical changes), or (*c*) negative for residual tumor. The MR images were then retrospectively reviewed to measure the thickness of the enhancing border of the seroma cavity. Because the outcome of re-excision or mastectomy was known at the time of review of the MR images, only the prospective readings were used. Evaluation of the enhancement of the biopsy cavity was qualitative. The thickness of the enhancing seroma border was noted, as was the presence of nodularity or irregularity of the border.

Table 1
Findings at Presentation

Finding	No. of Patients
Nonpalpable lesions (n = 16)	
Mammography	15
Mammography and US*	1
Palpable lesions (n = 31)	
Physical examination only	11
Mammography and physical examination	9
Mammography, physical examination, and US*	7
Physical examination and US*	4

* US = ultrasound.

Table 2
Mammographic Findings at Presentation

Finding	No. of Patients
Mass	15
Microcalcifications	12
Mass and microcalcifications	5

Table 3
Initial Histopathologic Findings

Histopathologic Finding	No. of Patients
Diagnosis	
Invasive ductal carcinoma and DCIS	15
Invasive ductal carcinoma	12
Invasive lobular carcinoma	8
DCIS	8
Tubular carcinoma	2
Medullary carcinoma	1
Papillary carcinoma	1
Initial margins	
Positive	30
Close	17

Note.—The range of the initial tumor sizes was 3–40 mm (mean, 15 mm) for all measurable lesions, 3–40 mm (mean, 18 mm) for all palpable lesions, and 3–25 mm (mean, 11 mm) for all mammographically detected lesions.

A regular, thin, enhancing rim (1–2 mm) around the seroma cavity was considered negative for residual disease (Figs 1, 2). An irregular and thicker (2–4 mm) enhancing rim was considered equivocal (residual disease vs granulation tissue) (Fig 3). A thick (>4–5 mm), nodular, and enhancing seroma cavity, enhancement of the tissue surrounding the biopsy cavity, or both were considered positive (Fig 4).

A lesion separate from the biopsy cavity was considered suspicious if it enhanced after contrast material administration and had at least partially irregular or ill-defined borders or had a linear or branching configuration suggestive of ductal enhancement. Scattered punctate (1–3 mm) foci of enhancement or patchy diffuse enhancement of fibroglandular tissue with no architectural distortion were considered benign findings. An enhancing lesion was classified as multifocal if there was intervening nonenhancing tissue between the lesion and the biopsy cavity. A lesion was considered multicentric if it was in a different quadrant than the biopsy cavity. Suspected carcinoma was classified as diffuse if the area of enhancement was extensive and distinct separate foci of enhancement were not visible.

In the pathology department, the re-excision specimen was measured and inked. The margins of the re-excision specimen were not routinely marked for orientation by the surgeon. If, however, the specimen was oriented by the surgeon, different colors of ink were used to correspond to the six margins (superior, inferior, medial, lateral, superficial, and deep). The specimen was then sectioned every 2–3 mm. The size of the biopsy cavity or any lesions identified grossly were measured. In most cases, the entire specimen was submitted for microscopic examination.

In those cases in which mastectomy was performed after excision of the primary tumor, the specimen was inked and sectioned and the biopsy cavity and any residual tumor were identified. If no tumor was grossly visible adjacent to (or within) the biopsy cavity, representative sections from the biopsy cavity were submitted for microscopic examination. A perpendicular section and a parallel section of the nipple and one to two random sections of breast tissue from the four quadrants were submitted. Any additional suspicious areas, with notation of the quadrant and the relationship to the primary tumor or the biopsy cavity, were submitted for histopathologic analysis. In those cases in which the specimen contained no discrete mass or biopsy cavity, three to four sections of breast tissue from each quadrant and all suspicious foci were submitted for examination.

For lesions that were localized with MR imaging, a diagram that delineated the relationship of the lesion to the hook wire accompanied the specimens. The area of concern was marked with ink of a different color from that used in the rest of the specimen. The specimen was then serially sectioned and submitted in its entirety for microscopic examination.

Tumors were considered histopathologically multifocal if they were distinct at gross examination or demonstrated separate microscopic foci with intervening normal breast tissue. Tumors were considered pathologically multicentric if they were in separate quadrants of the breast. Large areas of dispersed intraductal, invasive, or both intraductal and invasive carcinoma were designated as diffuse disease.

A receiver operating characteristic (ROC) analysis of the correlation between

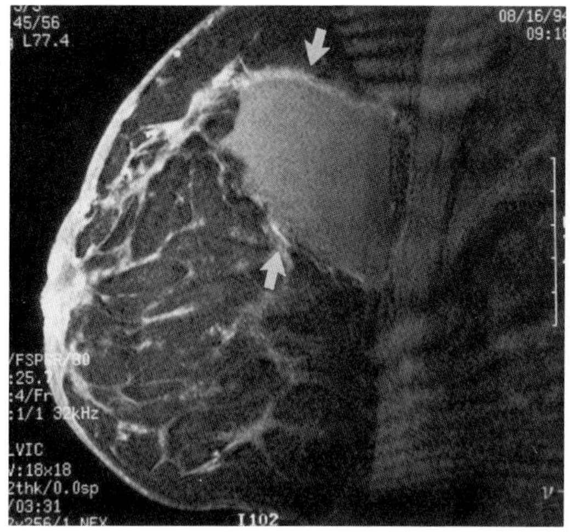

1.

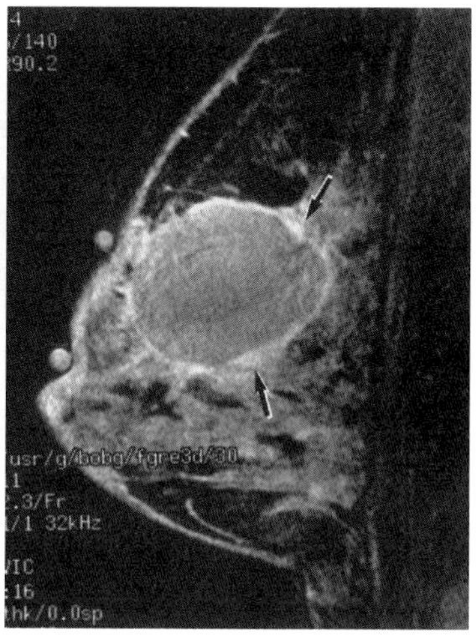

2.

Figures 1, 2. **(1)** True-negative MR imaging findings. Image obtained in a 33-year-old woman after excisional biopsy of a palpable mass that was also depicted with both mammography and US. A 3.5-cm invasive ductal carcinoma with close margins was found at excisional biopsy. Sagittal, gadolinium-enhanced, fat-suppressed, fast SPGR MR image (25.7/4) demonstrates a biopsy cavity with a thin, enhancing rim (arrows). No residual tumor was found at re-excision. **(2)** False-negative MR imaging findings. Image obtained in a 54-year-old woman after excisional biopsy of a palpable mass, which revealed a 9-mm invasive ductal carcinoma with positive margins. Sagittal, gadolinium-enhanced, fat-suppressed, fast SPGR MR image (11/2.3) demonstrates a thin, enhancing rim (arrows) that surrounds the biopsy cavity. At re-excision, focal invasive and intraductal carcinoma was found, and the margins of resection were negative. The patient underwent breast-conservation therapy.

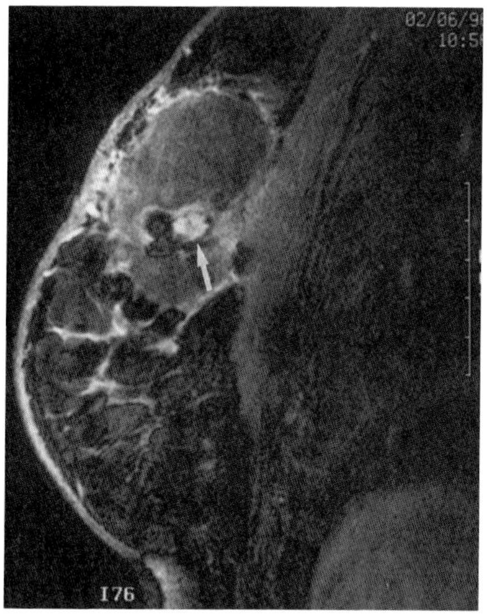

Figure 3. Equivocal MR imaging findings. Image obtained in a 55-year-old woman who had a mammographically detected 2-cm mass at presentation. Excisional biopsy revealed a 2.3-cm invasive ductal carcinoma with positive margins. Sagittal, gadolinium-enhanced, fat-suppressed, fast SPGR MR image (9.2/2.2) demonstrates a thin, enhancing rim that surrounds the biopsy cavity; however, a more focal enhancing area is identified centrally (arrow). The MR image was read as enhancing granulation tissue versus residual tumor. No residual tumor was found at re-excision.

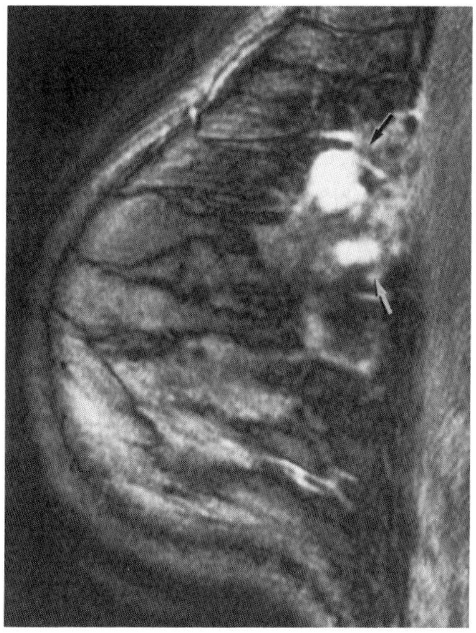

Figure 4. True-positive MR imaging findings. Image obtained in a 40-year-old woman after excisional biopsy of a 1.7-cm invasive lobular carcinoma with positive margins. Sagittal, gadolinium-enhanced, fat-suppressed, fast SPGR MR image (15/2.2) demonstrates nodular enhancing areas (arrows) in the biopsy cavity. Residual infiltrating lobular carcinoma was found at re-excision. The patient underwent breast-conservation therapy.

the MR imaging findings (positive, equivocal, or negative) and the histopathologic findings (residual tumor or no residual tumor) was performed by using the ROCFIT program (Apple Macintosh version; CE Metz, University of Chicago, 1991). Results are expressed as the area under the ROC curve (A_z). When calculating sensitivity, equivocal cases were included with the false-negative cases. When calculating specificity, equivocal cases were included with the false-positive cases.

RESULTS

Thirty patients underwent re-excision only, nine patients underwent re-excision followed by mastectomy, and eight patients underwent mastectomy only. The surgical procedures and the histopathologic results are summarized in Table 4. The correlation between MR imaging findings and histopathologic findings are summarized in Table 5.

A total of 54 "lesions" were identified on MR images in the 47 patients: 47 biopsy cavities in the 47 patients and seven additional lesions separate from the biopsy cavity in seven of the 47 patients. Twenty-eight (60%) of the 47 patients had histopathologic findings of residual tumor in the re-excision specimen, the mastectomy specimen, or both. Of the 28 patients with residual tumor, 23 patients had residual tumor at the biopsy site, three patients had residual tumor at the biopsy site and elsewhere in the breast, and two patients had no residual tumor at the biopsy site but did have tumor elsewhere in the breast.

The positive predictive value (PPV) of MR imaging for predicting residual disease in the breast was 82% (18 of 22) and the negative predictive value (NPV) was 61% (11 of 18). The MR imaging false-negative rate was 25% (seven of 28 patients) and the MR imaging false-positive rate was 21% (four of 19 patients). For predicting residual disease in the breast, the MR imaging sensitivity, specificity, and A_z were 64%, 58%, and 0.76, respectively (Table 5).

Twenty-six (55%) of the 47 patients had residual tumor at the biopsy site. The PPV for positive margins or close margins of the initial excisional biopsy specimen was 67% (20 of 30) or 35% (six of 17), respectively. The PPV of MR imaging for predicting residual tumor at the margins of resection was 78% (14 of 18). The NPV of MR imaging was 65% (13 of 20). The false-positive rate was 19% (four of 21 patients) and the false-negative rate was 27% (seven of 26 patients). For predicting residual tumor at the margins of resection, the MR imaging sensitivity, specificity, and A_z were 54%, 62%, and 0.75, respectively (Table 5).

Postbiopsy mammography was performed in 15 (88%) of the 17 patients with mammographic lesions that contained microcalcifications to rule out residual microcalcifications. The PPV for residual microcalcifications at mammography was 50% (four of eight). Of the four patients in whom postbiopsy mammography revealed residual microcalcifications and residual tumor was found at re-excision, the mammographic and MR imaging findings were concordant in two patients and discordant in two patients. In the first of the two patients with discordant findings, mammography revealed extensive residual microcalcifications and MR imaging findings were negative (Fig 5). Residual invasive and intraductal carcinoma was found at re-excision and subsequent mastectomy. In the second patient with discordant findings, postbiopsy mammography revealed only a few residual microcalcifications, while MR imaging revealed extensive contrast material enhancement both in the biopsy cavity and elsewhere in the breast. Extensive residual invasive and intraductal carcinoma was confirmed at mastectomy (Fig 6).

The NPV of the absence of microcalcifications was 29% (two of seven). In all five cases in which postbiopsy mammographic findings were false-negative, MR imaging demonstrated residual enhancing tumor (Fig 7). The histopathologic findings in these five cases were DCIS in three cases and invasive and intraductal carcinoma in two cases.

There were seven cases with false-negative MR imaging findings in the biopsy site. In six of the seven cases, residual tumor was found only in the original biopsy site (Fig 2). In three of the six cases, there was extensive residual invasive ductal carcinoma, DCIS, or both (Fig 5). In two of the six cases, there was a 1–5-mm focus of residual invasive carcinoma, and in one of the six cases, there was focal residual DCIS. In the seventh case, focal DCIS was found at the biopsy site and in one subareolar duct at mastectomy. Mastectomy was performed in four of the seven cases (re-excision before mastectomy was performed in two cases); residual DCIS was found at mastectomy in three of the four cases. Breast-conservation therapy was performed in the other three cases.

There were four false-positive MR imaging findings in the biopsy site. The histopathologic findings in these cases were atypical lobular hyperplasia, sclerosing adenosis, fat necrosis and granulation tissue (Fig 8), and fibrocystic changes. In the case of fat necrosis and granulation tissue, the time between initial excisional biopsy and MR imaging was 27 days.

There were a total of seven cases in which a suspiciously enhancing lesion outside of the biopsy site was identified with MR imaging. Histopathologic analysis showed that four lesions were malignant and three were benign. In three of the seven cases, the MR imaging–detected lesion was in the same quadrant as the original biopsy site. MR-guided localization and excisional biopsy in these three cases revealed a 10-mm invasive ductal carcinoma (Fig 7), a 4-mm DCIS, or apocrine metaplasia. In both cases in which the MR imaging–localized lesion proved to be malignant, residual tumor was also found at the biopsy site. In the remaining four cases, the MR imaging–detected lesion was in a different quadrant than the original biopsy site. MR-guided localization was performed in three of these four cases and revealed 4-mm DCIS, 10-mm DCIS, or ductal hyperplasia. In one of the two cases in which DCIS was found, the identification at MR imaging of the DCIS resulted in a change in management from breast-conservation therapy to mastectomy. In the fourth case, multiple fibroadenomas were found with no evidence of residual tumor.

In 14 (30%) of the 47 patients, either multifocal (n = 6) or diffuse (n = 8) carcinoma was found at re-excisional biopsy, mastectomy, or both. The initial method of detection in these cases was physical examination alone (n = 6), mammography and physical examination (n = 5), or mammography alone (n = 3). The tumor histopathologic findings in these cases were invasive and intraductal carcinoma (n = 6), DCIS only (n = 3), invasive lobular carcinoma (n = 2), invasive ductal carcinoma (n = 2), and tubular carcinoma (n = 1). Surgical management in these 14 patients was re-excision followed by mastectomy in seven patients, mastectomy in six patients, and re-excision alone in one patient.

Multifocal or diffuse residual tumor was correctly identified with MR imaging alone in nine (64%) of the 14 cases, with both mammography and MR imaging in three cases (21%), with mammography alone in one case (7%), and with neither modality in one case (7%) (Figs 9–12). The identification of clinically unsuspected dif-

Table 4
Findings at Re-excision and Mastectomy

Surgical Procedure	Residual Cancer	No Residual Cancer
Re-excision only (n = 30)	12	18
Re-excision and mastectomy (n = 9)	9*	0†
Mastectomy only (n = 8)	7	1
Total (N = 47)	28	19

Note.—Data are numbers of patients.
* Seven had residual cancer in mastectomy specimen.
† Two had residual cancer in mastectomy specimen.

Table 5
Correlation between MR Imaging and Histopathologic Findings

MR Imaging Finding	Residual Cancer	No Residual Cancer
Biopsy site and elsewhere in breast*		
Positive	18 (64)	4 (21)
Negative	7 (25)	11 (58)
Equivocal	3 (11)	4 (21)
Total	28 (100)	19 (100)
Biopsy site only†		
Positive	14 (54)	4 (19)
Negative	7 (27)	13 (62)
Equivocal	5 (19)	4 (19)
Total	26 (100)	21 (100)

Note.—Data are numbers of patients. Numbers in parentheses are percentages.
* A_Z = 0.76.
† A_Z = 0.75.

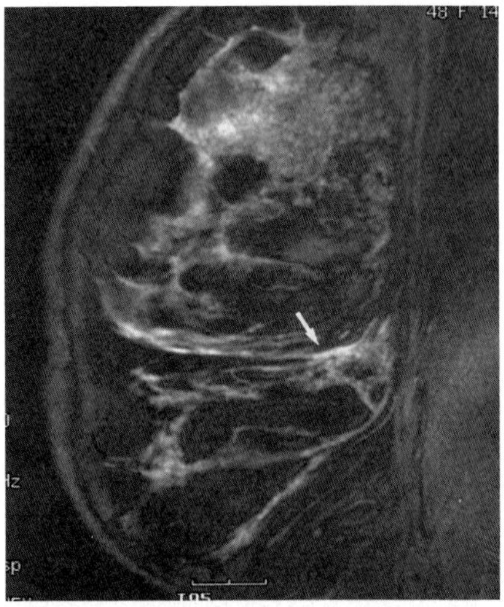

Figure 5. False-negative MR imaging findings. True-positive postbiopsy mammographic findings. Image obtained in a 48-year-old woman after excisional biopsy of mammographically detected microcalcifications, which revealed a 4-mm area of DCIS with a 2-mm area of invasive ductal carcinoma and positive margins. Postbiopsy mammogram revealed residual microcalcifications. Sagittal, gadolinium-enhanced, fat-suppressed, fast SPGR MR image (9.2/2.2) demonstrates minimal enhancement (arrow) along the border of the biopsy cavity. Residual invasive and intraductal carcinoma was found at re-excision, and residual DCIS was found at mastectomy.

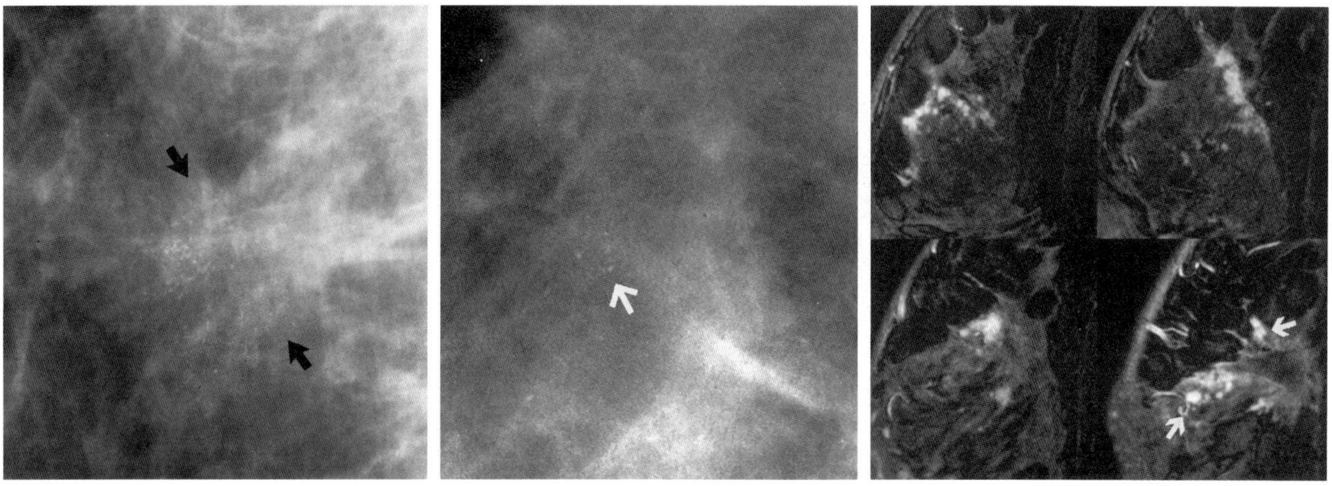

a. b. c.

Figure 6. MR imaging–detected multicentric disease. **(a)** Spot-compression magnification mammogram obtained in a 59-year-old woman with a palpable mass demonstrates a cluster of pleomorphic microcalcifications and associated architectural distortion (arrows). At excisional biopsy, a 3.5-cm invasive and intraductal carcinoma was found, and the margins were positive. **(b)** Postbiopsy mammogram reveals a few residual microcalcifications (arrow). Physical examination findings after excisional biopsy were normal. **(c)** Sagittal, gadolinium-enhanced, fat-suppressed, fast SPGR images (15/2.2) demonstrate multiple areas of enhancement both adjacent to the biopsy cavity (arrows in bottom right image) and extending several centimeters away from the biopsy site. On the basis of the MR imaging appearance, mastectomy was recommended. Extensive residual tumor that involved two quadrants of the breast was found at mastectomy.

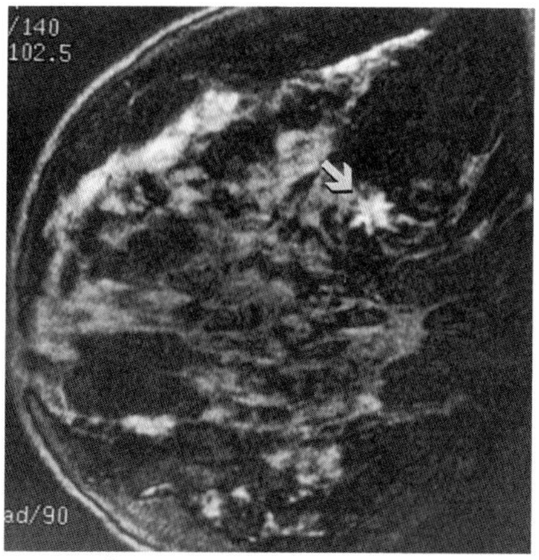

Figure 7. True-positive MR imaging findings. False-negative postbiopsy mammographic findings. Image obtained in a 44-year-old woman after excisional biopsy of a palpable lesion, which was depicted at mammography as a mass with microcalcifications. Histopathologic findings revealed a 1.4-cm invasive and intraductal cancer with positive margins. Postbiopsy mammogram revealed no residual microcalcifications. Sagittal, gadolinium-enhanced, fat-suppressed, fast SPGR MR image (15/2.2) demonstrates an enhancing 1-cm spiculated lesion (arrow), which was 2-cm superior and posterior to the biopsy cavity. MR-guided wire localization and re-excision demonstrated a 1-cm invasive ductal carcinoma, and the margins were positive. Residual tumor was found at mastectomy.

fuse residual disease with MR imaging altered management from re-excisional biopsy to mastectomy in three of the 14 cases (Figs 6, 9). In one of the 14 cases, the identification of multifocal DCIS altered management from breast-conservation therapy to mastectomy.

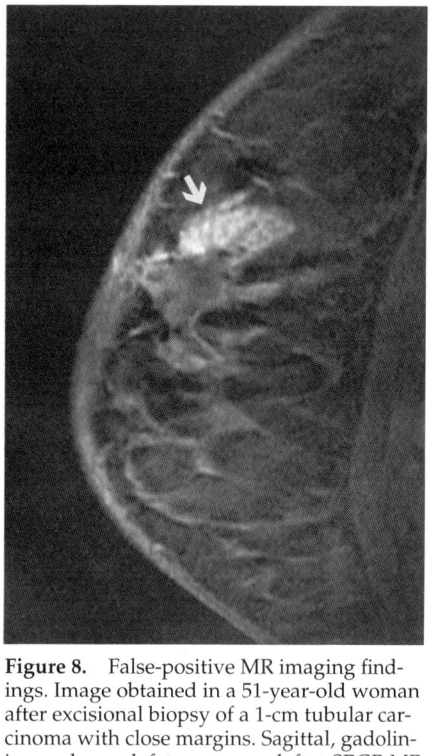

Figure 8. False-positive MR imaging findings. Image obtained in a 51-year-old woman after excisional biopsy of a 1-cm tubular carcinoma with close margins. Sagittal, gadolinium-enhanced, fat-suppressed, fast SPGR MR image (9/2.2) demonstrates enhancement along the superior aspect of the biopsy cavity (arrow). Re-excision revealed fat necrosis and granulation tissue.

DISCUSSION

After excisional biopsy of breast carcinoma, residual tumor is left in the breast in a reported 32%–63% of cases (13–17). Detecting the residual disease and determining its extent are important for further treatment planning. In patients considering breast-conservation therapy, complete removal of all gross tumor has been associated with improved local control rates (18). If there is no residual disease in the breast, further surgery would be unnecessary. If there is a small amount of residual disease, the patient might benefit from re-excision before radiation therapy. If extensive residual disease remains in the breast, then mastectomy might be the treatment of choice.

Assessment of the completeness of surgical excision, however, can be very difficult. Several factors have been associated with residual tumor in the breast after excisional biopsy; these factors include positive margins of resection, residual microcalcifications on postbiopsy mammograms, large tumors, histopathologic findings of invasive lobular carcinoma, tumors with an extensive intraductal component (or EIC), and tumors detected at physical examination (13–17). It is traditional that the two main methods of predicting the presence of residual disease after excisional biopsy are evaluating the margins of the excisional biopsy specimen for the presence of tumor and using postbiopsy mammography to identify residual microcalcifications.

Re-excision at the initial biopsy site is commonly performed when the initial margins of resection are positive or unknown. However, several investigators have observed that neither positive nor negative margins of resection are reliable indicators of the

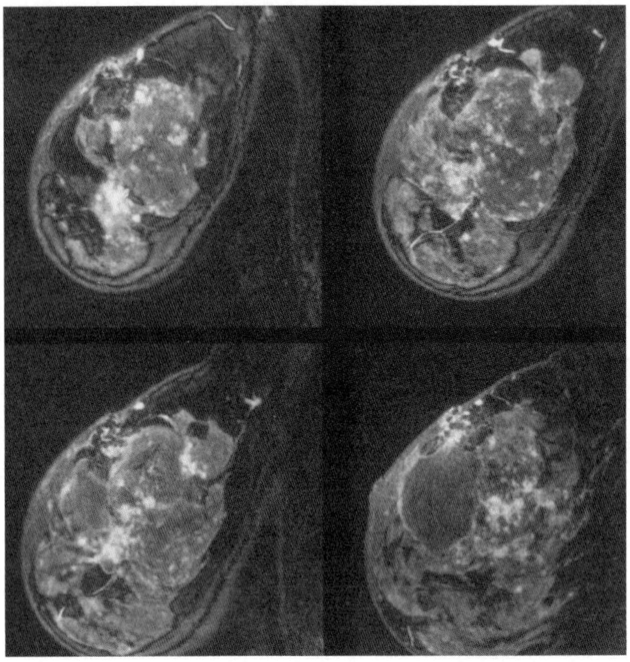

Figure 9. MR imaging–depicted residual diffuse carcinoma. Images obtained in a 49-year-old woman after excisional biopsy of a palpable mass, which revealed invasive lobular carcinoma with positive margins. Sagittal, gadolinium-enhanced, fat-suppressed, fast SPGR MR images (15/2.2) demonstrate multiple enhancing lesions, some adjacent to the biopsy cavity (bottom right image) and others at a distance from the biopsy cavity. At mastectomy, extensive residual invasive lobular carcinoma was found in all quadrants.

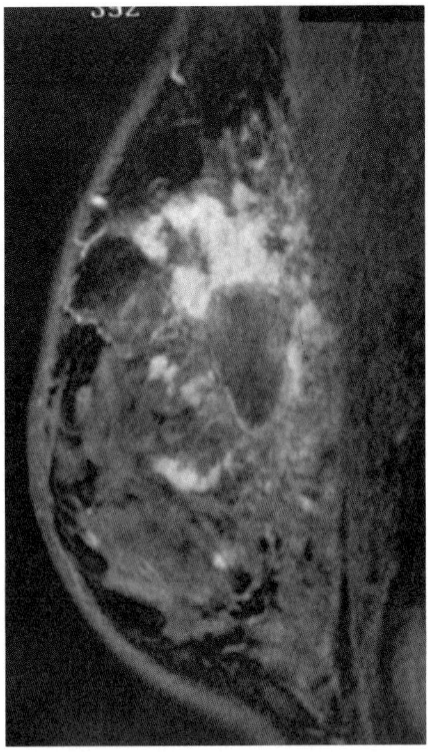

Figure 10. MR imaging–depicted residual tumor. Image obtained in a 42-year-old woman after excisional biopsy of a 2.5-cm invasive ductal carcinoma with close margins. Sagittal, gadolinium-enhanced, fat-suppressed, fast SPGR MR image (15/2.2) demonstrates multiple areas of enhancement that are most marked along the superior aspect of the biopsy cavity. Residual invasive and intraductal carcinoma was found at mastectomy.

completeness of surgical excision, probably owing to the difficulty in assessing all margins of resection (13–17,19). In cases in which the margins of the initially resected specimen are positive or unknown, reported rates of finding residual tumor are 23%–69%, with the higher rates in those cases with positive margins (13–17). In our study, we found similar rates, where the PPV of positive or of close margins of resection of the initial excisional biopsy specimen was 67% or 35%, respectively. In comparison, the PPV of MR imaging for predicting residual tumor anywhere in the breast was 82%, and that for predicting tumor at the margins of resection was 78%.

In addition to margin assessment, mammographic evaluation, specifically specimen radiography and postbiopsy mammography, has been used to identify or predict the presence of residual disease (19–22). Both mammographically visible tumor at the margins of the specimen and residual microcalcifications on postbiopsy images have a high PPV, reportedly 69%–98% (19–21). In our series, the PPV of mammography was 50%. In one of the cases in which mammography revealed residual microcalcifications, which reflected residual invasive and in situ carcinoma, MR imaging findings were false-negative. This represented the only case in this series in which the presence of residual tumor was predicted with mammography but not with MR imaging.

While specimen radiography and postbiopsy mammography have a high PPV, the NPV of the absence of tumor at the margins of a specimen or the NPV of the absence of residual microcalcifications is low, reportedly 32%–64% (19–21). In our series, the NPV of the absence of microcalcifications was 29%. In the five cases with false-negative mammographic findings, MR imaging depicted residual tumor in each case, DCIS in three cases, and invasive carcinoma in two cases. Among these five cases, mastectomy was performed in three cases and breast-conservation therapy was performed in two cases.

The low NPV of both specimen radiography and postbiopsy mammography may be the result of several factors, which include imaging the specimen in only one view, lack of routine magnification imaging, and, perhaps most important, tumor that is not radiographically visible (19–21). With its high PPV, postbiopsy mammography before re-excision is critical

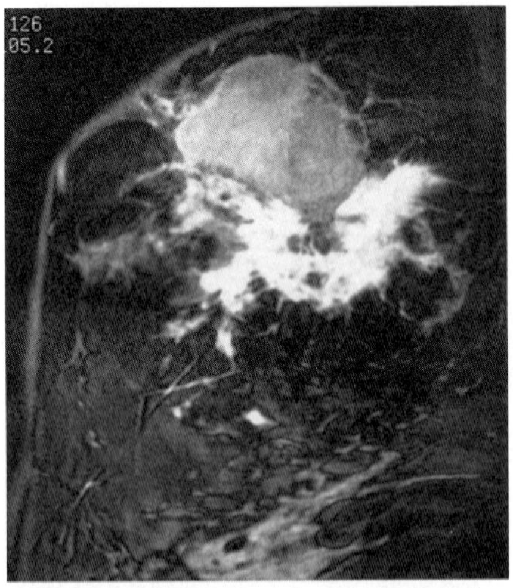

Figure 11. MR imaging–depicted residual tumor. Image obtained in a 51-year-old woman after excisional biopsy of a 3-cm invasive lobular carcinoma with positive margins. Sagittal, gadolinium-enhanced, fat-suppressed, fast SPGR MR image (15/2.2) demonstrates enhancement along the inferior aspect of the biopsy cavity. At re-excision, residual invasive lobular carcinoma was identified with positive margins. Residual invasive tumor in the biopsy cavity also was found at mastectomy.

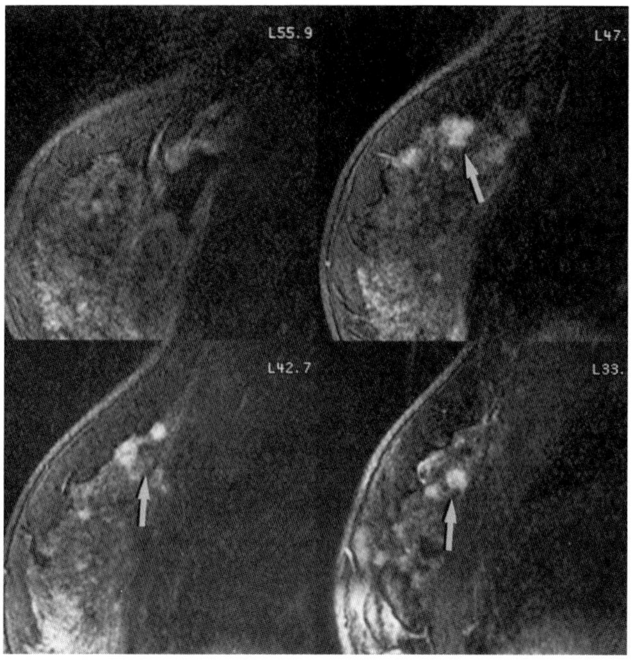

Figure 12. MR imaging–depicted extensive residual tumor. Images obtained in a 40-year-old woman who presented with a palpable mass, which was clinically thought to be benign. Three foci (9 mm each) of invasive ductal carcinoma with positive margins were identified at excisional biopsy. Sagittal, gadolinium-enhanced, fat-suppressed, fast SPGR MR images (9/2) demonstrate multiple, enhancing nodules (arrows) that extend from the medial side of the biopsy cavity in the upper outer quadrant (top left image) into the upper inner quadrant (bottom right image). At re-excision, extensive residual invasive ductal carcinoma was found with positive margins; at mastectomy, residual invasive tumor was present.

in the examination of patients with lesions that contain microcalcifications, even when the margins of resection are negative (19). However, postbiopsy mammography is limited in the assessment of the adequacy of excision of noncalcified lesions caused by postsurgical changes that include architectural distortion and hematoma and seroma formation. In addition, even in those cases in which the tumor does contain calcifications, residual tumor that is not calcified may also not be detected. In our series, there was one case in which mammography revealed a few residual microcalcifications, but MR imaging revealed extensive residual invasive carcinoma, confirmed at mastectomy, that was mammographically and clinically occult.

In contrast with mammography, MR imaging after excisional biopsy is not limited to the evaluation of lesions that contain calcifications. With its inherently high soft-tissue contrast and the intravenous administration of contrast material, MR imaging can depict mammographically visible calcified and noncalcified tumors, as well as mammographically occult tumors (1–9). In addition to the six cases described above in which MR imaging depicted residual tumor when postbiopsy mammographic findings were either negative or revealed only a few residual calcifications, there were nine cases in which MR imaging depicted residual disease that could not be predicted with mammography. In all nine cases, patients presented with a palpable abnormality; two cases were noncalcified lesions identified with mammography, and two cases were masses identified with US. Among the 18 cases in which the presence of residual tumor in the breast was correctly predicted with MR imaging, the extent of residual tumor was correctly predicted with mammography in only three cases: two cases of extensive residual microcalcifications and one case of multiple masses.

In our study, US was performed in 12 patients preoperatively but was not performed postoperatively to identify residual tumor. The role of US in preoperative carcinoma staging and, potentially, in postbiopsy evaluation has yet to be defined.

While the PPV of MR imaging was high, the NPV was lower (61%), with a 25% false-negative rate. Possible explanations for the false-negative findings include postsurgical changes, which can obscure enhancing residual tumor, and small, dispersed, or both small and dispersed foci of residual tumor, which do not demonstrate perceptible enhancement. However, the false-negative rate for MR imaging in this study is comparable to the reported false-negative rate for negative margins of resection, which was 26%–33% (13–17), and is lower than the reported false-negative rate for specimen radiography or postbiopsy mammography, which was 33%–72% (19–21). Nevertheless, owing to the high false-negative rate for MR imaging after excisional biopsy, negative MR imaging findings, like negative postbiopsy mammographic findings, cannot be used to reliably predict the removal of all tumor.

The results of our preliminary investigation into the use of MR imaging before re-excisional biopsy indicate that the PPV of MR imaging for predicting residual tumor is high, slightly higher than the PPV for positive margins and much higher than the PPV for close margins. In addition, MR imaging can depict residual tumor that is mammographically occult on preoperative, postbiopsy, or both preoperative and postbiopsy mammograms.

These results suggest that MR imaging could play a role complementary to the traditional methods of margin evaluation and mammographic imaging in assessing the adequacy of tumor removal. In patients with positive or close margins of resection, MR imaging, by indicating the presence of residual disease and defining its extent, could be used to triage patients either for re-excision or for mastectomy. If the MR imaging findings suggest the presence of a limited extent of residual tumor, this may lend support for limited re-excision.

However, a potentially more clinically important role of MR imaging would be to identify a subgroup of patients with clinically and mammographically unsuspected extensive or multifocal residual tumor who would be better served by undergoing mastectomy rather than re-excision. When extensive residual tumor is present and there are diffusely positive margins or multiple positive margins, the patient most likely is not a candidate for breast-conservation therapy, and mastectomy is recommended (13).

Little data are available on factors that correlate with final positive margins at the time of re-excision (13). In a study that evaluated factors associated with a positive finding of cancer at re-excision after excisional biopsy, Jardines and colleagues (13) reported that 9% of patients had positive margins at the time of re-excision and were considered for mastectomy. Factors associated with a final positive margin were tumors detected with physical examination, young age

(36–50 years), and histopathologic findings of invasive lobular carcinoma (13).

In our series, 14 (30%) of the 47 patients had either multifocal or diffuse carcinoma. The extent of disease was correctly identified with MR imaging alone in nine (64%) of the 14 patients. In only one patient (7%) was the extent of disease correctly identified with mammography alone. In three of the six patients who underwent mastectomy without re-excision, the MR imaging findings altered surgical treatment from re-excision to mastectomy.

The majority of patients in our series initially presented with a palpable mass. Of the 14 patients with multifocal or diffuse carcinoma, 10 patients presented with a palpable mass. The preponderance of patients who underwent re-excision who initially presented with a palpable mass has also been present in other reported series (13,14). The cause of the large number of palpable carcinomas in these series is not known; however, this could reflect a more frequent need for re-excision when a carcinoma is palpable and, often, larger than when a carcinoma is detected with screening mammography (1.8 cm vs 1.1 cm in this series). MR imaging may prove to be most valuable in those cases in which the carcinoma is palpable and not mammographically detected and may prove to have less value in those cases of screening-detected carcinomas. Continued investigation will be needed to address this issue.

It appears, on the basis of these initial results, that the identification of extensive or multifocal disease with MR imaging could be used to avoid multiple surgical procedures. However, if MR imaging is used in this capacity, the pitfall of false-positive enhancement must be addressed. While there were no false-positive findings in this group of 14 cases, there were false-positive findings in other cases in this series. Two of these cases resulted in unnecessary additional tissue removal: In the first case, a second incision was required; in the second case, mastectomy was performed when the patient may have been a candidate for breast-conservation therapy. The problem of false-positive enhancement, however, could potentially be overcome with the availability of MR imaging–compatible 14-gauge core biopsy needles so that enhancing areas could be sampled before re-excision. Such needles are now becoming available.

The patients in our study underwent initial excisional biopsy rather than core biopsy. An approach that could decrease the number of surgical procedures required for definitive treatment and, at the same time, avoid the MR imaging pitfalls of false-positive and false-negative cases caused by postsurgical change, is the use of imaging-guided core biopsy. With core biopsy, the diagnosis of carcinoma could be made without initial diagnostic excisional biopsy. After core biopsy, MR imaging could be performed to identify the extent of disease and guide surgical planning.

While the results of our study suggest a potential role for MR imaging in the detection and staging of residual tumor after excisional biopsy, MR imaging remains costly. Just as the use of MR imaging will probably not be realistic or cost-effective for staging suspected or newly diagnosed breast carcinoma in all patients, so it may not be realistic or cost-effective for identifying residual tumor after excisional biopsy in all patients. Identifying those patients at risk of clinically and mammographically unsuspected multifocal or diffuse disease that remains in the breast after excisional biopsy will have to be determined with further clinical research. In addition, cost-effectiveness studies will be required to define the cost-benefit ratio of this emerging technology as a method for detecting and staging breast carcinoma. In the case of re-excision versus mastectomy, positive MR imaging findings of extensive or multifocal tumor that result in mastectomy would be less costly and have less morbidity than multiple surgical procedures that result in mastectomy. Analyses that take many of these issues into consideration are needed. ■

Acknowledgments: We thank Harold L. Kundel, MD, for assistance with statistical analysis, Jean McDermott, RN, for coordinating the breast MR imaging project, and Norman S. Butler, RT-MR, and Tanya Kurtz, BSRT, for technical assistance.

References

1. Harms SE, Flamig DP, Hesley KL, et al. MR imaging of the breast with rotating delivery of excitation off resonance: clinical experience with pathologic correlation. Radiology 1993; 187:493–501.
2. Gilles R, Guinebretiere JM, Lucidarme O, et al. Nonpalpable breast tumors: diagnosis with contrast-enhanced subtraction dynamic MR imaging. Radiology 1994; 191:625–631.
3. Kaiser WA, Zeitler E. MR imaging of the breast: fast imaging sequences with and without Gd-DTPA. Radiology 1989; 170:681–686.
4. Heywang SH, Wolf A, Pruss E, Hilbertz T, Eiermann W, Permanetter W. MR imaging of the breast with Gd-DTPA: use and limitations. Radiology 1989; 171:95–103.
5. Gilles R, Zafrani B, Guinebretiere JM, et al. Ductal carcinoma in situ: MR imaging–histopathologic correlation. Radiology 1995; 196: 415–419.
6. Piccoli CW, Matteucci T, Outwater EK, Siegelman ES, Mitchell DG. Breast carcinoma diagnosis with MR imaging: effect of clinical and mammographic findings on recommendations for biopsy. Radiology 1995; 197(P):372.
7. Heywang-Köbrunner SH. Contrast-enhanced magnetic resonance imaging of the breast. Invest Radiol 1994; 29:94–104.
8. Orel SG, Mendonca MH, Reynolds C, Schnall MD, Solin LJ, Sullivan DC. MR imaging of ductal carcinoma in situ. Radiology 1997; 202: 413–420.
9. Orel SG, Schnall MD, Powell CM, et al. Staging of suspected breast cancer: effect of MR imaging and MR-guided biopsy. Radiology 1995; 196:115–122.
10. Orel SG, Hochman MG, Schnall MD, Reynolds C, Sullivan DC. High-resolution MR imaging of the breast: clinical context. RadioGraphics 1996; 16:1385–1401.
11. Insko EK, Schnall MD, Connick TJ, Orel SG. Multi-coil array for high resolution imaging of the breast. Magn Reson Med 1997; 37:778–786.
12. Orel SG, Schnall MD, Newman RW, Powell CM, Torosian MH, Rosato EF. MR imaging-guided localization and biopsy of breast lesions: initial experience. Radiology 1994; 193: 97–102.
13. Jardines L, Fowble B, Schultz D, et al. Factors associated with a positive reexcision after excisional biopsy for invasive breast cancer. Surgery 1995; 118:803–809.
14. Gwin JL, Eisenberg BL, Hoffman JP, Ottery FD, Boraas M, Solin LJ. Incidence of gross and microscopic carcinoma in specimens from patients with breast cancer after re-excision lumpectomy. Ann Surg 1993; 218:729–734.
15. Solin LJ, Fowble B, Martz K, Pajak TF, Goodman RL. Results of re-excisional biopsy of the primary tumor in preparation for definitive irradiation of patients with early stage breast cancer. Int J Radiat Oncol Biol Phys 1985; 12: 721–725.
16. Schnitt SJ, Connolly JL, Khettry U, et al. Pathologic findings on re-excision of the primary site in breast cancer patients considered for treatment by primary radiation therapy. Cancer 1987; 59:675–681.
17. McCormick B, Kinne D, Petrek J, et al. Limited resection for breast cancer: a study of inked specimen margins before radiotherapy. Int J Radiat Oncol Biol Phys 1987; 13:1667–1671.
18. Solin LJ, Fowble BL, Schultz DJ, Goodman RL. The significance of the pathology margins of the tumor excision on the outcome of patients treated with definitive irradiation for early stage breast cancer. Int J Radiat Oncol Biol Phys 1991; 21:279–287.
19. Lee CH, Carter D. Detecting residual tumor after excisional biopsy of impalpable breast carcinoma: efficacy of comparing preoperative mammograms with radiographs of the biopsy specimen. AJR 1995; 164:81–86.
20. Graham RA, Homer MJ, Sigler CJ, et al. The efficacy of specimen radiography in evaluating the surgical margins of impalpable breast carcinoma. AJR 1994; 162:33–36.
21. Gluck BS, Dershaw DD, Liberman L, Deutch BM. Microcalcifications on postoperative mammograms as an indicator of adequacy of tumor excision. Radiology 1993; 188:469–472.
22. Beron PJ, Horwitz EM, Martinez AA, et al. Pathologic and mammographic findings predicting the adequacy of tumor excision before breast-conserving therapy. AJR 1996; 167:1409–1414.

Elizabeth A. Morris, MD • Lawrence H. Schwartz, MD • D. David Dershaw, MD
Kimberly J. Van Zee, MD • Andrea F. Abramson, MD • Laura Liberman, MD

MR Imaging of the Breast in Patients with Occult Primary Breast Carcinoma[1]

PURPOSE: **To evaluate the utility of contrast material–enhanced magnetic resonance (MR) imaging of the breast for localization of the site of primary breast carcinoma in patients with isolated ipsilateral axillary metastasis, without other focal findings at physical examination or mammography.**

MATERIALS AND METHODS: **Twelve women with biopsy-proved metastatic adenocarcinoma to axillary lymph nodes and occult primary tumor underwent MR imaging at 1.5 T with a three-dimensional spoiled gradient-echo pulse sequence before and after administration of gadopentetate dimeglumine. Enhancing areas were correlated with histopathologic findings at mastectomy (n = 8) or breast-conserving treatment (n = 4).**

RESULTS: **In nine (75%) of the 12 patients, enhancement was seen on MR images that represented the site of the primary tumor at surgery. Eight had focal masses, and one had an area of regional enhancement. Two patients had negative MR findings, and no tumor was found at mastectomy. One patient with regional enhancement on MR images had no corresponding tumor at surgery.**

CONCLUSION: **Breast MR imaging enables identification of the site of primary tumor in most patients suspected of having occult primary breast cancer, and MR findings can influence surgical treatment.**

Occult primary breast cancer manifesting as isolated ipsilateral axillary metastases without evidence of tumor in the breast on a mammogram or at physical examination accounts for 0.3%–0.8% of operable breast carcinomas (1–6). First described by Halsted in 1907 (7), this uncommon clinical entity can be a diagnostic and therapeutic dilemma. Histopathologic assessment of the axillary nodes in these patients yields adenocarcinoma consistent with primary breast carcinoma. Other potential primary adenocarcinomas (such as thyroid, lung, gastric, pancreatic, and colon cancer) do not generally have isolated axillary metastasis as the only site of disease at presentation. It is for this reason that an extensive search for a primary tumor other than breast cancer has not been advocated (5,6). However, since the site of the primary tumor in the breast is not known, breast-conserving treatment traditionally has not been an option for these patients; therefore, treatment has been mastectomy (1). Histopathologic evaluation of mastectomy specimens in these patients has demonstrated carcinoma in two-thirds of patients. The other one-third of patients have either a different primary tumor or a small breast lesion that is not detected at histopathologic analysis (1).

Orel and colleagues (8) previously reported that breast cancers not seen on mammograms can be demonstrated on contrast material–enhanced breast magnetic resonance (MR) images. These reports and the high sensitivity for detection of breast lesions with contrast-enhanced MR imaging suggest that this modality might be useful for detecting lesions in patients with otherwise occult primary tumors. This study was undertaken to determine the clinical utility of contrast-enhanced breast MR imaging in patients with adenocarcinoma in ipsilateral axillary nodes that is suggestive of a primary carcinoma within the ipsilateral breast.

MATERIALS AND METHODS

From March 1995 to September 1996, preoperative breast MR imaging was prospectively performed at a single institution in 12 women with axillary nodal metastases consistent with breast carcinoma but without tumor evident on mammogram or at physical examination. All the women had palpable axillary adenopathy at initial presentation; biopsy was performed, and metastatic adenocarcinoma was the diagnosis. None had a history of breast cancer. The women ranged in age from 29 to 66 years (mean age, 53 years). Axillary adenopathy was left-sided in seven women and right-sided in five women. The time from initial presentation to MR imaging ranged from 2 to 48 days (mean, 21 days). Physical examination performed by a breast surgeon (including K.J.V.Z.) failed to reveal focal findings in any case. All patients underwent mammography with either a model M-III (Lorad Medical Systems, Danbury, Conn) or a model 600T or a model DMR (GE Medical Systems, Milwaukee, Wis) mammography system,

Index terms: Breast neoplasms, diagnosis, 00.32 • Breast neoplasms, localization, 00.32 • Breast neoplasms, metastases, 00.339, 997.33 • Gadolinium • Magnetic resonance (MR), utilization, 00.3247, 00.3248

Radiology 1997; 205:437–440

[1] From the Departments of Radiology (E.A.M., L.H.S., D.D.D., A.F.A., L.L.) and Surgery (K.J.V.Z.), Memorial Sloan Kettering Cancer Center, 1275 York Ave, New York, NY 10021. From the 1996 RSNA scientific assembly. Received March 4, 1997; revision requested April 30; revision received July 11; accepted July 14. **Address reprint requests to** E.A.M.

within 0–15 days (mean, 13 days) before the MR examination. All mammography examinations were performed at a facility certified by the Mammography Quality Standards Act. All mammograms were reviewed independently by a single mammographer (E.A.M.) before MR imaging to confirm that there were no suspicious findings.

MR imaging was performed with a 1.5-T commercially available system (Signa; GE Medical Systems). After we obtained informed consent, the patients underwent imaging in the prone position with use of a dedicated breast coil. Sagittal fat-suppressed volumetric spoiled gradient-echo images were obtained of the entire breast by using the following parameters: 24.6/6 (repetition time msec/echo time msec), 30° flip angle, 16-cm field of view (range, 16–20 cm), 2-mm section thickness without gap, and 256 × 192 matrix. Images were obtained before and after administration of gadopentetate dimeglumine (Magnevist; Berlex Laboratories, Wayne, NJ). Contrast material was administered by rapid bolus injection through an indwelling intravenous line without removing the patient from the magnet bore. Image acquisition started immediately after injection. Total examination acquisition time was 5–10 minutes. Subtraction images were obtained to ensure that small lesions were not missed. The unenhanced images were subtracted from the contrast-enhanced images on a pixel-by-pixel basis by using a GE Advantage Windows workstation (GE Medical Systems).

Breast MR images were interpreted before surgery by two radiologists experienced in MR imaging (E.A.M., L.H.S.). The MR images were reviewed with knowledge of the clinical history, and a consensus was reached. Enhancing lesions were categorized on the basis of lesion geometry as a focal enhancing mass or an area of regional enhancement. Regional enhancement was defined as an area of inhomogeneous enhancement without discrete borders. Focal enhancing lesions were defined as discrete lesions with border characteristics.

Because MR localization capabilities are under development at our institution, it was decided to perform ultrasound (US) of the breast in nine patients with positive MR findings. The US examination served to determine whether a lesion could be localized with US for breast-conserving surgery. The US examination was directed toward the region of abnormality noted on the MR image and was performed with a commercially available US system (Ultramark 4 Plus; Advanced Technology Laboratories, Bothell, Wash) with a 7.5-MHz linear-array transducer.

All patients underwent surgery, and the MR findings were correlated with surgical histopathologic findings. Mastectomy specimens were serially sliced into 5-mm sections. Close communication was maintained between the surgeon, pathologist, and radiologist as to the location and size of the enhancing lesions so that careful radiologic-histopathologic correlation could be made. Eight patients underwent mastectomy, and four patients underwent breast-conserving treatment. Three patients underwent preoperative US-guided needle localization, and one patient underwent wide excision (quadrentectomy) without preoperative localization.

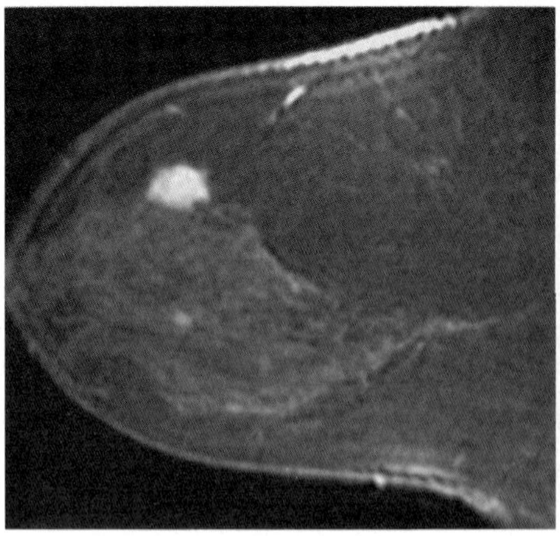

1.

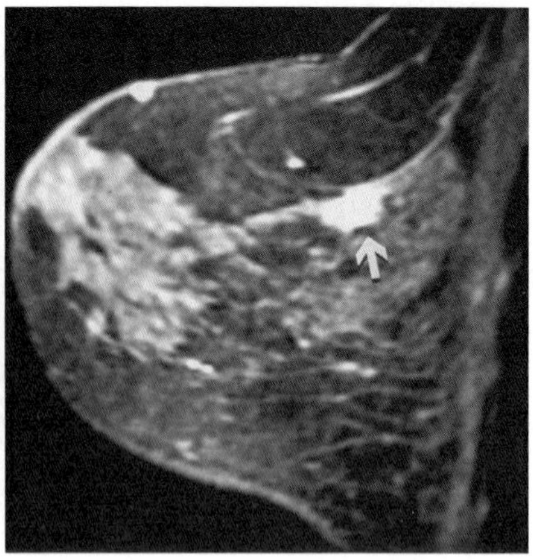

2.

Figures 1, 2. **(1)** MR image shows a focal, enhancing, irregular mass with discrete borders in a 65-year-old woman who had a negative mammogram and results of breast examination. The mass was visible on a US scan and proved to be invasive ductal carcinoma at histopathologic examination after lumpectomy. **(2)** Case of a 60-year-old woman who had a negative mammogram and results of breast examination and, at clinical presentation, had a palpable axillary node that proved to be adenocarcinoma consistent with primary breast carcinoma. MR image shows a focal irregular mass (arrow) that was subsequently identified on a US scan. The patient underwent lumpectomy, and histopathologic examination disclosed invasive ductal carcinoma.

RESULTS

Breast MR imaging enabled identification of the site of primary breast cancer in nine (75%) of the 12 women. Areas of abnormal enhancement were identified in ten women (83%), and no enhancement was identified in two women (17%). One woman with abnormal enhancement had no cancer discovered at surgery. The two women whose breast MR images demonstrated no enhancement underwent mastectomy, and histopathologic examination failed to discover tumor in the breast.

Of the 10 women with abnormal MR examinations, seven patients had a single enhancing discrete mass (Figs 1, 2); one patient had two separate, adjacent, enhancing masses (Fig 3); and two patients had areas of regional enhancement (Fig 4).

The borders of the masses were indistinct in six patients and spiculated in three patients. The sizes of the masses ranged from 9 to 20 mm (mean, 13 mm). All masses demonstrated homogeneous enhancement. All lesions were readily identified on contrast-enhanced MR images. No additional enhancing lesions were found on subtraction images that were not identified on contrast-enhanced MR images.

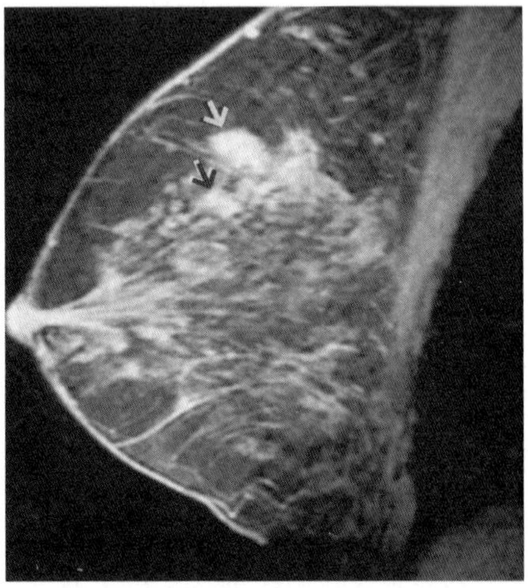

Figure 3. MR image shows two separate, adjacent, enhancing masses (arrows) in a 55-year-old woman. Both of these masses were visualized on a US scan. Preoperative US-guided core biopsy or needle localization was offered to the patient, who preferred to undergo mastectomy. Histopathologic examination yielded ductal carcinoma in situ, without evidence of invasion, and fibroadenoma (white arrow).

Among the eight women in whom enhancing masses consistent with primary carcinoma were identified, mastectomy was performed in five and breast-conserving therapy was performed in three. Histopathologic diagnosis revealed infiltrating ductal carcinoma in six patients and infiltrating lobular carcinoma in one patient. The single patient with two adjacent but separate enhancing lesions underwent mastectomy; histopathologic examination disclosed a 1.5-cm focus of ductal carcinoma in situ, solid and cribriform

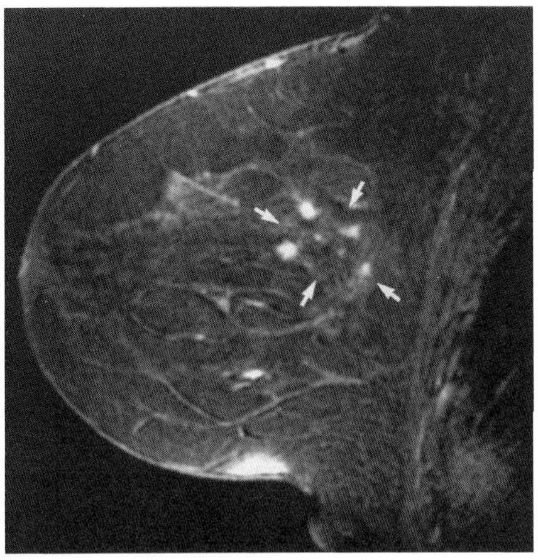

Figure 4. MR image shows regional enhancement (arrows) without discrete borders in a 55-year-old woman who refused mastectomy. The enhancement pattern was stippled and proved to represent fibrous mammary tissue at histopathologic examination after quadrantectomy, resulting in a single false-positive case.

type, without evidence of invasion, and a fibroadenoma.

Isolated areas of regional enhancement encompassing 11 and 25 mm, respectively, were noted in two patients. The patient with the larger area of regional enhancement underwent quadrentectomy, with no tumor found at histopathologic assessment. The patient with the smaller area of regional enhancement underwent mastectomy, and a 4-mm focus of invasive ductal carcinoma was found within the area of regional enhancement.

US examination of the breast in nine of the 10 patients with enhancing lesions was negative in three, including both women with areas of regional enhancement. In the other six patients, including the patient with two lesions, US enabled identification of solid masses that correlated with the MR findings. Three women elected to undergo lumpectomy with preoperative US-guided needle localization, and the other three women (including the woman with two lesions) chose to undergo mastectomy. The lesions removed with US-guided needle localization all proved to correspond to the site of primary tumor at surgery.

DISCUSSION

Although breast MR imaging has been shown to be sensitive in the detection of cancer, in the range of 86%–100%, the specificity for cancer is lower and more variable, in the range of 37%–97% (9–15). Because of both the low specificity and the costs of breast MR imaging, it is not applicable for evaluation of the breast in all patients. In certain specific subsets of patients, however, such as those with occult primary breast cancer, it is advantageous to have a test that is highly sensitive. A lower specificity may be acceptable when searching for a breast carcinoma that has evaded detection with conventional diagnostic means. Because occult primary breast cancer is a rare clinical event, reported series have been small. Harms and Flamig (16) and Davis et al (17) previously reported individual cases in which MR has proved valuable at identifying the primary site. Beatty and colleagues (18) confirmed the utility of breast MR imaging in 20 patients with positive axillary adenopathy and negative mammograms and physical examinations at four different centers. Porter et al (19) reported on the efficacy of varying breast MR imaging parameters at a single institution in six patients with occult primary breast cancer. To our knowledge, there has been no assessment of the utility of breast MR imaging in these patients at a single institution by using a uniform imaging protocol.

Treatment of occult breast cancer remains controversial. Overall survival is similar to that of other stage II breast cancers. Recent trials have shown equal survival after mastectomy or local radiation treatment; however, recurrence is higher in the irradiated group (20,21). Mastectomy remains the traditional treatment for best local control, and for this reason is still recommended in most cases. MR imaging can be important in these patients because identification of the primary tumor allows breast conservation to be offered in selected cases. In this study, breast conservation was offered to patients if the lesion was solitary and well visualized on US scans. In only one patient were multiple enhancing lesions found, and this patient underwent mastectomy. Previous authors have reported unsuspected multifocal disease in 34%–37% of patients whose disease was being staged with MR imaging before surgery (11,22). This was not the case among our patients, possibly related to the biologic difference of occult primary breast carcinoma or the small number of patients in the series.

Morphologic features of occult primary breast carcinomas resembled those of cancers previously described on MR images (15). An enhancing spiculated or irregular mass proved to correspond to the site of cancer in all patients except for one patient who demonstrated a small solitary area of stippled enhancement. Stippled regional enhancement may not correspond to the site of primary tumor and may be a cause of false-positive examinations. The one false-positive case occurred in a patient with stippled regional enhancement that was subtle and equivocal at interpretation. At histopathologic examination, this area represented fibrocystic changes.

In this series, two patients with no abnormal areas of enhancement on the MR images had no identifiable tumor at mastectomy. Despite the fact that histopathologic analysis fails to reveal the primary site, these patients are nevertheless considered to have breast cancer and are treated as such. In neither of the two patients with negative MR examinations was the opposite breast studied. No false-negative cases were identified. These results, however, should be interpreted cautiously, as previous authors have shown that false-negative examinations can occur with lobular carcinoma, tubular carcinoma, mucinous carcinoma, and ductal carcinoma in situ (23). As the actual false-negative rate of MR imaging is unknown, it is uncertain on the basis of this small series how patients with negative MR examinations should be treated. In the absence of identifiable tumor on MR images, breast conservation is not an option. It is uncertain, however, if these patients should undergo mastectomy. This question will need to be addressed with future studies.

Once the primary tumor site is identified, breast conservation may be offered to a select group of patients, depending on the localizing capabilities at the institution. At the time of this writing, localization with MR imaging was not available at our institution. Among our patients, we found that US was useful in preoperative localization of lesions that were sonographically visible. Unfortunately, not all lesions could be identified with US in this study. Many of the lesions detected on US scans were subtle and probably would not have been detected without the MR finding directing the radiologist to a specific region of the breast. Two patients in this study who had sonographically visible cancers after MR imaging had already undergone negative sonographic evaluation of the breast before referral to our institution. This emphasizes the operator variability of US and the need for a directed US examination. Ideally, a lesion identified on MR images should be localized with

MR imaging. Currently, however, such technology is not widely available on all systems. Until MR localization devices become more ubiquitous, directed breast US after the MR examination may be helpful in this group of patients.

MR imaging did not depict occult primary tumors in all women in this series, indicating either that the primary tumor was not in the breast or was not detectable with MR imaging. However, the results of this study demonstrate that breast MR imaging enables localization of the site of primary cancer with high sensitivity in patients with occult neoplasms. In this group of patients, breast MR imaging was found to be of value and may be worthwhile as a routine test in those women in whom the primary cancer site cannot be identified on the mammogram and at physical examination. This may allow breast conservation to be offered to the patient, instead of mastectomy. ■

Acknowledgments: We thank Richard Fischer, RMRIT, and Charles Gregory Nyman, RMRIT, for imaging; Nearlene Dillon for scheduling; and Susan M. Curley-Kikoler for manuscript preparation.

References

1. Fourquet A, De la Rochefordiere A, Campana F. Occult primary cancer with axillary metastases. In: Harris JR, Hellman S, Henderson CI, et al, eds. Breast diseases. 3rd ed. Philadelphia, Pa: Lippincott, 199: 892–896.
2. Baron PL, Moore MP, Kinne DW, et al. Occult breast cancer presenting with axillary metastases: updated management. Arch Surg 1990; 125:210–215.
3. Owen HW, Dockerty MB, Gray HK. Occult carcinoma of the breast. Surg Gynecol Obstet 1954; 98:302–308.
4. Rosen PP. Axillary lymph node metastases in patients with occult noninvasive breast carcinoma. Cancer 1980; 46:1298–1306.
5. Copeland EM, McBride CM. Axillary metastases from unknown primary sites. Ann Surg 1973; 178:25–27.
6. Patel J, Nemoto T, Rosner D, et al. Axillary lymph node metastasis from an occult breast cancer. Cancer 1981; 47:2923–2927.
7. Halsted W. The results of radical operations for the cure of carcinoma of the breast. Ann Surg 1907; 46:1–19.
8. Orel SG, Hochman MG, Schnall MD, Reynolds C, Sullivan DC. High-resolution MR imaging of the breast: clinical context. RadioGraphics 1996; 16:1385–1401.
9. Stomper PC, Herman S, Klippenstein DL, et al. Suspect breast lesions: findings at dynamic gadolinium-enhanced MR imaging correlated with mammographic and pathologic features. Radiology 1995; 197: 387–395.
10. Hulka CA, Smith BL, Sgroi DC, et al. Benign and malignant breast lesions: differentiation with echo-planar MR imaging. Radiology 1995; 197:33–38.
11. Harms SE, Flamig DP, Hesley KL, et al. MR imaging of the breast with rotating delivery of excitation off resonance: clinical experience with pathologic correlation. Radiology 1993; 187:493–501.
12. Gilles R, Guinebretiere JM, Lucidarme O, et al. Nonpalpable breast tumors: diagnosis with contrast-enhanced subtraction dynamic MR imaging. Radiology 1994; 191: 625–631.
13. Kaiser WA, Zeitler E. MR imaging of the breast: fast imaging sequences with and without Gd-DTPA—preliminary observations. Radiology 1989; 170:681–686.
14. Heywang SH, Wolf A, Pruss E, Hilbertz T, Eiermann W, Permanetter W. MR imaging of the breast with Gd-DTPA: use and limitations. Radiology 1989; 171:95–103.
15. Orel SG, Schnall MD, LiVolsi VA, Troupin RH. Suspicious breast lesions: MR imaging with radiologic-pathologic correlation. Radiology 1994; 190:485–493.
16. Harms SE, Flamig DP. Staging of breast cancer with MR imaging. Magn Reson Imaging Clin N Amer 1994; 2:573–584.
17. Davis PL, Julian TB, Staiger M, et al. Magnetic resonance imaging detection and wire localization of an "occult" breast cancer. Br Cancer Res Treat 1994; 32:327–330.
18. Beatty SM, Orel SG, Schnall MD, Weinreb JC, Harms SE, Stomper PC. MR imaging detection of occult breast carcinoma manifesting as axillary metastases (abstr). Radiology 1996; 201(P):129.
19. Porter BA, Smith JP, Borrow JW. MR depiction of occult breast cancer in patients with malignant axillary adenopathy (abstr). Radiology 1995; 197(P):130.
20. Fortunato L, Sorrento JJ, Golub RA, Cantu R. Occult breast cancer. NY State J Med 1992; 92:555–557.
21. Knapper WH. Management of occult breast cancer presenting as an axillary metastasis. Semin Surg Oncol 1991; 7:311–313.
22. Orel SG, Schnall MD, Powell CM, et al. Staging of suspected breast cancer: effect of MR imaging and MR-guided biopsy. Radiology 1995; 196:115–122.
23. Orel SG, Mendonca MH, Reynolds C, Schnall MD, Solin LJ, Sullivan DC. MR imaging of ductal carcinoma in situ. Radiology 1997; 202:413–420.

Nicholas A. Hanchak, MD • Howard B. Kessler, MD • Shawn MacPherson
Sherry Xuan, MS • Lawrence J. Solin, MD

Screening Mammography: Experience in a Health Maintenance Organization[1]

PURPOSE: **To evaluate (*a*) the relationship between mammogram interpretation and diagnosis of new breast cancer and (*b*) interprovider variation in mammogram interpretation.**

MATERIALS AND METHODS: **Interpretations of screening mammograms (133,668 mammograms in 114,899 women) acquired during 21 months in a large health maintenance organization were categorized (categories 1–5) with use of a standard format. During 1 year after mammography, new breast cancer was identified with use of claims data. Interprovider variation in the categories read was evaluated, and percentages of these categories were correlated with breast cancer detection.**

RESULTS: **Over the 21 months, 1,018 mammograms were followed by a diagnosis of new breast cancer. The category of mammogram interpretation was strongly associated with the diagnosis of new breast cancer; in 47.5% cases of category 5 mammograms, breast cancer was diagnosed. There was substantial interprovider variation in the percentages of category 3, 4, or 5 mammograms read. The percentage of category 4 and 5 mammograms read correlated inversely with the likelihood of cancer detection (Pearson correlation coefficient [*r*] = −.4778 after log-log transformation, *P* < .001).**

CONCLUSION: **A strong correlation existed between a mammographic abnormality suggestive of cancer and its detection; however, substantial interprovider variation in the reading of category 3, 4, and 5 mammograms and their positive predictive values existed. Reduction of interprovider variation should improve quality of care because the number of false-negative and false-positive mammograms should decrease.**

For women over 50 years of age, compelling evidence supports the use of screening mammography as part of a comprehensive program to reduce mortality of breast cancer (1–6). Despite multiple studies that document the benefits of mammography, the characteristics of mammography in different subsets of patients and the quality of interpretations by individual radiologists are less well understood. Many women do not undergo regular screening mammography (7). Yet, various outreach programs of health maintenance organizations (HMOs) have shown an improvement in screening rates by the independent providers in their networks (8). These outreach programs have resulted in cancers being diagnosed at lower stages (9,10) and the increased use of breast-conserving therapy (11). Although the benefits of screening mammography are persuasive, the procedure is not without its costs. These costs are, in particular, the related emotional, medical, and economic costs that result from (*a*) false-positive and false-negative mammogram interpretations, (*b*) surgery, (*c*) protracted follow-up for equivocal studies, including sonography and diagnostic mammograms, and (*d*) hidden costs related to missed work, anxiety, and the uncertainty surrounding the diagnosis of in situ carcinoma (12,13).

HMOs provide a unique opportunity to study the effects of screening mammography. The strengths of the HMO setting include (*a*) a large, defined-member population base, (*b*) a group of participating providers who follow the same administrative and data-reporting procedures, (*c*) a high rate of screening examinations because of various outreach programs, and (*d*) a large, administrative set of data that can be used to evaluate the effectiveness of screening mammography.

The goals of population-based breast cancer detection programs are to (*a*) reach out to members and encourage screening, (*b*) offer incentives to providers for improving compliance with screening, and (*c*) measure and improve the cognitive and technical aspects of performance so that the accuracy of radiologists' readings of mammograms is enhanced (14).

Although breast cancer detection is optimized with use of the triad of mammography, breast examination by a trained medical practitioner, and breast self-examination, small clinically occult breast cancers can be identified only with screening mammography. Some limitations of screening mammography include the following (15): (*a*) Radiologists show varying levels of interpretive expertise. (*b*) Expertise is often a function of the volume of studies interpreted. (*c*) There is considerable variation among radiologists about what constitutes a normal or abnormal study. (*d*) A threshold

Index terms: Breast neoplasms, diagnosis, 00.32 • Breast radiography, utilization, 00.11 • Diagnostic radiology, observer performance

Abbreviation: HMO = health maintenance organization.

Radiology 1997; 205:441–445

[1] From Aetna U.S. Healthcare, U.S. Quality Algorithms, 980 Jolly Rd, PO Box 1210, Blue Bell, PA 19422 (N.A.H., S.M., S.X.); the Department of Breast Imaging, Fox Chase Cancer Center, Philadelphia, Pa (H.B.K.); and the Department of Radiation Oncology, University of Pennsylvania School of Medicine, Philadelphia (L.J.S.). Received March 11, 1997; revision requested April 14; revision received July 10; accepted July 14. **Address reprint requests to** N.A.H.

that is too low for defining an abnormal study may lead to increased emotional and medical costs because false-positive interpretations will trigger the request for additional diagnostic studies and biopsies. (*e*) Failure to perceive an abnormality or ascribe importance to a finding (ie, a false-negative study) may result in breast cancer being missed at an early and treatable stage.

There are economic and legal implications of improperly interpreted studies. Missed abnormalities on mammograms are cited frequently as the most common cause of litigation when a diagnosis of cancer has been allegedly delayed (16). The costs of additional studies can be considerable for the provider of the radiologic study. Extra studies exact a toll on patients as well. Radiologists use varying thresholds when they interpret mammograms because they do not want to miss a cancer. Unnecessary examination (because of false-positive readings) creates emotional hardship, necessitates other needless tests and surgery, and can lower a woman's confidence in the medical-delivery system. In this system, variation in radiologists' performances leads to variable quality of care and potentially increased costs.

We evaluated the characteristics of standardized interpretive formats that are similar to the breast imaging reporting and data system, or BIRADS, format of the American College of Radiology (17). This format is used to classify mammographic findings—specifically, normal findings versus those suspected to indicate disease.

With use of a population-based breast cancer screening program of a large, independent-practice (direct-contract) HMO, we attempted to determine the characteristics of standardized, categorical interpretations when new breast cancers are detected in the aggregate HMO population and assess the performance of individual radiologic practices when the various formats are used. Correlations among individual radiologic practices regarding the interpreted categories and the detection of breast cancer were also assessed.

Interpretation Categories and U.S. Healthcare Mammography Study Results

Category	Interpretation	Distribution*
1	Negative. No radiographic evidence of malignancy and/or no change in interpretation of previous study.	73.8
2	Benign finding. No calcifications, benign mass, or benign architectural distortion.	15.4
3	Probably benign finding. Short-interval follow-up is suggested with magnified and/or additional views, repeat mammography in 6 months, or ultrasound examination and/or cytologic examination of aspirated fluid.	8.7
4	Suspected abnormality. Biopsy should be considered.	1.6
5	Probable malignancy. Biopsy is necessary.	0.3

* Numbers are percentages of total mammograms (n = 133,668).

MATERIALS AND METHODS

Setting

U.S. Healthcare is a large, independent-practice HMO operating in 13 eastern states and the District of Columbia. The number of members during the study period was in excess of 2 million. U.S. Healthcare has capitation agreements with most of its participating primary-care physicians and radiologists.

Screening-Mammography Program

U.S. Healthcare initiated its U.S. Healthcare Check breast cancer screening program in April 1987. The program has several components: Women receive a breast cancer risk-assessment survey and educational brochure when they are 40 years of age (or at the time of joining U.S. Healthcare if they are 40 years or older). If a family history or other factors indicate a high risk of breast cancer, these women receive an annual direct referral and a reminder to undergo mammography. Women with a normal risk receive a biennial direct referral until 50 years of age, after which time they receive an annual reminder and referral to undergo mammography. Repeat reminder notices are sent to noncompliant members. The screening component of the program is supplemented with physician-directed programs in which breast self-examination is taught and educational information about the benefits of early breast cancer detection is provided. Physician-education programs are established to persuade physicians to encourage breast cancer screening among female patients, participate in clinical breast-examination courses taught by trained medical personnel, and overcome physician-related barriers to screening mammography (Fig 1) (18).

All participating radiologists are required to submit results of mammographic studies on a standardized form with identifying member information and the category of the reading. This form is submitted to U.S. Healthcare, and the information is entered into a database. Compliance with this approach was approximately 90%, and radiologists and primary-care physicians receive feedback on their performances.

- Fully covered mammographic screening for all age-eligible members.
- Risk assessment of all members of U. S. Healthcare who are women aged 40–49 years.
- Certification program (with ACR accreditation and FDA certification) for participating radiologists to perform mammography.
- Educational material for members.
- Educational materials and a continuing education course developed jointly with Fox Chase Cancer Center for U.S. Healthcare primary-care physicians.
- Instructional course for physicians on clinical breast examination with use of silicone breast models.
- Follow-up of patients with abnormal mammograms.
- Prompt notification of mammographic results to physicians and participants.

Figure 1. Components of the U.S. Healthcare Check breast cancer screening program. ACR = American College of Radiology, FDA = U.S. Food and Drug Administration.

Study Design

The mammograms of 114,899 women who participated in this screening study between April 1, 1993, and December 31, 1994, were evaluated. The mean age of the women was 52.6 years. Among the subjects, 7,000 (6%) were younger than 40 years of age.

Information in the database about each woman was analyzed for 1 year after mammography to determine if a new diagnosis of breast cancer was made with use of a published, claims-based breast cancer algorithm (19). This algorithm (with use of the U.S. Healthcare claims and encounter databases and combinations of *International Classification of Diseases*-9, or ICD-9, diagnosis codes [20] and *Current Procedural Terminology*-4, or CPT-4, procedure codes [21]) was used to identify patients with common clinical presentations of breast cancer. This algorithm, shown in the Appendix, has a positive predictive value of 88% (19). In a more recent analysis of only women 65 years or older during 1993–1994, this algorithm had a positive predictive value of 83% (22).

A diagnosis of new breast cancer and its association with a category of mammogram interpretation were evaluated at the level of the aggregate health plan and that of the individual radiologic practice. During the reporting period, the total number of mammograms acquired by individual radiologic practices in U.S. Healthcare was calculated. Variation among providers in the percentages of interpreted categories was evaluated. These percentages were correlated to the detection of breast cancer.

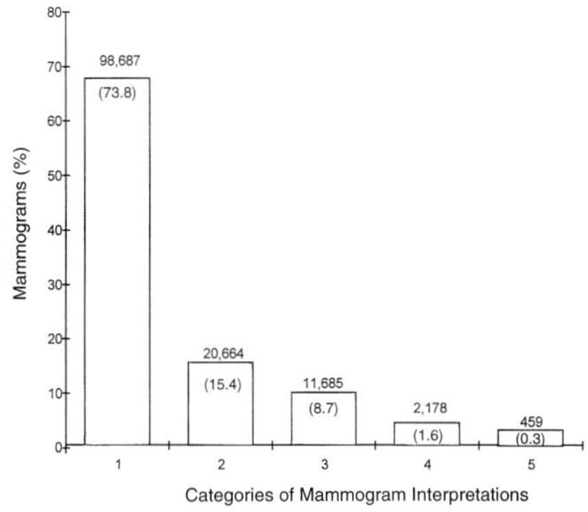

Figure 2. Percentages of mammograms in categories 1–5. Numbers above bars are total mammograms in that category. Numbers in parentheses are percentages of total mammograms obtained (n = 133,668).

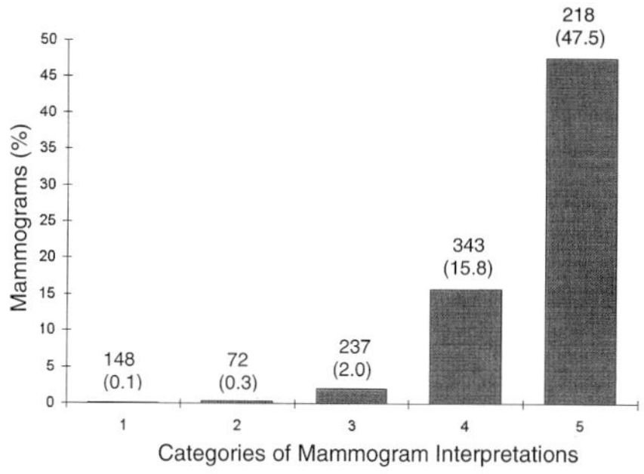

Figure 3. Percentages of mammograms in each category that subsequently led to a diagnosis of breast cancer within 1 year of mammography. Numbers above bars are numbers of mammograms. Numbers in parentheses are percentages of total mammograms in each category (Fig 2).

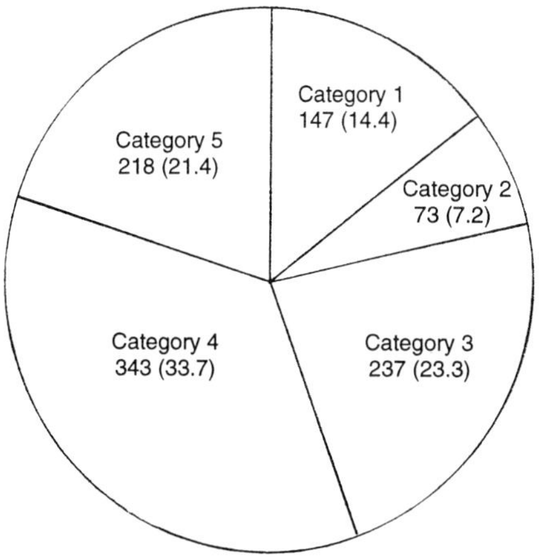

Figure 4. Distribution of identified breast cancers according to interpretation category. Numbers are numbers of breast cancers. Numbers in parentheses are percentages of total number of breast cancers (n = 1,018).

Statistical Analysis

The predictive value of the categorical reading for the diagnosis of new breast cancer was determined with a maximum likelihood analysis of variance. A correlation analysis with use of Pearson correla-

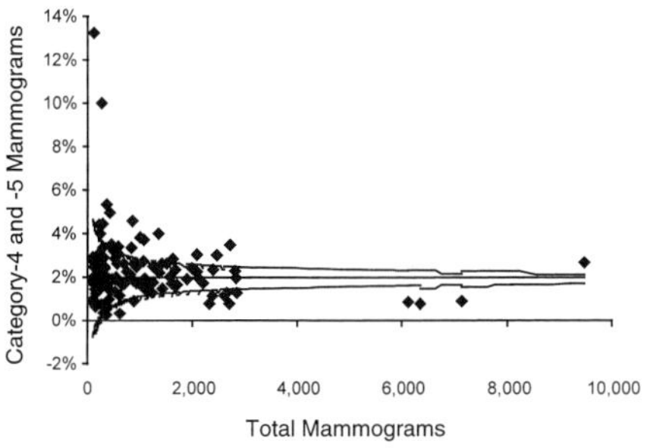

Figure 5. Graph shows the relationship between the total number of mammograms obtained for each participating radiology practice ◆ and the percentage of category 4 and 5 interpretations.

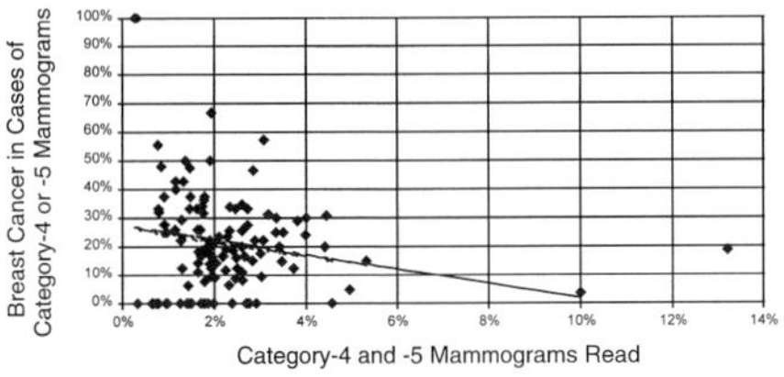

Figure 6. Graph shows the relationship between the percentage of mammograms read as category 4 or 5 and the percentage of women with category 4 or 5 mammograms in whom breast cancer was diagnosed (◆).

tion coefficients and the claims-based algorithm was used to determine the linear relationship between the percentage of category 4 and 5 interpretations and the likelihood of detecting a new case of breast cancer.

RESULTS

Predictive Properties of the Category of Mammogram Interpretation

Interpretations are shown in the Table and Figure 2. A total of 114,899 women underwent 133,668 mammographic examinations during the 21-month study period. The readings of 98,687 (73.8%) mammograms were normal (category 1 of the American College of Radiology). The interpreted categories of the other mammograms were the following: 20,664 (15.4%), category 2; 11,685 (8.7%), category 3; 2,178 (1.6%), category 4; and 459 (0.3%), category 5.

Figure 3 shows the percentages of interpreted categories in patients who were diagnosed with breast cancer during the 12 months after mammography. The likelihood of a diagnosis of breast cancer depended on the interpreted category. Women with a category 4 or 5 mammogram were more likely to be diagnosed with breast cancer than those with a category 1 or 2 mammogram ($P < .001$). The percentages of interpreted categories ranged from 0.1% (n = 148) (category 1) to 47.5% (n = 218) (category 5). In 84.2% and 52.5% cases of category 4 and 5 mammograms, respectively, breast cancer was *not* diagnosed.

For category 4 and 5 interpretations, there was a high correlation with the subsequent diagnosis of breast cancer. However, breast cancers were diagnosed in women with normal (category 1 and 2) mammograms and in those with probably benign findings (category 3 mammograms). Figure 4 shows the distribution of breast cancers by means of the interpreted categories. The number of breast cancers (n = 457) diagnosed in women with category 1, 2, and 3 mammograms was nearly equal to the number (n = 561) in women with category 4 and 5 mammograms.

Variation among Radiologic Practices in Mammogram Interpretations

The total number of mammographic studies performed by each participating radiologic practice was calculated. Figure 5 shows the variation in the percentage of category 4 and 5 mammograms as a function of the total number of mammographic studies performed.

The relationship between the percentage of category 4 and 5 mammograms and their positive predictive values are shown in Figure 6. The percentage of category 4 and 5 readings correlated negatively with the likelihood of breast cancer diagnosis (Pearson correlation coefficient [r] = −.4778 after the log-log transformation, $P < .001$). In other words, the more mammograms a radiologist read as category 4 or 5, the less likely cancer was diagnosed in those patients.

DISCUSSION

To understand fully the value of screening mammography and identify opportunities for improvement in quality of care, we (*a*) evaluated (with use of a claims-based algorithm) all breast cancers diagnosed, (*b*) assessed how the interpreted category aided the stratification of risk for breast cancer, and (*c*) examined differences in the quality of providers by analyzing variations in the frequencies and accuracies of their readings. Our study supports the value of categorical mammographic readings for identifying breast cancers; however, we also showed that 44.9% (n = 457) of breast cancers were identified in women without obvious signs of malignancy on the initial screening study (category 1, 2, and 3 mammograms).

We also demonstrated differences in the quality of interpretations of individual radiologic practices; there was a wide variation in the percentages of mammograms read as category 4 or 5. The variation among providers in the percentages of category 4 and 5 mammograms may have occurred for several reasons. These reasons can be classified broadly as differences in the referred patient population or differences in the thresholds providers used to identify an abnormality suggestive of malignancy. The variation among providers is not entirely explained with differences in the referred population because there was a strong inverse relationship between the percentage of mammograms read as category 4 or 5 and the likelihood of breast cancer being diagnosed. The interprovider variation was likely related to two different aspects, namely technical and cognitive aspects, of the quality of care provided. Technical performance can be described as the attributes of tests and procedures—such as proper positioning of the breast on the machine and the quality of the mammogram image—that maximize the likelihood of accurate diagnosis. Cognitive performance refers to the aspects of interpretation (such as accuracy) that influence treatment decisions. In our study, we were not able to distinguish between technical and cognitive aspects.

Many implications can be made about the variation of mammogram readings among radiologists. In terms of outcomes of care, underdiagnosis and missed identification of breast cancer at a potentially more treatable stage are costly. A large number of false-positive readings, however, cause (*a*) added emotional suffering as women await definitive work-up and its results, (*b*) greater economic costs because of repeated mammography and possible surgery with its complications, and (*c*) lost time from work and other intangible costs.

Any study that is based solely on administrative data has certain limitations. Analysis with use of a claims-data algorithm can never be completely accurate in positive or negative cases. In claims-data analysis, however, use of an algorithm can enable a rapid, inexpensive, and reasonably accurate evaluation of a large database. Similar, but not identical methodologies have been used by other investigators in breast cancer research (23,24). Other limitations of our study relate to assumptions made when only administrative data are used in the evaluation of practice patterns. With a claims-based approach, the accuracy of mammogram readings cannot be ensured to the same extent as the accuracy of readings with other methods, such as double-blind readings by an expert panel.

First, to reduce interprovider variation and thereby improve quality of care, this performance information must be shared with participating radiologists. The information should include group performance and the implications of interpretive skill as a function of cost. Possible remedies include an analysis of how care may be improved with teaching programs sponsored by the American College of Radiology. Internal tutorial programs for physicians can be used to help radiologists alter their threshold for interpreting examinations. U.S. Healthcare has developed a one-on-one educational program between its associate radiologic medical directors and its participating radiologists; individual results from this analysis are shared (and compared with results from other unidentified providers). Providers who are outliers are identified, and a discussion between the the medical directors and outliers is conducted. This intervention is for informational purposes only; there are no punitive actions or financial implications. Merely, information about relative performance—which most providers cannot obtain—is demonstrated. The premise is that information about relative performance will help radiologists improve the accuracy of their readings.

The breast cancer outreach program within this HMO has resulted in a high percentage of screening mammography in eligible women. According to the National Health Interview Survey (8,25), the biennial rate of screening mammography (72.1%) in this HMO surpasses the national rate (54%) in women aged 40 years and older who have undergone mammography in the last 2 years. The program has not only improved compliance with the process measure of improved performance of screening mammography; the program has also led to improved outcomes, demonstrated with a downstaging of breast cancer at diagnosis. Our study demonstrates the value of standardized categories to help stratify the likelihood of cancer in a woman with an abnormal mammogram. Our study also demonstrates how data on interprovider variation can be used to construct an educational program for radiologic providers. With the systems-of-care view and information systems used by managed-care providers, the important aspects of quality of care can be identified. These aspects, when improved in the aggregate HMO population, help optimize patient outcomes.

APPENDIX

Selection-Criteria Algorithms

With the algorithm (19), a new case of breast cancer was defined if a woman's claims data included one or more of the following six criteria: (*a*) mastectomy, (*b*) partial mastectomy with lymphadenectomy, (*c*) excision, breast biopsy, or partial mastectomy and lymphadenectomy, (*d*) excision, breast biopsy, or partial mastectomy and the diagnosis of breast cancer, (*e*) excision, breast biopsy, or partial mastectomy followed with radiation therapy, (*f*) excision, breast biopsy, or partial mastectomy followed with chemotherapy.

With criterion *c*, two events could occur sequentially or simultaneously. With criteria *e* and *f*, the two events had to occur sequentially.

Codes from the *International Classification of Diseases*-9 and *Current Procedural Terminology*-4

The codes from the *International Classification of Diseases*-9 used for the diagnosis of breast cancer were 174.0–174.9, inclusive, or 233.0. The codes from the *Current Procedural Terminology*-4 were the following: (*a*) mastectomy, 19180–19240, inclusive, (*b*) partial mastectomy with lymphadenectomy, 19162, (*c*) excision, 19120, 19125, 19126, (*d*) breast biopsy, 19100 or 19101, (*e*) partial mastectomy, 19160, (*f*) lymphadenectomy, 38740 or 38745, (*g*) radiation therapy, 77261–77499, inclusive, and (*h*) chemotherapy, 96400–96549, inclusive. ■

References

1. Tabar L, Gad A, Ljungquist U, et al. Reduction in mortality from breast cancer after mass screening with mammography. Lancet 1985; 8433:829–832.
2. Verbeek AL, Hendricks JH, Holland R, et al. Reduction of breast cancer mortality through mass screening with modern mammography: first results of the Nijmegen Project, 1975–1981. Lancet 1984; 1:1222–1224.
3. Lindfors KK, Rosenquist JC. The cost-effectiveness of mammographic screening strategies. JAMA 1995; 274:881–884.
4. Boer R, Verbeek ALM, Collette HJA, et al. Nationwide breast cancer screening in the Netherlands: support for breast cancer mortality reduction. Int J Cancer 1995; 60: 777–780.
5. Kerlikowske K, Grady D, Rubin S, et al. Efficacy of screening mammography: a meta-analysis. JAMA 1995; 273:149–154.
6. Eddy DM. Screening for breast cancer. Ann Int Med 1989; 111:389–399.

7. The NCI Breast Cancer Screening Consortium. Results of the NCI Breast Cancer Screening Consortium and National Health Interview survey studies. JAMA 1990; 264: 54–58.
8. Hanchak NA. Managed care, accountability, and the physician. Med Clin North Am 1996; 80:245–261.
9. Solin LJ, Schultz DJ, Legorreta AP, Goodman RL. Downstaging of breast carcinomas associated with mammographic screening. Breast Dis 1995; 8:45–56.
10. Riley GF, Potosky AL, Lubitz JD, Brown ML. Stage of cancer at diagnosis for Medicare HMO and fee-for-service enrollees. Am J Public Health 1994; 84:1598–1604.
11. Solin LJ, Legorreta A, Schultz DJ, Zatz S, Goodman RL. The importance of mammographic screening relative to the treatment of women with carcinoma of the breast. Arch Intern Med 1994; 154:745–752.
12. Miller AB, Baines CJ, To T, et al. Canadian National Breast Screening study. I. Breast cancer detection and death rates among women aged 40 to 49 years. Can Med Assoc J 1992; 147:1459–1476.
13. Hurley SF, Daldor JM. The benefits and risks of mammographic screening for breast cancer. Epidemiol Rev 1992; 14:101–130.
14. Hanchak NA, Schlackman N. The measurement of physician performance. Qual Manage Health Care 1995; 4:1–12.
15. Elmore JG, Wells KW, Lee CH, et al. Variability in radiologists' interpretations of mammograms. N Eng J Med 1994; 331:1493–1499.
16. Physician Insurers Association of America. 1995 report: the international classification of diseases—clinical modification. 9th rev. Vol 1–3. Baltimore, Md: HCIA, 1992.
17. American College of Radiology. Breast imaging reporting and data system (BI-RADS). Reston, Va: American College of Radiology, 1993.
18. Rimer BK, Keintz MK, Kessler HB, Engstrom PF, Rosan JR. Why women resist mammograms: understanding patient-related barriers to acceptance of screening mammography. Radiology 1989; 172:243–246.
19. Solin LJ, Legorreta A, Schultz DJ, Levin HA, Zatz S, Goodman RL. Analysis of a claims database for the identification of patients with carcinoma of the breast. J Med Sys 1994; 18:23–32.
20. The international classification of diseases—clinical modification. 9th rev. 3rd ed. Public Health Service Publication No. 89-1260. Washington, DC: Government Printing Office, 1989.
21. American Medical Association. Current Procedural Terminology. 4th ed. Chicago, Ill: American Medical Association, 1995.
22. Solin LJ, MacPherson S, Schultz DJ, Hanchak NA. Evaluation of an algorithm to identify women with carcinoma of the breast. J Med Syst (in press).
23. Nattinger AB, Gottlieb MS, Veum J, Yahnke D, Goodwin JS. Geographic variation in the use of breast-conserving treatment for breast cancer. N Engl J Med 1992; 326:1102–1107.
24. Farrow DC, Hunt WC, Samet JM. Geographic variation in the treatment of localized breast cancer. N Engl J Med 1992; 326: 1097–1101.
25. Brown ER, Wyn R, Cumberland WG, et al. Women's health-related behaviors and use of clinical preventive services: a special report. The Commonwealth Fund Commission on Women's Health, UCLA Center for Health Policy Research, October 1995.

Book Review

Differential Diagnosis in Conventional Gastrointestinal Radiology. Excerpt from Differential Diagnosis in Conventional Radiology. 2nd ed.

Francis A. Burgener, MD, and Martti Kormano, MD

New York, NY: Thieme Medical, 1997. ISBN 0-86577-676-8 (New York), 3-13-107621-6 (Stuttgart). Cloth, $69.00; pp 233; 521 figures; tables.

Differential Diagnosis in Chest X-rays. Excerpt from Differential Diagnosis in Conventional Radiology. 2nd ed.

Frances A. Burgener, MD, and Martti Kormano, MD

New York, NY: Thieme Medical, 1997. ISBN 0-86577-677-6 (New York), 3-13-107611-9 (Stuttgart). Cloth, $69.00; pp 190; 421 figures; tables.

Differential Diagnosis in Conventional Gastrointestinal Radiology and *Differential Diagnosis in Chest X-rays* are excerpts from *Differential Diagnosis in Conventional Radiology*, 2nd ed, by Dr Burgener and Dr Kormano. In the parent textbook, the authors state the book is "for physicians with some experience in radiology who wish to strengthen their diagnostic acumen. [The book] is a comprehensive outline of radiology findings and we expect it to be particularly useful to radiology residents preparing for their specialist examinations." Both excerpts are written in summary format on high-gloss paper with excellent radiographic reproductions. The excerpts are divided logically into chapters that provide a quick, efficient review of the subject. Graphics and illustrations are top-notch.

Differential Diagnosis in Conventional Gastrointestinal Radiology and *Differential Diagnosis in Chest X-rays* are reasonably priced. I recommend that both be added to your library; they provide excellent reviews for radiology residents or practicing radiologists.

Reviewed by Stanley L. Parker, MD

John R. Mayo, MD • Martine Remy-Jardin, MD, PhD • Nestor L. Müller, MD, PhD
Jacques Remy, MD • Daniel F. Worsley, MD • Claude Hossein-Foucher, MD
J. Stephen Kwong, MD • Maura J. Brown, MD

Pulmonary Embolism: Prospective Comparison of Spiral CT with Ventilation-Perfusion Scintigraphy[1]

PURPOSE: **To compare prospectively the accuracy of spiral computed tomography (CT) with that of ventilation-perfusion scintigraphy for diagnosing pulmonary embolism.**

MATERIALS AND METHODS: **Within 48 hours of presentation, 142 patients suspected of having pulmonary embolism underwent spiral CT, scintigraphy, and (when indicated) pulmonary angiography. Pulmonary angiography was attempted if interpretations of spiral CT scans and of scintigrams were discordant or indeterminate and intermediate-probability, respectively.**

RESULTS: **In the 139 patients who completed the study, interpretations of spiral CT scans and of scintigrams were concordant in 103 patients (29 with embolism, 74 without). In 20 patients, intermediate-probability scintigrams were interpreted (six with embolism at angiography, 14 without); diagnosis with spiral CT was correct in 16. Interpretations of spiral CT scans and those of scintigrams were discordant in 12 cases; diagnosis with spiral CT was correct in 11 cases and that with scintigraphy was correct in one. Spiral CT and scintigraphic scans of four patients with embolism did not show embolism. Sensitivities, specificities, and κ values with spiral CT and scintigraphy were 87%, 95%, and 0.85 and 65%, 94%, and 0.61, respectively.**

CONCLUSION: **In cases of pulmonary embolism, sensitivity of spiral CT is greater than that of scintigraphy. Interobserver agreement is better with spiral CT.**

PULMONARY embolism is a common condition with considerable morbidity and mortality (1). Prompt and accurate diagnosis is important because the mortality of untreated pulmonary embolism is high and serious complications can occur with its treatment, long-term anticoagulation (2).

Currently, ventilation-perfusion (V-P) scintigraphy is the most commonly used first-line examination in cases of clinically suspected pulmonary embolism. A normal or low-probability scan has a high negative predictive value when the clinical suspicion of pulmonary embolism is low (4% prevalence); a high-probability scan has a high positive predictive value when the clinical suspicion of pulmonary embolism is high (97% prevalence) (3). Unfortunately, at the typical tertiary-referral center, only 34% of cases correspond to these two categories (3). In addition, large differences (25%–30%) in interpretation among expert readers have been reported—especially in the classification of low- or intermediate-probability scans (4). Doppler ultrasound (US) and impedance plethysmography of the lower-extremity veins have often been used as adjuncts to V-P scintigraphy. Results of a large outcome-based study (5) demonstrated that the combination of V-P scintigraphic and noninvasive studies of lower-extremity veins enabled identification of 71% of patients who needed anticoagulation.

Pulmonary angiography is considered to be the definitive study for the diagnosis of pulmonary embolism because pulmonary angiography provides direct assessment of the pulmonary vasculature with a high sensitivity and specificity. However, pulmonary angiography is invasive and has a 6% morbidity and a 0.5% mortality (6). Furthermore, surveys have shown that physicians are reluctant to order pulmonary angiography, even when the procedure is appropriate (7).

Results of recent studies (8–12) have shown that spiral computed tomography (CT) is useful for detecting central and segmental pulmonary embolism. However, questions remain regarding the clinical role of spiral CT in pulmonary embolism (13). We therefore performed a prospective clinical study to compare spiral CT with V-P scintigraphy in patients who were suspected clinically of having pulmonary embolism.

MATERIALS AND METHODS

The prospective study was performed in 142 patients with suspected pulmonary

Index terms: Computed tomography (CT), comparative studies, 60.12115 • Computed tomography (CT), helical, 564.12115, 60.12115 • Embolism, pulmonary, 60.721 • Lung, radionuclide studies, 60.1217 • Pulmonary arteries, CT, 564.12115 • Pulmonary arteries, stenosis or obstruction, 564.721 • Radionuclide imaging, comparative studies, 60.12115, 60.1217

Abbreviations: PIOPED = Prospective Investigation of Pulmonary Embolism Diagnosis, V-P = ventilation-perfusion.

Radiology 1997; 205:447–452

[1] From the Department of Radiology, Vancouver Hospital and Health Sciences Centre and University of British Columbia, 855 W 12th Ave, Vancouver, British Columbia, Canada V5Z 1M9 (J.R.M., N.L.M., D.F.W., J.S.K., M.J.B.); the Department of Radiology, Hôpital Calmette, Lille, France (M.R.J., J.R.); and the Department of Nuclear Medicine, Hôpital B, Lille, France (C.H.F.). Received April 25, 1997; revision requested June 10; revision received July 15; accepted July 21. J.R.M. supported by a Career Scientist Grant from the British Columbia Lung Foundation. **Address reprint requests to** J.R.M.

embolism who were referred to the imaging departments of two academic medical centers (Vancouver Hospital, Vancouver, British Columbia, Canada; and Hôpital Calmette, Lille, France). There were 74 men and 68 women, aged 18–85 years (mean, 54.5 years). Pulmonary embolism was suspected clinically on the basis of subjective criteria. Patients were enrolled in the study from May 5, 1995, to November 13, 1996. Ethical approval was obtained from the institutions' respective review boards.

All patients underwent V-P scintigraphy, contrast material–enhanced spiral CT and, when indicated, pulmonary angiography within 48 hours of clinical presentation. The V-P scintigraphic and spiral CT studies were initially interpreted independently and tabulated by a nuclear medicine specialist and chest radiologist (J.R.M., N.L.M., M.R.J., J.R.), respectively. After initial independent interpretation, the need for pulmonary angiography was determined by comparing the results of V-P scintigraphy and those of spiral CT with the level of clinical suspicion for pulmonary embolism.

The combination of a high-probability V-P scintigram and a spiral CT finding of pulmonary embolism was considered diagnostic of pulmonary embolism, and no further imaging studies were performed. In these concordant positive cases, treatment was instituted without pulmonary angiography.

The combination of a normal, very low–, or low-probability V-P scintigram, a spiral CT scan without findings of pulmonary embolism, and a low clinical suspicion of pulmonary embolism was considered sufficient to exclude pulmonary embolism. In these concordant negative cases, anticoagulation was not instituted and pulmonary angiography was not performed. In these cases, patients with very low– or low-probability V-P scintigrams were followed up clinically for at least 3 months to ensure that the diagnosis of pulmonary embolism was not made subsequently. Clinical follow-up was performed by telephone with the patient's primary-care physician, who was asked if a diagnosis of pulmonary embolism had been made during follow-up. If pulmonary embolism was diagnosed during follow-up, the concordant negative case was labeled false-negative for V-P scintigraphic and spiral CT studies. In the concordant negative cases, patients with a normal V-P scan were not followed up clinically because the documented prevalence of pulmonary embolism is low in this population (3).

Patients who were highly suspected clinically of having pulmonary embolism underwent angiography even if V-P scintigraphic and spiral CT study findings were not strongly suggestive of pulmonary embolism. All patients whose V-P scintigraphic or spiral CT studies were interpreted to be intermediate or indeterminate, respectively, underwent pulmonary angiography. If interpretations of V-P scintigrams and those of spiral CT scans were discordant, pulmonary angiography was also performed.

CT Protocol

CT scans were acquired with a GE Hi-Speed Advantage (GE Medical Systems, Milwaukee, Wis) or a Somatom Plus S (Siemens Medical Systems, Erlangen, Germany) scanner. A contrast-enhanced spiral CT evaluation of the central and segmental pulmonary arteries was performed from the level of the aortic arch to 2 cm below the inferior pulmonary veins. Scans were acquired with suspended inspiration or during shallow breathing, depending on the patient's level of dyspnea. Technical parameters included 3-mm collimation, 1.8–2.0 pitch, 120–137 kVp, 180–320 mA, and 1-second scan time. Images were reconstructed at 1.5–3.0-mm intervals with use of the standard reconstruction algorithm and a field of view appropriate for the size of the patient. A 180° linear-interpolation algorithm was used for all helical data sets.

Contrast material was injected at 3–5 mL/sec with a power injector (Medrad, Pittsburgh, Pa) through an 18–20-gauge catheter in the antecubital fossa or (if available) a central venous catheter. The size and position of the catheter determined the flow rate used: A rate of 4–5 mL/sec was used in central catheters and 18-gauge peripheral catheters, and a rate of 3 mL/sec was used in 20-gauge peripheral catheters. There was no attempt to tailor the rate of contrast material injection to the size of the patient. To eliminate kinking of the subclavian vein at the thoracic inlet during injection, the arm was placed at the patient's side. The other arm was placed above the patient's head. A total volume of 140–180 mL of nonionic contrast material (meglumine ioxitamalate [Telebrix 30; Guerbet, Aulnay-sous-Bois, France], iohexol [Omnipaque 240; Nycomed Ingenor, Paris, France], or a mixture of 50% ioversol [Optiray 320; Mallinckrodt, Pointe Claire, Quebec, Canada] and 50% sterile normal saline) was injected. A timing bolus was not used, and scanning began 15–20 seconds after the initiation of injection. The scan delay and arm position allowed direct visualization of the intravenous site for the first phase of injection and minimized the risk of interstitial injection.

Images were viewed at settings for pulmonary vasculature (window width, 250 HU; window level, 35 HU) and lung parenchyma (window width, 1,500 HU; window level, −700 HU) at a workstation. Images were assessed initially by one of the two study radiologists (J.R.M., N.L.M, M.R.J., J.R.) who were on clinical service at each of the two institutions and who were unaware of the V-P scintigraphic results. The presence or absence of an occlusive or nonocclusive clot in the main and segmental pulmonary arteries was recorded on a study data sheet. Spiral CT studies were categorized as (*a*) positive for pulmonary embolism if a central or segmental clot was observed, (*b*) negative for pulmonary embolism if no clot was observed, or (*c*) indeterminate if poor signal-to-noise ratios, inadequate enhancement, or motion artifacts in any central or segmental vessel precluded confident interpretation of the study. Determination of the location and course of the pulmonary arteries at the segmental level was aided with knowledge of anatomic structure and identification of the accompanying bronchus on the corresponding lung-window image. Acute pulmonary embolism was diagnosed if (*a*) a normal-sized or enlarged pulmonary artery was obstructed completely by an unenhancing thrombus or (*b*) nonocclusive filling defects were apparent centrally in the vessel.

The initial reading was used to assess the need for pulmonary angiography and the calculation of sensitivity and specificity. Subsequently, the images were independently interpreted by the second chest radiologist at the same institution (J.R.M., N.L.M., M.R.J., J.R.) for calculation of interobserver variation.

Table 1
Accuracy of V-P Scintigraphy for the Diagnosis of Pulmonary Embolism

V-P Scintigraphy Interpretation	Pulmonary Embolism*: Present	Absent
High probability	30	6
Intermediate probability	6	14
Low probability	8	50
Very low probability or normal	2	23

* Standards of reference used for final diagnosis are given in text.

Table 2
Accuracy of Spiral CT for the Diagnosis of Pulmonary Embolism

Spiral CT Interpretation	Pulmonary Embolism*: Present	Absent
Positive	40	2
Indeterminate	1	3
Negative	5	88

* Standards of reference used for final diagnosis are given in text.

V-P Scintigraphy

Ventilation studies were performed after inhalation of 1 mCi (37 MBq) of technetium-99m phytate aerosol or 5 mCi (185 MBq) of xenon-133 gas. In Tc-99m phytate studies, six views were acquired with a minimum of 200,000 counts per view. In Xe-133 studies, a posterior 150,000-count single-breath image was acquired before four 1–2-minute equilibrium images. The washout consisted of four 60-second posterior views.

Perfusion studies were performed after intravenous administration of 3–5 mCi (111–185 MBq) of Tc-99m–labeled macroaggregated serum albumin. In patients who underwent Xe-133 ventilation imaging,

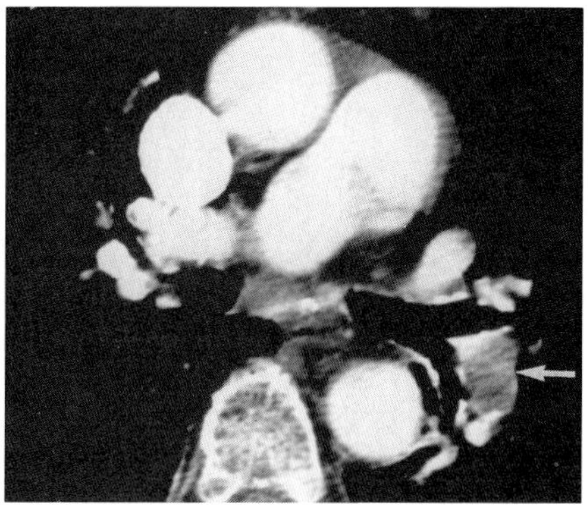

Figure 1. Contrast-enhanced spiral CT image obtained at the level of the intermediate bronchus shows occlusive thrombus (arrow) in the left interlobar pulmonary artery. The interpretation of the corresponding V-P scintigram (not shown) was high probability; there were multiple mismatched segmental defects in the left lower lobe.

perfusion images were acquired with a minimum of 400,000 counts per view except in the lateral position in which a minimum of 320,000 counts were acquired. In patients who underwent ventilation imaging with Tc-99m phytate aerosol, perfusion images were acquired with 800,000 counts per view. Perfusion images were acquired in six projections. Ventilation and perfusion studies were performed with a large field-of-view gamma camera (Siemens Medical Systems, Hoffman Estates, Ill; or SP4; Elscint, Bagnolet, France) equipped with a parallel-hole low-energy all-purpose collimator.

All patients underwent chest radiography the same day of V-P scintigraphy. The V-P scintigrams were interpreted in conjunction with the chest radiograph by the nuclear medicine physician on clinical service that day, and the results were tabulated. V-P scintigrams acquired in Lille and those acquired in Vancouver were classified with use of the original (4) and revised (Vancouver) (3) criteria, respectively, of the Prospective Investigation of Pulmonary Embolism Diagnosis (PIOPED). Like the interpretations of the spiral CT studies, the initial interpretation of the V-P scintigram was used to determine the need for pulmonary angiography and the calculation of specificity and sensitivity. The scans were later interpreted independently by a second blinded observer at the same institution with use of the same interpretation criteria.

Pulmonary Angiography

When indicated, selective bilateral pulmonary angiography was performed with film or digital recording. In all cases, multiple projections were acquired in the left posterior oblique, right posterior oblique, anteroposterior, or lateral projections. The selection of the imaging plane was the angiographer's choice. If there was inadequate visualization of the pulmonary arterial tree with standard views, selective lobar or segmental angiograms were acquired. A straight NIH or Grollman pigtail catheter was placed selectively in the right or left pulmonary artery and contrast material was injected at 20–22 mL/sec to a total of 40–45 mL. A total of 100–200 mL of 35% iodinated contrast material (iohexol [Omnipaque 350] or ioversol [Optiray 320]) was used. If pulmonary emboli were identified in the first lung (left or right) studied, the contralateral lung was not examined. The angiographers were aware of the results of all previous imaging studies and the level of clinical suspicion of pulmonary embolism.

Angiograms were independently interpreted and tabulated by two experienced angiographers. In the event of a discordant interpretation, a decision was made by consensus. Acute emboli were identified if a persistent intraluminal filling defect or a vascular cutoff of a pulmonary artery was seen on at least two projections.

Statistical Analysis

Differences in the diagnostic accuracy between V-P scintigraphic and spiral CT findings were assessed with the McNemar statistic. With use of the χ^2 statistic, the prevalence of pulmonary embolism detected with V-P scintigraphic results and that with spiral CT findings were compared with the prevalence detected with pulmonary angiography. Statistical significance was defined at the .05 level. Interobserver agreement was calculated with the κ statistic, with three categories for spiral CT results and five categories for V-P scintigraphic results.

RESULTS

In three concordant negative cases, patients were not available for follow-up. Therefore, 139 of 142 patients completed the study. The numbers of inpatients and outpatients in the study were the following: 113 (81%) inpatients in the medical or surgical ward, four (3%) patients in the intensive care or coronary care units, and 22 (16%) outpatients. Pulmonary embolism was diagnosed in 46 (33%) of 139 subjects on the basis of findings from the following modalities: angiography (n = 12), Doppler US of thigh veins in patients who refused pulmonary angiography (n = 3), high-probability V-P scintigraphy and positive spiral CT (n = 29), and clinical follow-up examination (n = 2). Pulmonary angiography was necessary in 44 cases and was performed in 41 (93%) cases. Three patients refused angiography after Doppler US studies showed noncompressible clot at the midthigh level. In these cases, categorized positive for pulmonary embolism on the basis of the Doppler US findings, patients received anticoagulant agents. In the 41 patients who underwent angiography, pulmonary embolism was identified in 12 (29%). The prevalence of pulmonary embolism in the patients who did not undergo pulmonary angiography (34 [35%] of 98) was not statistically significantly different from that in patients who underwent pulmonary angiography (12 [29%] of 41 patients) ($P > .05$). There was no statistically significant difference between the prevalence of pulmonary embolism at the two institutions (Vancouver, 34%; Lille, 31%) ($P > .05$). The mean time between V-P scintigraphy and spiral CT was 0.38 day ± 0.78 (median, 0 days). The duration of follow-up was 101–548 days (median, 175 days).

High-probability V-P scintigraphic studies (Table 1) were interpreted in 30 of 46 cases of pulmonary embolism (sensitivity, 65%). V-P scintigraphic studies that were not interpreted to be high-probability were obtained in 87 of 93 subjects without pulmonary embolism (specificity, 94%). Intermediate-probability V-P scintigrams were interpreted in 20 (14%) of the 139 cases; further imaging results demonstrated pulmonary embolism in six (30%) of these 20 cases and enabled exclusion of pulmonary embolism in the other 14 (70%).

Positive spiral CT scans were interpreted in 40 of 46 patients with pulmonary embolism (sensitivity, 87%) (Table 2). Negative spiral CT studies were interpreted in 88 of 93 patients without pulmonary embolism (specificity, 95%). The interpretation of four (3%) CT scans was indeterminate; subsequent pulmonary angiograms demonstrated pulmonary embolism in one patient and enabled exclusion of pulmonary embolism in the other three. No correlation was found between interpretation of indeterminate spiral CT scans and the tube current, reconstruction interval, or contrast material flow rate used.

By comparing V-P scintigraphic and spiral CT interpretations, concordant positive results were found in 29 (21%) of 139 cases (Fig 1), and concordant negative results were found in 74 (53%) of 139 cases. In the 20 cases with intermediate-probability V-P scintigrams, spiral CT results enabled correct identification of five patients with emboli (Fig 2) and 11 without. In this group, however, there were two false-positive and two indeterminate spiral CT studies. Interpretations of V-P scintigrams and those of spiral CT studies were discordant in 12 cases. Interpretation of the spiral CT study was correct in 11 (92%) of the 12 discordant cases. In these 11 cases, partially occlusive thrombus was confirmed in six and was excluded in five. In the other case correctly identified with V-P scintigraphy, the spiral CT study (which was incorrectly interpreted to be negative) was markedly limited because of the patient's large size.

Concordant negative V-P scintigraphic and spiral CT studies were obtained in four (3%) patients; these studies, however, were shown to be falsely negative at pulmonary angiography ($n = 2$) or during follow-up ($n = 2$). In two of these cases, there was a high clinical suspicion of pulmonary embolism at presentation; these patients underwent pulmonary angiography, which showed subsegmental emboli in the lingula (Fig 3) and the right middle lobe. In the two cases in which pulmonary embolism was detected during follow-up, one patient returned 3 months after concordant negative studies were acquired and reentered the study. At this second presentation, interpretation of the V-P scintigram (low probability) and that of the spiral CT scan (positive) were discordant. Pulmonary angiography confirmed embolism. The other patient returned 1 month after concordant negative studies. At this time, a repeat V-P scintigram was interpreted as high probability, and perfusion abnormalities resolved at follow-up V-P scintigraphy 1 week later. Spiral CT was not performed in this patient at the second presentation because the equipment was unavailable.

Between observers, interpretations of pulmonary angiograms were concordant in 36 (88%) of 41 cases. In one case, a single distal segmental arterial clot was not identified by one observer. At consensus reading, this case was correctly classified positive. In four cases, the pulmonary angiogram was classified negative by one of the two observers; the other observer classified the pulmonary angiogram indeterminate. At consensus reading, all four cases were classified negative. In two of these four cases, the corresponding spiral CT study acquired the same day was classified to be indeterminate by both observers. Both studies were suboptimal because the patients were unable to cooperate with examination.

Overall, interpretations of V-P scintigraphic studies were correct in 103 (74%) of 139 cases, whereas interpretations of spiral CT studies were correct in 128 (92%) of 139 cases. With the McNemar test, a statistically significant difference between the rate of correct interpretations of V-P scintigraphic studies and that of spiral CT studies was demonstrated ($P < .01$).

Interobserver agreement (κ statistic) for V-P scintigraphic interpretations (Table 3) was 0.61; for spiral CT interpretations (Table 4), the κ was 0.85. In three cases, V-P scintigrams were not interpreted by the second observer because the images could not be found.

DISCUSSION

The overall prevalence of pulmonary embolism in our study was 33% and was the same as that in the PIOPED study (4). In the PIOPED study, the sensitivity of a high-probability V-P scintigram (40%) was slightly lower than that (65%) in our study. Similar specificities of a high-probability V-P scintigram were obtained in our study (94%) and in the PIOPED study (98%) (3).

In earlier studies (8–12) with spiral CT, a similar sensitivity (87%) was obtained. In our study, the sensitivity with spiral CT findings was reduced because the V-P scintigraphic and spiral CT studies in two patients with pulmonary embolism diagnosed at follow-up were false-negative. The specificity (95%) with spiral CT findings in our study was also similar to that in previous reports (8–12). With the McNemar test, the statistically significant improvement in diagnosis with spiral CT (compared with that with V-P scintigraphic) findings is confirmed. This diagnostic difference occurred largely because spiral CT findings enabled a correct diagnosis in 80% of cases in which the V-P scintigram was interpreted intermediate probability. The decreased rate of indeterminate spiral CT studies compared with that of intermediate-probability V-P scintigrams will also influence the cost-effectiveness of spiral CT when screening for pulmonary embolism.

Spiral CT, however, does not enable diagnosis as effectively as pulmonary angiography. Spiral CT results were false-positive in two cases, false-negative in five cases, and indeterminate in four cases. The two false-positive studies were due to volume averaging of enhancing vessels with adjacent lymphadenopathy or atelectatic lung. One false-negative spiral CT study showed a low signal-to-noise ratio due to the patient's large size. In retrospect, this study should have been considered to be indeterminate. The other four false-negative spiral CT studies, which occurred in cases of low-probability V-P scintigrams, are more problematic. At pulmonary angiography, acute subsegmental clot in the lingula or in the right middle lobe was demonstrated in two of these cases. These results demonstrate the limitation of V-P scintigraphic and spiral CT findings for detection of subsegmental emboli. In the other two concordant false-negative cases noted during follow-up, subsegmental clot may have been present initially. Although these concordant false-negative cases were uncommon (3%), they underscore the need for pulmonary angiography when V-P scintigraphic and spiral CT studies do not demonstrate pulmonary embolism in patients who are highly suspected to have disease. However, further advances in spiral CT techniques (eg, narrower collimation or optimized delivery of contrast material) may improve visualization of subsegmental clot.

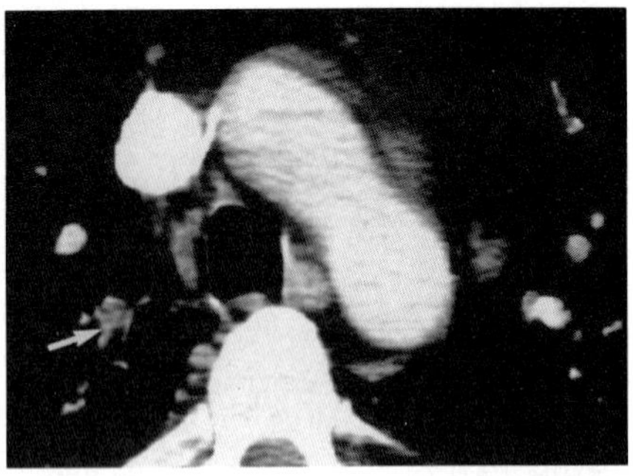
a.

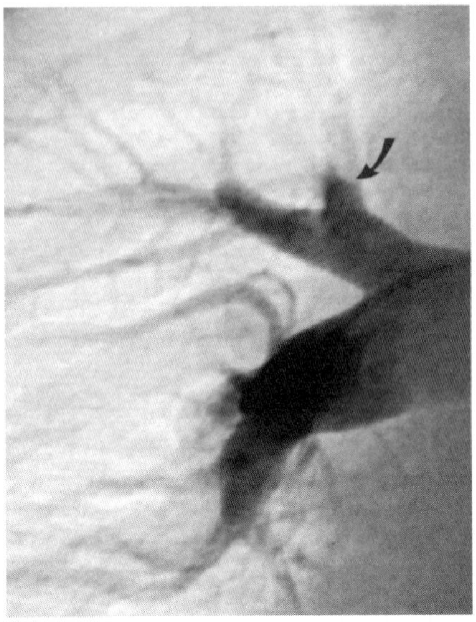
b.

Figure 2. **(a)** Contrast-enhanced spiral CT image obtained at the level of the aortic arch demonstrates occlusive thrombus (arrow) in the proximal apical segmental artery of the right upper lobe. The V-P scintigram (not shown) showed a single mismatched defect in the apical segment of the right upper lobe; with use of PIOPED criteria, this study was interpreted to be intermediate probability for pulmonary embolism. **(b)** Selective right frontal pulmonary angiogram shows vascular cutoff (arrow) of the apical segmental branch of the right upper lobe.

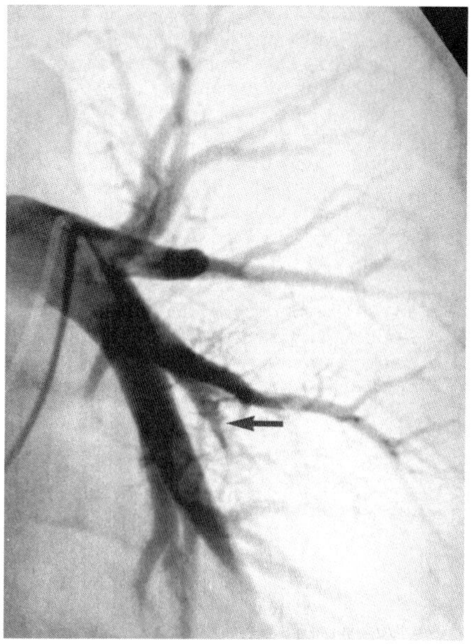

a.

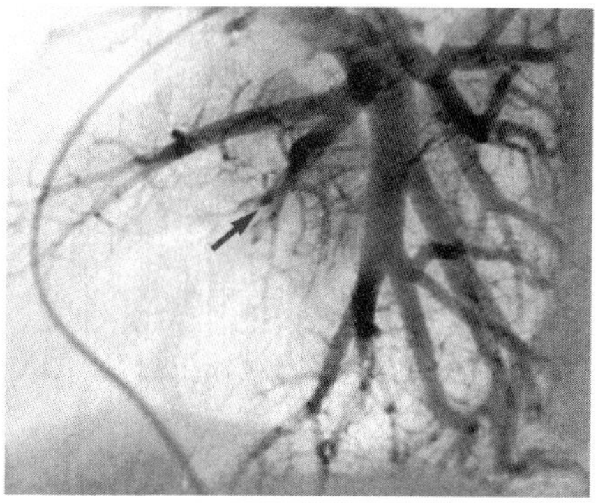

b.

Figure 3. **(a)** Frontal and **(b)** lateral views from a selective left pulmonary angiogram demonstrate vascular cutoff (arrow in **a** and **b**) in a subsegmental branch of the inferior lingular artery. The interpretation of the corresponding spiral CT study (not shown) was negative, and the V-P scintigram (not shown) was interpreted as low probability for pulmonary embolism.

Table 3
Comparison of Independent Interpretations of V-P Scintigraphy Studies

Reader 1 Interpretations	Reader 2 Interpretations: High Probability	Intermediate Probability	Low Probability	Very Low Probability	Normal
High probability	23	8	0	0	0
Intermediate probability	1	11	7	0	0
Low probability	0	7	53	2	3
Very low probability	1	1	3	0	0
Normal	0	0	2	1	13

Table 4
Comparison of Independent Interpretations of Spiral CT Studies

Reader 1 Interpretations	Reader 2 Interpretations: Positive	Indeterminate	Negative
Positive	42	0	1
Indeterminate	0	2	3
Negative	1	5	85

Four (3%) of 139 spiral CT studies were interpreted to be indeterminate because of poor enhancement, poor signal-to-noise ratio, or excessive patient motion. These cases highlight the technical limitations of current spiral CT scanners. Inadequate enhancement should occur less frequently with real-time measurement of the attenuation in blood in the pulmonary artery; this measurement would allow optimal timing of image acquisition. Further research is also needed to optimize the iodine dose and flow rate of contrast material at spiral CT for pulmonary embolism. In our study, prospective data about the relationship between the attenuation in contrast material and scan-acquisition delay, iodine dose, and flow rate and injection site of contrast material were not obtained. Therefore, we cannot address these important technical questions. More powerful tubes will improve image quality in patients with hyperattenuating areas on studies (caused by large size or large pleural effusions). The development of postprocessing respiratory-motion correction techniques would also be useful for improving image quality in dyspneic patients. This study has limitations that are intrinsic to the experimental design. For practical and ethical reasons, we elected prospectively to perform pulmonary angiography only in patients with inconclusive or discordant scintigraphic and CT results. As a consequence, the current definitive examination—pulmonary angiography—was performed in only 41 patients. However, data about the positive predictive value of high-probability V-P scintigrams and about the negative predictive value of normal V-P scintigrams support this approach (3). In the concordant negative cases with very low– or low-probability V-P scintigraphic studies, follow-up data support the assumption of no emboli. The validity of our experimental design is also strengthened because of the observation of no statistically significant difference between the rate (29%) of pulmonary embolism in those patients who underwent pulmonary angiography and the rate (35%) in patients who did not undergo pulmonary angiography ($P > .05$). Emboli may have been overlooked during the study period, however. The limited availability of spiral CT equipment prevented the examination of consecutive patients and introduced an inherent bias. As a result of this bias, there were no patients who did not undergo spiral CT examination because of allergy to contrast material, limited renal function, inability to lie supine, inability to be transported to the spiral CT scanner, or inadequate intravenous access. These restrictive entry criteria may have contributed to the low rate of indeterminate spiral CT examinations in our series.

In summary, for the diagnosis of pulmonary embolism, the sensitivity of spiral CT is greater than that of V-P scintigraphy. Interobserver agreement is also better with spiral CT. In patients who are candidates for spiral CT examination, it is reasonable to screen directly for pulmonary embolism with spiral CT or use spiral CT as an alternative, minimally invasive imaging modality after an intermediate-probability V-P scintigraphic study is obtained. Our results support the recent proposal (14) that spiral CT may be the initial imaging modality of choice in patients with a high rate of indeterminate V-P scintigraphic studies (eg, all inpatients and patients with chronic obstructive pulmonary disease). However, the choice of imaging modality is also influenced by the relative availability of V-P scintigraphy and spiral CT, as well as observer experience. If interpretation of a V-P scintigraphic or spiral CT study is negative, venous Doppler US or impedance plethysmography of the veins of the lower leg may be useful. However, if clinical suspicion of pulmonary embolism remains high, pulmonary angiography is indicated. Further technologic developments in spiral CT scanners and display devices may result in improved diagnostic accuracy with this examination in the near future. ■

References

1. Moser KM. State of the art: venous thromboembolism. Am Rev Respir Dis 1990; 414: 235–249.
2. Caranasos GJ, Stewart RB, Cluff LE. Drug-induced illness leading to hospitalization. JAMA 1974; 228:713–717.
3. Worsley DF, Alavi A. Comprehensive analysis of the results of the PIOPED study. J Nucl Med 1995; 36:2380–2387.
4. The PIOPED Investigators. Value of the ventilation/perfusion scan in acute pulmonary embolism: results of the Prospective Investigation of Pulmonary Embolism Diagnosis (PIOPED). JAMA 1990; 263:2753–2759.
5. Stein PD, Hull RD, Pineo G. Strategy that includes serial noninvasive leg tests for diagnosis of thromboembolic disease in patients with suspected acute pulmonary embolism based on data from PIOPED. Arch Intern Med 1995; 155:2101–2104.
6. Stein PD, Athanasoulis C, Alavi A, et al. Complications and validity of pulmonary angiography in acute pulmonary embolism. Circulation 1992; 85:462–468.
7. Henschke CI, Mateescu I, Yankelevitz DF. Changing practice patterns in the workup of pulmonary embolism. Chest 1995; 107: 940–945.
8. Remy-Jardin M, Remy J, Wattinne L, Giraud F. Central pulmonary thromboembolism: diagnosis with spiral volumetric CT with the single-breath-hold technique—comparison with pulmonary angiography. Radiology 1992; 185:381–387.
9. Remy-Jardin M, Remy J, Deschildre F, et al. Diagnosis of pulmonary embolism with spiral CT: comparison with pulmonary angiography and scintigraphy. Radiology 1996; 200:699–706.
10. Goodman LR, Curtin JJ, Mewissen MW, et al. Detection of pulmonary embolism in patients with unresolved clinical and scintigraphic diagnosis: helical CT versus angiography. AJR 1995; 164:1369–1374.
11. Teigen CL, Maus TP, Sheedy PF, et al. Pulmonary embolism: diagnosis with contrast-enhanced electron-beam CT and comparison with pulmonary angiography. Radiology 1995; 194:313–319.
12. van Rossum AB, Pattynama PMT, Tjin A Ton ER, et al. Pulmonary embolism: validation of spiral CT angiography in 149 patients. Radiology 1996; 201:467–470.
13. Hansell DM, Padley SPG. Continuous volume computed tomography in pulmonary embolism: the answer or just another test (editorial)? Thorax 1996; 51:1–2.
14. Goodman LR, Lipchik RJ. Diagnosis of acute pulmonary embolism: time for a new approach (editorial). Radiology 1996; 199: 25–27.

Gilbert R. Ferretti, MD • Jean-Luc Bosson, MD, PhD • Pierre-Denis Buffaz, MD
David Ayanian, MD • Christophe Pison, MD, PhD • François Blanc, MD
Françoise Carpentier, MD • Patrick Carpentier, MD • Max Coulomb, MD

Acute Pulmonary Embolism: Role of Helical CT in 164 Patients with Intermediate Probability at Ventilation-Perfusion Scintigraphy and Normal Results at Duplex US of the Legs[1]

PURPOSE: To assess prospectively the clinical effectiveness of helical computed tomography (CT) in the evaluation of patients with unresolved suspicion for pulmonary embolism (PE).

MATERIALS AND METHODS: Helical CT was performed in 164 consecutive patients suspected of having acute PE, intermediate probability at ventilation-perfusion (V-P) scintigraphy, and normal findings at duplex ultrasonography (US) of the legs. Fifteen patients also underwent pulmonary angiography. Helical CT results were analyzed immediately to help plan anticoagulant treatment. If helical CT did not show PE, anticoagulant treatment was not indicated. Clinical outcome for these patients was assessed during 3-month follow-up.

RESULTS: In 40 (24.4%) of 164 patients, the diagnosis of PE was based on results at helical CT (n = 39) or pulmonary angiography (n = 1). Repeated Doppler US of the legs depicted one thrombus in the calf of three patients with normal results at helical CT that could have been responsible for PE. During 3-month follow-up, three patients experienced recurrent PE (one death, two recurrences). Therefore, PE occurred in six (5.4% [95% confidence interval, 1.3%, 9.7%]) of 112 patients with normal findings at helical CT who did not receive anticoagulant treatment.

CONCLUSION: Findings at helical CT allowed accurate diagnosis of acute PE in patients with intermediate probability at V-P scintigraphy and without deep venous thrombosis at duplex sonography of the legs.

Clinical diagnosis of pulmonary embolism (PE) offers many challenges that are not met despite the use of numerous imaging modalities and various diagnostic schemes (1,2). In recent years, ventilation-perfusion (V-P) lung scintigraphy was used extensively as the primary imaging method for evaluating patients suspected of having PE. In approximately 70% of the patients, however, results at V-P scintigraphy were nondiagnostic (3). Such results necessitate further investigation to exclude or confirm the diagnosis of PE (4). As deep venous thrombosis and PE are manifestations of the same process, noninvasive explorations of the veins have been included in algorithms for the diagnosis of PE, in addition to V-P scintigraphy (5,6). Noninvasive explorations of the legs, however, help detection of deep venous thrombosis in approximately 50% of patients with angiographically proved PE (7). As the treatment for both conditions is similar, the presence of deep venous thrombosis justifies anticoagulant therapy and therefore obviates a search for pulmonary artery clots (8). In patients with nondiagnostic results at V-P scintigraphy and normal findings at duplex ultrasound (US) of the veins, pulmonary angiography is the next imaging method recommended for the diagnosis of PE (4). Despite the low mortality rate (<1%) and morbidity rate (2%–5%) associated with pulmonary angiography (9), clinicians are reluctant to prescribe it because it is invasive. Sostman et al (10) found that pulmonary angiography was performed in only 50 (12%) of 434 patients suspected of having PE and in whom it should have been performed because the question was not resolved after V-P scintigraphy. Therefore, in some institutions such patients do not undergo pulmonary angiography to rule out or confirm PE before treatment decisions are made (11).

Helical computed tomography (CT) is a minimally invasive technique that has shown great promise for diagnosis of central PE. Its sensitivity and specificity vary from 86% to 95% and from 92% to 97%, respectively (12–14). Current helical CT technology, however, limits visualization to fourth-generation pulmonary arteries (12–14). The place of helical CT in the diagnostic strategy for PE is not yet defined (1). Because pulmonary angiography is rarely performed in our institution, as in others (10,11), we conducted this prospective study in which helical CT replaced pulmonary angiography in the diagnosis-decision algorithm for patients with unresolved suspicion for PE after V-P scintigraphy and duplex sonography of the legs.

Index terms: Computed tomography (CT), helical, 944.12915 • Embolism, pulmonary, 944.77 • Lung, radionuclide studies, 60.1217 • Pulmonary arteries, CT, 944.12915 • Pulmonary arteries, thrombosis, 944.751

Abbreviations: PE = pulmonary embolism, PIOPED = Prospective Investigation of Pulmonary Embolism Diagnosis, V-P = ventilation-perfusion.

Radiology 1997; 205:453–458

[1] From the Departments of Radiology (G.R.F., D.A., F.B., M.C.), Biostatistics (J.L.B.), Nuclear Medicine (P.D.B.), Respiratory Disease (C.P.), Emergency Medicine (F.C.), and Internal Medicine and Angiology (P.C.), Centre Hospitalier Universitaire (CHU) Grenoble, BP 217, F-38043 Grenoble Cedex 09, France. Received March 24, 1997; revision requested May 19; revision received July 7; accepted July 8. Supported in part by a grant from the Délégation à la Recherche Clinique, CHU Grenoble, France. **Address reprint requests to** G.R.F.

The purpose of our study was to prospectively evaluate the immediate clinical usefulness of helical CT and to assess the outcome during 3-month follow-up in patients who did not receive anticoagulant treatment because of normal findings at helical CT.

MATERIALS AND METHODS

Patients

From October 1994 through March 1996, patients with clinical evidence of acute PE who were referred to undergo V-P scintigraphy were eligible for inclusion in our study. For each of these patients, the clinical probability of PE was scored on a graduated scale (0%–100%) on the basis of clinical data (ie, dyspnea, chest pain, hemoptysis, signs of right ventricular failure, syncope); risk factors for venous thromboembolism (history of thromboembolism, recent surgery, immobilization, malignancy, preexisting cardiac disease); abnormal blood gas levels; and abnormal findings at electrocardiography and chest radiography as determined by the physician in charge (15). Clinical probability was considered to be high if the score was 25% or greater and was considered to be low if the score was less than 25%. Exclusion criteria included severe PE (hemodynamic criteria), mean time greater than 72 hours between clinical suspicion for PE and helical CT, contraindications to the use of intravenous contrast material (eg, hypersensitivity, renal failure, heart failure), pregnancy, and age less than 18 years.

In 502 patients, findings were intermediate probability at V-P scintigraphy and normal at Doppler US of the legs, and they were eligible for inclusion in the study. Doppler US showed a thrombus in 211 (42%) of these patients; therefore, 291 (58%) patients could be included in the study. One hundred twenty-seven (44%) of these patients were excluded: 32 because of severe PE, 31 because the mean time between clinical suspicion and helical CT was greater than 72 hours, 35 because of contraindication to use of contrast material, 19 because images obtained at V-P scintigraphy were not satisfactory, and 10 because follow-up was not possible.

A total of 164 consecutive patients (109 women and 55 men, aged 21–90 years [mean, 63 years]) were entered into the study. At the time of presentation, 58 (35%) were outpatients from the emergency department and 106 (65%) were inpatients from various departments in our institution: 50 from internal medicine, 23 from surgery, 14 from respiratory medicine, 15 from cardiology, and four from intensive care. Clinical probability of PE was low in 41 (25%) patients and high in 123 (75%) patients.

Study Design

All patients with intermediate probability at V-P scintigraphy underwent duplex US of the legs (Figure). Patients with positive findings at US received anticoagulant therapy (8). All patients for whom the diagnosis of PE was inconclusive were included in our study. Inclusion criteria were (*a*) intermediate probability at V-P scintigraphy and (*b*) negative findings at Doppler US of the legs. We did not include patients with low probability at V-P scintigraphy because, in our institution, these patients are not candidates for pulmonary angiography.

Patients who were eligible to be included in the study were examined with helical CT. V-P scintigraphy, duplex US, and helical CT were performed within 72 hours after the patient's initial presentation with clinical evidence that suggested acute PE. Helical CT scans were analyzed immediately, and the diagnosis was based on the consensus of two radiologists. Helical CT results provided the basis for decisions regarding administration of anticoagulants. When helical CT demonstrated a thrombus within the pulmonary arteries, anticoagulants were administered. When helical CT did not depict any thrombus, anticoagulant therapy was not started or was suspended if previously initiated because of the clinical suspicion for PE. Clinicians were responsible for referring patients to undergo pulmonary angiography if they did not want to withdraw treatment when clinical suspicion for PE was high but results at helical CT were negative. Pulmonary angiography was then performed within 24 hours after helical CT to avoid incorrect analysis of results in case of spontaneous thrombolysis of PE. If pulmonary angiography demonstrated PE, anticoagulant therapy was started.

Three-month Follow-up

The usefulness of results at helical CT as an indicator of the need for anticoagulants was assessed in terms of occurrence of PE in patients who did not receive anticoagulant treatment because helical CT did not show any thrombus within the pulmonary arteries. Patients were followed up for 3 months after inclusion in the study to detect any clinical events or imaging abnormalities that could represent PE. Patients were asked to return to the hospital if they experienced symptoms or signs that suggested PE. Patients with clinical evidence of PE underwent V-P scintigraphy and duplex US of the legs. All patients were reevaluated at the end of 3 months. Ideally, clinical examination, duplex US, and V-P scintigraphy were performed in our institution. If the follow-up examination could not be performed in our institution, we contacted the patients or their family physicians by telephone and asked about the occurrence of any clinical events that could be related to PE. These patients, however, did not undergo V-P scintigraphy or US of the legs. If the patient had died, the cause of death was determined by means of discussion with the physician in charge at the time of death.

Imaging Evaluation

V-P scintigraphy.—In all patients, V-P scintigraphy was performed before helical CT. First ventilation imaging was performed with technetium 99m-labeled phytate aerosol (37 MBq) generated by a jet nebulizer. Next, perfusion imaging was performed with intravenous injection of 185 MBq of Tc-99m–labeled macroaggregates of human serum albumin. Images were acquired in six views: anterior, posterior, right and left anterior oblique, and right and left posterior oblique. V-P scintigraphy results were analyzed by an experienced nuclear medicine physician (P.D.B.) according to the modified Biello criteria (16).

V-P scintigraphy results were classified as normal if no perfusion defects were present, as low probability (<10%) if three or fewer subsegmental matches or one segmental or lobar match was present, and as high probability (>90%) if more than one segmental mismatch was present. Results were considered to be of intermediate probability (10%–90%) for PE in all other cases.

Venous duplex US.—All US examinations were performed by experienced angiologists (J.L.B. and another angiologist) with a Doppler US scanner (128XP; Acuson, Mountain View, Calif) with 7.5- and 3.5-MHz linear-display probes. The veins of both legs were examined with duplex sonography, from the calf to the inferior vena cava. The criterion for deep venous thrombosis was the presence of an intraluminal thrombus or incomplete compressibility of the vein, or both.

Helical CT.—All helical CT examinations (HiSpeed Advantage; GE Medical Systems, Milwaukee, Wis) were performed at 120 kVp and 200–250 mA with 5-mm-thick sections and a pitch of 1, as previously described by Rémy-Jardin et al (12). All scans were obtained in a caudocranial direction, starting at the level of the lower hemidiaphragm and ending at the top of the aortic arch. The length of the scanned volume, 12–15 cm, permitted imaging of the main, lobar, and segmental arteries of the upper, middle, and lower lobes. Breath holding lasted from 24 to 30 seconds. Acquisitions were performed during a single breath hold when possible or during quiet breathing when patients were short of breath. Images were reconstructed at 2.5-mm intervals with a standard reconstruction algorithm. Patients received 120 mL of 30% iodinated contrast material (Telebrix 30, Laboratoires Guerbet, Aulnay-sous-Bois, France; or Ivepaque 300, Nycomed Ingenor, Paris, France) administered through a 20-gauge catheter placed in an antecubital vein by using an automated injector (Medrad, Pittsburgh, Pa). The injection rate was 3 mL/sec with a 15–20-second delay. All images were analyzed with mediastinal (window width, 350 HU; window center, 50 HU) and lung (window width, 1,500 HU; window center, −500 HU) window settings on the CT monitor with use of the page mode and on hard copies.

Helical CT scans were analyzed during the course of clinical work-up by two radiologists, one of whom was an experienced thoracic radiologist, in consensus. The readers were unaware of the results at V-P scintigraphy when they read the helical CT scans. The pulmonary arteries were analyzed as far as the fourth generation. For

Table 1
Frequency of Identification of Segmental Arteries and the Number of Pulmonary Emboli per Segment in 164 Patients

Segmental Artery Location	No. of Analyzable Arteries (n = 164)	No. of Arteries with Thrombus
	Left Lung (LA)	
1	151 (92)	3 (2.0)
2	159 (97)	5 (3.1)
3	115 (70)	1 (0.9)
4	60 (37)	1 (1.7)
5	80 (49)	2 (2.5)
6	91 (55)	5 (5.5)
7	153 (93)	12 (7.8)
8	153 (93)	12 (7.8)
9	150 (91)	6 (4.0)
10	150 (91)	6 (4.0)
Total (N = 1,640)	1,262 (77)	53 (4.2)
	Right Lung (RA)	
1	153 (93)	4 (2.6)
2	131 (80)	3 (2.3)
3	113 (69)	1 (0.9)
4	87 (53)	2 (2.3)
5	95 (58)	2 (2.1)
6	135 (82)	13 (9.6)
7	140 (85)	12 (8.6)
8	140 (85)	14 (10.0)
9	151 (92)	21 (13.9)
10	153 (93)	22 (14.4)
Total (N = 1,640)	1,298 (79)	94 (7.2)

Note.—Numbers in parentheses are percentages.

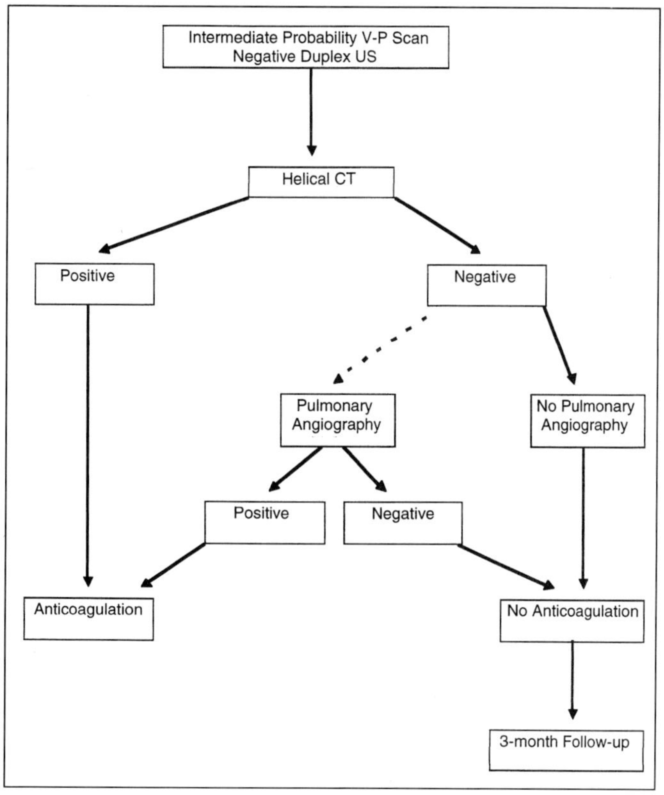

Study design.

each patient, 20 segmental pulmonary arteries according to the classification of Boyden (RA1–RA10 and LA1–LA10) (17) were analyzed separately. We followed the criteria proposed by Rémy-Jardin et al (17): The pulmonary arteries were considered analyzable when the vessel of interest was depicted without partial volume effects from its proximal to its distal portions on a single axial CT scan or on successive axial CT scans and as nonanalyzable when the segmental artery was not clearly depicted. We did not attempt to identify the subsegmental arteries, on the basis of results in the study of Goodman et al (13), who found that subsegmental arteries cannot be reliably identified on CT scans obtained with 5-mm-thick sections. The diagnosis of PE was based on the presence of complete or partial filling defects in the pulmonary arteries, according to the criteria proposed by Rémy-Jardin et al (12). Other ancillary findings were scored separately.

Pulmonary angiography.—Pulmonary angiography was indicated for patients whose clinicians did not consider the normal results at helical CT to be accurate and therefore refused to withdraw anticoagulants. Digital angiograms were obtained from a femoral-vein approach with use of the Seldinger technique. A 5-F angled pigtail catheter was used for selective angiography of the right and left pulmonary arteries. The V-P scintigraphy results were used to guide each pulmonary angiographic examination. Superselective views were acquired, when indicated, with use of a 5-F multipurpose catheter. Pulmonary angiograms were analyzed by consensus of two radiologists on the basis of the criteria of Sagel and Greenspan (18).

Data Analysis

Events during the 3-month follow-up of patients without PE at helical CT and pulmonary angiography who did not receive anticoagulants were used to calculate the false-negative rate for initial helical CT scans. The 95% confidence limits for the true incidence of PE during follow-up were calculated from the binomial distribution.

RESULTS

Initial Results

Opacification of the pulmonary arteries was satisfactory on all helical CT scans, and they were all adequate for interpretation. A total of 3,280 segmental arteries should be depicted theoretically, according to our criteria. Helical CT depicted 2,558 (78%) segmental pulmonary arteries; 1,262 (77%) of 1,640 segmental arteries were analyzable in the left lung and 1,298 (79%) of 1,640 segmental arteries were analyzable in the right lung (Table 1). Consequently, the mean number of segmental pulmonary arteries analyzable per patient was 15.6 of 20 (right segmental arteries, 7.9; left segmental arteries, 7.7). The frequency of identification of segmental arteries varied between 80% and 100% except for LA3 (70%), LA4 (37%), LA5 (49%), LA6 (55%), RA4 (53%), RA5 (58%), and RA3 (69%).

Of the 164 patients included in the study, helical CT depicted PE in 39 (23.8% [95% confidence interval, 18%, 30%]) and did not show PE in 125 (76.2%). The diagnosis of PE was based on the evaluation of analyzable central pulmonary arteries. Thrombi within the main pulmonary arteries were identified in four patients (left main pulmonary artery in three, right main pulmonary artery in one). Twenty-one thrombi were identified in the lobar pulmonary arteries (left lobar pulmonary arteries in 10, right lobar pulmonary arteries in 21). We identified 147 segmental emboli (94 [64%] in the segmental arteries of the right lung, 53 [36%] in the segmental arteries of the left lung) (Table 2). The mean number of segmental emboli (3.8) was higher in the right segmental arteries (2.4) than in the left segmental arteries (1.4). Thrombi were more frequently located in the segmental arteries of the right lower lobe (RA8–RA10).

Of 123 patients with high clinical probability, 33 (27%) had PE diagnosed at helical CT; of 41 patients with low clinical probability, six (15%) (P = .02) had PE diagnosed at helical CT. No immediate complications were associated with helical CT.

Pulmonary angiography was performed in 15 patients with high clinical probability (average, 50%; standard deviation, 15%) and normal results at helical CT. Results at pulmonary angiography were positive for PE in one patient and showed an isolated subsegmental thrombus that was not visible in retrospect at helical CT. Altogether, acute PE was diagnosed in 40 (24.4%) of the 164 patients.

In 18 (10.9%) of the 164 patients, alternative diagnoses were considered that could explain the clinical presentation but were unrelated to PE (infectious pneumonia in 10, bronchial dilatation in two, lung carcinoma in two, pneumothorax in two, and atelectasis in two). Findings at chest radiography were abnormal in 15 patients and were normal in three (bronchial dilatation in one, pneumothorax in one, and lung consolidation in one).

The 40 patients with PE and 14 patients without PE received anticoagulant drugs (heparin). Of the 14 latter patients, six received anticoagulant drugs because of heart disease (four because results at US of the legs repeated in the 48 hours after helical CT were positive for deep venous thrombosis). Repeat US was not included in our protocol but was ordered by the physician in charge of each of the four patients because they had developed clinical signs of deep venous thrombosis. Three of the 14 patients developed venous thrombosis in the calf (one developed femoral thrombosis after catheterization for pulmonary angiography), but PE was not depicted at repeat V-P scintigraphy. In the remaining five patients, anticoagulant therapy was initiated on the basis of clinical judgment exclusively, despite normal results at helical CT.

Of the 164 patients initially included in the study, 163 (99.4%) patients were followed up for 3 months, and one patient who received anticoagulants was lost to follow-up. Follow-up clinical examination, venous duplex US, and V-P scintigraphy were performed for 98 (59.8%) patients, and the patient or his physician was contacted by telephone for 65 (39.6%) patients.

Three-month Follow-up

One hundred nine patients with unresolved suspicion for PE and without demonstration of PE at helical CT or pulmonary angiography did not receive anticoagulant drugs. During the 3-month follow-up period, 10 (9.1%) of them died. Unfortunately, autopsy was not performed in any case. The cause of death was clearly defined in nine of the charts (end-stage cancer in seven, suicide in one, and myocardial infarction in one), and PE was highly suspected clinically in the other patient, who died 10 days after inclusion in the study.

Of the 99 patients who were alive at 3-month follow-up, PE was diagnosed in two (2% [95% confidence interval, 0%, 6.5%]) at 2- and 3-month follow-up, respectively. In both patients, clinical presentation including recent dyspnea was highly suggestive of the diagnosis. Results at V-P scintigraphy were high probability in both patients, and duplex US showed deep venous thrombosis in one patient.

Of the 97 patients who were alive without PE at 3-month follow-up, 54 (56%) underwent clinical examination, V-P scintigraphy, and venous duplex US; in the remaining 43 patients, follow-up consisted of contacting the physician or the patient by telephone. None of the 97 patients experienced deep venous thrombosis. Of the 18 patients with an alternative diagnosis on the basis of results at helical CT, none had PE.

In summary, our initial results show that helical CT did not depict an isolated subsegmental thrombus. With the technique we used (5-mm-thick sections), however, we were able to analyze the pulmonary arteries at the segmental level. Repeat Doppler US of the legs depicted a thrombus in the calf of three patients with normal results at helical CT that could have been responsible for the diagnosis of PE. At 3-month follow-up, three of 109 patients had experienced recurrent PE (one death, two recurrences). Therefore, initial helical CT results were found to be false-negative in six (5.4% [95% confidence interval, 1.3%, 9.7%]) of the 112 patients without PE at initial helical CT.

Table 2
Location of 147 Thrombi in 39 Patients with Abnormal Helical CT Results

Segmental Artery (A)	No. of Thrombi (n = 147) In Left Lung (N = 1,262)	In Right Lung (N = 1,298)
1	3 (2.0)	4 (2.7)
2	5 (3.4)	3 (2.0)
3	1 (0.7)	1 (0.7)
4	1 (0.7)	2 (1.4)
5	2 (1.4)	2 (1.4)
6	5 (3.4)	13 (8.8)
7	12 (8.2)	12 (8.2)
8	12 (8.2)	14 (9.5)
9	6 (4.1)	21 (14.3)
10	6 (4.1)	22 (15.0)
Total	53 (4.2)	94 (7.2)

Note.—Mean, 3.8 thrombi per patient. Numbers in parentheses are percentages.

DISCUSSION

This study was designed to assess the clinical accuracy of helical CT as a replacement for pulmonary angiography in patients with unresolved suspicion for PE because results at V-P scintigraphy indicate intermediate probability and duplex US of the legs did not show deep venous thrombosis. These patients account for about 30% of those clinically suspected of having acute PE who are evaluated with V-P scintigraphy and noninvasive venous studies; 20%–30% of them are seen to have acute PE at pulmonary angiography (19). Before deciding whether to treat these patients, the presence of clots in the pulmonary arteries must be confirmed or excluded.

Clinicians in our hospital, as in other institutions (10,11), are reluctant to prescribe pulmonary angiography. Therefore, treatment is often based on clinical probability of PE rather than on a definite diagnosis or ruling out of PE (3). Consequently, some patients receive anticoagulant drugs without proof of PE and other patients are not treated although they may have PE. In either situation, the chance for proper disease management may be lost. This clinical situation explains why we, as did others (12–14), chose to evaluate helical CT for the demonstration of clots in the pulmonary arteries in patients with theoretical indication for pulmonary angiography and why we did not perform pulmonary angiography systematically to compare results with the two techniques. Therefore, to validate our strategy that did not include pulmonary angiography in all patients, we assessed the outcome in a cohort of patients in whom the decision not to prescribe anticoagulant drugs was based on the absence of thrombus within the pulmonary arteries at helical CT. Our study included the most difficult cases to diagnose: patients with persistent unresolved clinical suspicion after V-P scintigraphy and duplex US of the legs.

Findings in our study confirmed that helical CT with 5-mm-thick sections and 2.5-mm interval reconstruction is limited in regard to depicting segmental pulmonary arteries. In the present study, 22% of the segmental arteries analyzed were inadequately demonstrated on axial scans. Our results are close to those of Teigen et al (20), who reported that 17% of segmental arteries were inadequately delineated on scans obtained with 6-mm-thick sections every 6 mm at electron-beam CT. The inability of helical CT with 5-mm-thick sections to show all the segmental arteries is the main limitation of our study because emboli located in segmental vessels could have been missed at helical CT. Helical CT depicted more than 85% of the segmental arteries A7–A10, however, where emboli are more likely to occur. Rémy-Jardin et al (17) used spiral CT with thinner 3- or 2-mm-thick sections to demonstrate the segmental arteries in 85% and 95%, respectively, of their study population. Scans obtained with thinner sections are particularly valuable to analyze segmental arteries in the axial or oblique planes, such as the right middle lobe and lingular segmental arteries, the anterior segmental arteries of the upper lobes, and the apical arteries of the lower lobes.

Our initial results showed that PE was diagnosed initially in 40 (24.4%) of the 164 patients with intermediate probability at V-P scintigraphy and normal results at duplex US. These results are similar to those of van Rooij et al (21), who found PE at digital pulmonary angiography in 51 (24.8%) of 206 patients who were clinically suspected of having PE but had normal results on sonograms of the legs. In the Prospective Investigation of PE Diagnosis (PIOPED) study (3), 22% of patients with nondiagnostic findings at V-P scintigraphy were found to have PE when examined with pulmonary angiography. Van Rossum et al (14) found a somewhat lower percentage of PE in patients with nondiagnostic findings at V-P scintigraphy (six [14%] of 42 patients). Evaluation of clinical probability in patients suspected of having PE offers a perspective: Among patients with a high clinical suspicion for PE, helical CT demonstrated PE in 33 (27%) of 123 patients but was positive for PE in only six (15%) of 41 patients with low clinical probability ($P < .02$). Pulmonary angiography is not performed in many institutions (10,11), however, and our initial results confirm that treatment decisions based on clinical probability in patients with unresolved suspicion at V-P scintigraphy are not reliable. Therefore, helical CT should be part of the diagnostic strategy in patients for whom pulmonary angiography would be recommended. In our study, PE was demonstrated at helical CT in 39 patients and at pulmonary angiography in one patient.

Our study was designed for routine clinical practice; therefore, pulmonary angiography was ordered by clinicians for only 15 (12.0%) of 125 patients with normal helical CT results. All patients who underwent pulmonary angiography (15 of 89) had a high clinical probability of PE. Femoral vein catheterization was responsible for one femoral thrombosis in a patient without PE. In one patient, pulmonary angiography demonstrated a thrombosis of the pulmonary artery that was not depicted at helical CT because of its subsegmental location, as we analyzed the pulmonary arteries up to only the segmental level. This situation illustrates one of the major limitations of helical CT. Thrombi within subsegmental vessels were better demonstrated with conventional angiography (22,23), although interobserver agreement is low, varying from 13% (24) to 66% (9) for the diagnosis of clots distal to segmental branches. Controversy exists concerning the frequency of subsegmental and isolated clots. In a recent report based on a retrospective analysis of pulmonary angiograms in patients with proved PE, Oser et al (25) found that 13 (17%) of 76 patients had isolated subsegmental clots and that PE would have been missed with helical CT. Goodman et al (13) found isolated subsegmental PE in four (36%) of 11 patients. Rémy-Jardin et al (22) found a lower incidence of subsegmental embolus (four [5%] of 75 patients), which supports the results of the PIOPED study (14 [5.6%] of 251 patients) (3). Moreover, the clinical importance of isolated subsegmental emboli remains controversial (1,26), although such emboli can be clinically important in patients with limited cardiopulmonary reserve. Among stable patients, as in those in this study, outcome is related to the risk of recurrence of PE. As we did not perform pulmonary angiography in all patients included in the study, we were limited in the immediate evaluation of subsegmental clots. Therefore, analysis of the outcome was of crucial importance in patients with negative results at helical CT and sonography of the legs in whom anticoagulant therapy was withdrawn (1,27).

One of the major advantages of helical CT over V-P scintigraphy is its ability to help evaluate the morphology of the mediastinum, the bronchial tree, the pleura, and the parenchyma. In our population, 18 (11%) patients had unequivocal abnormalities of lung parenchyma on initial helical CT scans that explained both the clinical presentation and the nondiagnostic results at V-P scintigraphy. Even though findings at chest radiography were abnormal in 15 of these patients, the clinical probability of PE remained sufficiently high to justify helical CT. As the results at helical CT were negative, treatment with anticoagulant drugs was not indicated. None of these patients experienced PE during the follow-up period. This ability of helical CT to help provide an immediate alternative diagnosis was emphasized by van Rossum et al (14), who found pleural or parenchymal abnormalities at helical CT that could explain defects seen at V-P scintigraphy in 24 (57%) of 42 patients with nondiagnostic findings at V-P scintigraphy. The difference in frequency could be explained by the fact that we considered abnormalities seen at helical CT that could explain both V-P scintigraphic findings and clinical presentation as alternative diagnoses.

Although findings at helical CT are highly accurate in the diagnosis of central PE, the precise place of helical CT in the diagnostic algorithm for PE remains to be defined. Because helical CT offers both greater specificity and greater sensitivity than V-P scintigraphy, helical CT might be used in place of V-P scintigraphy as a primary modality in the evaluation of PE (1,27). If so, normal results at helical CT would exclude PE, and a search for deep venous thrombosis would determine whether patients would be treated. If results at helical CT were positive for PE, treatment would be initiated. On the other hand, Gefter et al (27) suggested that helical CT might replace pulmonary angiography to evaluate clinically stable patients with nondiagnostic findings at V-P scintigraphy and negative results in deep venous thrombosis examinations.

To our knowledge, no prospective studies have been published that were performed to evaluate the clinical validity of use of results at helical CT to determine patient treatment. Our results show that replacement of pulmonary angiography with helical CT in the diagnosis of PE is safe: Among patients with negative results at helical CT, the absence of anticoagulant treatment was associated with a low incidence of later PE (three [2.8%] of 109 patients) during 3-month follow-up. However, we must emphasize that one patient died presumably of recurrent PE. PE occurred in two (3%) of 74 patients with high clinical probability of PE, as well as in one (3%) of 35 patients with low clinical probability. In addition to these three patients with late recurrence of PE, we must add three patients in whom findings at Doppler US repeated in the 48 hours after helical CT showed a thrombus in the calf. Then, six (5.4%) of 112 patients had false-negative findings at helical CT. This incidence is similar to that reported in follow-up studies that involved patients clinically suspected of having acute PE but without PE depicted at pulmonary angiography. These studies showed PE in 0.6%–4.2% of the patients during the year after pulmonary angiography (9,19,28–30). The original study data showed that during a 1-year follow-up in patients with negative results at pulmonary angiography, four (0.6%) of 681 patients experienced clinically recurrent PE (9). PE occurred in six (1.6%) of 380 patients followed up for 1 year in the series of Henry et al (28), in six (4.2%) of 144 patients followed up for an average of 13 months by Cheely et al (29), in one (2%) of 44 patients in the study of Hull et al (19), and in three (1.8%) of 167 untreated patients in the study of Novelline et al (30).

One of the limitations of our study could be the duration of follow-up, which was limited to 3 months. Several investigators (25,29) have found, however, that PE is more likely to occur in the 1st weeks after the initial clinical events. In the three patients who experienced recurrent PE, one recurrence was at 10 days after inclusion in the study, another at 8 weeks, and one at 12 weeks. Our results are close to those of Hull et al (31), who followed up 627 patients with nondiagnostic results at V-P scintigraphy and who did not take anticoagulant drugs because of negative results at serial impedance plethysmography on days 1, 3, 5–7, 10, and 14. Twelve (1.9% [95% confidence interval, 0.8%, 3%]) patients experienced venous thromboembolism during 3-month clinical follow-up. Helical CT was easy to implement, however, and allowed us to formulate an immediate diagnosis of PE, as well as an alternative diagnosis in 11% of the patients.

In a 1996 article, van Erkel et al (32) reported a cost-effectiveness analysis for 15 diagnostic strategies for PE, four of which included pulmonary angiography and eight of which included helical CT. Three outcome parameters were assessed: (*a*) mortality at 3 months (as a measure of effectiveness); (*b*) morbidity at 3 months (as a measure of effectiveness) based on the morbidity of helical CT (0.22%), angiography (1%), heparin treatment (10%), and Coumarin treatment (1.8%); and (*c*) the average realistic cost of diagnosis and therapy for PE. The diagnostic algorithm we used in this study was tested in that study and found to have (*a*) one of the lowest mortality rates, (*b*) one of the highest morbidity rates, and (*c*) lower expense than strategies that included pulmonary angiography. In our study, which was designed before the study of van Erkel et al was published, helical CT was implemented after V-P scintigraphy and duplex US because one of our main goals was to determine whether clinicians could reliably use helical CT, a noninvasive test, to replace pulmonary angiography (which is seldom prescribed in our institution) as a diagnostic tool in cases of inconclusive diagnosis of PE.

In conclusion, our results indicate that helical CT could replace pulmonary angiography as the technique to demonstrate thrombi within the pulmonary arteries in a majority of patients with intermediate probability at V-P scintigraphy and the absence of deep venous thrombosis in the legs. Helical CT is easy to implement, gives quick results, and can help provide alternative diagnoses. The outcome for patients without PE at helical CT during 3-month follow-up demonstrates the effectiveness of the technique, as the risk of recurrent PE was close to that of patients with suspected PE but with normal results at pulmonary angiography or at serial impedance plethysmography. Our experience indicates that pulmonary angiography should be reserved for use in patients in whom clinical suspicion for PE remains high despite normal results at helical CT and duplex sonography of the legs. ■

Acknowledgments: The authors thank Elisabeth Joubin for her help in conducting this study, Murielle Gousset for her statistical assistance, and Martine Rémy-Jardin, MD, PhD, for her critical review of the manuscript.

References

1. Goodman LR, Lipchik RJ. Diagnosis of acute pulmonary embolism: time for a new approach. Radiology 1996; 199:25–27.
2. Kelley MA, Carson JL, Palevsky HI, Schwartz JS. Diagnosing pulmonary embolism: new facts and strategies. Ann Intern Med 1991; 114: 300–306.
3. The PIOPED Investigators. Value of the ventilation/perfusion scan in acute pulmonary embolism: results of the Prospective Investigation of Pulmonary Embolism Diagnosis (PIOPED). JAMA 1990; 263:2753–2759.
4. Hull RD, Raskob GE, Pineo GF, Brant RF. The low-probability lung scan: a need for change in nomenclature. Arch Intern Med 1995; 155:1845–1851.
5. Cronan JJ. Venous thromboembolic disease: the role of US. Radiology 1993; 186:619–630.
6. Hull RD, Raskob GE, Coates G, Panju AA, Gill GJ. A new noninvasive management strategy for patients with suspected pulmonary embolism. Arch Intern Med 1989; 149:2549–2555.
7. Stein PD, Hull RD, Saltzman HA, Pineo G. Strategy for diagnosis of patients with suspected acute pulmonary embolism. Chest 1993; 103:1553–1559.
8. Moser KM. Venous thromboembolism. Am Rev Respir Dis 1990; 141:235–249.
9. Stein PD, Athanasoulis C, Alavi A, et al. Complications and validity of pulmonary angiography in acute pulmonary embolism. Circulation 1992; 85:462–468.
10. Sostman HD, Ravin CE, Sullivan DC, Mills SR, Glickman MG, Dorfman GS. Use of pulmonary angiography for suspected pulmonary embolism: influence of scintigraphic diagnosis. AJR 1982; 139:673–677.
11. Schluger N, Henschke C, King T, et al. Diagnosis of pulmonary embolism at a large teaching hospital. J Thorac Imaging 1994; 9:180–184.
12. Rémy-Jardin M, Rémy J, Wattinne L, Giraud F. Central pulmonary thromboembolism: diagnosis with spiral volumetric CT with the single-breath-hold technique—comparison with pulmonary angiography. Radiology 1992; 185:381–387.
13. Goodman LR, Curtin JJ, Mewissen MW, et al. Detection of pulmonary embolism in patients with unresolved clinical and scintigraphic diagnosis: helical CT versus angiography. AJR 1995; 164:1369–1374.
14. van Rossum AB, Treurniet FEE, Kieft GJ, Smith SJ, Schepers-Bok R. Role of spiral volumetric computed tomographic scanning in the assessment of patients with clinical suspicion of pulmonary embolism and an abnormal ventilation/perfusion lung scan. Thorax 1996; 51: 23–28.
15. Perrier A, Bounameaux H, Morabia A, et al. Contribution of D-dimer plasma measurement and lower-limb venous ultrasound to the diagnosis of pulmonary embolism: a decision analysis model. Am Heart J 1994; 127:624–635.
16. Alderson PO, Martin EC. Pulmonary embolism: diagnosis with multiple imaging modalities. Radiology 1987; 164:297–312.
17. Rémy-Jardin M, Rémy J, Artaud D, Deschildre F, Duhamel A. Peripheral pulmonary arteries: optimization of the spiral CT acquisition protocol. Radiology 1997; 204:157–163.
18. Sagel SS, Greenspan RH. Nonuniform pulmonary arterial perfusion: pulmonary embolism. Radiology 1971; 99:541–548.
19. Hull RD, Hirsh J, Carter CJ, et al. Pulmonary angiography, ventilation lung scanning, and venography for clinically suspected pulmonary embolism with abnormal perfusion lung scan. Ann Intern Med 1983; 98:891–899.
20. Teigen CL, Maus TP, Sheedy PF II, et al. Pulmonary embolism: diagnosis with contrast-enhanced electron-beam CT and comparison with pulmonary angiography. Radiology 1995; 194:313–319.
21. van Rooij WJ, den Heeten GJ, Sluzewski M. Pulmonary embolism: diagnosis in 211 patients with use of selective pulmonary digital subtraction angiography with a flow-directed catheter. Radiology 1995; 195:793–797.
22. Rémy-Jardin M, Rémy J, Deschildre F, et al. Diagnosis of pulmonary embolism with spiral CT: comparison with pulmonary angiography and scintigraphy. Radiology 1996; 200:699–706.
23. van Rossum AB, Pattynama PMT, Ton ERTA, et al. Pulmonary embolism: validation of spiral CT angiography in 149 patients. Radiology 1996; 201:467–470.
24. Quinn MF, Lundell CJ, Klotz TA, et al. Reliability of selective pulmonary arteriography in the diagnosis of pulmonary embolism. AJR 1987; 149:469–471.
25. Oser RF, Zuckerman DA, Gutierrez FR, Brink JA. Anatomic distribution of pulmonary emboli at pulmonary angiography: implications for cross-sectional imaging. Radiology 1996; 199:31–35.
26. Gurney JW. No fooling around: direct visualization of pulmonary embolism (editorial). Radiology 1993; 188:618–619.
27. Gefter WB, Hatabu H, Holland GA, Gupta KB, Henschke CI, Palevsky HI. Pulmonary thromboembolism: recent developments in diagnosis with CT and MR imaging. Radiology 1995; 197:561–574.
28. Henry JW, Relyea B, Stein PD. Continuing risk of thromboemboli among patients with normal pulmonary angiograms. Chest 1995; 107:1375–1378.
29. Cheely R, McCartney WH, Perry JR, et al. The role of noninvasive tests versus pulmonary angiography in the diagnosis of pulmonary embolism. Am J Med 1981; 70:17–22.
30. Novelline RA, Baltarowich OH, Athanasoulis CA, Waltman AC, Greenfield AJ, McKusick KA. The clinical course of patients with suspected pulmonary embolism and a negative pulmonary arteriogram. Radiology 1978; 126: 561–567.
31. Hull RD, Raskob GE, Ginsberg JS, et al. A noninvasive strategy for the treatment of patients with suspected pulmonary embolism. Arch Intern Med 1994; 154:289–297.
32. van Erkel AR, van Rossum AB, Bloem JL, Kievit J, Pattynama PMT. Spiral CT angiography for suspected pulmonary embolism: a cost-effectiveness analysis. Radiology 1996; 201:29–36.

Sandro Morassut, MD • Emanuela Vaccher, MD • Luca Balestreri, MD • Annunziata Gloghini, PhD
Gianluca Gaidano, MD, PhD • Rachele Volpe, MD • Umberto Tirelli, MD • Antonino Carbone, MD

HIV-associated Human Herpesvirus 8–Positive Primary Lymphomatous Effusions: Radiologic Findings in Six Patients[1]

PURPOSE: **To define the imaging features of body cavity–based lymphoma (BCBL) related to the acquired immunodeficiency syndrome. This is a peculiar type of non-Hodgkin lymphoma harboring infection by human herpesvirus 8 (HHV-8) and displaying a peculiar tropism for the serous body cavities.**

MATERIALS AND METHODS: **At diagnosis of BCBL, six consecutive patients were investigated with radiography of the chest and conventional computed tomography (CT) of the chest and abdomen. For all patients, clinical features and results of biologic characterization of the lymphoma were also available.**

RESULTS: **In all patients, chest radiographs displayed bilateral or unilateral pleural effusion in the absence of parenchymal opacities or mediastinal enlargement. CT scans confirmed chest radiographic findings and revealed a slight thickening of the parietal pleura in all patients and a pericardial thickening in four patients. CT also depicted pericardial and abdominal effusions in five and two patients, respectively, in the absence of solid tumor masses or parenchymal abnormalities.**

CONCLUSION: **BCBL must be included among the differential diagnoses of serous effusions detected radiologically in individuals infected with the human immunodeficiency virus (HIV). Since the combination of serous effusion, slight serosal thickening, and absence of solid masses is compatible with, though not specific for, BCBL in the context of HIV infection, radiologic findings need to be complemented by a detailed biologic and virologic characterization of tumor cells.**

The broad category of lymphomas that involve the serous body cavities comprises all non-Hodgkin lymphomas (NHLs) associated with a malignant effusion. NHLs that manifest in the serous body cavities in the absence of clinically identifiable tumor masses are defined as primary lymphomatous effusions, whereas secondary lymphomatous effusions represent malignant effusions that complicate a clinically evident solid NHL through contiguous spread of tumor cells into the body cavities (1).

Recently, both in the United States and Europe, a peculiar type of primary lymphomatous effusion has been recognized as an individual entity on the basis of its distinctive biologic features and its consistent infection by a novel member of the herpesvirus family—human herpesvirus 8 (HHV-8) (2–6). Because of its peculiar and predominant tropism for the serous cavities of the body, this type of B-cell NHL has been provisionally designated "body cavity–based lymphoma" (BCBL). In the United States, BCBL has also been termed *primary effusion lymphoma* (5).

The epidemiology of BCBL is peculiar, since this lymphoma is found preferentially, though not exclusively, in association with human immunodeficiency virus (HIV) infection (3–5). At the clinical level, BCBL displays a marked production of fluid with tumor cellularity in the serous cavities of the body and usually occurs without any identifiable tumor mass (1–3,5–11). At the pathologic level, however, the basic feature of BCBL is a striking predilection for diffuse spreading along the serous membranes without infiltrative or destructive growth patterns (1,12).

Although the clinical features of BCBL, as well as its immunophenotypic and molecular characteristics, have been clarified to a certain extent, little is known about the specific imaging findings of this NHL. Indeed, to our knowledge, for all cases reported in the literature so far detailed imaging information is lacking.

We have observed eight cases of HIV-associated HHV-8–positive BCBL over a 7-year period. In six of these cases, a complete clinical staging for NHL was performed and complete imaging data were available. In this study, we wished to define the spectrum of imaging findings detected in these six patients and to assess the potential utility of radiology for the diagnosis of BCBL.

Index terms: Acquired immunodeficiency syndrome (AIDS), 60.2518, 70.2068, 80.2068 • Lymphoma, AIDS-related, 60.3439, 70.3439, 80.3439 • Pericardium, fluid, 55.6991 • Peritoneum, fluid, 791.77 • Pleura, fluid, 66.76 • Pleura, neoplasms, 66.329

Abbreviations: AIDS = acquired immunodeficiency syndrome, BCBL = body cavity–based lymphoma, HHV-8 = human herpesvirus 8, HIV = human immunodeficiency virus, NHL = non-Hodgkin lymphoma.

Radiology 1997; 205:459–463

[1] From the Departments of Radiology (S.M., L.B.), Medical Oncology and AIDS Program (E.V., U.T.), and Pathology (A.G., R.V., A.C.), Centro di Riferimento Oncologico, Istituto Nazionale di Ricovero e Cura a Carattere Scientifico, Via Pedemontana Occidentale 12, 33081 Aviano (PN), Italy; and the Division of Internal Medicine, Department of Medical Sciences, University of Torino at Novara, Italy (G.G.). Received May 9, 1997; revision requested June 19; revision received July 10; accepted July 14. Supported by grants from Ministero della Sanità, Ricerca Finalizzata IRCCS, Rome, Italy; Associazione Italiana per la Ricerca sul Cancro, Milan, Italy; IX Progetto AIDS, ISS, Rome, Italy (grants 9404-33 and 9404-04); and from Fondazione Piera, Pietro e Giovanni Ferrero, Alba, Italy. **Address reprint requests to** S.M.

Table 1
Clinical Characteristics and Findings at Chest Radiography and Body CT in Six Patients with HHV-8–Positive BCBL

Patient No./Sex/Age (y)	Radiologic Findings (Initial Presentation)*: Pleural Effusion	Unilateral Pleural Thickening	Diffuse Pleural Thickening	Pericardial Thickening and Effusion	Peritoneal Effusion	Treatment	Response to Treatment	Survival (mo)	Outcome†
1/M/27	Unilateral	+	−	+	−	Chemotherapy	Not able to evaluate	4	Dead
2/M/34	Bilateral	+	−	−	−	Chemotherapy	Not able to evaluate	4	Dead
3/M/44	Bilateral	−	+	+	−	Chemotherapy	Progressive disease (myocardium, meninges)	6	Dead
4/M/49	Unilateral	+	−	−	+ moderate	None	. . .	1	Dead
5/M/35	Unilateral	+	−	+	−	None	. . .	2+	Alive
6/M/42	Bilateral	+	−	+	+ severe	None	. . .	2+	Alive

* + = present, − = absent.
† Cause of death was NHL in patients 1, 2, and 4 and toxicity in patient 3.

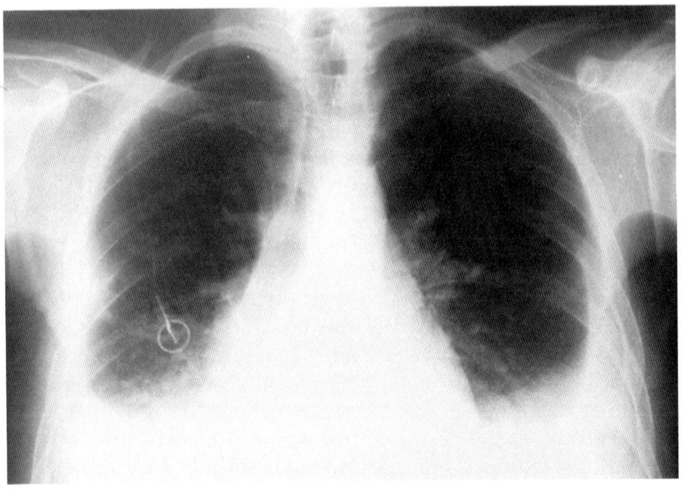

1.

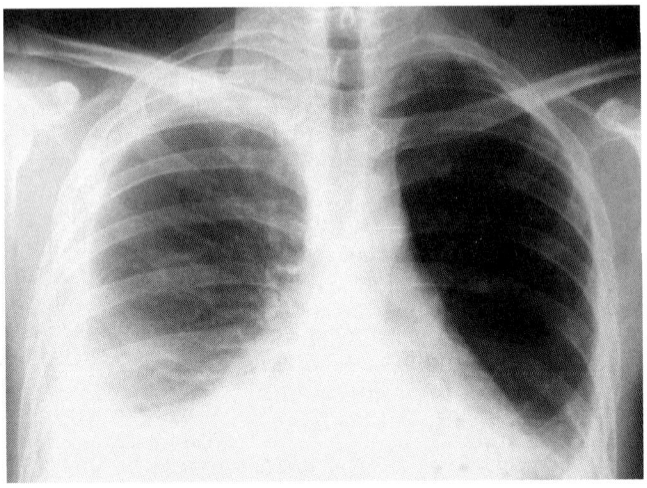

2.

Figures 1, 2. **(1) Patient 2.** Chest radiograph obtained in the upright position demonstrates bilateral pleural effusions. Neither mediastinal nor parenchymal abnormalities are detectable. **(2) Patient 3.** Chest radiograph obtained with the patient in supine position shows a large amount of free pleural effusion in the right hemithorax and small fluid on the left. The lungs and the mediastinum appear normal.

MATERIALS AND METHODS

For our retrospective review, the following criteria were used to identify cases of BCBL among lymphomatous effusions: (*a*) absence of identifiable tumor masses in the body cavities and (*b*) absence of systemic or nodal disease at initial examination. These imaging criteria were used in conjunction with the phenotypic and molecular characteristics of effusion lymphoma cells according to Nador et al (5). This study is based on six cases of HIV-associated B-cell NHL manifesting as lymphomatous effusions at diagnosis. According to the aforementioned criteria, these cases were classified as HHV-8–positive BCBL. All cases were consecutively observed at a single institution between October 1989 and March 1997. During the same period, 157 consecutive patients with HIV infection and systemic, diffuse, large cell and high-grade NHL were evaluated at the same center.

All six patients included in this study were evaluated with radiography of the chest and with conventional computed tomography (CT) of the chest and abdomen typically with 10-mm sections at 10-mm intervals before and during intravenous infusion of iodinated contrast medium (iopamidol, Iopamiron 300; Bracco, Milan, Italy). For interpretation of the chest CT scans, the imaging criteria used were circumferential pleural thickening, nodular pleural thickening, and mediastinal pleural involvement, as suggested by Müller (13). Abdominal CT investigation focused on lymphadenopathy, splenic or hepatic focal lesions, extranodal masses, and bowel involvement, according to Nyberg et al (14).

The Centers for Disease Control and Prevention revised classification system for HIV infection was used (15). As suggested by the World Health Organization, diagnosis of acquired immunodeficiency syndrome (AIDS) was performed according to clinical criteria of the Centers for Disease Control and Prevention (16). CD4+ cell count at the time of diagnosis was determined with flow cytometry. Necropsy was performed in one patient (patient 4).

Samples of lymphomatous effusions were collected under sterile conditions during standard diagnostic procedures. After centrifugation, the effusion sediments were used to prepare smears and cell blocks. For morphologic studies, cytospin preparations were routinely fixed and stained according to the Papanicolaou method. For cell block preparations (17), cell pellets were fixed in Bouin fluid and treated according to a standard regimen used in the division of pathology. The sectioned material from cell blocks was stained with hematoxylin-eosin. In all cases, the cytospin preparations and cell blocks showed a tumor cell population of 95% or greater as evaluated with morphologic and immunophenotypic analysis.

All samples were also subjected to immunophenotypic and immunogenotypic characterization, as well as determination of tumor infection by Epstein-Barr virus and HHV-8, according to previously reported strategies (3,18,19). The immunophenotypic and molecular results of some of the cases included in the present study have been described previously (3). In particular, four of the six patients with BCBL (patients 1–4) have been included in previous studies (3,19).

RESULTS

Clinical Features

The age range of the patients with BCBL was 27–49 years (Table 1). Risk membranes, including the omentum and the outer parts of the gastrointestinal tract wall, was noticed. Retroperitoneal lymph nodes were also involved by lymphoma. Tumor masses, however, were absent.

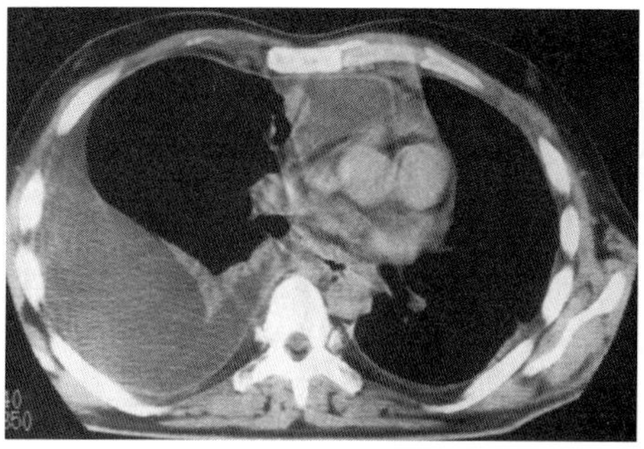

3.

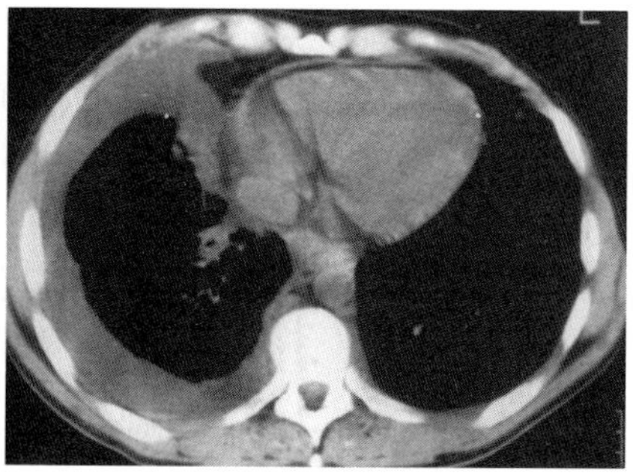

4.

Figures 3, 4. **(3) Patient 3.** Contrast material–enhanced CT scan obtained in the same patient as in Figure 2 confirms the large fluid collection and retrosternal loculated effusion in the right hemithorax and small effusion on the left. Diffuse smooth thickening of the parietal pleura is visible on both side. **(4) Patient 5.** CT scan of the thorax demonstrates discrete pleural effusion extending anteriorly. The underlying parietal pleura and the right pericardium are slightly thickened.

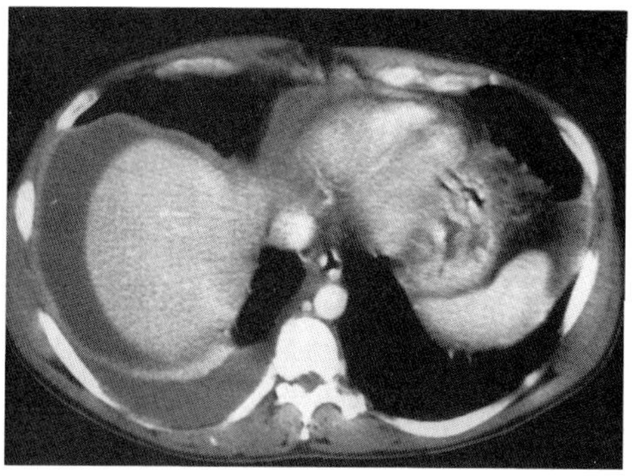

5.

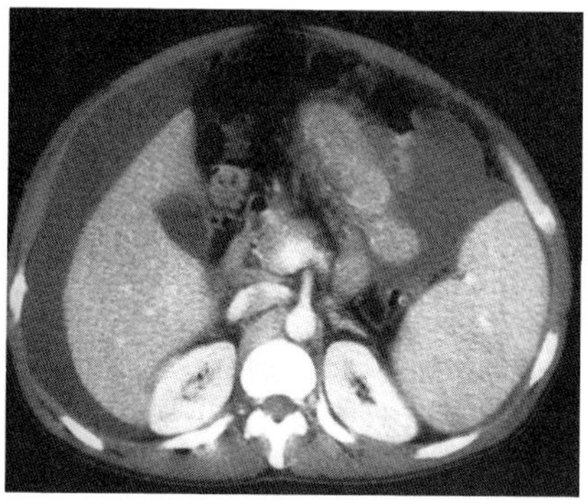

6.

Figures 5, 6. **Patient 6. (5)** Contrast-enhanced CT scan shows pleural and pericardial effusions along with ascites. The right hemidiaphragm and the anterior portion of the pericardium are moderately thickened. **(6)** CT section obtained more caudally in the same patient confirms a large amount of ascites. No peritoneal thickening is detectable. No tumor masses or parenchymal abnormalities are seen.

factors for HIV infection were intravenous drug use in three patients, homosexuality in two patients, and both factors in one patient. At diagnosis of lymphoma, two patients had Kaposi sarcoma and one of these two patients (patient 5) had concomitant intrathoracic Kaposi sarcoma disease. Pleural lymphomatous effusion was diagnosed in concomitance with *Pneumocystis carinii* pneumonia in one patient (patient 2). The median CD4+ cell count was 48/µL (range, 2–206/µL).

Clinical symptoms at presentation included fever (six patients); cough, chest pain, and dyspnea (five patients); and abdominal pain (one patient). The lag time between initial symptoms and diagnosis of lymphoma was 10, 2, and 11 months, respectively, for the first three patients evaluated from 1989 to 1993; for the other 3 patients evaluated in more recent years (1996–1997), lag time between initial symptoms and diagnosis of lymphoma was only 1 month.

In all BCBL patients, the lymphoma manifested exclusively (patients 1, 2, 4, 5, 6) or predominantly (patient 3) as a malignant effusion (Table 1). In the latter patient, localization of a lymphoma in the soft tissues of the neck was also found at diagnosis. In this same patient, systemic lymph node involvement was ruled out at both physical and radiologic examinations. This patient showed extension to contiguous visceral and distant sites during the course of the disease. In the other five BCBL patients, the lymphoma remained confined to body cavities.

Overall, the clinical outcome was poor (Table 1). Four patients died (patients 1–4). In three of them (patients 1, 2, and 4), the cause of death was attributed to tumor progression. Autopsy was performed in one patient (patient 4). At autopsy, the lymphoma manifested as multiple small tumor foci involving the serous membranes, which appeared irregularly thickened. It was difficult to define whether the neoplasm had originated in the pleura, pericardium, or peritoneum. Extension into tissue underlying the serous

Radiologic Findings

The imaging findings of chest radiography and CT are summarized in Table 1.

In all six BCBL patients, bilateral or unilateral pleural effusion was evident on chest radiographs and no parenchymal opacities or mediastinal enlargement was detectable (Figs 1, 2).

CT scans confirmed the presence of the pleural effusions and helped rule out the occurrence of solid lymphomatous masses within the lungs, mediastinum, or thoracic wall. No plaquelike or nodular thickening of the pleura was visible, although a unilateral or diffuse slight thickening of the parietal pleura was noticed in all patients (Figs 3–5). Extrapleural subcostal tissues had attenuation values within normal range.

A pericardial thickening with a small amount of pericardial effusion was detectable on CT scans in four patients (patients 1, 3, 5, 6) (Figs 4, 5).

Abdominal CT scans showed different degrees of peritoneal effusion in two patients (patients 4, 6): One patient (patient 4) had a small amount of peritoneal fluid, whereas severe ascites affected the other patient (patient 6). No peritoneal thickening was visible at CT. In all cases, there was no evidence of abdominal masses or liver cirrhosis (Figs 5, 6).

One patient (patient 3) had slight retroperitoneal nodal enlargement (1.0–1.5 cm); another patient (patient 6) displayed splenomegaly with homogeneous attenuation of the parenchyma.

Biologic Characterization of Lymphomatous Effusions

All BCBL were composed of large neoplastic cells with abundant cytoplasm, and irregularly shaped, variably chromatic and pleomorphic nuclei. The main immunophenotypic and viral features of the patient samples of lymphomatous effusions included in this study are summarized in Table 2. Briefly, all lymphomatous effusions were B-cell monoclonal proliferations as derived from immunophenotypic and/or immunogenotypic studies. Infection of the tumor clone by Epstein-Barr virus was identified in three patients with BCBL (patients 1, 4, 5), whereas infection by HHV-8 was detected in all cases (Table 2) by means of conventional polymerase chain reaction and in situ hybridization.

DISCUSSION

Secondary lymphomatous effusions may represent one of the localizations of systemic NHL or they may occur as a complication of NHLs that originate in extranodal sites and are strictly localized to the body cavities (1). Although less frequent than secondary lymphomatous effusions (3,5), primary lymphomatous effusions represent a distinct subset of NHL characterized by exclusive or predominant involvement of the serous body cavities throughout the entire course of the disease (2,3,5,8). Among primary effusions, the diagnosis of BCBL depends on special techniques such as immunocytohistochemical studies and molecular analyses, since the malignant cells in this disease are selectively infected by HHV-8 and typically lack c-*MYC* rearrangements and other known genetic lesions (2–4,8,10–12,20). Recently, autopsy studies have demonstrated that the basic pathologic feature of BCBL is a lymphomatous infiltration of serosal surfaces adjacent to the site of primary malignant effusion (1,12,19). At the clinical level, however, the correlative imaging findings of the basic anatomic pathologic findings of the disease have not been documented, to our knowledge.

Our evaluation of BCBL is limited by the rarity of the disease and the retrospective nature of this study. To our knowledge, however, our group of six patients constitutes the largest single series of patients for whom complete and detailed imaging information has been presented. Notably, in these patients with clinically, cytologically, phenotypically, and molecularly proved HHV-8–positive BCBL, we observed a common pattern of radiologic findings at initial examination. Review of our imaging studies showed pleural and pericardial or peritoneal effusions in the absence of tumor masses and node- or tissue-based lymphoma. In addition, slight pleural and pericardial thickening was a consistent imaging finding. Thus, the combination of serous effusion, slight serosal thickening, and absence of solid masses may be compatible with BCBL in the context of HIV infection.

Although these findings are not specific for a diagnosis of lymphoma, the presence of an isolated serosal effusion in an HIV-positive patient has a limited differential diagnosis (21–24) if infectious diseases are excluded. Kaposi sarcoma may be complicated by an effusion, but, like systemic NHL, these effusions are accompanied by parenchymal infiltrates (25,26). Moreover, on CT scans, systemic NHL involving the body cavities can manifest as plaquelike or nodular serosal thickening or as large serosal-based masses, in addition to the finding of different degrees of serous effusion (27).

Table 2
Phenotypic and Viral Features of Tumor Cells in Six Patients with HHV-8–Positive BCBL

Patient No.	Phenotype*	HIV Status†	EBV‡	HHV-8 ‡
1	B	+	+	+
2	Indeterminate	+	−	+
3	Indeterminate	+	−	+
4	Indeterminate	+	+	+
5	Indeterminate	+	+	+
6	Indeterminate	+	−	+

Note.—+ = positive, − = negative.
* Indeterminate phenotype was attributed to cases lacking antigens restricted to the B-cell and T-cell lineage.
† Host HIV status as defined by standard serologic assays.
‡ EBV = Epstein-Barr virus. Tumor cell infection as defined by a combination of in situ hybridization, Southern blot analysis, and polymerase chain reaction studies.

In addition to the diseases reported above, BCBL should also be differentiated from the cases of HIV-related lymphomatosis of the serous cavities described by Lynch et al (28). Both entities are relatively rare. BCBL represents approximately 3% of HIV-associated NHLs in southern Europe (3). Although the precise frequency of peritoneal lymphomatosis in AIDS patients has not been defined, it has been reported to be uncommon (28). Both BCBL and lymphomatosis of the serous cavities are associated with the presence of serous effusion; however, several features, including both radiologic and clinicopathologic aspects, may help to distinguish these two disorders. First, cases of lymphomatosis of the serous cavities described by Lynch et al (28) are associated with radiologic findings of peritoneal nodules and omental masses, whereas cases of BCBL are generally devoid of nodules or masses in the involved serous cavity. Second, effusion samples are generally negative for lymphoma in cases of lymphomatosis of the serous cavities, consistent with the solid growth pattern of these disorders. Consequently, surgery or guided needle aspiration is required for diagnosis of lymphomatosis of the serous cavities. Conversely, in the instance of BCBL, effusion samples are positive for tumor cells in all cases, consistent with the liquid phase growth pattern typical of BCBL. Finally, lymphomatosis of the serous cavities is morphologically heterogeneous encompassing the main histologic subtypes of systemic HIV-associated NHL, whereas BCBL represents a morphologically homogeneous group of lymphomas.

In conclusion, according to the findings of the present study, BCBL is associated with the following peculiar imaging features: (*a*) bilateral or unilateral pleural effusions, usually associated with pericardial effusion; (*b*) normal mediastinal and parenchymal imaging findings; and (*c*) slight serosal surface thickening at CT. Overall, these features would indicate a primary serous membrane neoplasm. Notably, these aspects correlate closely with anatomic pathologic findings of BCBL observed at autopsy in this and previous studies (12). Thus, the aforementioned clinical and gross pathologic features suggest that BCBL is a lymphoma of the serous membranes typically giving rise to lymphomatous effusions without mass formation. According to the results of this retrospective study, imaging patterns are identified that should lead to the inclusion of BCBL in the differential diagnosis of serous effusions, thus mandating the application of specific molecular and biologic techniques to the tumor samples to ensure accurate diagnosis and optimal clinical management. ■

References

1. Carbone A, Gaidano G. HHV-8-positive body cavity–based lymphoma: a novel lymphoma entity. Br J Haematol 1997; 97: 515–522.
2. Cesarman E, Chang Y, Moore PS, Said JW, Knowles DM. Kaposi's sarcoma–associated herpesvirus-like DNA sequences in AIDS-related body cavity–based lymphomas. N Engl J Med 1995; 332:1186–1191.
3. Carbone A, Gloghini A, Vaccher E, et al. Kaposi's sarcoma–associated herpesvirus DNA sequences in AIDS-related and AIDS-

unrelated lymphomatous effusions. Br J Haematol 1996; 94:533–543.
4. Nador RG, Cesarman E, Knowles DM, Said JW. Herpes-like DNA sequences in a body cavity–based lymphoma in an HIV-negative patient (letter). N Engl J Med 1995; 333: 943.
5. Nador RG, Cesarman E, Chadburn A, et al. Primary effusion lymphoma: a distinct clinicopathologic entity associated with the Kaposi's sarcoma–associated herpes virus. Blood 1996; 88:645–656.
6. Said JW, Tasaka T, Takeuchi S, et al. Primary effusion lymphoma in women: report of two cases of Kaposi's sarcoma herpes virus–associated effusion-based lymphoma in human immunodeficiency virus–negative women. Blood 1996; 88:3124–3128.
7. Said JW, Chien K, Tasaka T, et al. Kaposi's sarcoma–associated herpesvirus (KSHV or HHV8) in primary effusion lymphomas: ultrastructural demonstration of herpesvirus in lymphoma cell lines. Blood 1996; 87: 4937–4943.
8. Ansari MQ, Dawson DB, Nador R, et al. Primary body cavity–based AIDS-related lymphomas. Am J Pathol 1996; 105:221–229.
9. Cesarman E, Nador RG, Aozasa K, Delsol G, Said JW, Knowles DM. Kaposi's sarcoma–associated herpesvirus in non-AIDS–related lymphomas occurring in the body cavities. Am J Pathol 1996; 149:53–57.
10. Gaidano G, Pastore C, Gloghini A, et al. Distribution of human herpesvirus-8 sequences throughout the spectrum of AIDS-related neoplasia. AIDS 1996; 10:941–949.
11. Jaffe ES. Primary body cavity–based AIDS-related lymphomas: evolution of a new disease entity. Am J Clin Pathol 1996; 105:141–143.
12. Komanduri KV, Luce JA, McGrath MS, Herndier BG, Ng VL. The natural history and molecular heterogeneity of HIV-associated primary malignant lymphomatous effusions. J Acquir Immune Defic Syndr 1996; 13:215–226.
13. Müller NL. Imaging of the pleura. Radiology 1993; 186:297–309.
14. Nyberg DA, Jeffery RB, Federle MP, Bottles K, Abrams DI. AIDS-related lymphomas: evaluation by abdominal CT. Radiology 1986; 159:59–63.
15. Centers for Disease Control and Prevention. 1993 revision classification system for HIV infection and expanded surveillance case definition for AIDS among adolescents and adults. Morbidity Mortality Weekly Rep 1992; 41(RR-17):1–19.
16. Ancelle-Park R, Kleni JP, Stroobant A, et al. Expanded European AIDS case definition (letter). Lancet 1993; 341:441.
17. Naylor B. Pleural, peritoneal and pericardial fluids. In Bibbo M, ed. Comprehensive cytopathology. Philadelphia, Pa: Saunders, 1991; 541.
18. Chang Y, Cesarman E, Pessin MS, et al. Identification of herpesvirus-like DNA sequences in AIDS-associated Kaposi's sarcoma. Science 1994; 266:1865–1869.
19. Carbone A, Cilia AM, Gloghini A, et al. Establishment of HHV-8 positive and HHV-8 negative lymphoma cell lines from primary lymphomatous effusions. Int J Cancer (in press).
20. Knowles DM, Inghirami G, Ubriaco A, Dalla-Favera R. Molecular genetic analysis of three AIDS-associated neoplasms of uncertain lineage demonstrates their B-cell derivation and the possible pathogenetic role of Epstein-Barr virus. Blood 1989; 73: 792–799.
21. Sider L, Horton ES. Pleural effusion as a presentation of AIDS-related lymphoma. Invest Radiol 1989; 24:150–153.
22. Joseph J, Strange C, Sahn SA. Pleural effusions in hospitalized patients with AIDS. Ann Intern Med 1993; 118:856–859.
23. Marchevsky A, Rosen MJ, Chrystal G, Kleinerman J. Pulmonary complications of the acquired immunodeficiency syndrome: a clinicopathologic study of 70 cases. Hum Pathol 1985; 16:659–670.
24. Malatskey A, Fields S, Libson E. CT appearance of primary pleural lymphoma. Comput Med Imaging Graph 1989; 13:165–167.
25. Cohen BA, Pomeranz S, Rabinowitz JG, et al. Pulmonary complications of AIDS: readiologic features. AJR 1984; 143:115–122.
26. Ognibene FP, Steis RG, Macher AM, et al. Kaposi's sarcoma causing pulmonary infiltrates and respiratory failure in the acquired immunodeficiency syndrome. Ann Intern Med 1985; 102:471–475.
27. Shuman LS, Libshitz HI. Solid pleural manifestations of lymphoma. AJR 1984; 142:269–273.
28. Lynch MA, Cho KC, Jeffrey RB Jr, Alterman DD, Federle MP. CT of peritoneal lymphomatosis. AJR 1988; 151:713–715.

Book Review

Kinderradiologie [Pediatric Radiology]

Edited by Gabriele Benz-Bohm, MD

Stuttgart, Germany: Thieme Verlag, 1997. ISBN 3-13-107491-4. Cloth, DM 148; pp 286; 356 figures.

Only an editor with insight, organizational skills, and influence could have produced such a fine distillation of the latest knowledge of medical imaging in the child. Congratulations, Professor Benz-Bohm. In *Kinderradiologie*, the talents of many leading German-speaking pediatric radiologists have been harnessed; the book offers a compact discussion of what the general radiologist should know in this specialized area of pediatrics.

In his chapter on technique and radiation protection, Karl Schneider, MD, provides useful lists of unnecessary examinations (this information is repeated elsewhere in the book) and practical hints for radiation reduction. The chapter on anatomic findings in the newborn and infant by Ernst Richter, MD, is full of important facts, which will likely be surprising to the nonpediatric radiologist; here, several important examples of the fine illustrations from Dr Richter's regrettably out-of-print, classic large book of 1990 are presented. In his chapter on the skull, his important insights continue. The chapter on skeletal abnormalities by Helmut Kemperdick, MD, is a nice précis of the most important findings of the most important dysplasias. Herbert Glöbl, MD, defends, in his chapter on the chest, the routine use of only one view of the chest except in special circumstances. In his chapter on gastrointestinal disorders, A. E. Horwitz, MD, gives ultrasound a primary role in the evaluation of many conditions. Brigitte Stöver, MD, Heinz Tschäppeler, MD, and Reinhard Schulz, MD, nicely discuss magnetic resonance imaging, computed tomography, and sonography, respectively, and consider which modality is most appropriate. Dr Benz-Bohm's teacher, Eberhard Willich, MD, succinctly emphasizes the thymus in his chapter on the mediastinum.

Throughout the book, the choice and reproduction of images are first-class. The German-language text is easy to follow and, incidentally, peppered with English words used everyday by the German pediatric radiologist. Because the text is brief and didactic, there is little contrary opinion. (For example, I missed the corkscrew sign of midgut volvulus on the upper gastrointestinal examination, and I would not classify Scheuermann disease as an osteochondrosis.) The line drawings (with the exception of the drawing on page 94 of the trachea buckling) by Christine Opfermann-Rüngeler are helpful. The one glaring omission of the book is the topic of torsion of the testis or ovary, which are important disorders in emergency pediatric radiologic practice. Cross-references between chapters, without unnecessary duplication, are handled nicely.

A unique book, *Kinderradiologie* succeeds as an up-to-date, short presentation of pertinent issues in pediatric radiology.

Reviewed by Alan E. Oestreich, MD

Sylvia A. Worthy, MRCP, FRCR • Nestor L. Müller, MD, PhD • Thomas E. Hartman, MD
Stephen J. Swensen, MD • Simon P. G. Padley, MRCP, FRCR
David M. Hansell, MRCP, FRCR

Mosaic Attenuation Pattern on Thin-Section CT Scans of the Lung: Differentiation among Infiltrative Lung, Airway, and Vascular Diseases as a Cause[1]

PURPOSE: **To determine whether infiltrative lung, airway, or vascular disease can be differentiated as the cause of mosaic attenuation on thin-section computed tomographic (CT) scans of the lung.**

MATERIALS AND METHODS: **Thin-section CT scans were reviewed in 70 patients examined at three institutions. A mosaic attenuation pattern and pathologic or clinical proof of a specific type of disease were demonstrated. Causes of the mosaic pattern included infiltrative lung disease (n = 37), airway disease (n = 22), and vascular disease (n = 11). Thin-section CT findings were assessed independently by two observers blinded to clinical findings.**

RESULTS: **The type of disease was identified correctly at CT in 58 (83%) of 70 patients by observer 1 and 57 (81%) of 70 patients by observer 2. Infiltrative lung disease was diagnosed correctly by both observers in 34 (92%) of 37 cases. Observer 1 identified 21 (95%) of 22 cases of airway disease and three (27%) of 11 cases of vascular disease. Observer 2 identified 19 (86%) of 22 cases of airway disease and four (36%) of 11 cases of vascular disease.**

CONCLUSION: **Infiltrative lung disease and airway disease may be differentiated reliably as the cause of mosaic attenuation on lung CT scans, whereas vascular disease is often misinterpreted as infiltrative lung disease or airway disease.**

A mosaic pattern of attenuation, with patchy areas of increased and decreased attenuation, is nonspecific and may be seen on thin-section computed tomographic (CT) scans of the lungs when various infiltrative lung, airway, or vascular diseases are present. When this pattern is caused by regional differences in perfusion due to vascular diseases, it is also known as mosaic perfusion (1) or mosaic oligemia (2). In cases of infiltrative lung disease, mosaic attenuation results from patchy areas of ground-glass attenuation and interposed normal lung parenchyma. In cases of airway disease, the mosaic pattern results from reflex vasoconstriction secondary to hypoventilation of alveoli distal to airway obstruction and blood flow redistribution to adjacent normal areas of lung. Air trapping in the abnormal lung may also contribute to the reduced attenuation.

It has been suggested that these three categories of disease that cause a mosaic attenuation pattern can be distinguished on the basis of thin-section CT findings (3). To our knowledge, however, no study has been performed previously to determine the diagnostic accuracy with thin-section CT in this setting.

The purpose of this study was to determine whether infiltrative, airway, or vascular lung disease can be differentiated as the cause of mosaic attenuation on thin-section CT scans of the lung.

MATERIALS AND METHODS

The retrospective study included 70 patients with a pattern of mosaic lung attenuation on thin-section CT scans. The 36 women and 34 men ranged in age from 30 to 81 years (median age, 55 years). The study population included consecutive patients in whom a pattern of mosaic attenuation was identified on thin-section CT scans and pathologic or clinical proof of one of the three types of disease was obtained at one of three institutions over the preceding 3 years (July 1993 to June 1996). Initial patient selection was based on a radiology database search, which included cases in which findings of areas of ground-glass attenuation, areas of decreased attenuation, airway disease, or vascular disease were reported. Only patients in whom mosaic attenuation was found on CT scans were included in the study. Patients with diffuse ground-glass attenuation or with associated fibrosis were excluded.

Of the 70 patients, 37 had chronic infiltrative lung disease, 22 had airway disease, and 11 had vascular disease (Table 1). The type of disease was confirmed at biopsy in all 37 patients with chronic infiltrative lung disease (open lung biopsy or video-assisted thoracoscopic biopsy in 32 patients and transbronchial biopsy in five patients), in 12 patients with bronchiolitis obliterans (open lung biopsy in four patients and transbronchial biopsy in eight patients), and in the three patients with pulmonary veno-occlusive disease and the one patient with polyarteritis nodosa (open lung biopsy in all four of these patients). All cases of chronic pulmonary thromboembolism and pulmonary arterial hypertension were proved angiographically.

In all other patients, the diagnosis was

Index terms: Bronchiolitis obliterans, 60.2191 • Lung, CT, 60.12118 • Lung, diseases, 60.2191, 60.6113, 60.62, 60.635 • Lung, interstitial disease, 60.6113 • Lung, vascular disease, 60.6123

Radiology 1997; 205:465–470

[1] From the Department of Radiology, Vancouver Hospital and Health Sciences Centre and University of British Columbia, 855 W 12th Ave, Vancouver, British Columbia, Canada V5Z 1M9 (S.A.W., N.L.M.); the Department of Radiology, Mayo Clinic, Rochester, Minn (T.E.H., S.J.S.); and the Department of Radiology, Royal Brompton National Heart and Lung Hospital, London, England (S.P.G.P., D.M.H.). Received May 29, 1997; revision requested June 25; revision received July 9; accepted July 10. **Address reprint requests to** N.L.M.

made according to clinical history and results from appropriate functional tests. Specifically, in three patients with asthma the diagnosis was based on the presence of reversible airway obstruction defined according to criteria proposed by the American Thoracic Society (4). In the remaining 10 patients, the diagnosis of bronchiolitis obliterans was based on the criteria established by Turton et al (5). These criteria include irreversible airflow obstruction; a predicted forced expiratory volume in 1 second of less than 60% at initial examination; and exclusion of emphysema, chronic bronchitis, asthma, or any other known cause of airway obstruction.

CT of the chest was performed with a 9800 scanner (GE Medical Systems, Milwaukee, Wis) in 28 patients, a HiSpeed Advantage scanner (GE Medical Systems) in six patients, a 1200SX scanner (Picker International, Highland Heights, Ohio) in 15 patients, and an electron-beam scanner (Imatron, San Francisco, Calif) in 21 patients. In all patients, thin-section CT scans (1.0–1.5 mm collimation) were reconstructed with a high-spatial-frequency algorithm. Inspiratory scans were obtained at 10-mm intervals with the patient in the supine position. Expiratory scans were obtained in 27 patients at five equally spaced levels from the aortic arch to the diaphragm. The expiratory CT scans in these 27 patients were obtained as part of the routine assessment of patients undergoing thin-section CT at one institution (n = 15), or as part of evaluation of patients with evidence of airway obstruction at the other two institutions (n = 12). The images were obtained at window levels of −550 to −700 HU and a window width of 1,500 HU.

The CT findings were interpreted randomly by two experienced chest radiologists from a different institution who were unaware of the diagnosis in each case. The assignment of each case to the category of infiltrative, airway, or pulmonary vascular disease was based on reports of diseases known to cause mosaic attenuation (Table 2) (6–11). In particular, the presence of areas of ground-glass attenuation, decreased attenuation, and increased or decreased vascularity were assessed. Ground-glass attenuation was defined as a hazy increase in attenuation not associated with obscuration of the underlying vessels (1).

Distinction of ground-glass attenuation caused by infiltrative lung disease from increased attenuation caused by vascular redistribution was based on comparison of vessel size in areas with increased attenuation with that in areas with normal or decreased attenuation. Ground-glass attenuation was considered to be caused by infiltrative lung disease if the size and number of vessels in the areas of increased attenuation were similar to those in areas of apparently normal or decreased attenuation (12). The areas of increased attenuation were considered to be attributable to blood flow redistribution (ie, mosaic perfusion related to airway or vascular disease when the size and number of vessels in the areas of increased attenuation were increased compared with those in the areas with normal or decreased attenuation) (7,11,12).

Table 1
Diseases That Cause Mosaic Attenuation on CT Scans and Types of Disease Found in the 70 Patients

Type of Disease	No. of Patients	Specific Diagnosis	No. of Patients
Infiltrative lung	37	Extrinsic allergic alveolitis	13
		Desquamative interstitial pneumonitis	10
		Alveolar proteinosis	4
		Bronchiolitis obliterans with organized pneumonia	3
		Bronchoalveolar cell carcinoma	2
		Nonspecific interstitial pneumonitis	1
		Lymphangitic carcinomatosis	1
		Sarcoidosis	1
		Pulmonary edema	1
		Atypical interstitial pneumonitis	1
Airway	22	Bronchiolitis obliterans	19
		Asthma	3
Vascular	11	Chronic pulmonary thromboembolism	4
		Pulmonary veno-occlusive disease	3
		Pulmonary arterial hypertension	3
		Polyarteritis nodosa	1
Total	70		70

Table 2
Distinguishing Features of the Various Diseases That May Cause Mosaic Lung Attentuation on CT Scans

Type of Disease	CT Findings: Attenuation	CT Findings: Vessels	CT Findings: Air Trapping
Infiltrative lung	Ground glass	Normal size and number throughout lung	Not seen
Airway	Reduced (hypoxic vasoconstriction)	Decreased in size and number in areas of reduced attenuation	Seen at expiratory CT
	Increased (regional hyperperfusion)		
Vascular	Reduced (obstructed blood flow)	Decreased in size and number in areas of reduced attenuation	Not seen
	Increased (regional hyperperfusion)	Increased in size and number in areas of increased attenuation	

Distinction of airway disease from vascular disease was based on the presence of bronchial dilatation on inspiratory CT scans or air trapping demonstrated on expiratory CT scans in patients with airway disease (3,10,12). Distinction of areas with increased attenuation from normal lung or areas of decreased attenuation was based on subjective criteria. By definition, patients in whom areas of ground-glass attenuation were considered to be caused by infiltrative lung disease were considered to have areas of normal lung attenuation and vascularity between the areas of ground-glass attenuation unless additional focal areas of decreased attenuation and vascularity were also identified. Patients in whom these additional focal areas were identified were considered to have areas of ground-glass attenuation, normal attenuation, and decreased attenuation. By defintion, patients in whom vascular or airway disease was diagnosed were considered to have areas of increased attenuation caused by blood flow redistribution and areas of decreased attenuation and vascularity caused by vascular or airway disease (11,12). The diagnosis of air trapping was based on the presence of areas of decreased attenuation, which showed an increase in attenuation less than normal at expiratory CT (1).

After assessment of CT findings, each observer concluded whether the diagnosis was infiltrative lung disease, airway disease, or vascular disease and gave the degree of confidence in that category as high, moderate, or low. The observers then attempted to make a specific diagnosis and graded the degree of confidence in that diagnosis as high, moderate, or low. Interobserver agreement was assessed with the κ statistic (13).

RESULTS

The type of disease was identified correctly at CT by observer 1 in 58 (83%) of the 70 patients and by observer 2 in 57 (81%) of the 70 patients. Observer 1 made a correct diagnosis at CT in 34 (92%) of the 37 cases of infiltrative lung disease, 21 (95%) of

Table 3
Number of Correct and Confident Diagnoses by the Two Observers according to Disease Category

Disease Category	Observer 1 Correct	Observer 1 Correct and Confident	Observer 2 Correct	Observer 2 Correct and Confident
Infiltrative lung (n = 37)	34 (92)	30 (81)	34 (92)	28 (76)
Airway (n = 22)	21 (95)	16 (73)	19 (86)	17 (77)
Vascular (n = 11)	3 (27)	1 (9)	4 (36)	3 (27)

Note.—Numbers in parentheses are the percentages of correct diagnoses.

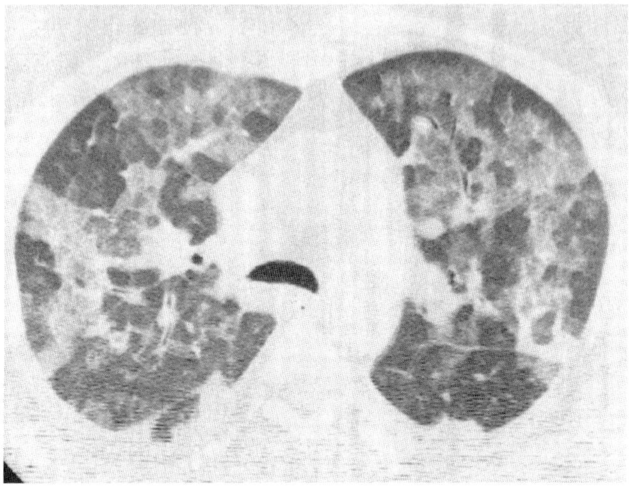

Figure 1. Mosaic attenuation caused by infiltrative lung disease in a 46-year-old woman with desquamative interstitial pneumonitis. Thin-section CT scan obtained at the level of the tracheal carina shows ground-glass attenuation and spared normal lung in a mosaic pattern.

the 22 cases of airway disease, and three (27%) of the 11 cases of vascular disease. Observer 2 made a correct diagnosis at CT in 34 (92%) of the 37 cases of infiltrative lung disease, 19 (86%) of the 22 cases of airway disease, and four (36%) of the 11 cases of vascular disease (Table 3).

Observer 1 made a correct diagnosis at CT with a high degree of confidence in 30 (81%) of the 37 cases of infiltrative lung disease, 16 (73%) of the 22 cases of airway disease, and one (9%) of the 11 cases of vascular disease. Observer 2 made a correct diagnosis at CT with a high degree of confidence in 28 (76%) of the 37 cases of infiltrative lung disease, 17 (77%) of the 22 cases of airway disease, and three (27%) of the 11 cases of vascular disease.

The two observers agreed as to the diagnosis made at CT in 34 (92%) of 37 cases of infiltrative lung disease, 19 (86%) of the 22 cases of airway disease, and two (18%) of the 11 cases of vascular disease.

The two observers agreed as to a highly confident diagnosis at CT in 28 (76%) of the 37 cases of infiltrative lung disease, 16 (73%) of the 22 cases of airway disease, and one (9%) of the 11 cases of vascular disease.

The κ statistic for agreement between the observers with regard to correct diagnosis of infiltrative disease, airway disease, and vascular disease at CT were 0.90, 0.46, and 0.87, respectively.

Observer 1 identified ground-glass attenuation in 35 (95%) of 37 patients with infiltrative lung disease, three (14%) of 22 patients with airway disease, and seven (64%) of 11 patients with vascular disease. Observer 2 identified ground-glass attenuation in 36 (97%) of 37 patients with infiltrative lung disease, one (5%) of 22 patients with airway disease, and six (55%) of 11 patients with vascular disease (Fig 1).

Observer 1 identified areas of decreased attenuation in 10 (27%) of 37 cases of infiltrative disease, 21 (95%) of 22 cases of airway disease, and six (55%) of 11 cases of vascular disease. Areas of decreased attenuation were seen by observer 2 in seven (19%) of 37 cases of infiltrative disease, 21 (95%) of the 22 cases of airway disease, and seven (64%) of the 11 cases of vascular disease (Figs 2, 3).

Observer 1 considered bronchial dilatation present in 17 (77%) of the 22 cases of airway disease, eight (21%) of the 37 cases of infiltrative lung disease, and three (27%) of the 11 cases of vascular disease. Observer 2 considered bronchial dilatation present in 16 (73%) cases of airway disease, 12 (32%) of 37 cases of infiltrative lung disease, and two (18%) of 11 cases of vascular disease (Fig 2).

Expiratory CT scans were available in 27 patients. Observer 1 determined the presence of air trapping in six (86%) of the seven patients with infiltrative lung disease, 12 (75%) of the 16 patients with airway disease, and two (50%) of the four patients with vascular disease. Observer 2 detected air trapping in five (71%) of the seven patients with infiltrative lung disease, 12 (75%) of the 16 patients with airway disease, and one (25%) of the four patients with vascular disease (Figs 2, 4).

On the basis of thin-section CT findings, correct diagnosis of a specific disease was made in 36 (51%) of the 70 patients by observer 1 and in 41 (59%) of the 70 patients by observer 2 (Fig 5). Bronchiolitis obliterans and extrinsic allergic alveolitis were the only two conditions diagnosed reliably by the two observers. Bronchiolitis obliterans was diagnosed correctly in all 19 (100%) patients by observer 1 and in 18 (95%) of the 19 patients by observer 2. Both observers made a correct diagnosis of bronchiolitis obliterans with a high degree of confidence in 16 (84%) of 19 patients. The diagnosis of extrinsic allergic alveolitis was made correctly in 10 (77%) of 13 patients by observer 1 and 11 (85%) of 13 patients by observer 2. However, the correct specific diagnosis of extrinsic allergic alveolitis was made with a high degree of confidence in only two (15%) of 13 patients by observer 1 and three (23%) of 13 patients by observer 2.

DISCUSSION

A pattern of mosaic attenuation may be caused by infiltrative lung disease and lead to patchy areas of ground-glass attenuation or be caused by primary airway or vascular abnormalities. In cases of infiltrative lung disease, the size of vessels within the areas of ground-glass attenuation is usually similar to that of uninvolved lung, allowing distinction from airway and vascular diseases in the majority of cases. In cases of airway and vascular

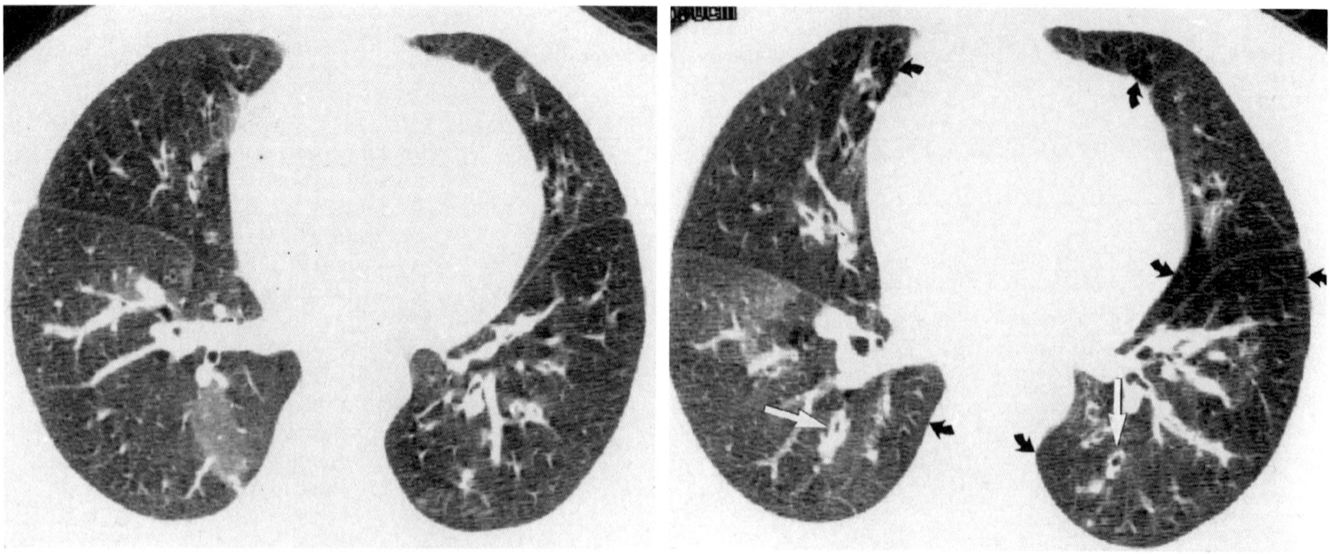

a. b.

Figure 2. Mosaic attenuation caused by airway disease in a 43-year-old woman with bronchiolitis obliterans. **(a)** Thin-section CT scan obtained through the lung bases at end inspiration shows a pattern of mosaic attenuation. **(b)** Thin-section CT scan obtained through the lung bases at end expiration shows air trapping (black arrows). Bronchial dilatation and bronchial wall thickening are seen (white arrows).

diseases, regional alteration in pulmonary blood flow is the final mechanism that causes the mosaic attenuation. Regional alterations in pulmonary blood flow are secondary to hypoxic vasoconstriction in cases of airway disease and to vascular occlusion in cases of vascular disease. In both categories of disease, areas of increased attenuation have relatively large vessels, while areas of decreased attenuation have small vessels (7).

Airway diseases that cause mosaic attenuation can usually be recognized by the presence of bronchial dilatation, seen in more than 70% of patients with airway abnormalities in our study. Bronchial dilatation has been shown previously to be associated with bronchiolitis obliterans (14). In all patients in whom bronchial dilatation and air trapping were identified, both observers confidently and correctly diagnosed airway disease. The combination of these findings on scans that show mosaic attenuation enables accurate diagnosis of airway disease. Although air trapping allows early recognition of airway abnormalities (3,6), it was not helpful as an isolated finding in the distinction of airway disease from other causes of mosaic attenuation in our study because it was also present in patients with infiltrative lung disease and vascular disease. Hansell et al (9) described the frequent association of areas of decreased perfusion in patients with extrinsic allergic alveolitis and suggested that this finding was related to the presence of bronchiolitis seen in these patients. Air trapping has been reported as a common finding in extrinsic allergic alveolitis (15), and in our study almost all patients with infiltrative lung disease who demonstrated air trapping at expiratory CT had extrinsic allergic alveolitis.

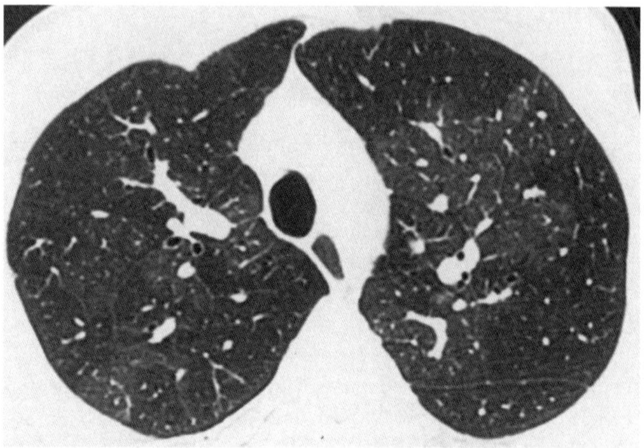

Figure 3. Mosaic attenuation caused by vascular disease in a 40-year-old man with chronic pulmonary thromboembolism. Thin-section CT scan obtained at the level of the aortic arch shows mosaic perfusion with enlarged vessels in the areas of increased attenuation.

In cases of vascular disease, it has been suggested that all areas of the lung, whether they show decreased or increased attenuation, demonstrate the expected increase in attenuation at expiration (3). Stern et al (3) suggested that air trapping is not present in cases of vascular lung disease and that this feature allows distinction from mosaic attenuation caused by airway disease. However, in our study air trapping did not allow reliable distinction of vascular and airway diseases. In patients in whom expiratory CT scans were available, air trapping was considered present in 12 (75%) of 16 patients with airway disease by both observers and in two (50%) of four and one (25%) of four (observers 1 and 2, respectively) patients with vascular disease. Acute vascular occlusion, resulting in a reduced arterial carbon dioxide concentration in the affected lung, can stimulate bronchoconstriction of small airways (16). Air trapping may then be expected in the affected areas of lung owing to the presence of bronchoconstriction. Bronchial dilatation has also been shown to be a common finding in patients with chronic pulmonary thromboembolism (17). In a recent study, bron-

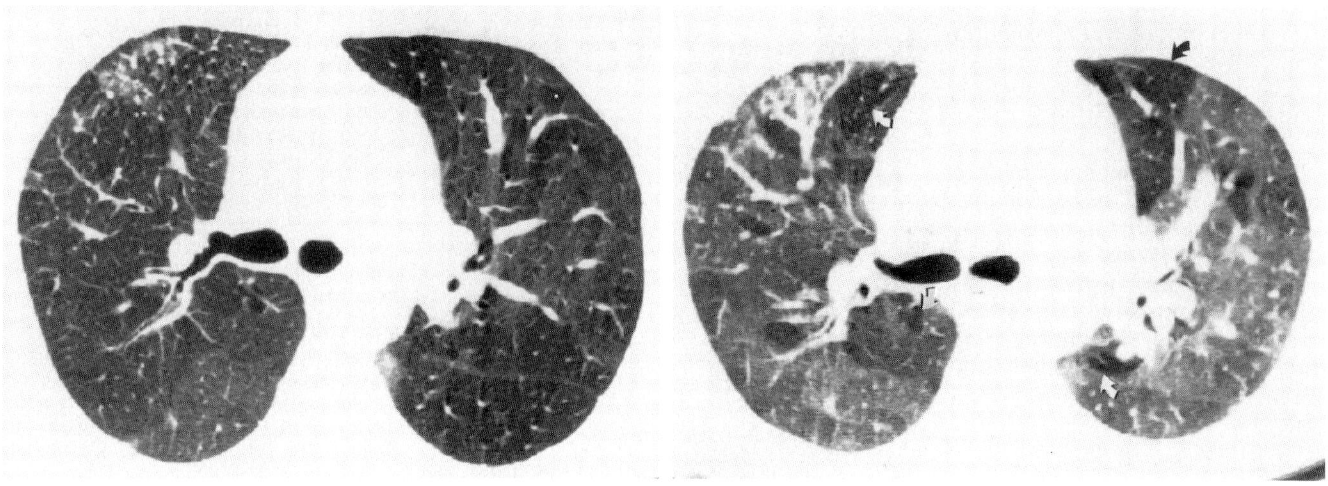

a. b.

Figure 4. Mosaic attenuation caused by vascular disease that was misinterpreted as airway disease in a 43-year-old woman with primary pulmonary arterial hypertension. **(a)** Thin-section CT scan obtained at the level of the tracheal carina at end inspiration shows a mosaic attenuation pattern. **(b)** Thin-section CT scan obtained at end expiration at the same level shows air trapping (arrows). In this case, both observers made the diagnosis of airway disease from interpretation of the scan.

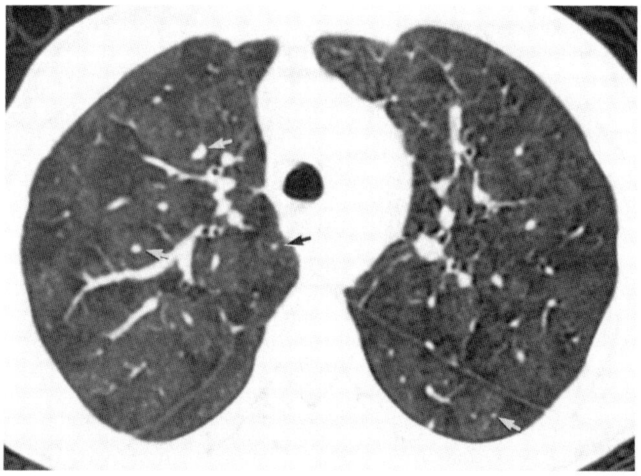

Figure 5. Mosaic attenuation caused by vascular disease that was misinterpreted as infiltrative lung disease in a 61-year-old woman with chronic pulmonary thromboembolism. Thin-section CT scan obtained at the level of the aortic arch shows a mosaic perfusion pattern with slightly enlarged vessels in the regions of increased attenuation (arrows). Both observers misinterpreted the findings as infiltrative lung disease.

chial dilatation was seen in 64% of patients with chronic thromboembolism; this condition was present in areas where the pulmonary arteries had been occluded completely by embolus (17).

In our study, vascular disease was the most difficult type of disease to identify correctly. It was identified correctly in only one-third of cases by each observer, and the observers seldom were confident in the diagnosis. Vascular disease was misinterpreted as infiltrative lung disease or airway disease. In the majority of cases of vascular disease, mosaic attenuation is caused by chronic pulmonary thromboembolism (10). This pattern may be seen less commonly in patients with primary pulmonary hypertension (Fig 4) or in patients with pulmonary capillary hemangiomatosis (11).

The specific diagnosis of the underlying disease was rarely identified, with the exception of bronchiolitis obliterans and extrinsic allergic alveolitis. Interpretations were performed in our study without the benefit of clinical history, investigation results, or reference to the course of any radiographic abnormalities. This additional information is clearly useful and is of assistance in interpretation of thin-section CT scans in clinical practice.

Furthermore, the study included only patients with infiltrative lung disease who demonstrated mosaic attenuation (ie, patchy distribution of areas of ground-glass attenuation). Patients who demonstrated diffuse ground-glass attenuation and patients who demonstrated ground-glass attenuation and had obvious fibrosis were excluded from the study. Therefore, in clinical practice the distinction of infiltrative lung disease from airway or vascular disease is probably easier to achieve than our results suggest.

A limitation of our study is the relatively high proportion of patients with bronchiolitis obliterans in whom expiratory CT scans were obtained compared with patients with infiltrative lung disease or vascular disease. This bias is based on the clinical practice of the institutions that participated in the study. Expiratory scans are obtained routinely in patients undergoing thin-section CT in only one of the three institutions; at the other two institutions, expiratory CT scans are obtained only as part of evaluation of patients in whom airway disease is suspected. The CT scans were interpreted by two independent observers from a different institution who were not aware of the study protocols being used, however; the results point out the difficulty in distinguishing air trapping associated with airway disease from persistent decreased attenuation seen on expiratory CT scans in patients with vascular disease.

Another limitation of the study is the subjective analysis of the data. It is possible that improved distinction of vascular disease from airway disease may be achieved with objective quantification of bronchial abnormalities, measurement of the diameter of the central pulmonary arteries, measurement of attenuation values, or use of dynamic CT.

In summary, in patients in our study with mosaic attenuation identified on thin-section CT scans, the diagnoses of infiltrative lung disease and airway disease were frequently correct and confident. Vascular disease was difficult to identify correctly and was often misinterpreted as infiltrative lung disease or airway disease. ■

References

1. Austin JHM, Müller NL, Friedman PJ, et al. Glossary of terms for CT of the lungs: recommendations of the Nomenclature Committee of the Fleischner Society. Radiology 1996; 200:327–331.
2. Martin KW, Sagel SS, Siegel BA. Mosaic oligemia simulating pulmonary infiltrates on CT. AJR 1986; 147:670–673.
3. Stern EJ, Swensen SJ, Hartman TE, Frank MS. CT mosaic pattern of lung attenuation: distinguishing different causes. AJR 1995; 165:813–816.
4. American Thoracic Society. Standards for the diagnosis and care of patients with chronic obstructive pulmonary disease (COPD) and asthma. Am Rev Respir Dis 1987; 136:225–244.
5. Turton CW, Williams G, Green M. Cryptogenic obliterative bronchiolitis in adults. Thorax 1981; 36:805–810.
6. Müller NL, Miller RR. Diseases of the bronchioles: CT and histopathologic findings. Radiology 1995; 196:3–12.
7. Remy-Jardin M, Remy J, Giraud F, Wattine L, Gosselin B. Computed tomography assessment of ground-glass opacity: semiology and significance. J Thorac Imaging 1993; 8:249–264.
8. Grenier P, Valeyre D, Cluzel P, et al. Chronic diffuse interstitial lung disease: diagnostic value of chest radiography and high-resolution CT. Radiology 1991; 179: 123–132.
9. Hansell DM, Wells AU, Padley SPG, Müller NL. Hypersensitivity pneumonitis: correlation of individual CT patterns with functional abnormalities. Radiology 1996; 199: 123–128.
10. King MA, Bergin CJ, Yeung DWC, et al. Chronic pulmonary thromboembolism: detection of regional hypoperfusion with CT. Radiology 1994; 191:359–363.
11. Primack SL, Müller NL, Mayo JR, Remy-Jardin M, Remy J. Pulmonary parenchymal abnormalities of vascular origin: high-resolution CT findings. RadioGraphics 1994; 14:739–746.
12. Stern EJ, Müller NL, Swensen SJ, Hartman TE. CT mosaic pattern of lung attenuation: etiologies and terminology. J Thorac Imaging 1995; 10:294–297.
13. Dawson-Saunders B, Trapp RG. Basic and clinical biostatistics. 2nd ed. Norwalk, Conn: Appleton & Lange, 1994; 41–63.
14. Lentz D, Bergin CJ, Berry GJ, Stoehr C, Theodore J. Diagnosis of bronchiolitis obliterans in heart-lung transplantation patients: importance of bronchial dilatation on CT. AJR 1992; 159:463–467.
15. Small JH, Flower CDR, Traill ZC, Gleeson FV. Air trapping in extrinsic allergic alveolitis on computed tomography. Clin Radiol 1996; 51:684–688.
16. Austin JHM, Sagel SS. Alterations of airway caliber after pulmonary embolization in the dog. Invest Radiol 1972; 3:135–139.
17. Remy-Jardin M, Remy J, Louvegny S, Artaud D, Deschildre F, Duhamel A. Airway changes in chronic pulmonary embolism: CT findings in 33 patients. Radiology 1997; 203:355–360.

Minming Zhang, MD • Michio Kono, MD

Solitary Pulmonary Nodules: Evaluation of Blood Flow Patterns with Dynamic CT[1]

PURPOSE: **To evaluate the efficacy of dynamic computed tomography (CT) for differentiating benign from malignant solitary pulmonary nodules (SPNs).**

MATERIALS AND METHODS: **Sixty-five patients with noncalcified SPNs (diameter, ≤30 mm; 42 malignant, 16 benign, seven inflammatory) underwent single-location dynamic contrast material–enhanced (100 mL, 4 mL/sec) serial CT. Peak height of time-attenuation curves and ratio of peak height of the SPN to that of the aorta were measured. Precontrast attenuation and enhancement pattern were recorded. Perfusion was calculated from the maximum gradient of the time-attenuation curve and the peak height of the aorta.**

RESULTS: **Peak heights of malignant (41.9 HU ± 2.8) and inflammatory (43.6 HU ± 7.7) SPNs were significantly higher than that (13.4 HU ± 2.2) of benign SPNs ($P < .001$; $P < .01$). SPN-to-aorta ratios in malignant and inflammatory SPNs were significantly higher than that in benign SPNs ($P < .001$, $P < .05$). No statistically significant differences in the peak height and SPN-to-aorta ratio were found between malignant and inflammatory SPNs. Precontrast attenuation of inflammatory SPNs was lower than that of malignant SPNs ($P < .05$). Perfusion values in malignant and inflammatory SPNs were significantly higher than that of the benign SPNs ($P < .01$).**

CONCLUSION: **Dynamic CT provides quantitative information about blood flow patterns of SPNs and is an applicable diagnostic method for differentiating SPNs.**

THE solitary pulmonary nodule (SPN) is one of the most common findings on chest radiographs (1–4). In clinical practice, the objectives are to differentiate malignant from benign nodules in the least invasive way and to make a specific diagnosis (1–8). Computed tomography (CT) has had a major influence on the evaluation of SPNs with regard to defining morphologic features, detecting calcification, and planning biopsy procedures (9–11). Despite advances in the assessment of SPNs with radiography, bronchoscopy, and transthoracic needle aspiration biopsy, a substantial proportion of SPNs remain radiographically indeterminate (1,9).

The blood supply and metabolism of malignant nodules are qualitatively and quantitatively different from those of most benign nodules (4,8, 12,13). Recently, investigators have exploited the differences in vascularity, pharmacodynamics, and metabolism between malignant and benign SPNs with imaging techniques. Littleton et al (5) reported that conventional tomographic analysis after intravenous infusion of contrast medium could potentially allow distinction between benign and malignant SPNs. Swensen et al (1–3) demonstrated that the degree of contrast medium enhancement of SPNs as measured with CT may indicate the likelihood of malignancy. The degree of enhancement on magnetic resonance (MR) images after administration of gadopentetate dimeglumine may be helpful in differentiating lung cancer from tuberculoma (14,15). Studies of positron emission tomography with 2-[fluorine-18]-fluoro-2-deoxy-D-glucose (FDG) showed that there was a substantial difference in FDG uptake between malignant and benign SPNs (4,8).

On the basis of attenuation changes in tissues after injection of contrast material, dynamic CT facilitates estimation of the pharmacokinetics of contrast material in organs or tissue (16–18). Blood flow patterns have been investigated with dynamic CT to delineate abnormal hemodynamic lesions in liver, brain, kidney, and lung (19–24). In the present study, we used dynamic CT to evaluate the blood flow patterns of SPNs and sought to determine the clinical efficacy of dynamic CT in the differential diagnosis of benign and malignant SPNs.

MATERIALS AND METHODS

Patient Population

Patients were selected according to the following criteria: (*a*) presence of an SPN with no calcification and smaller than 30 mm in diameter, (*b*) absence of contraindications to the administration of contrast medium, and (*c*) probable ability to cooperate with the procedure. The diameter was defined as the average value of the anteroposterior and lateral diameters on conventional radiographs or on CT scans obtained with a mediastinal window setting, or on both images. No calcification

Index terms: Aorta, flow dynamics, 943.91 • Computed tomography, contrast enhancement • Lung, nodule, 60.332 • Lung neoplasms, CT, 60.12113 • Lung neoplasms, diagnosis, 60.332

Abbreviations: FDG = 2-[fluorine-18]fluoro-2-deoxy-D-glucose, SPN = solitary pulmonary nodule.

Radiology 1997; 205:471–478

[1] From the Department of Radiology, Kobe University School of Medicine, Kusunoki-cho, 7-Chome, Chuo-ku, Kobe 650, Japan. Received December 20, 1996; revision requested February 19, 1997; final revision received July 14; accepted July 21. **Address reprint requests to** M.Z.

meant SPNs with no visible calcification on conventional CT scans (ie, 10- or 3-mm section thickness) obtained with a mediastinal window setting. Sixty-nine patients with SPN met the criteria and were referred for dynamic CT examination. Four patients (6%) were excluded from the study because of respiratory misregistration at the second series of scanning. These four patients all had SPNs at the base portion of the lung.

Sixty-five patients (40 men, 25 women; age range, 28–85 years; mean age, 64 years ± 12.2 [standard deviation]) with SPNs 5–30 mm (mean, 19.1 mm ± 8.4) in diameter were studied. Final diagnoses were confirmed histologically or cytologically by means of surgery, CT-guided transthoracic needle aspiration biopsy, or transbronchial lung biopsy in 54 patients. In the other 11 patients, the diagnoses were based on clinical data such as no radiologic evidence of nodular growth during 2 or more years of follow-up or resolution of the lesion on serial chest radiographs after antibiotic treatment. Some patients had definite diagnoses made on the basis of one or more examinations listed above. Among the 65 patients, the diagnosis was malignant in 42 (adenocarcinoma in 26 patients, squamous cell carcinoma in nine patients, small cell carcinoma in four patients, large cell carcinoma in two patients, and metastatic tumor from pleural malignant mesothelium in one patient) and benign in 23 patients (including granuloma or tuberculoma in 12 patients, bronchogenic cyst in two patients, and hamartoma in two patients). The other seven benign cases were labeled as active inflammatory nodules, of which three were organizing pneumonia, three were tuberculosis, and one was resolved after antibiotic treatment. We separated the active inflammatory nodules from the other benign nodules for analysis. In this way, all patients were divided into three groups: malignant group (n = 42), which comprised the patients with malignant neoplasm; benign group (n = 16), which comprised the patients with granulomas or benign neoplasm; and inflammatory group (n = 7), which comprised the patients with active inflammatory nodules.

Protocol

Before the examination began, patients were carefully instructed in and practiced the breath-holding technique to reproduce precisely the same degree of inspiration or expiration for each scan series and were given oxygen inspiration in 4 L^3/min. Scans were obtained after breath holding either in inspiration or in expiration.

Before dynamic scanning, control scans were obtained from which the scan level that best demonstrated the SPN, close to the nodule equator, was selected. Single-location dynamic scans were obtained at the selected section with use of a CT 9800 QUICK (n = 28) or HiSpeed Advantage RP (n = 41) scanner (GE Yokogawa Medical Systems, Osaka, Japan). Iodinated, low-osmolar, nonionic contrast material (iopamidol 300 [Iopamiron; Schering, Osaka, Japan] or iohexol 300 [Omnipaque; Daiichi Pharmaceutical, Tokyo, Japan]) was administered via the antecubital vein at a rate of 4 mL/sec for a total of 100 mL by using an autoinjector (Auto Enhance A50; Nemoto Kyolindou, Tokyo, Japan). The section thickness was 5 mm, and scanning time was 1.5 seconds with the 9800 QUICK scanner or 1 second with the HiSpeed Advantage RP scanner. For the first 25 patients, three series of CT scans (10 scans each for the first and second series and four scans for the third series) were obtained beginning at 15, 75, and 135 seconds after injection of contrast medium. For the first two series, the scanning interval was 2 seconds, and for the third series the scanning interval was 6 seconds. Interseries delay was 30 seconds. The preliminary results (25 patients) showed that the peak level of enhancement was almost executing in the 1st minute; therefore, for the subsequent 44 patients, the third series of scans was not obtained (Fig 1). One image without contrast material enhancement and 20 or 24 dynamic contrast material–enhanced images were obtained during a 105- or 165-second scanning period for each patient. A normal reconstruction algorithm without edge enhancement (window width, 350 HU; window level, 40 HU) was used for dynamic scanning.

Data Analysis

Time-attenuation curves were created from circular or oval (occasionally the cross-section of nodules were nonspherical) regions of the interest drawn over the SPN, aorta (or common carotid artery if the aorta was not included in the section), muscle, and opposite normal lung. The region of interest was as large as possible to minimize noise but with care to avert partial-volume effect. According to this criterion, the diameter of the region of interest was about 70%–80% of the diameter of the lung nodule. If there was substantial artifact from cardiac motion or beam hardening from adjacent bone to create rapid changes of attenuation or if the proper scan level was not attained due to improper respiration, the image was eliminated from data analysis.

Gamma variate fits were performed to the time-attenuation curves to remove recirculation (25,26) on the same data on two separate occasions to confirm reproducibility. The gamma variate curve used in this study was expressed by the following equation: $C(t) = K(t - At)^{\alpha}\exp(-(t - At)/\beta)$, where $C(t)$ = increasing value of the CT number, t = time after the start of injection, K = constant scale factor, α and β = fitting parameters, and At = appearance time. This technique was performed with DeltaGraph Pro 3 software (version 3.0.4, serial no. JAPM 301470; Delta Point, Monterey, Calif) and a commercially available computer (Power Macintosh 7100/66 AV; Apple Computer, Tokyo, Japan).

Peak height (ie, the maximum value of the time-attenuation curve), defined as total attenuation minus baseline precontrast attenuation, was determined and the following ratio of peak height of the SPN to peak height of the aorta was calculated: $(PH_{SPN}/PH_{aorta}) \times 100\%$.

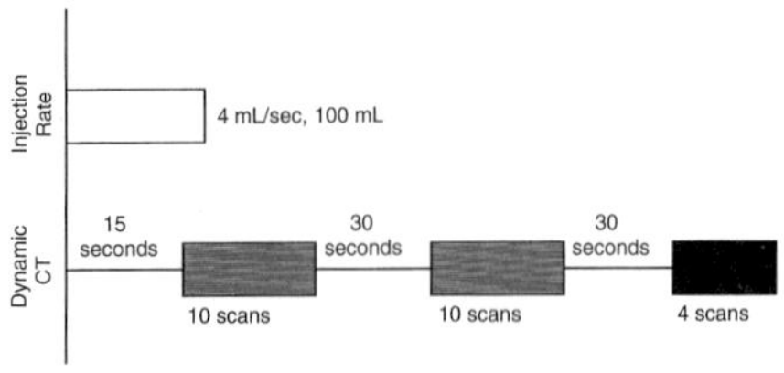

Figure 1. Dynamic scan program and injection rate of contrast medium. Scanning time was 1.0 or 1.5 seconds. Gray box = 2-second interval, black box = 6-second interval.

Perfusion of the SPNs was calculated by applying a nuclear medicine data processing technique to the time-attenuation data; this technique was based on the general equation as described by Miles (17): $P = TAC_{SPN}/PH_{AA}$, where P = perfusion in milliliters of blood flow per minute per milliliter of tissue, TAC_{SPN} = maximum gradient of the SPN time-attenuation curve in Hounsfield units per minute, and PH_{AA} = peak height of aortic attenuation in Hounsfield units (16,17).

Enhancement pattern was evaluated on the image that was maximally enhanced and was classified as follows: homogeneous, if enhancement of the nodule was completely homogeneous; heterogeneous, if enhancement of the nodule was completely heterogeneous; central, if enhancement was at the inner area of the nodule; peripheral, if enhancement was at the outer area of the nodule; and no enhancement, if a nodule showed no apparent enhancement. If a nodule tended to go from heterogeneous to homogeneous enhancement with time, the enhancement pattern was determined on the image at the time of peak height of enhancement. Two or three of seven experienced chest radiologists were involved in determining the enhancement pattern of SPNs. When a discrepancy occurred, consensus was reached by discussion.

All values were expressed as a mean ± standard error. The significance of the difference between groups was analyzed by means of an unpaired Student t test. A P value less than .05 was considered statistically significant. The relationships between peak height of the aorta and the parameters of the SPNs (peak height, SPN-to-aorta peak height ratio, and perfusion) were assessed by means of linear regression analysis. Statistical analysis of the enhancement patterns between groups was performed by means of the Kruskal-Wallis rank test. All the statistical analyses were performed with StatView software, version J4.02 (Abacus Concepts, Berkeley, Calif) and a commercially available computer (Power Macintosh 7100/66 AV; Apple Computer).

RESULTS

The time-attenuation curves appeared different for the malignant,

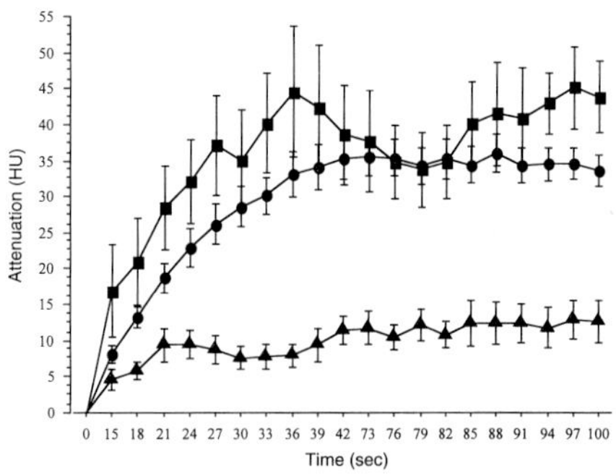

Figure 2. Time-attenuation curves of inflammatory (■), malignant (●), and benign (▲) SPNs.

benign, and inflammatory SPNs. The time-attenuation curve of the malignant nodules usually showed a moderate increase as contrast medium appeared in the thoracic aorta and a progressive increase to the peak height where it maintained a plateau. The time-attenuation curve of the benign nodules showed some or no increase after injection of contrast medium. Conversely, inflammatory nodules showed a rapid increase in enhancement after injection of contrast medium; after the nodule reached maximum enhancement, the time-attenuation curve declined then rose again thereafter (Fig 2).

Excellent curve fits for time-attenuation curves were obtained. Both the raw data and corresponding extrapolated values were reviewed for reproducibility; if doubt arose, data were excluded. Among the 65 patients, 17 images in 10 patients were eliminated from data analysis because of substantial cardiac motion or beam-hardening artifact. No patient was excluded from analysis because of the artifact. The characteristics of the SPNs are summarized in the Table.

Peak heights of the malignant nodules and the inflammatory nodules were significantly higher than that of the benign nodules ($P < .001$ and $P < .01$, respectively) (Table, Fig 3). Both the malignant and inflammatory nodules had higher SPN-to-aorta peak height ratios than that of the benign nodules ($P < .001$ and $P < .05$, respectively) (Table, Fig 4). No significant differences in the peak heights and the SPN-to-aorta peak height ratios were found between the malignant and the inflammatory nodules ($P = .52$ and $P = .14$, respectively). The peak heights of the SPN relative to the peak heights of muscle and opposite normal lung were recorded by means of normalization. The normalization proved to be not helpful, because the attenuation of muscle was quite constant during dynamic scanning and the attenuation of the opposite normal lung was considerably variable from scan to scan and from one region to another.

Precontrast attenuation of the inflammatory nodules was significantly lower than that of the malignant nodules ($P < .05$). Precontrast attenuation of the benign nodules was also higher than that of the inflammatory nodules, but the difference in attenuation did not reach statistical significance ($P = .25$) (Table, Fig 5).

Perfusion values of both the malignant and inflammatory nodules were significantly higher than that of the benign nodules (both $P < .01$); however, the difference of the perfusion between the malignant nodules and the inflammatory nodules was not significant ($P = .36$) (Table, Fig 6).

The mean aortic peak height value was 297.1 HU ± 99.1 (standard deviation). The correlation between the SPN peak height and the aortic peak height was significant ($r = .51$, $P < .001$). A less strong relationship was found between the aortic peak height and the SPN-to-aorta peak height ratio ($r = .34$, $P = .03$). No significant correlation was found between the aortic peak height and SPN perfusion ($r = .03$, $P = .84$).

The contrast material enhancement patterns of the SPNs were extremely complex. Of the 42 malignant nodules, 23 showed complete homogeneous enhancement (Fig 7), 13 showed heterogeneous enhancement (however, series delayed scans revealed the tendency of these nodules to become homogeneous [Fig 8]), and six showed peripheral enhancement owing to central small necrosis (Fig 9). One benign nodule showed homogeneous enhancement, one had slightly central enhancement, five enhanced in a peripheral or ringlike fashion, and nine showed no or little enhancement (Fig 10). Of the inflammatory nodules, one showed homogeneous enhancement, two showed heterogeneous enhancement, and four showed peripheral enhancement (Fig 11). The inflammatory nodules showed much more irregular peripheral enhancement, as compared with the peripheral enhancement pattern of some malignant nodules. The differences in the enhancement patterns within the three groups were statistically significant (all $P < .001$).

DISCUSSION

The increase in tissue attenuation after contrast material enhancement depends on the blood supply and the volume of the extravascular fluid in the tissue (27,28). Early changes in the time-attenuation curve in a region of interest correlate with blood flow per unit of tissue, and the latter changes mainly correlate with interstitial extravascular space (29). The different appearances of the time-attenuation curves between the malignant and benign SPNs mainly represented the differences in the volume of extracellular fluid and the diffusing spread of contrast medium. Lesser contrast material is delivered in hypovascular benign nodules than in malignant nodules, and the diffusion is a slower process in the benign nodules.

Our results indicate that the peak heights and SPN-to-aorta peak height ratio might be helpful in distinguishing benign nodules from malignant nodules. Malignant nodules tended to enhance significantly more than benign nodules. These results corroborate the findings of others (1–3,6). Swensen et al (1–3) evaluated SPNs with enhanced CT and suggested that a diagnostic enhancement threshold should be 20 HU. Yamashita et al (6) described the differentiation in maximum attenuation between malignant and benign nodules with incremental dynamic CT and concluded that maximum attenuation ranging from 20 to 60 HU appeared to be a good indicator of malignancy. If we consider 20 HU as a threshold to evaluate the nodules in this study (nodules with a peak height higher than 20 HU were considered malignant), there would be 40 of the 42 malignant nodules with peak height higher than this threshold and 16 of the total 23 benign nodules with peak height lower than this threshold. Sensitivity would be 95%, specificity 70%, and accuracy 89%. The positive predictive value would be 85%, and negative predictive value would be 89%. The specificity would be a little bit lower than the results of Swensen et al (1,2), because seven nodules of active inflammatory disease were included in our study; these nodules seemed to have high peak heights, although they are benign nodules.

In the studies by Swensen et al, four spiral acquisitions at 1-minute intervals (1) or six single scans at 30-second intervals (2) were obtained. Yamashita et al (6) obtained six serial CT scans at 30-second, 2-minute, and 5-minute intervals with incremental scans. They both took a limited number of data points with a long scan-to-scan interval time. The maximum enhancement may be underestimated if no scan in the series coincides exactly with the peak concentration of the contrast medium in the SPNs. The scanning procedure performed in our study has two distinct merits: First, high frequency recorded data with 1-second scanning time and 2-second intervals (20–24 scans) suffice to determine the exact peak height of the enhancement. Since at an injection rate of 4 mL/sec, average transit time in the thoracic vasculature is within 30 seconds and average time of arrival at peak contrast medium enhancement in masses is within 60 seconds, changes in the time-attenuation curve within the first 2 minutes appear to be diagnostically important (27). A reduction of the scan-to-scan interval to less than 1 second will be more ideal theoretically, whereas the high radiation exposure associated with obtainment of 60–120 scans is not acceptable in clinical practice. We considered that if the number of scans obtained either was sufficient for depiction of the dynamic change in enhancement in the first 2 minutes or was suitable for the patient with regard to radiation exposure and breath holding, the scan program would be optimal. Therefore, maintaining scanning intervals of 2–3 seconds and a scanning period of 1–2 minutes may be preferable. Second, fitting the measured data to a gamma variate curve and basing the further calculations from the gamma variate curve might improve the accuracy of the method.

Many researchers have found that a higher injection rate is more effective in increasing peak and overall contrast enhancement (30–32). Very shortly after injection (1–2 minutes), most iodine molecules will be distributed in the extravascular space of tissue rather than in vessels (27,33). Thus, a bolus injection will provide sufficient vascular characterization only on the first few scans after injection (27,28). In this study, we chose to use a technique of intermittent bolus injection of 4 mL/sec to achieve high-quality studies with purely intravascular agents, without extravascular distribution in early-phase scanning. A lower rate of injection, as other researchers have used (1–3,6), is tolerable for more patients but provides a slightly lower and later peak. The attenuation on CT scans at a lower rate of injection will not represent intravascular circulation only but will represent a mixture of intravascular and extravascular concentration of contrast medium. We used flexible 18- or 20-gauge intravenous catheters rather than a butterfly needle; by monitoring the progress of the injection visually and with palpation, no extravasation occurred. Therefore, no patient failed to receive the intravenous injection of 4 mL/sec in this study.

Yamashita et al (6) observed that some lung carcinomas reach peak enhancement late, at 5 minutes, with an injection rate of 2 mL/sec. This finding may represent that some lung carcinomas have a wide extravascular fluid pool. Because the total iodine concentration in tissue is measured on CT scans,

Nodule Characteristics of the Various Groups

Parameter*	Malignant (n = 42)	Benign (n = 16)	Inflammatory (n = 7)
Peak height (HU)			
Mean ± SE	41.9 ± 2.8	13.4 ± 2.2†	43.6 ± 7.7
Range	11.0–82.6	4.6–20.0	20.5–71.1
SPN-to-aorta ratio (%)			
Mean ± SE	14.6 ± 1.0	4.8 ± 0.7†	19.7 ± 5.8
Range	6.2–34.8	1.6–7.4	6.6–49.1
Perfusion (mL/min/mL)			
Mean ± SE	0.7 ± 0.1	0.1 ± 0.02†	1.0 ± 0.2
Range	0.04–3.5	0.0–0.2	0.5–1.6
Precontrast attenuation (HU)			
Mean ± SE	29.1 ± 1.9	28.4 ± 3.9	20.7 ± 2.4‡
Range	13.6–69.2	4.8–51.5	12.2–26.0
Enhancement pattern§			
Homogeneous	23 (55)	1 (6)	1 (14)
Heterogeneous	13 (30)	0 (0)	2 (28)
Central	0 (0)	1 (6)	0 (0)
Peripheral	6 (14)	5 (31)	4 (57)
No enhancement	0 (0)	9 (56)	0 (0)
Diameter (mm)			
Mean ± SE	22.0 ± 1.3	14.0 ± 1.3	13.7 ± 3.9
Range	8–30	5–20	5–30

* SE = standard error.
† Differences between the benign group and malignant group ($P < .001$, $P < .01$ [perfusion]) and the benign group and inflammatory group ($P < .01$, $P < .05$ [SPN-to-aorta ratio]) were statistically significant.
‡ Difference between the inflammatory group and malignant group was statistically significant ($P < .05$).
§ Data are number of patients. Numbers in parentheses are percentages.

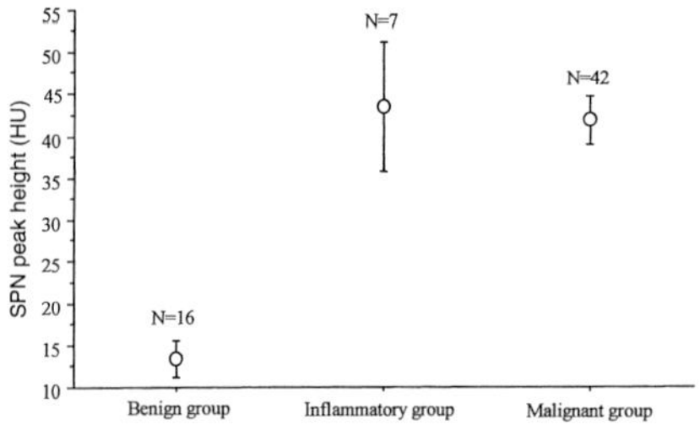

3.

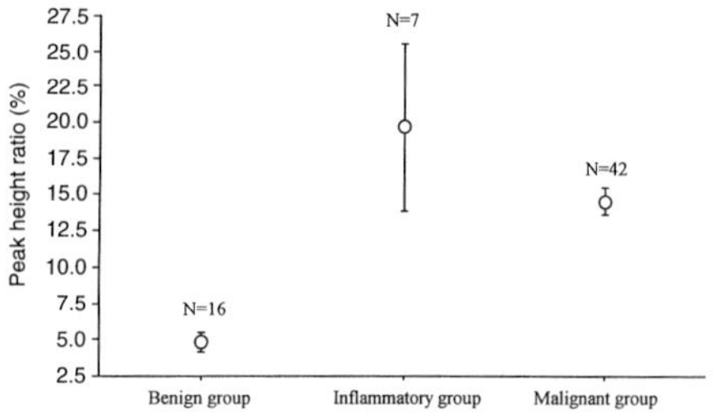

4.

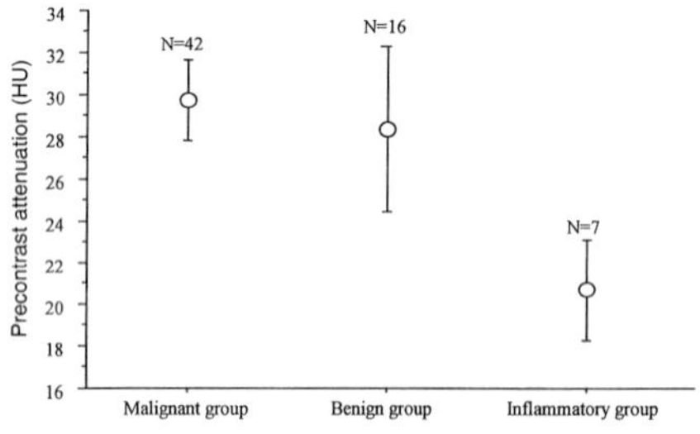

5.

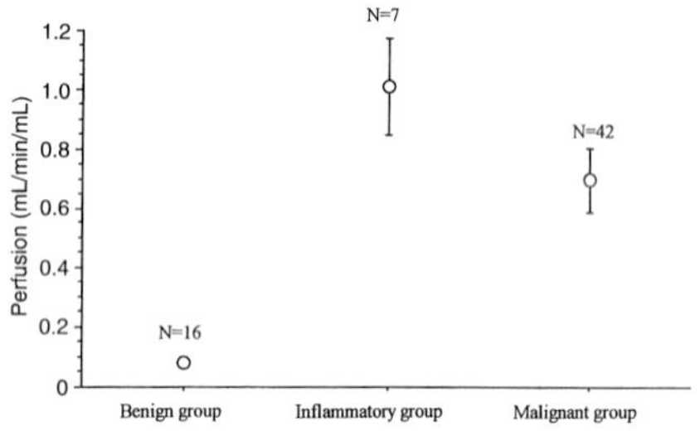

6.

Figure 3–6. Mean values ± 1 standard error for **(3)** the SPN peak height, **(4)** the SPN-to-aorta peak height ratio, **(5)** the precontrast attenuation, and **(6)** the perfusion for each group.

the contrast enhancement values obtained are a summation of the intra- and extravascular concentration of contrast medium. At 5 minutes, the distribution of contrast material approaches a balance that is directly related to the volume of the extracellular space, with more than 80% of the contrast medium remaining outside the blood vessels (29). A relative lower injection rate and longer scanning intervals may be responsible for such a late enhancement in some lung cancers, since a slower injection rate results in a longer time to peak enhancement and a more proportional extravascular distribution at peak enhancement. A series of consecutive CT scans at a injection rate of 4 mL/sec with a 2-second scanning interval and 105-second scanning period, as performed in this study, would best assess the blood flow at the first circulation rather than a certain equilibrium of intravascular and interstitial concentration.

Two false-negative cases of the malignant nodules were found in this study,

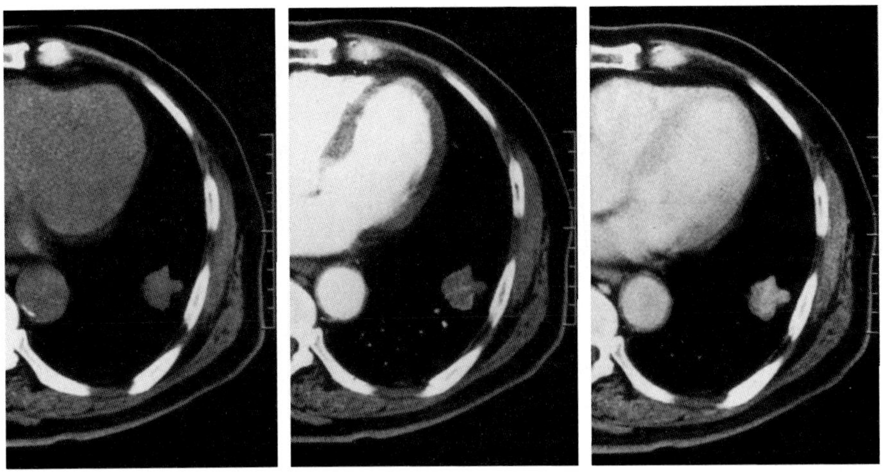

a. b. c.

Figure 7. Dynamic CT scans in an 82-year-old man with adenocarcinoma of the left lower lobe. The SPN shows homogeneous enhancement. The attenuation value is 26.1 HU on the precontrast scan **(a)**, 44.5 HU on the scan obtained 21 seconds after injection of contrast medium **(b)**, and 72.2 HU on the scan obtained 100 seconds after injection **(c)**.

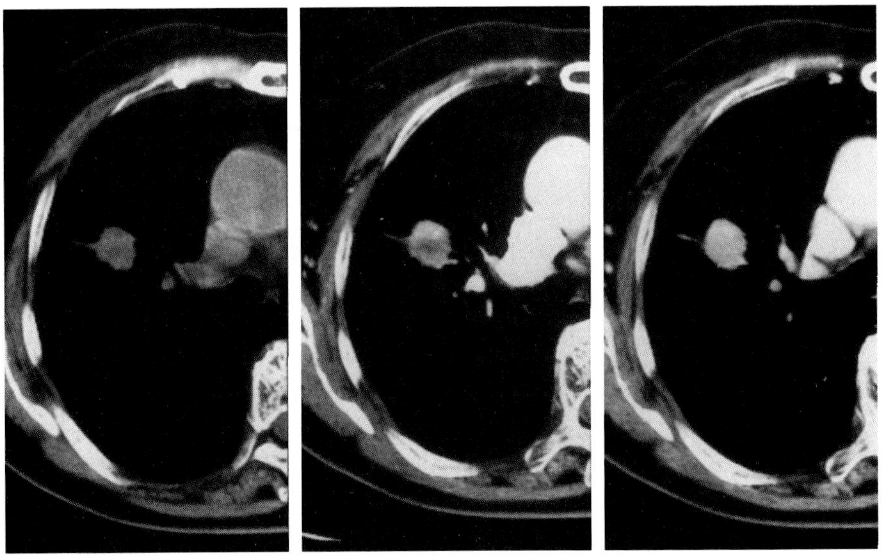

a. b. c.

Figure 8. Dynamic CT scans in a 79-year-old man with adenocarcinoma of the right upper lobe. The SPN shows heterogeneous to homogeneous enhancement. The attenuation value is 26.5 HU on the precontrast scan **(a)**, 70.7 HU on the scan obtained 24 seconds after injection of contrast medium **(b)**, and 109.1 HU on the scan obtained 85 seconds after injection **(c)**.

when considering 20 HU of peak height as the threshold. The peak heights of these two nodules were 11 and 17.5 HU, respectively. The enhancement pattern of these two nodules was heterogeneous. One case (with a peak height of 11 HU) was an adenocarcinoma that showed a low-attenuation area near the center of the nodule on dynamic enhanced images. The precontrast attenuation was slightly low (17 HU). The low-attenuation area on dynamic enhanced images was because of a small necrosis that was proved with histopathologic examination. The other case (with a peak height of 17.5 HU) was a small cell carcinoma that showed spokelike low attenuation on dynamic enhanced CT scans. The precontrast attenuation in this case was 27.7 HU. Also, we noticed that the peak heights of aortic enhancement in these two cases were 178.6 and 186.4 HU, respectively, which were much lower than the mean aortic peak height value (297.1 HU). We conjectured that factors contributing to the false-negative results may include small central necrosis and relative low cardiac output.

Tuberculomas could have small cavitation or heterogeneity on unenhanced scans and lack of central enhancement because of the central caseous necrosis (34), but cavitation or heterogeneity could not be considered as a sign of benignity for exclusion. Some malignant nodules with central necrosis, such as the false-negative cases in this study, or some adenocarcinomas filled with mucus could have heterogeneous enhancement. We noticed that the low-attenuation area of necrosis or mucus could diminish the mean value of peak height of enhancement when the region of interest was constructed to approximate 70%–80% of the nodule diameter in a dynamic study.

If care was taken not to include the area of necrosis when measuring the enhancement of nodules with central cavitation or central low attenuation, false-negative cases might be prevented. The value of peak height (an absolute measurement of nodule enhancement) would be simple and ideal, but this is complicated by a variety of physical factors (35,36). Especially since primary lung tumors appear to derive their blood supply almost entirely from the systemic circulation (12), absolute tumor enhancement would be expected to be in proportion to cardiac output. The statistically significant correlation between the peak height for the SPNs and that for the aortas in our study may demonstrate this inference. To minimize the differences in cardiac output by individuals, we calculated a ratio of SPN peak height to aortic peak height of enhancement. The data taken in this way would be more objective and corrective. In our study, no malignant nodule had an SPN-to-aorta ratio less than 6%. If we consider a 6% SPN-to-aorta ratio as a threshold complementary to the 20-HU peak height threshold to evaluate the nodules, there would be no false-negative results. This information might be useful clinically.

Some complex biologic factors, such as cardiac output, pulmonary blood flow, and body weight, are patient dependent and can result in a wide range of enhancement among different individuals, even when identical techniques are used. To avoid the pitfalls of interpatient physiologic variability, we planned to record SPN enhancement relative to that of muscles or opposite normal lung for adjustment or normalization. The normalization proved to be not helpful, because the attenuation of muscle was quite constant during dynamic scanning and the attenuation of the opposite normal lung was considerably variable from scan to scan and from one region to another.

In this study, we measured muscles of the posterior chest wall, such as the supraspinatus muscle, subscapularis muscle, infraspinatus muscle, and erector spinalis muscle. Data from some experimental research studies showed that blood flow to resting muscles was considerable lower in volume and rate than that in other tissues. In the study by Newhouse and Murphy (28), the blood volume measured in rats was 122 mL/kg in lung, 40.9 mL/kg in liver, and only 7.1 mL/kg in muscle. Cherry et al (37) found that tumor tissue displayed an average perfusion of three times greater than resting muscle. Dean et al (18) found in an experimental study of rats that a lower rate of uptake of contrast agent in muscle delayed the attainment of peak tissue concentrations until 2–5 minutes. These findings corroborate our result and, thus, may explain why the attenuation of muscle was quite constant during a short period of dynamic scanning.

In the literature, investigators describe the relationship between hepatic contrast enhancement and patient weight, but the published results are controversial. Some studies found an inverse linear relationship between hepatic contrast enhancement at CT and patient weight (38,39), whereas another study found no correlation between the peak enhancement and body weight and body surface (40). Most radiologists administer a uniform dose of intravenous contrast medium to all patients undergoing pulmonary CT, regardless of their size (2,3,6). Swensen et al (1), however, began to calculate dose of contrast material on the basis of patient weight in a recent pulmonary CT study; they hoped to reduce false-negative results and obtain high sensitivity. In this study, we did not record the weight of the patients but administered the same dose to all patients regardless of size. In the two false-negative cases, however, we know the patients' weight was under 70 kg. Weight, therefore, might not be the reason for the false-negative results in these two patients. Although for large patients the dose of contrast material should be modified according to the patient's size, for small patients (eg, a cohort of Japanese patients who rarely weigh over 100 kg, as in our study), it may not be necessary to relate the dose of contrast medium to patient weight.

False-positive results in our study mostly involved an inflammatory process. This finding is consistent with some other radiologic studies. Swensen et al (1,2) describe that an "active" granuloma will be more vascular and enhance more than an old granuloma. Littleton et al (5) found one false-positive case, a pneumonia mass that enhanced relatively high. Stark et al (41) reported a solitary pulmonary granuloma due to coccidioidomycosis with a vivid enhancement. In their research of SPNs with FDG positron emission tomography, Dewan et al (4) found two false-positive cases, both of which had caseous granulomas with active inflammation and histoplasma. To our knowledge, little particular attention has been paid to these findings. In our analysis of SPNs, we chose to separate active inflammatory nodules from the benign group in an effort to find a way to manage active inflammatory nodules. In this study, peak height and SPN-to-aorta peak height ratio of the inflammatory nodules were statistically significantly higher than those of the benign nodules, and no significant differences were found as compared with the malignant nodules. Almost all of the active inflammatory nodules would become false-positive cases if we evaluate SPNs simply on the basis of peak height or SPN-to-aorta peak height ratio. The fact that active inflammatory SPNs appear to have high blood flow patterns indicated that not all patients with high perfusion will have malignant tumors.

The vascular supply of most pulmonary cancers is from the bronchial arterial system (5,12). A large interstitial space has been found in some human and experimental malignant tumors (42). Most important, in the washout phase from the interstitial space, a near absence or substantial reduction of lymphatic flow is noted (5). The retarded flow in the intravascular and interstitial spaces would contribute to retention of contrast medium in malignant nodules. In most of the inflammatory pulmonary processes, because of diffuse thrombosis at the arterioles of the pulmonary circulation, the vascular supply is actually from the bronchial arteries, which are shown to be increased in size and number (43). Flow of contrast medium through the intravascular space in an inflammatory situation is taking place through relatively straight vessels with a normal configuration and is accelerated

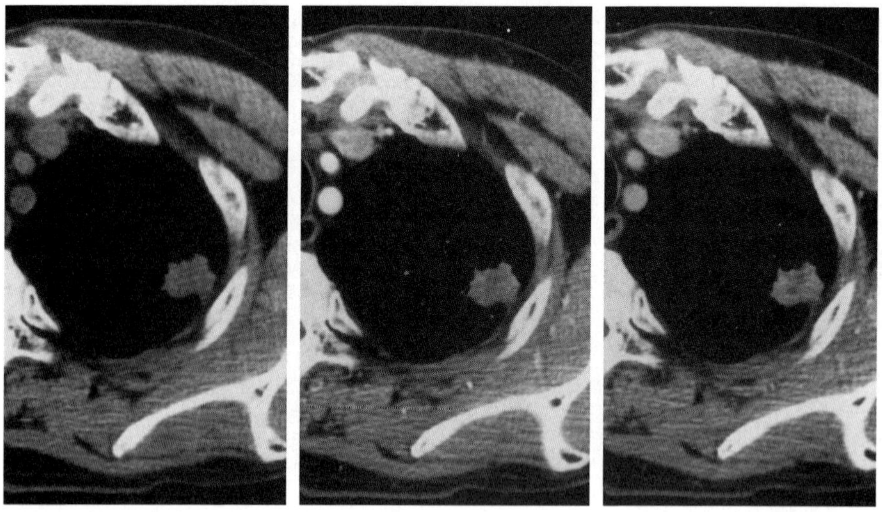

a. b. c.

Figure 9. Dynamic CT scans in a 59-year-old man with adenocarcinoma of the left upper lobe. The SPN shows peripheral enhancement owing to central necrosis. The attenuation value is 13.6 HU on the precontrast scan **(a)**, 26.6 HU on the scan obtained 27 seconds after injection of contrast medium **(b)**, and 38.0 HU on the scan obtained 82 seconds after injection **(c)**.

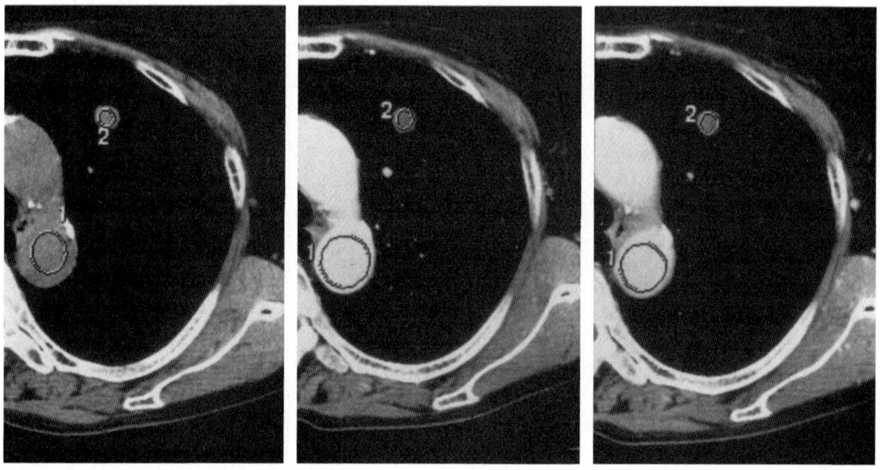

a. b. c.

Figure 10. Dynamic CT scans in a 69-year-old woman with granuloma of the left upper lobe. The SPN (circle 2) shows little enhancement. The attenuation value is 36.0 HU on the precontrast scan **(a)**, 34.6 HU on the scan obtained 36 seconds after injection of contrast medium **(b)**, and 39.7 HU on the scan obtained 100 seconds after injection **(c)**. Circle 1 = aorta.

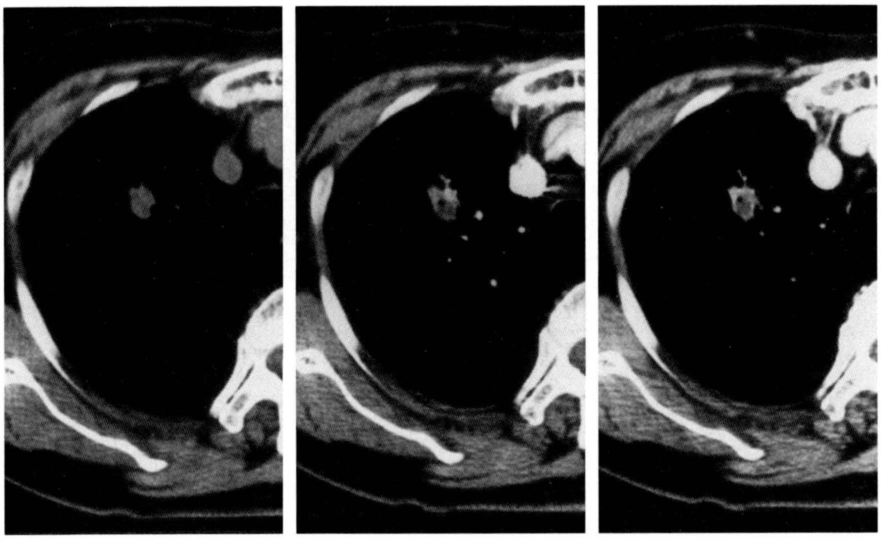

a. b. c.

Figure 11. Dynamic CT scans in a 70-year-old woman with tuberculosis of the right upper lobe. The SPN shows irregular peripheral enhancement with a small cavity. The attenuation value is 20.4 HU on the precontrast scan **(a)**, 41.7 HU on the scan obtained 27 seconds after injection **(b)**, and 34.0 HU on the scan obtained 94 seconds after injection **(c)**.

by active lymphatic flow (4). Contrarily, in instances of a quiescent fibrotic granuloma, there is no blood supply and retention of contrast medium would not be expected (5).

The pathologic nature of SPNs may be a reasonable explanation for why the enhancement of inflammatory nodules is as high as that of malignant nodules. In the inflammatory nodules, the time-attenuation curve declined after reaching peak height because of normal washout. In malignant nodules, the curve changed little after reaching peak height because of the retarded flow in the washout phase. This finding indicated that the time-attenuation curve may depict the hemodynamic characteristics of the malignant and inflammatory nodules and may be helpful in the differentiation of active inflammatory nodules and malignant nodules. Moreover, active inflammatory nodules appeared to have lower attenuation than that of malignant nodules on plain CT scans ($P < .05$) and usually have infiltrative margins. Some contrast enhancement patterns of the inflammatory nodules (Fig 11), such as irregular peripheral enhancement, may also be a characteristic of the active inflammatory nodule, whereas almost all of the malignant nodules appeared as complete homogeneous enhancement or as heterogeneous tending to homogeneous enhancement. Thus, it would seem that further discrimination between active inflammatory and malignant nodules in patients with high peak height and high SPN-to-aorta peak height ratio might be possible by taking into account the precontrast attenuation, enhancement patterns on dynamic CT scans, and appearance of the time-attenuation curve, as well as morphologic features. Large numbers of patients need to be studied to assess the validity of this proposal.

Determination of organ blood flow during the first pass of incompletely extracted radiotracers has been described and validated by Peters et al (44,45). Contrast media have similar pharmacokinetics to that of radiopharmaceuticals (16,17). Measurement of regional tissue perfusion with dynamic CT by applying a nuclear medicine data processing technique is possible (17). With the application of this technique, Blomley et al (16) and Miles (17) studied perfusion of some solid organs and obtained encouraging results. This technique has also been used to demonstrate changes in liver perfusion in disease states (20).

This study provided quantitative information about tissue perfusion of malignant, benign, and inflammatory SPNs. As would be expected, measured perfusion was higher in the malignant nodules than in the benign nodules ($P < .01$). The malignant nodule perfusion of 0.7 mL/min/mL is close to the value of 0.59–0.70 mL/min/mL obtained in hepatocellular carcinoma (20), although the tumors were in different sites. In the literature, with the studies of a single photon emission CT technique, tumor blood flow was reported to vary between 13.6 and 29.8 mL/min/100 g (37,46–48). The value in the present study appeared to be a little bit higher. There are many possible explanations. Vasodilatory effect of contrast media (20) and oxygen inspiration may increase the tumor perfusion (49). A further explanation would be that the tumor size in their research was larger than that in the present study. Raised interstitial pressure, necrosis in the center of the tumor, and heterogeneous blood flow in large tumors may reduce the perfusion (50). Furthermore, the limited resolution of the gamma camera may enable the study of only large regions of interest over the SPN, thereby easily including some nontumor tissue.

The availability of this technique has given us the opportunity to directly study and quantitate the blood flow of SPNs. To our knowledge, absolute values for SPN perfusion with dynamic CT have not been described previously. This technique is simple, requiring only the maximum gradient of the time-attenuation curve of the SPN and peak enhancement of the aorta, and can be performed in an ordinary department of radiology equipped with conventional CT. The quantifiable hemodynamic changes are considered helpful not only in differential diagnosis but also in planning further therapy, in assessing the result of therapy, and in suggesting prognosis of patients with pulmonary tumors.

The main limitation of the CT technique is that only one section level can be readily studied. A technique for the calculation of blood flow through a three-dimensional reconstruction of SPNs would have produced a result more representative than that reported.

The greatest potential source of error is patient variation in breath holding; this could result in measurement not representing the enhancement because of the varying partial-volume effect. If the nodule was situated in the upper or middle field of the lung, it would be easy to obtain the same central portion of the nodule, whereas if the nodule was located at the lower portion, that would be a little bit difficult. Four patients with SPNs at the base portion of the lung were excluded from this study because of respiratory misregistration. This can be minimized, however, by carefully instructing patients and maintaining oxygen inspiration. Before the examination began, we instructed patients to practice the breath-holding technique and scanned one or two sections repeatedly to confirm that the patients could hold their breath in the same degree of inspiration or expiration. Especially, we instructed patients with SPNs at the base portion of the lung to hold their breath in the expiration stage, which seams easy to prevent the nodules moving more at the second series of scanning. Administration of oxygen could help the patients with their breath holding.

Dynamic CT offers an alternate noninvasive option in the evaluation and management of SPNs. Lesions demonstrating high peak height or a high SPN-to-aorta peak height ratio and with high perfusion should be considered as a high possibility for malignancy until proved otherwise. Meanwhile, in this setting, to eliminate the possibility of an active inflammatory process, attention should be paid to investigating the precontrast attenuation, the enhancement pattern, and the appearance of the time-attenuation curve. More important, lesions with low peak height, low SPN-to-aorta peak height ratio, and low perfusion were always benign. ■

Acknowledgments: We appreciate the assistance of our colleagues in the department of radiology: Shuji Adachi, MD, Eiichiro Itouji, MD, Masahiko Kusumoto, MD, Kazuhiko Kimura, MD, and Fumitoshi Mimura, MD.

References

1. Swensen SJ, Brown LR, Colby TV, Weaver AL. Midthun DE. Lung nodule enhancement at CT: prospective findings. Radiology 1996; 201:447–455.
2. Swensen SJ, Brown LR, Colby TV, Weaver AL. Pulmonary nodules: CT evaluation of enhancement with iodinated contrast material. Radiology 1995; 194:393–398.
3. Swensen SJ, Morin RL, Schueler BA, et al. Solitary pulmonary nodule: CT evaluation of enhancement with iodinated contrast material—a preliminary report. Radiology 1992; 182:343–347.
4. Dewan NA, Gupta NC, Redepenning LS, Phalen JJ, Frick MP. Diagnostic efficacy of PET-FDG imaging in solitary pulmonary nodules: potential role in evaluation and management. Chest 1993; 104:997–1002.
5. Littleton JT, Durizch ML, Moeller G, Herbert DE. Pulmonary masses: contrast enhancement. Radiology 1990; 177:861–871.
6. Yamashita K, Matsunobe S, Tsuda T, et al. Solitary pulmonary nodules: preliminary study of evaluation with incremental dynamic CT. Radiology 1995; 194:399–405.
7. Patz EF Jr, Lowe VJ, Hoffman JM, et al. Focal pulmonary abnormalities: evaluation with F-18 fluorodeoxyglucose PET scanning. Radiology 1993; 188:487–490.
8. Gupta NC, Frank AR, Dewan NA, et al. Solitary pulmonary nodules: detection of malignancy with PET with 2-[F-18]-fluoro-2-deoxy-D-glucose. Radiology 1992; 184: 441–444.
9. Webb WR. Radiologic evaluation of the solitary pulmonary nodule. AJR 1990; 154: 701–708.
10. Li H, Boiselle PM, Shepard JAO, Trotman-Dickenson B, McLoud TC. Diagnostic accuracy and safety of CT-guided percutaneous needle aspiration biopsy of the lung: comparison of small and large pulmonary nodules. AJR 1996; 167:105–109.
11. Gaeta M, Barone M, Russi EG, et al. Carcinomatous solitary pulmonary nodules: evaluation of the tumor-bronchi relationship with thin-section CT. Radiology 1993; 187:535–539.
12. Milne ENC. Circulation of primary and metastatic pulmonary neoplasm: a postmortem microarteriographic study. AJR 1967; 100:603–619.
13. Milne ENC, Zerhouni EA. Blood supply of pulmonary metastases. J Thorac Imaging 1987; 2:15–23.
14. Kusumoto M, Kono M, Adachi S, et al. Gadopentetate dimeglumine–enhanced magnetic resonance imaging for lung nodules: differentiation of lung cancer and tuberculoma. Invest Radiol 1994; 29:S255–S256.
15. Guckel C, Schnabel K, Deimling M, Steinbrich W. Solitary pulmonary nodules: MR evaluation of enhancement patterns with contrast-enhanced dynamic snapshot gradient-echo imaging. Radiology 1996; 200: 681–686.
16. Blomley MJK, Coulden R, Bufkin C, Lipton MJ, Dawson P. Contrast bolus dynamic computed tomography for the measurement of solid organ perfusion. Invest Radiol 1993; 28:S72–S77.
17. Miles KA. Measurement of tissue perfusion by dynamic computed tomography. Br J Radiol 1991; 64:409–412.
18. Dean PB, Kivisaari L, Kormano M. The diagnostic potential of contrast enhancement pharmacokinetics. Invest Radiol 1978; 13:533–540.
19. Miles KA, Hayball M, Dixon AK. Colour perfusion imaging: a new application of computed tomography. Lancet 1991; 337: 643–645.
20. Miles KA, Hayball MP, Dixon AK. Functional images of hepatic perfusion obtained with dynamic CT. Radiology 1993; 188:405–411.
21. Sugano S, Okajima T, Kubo S, Yamazaki Y, Sumino Y, Abei T. Evaluation of hepatic density change by dynamic CT in healthy humans and in patients with chronic liver diseases. Dig Dis Sci 1992; 37:220–224.
22. Steiger HJ, Aaslid R, Stooss R. Dynamic computed tomographic imaging of regional cerebral blood flow and blood volume: a clinical pilot study. Stroke 1993; 24:591–597.
23. Satoh S, Togami I, Murakami K, Kitagawa T, Kimoto S, Hiraki Y. Evaluation of renal function by dynamic CT. Nippon Acta Radiol 1991; 51:1346–1351.
24. Oguchi K, Sone S, Kasuga T, et al. Methodological study of hemodynamic analysis of lung mass by contrast enhanced dynamic CT. Nippon Acta Radiol 1996; 56: 496–501.
25. Thompson HK, Starmer F, Whalen RE, Mclntosh HD. Indicator transit time considered as a gamma variate. Circ Res 1964; 14:502–515.
26. Starmer CF, Clark DO. Computer computations of cardiac output using the gamma function. J Appl Physiol 1970; 28:219–220.
27. Young SW, Turner RJ, Castellino RA. A strategy for the contrast enhancement of malignant tumors using dynamic computed tomography and intravascular pharmacokinetics. Radiology 1980; 137:137–147.
28. Newhouse JH, Murphy RX Jr. Tissue distribution of soluble contrast: effect of dose variation and changes with time. AJR 1981; 136:463–467.
29. Naidich DP, Zerhouni EA, Siegelman SS. Principles and techniques of chest computed tomography. In: Naidich DP, Zerhouni EA, Siegelman SS, ed. Computed tomography of the thorax. 1st ed. New York, NY: Raven, 1984; 9–12.
30. Berland LL, Lee JY. Comparison of contrast media injection rates and volumes for hepatic dynamic incremented computed tomography. Invest Radiol 1988; 23:918–922.
31. Garcia PA, Bonaldi VM, Bret PM, Liang L, Reinhold C, Atri M. Effect of rate of contrast medium injection on hepatic enhancement at CT. Radiology 1996; 199:185–189.
32. Chambers TP, Baron RL, Lush RM. Hepatic CT enhancement. II. Alterations in contrast material volume and rate of injection within the same patients. Radiology 1994; 193:518–522.
33. Kormano M, Dean PB. Extravascular contrast media: the major component of contrast enhancement. Radiology 1976; 121: 379–382.
34. Murayama S, Murakami J, Hashimoto S, Torii Y, Masuda K. Noncalcified pulmonary tuberculomas: CT enhancement patterns with histological correlation. J Thorac Imaging 1995; 10:91–95.
35. Claussen CD, Banzer D, Pfretzschner C, Kalender WA, Schorner W. Bolus geometry and dynamics after intravenous contrast medium injection. Radiology 1984; 153:365–368.
36. Cox IH, Foley WD, Hoffmann R. Right window for dynamic hepatic CT. Radiology 1991; 181:18–21.
37. Cherry SR, Carnochan P, Babich JW, Serafini F, Rowell NP, Watson IA. Quantitative in vivo measurements of tumor perfusion using rubidium-81 and positron emission tomography. J Nucl Med 1990; 31:1307–1315.
38. Heiken JP, Brink JA, MacClennan BL, Sagel SS, Crowe TM, Gaines MV. Dynamic incremental CT: effect of volume and concentration of contrast material and patient weight on hepatic enhancement. Radiology 1995; 195:353–357.
39. Kormano M, Partanen K, Soimakallio S, Kivimäki T. Dynamic contrast enhancement of the upper abdomen: effect of contrast medium and body weight. Invest Radiol 1983; 18:364–367.
40. Thorstensen Ö, Isberg B, Aspelin P. Contrast enhancement of the upper abdomen evaluated by CT: a comparison between iohexol 350 mg I/ml and iopamidal 370 mg I/ml. Acta Radiol 1995; 36:549–551.
41. Stark K, Wong V, Gold P. Solitary pulmonary granuloma with marked enhancement on dynamic CT scanning. Radiologe 1988; 28:489–490.
42. Peterson HI. Vascular and extravascular spaces in tumors: tumor vascular permeability. In: Peterson HI, ed. Tumor blood circulation: angiogenesis, vascular morphology and blood flow of experimental and human tumors. Boca Raton, Fla: CRC, 1979; 77–86.
43. Deffebach ME, Charan NB, Lakshminarayan S, Butler J. The bronchial circulation: small, but a vital attribute of the lung. Am Rev Respir Dis 1987; 135:463–481.
44. Peters AM, Gunasekera RD, Henderson BL, et al. Non-invasive measurement of blood flow and extraction fraction. Nucl Med Commun 1987; 8:823–827.
45. Peters AM, Brown J, Hartnell GG, Myers MJ, Haskell C, Lavender JP. Non-invasive measurement of renal blood flow with 99mTc DTPA: a comparison with radiolabelled microspheres. Cardiovasc Res 1987; 21:830-834.
46. Wheeler RH, Ziessman HA, Medvec BR, et al. Tumor blood flow and systemic shunting in patients receiving intraarterial chemotherapy for head and neck cancer. Cancer Res 1986; 46:4200–4204.
47. Rowell NP, Flower MA, Cronin B, McCready VR. Quantitative single-photon emission tomography for tumour blood flow measurement in bronchial carcinoma. Eur J Nucl Med 1993; 20:591–599.
48. Wilson CBJH, Lammertsma AA, McKenzie CG, Sikora K, Jones T. Measurements of blood flow and exchanging water space in breast tumours using potron emission tomography: a rapid and noninvasive dynamic method. Cancer Res 1992; 52:1592–1597.
49. Yamashita K, Matsunobe S, Takahashi R, et al. Small peripheral lung carcinoma evaluated with incremental dynamic CT: radiologic-pathologic correlation. Radiology 1995; 196:401–408.
50. Jain RK. Determinants of tumor blood flow: a review. Cancer Res 1988; 48:2641–2658.

Rajiv Mallick, PhD • Shelah G. Leader, PhD • Jonathan H. Sunshine, PhD • Katherine A. Shaffer, MD

Hiring by Radiology Groups in 1996[1]

PURPOSE: To determine the hiring activity of radiology groups in 1996.

MATERIALS AND METHODS: A survey was mailed to a stratified, random sample of 794 radiology groups in autumn 1996. The response rate was 78%. Responses were weighted to be representative of all of the approximately 3,300 groups in the United States. Findings were compared with those of previous, similar surveys.

RESULTS: In the 12 months before the survey, groups sought to hire 1,732 ± 155 (±1 standard error) diagnostic radiologists and radiation oncologists; 788 ± 105 of these positions were to fill expansion positions, 562 ± 86 were replacements for persons who had left the profession, and 382 ± 78 were replacements for persons who moved to other radiology positions. During the year, an additional 500 ± 119 positions were vacated that groups did not seek to refill. Groups succeeded in hiring 1,438 ± 143 radiologists. The percentage of available positions that were filled did not differ across fields. Managed health care reduced the probability a group was expanding but did not otherwise affect hiring activity.

CONCLUSION: The 1991–1995 decline in hiring has ceased and perhaps even reversed. There were approximately as many positions available in 1996 as were needed by graduates, although there may have been a small shortfall.

Since 1991, The American College of Radiology (ACR) has been closely monitoring the employment situation of diagnostic radiologists and radiation oncologists (1–14). As part of this ongoing commitment to documenting the demand for radiologists' services, the ACR has periodically conducted surveys of stratified, random samples of radiology groups about recruitment and hiring activities (4,6,7).

This article presents the results of the fourth such survey, which was conducted in late 1996. The 1996 survey, in addition to established questions about the number of openings groups wanted to fill, the success of these groups in hiring for these positions, the characteristics of job seekers, and changes in the job market, also contained a question about the number of departing radiologists for whom the group did not seek a replacement. Additionally, the 1996 survey obtained data not only on a calendar year–to-date basis, as was the case with previous surveys, but also on hiring activity over the full 12 months that preceded the survey.

In 1996, as in the past, we compared the number of positions available with the number of graduates who were seeking positions. Because the total number of graduates is a full-year statistic, the 12-month hiring data are more appropriate for this purpose than the calendar year–to-date data previously available. To measure trends, we also compared hiring in 1996 with that in earlier years. For this purpose, the calendar year–to-date data are appropriate, for these data are comparable with the data from surveys conducted in previous years.

MATERIALS AND METHODS

The Survey

In August 1996, the hiring survey was mailed to a stratified random sample of 794 radiology practice groups in the United States, which constituted 24% of the estimated 3,286 groups in the country. Up to three follow-up mailings were sent between then and October to groups that did not initially respond; the last was sent by means of Priority Mail. Telephone calls were made to clarify ambiguous responses to the most important questions. As in previous years, in the 1996 hiring survey we asked about the characteristics of each group, the number of positions each group sought to fill, the subspecialty areas the positions covered, the number and subspecialty areas of positions actually filled, and the self-perceived extent to which managed health care has affected the practice.

The practices surveyed encompassed all types of radiology groups, including radiology units of multispecialty groups and government facilities, as well as academic groups and private nonacademic groups. Respondents self-designated the type of their group by answering the question: "Is your group (check the *first* that applies) primarily academic, part of a private multispecialty group, government employees (ie, VA, military), or private radiology

Index terms: Economics, medical • Radiology and radiologists • Radiology and radiologists, socioeconomic issues

Abbreviations: ACR = American College of Radiology, FTE = full-time equivalent.

Radiology 1997; 205:479–486

[1] From PraCon, a division of Excerpta Medica, Reston, Va (R.M., S.G.L.); the Department of Research (J.H.S.) and the Committee on Radiologist Resources (K.A.S.), American College of Radiology, 1891 Preston White Dr, Reston, VA 20191-4397; and the Department of Radiology, Medical College of Wisconsin, Milwaukee (K.A.S.). Received June 4, 1997; revision requested July 7; revision received July 24; accepted August 4. **Address reprint requests to** J.H.S.

group." Responses from nine individuals who indicated that they were engaged in solo practice at the time of the survey were excluded from the analysis.

An important new feature of the 1996 survey was the use of two slightly different survey instruments. With form A, respondents were asked about recruitment during the most recent 12 months, whereas form B mirrored the 1995 and earlier surveys in which respondents were asked about recruitment during the calendar year to date. Half of the groups in the sample received form A, and half received form B.

The sample was drawn from the ACR's master list of radiology practices in the United States and was stratified to reflect the known distribution of groups according to size and census region. The sample was stratified on the basis of the four census regions—Northeast, Midwest, South, and West—and five size categories in each region—two radiologists, three or four radiologists, five to seven radiologists, eight to 10 radiologists, and 11 or more radiologists. Usable responses were weighted to reflect what the response would have been if all of the estimated 3,286 radiology groups in the United States had been surveyed and had responded.

We received 617 responses; an additional seven groups told us they no longer existed. Thus, the overall response rate was 78% after subtracting the seven groups that were definitively found to no longer exist (617/[794 − 7] × 100 = 78%). The previous survey response rates were 78% (150 of 192) in 1991, 92% (341 of 370) in 1994, and 85% (505 of 593) in 1995. The 617 responding groups comprised 459 diagnostic radiology–only groups, 57 radiation oncology–only groups, and 101 groups that provided both diagnostic radiology and radiation oncology services.

With the 1996 survey, we continued to use a rule, applied in 1994 and 1995, that no single position or radiologist hired could be associated with position responsibilities in more than three fields. When more than three fields were reported, we retabulated the information to reassign the smallest fraction(s) of the position(s) (or radiologist hired) to general diagnostic radiology so that the position (or radiologist) covered only three fields, including general diagnostic radiology. For example, suppose a group reported that it sought or hired a radiologist with the following division of responsibilities: general diagnostic radiology, 0.4 full-time–equivalent (FTE) responsibilities; pediatric radiology, 0.2 FTE; neuroradiology, 0.2 FTE; magnetic resonance (MR) imaging, 0.1 FTE; and computed tomography (CT), 0.1 FTE. The last two fields were then reassigned to the general diagnostic category, which yielded an FTE of 0.6 for that category. Thus, general diagnostic radiology included both plain radiography and fluoroscopy and work that involved relatively small amounts of time in a large number of fields.

We compared results from the 1996 survey with those from the 1994 and 1995 surveys, which were also mail surveys, and the 1991 survey, which was a telephone survey.

Statistical Analysis

As was the case with past surveys, each response was weighted so that the respondents reflected the universe of groups according to size and census region. Because responses are from a sample, there is a degree of uncertainty as regards the representativeness of responses received relative to the universe of all groups. Hence, for most findings we report the standard error, which is the usual measure of the degree of uncertainty in projections from sample responses to the universe.

To compare calendar year–to-date hiring, which was reported on form B and was the measure used in previous surveys, with hiring in the most recent 12 months, which was reported on form A and is a conceptually superior measure, we performed two comparisons. First, we simply compared totals from form B with those from form A. If these were equal, we would know that (essentially) all hiring occurred during the first 9 or so months of the calendar year, which was the assumption in previous surveys. Second, because most survey forms were returned about September, we multiplied form B totals by 12/9, because form B contained hiring information for approximately 9 of the previous 12 months of the year. We compared these adjusted form B totals with form A totals. If the totals were approximately equal, that would indicate fairly uniform hiring throughout the year.

After these comparisons of form A and form B totals, several hiring variables were measured for the universe of radiology groups and were compared with previous survey data. The outcomes compared with those of past years were (*a*) the total number of positions groups sought to fill, (*b*) the total number of radiologists hired, (*c*) the hiring success rate, and (*d*) the remaining vacancy rate. Because with past surveys we had obtained year-to-date data, these comparisons were made with form B responses.

Furthermore, the total number of position openings were categorized on the basis of the following components: (*a*) expansion positions, (*b*) replacements of radiologists who left the profession, (*c*) replacements of radiologists who left for another position in the profession, (*d*) total number of vacated positions that groups did not seek to fill, and (*e*) the number of FTEs sought and hired in each subspecialty field. In general, data on these components are shown in Table 1 and were derived from form A, because 12-month data are conceptually preferable.

The association between hiring activity and group type, group size, census region, degree of urbanization of the group's location, use of part-time or locum tenens radiologists, and the perceived effect of managed care was also tested (Table 2). The paired association of group characteristics and whether or not a group was hiring was tested by using χ^2 tests.

Table 1
Recruitment by Radiology Groups in the Most Recent 12 Months

Recruitment Variable	No. of Positions
Total no. of openings	1,732 ± 155
Total no. of radiologists hired	1,438 ± 143 (83)*
No. of radiologists who left group for whom no replacement was sought	500 ± 119
No. of openings for candidates with fellowship training	1,149 ± 120 (66)*
No. of expansion positions	788 ± 105 (46)*
No. of positions to replace those who left profession	562 ± 86 (32)*
No. of positions to replace those who moved within profession	382 ± 78 (22)*
No. of hires with fellowship training	1,051 ± 119 (73)†
No. of interviews conducted for all openings	6,427 ± 781
Ratio of interviews to openings	3.7‡
Ratio of interviews to hires	4.5‡
No. of offers made	2,130 ± 227
Ratio of offers to openings	1.2‡
Ratio of offers to hires	1.5‡
Remaining vacancy rate (%)	1.2
Effect of managed care	
None	5§
A little	33§
Moderate	34§
Significant	19§
Great	9§

Note.—Data are based on responses to form A and are weighted to reflect the answers that would have been given had all 3,286 groups in the United States been surveyed and responded. Unless otherwise indicated, data are number of positions ± 1 standard error. Numbers in parentheses are weighted percentages.
* Percentage is based on the total number of openings.
† Percentage is based on the total of all hires.
‡ Number is the ratio.
§ Number is the weighted percentage of groups.

In all of the statistical tests used (Student *t* tests or χ^2 tests), a two-tailed, 95% level of statistical significance was used to classify associations as statistically significant ($P \leq .05$). With one exception, "significant" is used in this article to indicate statistical significance. (The exception is the verbatim reporting of the response "significant" to a survey question about the effect of managed care, which appears in Tables 1 and 2.)

We conducted multivariate analysis to ascertain which group characteristics were independently predictive of four of the hiring activity variables: (*a*) the total number of positions a group sought to fill, (*b*) the number of expansion positions a group sought to fill, (*c*) whether or not a group that was hiring filled all open posi-

Table 2
Percentage of Groups Actively Hiring in the Most Recent 12 Months according to Group Characteristics

Characteristic	Hiring (%)
All groups	37
Group type*	
Academic	75
Private nonacademic multispecialty	55
Private nonacademic radiology	34
Group size*	
Two to four radiologists	29
Five to seven radiologists	31
Eight to 10 radiologists	42
11 or more radiologists	63
Urbanization of group's location*	
Main city–area population > 1 million	47
Suburbs-area population > 1 million	29
Main city–area population = 100,000 to 1 million	38
Suburbs-area population = 100,000 to 1 million	49
Area population < 100,000	25
Census region	
Northeast	43
Midwest	37
South	35
West	32
Employed part-time radiologists*	
No	30
Yes	48
Employed locum tenens radiologists	
No	35
Yes	40
Effect of managed care	
None	38
A little	34
Moderate	40
Significant	34
Great	38

Note.—Data are based on responses to form A and are weighted to reflect the answers that would have been given had all 3,286 radiology groups in the United States been surveyed and responded.
* Percentage differences for the characteristic were statistically significant at the 95% confidence interval.

tions, and (*d*) whether or not a group that was hiring offered any positions on a partnership-track basis.

For all four of these group hiring variables, the following group characteristics were examined to determine if they affected the variable in question: (*a*) group type (academic, nonacademic government, nonacademic private multispecialty, and nonacademic private radiology), (*b*) types of services provided (diagnostic radiology, radiation oncology, or both), (*c*) use of any part-time radiologists in the past year, (*d*) use of any locum tenens radiologists in the past year, (*e*) geographic region (Northeast, Midwest, South, or West), (*f*) degree of urbanization of the group's location, (*g*) group size, and (*h*) self-assessed effect of managed care on the group. To examine whether the group was able to fill all positions, the total number of positions the group sought to fill were also considered.

To attain greater statistical power to discern independent influences on hiring, we pooled responses from form A and form B for the multivariate analyses. Because form B covered only the year to date, we used a categorical variable to indicate whether a response was from form B.

For the total number of positions to be filled and the number of expansion positions to be filled, we conducted a regression analysis by using the Heckman two-step model (15) to determine if groups that did not have any positions to fill were systematically different from groups that did, and then to determine which factors affected the number of positions that groups sought to fill, if they were hiring. The regressions on the other two hiring-activity variables noted above were estimated with logistic modeling techniques because the variables of interest were dichotomous—that is, "yes" or "no".

RESULTS

Results throughout are reported as weighted or unweighted data ± 1 standard error.

1996 Findings

When unadjusted calendar year–to-date responses (which covered approximately the first 9 months of 1996) were compared with 12-month responses, no significant differences were found with regard to the total number of positions sought and filled (Fig 1, Table 3). In contrast, when we adjusted calendar year–to-date data by multiplying these responses by 12/9, the adjusted year-to-date totals of positions sought and positions filled were significantly greater than the corresponding 12-month totals. Thus, hiring in the first 9 months of the calendar year accounted for almost all hiring in a calendar year.

In the 12 months before the autumn 1996 date of the survey, 37% ± 3 of all groups actively recruited for a total of 1,732 ± 155 positions (Table 1). Radiologists with fellowship training were sought for 1,149 ± 120 (66% ± 7) of these positions. Furthermore, of these 1,732 positions, 788 (46%) were new positions, 562 (32%) were positions vacated by radiologists who left the profession (usually because of retirement or death), and the remaining 382 (22%) were positions vacated by radiologists who had moved to another position within the profession.

Groups also reported a total of 500 ± 119 vacated positions that they did not seek to fill. Of these, 241 ± 80 positions had been vacated by radiologists who left for another position within the profession. This number may include radiologists who were "downsized" or discharged. The remaining 259 ± 65 positions were vacated by radiologists who had left the profession (again, principally because of retirement or death). Some of these radiologists may have left the group involuntarily.

A total of 1,438 ± 143 radiologists were hired in the 12-month period, 1,051 (73%) of whom had fellowship training. The hiring success rate—that is, the ratio of the number hired to the number sought, expressed as a percentage—was 83%.

The remaining vacancy rate—that is, the total number of unfilled positions at the end of the hiring season as a proportion of the total number of radiologists employed before the hiring season plus those sought—was approximately 1%.

In the 12-month period covered by the survey, 6,427 ± 781 candidates were interviewed, which yielded an average of about four interviews per opening. This led to 2,130 ± 227 firm offers, or 1.3 offers per opening and 1.5 offers for each radiologist actually hired.

For nonacademic, private groups (both multispecialty and radiology-only), 1,023 ± 118 (73%) of all full-time positions that these groups sought to fill were partnership-track positions.

Table 2 lists the percentage of groups that actively recruited in the last twelve months according to group characteristics. Academic groups were more likely to recruit than nonacademic groups (recall that the academic vs nonacademic distinction was self-designated by respondents), larger groups were more apt to recruit than smaller groups, and groups that employed part-time radiologists during the preceding year were more likely to recruit than those that had not employed part-time radiologists. On the other hand, groups located in a nonmetropolitan area were significantly less likely to recruit than others.

1991–1996 Trends

Figures 1–4 depict trends in hiring. To update hiring trend lines by using the 1996 survey and to remain consistent with data from previous years, only the calendar year–to-date (form B) responses were used. (In previous years, as on form B, we had asked about hiring "in 1991," for example, and thus received calendar year–to-date information, rather than information about an entire 12-month period.) However, 12-month (form A) responses

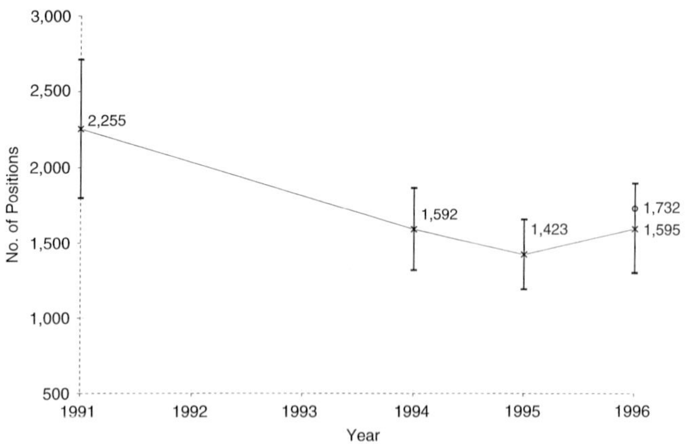

1.

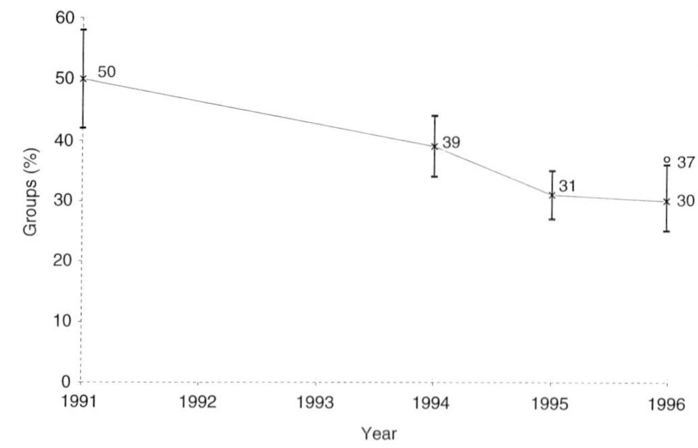

2.

Figures 1, 2. **(1)** Graph shows the number of positions that radiology groups sought to fill in 1991 and 1994–1996 on a year-to-date (×) and 12-month (O) basis. Error bars = 95% confidence interval. **(2)** Graph shows the percentage of radiology groups that were actively recruiting in 1991 and 1994–1996 on a year-to-date (×) and 12-month (O) basis. Error bars = 95% confidence interval.

are also shown in Figures 1–4, because data about a full 12 months are conceptually more relevant. The 95% confidence intervals associated with the hiring trend lines are also depicted.

The percentage of groups that were actively recruiting (Fig 2) and the remaining vacancy rate (Fig 3) did not improve over 1995. The number of position openings appear to have been higher than in 1995 (Fig 1), although the difference was not significant. Similarly, the hiring success rate (Fig 4) appears to have continued to rise, but the difference was not significant.

Table 3
Available Positions and Hiring in Radiation Oncology and Diagnostic Radiology Fields

Field	No. of Positions with Nearly Full-Time Responsibility in Single Field*	Total No. of Radiology Positions†	Total No. of FTEs Sought‡	Ratio of FTE Hired to FTE Sought (%)	No. of Groups Recruiting
Radiation oncology§	226 ± 56	301 ± 68	226 ± 50	90	180 ± 39
General diagnostic radiology	763 ± 80	1,066 ± 96	776 ± 69	79	708 ± 59
Pediatric radiology	44 ± 16	61 ± 19	47 ± 16	63	44 ± 15
Nuclear medicine/radiology	28 ± 9	96 ± 19	48 ± 10	100	85 ± 17
Neuroradiology	88 ± 19	145 ± 27	101 ± 19	83	114 ± 21
MR imaging	27 ± 10	101 ± 23	47 ± 12	73	87 ± 20
Interventional and vascular radiology	177 ± 27	300 ± 41	203 ± 27	90	223 ± 29
Ultrasound	14 ± 6	88 ± 19	36 ± 8	75	85 ± 18
CT	11 ± 5	78 ± 18	29 ± 8	88	72 ± 17
Mammography	61 ± 17	123 ± 25	77 ± 16	84	100 ± 20
Other	24 ± 8	59 ± 16	32 ± 9	86	42 ± 11

Note.—Data are based on combined responses (±1 standard error) from form A and form B. Form B responses about number of positions sought year to date were multiplied by 1.08 (the ratio of positions sought on form A to those on form B). Form B responses about number of positions filled were multiplied by 1.02 (the ratio of form A responses to form B responses with regard to positions filled).

* Nearly full time is defined as 70% or more of FTE.

† Includes both nearly full-time positions and positions with only part-time responsibilities in the field. No one position could be reported as including responsibilities in more than three fields.

‡ FTEs of the total number of positions.

§ The appearance of the number 226 twice in this row is coincidental.

Recruitment and Hiring in Specific Fields of Radiology

In 1996, a total of 1,622 FTE positions were sought, and positions in general diagnostic radiology accounted for 48% of these FTEs. Positions in radiation oncology accounted for 14% of the FTEs, and positions in interventional and vascular radiology accounted for 13% (Table 3).

To estimate the number of positions for radiologists to practice nearly full time in a single field (see the first column of Table 3), we separately analyzed recruitment for positions that necessitated at least 70% of the radiologist's time in a single field. We also measured the number of positions that necessitated any percentage of time in a field, after reclassification of the allocation of responsibilities so that no position was allocated to more than three fields (see the second column of Table 3). For example, Table 3 shows that there were 226 ± 56 (1 standard error) positions available in which the radiologist would work at least 70% of full time in radiation oncology and 301 ± 68 positions in which the radiologist would work in radiation oncology at all.

By further examining the data, we found that all these radiation oncology positions were radiation oncology–only positions; none also involved diagnostic radiology work. Thus, to the extent that the 226 nearly full-time positions did not involve full-time work in radiation oncology, the positions were part-time positions that involved, say, a 3½- or 4-d/wk work schedule. Similarly, the approximately 75 positions (301 positions minus 226 positions) that involved radiation oncology work for less than 70% of full time were radiation oncology–only part-time positions, with a work schedule of less than 70% of full time.

In the fields of radiation oncology, general diagnostic radiology, pediatric radiology, neuroradiology, and interventional radiology, more than half of the positions that involved any work in the field required radiologists to work at least 70% of full time in that single field. However, in the fields of nuclear medicine (and nuclear radiology), MR imaging, ultrasound, and CT, fewer than one third of the positions that involved work in the field required the radiologist to work at least 70% of full time in the field.

Table 3 also shows, for each field,

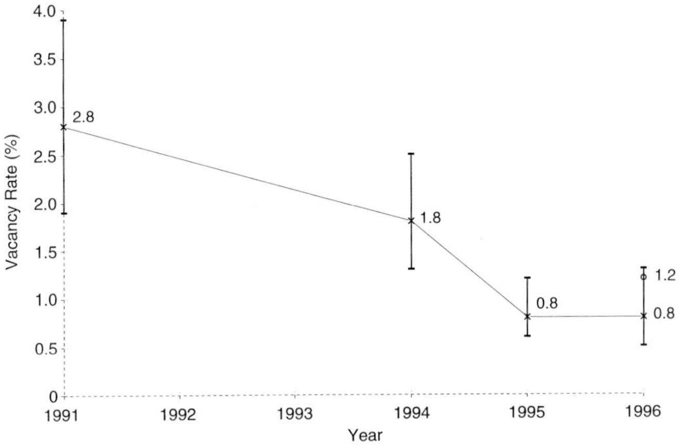

3.

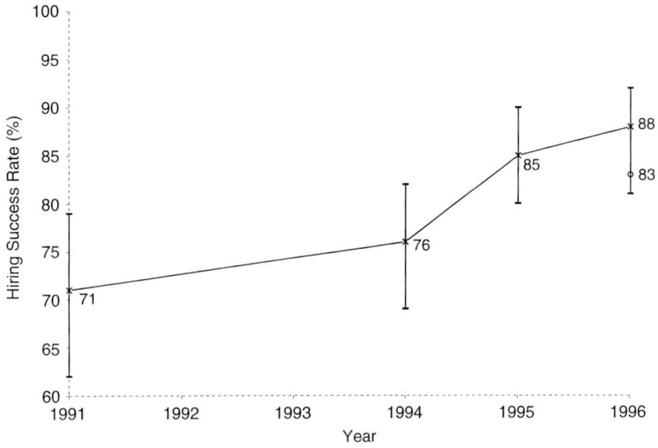

4.

Figures 3, 4. **(3)** Graph shows the percentage of positions that were not filled (remaining vacancy rate) in 1991 and 1994–1996 on a year-to-date (×) and 12-month (O) basis. Error bars = 95% confidence interval. **(4)** Graph shows the hiring success rate in 1991 and 1994–1996 on a year-to-date (×) and 12-month (O) basis. Error bars = 95% confidence interval.

the ratio of FTE radiologists actually hired to those sought. Although this ratio ranged from a low of 63% in pediatric radiology to 100% in nuclear medicine, no field differed by a significant amount from the average of all other fields in terms of this hiring success rate. The hiring success rate among all diagnostic subspecialties combined (not shown separately in Table 3) was 84%, which was not significantly different from the 81% rate among the fields of general diagnostic radiology and radiation oncology combined.

Groups with Unfilled Positions

We studied groups that were unable to hire all the radiologists they had sought to determine how such groups differed from actively recruiting groups that were able to fill all available positions. Those in the former category apparently interviewed fewer candidates on average (4.4 vs 5.5) than the latter. They also apparently had a slightly lower ratio of interviews to available openings (3.4 vs 3.8) than did groups that filled all positions. However, neither of these differences were statistically significant.

Groups that were unable to fill all their positions made a total of 1.4 offers, on average, compared with a total of 1.9 offers, on average, by groups that did fill all positions. The ratio of offers to available positions was significantly lower for the former than for the latter (1.07 vs 1.27).

Of the groups with remaining vacancies at the end of the 1996 hiring season, 6% had interviewed fewer candidates than the number of available positions, and 38% had made fewer offers than the total number of positions. Fifty-four percent of groups with remaining vacancies indicated that they were still seeking to fill those positions.

We asked groups that were unable to fill all vacancies why they thought they had been unable to do so. Of the 51 groups (unweighted) with remaining vacancies, the most frequently cited reason was that candidates had found the group's location unattractive (24%, on a weighted basis). Other frequently cited reasons were salary demands of candidates (12%) and dissatisfaction with quality of applicants (11%).

Multivariate Analysis of 1996 Data

As described in the Materials and Methods section, we used the Heckman two-step technique (15) to identify which group characteristics were significantly predictive of the total number of positions a group sought to fill, with other factors controlled for. The analysis showed, first, that groups that sought to hire any radiologists were systematically different from groups that did not. Specifically, with other factors held equal, hiring groups were more likely to be academic than nonacademic; were either radiation oncology–only groups or both radiation oncology and diagnostic radiology groups, rather than diagnostic radiology–only groups; were located in the Midwest; had used locum tenens or part-time radiologists; were generally larger in size; were not located in a suburb of a large metropolitan area or the main city of a small metropolitan area; and reported about recruitment activity for the previous 12 months (ie, responded to Form A) rather than for the calendar year to date (ie, responded to Form B).

By adjusting for these differences between groups that were hiring and those that were not, we found that, with other factors (including group size) held equal, academic groups and nonacademic private multispecialty groups recruited for a larger number of positions than did nonacademic private radiology groups. Furthermore, groups that had employed any locum tenens radiologists in the past year were seeking to fill 0.5 more positions than otherwise identical groups that did not use any locum tenens radiologists. Similarly, with other factors controlled for, groups that had employed any part-time radiologists sought to fill 0.6 more positions than did groups that had not employed any part-time radiologists. Finally, group size had a significant but nonlinear effect on the number of positions groups sought to fill. With other group characteristics controlled for, larger groups sought more radiologists; however, this effect decreased as group size increased.

None of the other group characteristics—degree of urbanization of the group's location, self-assessed effect of managed care, whether the group was engaged in radiation oncology either alone or in conjunction with diagnostic radiology rather than only in diagnostic radiology, and region of the country—were significantly predictive of how many radiology positions a recruiting group sought to fill.

The multivariate Heckman regression analysis of the number of expansion (rather than total) positions that groups sought to fill indicated that groups that recruited radiologists for expansion positions differed from groups that did not. With other factors held equal, groups that reported a greater self-assessed effect of managed care on their practice were less likely to recruit for expansion positions. Also, with other factors held equal, the groups that recruited for expansion positions were more likely to be private multispecialty groups, to have used locum tenens or part-time radiologists, to practice radiation oncology only, to be generally larger in size, to be located in the Midwest, and to be located in the suburbs of a small metropolitan area. However, no group characteristic was significantly associated with the number of expansion positions groups sought to fill.

Of the estimated 1,083 groups that actively recruited in 1996, approximately 22% were unable to fill all their vacancies. We conducted a multivariate analysis to determine which group characteristics had a significant, independent association with the presence of unfilled vacancies at the end of the hiring season. By adjusting for all other group characteristics, we found that groups in the South and in the West were significantly less likely to have remaining unfilled positions than were groups in the Midwest. Groups that had employed any locum tenens radiologists in the most recent 12-month period were more likely to have remaining unfilled positions. Other group characteristics—degree of urbanization, practice type, group size, whether or not the group had any part-time radiologists, and self-assessed effect of managed care—did not have significant, independent associations with the presence of remaining unfilled positions.

We also conducted a multivariate analysis of all private, nonacademic groups that actively recruited in 1996 to learn which group characteristics were independently associated with the offering of positions on a partnership-track basis. By controlling for other characteristics, we found that multispecialty groups were significantly less likely to offer full-time positions on a partnership-track basis than radiology groups. Groups located in the main city of a metropolitan area with a population of fewer than 1 million were more likely to offer positions on a partnership track than those located elsewhere; the same was true (marginally) of groups located in a nonmetropolitan area. No other group characteristic was independently associated with the offering of positions on a partnership-track basis.

DISCUSSION

Strengths and Weaknesses of the Data

Our survey data, like all data sets, have strengths and weaknesses. The strength of the data derives from the large, carefully drawn sample (n = 794), which comprised approximately 24% of all U.S. radiology groups. The high response rate to the survey (78%) and the accurate weighting of responses to reflect the known universe of radiology groups enhance our confidence in the findings. Another strength of the data derives from the increased understanding of the employment market gained from the two innovations in the 1996 survey, namely, (*a*) the question about vacancies for which no replacement was sought and (*b*) the acquisition of information about a full 12 months of hiring activity. Finally, we made follow-up telephone calls to respondents to clarify ambiguous responses to high-priority questions.

Despite these efforts, some data weaknesses remain. In particular, although a large number of groups responded, the actual number of responses on some points was small. As a result, there was considerable uncertainty about some specific findings that might otherwise be worthy of attention but did not attain statistical significance. Most notably, the ratio of FTE radiologists actually hired to those sought ranged from 63% for pediatric radiology positions to 100% for nuclear medicine positions. However, because the actual survey responses involved only eight unweighted FTE positions in pediatric radiology and only nine in nuclear medicine, there was insufficient statistical power to enable such differences to attain the requisite level of statistical significance that would permit 95% confidence that there was a difference between hiring success rates in these two fields. Somewhat similarly, although our findings about the ratio of offers to positions available showed that this ratio was significantly lower for groups that did not fill all positions than for groups that did, we were unable to pursue this intriguing finding because of an insufficient number of responses to the question about why groups thought they had not been able to fill all positions. Finally, because we surveyed only groups, we have no information on the movement of radiologists into solo practice. Eight percent of all radiologists are in solo practice.

Core Findings

The most important question we sought to answer was whether the number of positions available in 1996 were enough—or too few or too many—for all the radiologists who graduated from training that year plus all the experienced radiologists who, for whatever reason, sought to move from one group to another. To answer this question, it was helpful to assume, initially, that all experienced radiologists found positions, so that any shortage or excess of positions therefore affected only new graduates. Given this assumption, analytic reasoning shows that the number of positions available to graduates is equal to (*a*) the number of expansion positions groups sought to fill plus (*b*) the number of radiologists groups sought to hire as replacements for radiologists who had retired, died, or otherwise left the workforce minus (*c*) the number of instances in which a radiologist left a group for some other position, and the group did not seek to fill the vacated position. (Table 4 displays the logic that leads to this formula.) Our data thus show that the number of positions available ($\pm$1 standard error) for graduates were approximately 788 (expansion positions) plus 562 (replacements for those leaving the profession) minus 241 (radiologists who left for another position and were not replaced), or 1,109 $\pm$ 173.

The recent average annual number of graduates who complete training has been approximately 1,160 (1,000 diagnostic radiologists plus 160 radiation oncologists) (8,12,14). (The number of graduates completing training each year is estimated on the basis of the number who finish residency training. In fact, some—or most—residents accept a 1- or 2-year fellowship, but that means there is an equal number of fellows completing training each year.)

With an estimated 1,109 positions available to graduates in 1996 and approximately 1,160 graduates who completed training, there appears to have been a 1996 shortfall of 51 positions. For three reasons, however, we cannot be sure there was actually a shortfall of positions for graduates. First, the estimated shortfall (51 positions) is well within the limits of uncertainty in the estimated number of positions available to graduates, as is reflected in the standard error of $\pm$173 of the latter. Second, the number of graduates fluctuates slightly from year to year, and may be declining by a few percent (14). Third, any shortfall may, in reality, primarily affect experienced radiologists, not new graduates.

Indeed, the results of a recent survey (11) showed that groups that were hiring diagnostic radiologists generally preferred recent graduates to radiologists with 10–20 years experience. If, for example, the estimated 623 experienced radiologists who moved between positions in 1996 spent an average of 1 month between positions, either because they deliberately took some time for a move or were involuntarily unemployed, that would absorb a shortfall of approximately 52 positions. In any case, in a survey of training program directors (14), it was found that by December 1996, unemployment among 1996 graduates was less than 1%, which indicated

Table 4
Effect of Various Events on the Number of Positions in the United States Available to Graduates

Event	Effect on Total No. of Positions	Effect on No. of Experienced Radiologists in Practice	Net Effect on No. of Positions Available to Graduates*
Group hires for expansion position	One additional position	None	One additional position
Group hires to replace radiologist who left profession	None	One fewer radiologist	One additional position
Group hires to replace radiologist who moved to another group	None	None	None
Group does not seek to replace radiologist who left profession	One fewer position	One fewer radiologist	None
Group does not seek to replace radiologist who moved to another group	One fewer position	None	One fewer position

* The number in this column is the number in the first column minus the number in the second column. We assume that all experienced radiologists who moved to another group obtained a job; therefore, any excess or shortfall of jobs affects only graduates.

that if there was a shortfall in the number of positions available to radiologists, its effect on employment of new graduates has been small.

The number of diagnostic radiologists and radiation oncologists who left active practice in the 12 months preceding the survey appears to be unusually high. The survey results indicate that 821 ± 108 left practice during this period. (Specifically, groups reported that they sought to replace 562 radiologists who left practice and did not seek to replace an additional 259 who ceased practicing, which means that the total who left practice was 562 + 259 = 821.) In contrast, by using models (8,12), we estimated that approximately 400 diagnostic radiologists and 40 radiation oncologists leave the workforce each year. These models assume that (*a*) the percentage in each age group (age of 50–54 years, 55–59 years, etc) who are in active practice (rather than retired) remains constant and (*b*) the age-specific death rate in diagnostic radiologists and radiation oncologists equals that of white men generally.

We would expect a reasonable match between the number who left the profession and the predictions of the models, because the models are well validated. Specifically, the models have been used to predict with reasonable accuracy the growth over time in the total number of diagnostic radiologists and radiation oncologists in practice, as reported each year by the American Medical Association (16). Also, in a 1995 ACR survey of radiologists (9), no difference was found in the percentage of radiologists in each age category who were retired in 1995 compared with the percentage in 1990.

One possibility is that a new, large wave of retirements occurred in 1996, which approximately doubled the usual annual number. Alternatively, different results may be produced by asking groups about whether departed members have ceased active practice than by asking individual radiologists if they are retired. Questions addressed to different types of respondents in somewhat different ways about the same subject often produce substantially different results. We intend to continue to collect and analyze data on this issue.

Managed Health Care

The self-perceived effect of managed care on a group was significantly correlated with whether or not the group was recruiting for expansion positions in 1996. Specifically, with other factors held equal, groups that perceived their practice to be heavily affected by managed care were less likely to be expanding. The results of multivariate regression analyses indicated, however, that the perceived effect of managed care was not associated with other aspects of hiring: whether a group was hiring at all, the number of positions to be filled, whether positions were offered on a partnership-track basis, or the probability that a group that was hiring had unfilled positions at the conclusion of the 1996 hiring season.

Partnerships

Findings from this survey indicate that 27% of full-time positions offered in 1996 by private, nonacademic groups were non–partnership-track positions. The results of the ACR Survey of 1995 Graduates (13) show that a similar percentage of graduates that were hired full time by these groups were hired on a non–partnership-track basis. These findings appear to represent a major change over the past decade. Unpublished tabulations from the ACR 1995 Survey of Radiologists show that, of those who graduated about a decade earlier and, in 1995, worked full time in a group in which the partnership concept was relevant, only 10% were not partners. However, the difference (10% vs 27%) may only reflect the ability of radiologists who started their careers in non–partnership-track positions to find partnership-track positions and shift into such positions during a decade in practice.

The results of the multivariate regression analysis indicate that geographic and practice characteristics influence, to some extent, whether or not a group offers positions on a partnership-track basis. With other factors held equal, groups located in the main city of a metropolitan area with a population of less than 1 million and those located in a nonmetropolitan area were more likely to offer positions on a partnership-track basis than groups located in the main city of a large metropolitan area. Also, nonacademic multispecialty groups were less likely to offer radiology positions on a partnership-track basis than were nonacademic radiology groups.

Other Results of Regression Analyses

The regression analyses provide useful insights about the dynamics of the hiring process. By controlling for size and other group characteristics, we found that academic groups and nonacademic, private multispecialty groups sought to fill more positions than did private radiology groups. However, after controlling for other group characteristics, we found that academic groups were no more likely to be hiring for expansion positions than private groups, whereas nonacademic multispecialty groups were more likely to be hiring for expansion positions. The combination of these two findings suggests that academic groups probably sought to do a relatively large amount of hiring primarily as a result of higher turnover, whereas nonacademic, private multispecialty groups sought, in contrast, to do a relatively large amount of hiring because they were more likely to be expanding.

Groups that used any locum tenens or part-time radiologists in the past year sought to fill more positions, with other factors held equal, than did groups that did not. However, groups that had used locum tenens radiologists were less successful in filling all of their open positions than were groups that had not. These findings suggest some tendency for groups to want to replace locum tenens and part-time radiologists with regular group members by hiring. However, at least when locum tenens radiologists were involved, the energy devoted to the hiring process may be reduced (because fill-in staff is readily available), which would result in a greater likelihood that some positions remain unfilled.

Remaining Vacancies

In 1996, as in previous years, there were a substantial number of vacancies at the end of the hiring season—approximately 300 vacancies in 1996. At first glance, this seems surprising in view of the evidence that, if anything, there may have been a small shortage of positions relative to the number of radiologists. However, several factors may explain this seeming paradox. The first factor is statistical: Because we studied only a sample of radiology groups, there is a degree of uncertainty to our estimates, and an actual surplus of positions is well within the bounds of probability.

Another explanation for the vacancies is the possibility of a structural mismatch between available positions and the kinds of positions that are sought by job-seeking radiologists. Results of our regression analysis showed that otherwise similar groups in the South and the West had significantly greater success in filling all of their positions than did groups in the Northeast and the Midwest. Together with the finding that groups reported location preferences of candidates to be the single most important constraint to the filling of all positions, this result suggests that regional factors may be a source of structural imbalance in the radiology job market. Job seekers may consider positions in the "sun belt" to be considerably more attractive than positions elsewhere.

Another source of a structural disequilibrium could be a mismatch between the skills that are sought and the skills that are available among job seekers. However, we found no significant differences in the percentage of available positions that were filled among radiation oncologists, general diagnostic radiologists, all diagnostic subspecialties combined, and each individual diagnostic subspecialty. Thus, there is no evidence of such a mismatch.

The conclusion that there is no mismatch in fields of skills is supported by the results of ACR studies (3,14) of the "other side" of the job market—namely, the situation of graduates who are seeking positions. Similar to the results of the present study and of previous studies (4,7) of groups' hiring, the results of studies of graduates who were seeking positions did not indicate that the job market was significantly better or worse in some fields than in others.

We also examined data about fellowship training. We found that the number of radiologists hired who had fellowship training accounted for 92% of the positions for which a fellowship-trained radiologist was sought. In contrast, the number of radiologists hired who did not have fellowship training accounted for 66% of the positions for groups that had not sought a fellowship-trained radiologist. This difference (92% vs 66%) was statistically significant and may in part indicate that groups filled some positions for which fellowship training was not necessary with candidates who did have fellowship training. This finding was not observed in past years, and we shall need to monitor results from future surveys to ensure that it does not represent a one-time aberration.

Another possible cause of vacancies in an employment market otherwise characterized by balance between positions available and the number of job seekers is a phenomenon economists call "frictional disequilibrium." This term refers to the facts that, even with positions available, job seekers require some time to obtain positions and, conversely, even with candidates available, employers require some time to fill their vacancies. The clearest evidence that the hiring process takes time is our finding that more than half of all groups with remaining vacancies were still actively recruiting at the time of the survey, although the principal hiring season was over. Also, our data about the number of interviews and offers show that three interviews took place for every hiring offer made. The interview process necessarily takes time. As well, radiologists exercised some selectivity in the job-search process. The data show that for every three offers made, approximately two radiologists were hired, which means that one of every three offers was rejected. In summary, because the hiring process takes time for both radiologists seeking positions and groups seeking radiologists, it is almost inevitable that, at any given point in time, a substantial number of vacant positions will coexist with of a substantial number of radiologists seeking positions. ■

Acknowledgments: Jacqueline Levdahl, RN, and Laura Weber, BA, carried out the survey operations and worked with energy and attention to detail on a task that often involved tedium. The ACR Committee on Radiologist Resources oversaw this study. Members of the committee provided helpful comments on a draft of the manuscript, as did Kay Vydareny, MD. Gerald Busheé, PhD, participated in numerous discussions of the analysis and manuscript.

References

1. Sunshine JH, Kassing P, Shaffer KA, Janower ML. The job market for radiology residents and fellows graduating in 1994. AJR 1994; 163:1305–1308.
2. Sunshine JH, Burkhardt JH, Deitch CH, Chan WC. The employment market for diagnostic radiologists and radiation oncologists: an update. AJR 1995; 165:797–801.
3. Sunshine JH, Burkhardt JH, Crewson PE, Shaffer KA, Janower ML. The employment market for 1995 graduates of diagnostic radiology and radiation oncology training. AJR 1996; 167:21–26.
4. Busheé GR, Sunshine JH, Chan WC, Shaffer KA. The demand side of the job market for diagnostic radiologists and radiation oncologists: hiring by physician groups in 1995. AJR 1996; 167:303–309.
5. Sunshine JH, Evens RG, Chan WC. How accurate was GMENAC? a retrospective review of supply projections for diagnostic radiologists. Radiology 1992; 182:365–368.
6. Deitch CH, Evens RG, Sunshine JH. Recruiting radiologists: the 1991 hiring survey. Radiology 1992; 185:47–51.
7. Deitch CH, Sunshine JH, Chan WC. Hiring by radiology groups in 1994. Radiology 1996; 198:359–364.
8. Janower ML, Sunshine JH. Too many radiologists? update. Radiology 1996; 200: 545–549.
9. Deitch CH, Chan WC, Sunshine JH, Shaffer KA. Profile of U.S. radiologists at middecade: overview of findings from the 1995 survey of radiologists. Radiology 1997; 202: 69–77.
10. Sunshine JH, Burkhardt JH. Employment status of physicians completing training (letter). JAMA 1996; 276:281.
11. Campbell S, Chan WC, Wallace KK, Sunshine JH, Gray S. Hiring preferences of diagnostic radiology groups: results of a 1994 survey. Acad Radiol 1995; 2:1005–1010.
12. Sunshine, JH. Too many radiation oncologists? an empirical report. Int J Radiat Oncol Biol Phys 1996; 35:851–854.
13. Sunshine JH, Busheé GR, Vydareny KH, Shaffer KA. Graduates speak: the employment experience of 1995 graduates of diagnostic radiology and radiation oncology training programs. Radiology 1997; 204: 695–704.
14. Burkhardt JH, Sunshine JH, Shaffer KA. The employment market for 1996 diagnostic radiology and radiation oncology graduates: training program directors' point of view. AJR 1997; 169:333–337.
15. Kmenta J. Elements of economometrics. 2nd ed. New York, NY: Macmillan, 1986; 563.
16. Randolph L, Seidman B, Pasko T. Physician characteristics and distribution in the US, 1996–1997. Chicago, Ill: American Medical Association, 1997.

Akira Kawashima, MD • Carl M. Sandler, MD • Joseph N. Corriere, Jr, MD
Brian M. Rodgers, MD • Stanford M. Goldman, MD

Ureteropelvic Junction Injuries Secondary to Blunt Abdominal Trauma[1]

PURPOSE: **To describe the clinical and imaging findings of ureteropelvic junction (UPJ) injuries caused by blunt trauma.**

MATERIALS AND METHODS: **In two children (aged 10 and 16 years) and eight adults (aged 23–82 years) with UPJ injuries, findings at computed tomography (CT) ($n = 10$), excretory urography ($n = 6$), and retrograde pyelography ($n = 8$) were retrospectively reviewed to identify the location and extent of contrast material extravasation. Clinical and follow-up data were correlated with radiologic findings.**

RESULTS: **CT and urography played complementary roles in diagnosis. UPJ avulsion, defined as complete transection of the ureter with no filling of the ipsilateral ureter below the level of the UPJ, was diagnosed in four patients. UPJ laceration, defined as contrast material extravasation from the UPJ with contrast material in the ipsilateral ureter distal to the point of injury, was diagnosed in six patients. Medial perirenal contrast extravasation was seen in all 10 patients but failed to help differentiate UPJ avulsion from laceration. A distinctive pattern of contrast material extravasation at CT termed "circumrenal urinoma" was present in five patients and was found to be specific for UPJ injury.**

CONCLUSION: **Medial perinephric contrast material extravasation was highly suggestive of UPJ injury. Demonstration of ureteral filling differentiated UPJ laceration from avulsion.**

RENAL parenchymal injuries are usually caused by direct blunt trauma to the flank. Such injuries may result in extravasation of contrast material when a renal parenchymal laceration is present that involves the collecting system. In contrast, injuries of the ureteropelvic junction (UPJ) typically result in contrast material extravasation with intact renal parenchyma; such injuries are usually caused by deceleration that creates tension on the renal pedicle (1). Because the ureter is fixed in the retroperitoneum while the kidney is relatively mobile, the ureter may be lacerated or avulsed from its attachment to the UPJ by this mechanism. Such injuries are rare and have traditionally been described predominantly in children, especially boys (2).

The diagnosis of UPJ injury may be delayed, however, because hematuria is absent in one-third of cases (2). UPJ injury is usually suggested by the presence of massive medial accumulations of contrast material at excretory urography or computed tomography (CT), especially when the renal parenchyma appears intact and the ipsilateral ureter fails to become opacified (3,4). The most consistently described UPJ injury is avulsion, in which the ureter is completely transected at its attachment to the UPJ. Surgical repair of the injury is necessary in all cases.

Incomplete UPJ laceration has been mentioned in urology texts (1), but, to our knowledge, there is little in the radiology literature that describes the relative frequency of UPJ avulsion and laceration and the importance of differentiating between the two. In contrast to treatment of avulsion, laceration may be treated conservatively or with stent placement. Herein, we report the clinical and imaging findings in 10 patients with UPJ injuries caused by blunt abdominal trauma who underwent CT, urography, and retrograde pyelography.

MATERIALS AND METHODS

Patients at our institutions were identified who had sustained blunt abdominal trauma and had imaging findings of UPJ injury. Their records were retrospectively reviewed. Patients with contrast material extravasation attributable to lacerations of the renal parenchyma were excluded. Our study population comprised 10 patients (eight male and two female patients [two aged 16 and 10 years and eight aged 23–82 years]). Of the 10 patients, all underwent abdominal CT, six underwent urography, and eight underwent retrograde pyelography.

CT Examination

Contrast material–enhanced CT was performed in all 10 patients. One of the 10 patients initially underwent unenhanced CT, which was followed up with contrast-enhanced CT 2 days later. In three other patients, CT was performed immediately after urography, which showed contrast material extravasation at the UPJ. In

Index terms: Genitourinary system, injuries, 821.41 • Kidney, injuries, 81.41 • Ureter, CT, 821.12112, 821.12115 • Ureter, injuries, 821.41 • Urography, 821.122

Abbreviation: UPJ = ureteropelvic junction.

Radiology 1997; 205:487–492

[1] From the Department of Radiology, Lyndon B. Johnson General Hospital, 5656 Kelley St, Houston, TX 77026 (A.K., C.M.S., B.M.R.); and the Departments of Radiology (A.K., C.M.S., S.M.G.) and Urology (C.M.S., J.N.C., S.M.G.), University of Texas Houston Medical School, Houston. From the 1995 RSNA scientific assembly. Received April 24, 1997; revision requested June 12; revision received July 9; accepted July 10. **Address reprint requests to** A.K.

Clinical, CT, Excretory Urographic, and Retrograde Pyelographic Findings in 10 Patients with UPJ Injuries

Patient No./Age (y)/Sex	Clinical Findings: Cause of Injury	Clinical Findings: Hematuria	Clinical Findings: Time to Diagnosis	Clinical Findings: Other Injuries	UPJ Injury: Type	UPJ Injury: Side	CT Findings	Excretory Urographic Findings	Retrograde Pyelographic Findings	Treatment and Follow-up
1/10/M	Auto-pedestrian injury	Gross	<24 h	Closed head injury	Avulsion	Right	Circumrenal urinoma, no ureteral filling, no renal injury	Medial extravasation, no ureteral filling	Avulsion	Surgical repair followed by urography
2/16/M	Go-cart accident	Gross	<24 h	None	Laceration	Left	Circumrenal urinoma, no ureteral filling, no renal injury	Medial extravasation, no ureteral filling	Laceration	Ureteral stent placement
3/37/M	Bumped into doorknob	Gross	<12 h	None	Laceration	Left	Medial extravasation, no ureteral filling, minimal renal laceration	Medial extravasation, ureteral filling	Not performed	Conservative treatment
4/23/F	Water-skiing accident	Microscopic	<24 h	Fracture of transverse processes of the lumbar spine, ribs, and pelvis	Avulsion	Right	Circumrenal urinoma, no ureteral filling, minimal renal laceration	Medial extravasation, no ureteral filling	Avulsion	Surgical repair followed by urography and CT
5/27/M*	Assault	Gross	2–3 d	None	Laceration	Left	Medial extravasation, ureteral filling, no renal injury	Medial extravasation, ureteral filling	Laceration	Ureteral stent placement
6/65/F	Motor-vehicle accident	Gross	<24 h	Fracture of T-11 to T-12 vertebrae and left hip	Laceration	Left	Medial extravasation, ureteral filling, minimal renal contusion	Not performed	Laceration	Ureteral stent placement followed by retrograde pyelography; patient died of acute respiratory distress syndrome
7/21/M†	Ran into a metal bar	Gross	3 d	None	Laceration	Left	Circumrenal urinoma, no ureteral filling, minimal renal laceration	Not performed	Not performed	Conservative treatment followed by urography, retrograde pyelography, and CT
8/22/M†	Assault	Microscopic	<24 h	None	Avulsion	Left	Medial extravasation, no ureteral filling, no renal injury	Not performed	Avulsion	Nephrostomy followed by CT and nephrostography, nephrectomy
9/83/M	Motor-vehicle accident	Microscopic	<12 h	Fracture of transverse processes of the lumbar spine	Laceration	Left	Medial extravasation, ureteral filling, minimal renal contusion	Medial extravasation, no ureteral filling	Laceration	Ureteral stent placement
10/23/M	Motor-vehicle accident	Microscopic	<12 h	Fracture of transverse processes of the lumbar spine and pelvis	Avulsion	Left	Circumrenal urinoma, no ureteral filling, moderate renal contusion and laceration	Not performed	Avulsion	Nephrostomy followed by nephrostography, surgical repair was not performed because of associated medical problems

* Bilateral congenital UPJ obstruction.
† Ipsilateral congenital UPJ obstruction.

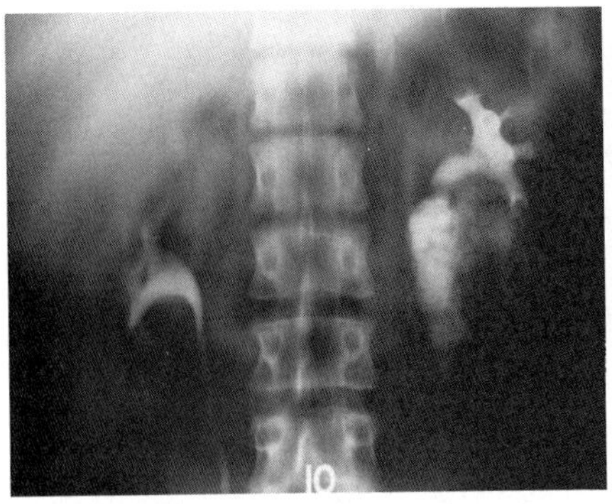

a.

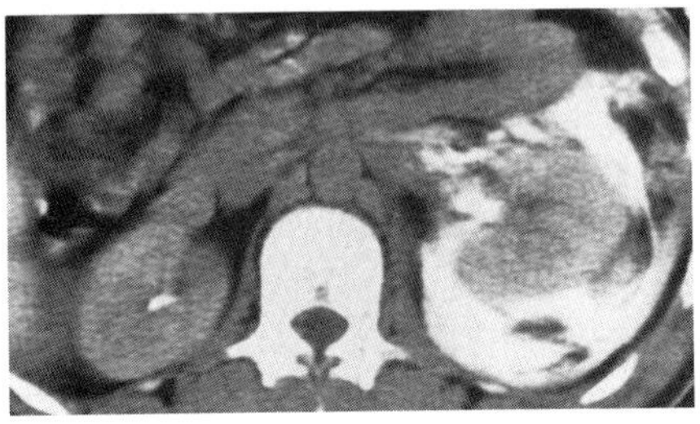

b.

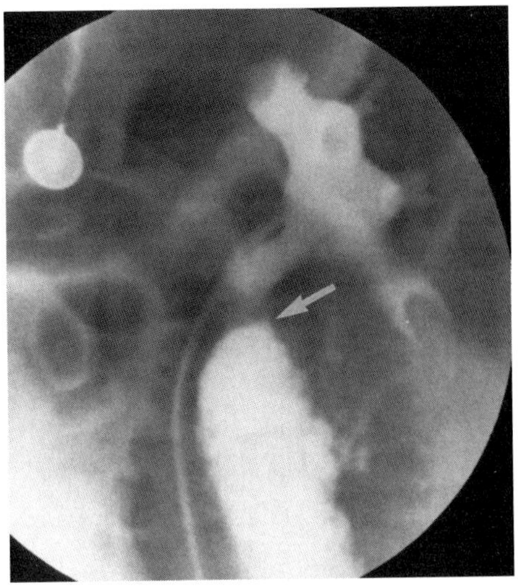

c.

Figure 1. Patient 2. UPJ laceration. **(a)** Nephrotomogram depicts an otherwise normal left renal collecting system with medial contrast material extravasation from the UPJ. **(b)** CT scan obtained after **a** depicts extensive extravasated contrast material surrounding the left kidney (circumrenal urinoma). **(c)** Spot radiograph obtained after retrograde pyelography and stent placement shows a partial tear at the left UPJ. Note the collection of extravasated contrast material (arrow) at the UPJ.

all 10 patients, delayed scanning depicted contrast material in the renal collecting system.

CT scans of the abdomen and pelvis were obtained with different scanners and techniques because the cases were collected over several years. The scanning mode was changed in 1994 from conventional axial technology (six cases) to helical technology (four cases). Ionic iodinated contrast material (Hypaque 50%; Nycomed, Princeton, NJ) and, more recently, nonionic iodinated contrast material (Omnipaque 300; Nycomed) were used for intravenous contrast enhancement. Contrast material was administered intravenously by means of either drip infusion or a mechanical power injector.

CT scans were reviewed retrospectively to determine (*a*) the presence or absence of associated renal parenchymal injuries; (*b*) the location of contrast material extravasation; (*c*) the degree of filling, if any, of the ipsilateral ureter; and (*d*) the presence of preexisting congenital renal anomalies. Contrast material extravasation was categorized as medial, lateral, or circumferential. Medial extravasation was defined as a collection of contrast material confined to the medial half of the perirenal space around the renal sinus that did not extend around the contour of the kidney for 360°. Lateral extravasation was defined as a collection of contrast material in the lateral perinephric space that did not extend beyond the medial contour of the kidney. Circumferential extravasation was defined as a perirenal collection that completely surrounded the kidney. Fluid was characterized as urine only when contrast material extravasation was associated with the fluid collection. In some patients, a variant of this pattern was noted that we termed a "circumrenal urinoma." This was defined as a fluid collection with at least some extravasated contrast material that completely surrounded the ipsilateral kidney.

Excretory Urographic Examination

Either routine or limited urography was performed in six patients. Delayed radiography was performed when necessary. The urograms were reviewed to determine (*a*) the presence or absence of an intact collecting system, (*b*) the location of extravasated contrast material in relation to the ipsilateral kidney, (*c*) filling or opacification of the ipsilateral ureter, and (*d*) the presence or absence of hydronephrosis.

Retrograde Pyelography Examination

Retrograde pyelography was performed in the cystoscopy suite with standard urologic technique. UPJ avulsion was defined as an abrupt termination of the ureter, contrast material extravasation at the UPJ without filling of the renal pelvis or collecting system, or both. UPJ laceration was defined as extravasation of contrast material at the UPJ with contrast material filling the renal pelvis and collecting system proximal to the site of extravasation.

RESULTS

The clinical and radiologic findings as well as the patient outcomes are summarized in the Table. Injuries were classified as complete ureteral avulsion in four patients or partial ureteral laceration in six patients. Findings at retrograde pyelography were used as the standard of reference for categorizing the nature of the injury in the eight patients who underwent this examination.

CT Findings

A circumferential pattern of contrast material extravasation, urinoma, or both was noted in five of the 10 patients (Figs 1, 2). Medial perinephric contrast material extravasation was noted in the other five patients (Fig 3). The extent of contrast material extravasation was most clearly depicted on delayed images. In no patient was contrast material extravasation found to be confined to the lateral perinephric space.

The distal ureter was opacified in three patients; in two of the three patients, the diagnosis of UPJ laceration was confirmed at retrograde pyelography. In one patient, the presence of extensive medial perinephric extravasation with intact renal parenchyma made accurate identification of the ureter difficult on axial CT images. In this patient, who did not undergo retrograde pyelography, urography clearly showed filling of the ipsilateral ureter distally; this finding indicated that the injury was a laceration rather than an avulsion (Fig 3). No ureteral filling was present in six other patients. Retrograde pyelography revealed UPJ avulsion in four of the six patients and laceration in one patient and was not performed in one patient.

CT showed ipsilateral renal parenchymal injuries in six patients; in five of these patients, the extent of the renal injury was less than 25% of the volume of the kidney, and in one patient, parenchymal injury involved approximately 40% of the kidney. Renal parenchymal laceration in proximity to the area of contrast material extravasation was not shown at CT in any of these patients.

Urographic Findings

Urography depicted medial perinephric extravasation in all six patients who underwent this examination. Distal ureteral opacification was noted in two patients; in the remaining four patients, the distal ureter could not be identified. These findings were correlated with the CT and retrograde pyelographic findings. In three of the four patients in whom the ureter could not be identified at urography, CT also did not depict the ureter (Fig 2). Two of these four patients had avulsion and one had laceration of the UPJ diagnosed at retrograde pyelography. In

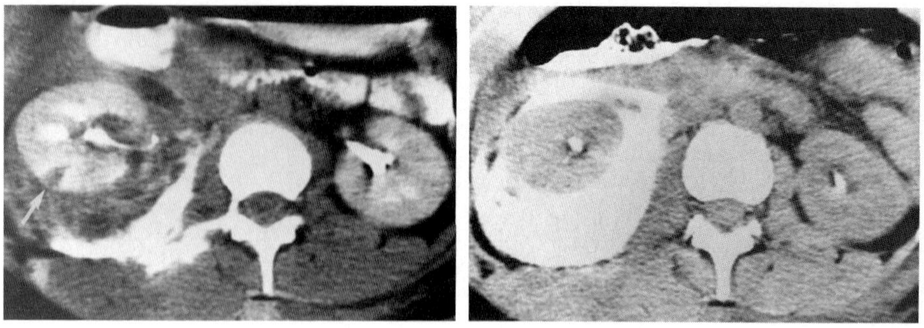

b. c.

Figure 2. Patient 4. Complete UPJ avulsion. **(a)** Urogram obtained 15 minutes after intravenous administration of contrast material shows a large amount of extravasated contrast material medial and inferior to the right kidney. No filling of the ureter is shown. **(b)** CT scan obtained after **a** depicts obvious contrast material extravasation from the UPJ. A moderate perirenal hematoma or urinoma is present. Note the small parenchymal laceration (arrow) not associated with contrast material extravasation. **(c)** Delayed CT scan shows a large circumrenal urinoma.

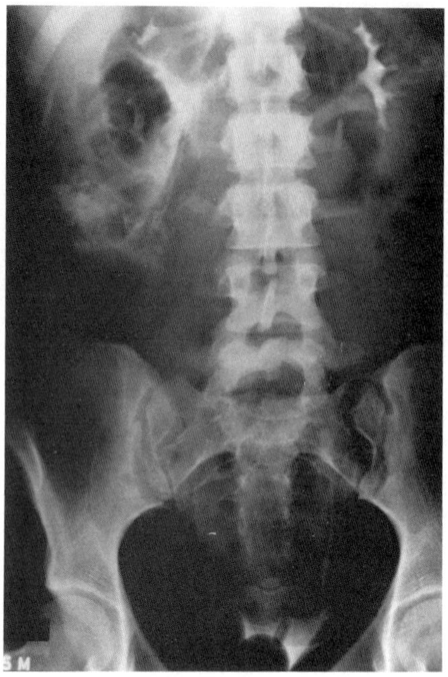

a.

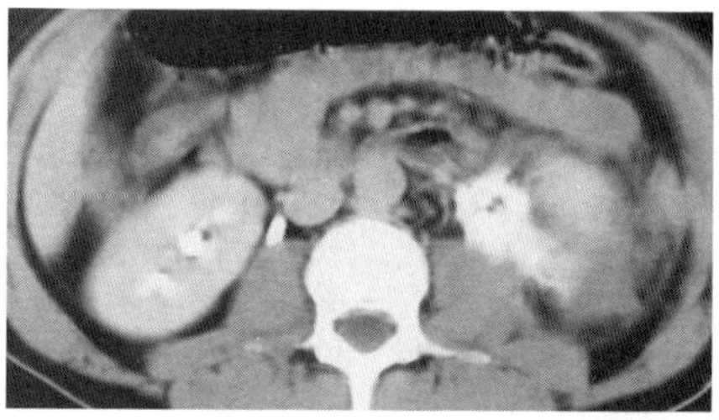

a.

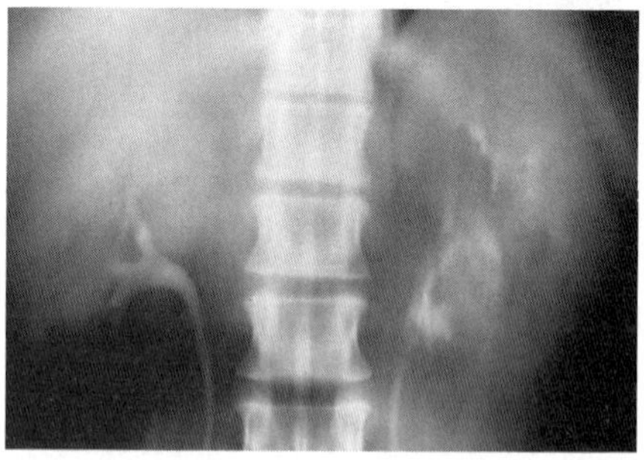

b.

Figure 3. Patient 3. UPJ laceration. **(a)** Axial CT scan shows a large amount of extravasated contrast material in the medial perinephric space. It is difficult to determine whether filling of the ureter is present. **(b)** Urogram shows medial extravasation from the UPJ and clearly depicts filling of the distal ureter.

one of the four patients, ureteral filling could be seen at CT but not at urography. In this patient, ureteral laceration was diagnosed at retrograde pyelography. In one patient, urography depicted filling of the ipsilateral ureter, which could not be clearly identified at CT, as described in the CT Findings section.

UPJ Injuries in Patients with Preexisting UPJ Obstruction

Three patients with UPJ injury had calicectasis and pelviectasis, which were attributed to preexisting congenital UPJ obstruction; two patients had laceration and one patient had avulsion. One of the patients with laceration was treated with ureteral stent placement (Fig 4). In the other patient with laceration, the initial CT scans showed medial urinoma without ipsilateral distal ureteral filling. This patient was treated conservatively, and follow-up CT, urography, and retrograde pyelography showed ipsilateral ureteral filling without extravasation and interval improvement of the urinoma. The third patient had avulsion and underwent nephrectomy because of marked renal parenchymal atrophy.

Other Injuries

Five patients had skeletal injuries including fracture of the transverse processes of the lumbar spine on the affected side ($n = 3$), pelvic fracture ($n = 2$), hip fracture ($n = 1$), lower rib fracture ($n = 1$), and compression fracture of the lower thoracic spine ($n = 1$). One patient had a closed head injury in addition to his renal injury. One patient with UPJ laceration due to trauma was successfully treated with ureteral stent placement but died of acute respiratory distress syndrome.

DISCUSSION

UPJ injuries are a rare consequence of blunt genitourinary trauma. This type of injury is usually caused by sudden deceleration, which creates tension on the renal pedicle (1,5). The ureter is retroperitoneal, and its only fixation points are at the UPJ and the ureterovesical junction. With sudden deceleration and the resulting hyperextension, the ureter is tensed like a bowstring across the transverse processes, which results in laceration or avulsion at the proximal point of fixation of the ureter (6). The presence of transverse process fractures has been correlated with UPJ injury (6).

When the UPJ is transected, hematuria may not be present. Gross or microscopic hematuria is seen in two-thirds of cases and may be transient (2). In a review by Boone et al (7) of 22 case reports of UPJ injury in 47 patients, only eight (53%) of 15 adults had either gross hematuria or microscopic hematuria with shock. These criteria were established by Nicolaisen et al (8) as indicators of the need for evaluation of the urinary tract in patients who have experienced blunt abdominal injury. Thus the correct diagnosis was delayed in approximately 50% of their patients. Similar findings were reported by LaBerge et al (9). In our study, gross hematuria was present in six of 10 patients, and microscopic hematuria was present in the remaining four patients. The correct diagnosis was established in less than 24 hours in eight of the 10 patients.

UPJ injury has been reported to occur predominantly in children, especially young boys, and it usually involves the right ureter. Of the cases reviewed by Boone et al (7), only 15 of the 47 patients were adults. In our series, eight of the 10 patients were adults, and the right ureter was involved in only two of the 10 patients. One of the pediatric patients was 16 years old and was the size of an adult at the time of injury. We assume that in the past, many of the injuries in

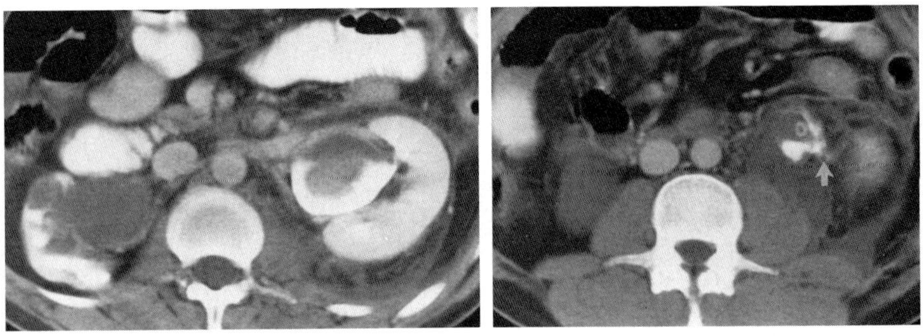

a. b.

Figure 4. Patient 5. UPJ laceration with preexisting UPJ obstruction. **(a)** Delayed CT scan depicts dilated renal pelves, consistent with bilateral UPJ obstruction. A large blood clot is present in the left renal pelvis. **(b)** Axial CT scan shows contrast material extravasation at the point of laceration of the UPJ (arrow). A large periureteral urinoma is present. The contrast-enhanced ureter contains a filling defect, presumably secondary to blood clot. **(c)** Urogram shows bilateral calicectasis and pelviectasis consistent with UPJ obstruction. Medial perinephric contrast material extravasation is present on the left, and a normal-caliber ureter is shown distally.

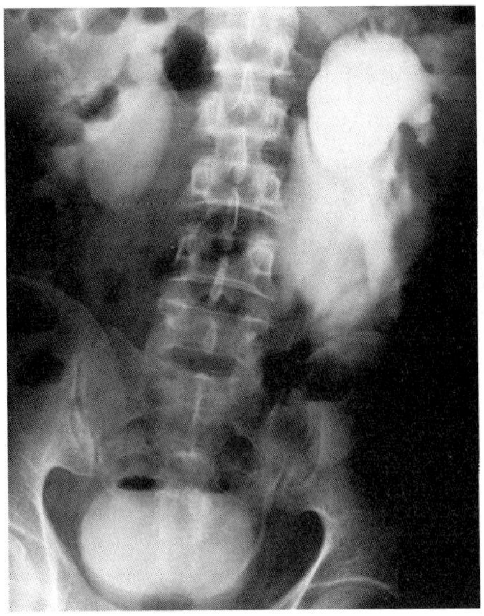

c.

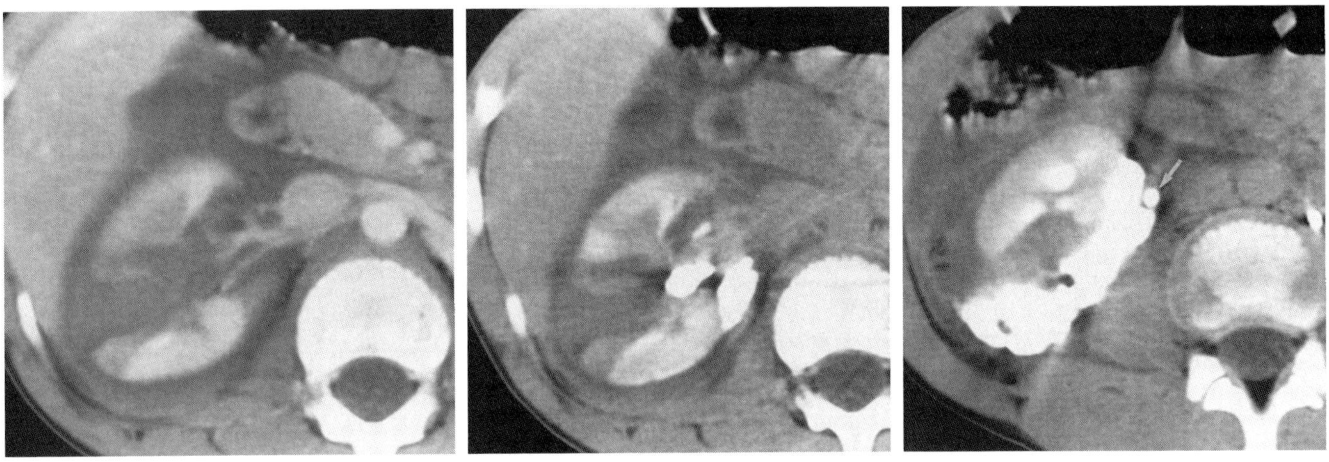

a. b. c.

Figure 5. Renal parenchymal laceration associated with medial perinephric contrast material extravasation in an 8-year-old boy (who was not included in our series) after a motor vehicle accident. **(a)** Nephrographic-phase CT scan shows a large distracted renal fracture through the midportion of the right kidney. Because this is an early-phase image, there is no contrast material in the collecting system. **(b)** Excretory-phase CT scan shows extravasation from a laceration of the renal pelvis into the medial perinephric space. **(c)** Delayed CT scan shows extensive extravasation. Note filling of the ureter (arrow).

adults were misdiagnosed as parenchymal lacerations that involved the collecting system.

The vast majority of cases of UPJ injury previously reported have involved complete UPJ avulsion. None of the cases reported by Boone et al (7) and only one case reported by Kenney et al (4) was a UPJ laceration. According to our data, lacerations account for 60% of injuries. In the past such injuries may have been overlooked if they were confused with contrast material extravasation associated with a renal fracture or with traumatic pyelosinus extravasation (10).

Avulsion of the UPJ should be suspected when massive urinary extravasation is detected after a patient has experienced blunt trauma. A tetrad of radiologic signs at urography have been previously described: (*a*) good renal excretion of contrast medium, (*b*) an intact calyceal system, (*c*) extravasation of contrast material in the region of the UPJ, and (*d*) nonfilling of the affected ureter (3). The same mechanism of injury may also result in damage to the renal vascular pedicle; when there is resultant thrombosis of the renal artery, contrast material extravasation will not be present as renal perfusion and excretion will be absent (9).

CT has become the imaging method of choice for the examination of patients with blunt abdominal injuries in major trauma centers in the United Sates. CT is more sensitive and specific than urography in the evaluation of suspected blunt genitourinary trauma (11). To our knowledge, Kenney et al (4) provided the first clear description of the CT findings of UPJ disruption. They described findings in three patients with avulsion and one patient with laceration of the UPJ in whom contrast material in the ipsilateral distal ureter was identified at CT. Their study population comprised three adults and one child. At CT as is found at urography, a finding of massive urinary extravasation is the rule, and the opacified urine tends to collect in the medial aspect of the perinephric space. In patients with a renal fracture that disrupts the collecting system, contrast material extravasation is usually seen in the dorsolateral perirenal space. All of the patients in the study of Kenney et al had intact renal parenchyma at CT, and none had associated perinephric hematoma. CT findings in our study support these observations; in six of 10 patients, however, CT showed evidence of some associated renal parenchymal injury not associated with disruption of the collecting system. Although coexisting parenchymal injuries are a potential source of confusion in determining the cause of contrast material extravasation, CT did not show contrast material extravasation in proximity to the laceration in any of our patients. Also, there were no patients in whom contrast material extravasation was found to be confined to the lateral perinephric space. Both of these findings are seen in association with contrast material extravasation from renal lacerations. The presence of medial contrast material extravasation is highly suggestive of UPJ injury but is not pathognomonic. In rare instances, large renal parenchymal lacerations may extend directly into the renal pelvis and produce medial perinephric contrast material extravasation (Fig 5).

A circumferential urinoma (circumrenal urinoma) was present in five of our 10 patients. Although this finding cannot be used to help distinguish between UPJ laceration and avulsion, we have not seen this pattern of contrast material extravasation in patients with renal parenchymal disruption without concomitant UPJ injury. A review of the illustrations published in previous reports of UPJ injury (6,12,13) also support the observation that a circumferential pattern of contrast material extravasation indicates UPJ injury.

Gary et al (14) described the case of a patient with traumatic rupture of the congenital hydronephrotic renal pelvis in whom CT depicted a dilated collecting system, contrast material extravasation anterior to the dilated renal pelvis, and a collection of urine and blood below the affected kidney. In our series, three patients had preexisting UPJ obstruction. This relatively high number suggests that patients with UPJ obstruction or a large extrarenal pelvis may be more susceptible to injury or may incur injury after experiencing less intense trauma. It is well known that the abnormal kidney is susceptible to injury from relatively minor trauma (15). Increased intrapelvic pressure from an abdominal injury may result in rupture of the dilated and thinned renal pelvis at the UPJ in a mechanism analogous to intraperitoneal bladder rupture.

The treatment of complete transection of the UPJ is definitive repair, usually with an end-to-end anastomosis and stent placement in the renal pelvis and ureter (1). We found that patients with ureteral laceration could be treated conservatively with stent placement alone. Therefore, the differentiation of UPJ avulsion from incomplete ureteral tear is crucial. We found that the diagnosis of partial ureteral tear can be established on the basis of ipsilateral ureteral filling distal to the UPJ at either contrast-enhanced CT or urography. In this regard, findings at urography and CT should be considered complementary. In one patient in our study, ureteral filling was shown at CT but not at urography; in another patient, the ureter was depicted at urography but not at CT.

CT should be performed with caution in patients with a history of blunt abdominal trauma, especially helical CT, because the kidneys may be scanned before the contrast material appears in the renal collecting system and ureter. Delayed CT through the kidneys must be performed during the excretory phase or later so that a collecting system injury will not be overlooked (Fig 5) (16). Extravasation of urine from the urinary tract can be subtle and may not be differentiated from perinephric hemorrhage unless the renal collecting system and ureter are filled with contrast material. When neither CT nor urography shows ipsilateral ureteral filling, retrograde pyelography should be performed. ■

References

1. Corriere JN Jr. Ureteral injuries. In: Gillenwater JY, Grayhack JT, Howards SS, Duckett JW, eds. Adult and pediatric urology. 3rd ed. St Louis, Mo: Mosby, 1996; 554–562.
2. Palmer JM, Drago JR. Ureteral avulsion from non-penetrating trauma. J Urol 1981; 125:108–111.
3. Beckly DE, Walters EA. Avulsion of the pelvi-ureteric junction: a rare consequence of non-penetrating trauma. Br J Radiol 1972; 45:423–426.
4. Kenney PJ, Panicek D, Witanowski LS. Computed tomography of ureteral disruption. J Comput Assist Tomogr 1987; 11:480–484.
5. Dunnick NR, Sandler CM, Amis ES Jr, Newhouse JH. Urinary tract trauma. In: Textbook of uroradiology. 2nd ed. Baltimore, Md: Williams & Wilkins, 1997; 297–324.
6. Toporoff B, Scalea TM, Abramson D, Scalafani SJA. Ureteral laceration caused by a fall from a height: case report and review of the literature. J Trauma 1993; 34:164–166.
7. Boone TB, Gilling PJ, Husmann DA. Ureteropelvic junction disruption following blunt abdominal trauma. J Urol 1993; 150: 33–36.
8. Nicolaisen GS, McAninch JW, Marshall GA, Bluth RF Jr, Carroll PR. Renal trauma: re-evaluation of the indications for radiographic assessment. J Urol 1985; 133:183–187.
9. LaBerge I, Homsy YL, Dadour G, Beland G. Avulsion of ureter by blunt trauma. Urology 1979; 13:172–178.
10. Cass AS, Lee JY, Smith CS. Perirenal extravasation with blunt trauma from rupture of a calyceal fornix. J Trauma 1993; 35:20–22.
11. Sandler CM, Toombs BD. Computed tomographic evaluation of blunt renal injuries. Radiology 1981; 141:461–466.
12. Siegel MJ, Balfe DM. Blunt renal and ureteral trauma in childhood: CT patterns of fluid collections. AJR 1989; 152:1043–1047.
13. Templeton PA, Mirvis SE, Whitley NO. Traumatic avulsion of the ureter: computed tomography correlation. J Comput Tomogr 1988; 12:159–160.
14. Gary R, Cass AS, Johnson CF. Computed tomography diagnosis of traumatic rupture of congenital hydronephrotic renal pelvis. Urology 1988; 32:65–66.
15. Rhyner P, Federle MP, Jeffrey RB. CT of trauma to the abnormal kidney. AJR 1984; 142:747–750.
16. Haker KM, Schilling VL, Van Allan RJ, Kallman CE. Pitfalls during spiral CT evaluation of blunt renal trauma (abstr). Radiology 1996; 201(P):149.

Hani B. Marcos, MD • Richard C. Semelka, MD • Suvipapun Worawattanakul, MD

Normal Placenta: Gadolinium-enhanced, Dynamic MR Imaging[1]

PURPOSE: **To establish the appearance of the normal placenta on dynamic, gadolinium-enhanced magnetic resonance (MR) images.**

MATERIALS AND METHODS: **Eleven patients underwent MR imaging for suspected uterine (four patients) or placental (seven patients) abnormalities (but not placental insufficiency or intrauterine growth retardation). Unenhanced or gadolinium-enhanced, T1-weighted, fat-suppressed, spoiled gradient-recalled-echo MR images and T2-weighted, half-Fourier, single-shot, spin-echo-train MR images were obtained. Two investigators retrospectively evaluated the images to determine the rate, pattern, and degree of placental contrast material enhancement with myometrial enhancement as a reference.**

RESULTS: **The diagnoses were normal placenta (six patients), abnormal placental position (four patients), and subchorionic hematoma (one patient). The placenta rapidly and intensely enhanced on images acquired immediately after contrast material administration and preceded substantial enhancement of the myometrium. Immediately postcontrast images showed closely packed 2–3-cm lobules of placental enhancement in third-trimester pregnancies and heterogeneous placental enhancement in second-trimester pregnancies. In all cases, placental enhancement became more homogeneous over time. The placenta could be readily distinguished from the myometrium. All neonates were healthy with no evidence of intrauterine growth retardation.**

CONCLUSION: **Normal placental enhancement is intense on immediately postcontrast images and precedes substantial myometrial enhancement. Third-trimester placentas exhibit a lobular pattern of enhancement, while second-trimester placentas exhibit heterogeneous enhancement.**

Ultrasonography (US) is the primary imaging modality for the evaluation of the pregnant uterus and fetus, because it acquires information on the fetus in real time and is biologically safe (1,2). US findings may be inconclusive, owing to limited soft-tissue characterization and technical difficulties caused by large patient size (1). For these reasons, magnetic resonance (MR) imaging has emerged as an adjunct to US when US findings are equivocal.

Recent innovations in MR sequences, which include breath-hold, T1-weighted (eg, spoiled gradient-recalled-echo [SPGR]) sequences and fat-suppressed, gadolinium-enhanced, breathing-independent, T2-weighted, half-Fourier, single-shot, spin-echo-train imaging sequences, have shown promising results in the evaluation of the maternal abdominopelvic organs and the fetus (3–6). The normal placenta is highly vascularized (7) and should enhance intensely on images obtained soon after contrast material administration.

A paucity of literature exists on evaluating the placenta with MR imaging. Prior articles have described the appearance of placental abnormalities, which include placenta accreta (4), retained placenta (4), and gestational trophoblastic disease (5,6). The appearances of the placenta on dynamic, gadolinium-enhanced images have been described in a simian model (8).

To our knowledge, no prior article has described the contrast material–enhancement characteristics of the normal human placenta. Knowledge of the MR appearance of the normal placenta may permit future comparison with compromised placentas. The purpose of the current study therefore was to demonstrate the appearance of the normal placenta on dynamic, gadolinium-enhanced MR images.

MATERIALS AND METHODS

Patients

Eleven pregnant patients (age range, 20–38 years; mean age, 28 years) underwent MR imaging between May 1995 and February 1997 and were included in our study. MR imaging was performed at 16–37 weeks of gestation (mean, 28 weeks). Three patients were examined during the second trimester and eight patients were examined during the third trimester. The clinical indications for MR imaging were suspected uterine (four patients) or suspected placental (seven patients) abnormalities. Suspected uterine abnormalities were uterine mass (one patient), uterine vascular abnormalities (one patient), and intrauterine hemorrhage (two patients). Suspected placental abnormalities were placenta accreta (six patients) and abruptio placenta (one patient).

All patients were examined for clinical indications on the basis of symptoms and US findings. All patients were informed about MR imaging and gadopentetate dimeglumine by a physician and gave their written consent. All patients underwent US before MR imaging. Referring obstetricians requested MR imaging to deter-

Index terms: Placenta, 857.121412, 857.121415, 857.12143 • Pregnancy, MR, 857.121412, 857.121415, 857.12143

Abbreviation: SPGR = spoiled gradient-recalled echo.

Radiology 1997; 205:493–496

[1] From the Department of Radiology, University of North Carolina, CB 7510, Chapel Hill, NC 27599-7510. Received May 20, 1997; revision requested June 24; revision received July 1; accepted July 8. **Address reprint requests to** R.C.S.

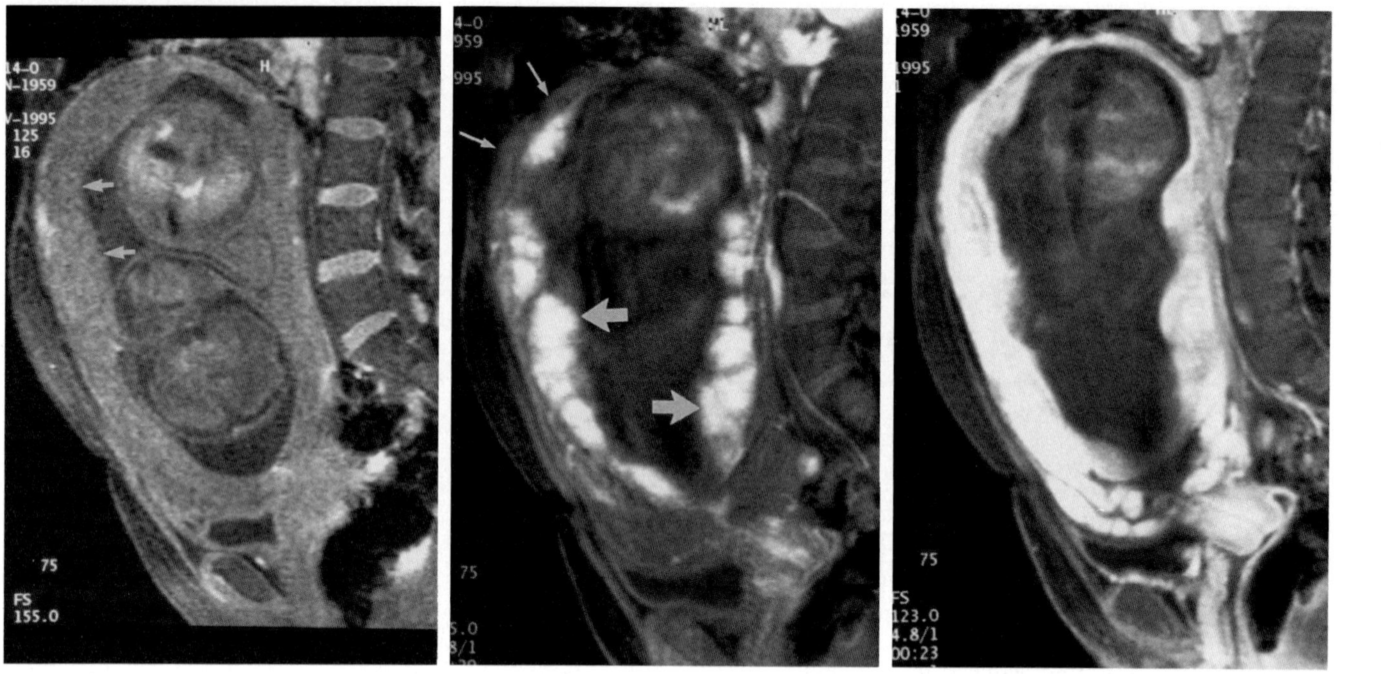

a. b. c.

Figure 1. Sagittal, T1-weighted, fat-suppressed SPGR MR images (155/4.8, 80° flip angle) obtained in a 38-year-old pregnant woman at 36 weeks of gestation (third trimester) **(a)** before, **(b)** immediately after, and **(c)** 45 seconds after gadopentetate dimeglumine administration. The placenta is at the lateral aspect of the uterus with anterior (arrows in **a**) and posterior extension and has mildly low signal intensity in **a. b** shows early, intense, and lobular placental enhancement (thick arrows in **b**) with closely packed nodules of enhancement that may represent cotyledons. Myometrial enhancement (thin arrows in **b**) is less than placental enhancement. **c** shows myometrial enhancement that is comparable with placental enhancement.

mine management, and all patients were referred to undergo MR imaging for the investigation of conditions that were considered potentially life-threatening to the mother. The gross appearance of the postpartum placenta was compared with MR findings. Clinical evaluation of fetal and maternal abnormalities was by means of patient clinical follow-up and chart review.

MR Technique

MR examinations were performed on a 1.5-T MR imager (Vision; Siemens Medical Systems, Iselin, NJ) with a phased-array body coil. All patients underwent axial and sagittal, T1-weighted, fat-suppressed, SPGR (140–170/2 [repetition time msec/echo time msec], 80° flip angle, 5–8-mm section thickness, 20% gap, 244 × 325 field of view, 129 × 256 matrix, 14–22 sections acquired in a 16–27-second breath hold) and coronal, axial, and sagittal, T2-weighted, half-Fourier, single-shot, spin-echo-train (single shot/90–103 [effective], 8-mm section thickness, 20% gap, 244 × 325 field of view, 129 × 256 matrix, 20 sections acquired in a 20–40-second breath hold). A bolus of gadopentetate dimeglumine (Magnevist; Berlex Imaging, Wayne, NJ) was rapidly injected by hand at a dose of 0.1 mmol/kg. Fat-suppressed, SPGR imaging was initiated immediately, 45 seconds, and 90 seconds after contrast material administration.

Image Interpretation

All MR images were retrospectively reviewed by two radiologists (H.B.M., R.C.S.). The following determinations were made: placental location; placental morphology; abnormal fluid collection; presence of placental abnormalities; and the rate, pattern, and degree of placental enhancement. The signal intensity of the placenta relative to the myometrium on pre- and postcontrast images was evaluated.

RESULTS

The diagnoses were normal placenta (six patients), abnormal placental position (four patients), and subchorionic hematoma (one patient). MR findings showed good correlation with postpartum examination findings of the placenta. No intrinsic placental abnormalities were found at MR imaging or histopathologic analysis. MR findings did not demonstrate placenta accreta or abruption, which was confirmed at the time of delivery and at subsequent histopathologic placental examination.

In all cases, the placenta was of mildly low signal intensity, minimally higher than the signal intensity of the myometrium, on T1-weighted, fat-suppressed SPGR images and of moderately high signal intensity, minimally higher than the signal intensity of the myometrium, on T2-weighted, half-Fourier, single-shot, spin-echo-train images. On immediately postcontrast, fat-suppressed, SPGR images, the placenta enhanced early and intensely. Three placentas imaged during the second trimester demonstrated heterogeneous enhancement on immediately postcontrast images, while eight placentas imaged during the third trimester demonstrated more clearly defined lobular enhancement.

On images acquired immediately after gadopentetate dimeglumine administration, placental enhancement was greater than myometrial enhancement in all cases (Fig 1). On images acquired 45 seconds after contrast material administration, the placental enhancement was comparable with the myometrial enhancement. On images acquired 90 seconds after contrast material administration, the placental enhancement was lower than the myometrial enhancement; this was observed in all cases.

The placenta was determined to be normal in six patients. One of these six patients had a large heterogeneous mass that extended from the right superolateral portion of the uterus with focal regions of necrosis and hemorrhage, which is consistent with a degenerating leiomyoma (Fig 2). Placenta previa was diagnosed in four patients. Subchorionic hemorrhage was diagnosed on MR images in one patient who had two lentiform, subchorionic regions. These regions were of low signal intensity with a periph-

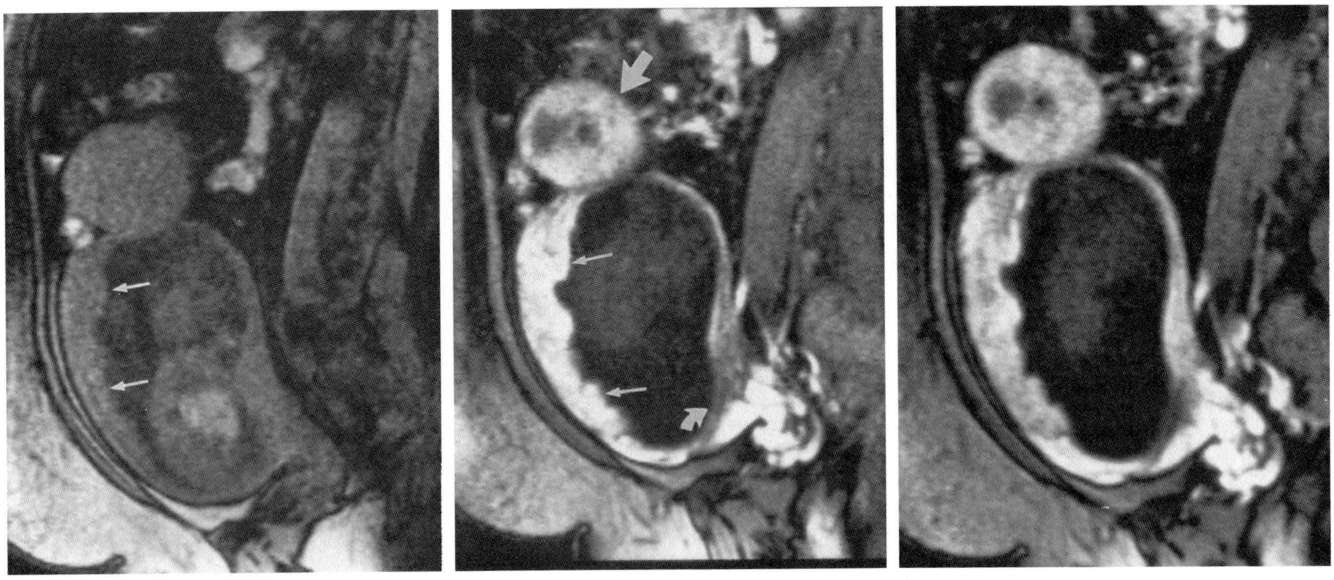

b. c. d.

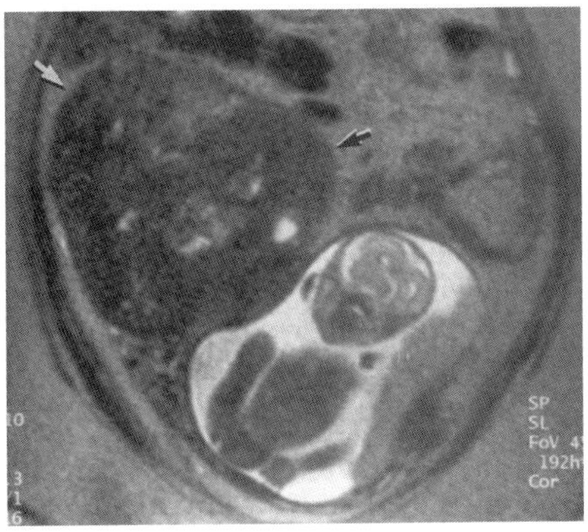

a.

Figure 2. **(a)** Coronal, T2-weighted, half-Fourier, single-shot, spin-echo-train (single shot/103) and **(b–d)** sagittal, T1-weighted, fat-suppressed, SPGR (152/2, 80° flip angle) MR images obtained in a 32-year-old pregnant woman with a leiomyoma at 23 weeks of gestation (second trimester) **(b)** before, **(c)** immediately after, and **(d)** 45 seconds after gadopentetate dimeglumine administration. **a** demonstrates a large mass that arises from a right superolateral portion of the uterus with focal regions of necrosis and hemorrhage (arrows). **b** demonstrates that the placenta (arrows) has an anterior location and mildly low signal intensity. **c** demonstrates early, intense placental enhancement (straight, thin arrows). Note that the placenta does not exhibit a lobular enhancement pattern. The myometrium enhances negligibly at this early phase (curved arrow in **c**). The large, degenerating leiomyoma also enhances minimally in **c** (straight, thick arrow). **d** demonstrates that the degrees of enhancement of the myometrium and of the degenerating leiomyoma are comparable to that of the placenta.

eral rim of higher signal intensity on both T1-weighted, fat-suppressed, SPGR images and T2-weighted, half-Fourier, single-shot, spin-echo-train images and showed a lack of enhancement on postcontrast, fat-suppressed, SPGR images (Fig 3); these imaging features were considered consistent with subacute subchorionic hemorrhage.

Clinical follow-up of the mothers and neonates revealed no abnormalities. All infants were healthy at birth.

DISCUSSION

This article describes the enhancement characteristics of nondiseased placenta. On immediately postcontrast, fat-suppressed SPGR images obtained in the arterial phase, the placenta has an early and intense pattern of enhancement consistent with its highly vascularized nature (7). Myometrial enhancement was less and was more delayed on gadolinium-enhanced, fat-suppressed SPGR images. The placenta could be distinguished from myometrium.

In the first and second trimesters, the placenta grows rapidly but is not differentiated, while in the third trimester the placenta grows slowly but exhibits villous differentiation (cotyledon formation) (9). The underlying anatomic changes were reflected in our study by the observation that second-trimester placentas enhanced heterogeneously without definition of lobules, while third-trimester placentas had lobular enhancement. Large, closely grouped lobules of placental enhancement on immediately postcontrast images reflect the organization of the placenta into cotyledons. This lobular enhancement has been considered to represent the presence of gadolinium-based contrast material in the intervillous spaces of placental lobules (8). Observation of changing placental morphology between the second and third trimesters has also been previously demonstrated in US studies (1).

Breath-hold SPGR and breathing-independent, half-Fourier, single-shot, spin-echo-train sequences have been described as demonstrating fetal anatomy in pregnancy (3). We also found this in our patient population. The placenta is also well depicted with these sequences, and distinction from the myometrium was well shown. Placenta previa was correctly diagnosed in four patients in our study by using SPGR and half-Fourier, single-shot, spin-echo-train imaging. Prior articles also have described the appearance of leiomyoma in pregnancy, which was found in one of our patients (10,11). Subchorionic hemorrhage is a disease process related specifically to the pregnant uterus; this was well shown on unenhanced, breath-hold, T1-weighted, fat-suppressed SPGR and breathing-independent, half-Fourier, single-shot, spin-echo-train images.

Recognition of the appearance of the normal placenta may provide a framework for understanding the appearance of the abnormal placenta. Intrauterine growth retardation is associated with decreased vascularity of the placenta (12), and placentas in patients with intrauterine growth retardation may have a distinctive MR appearance. This may be one group of patients in whom placental enhancement may correlate with clinical status.

To our knowledge, there are no series or reports that describe the safety of gadolinium-containing contrast material administration in human

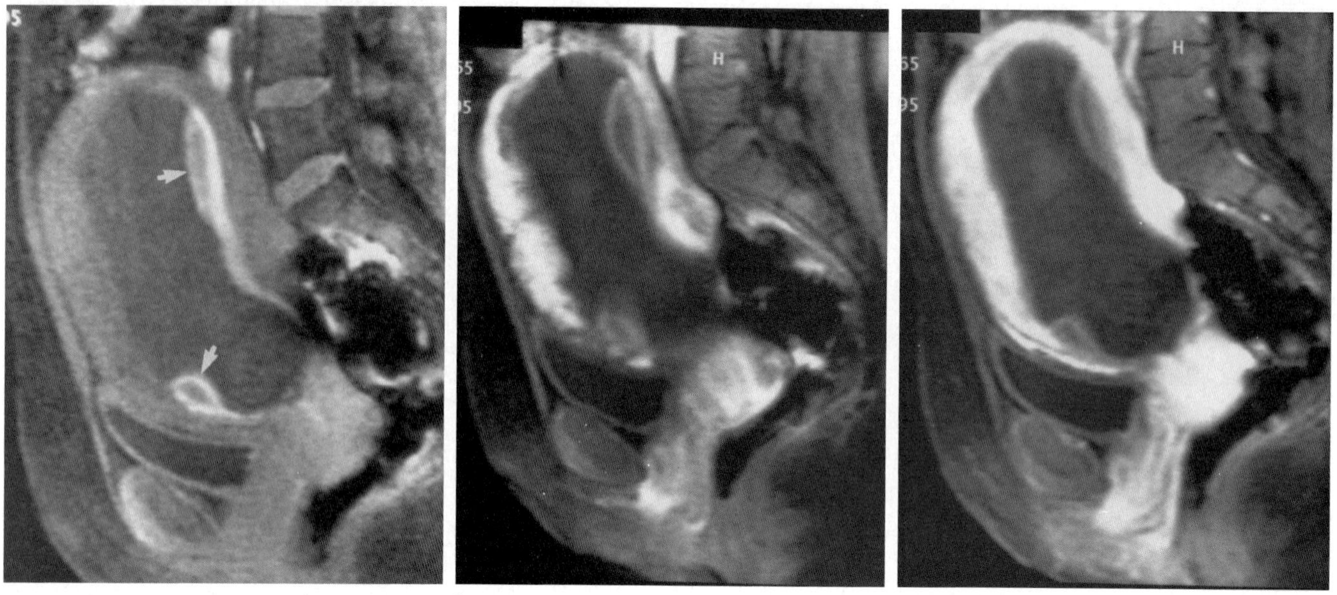

a. b. c.

Figure 3. Sagittal, T1-weighted, fat-suppressed, SPGR (155/4.8, 80° flip angle) MR images obtained in a 32-year-old pregnant woman at 16 weeks of gestation (second trimester) with subchorionic hemorrhage **(a)** before, **(b)** immediately after, and **(c)** 45 seconds after gadopentetate dimeglumine administration. **a** shows two lentiform regions in a subchorionic location that have low signal intensity with a peripheral rim of higher signal intensity (arrows), which is consistent with subacute hemorrhage. **b** shows intense placental enhancement with a heterogeneous pattern of enhancement, which is greater than the myometrium. **c** shows comparable placental and myometrial signal intensities by 45 seconds after contrast material administration. The regions of subchorionic hemorrhage do not enhance on the early and late gadolinium-enhanced images.

pregnancy. Prior case reports have shown no adverse effects (13,14). Gadolinium-based contrast material administration in pregnant mice has been shown to have no demonstrable harmful effects (15). It should be noted that the small number of patients in our study is insufficient to document the safety of intravenous gadolinium-based contrast material use in pregnancy.

In conclusion, intense, early enhancement was a consistent finding in the normal placenta. Heterogeneous enhancement was observed in the second-trimester and lobular enhancement was observed in the third-trimester placentas. ■

References

1. Kuhlmann RS, Warsof S. Ultrasound of the placenta. Clin Obstet Gynecol 1996; 39: 519–534.
2. Grannum PA, Hobbins JC. The placenta. Radiol Clin North Am 1982; 20:353–365.
3. Levine D, Hatabu H, Gaa J, Atkinson MW, Edelman RR. Fetal anatomy revealed with fast MR sequences. AJR 1996; 167:905–908.
4. Amoh Y, Watanabe Y, Saga T, et al. Retained placenta accreta: MRI and pathologic correlation. J Comput Assist Tomogr 1995; 19:827–829.
5. Barton JW, McCarthy SM, Kohorn EI, Scoutt LM, Lange RC. Pelvic malignancy imaging findings in gestational trophoblastic disease, incomplete abortion, and ectopic pregnancy: are they specific? Radiology 1993; 186:163–168.
6. Yamashita Y, Torashima M, Takahashi M, et al. Contrast-enhanced dynamic MR imaging of postmolar gestational trophoblastic disease. Acta Radiol 1995; 36:188–192.
7. Teasdale F, Jean-Jacques G. Morphometric evaluation of the microvillous surface enlargement factor in the human placenta from mid-gestation to term. Placenta 1985; 6:375–378.
8. Panigel M, Dixon T, Constantinidis I, et al. Fast scan magnetic resonance imaging and Doppler ultrasonography of uteroplacental hemodynamics in the rhesus monkey (*Macaca mulatta*). J Med Primatol 1993; 22:393–399.
9. Castellucci M, Kaufmann P. Hofbuer cells. In: Benirschke K, Kaufmann P, eds. Pathology of the human placenta. 2nd ed. New York, NY: Springer-Verlag, 1990; 71–80.
10. Kier R, McCarthy SM, Scoutt LM, Viscarello RR, Schwartz PE. Pelvic masses in pregnancy: MR imaging. Radiology 1990; 176:709–713.
11. Curtis M, Hopkins MP, Zarlingo T, Martino C, Graciansky-Lengyl M, Jenison EL. Magnetic resonance imaging to avoid laparotomy in pregnancy. Obstet Gynecol 1993; 82:833–836.
12. Altshuler G, Hyde SR. Clinicopathologic implication of placental pathology. Clin Obstet Gynecol 1996; 39:549–570.
13. Barkhof F, Hiijboer RJ, Algra PR. Inadvertent i.v. administration of gadopentetate dimeglumine during early pregnancy (letter). AJR 1992; 158:1171.
14. Shoenet JP, Semelka RC, Silverman R, Yaffe CS, Micflikier AB. MRI in the diagnosis of Crohn's disease in two pregnant women. J Clin Gastroenterol 1993; 17:244–247.
15. Rofsky NM, Pizzrello DJ, Weinreb JC, Ambrosino MM, Rosenberg C. Effect on fetal mouse development of exposure to MR imaging and gadopentetate dimeglumine. JMRI 1994; 4:805–807.

Masahiro Jinzaki, MD • Akihiro Tanimoto, MD • Yoshiaki Narimatsu, MD
Kiyoshi Ohkuma, MD • Tadayoshi Kurata, MD • Hiroshi Shinmoto, MD
Kyoichi Hiramatsu, MD • Makio Mukai, MD • Masaru Murai, MD

Angiomyolipoma: Imaging Findings in Lesions with Minimal Fat[1]

PURPOSE: To investigate a method of diagnosing angiomyolipoma that contains minimal fat.

MATERIALS AND METHODS: In six cases of angiomyolipoma with minimal fat, the attenuation on contrast material–enhanced and unenhanced computed tomographic (CT) images, the echogenicity on sonograms, the signal intensity on T2-weighted magnetic resonance (MR) images, and the gross configuration of the lesion were retrospectively analyzed. In 100 cases of renal cell carcinoma, the same parameters were analyzed, and results were compared with those of angiomyolipoma.

RESULTS: When compared with the surrounding renal parenchyma, all six angiomyolipomas showed homogeneously high attenuation on unenhanced CT images, homogeneous enhancement on contrast-enhanced CT images, and homogeneous isoechogenicity on sonograms. Of the five angiomyolipomas examined with MR imaging, four were hypointense and one was isointense on T2-weighted images. All six angiomyolipomas protruded from the renal margin. None of the 100 renal cell carcinomas showed homogeneously high attenuation on unenhanced CT images, homogeneous enhancement on contrast-enhanced CT images, or homogeneous isoechogenicity on sonograms.

CONCLUSION: In the kidney, homogeneously high attenuation on unenhanced CT images, homogeneous enhancement on contrast-enhanced CT images, and homogeneous isoechogenicity on sonograms are suggestive of angiomyolipoma that contains abundant muscle and minimal fat.

Angiomyolipoma is a benign renal lesion composed of variable amounts of fat, smooth muscle, and abnormal blood vessels. An angiomyolipoma that does not cause symptoms may not need to be surgically removed; this lesion may be treated conservatively. For renal cell carcinoma, nephrectomy is standard treatment. Therefore, definitive distinction between angiomyolipoma and renal cell carcinoma is essential.

Angiomyolipoma can be diagnosed noninvasively with great accuracy by detecting a fat component (1–6). However, in those lesions composed primarily of smooth muscle or with intratumoral hemorrhage (which obscures the fatty part of the lesion), the diagnosis of angiomyolipoma is difficult (4,7–9). When angiomyolipoma is suspected because an area of low attenuation on computed tomographic (CT) scans or hyperechogenicity on sonograms is seen, Bosniak et al (10) have advocated the use of unenhanced thin-section CT for improving the detection of small amounts of fat.

The purpose of this study was to (*a*) analyze retrospectively angiomyolipomas in which fat was not identified with the conventional imaging method used to detect fat and (*b*) investigate a method of diagnosing angiomyolipomas that contain minimal fat.

MATERIALS AND METHODS

Between January 1989 and December 1994, 175 renal lesions diagnosed preoperatively as renal cell carcinoma were surgically resected. Maximum diameters of lesions were 1.0–11.2 cm (mean, 5.1 cm). Ages of patients with these lesions ranged from 35 to 78 years (mean, 56 years). The lesions included 156 renal cell carcinomas, six angiomyolipomas, six oncocytomas, two multilocular cysts, one transitional cell carcinoma, one malignant fibrous histiocytoma, one medullary fibroma, one infectious cyst, and one case of xanthogranulomatous pyelonephritis.

We analyzed the findings on sonograms, CT scans, and magnetic resonance (MR) images of the six angiomyolipomas. Three men and three women had these lesions. Their ages ranged from 48 to 69 years (mean, 62 years). No patient had tuberous sclerosis or lymphangiomyomatosis.

During this same time (between 1989 and 1994), angiomyolipoma was diagnosed in 132 patients at our institution. These patients' ages ranged from 18 to 86 years (mean, 52 years). Maximum diameters of lesions were 0.5–28.5 cm. Renal cell carcinoma (which was resected) was diagnosed in six of these patients, and 10 patients' lesions were resected because of symptoms such as hematuria or flank pain. One patient underwent nephrectomy because of accompanying transitional cell carcinoma, and 115 patients' lesions were diagnosed on the basis of attenuation on CT scans consistent with fat. Among the 132 patients, 107 had one lesion, 16 had two lesions, four had three lesions, and five had more than three lesions. Three of these patients had tuberous sclerosis.

CT was performed with commercially available units (Quantex or ProSeed; Yokogawa Medical Systems, Tokyo, Japan) before and after intravenous administration of contrast material. Section thickness

Index terms: Kidney neoplasms, 81.3141, 81.324 • Kidney neoplasms, CT, 81.12111, 81.12112 • Kidney neoplasms, MR, 81.121411, 81.121416 • Kidney neoplasms, US, 81.1298

Radiology 1997; 205:497–502

[1] From the Departments of Diagnostic Radiology (M.J., A.T., Y.N., K.O., T.K., H.S., K.H.), Pathology (M. Mukai), and Urology (M. Murai), Keio University School of Medicine, 35 Shinanomachi, Shinjuku-ku, Tokyo 160, Japan. Received March 3, 1997; revision requested April 21; revision received June 26; accepted June 30. **Address reprint requests to** M.J.

was 5 or 10 mm. All images were acquired with cluster scanning. If areas (when compared with renal parenchyma) were hypoattenuating on unenhanced CT images or hyperechoic on sonograms, unenhanced CT images of 3- or 5-mm-thick sections were acquired. The 100 mL of intravenous contrast material (iohexol [Omnipaque 300]; Daiichi Pharmaceutical, Tokyo, Japan) was administered as a 60-mL bolus (1.5–2.0 mL/sec) followed by a rapid drip infusion of the remaining 40 mL. Scanning was initiated approximately 120 seconds after the beginning of the injection. Technical factors were 120 kVp and 200 mAs with 10-mm sections and 120 kVp and 250 mAs with 3- or 5-mm sections.

Sonography was performed with commercially available real-time units (RT 2800, Yokogawa Medical Systems; EUB 430, Hitachi, Tokyo, Japan; or model 270A, Toshiba, Tokyo, Japan) with a 3.5- or 3.75-MHz convex transducer. MR imaging was performed with a 1.5-T superconducting unit (Signa; GE Medical Systems, Milwaukee, Wis). T1-weighted spin-echo images (400–500/14–25 [repetition time msec/echo time msec]) and T2-weighted spin-echo images (2,000/80) or fast spin-echo images (4,000/90) were acquired in the axial plane with a matrix size of 256 × 192. Section thickness was 5–6 mm with a 2–3 mm intersection gap. Fat-saturated images were not acquired in these patients.

All images were reviewed and analyzed by consensus by two radiologists (M.J., A.T.). The attenuation on contrast material–enhanced and unenhanced CT images, the echogenicity on sonograms, and the signal intensity on MR images of lesions and those of surrounding renal parenchyma were compared. The range of lesion attenuation on CT images was obtained with multiple measurements of pixel value. On CT images that showed the maximum areas of the lesion and renal parenchyma, the mean attenuation of the lesion and that of renal parenchyma were obtained by measuring the largest possible region of interest. The mean attenuation of skeletal muscle was obtained by measuring the largest possible region of interest in the erector muscle of the spine. The homogeneity of attenuation was evaluated by visual inspection. An increase in attenuation of more than 10 HU was defined as "enhancement" (11). CT scanners were calibrated daily with a phantom. We also checked the gross configuration of the lesion and classified the configuration into the following patterns: pattern 1, protrusion from the kidney without beak appearance; pattern 2, protrusion with beak appearance on only one side; pattern 3, protrusion with beak appearance on both sides; and pattern 4, no protrusion. This classification was made with use of the comprehensive interpretation of three modalities: sonography, CT, and MR imaging. Examples of these configuration patterns are shown in Figure 1.

In a similar fashion, we attempted to review retrospectively renal cell carcinomas smaller than 5 cm (among the 175 renal lesions resected between 1989 and

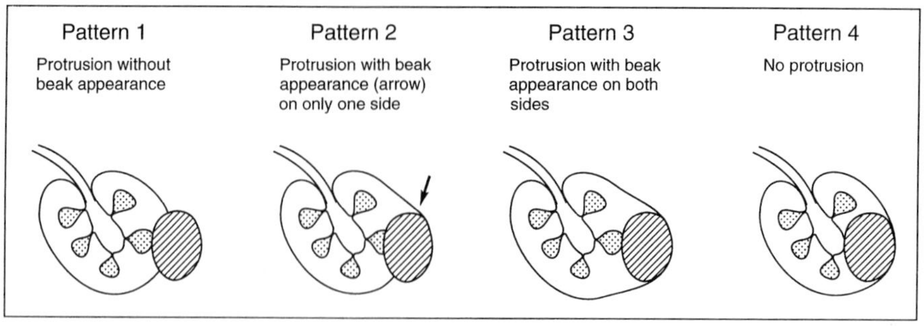

Figure 1. Schematic representation of the gross configurations of lesions.

1994) to ascertain any pattern of renal cell carcinoma that may have been similar to that of the six angiomyolipomas. Among the 175 renal lesions, 106 consecutive renal cell carcinomas were smaller than 5 cm; however, sonographic, CT, and MR imaging data were available in only 100 of these renal cell carcinomas.

RESULTS

Histopathologic Findings of Angiomyolipoma

All six angiomyolipomas were composed mostly of smooth muscle and only minimal, scattered fat. At immunohistochemical examination, the smooth-muscle component contained actin, desmin, S-100 protein, and HMB-45 antigen. One angiomyolipoma (in patient 5) contained many blood vessels, and the other five angiomyolipomas contained a few blood vessels.

Radiologic Findings of Angiomyolipoma

On sonograms, all six angiomyolipomas appeared homogeneously isoechoic (Figs 2–4). On unenhanced CT images, the attenuation of all six angiomyolipomas was homogeneously high compared with that of normal renal parenchyma (Figs 2–4, Table 1). Attenuation consistent with fat was not detected with pixel-value analysis, and the mean attenuation of each lesion was similar to that of skeletal muscle ($P > .05$, paired Student t test). Because the six angiomyolipomas were not hypoattenuating on unenhanced CT images or hyperechoic on sonograms, thinner-section CT was not performed in these patients. In four of these cases, 10-mm-thick sections were imaged initially; in two cases, 5-mm-thick sections were imaged initially (Table 1).

On contrast-enhanced CT images, the attenuation of all six angiomyolipomas was low compared with that of normal renal parenchyma; however, the attenuation of the angiomyolipomas increased homogeneously more than 20 HU (mean, 31 HU) from the attenuation of the lesions on unenhanced CT images. The mean increase in the attenuation of skeletal muscle on contrast-enhanced CT images was 17 HU. The difference between the mean increase in the attenuation of angiomyolipoma and that of skeletal muscle was significant ($P < .05$, paired Student t test). On T1-weighted MR images, five angiomyolipomas were isointense without any distinct areas of high signal intensity. On T2-weighted MR images, the signal intensity of four angiomyolipomas was low compared with that of normal renal parenchyma and slightly high compared with that of skeletal muscle. One angiomyolipoma was isointense with normal renal parenchyma (Figs 2–4). One angiomyolipoma was not examined with MR imaging.

Five angiomyolipomas demonstrated pattern 1 (protrusion of the lesion beyond the renal margin without a beak appearance), and one angiomyolipoma (patient 3) demonstrated pattern 2 (protrusion of the lesion with a beak appearance on only one side) (Fig 3).

Radiologic Findings of Renal Cell Carcinoma

We reviewed the frequencies of the following features in the 100 renal cell carcinomas in the same manner as described: feature 1, homogeneously high attenuation on unenhanced CT images and homogeneous enhancement on contrast-enhanced CT images; feature 2, homogeneous isoechogenicity on sonograms; and feature 3, homogeneous hypo- or isointensity on T2-weighted MR images. The frequency of each finding was 2%, 17%, and 21%, respectively (Tables 2–5). Among the five renal cell carcinomas that showed homogeneously high attenuation on unenhanced CT images, three showed diffuse intratumoral

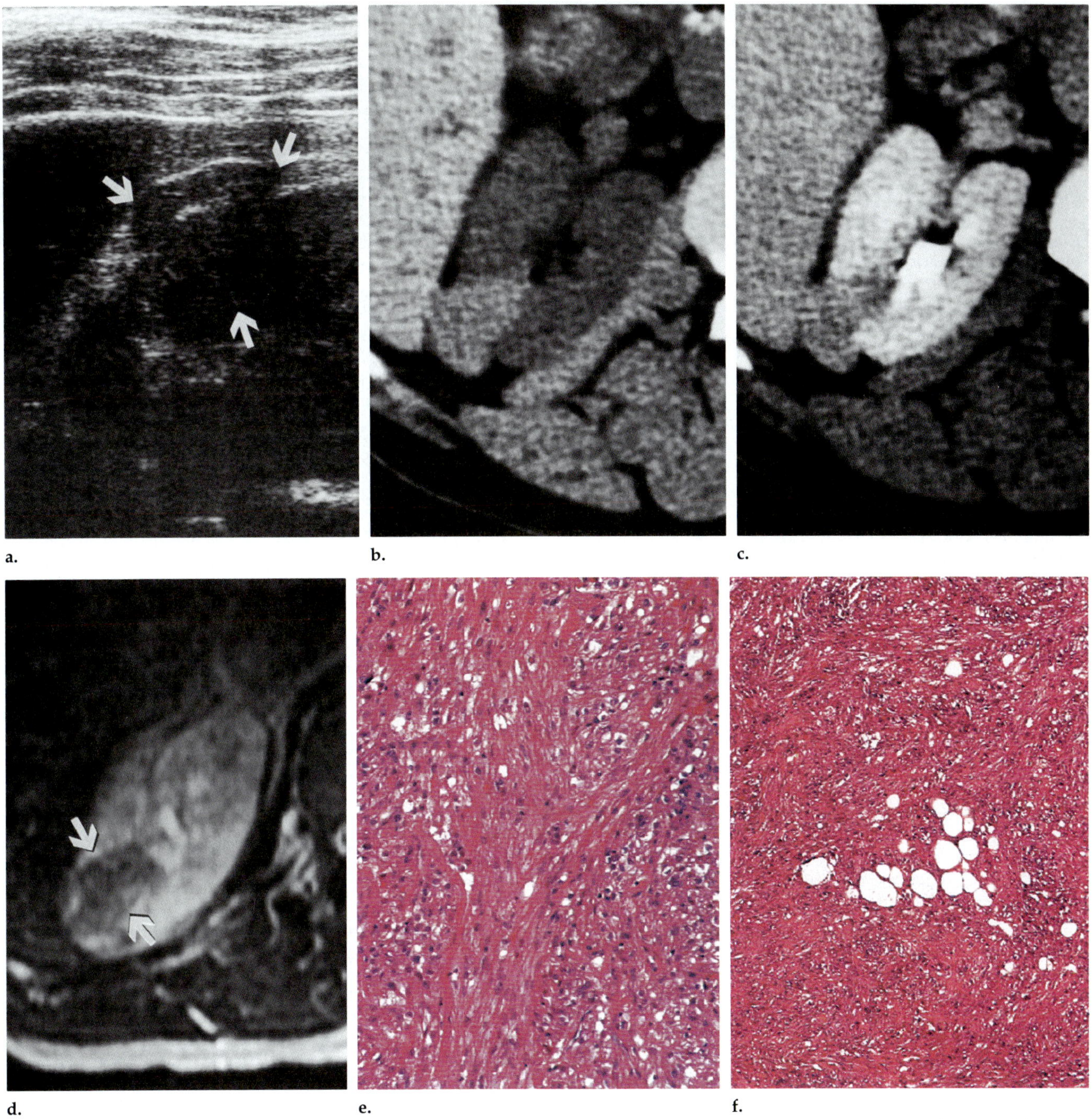

Figure 2. Angiomyolipoma in patient 1. **(a)** Transabdominal sonogram shows an isoechoic lesion (arrows) that is 3.0 cm in diameter. **(b)** Unenhanced CT image (5-mm section) shows a homogeneously hyperattenuating lesion that is protruding from the renal margin without a beak appearance (pattern 1). **(c)** Attenuation of a well-marginated lesion on the contrast-enhanced CT image is low compared with that of the surrounding renal parenchyma. Lesion attenuation on **c** increased 24 HU from that on **b.** **(d)** T2-weighted MR image (2,000/80) shows a hypointense lesion (arrows) in the right kidney. **(e)** Photomicrograph of the lesion shows abundant muscle, which occupied almost all portions of the lesion. (Hematoxylin-eosin stain; original magnification, ×50.) **(f)** Photomicrograph of the lesion shows minimal amounts of fat, which were seen in some portions of the lesion. (Hematoxylin-eosin stain; original magnification, ×20.)

hemorrhage at histopathologic examination, heterogeneous enhancement on contrast-enhanced CT images, and heterogeneous hyperechogenicity on sonograms. The other two renal cell carcinomas showed papillary architecture without hemorrhage or degeneration at histopathologic examination, homogeneous enhancement on contrast-enhanced CT images, and homogeneous hyperechogenicity on sonograms. Thus, no renal cell carcinoma had features 1 and 2 or 1, 2, and 3. Two renal cell carcinomas had features 1 and 2, and seven renal cell carcinomas had features 2 and 3. With regard to the gross configuration of the lesion, the frequencies of patterns 1 and 2 were 3% and 15%, respectively (Table 5).

DISCUSSION

Generally, renal angiomyolipoma can be diagnosed with great accuracy with modern imaging techniques owing to the fat component of the lesion. This fat component accounts for the areas of negative attenuation on CT images and increased echogenicity on sonograms (1–6). In our retrospective

Figure 3. Angiomyolipoma in patient 3. **(a)** Transabdominal sonogram shows an isoechoic lesion (arrows) that is 3.5 cm in diameter. **(b)** Unenhanced CT image (10-mm section) shows a homogeneously hyperattenuating lesion that is protruding from the renal margin with a beak appearance on only one side (pattern 2). **(c)** Attenuation of a well-marginated lesion on the contrast-enhanced CT image is low compared with that of the surrounding renal parenchyma. Lesion attenuation on **c** increased 22 HU from that on **b.** **(d)** T2-weighted MR image (2,000/80) shows a hypointense lesion in the left kidney.

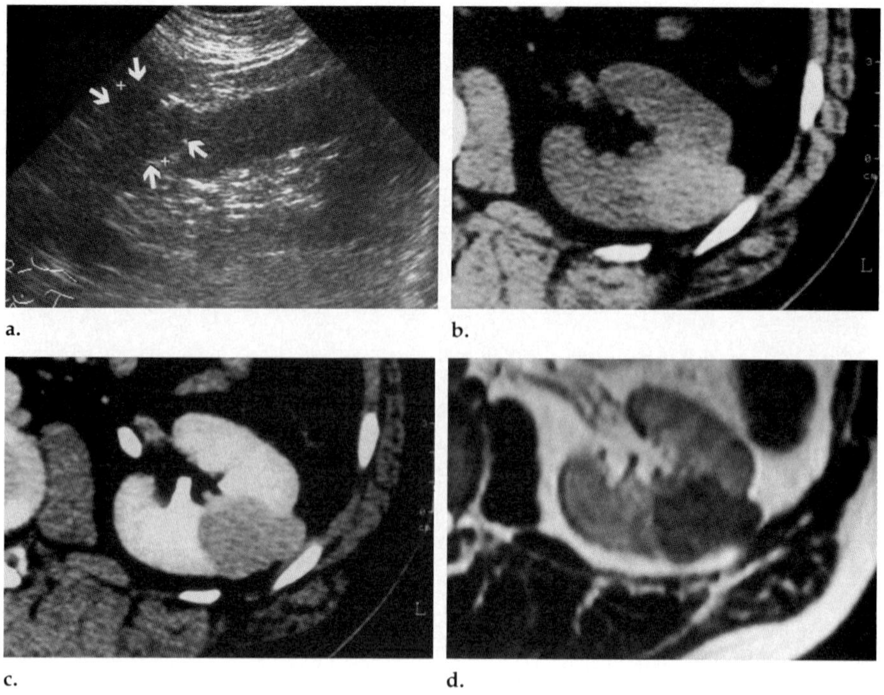

study of six patients with angiomyolipoma, not one lesion showed these characteristics, but all lesions showed homogeneously high attenuation on unenhanced CT images, homogeneous enhancement on contrast-enhanced CT images, and isoechogenicity on sonograms. Because six of the 132 patients in our retrospective study had these characteristics, we calculated the frequency of this angiomyolipoma to be 4.5%. On reviewing the data of previous case reports, we found only one report that concerned two angiomyolipomas with similar characteristics (9).

At histopathologic examination, the six angiomyolipomas were composed mostly of smooth muscle that contained the HMB-45 antigen. The HMB-45 antigen is associated with melanoma and is known to be in the smooth muscle of angiomyolipoma and lymphangiomyomatosis; however, the HMB-45 antigen has not been shown in other smooth-muscle tumors such as leiomyoma (12–14).

In our study, sonograms and CT images of angiomyolipomas showed signs of abundant muscle. For example, the attenuation of lesions on unenhanced CT images was high compared with that of the renal parenchyma and similar to that of muscle. This finding suggests that the lesions contained a rich muscle component. On sonograms, the lesions were isoechoic, not hyperechoic. The coexistence of fat and muscle would result in hyperechogenicity owing to the difference between the acoustic impedances of each component (15,16). Therefore, a homogeneous muscle component with minimal or no fat would account for the isoechoic pattern that was seen on the sonograms of the six angiomyolipomas in our study. Only the mean enhancement of the six renal angiomyolipomas differed from that of skeletal muscle; this difference could be the result of the vasculature of the lesion and not the smooth-muscle component.

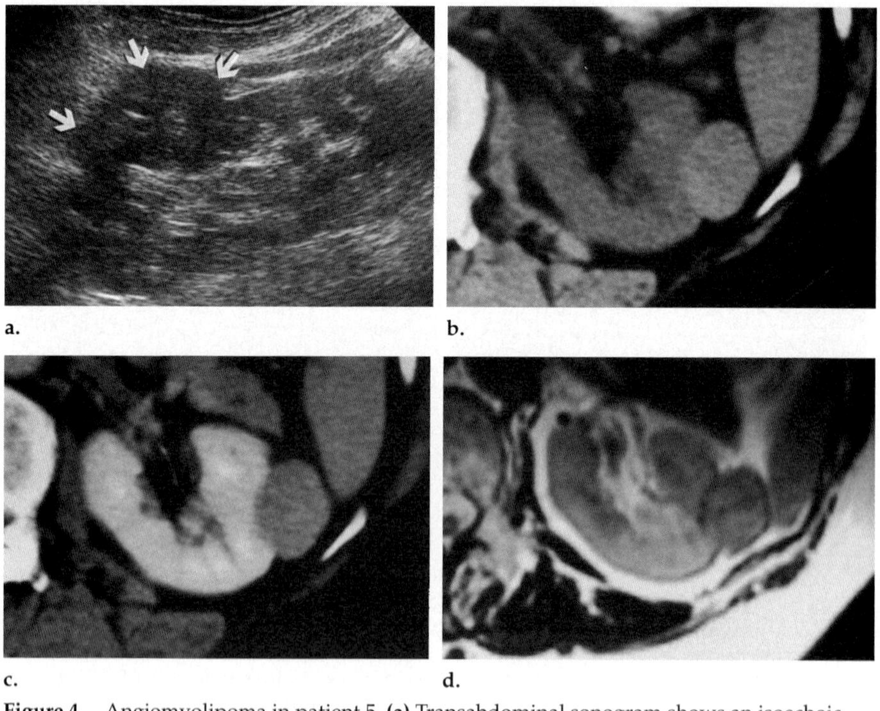

Figure 4. Angiomyolipoma in patient 5. **(a)** Transabdominal sonogram shows an isoechoic lesion (arrows) that is 2.7 cm in diameter. **(b)** Unenhanced CT image (10-mm section) shows a homogeneously hyperattenuating lesion that is protruding from the renal margin without a beak appearance (pattern 1). **(c)** The attenuation of the well-marginated lesion on the contrast-enhanced CT image is low compared with that of the surrounding renal parenchyma. Lesion attenuation on **c** increased 41 HU from that on **b.** **(d)** T2-weighted MR image (2,000/80) shows an isointense lesion in the left kidney.

The conventional method of detecting fat is still being used in the diagnosis of angiomyolipoma. Some problems with the use of this conventional method, however, have been reported. Episodically, CT may not enable the identification of fat in angiomyolipoma if there is a predominance of smooth muscle and blood vessels (4,7–9). These angiomyolipomas cannot be distinguished from other solid renal lesions with CT. Bosniak et al recommended the use of unenhanced thin-section (5-mm) CT to increase

Table 1
Characteristics of Six Patients and Their Angiomyolipomas

Patient No./ Patient Age (y)/ Sex	Lesion Size (cm)	Section Thickness on Unenhanced CT Images (mm)	Attenuation of Lesion on Unenhanced CT Images*	Mean Attenuation of Lesion on Contrast-enhanced CT Images† (HU)	Mean Attenuation of Normal Kidney on Unenhanced CT Images (HU)	Mean Attenuation of Skeletal Muscle (HU)		Echogenicity of Lesions on Sonograms	Signal Intensity of Lesions on T2-weighted MR Images
						Unenhanced CT	Contrast-enhanced CT†		
1/59/M	3.0	5	High (29–57; mean, 41)	65 (24)	24	43	58 (15)	Isoechoic	Hypointense
2/66/F	2.2	5	High (39–66; mean, 51)	86 (35)	35	45	67 (22)	Isoechoic	Hypointense
3/48/M	3.5	10	High (32–61; mean, 44)	66 (22)	26	44	59 (15)	Isoechoic	Hypointense
4/65/F	5.0	10	High (31–52; mean, 45)	82 (37)	25	47	65 (18)	Isoechoic	Hypointense
5/69/F	2.7	10	High (30–54; mean, 43)	84 (41)	34	44	64 (20)	Isoechoic	Isointense
6/66/F	2.5	10	High (31–58; mean, 48)	77 (29)	32	50	62 (12)	Isoechoic	NP‡

* Numbers in parentheses are ranges and means of attenuation in Hounsfield units (HU).
† Numbers in parentheses are increases (in Hounsfield units) of lesion attenuation on contrast-enhanced CT images.
‡ NP = MR imaging not performed.

Table 2
Pattern of Attenuation of Angiomyolipoma and Renal Cell Carcinoma on Unenhanced CT Images

Lesion	Homogeneous Hyperattenuation	Homogeneous Isoattenuation	Homogeneous Hypoattenuation	Heterogeneous Attenuation
Angiomyolipoma	6 (6)	0	0	0
Renal cell carcinoma	5 (2)	27 (12)	6 (4)	62 (0)

Note.—Numbers are numbers of cases. Numbers in parentheses are cases showing homogeneous enhancement after administration of contrast material.

Table 3
Pattern of Echogenicity of Angiomyolipoma and Renal Cell Carcinoma on Sonograms

Lesion	Homogeneous Hyperechogenicity	Homogeneous Isoechogenicity	Homogeneous Hypoechogenicity	Heterogeneous Echogenicity
Angiomyolipoma	0	6	0	0
Renal cell carcinoma	22	17	0	61

Note.—Numbers are numbers of cases.

Table 4
Pattern of Signal Intensity of Angiomyolipoma and Renal Cell Carcinoma on T2-weighted MR Images

Lesion	Homogeneous Hyperintensity	Homogeneous Isointensity	Homogeneous Hypointensity	Heterogeneous Signal Intensity
Angiomyolipoma	0	1	4	0
Renal cell carcinoma	24	15	6	55

Note.—Numbers are numbers of cases.

Table 5
Pattern of Gross Configuration of Angiomyolipomas and Renal Cell Carcinomas

Lesion	Pattern 1	2	3	4
Angiomyolipoma	5 (83)	1 (17)	0 (0)	0 (0)
Renal cell carcinoma	3 (3)	15 (15)	70 (70)	12 (12)

Note.—Numbers are numbers of lesions. Numbers in parentheses are percentages.

the detection of fat when angiomyolipoma was suspected (10). However, if the lesion does not show the distinguishing signs of angiomyolipoma—such as (in our patients) isoechogenicity on sonograms and homogeneously high attenuation on CT images—the procedure of using unenhanced, thin-section CT may not be considered, which leads to incorrect diagnosis. Thus, unenhanced thin-section CT of a larger group of renal lesions may need to be performed; sole reliance on finding hyperechogenicity on sonograms or low attenuation on unenhanced CT images may result in some lesions not being imaged in a way that would enable diagnosis. In four of our patients, use of unenhanced thin-section CT may have revealed fat; however, fat in two angiomyolipomas (in patients 1 and 2) was not detected with imaging of 5-mm-thick sections. Thus, in the other four patients, the detection of fat also may have been difficult because the amount or distribution of fat in these lesions was similar to that in the lesions of patients 1 and 2. In such cases, the findings we described on unenhanced CT images, contrast-enhanced CT images, and sonograms may be useful for detecting angiomyolipoma.

The most important disease to differentiate from angiomyolipoma is renal cell carcinoma. We have identified some characteristics that may enable this differentiation. In our study, no renal cell carcinoma showed homogeneously high attenuation on unenhanced CT images, homogeneous enhancement on contrast-enhanced CT images, or homogeneous isoechogenicity on sonograms. In renal cell carcinoma, homogeneously high attenuation on unenhanced CT images is very rare (17,18). High attenuation is thought to be caused by intratumoral hemorrhage or papillary or tubular architecture (17,18). Because these features also cause hyperechogenicity on sonograms (17,19), renal cell carcinoma rarely shows both homogeneously high attenuation on unenhanced CT images and homogeneous isoechogenicity on sonograms. However, these findings are merely suggestive of angiomyolipoma; thus, a biopsy should be performed before surgery if angiomyolipoma with minimal fat is suspected on CT images and sonograms.

On T1-weighted MR images, none of the angiomyolipomas showed signal intensity that was similar to that of fat. By contrast, on T2-weighted MR images, the lesions frequently showed low signal intensity (four [80%] of five cases of angiomyolipoma compared with six [6%] of 100 renal cell carcinomas). Further studies, however, will be necessary to determine the importance of this finding.

The most striking feature of angiomyolipoma with minimal fat is its high attenuation on unenhanced CT images. The differential diagnosis of a hyperattenuating renal lesion on unenhanced CT images includes a (*a*) complicated benign cyst, such as a hemorrhagic, protein-rich, or gelatinous cyst, (*b*) renal metastasis from thyroid carcinoma, (*c*) thrombosed renal vein, (*d*) leiomyoma, and (*e*) renal cell carcinoma (17,18,20–23). The first three lesions do not show homogeneous enhancement; thus, they may be differentiated from renal angiomyolipoma that contains minimal fat (18,20–22). On the other hand, the appearance of leiomyoma may mimic that of angiomyolipoma because both are composed of muscle. To our knowledge, there are three reports of leiomyomas that protruded from renal parenchyma and showed a homogeneously solid pattern (23–25). The sonographic findings of Selli et al (23) differed from ours. The imaging findings in the other two reports were not described in enough detail to determine whether these findings are consistent with ours (24,25). Thus, imaging findings of leiomyoma that match those of our angiomyolipomas have not been reported. Further studies are needed to evaluate whether the findings we describe are also seen in cases of leiomyoma.

Our study is limited by the small number of patients with angiomyolipoma and the limited use of unenhanced thin-section CT (only two of six patients). However, these limitations do not affect our findings of the following: Abundant muscle shows high attenuation on unenhanced CT images, and angiomyolipoma must be included in the differential diagnosis of a hyperattenuating renal lesion on unenhanced CT images.

On images, the well-known beak, or claw, sign suggests that the lesion originates from the renal parenchyma (26,27). A protrusion from the renal margin without the beak sign may indicate a capsular or subcapsular origin of the lesion. It is not known whether homogeneously high attenuation on unenhanced CT images, homogeneous enhancement on contrast-enhanced CT images, and homogeneous isoechogenicity on sonograms are specific for capsular or subcapsular origin, or whether these findings are also seen in intrarenal angiomyolipoma. Angiomyolipoma with minimal fat, however, may commonly protrude from the renal margin without showing the beak sign on one or both sides; this pattern (1 or 2) was seen in all six angiomyolipomas but in only 18 of the 100 renal cell carcinomas. Colvin (28) reported that the frequency of benign mesenchymal neoplasms ("capsulomas") arising from the renal capsule and subcapsular zone was 5.5% at autopsy. These capsulomas have been considered to represent a kind of angiomyolipoma (choristoma) because a large number of these lesions contain fat and smooth muscle (29,30). Patients with these lesions are usually asymptomatic, and these lesions have not been found frequently clinically. Because more capsulomas may be found with advanced imaging modalities, however, the recognition of the findings described are important.

In conclusion, findings in renal lesions of homogeneously high attenuation on unenhanced CT images, homogeneous enhancement on contrast-enhanced CT images, and homogeneous isoechogenicity on sonograms are suggestive of angiomyolipoma that contains minimal fat and abundant muscle. These angiomyolipomas tend to protrude from the renal margin without showing the beak sign, and these lesions frequently show low signal intensity on T2-weighted MR images. In such cases, biopsy is recommended to enable determination of treatment. ■

References

1. Bosniak NA. Angiomyolipoma (hamartoma) of the kidney: a preoperative diagnosis is possible in virtually every case. Urol Radiol 1981; 3:135–142.
2. Raghavendra BN, Bosniak MA, Megibow AJ. Small angiomyolipoma of the kidney: sonographic-CT evaluation. AJR 1983; 141:575–578.
3. Bret PM, Bretagnolle M, Gaillard D, et al. Small, asymptomatic angiomyolipomas of the kidney. Radiology 1985; 154:7–10.
4. Hanson GE, Hoffman RB, Sample WF, Becker R. Computed tomography diagnosis of renal angiomyolipoma. Radiology 1978; 128:789–791.
5. Totty WG, McClennan BL, Melson GL, Patel R. Relative value of computed tomography and ultrasonography in the assessment of renal angiomyolipoma. J Comput Assist Tomogr 1981; 5:173–178.
6. Friedman AC, Hartman DS, Sherman J, Lautin EM, Goldman SM. Computed tomography of abdominal fatty masses. Radiology 1981; 139: 415–429.
7. Sherman JL, Hartman DS, Friedman AC, Madewell JE, Davis CJ, Goldman SM. Angiomyolipoma: computed tomographic–pathologic correlation of 17 cases. AJR 1981; 137:1221–1226.
8. Sant GR, Heaney JA, Ucci AA, Sarno RC, Meares EM. Computed tomographic findings in renal angiomyolipoma: a histologic correlation. Urology 1984; 24:293–296.
9. Trigaux JP, Pauls C, Van Beers B. Atypical renal hamartomas: ultrasonography, computed tomography, and angiographic findings. JCU 1993; 21:41–44.
10. Bosniak MA, Megibow AJ, Hulnick DH, Horii S, Raghavendra BN. CT diagnosis of renal angiomyolipoma: the importance of detecting small amounts of fat. AJR 1988; 151:497–501.
11. Bosniak MA. The small (≤3.0 cm) renal parenchymal tumor: detection, diagnosis, and controversies. Radiology 1991; 179:307–317.
12. Pea M, Bonetti F, Zamboni G, et al. Melanocyte-marker-HMB-45 is regularly expressed in angiomyolipoma of the kidney. Pathology 1991; 23:185–188.
13. Hoon V, Thung SN, Kaneko M, Unger PD. HMB-45 reactivity in renal angiomyolipoma and lymphangioleiomyomatosis. Arch Pathol Lab Med 1994; 118:732–734.
14. Enzinger FM, Weiss SW. Benign lipomatous tumors. In: Soft tissue tumors. 3rd ed. St Louis, Mo: Mosby–Year Book, 1995; 405–409.
15. Behan M, Kazan E. The echogenic characteristics of fatty tissues and tumors. Radiology 1978; 129:143–151.
16. Lee TG, Henderson SC, Freeny PC, Raskin MM, Benson EP, Pearse HD. Ultrasound findings of renal angiomyolipoma. JCU 1978; 6: 150–155.
17. Yamashita Y, Takahashi M, Watanabe O, et al. Small renal cell carcinoma: pathologic and radiologic correlation. Radiology 1992; 184:493–498.
18. Coleman BG, Arger PH, Mintz MC, Pollack HM, Banner MP. Hyperdense renal masses: a computed tomographic dilemma. AJR 1984; 143:291–294.
19. Jinzaki M, Hisa N, Fujikura Y, Ohkuma K, Tashiro M, Sugiura H. Comparative study between ultrasonographic and pathological findings of small renal cell carcinoma. Jpn J Med Ultrasonics 1990; 17:68–75.
20. Sussman S, Cochran ST, Pagani JJ, et al. Hyperdense renal masses: a CT manifestation of hemorrhagic renal cysts. Radiology 1984; 150: 207–211.
21. Ro HJ, Ha HK, Kim HS, Shinn KS. Renal metastasis from thyroid carcinoma visible as a hyperdense lesion on unenhanced CT. AJR 1995; 165:1018.
22. Fukuda T, Matsuoka Y, Sakamoto I, Nagayoshi K, Hayashi K, Okimoto T. CT of thrombosed renal vein presenting as a hyperdense mass. J Comput Assist Tomogr 1995; 19:814–816.
23. Selli C, Masi A, Vanni L, et al. Conflicting aspects of renal leiomyoma with different imaging techniques. Urol Int 1992; 48:219–222.
24. Steiner M, Quinlan D, Goldman SM, et al. Leiomyoma of the kidney: presentation of 4 new cases and the role of computerized tomography. J Urol 1990; 143:994–998.
25. Zollikofer C, Castaneda-Zuniga W, Nath HP, et al. The angiographic appearance of intrarenal leiomyoma. Radiology 1980; 136:47–49.
26. Dautrebande JG, Duckett G, Roy P. The claw sign of cortical cysts in renal arteriography: a contribution to the differential diagnosis of renal space-occupying lesions. J Canad Assoc Radiol 1967; 18:240–250.
27. Pfister RC, Shea TE. Nephrotomography: performance and interpretation. Radiol Clin North Am 1971; 54:41–62.
28. Colvin SH. Certain capsular and subcapsular mixed tumors of the kidney herein called "capsuloma." J Urol 1942; 48:585–600.
29. Petersen RO. Kidney. In: Urologic pathology. 2nd ed. Philadelphia, Pa: Lippincott, 1992; 112.
30. Bennington JL, Beckwith JB, eds. Atlas of tumor pathology: tumors of the kidney, renal pelvis, and ureter, 2nd ser, fasc 12. Washington, DC: Armed Forces Institute of Pathology, 1975; 202.

Jean A. Pradel, MD • Jean-François Adell, MD • Patrice Taourel, MD • Mounir Djafari, MD
Elisabeth Monnin-Delhom, MD • Jean-Michel Bruel, MD

Acute Colonic Diverticulitis: Prospective Comparative Evaluation with US and CT[1]

PURPOSE: To compare the accuracy of ultrasonographic (US) and computed tomographic (CT) findings for diagnosis of acute colonic diverticulitis.

MATERIALS AND METHODS: US and CT were prospectively performed in 64 consecutive patients suspected of having acute colonic diverticulitis. Images were interpreted independently in a blinded fashion. Imaging data were compared with the final diagnosis, which was based on initial clinical and follow-up examination results (n = 64) and pathologic (n = 22), endoscopic (n = 21), and contrast enema (n = 15) examination findings.

RESULTS: Final diagnosis was acute colonic diverticulitis (n = 33), other acute abdominal condition (n = 24), or unknown (n = 7). Both CT and US findings yielded 84% accuracy. US and CT findings were not statistically significant different in terms of sensitivity (85% and 91%, respectively) and specificity (84% and 77%, respectively). Positive predictive value was 85% for US and 81% for CT; negative predictive value was 84% for US and 88% for CT. When determining alternative diagnoses, US and CT findings yielded sensitivity of 33% and 50%, respectively (difference not statistically significant). CT scans depicted a small pneumoperitoneum overlooked on plain radiographs and US scans. Six pericolic abscesses were depicted with both techniques; three were depicted with CT only.

CONCLUSION: US and CT findings result in similar accuracy for the evaluation of patients suspected of having diverticulitis.

In recent years, the use of cross-sectional imaging in the evaluation of complicated colonic diverticular disease has gained increasing acceptance. In a number of studies (1–3), findings from computed tomography (CT) have been shown to be more suitable than those from contrast enema examination when assessing mural and pericolic inflammatory changes in acute colonic diverticulitis.

Potential advantages of ultrasonography (US) over CT in the evaluation of the bowel wall and its environment include wider availability, lower cost, and absence of intravenous injection of iodinated contrast material. Since the initial report of Parulekar (4), the value of US findings in the diagnosis of acute colonic diverticulitis has been evaluated in a small number of studies (5–7) in which the sensitivity of US findings ranged from 84% to 100%, which was similar to that reported for CT findings. Despite these promising results, the consensus at present is that US cannot be used as a substitute for CT in the assessment of acute colonic diverticulitis (8). To our knowledge, a prospective comparison of US and CT accuracy has not been previously reported. The aim of our study was to prospectively compare the diagnostic value, advantages, and limitations of US and CT for assessing patients suspected of having acute colonic diverticulitis.

MATERIALS AND METHODS

During a 20-month period (August 1994 to April 1996), all patients referred to our imaging department because they were suspected of having acute colonic diverticulitis were evaluated with US and CT. Radiologic evaluation was requested entirely on the basis of clinician's judgment. Sixty-four patients were included, aged 38–87 years (mean, 64 years). Informed consent for the additional US evaluation was obtained orally.

Sixty-three of 64 patients presented with abdominal pain localized or predominant in the left lower quadrant; in one patient, the pain was localized in the right lower quadrant, but acute colonic diverticulitis was clinically suspected on the basis of a history of recurrent cecal diverticulitis.

The temperature in 50 of the 64 (78%) patients was above 37.5°C, and the white blood cell count was greater than 10,000 cells per cubic millimeter (10×10^9/L) in 47 of 63 (75%) patients (the count was unknown in one patient). In eight patients, both temperature and white blood cell count were within the normal range; nevertheless, a final diagnosis of acute colonic diverticulitis was rendered in four of these eight patients.

The interval between the CT and US examinations was as short as possible (less than 2 hours, in most cases, and never more than 24 hours), and the findings were independently interpreted by two of five radiologists (J.A.P., J.F.A., P.T., M.D., E.M.D.), who were blinded, in all cases, to the results of the other imaging examination.

The operator was randomly selected from among five radiologists (J.A.P., J.F.A., P.T., M.D., E.M.D.), all of whom had 3–5

Index terms: Colon, CT, 75.12111, 75.12112, 75.12113 • Colon, diseases, 75.273, 75.274 • Colon, US, 75.12981 • Computed tomography (CT), comparative studies, 75.12111, 75.12112, 75.12113 • Ultrasound (US), comparative studies, 75.12981

Radiology 1997; 205:503–512

[1] From the Department of Radiology, Hôpital Saint-Eloi, ave Bertin Sans, F-34295 Montpellier 5, France. Received March 3, 1997; revision requested April 2; revision received June 25; accepted June 27. **Address reprint requests to** J.A.P.

Table 1
Diagnosis, Treatment, and Examination Findings in 64 Patients with Abdominal Symptoms

Patient	Final Diagnosis	Treatment	Surgical or Histopathologic Findings	Colonoscopic Findings	Contrast Enema Findings
1	ACD	Emergency surgery (0)	ACD	NA	NA
2	ACD	Medical	NA	NA	NA
3	ACD	Medical	NA	Normal (30)	NA
4	ACD	Delayed surgery (7)	ACD	NA	NA
5	ACD	Medical	NA	NA	NA
6	ACD	Medical	NA	NA	NA
7	ACD	Delayed surgery (30)	ACD	NA	ACD
8	ACD	Medical	NA	Normal (30)	NA
9	ACD	Medical	NA	ACD (60)	NA
10	ACD	Delayed surgery (7)	ACD	NA	NA
11	ACD	Delayed surgery (110)	Diverticulosis	NA	ACD
12	ACD	Delayed surgery (40)	ACD	NA	ACD
13	ACD	Medical	NA	NA	NA
14	ACD	Delayed surgery (30)	ACD	NA	ACD
15	ACD	Delayed surgery (28)	ACD	NA	ACD
16	ACD	Medical	NA	ACD (15)	NA
17	ACD	Delayed surgery (90)	Diverticulosis	Normal (45)	NA
18	ACD	Medical	NA	NA	NA
19	ACD	Delayed surgery (60)	NA	ACD (60)	ACD
20	ACD	Delayed surgery (40)	ACD	NA	ACD
21	ACD	Delayed surgery (180)	Diverticulosis	NA	NA
22	ACD	Delayed surgery (30)	ACD	Normal (25)	NA
23	ACD	Delayed surgery (70)	Diverticulosis	NA	NA
24	ACD	Emergency surgery (1)	ACD	NA	NA
25	ACD	Delayed surgery (60)	ACD	Normal (30)	ACD
26	ACD	Medical	NA	NA	NA
27	ACD	Delayed surgery (10)	ACD	NA	ACD
28	ACD	Medical	NA	NA	NA
29	ACD	Delayed surgery (30)	ACD	ACD (25)	NA
30	ACD	Medical	NA	NA	NA
31	ACD	Delayed surgery (40)	ACD	ACD (8)	ACD
32	ACD	Medical	NA	Normal (30)	NA
33	ACD	Medical	NA	NA	NA
34	Unknown origin	Medical	NA	NA	NA
35	Unknown origin	Medical	NA	NA	NA
36	Unknown origin	Medical	NA	Normal (2)	NA
37	Unknown origin	Medical	NA	Normal	NA
38	Unknown origin	Medical	NA	NA	Normal
39	Unknown origin	Medical	NA	NA	NA
40	Unknown origin	Medical	NA	NA	NA
41	Ischemic colitis	Medical	NA	Ischemic colitis (20)	Ischemic colitis
42	Ischemic colitis	Medical	NA	Ischemic colitis (4)	NA
43	Small bowel obstruction	Medical	NA	NA	NA
44	Small bowel obstruction	Emergency surgery (1)	Small bowel obstruction	NA	NA
45	Ureterolithiasis	Medical	NA	NA	NA
46	Ureterolithiasis	Medical	NA	NA	NA
47	Adenocarcinoma	Delayed surgery	Adenocarcinoma	NA	NA
48	Adenocarcinoma	Delayed surgery (120)	Adenocarcinoma	Adenocarcinoma (120)	Normal
49	Appendagitis	Medical	NA	NA	NA
50	Endometritis	Medical	NA	NA	NA
51	Jejunal hematoma	Medical	NA	NA	NA
52	Urinary tract infection	Medical	NA	NA	NA
53	Bacterial enteritis	Medical	NA	Bacterial enteritis (7)	NA
54	Left kidney carcinoma	Medical	NA	NA	Normal
55	Indeterminate colitis	Medical	NA	Colitis (3)	NA
56	Indeterminate colitis	Medical	NA	Colitis (1)	NA
57	Indeterminate colitis	Medical	NA	Colitis (4)	NA
58	Irritable bowel syndrome	Medical	NA	Normal (5)	Normal
59	Irritable bowel syndrome	Medical	NA	NA	NA
60	Abdomen wall hematoma	Medical	NA	NA	NA
61	Pyelonephritis	Medical	NA	NA	NA
62	Epididymo-orchitis	Medical	NA	NA	NA
63	Appendicitis	Emergency surgery (2)	Appendicitis	NA	NA
64	Abdomen wall abscess	Medical	NA	NA	NA

Note.—Numbers in parentheses are number of days after presentation. ACD = acute colonic diverticulitis, NA = not applicable.

years experience in both US and CT of the gastrointestinal tract. No US examination was performed by a technologist. The results of this initial real-time evaluation were later compared with the final diagnosis. The final diagnosis in four patients was established on the basis of the findings obtained at emergency surgery performed less than 24 hours after radiologic assessment. In the other patients, the final diagnosis was based on the data from clinical and radiologic follow-up and response to medical treatment ($n = 60$), pathologists' reports of surgical specimens ($n = 18$) obtained 7–180 days (mean, 63 days) after presentation, and various diagnostic procedures, including contrast enema examination ($n = 15$) and colonoscopy ($n = 21$). These data are presented on a patient-by-patient basis in Table 1.

Contrast enema examinations were con-

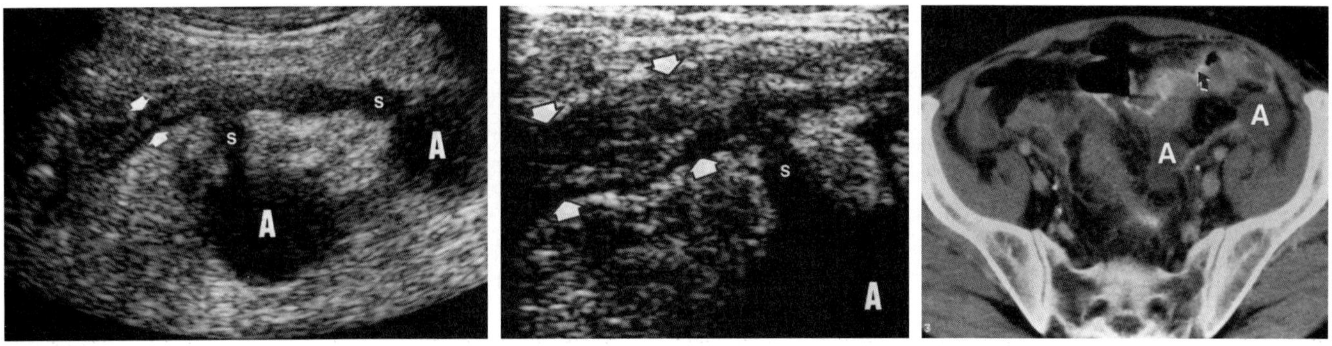

a. b. c.

Figure 1. Acute colonic diverticulitis. True-positive US scans obtained at the same level with **(a)** a 2–4-MHz convex-array transducer and **(b)** a 5–10-MHz linear-array transducer and **(c)** a concordant true-positive CT scan obtained after rectal administration of barium sulfate. **(a, b)** On US images obtained in the axial plane, the sigmoid colon (arrows) is thickened and the pericolic fat is enlarged and hyperechoic and contains ill-defined zones of moderate hypoechogenicity. The well-defined, markedly hypoechoic masses are pericolic abscesses (*A*). Sinus tracts (*S*) connecting the abscesses and the colonic wall are also visible. **(c)** On the CT scan, the lumen (arrow) is distended by means of the dilute barium sulfate suspension. Bowel wall thickening and inflammatory pericolic fat are well demonstrated, and pericolic abscesses (*A*) are visible.

sidered positive for acute colonic diverticulitis when at least two of the following findings were present: localized extravasation of contrast material, marked and distorted colonic fold thickening, localized mass effect, and mucosal tethering (3,6). The interval between contrast enema examination and US and CT assessment never exceeded 2 days. Endoscopic findings were considered to be indicative of acute colonic diverticulitis in the presence of segmental luminal narrowing of the diverticular bowel segment, with signs of inflammatory mucosal changes (5); the colonoscopic evaluation was performed 1–120 days (mean, 26 days) after cross-sectional imaging. When colonoscopic, surgical, or pathologic data were obtained with a delay after the resolution of clinical symptoms after medical treatment, the absence of positive signs of acute colonic diverticulitis was not considered to exclude this diagnosis, and the main contribution of these data for establishment of the final diagnosis was to confirm the absence of any other colonic pathologic condition, especially cancer.

The final diagnosis was acute colonic diverticulitis in 33 patients, which was localized in the sigmoid colon ($n = 31$), in the left part of the transverse colon ($n = 1$), and in the cecum ($n = 1$). In the other patients, the final diagnosis was abdominal pain of unknown cause ($n = 7$) or other abdominal condition ($n = 24$), including indeterminate colitis ($n = 3$), ischemic colitis ($n = 2$), irritable bowel syndrome ($n = 2$), appendicitis ($n = 1$), adenocarcinoma of the sigmoid colon ($n = 2$), small bowel obstruction ($n = 2$), bacterial enteritis ($n = 1$), jejunal hematoma ($n = 1$), primary epiploic appendagitis ($n = 1$), abdominal wall abscess ($n = 1$) and hematoma ($n = 1$), ureterolithiasis ($n = 2$), pyelonephritis ($n = 1$), urinary tract infection ($n = 1$), left kidney carcinoma ($n = 1$), epididymo-orchitis ($n = 1$), and endometritis ($n = 1$).

All CT examinations were performed with a Somatom DRH unit (Siemens Medical Systems, Erlangen, Germany) by using a nonspiral dynamic sequential data acquisition mode. Scans were obtained with 8-mm collimation, 12–16-mm intervals in the upper abdomen (above the iliac crests), and 8-mm intervals in the lower abdomen. If necessary, repeated 4-mm sections at 4-mm intervals of the lower abdomen were obtained at the end of the examination. In 56 of 64 (88%) patients, 2 mL per kilogram of body weight of ionic (ioxithamalate meglumine, Telebrix 350; Guerbet, Aulnay-sous-bois, France) or nonionic (iohexol, Omnipaque; Nycomed, New York, NY) iodinated contrast material were intravenously administered at a rate of 2 mL/sec with an injection delay of 40 seconds. Contrast material was not administered in eight patients because of renal failure ($n = 3$), difficulties in the positioning of the venous catheter ($n = 2$), or unknown reason ($n = 3$). In 41 (64%) patients, 500–800 mL of 2.5% dilute ioxithamalate meglumine (Telebrix Gastro; Guerbet) were orally administered. Patients received contrast material by way of the rectum (air or dilute barium sulfate suspension) only in selected cases, when identification of the colon or assessment of bowel wall thickness was considered to be unsatisfactory with the standard CT technique.

All US studies were obtained with an Ultramark 9 high-definition imaging unit (Advanced Technology Laboratories, Bothell, Wash). In each patient, the colon and its environment were initially examined by using a broad-band 2–4-MHz convex-array transducer. This evaluation was completed with a sonographic assessment of the colonic wall performed with a broad-band 5–10-MHz linear-array transducer and the graded-compression technique described by Puylaert (9).

In the patients who presented with clinical symptoms that were localized or predominating in the left lower quadrant, US was initiated by scanning of the area of left iliac fossa, which usually allowed easy identification of the sigmoid colon as an oblique intestinal segment located between the left iliac crest and the bladder dome anterior to and above the left iliac vessels. In continuity with this segment, the descending colon was easily followed by scanning above the iliac crest up to the splenic flexure. Special attention was paid to the specifically painful area described by the patient. In the one patient who was referred because of the suspicion of cecal acute colonic diverticulitis, the sonologist began with scanning of the area below the tip of the right hepatic lobe, which allowed identification of the ascending colon and cecum as the most lateral intestinal segment that ran lengthwise in the right flank. US evaluation of the colon was completed in each patient with an overall abdominal examination performed with the 2–4-MHz convex-array transducer, including a search for intraperitoneal free fluid (especially in the left paracolic gutter, lower pelvic recesses, and perihepatic and perisplenic spaces), and for a pneumoperitoneum (seen as an echogenic line with a posterior ring-down or reverberation artifact between the anterior abdominal wall and the anterior surface of the liver) (10). An especially detailed overall evaluation of the abdomen was performed to determine an alternative diagnosis when the colon appeared to be normal. The whole US examination routinely took about 30 minutes.

Our assessment of the colonic wall and local environment, which we derived from reports in the literature (1,2,5–7), was based on a set of four criteria, defined before the beginning of the study and matched for CT and US evaluation: (*a*) thickening of the bowel wall and (*b*) presence of diverticula, (*c*) inflammatory pericolic fat, and (*d*) pericolic abscess.

For CT evaluation, these criteria were determined as follows: (*a*) Thickening of the bowel wall was considered to be present when the thickness of the colonic wall exceeded 4 mm (Figs 1, 2, 4) on a scan obtained perpendicular to or through the long axis of a slightly distended colonic lumen (2). (*b*) Diverticula were identified as flask-shaped structures filled with air, barium, or fecal material (Figs 2–5) that projected through the colonic wall (2). (*c*) Inflammatory pericolic fat was defined as a poorly marginated, hazy area of increased attenuation, with or without linear stranding (Figs 1–4), in the fat adjacent to or surrounding the colonic wall (1,2). (*d*) A pericolic abscess was considered to be present when CT scans depicted a well-defined mass that was localized in the pericolic environment and contained central liquid and/or gas components (Figs 1, 2, 4) (2).

For US evaluation, the same four criteria were defined as follows: (*a*) Thickening of the bowel wall was considered to be present when the distance from the echogenic lumen interface to the hyperechoic serosa and pericolic fat exceeded 4 mm on a scan obtained through the long axis of or perpendicular to the colonic lumen (Figs 1, 2, 4) (5,6). (*b*) Diverticula were defined as round or oval foci that protruded from the colonic wall, with focal disruption of the normal layer continuity (5–7); the echogenicity of these foci varied from hypoechoic to hyperechoic, with or without internal acoustic shadowing (Fig 3). (*c*) Inflammatory pericolic fat was defined as the presence of an area of regionally increased echogenicity (hyperechoic halo), adjacent to or surrounding the colonic wall (6,7), that possibly contained ill-defined hypoechoic zones (6) (Figs 1–4). (*d*) Pericolic abscess was identified as a well-defined hypoechoic mass that was localized in the pericolic environment (Figs 1, 2, 4) and possibly contained central liquid and/or gas; gas was considered to be present when dense echoes with acoustic shadowing were seen in the mass (6,7). The differentiation of abscesses from the adjacent bowel loops was based on the absence of mural layering and of internal peristalsis.

The authors of previous reports have questioned the diagnostic value of each of these US and CT criteria, considered individually: None of the criteria were considered to be sensitive and specific enough to allow confident diagnosis of acute colonic diverticulitis. Particularly, several authors (1,5–7,11) have pointed out that mural abnormalities (ie, diverticula and thickening of the bowel wall) can be observed in patients with noncomplicated diverticulosis, as well as in patients with a colonic nondiverticular disease. Similarly, extramural abnormalities (ie, inflammatory pericolic fat and pericolic abscess) can be due to an extracolic pathologic condition with an inflammatory component located in the pericolic area. For these reasons, we divided our four criteria into two subgroups: mural signs (thickening of the bowel wall and diverticula), and extramural signs (inflammatory pericolic fat and pericolic abscess). At our prospective evaluation, we considered the examination result to be positive for acute colonic diverticulitis when at least one mural sign was present and was associated with at least one extramural sign (ie, when at least one sign from each subgroup was present). These criteria were established prospectively at the outset of the study so that US and CT studies could be categorized in real time by the physician-investigator who performed the examination and interpreted the results.

Statistical analysis was performed by using SAS/STAT software (SAS Institute, Cary, NC). The McNemar test for paired data was used to investigate differences between the sensitivities, specificities, and accuracies of US and CT findings in the detection of acute colonic diverticulitis, and to compare the ability to establish an alternative diagnosis when using US and CT findings. Differences were considered to be statistically significant when *P* values were less than .05. The κ statistic was used to measure the degree of agreement between the two imaging modalities in the depiction of the four diagnostic criteria that were the basis of the comparative evaluation. A κ of less than 0.40 indicated poor agreement; a value of 0.40–0.59, fair agreement; a value of 0.60–0.74, good agreement; and a value of 0.75 or greater, excellent agreement.

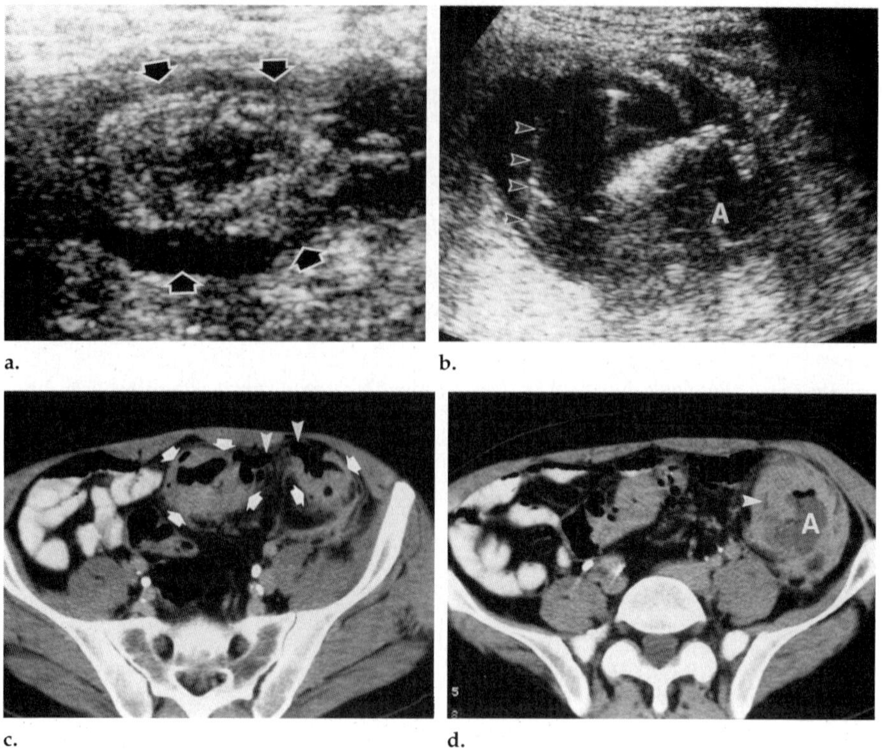

Figure 2. True-positive images in a patient with acute colonic diverticulitis. **(a, b)** The US scans were obtained with **(a)** a 5–10-MHz linear-array transducer and **(b)** a 2–4-MHz convex-array transducer. **(c, d)** CT scans were obtained after intravenous administration of iodinated contrast material and rectal air insufflation. **(c)** CT scan obtained at the same level as in **a** shows the lumen, which is distended after rectal air insufflation. **(d)** CT scan obtained at the same level as in **b** shows that the lumen is collapsed (arrowheads). **(a, c)** The sigmoid colon (arrows) is thickened, with diverticula evident on CT image (arrowheads in **c**). The pericolic fat is enlarged and heterogeneous on the axial US image, with stranding of the pericolic fat. **(b, d)** Transverse images obtained at a more cephalic level than **a** and **c** show a pericolic abscess (*A*), with air and fluid components, abutting the thickened colonic wall and collapsing the lumen (arrowheads).

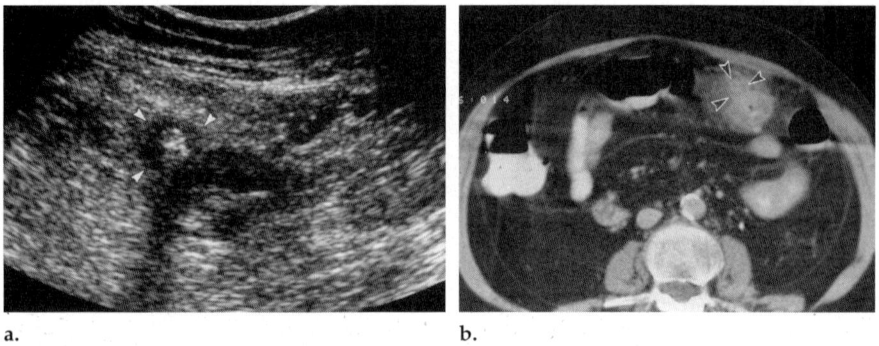

Figure 3. Acute colonic diverticulitis. **(a)** Axial US scan obtained with a 2–4-MHz convex-array transducer was initially falsely interpreted to be negative (false-negative) for acute colonic diverticulitis. **(b)** On a subsequently obtained CT scan enhanced with intravenously administered iodinated contrast material, circumferential mural thickening of the left part of the transverse colon was noted, and the scan was interpreted to be positive (true-positive) for acute colonic diverticulitis. On both US and CT scans, the inflamed diverticulum (arrowheads) of the anterior colonic wall is well demonstrated and is surrounded by inflammatory fat (hyperechoic halo in **a**, poorly marginated, hazy area of increased attenuation in **b**).

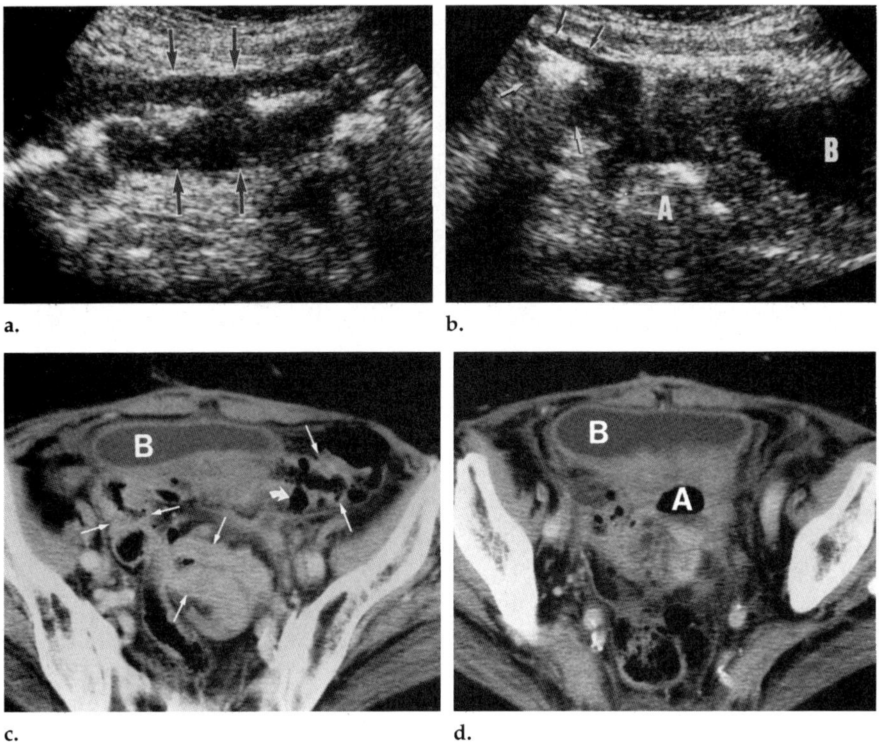

Figure 4. Perforated, infected colon cancer. **(a, b)** US scans obtained with a 2–4-MHz convex-array transducer and **(c, d)** concordant CT scans (enhanced with intravenously administered iodinated contrast material) were falsely interpreted to show acute colonic diverticulitis. The sigmoid colon (straight arrows in **a–c**) appears to be thickened on **(a)** sagittal oblique and **(b)** sagittal US images and on **(c, d)** axial CT images. There is evidence of diverticula on a CT image (curved arrow in **c**). Inflammatory pericolic fat with pericolic abscess (*A* in **b** and **d**) is seen on the sagittal US and axial CT images (**d** was obtained at a level more caudal than **c**) abutting the thickened wall bladder lumen (*B* in **b–d**).

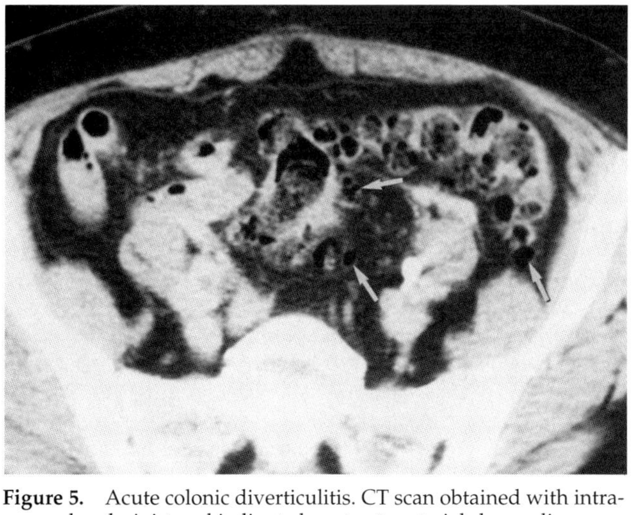

Figure 5. Acute colonic diverticulitis. CT scan obtained with intravenously administered iodinated contrast material shows diverticula of the sigmoid colon (arrows). No perimural signs are present. The US scan (not shown) was initially interpreted to be negative for diverticulitis (false-negative).

RESULTS

Table 2 details the sensitivity and specificity, in terms of our four diagnostic criteria considered individually, for CT and US findings of acute colonic diverticulitis. The agreement between the CT and US results was excellent for depiction of inflammatory pericolic fat ($\kappa = 0.78$), good for the depiction of both bowel wall thickening ($\kappa = 0.69$) and pericolic abscess ($\kappa = 0.69$), and poor for the depiction of diverticula ($\kappa = 0.35$).

Sensitivity, specificity, accuracy, and positive and negative predictive values for US and CT findings in the diagnosis of acute colonic diverticulitis are summarized in Table 3. In the overall study population, CT and US evaluation yielded the same number of incorrect results (in 10 of 64 patients), which resulted in an identical accuracy of 84% for findings from both techniques. In the 33 patients with a final diagnosis of acute colonic diverticulitis, false-negative CT results were obtained in three patients, and false-negative US results were obtained in five patients. The sensitivity for CT and US findings was 91% and 85%, respectively; this difference was not statistically significant ($P = .16$).

The US and CT results were in agreement in 31 of these 33 patients: True-positive US and CT results were concordant in 28 patients (Figs 1–4), and false-negative US and CT results were concordant in three patients. In the latter three patients, both CT (Fig 5) and US scans demonstrated mural signs (diverticula in two patients, bowel wall thickening in the third patient) but failed to demonstrate any extramural signs.

US and CT results were discordant in two of the 33 patients with acute colonic diverticulitis; in these two patients, the CT study was true-positive, and the US study was false-negative. In the first patient, CT scans demonstrated subtle inflammatory changes in the pericolic fat around a cecal diverticulum, whereas US scans showed no extramural signs. In the second patient, the initial abdominal US results were considered to be normal. CT results demonstrated an inflamed diverticulum located in the left part of the transverse colon, which was easily identified with further US evaluation performed with knowledge of the CT results (Fig 3).

In the 31 patients without acute colonic diverticulitis, the CT study was false-positive in seven patients, and the US study was false-positive in five patients. The specificity of CT and US findings was 77% and 84%, respectively; this difference was not statistically significant ($P = .32$). US and CT results were in agreement in 27 of these 31 patients for exclusion of the diagnosis of acute colonic diverticulitis: Concordant US and CT true-negative results were obtained in 23 patients, and concordant false-positive results were obtained in four patients. In these latter four patients, the final diagnosis was ischemic colitis ($n = 2$), indeterminate colitis ($n = 1$), and adenocarcinoma of the sigmoid colon ($n = 1$) (Fig 4).

In four of the 31 patients, CT and US results were not in agreement with regard to the absence of acute colonic diverticulitis. In three of these four patients, the US results were true-negative, and the CT findings were false-positive; the final diagnosis in these patients was abdominal pain of unknown origin ($n = 1$), indeterminate colitis ($n = 1$), and adenocarcinoma of the sigmoid colon ($n = 1$). In these three patients, US scans demonstrated only mural signs without evidence of extramural inflammation, whereas CT scans showed both mural and extramural changes. One of these four patients had false-positive US results and true-negative CT results (the disagreement concerned the presence of inflammation in the pericolic fat).

Table 2
Sensitivity and Specificity of the Four Diagnostic Criteria Used for Diagnosis of Acute Colonic Diverticulitis

	CT		US	
Criterion	Sensitivity (%)	Specificity (%)	Sensitivity (%)	Specificity (%)
Bowel wall thickening	82 (27/33) 69–95	71 (22/31) 55–87	76 (25/33) 62–90	77 (24/31) 62–92
Diverticula	82 (27/33) 69–95	51 (16/31) 33–69	79 (27/33) 65–93	68 (21/31) 51–85
Inflammatory pericolic fat	91 (30/33) 81–100	71 (22/31) 55–87	85 (28/33) 72–98	81 (25/31) 67–95
Pericolic abscess	27 (9/33) 12–42	100 (31/31) 100–100	18 (6/33) 5–31	97 (30/31) 91–100

Note.—Numbers in parentheses are actual values; the range is the 95% confidence interval for the percentages.

CT scans demonstrated a pericolic abscess in nine of the 33 (27%) patients with a final diagnosis of acute colonic diverticulitis (Figs 2, 3). The abscess was 1.5–7.0 cm in diameter (mean, 3.3 cm). US scans were positive for the presence of a pericolic abscess in six of these nine patients and negative in three patients. The collections seen on CT scans in three patients but overlooked on US scans were 2.5 cm in diameter or smaller and did not necessitate any specific treatment (one patient underwent emergency surgery for peritonitis, and two were treated successfully with medical treatment alone). In one patient, US scans showed a 3.5-cm-diameter pericolic mass that was not depicted on CT scans. This patient was treated medically, and a final diagnosis of indeterminate colitis was rendered; on the basis of the comparison between US and CT images, we retrospectively assumed the US evaluation to be false-positive due to fluid-filled enlarged bowel loops that mimicked pericolic abscess. The presence of a pericolic abscess was confirmed at immediate surgery for peritonitis in one patient and at percutaneous drainage in one patient; the other seven patients were successfully treated with initial medical treatment. The collections were no longer present in these seven patients at follow-up CT, delayed surgery, or both.

In the 31 patients without acute colonic diverticulitis, 24 had another acute intraabdominal condition finally determined to be responsible for the clinical symptoms. Table 4 shows the comparison of CT and US findings for determination of these nonacute colonic diverticulitis conditions. The alternative diagnosis could be established with CT findings in 12 (50%) patients and with US findings in eight (33%) patients; this difference was not statistically significant. The alternative diagnosis was determined on the basis of both US and CT findings in seven patients. CT findings enabled determination of the alternative diagnosis in five patients with negative US results; the pathologic condition was pyelonephritis, ureterolithiasis, renal adenocarcinoma, abdominal wall hematoma, and primary epiploic appendagitis. In the latter three of these five patients, suggestive findings were retrospectively seen on US scans obtained with knowledge of CT results. In one patient with a low-grade small bowel obstruction, the diagnosis was correctly rendered on the basis of US findings, whereas the CT results were negative.

Free intraperitoneal fluid was seen in two patients (one with jejunal hematoma and one with indeterminate colitis) and was noted on both US and CT scans in each case. CT scans showed intraperitoneal air in two patients; in one of these patients, the pneumoperitoneum was demonstrated on US scans and plain radiographs, as well. In the other patient, however, a small amount of intraperitoneal air in the right subphrenic space was visible only on the CT scans.

Table 3
Sensitivity, Specificity, Accuracy, and Predictive Values of CT and US Findings for Diagnosis of Acute Colonic Diverticulitis

Parameter	CT Findings	US Findings
Sensitivity (%)	91 (30/33) 81–100	85 (28/33) 73–97
Specificity (%)	77 (24/31) 62–92	84 (26/31) 71–97
Accuracy (%)	84 (54/64) 75–93	84 (54/64) 75–93
Positive predictive value (%)	81 (30/37) 68–94	85 (28/33) 73–97
Negative predictive value (%)	88 (24/27) 75–100	84 (26/31) 71–97

Note.—Numbers in parentheses are actual values; ranges are 95% confidence intervals for the percentages.

DISCUSSION

Colonic diverticulosis affects approximately 5% of the population (12); acute inflammation secondary to colonic diverticula occurs in 10%–35% of these patients (12,13) and increases in frequency with advancing age. Acute colonic diverticulitis is, therefore, a common cause of acute abdominal symptoms, especially in elderly patients.

The clinical diagnosis and assessment of acute colonic diverticulitis can be difficult (12,13); the classic pattern of left lower quadrant pain, tenderness, fever, and leukocytosis is, in theory, suggestive of acute colonic diverticulitis but can be mimicked by numerous acute abdominal conditions. Besides, the complete combination of these signs is actually seldom found in cases of acute colonic diverticulitis. In one study (14), fever was present in only 35 of 140 (25%) patients, and up to 90 (64%) patients had a white blood cell count within the normal range. Furthermore, clinical evaluation results are limited for the purpose of prediction of the extent of the pericolic inflammatory process, which can lead to inaccurate management of acute colonic diverticulitis (13). Thus, the role of the radiologic evaluation of patients suspected of having acute colonic diverticulitis is twofold (13,15): (*a*) to confirm the diagnosis and to distinguish patients with acute colonic diverticulitis from those with another acute abdominal condition that produces similar symptoms and (*b*) to assess the site and severity of the pericolic extension to determine which patients are less likely to respond to

Table 4
Agreement of Imaging Findings and Final Alternative Diagnosis

Diagnosis	CT Findings	US Findings
Indeterminate colitis	Yes	Yes
Indeterminate colitis	Yes	Yes
Indeterminate colitis	No	No
Ischemic colitis	No	No
Ischemic colitis	No	No
Irritable bowel syndrome	No	No
Irritable bowel syndrome	No	No
Appendicitis	No	No
Colonic adenocarcinoma	No	No
Colonic adenocarcinoma	No	No
Small bowel obstruction	Yes	Yes
Small bowel obstruction	No	Yes
Bacterial enteritis	No	No
Jejunal hematoma	Yes	Yes
Primary epiploic appendagitis	Yes	No
Abdominal wall abscess	Yes	Yes
Abdominal wall hematoma	Yes	No
Ureterolithiasis	Yes	Yes
Ureterolithiasis	Yes	No
Pyelonephritis	Yes	No
Urinary tract infection	No	No
Left kidney carcinoma	Yes	No
Epididymo-orchitis	No	No
Endometritis	Yes	Yes

Note.—Data indicate whether the alternative diagnosis (based on colonoscopic, surgical, and/or histopathologic findings) could be established by using CT and US findings.

conservative treatment and should therefore be considered candidates for initial surgical treatment or percutaneous drainage.

Traditionally, the contrast enema examination has been the mainstay in the evaluation of patients suspected of having acute colonic diverticulitis. However, only mucosal changes can be directly evaluated with this technique, which represents an inherent limitation in the assessment of acute colonic diverticulitis because the location of the pathologic process is mainly extramucosal (11). Thus, the sensitivity of the results of a contrast enema examination in the diagnosis of acute colonic diverticulitis does not exceed 77%–86% (1,3,16). Besides, the use of findings from this technique has been shown to result in underestimation of the extent of pericolic inflammation in up to 41% of patients (2). Conversely, with cross-sectional imaging, direct visualization of both the intramural component (abnormal colonic wall) and the extramural component (inflammatory changes in the pericolic fat) of the diverticular disease is possible.

The authors of previous studies (1,3) in which CT and contrast enema examination were used for evaluation of acute colonic diverticulitis reported the sensitivity for CT findings to be 79%–93%, which is equal or superior to the sensitivity for contrast enema examination findings, and determined that CT was more suitable for grading the severity of pericolic inflammation (2). Particularly, CT scans more accurately depicted the presence, location, and size of pericolic abscesses—findings that are considered to have a marked effect on patient care (17,18). Besides, the use of CT findings has been shown (7) to be more effective than the use of contrast enema examination results for the determination of alternative diagnoses (ie, for identification of other acute intraabdominal conditions that mimic acute colonic diverticulitis), especially when the pathologic process is extracolic. For these reasons, many authors (1,11,17–18) advocate the use of CT as the initial procedure for radiologic evaluation in patients suspected of having acute colonic diverticulitis. At our institution, CT is routinely used as the initial imaging modality in patients suspected of having acute colonic diverticulitis. However, the wide use that is made of US as a "first-line" imaging method in patients with acute abdomen (19) and the impressive results reported (5–7) in the small number of prospective studies in which US findings were used for the diagnosis of acute colonic diverticulitis are inducements to include assessment of complicated diverticular disease in the field of abdominal US imaging, if diagnostic accuracy similar to that of CT findings can be achieved.

Our experience confirms the difficulties encountered at clinical evaluation in the diagnosis of acute colonic diverticulitis: In our series, a final diagnosis of complicated diverticular disease was established in only 33 of the 64 (52%) patients suspected of having acute colonic diverticulitis, whereas a final diagnosis of another disease was rendered in 24 (38%) patients.

These data stress the importance of the use of findings from a widely available and accurate imaging method for establishing the correct diagnosis when the clinical data are inconclusive. The results we obtained with the two imaging modalities are in agreement with those of previous studies (1–3,5–7) in which the value of US and CT findings for the diagnosis of acute colonic diverticulitis have been independently reported. In our series, CT findings enabled the correct diagnosis in 30 of 33 (91%) patients with acute colonic diverticulitis; this result is similar to the 93% sensitivity reported by Cho et al (1) in a prospective evaluation of the efficacy of CT versus that of barium enema examination.

The three false-negative CT studies we obtained depicted mural changes in the colonic wall but failed to demonstrate any sign of pericolonic inflammation (Fig 5). This pitfall in the CT diagnosis of acute colonic diverticulitis has been well documented in a study by Balthazar et al (20), who demonstrated that this CT finding was seen in less severe forms of diverticulitis that were confined mainly to the wall of the colon. In their series, pathologic correlation showed infected intramural diverticula, microabscesses, intramural inflammatory reaction, and small amounts of fibropurulent exudate that coated the serosa. In our series, the three patients in whom false-negative CT scans were obtained were successfully treated with medical treatment alone, and thus no pathologic correlation was available; however, it is likely that these patients had a mild, purely intramural form of acute colonic diverticulitis that was overlooked at CT because of the lack of inflammatory changes in the pericolic fat.

The sensitivity of US findings, in our series, was 85% (28 true-positive studies in 33 patients with acute colonic diverticulitis) and was therefore identical to that reported by Verbanck et al (5) for their prospective evaluation. Schwerk et al (7) achieved a sensitivity of 98% with US findings, and Wilson and Toi (6) reported no false-negative US results in 46 patients with acute colonic diverticulitis. In the three patients in whom we obtained false-negative CT results, false-negative US studies were also obtained; the US scans demonstrated only mural changes without evidence of pericolic involvement. Therefore, subtle pericolic inflammatory changes may be no better depicted on US scans than on CT scans.

US findings were less effective than CT results for the identification of pericolic inflammation in two patients. One of these patients had focal acute colonic diverticulitis of the transverse colon, which was readily demonstrated at a retrospective US evaluation performed with knowledge of CT data (Fig 3). In this patient, the failure to detect the pathologic condition on the initial US study was probably related to an insufficiently careful evaluation of the transverse colon, which is an unusual site of involvement in cases of acute colonic diverticulitis. This case stresses the importance of meticulous assessment of the entire large bowel in patients referred for US evaluation of possible acute colonic diverticulitis.

The specificity of CT findings for the diagnosis of acute colonic diverticulitis was only 77% (seven false-positive results in 31 patients without acute colonic diverticulitis) in our study. Because many reports about CT assessment of acute colonic diverticulitis are retrospective, the specificity of CT findings cannot be considered to be definitely established. At a prospective evaluation, Cho et al (1) did not report any false-positive CT results; however, other authors (11,17,20) have pointed out the existence of a substantial overlap between the CT appearance of acute colonic diverticulitis and that of colon cancer. This was the case in two patients in our series who had colon cancer; CT scans showed mural thickening and inflammatory pericolic fat, as well. One of these two patients had a perforated and infected cancer with pericolic abscess (Fig 4).

Given the presence of both mural and extramural signs, we observed that the differential diagnosis was not limited to colon cancer. CT scans in two patients with colonic ischemia and in two patients with indeterminate colitis demonstrated association of a thickened colonic wall and mild inflammation of pericolic fat, which resulted in false-positive CT evaluations.

Evaluation of US findings yielded a specificity of 84% (five false-positive results in 31 patients without acute colonic diverticulitis) in our series. The reported specificity of US findings for diagnosis of acute colonic diverticulitis varies from 80% (5) to 97% (7). False-positive results are related to the presence of tumoral (adenocarcinoma, lymphoma), inflammatory (Crohn disease), or ischemic colonic diseases and to extracolic inflammatory conditions adjacent to the colonic wall (5–7). We did not encounter any extracolonic pathologic process that mimicked acute colonic diverticulitis. Four of the five false-positive US studies in our series could be related to another colonic disease: ischemic colitis (n = 2), adenocarcinoma (n = 1), and indeterminate colitis (n = 1). In these four patients, both US and CT results were false-positive owing to the presence of both a mural sign (thickening of the bowel wall) and an extramural sign (inflammatory pericolic fat); this combination is therefore nonspecific for diagnosis of acute colonic diverticulitis, regardless of the method of cross-sectional imaging used.

Accurate diagnosis of pericolic abscesses is considered to have a marked impact on the management of acute colonic diverticulitis; especially, several authors (15–21) have emphasized the usefulness of CT-guided percutaneous abscess drainage, which can be used to change a two-stage or multistage surgical procedure into a single-stage procedure. However, Ambrosetti et al (18) reported that 15 of 22 (68%) cases of peridiverticular abscess were successfully managed with antibiotic drugs alone.

In the 33 patients with acute colonic diverticulitis in our series, nine had a pericolic abscess identified at CT; the abscess (diameter ≤ 2.5 mm) in three of these patients was overlooked at US, but the identification of an abscess had no effect on the care of these three patients (one patient underwent immediate surgery for peritonitis, and two patients were successfully treated medically). In the six other patients, who had an abscess depicted on both US and CT scans, the effect on the treatment was also limited: only one patient underwent percutaneous drainage; the rest were successfully treated with antibiotic drugs alone. Therefore, even if the number of abscesses in our series was too small to allow definitive conclusions, our experience suggests that US and CT may provide data of similar usefulness as regards the care of patients with acute colonic diverticulitis that is complicated by the presence of abscess.

CT guidance was used in the patient who underwent percutaneous drainage; US-guided percutaneous aspiration or catheter drainage of complicating abscesses has been demonstrated to be feasible (7), although some authors (5) have suggested that CT guidance allows more accurate delineation of abscesses and identification of a safe pathway for drainage. We did not attempt a qualitative assessment of the morphologic features of the pelvic abscesses that complicated acute colonic diverticulitis, and our experience is too limited to ascertain whether US can be as useful as CT for the evaluation of the full extent of these abscesses.

The false-positive US diagnosis of pericolic abscess that we encountered in our study is another argument for performing CT if a pericolic abscess is depicted at US and percutaneous drainage is considered. Definitive assessment of the roles of US and CT in the anatomic delineation and the drainage technique for pericolic abscesses, as well as analysis of the merits of percutaneous treatment compared with those of conservative and surgical treatment of acute colonic diverticulitis, await dedicated prospective comparative evaluation, which was beyond the scope of this study.

Accurate determination of alternative diagnoses is one of the major goals of imaging in patients with acute colonic diverticulitis. In our study, CT scans were more useful than US scans for determination of the alternative diagnosis in five patients, whereas US findings were superior to CT findings in only one patient. For each of these six patients, the treatment determined on the basis of positive imaging findings differed from that of acute colonic diverticulitis. The ability to determine the alternative diagnosis with US findings and with CT findings did not statistically significantly differ, but we must recognize that the number of alternative diagnoses encountered in our study is relatively small. Nevertheless, CT findings are clearly ideal for determination of alternative diagnoses because this modality permits a quick, overall assessment of the intraperitoneal, retroperitoneal, and pelvic organs and the abdominal wall, which can be achieved with US only at the expense of a careful, methodic examination of the entire abdomen, the accuracy of which depends largely on the sonologist's experience and patience. We did not carefully compare the amount of physician time needed for a complete examination of the colon and the entire abdomen versus that needed to interpret a CT study of the abdomen, but US would undoubtedly seem to be the more time-consuming technique.

In our series, two patients with acute colonic diverticulitis required emergency surgery for peritonitis. CT findings had an effect on the care of one of the patients owing to the demonstration of a small pneumoperitoneum that was not seen on plain radiographs or US scans. The circumstances of this case suggest that CT may be more suitable than US in the evaluation of a patient for acute colonic diverticulitis when clinical examination results are suggestive of free perforation in the peritoneal cavity.

A number of limitations of our study must be considered. The design of our study was based on the prospective use of a limited number of diagnostic criteria, which were as clearly defined as possible, were matched for US and CT evaluation, and the diagnostic value of which had been validated in previous studies. However, we are aware that some additional criteria not included in our evaluation protocol could have improved the diagnostic value of CT and/or US findings with regard to both acute colonic diverticulitis and nondiverticular colonic disease. For instance, in the two patients with colonic ischemia, both US and CT studies demonstrated involvement of the left colon that extended to the splenic flexure and the left part of the transverse colon; this feature is common in ischemic colitis but is extremely unusual in acute colonic diverticulitis (5) and should have led to a more specific diagnosis.

During this study, we found local tenderness induced by means of graded compression to be useful in specifically relating the pain described by the patient to the colon; however, the sensitivity and the specificity of this criterion (considered separately from the morphologic sonographic features of acute colonic diverticulitis) have not been established in the literature, so we did not include it in our prospective evaluation.

Analysis of mural vascularity with color Doppler US could potentially improve the sensitivity of US findings for diagnosis of acute colonic diverticulitis, although results of preliminary studies (22) have suggested that Doppler US scans demonstrate only mildly increased mural flow in patients with early acute colonic diverticulitis. Besides, in a recent study, the absence of color Doppler signal in the thickened bowel wall was found to be a useful clue for differentiating colonic ischemia from nondiverticular inflammatory colitis. We did not include color Doppler US assessment of the colonic wall in our evaluation, and we were unable to ascertain whether this criterion is useful for determining mild intramural forms of acute colonic diverticulitis and/or for differentiating colonic ischemia from acute colonic diverticulitis.

Similarly, some ancillary CT findings have been reported (24) to be helpful for differentiation of acute colonic diverticulitis from carcinoma of the sigmoid colon; these findings include the presence of fluid at the root of the mesentery and vascular engorgement. Currently, our experience does not allow us to compare the accuracy of US and CT findings for differentiating acute colonic diverticulitis from cancer, owing to the small number of patients with colonic adenocarcinoma included in our series; however, the fact that the colon cancer found in two patients in our series was overlooked at both US and CT may indicate that neither modality can be used to exclude the presence of underlying carcinoma in a patient suspected of having acute colonic diverticulitis, at least on the basis of the diagnostic criteria we used. Consequently, we currently consider that patients with a diagnosis of acute colonic diverticulitis rendered on the basis of cross-sectional imaging findings obtained during the acute phase should be evaluated with a follow-up colonoscopic or barium study.

We performed CT with a conventional scanner and 8-mm collimation. Some authors (25) have suggested that the use of helical thin-section CT will improve accuracy in the assessment of the right lower quadrant digestive inflammatory processes (25). Further experience is needed to ascertain whether the use of helical CT findings will result in better identification of mild forms of acute colonic diverticulitis with minimal pericolic inflammation.

Another technical limitation of our study is the lack of intravenously administered contrast material in a small number (eight [13%] patients) of our patients; however, there were no false-positive or false-negative CT results in this subgroup.

Systematic administration of contrast material by way of the rectum might have improved the assessment of wall thickness in some patients. We believe, however, that this potential technical limitation had no notable effect on our results. In the three false-negative CT studies, the lack of perimural signs would have resulted in a false-negative evaluation regardless of the wall-thickness assessment; besides, of the seven false-positive CT studies that depicted a thickened bowel wall, only one was obtained in a patient with no colonic disease. The six other patients in whom false-positive CT studies were obtained had a colonic pathologic condition that accounted for the thickened bowel wall; thus, the diagnostic error was due not to defective assessment of wall thickness, but to the lack of specificity of this criterion (and of the extramural signs) for differentiation of acute colonic diverticulitis from other pathologic conditions. Clearly, further studies are needed to define additional criteria that could help in the differentiation of mural and extramural abnormalities seen in cases of acute colonic diverticulitis from those observed in cases of other inflammatory and tumoral colonic diseases. Further research is also needed to determine whether specific technical modalities (the use of intraluminal contrast material or others) are helpful in the depiction of these additional criteria.

One other limitation of our study is the lack of pathologic correlation obtained a short time after the initial imaging assessment in almost all patients; these correlations would have been the most accurate reference standard to use in our evaluation. As is the case at many institutions (13,17,18), however, the current trend among surgeons is promotion of initial conservative management of acute colonic diverticulitis, which usually results in longer delay between initial imaging and surgical intervention (if performed).

In summary, we found that US and CT findings provide similar accuracy for the diagnosis of acute colonic diverticulitis, and our results suggest that US may be a valuable alternative to CT for the radiologic evaluation in patients with this disease. Our data may serve as a basis for a cost-benefit analysis to assess definitively whether US could replace CT as the first-line examination in patients suspected of having acute colonic diverticulitis. ■

References

1. Cho KC, Morehouse HT, Alterman DD, Thornhill BA. Sigmoid diverticulitis: diagnostic role of CT—comparison with barium enema studies. Radiology 1990; 176:111–115.
2. Hulnick DH, Megibow AJ, Balthazar EJ, Naidich DP, Bosniak MA. Computed tomography in the evaluation of diverticulitis. Radiology 1984; 152:491–495.
3. Johnson CD, Baker ME, Rice RP, Silverman P, Thompson WM. Diagnosis of acute colonic diverticulitis: comparison of barium enema and CT. AJR 1987; 148:541–546.
4. Parulekar SG. Sonography of colonic diverticulitis. J Ultrasound Med 1985; 4:659–666.
5. Verbanck J, Lambrecht S, Rutgeerts L, et al. Can sonography diagnose acute colonic diverticulitis in patients with acute intestinal inflammation? a prospective study. JCU 1989; 17:661–666.
6. Wilson SR, Toi A. The value of sonography in the diagnosis of acute diverticulitis of the colon. AJR 1990; 154:1199–1202.
7. Schwerk WB, Schwarz S, Rothmund M. Sonography in acute colonic diverticulitis. Dis Colon Rectum 1992; 35:1077–1084.
8. Yacoe ME, Jeffrey RB Jr. Sonography of appendicitis and diverticulitis. Radiol Clin North Am 1994; 32:899–912.
9. Puylaert JBCM. Acute appendicitis: US evaluation using graded compression. Radiology 1986; 158:355–360.
10. Lee DH, Lim JH, Ko YT, Yoon Y. Sonographic detection of pneumoperitoneum in patients with acute abdomen. AJR 1990; 154:107–109.
11. Birnbaum BA, Balthazar EJ. CT of appendicitis and diverticulitis. Radiol Clin North Am 1994; 32:885–898.
12. Chappuis CW, Cohn I. Acute colonic diverticulitis. Surg Clin North Am 1988; 68: 301–313.
13. McKee RF, Deignan RW, Krukowski ZH. Radiological investigation in acute diverticulitis. Br J Surg 1993; 80:560–565.
14. Hackford AW, Schoetz DJ, Coller JA, Veidenheimer MC. Surgical management of complicated diverticulitis. Dis Colon Rectum 1985; 28:317–321.

15. Neff CC, vanSonnenberg E, Casola G, et al. Diverticular abscesses: percutaneous drainage. Radiology 1987; 163:15–18.
16. Nicholas GG, Miller WT, Fitts WT, Tondreau RL. Diagnosis of diverticulitis of the colon: role of the barium enema in defining pericolic inflammation. Ann Surg 1972; 176:205–209.
17. Hachigian MP, Honickman S, Eisenstat TE, Rubin RJ, Salvati EP. Computed tomography in the initial management of acute left-sided diverticulitis. Dis Colon Rectum 1992; 35:1123–1129.
18. Ambrosetti P, Robert J, Witzig JA, et al. Incidence, outcome, and proposed management of isolated abscesses complicating acute left-sided colonic diverticulitis. Dis Colon Rectum 1992; 35:1072–1076.
19. Puylaert JBCM. When in doubt, sound it out (editorial). Radiology 1994; 191:320–321.
20. Balthazar EJ, Megibow A, Schinella RA, Gordon R. Limitations in the CT diagnosis of acute diverticulitis: comparison of CT, contrast enema and pathologic findings in 16 patients. AJR 1990; 154:281–285.
21. Mueller PR, Saini S, Wittenberg J, et al. Sigmoid diverticular abscesses: percutaneous drainage as an adjunct to surgical resection in 24 cases. Radiology 1987; 164: 321–325.
22. Jeffrey RB Jr, Sommer FG, Debatin JF. Color doppler sonography of focal gastrointestinal lesions: initial clinical experience. J Ultrasound Med 1994; 13:473–478.
23. Teefey AS, Roarke MC, Brink JA, et al. Bowel wall thickening: differentiation of inflammation from ischemia with color doppler and duplex US. Radiology 1996; 198:547–551.
24. Padidar AM, Jeffrey RB, Mindelzun RE, Dolph JF. Differentiating sigmoid diverticulitis from carcinoma on CT scans: mesenteric inflammation suggests diverticulitis. AJR 1994; 163:81–83.
25. Rao PM, Rhea JT, Novelline RA, et al. Helical CT technique for the diagnosis of appendicitis: prospective evaluation of a focused appendix CT evaluation. Radiology 1997; 202:139–144.

Mary T. Keogan, MD • Vincent G. McDermott, MD • Erik K. Paulson, MD • Douglas H. Sheafor, MD
M. Gena Frederick, MD • David M. DeLong, PhD • Rendon C. Nelson, MD

Pancreatic Malignancy: Effect of Dual-Phase Helical CT in Tumor Detection and Vascular Opacification[1]

PURPOSE: **To determine the relative value of hepatic arterial and portal venous phase helical computed tomographic (CT) scans for tumor detection and vascular opacification in patients with pancreatic malignancy.**

MATERIALS AND METHODS: **Ninety-five patients who had or were suspected of having pancreatic disease underwent dual-phase helical CT. Arterial phase scans were acquired 20–40 seconds after contrast material administration; venous phase scans, 70–100 seconds after administration. Three readers independently scored images in a blinded fashion for the presence of tumor, for lesion attenuation relative to normal pancreas, and for vascular opacification.**

RESULTS: **The final diagnosis was pancreatic malignancy (n = 60), acute or chronic pancreatitis (n = 22), and normal pancreas (n = 13). The readers identified possible or definite tumors on arterial phase studies in 47–50 patients and on venous phase studies in 48–53 patients ($P > .10$). There was no statistically significant difference in tumor attenuation between scans from the two phases ($P > .05$). Agreement between the readers for tumor detection was not affected by the scanning phase ($P > .10$). Opacification of arteries and of veins was greater on arterial phase scans and on venous phase scans, respectively ($P < .001$).**

CONCLUSION: **The acquisition of arterial phase scans in addition to venous phase scans does not result in improved detection of pancreatic malignancies.**

Dual-phase imaging of the pancreas and other organs is a new application of helical computed tomographic (CT) technology (1–3). By using this technique, it is possible to image the pancreas twice during a single injection of contrast material, once during the earlier hepatic arterial–predominant phase, and once during the later portal venous–predominant phase. In recent reports (4,5), it has been shown that pancreatic parenchymal and vascular enhancement is improved if scanning is performed during an early phase (20–70 seconds after the start of contrast material injection) compared with a later phase (70–100 seconds after the start of the injection). To the extent that the conspicuity of pancreatic lesions is based on differences in attenuation between tumor and adjacent normal parenchyma, it has been suggested (4,5) that pancreatic tumors would be easier to detect during the early phase than during the later phase. Additionally, improved definition of pancreatic vessels is expected at early-phase imaging (5).

The reports to date, however, have been concerned solely with quantitative differences in pancreatic parenchymal, tumor, and vascular attenuation between the early and late phases. To the best of our knowledge, there has been no qualitative assessment of the value of dual-phase helical CT in patients with malignant pancreatic tumors. As such, it is unknown as to what extent changes in enhancement in the early phase will affect assessment of tumor and vascular structures. The purpose of this study, therefore, was to perform a qualitative evaluation of a dual-phase helical CT protocol with regard to tumor detection and vascular opacification.

MATERIALS AND METHODS

Between October 1994 and January 1996, all patients who were suspected of having or were known to have pancreatic disease and who were referred for CT evaluation underwent imaging with a dual-phase pancreatic CT protocol. The first 95 patients studied during this time in whom a specific diagnosis of normal or abnormal pancreas was determined composed the study group. These patients were 53 men and 42 women, aged 21–83 years (mean 61, years). The final diagnosis, which was based on review of histopathologic (n = 70) or follow-up clinical (n = 25, minimum of 18 months) examination findings, was malignancy (n = 60), acute or chronic pancreatitis (n = 22), or normal pancreas (n = 13). Pancreatic malignancy was confirmed with findings from fine-needle aspiration biopsy (n = 43) or at surgery (n = 17). Histologic types of tumors were adenocarcinoma (n = 52), islet cell tumor (n = 5), and mucinous cystic tumor (n = 3). Tumor location was the pancreatic head (n = 40), pancreatic body (n = 17), pancreatic tail (n = 2), and entire pancreas (n = 1).

The CT examinations were performed (HiSpeed Advantage; GE Medical Systems, Milwaukee, Wis) after oral and intravenous administration of contrast material. Patients received 175 mL of iopamidol (Isovue 300; Bracco Diagnostics, Princeton, NJ) injected intravenously at the rate of 4 mL/sec and 450 mL of a 1.2% barium sulfate suspension (Readi-CAT; E-Z-Em,

Index terms: Computed tomography (CT), helical, 770.12115 • Pancreas, CT, 770.12112, 770.12113, 770.12115 • Pancreas, neoplasms, 770.32 • Pancreatitis, 770.291

Radiology 1997; 205:513–518

[1] From the Department of Radiology, Duke University Medical Center, Erwin Rd, Box 3808, Durham, NC 27710. Received October 4, 1996; revision requested November 19; revision received June 26, 1997; accepted June 30. **Address reprint requests to** M.T.K.

Westbury, NY). Glucagon was not administered. The craniocaudal extent of the pancreas was initially determined at non–contrast-enhanced CT. Arterial phase images were obtained with 3-mm collimation and 1-mm reconstruction intervals through the entire pancreas (beginning above the celiac axis and scanning in the craniocaudal direction) after an initial delay of 20 seconds. Venous phase images were obtained after a total delay of 70 seconds. Venous-phase scanning began at the dome of the liver; 7-mm collimation (7-mm reconstruction intervals) was used through the liver, and 5-mm collimation (5-mm reconstruction intervals) was used through the pancreas. The acquisition of larger sections through the pancreas during the venous phase was necessary so that hepatic scanning could be completed during a 70–100-second time frame to optimize detection of any hepatic lesions. All images were obtained with a pitch of 1:1 and were reconstructed at 3–7-mm intervals, depending on the section thickness. Arterial- and venous phase images were each acquired during a single breath hold, with a 20–30-second interval for breathing between the phases.

Arterial and venous phase images were interpreted independently and in random order by three radiologists (V.G.M., E.K.P., D.H.S.) experienced in abdominal CT. Readers were blinded to patient identity, clinical history, and surgical or histopathologic findings. Although an attempt was made to blind readers to the phase of imaging, obvious differences in vascular enhancement made this difficult. For both phases of imaging, readers scored the presence or absence of tumor with a five-point scale (1 = normal, 2 = acute or chronic pancreatitis, 3 = equivocal [radiologist would suggest follow-up imaging], 4 = possible tumor [radiologist would suggest biopsy], and 5 = definite tumor). When a mass was identified, the maximum diameter was noted, and the mass was described as hypo-, iso-, or hyperattenuating relative to adjacent pancreatic parenchyma. In cases in which a tumor was thought to be present (grade 4 or 5), the maximum diameter of the mass or abnormality was recorded, and three diameter ranges were subsequently considered for analysis (smaller than 2 cm, 2–3 cm, or larger than 3 cm).

Vascular opacification of the celiac axis, superior mesenteric artery, and the portal and splenic veins was qualitatively assessed. Readers graded vascular opacification with a three-point scale (1 = not opacified, 2 = well opacified, 3 = brightly opacified).

Statistical analysis was performed as follows: (*a*) Sensitivity and specificity for tumor detection with scans from both phases for each of the four confidence grades (grades 2–5) were compared for each reader; (*b*) agreement among the three readers with regard to tumor detection on images from both phases was compared by using the Cohen κ statistic (perfect agreement = 1.0, expected chance agreement = 0, perfect disagreement = −1.0); (*c*) relative tumor attenuation on images from the two phases was compared for each reader by using the McNemar test; (*d*) the relationship of size to attenuation was analyzed with the analysis of variance, and (*e*) vascular opacification was compared by means of a signed rank test. A *P* value of less than .05 was considered to be indicative of a statistically significant difference.

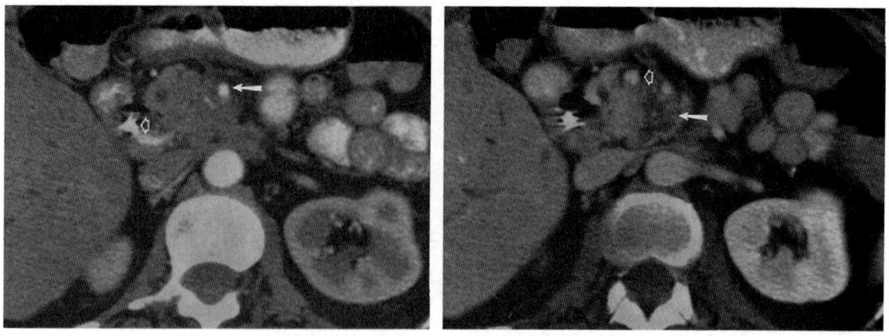

a. **b.**

Figure 1. Adenocarcinoma of the head of the pancreas in a 62-year-old woman. **(a)** Arterial phase CT image shows a low-attenuating mass in the region of the pancreatic head. Note encasement of the brightly opacified superior mesenteric artery (solid arrow). A biliary stent is in situ (open arrow). **(b)** Venous phase CT image obtained at the same level as in **a** shows improved tumor-to–pancreatic parenchymal enhancement (solid arrow) and opacification of the superior mesenteric vein (open arrow).

Table 1
Sensitivity for Tumor Detection on Dual-Phase Helical CT Scans in 60 Patients with Pancreatic Malignancy

	Reader 1		Reader 2		Reader 3	
Confidence Grade	Arterial Phase	Venous Phase	Arterial Phase	Venous Phase	Arterial Phase	Venous Phase
1	4 (7)	1 (2)	1 (2)	2 (3)	2 (3)	1 (2)
2	2 (3)	2 (3)	1 (2)	2 (3)	4 (7)	6 (10)
3	7 (12)	4 (7)	10 (17)	3 (5)	4 (7)	5 (8)
4	15 (25)	25 (42)	14 (23)	15 (25)	8 (13)	10 (17)
5	32 (53)	28 (47)	34 (57)	38 (63)	42 (70)	38 (63)

Note.—Data are number of patients with tumor detected on CT scans. Numbers in parentheses are percentages.

Table 2
Tumor Diagnosis on Dual-Phase Helical CT Scans in Patients with Normal (n = 13) or Inflamed (n = 22) Pancreas

	Reader 1		Reader 2		Reader 3	
Confidence Grade	Arterial Phase	Venous Phase	Arterial Phase	Venous Phase	Arterial Phase	Venous Phase
1	12 (34)	13 (37)	9 (26)	9 (26)	7 (20)	12 (34)
2	7 (20)	8 (23)	9 (26)	11 (31)	10 (29)	10 (29)
3	9 (26)	5 (14)	7 (20)	4 (11)	10 (29)	7 (20)
4	5 (14)	7 (20)	7 (20)	7 (20)	2 (6)	0 (0)
5	2 (6)	2 (6)	3 (9)	4 (11)	6 (17)	6 (17)

Note.—Data are number of patients with tumor detected on CT scans. Numbers in parentheses are percentages.

RESULTS

Overall tumor detection rates with arterial and venous phase images (ie, grades 4 and 5 vs grades 1, 2, and 3) were not statistically significantly different for any of the three readers. Readers 1, 2, and 3 detected 47, 48, and 50 tumors, respectively, on the arterial phase images and 53, 53, and 48 tumors, respectively, on venous phase images ($P > .05$) (Fig 1). Table 1 shows the sensitivity for tumor detection and, again, there was no statistically significant difference in detection with images obtained at the two phases ($P > .05$). Agreement between the three readers for tumor detection

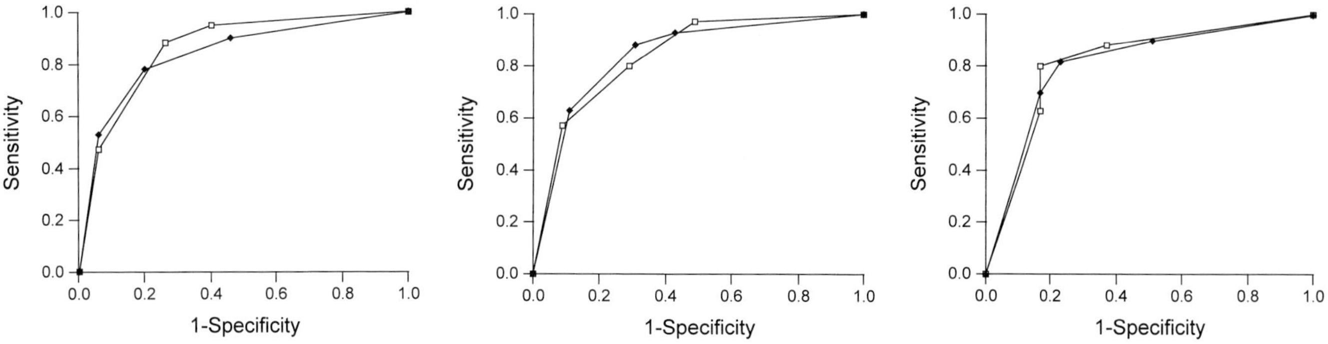

2. 3. 4.

Figures 2–4. Receiver operating characteristic curves for tumor detection with arterial phase (◆) and venous phase (□) images by **(2)** reader 1, **(3)** reader 2, and **(4)** reader 3. Note that for each reader, there is close approximation between the curves for arterial and venous phase images.

Table 3
Assessment of Degree of Tumor Attenuation

	Hypoattenuating		Isoattenuating		Hyperattenuating	
Reader	Arterial Phase	Venous Phase	Arterial Phase	Venous Phase	Arterial Phase	Venous Phase
1	69	73	25	23	6	4
2	60	61	35	36	5	3
3	75	79	21	15	4	6

Note.—Numbers are percentage of grade 4 and 5 tumors. Each reader detected a different total number of tumors.

was not statistically significantly different with images obtained during the arterial phase compared with those obtained during the venous phase (P range, .41–.98).

Table 2 shows the confidence grades for nontumor cases (inflamed and normal pancreas) for each reader. No statistically significant difference was seen in diagnosis with images obtained during the two phases ($P > .05$).

Empirical receiver operating characteristic curves for each reader for the diagnosis of malignancy on the basis of findings from images obtained during both phases are shown in Figures 2–4. The curves do not statistically significantly differ for images obtained during the arterial or venous phases. The degree of tumor attenuation relative to normal pancreas for each reader is shown in Table 3. No statistically significant differences were found with regard to the assessment of attenuation on arterial versus venous-phase images ($P > .05$). The diameter of detected tumors was 1.0–15.0 cm; the mean diameter among the readers ranged from 3.6 to 4.8 cm, and the standard deviation ranged from 1.6 to 2.3 cm. For readers 1 and 3, there was no relationship between tumor diameter and attenuation with images obtained during either phase (P range, .11–.77). For reader 2, however, an increase in tumor diameter was associated with a decrease in tumor attenuation on images obtained during both the arterial ($P < .02$) and the venous ($P < .001$) phase. Tumor diameter was correlated with confidence in tumor detection (grades 4 and 5) with images from both phases by pooling the data for the three readers. By using this pooled data, two tumors with a diameter smaller than 2 cm, nine tumors with a diameter of 2–3 cm, and 41 tumors with a diameter larger than 3 cm were detected on arterial phase images; one tumor smaller than 2 cm in diameter, 12 tumors of 2–3 cm in diameter, and 40 tumors larger than 3 cm in diameter were detected on venous phase images. With images from both phases, tumors with a diameter larger than 3 cm were statistically significantly associated with a confidence grade of 5 by all readers, compared with tumors 3 cm or smaller in diameter ($P < .001$). A tendency was noted for the venous phase image findings to result in better tumor detection confidence levels at smaller sizes, although this tendency was not statistically significant (Table 4).

The study group included five patients with an islet cell tumor; the findings in these patients were analyzed with findings in the other patients. By considering findings in these five patients separately, four of five tumors were considered to be definitely present (grade 5) by all readers on both the arterial and the venous phase images. In the remaining patient, the pancreas was considered by all readers to be normal on the basis of findings from images obtained during both phases. All three readers considered only two of five tumors to be hyperattenuating on arterial phase images, whereas their assessment of tumor attenuation varied when venous phase images were used (Fig 5).

For all three readers, there was a statistically significant difference in arterial (celiac axis and superior mesenteric) and venous (portal and splenic) opacification on images obtained during the two phases ($P < .001$) (Fig 6). A statistically significantly greater degree of arterial opacification was present on arterial phase images, whereas a statistically significantly greater degree of venous opacification was present on venous phase images (Table 5).

DISCUSSION

Despite technical advances in other imaging modalities, CT continues to be the primary technique for imaging in patients suspected of having a pancreatic malignancy (6). With a dynamic contrast-enhanced technique and thin collimation (by using either incremental or helical scanners), the detection rates for pancreatic cancer have been reported (7–9) to be as high as 89%–94%. Although CT findings are also reported (6,10) to result in high accuracy for the determination of nonresectability (100%), such findings result in less accuracy for determination of resectability (72%) owing to the difficulty in detecting the spread of local small-volume tumor to lymph nodes, vessels, and the liver.

Surprisingly, accuracy for detection and staging has not been markedly improved by the use of the helical technique, despite improvements in pancreatic image quality (9,11). It has been suggested (3,9) that modification of the helical technique to include both an early and a late imaging phase may offer a mechanism to improve the accuracy of helical imaging by allowing optimal demonstration of parenchymal and vascular structures. It has also been suggested (4,9) that imaging during a phase earlier than that typically used for hepatic imaging (ie, earlier than 70 seconds after injection) may result in improved enhancement of normal pancreatic tissue and, therefore, in improved tumor-to-parenchyma contrast, which would consequently result in the improved ability to detect pancreatic carcinoma. Conversely, in patients with an islet cell tumor (which characteristically has a hypervascular appearance on angiograms), increased detection rates are anticipated on the basis of increased enhancement of the tumor relative to pancreas during the arterial phase (12,13).

Helical dual-phase CT has several disadvantages. The imaging protocol is more complicated and time consuming for the technologist in terms of both image acquisition and recording on film. Film costs, demands on the equipment, and radiation dose to the patient are also increased. At our institution, we use 175 mL of contrast material for our dual-phase studies, compared with 150 mL for our routine helical studies. We chose a higher volume because, in theory, it allows a wider "window" of optimal enhancement, particularly when using a faster infusion rate. However, an increase in the volume of contrast material has not been shown to be an absolute requirement.

For these reasons, it is important to establish whether imaging during the arterial phase results in a clear benefit in terms of tumor detection, vascular opacification, or both. In the patient group as a whole in our study, we did not achieve a statistically significant improvement in the detection rate of tumors on scans from the arterial phase compared with those from the venous phase. This result suggests that the previous reports about the value of early-phase imaging, in terms of quantitative changes in pancreatic parenchymal and tumor enhancement, may not equate with improved tumor detection in the clinical situation. It is important to note, however, that Lu et al (5) used a longer delay time for the arterial phase images (40–70 seconds), which may have optimized their ability to detect tumors.

Table 4
Probability of Confidence Grade for Tumor Detection according to Tumor Diameter

Diameter	Grade 4 Arterial Phase	Grade 4 Venous Phase	Grade 5 Arterial Phase	Grade 5 Venous Phase
Smaller than 2 cm	50 (1/2)	0 (0/1)	50 (1/2)	100 (1/1)
2–3 cm	67 (6/9)	50 (6/12)	33 (3/9)	50 (6/12)
Larger than 3 cm	12 (5/41)	5 (2/40)	88 (36/41)	95 (38/40)

Note.—Data are percentages based on pooled data from all three readers. Numbers in parentheses are raw data; the denominator is the total number of tumors detected on images from each phase.

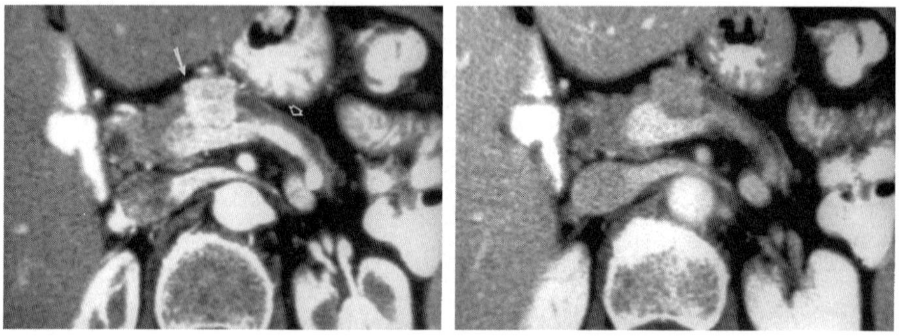

a. b.

Figure 5. Gastrinoma in the body of the pancreas in a 44-year-old woman. **(a)** Arterial phase CT image demonstrates a brightly enhancing mass (solid arrow) obstructing the pancreatic duct (open arrow). This finding is indicative of an islet cell tumor. **(b)** Venous phase CT image obtained at the same level as in **a** demonstrates a contour deformity caused by the mass, which now appears isoattenuating relative to normal pancreas.

A related issue is the degree of agreement between the three readers in grading the presence of tumor. We found that agreement was not improved with the arterial phase scans compared with the venous phase scans. Thus the addition of an arterial phase does not appear to reduce the variability between readers.

In the small group of five patients with an islet cell tumor, there was no evidence of improved detection of tumor on arterial phase scans. Surprisingly, areas of hyperattenuation were present on arterial phase scans in only two of these patients. The reason for this is unclear; however, our results are similar to those of Van Hoe et al (13), who found that of 11 patients with islet cell tumors who underwent dual-phase scanning, two patients had tumors that were hypoattenuating relative to pancreas, three had isoattenuating tumors, and six had slightly to markedly hyperattenuating tumors on the arterial phase scans. Also in their study, an islet cell tumor in one patient was seen only on images from the later phase. It may be that islet cell tumors are not uniformly hyperattenuating on arterial phase scans, as was previously thought. The marked hypervascularity frequently seen at angiography may be related to the higher iodine dose delivered to the tumor by means of selective injections of contrast material. Further study with a larger group of patients with an islet cell tumor is needed to address fully the potential of dual-phase scanning for this type of pancreatic malignancy.

The relationship of initial tumor size to outcome is controversial. It has been claimed (14–16) that survival is improved in patients with tumors smaller than 2 cm in diameter compared with those with larger tumors and that, for this reason, detection of smaller tumors may be important. In our study, there were few tumors smaller than 3 cm in diameter; however, an analysis of tumor size and confidence for tumor detection showed, not surprisingly, improved confidence for detection of tumors larger than 3 cm in diameter on images from both phases compared with the confidence associated with tumors that were smaller than 3 cm in diameter. There was no evidence, however, for improved detection of smaller tumors on arterial-phase scans compared with that on venous phase scans; however, because our sample size was small, firm conclusions should not be drawn, particularly with regard to tumors smaller than 2 cm in diameter.

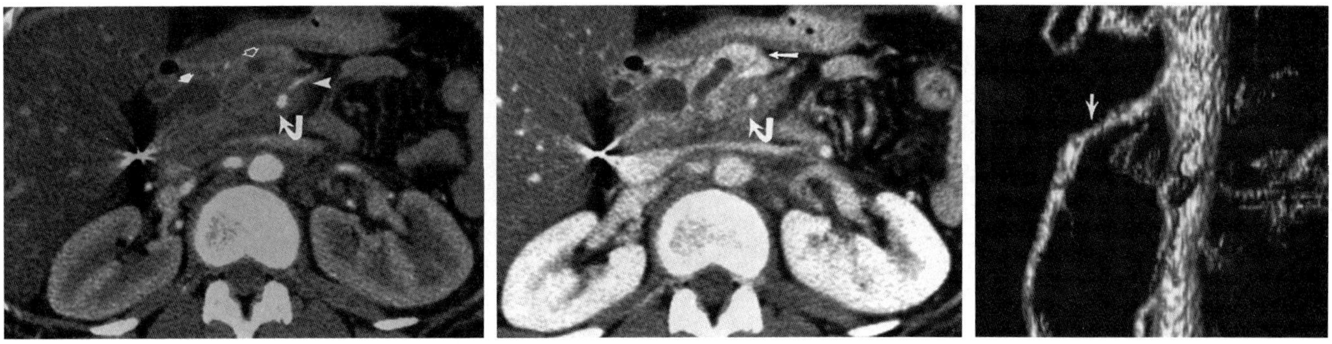

a. b. c.

Figure 6. Adenocarcinoma of the head of the pancreas in a 60-year-old woman. **(a)** Arterial phase CT image shows a dilated pancreatic duct (open straight arrow) and common bile duct (solid straight arrow) in the pancreatic head. There is encasement of the superior mesenteric artery by the pancreatic mass (curved arrow) and opacification of a branch of the jejunal artery (arrowhead). **(b)** Venous phase CT image obtained at the same level as in **a** shows improved tumor-to-pancreas contrast due to increased enhancement of the pancreas (straight arrow) and the mass (curved arrow). The superior mesenteric artery is less well seen. **(c)** Lateral volume rendering from a noninvasive CT arteriogram confirms encasement (arrow) of the superior mesenteric artery.

Table 5
Qualitative Assessment of Vascular Opacification in 60 Patients with Pancreatic Malignancy

Reader	Not Opacified: Arterial Phase	Not Opacified: Venous Phase	Well Opacified: Arterial Phase	Well Opacified: Venous Phase	Brightly Opacified: Arterial Phase	Brightly Opacified: Venous Phase
Celiac Axis						
1	2	2	8	49	50	9
2	0	4	5	42	55	14
3	1	2	6	47	53	11
Portal Vein						
1	41	4	19	48	0	8
2	42	4	15	37	3	19
3	38	3	20	48	2	9

Note.—Data are number of patients.

Experience with contrast-enhanced CT has shown that pancreatic adenocarcinoma is typically hypoattenuating relative to normal pancreas (7,16,17). However, Bluemke et al (9) have shown that up to 42% of pancreatic adenocarcinomas may be isoattenuating relative to pancreas on helical CT scans. On the basis of expected improvements in tumor-to-parenchyma contrast, there should be fewer isoattenuating tumors on arterial-phase scans than on venous phase scans. Interestingly, however, in our study, the proportions of hypo-, iso-, and hyperattenuating tumors were the same on scans from both phases. Furthermore, although by design we did not perform a quantitative analysis of differential tumor or pancreatic enhancement, no statistically significant difference was found among the three readers in terms of their visual assessment of attenuation on images from the two phases.

A criticism of our study may relate to the timing of the early phase. On the basis of single-phase studies, it has been previously suggested (18–20) that at single-phase CT of the pancreas, image acquisition is optimal 30–40 seconds after initiation of the contrast material injection. Conversely, in patients who may have malignant disease, the optimal timing for both phases of a dual-phase pancreatic study remains unclear and is more controversial. It is accepted that timing of the later phase is based on the need to optimally depict hepatic metastases, because overlooked hepatic metastatic disease is a substantial cause of error when determining if a patient is a candidate for resection (9). Because metastases from adenocarcinoma are typically hypovascular, imaging is optimal 70–100 seconds after initiation of the bolus injection (21,22). This delay will also result in maximum opacification of the superior mesenteric vein and splenoportal confluence (23).

The timing of the early phase, however, is more difficult. The first quantitative report (4) of differential pancreatic attenuation during a dual-phase study was based on an "arterial phase" and "portal venous phase" that began 20 and 49–71 seconds, respectively, after injection of 150 mL of contrast material at a rate of 5 mL/sec. This protocol resulted in arterial phase images that depicted a 20 HU increase in normal pancreatic parenchymal enhancement and a 28% increase in tumor-to-pancreas contrast, relative to the enhancement and contrast on venous phase images. Lu et al (5), however, suggested that the early phase should begin later (40–70 seconds after injection of 150 mL of contrast material at a rate of 3 mL/sec). They argued that this longer delay (which they called the "pancreatic phase") resulted in better pancreatic enhancement and maximum vascular—especially venous—enhancement. By using the technique of Lu et al, the mean difference in parenchymal attenuation between scans obtained at the early (pancreatic) phase and those obtained at the late phase was 28 HU, which was similar to that seen with the previously reported (4) "arterial phase" technique; however, Lu et al reported a 70% increase in tumor-to-pancreas contrast.

In our study, timing of the two imaging phases was similar to that of Hollett et al (4), although we used a larger bolus of contrast material (175 mL at 4 mL/sec) to optimize visualization of arterial structures. Our results confirm that arterial opacification is maximized during the arterial phase, as expected. Furthermore, this technique lends itself to two- or three-dimensional reconstruction with noninvasive arteriograms of the celiac axis and superior mesenteric artery by using maximum intensity projections, shaded surface displays, or volume rendering. These views may be particularly useful in cases under consideration for resection, in which arteriography is sometimes necessary to determine tumor encasement or occlusion (6). Whether arterial encasement is better appreciated on two- or three-dimensional images obtained during the arterial phase as compared with images obtained during the venous phase has yet to be determined.

Opacification of the peripancreatic venous structures on the venous-phase images was generally good, although predictably these structures were rarely as "bright" as the arteries on the earlier-phase images. It is certainly likely that, owing to the timing of our arterial phase, we may not have maximized tumor-to-pancreas contrast; however, our detection rates for tumor ranged from 87% to 98% on arterial phase scans and from 88% to 93% on venous phase scans. These detection rates are virtually the same as those previously reported (7,8,10) for optimal dynamic CT findings. In addition, further delay of the arterial phase may reduce the sensitivity for detecting islet cell tumors by increasing surrounding parenchymal enhancement. Much of the concern regarding the exact timing of the early phase may not in fact be warranted, because it is likely that physiologic patient variables would cause as much variability in enhancement as would be expected with different injection protocols.

Some potential limitations of our study should be mentioned. First, the study was a retrospective review of a prospective imaging protocol rather than a formal prospective study. Second, the timing of our early phase was fixed and we did not attempt to correct for physiologic patient differences by means of a test-dose technique (which we believed would unduly lengthen the duration of the study) or by using a semiautomated scanning delay. In our experience, current techniques for automating the scanning delay (24) do not work well for triggering the arterial phase because the entire process is too slow. Third, the arterial phase images are acquired at 3-mm increments compared with 5-mm increments for the venous phase images. The thin-section arterial phase images may therefore be expected to improve tumor detection relative to the venous phase images (particularly for small tumors). Fourth, the small number of patients with an islet cell tumor in our study makes it difficult to draw any firm conclusions about this patient group. Finally, we did not address the effect of dual-phase imaging on tumor staging. Unfortunately, a minority of patients with pancreatic malignancy actually undergo surgery for staging, resection, or both; however, correlation with surgical findings—particularly with relevance to vascular involvement—will be important for further assessment of the dual-phase technique.

We conclude that the addition of arterial phase to venous phase helical CT does not result in improved detection of pancreatic carcinoma. Nonetheless, because the dual-phase technique provided improved arterial definition, we routinely use a dual-phase protocol for evaluation of patients who are known to have or are suspected of having pancreatic malignancy. Additionally, we use a dual-phase protocol for evaluation of patients suspected of having an islet cell tumor. A larger series that substantiated these results would be welcome. ■

References

1. Bonaldi VM, Bret PM, Reinhold C, Atri M. Helical CT of the liver: value of an early hepatic arterial phase. Radiology 1995; 197: 357–363.
2. Frederick MG, McElaney BL, Singer A, et al. Timing of parenchymal enhancement on dual-phase dynamic helical CT of the liver: how long does the hepatic arterial phase predominate? AJR 1996; 166:1305–1310.
3. Hollett MD, Jeffrey RB Jr, Nino-Murcia M, Jorgensen MJ, Harris DP. Dual-phase helical CT of the liver: value of arterial phase scans in the detection of small (≤1.5 cm) malignant hepatic neoplasms. AJR 1995; 164:879–884.
4. Hollett MD, Jorgensen MJ, Jeffrey RB Jr. Quantitative evaluation of pancreatic enhancement during dual-phase helical CT. Radiology 1995; 195:359–361.
5. Lu DS, Vedantham S, Krasny RM, Kadell B, Berger WL, Reber HA. Two-phase helical CT for pancreatic tumors: pancreatic versus hepatic phase enhancement of tumor, pancreas, and vascular structures. Radiology 1996; 199:697–701.
6. Freeny PC, Traverso LW, Ryan JA. Diagnosis and staging of pancreatic adenocarcinoma with dynamic computed tomography. Am J Surg 1993; 165:600–606.
7. Freeny PC, Marks WM, Ryan JA, Traverso LW. Pancreatic ductal adenocarcinoma: diagnosis and staging with dynamic CT. Radiology 1988; 166:125–133.
8. Megibow AJ. Pancreatic adenocarcinoma: designing the examination to evaluate the clinical questions. Radiology 1992; 183: 297–303.
9. Bluemke DA, Cameron JL, Hruban RH, et al. Potentially resectable pancreatic adenocarcinoma: spiral CT assessment with surgical and pathologic correlation. Radiology 1995; 197:381–385.
10. Megibow AJ, Zhou XH, Rotterdam H, et al. Pancreatic adenocarcinoma: CT versus MR imaging in the evaluation of resectability—report of the Radiology Diagnostic Oncology Group. Radiology 1995; 195:327–332.
11. Dupuy DE, Costello P, Ecker CP. Spiral CT of the pancreas. Radiology 1992; 183: 815–818.
12. Fishman EK, Wyatt SH, Ney DR, Kuhlman JE, Siegelman SS. Spiral CT of the pancreas with multiplanar display. AJR 1992; 159:1209–1215.
13. Van Hoe L, Gryspeerdt S, Marchal G, Baert A, Mertens L. Helical CT for the preoperative localization of islet cell tumors of the pancreas: value of arterial and parenchymal phase images. AJR 1995; 165:1437–1439.
14. Tsuchiya R, Noda T, Harada N, et al. Collective review of small carcinomas of the pancreas. Ann Surg 1986; 203:77–81.
15. Connolly MM, Dawson PJ, Michelassi F, Moossa AR, Lowenstein F. Survival in 1001 patients with carcinoma of the pancreas. Ann Surg 1987; 206:366–370.
16. Ward EM, Stephens DH, Sheedy PF. Computed tomographic characteristics of pancreatic carcinoma: an analysis of 100 cases. RadioGraphics 1983; 3:547–565.
17. Thoeni RF, Blankenberg F. Pancreatic imaging: computed tomography and magnetic resonance imaging. Radiol Clin North Am 1993; 31:1085–1113.
18. Foley WD, Oneson SR. Helical CT: clinical performance and imaging strategies. RadioGraphics 1994; 14:894–904.
19. Anderson DJ, Berland L. CT techniques. In: Lee JKT, Stanley RJ, Sagel SS, eds. Computed body tomography with MRI correlation. 2nd ed. New York, NY: Raven, 1989; 31–60.
20. Bonaldi VM, Bret PM, Atri M, Garcia P, Reinhold C. A comparison of two injection protocols using helical and dynamic acquisitions in CT examinations of the pancreas. AJR 1996; 167:49–55.
21. Baron RL. Understanding and optimizing use of contrast material for CT of the liver. AJR 1994; 163:323–331.
22. Silverman PM, Cooper C, Trock B, Garra BS, Davros WJ, Zeman RK. The optimal temporal window for CT of the liver using a time-density analysis: implications for helical (spiral) CT. J Comput Assist Tomogr 1995; 19:73–79.
23. Zeman RK, Davros WJ, Berman P, et al. Three-dimensional models of the abdominal vasculature based on helical CT: usefulness in patients with pancreatic neoplasms. AJR 1994; 162:1425–1429.
24. Silverman PM, Roberts SC, Ducic I, et al. Assessment of a technology that permits individual scan delays on helical hepatic CT: a technique to improve efficiency in use of contrast material. AJR 1966; 167:79–84.

Emil J. Balthazar, MD • Marc E. Liebeskind, MD • Michael Macari, MD

Intestinal Ischemia in Patients in Whom Small Bowel Obstruction Is Suspected: Evaluation of Accuracy, Limitations, and Clinical Implications of CT in Diagnosis[1]

PURPOSE: To determine the accuracy of computed tomography (CT) in diagnosis of intestinal ischemia in patients with possible intestinal obstruction and the limitations and clinical implications of use of CT.

MATERIALS AND METHODS: In 100 patients in whom intestinal obstruction was suspected clinically, CT findings were correlated with surgical findings in 77 patients and with follow-up clinical findings after nasogastric suction in 23 patients. The interval between CT and surgical exploration in patients with ischemic bowel was 1–98 hours (mean, 13 hours).

RESULTS: Correlation of CT findings of strangulation obstruction with surgical findings revealed 72 true-negative, 19 true-positive, five false-positive, and four false-negative CT results. Sensitivity was 83%, specificity was 93%, accuracy was 91%, positive predictive value was 79%, and negative predictive value was 95%.

CONCLUSION: CT enables accurate detection of bowel ischemia, particularly when small bowel obstruction is present. Exploratory laparotomy should be performed when unexplained disparities exist between equivocal CT findings and a deteriorating clinical condition in patients with possible small bowel obstruction or mesenteric infarction.

Abdominal computed tomographic (CT) examinations have been used successfully to diagnose disease and evaluate patients in whom intestinal obstruction is suspected (1–5). Examination with CT is useful particularly in cases of acute disease and in patients in whom findings from emergent plain abdominal radiographic studies are equivocal or nonspecific. The potential ability of CT to enable detection or exclusion of strangulation obstruction or mesenteric infarction is important, since definite diagnosis can drastically alter surgical management and decrease mortality in this group of patients. Previous reports have described the expected findings and preliminary encouraging data regarding the ability of CT to enable diagnosis of strangulation obstruction (6–11) and primary mesenteric ischemia (12–16).

The purpose of this prospective study was to assess the accuracy of CT in diagnosis of these acute abdominal conditions and to evaluate the pitfalls, limitations, and clinical implications of use of CT.

MATERIALS AND METHODS

Between July 1994 and June 1996, abdominal CT examinations were performed in 100 consecutive patients in whom small bowel obstruction was suspected clinically, and findings from these examinations form the basis of the study. The initial CT findings were correlated with the surgical findings in 77 patients and with clinical follow-up findings after nasogastric suction in 23 patients. The 40 women and 60 men ranged in age from 19 to 90 years (mean, 52 years).

Abdominal CT was performed with a Hilite or HiSpeed Advantage unit (GE Medical Systems, Milwaukee, Wis). In all patients, 600–800 mL of a 2% diluted solution of diatrizoate meglumine (Gastrografin; Bristol-Myers Squibb, Princeton, NJ) was administered orally 30–60 minutes before the study, and then contrast material was administered intravenously with a power injector in 91 patients. Contrast material was not administered intravenously in nine patients because of contraindications. In 64 of the 91 patients who received intravenous contrast material, scanning was performed with a dynamic sequential incremental technique with 10-mm collimation after an intravenous bolus of 150 mL of meglumine 60% (Conray; Mallinckrodt Medical, St Louis, Mo) (50 mL at a rate of 1.5 mL/sec followed by a rate of 0.8 mL/sec for the remainder of the injection). Helical scanning was performed with 7-mm collimation and a pitch of 1 after administration of 150 mL of meglumine 60% at a single rate (2 mL/sec) in the remaining 27 patients. Additional 5 × 5-mm sections were obtained over the region of interest in 28 patients.

CT scans were interpreted by members of our abdominal imaging section who were familiar with the CT signs of strangulation obstruction (6–11) and ischemic bowel disease (12–16). Official prospective critera were used to diagnose closed-loop and strangulation obstruction (8,10,11). The criteria for diagnosis of closed-loop obstruction were incarcerated small bowel (radial distribution with stretched mesenteric vessels converging toward torsion and a U- or C-shaped dilated bowel loop); and at the site of torsion, the presence of two adjacent collapsed, round, oval, or triangular loops, the Beak sign, and the

Index terms: Intestines, CT, 74.12112 • Intestines, infarction, 74.795 • Intestines, ischemia, 95.7145, 95.761 • Intestines, stenosis or obstruction, 74.721, 74.724

Radiology 1997; 205:519–522

[1] From the Department of Radiology, New York University Tisch Medical Center, 550 First Ave, New York, NY 10016. Received March 11, 1997; revision requested May 5; final revision received July 7; accepted July 8. **Address reprint requests to** E.J.B.

Whirl sign. CT criteria for strangulation included slight circumferential thickening of the bowel wall, increased attenuation, target or halo sign, pneumatosis intestinalis, lack of enhancement of the wall of the incarcerated small bowel during intravenous administration of contrast material; and blurring and haziness of the mesenteric vessels, or obliteration of the mesenteric vessels with hemorrhage in the attached mesentery.

The prospective CT signs of mesenteric ischemia were arterial occlusion, mesenteric or portal vein thrombosis, thick bowel wall, lack of enhancement of bowel wall, intestinal pneumatosis, and mesenteric and/or portal gas (12–16). In addition, the presence of intraperitoneal air and fluid or blood in the peritoneal cavity was determined. In each case, an attempt was made to confirm the clinical diagnosis of small bowel obstruction, to detect the actual cause of obstruction, and to diagnose closed-loop obstruction, strangulation obstruction, or nonobstructive ischemic bowel disease. In cases in which the cause of small bowel obstruction was not apparent, the obstruction was considered to be caused by adhesions.

The initial CT interpretation with regard to the presence of small bowel obstruction, cause of obstruction, and presence of closed-loop obstruction, strangulation, or primary mesenteric ischemia was considered official and was used for statistical analysis. In addition, CT scans were reviewed by two gastrointestinal radiologists (E.J.B., M.M.) who paid particular attention to false-positive and false-negative CT results.

The study group was a selected group of patients with clinical findings of acute small bowel obstruction in whom CT evaluation was requested, on the basis of clinical judgment of the emergency department physician and/or surgical staff, in an attempt to confirm the clinical diagnosis and contribute to the surgical or medical care of these patients. The interval between CT and abdominal exploration was 1–98 hours (mean, 13 hours) in 25 patients who had surgically proved ischemic bowel disease. However, only four patients had a delay of more than 12 hours. The mean interval between CT and surgery was 4 hours when calculated without data from these four patients.

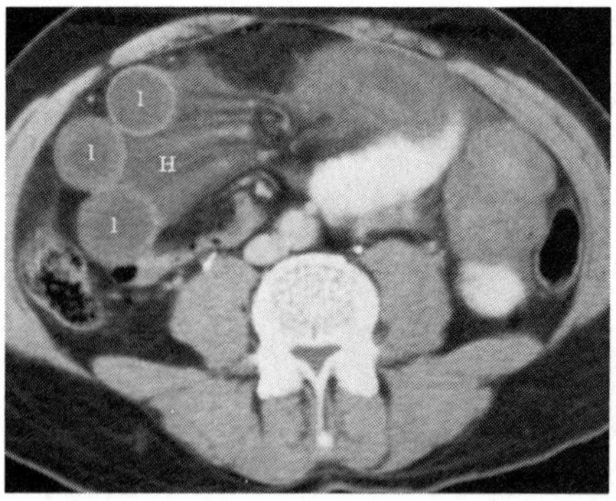

1.

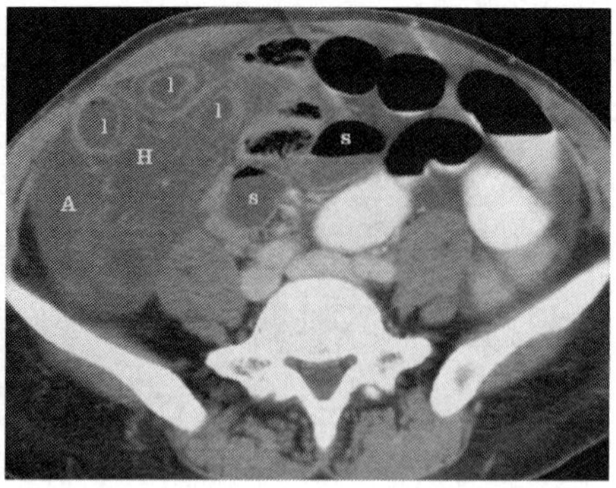

2.

Figures 1, 2. Strangulation small bowel obstruction in **(1)** a 54-year-old man and **(2)** a 54-year-old woman with typical CT findings. **(1)** CT scan shows distended fluid-filled intestinal loops (*I*) in a radial distribution with stretching of attached mesenteric folds and mesenteric hemorrhage (*H*). Mild thickening of the bowel wall is present. Surgery performed 90 minutes later revealed strangulated obstruction with nonviable bowel. These were true-positive CT findings. **(2)** CT scan reveals distended fluid-filled intestinal loops in the right lower quadrant (*I*) that show a target configuration with fluid in the attached mesentery (*H*) and ascites (*A*). Marked distention of the proximal small bowel loops (*s*) is present, with the bowel filled with fluid and air. Surgery performed 1 hour later revealed internal hernia with strangulated obstruction and nonviable bowel. These CT findings were true-positive.

RESULTS

CT showed small bowel obstruction in 90 patients and a nonobstructive ileus pattern in 10 patients. There were two false-negative CT results and no false-positive CT results of small bowel obstruction. One patient in whom ileus was diagnosed initially had adhesions and one patient had ischemic bowel disease detected at surgery. Conservative treatment with nasogastric suction was successful in 23 patients, and surgical exploration was performed in the remaining 77 patients. On the basis of clinical history and CT findings, the causes of the clinical symptoms in the 23 patients treated conservatively were ileus in eight patients, Crohn disease in four patients, recurrent abdominal tumor in two patients, radiation ileitis in one patient, and unconfirmed adhesions in eight patients. Documented histories of Crohn disease, primary colon neoplasm, and pelvic irradiation were available to reinforce the CT diagnosis.

Rapid resolution of clinical symptoms and marked improvement observed at clinical evaluation after nasogastric suction excluded the presence of mesenteric infarction or strangulation obstruction in the 23 patients treated conservatively.

Surgical exploration in 77 patients revealed intestinal obstruction in 75 patients and nonobstructive mesenteric infarction in two patients. The cause of obstruction was adhesions in 53 patients, primary or secondary tumors in seven patients, external hernia in six patients, internal hernia in two patients, appendicitis in two patients, hematoma in two patients, foreign bodies in two patients, and intussusception in one patient. CT enabled correct identification of the cause of obstruction in 65 patients and did not enable identification of the cause of obstruction in 12 patients. The underlying pathologic process that caused intestinal obstruction was missed at CT in four cases of adhesions, two cases of appendicitis, two cases of a foreign body (bezoar), two cases of internal hernia, and two cases of primary mesenteric ischemia. Thus, CT enabled accurate prediction of the cause of intestinal obstruction in 65 (84%) patients.

CT showed strangulation small bowel obstruction in 24 patients and did not depict primary mesenteric ischemia in any of the patients.

At surgery, 23 patients were found to have strangulation obstruction; 12 required bowel resection and 11 were found to have viable bowel in the incarcerated intestinal loop. The results of CT in detection of strangulation obstruction were 73 true-negative findings, 19 true-positive findings (Figs 1, 2), five false-positive findings (Fig 3), and four false-negative findings. One patient had bowel perforation with free air and peritonitis secondary to strangulation obstruction (Fig 4). Findings in one patient with a cecal volvulus missed at CT were included as false-negative for strangulation.

Among the 19 true-positive CT findings, one or more of the following findings were demonstrated at CT: segmental mild homogeneous thickening of bowel wall in seven patients (Fig 1), target configuration of bowel wall in five patients (Fig 4), congestion of mesentery attached to the closed loop in nine patients (Fig 1), radial distribution of loops of bowel and/or U-shaped or C-shaped dilated bowel loop with engorged mesenteric vessels in 17 patients (Fig 4), and two adjacent collapsed loops of bowel at the site of torsion in four patients. Signs of closed-loop obstruction alone were detected in five patients, of ischemia alone in two patients, and of both closed-loop obstruction and ischemia in 12 patients (Fig 1).

Among the five false-positive CT findings, mild bowel wall thickening was detected in two patients (Fig 3),

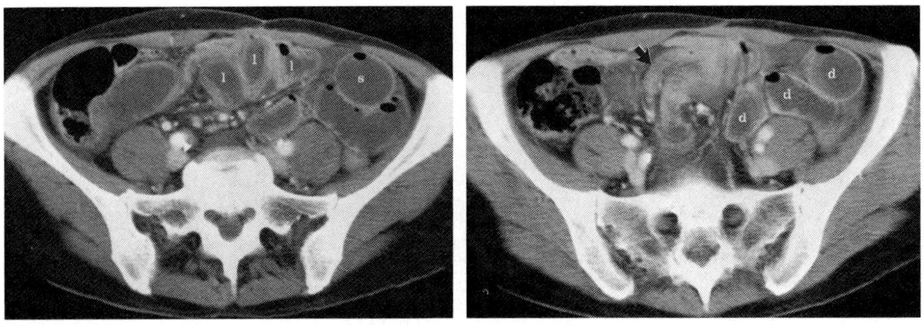

a. b.

Figure 3. CT signs of strangulation obstruction in a 51-year-old woman. **(a)** CT scan shows distended fluid-filled intestinal loops (*l*) in midpelvis with bowel wall thickening. Dilatation of fluid-filled proximal loops (*s*) was present, with normal bowel wall thickness. **(b)** CT scan shows collapsed loops of bowel (arrow) at the transition zone, indicating a high degree of mechanical obstruction. The proximal portion of bowel is distended (*d*). The patient had improvement of symptoms after nasogastric suction, and surgery was not performed. These CT findings were considered false-positive.

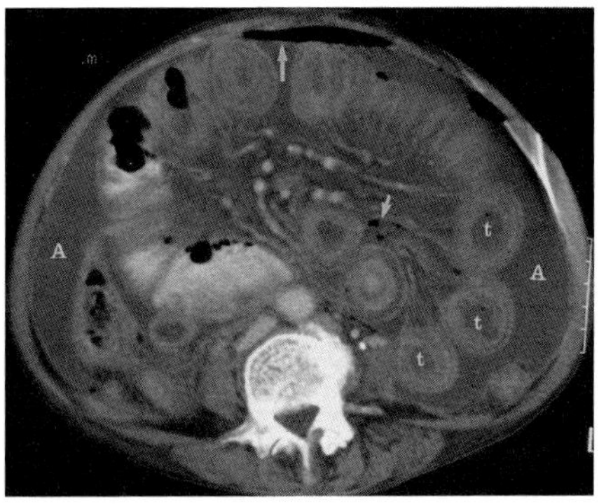

Figure 4. Strangulation obstruction with perforation and peritonitis in a 60-year-old woman. CT scan shows radial distribution of fluid-filled bowel loops with a target sign configuration (*t*). Free air is seen in the adjacent mesentery (short arrow) and in the peritoneal cavity (long arrow). Ascites (*A*) and thickening of the parietal peritoneum are present. Findings were confirmed at surgery performed 4 hours later. These CT findings were considered true-positive.

target configuration in one patient, and a distribution of fluid-filled distended bowel loops suggestive of closed-loop obstruction in five patients. Mild to moderate ascites was present in five of the 19 cases of true-positive findings and in two of the five cases of false-positive findings. In all patients with strangulation obstruction, CT showed a high degree of small bowel obstruction.

Analysis of the statistical data yielded a sensitivity of 83%, specificity of 93%, positive predictive value of 79%, negative predictive value of 95%, and accuracy of 91% for strangulation obstruction. However, two additional cases of primary bowel infarction (small bowel ischemia without bowel obstruction) were detected at surgery but were missed at CT. One case was reported as partial small bowel obstruction (Fig 5) and the second case in which intravenous contrast material was not used was reported as a nonobstructive ileus pattern (Fig 6). When these two cases of primary mesenteric infarction were added to the false-negative results in this series (100 patients), the sensitivity of CT in detection of ischemic bowel decreased to 76%, negative predictive value decreased to 92%, and accuracy decreased to 89%. Specificity (93%) and positive predictive value (79%) remained unchanged. If the analysis included only the 77 patients who underwent surgery, similar statistical values would have been obtained.

DISCUSSION

In patients with possible acute small bowel obstruction, CT has been useful in confirmation of the clinical diagnosis, in establishment of the cause of obstruction, and in correct alteration of treatment of the patients (1–5). In our study, surgery was performed in 77 patients, and CT enabled correct prediction of the cause of obstruction in 65 (84%) patients and the presence of obstruction in all patients except one. On the basis of these factors and on the ability of CT to depict strangulation obstruction, the clinical treatment of patients who underwent CT was modified in 12 (21%) of 57 cases reported by Taourel et al (5).

Accurate detection with CT of ischemic bowel caused by strangulation obstruction or mesenteric infarction remains controversial, however, having shown wide variations in the few reported series. The detection rate of strangulation obstruction has been reported to be 63%–100% (5,8,11) and that of mesenteric infarction was reported to be 26%–82% (12–16). Both conditions are considered surgical emergencies, are difficult to diagnose clinically, and manifest with signs of small bowel obstruction. Early detection followed by surgery would reduce current mortality rates of 10%–37% that are reported to occur in about 10% of patients with small bowel obstruction in whom strangulation develops (17–22).

Since the occurrence of closed-loop obstruction is responsible for and precedes the development of strangulation (ischemia), we have included CT signs of closed-loop obstruction with those of bowel ischemia in our attempt to differentiate patients who may be treated conservatively initially from those who require emergency laparotomy. However, our efforts were only partially successful, resulting in a detection rate of 79% (19 of 24 patients) for strangulation obstruction and 73% (19 of 26 patients) for bowel ischemia (strangulation and mesenteric infarction combined) diagnosed in this series. Retrospective analysis of the CT images showed that in two patients, one with strangulation and one with primary mesenteric ischemia (Fig 6), the correct diagnosis could have been suspected. Even without these two cases, however, our rate of detection would have been 83%. Our overall detection rate of 73% is similar to the 75% detection rate of strangulation reported by Taourel et al (5) but substantially lower than the 100% detection rate reported by Frager et al (11).

Several parameters variable in substance and number are responsible for the discrepancies in the detection rates reported in published studies. Substantial advances in image quality, helical scanning, and better techniques that use high rates of intravenous bolus administration of contrast material have improved resolution and have led to an increase in the detection rates of bowel ischemia (5,11). With increased experience, the interpretation of images and the detection of better-known CT signs have improved simultaneously, although they continue to represent uneven and somewhat capricious factors. Subtle CT findings that are often only suspected can be interpreted differently by various readers, leading to inconsistent results. A rigid interpretation of less specific and questionable changes increase sensitivity to the detriment of specificity. The 100% sensitivity in the series of Frager et al (11) of 60 patients was associated with a 61% specificity, while the higher specificity of 93% achieved in our prospective series was accompanied by a sensitivity of 83% for strangulation and 76% for bowel isch-

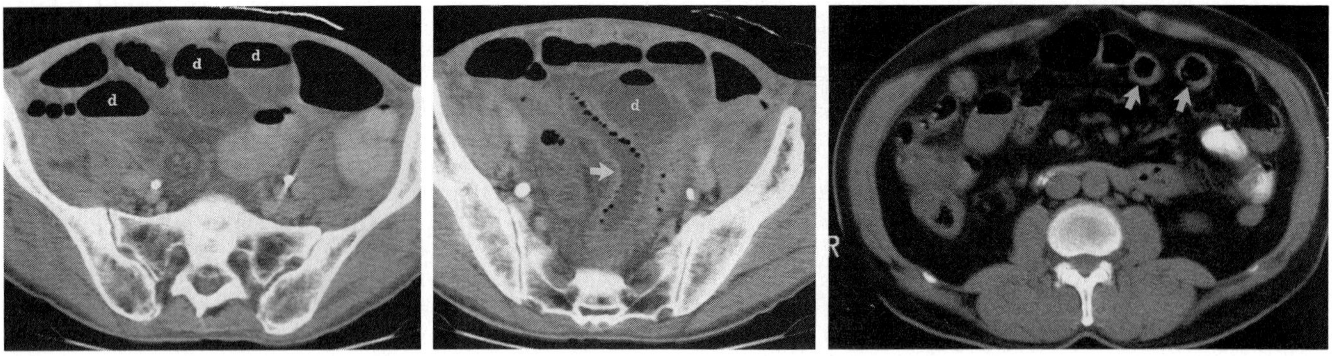

5a. 5b. 6.

Figures 5, 6. Mesenteric infarction in **(5)** a 75-year-old man with a history of atrial fibrillation and **(6)** a 69-year-old man with diabetes and renal failure. **(5a)** CT scan obtained after administration of contrast material shows marked dilatation of proximal intestinal loops (*d*) with multiple air-fluid levels. **(5b)** Contrast-enhanced CT scan shows a partially collapsed loop of bowel containing fluid and air (arrow) in the midpelvis. There were no signs of arterial or venous occlusion. CT findings were interpreted as partial small bowel obstruction. Surgery performed 5 hours later revealed massive infarction of the distal small bowel with only the proximal 55 cm of the jejunum viable. These CT findings were false-negative. *d* = dilated proximal intestinal loops. **(6)** Unenhanced CT scan shows dilatation of air-filled bowel loops and mild circumferential wall thickening of two adjacent loops of bowel in the middle portion of the abdomen (arrows). CT findings were interpreted as adynamic ileus. Surgery performed 3 hours later revealed mesenteric infarction of 260 cm of the small bowel and a thrombus in the distal trunk of the superior mesenteric artery. These CT findings were false-negative.

emia, or strangulation combined with mesenteric infarction.

Other intrinsic pathophysiologic factors explain the remaining CT limitations and the discrepancies between CT and surgical findings in patients with bowel ischemia. Strangulation obstruction is a dynamic changing process, imaged at a single given point during development, about which false assumptions are being made. Strangulation obstruction can develop at any time during an episode of small bowel obstruction; hence, it does not need to be the initial manifestation. The occurrence of strangulation after a closed-loop obstruction develops varies in time and severity; it is unpredictable but it can occur in only a few hours and can progress rapidly to bowel infarction. However, this process is not always irreversible. Decompression of proximal bowel loops with untwisting of the closed loop may lead to resolution of CT and clinical findings as we believe occurred in one of our false-positive cases (Fig 3). Thus, a short interval (6 hours) between CT and surgical exploration is crucial for determining the efficacy and inherent limitations of CT in the diagnosis of intestinal ischemia.

On the basis of our data and previous reports, CT is an accurate, noninvasive presurgical modality for detection of intestinal ischemia. In our study, CT had an accuracy of 91%, a specificity of 93%, and a sensitivity of 83% for strangulation obstruction. However, CT had an accuracy of 89% and a specificity of 76% for diagnosis of combined strangulation obstruction and nonobstructive mesenteric infarction. Because of these remaining limitations associated with CT, the clinical implications of the data presented in our study should be interpreted with caution. The 79% positive predictive value demonstrated by CT should lead to emergent exploratory laparotomy in all patients in whom CT signs of ischemia or closed-loop obstruction are detected. Laparotomy should be performed with the understanding that among this group of patients, about one-fifth (20% in our series) would be found to have simple mechanical small bowel obstruction at surgery. The 95% negative predictive value indicates that a more conservative initial approach may be considered unless other CT findings (intestinal tumor, hernia, abscess) or a rapidly deteriorating clinical condition dictate surgical intervention. It must be stressed that the diagnosis of intestinal ischemia can be missed with state-of-the-art CT, and that obvious discrepancies between CT findings and clinical findings in patients in whom small bowel obstruction or mesenteric infarction is suspected should lead to exploratory laparotomy. ■

References

1. Megibow AJ, Balthazar EJ, Cho KC, et al. Bowel obstruction: evaluation with CT. Radiology 1991; 180:313–318.
2. Maglinte DD, Gage SN, Harmon BH, et al. Obstruction of the small intestine: accuracy and role of CT in diagnosis. Radiology 1993; 188: 61–64.
3. Fukuya T, Hawes DR, Lu CC, et al. CT diagnosis of small-bowel obstruction: efficacy in 60 patients. AJR 1992; 158:765–769.
4. Frager D, Medwid SW, Baer JW, et al. CT of small-bowel obstruction: value in establishing the diagnosis and determining the degree and cause. AJR 1994; 162:37–41.
5. Taourel PG, Fabre JM, Pradel JA, et al. Value of CT in the diagnosis and management of patients with suspected acute small-bowel obstruction. AJR 1995; 165:1187–1192.
6. Balthazar EJ, Bauman JS, Megibow AJ. CT diagnosis of closed loop obstruction. J Comput Assist Tomogr 1985; 9:953–955.
7. Cho KC, Hoffman-Tretin JC, Alterman DD. Closed-loop obstruction of the small bowel: CT and sonographic appearance. J Comput Assist Tomogr 1989; 13:256–258.
8. Balthazar EJ, Birnbaum BA, Megibow AJ, et al. Closed-loop and strangulating intestinal obstruction: CT signs. Radiology 1992; 185:769–775.
9. Balthazar EJ. CT of small-bowel obstruction. AJR 1994; 162:255–261.
10. Ha HK, Park CH, Kim SK, et al. CT analysis of intestinal obstruction due to adhesions: early detection of strangulation. J Comput Assist Tomogr 1993; 17:366–389.
11. Frager D, Baer JW, Medwid SW, et al. Detection of intestinal ischemia in patients with acute small-bowel obstruction due to adhesions or hernia: efficacy of CT. AJR 1996; 166: 67–71.
12. Federle MP, Chun G, Jeffrey RB, et al. Computed tomographic findings in bowel infarction. AJR 1984; 142:91–95.
13. Alperm MB, Glazer GM, Francis IR. Ischemic or infarcted bowel: CT findings. Radiology 1988; 166:149–152.
14. Smerud MJ, Johnson CD, Stephens DH. Diagnosis of bowel infarction: a comparison of plain films and CT scans in 23 cases. AJR 1990; 154:99–103.
15. Balthazar, EJ, Hulnick D, Megibow AJ, et al. Computed tomography of intramural intestinal hemorrhage and bowel ischemia. J Comput Assist Tomogr 1987; 11:67–72.
16. Klein H-M, Lensing R, Klosterhalfen B, et al. Diagnostic imaging of mesenteric infarction. Radiology 1995; 197:79–82.
17. Laws HL, Aldrete JS. Small bowel obstruction: a review of 465 cases. South Med J 1976; 69: 733–734.
18. Waldon GW, Hampton JM. Intestinal obstruction: a half century comparative analysis. Ann Surg 1961; 153:839–850.
19. Bizer LS, Liebling RW, Delany HM, et al. Small bowel obstruction: the role of nonoperative treatment in simple intestinal obstruction and predictive criteria for strangulation obstruction. Surgery 1981; 89:407–413.
20. Sarr MG, Bulkley GB, Zuidema GD. Preoperative recognition of intestinal strangulation obstruction: prospective evaluation of diagnostic capability. Am J Surg 1983; 145:176–182.
21. Barnett WO, Petro AB, Williamson JW. A current appraisal of problems with gangrenous bowel. Ann Surg 1976; 183:653–659.
22. Shatila AH, Chamberlain BE, Webb WR. Current status of diagnosis and management of strangulation obstruction of the small bowel. Am J Surg 1976; 132:299–303.

Christoph D. Becker, MD • Marianne Grossholz, MD • Minerva Becker, MD
Gilles Mentha, MD • Raymond de Peyer, MD • François Terrier, MD

Choledocholithiasis and Bile Duct Stenosis: Diagnostic Accuracy of MR Cholangiopancreatography[1]

PURPOSE: To evaluate the accuracy of magnetic resonance (MR) cholangiopancreatography for detecting bile duct calculi and stenosis.

MATERIALS AND METHODS: At MR cholangiopancreatography, 108 patients suspected of having bile duct calculi or stenosis were examined with two-dimensional fast spin-echo MR sequences and respiratory gating. On the basis of findings at surgery and/or intraoperative, endoscopic retrograde, and/or percutaneous cholangiography, final diagnoses were normal bile ducts ($n = 38$), choledocholithiasis ($n = 23$), Mirizzi syndrome ($n = 3$), benign or malignant bile duct stenosis ($n = 40$), choledochal cyst ($n = 1$), and bile duct dilatation without calculi or stenosis ($n = 3$). MR cholangiopancreatographic images were analyzed retrospectively by three reviewers who were unaware of final diagnoses.

RESULTS: Choledocholithiasis was diagnosed with a sensitivity of 88%–92% and a specificity of 91%–98%. False-negative readings occurred because small or impacted calculi at the distal common bile duct or ampulla were difficult to detect or distinguish from stenosis. Bile duct stenosis was diagnosed with a sensitivity of 93%–100% and a specificity of 98%. Presence or absence of bile duct abnormality was assessed with a sensitivity of 97%–99% and a specificity of 95%–97%. Interobserver agreement was very good ($\kappa = 0.86$–0.96).

CONCLUSION: With MR cholangiopancreatography, bile duct calculi and stenoses can be diagnosed with high accuracy and good interobserver agreement.

Magnetic resonance (MR) cholangiopancreatography is a noninvasive method used to visualize the bile ducts and pancreatic ducts without use of contrast material. MR cholangiopancreatography is based on the principle that stationary fluids are hyperintense on heavily T2-weighted images. MR cholangiopancreatography has several advantages over the established noninvasive imaging techniques and has no known side effects. Endoscopic retrograde cholangiopancreatography (ERCP) is currently the standard method for delineating the bile duct system. Because diagnostic ERCP is associated with a small but substantial risk of complications (1,2), it is desirable to use MR cholangiopancreatography for diagnostic purposes and to restrict ERCP to those cases in which endoscopic interventions are anticipated.

MR cholangiopancreatographic images of adequate quality may be obtained with many different types of equipment and varieties of pulse sequences (3,4). The diagnostic value of MR cholangiopancreatography is still under investigation; however, the results of recent studies have been promising and suggest that MR cholangiopancreatography may accurately demonstrate choledocholithiasis, stenoses, and anatomic variants of the bile ducts and pancreatic ducts (5–9). To evaluate further the clinical usefulness of MR cholangiopancreatography in suspected bile duct disorders, we analyzed the diagnostic accuracy of the technique in a series of 108 patients with confirmed diagnoses.

MATERIALS AND METHODS

Patients

Between July 1995 and May 1997, 188 MR cholangiopancreatographic examinations were performed at our institution in 183 patients who had clinical symptoms or showed biochemical evidence consistent with bile duct or pancreatic disorders. During the same time, 721 patients underwent surgery of the bile duct system and/or pancreas, 202 patients underwent diagnostic or therapeutic ERCP, and 96 patients underwent percutaneous transhepatic cholangiography with or without interventional procedures. Regardless of the suspected pathologic diagnosis, patient selection for MR cholangiopancreatography was based on the availability of abdominal MR imaging within 48 hours for inpatients and within a reasonable time (usually 3–4 days) for outpatients. Patients who needed urgent treatment, however, were selected for MR cholangiopancreatography only if the study could be scheduled immediately without delay of the therapeutic procedure. MR cholangiopancreatography was always performed in addition to sonogra-

Index terms: Bile ducts, calculi, 76.289 • Bile ducts, MR, 76.121411, 76.121412, 76.121419 • Bile ducts, neoplasms, 76.32 • Bile ducts, stenosis or obstruction, 76.28 • Endoscopic retrograde cholangiopancreatography (ERCP), 76.1222 • Gadolinium • Mirizzi syndrome, 764.28 • Pancreas, neoplasms, 774.321 • Pancreatic ducts, 774.321, 774.921 • Pancreatic ducts, MR, 774.121411, 774.121412

Abbreviations: ERCP = endoscopic retrograde cholangiopancreatography, MIP = maximum intensity projection.

Radiology 1997; 205:523–530

[1] From the Department of Radiology, Division of Diagnostic and Interventional Radiology (C.D.B., M.G., M.B., F.T.), the Department of Surgery (G.M.), and the Division of Gastroenterology (R.D.), University Hospital, 24, Rue Micheli-du-Crest, CH-1211 Geneva 14, Switzerland. From the 1996 RSNA scientific assembly. Received January 24, 1997; revision requested March 25; revision received June 25; accepted June 30. **Address reprint requests to** C.D.B.

Table 1
Final Diagnoses in 108 Patients

Diagnoses	Patients
Normal bile ducts	38
Bile duct dilatation without stenosis or calculi*	3
Choledocholithiasis	23
Choledocholithiasis and common duct stenosis (Mirizzi syndrome)	3
Stenoses, benign causes	
Sclerosing cholangitis	1
Common bile duct stenosis†	1
Chronic pancreatitis	9
Papillary stenosis	2
Stenoses, malignant causes	
Intrahepatic metastases	2
Neoplasm of the common bile duct‡	9
Neoplasm of the pancreatic head§	12
Ampullar carcinoma	4
Choledochal cyst	1
Total	108

* Dilatation was attributable to ampullar anomaly (duodenal diverticulum), papillary edema, or previous endoscopic sphincterotomy.
† Common bile duct stenosis was diagnosed with ERCP. Autopsy (death was due to an unrelated cause) did not reveal malignancy.
‡ Including neoplasm at the hepatic bifurcation.
§ Primary or metastatic neoplasm.

Table 2
Choledocholithiasis: Diagnostic Value of MR Cholangiopancreatography in 108 Patients

Test Parameters	Reviewer 1	Reviewer 2	Reviewer 3
Findings*			
True-positive	23	23	24
True-negative	76	75	80
False-positive	6	7	2
False-negative	3	3	2
Statistical measures			
Sensitivity (%)	88	88	92
Specificity (%)	93	91	98
Accuracy (%)	92	91	96
Positive predictive value (%)	79	77	92
Negative predictive value (%)	96	96	98

Note.—Interobserver agreement was very good (κ = 0.86).
* Standards of reference used for final diagnoses are given in text. Numbers are numbers of patients.

Table 3
Bile Duct Stenosis: Diagnostic Value of MR Cholangiopancreatography in 108 Patients

Test Parameters	Reviewer 1	Reviewer 2	Reviewer 3
Findings*			
True-positive	42	40	43
True-negative	64	64	64
False-positive	1	1	1
False-negative	1	3	0
Statistical measures			
Sensitivity (%)	98	93	100
Specificity (%)	98	98	98
Accuracy (%)	98	96	99
Positive predictive value (%)	98	98	98
Negative predictive value (%)	98	96	100

Note.—Interobserver agreement was very good (κ = 0.96).
* Standards of reference used for final diagnosis are given in text. Numbers are numbers of patients.

phy or computed tomography (CT), and informed consent to undergo MR cholangiopancreatography was obtained from all patients. Ten patients were excluded because their MR cholangiopancreatographic examinations were considered nondiagnostic owing to motion artifacts. In five patients who were examined twice, only results of the first examination were analyzed. After we reviewed the radiologic, surgical, and medical records of the 168 patients with MR cholangiopancreatographic studies of adequate diagnostic quality, we identified all patients who underwent surgery, ERCP, or percutaneous transhepatic cholangiography. We excluded all patients with morphologically distorted bile ducts owing to previous surgical bile duct anastomoses.

Among these 168 patients, 108 fulfilled the selection criteria and formed the basis of our study. There were 48 women, 59 men, and a 2-year-old girl. Ages of adult patients ranged from 22 to 92 years (mean, 60.6 years). Fourteen patients had undergone cholecystectomy; 94 patients had their gallbladders in place. Final diagnosis was always based on the complete surgical, medical, radiologic, and pathologic records. The standards of reference for assessing bile duct stenosis, choledocholithiasis, or other bile duct abnormalities were surgical and intraoperative cholangiographic findings in 48 patients, surgical and preoperative ERCP or percutaneous transhepatic cholangiographic findings in 14 patients, ERCP and autopsy findings in two patients, percutaneous transhepatic cholangiographic findings alone in 11 patients, and ERCP findings alone in 28 patients. In five patients with incomplete or unsuccessful ERCP, the common bile duct was clearly visualized with endoscopic ultrasound examination. Bile ducts were considered abnormal if the final diagnosis included choledocholithiasis or benign or malignant bile duct stenosis or if bile duct dilatation due to other causes was documented. Final diagnoses of all 108 patients are summarized in Table 1.

MR Examination Technique

MR cholangiopancreatography was performed on a 1.5-T system (Edge; Picker International, Cleveland, Ohio) with a two-dimensional fast spin-echo sequence with respiratory gating. The body coil was used in all patients except the 2-year-old child who was examined with the head coil. Imaging parameters were the following: repetition time (adapted automatically with the software according to the patient's breathing pattern), 9,000–18,000 msec; echo time, 256 msec; echo-train length, 16; matrix size, 256 × 192 pixels; field of view, 28; signals acquired, two. Because respiratory gating was not available at the beginning of our study, the first 17 patients of our study group were examined without gating. When all MR cholangiopancreatographic examinations in the entire group of 183 patients were considered, the percentage of nondiagnostic examinations was 20% without respiratory gating and only 4% with respiratory gating.

Patients fasted at least 4 hours before MR examination to enhance gallbladder demonstration. Patients received 20 mg of scopolamine butylbromide (Buscopan; Boehringer Ingelheim, Basel, Switzerland) or 1 mg of glucagon hydrochloride (GlucaGen; Novo, Küsnacht, Switzerland) intramuscularly immediately before MR examination. Patients were instructed to breathe quietly and in a constant rhythm during the examination. After the common bile duct was localized in the transverse plane, a typical MR cholangiopancreatographic examination included 20–24 coronal images with a section thickness of 3 mm and no intersection gap. An oblique coronal plane (10°–30°) was chosen in 82 patients to include the hepatic bifurcation; true coronal images were acquired in 26 patients in whom demonstration of the entire pancreatic duct was of particular interest. Another series of 12–24 axial images was acquired at the level of interest (eg, at the level of the distal common bile duct for detection of calculi). The acquisition time for each MR cholangiopancreatographic

Table 4
Bile Duct Abnormality: Diagnostic Value of MR Cholangiopancreatography in 108 Patients

Test Parameters	Reviewer 1	Reviewer 2	Reviewer 3
Findings*			
True-positive	69	68	69
True-negative	37	36	37
False-positive	1	2	1
False-negative	1	2	1
Statistical measures			
Sensitivity (%)	99	97	99
Specificity (%)	97	95	97
Accuracy (%)	98	96	98
Positive predictive value (%)	99	97	99
Negative predictive value (%)	97	95	97

Note.—Interobserver agreement was very good (κ = 0.96).
* Standards of reference used for final diagnoses are given in text. Numbers are numbers of patients.

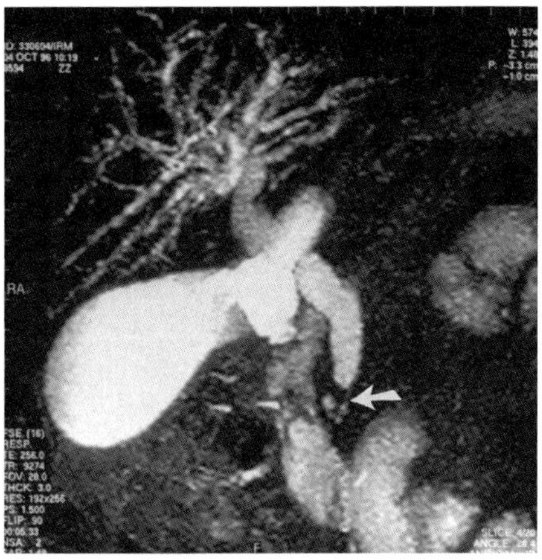

1.

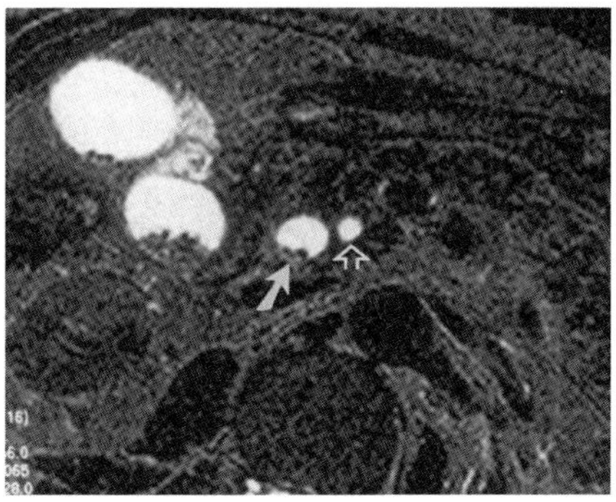

2.

Figures 1, 2. **(1)** Choledocholithiasis. MR cholangiopancreatographic coronal MIP image (9,274/256 [repetition time msec/echo time msec]) demonstrates the signal void (arrow) of calculi in the distal common bile duct with surrounding hyperintense bile. **(2)** Choledocholithiasis. MR cholangiopancreatographic axial source image (9,065/256) shows two 2-mm-diameter calculi (solid arrow) in the common bile duct. Note multiple small calculi in the gallbladder and dilatation of pancreatic duct (open arrow).

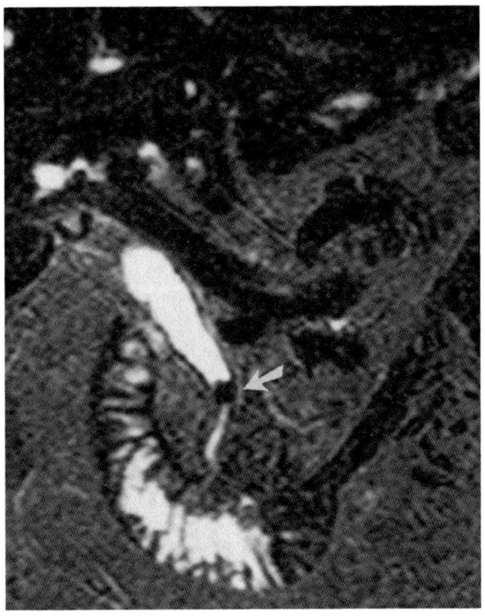

Figure 3. Partially impacted calculus. MR cholangiopancreatographic coronal MIP image (15,720/256) shows an impacted calculus (arrow) causing dilatation of the suprapancreatic common bile duct.

sequence varied according to the examined volume and the patient's breathing pattern; however, 6–8 minutes was required for a typical MR cholangiopancreatographic sequence. In 23 patients, additional T1-weighted axial MR images with spin-echo or gradient spin-echo sequences were acquired before and after intravenous administration of 0.2 mL/kg gadopentetate dimeglumine (Magnevist; Schering, Berlin, Germany) to better demonstrate parenchymal structures and differentiate soft-tissue masses from calculi at the level of obstruction. In all patients, postprocessing of the MR cholangiopancreatographic images was performed at a separate Vistar workstation (Picker International); maximum-intensity-projection (MIP) reconstructions were acquired in all cases, but multiplanar reconstructions were not acquired.

MR Image Interpretation

All MR cholangiopancreatographic studies were reviewed independently by three radiologists (M.B., M.G., C.D.B.) according to uniform criteria that were predefined before the readings. Reviewer 1 had not participated in the prospective clinical readings; reviewer 1 had no practical experience with MR cholangiopancreatography but was familiar with MR imaging. Reviewers 2 and 3 were familiar with MR cholangiopancreatography and had participated in the original, prospective clinical readings in approximately 30% and 70% of cases, respectively; however, with the exception of the last six cases, there was a minimum delay of 3 months between the times of the prospective and retrospective readings by each reviewer. The reviewers were unaware of the final diagnosis and the cholangiographic findings at the time of retrospective analysis. Image interpretation was based on hard copies. The following criteria for retrospective image interpretation were listed on each reviewer's evaluation sheet: The common bile duct was considered to be dilated if its maximum diameter exceeded 7 mm in patients who had not undergone cholecystectomy or 10 mm in patients who had undergone cholecystectomy. Calculi were diagnosed when round, ovoid, or irregularly shaped signal voids were identified within or immediately next to a dilated or nondilated bile duct. All MR cholangiopancreatographic images were examined together; however, if there was a discrepancy in interpretations regarding calculi between source images and MIP images, interpretation of source images took precedence. Stenosis was defined as a transition from ductal dilatation to signal void or a tapered appearance of the common bile duct. Stenosis of the intrahepatic bile ducts was diagnosed if there was a major asymmetry between appearances of the right and left intrahepatic bile ducts or if there was an abrupt difference in caliber between the bile ducts at the hepatic bifurcation. On the basis of their most cephalad, longitudinal extent, stenoses were located at one of three anatomic levels: intrahepatic and/or hilar level, level of the suprapancreatic common bile duct, and intrapancreatic level and/or level of the ampulla. Again, all MR images were evaluated together; however, if there was a discrepancy in interpretation regarding stenosis between source images and MIP images, interpretation of source images took precedence. Because coexisting changes in the pancreatic duct could possibly influence the reviewers' decisions regarding coexisting bile duct abnormalities, each reviewer noted if the pancreatic duct appeared dilated (>3 mm) or normal or if the pancreatic duct was not seen. Each reviewer also assessed any abrupt caliber change that indicated obstruction or stenosis at the level of the pancreatic head or ampulla. On the basis of these criteria, each reviewer noted the presence or absence of bile duct calculi or bile duct stenosis and any abnormality in general (so that cases of bile duct dilatation without visible calculi or stenosis were included).

In the case of apparent stenosis, diagnostic features on MR cholangiopancreatographic images that permitted characterization of the underlying cause (eg, an inflammatory or neoplastic lesion) were noted. The diagnostic information from the T1-weighted MR images obtained in 23 patients was listed separately from that of the other MR cholangiopancreatographic images. Each reviewer also commented on whether these images were helpful for assessing the cause of bile duct dilatation (such as an unenhancing calculus or an enhancing mass).

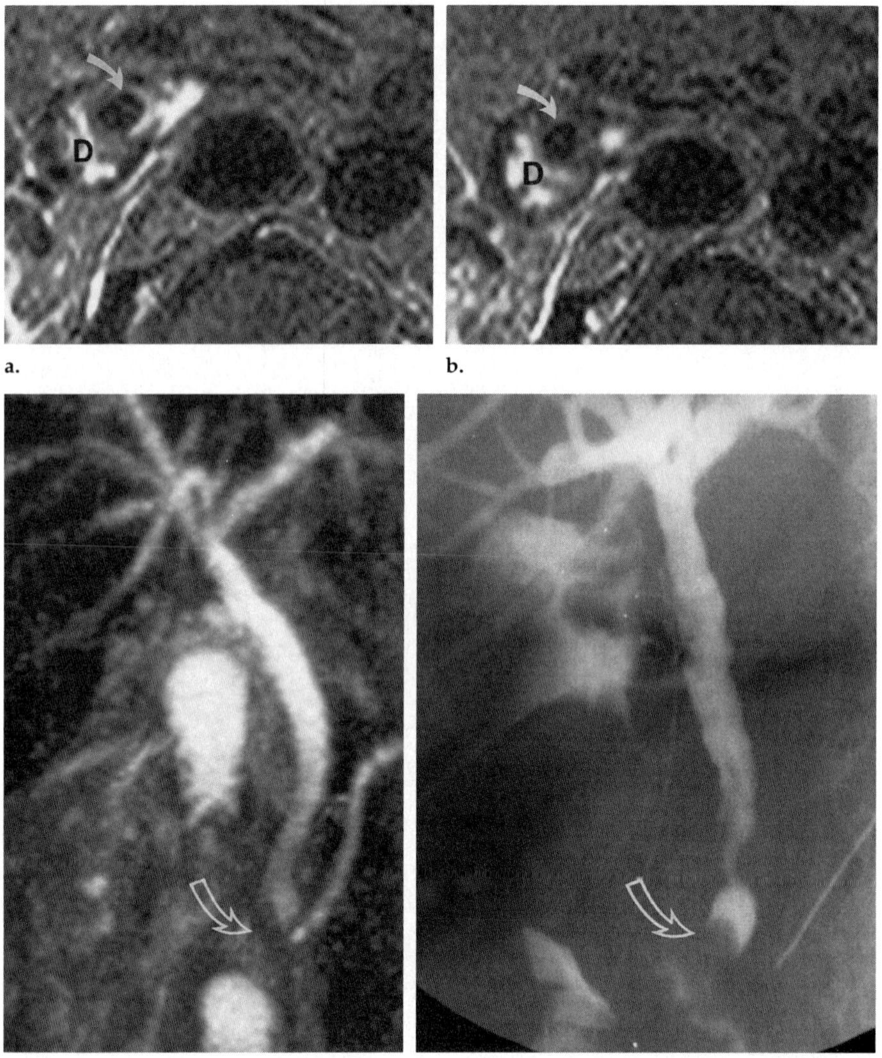

a. b. c. d.

Figure 4. Impacted bile duct calculus. **(a, b)** MR cholangiopancreatographic transverse source images (15,420/256) at different levels show a calculus (arrow) that is partially impacted in the distal ampulla. At the level in **a**, the calculus is partially surrounded by hyperintense bile. At the level in **b**, the calculus is surrounded by the sphincter of Oddi, which is hypointense. *D* = duodenal lumen. **(c)** Partial coronal MIP image (15,720/256) shows a moderately dilated common bile duct and a slightly dilated pancreatic duct. Although the level of obstruction (arrow) is localized at the ampulla, the cause of obstruction cannot be defined correctly with this image. **(d)** Intraoperative cholangiogram confirms an impacted calculus (arrow) within the ampulla.

Statistical Analysis

The MR cholangiopancreatographic findings of each reviewer were compared with the cholangiographic findings and the final diagnoses (Tables 2–4). Sensitivity, specificity, negative and positive predictive values, and overall accuracy of MR cholangiopancreatography for detection of choledocholithiasis, bile duct stenosis, and abnormality in general were calculated for each reviewer. Interobserver variability was assessed by means of the κ statistic with use of the STATA release 3 program for Unix (Stata Corp, College Station, Tex). Interobserver agreement was expressed as a two-outcomes κ result for multiple reviewers; MR images were reported as positive or negative for choledocholithiasis, bile duct stenosis, and abnormality in general. Interobserver agreement was interpreted as very good ($\kappa > 0.80$), good ($\kappa = 0.80$–0.61), moderate ($\kappa = 0.60$–0.41), fair ($\kappa = 0.40$–0.21), and poor ($\kappa \leq 0.20$) (10).

RESULTS

Choledocholithiasis

On the basis of the final diagnosis, 26 patients had choledocholithiasis and 82 patients did not. Six patients had calculi less than 5 mm, and 17 patients had 5–10-mm calculi. Three patients had at least one calculus greater than 10 mm that was located partially outside the common bile duct. In one of these patients, a stone was impacted partially in the cystic duct and partially in the common hepatic duct. In the other two patients, a large calculus had eroded through the pouch of Hartmann into the common hepatic duct; this calculus caused partial bile duct obstruction, by compressing and eroding through the ductal wall, and a chronic fibrotic reaction (Mirizzi syndrome). In these cases, a gallbladder–to–bile-duct fistula was found at surgery.

The diagnostic value of MR cholangiopancreatography for detecting choledocholithiasis is presented in Table 2. In 96 cases, all three reviewers correctly assessed the presence or absence of calculi. Calculi were associated with mild or distinct bile duct dilatation in 23 cases and with nondilated bile ducts in three cases. The diagnosis of calculi was straightforward in 17 cases because MR cholangiopancreatographic images revealed the typical findings of a signal void with surrounding hyperintense bile (Figs 1–3). Diagnosis, however, was more difficult in the other nine cases because calculi were only partially outlined or not outlined at all by hyperintense bile (Figs 4, 5). The diagnostic features of Mirizzi syndrome were recognized by all three reviewers in all three cases (Fig 5). All three reviewers agreed that the source images—particularly those acquired in the transverse plane—were crucial for the diagnosis of small calculi because these calculi were often obscured by surrounding hyperintense bile or adjacent soft-tissue structures (Figs 4, 5). False-negative readings occurred in three cases. No reviewer detected a prepapillary calculus of 3 mm that was in a nondilated bile duct. All three reviewers misread an impacted distal calculus of 4 mm as a stenosis. Two reviewers did not detect an ampullar calculus of 5 mm in a slightly dilated bile duct. False-positive readings of choledocholithiasis occurred in nine cases. In one case, all three reviewers diagnosed a calculus that was not detected with ERCP before or intraoperative cholangiography after MR cholangiopancreatography; endoscopic findings suggested recent stone passage in this case (Fig 6). In four cases, two reviewers interpreted a signal void at the pancreatic level as a calculus; however, short circumscribed stenoses at the pancreatic level due to chronic pancreatitis ($n =$

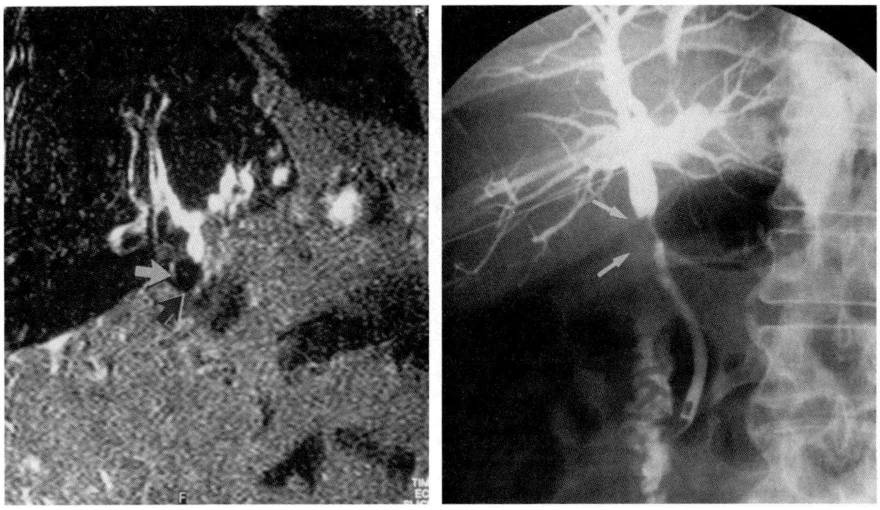

a. b.

Figure 5. Impacted calculus (Mirizzi syndrome). **(a)** MR cholangiopancreatographic coronal source image (10,695/256) shows a calculus (arrows) that is situated partially outside the common hepatic duct and is causing dilatation of the proximal common hepatic duct. **(b)** Percutaneous transhepatic cholangiogram shows an eccentric stenosis of the common hepatic duct that is caused by the radiolucent stone (arrows), which is mainly extraluminal. Also note two small intraluminal calculi in the distal bile duct. At surgery, a calculus was found that had eroded from the pouch of Hartmann directly into the common hepatic duct and thus had caused a gallbladder–to–bile-duct fistula.

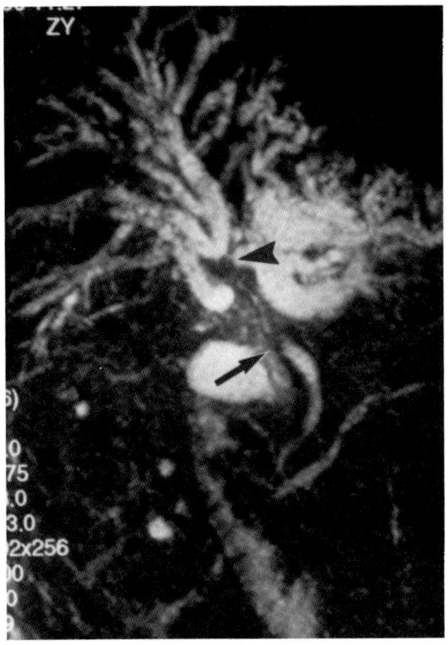

Figure 8. Cholangiocarcinoma of the common hepatic duct and hepatic bifurcation. MR cholangiopancreatographic coronal MIP image (17,475/256) shows dilated intrahepatic bile ducts, stenoses of the intrahepatic bile ducts (arrowhead) and the entire suprapancreatic common bile duct (from arrowhead to arrow), and a normal-sized common bile duct below the stenosis. There is a separation between the right and left hepatic ducts (arrowhead).

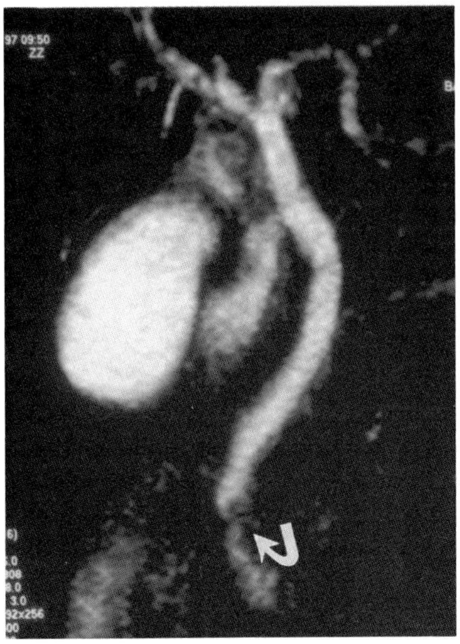

Figure 6. Impacted calculus (arrow) at the ampulla suggested on an MR cholangiopancreatographic image (13,808/256). A false-positive diagnosis was made by all three reviewers. ERCP and endoscopic findings before MR cholangiopancreatography suggested recent passage of a bile duct stone through the papilla but no intraductal calculus. At intraoperative cholangiography after MR cholangiopancreatography, choledocholithiasis was not detected.

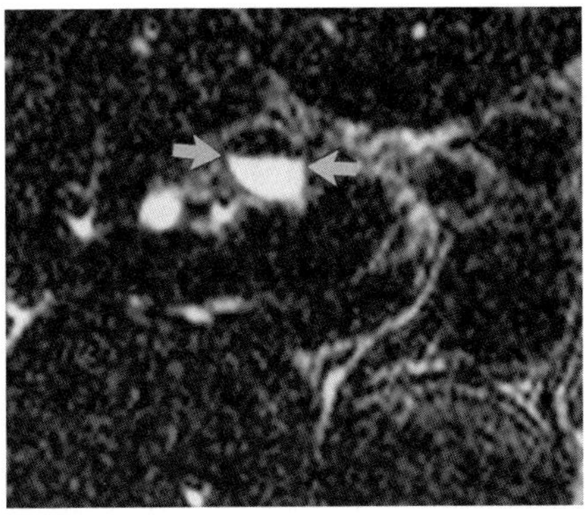

Figure 7. Pneumobilia in a patient who underwent cholecystectomy and endoscopic sphincterotomy. MR cholangiopancreatographic axial source image shows an air-fluid level (arrows) between the signal void of air and dependent hyperintense bile.

3) or carcinoma (n = 1) were proved later. In four cases, one reviewer diagnosed a calculus; however, final diagnoses were normal findings (n = 2), stenosis due to chronic pancreatitis (n =1), or intraductal signal void due to pneumobilia (n =1) (Fig 7). Interobserver agreement regarding diagnosis of choledocholithiasis was very good (κ = 0.86).

Bile Duct Stenosis

On the basis of the final diagnoses, 43 patients had stenoses; causes of stenoses were benign in 16 patients (including the three patients with Mirizzi syndrome) and malignant in 27 patients (Table 1). The stenoses were localized at the intrahepatic or hilar level in 10 patients, the suprapancreatic portion of the common bile duct in seven patients, and the intrapancreatic or ampullar level in 24 patients. One patient had multiple intra- and extrahepatic stenoses due to sclerosing cholangitis. One patient with a pancreatic tumor had bile duct obstruction due to metastases not only at the pancreatic level but also at the hilar level.

The diagnostic value of MR cholangiopancreatography for detecting bile duct stenosis is presented in Table 3. In 40 cases (including the three cases of Mirizzi syndrome), stenosis was correctly identified by all three reviewers. False-negative readings of bile duct stenosis occurred in three cases. Bile duct stenoses were misinterpreted as calculi in two cases by two reviewers and in the other case by one reviewer. In one case, a short stenosis of the intrapancreatic portion of the bile duct was not detected by one reviewer. One case of an impacted calculus was misinterpreted as a stenosis by all three reviewers. Interobserver agreement regarding the presence or absence of stenosis was very good (κ = 0.96).

The level of stenosis was correctly assessed by all three reviewers in 37 cases (Figs 8–11). In 17 of 24 patients with bile duct stenosis at the pancreatic or ampullar level, the pancreatic duct appeared dilated on MR cholangiopancreatographic images; however,

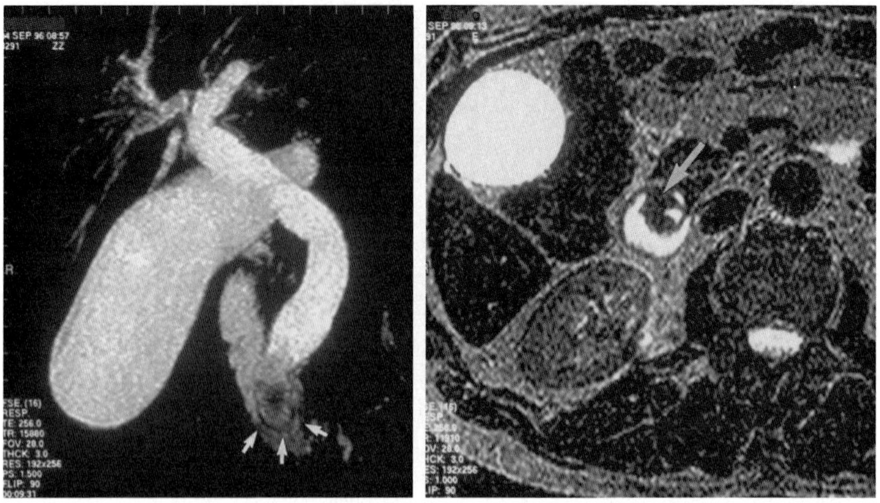

a. b.

Figure 9. Ampullar carcinoma within a choledochocele. **(a)** MR cholangiopancreatographic coronal MIP image (15,880/256) shows dilatation of the common bile duct and protrusion of its ampullar portion into the duodenal lumen consistent with a choledochocele (arrows). There is a signal void measuring 12 mm in diameter within the choledochocele. **(b)** Axial source MR image (11,910/256) shows that the signal void (arrow) within the choledochocele is irregularly shaped and not in a dependent position.

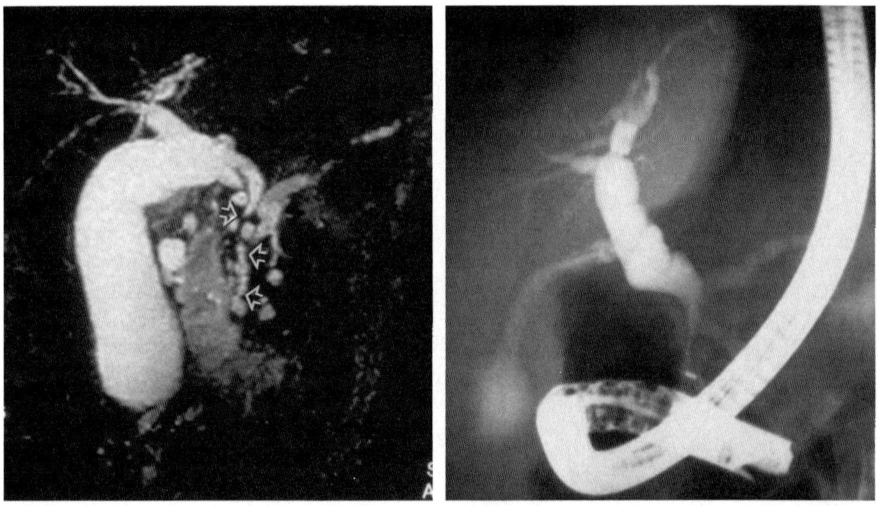

a. b.

Figure 10. Bile duct stenosis due to chronic pancreatitis. **(a)** MR cholangiopancreatographic coronal MIP image (12,368/256) shows a dilated common bile duct due to a long stenosis at the pancreatic level (arrows). The pancreatic duct is also dilated and has an irregular lumen. Multiple, small, round hyperintense structures throughout the pancreatic head are consistent with pancreatic pseudocysts. **(b)** ERCP image shows a long, smooth stenosis of the intrapancreatic bile duct and prestenotic dilatation. There is also dilatation of the pancreatic duct.

in all patients with stenosis at the suprapancreatic level (except the patient with two-level obstruction due to metastatic carcinoma of the pancreas), the width of the pancreatic duct appeared normal or the duct was not visualized. In a case of benign common duct stenosis, hilar involvement was erroneously diagnosed by one reviewer. In two cases of malignant stenosis due to pancreatic carcinoma, the observers disagreed on the involvement of the suprapancreatic portion of the common bile duct.

In 20 of the 43 cases of proved stenosis, MR cholangiopancreatographic findings strongly suggested a malignant cause: neoplasm involving the intrahepatic bile ducts or the hepatic bifurcation (Fig 8), 10 cases; neoplasm of the extrahepatic bile ducts, six cases; and neoplasm involving the intrapancreatic bile duct or the ampulla (Fig 9), four cases. In five cases, MR cholangiopancreatographic findings were consistent with benign causes: Mirizzi syndrome, three cases; and chronic pancreatitis with multiple or large pseudocysts (Fig 10), two cases. In the other 15 cases, however, MR cholangiopancreatography did not enable identification of a benign or malignant cause. In one patient with stenoses at the intrahepatic and intrapancreatic levels, the diagnosis of sclerosing cholangitis was suggested; however, the reviewers could not determine if the dominant distal stenosis was due to inflammation or neoplastic degeneration. In 14 cases of stenoses at the pancreatic and ampullar levels, the reviewers could not differentiate chronic pancreatitis from pancreatic cancer or benign papillary stenosis from ampullar carcinoma. Comparison of the MR cholangiopancreatographic diagnosis with the final diagnosis showed that small pseudocysts due to chronic pancreatitis were visible on MR images in not only three patients with bile duct stenosis due to inflammation or reactive fibrosis (Fig 10) but also in two patients with pancreatic neoplasm. In one patient, MR cholangiopancreatographic images showed a stenosis at the ampullar level. In this patient, a benign papillary stenosis was subsequently diagnosed with ERCP, and endoscopic sphincterotomy was performed. One year later, however, the patient returned with obstructive jaundice, and adenocarcinoma of the ampulla was diagnosed at histologic examination. In one patient, ERCP findings suggested cholangiocarcinoma of the intrapancreatic bile duct. This patient died of an unrelated cause, and no malignancy was revealed at autopsy.

T1-weighted MR images before and after administration of contrast material were acquired in 23 cases. In three instances, the T1-weighted MR images were considered helpful because enhancement enabled additional differentiation between a soft-tissue mass and an impacted calculus. However, the information provided with the T1-weighted MR images did not alter the diagnosis made with only the MR cholangiopancreatographic images. In the remaining 20 cases, the T1-weighted MR images gave no relevant diagnostic information in addition to that provided with the MR cholangiopancreatographic images.

Detection of Normal and Abnormal Bile Ducts

On the basis of the final diagnosis, bile ducts were normal in 38 cases whereas pathologic changes were detected in 70 cases (Table 1). The diagnostic value of MR cholangiopancreatography for distinguishing normal

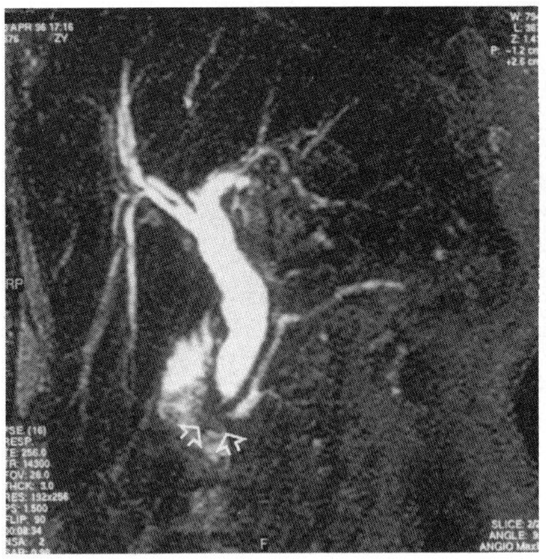

11.

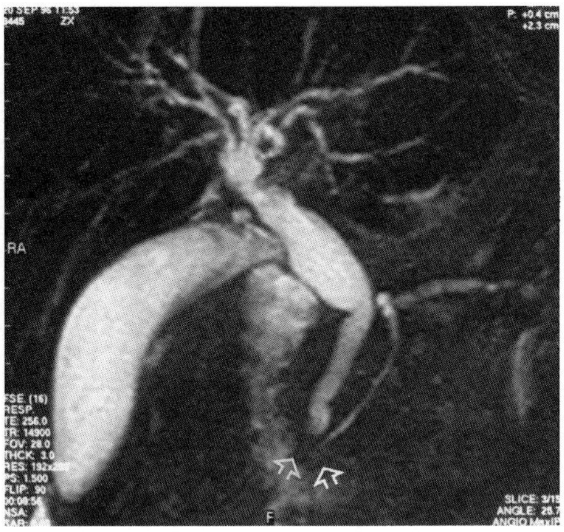

12.

Figures 11, 12. **(11)** Benign papillary stenosis. MR cholangiopancreatographic coronal MIP image (15,720/256) shows a stenosis at the ampulla of Vater with prestenotic bile duct dilatation. A soft-tissue mass (arrows) is seen at the level of the ampulla. No tumor was seen with endoscopy, and ERCP revealed no calculi. **(12)** Papillary edema as a result of recent passage of a bile duct calculus in a patient with acute biliary pancreatitis. MR cholangiopancreatographic coronal MIP image (15,648/256) shows dilatation of the bile duct and pancreatic duct at the level of the ampulla. These findings suggest a stenosis (arrows), but the cause of dilatation is not evident. ERCP images showed papillary edema but no stenosis or calculi.

and abnormal bile ducts is given in Table 4. In 104 cases, the presence or absence of pathologic changes was assessed correctly by all three reviewers. False-negative readings occurred in two cases: A stone in a nondilated bile duct was missed by all three reviewers, and a stenosis was missed by one reviewer. False-positive readings occurred in two cases in which calculi were erroneously diagnosed by all three reviewers in one case and by one reviewer in the other. In four patients, MR cholangiopancreatographic images showed dilatation of the entire common bile duct but no stones or stenosis. In these patients, the causes of bile duct dilatation were a choledochal cyst, an abnormal position of the ampulla within a duodenal diverticulum, papillary edema due to recent stone passage (Fig 12), and previous endoscopic sphincterotomy after cholecystectomy (Fig 7). Interobserver agreement regarding the presence or absence of bile duct abnormality was very good ($\kappa = 0.96$).

DISCUSSION

No established noninvasive imaging method is sufficiently reliable to answer the clinically important questions that arise when bile duct disorders are suspected because each imaging method has inherent limitations. Ultrasonography is an operator-dependent method and often fails to demonstrate the distal bile duct (11,12), CT cannot reliably show noncalcified stones (13), and intravenous cholangiography (including CT cholangiography) is of limited value with elevated bilirubin levels (14,15). Thus, ERCP often is needed to delineate the bile duct system. Diagnostic ERCP is, however, a relatively costly examination and may cause transient acute pancreatitis in approximately 5% of cases (1,2) (in addition to the relatively low risk associated with endoscopy in general). The cost and risk may be acceptable in patients who are likely to benefit from a definitive therapeutic procedure in the same session (eg, sphincterotomy and stone removal). For other patients, however, it appears desirable to replace diagnostic ERCP with a noninvasive test that has a similar accuracy.

A variety of pulse sequences have been proposed for MR cholangiopancreatography. With most current protocols, coronal source images and MIP reconstructions are acquired from two- or three-dimensional data sets. Respiratory motion artifacts may be overcome with multiple short acquisitions (breath-hold imaging techniques) or compensated for during quiet respiration with signal averaging or respiratory gating (non–breath-hold imaging techniques). Early MR cholangiopancreatographic protocols included multiple gradient-recalled echo acquisitions of approximately 20 seconds (16–18). More recently, fast spin-echo sequences have been preferred increasingly because they offer better signal-to-noise and contrast-to-noise ratios and are more resistant to artifacts due to motion, intestinal gas, and surgical clips (19,20). Fast spin-echo sequences are suitable for non–breath-hold examination protocols, which are easier to accomplish than breath-hold protocols although examination times may be longer (3–8,21,22). Results of our study indicate that, with our current two-dimensional fast spin-echo technique, we can acquire images of consistent quality in the vast majority of patients (including the elderly who are often unable to cooperate well). We found respiratory gating very useful because it increased the yield of diagnostic studies from 80% to 96%, whereas the resulting acquisition time remained within acceptable limits. We also recommend antiperistaltic agents to minimize bowel motion, but fat saturation is unnecessary with the heavily T2-weighted MR imaging parameters we used. Although the resolution on MR cholangiopancreatographic images is currently inferior to that of conventional cholangiographic images, MR cholangiopancreatography is still undergoing a rapid technical evolution. Further improvement of image quality may be possible with use of phased-array body coils and an increased matrix (23) or by acquiring three-dimensional data sets, which permit reduction of section thickness (24). Early experience with sequences (such as rapid acquisition with relaxation enhancement or half-Fourier turbo spin echo) that can be implemented with the new strong-gradient systems suggests that high-quality MR cholangiopancreatographic images may also be acquired with short breath-hold intervals, which may shorten considerably the examination time. To date, however, preliminary studies have focused mainly on the evaluation of image quality achieved with these new sequences, and diagnostic data from clinical series have been limited (9,20,25,26).

For practical reasons, hard-copy images were interpreted in our study. Prospective clinical assessments, however, are usually made at the workstation; thus, the radiologist may obtain additional information with use of postprocessing if necessary. Some errors could perhaps have been avoided by reviewing all images directly on the computer screen with variable window settings; however, we do not believe that hard-copy image interpretation substantially negatively influenced our data. All source and MIP images were interpreted together, and the postprocessed (MIP) images were available in all cases. Although one of the reviewers had no practical experience with MR cholangiopancreatography, interobserver agreement was very good.

Choledocholithiasis is a common disorder and may be associated with bile duct dilatation. The frequency of bile duct calculi in our series of patients was 24%. Although bile duct calculi were associated with bile duct dilatation in 23 (88%) of 26 patients, MR cholangiopancreatography enabled detection of calculi as small as 2 mm in diameter in two of the three patients without bile duct dilatation. Small calculi were best displayed on axial source images because they are perpendicular to the axis of the bile duct. Small calculi may be obscured on MIP images because of volume averaging with surrounding hyperintense bile. In our study, the sensitivity of MR cholangiopancreatography for detecting choledocholithiasis varied from 88% to 92%, and the specificity ranged from 91% to 98%. Guibaud et al (5) reported a sensitivity of 81%. Other recent studies have yielded sensitivities of 90%–100% (3,6,7). Although the specificities reported in these studies have been very high (ie, 98%–100%), some conditions may occasionally mimic calculi and thus result in false-positive diagnoses. In our study, such conditions included pneumobilia and short bile duct stenosis, but intraluminal clot, surgical clips or suture material, and metallic stents should also be mentioned. For practical reasons, most investigators have used ERCP as a standard of reference when evaluating MR cholangiopancreatography results. One must consider, however, that ERCP is an operator-dependent technique and may be associated with false-negative and false-positive findings (27,28). Although our results were based in part on ERCP findings, most patients in our series underwent surgery—including intraoperative cholangiography, which is considered to be a very reliable technique and less operator-dependent than ERCP.

With MR cholangiopancreatography, bile duct stenosis was detected with a high sensitivity and specificity. The level of stenosis was defined precisely in the vast majority of cases. Although MR cholangiopancreatographic findings suggested the underlying cause of stenosis in two-thirds of cases, the distinction between benign and malignant strictures could not be determined in approximately one-third of these cases; mainly, pancreatic carcinoma could not be differentiated from chronic pancreatitis and benign ampullar stenosis could not be differentiated from ampullar carcinoma. These differentiations, however, were also sometimes difficult to make with ERCP or even at surgery. In our study, a more complete examination of the pancreatic region with dedicated sequences may have added diagnostic information; however, the limited number of MR studies that included T1-weighted images and contrast enhancement did not allow definite conclusions regarding the usefulness of these sequences. In some cases, these sequences facilitated differentiation of an unenhancing impacted calculus from an enhancing tumor, but these sequences did not add substantial diagnostic information to that provided with the MR cholangiopancreatographic images in most cases. For economic reasons, we therefore recommend use of contrast–enhanced T1-weighted MR images selectively instead of routinely. Further studies are needed to address this issue.

Although calculi and stenoses were not always identified correctly, the presence or absence of abnormality was identified with a very high accuracy by all reviewers. On the basis of our study, MR cholangiopancreatography allows prediction of bile duct abnormality in at least 97% of cases and exclusion of abnormality in at least 95% of cases.

In summary, MR cholangiopancreatography can provide nearly similar diagnostic information about choledocholithiasis and bile duct stenosis as that provided with direct cholangiography. With the protocol used in our series, images of consistent diagnostic quality can be acquired even in the elderly and debilitated patient. MR cholangiopancreatography appears sufficiently accurate to be recommended as a noninvasive method in patients with suspected bile duct disorders. In fact, we have begun to restrict the use of ERCP, whenever possible, to cases in which therapeutic procedures are anticipated or MR cholangiopancreatographic findings are equivocal. The clinical role of MR cholangiopancreatography, however, will depend not only on its diagnostic accuracy but on its availability and cost-effectiveness. Outcome studies will be needed to determine the diagnostic value of MR cholangiopancreatography in specific clinical settings. ■

Acknowledgments: We thank Paul Margosian, PhD, and Frank Henri, RT, for help with the imaging protocol; Patricia Villoz for assistance with clinical data collection; and Shu-Fang Hsu-Schmitz, PhD, for performing the statistical analysis.

References

1. Sherman S, Lehman G. ERCP- and endoscopic sphincterotomy–induced pancreatitis. Pancreas 1991; 3:350–367.
2. Cohen SA, Siegel JH, Kasmin FE. Complications of diagnostic and therapeutic ERCP. Abdom Imaging 1996; 21:385–394.
3. Reinhold C, Bret PM. Current status of MR cholangiopancreatography. AJR 1996; 166:1285–1295.
4. Becker CD, Grossholz M, Mentha G, de Peyer R, Terrier F. MR cholangio-pancreatography: technique, potential indications, and diagnostic features of benign, malignant, and postoperative conditions. Eur Radiol 1997;7:865–874.
5. Guibaud L, Bret PM, Reinhold C, Atri M, Barkun ANG. Bile duct obstruction and choledocholithiasis: diagnosis with MR cholangiography. Radiology 1995; 197:109–115.
6. Soto JA, Barish MA, Yucel EK, Siegenberg D, Ferrucci JT, Chuttani R. Magnetic resonance cholangiography: comparison with endoscopic retrograde cholangiopancreatography. Gastroenterology 1996; 110:589–597.
7. Pavone P, Laghi A, Catalano C, et al. MR cholangio-pancreatography (MRCP) at 0.5 T: technique optimisation and preliminary results. Eur Radiol 1996; 6:147–152.
8. Taourel P, Bret PM, Reinhold C, Barkun A, Atri M. Anatomic variants of the biliary tree: diagnosis with MR cholangiography. Radiology 1996; 199:521–527.
9. Reuther G, Kiefer B, Tuchmann A. Cholangiography before biliary surgery: single-shot MR cholangiography versus intravenous cholangiography. Radiology 1996: 198:561–566.
10. Davies M, Fleiss JL. Measuring agreement for multinomial data. Biometrics 1982; 38:1047–1051.
11. Gross BH, Harter L, Gore RM, et al. Ultrasonic evaluation of common bile duct stones: prospective comparison with endoscopic retrograde cholangiopancreatography. Radiology 1983; 146:471–475.
12. Mitchell SE, Clark RA. A comparison of computed tomography and sonography in choledocholithiasis. AJR 1984; 142:729–733.
13. Baron RL. Common bile duct stones: reassessment of criteria for CT diagnosis. Radiology 1987; 162:419–424.
14. Van Beers BE, La Crosse M, Trigaux JP, de Canniére L, de Ronde TD, Pringot J. Noninvasive imaging of the biliary tree before and after laparoscopic cholecystectomy: use of three-dimensional spiral CT cholangiography. AJR 1994; 162:1331–1335.
15. Fleischmann D, Ringl H, Schöfl R, et al. Three-dimensional spiral CT cholangiography in patients with suspected obstructive biliary disease: comparison with endoscopic retrograde cholangiography. Radiology 1996; 198:861–868.
16. Wallner BK, Schumacher KA, Weidenmaier W, Friedrich JM. Dilated biliary tract: evaluation with MR cholangiography with a T2-weighted contrast-enhanced FAST sequence. Radiology 1991; 181:805–808.
17. Morimoto K, Shimoi M, Shirakawa T, et al. Biliary obstruction: evaluation with three-dimensional MR cholangiography. Radiology 1992; 183:578–580.
18. Hall-Craggs MA, Allen CM, Owens CM, et al. MR cholangiography: clinical evaluation in 40 cases. Radiology 1993; 189:423–427.
19. Reinhold C, Guibaud, L, Genin G, Bret PM. MR cholangiopancreatography: comparison between two-dimensional fast spin-echo and three-dimensional gradient-echo pulse sequences. J Magn Reson Imaging 1995; 4:379–384.
20. Ichikawa T, Nitatori T, Hachiya J, Mizutani Y. Breath-held MR cholangiopancreatography with half-averaged single-shot hybrid rapid acquisition with relaxation enhancement sequence: comparison of fast GRE and SE sequences. J Comput Assist Tomogr 1996; 20:798–802.
21. Macaulay SE, Schulte SJ, Sekijima JH, et al. Evaluation of a non-breath-hold MR cholangiography technique. Radiology 1995; 196:227–232.
22. Guibaud L, Bret PM, Reinhold C, Atri M, Barkun A. Diagnosis of choledocholithiasis: value of MR cholangiography. AJR 1994; 163: 847–850.
23. Bret PM, Reinhold C, Taourel P, Guibaud L, Atri M, Barkun AN. Pancreas divisum: evaluation with MR cholangiopancreatography. Radiology 1996; 199:99–103.
24. Soto JA, Yucel EK, Barish MA, Chuttani R, Ferrucci JT. MR cholangiopancreatography after unsuccessful ERCP. Radiology 1996; 199:91–98.
25. Laubenberger J, Büchert M, Schneider B, Blum U, Hennig J, Langer M. Breath-hold projection magnetic resonance-cholangio-pancreatography (MRCP): a new method for the examination of the bile and pancreatic ducts. Magn Reson Med 1995; 33:18–23.
26. Miyazaki T, Yamashita Y, Tsuchigame H, Urata J, Takahashi M. MR cholangiography using HASTE (half-Fourier acquisition single-shot turbo spin-echo) sequences. AJR 1996; 166:1297–1303.
27. Pasanen P, Partanen K, Pikkarainen P, Alhava E, Pirinen A, Janatuinen E. Ultrasonography, CT, and ERCP in the diagnosis of choledochal stones. Acta Radiol 1992; 33:53–56.
28. Frey CF, Burbige EJ, Meinke WB, et al. Endoscopic retrograde cholangiopancreatography. Am J Surg 1982; 144:109–114.

Yutaka Inoue, MD • Hironobu Nakamura, MD

Aplasia or Hypoplasia of the Pancreatic Uncinate Process: Comparison in Patients with and Patients without Intestinal Nonrotation[1]

PURPOSE: To investigate whether the pancreatic uncinate process is hypoplastic in patients with intestinal nonrotation, and to evaluate the association of hypoplasia or aplasia of the uncinate process with mesenteric vascular inversion.

MATERIALS AND METHODS: Computed tomographic (CT) scans of the pancreas in five patients with intestinal nonrotation and in 101 patients with normal intestinal rotation were reviewed to assess the morphology of the uncinate process. The transverse diameter of the uncinate process was measured, and the relationship with the superior mesenteric artery and vein was defined.

RESULTS: The uncinate process was absent in three and unusually small in two of the five patients with nonrotation. The uncinate process was clearly present in all patients with normal rotation. The mean transverse diameter (2.60 mm ± 2.61 [standard deviation]) of the uncinate process in patients with nonrotation was significantly smaller than that (15.1 mm ± 5.0) in the patients with normal rotation ($P < .001$). Four of the five patients with nonrotation had mesenteric vascular inversion, and three of these patients had no uncinate process. None of the patients with normal rotation had mesenteric vascular inversion.

CONCLUSION: The uncinate process was aplastic or hypoplastic in patients with nonrotation, which may have been associated with incomplete rotation of the ventral bud of the pancreatic primordium, as well as mesenteric vascular inversion.

INTESTINAL malrotation is an important cause of gastrointestinal obstruction in the neonate (1). Adolescents and adults with intestinal malrotation may experience abdominal pain or vomiting secondary to chronic intestinal obstruction from Ladd bands or volvulus (2). Inverse relationships of the superior mesenteric artery and the superior mesenteric vein have been reported at computed tomography (CT) or ultrasonography (US) in some patients with malrotation (3–6). During the past several years, we have observed that the pancreatic uncinate process is not depicted or is unusually small at CT in patients with intestinal nonrotation. Because development of the pancreas is intimately related to rotation of the duodenojejunal loop in the embryo, intestinal malrotation may be expected to be associated with abnormal pancreatic morphology (7–9). The uncinate process develops from the ventral pancreas (8), and faulty rotation of the ventral pancreas may result in a paucity of pancreatic tissue in the usual location of the uncinate process.

The purpose of this study was to assess the morphology of the pancreatic uncinate process in patients with intestinal nonrotation and to compare the morphology with that in patients with normal intestinal rotation. More specifically, we wanted to determine whether aplasia or hypoplasia of the uncinate process may be associated with intestinal nonrotation.

MATERIALS AND METHODS

We retrospectively reviewed abdominal CT scans obtained in 10 consecutive patients with intestinal malrotation who were examined at Minoo City Hospital from May 1992 through July 1995. We excluded five patients from the study population because of the presence of situs ambiguous, heterotaxia with polysplenia, or situs inversus. Our study population comprised five patients (two men and three women aged 20–66 years [mean, 47.6 years]), who weighed 43–70 kg (mean, 51.0 kg). These patients had normal situs of organs, with the heart, stomach, and spleen on the left in the chest and abdomen and the liver and gallbladder on the right. No patient had pancreatic disease, including diabetes mellitus. In these patients, a barium study was performed routinely ($n = 2$) or because of abdominal pain ($n = 3$). In all the patients, intestinal nonrotation was confirmed by means of the barium study, with the small bowel on the right side in the abdomen and the large bowel on the left. CT was performed because volvulus was suspected on the basis of results of the barium study in three patients and peritoneal tumor was suspected on the basis of results at US in one patient.

To select patients for the control group, we reviewed helical CT scans that included the entire pancreas and were obtained in 108 consecutive patients at Minoo City Hospital who had no history of abdominal surgery and were confirmed to have normal situs by means of chest radiography and CT and normal intestinal rotation by means of barium study. Seven of these patients were excluded because of the presence of primary or secondary pancreatic disease. The control group comprised 101

Index terms: Intestines, malrotation, 75.146 • Pancreas, abnormalities, 75.14, 770.14 • Pancreas, anatomy, 770.92 • Pancreas, CT, 77.12114, 77.12115

Radiology 1997; 205:531–533

[1] From the Department of Radiology, Minoo City Hospital, 5-7-1 Kayano, Minoo, Osaka 562, Japan (Y.I.); and the Department of Radiology, Osaka University Medical School, Osaka, Japan (H.N.). Received March 17, 1997; revision requested April 30; revision received July 14; accepted July 21. **Address reprint requests to** Y.I.

patients without diabetes mellitus (65 men and 36 women aged 21–83 years [mean, 61.4 years]), who weighed 37–78 kg (mean, 55.6 kg). CT was performed to exclude or evaluate the following conditions: gastric carcinoma (n = 42), chronic liver disease alone or with hepatocellular carcinoma (n = 37), extrapancreatic biliary disease (n = 7), renal neoplasm (n = 10), and intestinal neoplasm (n = 5). Barium studies were performed routinely (n = 14) or preoperatively (n = 87) to exclude or evaluate gastrointestinal disease.

In four of the patients with intestinal nonrotation and in all control patients, dynamic helical CT that included the pancreas was performed with a beam collimation of 5 mm and a table speed of 5 mm/sec, with reconstruction increments of 2 or 3 mm. Scanning was started 30 seconds after initiation of intravenous injection of 100 mL of iopamidol (Iopamiron 300 [300 mg of iodine per milliliter]; Nihon Schering, Osaka, Japan) at a rate of 3 mL/sec. Conventional delayed CT was performed after dynamic helical CT to obtain venous phase images, with section thickness of 5 mm and scan intervals of 5 mm. Patient 1 underwent unenhanced and contrast material–enhanced conventional CT, with section thickness of 5 mm and scan intervals of 5 mm. In that patient, CT was started after initiation of the injection of 100 mL of iopamidol at a rate of 2 mL/sec. All CT examinations were performed with a commercially available scanner (TCT 900S; Toshiba, Tokyo, Japan).

For the purpose of this study, we defined the uncinate process as constituting that portion of the inferior aspect of the pancreatic head that is dorsal to the superior mesenteric vein and artery and medial to the remaining portion of the head of the pancreas. The pancreatic head was traced to the caudal end to define the uncinate process throughout the serial axial CT images. The transverse diameter of the uncinate process was measured if it was depicted, as indicated in Figure 1. A value of 0 was assigned when the uncinate process was not seen. The uncinate process was defined as hypoplastic when the transverse diameter was within the 5th percentile of the diameter measured in patients with normal intestinal rotation. The relationships of the superior mesenteric artery and vein were defined within 3 cm below the portal venous confluence.

Data were analyzed with commercially available software (StatView; Abacus Concepts, Berkeley, Calif). We used the Fisher r to z transformation to assess the statistical significance of the correlation between the transverse diameters of the uncinate process and the ages or weights of the patients with normal intestinal rotation. We used the Welch test to determine the significance of the difference in transverse diameters of the uncinate process between the two groups of patients. A P value less than .05 was considered statistically significant.

RESULTS

At CT in all control patients, the superior mesenteric vein was located to the right of the superior mesenteric artery and the uncinate process projected leftward from the right lateral margin of the superior mesenteric vein, with transverse diameters of 4–28 mm (mean, 15.1 mm ± 5.0 [standard deviation]; 95% confidence interval, 14.1 mm, 16.1 mm) (Figs 2, 3). There was no statistically significant correlation between transverse diameter and age (P = .06) or weight (P = .22). The 5th percentile of the transverse measurements was 7 mm. In three patients, the diameter of the uncinate process was less than 7 mm (4, 4, and 5 mm); thus, according to our definition, the uncinate process was hypoplastic in these patients.

The results for the five patients with intestinal nonrotation are displayed in the Table. Three of these patients had no uncinate process (Fig 4), and the remaining two patients had a hypoplastic uncinate process with a transverse diameter of not more than 6 mm (Fig 5). In these latter two patients, the uncinate process was defined as a small leftward projection from the right lateral margin of the superior mesenteric vein; the pancreatic head appeared normal except for aplasia or hypoplasia of the uncinate process. The mean transverse diameter of the uncinate process in the five patients with intestinal nonrotation (2.60 mm ± 2.61) was statistically significantly smaller than that in the control group (P < .001).

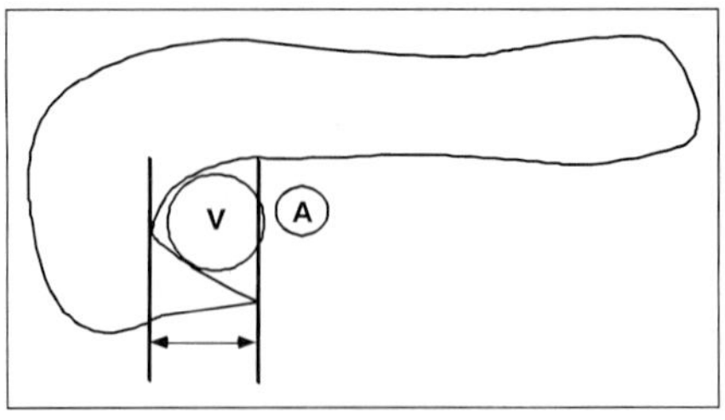

Figure 1. Schematic representation of measurement of the transverse diameter of the pancreatic uncinate process. The maximal value throughout the serial images was defined as the transverse diameter of the uncinate process. A = superior mesenteric artery, V = superior mesenteric vein.

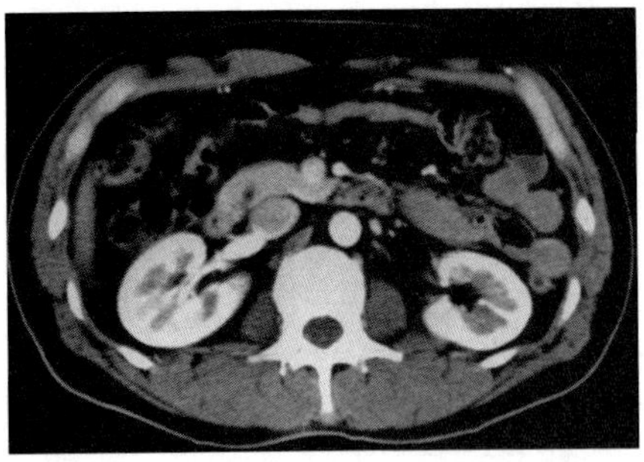

Figure 2. CT scan depicts the uncinate process in a 48-year-old man with normal intestinal rotation. The uncinate process is adequately seen, with a transverse diameter of 19 mm.

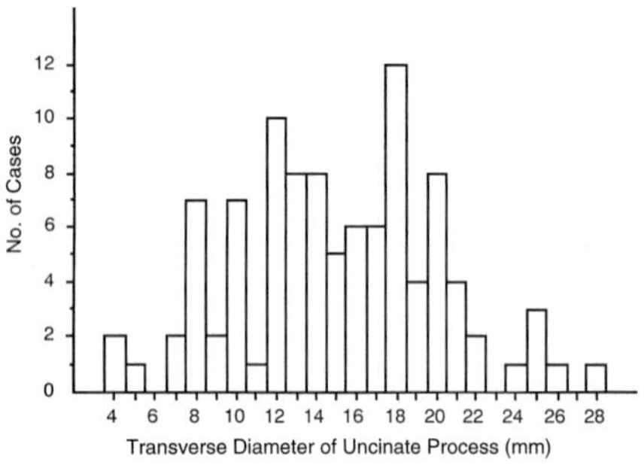

Figure 3. Histogram depicts the transverse diameter of the uncinate process in 101 patients with normal intestinal rotation.

Results for Patients with Intestinal Nonrotation

Patient No./ Age (y)/Sex	Transverse Diameter (mm) of Uncinate Process	Inversion of Superior Mesenteric Vein and Artery
1/26/F	0	Yes
2/62/F	0	Yes
3/66/M	0	Yes
4/23/M	4	Yes
5/61/F	6	No

DISCUSSION

The pancreatic primordium consists of a dorsal bud in the mesoduodenum and a ventral bud below the primordial liver. The ventral bud is composed of right and left lobes. These primordia rotate in accordance with the rotation of the bowel loop and finally occupy the expected location. The dorsal bud gives rise to the upper part of the head, the isthmus, the body, and the tail of the pancreas. The left ventral bud regresses completely. The right ventral bud develops into the lower part of the head and the uncinate process (7,8). The pancreatic uncinate process is a lower portion of the pancreatic head that lies dorsal to the superior mesenteric vessels.

Congenital abnormalities of the pancreas include pancreas divisum, annular pancreas, and agenesis of the dorsal pancreas (9,10). These abnormalities may occur in association with abnormal situs, polysplenia, or intestinal malrotation (9). Because the development of the pancreas is intimately related to rotation of the duodenojejunal loop in the embryo (7–9), abnormal rotation of the intestine may interrupt the normal rotation of the pancreatic primordia, with malpositioning of the pancreatic buds. Malpositioning of the

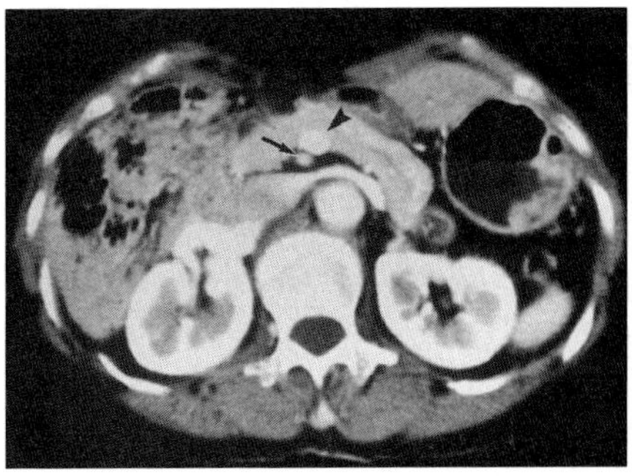

4.

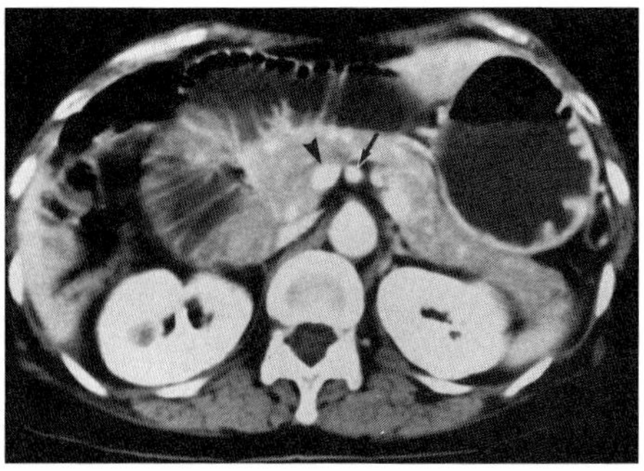

5.

Figures 4, 5. **(4) Patient 2.** CT scan does not depict the uncinate process. Note that the superior mesenteric artery (arrow) is slightly to the right of the superior mesenteric vein (arrowhead). **(5) Patient 5.** CT scan depicts an unusually small uncinate process, with a transverse diameter of 6 mm. The superior mesenteric artery (arrow) is in the normal position to the left of the superior mesenteric vein (arrowhead).

ventral buds may result in abnormal morphology of the uncinate process.

Among the control group in this study, only three (3%) of 101 patients had hypoplasia of the uncinate process, and no patient had aplasia. In contrast, all five (100%) patients with intestinal nonrotation had aplasia and hypoplasia of the uncinate process. These results suggest a close association between intestinal nonrotation and aplasia or hypoplasia of the uncinate process. The pancreatic head appeared normal except for the presence of aplasia and hypoplasia of the uncinate process in the patients with intestinal nonrotation. This finding may reflect partial rotation of the ventral buds.

The superior mesenteric vein is usually positioned to the right of the superior mesenteric artery. Although inversion of this relationship may be associated with intestinal malrotation, this sign is not always pathognomonic for malrotation (4,5). Four (80%) of our five patients with intestinal nonrotation had mesenteric vascular inversion. In three (75%) of these four patients, no uncinate process was depicted at CT. Patient 5 had a normal mesenteric vascular relationship but a small uncinate process. Mesenteric vascular inversion may further effect malpositioning of the pancreatic ventral bud in patients with intestinal nonrotation.

Various factors may influence the contour and thickness of the pancreas. Uneven fatty replacement of the pancreas is a pathologic finding seen increasingly in adults as their age and weight increase and may result in morphologic changes in the uncinate process. The posterior aspect of the head and the uncinate process of the pancreas, however, tend to be spared from fatty replacement (11). All parts of the pancreas tend to be smaller in diabetic patients than in healthy subjects. This reduction in size is not caused by diffuse atrophy. The pancreatic polypeptide-rich part of the head of the pancreas, which is derived from the embryologic ventral bud, is entirely preserved, and the atrophy is limited to the pancreatic polypeptide-poor lobe derived from the dorsal bud. In healthy subjects, the size of the pancreas does not change with age (12,13). In pancreas divisum, the most common abnormality of the pancreas, the dorsal and ventral pancreatic ducts fail to fuse, but the head and uncinate process are normal or enlarged (14). In our study, patient age and weight had no statistically significant effect on the transverse diameter of the uncinate process. Therefore, the uncinate process may be the portion of the pancreas that is least affected by atrophy.

A spectrum of patterns of fusion of the dorsal and ventral pancreatic buds may cause normal variation in the lateral contour of the pancreatic head and neck. These variants, which were seen in 34.5% of 119 healthy subjects, include discrete lobulation oriented posteriorly (19%), anteriorly (10%), and horizontally (5%) (15). In our study, there was a great difference in the rate of hypoplasia or aplasia of the uncinate process between the study and control groups. Therefore, although an absent or small uncinate process can be a normal variant, we think that hypoplasia or aplasia of the uncinate process in patients with intestinal nonrotation is not just a normal variant but rather is associated with the nonrotation.

In our study, no patient underwent endoscopic retrograde cholangiopancreatography because there was no indication for this study. The diagnosis of aplasia or hypoplasia of the uncinate process was made on the basis of the contour of the pancreatic head at CT. Findings at endoscopic retrograde cholangiopancreatography may help to further confirm a diagnosis of aplasia or hypoplasia of the uncinate process by enabling observation of the pancreatic ductal system.

The findings in this study, which focused on the uncinate process in patients with intestinal nonrotation, may not be applicable to patients with other types of malrotation. We believe that the morphology of the pancreatic uncinate process should be evaluated in patients with other types of nonrotation and in association with mesenteric vascular relationships. ■

References

1. Andrassy RJ, Mahour GH. Malrotation of the midgut in infants and children: a 25-year review. Arch Surg 1981; 116:158–160.
2. Wang CA, Welch CE. Anomalies of intestinal rotation in adolescents and adults. Surgery 1963; 54:839–855.
3. Nichols DM, Li DK. Superior mesenteric vein rotation: a CT sign of midgut malrotation. AJR 1983; 141:707–708.
4. Zerin JM, DiPietro MA. Mesenteric vascular anatomy at CT: normal and abnormal appearances. Radiology 1991; 179:739–742.
5. Zerin JM, DiPietro MA. Superior mesenteric vascular anatomy at US in patients with surgically proved malrotation of the midgut. Radiology 1992; 183:693–694.
6. Weinberger E, Winters WD, Liddell RM, Rosenbaum DM, Krauter D. Sonographic diagnosis of intestinal malrotation in infants: importance of the relative positions of the superior mesenteric vein and artery. AJR 1992; 159:825–828.
7. Snyder Jr WH, Chaffin L. Embryology and pathology of the intestinal tract: presentation of 40 cases of malrotation. Ann Surg 1954; 140:368–379.
8. Adda G, Hannoun L, Loygue J. Development of the human pancreas: variations and pathology—a tentative classification. Anat Clin 1984; 5:275–283.
9. Adeyemi SD. Combination of annular pancreas and partial situs inversus: a multiple organ syndrome associated with duodenal obstruction. J Pediatr Surg 1988; 23: 188–191.
10. Rizzo RJ, Szucs RA, Turner MA. Congenital abnormalities of the pancreas and biliary tree in adults. RadioGraphics 1995; 15: 49–68.
11. Matsumoto S, Mori H, Miyake H. Uneven fatty replacement of the pancreas: evaluation with CT. Radiology 1995; 194:453–458.
12. Rahier J, Wallon J, Loozen S, Lefevre A, Gepts W, Haot J. The pancreatic polypeptide cells in the human pancreas: the effect of age and diabetes. J Clin Endocrinol Metab 1983; 56:441–444.
13. Gilbeau JP, Poncelet V, Libon E, Derue G, Heller FR. The density, contour, and thickness of the pancreas in diabetics: CT findings in 57 patients. AJR 1992; 159:527–531.
14. Soulen MC, Zerhouni EA, Fishman EK, Gayler BW, Milligan F, Siegelman SS. Enlargement of the pancreatic head in patients with pancreas divisum. Clin Imaging 1989; 13:51–57.
15. Ross BA, Jeffrey RB, Mindelzun RE. Normal variations in the lateral contour of the head and neck of the pancreas mimicking neoplasm: evaluation with dual-phase helical CT. AJR 1996; 166:799–801.

Sum & Substance

Polyposis: The Peutz-Jeghers Syndrome.
A. D. Spigelman, P. Arese, R. K. S. Phillips. *Br J Surg* 1995; 82:1311–1314. (R.K.S.P., Polyposis Registry, St Mark's Hospital, Northwick Park, Harrow, Middlesex HA1 3JU, England.)

Peutz-Jeghers syndrome is a rare, inherited condition (probably autosomal dominant), characterized by melanin spots. These flat cutaneous lesions, located mainly in the perioral region, buccal mucosa, hands, and feet, become noticeable in the first few years of life.

Hamartomatous polyps are the predominant gastrointestinal manifestation. They may bleed, acutely or chronically, and they frequently intussuscept. Polyps have been found in the entire gastrointestinal tract, except for the mouth; those reported in the esophagus have not been sampled for biopsy. The site most frequently affected is the small bowel. The polyps are hamartomas of the smooth muscle, which extends, treelike, into the lamina propria. They are usually broad based, varying in size from a few millimeters to several centimeters.

About 10% of polyps in the small bowel show epithelial islands within and deep to the submucosa, suggesting an invasive lesion. This benign "pseudoinvasion" can be diagnosed without accompanying irregularities, in the presence of normal epithelial subtypes with a brush border.

Two large studies have shown a high relative risk for both intestinal and gastrointestinal malignancy. Survival was affected, with the risk of death from cancer approaching 40% by 40 years of age. The transformation of some hamartomas into dysplastic (adenomatous) polyps and cancer was clearly documented, suggesting the possibility of a hamartoma-adenoma-carcinoma sequence. Malignant tumors may also arise de novo or from coexisting adenomas. The relative importance of hamartomas and these other mechanisms in intestinal carcinogenesis remains unclear.

An increased risk of extraintestinal tumor development has also been described in studies using life-table analysis. This finding suggests an associated diffuse cancer risk. Gynecologic tumors have a genuine association with Peutz-Jeghers syndrome, especially sex cord tumors of the annular tubules and adenoma malignum of the cervix. Feminizing Sertoli cell tumor of the testis, otherwise rare, also occurs in this syndrome, as do bilateral breast cancer and pancreatic cancer. The cancer risk will be better understood after the sites of inherited abnormality in Peutz-Jeghers syndrome are identified.

Surgical management typically consists of multiple laparotomies performed at frequent intervals. Polypectomy performed through small enterotomies has been made more effective by the use of perioperative enteroscopy. Endoscopy is also used in the treatment of gastroduodenal and colonic polyps; "top and tail" endoscopy is generally performed every 2 years, with removal of polyps larger than 0.5 cm.

RSNA Publications

Moon-June Cho, MD • Chul S. Ha, MD • Pamela K. Allen, MPH • Lillian M. Fuller, MD
Fernando Cabanillas, MD • James D. Cox, MD

Primary Non-Hodgkin Lymphoma of the Large Bowel[1]

PURPOSE: **To characterize the natural history of primary non-Hodgkin lymphoma of the large bowel and identify prognostic factors.**

MATERIALS AND METHODS: **Twenty-three patients with primary non-Hodgkin lymphoma according to strict criteria were identified. Seventeen patients underwent resection, and six patients underwent biopsy. Among 19 patients with intermediate- or high-grade lymphoma, 13 had diffuse large cell lymphoma. Ann Arbor stage was I in 15 cases, II in seven cases, and IV in one case. In 15 patients, the International Prognostic Index was available: 0, eight patients; 1, six patients; and 3, one patient. Postoperatively, six patients received combined chemotherapy and radiation therapy, eight patients received chemotherapy, and six patients received radiation therapy. Overall and relapse-free survival were calculated actuarially, and univariate analysis was performed with regard to stage, treatment, extent of surgery, and the International Prognostic Index.**

RESULTS: **Median follow-up was 144 months. Two patients' disease recurred. Overall and relapse-free survival at 10 years were 61% and 82%, respectively. The International Prognostic Index was the only significant prognostic factor for overall survival (*P* = .03, log-rank test).**

CONCLUSION: **The prognosis of primary non-Hodgkin lymphoma appears to be as good as that of low- or intermediate-grade lymphoma. The only significant prognostic factor for overall survival is the International Prognostic Index.**

PRIMARY non-Hodgkin lymphoma of the large bowel is rare; secondary involvement of this disease in the large bowel is undoubtedly more frequent. Primary gastrointestinal lymphoma accounts for 4%–20% of all cases of non-Hodgkin lymphoma, and large-bowel involvement accounts for about 10%–20% of cases in most studies of gastrointestinal lymphoma (1–5). The most common treatment has been resection of the primary disease followed with adjuvant radiation therapy, chemotherapy, or both (1,4,6–10). However, a substantial number of studies have reported on primary large-bowel lymphoma as only a subset of a larger series of gastrointestinal lymphoma or have included patients with secondary large-bowel involvement of more diffuse and generalized lymphomas (7). Only a few small studies of patients with primary large-bowel lymphoma defined with more strict criteria have been reported (5,11). The purpose of this study was to clarify the natural history of primary large-bowel lymphoma, identify preferred treatments of the disease, and delineate major prognostic factors.

MATERIALS AND METHODS

Patient Selection

The medical records of all patients with lymphomatous involvement of the large bowel evaluated at our institution between 1946 and 1993 were reviewed; 54 patients were identified. Patients with antibodies to human immunodeficiency virus and patients with primary mesenteric lymphoma in the colon were excluded. Patients with lymphoma in the ileocecal region were also excluded because their lesions more likely arose from the ileum than the cecum. In 29 patients, the features of disease met the criteria of Dawson et al (12) for primary large-bowel lymphoma; these criteria were no superficial adenopathy at the time of diagnosis, no mediastinal adenopathy seen on chest radiographs, a normal blood cell count, no liver or spleen involvement, and disease in only regional lymph nodes at laparotomy. Patients with inguinal lymph-node involvement were included on the basis of the recommendation at the Fifth International Conference on Malignant Lymphoma (13). Excluded from the study were six patients who received radiation therapy outside our institution or chemotherapy outside our institution in a manner not in accordance with our institutional policies and/or recommendations at the time. Patients who received chemotherapy at another institution in a manner in accordance with our policies and/or recommendations were included. Therefore, 23 patients were included in this study.

Pretreatment Evaluation and Staging

All patients underwent resection or biopsy of the primary lesion at our institution. All pathologic specimens were reviewed and classified with use of the Working Formulation (14). The staging of disease evolved over the time of the study. A thorough medical history was obtained from all patients. All patients underwent physical examination, chest radiography, and analysis of serum chemistry levels and complete blood cell count. Sixteen patients

Index terms: Intestinal neoplasms, 75.343 • Lymphoma, 75.343 • Lymphoma, therapy, 75.343

Radiology 1997; 205:535–539

[1] From the Departments of Radiation Oncology (M.J.C., C.S.H., P.K.A., L.M.F., J.D.C.) and Hematology (F.C.), The M.D. Anderson Cancer Center, University of Texas, 1515 Holcombe Blvd, Box 97, Houston, TX 77030. From the 1996 RSNA scientific assembly. Received February 21, 1997; revision requested March 26; revision received June 16; accepted June 19. **Address reprint requests to** C.S.H.

underwent bone marrow biopsy and/or aspiration. All but one patient underwent evaluation of the abdomen and pelvis with laparotomy ($n = 13$), lymphangiography ($n = 18$), or computed tomography (CT) ($n = 11$). The patient who did not undergo imaging of the abdomen and pelvis had a rectal polyp, which was removed completely.

The Ann Arbor staging system was used (15). The International Prognostic Index was assigned as described (16). This index is the number of the following prognostic variables exhibited at the time of patient presentation: age, greater than 60 years; Ann Arbor stage, III or IV; number of extranodal sites with disease, greater than one; performance status score according to the Eastern Cooperative Oncology Group, 2 or greater; and serum lactate dehydrogenase level, above the upper limit of normal. In 15 cases, there was sufficient information to determine the International Prognostic Index.

Patient Characteristics

The patient characteristics, treatments received, and outcomes are summarized in the Table. There were 17 male and six female patients in this study. Patient ages ranged from 11 to 86 years (median, 44 years). The most common presenting symptoms were blood in the stool ($n = 10$ [43%]); abdominal pain ($n = 7$ [30%]); weight loss ($n = 2$ [9%]); and diarrhea, constipation, or change in bowel habit ($n = 4$ [17%]). One patient had had ulcerative colitis; another patient had had squamous cell carcinoma of the anus and uterine cervix and adenocarcinoma of the colon.

The histologic grades of most lesions were intermediate to high. The histologic subtypes were diffuse large cell lymphoma ($n = 13$ [57%]); diffuse small noncleaved cell lymphoma ($n = 4$ [17%]); follicular lymphoma ($n = 3$ [13%]); lymphoblastic lymphoma ($n = 1$ [4%]); diffuse small cleaved cell lymphoma ($n = 1$ [4%]); and small lymphocytic lymphoma ($n = 1$ [4%]). The primary sites of involvement were the rectum ($n = 8$ [35%]), the cecum ($n = 4$ [17%]), the appendix ($n = 3$ [13%]), and the rest of the colon ($n = 8$ [35%]). In two patients, disease was in multiple areas of the large bowel. Staging with the Ann Arbor system was as follows: stage I, 15 patients; stage II, seven patients; and stage IV (owing to bone marrow involvement with divergent histologic findings), one patient.

Treatment

Seventeen patients underwent resection of all gross disease, and six patients underwent biopsy only. Postoperative treatments were the following: combined chemotherapy and radiation therapy ($n = 6$), chemotherapy alone ($n = 8$), and radiation therapy alone ($n = 6$). The three patients who did not undergo chemotherapy or radiation therapy were observed: One patient underwent complete resection of primary diffuse large cell lymphoma at the hepatic flexure of the colon; one patient underwent abdominoperineal resection of primary diffuse large cell lymphoma of the rectum; and one patient underwent polypectomy of small lymphocytic lymphoma. When combined chemotherapy and radiation therapy was given, chemotherapy was always administered first. Radiation therapy was sometimes administered between treatment cycles of chemotherapy. Radiation was delivered with either cobalt-60 gamma rays or linear accelerators in all but one case. In this case (before 1960), 220-kVp x rays were administered. The strip-field technique or opposed anterior-posterior fields were used as described (17) (Table). Every patient but two with disease above the peritoneal reflection line underwent whole abdominopelvic radiation therapy; the other two patients underwent involved-field radiation therapy or involved-field and paraaortic-field radiation therapy. Every patient but one with disease below the peritoneal reflection line underwent whole-pelvic radiation therapy; the other patient underwent paraaortic-field radiation therapy. The radiation doses ranged from 20 to 60 Gy (median, 30 Gy) at 1.5–2.0 Gy per fraction, 5 days a week. A boost dose was administered to four patients.

Several different chemotherapy regimens were used. Regimens with doxorubicin were administered to 13 of the 14 patients who received chemotherapy. Regimens used were the following: cyclophosphamide, doxorubicin, vincristine, and prednisone (or CHOP) (18), three patients; cyclophosphamide, doxorubicin, vincristine, prednisone, and bleomycin (or CHOP-bleo) (19), five patients; cyclophosphamide, doxorubicin, vincristine, prednisone, and bleomycin (or CHOP-bleo) alternating with vincristine, prednisone, etoposide, and mitoxantrone (or OPEN) (20), one patient; cyclophosphamide, doxorubicin, vincristine, dexamethasone, and bleomycin (or CHOD-bleo) alternating with dexamethasone, cytosine arabinoside, and cisplatin (or DAP) (21), one patient; methotrexate, cyclophosphamide, vincristine, and prednisone (or MCOP) alternating with (*a*) cyclophosphamide, methotrexate, etoposide, and dexamethasone (or CMED) and (*b*) doxorubicin, vincristine, cytosine arabinoside, prednisone, and bleomycin (or HOAP-bleo) (22), one patient; methotrexate, cyclophosphamide, vincristine, and prednisone (or MCOP) alternating with (*a*) ifosfamide, methotrexate, and etoposide (or IMVP-16) and (*b*) doxorubicin, vincristine, cytosine arabinoside, prednisone, and bleomycin (or HOAP-bleo) (22), one patient; doxorubicin, methylprednisolone, cytosine arabinoside, and cisplatin (or ASHAP) alternating with (*a*) methotrexate, bleomycin, doxorubicin, cyclophosphamide, vincristine, and methylprednisolone (or MBACOS) and (*b*) mesna, ifosfamide, mitoxantrone, and etoposide (or MINE), one patient; and cyclophosphamide, vincristine, and prednisone (or COP) (23), one patient. The number of treatment cycles of chemotherapy ranged from one to 16 (median, six). Only one patient underwent fewer than three treatment cycles.

Assessment of Response to Treatment

Patients were followed up at regular intervals after completion of treatment according to our institution's lymphoma-service policy.

The follow-up intervals were usually every 3–4 months during the first 2 years, every 6 months during the next 2 years, and yearly thereafter. At follow-up, a complete medical history was obtained and the patient underwent physical examination, analysis of serum chemistry levels and complete blood cell count, chest radiography, and abdominopelvic imaging with CT or lymphangiography. If patients could not return for follow-up visits, follow-up information was obtained by correspondence or telephone.

Statistical Analysis

Survival data were calculated actuarially with use of the Kaplan-Meier survival curve (24). A relapse-free survival of zero was assigned to patients who never achieved complete remission. Univariate analyses of overall survival data and relapse-free survival data were performed to determine prognostic factors. The log-rank test was used to determine significant differences between subgroups. Multivariate analysis could not be performed due to the small number of patients.

RESULTS

Fourteen patients were alive at the time of the last follow-up. Median follow-up for living patients was 144 months (range, 14–413 months). The disease of two patients recurred. One patient had diffuse large cell lymphoma of the rectum that extended to the pelvic wall, which did not respond to initial chemotherapy after biopsy. This patient's disease responded considerably to pelvic radiation therapy; however, the disease progressed locally soon thereafter. The other patient underwent surgical resection of a diffuse large cell lymphoma of the appendix that progressed locally during chemotherapy. This patient then underwent regional radiation therapy and additional chemotherapy; however, spinal metastases developed during chemotherapy. Both patients died of lymphoma. The cause of death was not well documented for two other patients. The disease of both of these patients responded completely to initial treatment. For the calculation of overall survival and relapse-free survival, however, we considered their disease to be recurrent at the time of death.

The 10-year overall and relapse-free survival rates for all patients were 61% and 82%, respectively (Fig 1). The

Patient Characteristics, Treatments, and Outcomes

Patient No.	Age (y)/ Sex	Presenting Symptom	Primary Site	IPI*	Lymphoma Type	Stage	Resection Performed	Chemotherapy†	Radiation Therapy	Status	Comments
1	50/F	Abdominal pain	Colon	NA	Diffuse large cell	I	Yes	None	None	No evidence of disease at 351 mo	
2	56/M	Bloody stool	Rectum	NA	Diffuse small cleaved cell	IA	Yes	None	Pelvic and paraaortic	Died with no evidence of disease at 268 mo	Died of duodenal perforation
3	30/F	Abdominal discomfort	Cecum	NA	Lymphoblastic	IIA	Yes	None	Whole abdominopelvic	No evidence of disease at 413 mo	
4	11/M	Weight loss	Colon	NA	Diffuse small noncleaved cell	IIB	Yes	None	Whole abdominopelvic	No evidence of disease at 375 mo	
5	25/M	Abdominal pain	Appendix	NA	Diffuse large cell	IA	Yes	None	Whole abdominopelvic with boost dose	No evidence of disease at 329 mo	
6	33/M	Bloody stool	Anorectum	NA	Diffuse large cell	IA	Yes	None	Pelvic with boost dose	No evidence of disease at 309 mo	
7	26/M	Abdominal pain	Colon	0	Diffuse large cell	IA	Yes	COP	Whole abdominopelvic with boost dose	Died with no evidence of disease at 110 mo	Died of cholangiocarcinoma
8	69/M	Bloody stool	Colon	NA	Follicular mixed‡	IIA	Yes	None	Whole abdominopelvic	Died with no evidence of disease at 8 mo	Died of upper gastrointestinal bleeding
9	68/M	Abdominal pain, bloody stool	Appendix	1	Diffuse large cell	IA	Yes	CHOP and bleomycin	Involved-field (right lower quadrant) and paraaortic	Died of disease at 35 mo	Disease recurred at primary site and spine§
10	86/F	Bloody stool	Rectum	1	Diffuse large cell	IA	No	CHOP	Pelvic and boost dose	Died with no evidence of disease at 30 mo	Died of fall and hip fracture
11	43/M	Bowel-habit change	Rectum	0	Diffuse small noncleaved cell	IA	No	CHOP and bleomycin	None	No evidence of disease at 197 mo	
12	59/M	Constipation, bloody stool	Rectum	0	Diffuse large cell	IA	Yes	None	None	Died at 7 mo	Cause of death unknown
13	22/M	Abdominal pain	Appendix	0	Diffuse small noncleaved cell	IA	Yes	MCOP, IMVP-16, HOAP-B	None	No evidence of disease at 80 mo	
14	55/M	Weight loss	Colon	0	Follicular mixed‡	IIB	Yes	CHOP and bleomycin	Whole abdominopelvic and inguinal	No evidence of disease at 148 mo	
15	18/M	Abdominal pain	Colon	0	Diffuse small noncleaved cell	IIA	Yes	MCOP, CMED, HOAP-B	None	No evidence of disease at 139 mo	
16	28/M	Abdominal mass	Cecum	NA	Diffuse large cell	IIA	Yes	CHOP and bleomycin	Involved-field	No evidence of disease at 52 mo	
17	63/M	Bloody stool	Rectum	1	Diffuse large cell	IA	No	CHOP and bleomycin	Pelvic	Died of disease at 6 mo	Disease progressed at primary site§
18	44/F	Bloody stool	Rectosigmoid colon	3	Follicular small cleaved cell‖	IVA	No	CHOD and bleomycin, DAP	None	Died with no evidence of disease at 32 mo	Died of cardiac disease and chronic obstructive pulmonary disease
19	47/F	Bloody stool, diarrhea	Rectum	1	Diffuse large cell	IIA	No	ASHAP, MBACOS, MINE	None	No evidence of disease at 68 mo	
20	59/F	Diarrhea	Rectum	1	Diffuse large cell	IB	No	CHOP	None	Died at 9 mo	History of squamous cell carcinoma of the anus and cervix and adenocarcinoma of the colon, cause of death unknown
21	39/M	Abdominal pain	Cecum	0	Diffuse large cell	IA	Yes	CHOP and bleomycin, OPEN	None	No evidence of disease at 46 mo	
22	40/M	Bloody stool	Rectum	0	Diffuse large cell	IA	Yes	CHOP	None	No evidence of disease at 15 mo	
23	70/M	Mild fever	Cecum	1	Small lymphocytic	IA	Yes	None	None	No evidence of disease at 21 mo	

* IPI = International Prognostic Index, NA = not available.

† ASHAP = doxorubicin, methylprednisolone, cytosine arabinoside, and cisplatin; CHOD = cyclophosphamide, doxorubicin, vincristine, and dexamethasone; CHOP = cyclophosphamide, doxorubicin, vincristine, and prednisone; CMED = cyclophosphamide, methotrexate, etoposide, and dexamethasone; COP = cyclophosphamide, vincristine, and prednisone; DAP = dexamethasone, cytosine arabinoside, and cisplatin; HOAP-B = doxorubicin, vincristine, cytosine arabinoside, prednisone, and bleomycin; IMVP-16 = ifosfamide, methotrexate, and etoposide; MBACOS = methotrexate, bleomycin, doxorubicin, cyclophosphamide, vincristine, and methylprednisolone; MCOP = methotrexate, cyclophosphamide, vincristine, and prednisone; MINE = mesna, ifosfamide, mitoxantrone hydrochloride, and etoposide; OPEN = vincristine, prednisone, etoposide, and mitoxantrone.

‡ Follicular mixed small cleaved and large cell.

§ Relapse-free survival = 0.

‖ Large cleaved cell lymphoma in bone marrow.

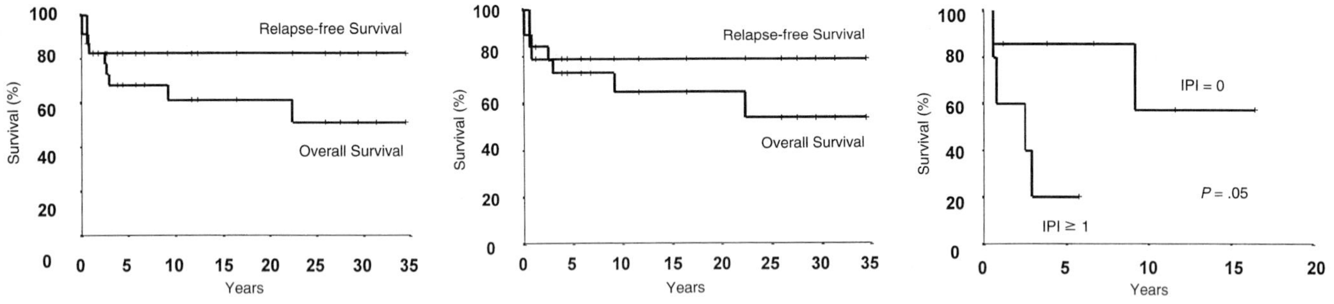

1. 2. 3.

Figures 1–3. **(1)** Overall and relapse-free survival of all patients. **(2)** Overall and relapse-free survival of patients with intermediate- and high-grade lymphoma. **(3)** Overall survival of patients with intermediate- and high-grade lymphoma as a function of the International Prognostic Index (*IPI*).

10-year overall and relapse-free survival rates for the 19 patients with intermediate- or high-grade lymphoma were 65% and 79%, respectively (Fig 2). Subgroup analyses were performed to compare the overall and relapse-free survival rates with respect to staging (I vs II), treatment modality, surgery (gross resection vs biopsy), and the International Prognostic Index. Comparison of survival rates with regard to the value of the International Prognostic Index was the only comparison that yielded a statistically significant result. The overall survival rate of patients with scores of 0 was significantly higher than that of patients with scores of 1 or greater (P = .03 for all patients, P = .05 for patients with intermediate- and high-grade lymphoma; log-rank test) (Fig 3).

Radiation therapy was generally well tolerated; treatment was not interrupted substantially as a result of side effects. The expected side effects of chemotherapy—such as low blood cell count and nausea and vomiting—were experienced, and doses were adjusted as indicated. Two patients died of possible gastrointestinal sequelae. One patient died of a perforated duodenal ulcer, and the other patient died of massive upper gastrointestinal bleeding; in this patient, there was no evidence of lymphoma at laparotomy. The patient who died of a perforated duodenal ulcer was the only patient who underwent radiation therapy with 220-kVp x rays. This patient received 24 Gy to the pelvis and paraaortic region in 26 fractions over 36 days. The patient who died of upper gastrointestinal bleeding received 30 Gy in 20 fractions to the upper two-thirds of the abdomen over 26 days and then to the pelvis over 29 days. A pair of opposed anterior-posterior fields was irradiated each day with Co-60 gamma rays. One patient died of cholangiocarcinoma 9 years after treatment. A fourth patient died of heart disease and chronic obstructive pulmonary disease. This patient had had hypertension. None of these deaths was clearly attributable to complications of treatment; however, the cholangiocarcinoma could have been radiation induced, and heart disease and chronic obstructive pulmonary disease could have resulted from chemotherapy toxicity.

DISCUSSION

We studied the experience at a single institution to define the natural history and optimum treatment of primary large-bowel lymphoma and delineate its prognostic factors. The histologic grade of most (83%) of our cases of primary large-bowel lymphoma was intermediate or high. This finding is corroborated with a number of other reports (1,5,7,11). We also noted a preponderance of male patients among our group of patients with primary large-bowel lymphoma; this finding is consistent with those in other series. Before the use of combination chemotherapy, surgical resection followed by radiation therapy was the cornerstone of treatment of regionally confined primary large-bowel lymphoma. However, the rate of distant failures was high with this treatment, and therapy has changed in the era of combined modalities (7,25,26).

Since its introduction, combined-modality therapy in patients with intermediate- or high-grade non-Hodgkin lymphoma has yielded superior survival to that associated with radiation therapy alone; this finding is supported with a number of other studies (27,28). Since the early 1970s, physicians at our institution have strongly favored use of combined-modality therapy in intermediate- or high-grade non-Hodgkin lymphoma—including primary large-bowel lymphoma. In our series, there were no apparent differences in overall and relapse-free survival rates among patients who received radiation therapy alone, chemotherapy alone, or combined-modality therapy. This observation could be due to the small number of patients in each group who were treated for a long time.

The only significant prognostic factor that allowed determination of overall survival was the International Prognostic Index; none of the variables we analyzed was significantly related to relapse-free survival. Factors such as local extension of disease, lymph-node involvement, and operability have been reported to be of prognostic importance (7,9,29). However, we could not perform a meaningful analysis with these variables owing to the small number of treatment failures in our study. The prognostic value of the International Prognostic Index in treatment of intermediate- and high-grade non-Hodgkin lymphoma has been demonstrated by Shipp et al (16). Our data concur with those of Shipp et al; overall survival of patients with a score of 0 was significantly different from that of patients with a score greater than 0. This difference can be attributed mainly to the older ages of the patients with an International Prognostic Index greater than 0.

Analysis of treatment failures revealed that one patient's disease recurred at the primary site only and another patient's disease recurred at the primary site and in the spine. Again, it is difficult to make any generalizations about the patterns of failures with regard to specific treatments because the number of failures were small.

Some authors have indicated that the prognosis of primary large-bowel lymphoma is worse than that of other types of non-Hodgkin lymphoma (5,7). However, our data suggest that the prognosis of primary large-bowel lymphoma is as good as that of any low- or intermediate-grade lymphoma when our data are compared with representative data from our institution and others (19,27,30). The reason for this discrepancy is not clear and could be simply statistical because of the small numbers of patients in each series, including ours. Also, different definitions of primary large-bowel lymphoma may have been used. The natural history of secondary large-bowel involvement of mesenteric, ileocecal, or more generalized lymphoma is probably different from that of primary large-bowel lymphoma (7).

The best treatment for primary large-bowel lymphoma has not been clearly established, but the current approach at our institution is the following: If the patient has surgically correctable symptoms (such as obstruction), laparotomy with surgical resection is the first choice of treatment (7). Resection provides tissue for pathologic diagnosis, alleviates symptoms, and reduces tumor burden (31). Otherwise, biopsy followed with combined-modality therapy is a reasonable option. Chemotherapy usually includes doxorubicin. Involved-field radiation is usually used; microscopic disease is treated to 30.6 Gy, and gross disease is treated to 39.6 Gy at 1.8 Gy per fraction. In recent years, a trend to treat primary large-bowel lymphoma with chemotherapy alone has been noted; in our study, no disease treated with chemotherapy alone has recurred to date. The follow-up of these patients, however, was shorter than that of the others. Longer observation of more patients would ensure that the prognosis of these patients is as good as that of those who undergo combined-modality therapy. ■

Acknowledgments: We thank James J. Butler, MD, William C. Pugh, MD, Barbara Osborne, MD, and John T. Manning, MD, for reviewing the pathologic specimens.

References

1. d'Amore F, Brincker H, Grønbaek K, et al. Non-Hodgkin's lymphoma of the gastrointestinal tract: a population-based analysis of incidence, geographic distribution, clinicopathologic presentation features, and prognosis. J Clin Oncol 1994; 12:1673–1684.
2. Herrmann R, Panahon AM, Barcos MP, Walsh D, Stutzman L. Gastrointestinal involvement in non-Hodgkin's lymphoma. Cancer 1980; 46:215–222.
3. Lewin KJ, Ranchod M, Dorfman RF. Lymphomas of the gastrointestinal tract. Cancer 1978; 42:693–707.
4. Salles G, Herbrecht R, Tilly H, et al. Aggressive primary gastrointestinal lymphomas: review of 91 patients treated with the LNH-84 regimen—a study of the Groupe d'Etude des Lymphomes Agressifs. Am J Med 1991; 90:77–84.
5. Zighelboim Z, Larson MV. Primary colonic lymphoma: clinical presentation, histopathologic features, and outcome with combination chemotherapy. J Clin Gastroenterol 1994; 18:291–297.
6. Renard TH, Morton RL, Mathews R, Poulos E. Primary lymphoma of the rectum. Am Surg 1992; 58:634–637.
7. Richards MA. Lymphoma of the colon and rectum. Postgrad Med J 1986; 62:615–620.
8. Wychulis A, Beahrs OH, Woolner LB. Malignant lymphoma of the colon. Arch Surg 1966; 93:215–225.
9. Blackledge G, Bush H, Dodge OG, Crowther D. A study of gastro-intestinal lymphoma. Clin Oncol 1979; 5:209–219.
10. Gospodarowicz MK, Sutcliffe SB. The extranodal lymphomas. Semin Radiat Oncol 1995; 5:281–300.
11. Shepherd NA, Hall PA, Coates PJ, Levison DA. Primary malignant lymphoma of the colon and rectum: a histopathological and immunohistochemical analysis of 45 cases with clinicopathological correlations. Histopathology 1988; 12:235–252.
12. Dawson IM, Cornes JS, Morson BC. Primary malignant lymphoid tumours of the intestinal tract. Br J Surg 1961; 49:80–89.
13. Rohatiner A, d'Amore F, Coiffier B, et al. Report on a workshop convened to discuss the pathological and staging classifications of gastrointestinal lymphoma. Ann Oncol 1994; 5:388–400.
14. The Non-Hodgkin's Lymphoma Pathologic Classification Project. National Cancer Institute sponsored study of classifications of non-Hodgkin's lymphomas: summary and description of a working formulation for clinical usage. Cancer 1982; 49:2112–2135.
15. Non-Hodgkin's lymphoma. In: Beahrs OH, Henson DE, Hutter RVP, Kennedy BJ, eds. Manual for staging of cancer. 4th ed. Philadelphia, Pa: Lippincott, 1992; 257–259.
16. The International Non-Hodgkin's Lymphoma Prognostic Factors Project (Shipp MA, Harrington DP, Anderson JR, et al). A predictive model for aggressive Non-Hodgkin's lymphoma. N Engl J Med 1993; 329:987–994.
17. Million R. Non-Hodgkin's lymphoma. In: Fletcher GH, ed. Textbook of radiotherapy. 3rd ed. Philadelphia, Pa: Lea & Febiger, 1980; 621–636.
18. Fisher RI, Gaynor ER, Dahlberg S, et al. Comparison of a standard regimen (CHOP) with three intensive chemotherapy regimens for advanced non-Hodgkin's lymphoma. N Engl J Med 1993; 14:1002–1006.
19. Fuller LM, Krasin MJ, Velasquez WS, et al. Significance of tumor size and radiation dose to local control in stage I–III diffuse large cell lymphoma treated with CHOP-BLEO and radiation. Int J Radiat Oncol Biol Phys 1995; 31:3–11.
20. Swan F, Velasquez W, Fuller L, et al. Successful outcome of patients (PTS) with good risk large cell lymphoma (LCL) with a shortened schedule of treatment (RX) (abstr). Proc Am Soc Clin Oncol 1991; 10:273.
21. Avilés A, Delgado S, Nambo MJ, Alatriste S, Díaz-Maqueo JC. Adjuvant radiotherapy to sites of previous bulky disease in patients with stage IV diffuse large cell lymphoma. Int J Radiat Oncol Biol Phys 1994; 30:799–803.
22. Lopez TM, Hagemeister FB, McLaughlin P, et al. Small noncleaved cell lymphoma in adults: superior results for stages I–III disease. J Clin Oncol 1990; 8:615–622.
23. Coltman CA, Luce JK, McKelvey EM, Jones SE, Moon TE. Chemotherapy of non-Hodgkin's lymphoma: 10 years' experience in the Southwest Oncology Group. Cancer Treat Rep 1977; 61:1067–1078.
24. Kaplan EL, Meier P. Nonparametric estimation from incomplete observations. J Am Stat Assoc 1958; 53:457–481.
25. Lewin KJ, Ranchod M, Dorfman RF. Lymphomas of the gastrointestinal tract: a study of 117 cases presenting with gastrointestinal disease. Cancer 1978; 42:693–707.
26. Gospodarowicz MK, Sutcliffe SB, Clark RM. Outcome analysis of localized gastrointestinal lymphoma treated with surgery and postoperative irradiation. Int J Radiat Oncol Biol Phys 1990; 19:1351–1355.
27. Shafman TD, Mauch PM. The large-cell lymphomas. Semin Radiat Oncol 1995; 5:267–280.
28. Nissen NI, Ersbøll J, Hansen HS, et al. A randomized study of radiotherapy versus radiotherapy plus chemotherapy in stage I–II non-Hodgkin's lymphomas. Cancer 1983; 52:1–7.
29. Azab MB, Henry-Amar M, Rougier P, et al. Prognostic factors in primary gastrointestinal non-Hodgkin's lymphoma: a multivariate analysis, report of 106 cases, and review of the literature. Cancer 1989; 64:1208–1217.
30. Mendenhall NP, Lynch JW Jr. The low-grade lymphomas. Semin Radiat Oncol 1995; 5:254–266.
31. Romaguera JE, Velasquez WS, Silvermintz KB. Surgical debulking is associated with improved survival in stage I–II diffuse large cell lymphoma. Cancer 1990; 66:267–272.

Sum & Substance

Fibrous Dysplasia.
Robert P. Stanton, MD, Ben E. Montgomery, BS. *Orthopedics* 1996; 19:679–685. (R.P.S., c/o Editorial Services, Alfred I. duPont Institute, PO Box 269, Wilmington, DE 19899.)

Fibrous dysplasia, described in 1937 by Albright, may occur as an isolated bone abnormality or as part of Albright syndrome, which also features endocrinopathies and skin lesions. Fibrous dysplasia occurs throughout life, but most often it manifests between early childhood and adolescence. Boys and girls are affected; however, when associated with endocrinopathies, fibrous dysplasia is more common in girls.

The cause has not been precisely determined. Some molecular biologists theorize that the condition results from a gene mutation that occurs early in embryogenesis. Increased levels of a mutated gene product, abnormal G protein, in affected endocrine tissues support this view.

Histologic examination of bone in fibrous dysplasia reveals an immature matrix and inadequate mineralization. The matrix is composed of collagen, and, within it, small and irregularly shaped trabeculae of immature "woven" bone are created by osteoblasts; the histologic pattern often resembles letters of the Chinese alphabet. Because abnormal immature bone is formed, during growth, this abnormal bone is not replaced by mature lamellar bone. Depending on the amount of woven bone and the extent of its mineralization, these lesions appear variably lucent on radiographs. In bone, the proliferation of fibrous tissue and the process of metaplasia result in the extension of old lesions and the appearance of new ones, which cause progressive weakness and deformity. There is also expansion of lesions within the medullary canal, formation of cysts, and resorption of cortex. Endosteal scalloping, appearing as areas of cortical thinning with intervening areas of normal cortex, is the radiographic hallmark of fibrous dysplasia.

The histologic and radiographic appearances of fibrous dysplasia change with pathologic fracture or surgery. Bleeding, dense fibrosis, or transformation of woven bone into lamellar bone may be seen. Subperiosteal healing may occur, but endosteal healing does not.

In fibrous dysplasia, there are several, potentially unrelenting, mechanical consequences of bone lesions. In affected bones, the stresses of normal weight bearing are compounded and may cause deformity of limbs. Not only do pain and limping result, but recurrent, poorly healing fractures and further deformity occur. In addition, the articular surface is compromised, leading to premature onset of arthritis.

The clinical spectrum of fibrous dysplasia is wide. In an adult with unrelated symptoms or a child with mild symptoms, fibrous dysplasia may be detected incidentally on radiographs. When associated with endocrinopathies, the disease may manifest dramatically with menarche in infancy. The clinical course may be limited, or it may include progressive, debilitating pain and deformity. Although fibrous dysplasia most commonly involves the bones of the extremities—particularly the proximal femur—it may also affect the ribs, pelvis, and skull. Monostotic involvement is most often seen, but extensive involvement of nearly the entire skeleton can occur with severe forms of the illness. Patients most commonly experience pain, limping, discrepancy of leg length, tibial bowing, and other deformities—such as the extreme varus deformity of the proximal femur that resembles a shepherd's crook. Multiple pathologic fractures are common. When the skull base and paranasal sinuses are affected, asymmetric facies, blindness, headache, anosmia, and upper respiratory symptoms can occur.

Irregular, pigmented macules on the face, nape, or lower back may be a sign of Albright syndrome. These cafe au lait spots may be accompanied by any of the following effects of endocrinopathy: precocious puberty, acromegaly, thyrotoxicosis, growth retardation, renal stones, abnormal calcium deposition, osteoporosis, diabetes mellitus, acne, hirsutism, obesity, and muscle wasting or poor muscle development and control.

Because fibrous dysplasia cannot be prevented or cured, detection and treatment of early disease are critical. Treatment has included drugs, radiation therapy, gland resection, cryotherapy, and various orthopedic procedures; results have varied. Intravenously administered pamidronate has been proved to be successful in a small series of patients—particularly in those with less severe disease—for decreasing pain and causing a reduction in lesion size and number. This agent, however, must be used with caution in children because it may affect the normal function of the growth plate. Radiation therapy is no longer recommended because it has been proved to be unsuccessful, and it substantially increases the risk of sarcomatous degeneration in this disorder. Endocrinopathies may be treated with hormonal therapies and surgery. Aromatase inhibitors (eg, testolactone) are used to treat precocious puberty. Hyperplastic adrenal glands or parathyroid glands can be removed surgically.

Goals of the orthopedist include pain relief, fracture union, and prevention of deformity. Orthopedic surgery is challenging because weakened bone does not provide sufficient support for fixation devices, lesions occur in areas typically chosen for bone grafting, affected bone cells may be transplanted into normal bone during surgery, and recurrent fracture and progressive deformity necessitate repeat surgery.

Tina Harris, MD
The Johns Hopkins Hospital
Baltimore, Md

Kiaran P. McGee, MS • Roger C. Grimm, MS • Joel P. Felmlee, PhD
John R. Rydberg, MD, PhD • Stephen J. Riederer, PhD • Richard L. Ehman, MD

The Shoulder: Adaptive Motion Correction of MR Images[1]

PURPOSE: To evaluate an adaptive-motion-correction technique to reduce global motion in shoulder magnetic resonance (MR) images.

MATERIALS AND METHODS: In the adaptive-motion-correction technique, interleaved navigator echoes are used to provide a measure of view-to-view displacement along the craniocaudal direction for each image echo in the acquisition. The information is then retrospectively applied to the k-space data to correct for global shoulder motion. This algorithm was evaluated in a series of 143 consecutive patient shoulder examinations by comparing the original image set for each patient with the same image set after retrospective correction by means of this algorithm.

RESULTS: The average amplitude of craniocaudal motion was 1.4 mm. Image degradation due to motion was apparent in 100 (70%) of the 143 examinations. Application of the adaptive-motion-correction technique improved image quality in 73 (73%) of these 100 examinations or 51% of all 143 examinations.

CONCLUSION: Adaptive motion correction improved image quality in approximately three-quarters of the examinations in which motion was present.

Shoulder imaging is a common application for musculoskeletal magnetic resonance (MR) imaging, primarily because of its efficacy for evaluating rotator cuff disease (1). These examinations necessitate high spatial resolution to adequately image structures such as the rotator cuff and glenoid labrum (2). Unfortunately, degradation of image quality due to motion is relatively common.

During MR imaging in the shoulder, patients typically lie supine with their arms placed alongside the thorax. This position tends to limit anteroposterior motion of the shoulder girdle but does little to restrain motion in the craniocaudal direction. Such motion can be due to voluntary movements in restless or uncomfortable patients. In addition, findings in our studies have shown that observable respiratory motion of the glenohumeral region is present in most patient examinations (3). Respiratory motion of the rib cage is transferred to the shoulder girdle, resulting in a cyclic displacement predominantly in the craniocaudal direction.

The effect of motion on the MR imaging process is often characterized by dividing the phenomena into "intraview" and "inter-view" (view-to-view) effects (4–11). Intraview effects result from motion during the interval between the application of the radiofrequency pulse and the readout gradient and typically cause phase shifts in the moving material that are proportional to velocity, which can be reduced or eliminated by means of gradient moment nulling techniques (6). Inter-view effects are caused by displacements of the object from one repetition of the sequence to the next. These phase shifts may cause artifacts and signal loss, especially in images obtained with long echo time. Inter-view effects are often manifested as blurring and ghosting in the reconstructed image along the phase-encoding direction (7,12). A variety of techniques including fast imaging (13–15), phase-encode reordering (16), respiratory gating (17), spatial and spectral presaturation (8,18), and navigator echo–based adaptive motion correction (3,7,10,12,19–25) have been developed to address this problem.

Findings in a preliminary study conducted by our group (3) suggested that adaptive-motion-correction techniques may be useful in the specific application of shoulder MR imaging. On the basis of this work, we developed the following hypotheses regarding shoulder MR imaging: (*a*) view-to-view motion of the rotator cuff is frequently present during image acquisition, (*b*) these displacements have an amplitude comparable to the in-plane resolution, and (*c*) use of a navigator echo–based adaptive-motion-correction technique can improve images obtained in the rotator cuff by correcting MR data for the craniocaudal component of such motion. The purpose of this study was to evaluate each of these hypotheses within an extended clinical trial.

Index terms: Magnetic resonance (MR), motion correction • Magnetic resonance (MR), reconstruction algorithms • Shoulder, MR, 41.121411

Radiology 1997; 205:541–545

[1] From the Department of Diagnostic Radiology, Mayo Clinic, 200 First St SW, Rochester, MN 55905. From the 1996 RSNA scientific assembly. Received April 25, 1997; revision requested June 18; revision received July 9; accepted July 10. Supported in part by National Institutes of Health grant CA51124. **Address reprint requests to** R.L.E.

MATERIALS AND METHODS

With most shoulder MR imaging protocols, images are acquired in the transverse, oblique coronal, and oblique sagittal planes (2). In a typical clinical protocol, a double spin-echo sequence is used to provide proton-density– and T2-weighted images in each of these planes. For the purpose of this study, a modified pulse sequence was developed for the oblique coronal acquisition that incorporated an interleaved navigator echo with frequency encoding in the superior-inferior direction. A diagram of this pulse sequence is shown in Figure 1.

Images were acquired on a 1.5-T imager (GE Medical Systems, Milwaukee, Wis). The resolution of the navigator echoes along the frequency-encoding direction was the same as that of the images. No phase encoding was applied to the navigator echo, yielding a simple projection of the shoulder along the superior-inferior axis. The image echoes were acquired with frequency encoding in the right-left direction. Pulse sequence parameters were repetition time of 2,000 msec and echo time of 23 and 69 msec, 16-cm field of view, 192 views, 3-mm section thickness, 1.5-mm section gap, two signals acquired, and no phase wrap.

The motion-corrected reconstruction requires two steps. The first step is to process the data from each navigator echo to determine the longitudinal position of the rotator cuff region relative to a reference projection obtained at the beginning of image data acquisition, by means of a least squares minimization technique. Figure 2 shows a motion-corrupted image and the corresponding navigator-echo projections after they have been Fourier transformed. Longitudinal motion of the rotator cuff region is clearly apparent. Once the longitudinal displacement for each view has been determined from the navigator-echo data, the image echo data are modified by means of phase correction according to the following algorithm, which has been previously described (7,24):

$$S^*_j\,(k_y) = S'_j(k_y)\exp\left(-i2\pi k_y \Delta y_j\right),$$

where $S'_j(k_y)$ represents an individual view of the motion-corrupted image data sampled in k space; $S^*_j\,(k_y)$, the inter-view motion-corrected data; Δy_j, the measured inter-view displacement (in pixels) for view j; and k_y, the k-space view number. With this algorithm, the frame of reference of the imaging process is adaptively shifted in synchrony with the measured longitudinal displacement in each view, thereby reducing the apparent motion of the rotator cuff.

The adaptive-motion-correction technique was evaluated in 143 consecutive clinical shoulder MR imaging examinations over a 14-month period (from September 1995 through November 1996). In all cases, imaging was performed with echo times of 23 and 69 msec and a navigator echo at 46 msec. The "conventionally reconstructed" images were considered to be those images reconstructed without use of the navigator–echo–derived view-to-view

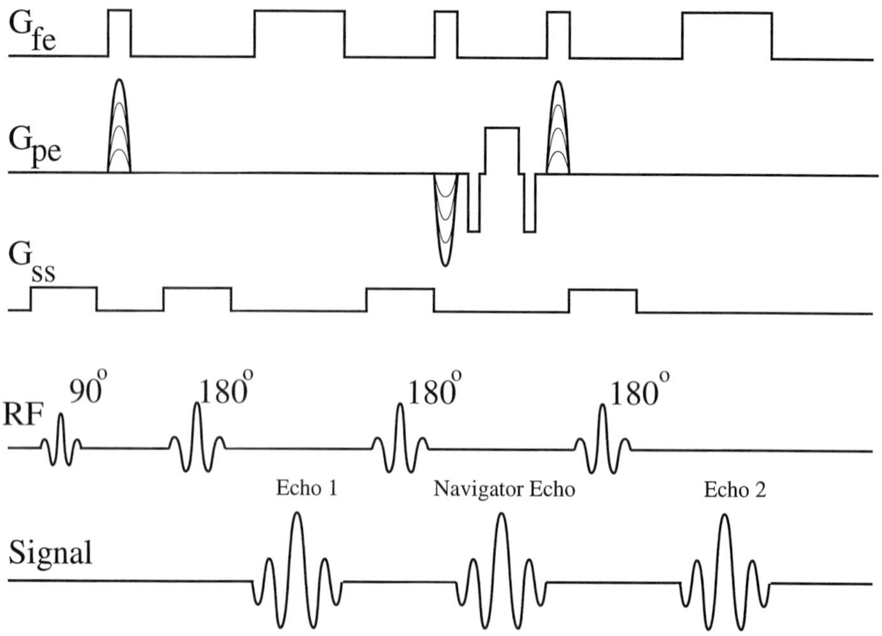

Figure 1. Double spin-echo pulse sequence with navigator echo acquired between the proton-density– and T2-weighted echoes. G_{fe}, G_{pe}, and G_{ss} represent the frequency-, phase-, and section-encoding axes, respectively. *RF* = radio frequency.

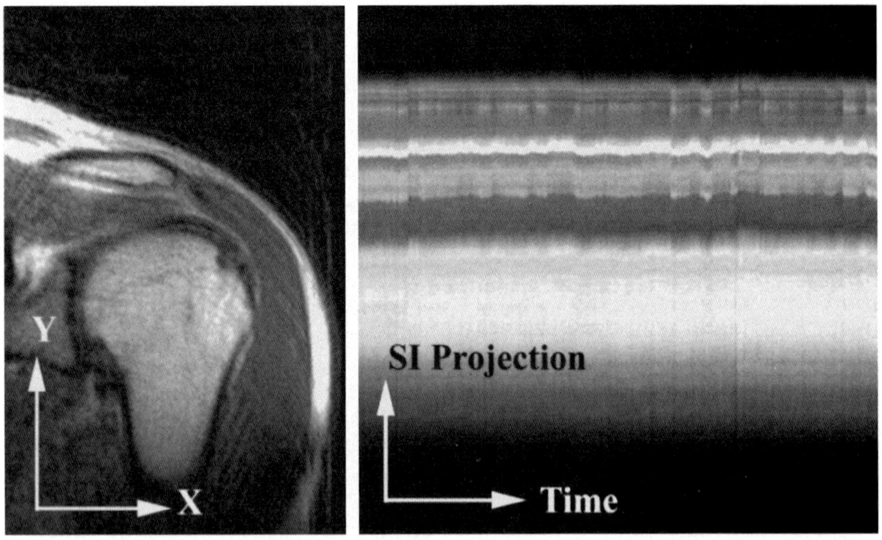

a. **b.**

Figure 2. **(a)** Proton-density–weighted image and **(b)** corresponding navigator-echo map from a typical shoulder MR examination. The cyclic displacements of the navigator echoes result from normal tidal breathing, which is directly transferred to the shoulder girdle. *SI* = superior-inferior.

phase corrections in the coronal plane. These images were used for clinical interpretation at the time of the examination. A second set of adaptively corrected reconstructions of the coronal images was obtained at a later time for side-by-side comparison with the uncorrected images. Because the navigator echo was centered between the proton-density (echo time, 23 msec) and T2-weighted (echo time, 69 msec) echoes, the conventional imaging time was not increased. For this study, reconstruction of the adaptively corrected set was performed off-line. The current implementation necessitates 1.7 seconds per image (the algorithm can readily be implemented on the MR system computer, with similar or better performance).

Four observers (K.P.M., J.P.F., R.L.E., and one other) experienced in reviewing shoulder MR images were asked to assess the degree of motion corruption in the original and adaptively corrected images in a paired comparison. An initial survey of the images demonstrated that when perceptible differences were present between the corrected and uncorrected images, the corrected images could be easily identified owing to their improved quality. Hence, in the formal paired comparison, we did not

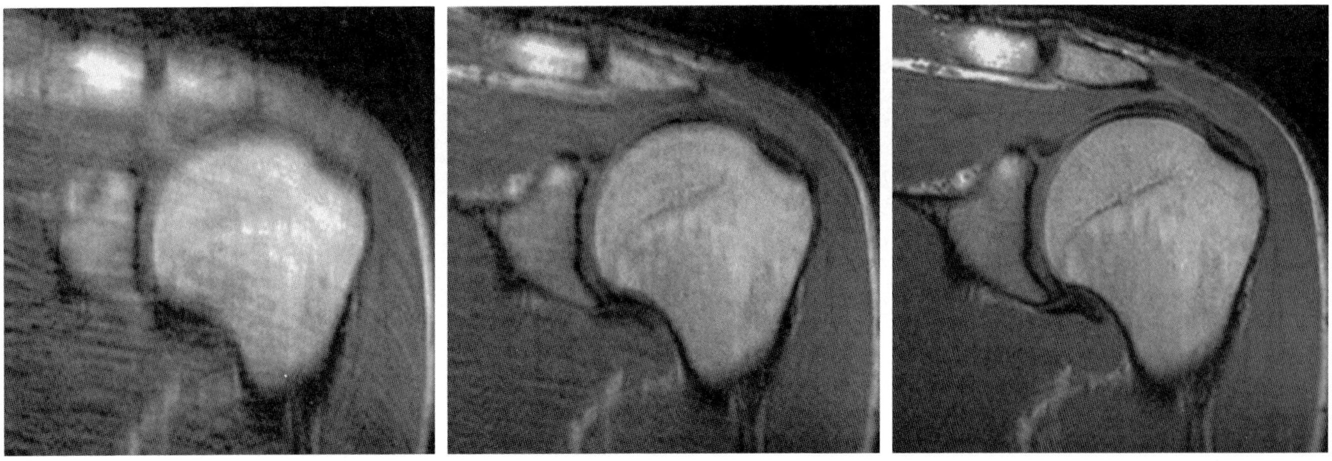

a. b. c.

Figure 3. Sample coronal images obtained in the rotator cuff illustrate motion effects ranging from **(a)** nondiagnostic (score, 1) to **(b)** moderate motion effect (score, 3) to **(c)** no motion effect (score, 5). Scores of 2 and 4 were assigned to images with diagnostic quality intermediate between that of images with correspondingly lower or higher scores.

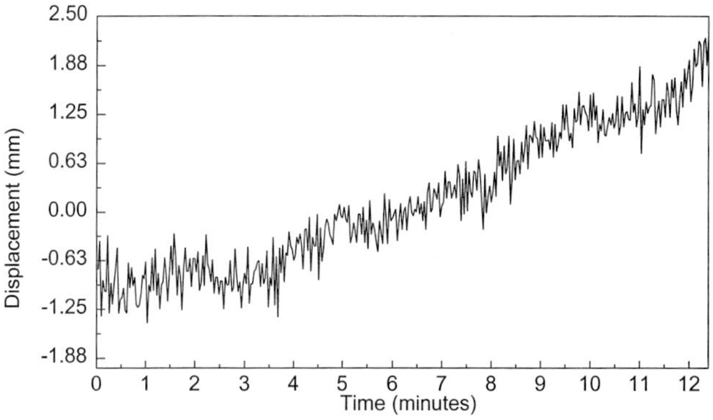

Figure 4. View-to-view displacement record obtained for a patient in this study. Displacements are plotted versus time and demonstrate that two components are present. The first is a periodic respiratory motion, and the second is probably due to the patient relaxing over the course of imaging.

attempt to blind the reviewers with regard to which of the images in each pair was uncorrected. Three coronal-oblique sections through the center of the supraspinatus tendon were chosen to represent overall image quality and were printed to film for review. The observers were then asked to review and score the original and corrected images according to the following scoring scale: 1 = nondiagnostic, 2 = severe motion effect, 3 = moderate motion effect, 4 = mild motion effect, and 5 = no visible motion effect. The images in Figure 3 were obtained by applying navigator-echo data from patient data sets to coronal images obtained in a healthy volunteer to acquire various degrees of motion corruption in the same section.

RESULTS

The superior-inferior motion of the shoulder during MR imaging was measured by means of the mean and standard deviation of view-to-view superior-inferior displacements calculated from the navigator-echo data for a coronal section that passed through the center of the supraspinatus tendon. The magnitude of the view-to-view displacements, averaged over all views and patients, was 0.2 mm. The average motion, as measured with the population-pooled standard deviation, was 1.4 mm (±1 standard deviation). Standard deviation values ranged from 0.06 to 4.14 mm over this patient population. Although not evident in these mean and standard deviation values, many of the navigator-echo data sets demonstrated some component of noncyclic motion in addition to cyclic motion attributed to respiration. Figure 4 shows navigator-echo data for such an acquisition. In this example, periodic respiratory motion is superimposed on a slow linear displacement during acquisition and is most likely due to gradual relaxation over the duration of imaging.

The average scores for the uncorrected images for the four observers as a percentage of all 143 examinations were as follows: nondiagnostic (score, 1), 9 (6.3%) of 143 examinations; severe motion effect (score, 2), 18 (12.6%); moderate motion effect (score, 3), 28 (19.6%); mild motion effect (score, 4), 45 (31.2%); no motion effect (score, 5), 43 (30.1%). The κ statistic was computed to be 0.4, indicating that there was fair agreement among the observers' scores (26). No motion corruption was seen in approximately 43 (30%) of 143 examinations, whereas the other 100 (70%) examinations demonstrated motion effects ranging from mild, through severe, to nondiagnostic. A total of 55 (38.5%) of cases had motion effects that ranged from moderate to nondiagnostic.

Changes in image-quality scores for the 143 examinations after application of the adaptive-motion-correction algorithm were as follows: degraded (−1), 1 [0.7%] of 143 examinations; no change (0), 70 (49.0%); improvement (+1), 55 (38.5%); marked improvement (+2), 16 (11.2%); and substantial improvement (+3), 1 (0.7%). The κ statistic was 0.5, indicating moderate interobserver agreement. In a single patient examination, two of the four observers determined image quality to be degraded by a score of 1 unit in the "corrected" images (original score, 5; processed score, 4). In approximately 73 (51%) of the 143 cases, however, adaptive motion correction improved image quality whereas the remaining 70 (49%) showed no change in score. The percentage distribution of examinations that showed no improvement after processing as a function of their original score is as follows: score 1, 1 (0.7%) of 143 examinations; 2, 2 (1.4%);

3, 2 (1.4%); 4, 22 (15.4%); and 5, 43 (30.0%). Fewer than 5 (3.5%) of 143 cases had motion effects graded as moderate or worse, whereas 22 (16%) of cases had mild motion effect. Almost 43 (30%) cases had an initial score of 5 (no visible motion corruption), and the adaptive-motion-correction technique had no effect on these images. In those examinations with an initial score of 4 or less, 73 (73%) of 100 examinations had observable improvement in image quality after adaptive correction. Overall, only 27 (19%) of all 143 examinations were not improved with the technique.

Figure 5a and 5b show proton-density–weighted oblique coronal images before and after adaptive motion correction. The uncorrected image was severely corrupted by motion. The corrected image was judged to be improved by 2 points. The corrected image clearly shows the absence of the supraspinatus tendon in the space between the humeral head and the acromion; this finding is consistent with a full-thickness tear of the rotator cuff. The depiction of the superior glenoid labrum is also markedly improved. Figure 5c and 5d shows the T2-weighted images of the same section, illustrating similar motion-corruption effects as are in the original image and improvement in the corrected image that is similar to that seen in the proton-density–weighted images.

Figure 6 shows a proton-density–weighted image with motion effects that were graded as moderate. The uncorrected image (Fig 6a) shows blurring of the supraspinatus tendon and spurious widening of the cortical line along the undersurface of the acromion. The corrected image (Fig 6b) was judged to be improved by 2 points. The laminated anatomy of the supraspinatus tendon is more clearly depicted and the cortical lines of the acromion and humeral head are sharper after adaptive motion correction.

DISCUSSION

The results of this study confirm the hypotheses that motion-induced artifacts are present in the majority (three of every four) of MR shoulder examinations with an average amplitude (population average, 1.4 mm) comparable to the in-plane resolution (1.25 mm). Furthermore, the results show that use of navigator-echo–based adaptive motion correction can reduce motion corruption artifact and improve image quality in these examinations. Although the initial motivation

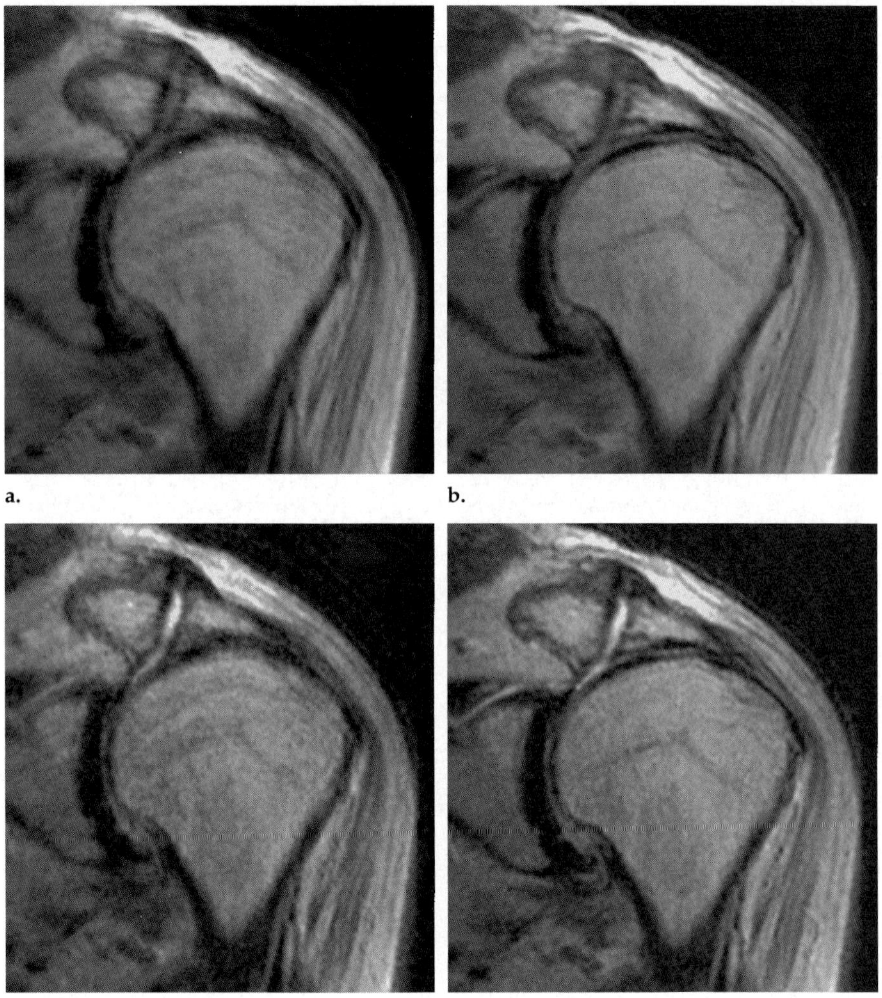

a. b. c. d.

Figure 5. **(a)** Proton-density–weighted patient image with marked motion degradation was classified as nondiagnostic (score, 1). **(b)** **a** after adaptive motion correction. The corrected image shows improvement in image quality of +2 points. Supraspinatus tendon substance is absent between the acromion and humeral head, which is consistent with a complete tear of the rotator cuff. **(c)** T2-weighted image obtained in the same patient. **(d)** **c** after adaptive motion correction. Both **a** and **c** show similar improvement in image quality in **b** and **d**, respectively.

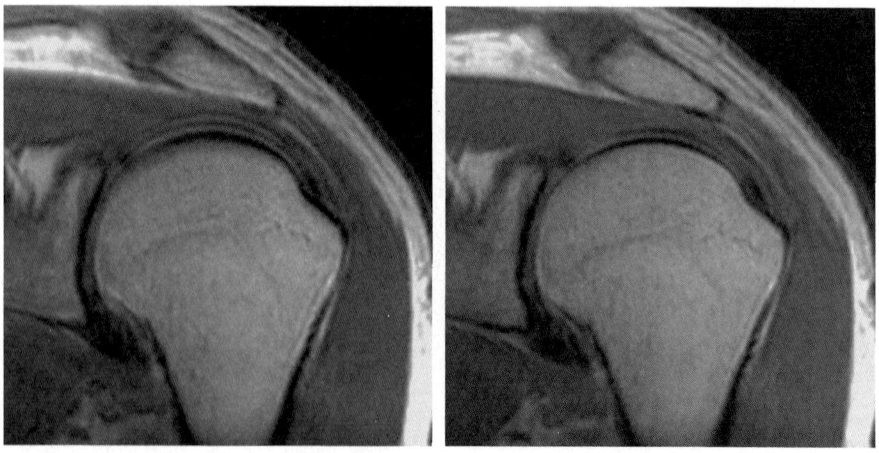

a. b.

Figure 6. **(a)** Proton-density–weighted patient image with moderate motion effects (score, 3). The supraspinatus tendon has a laminated appearance owing to motion, not anatomy. The cortical line of the superior humerus is widened, and the subacromial fat planes are blurred. **(b)** **a** after adaptive motion correction. The corrected image score improved by 2 points. It depicts the supraspinatus tendon with a more homogeneous appearance, and the cortical lines of the superior humerus, the physeal scar, and the subacromial fat plane with improved sharpness.

for implementing adaptive motion correction was to address the effects of respiratory motion transmitted to the shoulder, our review of the motion data showed that other, nonrespiratory-related, motion is also a major contributor to image degradation that can also be corrected. The technique should be equally useful for improving the sagittal images acquired in rotator cuff examinations. As implemented, the technique is not applicable to correcting superior-inferior motion effects in transverse images. Fortunately, such motion causes less degradation in these images because it is relatively small compared with the z-axis dimensions of the voxels.

A potential limitation of this study is that we did not specifically measure the effect of adaptive motion correction on the *diagnostic accuracy* of shoulder MR images. This limitation was necessitated by the difficulty in obtaining an independent test to establish the diagnosis in all patients in this series. Nevertheless, the improved image quality provided with the technique is readily apparent and is obtained without additional acquisition time or other disadvantages when compared with the conventional technique. The motion-correction technique evaluated in this study addresses only global longitudinal motion and does not account for lateral, through-plane, or rotational motion. Yet the majority of images in this study were improved when the technique was applied, which supports the hypothesis that longitudinal motion is a dominant problem at coronal MR imaging in the rotator cuff.

In summary, observable motion corruption was present in the majority of the 143 MR examinations in the shoulder that were evaluated in this study. Adaptive motion correction effectively improved image quality in most of these examinations. ■

Acknowledgments: The authors thank John V. Crues, MD, who initially suggested this application of adaptive motion correction, and David J. Lomas, MD, for reviewing the images in this series.

References

1. Feller JF, Tirman PF, Steinbach LS, Zucconi F. Magnetic resonance imaging of the shoulder: review. Semin Roentgenol 1995; 30:224–240.
2. Stoller DW. Magnetic resonance imaging in orthopaedics and sports medicine. Philadelphia, Pa: Lippincott, 1993.
3. Fu JZW, Burkart DJ, Felmlee JP, Grimm RC, Ehman RL. Clinical trial of adaptive correction of motion in shoulder MR imaging (abstr). Magn Reson Imaging 1994; 4(P):61.
4. Butts K, Riederer SJ, Ehman RL. The effect of respiration on the contrast and sharpness of liver lesions in MRI. Magn Reson Med 1995; 33:1–7.
5. Ehman RL, McNamara MT, Brasch RC, Felmlee JP, Gray JE, Higgins CB. Influence of physiologic motion on the appearance of tissue in MR images. Radiology 1986; 159:777–782.
6. Ehman RL, Felmlee JP. Flow artifact reduction in MRI: a review of the roles of gradient moment pulling and spatial presaturation. Magn Reson Med 1990; 14:293–307.
7. Ehman RL, Felmlee JP. Adaptive technique for high-definition MR imaging of moving structures. Radiology 1989; 173: 255–263.
8. Felmlee JP, Ehman RL. Spatial presaturation: a method for suppressing flow artifacts and improving depiction of vascular anatomy in MR imaging. Radiology 1987; 164:559–564.
9. Korin HW, Farzaneh F, Wright RC, Riederer SJ. Compensation for effects of linear motion in MR imaging. Magn Reson Med 1989; 12:99–113.
10. Korin HW, Felmlee JP, Ehman RL, Riederer SJ. Adaptive technique for three-dimensional MR imaging of moving structures. Radiology 1990; 177:217–221.
11. Wang Y, Riederer SJ, Ehman RL. Respiratory motion of the heart: kinematics and the implications for the spatial resolution in coronary imaging. Magn Reson Med 1995; 33:713–719.
12. Ordidge RJ, Helpern JA, Qing ZX, Knight RA, Nagesh V. Correction of motion artifacts in diffusion-weighted MR images using navigator echoes. Magn Reson Imaging 1994; 12:455–460.
13. Wright RC, Riederer SJ, Faraneh F, Rossman PJ, Liu Y. Real-time MR fluoroscopic data acquisition and image reconstruction. Magn Reson Med 1989; 12:407–415.
14. Hennig J, Nauerth A, Friedburg H. RARE imaging: a fast imaging method for clinical MR. Magn Reson Med 1986; 3:823–833.
15. Frahm J, Haase A, Matthaei D. Rapid NMR imaging of dynamic processes using the FLASH technique. Magn Reson Med 1986; 3:321–327.
16. Bailes DR, Gilderdale DJ, Bydder GM, Collins AG, Firim DN. Respiratory ordered phase encoding (ROPE): a method for reducing respiratory motion artifacts in MR imaging. J Comput Assist Tomogr 1985; 9:835–838.
17. Runge VM, Clanton JA, Partain CL, James AK Jr. Respiratory gating in magnetic resonance imaging at 0.5 T. Radiology 1984; 151:521–523.
18. Edelman RR, Atkinson DJ, Silver MS, Loaiza FL, Warren WS. FRODO pulse sequences: a new means of eliminating motion, flow, and wraparound artifacts. Radiology 1988; 166:231–236.
19. Felmlee JP, Ehman RL, Riederer SJ, Korin H. Adaptive motion compensation in MRI: accuracy of motion measurement. Magn Reson Med 1991; 18:207–213.
20. Fu ZW, Wang Y, Grimm RC, et al. Orbital navigator echoes for motion measurements in magnetic resonance imaging. Magn Reson Med 1995; 34:746–753.
21. Lee CL, Jack CR, Grimm RC, et al. Real-time adaptive motion correction in functional MRI. Magn Reson Med 1996; 36:436–444.
22. Liu YL, Riederer SJ, Rossman PJ, Grimm RC, Debbins JP, Ehman RL. A monitoring, feedback, and triggering system for reproducible breath-hold MR imaging. Magn Reson Med 1993; 30:507–511.
23. Sachs TS, Meyer CH, Hu BS, Kohli J, Nishimura DG. Real-time detection in spiral MRI using navigators. Magn Reson Med 1994; 32:639–645.
24. Wang Y, Grimm RC, Felmlee JP, Riederer SJ, Ehman RL. Algorithms for extracting motion information from navigator echoes. Magn Reson Med 1996; 36:117–123.
25. Wang Y, Rossman PJ, Grimm RC, Riederer SJ, Ehman RL. Navigator-echo–based real-time respiratory gating and triggering for reduction of respiration effects in three-dimensional coronary MR angiography. Radiology 1996; 198:55–60.
26. Woolson RF. Statistical methods for the analysis of biomedical data. New York, NY: Wiley, 1987.

Bernard J. Dardzinski, PhD • Timothy J. Mosher, MD • Shizhe Li, PhD
Mark A. Van Slyke, MD • Michael B. Smith, PhD

Spatial Variation of T2 in Human Articular Cartilage

PURPOSE: **To determine the spatial variation of in vivo cartilage T2 in young asymptomatic adults.**

MATERIALS AND METHODS: **Quantitative T2 maps of seven asymptomatic young male adults and one male volunteer with a history of previous intraarticular chondroid fragments were calculated by using a multiecho, spin-echo magnetic resonance imaging sequence at 3.0 T. The T2 maps were bilinearly interpolated to generate T2 profiles across the thickness of cartilage.**

RESULTS: **All seven asymptomatic volunteers demonstrated a monotonic increase in T2, which increased from 32 msec ± 1 in the deep radial zone and 48 msec ± 1 in the deep transitional zone to 67 msec ± 2 in the outer transitional superficial zone. The T2 profile of the volunteer with superficial fibrillation observed at arthroscopy demonstrated marked spatial heterogeneity and a statistically significant increase in cartilage T2.**

CONCLUSION: **There is a reproducible pattern of increasing T2 that is proportional to the known spatial variation in cartilage water and is inversely proportional to the distribution of proteoglycans. The authors postulate that these regional T2 differences are secondary to the restricted mobility of cartilage water within an anisotropic solid matrix.**

An important component of osteoarthritis is the degeneration and loss of articular cartilage. Ongoing research to characterize the process of cartilage degeneration and evaluate the effectiveness of chondroprotective agents for preserving and repairing damaged cartilage requires noninvasive techniques to identify early, reversible degeneration. Most previous magnetic resonance (MR) imaging studies have focused on techniques for assessing the morphology of articular cartilage to accurately measure the thickness and volume of cartilage (1,2). The results of early studies on isolated cartilage samples suggest an ability of MR imaging to depict changes in cartilage structure that precede cartilage loss (3,4). The ability of MR imaging and MR spectroscopy to enable noninvasive investigation of the macromolecular environment of cartilage water provides unique information that can potentially lead to a better understanding of cartilage degeneration.

Two previous studies with use of MR microscopy of isolated cartilage plugs demonstrate a spatial dependence of T2 in articular cartilage, with values increasing from the subchondral bone towards the articular surface (5,6). This pattern is proportional to the known distribution of water content in cartilage and is inversely proportional to the distribution of proteoglycans (7). Because tissue T2 is dependent on the slow molecular motion of water, we assumed that these regional differences reflect inherent differences in water mobility secondary to the surrounding macromolecular matrix. It is likely that early degenerative change in the cartilage matrix will alter the mobility, and thus the T2, of cartilage water. Thus far, to our knowledge, these techniques have not been applied in vivo. In this study, we evaluated the spatial variation of T2 in the patellar cartilage of young asymptomatic volunteers.

MATERIALS AND METHODS

MR Imaging

From January 1996 to July 1996, we evaluated the right knee of seven asymptomatic male volunteers (mean age, 34 years; age range, 24–40 years) and of one male volunteer (aged 35 years) who demonstrated superficial fibrillation at arthroscopy. Informed written consent was obtained from all volunteers after the nature of the procedure had been fully explained.

MR imaging experiments were performed on a Medspec S300 3.0-T imaging-spectrometer (Bruker Instruments, Karlsruhe, Germany) operating at 125 MHz for protons (hydrogen-1). A 33-cm-diameter asymmetric gradient insert, capable of delivering ±6 G/cm, was used in all imaging experiments. B_1 field generation and signal reception was accomplished with a 9-cm transmit-receive surface coil. Data were acquired in the axial plane through the middle of the patella prescribed from a sagittal locator image. Proton-density and

Index terms: Cartilage, MR, 4521.121411 • Magnetic resonance (MR), high-field-strength imaging, 4521.121411, 4521.12146 • Magnetic resonance (MR), relaxometry, 4521.12146 • Magnetic resonance (MR), tissue characterization, 4521.12146

Radiology 1997; 205:546–550

[1] From the Departments of Radiology, Center for NMR Research (B.J.D., T.J.M., S.L., M.A.V.S., M.B.S.), and Cellular and Molecular Physiology (M.B.S.), Pennsylvania State University College of Medicine, Milton S. Hershey Medical Center, 500 University Dr, Hershey, PA 17033. From the 1996 RSNA scientific assembly. Received May 8, 1997; revision requested June 19; revision received July 9; accepted July 10. **Address reprint requests to** T.J.M.

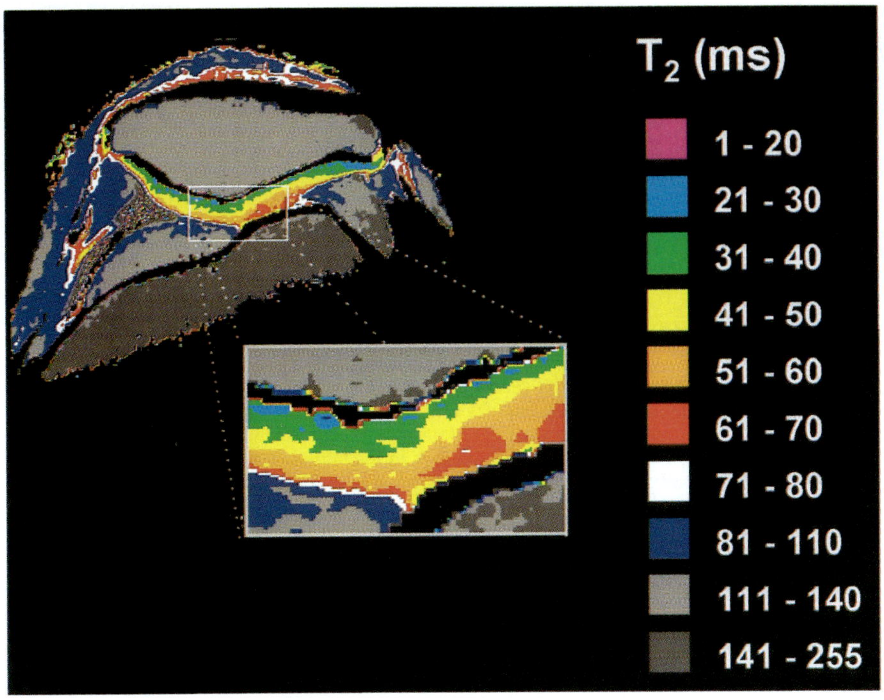

Figure 1. Color map of T2 in patellar cartilage from an asymptomatic young adult demonstrates a progressive increase in the T2 from the radial to the superficial zone.

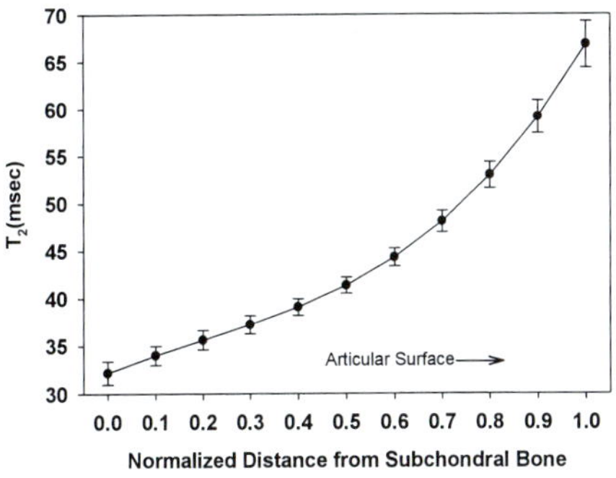

Figure 2. Mean T2 (± standard error of the mean) versus normalized distance from subchondral bone for seven asymptomatic young male volunteers demonstrates a smooth monotonic increase in T2 from the deep radial zone to the superficial zone. Values are averaged from the middle of the medial and lateral facets and the median ridge.

T2 maps were calculated from 11 axial spin-echo images simultaneously acquired through the middle of the patella with a multiecho spin-echo imaging sequence. Imaging parameters were as follows: repetition time of 1,500 msec, echo time from 9 to 99 msec in 9-msec increments, 3-mm section thickness, 8-cm field of view, 128 × 128 matrix, 50-kHz bandwidth, section-selection and refocusing pulse widths of 2,000 msec, two signals acquired, total acquisition time of 6.5 minutes. The read-encoding (frequency) axis was chosen in the left-to-right direction, across the patella, to minimize chemical shift artifact at the patellar cartilage-bone interface. Cartilage thickness was calculated from axial gradient-echo images with the following parameters: 200/13 (repetition time msec/echo time msec), 45° flip angle, 3-mm section thickness, 8-cm field of view, 256 × 256 matrix, 25-kHz bandwidth, section-selection pulse width of 4,000 msec, four signals acquired, total acquisition time of 3.5 minutes.

Data Analysis

Proton-density and T2 maps were calculated from the 11 spin-echo images by using nonlinear least squares curve fitting, on a pixel-by-pixel basis, with Interactive Data Language (IDL Research Systems, Boulder, Colo). Fitting the signal intensity, SI, for the ith, j^{th} pixel as a function of time, t, can be expressed as follows: $SI_{i,j}(t) = S0_{i,j} \cdot \exp(-t/T2_{i,j})$, where $S0_{i,j}$ is the pixel intensity at $t = 0$, and $T2_{i,j}$ is the T2 time constant of pixel i, j. A proton-density map is generated from the pixel $S0_{i,j}$ data, and a T2 map (image) is generated from the $T2_{i,j}$ data. The T2 map was then bilinear interpolated to a 512 × 512 image matrix. T2 profiles were acquired through the median ridge and the middle of the medial and lateral facets of the patellar cartilage. Each profile was normalized for distance and fit with a cubic polynomial for comparison between volunteers. The mean and standard deviation of T2 was then plotted as a function of normalized distance for the seven asymptomatic volunteers. The T2 maps were color coded to represent a specific range of values. With the gradient-echo images, cartilage thickness was measured perpendicular to the bone-cartilage interface of the middle of the medial and lateral facets and the median ridge.

RESULTS

Figure 1 depicts the color-coded T2 map of an axial section through the patellar cartilage from a representative asymptomatic volunteer. T2 values range from 30 to 70 msec within the cartilage and greater than 100 msec in the patellar marrow space. The laminar appearance of T2 values within the cartilage is a function of the color coding used for illustration. T2 values as a function of normalized distance from the subchondral bone are illustrated in Figure 2. Each point in this graph represents the mean ± standard error of the mean of the three profiles for seven asymptomatic volunteers for all three locations. All volunteers demonstrated a monotonic increase in T2, increasing from 32 msec ± 1 in the deep radial zone and 48 msec ± 1 in the deep transitional zone to 67 msec ± 2 in the outer transitional zone ($P < .001$). Due to the spatial resolution of the T2 measurement, the histologic superficial zone was not resolved. For the symptomatic volunteer, the monotonic increase in T2 was not observed. In the median ridge, the T2 measured 51 msec in the deep radial zone, 56 msec in the deep transitional zone, and 41 msec in the outer transitional zone. Mean cartilage thickness (± standard error of the mean) measured on gradient-echo images of the seven asymptomatic volunteers was 4.2 mm ± 0.4, 4.1 mm ± 0.4, and 4.2 mm ± 0.3 for the medial facet, median ridge, and lateral facet, respectively.

DISCUSSION

Current theories on the biomechanical properties of articular cartilage stress the importance of fluid transport and cartilage permeability in determining the response to compressive stress (8). The viscoelastic behavior of cartilage, which is determined by the mobility of cartilage water, has been previously studied with use of destructive techniques. Biophysical techniques such as compression creep experiments provide information on the material properties of excised cartilage tissue, and characterize the bulk properties of fluid flux (9). The measurement of streaming potentials, which are generated by ionic fluid flux through cartilage with compression, has poor spatial resolution and is limited to excised samples (10,11). Combined histologic-compression techniques have been described to evaluate regional strain (12,13) and thus can indirectly characterize the movement of cartilage fluid. The information obtained noninvasively through MR imaging and MR spectroscopy is unique in its ability to facilitate characterization of the macro-

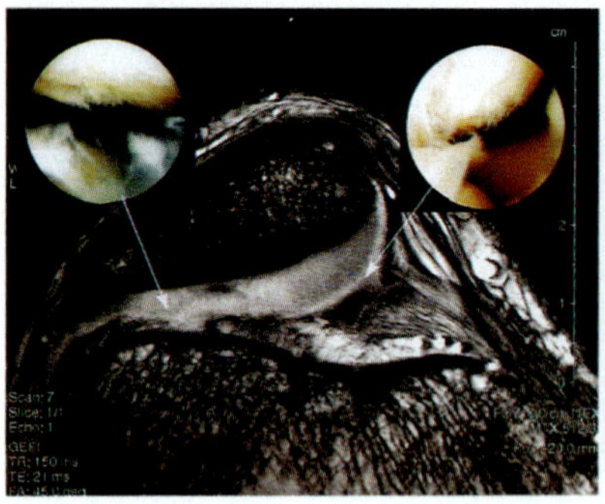

3.

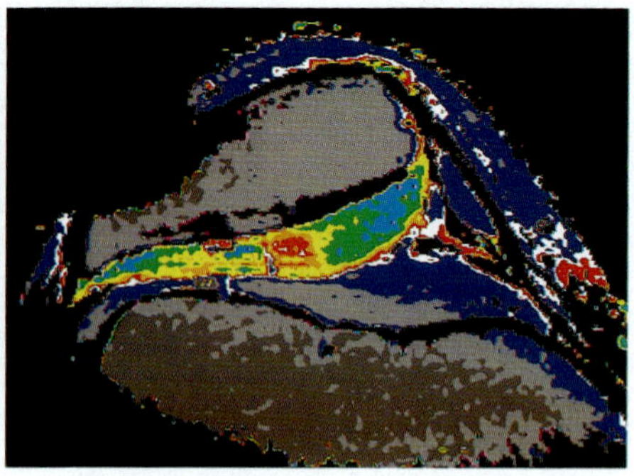

4a.

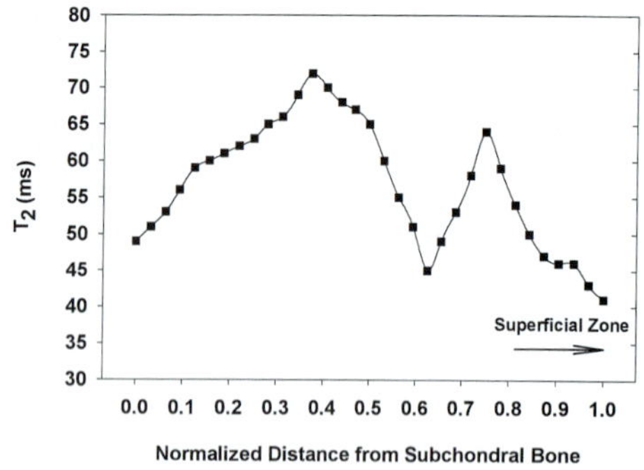

4b.

Figures 3, 4. **(3)** Gradient-echo MR image (150/21, 45° flip angle) in a symptomatic 35-year-old man and the corresponding arthroscopic images (insets). The lateral facet contains heterogeneous internal signal intensity, with irregularity of the surface. Arthroscopic visualization (right inset) confirms moderate fibrillation and superficial erosion. The medial facet has an indistinct hyperintense superficial zone. At arthroscopy (left inset), there was evidence of mild fibrillation. **(4a)** T2 map of the patellofemoral joint shown in **3**. In the lateral facet, there is an overall increase in the T2 values and loss of the normal laminar appearance. The medial facet, which demonstrated superficial fibrillation at arthroscopy, shows uncharacteristically low T2 values in the deep and radial zones. **(4b)** T2 profile across the median ridge demonstrates the increased T2 values in the deep and transitional zones.

molecular environment of water protons and probe the important interaction of cartilage fluid with the solid matrix. As MR imaging is nondestructive, it is the only technique available to monitor long-term temporal changes in cartilage water mobility.

The results of several previous studies indicate that regional differences in the solid matrix affect the relaxation properties of cartilage water. Initial studies by Lehner et al (14) and later studies by Modl et al (15) and Rubenstein et al (16) demonstrate zonal differences in signal intensity that are postulated to be secondary to regional differences in collagen and proteoglycan concentrations identified at histologic examination. Paul and co-workers (17) suggest that the variation in signal intensity of human patellar cartilage is secondary to zonal variation in proteoglycan concentration but does not correlate with the known distribution of collagen or free water concentration.

T2 of Normal Articular Cartilage

In this study, the observed spatial dependence of T2 is in excellent agreement with two previous studies obtained at high magnetic field strength (7 T). With use of H-1 MR microscopy of excised canine articular cartilage plugs, Xia and colleagues (5) demonstrated a relatively uniform distribution of T1 values; however, the T2 values are nonuniform, with the T2 increasing from 10 msec at the subchondral bone layer to 50 msec at the articular surface. They postulate that the spatial variation in T2 is secondary to the known distribution of proteoglycan concentration. A similar pattern recently has been described in excised cartilage plugs from human femoral head samples (6). The pattern of increasing T2 from the deep radial zone to the articular surface closely resembles the known spatial variation of water content in articular cartilage (18,19). We postulate that these regional differences in cartilage T2 are secondary to the restricted mobility of cartilage water within an anisotropic solid matrix.

Tissue T2 is sensitive to the slow molecular motions of the water protons and the macromolecular environment. In cartilage, the highly structured architecture of the collagen framework results in anisotropy of the dipole-dipole interactions. The large biopolymers reduce the rotational and translational motion of water protons. Because of the restricted mobility, the dipole-dipole interactions are not averaged. This produces an efficient mechanism for spin-spin relaxation (20), which reduces the T2 of cartilage water.

Several factors can limit the accuracy and precision of the T2 measurements. There is a radio-frequency flip angle dependence for surface coils as a function of depth perpendicular to the plane of the surface coil. Due to the geometry of the patellofemoral joint, the patellar cartilage is positioned in the isocenter of the surface coil where there is maximal B_1 homogeneity (21). At the beginning of each study, the 90° and 180° section-selective pulses are optimized by maximizing the signal intensity. The maximum signal intensity originates from the cartilage providing confidence that the flip angles were set properly for accurate T2 quantification. Imperfection in the 180° refocusing pulse gives rise to the formation of stimulated echoes with accumulation of magnetization along the z axis. As this component decays as a function of T1 rather than T2 decay, this will lead to an overestimation of the T2 value (22). To minimize the formation of stimulated echoes, spoiler gradients were used to disperse the unfocused magnetization. Off-resonance effects were minimized by acquiring the data as a single section. Previous reported values of cartilage T2 range from 24 to 77 msec, with longer values observed in the more superficial layers (14,23–26). Given the excellent agreement of our measured T2 with that of previous studies, in which T2 was measured with both MR spectroscopic and MR imaging techniques, the error due to T1 contamination is believed to be small. As there is little variation in T1 across the layers of articular cartilage (5,27), the effect of T1 contamination should have a negligible effect on the observed spatial variation in T2.

Pixel resolution was chosen as 625 µm in-plane (80 mm/128 pixels) with a 3-mm section thickness (1.2-µL voxels) to limit the total acquisition time of the experiment to 6.5 minutes and to provide an adequate signal-to-noise ratio. A bandwidth of 50 kHz was chosen to ensure adequate signal-to-noise ratio in the 11 spin-echo images while minimizing the interecho delay to 9 msec. This short delay is necessary to accurately fit the data for regions of relatively short T2 (T2 $<$ 30 msec). For several volunteers, T2 maps were acquired with a 256 $\times$ 256 matrix. Although the measured T2 values and spatial dependency were equivalent to the reported measurements obtained with a 128 $\times$ 128 matrix, the lower signal-to-noise ratio and increased interecho time produced greater uncertainty in the calculated T2 value. For quantification, the calculated T2 maps were interpolated to a 512 × 512 matrix to increase the average number of pixels in the profile across the patellar cartilage to 26. Interpolating and fitting the profile with a cubic polynomial smooths the monotonically increasing T2 profiles across the patellar cartilage.

For calculation of T2, data were fit to a single exponential. We recently used a multiecho, spin-echo MR spectroscopy technique to demonstrate the multiexponential T2 decay of cartilage water (28). A second, tightly bound compartment of water with a mean T2 of 250 µsec is observed. Given the short T2, this population of water protons does not contribute to the calculated T2 values reported in this study. For measurements made within a small voxel, there is little volume averaging, and a single exponential fit agrees best with the observed data. Evaluating the decaying signal intensity with a two or three exponential fit requires more images with echo times substantially less than 1 msec.

Although this study does not address the orientation dependence of T2 in cartilage, previous studies on excised samples suggest that the T2 values of the deep radial zone will be longer at sites where the surface is oriented 55° relative to the constant magnetic induction field (B_0) (6,29). Investigators attribute these findings to the "magic angle effect," which can be seen in highly structured anisotropic tissues (16,30–32). In addition, Rubenstein et al (33) recently demonstrated that the zonal appearance is dependent on the degree of compression applied to the cartilage sample and is hypothesized to result from a combination of net water loss and change in the orientation of the collagen fibers. Most of these observations were made in disarticulated samples. It is not as clear if intact living joints, which experience an intrinsic degree of compression due to the tension of ligaments and muscles, will demonstrate the same degree of orientation dependence. A quantitative evaluation of the orientation dependence of cartilage T2 in the intact living joint, to our knowledge, has not yet been reported. Results from excised samples and qualitative observations from clinical images support the theory that the spin-spin relaxation behavior of cartilage water is strongly influenced by the orientation of the collagen framework and suggest that dipole-dipole anisotropy in the presence of restricted water mobility is a major pathway for spin-spin relaxation in the deep layers of cartilage.

T2 of Damaged Articular Cartilage

Previous studies with use of excised cartilage plugs demonstrate the permeability of cartilage is increased with the onset of cartilage degeneration (34). The earliest detectable change in degeneration is an increase in water content, associated with an increase in cartilage permeability (35). As the permeability increases, hydrodynamic fluid pressure is unable to maintain load support, and greater stress is generated in the solid matrix. This stress leads to the degeneration and fragmentation of the proteoglycan-collagen matrix and a subsequent loss of cartilage tissue.

Initial observations demonstrate an increase in cartilage T2 with early degenerative change. Gradient-echo images and T2 maps were obtained for a 35-year-old volunteer with a history of prior arthroscopic surgery for free chondroid fragments. As presented in Figure 3, the gradient-echo images demonstrate heterogeneity and superficial irregularity in the lateral patellar facet; this finding corresponded to moderate fibrillation and superficial erosion at arthroscopy performed 2 days after the MR imaging examination (Fig 3, right inset). The medial facet demonstrates an indistinct superficial hyperintense zone that corresponded to mild superficial fibrillation at arthroscopy. The T2 map and T2 profile of the median ridge are presented in Figure 4. In comparison to the normal pattern of T2 spatial dependency shown in Figures 1 and 2, there is marked heterogeneity in the distribution of T2 values of the lateral facet with a substantial increase in T2 of the radial and transitional zones. This observation is compatible with an increased mobility of water protons and may also reflect the loss of normal anisotropy present in the radial zone of cartilage due to damage to the collagen-proteoglycan matrix.

In conclusion, our results demonstrate a reproducible spatial dependence of cartilage water T2. As these results were obtained from a selected population of young asymptomatic volunteers, they should not be extrapolated to older populations. Additional studies are needed to determine how normal aging changes will alter the T2 values and distribution. The results of previous studies conducted on animal models and excised human cartilage samples suggest that degenerative changes in cartilage increase water content and produce a measurable increase in cartilage T2. Our initial observations support these preliminary studies and demonstrate that these experiments can be performed in vivo. Noninvasive methods such as MR imaging provide unique information on the mobility of cartilage water and allow repeatable measurements to be made in the intact joint. This information will aid in the understanding and treatment of osteoarthritis and traumatic cartilage injury and in monitoring the maturation of cartilage transplants. ■

Acknowledgments: The authors express their gratitude to Salvatore Larusso, BS, RDMS, RTR, and Wayne Conrad, MD, for their assistance with acquisition of the arthroscopic images.

References

1. Peterfy CG, van Dijke CF, Ying L, et al. Quantification of the volume of articular cartilage in the metacarpophalangeal joints of the hand: accuracy and precision of three-dimensional MR imaging. AJR 1995; 165:371–375.
2. Sittek H, Eckstein F, Gavazzeni A, et al. Assessment of normal patellar cartilage volume and thickness using MRI: an analysis of currently available pulse sequences. Skeletal Radiol 1996; 25:55–62.
3. Bashir A, Gray ML, Burstein D. Gd-DTPA as a measure of cartilage degradation. Magn Reson Med 1996; 36:665–673.
4. Xia Y, Farquhar T, Burton-Wurster N, Vernier-Singer M, Lust G, Jelinski LW. Self-diffusion monitors degraded cartilage. Arch Biochem Biophys 1995; 323:323–328.
5. Xia Y, Farquhar T, Burton-Wurster N, Ray E, Jelinski LW. Diffusion and relaxation mapping of cartilage-bone plugs and excised disks using microscopic magnetic resonance imaging. Magn Reson Med 1994; 31:273–282.
6. Mlynarik V, Degrassi A, Toffanin R, Vittur F, Cova M, Pozzi-Mucelli RS. Investigation of laminar appearance of articular cartilage by means of magnetic resonance microscopy. Magn Reson Imaging 1996; 14: 435–442.
7. Mankin HJ, Brandt KD. Biochemistry and metabolism of articular cartilage in osteoarthritis. In: Moskowitz RW, Howell DS, Goldberg VM, Mankin HJ, eds. Osteoarthritis: diagnosis and medical/surgical management. 2nd ed. Philadelphia, Pa: Saunders, 1992; 109–154.
8. Mow VC, Holmes MH, Lai WM. Fluid transport and mechanical properties of articular cartilage: a review. J Biomechanics 1984; 17:377–394.
9. Mow VC, Zhu W, Ratcliffe A. Structure and function of articular cartilage and meniscus. In: Mow VC, Hayes WC, eds. Basic orthopedic biomechanics. New York, NY: Raven, 1991; 143–198.
10. Kim YJ, Bonassar LJ, Grodzinsky AJ. The role of cartilage streaming potential, fluid flow and pressure in the stimulation of chondrocyte biosynthesis during dynamic compression. J Biomech 1995; 9:1055–1066.
11. Garon M, Guardo R, Savard P, Buschmann P. Spatially resolved detection of streaming potentials in articular cartilage (abstr). In: Transactions of the 43rd Annual Meeting of the Orthopedic Research Society. Palatine, Ill: Orthopedic Research Society, 1997; 80–14.
12. Guilak F, Ratcliffe A, Mow VC. Chondrocyte deformation and local tissue strain in articular cartilage: a confocal microscopic study. J Orthop Res 1995; 13:410–421.

13. Broom ND, Myers DB. A study of the structural response of wet hyaline cartilage to various loading situations. Conn Tissue Res 1980; 7:227–237.
14. Lehner KB, Rechl HP, Gmeinwiesser JK, Heuck AF, Lukas HP, Kohl HP. Structure, function, and degeneration of bovine hyaline cartilage: assessment with MR imaging in vitro. Radiology 1989; 170:495–499.
15. Modl JM, Sether LA, Haughton VM, Kneeland JB. Articular cartilage: correlation of histologic zones with signal intensity at MR imaging. Radiology 1991; 181:853–855.
16. Rubenstein JD, Kim JK, Morava-Protzner I, Stanchev PL, Henkelman RM. Effects of collagen orientation on MR imaging characteristics of bovine articular cartilage. Radiology 1993; 188:219–226.
17. Paul PK, Jasani MK, Sebok D, Rakhit A, Dunton AW, Douglas FL. Variation in MR signal intensity across normal human knee cartilage. Magn Reson Imaging 1993; 3:569–574.
18. Lipshitz H, Etheridge R, Glimcher MJ. Changes in hexosamine content and swelling ratio of articular cartilage as a function of depth from the surface. J Bone Joint Surg [Am] 1976; 58:1149–1153.
19. Maroudas A, Venn M. Chemical composition and swelling of normal and osteoarthritic femoral head cartilage. Ann Rheum Dis 1977; 36:399–406.
20. Packer KJ. The dynamics of water in heterogeneous systems. Phil Trans R Soc Lond B 1977; 278:59–87.
21. Styles P, Smith MB, Briggs RW, Radda GK. A concentric surface-coil probe for the production of homogeneous B1 fields. J Magn Reson 1985; 62:397–405.
22. Poon CS, Henkelman RM. Practical T_2 quantitation for clinical applications. JMRI 1992; 2:541–553.
23. Gahunia HK, Lemaire C, Babyn PS, Cross AR, Kessler MJ, Pritzker KPH. Osteoarthritis in rhesus macaque knee joint: quantitative magnetic resonance imaging tissue characterization of articular cartilage. J Rheumatol 1995; 22:1747–1756.
24. Kim DK, Ceckler TL, Hascall VC, Calabro A, Balaban RS. Analysis of water-macromolecule proton magnetization transfer in articular cartilage. Magn Reson Med 1993; 29:211–215.
25. Duewell SH, Ceckler TL, Ong K, et al. Musculoskeletal MR imaging at 4 T and 1.5 T: comparison of relaxation times and image contrast. Radiology 1995; 196:551–555.
26. Kaufman JH, Cecil KM, Kneeland JB, Bolinger L. Structure in image of articular cartilage at 4T (abstr). In: Proceedings of the Fourth Meeting of the International Society for Magnetic Resonance in Medicine. Berkeley, Calif: International Society for Magnetic Resonance in Medicine, 1996; 834.
27. Freeman DM, Bergman G, Glover G. Short TE microscopy: accurate measurement and zonal differentiation of normal hyaline cartilage. Magn Reson Med 1997; 38:72–81.
28. Mosher TJ, Dardzinski BJ, Smith MB. Characterization of multiple T_2 components in articular cartilage (abstr). In: Proceedings of the Fifth Meeting of the International Society for Magnetic Resonance in Medicine. Berkeley, Calif: International Society for Magnetic Resonance in Medicine, 1997; 1331.
29. Xia Y, Farquhar T, Burton-Wurster N, Lust G. T_2 relaxation anisotropy as a sensitive signature for the orientation of molecular networks in cartilage (abstr). In: Transactions of the 43rd Annual Meeting of the Orthopedic Research Society. Palatine, Ill: Orthopedic Research Society, 1997; 218–237.
30. Henkelman RM, Stanisz GJ, Kim JK, Bronskill MJ. Anisotropy of NMR properties of tissues. Magn Reson Med 1994; 32:592–601.
31. Dunn JF, Goodwin DW. Micro-imaging and the magic angle effect in cartilage (abstr). In: Proceedings of the Fourth Meeting of the International Society for Magnetic Resonance in Medicine. Berkeley, Calif: International Society for Magnetic Resonance in Medicine, 1996; 206.
32. Shinar H, Eliav U, Schneiderman R, Maroudas A, Navon G. ^{2}H and ^{23}Na Multiple quantum filtered NMR spectroscopy and diffusion measurements of human articular cartilage (abstr). In: Proceedings of the Third Meeting of the International Society for Magnetic Resonance in Medicine. Berkeley, Calif: International Society for Magnetic Resonance in Medicine, 1995.
33. Rubenstein JD, Kim JK, Henkelman RM. Effects of compression and recovery on bovine articular cartilage: appearance on MR images. Radiology 1996; 201:843–850.
34. Armstrong CG, Mow VC. Variations in the intrinsic mechanical properties of human articular cartilage with age, degeneration, and water content. J Bone Joint Surg [Am] 1982; 64:88–94.
35. McDevitt CA, Muir H. Biochemical changes in the cartilage of the knee in experimental and natural osteoarthritis in the dog. J Bone Joint Surg [Br] 1976; 58:94–101.

Adil Bashir, SM • Martha L. Gray, PhD • Robert D. Boutin, MD • Deborah Burstein, PhD

Glycosaminoglycan in Articular Cartilage: In Vivo Assessment with Delayed $Gd(DTPA)^{2-}$–enhanced MR Imaging[1]

PURPOSE: **To investigate the feasibility of applying magnetic resonance (MR) imaging with use of an anionic compound, $Gd(DTPA)^{2-}$ (gadolinium diethylenetriamine-pentaacetic acid), for measuring glycosaminoglycan concentration in human cartilage in clinical studies.**

MATERIALS AND METHODS: **Penetration of $Gd(DTPA)^{2-}$ into cartilage was monitored through sequential T1-calculated images obtained after intraarticular (n = 2) or intravenous (n = 2) injection. T1-weighted and T1-calculated image series were then obtained in seven volunteers (nine knees) after penetration of $Gd(DTPA)^{2-}$ into cartilage. If T1 was heterogeneous on $Gd(DTPA)^{2-}$-enhanced images, images were also obtained after penetration of the cartilage with the nonionic contrast agent, gadoteridol.**

RESULTS: **$Gd(DTPA)^{2-}$ penetrated cartilage from the articular surface after intraarticular injection and from both the articular surface and the subchondral bone after intravenous injection. The latter resulted in shorter overall penetration time. T1 values on $Gd(DTPA)^{2-}$-enhanced images were homogeneous in four knees, but in five knees T1 differences of up to 30% were observed. These T1 differences were not seen in the presence of gadoteridol. These variations in T1 reflected about 50% variations in glycosaminoglycan.**

CONCLUSION: **The data suggest that $Gd(DTPA)^{2-}$-enhanced MR imaging has potential for monitoring glycosaminoglycan content of cartilage in vivo.**

Osteoarthritis, commonly referred to as degenerative joint disease, currently affects the lives of over 16 million people in the United States (1). This disease process tends to begin in midadult life, with autopsy studies demonstrating degenerative changes in the weight-bearing joints of 90% of people over age 40 years (2). Early osteoarthritis is characterized by a loosening of the cartilage extracellular collagen matrix and a substantial loss of glycosaminoglycan (3–6). Later degenerative changes manifest as gross anatomic abnormalities, including cartilage edema, fibrillation, fissuring, fragmentation, and denudation (7,8). Although magnetic resonance (MR) imaging can depict cartilage abnormalities earlier and more accurately than any other imaging modality (9), it has been an unreliable and insensitive means of detecting early cartilage degeneration. The general consensus among musculoskeletal radiologists, orthopedists, and rheumatologists is that substantial radiologic advances still are necessary (10,11).

With the aim of developing a more sensitive and specific MR imaging technique for evaluating cartilage abnormalities, during the past several years we have been developing MR techniques for monitoring the concentration of glycosaminoglycan in cartilage (12–14). We focus on glycosaminoglycan for several reasons: Glycosaminoglycans are lost early in the course of cartilage degeneration and would likely need to be replenished in the course of any effective therapy for cartilage disorders. Glycosaminoglycans also play a major role in the mechanical support function in normal cartilage and thereby provide a sensitive and specific measure of cartilage integrity (15–18). Effectively imaging the concentration of glycosaminoglycan would have a major influence on the ability to assess the natural progression of the disease, the timing of therapeutic interventions and the efficacy of these therapeutic measures, and the ability to provide an indication of the functional state of the tissue.

Our approach follows a paradigm pioneered by Maroudas and colleagues (19,20). It depends on the fact that glycosaminoglycan macromolecules contain numerous, highly negatively ionized side groups. We use the principle that a negatively charged ion is relatively excluded from normal cartilage containing a high concentration of (the highly negatively charged)

Index terms: Arthritis, degenerative, 4521.77 • Cartilage, 4521.91 • Gadolinium • Gadoteridol • Magnetic resonance (MR), contrast enhancement, 4521.12143

Abbreviation: DTPA = diethylenetriaminepentaacetic acid.

Radiology 1997; 205:551–558

[1] From the Department of Radiology, Charles A. Dana Research Institute, Beth Israel Deaconess Medical Center and Harvard Medical School, 330 Brookline Ave, Boston, MA 02215 (A.B., R.D.B., D.B.); the Department of Electrical Engineering and Computer Science, Continuum Electomechanics Group, Laboratory for Electromagnetic and Electronic Systems, Massachusetts Institute of Technology, Cambridge (A.B., M.L.G.); the Arthritis Unit, Massachusetts General Hospital, Boston (M.L.G.); the Division of Health Sciences and Technology, Harvard-Massachusetts Institute of Technology, Cambridge (M.L.G., D.B.). Received May 7, 1997; revision requested June 16; revision received July 7; accepted July 8. Supported in part by the J. W. Kieckhefer Foundation, the Procter and Gamble Company (PYI matching program), National Science Foundation PYI BCS9158507, National Institutes of Health grants AR41713 and AR42773, and the Arthritis Foundation. A.B. supported by the Poitras Foundation. R.D.B. supported by an RSNA Seed Grant. **Address reprint requests to** D.B.

glycosaminoglycan. This relative exclusion would not occur when glycosaminoglycans are lost as part of the degenerative process, since the negative charge that they confer to cartilage also is lost (6,20). In particular, we looked at the distribution in tissue of the anionic compound $Gd(DTPA)^{2-}$ (gadolinium diethylenetriaminepentaacetic acid), obtained from the dissociation of the contrast agent gadopentetate dimeglumine (Magnevist; Berlex Laboratories, Wayne, NJ) in solution (21). A measurement of $Gd(DTPA)^{2-}$ concentration should serve as a surrogate for a measurement of glycosaminoglycan concentration as $Gd(DTPA)^{2-}$ is expected to distribute into degraded areas at a higher concentration than that in nondegraded areas (Fig 1). Since the concentration of gadolinium compounds can be determined from an MR measurement of T1, contrast on a T1-weighted image in the presence of $Gd(DTPA)^{2-}$, or on a T1-calculated image, should reflect variations in tissue glycosaminoglycan concentration. It is important to note that such a differential distribution pattern would not be expected to be seen with a nonionic compound such as gadoteridol (ProHance; Bracco Diagnostics, Princeton, NJ) (formerly Gd-HP-DO3A [gadolinium 2-tetraazacyclododecanetriacetate]).

This technique has already been validated in excised bovine and human samples (13,14). It has been applied to bovine cartilage cultured in interleukin-1β to demonstrate near-histologic level resolution of glycosaminoglycan loss (13) and to excised human cartilage samples to demonstrate that morphologically intact tissue may still have substantially lowered glycosaminoglycan concentration (22). To our knowledge, however, the technique has not yet been applied in vivo. The main goal of the current work was to determine the feasibility of applying this MR technique for evaluating cartilage glycosaminoglycan concentration in vivo in humans. Toward this end, the specific objectives of this work were to (*a*) calculate the theoretic sensitivity of the technique to expected variations in glycosaminoglycan concentration under clinical conditions; (*b*) compare delivery of $Gd(DTPA)^{2-}$ to articular cartilage in vivo by means of intraarticular and intravenous administration; (*c*) obtain T1-weighted and T1-calculated images after tissue penetration with an ionic contrast agent, $Gd(DTPA)^{2-}$; and (*d*) obtain T1-weighted and T1-calculated images after tissue penetration with the nonionic contrast agent, gadoteridol. Variations in T1 in the presence of $Gd(DTPA)^{2-}$ would be interpreted as variations in glycosaminoglycan concentration. This interpretation would be supported if the variations did not occur in the presence of gadoteridol, because the distribution of gadoteridol should not be affected by the charged glycosaminoglycan molecule.

MATERIALS AND METHODS

Theoretic Calculations

Normal human cartilage has a glycosaminoglycan concentration on the order of 60 mg/mL, whereas in osteoarthritis glycosaminoglycan concentration can decrease to nearly 0 mg/mL (5). As just described, the charge on the glycosaminoglycan will affect the tissue concentration of a charged contrast agent, in this case $Gd(DTPA)^{2-}$. The $Gd(DTPA)^{2-}$ concentration in turn determines the tissue T1. The goal of this section was to calculate the theoretic dependence of T1 on $Gd(DTPA)^{2-}$ concentration in the tissue, and hence tissue glycosaminoglycan concentration, to determine the sensitivity of the MR measurement to glycosaminoglycan variation expected in degenerating cartilage. The details of the calculations, which were performed according to previously validated relationships (13,14,23), are given in the Appendix and were performed for concentrations of $Gd(DTPA)^{2-}$ of 1 and 4 mmol/L, in the range of that expected clinically.

Similar relationships were calculated for the nonionic contrast agent, gadoteridol. In this case, the tissue gadoteridol concentration should not be affected by the tissue glycosaminoglycan concentration and was assumed to be equal to the concentration of gadoteridol outside the tissue. (This was validated in our laboratory [unpublished data]). The T1 was then calculated from the gadoteridol concentration, as given in the Appendix.

Intraarticular versus Intravenous Administration of Contrast Material

To characterize the effectiveness of intraarticular versus intravenous administration in achieving penetration of $Gd(DTPA)^{2-}$ into hyaline cartilage, T1-calculated images of articular cartilage were obtained at selected time points after intraarticular and intravenous administration of the contrast agent. Institutional review board approval was obtained for all studies described here, and informed consent was obtained from all participants after the nature of the procedure was fully explained.

General imaging methods.—All in vivo studies were performed at 1.5 T with a commercially available MR imager (Vision; Siemens, Iselin, NJ) and a dedicated knee coil or a small flex coil. To establish orientation, a sagittal scout image was obtained, from which multisection axial images were prescribed.

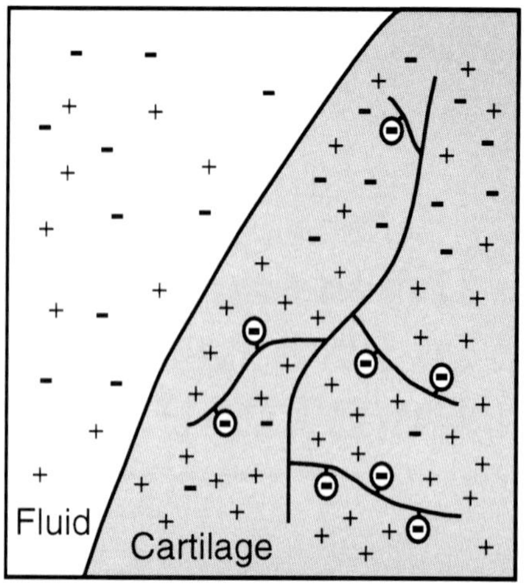

Figure 1. Schematic of synovial fluid and cartilage to demonstrate the distribution of charged ions in the tissue. The proteoglycan component of the tissue is represented by a black backbone with the glycosaminoglycan represented as charged negative side groups fixed to the matrix. Because of these negative ions "fixed" to the matrix, the concentration of free negative ions such as $Gd(DTPA)^{2-}$ will be in lower concentration in the normal cartilage (lower part of the Figure) than in synovial fluid. In cartilage that has lost much of the glycosaminoglycan (upper part of the Figure), the concentration of fixed negative charge is lower, and hence, the concentration of free negative ions will be higher than in the normal cartilage.

T1-weighted images were obtained with an inversion-recovery turbo spin-echo sequence with the following parameters: 350 × 400-μm in-plane resolution, 2- or 3-mm section thickness, 1,000/30/25–850 (repetition time msec/echo time msec/inversion time msec) for intraarticular studies or 1,800/14/25–1,680 for intravenous studies, four signals acquired (intraarticular) or one signal acquired (intravenous). The T1-weighted image series were transferred to a commercially available workstation (Indy; Silicon Graphics, Mountain View, Calif), and the T1 values from 10 to 20 voxels in a region of interest were calculated from selected areas in the images, as described in the next section.

Intraarticular administration.—In two subjects (one 35-year-old man and one 26-year-old woman), 40 mL of a 4 mmol/L $Gd(DTPA)^{2-}$ solution (diluted with normal saline) containing 0.3 mL of epinephrine (1:1,000) was injected intraarticularly with a sterile technique. Epinephrine was used since in two pilot studies without epinephrine, the $Gd(DTPA)^{2-}$ cleared from the joint space before full penetration of patellar cartilage was achieved; thus, epinephrine was used to slow resorption of the contrast medium, as has been previously described (24). In these subjects, each time point involved five T1-weighted images with the inversion delays varying between 25 and 850 msec, for a total imaging time of 16 minutes for the series, from which T1-calculated images were obtained.

Intravenous administration.—In two sub-

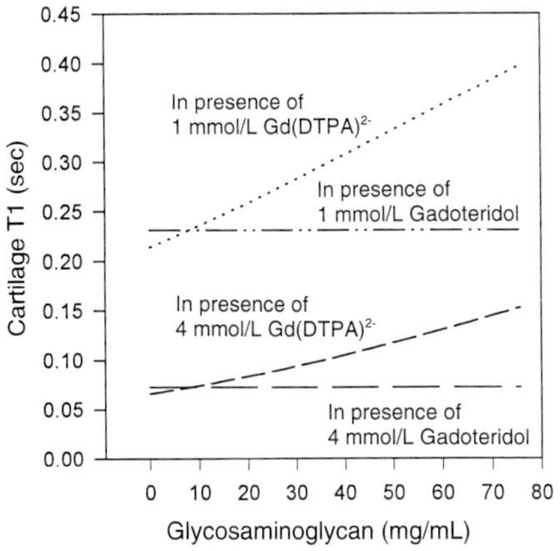

Figure 2. Calculated T1 of cartilage as a function of glycosaminoglycan concentration for tissue equilibrated in 4 mmol/L Gd(DTPA)$^{2-}$, 4 mmol/L gadoteridol, 1 mmol/L Gd(DTPA)$^{2-}$, and 1 mmol/L gadoteridol. The concentration of Gd(DTPA)$^{2-}$ within cartilage is dependent on the concentration in the surrounding fluid (blood, synovial fluid) but varies with the tissue glycosaminoglycan concentration. The concentration of the nonionic contrast agent, gadoteridol, in tissue is the same as that in the surrounding fluid, independent of glycosaminoglycan concentration. Therefore, note the large variation in T1 values in the presence of Gd(DTPA)$^{2-}$ with differing glycosaminoglycan concentration, as compared with the constant T1 values in the presence of gadoteridol with differing glycosaminoglycan concentration. The crossover of the T1 values near 0 mg/mL glycosaminoglycan, where the concentration of Gd(DTPA)$^{2-}$ should equal that of gadoteridol, is due to the slightly higher relaxivity of Gd(DTPA)$^{2-}$ relative to that of gadoteridol (3.5 vs 3.2 L · mmol^{-1} · sec^{-1}).

jects (two men aged 29 and 34 years, respectively), 40 mL of a 0.5 mmol/L Gd(DTPA)$^{2-}$ solution was administered over 3–5 minutes in a single bolus intravenously. Immediately after the bolus, volunteers exercised their lower extremity for 10 minutes (5 minutes of walking and 5 minutes of active knee flexion-extension while sitting on the edge of a table); the results of previous studies have suggested that this exercise increased the rate of delivery of Gd(DTPA)$^{2-}$ to the joint (25,26). A set of images were obtained in which each time point involved seven T1-weighted images with the inversion delays varying between 25 and 1,680 msec, for a total imaging time of 12 minutes. T1-calculated images were then computed for each time point.

T1 Imaging after Tissue Penetration with Gd(DTPA)$^{2-}$

MR imaging of the knee was performed in nine knees of seven volunteers (two women, five men; age range, 21–39; mean age, 31 years), which included three of the previously mentioned subjects. Unenhanced MR imaging employed conventional MR techniques currently used to image knee cartilage, that is, fast low-angle shot axial imaging with the following parameters: 480/15, 80° flip angle, 550 × 550-μm resolution, and 3-mm section thickness.

The volunteers each underwent T1-calculated imaging after penetration of the tissue with Gd(DTPA)$^{2-}$ (5–7 hours for intraarticular injection in two knees and 1½–3 hours for intravenous injection in seven knees). The T1-weighted images were obtained with the parameters described in the previous section.

T1 Imaging after Tissue Penetration with Gadoteridol

Gadoteridol-enhanced images were obtained in five knees that had previously demonstrated abnormalities on Gd(DTPA)$^{2-}$–enhanced images. The gadoteridol-enhanced images were obtained under the same conditions and at approximately the same time point as the Gd(DTPA)$^{2-}$-enhanced images. Landmarks on the patella, femur, and tibia were used to ensure consistency in image selection for the T1-weighted series performed on different days (which were up to 3 months apart for different volunteers).

RESULTS

Theoretic Calculations

The predicted dependence of T1 on glycosaminoglycan (Fig 2) illustrates the large differences in T1 that would be expected between normal and osteoarthritic cartilage. If we assume the cartilage is in equilibrium with a 4-mmol/L Gd(DTPA)$^{2-}$ solution (similar to that of the intraarticular cases [see next section]), cartilage with a relatively normal glycosaminoglycan concentration of 60 mg/mL would have a T1 of 120 msec. Cartilage with a concentration of 0 mg/mL, as might be seen in severely arthritic tissue, would have a T1 of 60 msec. Therefore, the ratio of T1 in healthy cartilage to that in severely osteoarthritic cartilage would be expected to be up to about 2:1. Similarly, with 1 mmol/L Gd(DTPA)$^{2-}$ surrounding the cartilage (similar to that of the intravenous cases described in the next section), the normal cartilage would have a T1 of 375 msec and the osteoarthritic cartilage would have a T1 of 210 msec, still approximately a 2:1 ratio.

A nonionic contrast agent like gadoteridol would be expected to distribute in the tissue water at the same concentration as the surrounding fluid, independent of the glycosaminoglycan concentration. Therefore, for the same surrounding concentration, the intratissue concentration of gadoteridol will be higher than the concentration of the negatively charged Gd(DTPA)$^{2-}$, and the resultant cartilage T1 values will be lower than those with Gd(DTPA)$^{2-}$ (given the almost equal relaxivities of the two compounds).

Intraarticular versus Intravenous Administration

Diffusion of Gd(DTPA)$^{2-}$ into cartilage in vivo was inferred from a decrease in T1 of the cartilage with time after administration of Gd(DTPA)$^{2-}$. We focused mainly on penetration of patellar cartilage, which (as one of the thickest cartilages in the human body) would take the longest to be penetrated.

After intraarticular administration, Gd(DTPA)$^{2-}$ diffused in from the articular surface. Penetration of the patellar cartilage (approximately 5 mm thick) occurred within approximately 7 hours after the intraarticular injection (Figs 3a–3c, 4a). Penetration of the cartilage on the femoral condyle (approximately 1 mm thick) occurred within 2½ hours (the earliest intraarticular image obtained in that plane).

Intravenous administration of the gadolinium compounds allowed the contrast agents to diffuse into patellar cartilage from both the articular surface and the subchondral bone. Penetration of the thick patellar cartilage after intravenous administration of Gd(DTPA)$^{2-}$ was achieved within 2½ hours (Figs 3d–3f, 4b). Penetration of the cartilage on the femoral condyle occurred within 45 minutes. The kinetics of gadoteridol penetration into cartilage was similar.

T1 Imaging after Tissue Penetration with Gd(DTPA)$^{2-}$

Although not explicitly validated in vivo, there is extensive evidence (see Discussion) to support the interpretation that these T1 values, Gd(DTPA)$^{2-}$ concentrations, are directly related to tissue glycosaminoglycan concentration. Therefore, for the purpose of presentation, we will directly refer to T1 variations in the presence of Gd(DTPA)$^{2-}$ as glycosaminoglycan variations.

In four of nine knees imaged, there was no visualized variation in signal intensity on the delayed Gd(DTPA)$^{2-}$-enhanced images. Two of these volunteers also underwent unenhanced MR imaging of the knee, which did not show any cartilage abnormalities. These data suggest that their cartilage had a uniform glycosaminoglycan content and was also morphologically intact. In one knee (knee 1, Table), the T1 was much lower than that of the

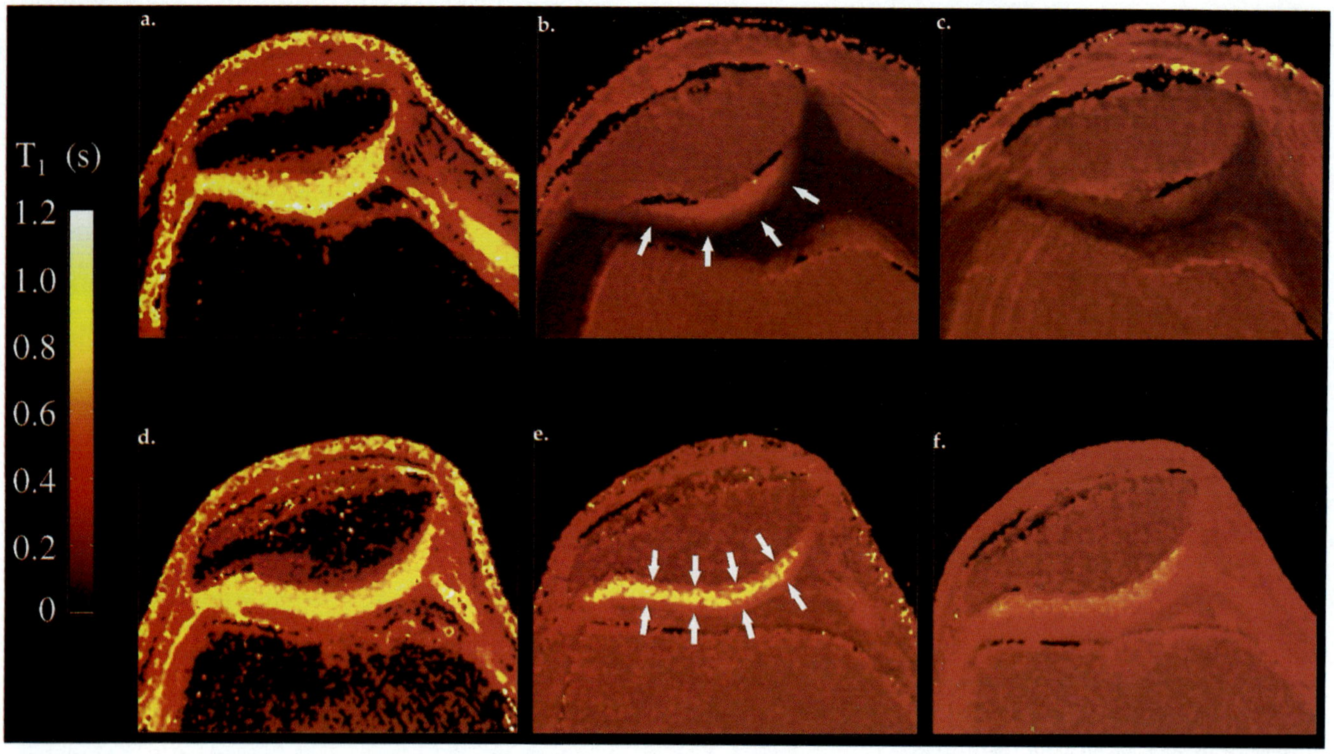

Figure 3. T1-calculated images obtained **(a)** before administration of contrast material and **(b)** 2½ hours and **(c)** 7 hours after intraarticular injection of $Gd(DTPA)^{2-}$. With intraarticular administration, diffusion of contrast material occurs from the articular surface only, as evidenced by the lower T1 values along the joint surface of the cartilage (arrows in **b**) as contrast agent penetrates over time. T1-calculated images obtained **(d)** before administration of contrast material and **(e)** 50 minutes and **(f)** 150 minutes after intravenous injection. With intravenous administration, $Gd(DTPA)^{2-}$ penetrates from both the articular surface and from the bone (arrows in **e**). Note the lower values for T1 with the intraarticular injection due to the higher concentration of $Gd(DTPA)^{2-}$ in this case. While the rate of penetration is the same for both, the overall penetration of the $Gd(DTPA)^{2-}$ takes less time with the intravenous injection, since $Gd(DTPA)^{2-}$ is penetrating the cartilage from both sides.

others. This patellar cartilage was particularly thin, on the order of 2 mm. It is possible that the glycosaminoglycan content was also low, although it was homogeneous across the patella. This example illustrates a situation in which absolute quantitation of glycosaminoglycan concentration would be particularly useful.

The $Gd(DTPA)^{2-}$-enhanced images in the other five knees showed visualizable T1 variations in the presence of $Gd(DTPA)^{2-}$. On all images, regions of interest were chosen from which to calculate T1 values for cartilage after penetration with $Gd(DTPA)^{2-}$ (Table). One region of interest was chosen in the "high T1" area and one in the "low T1" area. At least 10 voxels were in each region of interest. The T1 values of these two regions were compared by means of the Student *t* test. In all cases, the *P* values were less than .05, indicating significantly different values of T1 in these areas and, hence, different concentrations of Gd-$(DTPA)^{2-}$. One knee (knee 6) was studied with both intraarticular and intravenous administration. Although the absolute values of T1 differed owing to the different concentrations surrounding the cartilage with intraarticular versus intravenous administration, the ratio

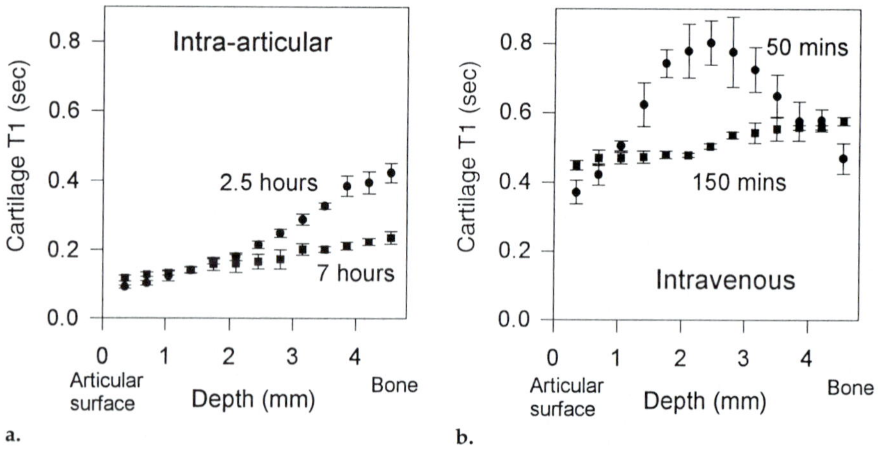

Figure 4. Plot of quantitative T1 values versus depth after **(a)** intraarticular and **(b)** intravenous administration of $Gd(DTPA)^{2-}$ from a study similar to that shown in Figure 3. The error bars represent the standard deviation of the T1 values of the voxels in the region of interest. The absolute values of T1 differ due to the different concentration of $Gd(DTPA)^{2-}$ in the body fluids in the intraarticular and intravenous cases. Note that with intraarticular injection, contrast material penetrates from the articular side only. With intravenous injection, contrast material penetrates from both the superficial and deep margins of the cartilage.

of the T1 values in the different regions of interest (A and B) were 24% and 25% for intraarticular and intravenous administration, respectively. These data confirm the prediction of Figure 2 that the contrast, and differences in T1, are not heavily dependent on the background level of $GD(DTPA)^{2-}$ (or absolute T1). While this study is too small to draw clinical conclusions, it is interesting to note that some volunteers (knees 1 and 6–9, Table) reported history of knee injury.

One volunteer (knee 5, Table; Fig 5) showed a focal lesion on the Gd-$(DTPA)^{2-}$-enhanced images evidenced

T1 Values Obtained from Regions of Interest in the Patellar Cartilage of Seven Volunteers (Nine Knees)

Knee No.	Delivery*	T1 Values (msec) with Gd(DTPA)$^{2-}$ ROI A	T1 Values (msec) with Gd(DTPA)$^{2-}$ ROI B	T1 Values (msec) with Gadoteridol ROI A	T1 Values (msec) with Gadoteridol ROI B
1	IV	237 ± 27	NP	NP	NP
2	IV	416 ± 76	NP	NP	NP
3	IV	469 ± 28	NP	NP	NP
4	IV	464 ± 19	NP	NP	NP
5	IA	280 ± 38	185 ± 39†	157 ± 22	159 ± 24
6	IA	168 ± 61	128 ± 16†	NP	NP
	IV	362 ± 59	269 ± 53†	243 ± 31	247 ± 39
7	IV	376 ± 60	273 ± 19†	310 ± 60	306 ± 60
8	IV	471 ± 9	313 ± 49†	248 ± 37	235 ± 18
9	IV	478 ± 96	374 ± 48†	319 ± 32	334 ± 42

Note.—NP = not performed, ROI = region of interest.
* IA = intraarticular, IV = intravenous.
† T1 values from ROI A and B were significantly different ($P < .05$).

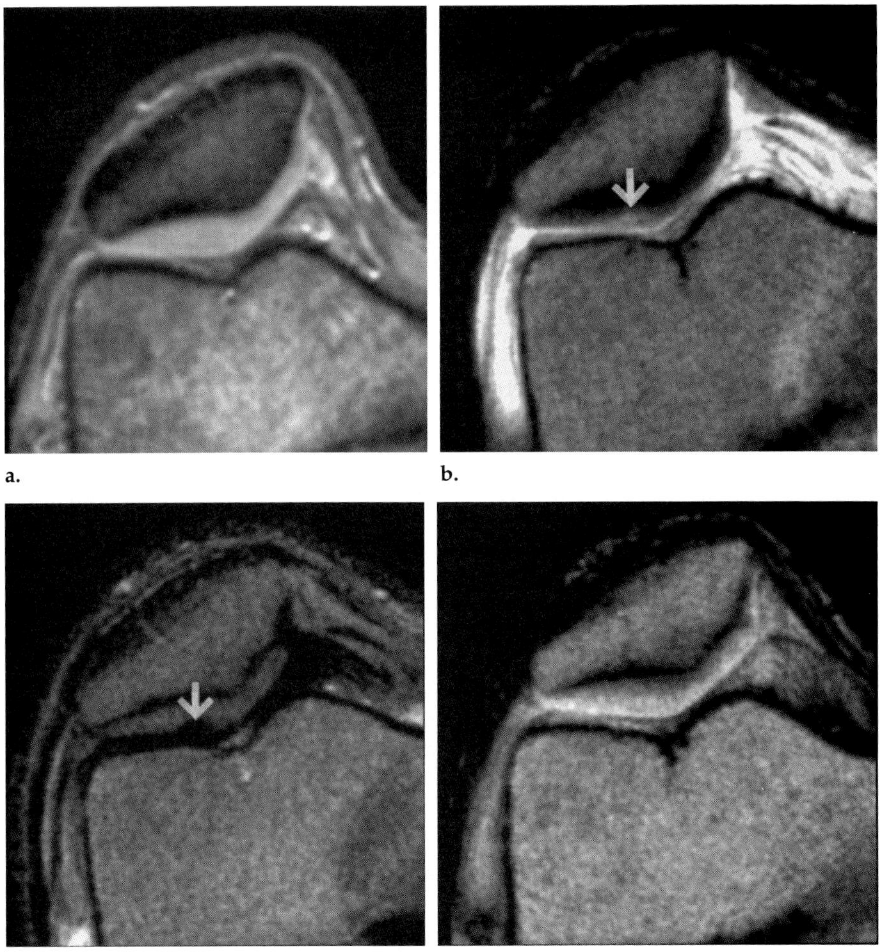

a. b. c. d.

Figure 5. **(a)** Unenhanced (fast low-angle shot) axial MR image shows a patella with no obvious abnormality. **(b)** Gd(DTPA)$^{2-}$-enhanced T1-weighted image (inversion time = 250 msec) from the T1-calculated series obtained 6 hours after intraarticular administration of contrast agent. A focal region of increased enhancement (arrow) can easily be seen. The T1 of the "lesion" is 185 msec ± 39 compared with a T1 of 280 msec ± 38 in a another region at the same depth from the articular surface. These values demonstrate a 34% difference in T1 in the lesion versus that in the surrounding tissue. **(c)** Image from the same T1-weighted series shown in **b** but with an inversion delay of 100 msec. The lesion here is seen with a lower signal intensity (arrow) than that of the surrounding tissue, illustrating the strong effect of the image parameters on the appearance of the image. **(d)** Gadoteridol-enhanced T1-weighted MR image (inversion time = 250 msec) obtained 7 hours after intraarticular administration of contrast agent. The T1 is relatively homogeneous with values of 159 msec ± 24 in the area of the "lesion" shown in **b** and **c** and 157 msec ± 22 in the surrounding tissue.

by regions of lower T1, or high Gd-(DTPA)$^{2-}$, suggesting a lower glycosaminoglycan content than that of the surrounding regions. The unenhanced images did not show any evidence of an anatomic defect or substantial signal variation. These data suggest that this subject had an area of morphologically intact cartilage with low glycosaminoglycan concentration, an area not seen with the conventional MR imaging method. Another volunteer (knee 6, Table) showed heterogeneous T1 across the patella, while the other volunteers demonstrated substantial medial to lateral differences in T1 in the presence of Gd(DTPA)$^{2-}$ (Fig 6).

On several images of knees penetrated with Gd(DTPA)$^{2-}$ (with both intraarticular and intravenous administration), the T1 of the articular surface was slightly (2%–10%) lower than that near the bone, suggesting a lower glycosaminoglycan content near the articular surface. This glycosaminoglycan profile with depth is consistent with previous literature reports of lower glycosaminoglycan at the articular surface (6). However, particularly for intraarticular administration, this T1 profile may also possibly be due to incomplete penetration by Gd(DTPA)$^{2-}$.

T1 Imaging after Tissue Penetration with Gadoteridol

In the five cases that were reimaged after administration of gadoteridol (Figs 5d, 6c) (Table), the heterogeneity observed with the negatively charged Gd(DTPA)$^{2-}$ was not observed with the nonionic contrast agent, gadoteridol. T1 values were calculated on the gadoteridol-enhanced images from approximately the same regions as those on the Gd(DTPA)$^{2-}$-enhanced images. No statistically significant difference was found in the T1 values on the gadoteridol-enhanced images.

DISCUSSION

The main goal of this work was to investigate the feasibility of an MR imaging technique for in vivo imaging of the glycosaminoglycan concentration of cartilage. One of the strengths of this approach is the large T1 difference expected between normal and diseased tissue in the presence of Gd-(DTPA)$^{2-}$. As illustrated by means of both the theoretic analysis and in vivo observations, T1 in the presence of Gd(DTPA)$^{2-}$ can differ by more than twofold when comparing regions of "normal" and "low" glycosaminoglycan concentration. Note that this study used T1-calculated images

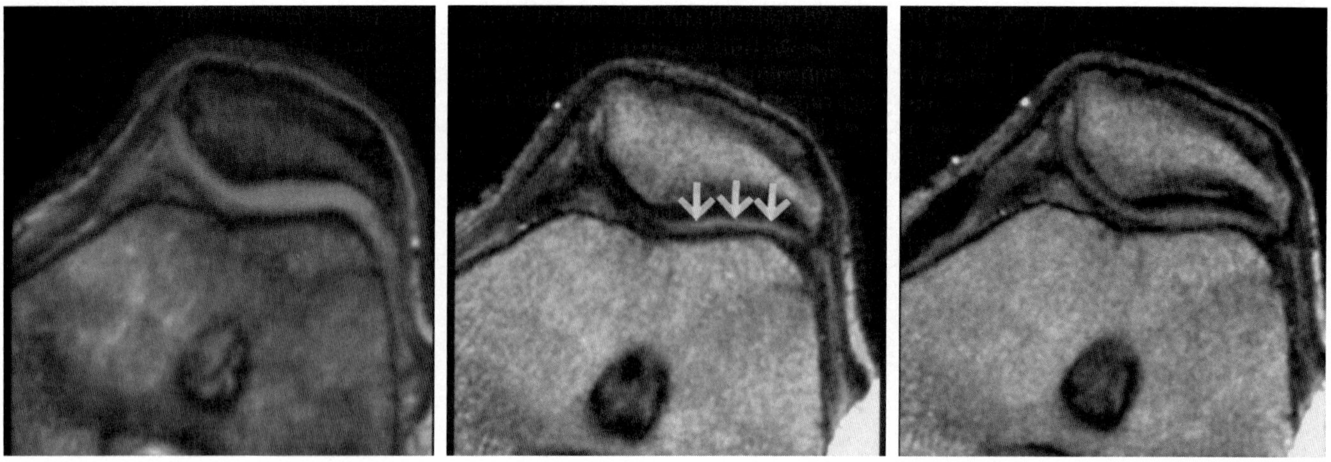

a. b. c.

Figure 6. **(a)** Unenhanced (fast low-angle shot) axial MR image shows a patella with no obvious abnormality. **(b)** T1-weighted image (inversion time = 250 msec) obtained 1½ hours after intravenous injection of $Gd(DTPA)^{2-}$. The T1 on the lateral aspect of the knee in the presence of $Gd(DTPA)^{2-}$ is 374 msec ± 48 (arrows), while it is 478 msec ± 96 on the medial aspect (22% difference). **(c)** Inversion-recovery turbo spin-echo image (inversion time = 350 msec) obtained 2 hours after intravenous injection of gadoteridol. The values of T1 are relatively homogeneous with a value of 334 msec ± 37 (lateral) and 319 msec ± 42 (medial). The actual signal intensity is hypointense in the deep zone of the cartilage due to the combined T1 and T2 weighting with this sequence.

(where the T1 values can be quantified and compared directly) as well as inversion-recovery T1-weighted images. The inversion-recovery images provided very high contrast between regions of differing T1 when the inversion time was set close to the null of the T1 of one part of the tissue (Figs 5b, 5c, 6b). Suboptimal image settings may be the reason that previous studies employing $Gd(DTPA)^{2-}$ penetration into cartilage did not observe contrast between regions of high and low glycosaminoglycan concentration (27,28).

Another strength of this technique is the specific interpretation of the resultant image T1, which is dominated by the $Gd(DTPA)^{2-}$ concentration, for cartilage glycosaminoglycan concentration. The basis for this interpretation is the extensive theoretic and experimental evidence showing that the charged glycosaminoglycans strongly influence the concentration of charged solutes (12,20,29). This interpretation that the charged glycosaminoglycan is the primary determinant of $Gd(DTPA)^{2-}$ distribution is further supported by our data showing that a similarly sized, uncharged agent (gadoteridol) has a uniform distribution within cartilage matrix. This finding strongly suggests it is the charge of the ionic contrast agent that enables it to distribute in accordance with tissue glycosaminoglycan concentration (as has been demonstrated previously through in vitro studies). Indeed, the measured T1s (Table) indicated that the concentration of the nonionic agent is higher than that of the ionic agent, a finding that is consistent with the notion that the ionic agent will be relatively excluded (ie, at a lower concentration) compared with a nonionic agent.

There are, however, disadvantages of this approach. First, it involves the administration of a contrast agent, thereby increasing the risk and expense of any study. Second, though the MR study itself can take less than 10 minutes, it is necessary to wait over 1 hour before initiating the MR study to allow the $Gd(DTPA)^{2-}$ to penetrate the tissue.

Contrast agent was found to penetrate the cartilage with both intraarticular and intravenous administration. With intraarticular delivery, $Gd(DTPA)^{2-}$ penetration appeared to proceed from the articular surface inward. Intraarticular administration of $Gd(DTPA)^{2-}$ has the advantage of providing a lower systemic dose of contrast agent, but has the disadvantages of both the discomfort associated with an intraarticular injection and the long time between intraarticular administration and the MR study. Intravenous delivery of $Gd(DTPA)^{2-}$ was notably quicker, as $Gd(DTPA)^{2-}$ was able to penetrate the cartilage from both the bone-cartilage and synovial fluid–cartilage interfaces. This would be expected to reduce penetration time by about a factor of 4, an expectation that was consistent with our observation of penetration of patellar cartilage within 2½ hours. (Penetration of the 1-mm-thick condylar cartilage occurred in less than 45 minutes.) Thus, intravenous administration of $Gd(DTPA)^{2-}$ has the advantage of achieving more rapid penetration of the cartilage and is a more comfortable route of administration, but it involves a higher systemic dose and is more costly.

The information on glycosaminoglycan content can be derived from the eventual distribution of contrast material within the cartilage. After allowing sufficient time for penetration of $Gd(DTPA)^{2-}$ into cartilage, in four of nine knees we saw homogeneous enhancement (and correspondingly normal unenhanced images), whereas in five knees we were able to observe variations in signal intensity that were not observable with standard unenhanced MR imaging or contrast material–enhanced MR imaging with a nonionic contrast agent. As noted above, we interpreted these variations as reflecting variations in tissue glycosaminoglycan concentration for two main reasons: (*a*) Extensive in vitro data with use of bovine and human cartilage have demonstrated a quantitative relationship between tissue glycosaminoglycan concentration and T1 in the presence of $Gd(DTPA)^{2-}$ (13,14,23), and (*b*) signal intensity in cartilage in the presence of the nonionic contrast agent, gadoteridol, was consistently homogeneous. At these late time points after injection, we believe it is unlikely that $Gd(DTPA)^{2-}$ transport could alone account for the signal intensity variations that we are referring to as "lesions." These variations are evident when comparing cartilage of the same depth, and they do not show up on images obtained with use of a nonionic contrast agent, which penetrated the tissue in the same time course as that of the ionic contrast agent.

The ability to image cartilage glycosaminoglycan concentration in vivo and to observe contrast indicating differences in glycosaminoglycan content in anatomically intact cartilage is exciting. Several caveats, however, are important to note. The prevalence and physiologic relevance of these "lesions" in the general population is unknown and would require more widespread studies. In addition, although we have extensive in vitro validation, including correlations between MR measures and histologic and biochemical analyses, we have no such direct validation for the in vivo studies to prove that the areas we are referring to as "lesions" are relatively low in glycosaminoglycan concentration. These studies, involving in vivo imaging and in vitro validation after total joint replacement surgery, are currently underway. Finally, we do not yet have enough information to quantify glycosaminoglycan concentration from these in vivo measurements. Such quantification requires that we measure (or know) the concentration of $Gd(DTPA)^{2-}$ in the blood and synovial fluid. We have not accounted for the fact that blood and synovial concentrations of $Gd(DTPA)^{2-}$ are not constant over time. The T1-calculated images should provide a relatively quantitative assessment of relative glycosaminoglycan concentration (eg, when comparing one region with another). Particularly in circumstances in which one wishes to compare data from one time with another (eg, annual examinations), quantification of glycosaminoglycan concentration may be more important.

In conclusion, these studies demonstrated that $Gd(DTPA)^{2-}$ will penetrate articular cartilage after intraarticular and intravenous injection. Variations in cartilage T1 in the presence of the ionic contrast agent $Gd(DTPA)^{2-}$ were interpreted as reflecting approximately 50% variations in the charged glycosaminoglycan constituent of cartilage. This interpretation is supported by the finding that T1 variations were not observed in the presence of the nonionic contrast agent gadoteridol and by previous in vitro work (13,14,23). Various aspects of the method must be more thoroughly investigated, in particular those pertaining to the pharmacokinetics of $Gd(DTPA)^{2-}$ delivery within cartilage and direct in vitro validation of the in vivo findings. To our knowledge, this is the first clinical study suggesting the ability to noninvasively monitor the concentration of glycosaminoglycan and, hence, early osteoarthritic changes, in humans.

APPENDIX

As described in the text, the goal of this section was to calculate the theoretic dependence of tissue T1 on glycosaminoglycan concentration in the presence of either an ionic contrast agent, $Gd(DTPA)^{2-}$, or a nonionic contrast agent, gadoteridol.

In the case of $Gd(DTPA)^{2-}$, the tissue T1, $T1_t$, is related to the tissue $Gd(DTPA)^{2-}$ concentration, $[Gd(DTPA)^{2-}]_t$, through the following relation:

$$T1_t = T1_{unenhanced} \div \{T1_{unenhanced} \cdot R \cdot [Gd(DTPA)^{2-}]_t + 1\},$$

where $T1_{unenhanced}$ = T1 of cartilage in the absence of contrast agent and R = relaxivity of the $Gd(DTPA)^{2-}$ in tissue, measured to be 3.5 L · $mmol^{-1}$ · sec^{-1} at 1.5 T and body temperature. R and $T1_{unenhanced}$ were assumed to be relatively constant and unaffected by tissue degradation (30). The small change in T1 with the hydration changes in the tissue would affect these calculations by 5% or less.

The tissue $Gd(DTPA)^{2-}$ concentration is then related to the tissue fixed charge density (FCD, the concentration of charge on the extracellular matrix). This is done through the empirically derived modification of a single-compartment ideal Donnan model of the tissue (13):

$$[Gd(DTPA)^{2-}]_t = \left\{\frac{FCD\sqrt{[Gd(DTPA)^{2-}]_o}}{4[Na^+]_o} + \sqrt{\frac{FCD^2[Gd(DTPA)^{2-}]_o}{16[Na^+]_o^2} + [Gd(DTPA)^{2-}]_o}\right\}^2,$$

where $[Na^+]_o$ and $[Gd(DTPA)^{2-}]_o$ refer to the concentration outside the tissue (eg, in the synovial fluid and surrounding tissue). $[Na^+]_o$ was assumed to be 0.15 mol/L, and $[Gd(DTPA)^{2-}]_t$ = 1 or 4 mmol/L as indicated in Figure 2.

Finally, we assume that glycosaminoglycans are the only macromolecules in cartilage that contribute to the net tissue fixed charge density. Collagen, the other predominant constituent of cartilage matrix, is net neutral (31). Tissue fixed charge density is then quantitatively related to glycosaminoglycan concentration assuming glycosaminoglycans have two negative charges per disaccharide (glycosaminoglycans are repeating disaccharides) and the predominant disaccharide (chondroitin sulfate) has a molecular weight of 502.5 g/mol. $FCD = -2[GAG]/502.5$, where FCD = fixed charge density and [GAG] = glycosaminoglycan concentration. The previous three equations were solved to relate cartilage T1 in the presence of $Gd(DTPA)^{2-}$ to tissue glycosaminoglycan concentration.

In the case of gadoteridol, the tissue T1, $T1_t$, is similarly related to the gadoteridol concentration, [gadoteridol], through the following equation:

$$T1_t = T1_{unenhanced} \div \{T1_{unenhanced} \cdot R \cdot [gadoteridol]_t + 1\},$$

where R was measured to be 3.2 L · $mmol^{-1}$ · sec^{-1} at 1.5 T and body temperature. Tissue gadoteridol concentration was assumed to be equal to the concentration of gadoteridol outside the tissue, independent of tissue glycosaminoglycan concentration:

$$[gadoteridol]_t = [gadoteridol]_o.$$

The previous two equations were solved to provide the value for cartilage T1 in the presence of gadoteridol. ■

Acknowledgment: The authors greatly appreciate the assistance of Chao-Wei Hwang, BS, in the image data analysis.

References

1. Pramer A, Furner S, Rice D. Musculoskeletal conditions in the United States. Park Ridge, Ill: American Academy of Orthopaedic Surgeons, 1992; 34–35.
2. Namba RS, Skinner HB. Adult reconstructive surgery. In: Skinner HB, ed. Current diagnosis and treatment in orthopedics. Norwalk, Conn: Appleton & Lane, 1995; 315–345.
3. Maroudas A. Balance between swelling pressure and collagen tension in normal and degenerate cartilage. Nature 1976; 260: 808–809.
4. Buckwalter JA, Roughley PJ, Rosenberg LC. Age-related changes in cartilage proteoglycans: quantitative electron microscopic studies. Microsc Res Tech 1994; 28:398–408.
5. Venn M, Maroudas A. Chemical composition and swelling of normal and osteoarthrotic femoral head cartilage. I. Chemical composition. Ann Rheum Dis 1977; 36:121–129.
6. Grushko G, Schneiderman R, Maroudas A. Some biochemical and biophysical parameters for the study of the pathogenesis of osteoarthritis: a comparison between the process of aging and degeneration in human hip cartilage. Connect Tissue Res 1989; 19:149–176.
7. Hayes CW, Sawyer RQ, Conway WF. Patellar cartilage lesions: in vitro detection and staging with MR imaging and pathologic correlation. Radiology 1992; 176:479–483.
8. Noyes RF, Stabler CL. A system for grading articular cartilage lesions at arthroscopy. Am J Sports Med 1989; 17:505–513.
9. Priedler KW, Resnick D. Imaging of osteoarthritis. Radiol Clin North Am 1996; 34:259–271.
10. Quinn SF, Rose PM, Brown TR, Demlow TA. MR imaging of the patellofemoral compartment. Magn Reson Imaging Clin N Am 1994; 2:425–440.
11. Bonamo JJ, Saperstein AL. Contemporary magnetic resonance imaging of the knee: the orthopedic surgeon's perspective. Magn Reson Imaging Clin N Am 1994; 2:481–495.
12. Lesperance LM, Gray ML, Burstein D. Determination of fixed charge density in cartilage using nuclear magnetic resonance. J Orthop Res 1992; 10:1–13.
13. Bashir A, Gray ML, Burstein D. $Gd(DTPA)^{2-}$ as a measure of cartilage degradation. Magn Reson Med 1996; 36:665–673.
14. Bashir A, Boutin RD, Gray ML, Burstein D. MRI of glycosaminoglycan distribution in cartilage using $Gd(DTPA)^{2-}$ in vivo. In: Proceedings of the Fifth Meeting of the International Society for Magnetic Resonance

in Medicine. Berkeley, Calif: International Society for Magnetic Resonance in Medicine, 1997; 345.
15. Kempson GE. Mechanical properties of articular cartilage. In: Freedman MAR, ed. Adult articular cartilage. 2nd ed. Kent, England: Pitman Medical, 1979; 333–413.
16. Frank EH, Grodzinsky AJ, Koob TJ, Eyre DR. Streaming potentials: a sensitive index of enzymatic degradation in articular cartilage. J Orthop Res 1987; 5:497–508.
17. Allen RG. Mechanical properties of selectively degraded cartilage explants: correlation to the spatiotemporal distribution of glycosaminoglycans. Thesis. Massachusetts Institute of Technology, Cambridge, Mass, 1996; 35–58.
18. Bonassar LJ, Frank EH, Murray JC, et al. Changes in cartilage composition and physical properties due to stromelysin degradation. Arthritis Rheum 1995; 38:173–183.
19. Maroudas A, Muir H, Wingham J. The correlation of fixed negative charge with glycosaminoglycan content of human articular cartilage. Biochim Biophys Acta 1969; 177:494–500.
20. Maroudas A. Physicochemical properties of articular cartilage. In: Freedman MAR, ed. Adult articular cartilage. 2nd ed. Kent, England: Pitman Medical, 1979; 215–290.
21. Tweedle MF. Nonionic or neutral. Radiology 1991; 178:891.
22. Boutin RD, Bashir A, Gray ML, Burstein D. MR imaging of early cartilage degeneration in the knee. AJR 1997; 168(suppl):58–59.
23. Bashir A, Paley D, Davidson SA, Gray ML, Burstein D. MRI measurements of fixed charge density as a measure of cartilage proteoglycan content (abstr). Proc Orthop Res Soc 1997; 217.
24. Corbetti F, Malatesta V, Camposampiero A, et al. Knee arthrography effects of various contrast media and epinephrine on synovial fluid. Radiology 1986; 161:195–198.
25. Drape JL, Thelen P, Gay-Depassier P, Silbermann O, Benacerraf R. Intraarticular diffusion of Gd-DOTA after intravenous injection in the knee: MR imaging evaluation. Radiology 1993; 188:227–234.
26. Winalski C, Aliabadi P, Wright RJ, Shortkroff S, Sledge CB, Weissman B. Enhancement of joint fluid with intravenously administered gadopentetate dimeglumine: technique, rationale, and implications. Radiology 1993; 187:179–185.
27. Kusaka Y, Grunder W, Rumpel H, Dannhauer KH, Gersonde K. MR microimaging of articular cartilage and contrast enhancement by manganese ions. Magn Reson Med 1992; 24:137–148.
28. Bacic G, Liu KJ, Goda F, Hoopes PJ, Rosen GM, Swartz HM. MRI contrast enhanced study of cartilage proteoglycan degradation in the rabbit knee. Magn Reson Med 1997; 37:764–768.
29. Buschmann MD, Grodzinsky AJ. A molecular model of proteoglycan associated electrostatic forces in cartilage mechanics. J Biomech Eng 1995; 117:179–192.
30. Donahue KM, Burstein D, Manning WJ, Gray ML. Studies of Gd-DTPA relaxivity and proton exchange rates in tissue. Magn Reson Med 1994; 32:66–76.
31. Li ST, Katz EP. An electrostatic model for collagen fibrils. Biopolymers 1976; 15: 1439–1460.

Suvimol Chirathivat Hill, MD • Alan R. Baker, MD • Norman W. Barton, MD, PhD
Leonard H. Wexler, MD • Leland J. C. Scott, MD, PhD

Sciatic Nerve: Paradoxic Hypertrophy after Amputation in Young Patients[1]

PURPOSE: To evaluate the appearance of the sciatic nerve after leg amputation.

MATERIALS AND METHODS: Magnetic resonance (MR) images were obtained in seven patients (age at amputation, 11–19 years) who underwent above-knee amputation to treat osteogenic sarcoma. Images were evaluated for sciatic nerve enlargement. Findings were correlated with the time after amputation.

RESULTS: All seven patients were found to have a markedly enlarged sciatic nerve in the stump of the amputated leg. The enlargement extended proximally from the point of nerve transection to a level posterior to the femoral neck (8–27 cm) depending on the length of the stump. No evidence of sciatic nerve enlargement was found in the opposite leg or on preoperative MR images that were available in three of the patients. Moreover, in one patient with a sarcoma who underwent a leg-sparing procedure, no sciatic nerve enlargement was seen postoperatively. The thickness of the distal sciatic nerve was related to the time after amputation.

CONCLUSION: Hypertrophy of the sciatic nerve occurred after above-knee amputation in young patients. This finding differed from atrophy of the nerve that has been reported previously in older patients.

One of the patients at our institution who underwent above-knee amputation at age 12 years to treat osteogenic sarcoma experienced phantom leg pain exacerbated by voiding 15 years after the amputation. Magnetic resonance (MR) imaging in the thighs showed unexpected enlargement of the sciatic nerve in the stump after amputation without the usual neuroma of the nerve. The purpose of this study was to determine if the phenomenon could also be detected in a group of similar patients.

MATERIALS AND METHODS

We evaluated the cases of seven patients seen at the National Institutes of Health who underwent MR imaging in their legs after above-knee amputation to treat osteogenic sarcoma. The patients included three female and four male patients aged 11–19 years at the time of amputation. MR imaging follow-up was performed from 6 months to 18 years after amputation. Sarcoma in six of the patients was in the distal femur and in one patient was in the proximal fibula. All patients underwent sciatic nerve ligation before transection. The patients' medical records were reviewed retrospectively to determine chemotherapy protocols.

Preoperative (n = 3) and postoperative (n = 7) MR imaging was performed with a 0.5-T unit (Vista; Picker International, Cleveland, Ohio) without gadolinium enhancement. Transaxial and coronal imaging were performed through the pelvis to include the lower thecal sac and the stump with the following sequences: T1-weighted spin echo (repetition time msec/echo time msec = 300–400/10) and short inversion time inversion recovery (STIR) (repetition time, 1,500–2,500 msec; inversion time, 100 msec). Contiguous coronal 3.5-mm-thick images were obtained through the lower spine and pelvis with use of a surface coil. Transaxial 10-mm-thick contiguous images were also obtained through the pelvis and stump with use of a body coil (128 × 256 matrix, two to four signals acquired, 35–45-cm field of view).

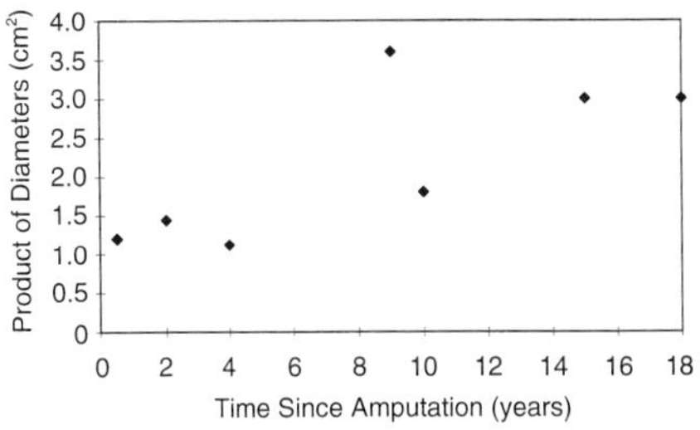

Figure 1. Scatter plot shows the correlation between the diameter of the distal end of the sciatic nerve with the time after amputation.

The images were evaluated for evidence of recurrent tumor, bone marrow and muscle changes, and sciatic nerve enlargement. For each enlarged sciatic nerve, the following were determined: (*a*) the anteroposterior and mediolateral diameters at the distal end and at the midpoint of the nerve in the stump, (*b*) the length of the nerve, and (*c*) the location

Index terms: Bone neoplasms, in infants and children, 45.322, 45.452 • Bone neoplasms, MR, 45.121411, 45.121413 • Bones, MR, 45.121411, 45.121413 • Sarcoma, 45.322

Abbreviation: STIR = short inversion time inversion recovery.

Radiology 1997; 205:559–562

[1] From the Department of Diagnostic Radiology, Warren Grant Magnuson Clinical Center, National Institutes of Health, Bldg 10, Rm 1C-660, 10 Center Dr, Mail Stop Code (MSC) 1182, Bethesda, MD 20892-1182 (S.C.H.); Virginia Medical Associates, Springfield, Va (A.R.B.); the Developmental and Metabolic Branch, National Institutes of Neurological Disorders and Stroke, National Institutes of Health, Bethesda, Md (N.W.B.); the Division of Pediatric Oncology, Columbia Presbyterian Medical Center, New York, NY (L.H.W.); and the Department of Neurology, University of Vermont, Burlington (L.J.C.S.). Received March 14, 1997; revision requested April 23; final revision received July 1; accepted July 8. **Address reprint requests to** S.C.H.

of the proximal end of the nerve. The presence or absence of enlargement of the transected sciatic nerve was determined by means of comparison with the intact nerve in the opposite thigh. The sign test was used to assess the statistical significance of the differences between the diameters of the transected and intact nerves.

The relationship between the size of the distal end of the sciatic nerve and the time after amputation was analyzed by generating a scatter plot and calculating a linear correlation coefficient (Fig 1).

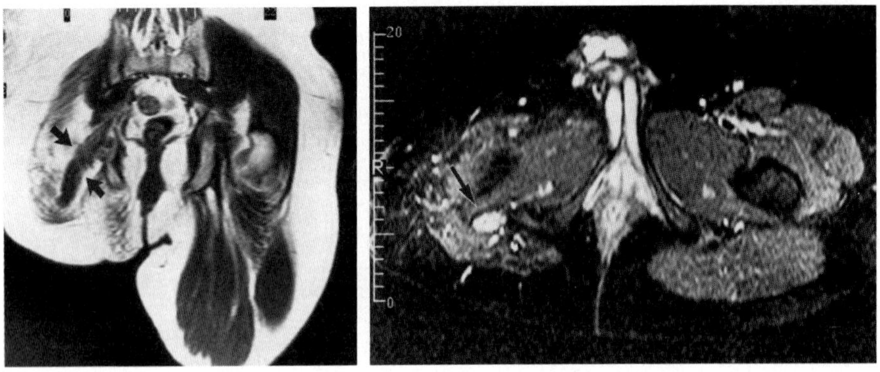

a. b.

Figure 2. Patient 3. Images obtained after above-knee right-leg amputation to treat osteogenic sarcoma. **(a)** Coronal T1-weighted (417/10) image in the right stump shows enlarged sciatic nerve (arrows) and muscle atrophy. **(b)** Axial STIR (3,067/100/30) image in the enlarged nerve (arrow) shows enlarged sciatic nerve posterior to the right femoral neck. The ruler indicates centimeters.

RESULTS

In all seven patients, diffuse enlargement of the entire sciatic nerve was apparent in the stump of the amputated leg (Fig 2). This was best seen on coronal and transaxial STIR images. The enlargement extended proximally from the end of the nerve for a minimum of 8 cm to a maximum of 27 cm (Table). In all cases, the enlargement ceased at the level of the femoral neck between the gemelli and gluteus maximus muscles. Patients with visible nerve roots exiting through the spinal foramina (n = 3) had no enlargement of the nerve roots. The distal end of the nerve was round in cross section and became elliptic or ribbonlike proximally. The enlargement was invariably greatest at the distal end and tapered proximally. In each case (Table), the diameter of the transected nerve was greater than that of the contralateral intact nerve at both the distal end and middle of the stump. At the distal end, maximal diameters ranged from 1.2 to 2.5 cm (mean, 1.8 cm) for the transected nerve versus from 0.5 to 1.0 cm (mean, 0.8 cm) for the intact nerve. At the middle of the stump, maximal diameters ranged from 1.0 to 1.5 cm (mean, 1.4 cm) for the transected nerve versus from 0.6 to 1.0 cm (mean, 0.8 cm) for the intact nerve.

These differences between the diameters of the transected nerves at the end and middle of the thigh were found to be statistically significant at $P \leq .02$ (two-tailed sign test).

In all patients, the appearance of the sciatic nerve on all MR images was identical to that of normal nerves (ie, hyperintense to muscle on STIR images and hypointense to muscle on T1-weighted images).

Three patients underwent MR imaging in the legs before amputation. Images in the region of the tumor and proximally revealed no evidence of sciatic nerve enlargement. Patient 4, who did not undergo MR imaging prior to above-knee amputation of his left leg to treat an osteosarcoma in the left femur, developed an osteosarcoma in the right femur 8 years later. Preoperative MR imaging in the second tumor showed dramatic enlargement of the left sciatic nerve but no enlargement of the right sciatic nerve (Fig 3). A leg-sparing procedure was performed to remove the tumor from his right femur; only the tumorous bone and contiguous soft tissues were removed, leaving the remainder of the leg including the sciatic nerve intact. No enlargement of the right sciatic nerve was observed at follow-up MR imaging 2 years after the second surgery.

Figure 1 shows the relationship between the size of the distal end of the sciatic nerve and the time after amputation. The diameter of the nerve increased with the time after amputation (r = .83 for maximal diameter, r = .61 for minimal diameter, and r = .83 for the product of the maximum diameter multiplied by the minimum diameter).

None of the patients had evidence of recurrence of osteogenic sarcoma or bone involvement, and all demonstrated muscle atrophy in the stump of the amputated leg.

All patients received chemotherapy to treat osteogenic sarcoma. The agents included bleomycin sulfate, cyclophosphamide, cisplatin, dactinomycin, doxorubicin hydrochloride, methotrexate sodium, and vincristine sulfate (Table). The treatment varied among the patients, but methotrexate sodium was included in every chemotherapy protocol.

DISCUSSION

In patients who undergo above-knee amputations to treat osteogenic sarcoma, findings in this study show that the portion of the sciatic nerve in the stump becomes enlarged in young patients rather than undergoing the atrophy that has come to be expected in older patients (Fig 4).

The changes that occur after a nerve is cut have been studied for most of this century, and the sequence of changes that normally occur has been well described (1–5). The portion of the nerve distal to the site of transection undergoes wallerian degeneration, whereas nerve fibers proximal to the site become atrophic. Nerve sprouts occur within hours of the damage (6), and the regenerating neurites grow in an effort to reestablish their original synaptic connections. If the atrophic fibers succeed in synapsing on an appropriate target, they regain most of their original caliber (3). If these fibers fail to reestablish connections, however, they will remain atrophic. Additionally, atrophy of the remaining nerve can be substantial because some of the neurons will die without target-derived trophic support (7).

In the case of leg amputations, the normal distal target for the fibers to reinnervate no longer exists, which frequently leads to a disorganized, tangled mass of outward growing axons, Schwann cells, fibroblasts, and connective tissue that form a neuroma. Grossly, a neuroma is a bulb-shaped enlargement of variable size at the distal end of a severed nerve. Its size depends on several factors, including the size of the parent nerve and the amount of pressure or irritation experienced by the neuroma. In sciatic neuromas, a cross-sectional diameter of 12 mm is common. Neuromas can often be symptomatic in patients, causing pain and local swelling. In patients with cancer who have undergone amputation to remove tumor, a symptomatic neuroma can mimic the symptoms of cancer recurrence.

Data in Seven Patients after Above-Knee Amputation to Treat Osteogenic Sarcoma

Patient No./ Sex/Age at Amputation	Time (y) from Amputation to MR Imaging	Length (cm) of Sciatic Nerve Stump Enlargement	Distal Sciatic Nerve Diameter (cm)		Middle Thigh Sciatic Nerve Diameter (cm)		Chemotherapy*
			Amputated Leg	Intact Leg	Amputated Leg	Intact Leg	
1/F/11 y 3 mo	0.5	8	1.5 × 0.8	0.8 × 0.2	1.5 × 0.5	0.8 × 0.2	CP, DH, MS
2/F/12 y 3 mo	10.0	20	1.8 × 1.0	0.8 × 0.1	1.2 × 0.6	0.8 × 0.2	BS, C, D, MS
3/M/13 y 3 mo	15.0	12	2.5 × 1.2	1.0 × 0.4	1.2 × 0.8	1.0 × 0.4	MS, VS
4/M/14 y 10 mo	9.0	27	2.0 × 1.8	0.5 × 0.2	2.0 × 0.8	0.5 × 0.2	BS, C, CP, D, MS
5/M/14 y 1 mo	18.0	18	2.0 × 1.5	0.8 × 0.2	1.0 × 0.6	0.8 × 0.2	DH, MS
6/M/17 y 6 mo	4.0	18	1.6 × 0.7	1.0 × 0.2	1.5 × 0.3	1.0 × 0.2	BS, C, CP, D, DH, MS
7/F/18 y 8 mo	2.0	10	1.2 × 1.2	0.6 × 0.2	1.2 × 0.6	0.6 × 0.2	BS, C, CP, D, DH, MS

* BS = bleomycin sulfate, C = cyclophosphamide, CP = cisplatin, D = dactinomycin, DH = doxorubicin hydrochloride, MS = methotrexate sodium, VS = vincristine sulfate.

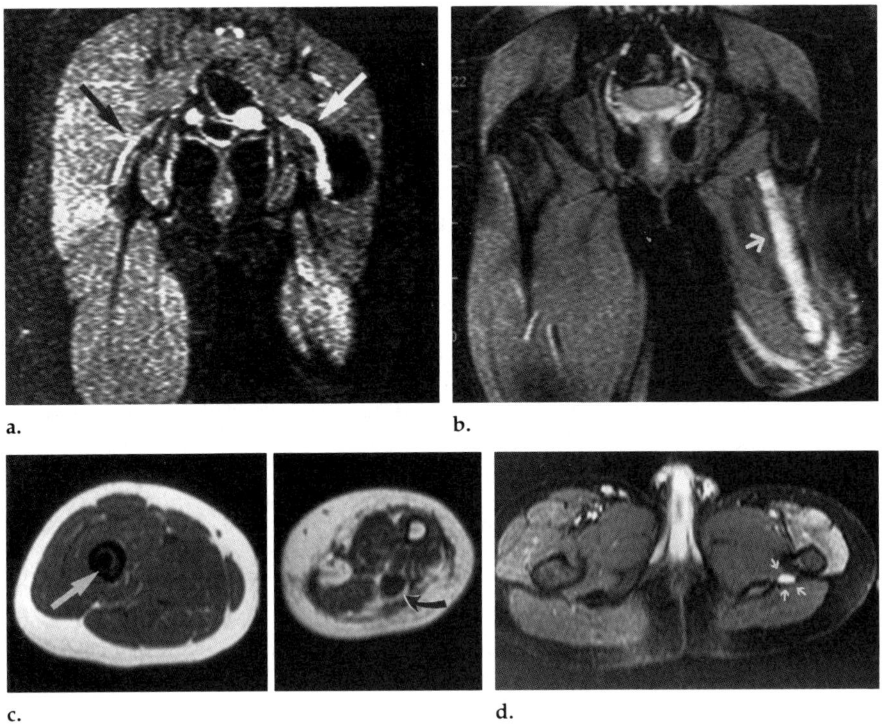

Figure 3. Patient 4. Images obtained after above-knee left-leg amputation and a right-leg–sparing procedure. **(a, b)** Coronal STIR (1,500/100/30) images demonstrate enlarged sciatic nerve (white arrow in **a** and **b**) and muscle atrophy of the left stump with no nerve enlargement on the right (black arrow in **a**). The enlargement of the sciatic nerve extends from the distal end of the stump proximally to the level behind the femoral neck. **(c)** Axial T1-weighted (400/10) images at the level of the distal end of the stump show the typical rounded distal end of the sciatic nerve (curved arrow). Note the prosthesis on the right femur (white arrow). **(d)** Axial STIR (2,850/100/30) image in the more proximal end of the stump shows typical elliptic shape of the enlarged sciatic nerve (arrows) at the level of the ischial tuberosity.

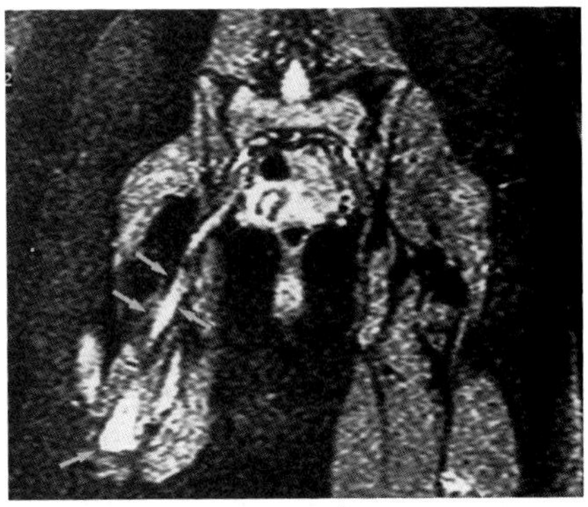

Figure 4. Patient 2. Images obtained after above-knee right-leg amputation to treat osteogenic sarcoma. Coronal STIR (1,633/100/30) image shows enlargement of the right sciatic nerve (arrows), which is largest at the end of the stump and tapered proximally.

Computed tomography and MR imaging are now being used to help distinguish between these two (8,9) alternatives.

In the patients in our study, nerve enlargement was generally greatest at the site of sciatic nerve transection with extension proximally for distances up to 27 cm. This observation was unexpected, as findings in previous investigations of nerve reactions to axotomy, in humans and in animals, have uniformly demonstrated atrophy of the proximal nerve (1,2,4,5,10–12). In contrast to what was observed in our patients, the most pronounced atrophy has been reported to occur in the portion of the nerve nearest the site of transection (7).

Variables that might be implicated in this unusual nerve reaction include the young age of the patients, the presence of osteosarcoma, and the chemotherapy regimen. Young age may account for this phenomenon; the bulk of the atrophy data have been acquired in older patients who underwent amputation to treat vascular insufficiency. Animal data suggest that age may not be a factor, however, as studies of amputation effects on the sciatic nerve in kittens showed nerve atrophy rather than hypertrophy (13).

In our study, MR imaging characteristics of the enlarged nerves were indistinguishable from those of normal peripheral nerves and neuromas. This argues that the enlargement is not the result of fat infiltration or residual sarcoma tissue. In the absence of histologic data, however, the pathogenesis of sciatic nerve enlargement in these patients is unclear. Enlargement may be the result of hypertrophy of the neural fascicles, but other causes of neural swelling should also be considered such as deterioration with disorganization and spreading of the nerve fibers and deposition of perineural fibrous tissue.

An alternative hypothesis is that the enlargement results from abnormal axonal transport. After axotomy, the synthesis and transport of neurofilaments—a cytoskeletal element thought to be important in determining normal axonal caliber—is diminished (14). This downward regulation may be responsible in part for the normal axonal atrophy seen after nerve transection. The enlargement seen in our patients, which extended proximally from the site of transection, could be due to an alteration in the normal cellular response in which neurofilaments (or other cytoskeletal constituents) continue to be synthesized and transported after nerve transection, which leads to their accumulation in the distal axon segment.

The potential role of osteosarcoma or subsequent chemotherapy in the development of nerve enlargement in our patients is unknown. Cancers in general, and sarcomas in particular, have been shown to synthesize a variety of trophic factors and cytokines, as well as their receptors (15–18). For example, insulinlike growth factor I, which has been implicated in peripheral nerve regeneration (19,20), has been shown to be synthesized by osteosarcomas (21). Such a tumor-derived factor may be responsible for the observed nerve enlargement, but the way this would occur after the tumor is removed is unclear.

The ultimate clinical consequences of nerve enlargement in these patients are unknown but seem to be innocuous. Of the seven patients in this study, only two were symptomatic with occasional phantom leg pain. Moreover, follow-up of up to 18 years showed no evidence that the sciatic nerve enlargement represented latent osteosarcoma or some other health threat. Thus, from a radiologic viewpoint, these observations are important only in that they demonstrate the benign nature of this phenomenon. Recognition of this phenomenon could obviate unnecessary painful biopsy. These results conflict, however, with previous observations and well-established neurobiologic theory. Pathologic studies of enlarged sciatic nerves, as well as studies of the effects that osteosarcomas and methotrexate sodium have on sciatic nerve regeneration, should be undertaken to clarify the issue. ■

Acknowledgments: The authors thank Andrew Dwyer, MD, Roscoe Brady, MD, and Lynne Schneider, PhD, for their helpful criticisms of the manuscript for this article.

References

1. Ranson SW. Retrograde degeneration in the spinal nerves. J Comp Neurol 1906; 16: 265–293.
2. Greenman MJ. Studies on the regeneration of the peroneal nerve of the albino rat: number and sectional areas of fibers—area relation of axis to sheath. J Comp Neurol 1913; 3:479–513.
3. Gutmann E, Sanders FK. Recovery of fibre numbers and diameters in the regeneration of peripheral nerves. J Physiol 1943; 101:489–518.
4. Cragg BG, Thomas PK. Changes in conduction velocity and fibre size proximal to peripheral nerve lesions. J Physiol 1961; 157:315–327.
5. Aitken JT, Thomas PK. Retrograde changes in fibre size following nerve section. J Anat 1962; 96:121–129.
6. Ramon Y, Cajal S; May RM, trans. Degeneration and regeneration of the nervous system. London, England: Oxford University Press, 1928.
7. Dyck PJ, Thomas PK, Lambert EH, Bunge R. Permanent axotomy: a model of chronic neuronal degeneration preceded by axonal atrophy, myelin remodeling, and degeneration. In: Peripheral neuropathy. Vol 1. Philadelphia, Pa: Saunders, 1984; 666–690.
8. Singson RD, Feldman F, Staron R, Fletchner D, Gonzalez E, Stein J. MRI of postamputation neuromas. Skeletal Radiol 1990; 19: 259–262.
9. Donnal JF, Blinder RA, Coblentz CL, Moylan JA, Fitzpatrick KP. MR imaging of stump neuroma. J Comput Assist Tomogr 1990; 14:656–657.
10. Gutmann E, Holumbar J. Atrophy of nerve fibres in the central stump following nerve section and the possibilities of its prevention. Arch Int Stud Neurol 1951; 1:1–11.
11. Hoffer JA, Stein RB, Gordon T. Differential atrophy of sensory and motor fibers following section of cat peripheral nerves. Brain Res 1979; 178:347–361.
12. Dyck PJ, Lais AC, Karnes JL, et al. Permanent axotomy, a model of axonal atrophy and secondary segmental demyelination and remyelination. Ann Neurol 1981; 9: 575–583.
13. Jorgensen D, Dyck PJ. Axonal underdevelopment from axotomy in kittens. J Neuropathol Exp Neurol 1979; 38:551–557.
14. Hoffman PN, Cleveland DW, Griffin JW, Landes PW, Cowan NJ, Price DL. Neurofilament gene expression: a major determinant of axonal caliber. Proc Natl Acad Sci USA 1987; 84:3472–3476.
15. Pekarek LA, Weichselbaum RR, Beckett MA, Nachman J, Schreiber H. Footprinting of individual tumors and their variants by constitutive cytokine expression patterns. Cancer Res 1993; 53:1978–1981.
16. Kloen P, Jennings CL, Gebhardt MC, Springfield DS, Mankin HJ. Expression of transforming growth factor-beta (TGF-beta) receptors, TGF-beta 1 and TGF-beta 2 production and autocrine growth control in osteosarcoma cells. Int J Cancer 1994; 58: 440–445.
17. Muller HL, Oh Y, Lehrnbecher T, Blum WF, Rosenfeld RG. Insulin-like growth factor–binding protein-2 concentrations in cerebrospinal fluid and serum of children with malignant solid tumors or acute leukemia. J Clin Endocrinol Metab 1994; 79:428–434.
18. Wang J, Coltrera MD, Gown AM. Cell proliferation in human soft tissue tumors correlates with platelet-derived growth factor B chain expression: an immunohistochemical and in situ hybridization study. Cancer Res 1994; 54:560–564.
19. Hansson HA, Dahlin LB, Danielsen N, et al. Evidence indicating trophic importance of IGF-I in regenerating peripheral nerves. Acta Physiol Scand 1986; 126:609–614.
20. Kanje M, Skottner A, Sjoberg J, et al. Insulin-like growth factor I (IGF-I) stimulates regeneration of the rat sciatic nerve. Brain Res 1987; 486:396–398.
21. Kappel CK, Velez-Yanguas MC, Hirschfield S, Helman LJ. Human osteosarcoma cell lines are dependent on insulin-like growth factor for in vitro growth. Cancer Res 1994; 54:2803–2807.

Francis G. Blankenberg, MD • Nyu-Nyu Loh, MD • Alexander M. Norbash, MD
Judith A. Craychee, MD • Daniel M. Spielman, PhD • Brenda L. Person, RDMS
C. Angela Berg, RDMS, RDCS • Dieter R. Enzmann, MD

Impaired Cerebrovascular Autoregulation after Hypoxic-Ischemic Injury in Extremely Low–Birth-Weight Neonates: Detection with Power and Pulsed Wave Doppler US[1]

PURPOSE: To evaluate regional cerebral blood flow with power and pulsed wave Doppler ultrasound (US) in extremely low–birth-weight neonates with periventricular leukomalacia (PVL), germinal matrix hemorrhage (GMH), or both.

MATERIALS AND METHODS: The lenticulostriate arteries of 17 preterm neonates (birth weight ≤ 1,100 g) were assessed daily with Doppler US during the first 5–6 days of life. The mean arterial pressure and bilateral peak velocity, resistive index, coronal vascular cross-sectional area, and product of the peak velocity and vascular cross-sectional area were measured.

RESULTS: Five neonates developed PVL, GMH, or both; results of follow-up examinations in 11 patients were normal. One neonate with severe intrauterine growth retardation and renal tubular acidosis was excluded. Neonates with PVL, GMH, or both showed significantly greater mean values and more variable values of vascular cross-sectional area and product of peak velocity and cross-sectional area than neonates without PVL or GMH ($P < .025$). Mean resistive index was significantly lower in neonates with PVL, GMH, or both than in neonates without ($P < .01$). There were no significant differences between mean arterial pressure in neonates with and those without PVL, GMH, or both.

CONCLUSION: By enabling the detection of autoregulatory fluctuations in cerebral blood flow associated with hypoxic-ischemic injury, power and pulsed wave Doppler US may enable identification of preterm neonates who are at risk of developing PVL, GMH, or both during the 1st week of life.

Impaired cerebrovascular autoregulation due to perinatal asphyxia is believed to often contribute to or be coexistent with germinal matrix hemorrhage (GMH) and periventricular leukomalacia (PVL) (1–7). Blunted or absent cerebrovascular responses in preterm neonates to changes in Pa_{CO_2}, Pa_{O_2}, and blood glucose concentration have been correlated with severe hypoxic-ischemic encephalopathy and poor neurologic outcome (2–7). Before loss of these autoregulatory mechanisms, there is a defective or absent cerebrovascular response (which may be a considerable cofactor in this pathophysiologic process) to changes in mean arterial pressure. In healthy preterm neonates, there is an intact vasoregulatory mechanism (termed "pressure-flow autoregulation" [5]), and global cerebral blood flow is well maintained with mean arterial pressures of 26–52 mm Hg. Hypoxic-ischemic injury results in attenuation or loss of pressure-flow autoregulation; this attenuation or loss results in an increase or decrease in global cerebral blood flow with a respective rise or fall in mean arterial pressure. Pyrds (5) found that a defective pressure-flow autoregulation in asphyxiated neonates results in exponential and disproportionate increases in cerebral blood flow with an increasing mean arterial pressure. Premature neonates who have experienced severe hypoxic-ischemic episodes can, therefore, demonstrate a marked increase in global cerebral blood flow despite a normal mean arterial pressure. This blood-flow increase, which may be up to four times the normal value, is known as "luxury perfusion" (8) and can be seen with a concomitant decrease in cerebral demand for oxygen and glucose (5). The mismatch of global cerebral blood flow and cerebral metabolic activity results in decreased cerebral oxygen extraction and increased cerebral venous P_{O_2}; these findings have been demonstrated with near infrared spectroscopy and direct venous sampling (4,6,7). The specific mechanisms of capillary recruitment and vasoparalysis appear to be important in the development of luxury perfusion and intracerebral shunting after hypoxic-ischemic injury (3,4,6,7).

In premature neonates, investigators have used a combination of xenon-133 clearance and near infrared spectroscopy to study global cerebral blood flow and oxygen extraction (1–7). The regional nature of luxury perfusion suggests that determining regional cerebral blood flow may be more important clinically than measuring global cerebral blood flow if regional cerebral blood flow can be correlated with more specific locations in the neonatal brain that are affected by focal hypoxic-ischemic injury. Recently, functional magnetic resonance (MR) imaging and positron emission tomography have been used to study regional cerebral blood flow (9). When used to examine severely ill preterm

Index terms: Arteries, middle cerebral, 1741.12989 • Infants, newborn, central nervous system, 13.5911, 13.8729, 1741.12989 • Leukomalacia, 13.5911, 13.8729 • Ultrasound (US), Doppler studies, 1741.12989 • Ultrasound (US), in infants and children, 1741.12989

Abbreviations: GMH = germinal matrix hemorrhage, PVL = periventricular leukomalacia.

Radiology 1997; 205:563–568

[1] From the Department of Radiology, Stanford University School of Medicine, 300 Pasteur Dr, Stanford, CA 94305. From the 1996 RSNA scientific assembly. Received March 11, 1997; revision requested April 30; revision received July 16; accepted July 21. **Address reprint requests to** F.G.B.

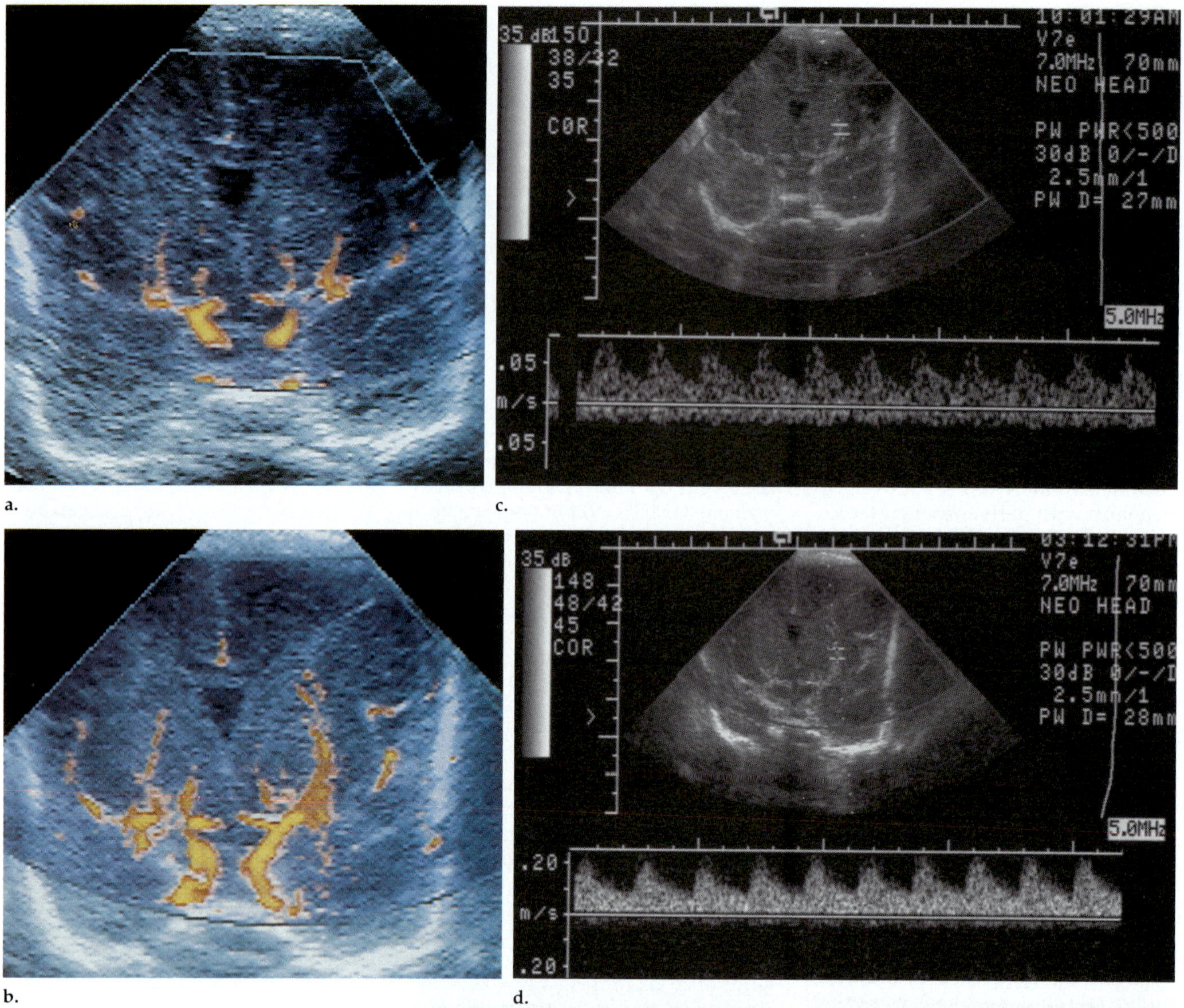

Figure 1. **(a–d)** Power and pulsed wave Doppler sonograms of a 26-week-old preterm neonate with developing PVL and left, grade 2 GMH. **(a, b)** Coronal power Doppler sonograms of the lenticulostriate arteries on **(a)** day 3 and **(b)** day 4 of life. On day 3, the left cross-sectional vascular area of 0.132 cm^2 was within the normal range of values and increased to 0.36 cm^2 on day 4. **(c, d)** Pulsed wave Doppler sonograms of the lenticulostriate arteries on **(c)** day 3 and **(d)** day 4 of life. On day 3, the left peak velocity of 8.0 cm/sec was within the normal range of values and increased to 23.0 cm/sec on day 4. On day 5, the patient developed a left, grade 2 GMH (not shown). **(e, f)** Coronal sonograms of the **(e)** frontal and **(f)** parietal regions at 4 weeks of age demonstrate bilateral PVL.

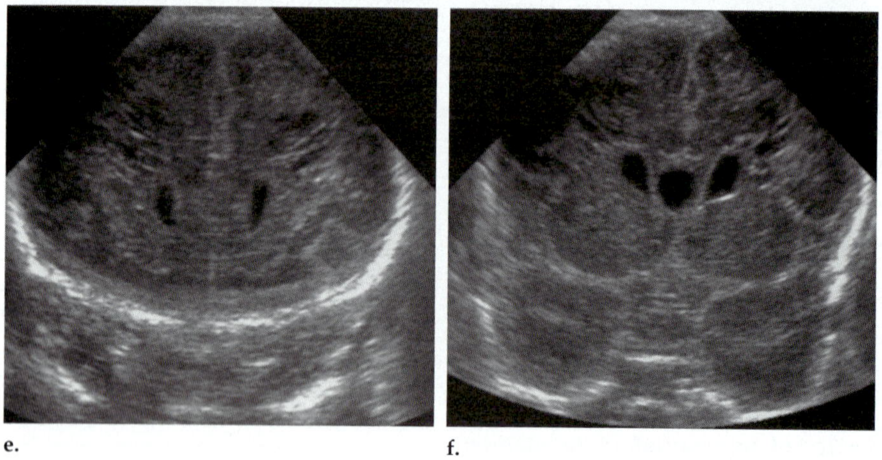

neonates, MR imaging and positron emission tomography are limited by their expense and lack of portability.

Duplex Doppler ultrasound (US) examination of the anterior and middle cerebral arteries can provide an approximate estimate of global cerebral blood flow (10). Color Doppler US has also been used in neonates to examine regional increases in mean blood-flow velocities in areas of acute infarction (11). The duplex and color Doppler US techniques are insensitive to very low velocity signals from small vessels and provide imprecise measurements of vessel diameter. Some of these technical difficulties are overcome with power Doppler US, which is less dependent on the angle of examination and more sensitive for the detection of low velocities (12).

We performed this study to evaluate blood flow in the lenticulostriate arteries in neonates with PVL, GMH, or both. We examined 17 extremely low–birth-weight (≤1,100 g) preterm neonates during the 1st week after birth. We specifically examined lenticulostriate arteries because they provide central perfusion to the periventricular white matter in premature neonates (13–15). This vascular bed may be affected most with regional hypoxic-ischemic injury after partial perinatal asphyxia (13,16,17).

MATERIALS AND METHODS

Patient Population

Preterm neonates were selected solely on the basis of *(a)* low birth weight (≤1,100 g) and *(b)* the procurement of parental consent to serial examination of neonates as approved by the in-house institutional human investigation review board. From April 1995 to June 1996, 17 low-birth-weight neonates (seven male and 10 female neonates) who were born in-house or transferred to the neonatal unit were consecutively entered into the study within the first 24 hours of life. Mean birth weight was 839 g ± 138 (± standard deviation). Mean estimated gestational age was 26.8 weeks ± 1.6 (range, 24–31 weeks). Mean Apgar scores were 3.9 ± 2.0 and 6.7 ± 2.0 at 1 and 5 minutes, respectively. The heart rate, blood pressure, and mean arterial pressure in the umbilical catheter (if available) were recorded at the time of power Doppler US examination. Examination results without simultaneous measurement of mean arterial pressure in the umbilical catheter were excluded from the final analysis. Simultaneous measurements of arterial blood gases from umbilical catheters were not performed, because this procedure was considered semi-invasive owing to the small blood volumes of premature neonates. All patients were followed up at 1–2 months after birth with routine US examination of the head and neurologic examination under the direction of neonatologists.

Among the 17 preterm neonates, five developed PVL, GMH, or both. One neonate showed profound intrauterine growth retardation with a birth weight of 588 g despite an estimated gestational age of 31 weeks. This neonate was diagnosed with Turner syndrome (with mosaicism) and type 2 renal tubular acidosis; findings of this neonate's examination were excluded from statistical calculations. The findings of routine follow-up US and neurologic examinations of the other 11 patients were normal 1–2 months after birth.

Gray-Scale US Examination

In each neonate, a routine gray-scale US examination was performed through the anterior and posterior fontanelles in the coronal and sagittal planes during the first 5 or 6 days of life with use of an Acuson 128XP/10 unit (Mountain View, Calif) and a 7-MHz electronic sector probe. Gray-scale US images were screened daily by a neurosonographer (F.G.B.) for GMH, PVL, or hydrocephalus; these results were promptly relayed to the staff of the neonatal intensive care unit. Routine sonography was performed immediately before power and pulsed wave Doppler US examinations by one of four neurosonographers (F.G.B., J.A.C., B.L.P., C.A.B.)

Power Doppler US Examination

Power Doppler US examinations were performed with color Doppler energy software and a 7-MHz sector arterial probe. Power Doppler US imaging of the right and left lenticulostriate arteries was performed in the coronal and sagittal planes with use of the following settings during each examination: power level, less than 500 mW/cm^2; preprocessing, 0; persistence, 4; postprocessing, E9 + 4; gate, 1 (smallest); filter, 1 (lowest-frequency wall filter); sensitivity, 0 (medium); depth, 6 cm; and screen color, full at 7.0 MHz with color gain set immediately below flash artifact. A power Doppler US examination was considered satisfactory if at least one lateral lenticulostriate artery was seen in the coronal plane from the level of the horizontal segment of the middle cerebral artery to at least the cephalic level of the cavity of the septum pellucidum (Fig 1). In all neonates, power Doppler US examination was performed in less than 10 minutes. Given the settings used, the thermal index for soft tissue was less than 1 for the entire range of pulsed repetition frequencies (highest, default, and lowest) as defined by published standards (18). Values of the thermal index for soft tissue of less than 1 have no reported biologic effect (18).

The brandy-glass configuration of the lenticulostriate vessels is shown in Figure 1a and 1b. The borders of lenticulostriate vessels (lateral and medial groups) in the coronal plane were manually traced, and the vascular cross-sectional areas within the tracings were obtained with graph analysis (19). The horizontal segment of the middle cerebral artery and other vessels were excluded. The cross-sectional areas of the right and left lenticulostriate vessels were analyzed separately. Different fields of view (depth) were normalized with reference to centimeter scales on each image. Tracings and measurements of coronal vascular cross-sectional areas were performed by F.G.B.

Pulsed Wave Doppler US Examination

Pulsed wave Doppler US examination of a single lenticulostriate vessel at the level of the cavity of the septum pellucidum was performed bilaterally during each examination (Fig 1c, 1d). Angle corrections were made during measurements of velocity. The mean Doppler angle (ie, the mean angle between the long axis of the examined vessel and the short axis of the electronic gate of the pulsed wave Doppler signal) was 7.5° ± 8.36. Peak velocity and resistive indexes were also measured bilaterally.

Statistical Analysis

Values of the peak velocity, coronal cross-sectional area of the lenticulostriate vasculature, product of the peak velocity and vascular cross-sectional area, and resistive index were compared with the standard Student two-tailed t test. Variances in these quantities were compared with use of the F test and 95th- and 99th-percentile tables (20). Values determined with the Student t test and F test that equaled or exceeded the 95th-percentile value were considered significant (ie, $P < .05$).

RESULTS

Gray-Scale US Examination

Among the 17 preterm neonates, patients 1 and 2 developed PVL, which was confirmed with follow-up US examination. At 1 month of age, patient 1 demonstrated cystic changes in the parietooccipital periventricular white matter bilaterally. This patient also showed neurologic evidence of cerebral palsy at the 6-month follow-up examination. On the 2nd day of life, patient 2 also developed a grade 1 GMH; on the 5th day of life, the hemorrhage increased in size with extension into the ipsilateral ventricle (grade 2). At 6 weeks of age, patient 2 showed extensive cystic changes of PVL that involved the frontoparietooccipital periventricular white matter bilaterally. At the 2-month follow-up neurologic examination, this patient showed increased muscle tone and clonus in the lower extremities and was considered to be at high risk for developing cerebral palsy. At 3 months of age, patient 2 underwent computed tomography of the brain; PVL of the bilateral frontoparietooccipital areas and a chronic left temporal lobe infarction were found.

Patient 3 developed bilateral grade 2 GMH; the first hemorrhage occurred on the 2nd day, and the second hemorrhage occurred on the 4th day of life. Despite multiple medical problems, including bronchopulmonary dysplasia and retinopathy of prematurity, patient 3 appeared neurologically healthy at the 6-month follow-up examination. Patient 4 showed a unilateral grade 2 GMH on the 6th day of life, and patient 5 developed a unilateral grade 1 GMH on the 3rd day of life. Patients 4 and 5 appeared neurologically healthy at their follow-up examinations.

In all 11 patients who did not show sonographic evidence of PVL or GMH, the results of follow-up neurologic examinations were normal. One of these neonates did experience a single, reported tonicoclonic seizure in the left lower extremity on the 1st day of life; however, at 2 months of age, US and MR imaging findings in this patient were normal. Neonates in both groups experienced multiple other chronic conditions associated with extreme prematurity, such as bronchopulmonary dysplasia ($n = 9$), retinopathy of prematurity ($n = 8$), gastrointestinal complications of necrotizing enterocolitis ($n = 2$), and gastroesophageal reflux and aspiration pneumonia ($n = 5$). Only three neonates—patient 4 with a right, grade 2 GMH and two neonates with normal findings at follow-up US and neurologic examinations—had patent arterial ducts that necessitated treatment with indomethacin or surgical closure.

Mean Daily Measurements with Power and Pulsed Wave Doppler US

The daily resistive indexes (right- and left-sided measurements were pooled for statistical analyses) in preterm neonates with PVL, GMH, or both ($n = 5$) were significantly lower than those in neonates with normal findings at US and neurologic examinations ($P < .025$) (Table 1). The mean daily vascular cross-sectional area and mean product of the peak velocity and vascular cross-sectional area in neonates with PVL, GMH, or both were significantly higher than those in neonates without PVL or GMH ($P < .01$ and $P < .05$, respectively). The mean daily peak velocity and mean arterial pressure in neonates with PVL, GMH, or both and those in neonates without PVL or GMH did not differ significantly.

Mean Maximum or Minimum Daily Measurements with Power and Pulsed Wave Doppler US

The mean value of the maximum daily resistive index (highest value for each examination [ie, right or left lenticulostriate vessel]) in neonates with PVL, GMH, or both were significantly lower than those in neonates without PVL or GMH ($P < .05$). The mean maximum daily vascular cross-sectional area and mean product of the peak velocity and cross-sectional area (irrespective of side measured) in neonates with PVL, GMH, or both were significantly higher than those in neonates without PVL or GMH ($P < .05$). The mean maximum and minimum daily peak velocities in the two groups did not differ significantly. The mean minimum daily resistive indexes, vascular cross-sectional areas, and products of the peak velocity and cross-sectional area in the two groups also did not differ significantly.

Table 1
Measurements with Power and Pulsed Wave Doppler US in Neonates

Parameters	Neonates with PVL and/or GMH	Neonates without PVL or GMH
Mean daily measurements*		
Resistive index	0.543 ± 0.087 (38)	0.586 ± 0.091 (104)
Peak velocity (cm/sec)	8.43 ± 4.04	8.0 ± 2.44
Vascular area (cm^2)	0.290 ± 0.175	0.205 ± 0.091
Velocity × area (cm^3/sec)	2.62 ± 2.45	1.69 ± 1.03
Mean arterial pressure (mm Hg)	36.9 ± 6.34 (19)	38.5 ± 5.57 (52)
Mean maximum daily measurements†		
Resistive index	0.577 ± 0.087 (19)	0.624 ± 0.082 (52)
Peak velocity (cm/sec)	9.97 ± 4.75	8.97 ± 2.24
Vascular area (cm^2)	0.33 ± 0.173	0.231 ± 0.093
Velocity × area (cm^3/sec)	3.36 ± 3.04	1.96 ± 1.07
Mean minimum daily measurements†		
Resistive index	0.508 ± 0.76 (19)	0.548 ± 0.084 (52)
Peak velocity (cm/sec)	6.89 ± 2.44	7.03 ± 2.24
Vascular area (cm^2)	0.249 ± 0.172	0.182 ± 0.082
Velocity × area (cm^3/sec)	1.87 ± 1.38	1.43 ± 0.92
Mean highest measurements in each neonate‡		
Resistive index	0.684 ± 0.073 (5)	0.709 ± 0.041 (11)
Peak velocity (cm/sec)	14.58 ± 6.59	11.35 ± 1.30
Vascular area (cm^2)	0.51 ± 0.20	0.33 ± 0.17
Velocity × area (cm^3/sec)	6.56 ± 3.29	3.27 ± 0.91
Mean lowest measurements in each neonate‡		
Resistive index	0.436 ± 0.050 (5)	0.452 ± 0.068 (11)
Peak velocity (cm/sec)	5.18 ± 1.81	4.96 ± 1.44
Vascular area (cm^2)	0.189 ± 0.192	0.119 ± 0.049
Velocity × area (cm^3/sec)	1.43 ± 1.43	0.76 ± 0.31

Note.—Numbers in parentheses are numbers of measurements averaged.
* Daily measurements of the right and left lenticulostriate arteries were pooled for statistical analysis.
† The maximum or minimum daily measurement during each examination (ie, from the right or left lenticulostriate artery).
‡ The highest or lowest measurement during the 1st week of life in each neonate.

Mean Highest or Lowest Measurements with Power and Pulsed Wave Doppler US

In each neonate, the mean highest product of the peak velocity and cross-sectional area during the first 5–6 days of life was significantly greater in those with PVL, GMH, or both than in those without ($P < .025$). The highest or lowest measurements of resistive index, peak velocity, and vascular cross-sectional area did not vary significantly between the two groups (Table 1).

Comparison of Product of Peak Velocity and Cross-sectional Area with Mean Arterial Pressure

The maximum daily products of peak velocity and cross-sectional area were plotted against mean arterial pressures (Fig 2). In the neonates with PVL, GMH, or both, there was significantly more variation of the product of the peak velocity and cross-sectional area than in those without PVL or GMH ($P < .001$); there was no significant difference in mean (and variance in mean) arterial pressure between the groups. The preterm neonates who developed PVL ($n = 2$) or grade 2 GMH ($n = 3$; note that patient 2 developed

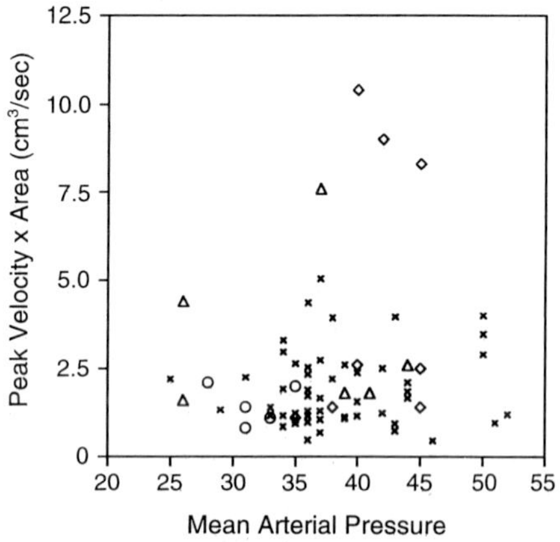

Figure 2. Product of peak velocity and cross-sectional area as a function of mean arterial pressure (in millimeters of mercury). Daily maximum products of peak velocity and cross-sectional area (from the right or left lenticulostriate vessels) are plotted against simultaneous measurements of mean arterial pressure from umbilical arterial catheters. The range of the products of peak velocity and cross-sectional area with respect to mean arterial pressure were wider in neonates with PVL or grade 2 GMH than in those with grade 1 GMH or normal imaging findings. × = neonates without PVL or GMH ($n = 11$), ◇ = neonates with PVL ($n = 2$), ○ = neonate with grade 1 GMH ($n = 1$), △ = neonates with grade 2 GMH ($n = 2$).

Table 2
Subgroup Analysis of Neonates with PVL and/or GMH

Parameters	Neonates with PVL (n = 2)	Neonates with Grade 2 GMH (n = 2)	Neonate with Grade 1 GMH (n = 1)
Mean daily measurements			
Resistive index	0.541 ± 0.088 (16)	0.554 ± 0.11 (12)	0.532 ± 0.051 (10)
Peak velocity (cm/sec)	9.74 ± 4.75	8.31 ± 2.98	5.55 ± 1.79
Vascular area (cm^2)	0.291 ± 0.22	0.343 ± 0.16	0.224 ± 0.08
Velocity × area (cm^3/sec)	3.16 ± 3.19	2.89 ± 2.0	1.24 ± 0.53
Mean arterial pressure (mm Hg)	41.3 ± 3.69 (8)	35.5 ± 3.0 (6)	31.6 ± 2.6 (5)
Minimum resistive index	0.509 ± 0.043 (8)	0.508 ± 0.13 (6)	0.508 ± 0.041 (5)
Maximum resistive index	0.573 ± 0.111	0.600 ± 0.091	0.556 ± 0.052
Maximum peak velocity (cm/sec)	12.4 ± 5.46	9.25 ± 3.06	6.24 ± 1.63
Maximum vascular area (cm^2)	0.328 ± 0.22	0.384 ± 0.18	0.27 ± 0.079
Maximum velocity × area (cm^3/sec)	4.56 ± 3.98	3.27 ± 2.35	1.44 ± 0.51
Mean maximum or minimum measurements in each neonate			
Minimum resistive index	0.465	0.395	0.46
Maximum resistive index	0.72	0.675	0.63
Maximum peak velocity (cm/sec)	20.5	10.5	8.5
Maximum vascular area (cm^2)	0.56	0.574	0.264
Maximum velocity × area (cm^3/sec)	9.39	5.95	2.0

Note.—Numbers in parentheses are numbers of measurements averaged.

PVL and grade 2 GMH) demonstrated the highest products of peak velocity and cross-sectional area (10.4, 8.3, and 7.6 cm^3/sec) with respect to mean arterial pressure. The products in the one patient who developed grade 1 GMH (range, 0.81–2.1 cm^3/sec) were within the normal range of values (0.32–5.0 cm^3/sec). The ranges of the maximum daily peak velocities and vascular cross-sectional areas also were significantly greater in neonates with PVL, GMH, or both than in those without ($P < .01$).

Subgroup Analysis of Neonates with PVL, GMH, or Both

There were no significant differences between any parameter measured in neonates who developed PVL and in neonates with subsequent grade 2 GMH (Table 2). Neonates with grade 2 GMH tended to show higher vascular cross-sectional areas, lower peak velocities, and lower products of peak velocity and cross-sectional area than those with PVL. Neonates with grade 2 GMH showed significantly higher daily peak velocities, vascular cross-sectional areas, and products of peak velocity and cross-sectional area than those who developed grade 1 GMH ($P < .025$). Neonates who developed PVL showed significantly higher daily peak velocities ($P < .005$) and products of peak velocity and cross-sectional area ($P < .01$) than those with grade 1 GMH; however, there was no significant difference between vascular cross-sectional areas in these two groups.

Grade 2 GMH occurred within 24 hours (patients 2 and 4) or was concurrent with the highest observed vascular cross-sectional area during the first 5 days of life (patient 3). With respect to the side of the GMH, there was no clear lateralization of peak velocities, vascular cross-sectional area, or products of peak velocity and cross-sectional area. In patient 2, however, the left side (with a temporal lobe infarction) demonstrated a larger mean daily peak velocity (12.52 cm/sec), vascular cross-sectional area (0.221 cm^2), and product of peak velocity and cross-sectional area (3.18 cm^3/sec) than the right side (7.66 cm/sec, 0.163 cm^2, and 1.30 cm^3/sec, respectively).

DISCUSSION

In preterm neonates with normal findings at follow-up US and neurologic examinations, the product of the peak velocity and cross-sectional area was remarkably constant despite variations in mean arterial pressure, which ranged from 25 to 55 mm Hg; the constancy of the product of peak velocity and cross-sectional area presumably reflects the autoregulatory capabilities of the uninjured cerebrovascular arterial bed. By contrast, this regulated plateau was lost in our preterm neonates who developed PVL, GMH, or both. Neonates in this group demonstrated significantly larger values and fluctuations in velocity and lenticulostriate vascular cross-sectional areas than those without PVL or GMH. In addition, the daily values and ranges of the product of the peak velocity and cross-sectional area (which indirectly reflects regional cerebral blood flow) were higher in neonates with PVL, GMH, or both than in those without. The resistive indexes in the neonates with PVL, GMH, or both also were significantly lower than those in neonates without PVL or GMH. The increase in the product of the peak velocity and cross-sectional area with a corresponding lower resistive index may reflect capillary recruitment, vasoparalysis, or both, which result in intracerebral vascular shunting after hypoxic-ischemic injury (3,4,6,7).

We postulate that our data reflect the loss or attenuation of pressure-flow autoregulation in preterm neonates who have experienced hypoxic-ischemic events. Because we did not simultaneously measure $Paco_2$ and Pao_2 owing to the semi-invasive nature of arterial blood sampling in premature neonates, we could not determine the effect of $Paco_2$ and Pao_2 on the peak velocity, resistive index, and coronal vascular cross-sectional area.

Pyrds (5), in his study of pressure-flow autoregulation in asphyxiated neonates, used a combination of Xe-133 clearance and near infrared spectroscopy measurements to determine cerebral blood flow and oxygen extraction. These methods necessarily only measure global cerebral blood flow and therefore may not sensitively measure regional changes or loss of cerebral blood flow and autoregulation. Recently, attention has been focused on regional measurements of cerebral blood flow with MR imaging, positron emission tomography, or both (9); however, these modalities are limited by their expense and lack of portability, which may severely curtail their use in the populations at risk.

Power Doppler US examination is a portable, noninvasive, and relatively inexpensive technique. In our hands, the additional time needed to perform power and pulsed wave Doppler measurements of the lenticulostriate vessels has been less than 10 minutes. Power Doppler US is a potentially useful new technique; in animals given potent vasodilators, power Doppler US examination has provided qualitative information about regional cerebral blood flow (12). In our study, the product of the peak velocity and cross-sectional area—although not a strictly quantitative measure—did allow the discrimination of cerebrally injured preterm neonates from those who were uninjured. Although the number of neonates with PVL, GMH, or both was small in our study, preliminary results demonstrate higher products of the peak velocity and cross-sectional area in PVL and in increasingly higher grades of GMH. The neonate who developed grade 1 GMH did not show significantly abnormal products of the peak velocity and cross-sectional area. The peak velocities and products of the peak velocity and cross-sectional area in neonates with PVL tended to be higher than those in neonates who developed grade 2 GMH; however, there were too few neonates (n = 4) for an adequate statistical comparison. The vascular cross-sectional area tended to be higher in neonates who developed grade 2 GMH. This finding may suggest that part of the pathophysiologic process of GMH is the result of hyperperfusion, as hypothesized by Volpe (21); however, again, there were too few patients in our study to permit adequate statistical comparison.

The two neonates who subsequently developed PVL and neurologic dysfunction showed maximum peak velocities (19.7 and 23.0 cm/sec) that exceeded, by 4–5 standard deviations, those in neonates without PVL or GMH. If this finding is observed in a larger study population, measurements of regionally increased lenticulostriate arterial velocities may prove useful in identifying the neonate who is at risk for developing PVL. It is unclear whether peak velocity, vascular cross-sectional area, product of the peak velocity and cross-sectional area, or resistive index individually could be predictive of GMH. In our study, the highest values of the peak velocity, the vascular cross-sectional area, the product of the peak velocity and cross-sectional area, or a combination of these occurred 24 hours before or at the time of the highest grade of GMH.

Variations in these measurements (and not a single threshold value) may better reflect an underlying hypoxic-ischemic insult. Use of fluctuations (and not absolute measurements) of peak velocities, vascular cross-sectional areas, and relative cerebral blood flow as indicators of hypoxic-ischemic injury obviates many difficulties in the quantitative assessment of blood flow with Doppler US, such as inaccurate measurement of vessel diameter and specific angle corrections for velocity measurement (11,12).

Observation of impaired pressure-flow autoregulation may be primarily useful for prognostication because changes in treatment may not change the pathophysiologic process of hypoxic-ischemic injury and the ultimate clinical outcome. The clinical trials of protective agents—including free-radical scavengers, glutamate antagonists, and specific inhibitors of neuronal apoptosis—may provide new therapeutic options in these selected neonates (5,22–24).

In summary, with power and pulsed wave Doppler US examination, extremely low–birth-weight preterm neonates who develop PVL, GMH, or both demonstrate significantly larger means and fluctuating values of peak velocity, vascular coronal cross-sectional areas, and products of the peak velocities and cross-sectional areas of the lenticulostriate vessels. Regional fluctuations of cerebral blood flow in the lenticulostriate vascular bed are associated with hypoxic-ischemic injury. Future studies will be necessary to assess the predictive value of power Doppler US for identifying the neonate who is at increased risk of developing PVL, GMH, or both. ■

Acknowledgments: We thank Doug Worth of Acuson for obtaining thermal-index measurements. We thank Ziv Molder, PhD, William D. Rhine, MD, and David K. Stevenson, MD, for identifying patients and obtaining parental consent.

References

1. Wyatt JS, Cope M, Delpy DT, Wray S, Reynolds EOR. Quantification of cerebral oxygenation and haemodynamics in sick newborn infants by near infrared spectrophotometry. Lancet 1986; 8515:1063–1066.
2. Pyrds O, Greisen G, Lou H, Friis-Hansen B. Heterogeneity of cerebral vasoreactivity in preterm infants supported by mechanical ventilation. J Pediatr 1989; 115:638–645.
3. Pyrds O, Greisen G, Lou H, Friss-Hansen B. Vasoparalysis associated with brain damage in asphyxiated term infants. J Pediatr 1990; 117:119–125.
4. Frewen TC, Kissoon N, Kronick J, et al. Cerebral blood flow, cross-brain oxygen extraction, and fontanelle pressure after hypoxic-ischemic injury in newborn infants. J Pediatr 1991; 118:265–271.
5. Pyrds O. Control of cerebral circulation in the high-risk neonate. Ann Neurol 1991; 30:321–329.
6. Skov L, Pyrds O, Greisen G, Lou H. Estimation of cerebral venous saturation in newborn infants by near infrared spectroscopy. Pediatr Res 1993; 33:52–55.
7. Pyrds O. Low neonatal cerebral oxygen delivery is associated with brain injury in preterm infants. Acta Paediatr 1994; 1233.
8. Lassen NA. The luxury-perfusion syndrome and its possible relation to acute metabolic acidosis localised within the brain. Lancet 1966; 2:1113–1115.
9. Toft PB, Leth H, Lou HC, Pyrds O, Peitersen B, Henriksen O. Local vascular CO_2 reactivity in the infant brain assessed by functional MRI. Pediatr Radiol 1995; 420–424.
10. Taylor GA, Trescher WA, Traystma RJ, Johnston MV. Acute experimental neuronal injury in the newborn lamb: US characterization and demonstration of hemodynamic effects. Pediatr Radiol 1993; 23:268–275.
11. Taylor GA. Alterations in regional cerebral blood flood in neonatal stroke: preliminary findings with color Doppler sonography. Pediatr Radiol 1992; 111–115.
12. Taylor GA. Regional cerebral blood flow estimates in newborn lamb using amplitude-mode color Doppler ultrasound. Pediatr Radiol 1996; 26:282–286.
13. Takashima S, Tanaka K. Development of the cerebrovascular architecture and its relationship to periventricular leukomalacia. Arch Neurol 1978; 35:11–16.
14. Volpe J, Herscovitch P, Perlman J, Raichle M. Positron emission tomography in the newborn: extensive impairment of regional blood flow with intraventicular hemorrhage and hemorrhagic intracerebral involvement. Pediatrics 1983; 72:589–595.
15. Wigglesworth J, Pape K. An integrated model for hemorrhage and ischemic lesions in the newborn brain. Early Hum Dev 1978; 2:179–199.
16. DeReuck J. The human periventricular arterial blood supply and the anatomy of cerebral infarctions. Eur Neurol 1971; 5: 321–334.
17. DeReuck J, Chattha AS, Richardson EP. Pathogenesis and evolution of periventricular leukomalacia in infancy. Arch Neurol 1972; 27:229–236.
18. Standards for real-time display of thermal and mechanical acoustic output indices on diagnostic ultrasound equipment. Laurel, Md: American Institute of Ultrasound in Medicine, 1992.
19. Blankenberg FG, Teplitz RL, Ellis W, et al. The influence of volumetric tumor doubling time, DNA ploidy, and histologic grade on the survival of patients with intracranial astrocytomas. AJNR 1995; 16:1001–1012.
20. Lindgren BW, ed. Statistical theory. 3rd ed. New York, NY: Macmillan, 1976; 347–350,577–578.
21. Volpe J. Neurology of the newborn. 3rd ed. Philadelphia, Pa: Saunders, 1995; 279–313,403–463.
22. Morrison FK, Patel NB, Howie PW, Mires GJ, Herd RM. Neonatal cerebral arterial flow velocity waveforms in term infants with and without metabolic acidosis at delivery. Early Hum Dev 1995; 42:155–168.
23. Mills EM, Gunasekar PG, Pavlakovic G, Isom GE. Cyanide-induced apoptosis and oxidative stress in differentiated PC12 cells. J Neurochem 1996; 67:1039–1046.
24. Matsuyama T, Hata R, Yamamoto Y, et al. Localization of Fas antigen mRNA induced in postischemic murine forebrain by in situ hybridization. Brain Res Mol Brain Res 1995; 34:166–172.

Tejas S. Mehta, MD • Deborah Levine, MD • Bruce Beckwith, MD

Treatment of Ectopic Pregnancy: Is a Human Chorionic Gonadotropin Level of 2,000 mIU/mL a Reasonable Threshold?[1]

PURPOSE: To determine whether a human chorionic gonadotropin (hCG) level of 2,000 mIU/mL is a reasonable threshold for diagnosing ectopic pregnancy in the absence of ultrasound (US) findings of intrauterine pregnancy (IUP) and thus to prevent inappropriate treatment that will result in the loss of an otherwise normal pregnancy in women with early IUPs.

MATERIALS AND METHODS: The authors reviewed the medical records of and US scans obtained in 676 patients in whom ectopic pregnancy was clinically suspected between January 1, 1994, and December 31, 1995.

RESULTS: Five hundred forty-eight patients had evidence of a normal or abnormal IUP. Fifty-one (40%) of the 128 patients without evidence of an IUP had an hCG level of more than 2,000 mIU/mL. Of these 51 patients, 15 (29%) were treated for ectopic pregnancy; 17 (33%) were not immediately treated for ectopic pregnancy and had a normal IUP at follow-up US.

CONCLUSION: An hCG level of 2,000 mIU/mL without US findings of IUP, while suggestive of an abnormal pregnancy, is not diagnostic. Per the results of recent studies, it is reasonable to closely follow up rather than treat many of these early, stable cases of ectopic pregnancy.

The number of diagnoses of ectopic pregnancy is increasing, owing to both the earlier diagnosis (of previously unsuspected cases) and an increase in the prevalence of this abnormality (1,2). In the United States, the leading causes of pregnancy-related deaths in the first trimester are complications of ectopic pregnancy (3). It has been tradition to treat ectopic pregnancy surgically; however, there is now a trend toward medical management when feasible. Local injections of methotrexate (4,5), prostaglandin (6), potassium chloride (7), or hyperosmolar glucose solution (8) have all been performed. Systemic intramuscular injection of methotrexate also has been used (9,10). Observation without treatment also has been advocated, because many ectopic pregnancies spontaneously resolve (2).

There are variable data on a discriminatory human chorionic gonadotropin (hCG) level at which an intrauterine pregnancy (IUP) should be depicted with transvaginal ultrasonography (US); however, hCG levels of 1,000–2,000 mIU/mL (international reference preparation) have been used (11–14). Our current institutional recommendations are that when an IUP is not visualized in a patient with an hCG level greater than 2,000 mIU/mL, she be treated as if she has an ectopic pregnancy. The purpose of this study was to review our experience to determine whether this threshold is appropriate and to make certain that women with early IUPs are not inappropriately treated.

MATERIALS AND METHODS

Static US scans obtained in all patients who were clinically suspected of having an ectopic pregnancy (because of positive pregnancy test results with pain, bleeding, or both) from January 1, 1994, to December 31, 1995, were reviewed by two of the authors (D.L., T.S.M.) without knowledge of pregnancy outcome. An intradecidual sign (15) (Fig 1), an intrauterine gestational sac with yolk sac, or a fetal pole with cardiac activity were considered to be signs of a normal IUP. An intradecidual sign was defined as a round or oval fluid collection within the decidua with an echogenic rim and located eccentrically in the endometrial cavity (15). An irregular or enlarged intrauterine sac without clear decidual reaction, embryonic demise, or molar pregnancy was considered an abnormal IUP. US scans with evidence of a normal or abnormal IUP were not evaluated further.

The medical records of the remaining patients, who did not have a definite intradecidual sign, yolk sac, or fetal pole or an obviously abnormal IUP, were reviewed. Only those patients with transvaginal US scans, adequate clinical and US follow-up, and an hCG level obtained within 24 hours of the initial US examination were included in the study. Six hundred seventy-six patients were referred for clinical suspicion of ectopic pregnancy. Five hundred forty-eight of these patients had normal or abnormal IUPs. One hundred twenty-eight patients (age range, 19–44 years; mean age, 31.0 years) without evidence of IUP (nor-

Index terms: Hormones • Pregnancy, ectopic, 856.823 • Pregnancy, US, 856.1298

Abbreviations: hCG = human chorionic gonadotropin, IUP = intrauterine pregnancy.

Radiology 1997; 205:569–573

[1] From the Departments of Radiology (T.S.M., D.L.) and Pathology (B.B.), Beth Israel Deaconess Medical Center, Harvard Medical School, 330 Brookline Ave, Boston, MA 02215. From the 1996 RSNA scientific assembly. Received April 4, 1997; revision requested May 13; revision received July 18; accepted July 21. **Address reprint requests to** D.L.

Table 1
US Findings in Women Treated for Ectopic Pregnancy

US Finding	hCG <2,000 mIU/mL (n = 27)* Methotrexate (n = 6)	hCG <2,000 mIU/mL (n = 27)* Surgery (n = 21)	hCG >2,000 mIU/mL (n = 16)† Methotrexate (n = 2)	hCG >2,000 mIU/mL (n = 16)† Surgery (n = 14)
Adnexal mass (not definite that it is a corpus luteum)	2	14	2‡	11‡,§
Free fluid	1	16	0	10
Endometrial fluid	2	5	0	4
None of the above	1	4	0	1

* Dilation and curettage (no villi) was performed in three patients treated with methotrexate and in five treated with surgery.
† None of the patients underwent dilation and curettage.
‡ Two patients did not respond to methotrexate therapy and were subsequently treated surgically. They are counted in both columns.
§ One patient had an IUP at follow-up.

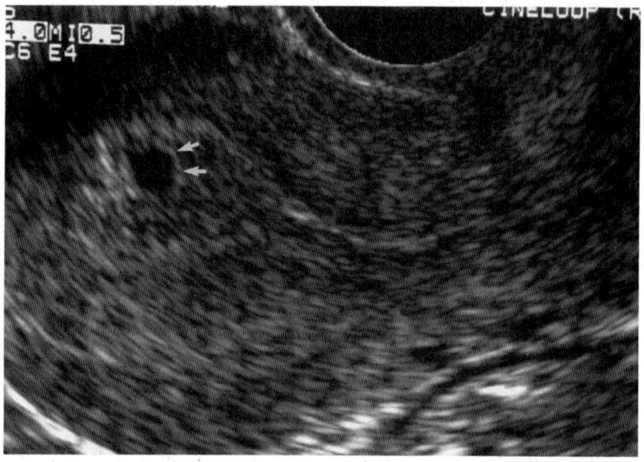

Figure 1. Intradecidual sign in a 26-year-old woman. Sagittal US scan of the uterus demonstrates a fluid collection eccentric to the endometrial stripe with an echogenic rim (arrows).

mal or abnormal) composed the study population.

The US scans were reviewed and evaluated for the presence of fluid within the endometrial cavity, presence of an adnexal mass, and presence of free fluid. The quality of the initial and subsequent images was assessed. Image quality was rated as good if the image was focused on the gestational sac or endometrium with the focal zone at or just below the area of interest. Image quality was rated as poor if the above standard was not met. Note was made of whether the examination was performed only by a resident on call (n = 27), only by a technologist (n = 6), by a technologist and a resident (n = 16), or during the day by a technologist with scanning supervision by an attending physician (n = 79).

Levels of hCG were determined by using a Stratus II analyzer (Baxter Diagnostics, Miami, Fla) in serum samples obtained before April 1995 or an Opus Magnum analyzer (Behring Diagnostics, Westwood, Mass) in serum samples obtained during or after April 1995.

The patients were divided into three categories on the basis of follow-up findings: IUP, spontaneous abortion, or ectopic pregnancy. IUP was diagnosed when US scans demonstrated at least a gestational sac with a yolk sac; most demonstrated a fetal pole with cardiac activity. Spontaneous abortion was diagnosed when serial hCG levels were decreasing, when US scans showed no or an irregular intrauterine sac, when a history of passage of fetal tissue was given, or when a combination of these occurred. Ectopic pregnancy was diagnosed with surgery, negative findings at dilation and curettage with a rising hCG level, an abnormally rising hCG level, US demonstration of an adnexal mass separate from the ovary without an IUP, or a combination of these (Fig 2).

The patients with ectopic pregnancy were separated into two groups: those who were treated with intramuscular injection of methotrexate and those who were treated surgically. Eight patients were treated with methotrexate. Four patients had adnexal masses at US; methotrexate therapy failed in two of the four patients, as determined with worsening pain or rising hCG levels. Those two patients were subsequently treated surgically. Another three of the eight patients underwent dilation and curettage, with negative findings for products of conception. The remaining patient had no proof of ectopic pregnancy and was treated on the basis of abnormally rising hCG levels. Decisions for clinical care, including whether to treat for ectopic pregnancy, were made by the clinical staff and varied according to physician preference and the physicians' assessment as to the reliability of the patient.

RESULTS

Figure 3 is a flow chart of the patients examined. Of the 128 patients without evidence of an IUP on the initial US scans, 43 (34%) were treated for ectopic pregnancy (one of whom had a normal IUP at follow-up), 34 (26%) had an IUP, and 52 (41%) had a spontaneous abortion.

Of the 43 women treated for ectopic pregnancy, 27 had an hCG level of less than 2,000 mIU/mL and 16 had an hCG level of greater than 2,000 mIU/mL. The sensitivity for the detection of ectopic pregnancy with an hCG level of 2,000 mIU/mL as a threshold (Fig 3) was 36% (15 of 42 women), and the specificity was 58% (50 of 86 women). The US findings in the patients treated for ectopic pregnancy are given in Table 1. The US findings in the patients with an hCG level greater than 2,000 mIU/mL and without a definite IUP are given in Table 2.

Of 51 patients without a definite IUP (normal or abnormal) and with an hCG level of greater than 2,000 mIU/mL, 17 (33%) had a normal IUP at follow-up US. Studies in 10 of these patients were performed by a technologist and supervised by an attending radiologist, and studies in seven were performed by medical personnel on call (by a resident only in four, by both a resident and a technologist in two, and by a technologist only in one).

A retrospective review of the US scans obtained in these 17 patients showed that six patients had a weak intradecidual sign. The hCG levels in these six patients were 3,344–9,159 mIU/mL (mean, 6,082 mIU/mL). Of the remaining 11 patients, one patient had an hCG level of 2,150 mIU/mL. This patient had no fluid within the endometrial cavity but had a small amount of free fluid. She underwent exploratory laparoscopy because of the presence of a questionable extraovarian mass at US, which, at surgery, was determined to be a corpus luteal cyst. A follow-up US scan obtained 24 hours after laparoscopy demonstrated an intradecidual sign (Fig 4). Another patient had undergone in vitro fertilization and was subsequently shown to have triplets. Her initial US scan, obtained when the hCG level was

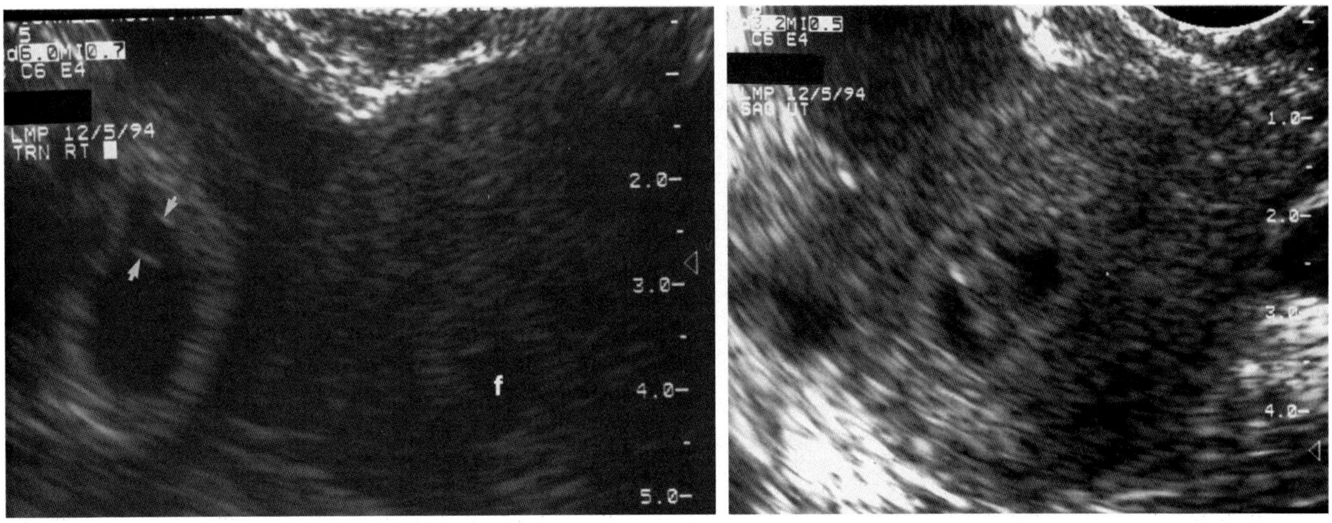

a. b.

Figure 2. Ectopic pregnancy in a 30-year-old woman. **(a)** Transverse US scan of the right adnexa demonstrates a mass with a yolk sac (arrows). A fluid collection (*f*) is seen in the endometrial cavity. **(b)** Sagittal US scan provides better definition of the intrauterine fluid collection.

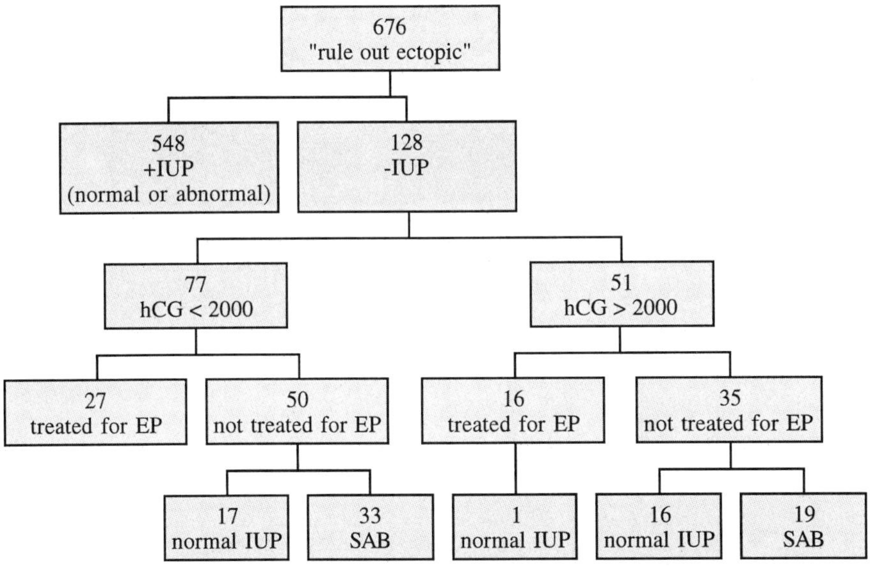

Figure 3. Flow chart of patients who underwent US for clinical suspicion of ectopic pregnancy. Seventeen (33%) of 51 patients with no definite IUP and an hCG level of greater than 2,000 mIU/mL had a normal IUP at follow-up. *EP* = ectopic pregnancy, *SAB* = spontaneous abortion.

Table 2
US Findings in Patients with an hCG Level Greater than 2,000 mIU/mL and without a Definite IUP on the Initial US Scan ($n = 51$)

US Finding	Ectopic Pregnancy ($n = 15$)	IUP ($n = 17$)	Spontaneous Abortion ($n = 19$)
Adnexal mass (not definite that it is a corpus luteum)	10	1*	0
Free fluid	10	2	1
Endometrial fluid	4	14	14
None of the above	1	2	5

* At US, this was believed to be separate from the ovary. At laparoscopy, however, this was shown to be a corpus luteum.

7,827 mIU/mL, demonstrated two small intrauterine fluid collections without a definite intradecidual sign. In one patient (with an hCG level of 11,500 mIU/mL), who presented in the evening and underwent US performed by a resident, the images were suboptimal. The image quality in the remaining eight patients with an hCG level of more than 2,000 mIU/mL was good (Figs 5, 6). The hCG levels in these patients were 2,710–12,430 mIU/mL (mean, 5,878 mIU/mL).

DISCUSSION

The prevalence of coexisting intrauterine and extrauterine pregnancies is very low (one in 7,000 pregnancies); thus, the depiction of an IUP with US virtually excludes the diagnosis of ectopic pregnancy (16). As part of the evaluation for ectopic pregnancy, there have been a number of studies performed to determine the discriminatory hCG level at which an IUP should be visible. In 1981, Kadar and colleagues (17) stated that nondepiction of an IUP at transabdominal US with an hCG level of greater than 6,500 mIU/mL was suggestive of an ectopic pregnancy. In more recent studies with transvaginal US, it has been determined that a normal IUP should be identifiable with threshold hCG levels of greater than 1,000–2,000 mIU/mL (11–14). Some of the variability in discriminatory hCG levels likely is due to the variability in the criteria for defining a definite IUP.

By using the second international standard for hCG (conversion factor, 2.2), Nyberg and colleagues (18) reported recognition of a gestational sac in 80% (four of five) of patients with an hCG level of 500–1,000 mIU/mL and in 100% (17 of 17) of patients with an hCG level of greater than 1,000 mIU/mL (2,200 mIU/mL, international reference preparation). In their study, a gestational sac was defined as an intrauterine fluid collection sur-

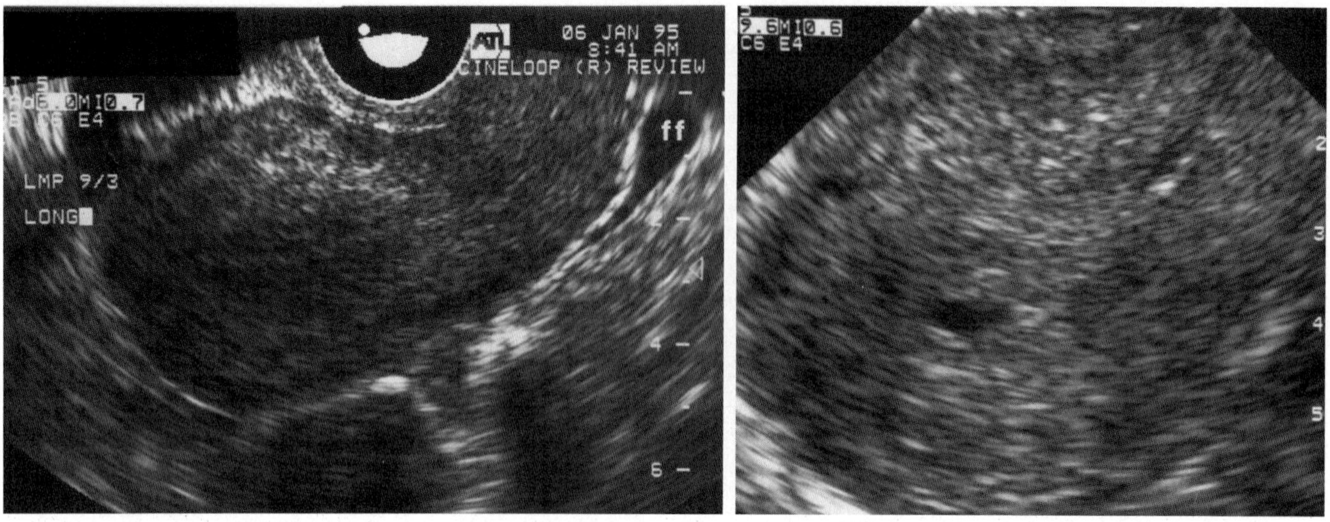

a. b.

Figure 4. Images obtained in a 28-year-old woman with an hCG level of 2,150 mIU/mL. **(a)** Initial US scan demonstrates no fluid within the endometrial cavity. There is a small amount of free fluid (*ff*). **(b)** US scan obtained the following day, after negative laparoscopic findings, shows an intradecidual sign.

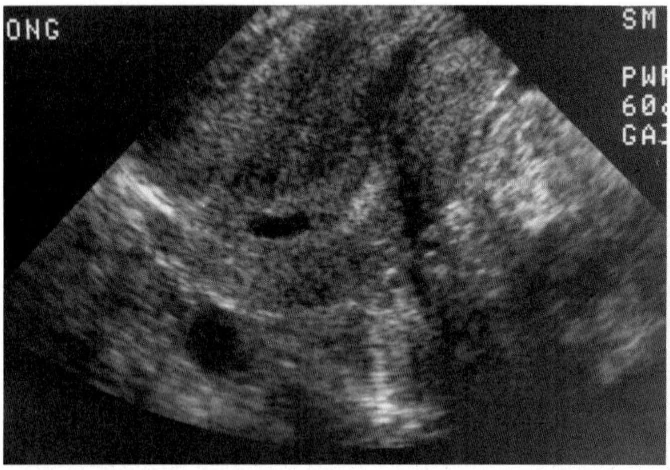

5.

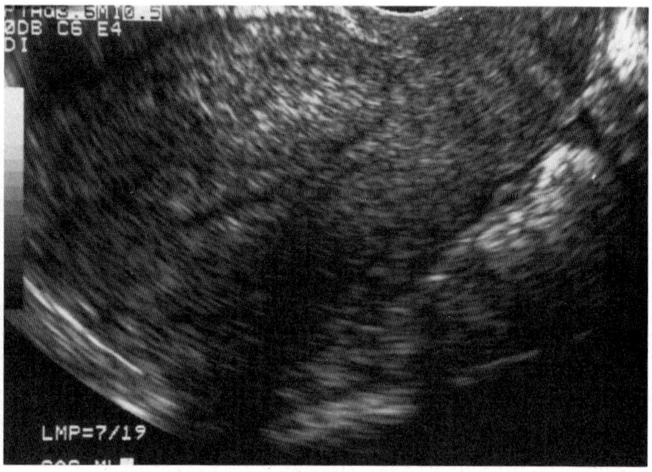

6.

Figures 5, 6. **(5)** Sagittal US scan demonstrates a fluid collection within the uterus, without a definite intradecidual sign, in a 24-year-old woman with an hCG level of 9,016 mIU/mL. An IUP was confirmed 2 days later. **(6)** Sagittal US scan of the uterus demonstrates a nonspecific fluid collection within the endometrial cavity in a 22-year-old woman with an hCG level of 3,000 mIU/mL. The patient was subsequently found to have a normal IUP.

rounded by an echogenic rim. Bernaschek and colleagues (19) reported consistent recognition of a sac with an hCG level of greater than 300 mIU/mL by using the second international standard of hCG; however, they defined a gestational sac as an intrauterine fluid collection and did not require criteria of eccentricity or surrounding echogenicity, which explains the lower hCG threshold. The risk of using such a definition for a normal pregnancy is that a pseudogestational sac of ectopic pregnancy will be mistaken for an IUP (Fig 2b). This also raises the important issue of knowing which standard for hCG is being used in a hospital laboratory. Knowledge of this is important because discriminatory levels can differ by a factor of more than 2.

We defined a normal IUP as at least having an intradecidual sign, which has been shown to be 91.7% sensitive and 100% specific (15). US scans without a clear IUP were deemed indeterminate; patients with these scans composed 18.9% of our patient population. This finding is similar to the 19% indeterminate rate found by Braffman and colleagues (14), who used an hCG threshold of 1,500 mIU/mL.

One potential problem with our study was our definition of spontaneous abortion as decreasing serial hCG levels, abnormal US scans that showed no or an irregular intrauterine sac, clinical passage of fetal tissue, or a combination of these. It is possible that tubal pregnancies in which tubal abortion was performed were included in this group. This potential bias would decrease even further the sensitivity of an hCG threshold of 2,000 mIU/mL for the detection of ectopic pregnancy.

An additional problem is that patients treated with methotrexate may not have had an ectopic pregnancy. Inclusion of these patients in our ectopic group could further decrease the specificity of an hCG threshold of 2,000 mIU/mL for the detection of ectopic pregnancy.

We demonstrated that 17 (33%) of 51 patients without a definite IUP (normal or abnormal) and with hCG levels of greater than 2,000 mIU/mL subsequently had normal IUPs at follow-up US. The explanations for the failure to identify an IUP with an hCG level of greater than 2,000 mIU/mL are varied. The technical quality of the examination is important. One image was obtained during the evening hours and, when retrospectively reviewed, was believed to be of suboptimal quality. Women with multiple gestations can have elevated hCG levels in relation to the intrauterine US findings (12). This was the case in one of our patients, who had triplets. Factors distorting the uterine cavity, such as leiomyomas, have also been reported to limit the US evaluation for early IUP (12,20). One patient had a large hemorrhage, which also limits our ability to diagnose an early IUP. These data emphasize potential pitfalls in the evaluation of early gestational sacs. The absence of a sac should be interpreted with caution in relation to the hCG level in patients with fibroids, patients who have undergone infertility treatment, and patients with inadequate-quality scans.

Other possible explanations for the failure to identify a definite IUP in patients with an hCG level of greater than 2,000 mIU/mL could include analytic issues in the measurement of hCG. All assays have an inherent imprecision that should be considered when interpreting individual values. In our laboratory, the method used for determining the hCG level had a coefficient of variation (standard deviation/mean) of approximately 8% for quality control materials. This is consistent with previously published data for between-run precision of other hCG assays, which were 6%–15% (21). Therefore, considering the inherent assay variation, the 95% confidence interval for a specimen with a measured value of 2,000 mIU/mL would be 1,680 mIU/mL, 2,320 mIU/mL (2,000 mIU/mL ± 16%). In addition, both hCG analyzers used during this study did not have results above 500 mIU/mL, so specimens with hCG levels of greater than 500 mIU/mL required dilution, which is another source of imprecision. One of our patients who did not demonstrate a definite IUP on the initial US scan had an hCG level of 2,150 mIU/mL, which clearly has a confidence interval that includes values of less than 2,000 mIU/mL.

An additional factor to consider is that in cases in which hCG levels were measured up to 24 hours after US, the level could have been increased by as much as 1.7 times (19).

In eight patients with hCG levels of greater than 2,000 mIU/mL, there was no obvious explanation for the failure to demonstrate a definite IUP. The hCG levels in these patients were 2,710–12,430 mIU/mL (mean, 5,878 mIU/mL). This suggests that if an hCG level of more than 2,000 mIU/mL is used as a threshold for visualization of an IUP in all cases, it is possible that women with early IUPs will be inappropriately treated and that these women may lose an otherwise normal pregnancy. Because many women with hCG levels of greater than 2,000 mIU/mL without an IUP will have had spontaneous abortion, it may be reasonable to attain another hCG level in these patients.

Our finding of such high hCG levels without definite IUPs is surprising and is likely due to our strict definition of IUP (a clear intradecidual sign with an echogenic rim). We used this definition so as to not miss any ectopic pregnancies. In a similar study, Braffman and colleagues (14) found fluid collections without an intradecidual sign in 40 of 90 patients with an hCG level of greater than 1,500 mIU/mL. Similarly, Bateman and colleagues (12), with a threshold of 2,004 mIU/mL, found that 29% of patients with sacs less than 5 mm in diameter did not demonstrate an echogenic rim.

In summary, we conclude that if all women with an hCG level of greater than 2,000 mIU/mL without US demonstration of an IUP were treated medically for ectopic pregnancy, it is possible that some women with early IUPs might be inappropriately treated and that these women might lose an otherwise normal pregnancy. We are not recommending a change in the threshold hCG level for the diagnosis of ectopic pregnancy, because that would decrease an already low sensitivity for the detection of this abnormality. Rather, we want to address the limitations of US in early pregnancy to improve our ability to counsel patients who have an indeterminate early study. ■

References

1. Centers for Disease Control. Ectopic pregnancy: United States, 1988–1989. MMWR 1992; 41:591–594.
2. Atri M, Bret PM, Tulandi T. Spontaneous resolution of ectopic pregnancy: initial appearance and evolution at transvaginal US. Radiology 1993; 186:83–86.
3. Goldner TE, Lawson HW, Xia Z, Atrash HK. Surveillance for ectopic pregnancy: United States, 1970–1987. MMWR 1993; 42:73–85.
4. Atri M, Bret PM, Tulandi T, Senterman MK. Ectopic pregnancy: evolution after treatment with transvaginal methotrexate. Radiology 1992; 185:749–763.
5. Tekay A, Martikainen H, Heikkinen H, Kivela A, Jouppila P. Disappearance of the trophoblastic blood flow in tubal pregnancy after methotrexate injection. J Ultrasound Med 1993; 12:615–618.
6. Paulsson G, Knut S, Labecker BM, Lofstraid T, Lindblom B. Laparoscopic prostaglandin injection of ectopic pregnancy: success rate according to endocrine activity. Fertil Steril 1995; 63:473–477.
7. Robertson DE, Hoye MAH, Hansen JN. Reduction of ectopic pregnancy by injection under ultrasound control. Lancet 1989; 2:974–975.
8. Lang P, Weiss PAM, Mayer HO. Local application of hyperosmolar glucose solution in tubal pregnancy. Lancet 1989; 2:922–923.
9. Stika CS, Anderson L, Frederiksen MC. Single-dose methotrexate for the treatment of ectopic pregnancy: Northwestern Memorial Hospital three-year experience. Am J Obstet Gynecol 1996; 174:1840–1848.
10. Henry MA, Gentry WL. Single injection of methotrexate for treatment of ectopic pregnancies. Am J Obstet Gynecol 1994; 171:1584–1587.
11. Cacciatore B, Stenman UH, Ylostalo P. Diagnosis of ectopic pregnancy by vaginal ultrasonography in combination with a discriminatory serum hCG level of 1000 IU/L (IRP). Br J Obstet Gynaecol 1990; 97:904–908.
12. Bateman BG, Nunley WC, Kolp LA, Kitchin JD, Felder R. Vaginal sonography findings and hCG dynamics of early intrauterine and tubal pregnancies. Obstet Gynecol 1990; 75:421–427.
13. Bree RL, Edwards M, Bohm-Velez M, Beyler S, Roberts J, Mendelson EB. Transvaginal sonography in the evaluation of normal early pregnancy: correlation with hCG level. AJR 1989; 153:75–79.
14. Braffman BH, Coleman BG, Ramchandani P, et al. Emergency department screening for ectopic pregnancy: a prospective US study. Radiology 1994; 190:797–802.
15. Yeh HC, Goodman JD, Carr L, Rabinowitz JG. Intradecidual sign: a US criterion of early intrauterine pregnancy. Radiology 1986; 161:463–467.
16. Hann LE, Bachman DM, McArdle CR. Coexistent intrauterine and ectopic pregnancy: a reevaluation. Radiology 1984; 152: 151–154.
17. Kadar N, DeVore G, Romero R. Discriminatory hCG zone: its use in the sonographic evaluation for ectopic pregnancy. Obstet Gynecol 1981; 58:156–160.
18. Nyberg DA, Mack LA, Laing FC, Jeffrey RB. Early pregnancy complications: endovaginal sonographic findings correlated with human chorionic gonadotropin levels. Radiology 1988; 167:619–622.
19. Bernaschek G, Rudelstorfer R, Csaicsish P. Vaginal sonography versus serum human gonadotropin in early detection of pregnancy. Am J Obstet Gynecol 1988; 158:608–612.
20. Goldstein SR, Snyder JR, Watson C, Danon M. Very early pregnancy detection with endovaginal ultrasound. Obstet Gynecol 1988; 72:200–204.
21. Ooi DS, Perkins SL, Claman P, Muggah HF. Serum human chorionic gonadotropin levels in early pregnancy. Clin Chem Acta 1989; 181:281–292.

Gel Tubes: A Method of Core-Specimen Retrieval and Transport[1]

Kenneth D. Hopper, MD
Thomas R. TenHave, PhD

The utility of saving core biopsy specimens in sterile gel tubes was evaluated with 30 liver and 30 kidney core specimens obtained at open biopsy with an 18-gauge needle during autopsy. The core specimens were saved with one of three methods: gel tube, formalin swirl, or scalpel retrieval. The combined-organ mean time for the radiologist to save core specimens was not statistically significantly different with gel tubes (3.8 seconds) and the formalin-swirl method (4.5 seconds). Both of these methods, however, were significantly faster than the scalpel-retrieval method (11.2 seconds) ($P < .001$). The combined radiologist and cytotechnologist time was greatest with the gel tubes (35.1 seconds vs 11.7 and 21.2 seconds, respectively). Core specimens were broken with the formalin-swirl and scalpel-retrieval methods but not with the gel-tube method.

Index terms: Biopsies, technology • Kidney, biopsy, 81.126 • Liver, biopsy, 761.126

Radiology 1997; 205:574–576

The use of automated biopsy devices (biopsy guns) to obtain high-quality core tissue for histopathologic analysis has become commonplace in image-guided percutaneous biopsy. Because the biopsy guns are simple, easy to use, and consistently obtain high-quality tissue cores, automated biopsy has largely replaced fine-needle biopsy in clinical radiology practice. Extensive attention has been given to how the core specimen is obtained (1–6) but, to our knowledge, no study has been performed to evaluate how core specimens should be saved and transported for pathologic examination.

In our experience, two methods are commonly used for formalin fixing of core tissue for transport: the formalin-swirl method and the scalpel-retrieval method. In the first method, the needle, with the core specimen exposed, is submerged and swirled in formalin; this action releases the core specimen but prohibits further use of the needle and biopsy gun. In an effort to save needles, it has become common practice to carefully remove the core specimen from the needle by using a scalpel (or needle) and then swirling the scalpel in the formalin to release the core specimen. Use of sterile gel (Histocare; Amedic, Sollentuna, Sweden [U.S. distributor, Jason, Huntington Beach, Calif]) allows easy removal of the core specimen from the needle (Fig 1) and continued use of the needle. Formalin is added to the gel after the biopsy is complete (Fig 2). The concentration of formalin (5%) is adequate to preserve the core specimen. At our institution, core specimens have been preserved in the formalinized gel for more than a year with no tissue degradation.

In this study, we evaluated the formalin-swirl, scalpel-retrieval, and gel-tube methods for the time needed by the radiologist and cytotechnologist and for breakage of the core specimens.

Materials and Methods

Fresh (not more than 4 hours after death) liver and kidneys were removed during routine autopsy. Sixty open biopsy procedures (30 of liver, 30 of kidney) were performed by using an 18-gauge-needle biopsy gun (Manan Medical Products, Northbrook, Ill) to obtain 1.7-cm-long core specimens. All biopsies were performed by one radiologist (K.D.H.), who had performed more than 7,000 percutaneous biopsy procedures (more than 500 with the Manan biopsy gun). The 60 core-biopsy specimens were assigned randomly to be saved with one of the three methods. (*a*) Gel tube: The needle was placed into the gel tube, the core specimen was exposed and released, the needle was removed, and the core specimen was suspended in gel. (*b*) Formalin swirl: The core specimen was submerged in formalin and exposed, and the needle was carefully swirled to release the core specimen. (*c*) Scalpel retrieval: The sharp end of a scalpel was used to remove the core specimen from the needle notch, and the scalpel tip was then swirled in formalin to release the core specimen.

The radiologist had extensive experience with the formalin-swirl and scalpel-retrieval methods, but he had not previously used gel tubes. Before the study was started, he was carefully instructed on their use by the manufacturer. He practiced using the gel tubes in 30 biopsies and was confident he could use them correctly and efficiently. Each needle was used for five biopsies and was then discarded. The time needed by the radiologist to save the core specimen was measured from the time the needle was removed from the organ to the time the core specimen was freely floating or suspended in formalin or gel. It was also noted whether the core specimen broke during the formalin-fixing process.

One cytotechnologist prepared the 60 core specimens in tissue blocks. He had previously prepared thousands of needle core specimens and was experienced in retrieving core specimens by using a bulb aspirator, but he had no previously retrieved core specimens from gel. The time needed to remove the core specimen from the formalin-gel solution and place it into tissue paper for preparation in a cell block was measured, and any further core-specimen breakage was noted. The results from both the radiologist and the cytotechnologist were forwarded separately for statistical analysis.

The times were analyzed by means of an analysis of variance, with log time used as the dependent variable and organ and method and their interaction used as the independent variables. Pairwise comparisons with 95% confidence intervals and P values were performed by means of the Tukey multiple comparisons procedure. Results of Cox regression analyses showed that censoring on the basis of breakage did not impact the analysis. Combined radiologist and cytotechnologist results were analyzed by means of linear mixed effects models, with biopsy as the cluster effect to account for repeated measures. Breakage analysis was performed with the Fisher exact test, and exact 95% intervals for odds ratios were determined with Bonferonni adjustments for pairwise comparisons among the three groups. The P values for the combined cytotechnologist and radiologist data and liver and kidney data were adjusted for physician type and tissue type, respectively.

[1] From the Department of Radiology (K.D.H.) and the Center for Biostatistics and Epidemiology (T.R.T.), Penn State University, 500 University Dr, PO Box 850, Hershey, PA 17033. Received May 29, 1997; revision requested June 13; revision received June 30; accepted July 8. **Address reprint requests to** K.D.H.

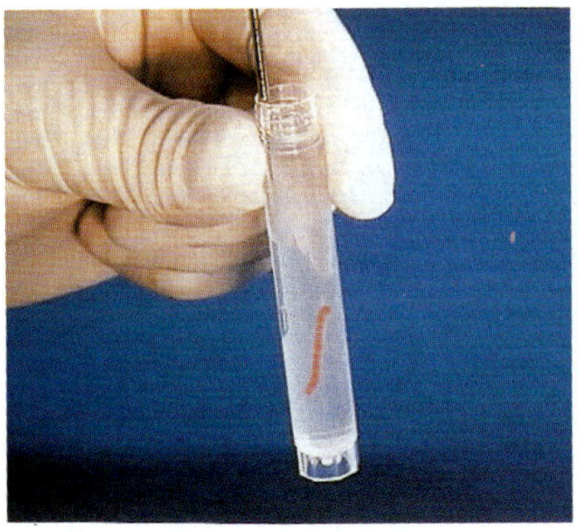

1.

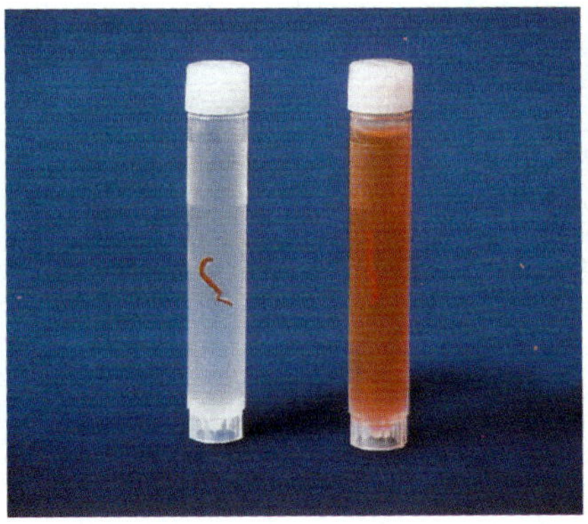

2.

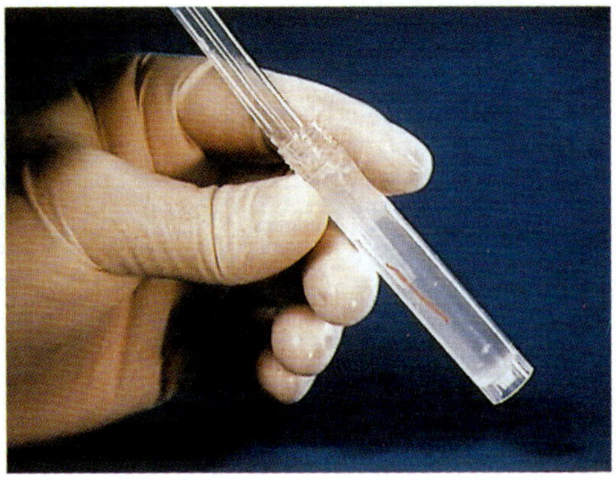

3.

Figures 1–3. Photographs of gel tubes that contain specimens. **(1)** The core needle is placed into the sterile gel, and the core specimen is exposed. The needle is rotated slightly side to side to release the specimen. The needle is then withdrawn, wiped free of gel with a gauze pad, and reused. **(2)** After all core specimens are placed into the gel (left tube), one to two drops of formalin fixative are added, and they quickly diffuse throughout the gel (right tube). An orange formalin mixture is used so the operator can be certain it has been added. **(3)** The cytotechnologist aspirates the core specimen, suspended in gel, into a bulb syringe. For illustrative purposes, the orange formalin was not added to the gel.

Results with Three Core-Biopsy Methods

	Gel Tube			Formalin Swirl			Scalpel Retrieval		
Operator	Kidney (n = 30)	Liver (n = 30)	Combined (n = 60)	Kidney (n = 30)	Liver (n = 30)	Combined (n = 60)	Kidney (n = 30)	Liver (n = 30)	Combined (n = 60)
Mean Time (sec)*									
Radiologist	4.1 (0.3)	3.5 (1.3)	3.8 (1.0)	4.0 (1.3)	5.0 (1.4)†	4.5 (1.4)	12.1 (3.1)‡	10.3 (3.5)‡	11.2 (3.3)‡
Cytotechnologist	25.8 (8.1)	36.7 (11.0)	31.3 (11.0)	6.6 (2.8)†	13.8 (8.7)‡	10.2 (7.3)‡	9.0(7.4)‡	11.0 (6.2)‡	10.0 (6.7)‡
Combined	29.9 (8.1)	40.2 (11.3)	35.1 (10.9)	10.6 (3.2)†	18.8 (8.1)	14.7 (7.3)†	21.1 (7.6)	21.3 (7.5)	21.2 (7.3)
No. of Specimens Broken§									
Radiologist	0	0	0	3 (10)	3 (10)	6 (10)	3 (10)	15 (50)$^{\|}$	18 (30)†
Cytotechnologist	6 (20)	6 (20)	12 (20)	0	0	0	0	0	0
Combined	6 (20)	6 (20)	12 (20)	3 (10)	3 (10)	6 (10)	3 (10)	15 (50)	18 (30)

* Numbers in parentheses are standard deviations.
† Significantly different from gel-tube method ($P < .05$).
‡ Significantly different from gel-tube method ($P < .001$).
§ Numbers in parentheses are percentages.
$^{\|}$ Significantly different from gel-tube method ($P = .09$).

Results

For the radiologist, the use of gel tubes to save core specimens was simple and fast, and no breakage occurred. The combined-organ mean time for the radiologist to save core specimens was not statistically significantly different with gel tubes (3.8 seconds) and the formalin-swirl method (4.5 seconds). Both of these methods, however, were significantly faster than the scalpel-retrieval method (11.2 seconds) ($P < .001$). With the formalin-swirl and scalpel-retrieval methods, breakage occurred in six (10%) and in 18 (30%) of the 60 core specimens, respectively (Table). Breakage occurred in 15 (50%) of the 30 liver core specimens with use of the scalpel-retrieval method; this difference was statistically significant ($P = .09$).

The cytotechnologist required significantly more time to remove core specimens from the gel than from the formalin (mean time with gel tubes, using a bulb aspirator, 31.3 seconds; formalin swirl, 10.2 seconds; scalpel retrieval, 10.0 seconds [$P < .001$]). Breakage occurred during preparation of tissue blocks of only core specimens suspended in gel. The cytotechnologist broke the specimen into two pieces in four (20%) of the 20 liver and kidney core specimens suspended in gel, but none of the specimens suspended in formalin were broken. This difference was not statistically significant ($P = .3$).

When findings for the radiologist and cytotechnologist were combined, the gel method was found to necessitate the most time (mean time for the combined organs with the gel method, 35.1 seconds; formalin swirl, 14.7 seconds; scalpel retrieval, 21.2 seconds) (Table). The breakage rates for the radiologist and cytotechnologist combined for the 60 core specimens from the combined liver and kidney were 20% (four gel-tube specimens), 10% (two formalin-swirl specimens), and 30% (six scalpel-retrieval specimens). None of these differences was statistically significant for the combined organs, but use of the scalpel-retrieval method in the liver resulted in a higher breakage rate (50%).

Discussion

There are several methods of retrieving core tissue at percutaneous biopsy. The simplest method is swirling the needle in formalin with the core specimen exposed. Although this method is easy, it adds substantially to the cost of the procedure when acquisition of more than one core specimen is desired, as the needle and disposable biopsy gun should not be reinserted once they have been swirled in formalin. Use of additional needles ($13–$15 each) or disposable biopsy guns ($30–$50 each) is then necessary.

An alternative is the manual removal of the core specimen from the notch of the needle by using a scalpel or needle or by touching the specimen to gauze. All three of these techniques frequently cause additional specimen breakage, but in the our experience careful use of a scalpel causes the least breakage. As shown by our data, even radiologists experienced in performing biopsy have some breakage with scalpel retrieval, especially when core specimens are from softer organs such as the liver.

Use of a gel tube allows the radiologist the possibility of less breakage of the core specimen and decreases the time needed for tissue retrieval. Because the gel tube is sterile, it also allows the unlimited use of a single needle or biopsy gun. In addition, unlike formalin, gel tubes do not have to be kept in an upright position during transport. Their use allows core specimens to be mailed or transported to remote laboratories.

Unfortunately, the cytotechnologist needs more time to prepare the tissue block when gel tubes are used. When core specimens are suspended in formalin, the cytotechnologist pours the formalin (plus the core specimen) onto the tissue paper. After the formalin drains through the tissue paper, the core specimen is left lying on top of the paper. When gel tubes are used, the cytotechnologist must first aspirate the core specimen into a bulb aspirator (Fig 3) and then express the core specimen onto the paper. Use of the bulb aspirator adds approximately 20 seconds to the time necessary to prepare the tissue block.

The finding that the scalpel-retrieval method causes substantially more breakage is not surprising. Single core-biopsy specimens are saved best with the formalin-swirl method. When multiple core specimens are needed, however, the use of gel tubes offers a cost-effective, simple alternative. Gel tubes also provide a convenient method of transporting tissue to remote laboratories. ■

References

1. Hopper KD, Abendroth CS, Sturtz KW, Matthews YL, Stevens LA, Shirk SJ. Automated biopsy devices: a blinded evaluation. Radiology 1993; 187:653–660.
2. Hopper KD, Abendroth CS, Sturtz KW, Matthews YL, Shirk SJ, Stevens LA. Blinded comparison of biopsy needles and automated devices in vitro. I. Biopsy of diffuse hepatic disease. AJR 1993; 161:1293–1297.
3. Hopper KD, Abendroth CS, Sturtz KW, Matthews YL, Shirk SJ, Stevens LA. A blinded comparison of biopsy needles and automated devices in vitro. II. Biopsy of medical renal disease. AJR 1993; 161:1299–1301.
4. Hopper KD, Abendroth CS, Sturtz KW, Matthews YL, Hartzel JS, Potok PS. Percutaneous biopsy guns: comparison of end-cut and side-notch devices in cadaveric specimens. AJR 1995; 164:195–199.
5. Hopper KD, Grenko RT, TenHave TR, Hartzel JS, Sturtz KW, Savage CS. Percutaneous biopsy of the liver and kidney by using coaxial technique: adequacy of the specimen obtained with three different needles in vitro. AJR 1995; 164:221–224.
6. Burbank F, Kaye K, Belville J, Ekuan J, Blumenfeld M. Image-guided automated core biopsies of the breast, chest, abdomen, and pelvis. Radiology 1994; 191:165–171.

Letters to the Editor

Endovascular Therapy for Intracranial Aneurysms

From:
David M. Pelz, MD, FRCPC,*,† Allan J. Fox, MD, FRCPC,*,† and Stephen P. Lownie, MD, FRCPC†
Departments of Diagnostic Radiology* and Clinical Neurological Sciences,† University of Western Ontario
339 Windermere Road, PO Box 5339, London, Ontario, Canada N6A 5A5

Editor:
Two recent articles from France, "Saccular Intracranial Aneurysms: Endovascular Treatment with Mechanical Detachable Spiral Coils" by Tournade and colleagues in the February 1997 issue of *Radiology* and "Intracranial Aneurysms: Endovascular Treatment with Mechanical Detachable Spirals in 60 Aneurysms" by Cognard and colleagues in the March 1997 issue, have reported on the use of mechanical detachable coils for the endovascular treatment of intracranial aneurysms (1,2). The results have been promising; however, the indications for endovascular rather than direct surgical therapy are confusing.

Tournade and colleagues (1) state that the indications for endovascular treatment include the presence of intracranial arterial vasospasm and anatomically difficult aneurysms such as carotid-ophthalmic, basilar bifurcation, and intracavernous aneurysms. Surgery or a combined approach is still used in most cases at their institutions. Cognard and colleagues (2) state that endovascular therapy is now the preferred primary treatment in France for both ruptured and unruptured intracranial aneurysms, with surgery reserved for those cases in which the coil treatment is unsuccessful.

These opinions should be read in light of a recent review (3) in the neurosurgical literature that reports on the anatomic and clinical outcome in what is to our knowledge the largest North American series of patients with intracranial aneurysms treated with the Guglielmi detachable coil (Target Therapeutics, Boston, Mass). In this series of 403 patients, the value of endovascular therapy is affirmed. The U.S. Food and Drug Administration–approved indications for this treatment, however, are clearly stated to include only those cases in which the aneurysm was considered to be unclippable by a vascular neurosurgeon or in which the surgical procedure was believed to carry an unacceptably high potential for morbidity or mortality.

Endovascular therapy for intracranial aneurysms is a powerful tool. Your readers should be aware that there are uncertainties in the indications for its use. Further investigation, perhaps a randomized controlled trial with surgery, is necessary before it can be considered to be the primary treatment for intracranial aneurysms.

References

1. Tournade A, Courtheoux P, Sengel C, Ozgulle S, Tajahmady T. Saccular intracranial aneurysms: endovascular treatment with mechanical detachable spiral coils. Radiology 1997; 202:481–486.
2. Cognard C, Pierot L, Boulin A, et al. Intracranial aneurysms: endovascular treatment with mechanical detachable spirals in 60 aneurysms. Radiology 1997; 202:783–792.
3. Vinuela F, Duckwiler G, Mawad N. Guglielmi detachable coil embolization of acute intracranial aneurysms: perioperative anatomical and clinical outcome in 403 patients. J Neurosurg 1997; 86:475–482.

Dr Tournade and colleagues respond:

We thank Dr Pelz very much for the letter on the endovascular treatment of intracranial aneurysms with mechanical detachable coils.

In our institution, on the basis of both the safety and the efficiency of the procedure, there has been a marked shift of opinion toward favoring endovascular treatment.

We always proceed with a team approach and gather neuroradiologists, neurosurgeons, and neuroanesthesiologists as we focus on the following considerations: (*a*) the clinical status, (*b*) the anatomic location of the aneurysm, (*c*) the size-neck ratio of the aneurysm, and (*d*) the general arterial accessibility. The treatment method is based on both how fast and how safely a cure can be achieved.

For instance, an aneurysm with a sylvian location associated with a sylvian valley hematoma is treated neurosurgically, as are wide-neck aneurysms.

With consideration of these facts, we use the endovascular route as a primary treatment in the majority of the aneurysm cases, that is, in those with as well as in those without subarachnoid hemorrhage.

Alain Tournade, MD,* Patrick Courtheoux, MD,† Christian Sengel, MD,* Sebnem Ozgulle, MD,* and Taghi Tajahmady, MD*
Department of Neuroradiology, Hôpital Pasteur, 39 avenue de la Liberté, 68024 Colmar, France,* and the Department of Interventional Neuroradiology, University Hospital, Caen, France†

Extreme Variability of Cerebrovascular US Results and Some Solutions

From:
J. Jay Crittenden, MD, FACR
Department of Diagnostic Imaging, West Florida Medical Center
8333 North Davis Highway, Pensacola, FL 32514-6049

Editor:
Many years ago my very capable and trusted chief sonographer resigned his position to start his own mobile ultrasound (US) service. Ensuing discussions with him introduced me to the fact that substantial variations occur between different US machines used to perform peripheral vascular studies. In this instance, there were marked variations in the velocity readings between his machine and our hospital-based machine. This was especially evident in carotid artery US. Even in high-degree stenoses in the hospital setting, we rarely saw peak systolic velocity readings of greater than 300 cm/sec, while he frequently saw peak systolic velocity readings of greater than 500 cm/sec. Similar disparities were present in all velocity ranges. We were both puzzled. We decided to pursue this problem by performing "no charge" examinations, cross-checking velocities, and comparing US findings with angiographic findings. It became apparent that a patient with a certain degree of angiographically proved stenosis could have very different velocity readings from machines with different manufacturers.

Over the years, I and others (1,2) have maintained an active interest in the variability of results from vascular laboratories. The manufacturer-to-manufacturer velocity variation is only the tip of the iceberg. Currently, there exists a serious multifactorial problem with vascular laboratory reliability that can, at the least, cause bothersome inconsistencies and, at the most, cause misdiagnoses and result in inappropriate therapy. This problem must be addressed.

The magnitude of this problem has been highlighted by recent media attention. A major news network recently sent a single patient to 10 vascular laboratories for carotid artery–cerebrovascular US ("Cerebrovascular Ultrasound Studies at Ten Vascular Laboratories, " *Primetime Live,* American Broadcasting Company, 1996 [to be broadcast on television]). I was asked to review the 10 studies while blinded to the laboratory and the specialty of the interpreting physician. I did know, however, that the first laboratory was accredited by the Intersocietal Commission for the Accreditation of Vascular Laboratories, Columbia, Md, and that findings from this laboratory were considered to be the reference or standard. At this laboratory, it was determined by using peak systolic velocity, end diastolic velocity, B-mode imaging, and color Doppler parameters that the patient had 30% diameter stenosis at the left internal carotid artery origin.

A tremendous variation in results from the other nine laboratories with regard to the left internal carotid artery origin was bothersome. At one extreme, two laboratories didn't mention any abnormality at the left internal carotid artery origin.

At the other extreme, one laboratory found 80%-diameter stenosis and another laboratory found "moderately severe stenosis and probably ulcerated plaque." These interpretations result in triaging patients for possible surgical treatment. The findings of the other five laboratories were everywhere in between these extremes and accompanied statements such as "less than 39%," "plaque, not hemodynamically significant," and "40% diameter stenosis." All nine laboratories used duplex US. Various combinations of peak systolic velocity, end diastolic velocity, internal carotid artery–common carotid artery ratios, and B-mode imaging parameters were used. Five laboratories used peak systolic velocity and B-mode imaging alone. Two laboratories asked for a brief history. No laboratory did any sort of physical examination or blood pressure determination. A physician did not see the patient in any of these nine laboratories.

One has to ask how these laboratories that used duplex equipment could arrive at such tremendously variable results. The variability, I believe, is due to several factors.

A major factor is the patient him- or herself. For example, certain cardiac (pump) problems such as cardiomyopathy and valvular diseases can cause considerable velocity variations at the carotid artery bifurcations. Blood pressure variations at the time of follow-up examination can cause substantial velocity changes, so the comparisons are not always exact.

Another important factor is inter- and intraobserver variation. This certainly applies to individual sonographers. Recently, I asked five experienced sonographers in my laboratory to determine the velocity in my proximal left internal carotid artery. Their peak systolic velocity determinations ranged from 54 cm/sec to 72 cm/sec. Because of patient and sonographer variations, exact velocity comparisons are inconsistent. For example, a peak systolic velocity of 200 cm/sec on one occasion and 225 cm/sec on another occasion may not indicate clinically important change.

The machine-to-machine variability mentioned earlier is a factor that may be able to be minimized. At the recent Ultrasound Summit Meeting (October 13 and 14, 1996, Las Vegas, Nev; sponsored by the American Institute of Ultrasound in Medicine, Laurel, Md), we asked the US machine manufacturers' representatives to consider some means of standardization of velocities. The discussants considered this a complex issue that will likely require considerable time for progress.

A more timely and practical approach is for each local laboratory to calibrate the machines to angiographic measurements of diameter stenosis. With a reasonable number of angiographic correlations, one can get a good idea of the velocities or other parameters required for a diagnosis of 60%–70% or greater diameter stenosis. This is a key range of percentages; the North American Symptomatic Carotid Endarterectomy Trial (3) used 70% stenosis and the Asymptomatic Carotid Atherosclerosis Study (4) used 60% stenosis to triage patients for potential surgical versus nonsurgical management. It is important that one know these locally calibrated velocities instead of using published data. While one could use a published table as a starting point, the local study will yield results much more reliable than those derived from a different machine and by a different sonographer in a remote center.

US laboratories can use other parameters to pick out the 60%–70% or greater diameter stenoses. Fortunately, this is the range at which hemodynamically significant changes occur distal to the stenosis; thus, ophthalmic artery–related studies, such as directional ophthalmic artery branch studies and ocular plethysmography, can be used. We have found these to be highly reliable in substantiating 60%–70% or greater diameter stenosis. Power Doppler has also proved useful. Owing to its increased signal-to-noise ratio and edge definition, we have found that the actual percentage of diameter stenosis can frequently be measured and compares favorably with angiographic measurements. While sensitivity settings are critical owing to the increased tendency for motion artifact, power Doppler should contribute greatly to the accurate diagnosis of carotid artery stenosis (5).

It is essential that some minimal standards and guidelines be established in this age of widespread use of high-technology US equipment. This is best done through an accreditation process. It would be desirable to have one accrediting body, but this is not politically possible at this time. There are, therefore, valid and excellent accreditation processes that were begun by the Intersocietal Commission for the Accreditation of Vascular Laboratories several years ago and more recently by the American College of Radiology and the American Institute of Ultrasound in Medicine. It is extremely important that training guidelines for physicians and sonographers be established and that vascular laboratories become accredited. Minimum standards for US equipment are also essential to prevent abusive practices. For example, I know of a carotid artery US examination that was performed by using a zero-crossing continuous wave machine in 1990. This examination was billed to and reimbursed by the Medicare carrier.

In this regard, reimbursement can be a control factor for improving quality in vascular laboratories. Ideally, quality should drive reimbursement. In a twisted way, the reverse may be true in vascular US. In several states, carriers have tied reimbursement to laboratory accreditation or sonographer registration. This seems onerous; however, in the long run this may help to drive out laboratories with poorly trained staff or those laboratories that perform examinations primarily for pecuniary reasons. In this regard, it is highly desirable for radiologists to meet with the insurance carriers on a state, regional, and national basis to help with these reimbursement and quality problems.

Organized radiology has been a leader in imaging quality. The status of mammography, for example, has taken a quantum leap because of the American College of Radiology standards. Likewise, radiologists should lead the process of standardization of vascular US to a high level. We should be sure that results in our own labs are accurate in the triaging of patients for potential surgery versus no surgery. In doing so, we cannot assume that a cookbook approach, in which we rely on published tables, will accurately reflect the percentage of diameter stenosis in our laboratories. Tests that measure hemodynamic events distal to stenoses are available and should be used in addition to velocity and anatomic parameters when possible. Power Doppler is a very useful imaging adjunct in estimating the percentage of diameter stenosis. Finally, vascular laboratories should seek accreditation by appropriate accrediting bodies to demonstrate minimum standards.

Through these means, radiologists can enhance the quality of cerebrovascular US performed in our laboratories and earn the "value-added" status we desire.

I thank William R. Scott, MD, for reviewing this letter and offering constructive suggestions.

References

1. Polak JF, Dobkin GR, O'Leary DH, Wang AM, Cutler SS. Internal carotid artery stenosis: accuracy and reproducibility of color-Doppler-assisted duplex imaging. Radiology 1989; 173:793–798.
2. Fillinger MF, Baker RJ, Zwolak RM, et al. Carotid duplex criteria for a 60% or greater angiographic stenosis: variation according to equipment. J Vasc Surg 1996; 24:856–864.
3. North American Symptomatic Carotid Endarterectomy Trial Collaborators. Beneficial effect of carotid endarterectomy in symptomatic patients with high-grade carotid stenosis. N Engl J Med 1991; 325:445–453.
4. Executive Committee for the Asymptomatic Carotid Atherosclerosis Study. Endarterectomy for asymptomatic carotid artery stenosis. JAMA 1995; 273:1421–1428.
5. Griewing B, Morgenstern C, Dreisner F, Kallwellis G, Walker ML, Kesslee C. Cerebrovascular disease assessed by color flow and power doppler ultrasonography. Stroke 1996; 27:95–100.

Future of Teleradiology

From:
John S. Wills, MD
Department of Radiology, Medical Center of Delaware
4755 Ogletown-Stanton Road, PO Box 6001, Newark, DE 19718

Editor:
In their discussion of the future of teleradiology in the June 1997 issue of *Radiology*, Dure-Smith and Fymat (1) envision the day when all radiologists, save angiographers and interventionalists, will perform their work from the lofty confines of the academic medical institution. As they see it, the increasingly sophisticated medical consumers of the future will be drawn inexorably toward the most highly specialized and best-known imaging experts, who are, of course, located in larger university centers. In this radiologic utopia, local community imaging services will be provided largely by "super technologists" under the direction of geographically distant radiologists, who will be supported by triage consultant radiologists (the authors do not indicate where the latter specialists will be located).

I agree that teleradiology is a tool with powerful potential. Without a doubt, this technology promises to bring quality radiologic services to underserved populations here and abroad, provide opportunities for radiologic consultation with experts in centers remote from the location of the point of service, and enhance the efficiency of radiologic practice in general. Teleradiology, along with other facets of telemedicine, will likely contribute in a major way to the transformation of the health care system in the United States early in the coming century.

Before accepting the vision of Dure-Smith and Fymat, however, there are unanswered questions to ponder. Is the best imaging service for all patients that provided by radiologists remote from the local community, with no accountability or commitment to that community? Is the highly specialized radiologist based at the university center, whose national reputation and expertise may be based wholly or in part on his or her research activities, necessarily better equipped to provide imaging consultation for most patients than the dedicated community-based radiologist with some general skills in addition to an area of special interest, who has devoted a career to patient care? Is there not a value to the community of the physical presence of radiologists who participate in the local heath care system, even if their skills are known to and appreciated by only the physicians in that locale? Does not the presence of the radiologist in the community help to guarantee the availability of imaging services to those who are less sophisticated and knowledgeable about "better" options at geographically distant sites? Does not a system of the kind proposed by Dure-Smith and Fymat potentially provide more opportunity for nonradiologic physicians in a community to assume an expanded role in the provision of imaging services, which would result in a lower quality of those services?

I suggest consideration of a different model for the future. Radiologists should promote and refine teleradiology for the medically underserved, for expert consultation, for continuing education, and to improve the quality and efficiency of their service, such as 24-hour hospital or remote office coverage. But, rather than looking for ways to eliminate radiologists at the community level, we should focus on encouraging more active and direct involvement locally in the selection of appropriate imaging studies and more timely provision of service. Our organizations must support and help develop more relevant quality assurance tools and systems of physician accountability. And we should work to develop more sophisticated and reliable methods of ensuring adequate continuing education for all radiologists. Rather than moving away from active involvement in the community environment, where most patients receive health care, we should increase our direct participation locally. It is in this manner that we will best prove our value as imaging specialists to patients, third-party payers, and our nonradiologic physician colleagues.

Reference

1. Dure-Smith P, Fymat AL. Teleradiology: will it transform the practice of radiology? Radiology 1997; 203(3):49A–50A.

Drs Dure-Smith and Fymat respond:

We thank Dr Wills for the thoughtful comments. We agree that the many questions raised by teleradiology need to be debated and a consensus opinion incorporated into immediate and long-term planning.

We clarify that we do not equate specialization with "super-specialists" working from academic centers. We believe that the competitive and economic factors in teleradiology will impose more specialization, that is, practice limited to a specific field or area. The extent and breakdown of this specialization is one of the many fascinating issues that need to be addressed. Like the correspondent, we are concerned that the changes that teleradiology is likely to impose will be under the control of or strongly influenced by our profession. We are especially concerned that this technology could be the Trojan horse invited into the heart of our profession only to break it up into attractive morsels to be gobbled up by eager, poorly qualified entrepreneurs. To highlight this point, let us trace a worst-case orwellian scenario that could result from the uncontrolled and unregulated growth of teleradiology, driven primarily by commercial forces and providing image production, management, and interpretation. It could be as follows.

Image production and management are taken over by large manufacturers of radiology equipment, entrepreneurs, or both, who own and manage image centers and employ technicians ("supertechs") to feed images into the global network.

Image interpretation is offered by competing national or international entities. The larger organizations, sited on uninhabited wasteland (cheap real estate), employ image interpreters (remember when they were called radiologists?) to sit in darkened rooms banked with workstations and work 8-hour shifts, 24 hours a day, and produce (like battery hens) a steady stream of interpretations. Smaller organizations, down to individuals who work from their homes, offer one-modality, single-organ or single–body part interpretation (eg, magnetic resonance imaging of the hand) for a very modest fee.

Is it even conceivable that the great inherent strength and cohesion of radiology today that has been built up through the acquisition of knowledge and skills and fused together by its professional organizations and journals could be so decimated by this technology? We believe the answer is "yes." This being so, what needs to be done? What specific questions need to be asked, and which of our professional organizations should address them? We believe the questions should include at least some of the following:

1. What fundamental organizational changes are likely to occur or should be sought and encouraged when global, networked radiology becomes a reality?

2. How may these changes affect the numbers of radiologists likely to be needed, assuming that current trends will continue in health care delivery (growth of capitation systems) and recognizing that teleradiology will make radiology available to many underserved parts of the United States and the world?

3. If the number of radiologists needs to be controlled, how will this be achieved, considering the potentially divergent interests of residency training programs, residents in training, and practicing radiologists?

4. How will radiology ensure strong representation in the development of legislation to regulate cyberspace, which includes legislation on the qualifications for providing imaging services, cross-state and cross-international licensing and credentialing, and other legal and liability issues?

5. Should changes be made in the residency training programs to respond to networked radiology? Will there be a need for more specialization (superspecialists) and a new breed of clinical radiologists ("triaging radiologists")? How should these changes be structured to support academic radiology?

6. Will there be a need for new teleradiology managers (new "technocrats") to develop and manage teleradiology imaging centers and systems, and how will they receive appropriate technical training and maintain qualifications?

7. Likewise, will there be a need for a new breed of technicians in teleradiology (supertechs), and how will they receive appropriate technical training and maintain qualifications?

Finally, while teleradiology conferences in recent years have proliferated, they tend to be focused on the "gee-whiz" technology (your friendly monster) and tend not to address the more contentious organizational issues, some of which are listed above. This may be an appropriate time for the international radiology fraternity to hold an international consensus conference. The horse has been built and is already in our midst.

Peter Dure-Smith, MD, and Alain L. Fymat, PhD
Radiology Service-114, Jerry L. Pettis Memorial Veteran Affairs Medical Center
11201 Benton St, Loma Linda, CA 92357

Enhancement Velocity Not Necessarily Reflective of Contrast Material Uptake in Breast MR Imaging

From:
Markus Pedevilla, MSc
Magnetic Resonance Institute, Karl Franzens University of Graz
Auenbruggerplatz 9, A-8036 Graz, Austria

Editor:

In their article in the January 1997 issue of *Radiology* on the use of T2* susceptibility contrast to differentiate between rapidly contrast material–enhancing fibroadenomas and malignant breast tumors, Dr Kuhl and colleagues (1) compared the signal intensity loss during T2-weighted, first-pass magnetic resonance (MR) imaging studies with the signal intensity increase during T1-weighted, dynamic MR imaging studies.

The distinct distribution of the T2*-induced signal intensity loss in the first 30 seconds, shown in figure 4b of Kuhl and colleagues' article, is impressive. If these encouraging results of perfusion imaging can be proved in a larger study, this technique seems to be an appropriate way to reduce false-positive findings and to improve the specificity of gadolinium-enhanced breast MR imaging.

For the evaluation of the signal intensity increase, the authors use an "enhancement velocity" (signal intensity increase within a certain time frame). This is the increase in the signal intensity in the 1st minute after the administration of gadopentetate dimeglumine normalized to the baseline signal intensity. A threshold of an 80% signal intensity increase within the 1st minute was used to indicate malignancy. However, the magnitude of signal intensity enhancement induced by gadopentetate dimeglumine is not only dependent on the gadopentetate dimeglumine concentration within the tissue in question, but also strongly dependent on the native relaxation times T1 and T2, which vary widely for benign and malignant tumors (2,3). This is totally neglected in the calculation of the enhancement velocity.

By using a signal intensity increase of 80% (malignancy threshold) and the imaging parameters published in the article of Kuhl and colleagues (fast field echo, 230/4.6 [repetition time msec/echo time msec], 80° flip angle), the concentration of gadopentetate dimeglumine in different tissue types can be calculated. Assuming the tissue in question is a malignant tumor with a native T1 of 880 msec yields a gadopentetate dimeglumine concentration of 0.297 mmol/L within the tumor tissue. Assuming the tissue in question is a benign tumor with a native T1 of 1,100 msec yields a gadopentetate dimeglumine concentration of 0.218 mmol/L within the tumor tissue. Hence, considering the different native longitudinal relaxation times, the gadopentetate dimeglumine concentration in the carcinoma is about 1.36 times higher than that in the benign tumor. This shows that the relative signal intensity increase that was used to calculate the enhancement velocity does not properly reflect the gadopentetate dimeglumine uptake in the tumor tissue and therefore cannot be a reliable parameter in describing the neovascularization of tumor lesions.

We want to stress that the evaluation of the contrast material uptake in a lesion by means of determining the signal intensity increase without considering the native longitudinal relaxation time is unreliable and should therefore not serve as a reference method.

However, the neglect of native relaxation times is a common problem and we want to state that all methods in which enhancement velocity is a criterion for malignancy are biased and have low specificity.

References

1. Kuhl CK, Bieling H, Gieseke J, et al. Breast neoplasms: T2* susceptibility-contrast, first-pass perfusion MR imaging. Radiology 1997; 202:87–95.
2. Merchant TE, Thelissen GR, de-Graaf PW, et al. Application of a mixed sequence for MR imaging characterization of human breast disease. Acta Radiol 1993; 34:356–361.
3. Kievit HCE, Sikkenk AC, Thelissen GR, et al. Magnetic resonance image appearance of hamartoma of the breast. Magn Reson Imaging 1993; 11:293–298.

Dr Kuhl and colleagues respond:

We thank Dr Pedevilla for his interest in our study (1) and for his interesting comments.

The comments may be summarized as four statements or assumptions. First, Dr Pedevilla states that plain enhancement values (ie, $[SI_c - SI]/SI$, where SI and SI_c are the baseline and the postcontrast signal intensities, respectively) are not useful in calculating tissue gadopentetate dimeglumine concentration. Second, he suggests that the gadopentetate dimeglumine concentration may be calculated by using the enhancement values and the tissue T1 relaxation times. Third, he states that the enhancement values thus gained yield better differentiation between benign and malignant lesions than plain enhancement values. Fourth, he concludes that the results of the T2*-

weighted, first-pass perfusion studies should be compared with these gadopentetate dimeglumine "concentration values" rather than with the plain enhancement values.

Dr Pedevilla states that "... the magnitude of signal intensity enhancement induced by gadopentetate dimeglumine is not only dependent on the gadopentetate dimeglumine concentration within the tissue in question, but also strongly dependent on the native relaxation times T1 and T2, which vary widely for benign and malignant tumors." This is absolutely correct. In fact, this is almost literally expressed in the introduction of our article. Thus, we completely agree that in T1-weighted pulse sequences, "... the relative signal intensity increase ... does not properly reflect the gadopentetate dimeglumine uptake in the tumor tissue and therefore cannot be a reliable parameter in describing the neovascularization of tumor lesions," as Pedevilla puts it. This lack of a straightforward correlation between the postcontrast signal intensity increase on the image and the amount of gadopentetate dimeglumine in the tissue is the reason we tried T2*-weighted pulse sequences at all. However, the problem is that the alternative Pedevilla suggests is not suitable for establishing this correlation, either.

The reason is that, unfortunately, Pedevilla's second assumption is not correct. It is not true that the concentration of gadopentetate dimeglumine in the tissue may be calculated by considering the imaging parameters, the tissue T1 relaxation times, and the postcontrast signal intensity increase. The relation between native T1 ($T1_0$), the T1 after injection of gadopentetate dimeglumine ($T1_c$), and the local concentration of gadopentetate dimeglumine in the tissue (C) is $1/T1_c = 1/T1_0 + \alpha C$, where α is tissue relaxivity. So, what can be calculated by using $T1_0$ and the enhancement is the product of α and C, not C. The relaxivity, however, is not known; it varies strongly from tissue to tissue in an unpredictable way. And even the calculation of α multiplied by C is correct only as long as certain conditions are fulfilled (no strong flow, no differences in perfusion, etc).

Accordingly, the third statement is clearly not correct because the proposed calculation does not yield the tissue gadopentetate dimeglumine concentration. Given the comparable contrast material enhancement in T1-weighted studies of fibroadenomas and breast cancers, the gain in specificity in the correspondent's calculation is based solely on his assumption that the fibroadenoma has a much longer T1 relaxation time than the breast cancer. There may be fibroadenomas with long T1 relaxation times, but this is not a consistent finding. If this were true, we could even restrict our breast MR imaging protocol to a single mixed- or multiple-repetition-time sequence to determine tissue T1 relaxation times and would not even need the enhancement values.

The specificity gain the correspondent predicts has not been documented in controlled studies so far, and—for the reasons mentioned above—we doubt that it ever will be. Others (including ourselves) have studied how the consideration of the T1 relaxation times affects the specificity of dynamic breast MR imaging. In our experience, there is no difference concerning specificity with this method as compared with the method in which plain, conventional enhancement velocities are used.

Finally, in Pedevilla's conclusion, we suppose that there is a misunderstanding about the study design. Once a novel imaging technique has been presented in the field of diagnostic imaging, we face two tasks: We must validate the technique (does it really measure what it intends to measure?), and we must evaluate its clinical usefulness (is it really better than what we already have?). These are two different tasks that have to be thoroughly distinguished.

It has not been our intention to validate the perfusion technique with the enhancement values (which is what Pedevilla suggests); we did not attempt to use the enhancement values as reference for the tissue gadopentetate dimeglumine concentration. Validation was attempted, as stated in the article, by counting tissue vessel densities; validation has yet to be completed (and is currently being done in our department) with further histopathologic or pathophysiologic correlative studies.

In fact, the comparison of the lesions' T2* perfusion values with the lesions' enhancement in T1-weighted studies helped in assessing the clinical value of perfusion imaging as a diagnostic tool. In our opinion, the introduction of a new technique (not only in the field of diagnostic imaging) is justified only if it offers statistically significant diagnostic gain with respect to established techniques. Therefore, to evaluate the usefulness of a new technique, it must be compared with an accepted reference technique that serves as the standard. In contrast-enhanced, dynamic breast MR imaging, the established diagnostic standard (for which extensive clinical experience exists) is to calculate enhancement by using the relative signal intensity increase that occurs in T1-weighted, gradient-echo imaging.

In our eyes, there is virtually no alternative to the comparison of the T2* perfusion values with relative enhancement values. A comparison with another experimental technique like the one Pedevilla suggests does not seem appropriate for validation or for clinical assessment of the T2* perfusion technique.

Reference

1. Kuhl CK, Bieling H, Gieseke J, et al. Breast neoplasms: T2* susceptibility-contrast, first-pass perfusion MR imaging. Radiology 1997; 202:87–95.

Christiane K. Kuhl, MD, Juergen Gieseke, PhD, and Hans H. Schild, MD

Department of Radiology, University of Bonn, Sigmund-Freud-Strasse 25, D-53105 Bonn, Germany

Vascular Rings and the Straight Trachea

From:

Alan E. Oestreich, MD

Department of Radiology, Children's Hospital Medical Center

3333 Burnet Avenue, Cincinnati, OH 45229-3039

Editor:

I read with interest the article in the May 1997 issue of *Radiology* by Pickhardt and colleagues (1), who emphasize the plain radiographic findings of vascular rings in symptomatic children. In their series, four frontal radiographs (10%) were "normal or indeterminate" for the radiographic signs being analyzed. In their discussion, they also emphasized the need for radiographs obtained at full inspiration.

Not discussed by the authors was a sign we have found useful in predicting the presence of double aortic arch: the straight trachea on frontal radiographs obtained during expiration in infants and young children (2). Most frontal chest radiographs obtained in young children (children not old enough to respond to a request to hold the breath at inspiration) are indeed obtained during expiration. Expiration radiographs, incidentally, are useful in patients with wheezing, because they permit assessment for air trapping.

In general, the frontal expiration radiographs obtained in such young subjects show the well-known buckle toward the side opposite the aortic arch. However, subjects with double aortic arches do not show any expiratory buckle on frontal views. A straight trachea on several (all) frontal radiographs obtained in the first years of life has been a helpful hint for the presence of a double aortic arch. I wonder how many of the four patients with normal frontal radiographs in the series of Pickhardt and colleagues were indeed subjects with double aortic arches and, repeatedly, a straight trachea at expiration. As more frontal radiographs obtained in a baby show a straight trachea, the likelihood of double aortic arch rises. The data on lateral radiographs reported by Pickhardt and colleagues (1) can thus be helpful once the suspicion of such a diagnosis has been raised. Nonetheless, I emphasize that repeated acquisition of apparently normal frontal radiographs (that show a straight trachea) are in themselves a sign of the double aortic arch vascular ring.

References
1. Pickhardt PJ, Siegel MJ, Gutierrez FR. Vascular rings in symptomatic children: frequency of chest radiographic findings. Radiology 1997; 203:423–426.
2. Oestreich AE. Pediatric radiology: medical outline series. 3rd ed. New Hyde Park, NY: Medical Examination, 1984; 74–75.

Dr Pickhardt and colleagues respond:

We appreciate the comments made by Dr Oestreich with regard to the straight trachea as a finding of a double aortic arch, but we remain skeptical of the diagnostic usefulness. Among children with double aortic arches in our series, a far more common and useful finding was tracheal buckling to the left, away from the larger right arch component, which was seen in 12 (75%) of 16 children. Four children with double arches without focal tracheal indentation had straight tracheas. Of perhaps more importance is that seven of 25 children with right aortic arch anomalies had straight tracheas, as did the majority of the healthy population. Thus, the straight trachea appears to be a nonspecific sign. We believe that focal indentation or deviation of the trachea represents a more specific finding for a vascular ring than does the straight trachea. We are unable to confirm Dr Oestreich's belief that a straight trachea is a sign of a double arch.

We maintain that the combination of frontal and lateral radiographs is a reliable screening tool for detecting the presence of vascular rings in symptomatic children. In our experience, the chest radiograph is not reliable for distinguishing between the double aortic arch and the right arch. Additional imaging studies, magnetic resonance imaging in particular, should be performed if this differentiation is clinically important.

References
1. Pickhardt PJ, Siegel MJ, Gutierrez FR. Vascular rings in symptomatic children: frequency of chest radiographic findings. Radiology 1997; 203:423–426.

Perry J. Pickhardt, MD, Marilyn J. Siegel, MD, and Fernando R. Gutierrez
Mallinckrodt Institute of Radiology, Washington University of Medicine
510 South Kingshighway Boulevard, St Louis, MO 63110

Percutaneous US-guided Ablation of Liver Metastases

From:
Alighieri Mazziotti, MD, and Antonino Cavallari, MD
Department of Surgery and Transplantation, Saint Orsola Hospital, University of Bologna
via Massarenti 9, 40138 Bologna, Italy

Editor:
The last few years have seen a great increase in the use of ablative, percutaneous methods for the treatment of hepatocellular carcinoma in patients with cirrhosis. Injection of alcohol has been the most widely used treatment in large clinical series both in the Far East and in Europe (1,2). The limits of excision in patients with cirrhosis justify resorting to this alternative treatment: The features of hepatocellular carcinomas in cirrhosis, most of which have a pseudocapsule, are less consistent with respect to the surrounding parenchyma, which favors the spread of the alcohol inside the lesion and the cytonecrotic effect.

The results of ablative, percutaneous, ultrasound-guided treatment in hepatocellular carcinoma have led radiology teams to extend the indications for this treatment to liver metastases. Treatment with radio frequency is an evolution of the ablative, percutaneous methods to effect coagulative necrosis of the tumor with heat. The two articles by Solbiati and colleagues (3) and Livraghi and colleagues (4) in the January 1997 issue of *Radiology* report results that the authors define as "potentially effective" because a "complete response for at least 9 months can be achieved in approximately 50% of patients" (3). These results are proposed as a "less invasive alternative to surgical therapy" in relation to the "high morbidity and mortality" of surgery (3). In the clinical series reported on in the two articles, the lesions all were small, most were solitary, and most originated from colorectal tumors.

As surgeons in a university hospital center with an overall experience of more than 800 liver resections, we need to comment on the evaluation of the results of these two studies.

In all the most recent surgical series, the rate of mortality due to hepatic resections in noncirrhotic livers has declined to around 1% both in Europe and in the Far East (5–8) and to 0.4% in 240 liver resections of metastases in our series (one patient died of digestive tract hemorrhage in 1984; since then, there have been no postoperative deaths), with a truly negligible morbidity rate (9). In the 1990s, liver surgery can be considered perfectly safe; it is performed routinely in a growing number of centers and more and more frequently without blood transfusions (5). It is appropriate to remember that the above-mentioned surgical series, like the series mentioned in the quotations from Solbiati and colleagues' article, includes a substantial percentage of patients with large lesions who underwent surgery and that the reported mortality rate refers only to mortality due to major hepatectomy for voluminous lesions. If one were to consider only the superficial metastases smaller than 3 cm in diameter, as those shown in the figures of the articles by Solbiati and colleagues (3) and Livraghi and colleagues (4) appear to be, then the surgical risk can be considered truly negligible.

The size of the tumor also plays a role in determining long-term results (10). Survival after surgical resection is greatly dependent on the size of the tumor. The surgical series reported on in Solbiati and colleagues' article (3) includes a high percentage of tumors larger than 5 cm in diameter, for which long-term survival after removal will certainly be worse than it is for tumors smaller than 3 cm.

The mean follow-up in the two studies was 6 months (Livraghi and colleagues [4]) and 16.6 months (Solbiati and colleagues [3]). These periods are not long enough to assess the long-term efficacy of treatment for liver metastases. It should be remembered that in untreated patients with 3-cm tumors the survival is around 100% after 1 year (11,12); we are amazed that as many as three patients with such an initially small tumor in Solbiati and colleagues' study (3) died of neoplastic dissemination a little more than 1 year after treatment.

In addition to the size of the tumor, the number of lesions, and the stage of the primary tumor, the prognostic factors involved in the surgical treatment of liver metastases include acquisition of an adequate margin of healthy tissue around the tumor. One fact that is commonly accepted in surgery for liver metastases is that only radical resection, with a margin of at least 1 cm, can ensure good long-term survival (10). Metastatectomies or cytoreductive surgery have now been abandoned in all surgical centers because they do not modify patient survival in any way. A "partial response" or cytoreduction makes no sense in therapy for liver metastases, and a longer follow-up than those in the two articles in *Radiology* will certainly show a progression of the disease in all cases of partial necrosis.

A final point that causes some perplexity with regard to these ablative, percutaneous treatments is our personal experience of liver resection in cases initially treated at other centers with percutaneous methods such as alcoholization (five cases) and radio frequency (two cases). These lesions were initially small and easily accessible for segmentary resection. In all these cases, multiple percutaneous treatments (up to 211 treatments) had been performed. At the time of surgery, the lesions were all much larger. Major hepatectomy was needed in four cases. In four cases, there was infiltration of the diaphragm, which was resected together with the tumor. In two cases, the diaphragm was infiltrated in an area where there was no tumor on the corresponding liver capsule; this infiltration was therefore a true tumoral seeding through the needle stab. In all the cases in which surgery was performed, histologic examination of the surgical specimen revealed completely vital tissue; only one case showed evidence of necrotic zones adjacent to the areas of disease recurrence (this was a case of carcinoid metastases, which are known to be highly vascularized and perhaps for this reason more sensitive to local treatment). Unfortunately, the hope that "diseases which are not cured by iron are cured by fire" (13) is not fulfilled in liver metastases.

The problems of liver resection for metastases are related to multiple or voluminous metastases or to those that extend from one half of the liver to other segments, which makes traditional hepatectomy problematic. In these cases, it is only through cooperation between surgeons, oncologists, and angioradiologists that treatment is possible in patients who until fairly recently were considered to have inoperable disease.

For individual small metastases, however, surgery must be considered as the standard treatment. All other therapeutic proposals must be considered as experimental trials. "Ars longa, iudicium difficile, experimentum periculosum" (Hippocrates, 400 BC).

References

1. Sheu JC, Sung L, Huang GT, et al. Intratumor injection of absolute ethanol under ultrasound guidance for the treatment of small hepatocellular carcinoma. Hepatogastroenterology 1987; 34:255–261.
2. Livraghi T, Bolondi L, Buscarini L, et al. No treatment, resection and ethanol injection in hepatocellular carcinoma in a retrospective analysis of survival in 391 patients with cirrhosis. J Hepatology 1995; 15:77–80.
3. Solbiati L, Ierace T, Goldberg SN, et al. Percutaneous US-guided radio-frequency tissue ablation of liver metastases: treatment and follow-up in 16 patients. Radiology 1997; 202:195–203.
4. Livraghi T, Goldberg SN, Monti F, et al. Saline-enhanced radio-frequency tissue ablation in the treatment of liver metastases. Radiology 1997; 202:205–210.
5. Gozzetti G, Mazziotti A, Grazi GL, et al. Liver resections without blood transfusion. Br J Surg 1995; 82:1105–1110.
6. Belghiti J, Di Carlo I, Sauvanet A, Uribe M, Fèkètè F. A ten years experience with hepatic resection in 338 patients: evolution in indication and operative mortality. Eur J Surg 1994; 160:277–282.
7. Miyagawa S, Makuuchi M, Kawasaki S, Kakawa T. Criteria for safe hepatic resection. Am J Surg 1995; 169:589–594.
8. Rees M, Plant G, Wells J, Bygrave S. One hundred and fifty hepatic resections: evolution of technique towards bloodless surgery. Br J Surg 1966; 83:1526–1529.
9. Mazziotti A, Cavallari A. Techniques in liver surgery. London, England: Greenwich Medical Media, 1997; 139.
10. Sheele J, Stang R, Alterndorf HA, Paul M. Resection for colorectal liver metastases. World J Surg 1995; 19:59–71.
11. Bengtsson G, Carlsson G, Hafstrom L, Jonsson P. The natural history of patients with untreated liver metastases from colorectal cancer. Am J Surg 1981; 141:586–589.
12. Wanebo HJ. Natural history of colorectal cancer metastasized to the liver. In: Wanebo HJ. Hepatic and biliary cancer. New York, NY: Dekker, 1987; 464–466.

Dr Solbiati and colleagues respond:

Drs Mazziotti and Cavallari have raised several important issues concerning our early reports of percutaneous ablation of liver metastases by using radio frequency (1,2). To begin with, these surgeons are critical of our proposal that percutaneous tumor ablation therapies such as radio frequency may be "less invasive alternative[s] to surgical therapy" because of the "high morbidity and mortality" of surgery (1). They point to recent series from large cancer centers that document the reduction to 1% in the rate of mortality due to hepatic resection.

While these results are remarkable, other recent, similar series (3–5) have suggested that major morbidity and perioperative mortality rates are closer to 9%–33% and 2.8%–4.6%, respectively, as suggested in our article. Regardless of the exact numbers, it is difficult to accept that even laparotomy alone, much less hepatic resection, could be less invasive than percutaneous needle insertion. Were this so, open laparotomy, and not the image-guided percutaneous technique, would have remained the standard for tissue biopsy. In addition, the length of the hospital stay and the attendant costs for surgery are much greater than those for percutaneous radio-frequency ablation, which is performed as an outpatient procedure.

Drs Mazziotti and Cavallari further stress that patient follow-up is limited. We certainly agree that these results are preliminary and have appropriately stressed this within the published articles. We have continued to report results of longer-term follow-up as they become available (6) and will continue to do so in the future. We also agree that at present surgical resection should be considered the standard treatment of small liver metastases. In both of our series, all patients were referred to us either because the patient was deemed to have inoperable disease or because the patient had refused surgery. Many of the patients we are currently treating have had recurrent hepatic metastases after hepatic resection and are not thought to be candidates for repeat hepatic resection.

Drs Mazziotti and Cavallari suggest that only with surgical margins of at least 1 cm is there any chance of long-term survival. We agree that a necessary aim of all ablation therapy should be to induce coagulation that extends at least 1 cm beyond the margin of the identified metastases and that alteration of outcome is highly unlikely if ablation of the entire metastasis is not accomplished. This was often difficult with the technology available at the time of our initial studies, as multiple electrode insertions were required to achieve large volumes of coagulation. More recent clinical studies with internally cooled radio-frequency electrodes have demonstrated the feasibility of inducing larger zones of necrosis with a single electrode insertion (7). We are confident that ongoing technical advances in radio-frequency technology will enable the creation of even greater volumes of coagulation necrosis. These advances may ultimately lead to successful treatment of larger hepatic metastases, such as adequate coagulation of appropriate margins.

Drs Mazziotti and Cavallari cite limited personal experience in two patients treated with radio frequency and in five patients treated with percutaneous ethanol instillation who they believe could have been easily treated with segmental resection. These patients ultimately required major hepatectomy for recurrent local disease. It is likely that these patients were treated with older radio-frequency technology, and it is possible that, had newer techniques been used, their lesions might have been adequately treated with percutaneous therapy. Nevertheless, until the efficacy of radio-frequency ablation has been better established, we agree that the treatment should be reserved primarily for patients who are not surgical candidates.

On the basis of their two specimens, Drs Mazziotti and Cavallari also doubt the efficacy of radio frequency in inducing coagulative necrosis, because only "completely viable tissue" was found. We have recently reported the histopathologic findings of radio-frequency–induced necrosis in 28 patients (8). These findings conclusively demonstrate that continuous coagulative necrosis is induced in hepatic tumor, but that special stains, such as those that detect lactate dehydrogenase activity, may be required to discern these changes in some cases.

Finally, while it is true that the development of new therapeutic techniques can entail certain risks—as undoubtedly did the development of many surgical techniques—it is also true that only through careful and dedicated clinical research can the frontiers of modern medicine be advanced. Our studies have been performed with careful planning and only after appropriate approval from our institutional ethics committees and informed patient consent. Furthermore, we have reported our early results not only to document the potential of the technique, but also so that others can learn from our experience and so that together we can better understand the ultimate role of radio frequency and other ablative therapies in the care of patients with liver metastases. Long-term and larger studies are certainly needed, but we believe that our preliminary clinical results, as well as recent technologic advances, do give reason for cautious optimism with regard to the future of radiofrequency ablation.

We thank Drs Mazziotti and Cavallari for their interest from a surgeon's perspective. Taking their lead, we finish with the remainder of Hippocrates' first aphorism: "Oportet autem non modo se ipsum exhibere quae oportet facientem, sed etiam aegrum, et praesentes, et externa" ("It is the duty of the physician not only to do that which immediately belongs to him, but likewise to secure the cooperation of the sick, of those who are in attendance, and of all the external agents") (9). This we have done and will continue to do.

References

1. Solbiati L, Ierace T, Goldberg SN, et al. Percutaneous US-guided radio-frequency tissue ablation of liver metastases: treatment and follow-up in 16 patients. Radiology 1997; 202:195–203.
2. Livraghi T, Goldberg SN, Monti F, et al. Saline-enhanced radio-frequency tissue ablation in the treatment of liver metastases. Radiology 1997; 202:205–210.
3. Sitzmann JV, Greene PS. Perioperative predictors of morbidity following hepatic resection for neoplasm: a multivariate analysis of a single surgeon experience with 105 patients. Ann Surg 1994; 219:13–17.
4. Ballantyne GH, Quin J. Surgical treatment of liver metastases in patients with colorectal cancer. Cancer 1993; 71(suppl):4252–4266.
5. Fong Y, Cohen AM, Fortner JG, et al. Liver resection for colorectal metastases. J Clin Oncol 1997; 15:938–946.
6. Solbiati L, Goldberg SN, Ierace T, Livraghi T, Sironi S, Gazelle GS. Follow-up of liver metastases treated with percutaneous radiofrequency ablation: clinical outcome and survival rates (abstr). Radiology 1996; 201:P268.
7. Solbiati L, Goldberg SN, Ierace T, et al. Hepatic metastases: percutaneous radio-frequency ablation with cooled-tip electrodes. Radiology 1997; 205:367–373.
8. Goldberg SN, Tanabe KK, Solbiati L, Gazelle GS, Hahn PF, Mueller PR. Treatment of intrahepatic malignancy with radiofrequency ablation: radiologic-pathologic correlation in 16 patients (abstr). AJR 1997; 168(suppl):121.
9. Coar T, trans. The aphorisms of Hippocrates. Classics of Medicine Library. Birmingham, Ala: Adams, 1982.

Luigi Solbiati, MD,* S. Nahum Goldberg, MD,† Tito Livraghi, MD,‡ and G. Scott Gazelle, MD, MPH†

Department of Radiology, General Hospital, Piazzale Solaro, 3, 21052 Busto, Arsizio (VA), Italy*; the Department of Radiology, Massachusetts General Hospital, Harvard Medical School, Boston, Mass†; and the Department of Radiology, Ospedale Civile, Vimercate, Italy‡

Erratum

"Meta-analysis of the Results of Percutaneous Transluminal Angioplasty and Stent Placement for Aortoiliac Occlusive Disease." Radiology 1997; 204:87–96.

The first sentence of Results in the abstract read as follows: "Stent placement and PTA yielded statistically significantly different immediate technical success rates of 96% and 91%, respectively (*z* test, $P < .05$)." It should have read as follows: **"The immediate technical success rate in the PTA group was 91%; the rate was higher in the stent group (96%), but the difference was not statistically significant ."**

Ramón Barreda, MD
1930–1997

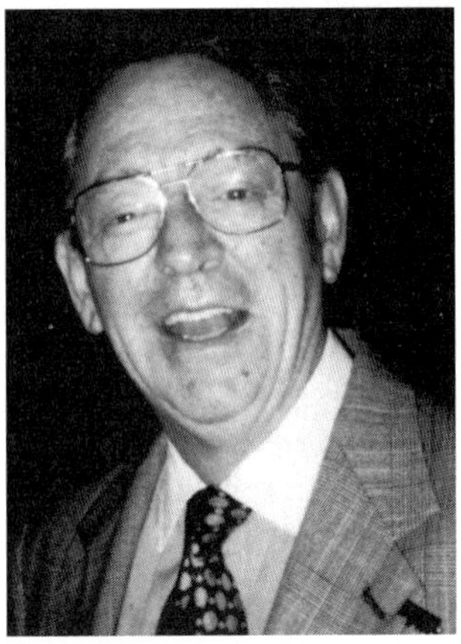

Dr Ramón Barreda, one of the most preeminent contributors to organized radiology in Mexico, died on March 20, 1997. He was born in Mexico City on August 30, 1930, and graduated from medical school at the National Autonomous University of Mexico in 1953. He pursued his residency at the Central Military Hospital and University Medical Center, Mexico City, completing his radiology training in 1961. In the same year, he opened his first office in Mexico City, beginning a longstanding tradition of excellence in the private practice of radiology that he maintained until his death. From 1967 until 1972, he was also a faculty member in the department of radiology at the General Hospital of Mexico, Mexico City. Dr Barreda was also a consultant radiologist to key institutions, such as the Mexican Federal Commission of Electricity, the United Nations office in Mexico, and the U.S. Embassy in Mexico City.

Since 1968, Dr Barreda served as treasurer, secretary, vice president, and, finally in 1974, as president of the Mexican Society of Radiology. During his presidency, he initiated the construction of the current building that houses the society and had the vision of uniting all the state and local Mexican societies under a common organization, becoming the founding president of the Mexican Federation of Radiology and Imaging (MFRI), a position he held until 1978. During his tenure as president, the *Mexican Journal of Radiology* became the official organ of the MFRI, and the Mexican Board (Consejo) of Radiology was founded. With the enthusiasm and intuition that characterized Dr Barreda, he became one of the key organizers of the Mexican Society of Radiology Annual International Course between 1976 and 1990. This is of interest for many radiology educators in the United States and Canada, since this meeting now attracts over 1,500 Mexican and Latin American radiologists and has been officially co-sponsored by the Radiological Society of North America since 1994. In 1994, he received the Gold Medal of the MFRI, the highest honor in Mexican radiology.

With Ramón Barreda's death, Mexican and North American radiology loses one of its key organizers—a man with faith in the future of Mexican radiology, convinced that a strong and united specialty in his country and throughout North America was the only way to succeed. The current vitality and strength of the institutions he was instrumental in creating are the best testimonial to his lifelong dedication to his profession.

He is survived by his wife, Esther; four children, Maria Esther, Ramón, Raúl, and Laura; and nine grandchildren.

—Pablo R. Ros, MD

Harold L. Shinall, MD
1909–1997

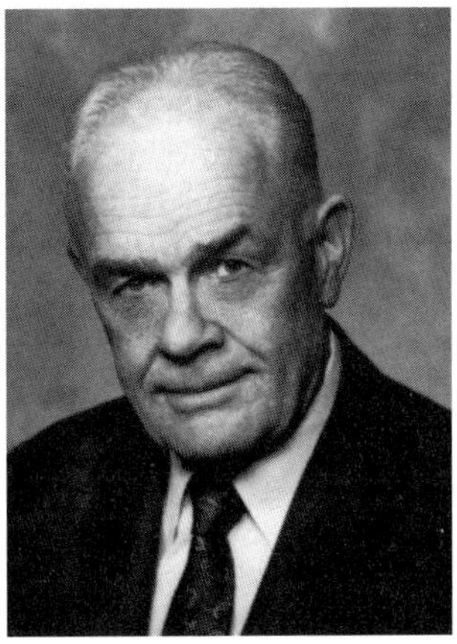

Dr Harold L. Shinall died on February 22, 1997, of complications related to leukemia. He was born on December 19, 1909, in St Louis, Mo. He obtained his bachelor's degree from the University of Illinois, Urbana, and his MD deegree from the University of Illinois College of Medicine, Chicago, where he also completed his internship in 1935. He completed his residency in radiology at St Louis City Hospital in 1946.

Harold did general practice in medicine from 1935 until he entered the U.S. Army during World War II to serve as a medical officer in the North African campaign. During his time in the army, Harold achieved the rank of major.

He had a distinguished practice in radiology in Bloomington, Ill, from 1946 until 1980. He founded the Bloomington-Normal School of Radiography in 1966. He was also a founding member of Bloomington Radiology, which continues today providing quality radiology service to the Bloomington-Normal community.

He was past president of the Illinois Radiological Society as well as the Ford County Medical Society, the McLean County Medical Society, St Joseph's Hospital Medical Staff, and the Mennonite Hospital Medical Staff. His professional associations in addition to local societies included the American College of Radiology, the Radiological Society of North America, and the American Roentgen Ray Society.

Harold was a true gentleman as well as a fine scholar and radiologist. His leadership in the Central Illinois medical community will be sorely missed.

—William E. Cooley, Jr, MD

Cesar H. Carrasco, MD

1948–1997

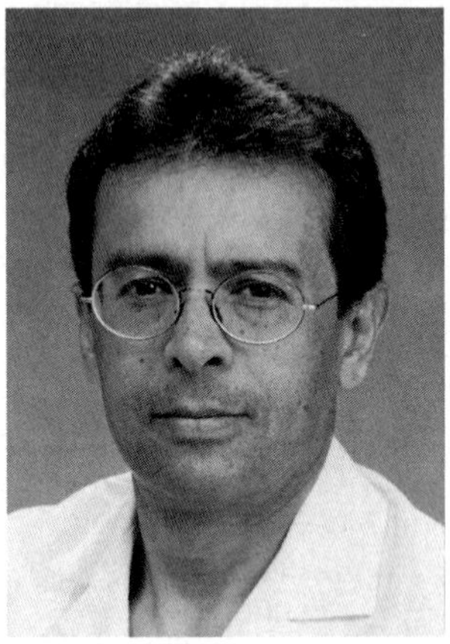

Dr Cesar Humberto "Tito" Carrasco died on May 24, 1997, in a rock slide while climbing El Potero Chico range near Monterrey, Mexico. Tito Carrasco died doing what he loved most. He was a man of excitement, enthusiasm, and excellence who had a passion for medicine. He came by that naturally from his father, Cesar Carrasco, Sr, who was a general radiologist in La Paz, Bolivia. Tito Carrasco came to the University of Texas M. D. Anderson Cancer Center, Houston, in 1981 for a fellowship in angiography and interventional radiology after completing his radiology residency at the Pennsylvania Hospital, Philadelphia. He demonstrated his academic, clinical, and technical expertise and, in 1982, was asked to join the staff at M. D. Anderson Cancer Center, where he remained his entire career. His adversary was cancer and, oh, what a battle he fought. In 1989, he earned the position of head of the section of interventional radiology and, in the following year, the rank of professor. Tito transmitted his tenacity for solving patient problems to his many residents and fellows. He documented his experiences in interventional radiology through his nearly 200 peer-reviewed original publications, invited articles, and book chapters.

Above all, the welfare of the cancer patient was his driving force. Tito was committed to excellence in medicine. He quietly commanded the same of all his associates. Tito was truly superb at his craft; few were as technically adept. He always reveled in the difficult challenge. He was the consultant's consultant—always ready, always willing, and so very able.

Tito Carrasco was no ordinary athlete. He biked the west coast of the United States and jogged daily in preparation for the heights of the Andes and the Canadian Rockies. He was the first to ascend the difficult snow- and ice-covered west face of Bolivia's Huayna Potosi peak. For all these endeavors, he was affectionately known as the "Bolivian Bullet." The ability to overcome the challenges of nature was his "high"—he was truly liberated by the rarefied air.

His relaxation was classical music and opera, which permeated his activities, creating the soothing background in which he operated at work and at play. He appreciated the great composers, particularly Richard Wagner and his opera "The Ring." Tito taught us to appreciate the finer things in life.

He encouraged all of us, by example, to achieve more than we thought we were capable of doing, but demanded even more of himself. Whether the endeavor was medicine, mountain climbing, or music, Tito Carrasco was an established expert. He was uncompromising in his quest for excellence from all those who were privileged to share his enthusiasm. He was committed to honesty in medicine, honesty to the patient, and especially honesty to oneself. He was extremely critical of himself and what he could accomplish through his intervention.

Dr Carrasco is survived by his mother, Mary Carrasco; his brother, Cesar Augusto Carrasco, of La Paz, Bolivia; and his sister and brother-in-law, Magda and Lee Arbuckle, and their sons, Anthony and Andrew, of Honduras.

The following most appropriately describes the life and death of Cesar Humberto Carrasco.

Out of the night that covers me
Black as the pit from pole to pole
I thank whatever Gods may be
For my unconquerable soul

In the fell clutch of circumstance
I have not winced nor cried aloud
Under the bludgeonings of chance
My head is bloody but unbowed

Beyond this place of wrath and tears
Looms but the horror of the shade
And yet the menace of the years
Finds and shall find me unafraid

It matters not how straight the gate
How charged with punishment the scroll
I am the master of my fate
I am the captain of my soul

(William Ernest Henley, "Invictus")

—Sidney Wallace, MD, Thomas S. Harle, MD, and William A. Murphy, Jr, MD

Abstracts of Current Literature

Abdomen and Gastrointestinal System

Desmoid Fibromatosis Is a Clonal Process. Maomi Li, Carlos Cordon-Cardo, William L. Gerald, et al. *Hum Pathol* 1997; 27:939–943. (Juan Rosai, Department of Pathology, Memorial Sloan-Kettering Cancer Center, 1275 York Ave, New York, NY 10021)

Desmoid fibromatosis is a locally aggressive proliferative soft tissue lesion of controversial nature. The authors investigated the clonality of this process by molecular genetic analysis of DNA methylation pattern at a polymorphic site at the human androgen–receptor gene (HUMARA) to examine the inactivation pattern of the X chromosome. Twenty desmoid fibromatoses, including primary and recurrent lesions from 11 female patients, were studied. Sixteen lesions from eight patients showed nonrandom X inactivation, consistent with a clonal origin and, therefore, a true neoplastic nature. Furthermore, multiple recurrent lesions from two patients exhibited the same inactivation pattern as the corresponding primary lesions, suggesting that they were derived from the same cell clone as the primary lesion. One patient was homozygous at the HUMARA locus, and two patients had the same skewed pattern in their normal and lesional tissues. The authors also found that digestion with *Hpa*II, but not *Hha*I, failed to generate a nonrandom X inactivation pattern in some of the cases, suggesting that the methylation status at the *Hpa*II sites was altered in some lesions, and that *Hha*I should be used to verify results and to avoid incorrect conclusions.
AUTHORS' ABSTRACT

Pancreatic Mucinous Ductal Ectasia and Intraductal Papillary Neoplasms: A Single Malignant Clinicopathologic Entity. Jaime A. Rivera, Carlos Fernández–del Castillo, Michael Pins, et al. *Ann Surg* 1997; 225:637–646. (Andrew L. Warshaw, Department of Surgery, WAC 336, Massachusetts General Hospital, Boston, MA 02114)

Objective: The purpose of the study is to review a single institutional experience with mucinous ductal ectasia (MDE) and intraductal papillary neoplasms (IPNs) and to compare the clinicopathologic features of the two groups of tumors. *Summary Background Data:* Mucinous ductal ectasia and IPNs represent newly recognized categories of pancreatic exocrine tumors, previously confused with pancreatic cystic neoplasms. The natural history of MDE and IPN is not well understood, and it is unclear whether MDE and IPN represent two distinct tumors or the same clinicopathologic entity. *Methods:* The authors reviewed the clinical presentation, treatment, histopathology, and outcomes of 23 patients diagnosed with MDE or IPN at their institution over the past 6 years. *Results:* The mean age at presentation for the cohort of patients with MDE and IPN was 62.5 years. The prevalence of abdominal pain was 75%, jaundice 25%, weight loss 42%, steatorrhea 37.5%, diabetes 37.5%, and history of pancreatitis 29%. Serum CA 19-9 levels ranged from 0 to 5,350 U/mL with high levels reflecting advanced disease. There were no significant differences between MDE and IPN with respect to these parameters. Both MDE and IPN comprised papillary villous epithelial neoplasms involving the main and large pancreatic ducts. The tumors ranged from a few millimeters in size to panductal and were distinguished easily from cystic neoplasms in all cases. Invasive carcinoma was present in 11 (46%) of 24 patients, carcinoma in situ in an additional 10 (42%) of 24 patients, and low grade dysplasia in the remaining three (12%) of 24 patients. Mucinous ductal ectasia and IPN differed histopathologically only in degree of mucin secretion and tumor location. Mucinous ductal ectasia, but not IPN, was characteristically mucin hypersecreting and more frequently involved the head of the gland than did IPN (11/16 vs 1/8, $P < .04$). All patients were explored surgically, and 20 (83%) of 24 of the tumors were resectable with frozen section control of the duct margins (nine pancreatoduodenectomies, four distal pancreatectomies, seven total pancreatectomies). Despite the 88% prevalence of cancer, the overall survival at a mean follow-up of 21 months was 13 (87%) of 15 for MDE and five (71%) of 7 for IPN. *Conclusion:* Intraductal papillary neoplasms with or without MDE represent a spectrum of main duct papillary tumors ranging from adenoma to carcinoma, with differing amounts of extracellular mucin production. Malignant IPNs with or without MDE typically exhibit extensive intraductal growth but are slow to invade the periductal tissues and slow to metastasize. The majority of patients with these tumors have resectable disease and a favorable prognosis; endoscopic therapy is inappropriate. The encompassing term intraductal papillary-mucinous tumors is appropriate.
AUTHORS' ABSTRACT

Serum Amylase Level on Admission in the Diagnosis of Blunt Injury to the Pancreas: Its Significance and Limitations. Tsunemasa Takishima, Katsuhiko Sugimoto, Mitsuhiro Hirata, et al. *Ann Surg* 1997; 226:70–76. (T.T., Department of Surgery, Kitasato University School of Medicine, 1-15-1 Kitasato, Sagamihara, Kanagawa 228, Japan)

Objective: The objective of this study was to elucidate the significance and limitations of serum amylase levels in the diagnosis of blunt injury to the pancreas. *Summary Background Data:* Several recently published reports of analyses of patients with blunt abdominal trauma have indicated that determination of the serum amylase level at admission seemed to be of little value in the diagnosis of acute injury to the pancreas. Few previous reports have described clearly the significance and the limitations of the serum amylase level in diagnosing injury to the pancreas. *Methods:* Retrospective analysis was performed in 73 patients with blunt injury to the pancreas during the 16-year period from February 1980 to January 1996. The factors analyzed in the current study included age, gender, time elapsed from injury until admission, hypotension at admission, type of injury to the pancreas, intraabdominal- and intracranial-associated injuries, and death. *Results:* The serum amylase level was found to be abnormal in all patients admitted more than 3 hours after trauma. Various comparisons between patients with elevated ($n = 61$, 83.6%) and nonelevated ($n = 12$, 16.4%) serum amylase levels showed the statistical significance solely of the time elapsed from injury to admission (7 hours ± 1.5 vs 1.3 hours ± 0.2, $P < .001$). The major factor that influences the serum amylase level at admission appeared to be the time elapsed between injury and admission. Determination of the serum amylase level is not diagnostic within 3 hours or fewer after trauma, irrespective of the type of injury. *Conclusion:* To avoid failure in the detection of pancreatic injury, the authors advocate determination of serum amylase levels more than 3 hours after trauma.
AUTHORS' ABSTRACT

Tc-99m-HMPAO White Blood Cell Scan for Diagnosis of Acute Appendicitis in Patients with Equivocal Clinical Presentation. Eric B. Rypins, David G. Evans, William Hinrichs, et al. *Ann Surg* 1997; 226:58–65. (Samuel L. Kipper, Department of Nuclear Medicine, Tri-City Medical Center, 4002 Vista Way, Oceanside, CA 92056)

Objective: The authors' goal was to evaluate the accuracy of technetium-99m-HMPAO–labeled leukocyte imaging for screening patients with atypically presenting appendicitis and to determine how availability of this test affected practice patterns of surgeons at the authors' medical center. *Summary Background Data:* Appendicitis can be difficult to diagnose and in equivocal cases usually requires inpatient observation. The delay may increase morbidity and costs. A test that rules out acute appendicitis could be cost effective if it allowed early discharge from the emergency department. Previously, there have been no simple, rapid, accurate, noninvasive methods for improving diagnostic accuracy in patients with equivocal presentations of appendicitis. *Methods:* Patients referred to rule out appendicitis were analyzed. Patients were imaged up to 3 hours after injection of 10 mCi of Tc-99m-HMPAO–labeled autologous leukocytes (Tc-WBCs); when the scans became positive, imaging was terminated, and the requesting physician was notified of the results. Diagnostic accuracy was established by means of surgical and histopathologic findings or by absence of symptoms after 1-month clinical follow-up. The

source of referral, hospital length of stay, disposition of patients, and ancillary tests (ultrasound, computed tomography, and barium enema) were analyzed. *Results:* One hundred twenty-four patients were studied from November 1991 through December 1995. Fifty-eight percent of positive scans showed uptake within 1 hour of injection, and 73% showed uptake by 2 hours. The Tc-WBC scan correctly depicted an inflammatory source of abdominal pain in 65 of 66 cases (sensitivity, 98%) and was correctly negative in 55 of 58 cases (specificity, 95%). The scan was correctly diagnostic for appendicitis in 50 of 51 cases (sensitivity, 98%) and correctly excluded appendicitis in 62 of 73 cases (specificity, 85%). Outpatient referrals increased from 38% to 87%. In those patients with negative scans, inpatient observation, number of adjunctive tests, and length of stay decreased significantly. *Conclusion:* The high sensitivity and negative predictive value of Tc-WBC imaging may permit patients to be screened and discharged from the emergency department. Focally positive scans often indicate disease requiring operation but not in all cases. The Tc-WBC imaging reduced the negative laparotomy rate to 3.9% while reducing admission rates and length of stay at the hospital.
Authors' Abstract

Management Outcomes in Splenic Injury: A Statewide Trauma Center Review. Thomas V. Clancy, David G. Ramshaw, J. Gary Maxwell, et al. *Ann Surg* 1997; 226:17–24. (T.V.C., Department of Surgery, Coastal Area Health Education Center, PO Box 9025, Wilmington, NC 28402-9025)

Objective: Clinical pathways now highlight both observation and operation as acceptable initial therapeutic options for the management of patients with splenic injury. The purpose of this study was to evaluate treatment trends for splenic injury in all North Carolina trauma centers over a 6-year period. *Methods:* Splenic injuries in adults over a 6-year period (January 1988 to December 1993) were identified in the North Carolina Trauma Registry by using ICD-9-CM codes. Patients were classified in four groups according to method of management: (*a*) no spleen operation, (*b*) splenectomy, (*c*) definitive splenorrhaphy, and (*d*) splenorrhaphy failure followed by splenectomy. The authors examined age, mechanism of injury, admitting blood pressure, and severity of injury by trauma score and injury severity score. *Summary Background Data:* Comparisons were made between adult (17–64 years of age) and geriatric (older than 65 years of age) patients and between patients with blunt and penetrating injuries. Resource utilization (length of stay, hospital charges) and outcome (mortality) were compared. *Results:* There were 1,255 patients with splenic injury. Rate of splenic preservation increased over time and was achieved in more than 50% of patients through nonoperative management (40%) and splenorrhaphy (12%). Splenorrhaphy was not used commonly in either blunt or penetrating injury. Overall mortality was 13%. Geriatric patients had a higher mortality and resource utilization regardless of their mechanism of injury or method of management. *Conclusion:* Nonoperative management represents the prevailing method of splenic preservation in both the adult and geriatric populations in North Carolina trauma center hospitals. Satisfactory outcomes and economic advantages accompany nonoperative management in this adult population.
Authors' Abstract

Breast

Morphological and Biological Characteristics of Mammogram-detected Invasive Breast Cancer. M. Moezzi, J. Melamed, E. Vamvakas, et al. *Hum Pathol* 1997; 27:944–948. (Helen Feiner, Department of Pathology, Tisch Hospital, New York University Medical Center, 560 First Ave, New York, NY 10016)

Thirty-nine small invasive carcinomas of the breast (diameter ≤ 5 mm) identified on mammograms were compared with 78 consecutive clinical cancers (diameter ≥ 10 mm) for a variety of morphologic and biologic markers of prognostic importance. There were more tubular carcinomas in the mammographically detected group (12.8% vs 3.8%), but this difference did not reach statistical significance. Incidences of other histologic types were similar. The types of associated in situ component were similar in the two groups. Mammographically detected cancers were of lower overall grade ($P < .001$), lower architectural and nuclear grades ($P = .0164$ and $P < .0001$, respectively), and had fewer mitotic cells ($P < .0001$). No positive lymph nodes were seen ($P < .0001$). Estrogen and progesterone receptor expression were similar in both groups. Mammographically detected cancers expressed the p53 nuclear protein less frequently than clinical cancers ($P = .0398$), had lower levels of microvessel density ($P = .0001$), and were more often diploid ($P = .0131$). The S-phase of diploid tumors in the two groups was similar, but the S-phase of aneuploid tumors was lower in the mammographically detected group ($P = .0057$). Ki67 expression was lower in mammographically detected cancers ($P < .0001$). In conclusion, small breast cancers detected on mammograms, although invasive, represent an evolutionary phase of breast cancer that generally lacks morphologic and biologic markers of aggressive behavior. The presence or absence of these markers, collectively, may explain the influence of tumor size on survival in patients with breast cancer.
Authors' Abstract

Genitourinary System

Conformal External Beam Treatment of Prostate Cancer. Gerald E. Hanks, Alexandra L. Hanlon, Timothy E. Schultheiss, et al. *Urology* 1997; 50:87–92. (G.E.H., Department of Radiation Oncology, Fox Chase Center, 7701 Burholme Ave, Philadelphia, PA 19111)

Objectives: This study reports the 5-year outcomes of treatment in patients with prostate cancer treated largely with conformal three-dimensional radiation therapy. *Methods:* Results are presented for 456 consecutive patients treated prior to December 31, 1993, whose pretreatment prostate-specific antigen (PSA) levels are known. Biochemical failure was defined as two consecutive rises in the PSA level that equals or exceeds 1.5 ng/mL. Kaplan-Meier product limit methods, the log rank test, and Cox regression models were used in evaluating the data. No patient was lost to follow-up. *Results:* The 5-year biochemically free of failure (bNED) rate for all patients was 61% and 57% at 7 years. In the group with pretreatment PSA level less than 10 ng/mL, the 5-year bNED rate for patients with localized disease (T1, 2AB disease; Gleason sum ≤ 6) was 85%, and for those with locally advanced disease (T2C, 3), the rate was 70%. In the group with pretreatment PSA level of 10–19.9 ng/mL, the 5-year bNED rate was 66% for patients with localized disease and 44% for those with locally advanced disease. In the group with pretreatment PSA level of 20 ng/mL or above, the patients with localized or locally advanced disease had 5-year bNED rates of 31% and 21%, respectively. *Conclusion:* The results of largely conformal three-dimensional beam treatment of localized prostate cancer produced 5-year bNED results that are comparable with those in recent reports of nerve-sparing prostatectomy. Preliminary 7-year bNED results in all patients and in patients with localized tumors indicated a modest decrease in the cancer-free rate from that observed at 5 years, suggesting the results are durable.
Authors' Abstract

The Exercise Renogram and Its Interpretation. John H. Clorius, Thomas Hupp, Ivan Zuma, et al. *J Nucl Med* 1997; 38:1146–1151. (J.H.C., Department of Oncological Diagnostics and Therapy, German Cancer Research Center, Im Neuenheimer Feld 280, FRG-69120 Heidelberg, Germany)

Objective: The exercise renogram is a rarely used diagnostic procedure, but it may depict an exercise-induced change in renal function related to the pathophysiology of essential hypertension, which could greatly increase interest in this examination. The aim of this study was to demonstrate the interpretative approach and the terminology used to describe results of exercise renography in a population of hypertensives with renovascular disease. *Methods:* The authors reviewed the examinations of 70 hypertensives who underwent supine renography as well as exercise renography with a 60–80-W work load. Forty-eight patients were examined with technetium-99m–MAG3, and 22 patients were examined with iodine-131 hippurate. The results of renography and angiography were recorded, as well as the antihypertensive drugs and the site of vascular lesions. *Results:* Thirty-three hyperten-

sive patients developed a bilateral-abnormal exercise renogram, which appears to be associated with primary hypertension. Eight individuals responded to exercise with a unilateral-abnormal exercise renogram, in a kidney behind a stenosis. Only 19 patients had a normal exercise renogram, and 10 had only one functioning kidney. Pathologic conditions recognized but unrelated to the intervention included nonfunctioning and small kidneys and pelvic retention. *Conclusion:* Exercise renography's only indication is for recognition of pathology unique to hypertension, since other function disturbances were recognized in resting renograms.
AUTHORS' ABSTRACT

Prevalence and Predictors of a Positive Repeat Transrectal Ultrasound Guided Needle Biopsy of the Prostate. Neil E. Fleshner, Maryellen O'Sullivan, William R. Fair. *J Urol* 1997; 158:505–509. (N.E.F., Urology Service, Memorial Sloan-Kettering Cancer Center, New York, NY)

Purpose: The authors determined the prevalence of and risk factors for carcinoma in patients with one previously negative finding at prostate gland biopsy. *Materials and Methods:* Transrectal prostate needle biopsy with ultrasound (US) guidance was repeated in 130 men. Risk factors analyzed included age, pathologic result of initial biopsy, interbiopsy interval, prostate specific antigen (PSA) level, PSA density, PSA velocity, digital rectal examination, abnormal transrectal US findings, and family history of prostate cancer. *Results:* Biopsy findings in a total of 39 patients (30%) were positive for cancer. Univariate analysis revealed that PSA level of more than 20 ng/mL and abnormal transrectal US results were more frequent in men with positive findings at second biopsy. At multivariate logistic regression analysis, only PSA level of more than 20 ng/mL was a significant risk factor (adjusted odds ratio = 4.48; 95% confidence interval = 1.02, 20.10). The authors determined that the incidence of carcinoma in patients who represent the lowest risk group was defined by PSA level less than 10 ng/mL, PSA density less than 0.15 mg/nL/cm^3, PSA velocity less than 0.75 ng/mL per year, no prostatic intraepithelial neoplasia plus negative transrectal US and digital rectal examination findings and family history. Of 21 patients who fit this cohort, five (23.8%) had carcinoma at repeated biopsy. *Conclusion:* A significant false-negative rate for initial transrectal ultrasound-guided prostate biopsies exists. Baseline risk in lowest-risk patients is sufficiently high that one cannot define a subset of patients for whom repeated biopsy is unnecessary. The authors recommend repeated biopsy in all patients who meet the criteria for a transrectal US-guided biopsy and in whom the initial biopsy result is negative.
AUTHORS' ABSTRACT

Traumatic Posterior Urethral Injury and Early Realignment Using Magnetic Urethral Catheters. James R. Porter, Thomas K. Taka-yama, Alfred J. Defalco. *J Urol* 1997; 158:425–430. (J.R.P., Department of Urology, Harborview Medical Center, Seattle, Wash)

Purpose: The authors determined the success of early urethral realignment by using magnetic urethral catheters. *Materials and Methods:* The authors retrospectively reviewed the records of 13 patients with complete urethral disruption treated 0–11 days after injury with endourologic realignment by using coaxial magnetic urethral catheters. *Results:* Urethral realignment was established in 11 of the 13 patients (85%) by using magnetic urethral catheters. In the 10 patients for whom follow-up findings were available, urethral strictures developed in five (50%) a mean of 6.1 months after realignment, which necessitated a mean of 1.4 corrective procedures per patient. Impotence was noted in one of seven (14%) patients, and no urinary incontinence developed after realignment. *Conclusion:* Urethral realignment accomplished within 2 weeks of injury by using magnetic urethral catheters is a safe and simple technique that results in minimal morbidity. The stricture formation, impotence, and incontinence rates of this technique are comparable to those reported for delayed urethroplasty. The authors advocate early realignment with magnetic urethral sounds as an alternative treatment for traumatic urethral disruption.
AUTHORS' ABSTRACT

The Impact of Sonography on the Diagnosis of Scrotal Disorders. Robert A. Older, Reed A. Omary, Laurence R. Watson. *J Urol* 1997; 158:479–480. (R.A.O., Department of Urology, University of Virginia Health Sciences Center, Charlottesville)

Purpose: The authors assessed the impact of ultrasound (US) findings on the referring urologist's diagnosis of scrotal disorders. *Materials and Methods:* University urologists (six attending physicians and three resident physicians) in a clinic setting completed questionnaires before and after about 35 patients with scrotal symptoms. The physicians were requested to eliminate the probability (0%–100%) of their most likely diagnosis before and after receiving sonographic information. The authors calculated both the mean change in percentage diagnostic confidence and the proportion of patients in whom presonographic diagnosis was changed. *Results:* Scrotal US findings resulted in a change in the initial diagnosis in 11 of 35 (32%) patients (95% confidence interval = 19%, 49%). The mean percentage gain in diagnostic certainty based on US findings was 29% (95% confidence interval = 20%, 39%; $P < .001$). *Conclusion:* Scrotal US findings have considerable impact on the referring urologist's diagnosis of scrotal abnormalities.
AUTHORS' ABSTRACT

Cardiovascular System

Thrombolysis of Occluded Infrainguinal Vein Grafts: Predictors of Outcome. Gary B. Nackman, Daniel B. Walsh, Mark F. Fillinger, et al. *J Vasc Surg* 1997; 25:1023–1032. (D.B.W., Section of Vascular Surgery, Dartmouth Hitchcock Medical Center, 1 Medical Center Dr, Lebanon, NH 03756)

Purpose: The purpose of this study was to identify factors that influence graft patency and limb salvage rates after thrombolysis of occluded infrainguinal vein grafts. *Methods:* The records of patients who underwent percutaneous catheter-directed thrombolysis of occluded infrainguinal vein bypass grafts at the authors' institution between 1985 and 1995 were reviewed. Life table analysis was used to determine survival and patency differences. Univariate and multivariate analyses were used to identify the patient-specific factors that affected outcomes. *Results:* Forty-four patients with a thrombosed infrainguinal vein graft underwent thrombolysis with urokinase. The thrombolysis-related mortality rate was 2%, and nonfatal complications occurred in 16% of patients. Thrombolysis was unable to restore graft patency in 11 of 44 (25%) of grafts. Of the remaining 33 successfully lysed grafts, 88% required adjunctive surgery or percutaneous transluminal angioplasty after thrombolysis. Overall, the primary graft patency rate was 25% at 1 year and 19% at 2 years after thrombolysis. By considering only successfully lysed grafts, the primary patency rate improved to 34% at 1 year and 25% at 2 years. Multivariate analysis showed that the graft-patency rate was substantially better in patients without diabetes and in vein grafts that had been in place for longer than 12 months ($P < .01$). The limb salvage rate was statistically significantly improved after successful thrombolysis (63% at 2 years vs 31% if lysis failed; $P < .01$). The patient survival rate was high—89% at 2 years after thrombolysis. *Conclusion:* Even with adjunctive therapy, vein graft thrombolysis is unlikely to yield durable patency overall. However, successful thrombolysis improves limb salvage rates and may be beneficial in patients without diabetes who have mature vein grafts but who do not have options for other autologous revascularization procedures.
AUTHORS' ABSTRACT

Pediatrics

Inhaled Nitric Oxide and Hypoxic Respiratory Failure in Infants with Congenital Diaphragmatic Hernia. The Neonatal Inhaled Nitric Oxide Study Group. *Pediatrics* 1997; 99:838–845. (Neil M. Finer, University of California, San Diego Medical Center, 200 W Arbor Dr, Box 8774, San Diego, CA 92103-8774)

Congenital diaphragmatic hernia (CDH) is a malformation occurring in approximately one in every 3,000–4,000 deliveries. The overall mortality for fetuses with isolated, potentially correctable CDH diagnosed before 24 weeks gestation is approximately 58%. Despite aggressive support required to maintain adequate gas exchange, there is a high rate of failure of conventional management. The underlying patho-

physiology in such infants appears to be a combination of lung hypoplasia and immaturity and persistent pulmonary hypertension, which may be further aggravated by left ventricular underdevelopment. A prospective, multicenter randomized controlled trial was conducted to evaluate the ability of inhaled nitric oxide to prevent death or the initiation of extracorporeal membrane oxygenation (ECMO) treatment in term and near-term infants with hypoxic respiratory failure unresponsive to aggressive conventional therapy. Infants with CDH and hypoxic respiratory failure were enrolled in a separate parallel study; the results of that trial are reported. Although the immediate short-term improvements in oxygenation in some treated infants may be of benefit in stabilizing responding infants for transport or initiation of ECMO, the study concludes that for term and near-term infants with CDH and hypoxemic respiratory failure unresponsive to conventional therapy, inhaled nitrate oxide therapy did not reduce the need for ECMO or the incidence of death.
Beverly P. Wood, MD
Childrens Hospital, Los Angeles, Calif

Randomized Trial of Varying Mineral Intake on Total Body Bone Mineral Accretion during the First Year of Life. Bonny L. Specker, Anne Beck, Heidi Kalkwarf, et al. *Pediatrics* 1997; 99:e12, *http://www.pediatrics.org*. (B.L.S., Department of Pediatrics, College of Medicine, University of Cincinnati, PO Box 670541, Cincinnati, OH 45267-0541)

The effect of varying mineral intakes on total body bone mass accretion during the 1st year of life in full-term newborn infants is unknown. This study was designed to determine whether total body bone mass accretion during the 1st year of life was influenced by the calcium and phosphorus intake of an infant and whether early differences in bone accretion persist through 1 year of age. A prospective randomized trial was conducted in two phases, with 67 infants randomized within the first 2 weeks of life into either a low- or moderate-mineral formula feeding group. An additional group of 34 infants fed human milk (low mineral) was also enrolled. Phase 2 involved an additional randomization of all infants at 6 months of age into a moderate-mineral formula, high-mineral formula, or cow milk feeding group. Anthropometric measurements and measurement of total body bone mineral content with dual x-ray absorptiometry were performed at 1, 3, 6, 9, and 12 months. The authors found that by 1 month of age there already were differences among the feeding groups. Findings indicate a dramatic effect of early feeding on bone metabolism or baseline differences between infants fed human milk and those fed formula. There was a significant effect of infant mineral intake on bone mass accretion on the first 6 months of life, but this effect was not evident during the second 6 months. Despite a significant difference in mineral content of formulas consumed during the second 6 months, bone mass accretion did not differ. It is possible that the mineral content of both moderate and high mineral formulas are high enough to have reached a "threshold" effect of these minerals on bone mass accretion already. The formulas used represent commercially available formulas that are marketed for 6–12-month-old infants.
Beverly P. Wood, MD
Childrens Hospital, Los Angeles, Calif

Resource Utilization among Neonatologists in a University Childrens Hospital. James M. Adams, Juan Moreno, Kim Reynolds, et al. *Pediatrics* 1997; 99:e2, *http://www.pediatrics.org*. (J.M.A., Department of Pediatrics, Baylor College of Medicine, 6621 Fannin, A340, Houston, TX 77030)

The purpose of this study was to evaluate factors affecting length of hospital stay and resulting in hospital charges among patients managed by two separate groups of neonatologists in the same academic health science center. Academic health science center hospitals, including children's hospitals and their associated medical school faculty, often are depicted as being unable to deliver cost-effective health care. These institutions are deemed costly because of high rates of uncompensated care and cost shifting, personnel background, and technology-oriented delivery systems, and their central role in development of innovative and expensive new medical techniques. Patient care by medical school physicians is viewed as costly and possibly inefficient compared with the private sector, because of participation of physicians in training, detailed testing, and unwillingness to consider approaches that may compromise perceived standards of care. Indicators most commonly used to analyze resource utilization are hospital charges and length of hospital stay. This study was designed to determine whether neonatal care by academic physicians was more costly than that delivered by other neonatologists and to gain further insight into this complex issue. Two groups of neonatologists were studied: an academic group consisting of 23 full-time faculty neonatologists and a private provider group consisting of three neonatologists associated with a large managed-care organization. Comparison of multiple demographic parameters between the two physician provider groups was performed by using the χ^2 method with continuity correction for categorical variables and a two-tailed t test for continuous variables. Three levels of analysis were performed. First, the authors compared multiple clinical variables among patients receiving care from the two physician groups. Analysis was used to assess factors determining length of stay. Analysis of covariants was used to compare physician groups, with variables including birth weight, gestation, sex, race, admission age, death, age at death, antenatal steroids, congenital anomalies, congenital heart disease, congenital diaphragmatic hernia, hyaline membrane disease, and related variables affecting level of care and length of stay. Patients in group A, treated by the academic neonatologists, were older at admission than those of the other group and exhibited characteristics of a sicker population. Differences in risk and acuity of illness between the two patient groups tended to bias the comparison of length of stay. Correcting for these variables demonstrated that the length of stay for group A was on average 7.8 days shorter than that for group B. Using the average difference in length of stay, corrected for risk factors, the authors calculated that net reduction of $3,114,969 in hospital charges might have been realized had group A physicians provided care for all study patients.
Beverly P. Wood, MD
Childrens Hospital, Los Angeles, Calif

New Renal Scars in Children with Urinary Tract Infections, Vesicoureteral Reflux and Voiding Dysfunction: A Prospective Evaluation. Shahida R. Naseer, George F. Steinhardt. *J Urol* 1997; 158:566–568. (S.R.N., Departments of Pediatrics and Surgery, Division of Urology, St Louis University Medical Center and Cardinal Glennon Children's Hospital, Mo)

Purpose: Established renal scarring represents areas of the kidney that imaging reveals to be damaged at presentation for medical management of urinary tract infection. New renal scarring represents new renal damage in parts of the kidney that imaging reveals to be normal at presentation. The authors attempted to characterize patients in whom new renal scars developed while they were under the authors' care. *Materials and Methods:* In 1988, a database was started to identify patients with new renal scarring. All patients presenting with urinary tract infections were enrolled. This database has 250 fields per event with multiple events per patient. More than 2,100 patients have been enrolled to date. All patients with pyelonephritis, defined as a febrile urinary tract infection with flank pain and tenderness, and all with reflux underwent dimercaptosuccinic acid (DMSA) scanning at least 4 months after presentation for assessment of established renal scars. New renal scars were identified when new renal defects were demonstrated on a second DMSA scan. *Results:* In the database, there are 1,426 patients with urinary tract infections, 685 (46%) with pyelonephritis, and 1,062 (74.5%) with vesicoureteral reflux, including 558 found to have bilateral vesicoureteral reflux and 504 with unilateral reflux. A history of daytime urinary incontinence was noted in 538 patients (37.7%), 192 (13.5%) had established scars at initial presentation, and in 31 (2.1%) patients, new renal scars developed while they were under the authors' care, including 30 with established scars, as well. Of the 25 patients in whom new renal scars developed during medical therapy, 11 underwent surgery. In six patients with dysfunctional voiding who were receiving medical treatment, renal scars developed postoperatively. Surgery was performed in 17 of the 31 patients, and 24 (77%) patients with new renal scars had a history of dysfunctional voiding. *Conclusion:* Previous characterizations of patients with new renal scars have relied on excretory urography for assessment of renal architecture and have ignored voiding patterns of the children affected. By

using DMSA scanning, 31 children were identified with reflux, urinary tract infection, and dysfunctional voiding in whom renal scars developed while they were under the authors' care.
AUTHORS' ABSTRACT

Correlation of Cystographic Bladder Morphology and Neuroanatomy in Boys with Posterior Urethral Valves. David A. Bloom, Robert L. Lebowitz, Stuart B. Bauer. *Pediatr Radiol* 1997; 27:553–556. (D.A.B., Department of Radiology, Children's Hospital, 700 Children's Dr, Columbus, OH 43205-2696)

Purpose: The authors have observed a difference in the radiographic appearance of the body of the bladder (trabeculated) and its base (smooth) in boys with severely obstructing posterior urethral valves. The authors wanted to determine if (*a*) this was a reproducible finding and (*b*) there was an anatomic and/or physiologic explanation for it. *Materials and Methods:* The authors reviewed the initial voiding cystourethrogram in 47 boys with severe posterior urethral valves. The interureteric ridge was used as the division between the body and the base of the bladder. The presence of trabeculation for each region was recorded. *Results:* Ages ranged from 1 day to 6 years at the time of initial cystographic evaluation (median, 14 days). The body of the bladder was trabeculated and the base was smooth in 34 (72%) patients. In the remaining patients, both the body and the base were smooth. In no patient was the base trabeculated. *Conclusion:* The cystographic morphology of the urinary bladder in boys with posterior urethral valves can be explained by its neuroanatomy. The body of the bladder, which contracts during voiding because of parasympathetic (cholinergic) stimulation, becomes trabeculated. The bladder base relaxes during voiding owing to sympathetic (α-adrenergic) stimulation and remains smooth. Thus, the difference in the cystographic appearance of the two parts of the urinary bladder reflects the normal innervation and the mechanics of micturition in boys with urethral obstruction.
AUTHORS' ABSTRACT

Primary Vesicoureteric Reflux: How Useful Is Postnatal Ultrasound? J. M. Tibballs, R. De Bruyn. *Arch Dis Child* 1996; 75:444–447. (J.M.T., Department of Radiology, Royal Free Hampstead NHS Trust, Pond St, Hampstead, London NW3 2QG, England)

Postnatal ultrasound (US) and micturating cystourethrographic (MCU) findings were assessed retrospectively in 177 patients (132 [75%] boys) with a diagnosis of antenatal hydronephrosis due to primary vesicoureteric reflux (VUR). Reflux was unilateral in 103 cases and bilateral in 74 (42%). Thirty-seven percent of boys and 33% of girls with a renal pelvic diameter of 10 mm or smaller had a grade III–V VUR. Caliceal and/or ureteric dilatation had a specificity of 87%–96% for grade III–V VUR but a sensitivity of only 37%–54%. Fifty-eight percent of male and 75% of female renal units with grade III VUR and 17% of male units with grade IV–V VUR were normal at US. Approximately 25% of sonographically normal renal units had grade III–V VUR at MCU. Postnatal US criteria correlate poorly with the presence and degree of VUR in children with prenatally diagnosed hydronephrosis and should not be used to direct the use of cystography.
PAULA W. BRILL, MD
New York Hospital–Cornell Medical Center, New York, NY

The Ultrasonographic Differentiation of Obstructive versus Nonobstructive Hydronephrosis in Children: A Multivariate Scoring System. Barbara M. Garcia-Peña, Marc S. Keller, Dana S. Schwartz, et al. *J Urol* 1997; 158:560–565. (B.M.G.P., Department of Diagnostic Radiology, Yale University School of Medicine, New Haven, Conn)

Purpose: The authors identified sonographic prognosticators to aid in distinguishing obstructive from nonobstructive hydronephrosis in children. *Materials and Methods:* Twelve sonographic variables were initially analyzed to determine significant associations between the variables and the presence of urinary tract obstruction as defined by diuretic radionuclide renography. The significant findings were subsequently analyzed with logistic regression models to identify potential predictors of obstructive hydronephrosis. *Results:* The seven variables associated with a significantly higher risk of urinary tract obstruction were increased echogenicity, parenchymal rims of 5 mm or smaller, contralateral hypertrophy, resistive index ratio of 1.10 or greater, and aperistaltic ureter. These variables were used for the development of a multivariate scoring system. *Conclusion:* The obstructive scoring system shows promise as a screening method for the sonographic differentiation of obstructive from nonobstructive hydronephrosis in children.
AUTHORS' ABSTRACT

Extremely Low-Birth-Weight Children and Their Peers: A Comparison of School-Age Outcomes. Carey L. Halsey, Marc F. Collin, Craig L. Anderson. *Arch Pediatr Adolesc Med* 1996; 150:790–794. (C.L.H., Department of Pediatrics, Loyola University Medical Center, 2160 S First Ave, Maywood, IL 60153)

The objective of the study was to document the 7-year developmental and educational outcomes in a cohort of predominantly white, middle class, extremely low-birth-weight (ELBW) (weight < 1,000 g) children. Fifty-four ELBW children and 58 comparison children were matched according to race, sex, and socioeconomic status. In the comparison group, there were 30 children with low birth weight (1,500–2,500 g) and 28 with a birth weight greater than 25,000 g. The ELBW cohort was drawn from 104 presurfactant survivors born between 1984 and 1986 and cared for at a single hospital. Twenty-seven (50%) of the ELBW children were in regular classrooms with no special services, compared with 70% of those in the group with a birth weight of 1,500–2,500 g and 93% of those in the full-term group. This result indicates a statistically significant trend toward increasing need for special services with decreasing birth weight across the three groups ($P <$ .001). The ELBW group scored significantly lower than the comparison group on all tests, although their scores were generally within the average range. Seventy-nine percent of ELBW children had a cognitive score within the average range but lower than the scores in children from the two comparison groups. Twenty percent of ELBW children had severe disabilities, including cerebral palsy, mental retardation, autism, and low intelligence with severe learning problems.
PAULA W. BRILL, MD
New York Hospital–Cornell Medical Center, New York, NY

Unilateral Multicystic Dysplastic Kidney: The Case for Nephrectomy. N. J. A. Webb, M. A. Lewis, J. Bruce, et al. *Arch Dis Child* 1997; 76:31–34. (M.A.L., Department of Nephrology, Manchester Children's Hospital, Pendlebury, Manchester M27 4HA, England)

Unilateral multicystic dysplastic kidney (MCDK) occurs with an incidence of one in 4,300 live births. Most cases are diagnosed at prenatal ultrasound (US). Many authors have recommended conservative nonsurgical treatment because of the low incidence of short-term complications. Surgery has been proposed by some authors because of the potential complications of hypertension, infection, and malignant change. This report describes three children at one institution who developed hypertension secondary to MCDK during a 4-year period. One of the children had been discharged at follow-up after "disappearance" at US of the cystic kidney. The authors believe that the risks of hypertension secondary to MCDK have been understated and that many children may be receiving suboptimal follow-up. They favor elective nephrectomy as the treatment of choice for this lesion.
PAULA W. BRILL, MD
New York Hospital–Cornell Medical Center, New York, NY

Ten-Year Clinical, Developmental, and Intellectual Follow-up of Children with Congenital Cytomegalovirus Infection without Neurologic Symptoms at One Year of Age. Sten-A. Ivarsson, Barbro Lernmark, Lars Svanberg. *Pediatrics* 1997; 99:800–803. (S.A. I., Department of Pediatrics, University Hospital, 205 02 Malmö, Sweden)

Congenital cytomegalovirus (CMV) infection is present in some 0.4%–2.3% of all live-born infants and is the most common viral infection known to be transmitted in utero. In up to 10% of congenitally infected infants, the clinically symptomatic form, cytomegalic inclusion disease, is manifest in the neonatal period. Both neonatally overt and asymptomatic infections can result in permanent neurologic sequelae. Of infants with silent infection at birth, 5%–17% suffer neurologic sequelae. This study was undertaken to ascertain whether children with congenital CMV infection at birth, but without neurologic symptoms at 1 year of age, differed in somatic, neurologic, developmental, or intellectual status from matched control children at long-term follow-up. Congenital CMV infection was diagnosed in 0.5% of infants in this study and, from this basic CMV-infected population, the authors excluded children who developed neurologic disturbances, including sensory neural deafness, before 1 year of age. Congenitally infected infants and matched control infants were followed up clinically and neurologically. Children with congenital CMV infection are unlikely to be at increased risk of subsequent neurodevelopmental or intellectual impairment if they show normal development at 12 months of age.

Beverly P. Wood, MD
Childrens Hospital, Los Angeles, Calif

Clinical Associations and Time of Onset of Cerebral White Matter Damage in Very Preterm Babies. Deirdre J. Murphy, Marian V. Squier, Peter L. Hope, et al. *Arch Dis Child* 1996; 75:F27–F32. (D.J.M., 22 Manor Pk, Redland, Bristol BS6 7HH, England)

Neuropathologic examinations were performed at necropsy in 83 very premature infants who died during their first hospital admission; 39 had ischemic white matter damage. The time of onset was thought to be prenatal in 31% and postnatal in another 31%. Exact timing could not be determined in 38%. In those infants who were studied with ultrasound, there was close correlation with pathologic findings. Review of clinical data showed no clear associations between adverse clinical factors and prenatal ischemic white matter damage. In contrast, preeclampsia, intrauterine growth retardation, and delivery without labor were associated with postnatal damage, as were neonatal sepsis, necrotizing enterocolitis, and seizures. The absence of a clear association between the timing of adverse clinical factors and the timing of ischemic damage suggest that cerebral damage in very premature infants may result from a sequence of events rather than from one specific insult.

Paula W. Brill, MD
New York Hospital–Cornell Medical Center, New York, NY

Postural Drainage and Gastro-oesophageal Reflux in Infants with Cystic Fibrosis. Brenda M. Button, Ralf G. Heine, Anthony G. Catto-Smith, et al. *Arch Dis Child* 1997; 76:148–150. (A.G.C.S., Department of Gastroenterology, Royal Children's Hospital, Flemington Rd, Parkville, Victoria 3052, Australia)

There is an increased incidence of gastroesophageal reflux in cases of cystic fibrosis. Twenty infants with cystic fibrosis underwent 30 hours of esophageal monitoring while they underwent standard physical therapy (SPT) with head-down tilt and modified physical therapy (MPT) without head-down tilt. The two techniques were compared with regard to their effect on the number and duration of reflux episodes. The number of reflux episodes per hour, but not their duration, was significantly increased during standard physical therapy (2.5/h) compared with modified physical therapy (1.6/h) and background (1.1/h). Fractional reflux time was also increased during standard therapy (11.7%) compared with background (6.9%) but not compared with modified therapy (10.7%). There was no significant difference between modified physical therapy and background for number of reflux episodes, their duration, or fractional reflux time. It was concluded that standard, but not modified, physical therapy was associated with a significant increase in gastroesophageal reflux in infants with cystic fibrosis.

Paula W. Brill, MD
New York Hospital–Cornell Medical Center, New York, NY

Gastric Emptying and Gastro-oesophageal Reflux in Preterm Infants. A. K. Ewer, G. M. Durbin, M. E. I. Morgan, et al. *Arch Dis Child* 1996; 75:F117–F121. (A.K.E., Neonatal Unit, Birmingham Women's Hospital, Edgbaston, Birmingham B15 2TG, England)

The purpose of the study was to determine whether delayed gastric emptying plays a causal role in gastroesophageal reflux in premature infants. Gastric emptying was measured on ultrasound (US) images in 19 healthy, premature infants (median gestational age, 32 weeks); 24-hour lower esophageal pH was measured concurrently. US measurements of antral cross-sectional area (ACSA) were made immediately before nasogastric feeding and then during subsequent gastric emptying until ACSA returned to the prefeeding value. Half-emptying time was calculated as the time for the ACSA to decrease to half the maximum postprandial increment. The mean reflux index (percentage of study time during which lower esophageal pH was less than 4.0) for the group was 11.9%. The mean number of reflux episodes per 24 hours was 15.4. The mean number of reflux episodes that lasted longer than 5 minutes was 5.5. Average half-emptying time for an individual infant was 46 minutes (range, 18–105 minutes). There were no associations between gastric emptying rates and any of the indexes of gastroesophageal reflux, during either the 24-hour period for which the lower esophageal pH was recorded or the periods after the feedings that were studied with US. Reflux was also unrelated to type and volume of feeding. The authors concluded that asymptomatic gastroesophageal reflux is common in premature infants, but gastric emptying time is not a determinant. Inappropriate relaxation of the lower esophageal sphincter or abnormal esophageal motility offer more plausible explanations.

Paula W. Brill, MD
New York Hospital–Cornell Medical Center, New York, NY

Delayed Gastric Emptying: A Novel Gastrointestinal Finding in Turner's Syndrome. Annamaria Staiano, Mariacarolina Salerno, Salvatore Di Maio, et al. *Arch Dis Child* 1996; 75:440–143. (A.S., Department of Pediatrics, Università Federico II, Via S Pansini 5, 80131 Naples, Italy)

Infants and young children with Turner syndrome have previously been reported to have a high incidence of feeding difficulties, including regurgitation and vomiting. The present study was undertaken to evaluate gastric emptying in girls with Turner syndrome to detect if gastrointestinal motor dysfunction was present. Thirteen girls (mean age, 8.1 years) with Turner syndrome, seven girls with familial short stature (mean age, 6.1 years), and eight control girls (mean age, 7.6 years) underwent gastric-emptying studies after administration of 500 μCi of technetium-99m–sulfur colloid bound to a scrambled egg. Scintigraphic measurements were performed for 60–90 minutes. Mean percentage gastric retention of isotope was significantly greater in girls with Turner syndrome than in children with short stature and in control children. In contrast with control subjects, in whom there was an inverse linear relationship between gastric-emptying rate and body-mass index, the delay in gastric emptying in children with Turner syndrome was independent of body mass. The results suggest that delayed gastric emptying is detectable in girls with Turner syndrome, independent of age, body-mass index, karyotype, and growth-promoting treatment.

Paula W. Brill, MD
New York Hospital–Cornell Medical Center, New York, NY

Japanese Experience with Micropremies Weighing Less Than 600 Grams Born between 1984 to 1993. Masaya Oishi, Hiroahi Nishida, Toshie Sasaki. *Pediatrics* 1997; 99:e7, *http://www.pediatrics.org*. (M.O., Maternal and Perinatal Center, Tokyo Women's Medical College, Kawada-cho 8-1, Shinjyuku-ku, Tokyo 162, Japan)

A survey involving infants with birth weights less than 600 g born from 1984 to 1993 was conducted by sending questionnaires to hospitals having tertiary and secondary neonatal intensive care units. Questionnaires were mailed to 205 hospitals with neonatal intensive care units, with an 80% response. Of 1,655 infants of less than 600 g birth weight admitted to neonatal intensive care units, 457 (28%) survived to hospital discharge. The majority (68%) died within 1 week after birth, and only 10% died after the neonatal period. The main causes of death were acute respiratory failure, intraventricular hemorrhage, infection, and heart failure. Of the 457 survivors, 65% did not have handicaps. The incidences of mental retardation, visual disturbance, and cerebral palsy were 15%, 14%, and 11%, respectively. The survival rate increased from 22% to 33% after generalized use of surfactant in 1988, but the handicap rate among survivors remained unchanged. A viability limit of 22 complete weeks of gestation was feasible because survival of infants born at less than 22 weeks was exceptional, whereas the survival rate of those born at 22–23 weeks was 18%.

Beverly P. Wood, MD
Childrens Hospital, Los Angeles, Calif

Scott J. Erickson, MD

High-Resolution Imaging of the Musculoskeletal System[1]

The history of musculoskeletal imaging begins with Roentgen's discovery of the x ray in 1895. Plain radiography has since become the initial, and in many cases the only, imaging modality used for diagnosis of osseous abnormalities. Over the years, however, radiologists have assumed a pivotal role in the diagnosis of not only bone conditions but also a diverse variety of soft-tissue entities. Each major technologic advance creates an initial upheaval in the status quo, requiring the imager to further refine his or her understanding of both human anatomic structure and disease and to learn or relearn the appropriate imaging principles involved. Even minor improvements (ie, hardware and/or software upgrades) will serve as a stimulus for the imager to revise existing protocols in an effort to achieve yet better performance. One must be on guard against imaging complacency. In the author's opinion, the "perfect" imaging protocol does not exist because imaging parameters will be both patient and disease specific.

Index terms: Bones • Computed tomography (CT), thin-section, **.12118[2] • Magnetic resonance (MR), thin-section, **.12149 • Muscles • Radiography, **.11 • State-of-art reviews • Ultrasound (US), **.12989

Radiology 1997; 205:593–618

[1] From the Department of Radiology, Froedtert Memorial Lutheran Hospital, 9200 W Wisconsin Ave, Milwaukee, WI 53226. Received June 17, 1997; revision requested July 21; revision received and accepted August 25. **Address reprint requests to** the author.

[2] ** indicates generalized anatomic involvement.

When assessing image quality, one must consider both contrast resolution and spatial resolution. Contrast resolution refers to the ability to distinguish different normal tissues and normal from abnormal tissue. Spatial resolution refers to the ability to depict and distinguish small objects that are in close proximity. An improvement in spatial resolution without adequate contrast resolution is meaningless. As a general rule, sufficient tissue contrast is required to fully exploit the spatial resolution capabilities of a given modality. The colloquial term "high resolution" has become trite to the point that one prominent editor suggested that it be omitted from the titles of future publications. Nevertheless, this phrase has become entrenched in the imaging lexicon.

In this article, the following imaging modalities are reviewed: plain radiography, computed tomography (CT), magnetic resonance (MR) imaging, and ultrasound (US). Radioisotope imaging, recognized as an important diagnostic modality in the evaluation of musculoskeletal abnormalities, will not be discussed because of its inherently low spatial resolution. For each modality, the pertinent technical aspects are discussed and the current achievable limits of resolution described (Table). Next, the essential anatomic and histologic features of the musculoskeletal tissues are presented. These descriptions are based on standard anatomic texts (1,2) as well as pertinent illuminating articles culled from the literature. Last, representative images of each of these tissues are presented with a focus on US and MR imaging. Though emphasis will be on the practical and attainable, there are occasional digressions to recount the findings of those performing both exciting in vivo imaging and in vitro specimen work.

Dimensions of Reference Tissues

Reference Tissue	Approximate Size (μm)
Red blood cell	7
Haversian canal	50–100
Calf (leg) epidermis	100
Glomus body	300
Humeral hyaline cartilage	1,000 (1 mm)

MODALITIES

Radiography

In 1975, Takahashi and Sakuma (3) stated that "magnification radiography should open up a new radiodiagnostic field and promote the establishment of much more accurate diagnosis." Years later, Buckland-Wright and Bradshaw (4) also extolled the merits of this technique, which they believed was capable of "permitting the identification of features virtually at the histological level." The latter investigators further stated that "the significant advantage of taking direct accurate measurements of radiographic features provides indisputable evidence of the extent of the disease process" (4). The enthusiasm conveyed by Buckland-Wright and Bradshaw in these statements from their 1989 article might seem surprising in this age of high-technologic cross-sectional imaging. One must, at times, be reminded that radiography remains an essential and, in many cases entirely sufficient, diagnostic technique.

Abbreviations: ETL = echo train length, FOV = field of view, GRE = gradient-recalled echo, RF = radio frequency, SE = spin echo, S/N = signal-to-noise ratio, STIR = short inversion time inversion recovery, TE = echo time, TR = repetition time, 2D = two-dimensional, 3D = three-dimensional.

There are two primary magnification techniques that have been espoused in the literature: optical magnification and radiographic magnification (4–10). Doi et al (8) and Genant et al (9) each compared these two in the mid-1970s by using then state-of-the-art techniques. Optical magnification was performed with fine-grain film *without screens* and a 1.2-mm focal spot; the images were viewed at four to 10 times normal size with a handheld lens, projector, or microscope. The authors noted that this technique occasionally suffers from motion unsharpness (attributable to long exposure times), requires manual or industrial film processing, may impart a higher radiation dose, and requires special viewing procedures. Radiographic magnification was performed with a slow screen-film system, four times geometric enlargement, and a grid-biased 50-μm micro–focal spot. In their studies, these investigators showed optical to be superior to radiographic magnification when imaging thin objects, such as the hand. More recent publications have employed micro–focal spot sources as small as 6–8 μm, which permit magnifications in the range of five to 15 times and reportedly yield greater spatial resolution than optical magnification techniques (6). With fast rare-earth screen-film systems, spatial resolution ranged between 10 line pairs per millimeter ([lp/mm] object diameter of 50 μm) to 20 lp/mm (object diameter of 25 μm) at magnifications of five and 10 times, respectively. Although local skin doses are larger than those with conventional radiography, total body radiation exposure is similar because the beam is much more collimated (4). Use of stereo technique, however, will result in a doubling of the radiation dose.

Clinical mammography is performed with single screen emulsions with small focal spots, permitting 50-μm spatial resolution. In this article, such a unit was used to evaluate normal osseous anatomic structures, perhaps to the level of the haversian canal.

Investigators have used high-resolution radiography to study cases of osteoarthritis, rheumatoid arthritis, calcium pyrophosphate deposition disease, scleroderma, and metabolic bone disease (4–7,10,11). For example, depiction of early, subtle subperiosteal resorption and intracortical tunneling is helpful in the clinical management of patients with hyperparathyroidism (10).

CT Scanning

General considerations.—Determination of in-plane spatial resolution with CT is dependent on multiple factors. One may compute pixel size merely by dividing the field of view (FOV) by the number of pixels in both dimensions (typically 512 × 512). For example, with a 50-cm FOV, a pixel would measure approximately 1 × 1 mm (50 cm × 10 mm/cm = 500 mm; 500 mm ÷ 512 pixels = ~1 mm). This will be the actual resolution limit for body scans that use a large FOV. At small FOVs, however, the effective sampling aperture becomes the primary limiting factor. Effective aperture is, in turn, determined by both focal spot size and detector aperture. The minimum computed pixel size may be on the order of 200 μm by using a 10-cm FOV. However, the actual spatial resolution limit as determined by the effective aperture is approximately 500 μm, over twice the computed pixel size.

The selection of reconstruction algorithm determines the point spread function for the image, the highest resolution algorithm design based on the resolution limit set by the CT scanner. A minor drawback associated with use of this algorithm is an increase in image noise.

Contrast resolution, though far superior to that of plain radiography, is inferior to that of MR imaging. With the exception of its use in trauma, tumor characterization, and the evaluation of fine cortical detail, in most institutions CT assumes a minor role in the evaluation of musculoskeletal abnormalities.

Quantitative CT and computerized microtomography.—Peripheral quantitative CT (also referred to as "noninvasive bone biopsy") has been used to study the architecture of the distal radius (12). With this modality, the degree of osteoporosis can be quantitated and the effectiveness of treatment monitored. Muller et al (12) achieved in-plane resolution of 250 μm and section thicknesses of 0.48 mm, permitting three-dimensional (3D) renderings of trabecular bone structure. Investigators now believe that trabecular connectivity and plate thickness may be as important as, or more important than, the actual mineral content in the identification of those patients at risk for fracture.

Computerized microtomography, which consists of a specialized setup using monoenergetic synchrotron radiation, has been used to image 5-mm, cubic iliac crest specimens (13). Spatial resolution of 8 μm can be achieved, which permits reconstruction of accurate 3D images of trabecular bone structure. Further modifications of the procedure, including use of optical premagnification, may permit spatial resolution on the order of 1 μm. Bonse et al (13) predict that with this technique "it should be possible to study tomographically the 3D distribution and amount of osteoclastic resorption in the surrounding bone structure."

MR Imaging

General considerations.—In MR imaging, improvement in spatial resolution is advantageous only if there is concomitant maintenance of an adequate signal-to-noise ratio (S/N). Without the latter, reduction in pixel size will result in "noisy images," which are at best merely unaesthetic and at worst uninterpretable. S/N is, in turn, dependent on magnetic field strength, coil selection, and choice of imaging sequence and imaging parameters.

Field strength.—One typically associates high-resolution MR imaging with high-field-strength systems (≥1.5 T). There is, in fact, a linear relationship between field strength and S/N. "Research MR systems" operating at field strengths of 2.4–9.4 T have been used by several investigators, but in many of these units, reduction in the size of the bore restricts clinical utility (14). Although the U.S. Food and Drug Administration recommends that the whole-body-averaged specific absorption rate be limited to 0.4 W/kg, Shellock et al (15) have shown that a specific absorption rate as high as 6.0 W/kg may be tolerated by persons with normal thermoregulatory function. This seemingly strong endorsement of high-field-strength units should be qualified—relatively high-resolution images *may* be obtained at mid–field strengths provided one uses appropriate coils and optimal imaging technique (Fig 1) (16). The MR images in this article, unless otherwise stated, were obtained with 1.5-T units.

Local (surface) coils.—Proper selection of local (surface) radio-frequency (RF) coils is paramount to image optimization. As alluded to previously, use of the proper coil may overcome what one might assume to be insurmountable S/N restrictions associated with field strength. *As a general rule, the local coil should only be large*

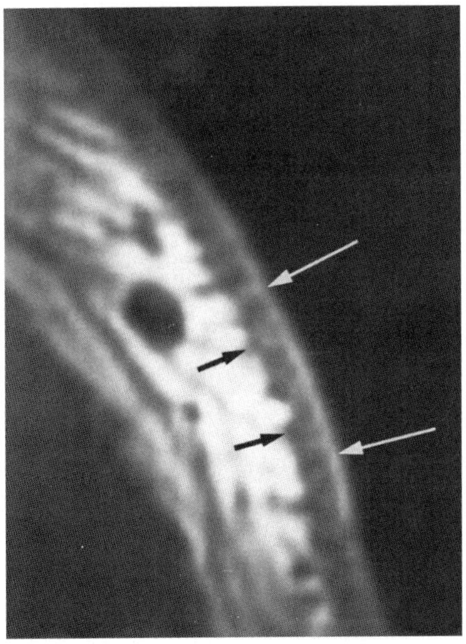

Figure 1. Three-dimensional spoiled gradient-recalled-echo (GRE) image (50/12 [repetition time {TR} msec/echo time {TE} msec], 45° flip angle, 1-mm section thickness, 9-cm FOV, 224 × 160 matrix, two signals acquired, imaging time of 8 minutes) obtained of normal facial skin with use of a 0.5-T MR unit. Note hyperintense epidermis (white arrows) and hypointense dermis (black arrows). (Reprinted, with permission, from reference 16.)

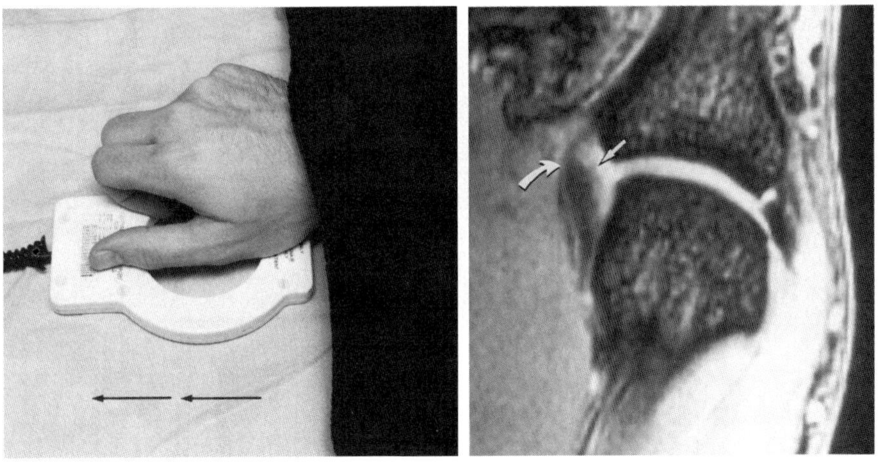

a. b.

Figure 2. Receive-only planar coil. **(a)** Configuration used for evaluation of the metacarpophalangeal joint and ligaments of the thumb. Arrows indicate the direction of B_0 (main magnetic field). **(b)** GRE MR image (600/17, 30° flip angle, 3-mm section thickness, 8-cm FOV, 256 × 192 matrix, two signals acquired, imaging time of 3 minutes 54 seconds) obtained of the thumb. Note ulnar collateral ligament tear (straight arrow) and overlying adductor aponeurosis (curved arrow).

enough to encompass the region of interest. Unnecessarily large coils detect noise outside the region of interest and, therefore, decrease the S/N (17).

Planar coils, which consist of a single loop of wire, act as receivers, with the body coil assuming the role of transmitter (Fig 2). There is an expected falloff of S/N with increasing distance from the coil surface, the effective imaging depth on the order of one coil radius. Maurer et al (18) used planar coils measuring on the order of 2.5 cm (1 inch) for the imaging of volunteers, patients, and specimens.

Saddle, birdcage, and solenoid designs act as both transmitter and receiver. These "whole-volume" coils encompass the region of interest and provide homogeneous images. Our group has found the solenoid design particularly useful because of its inherently superior S/N (19–23). The pattern of its flux lines mandates that this coil be oriented perpendicular to B_0. As such, the solenoid design is seldom used by manufacturers of superconducting magnets in which the direction of B_0 is oriented parallel to the bore, but this design is routinely employed by manufacturers of vertical field magnets, in which B_0 is perpendicular to the direction of the bore. Nevertheless, solenoid coils can be used with superconducting magnets for examinations of the foot, wrist, hand, and fingers, provided the patient is appropriately positioned (Fig 3) (19–24). Totterman et al (25) have designed a specialty coil for evaluation of the wrist that similarly requires careful positioning of the patient.

Creative use of commercially available coils can substantially improve image quality. For example, both the 5- and 3-inch planar coils may be oriented perpendicular to the long axis of the extremity, thereby producing "bracelet" coils that perform nearly as well as single-turn solenoid coils (Fig 4).

Coils may also be used in combination to improve image quality. The Helmholtz pair consists of two loops—either fixed or adjustable—placed on either side of the region of interest (17). Two to four coils may be used simultaneously with phased-array techniques to increase image coverage while achieving optimal spatial resolution (Fig 5). Since one is encompassing a larger area of interest with multiple coils, each of the coils may, in turn, be made smaller with resultant increased S/N as compared with larger single-coil configurations.

Another variation is achieved by using a local RF coil in combination with a "local gradient" coil (Fig 6). The local gradient coil can increase gradient strength in a region restricted to the area of interest, providing many inherent advantages (26–32). For example, one may prescribe smaller FOVs (improving spatial resolution), thinner section thicknesses (decreasing partial volume effects), and reduced TEs (improving the S/N and providing "truer" T1 and proton-density contrast). In fact, these inherent improvements are now being offered on a global scale in newer commercial platforms that feature body coil gradient strengths as high as 2.5 G/cm and faster slew rates (the measure of the time required to go from 0 to maximum gradient strength).

Sequences and parameters.—Commercially available sequences include conventional spin-echo (SE), fast (turbo) SE, two-dimensional (2D) GRE, 3D GRE and fast SE, inversion recovery, and magnetization transfer techniques. At our institution, we use conventional SE for T1-weighted sequences and fast SE for all proton (spin)-density– and T2-weighted sequences. Three-dimensional sequences permit acquisition of thinner sections and the opportunity for subsequent reformation in other planes. Inversion-recovery technique has been used primarily to achieve fat suppression (short inversion time inversion recovery [STIR] or fast SE STIR). Magnetization transfer techniques have been applied to the imaging of hyaline cartilage, but other musculoskeletal uses have yet to be developed (33).

In addition to specification of the coil and imaging sequence, the imaging protocol must further include TR, TE, FOV, matrix size, section thickness, number of signals acquired, and bandwidth. The choice of TR and TE depends, of course, on whether one is interested in obtaining T1-, proton-density–, or T2-weighted images. The TR also affects coverage, because the

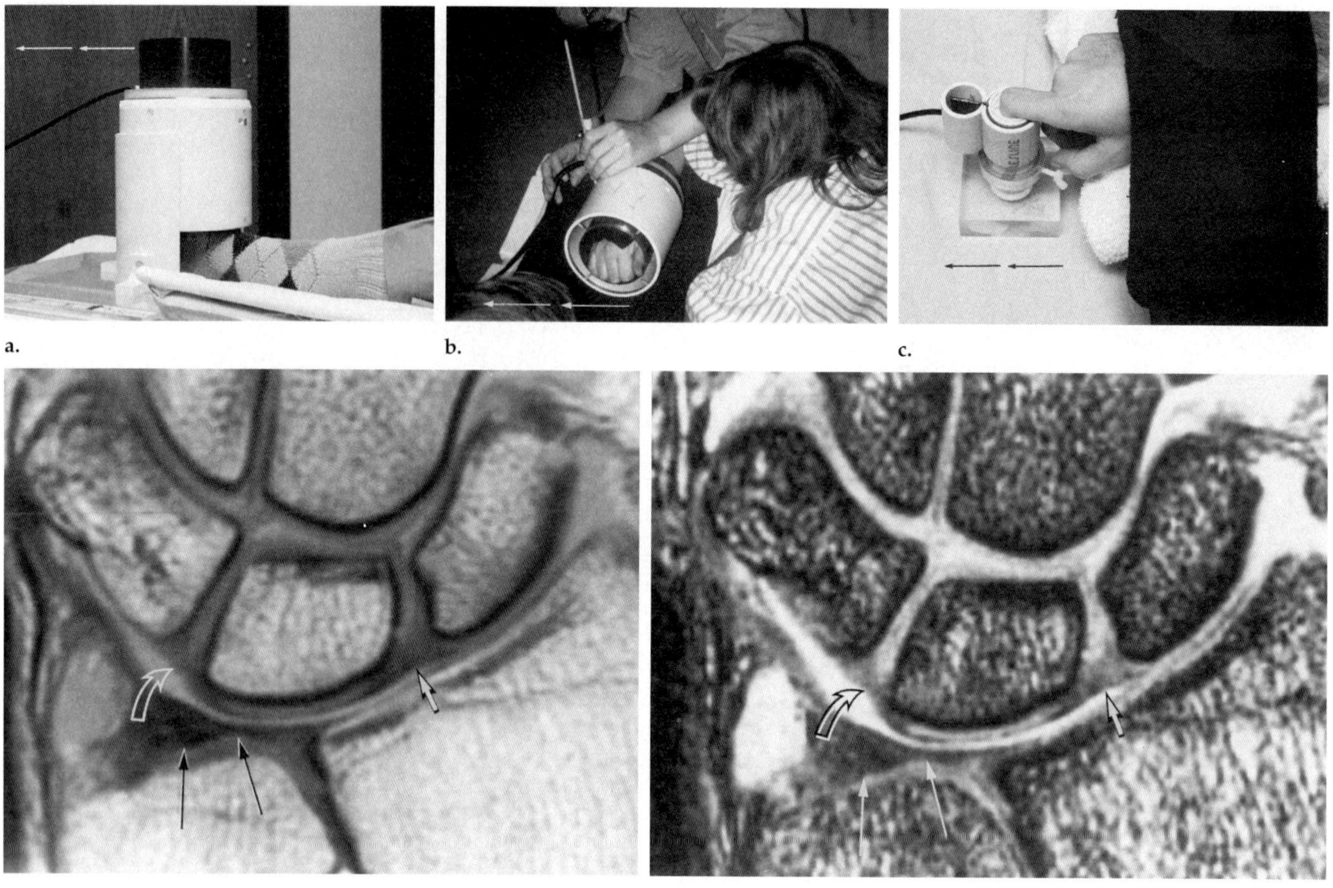

Figure 3. Solenoid local coils. For **a–c**, arrows indicate the direction of B_0. **(a)** Four-inch solenoid coil used for evaluation of the foot with the patient supine and the ankle in neutral position. **(b)** Four-inch solenoid coil used for evaluation of the wrist with the patient prone, the arm abducted 180°, and the elbow flexed 90°. This setup has been used successfully at our institution in the evaluation of over 1,000 wrists. **(c)** One-inch solenoid coil used for evaluation of the nail apparatus with the patient prone and arm positioned overhead. **(d)** Proton-density–weighted MR image (2,200/16, 2.5-mm section thickness, 8-cm FOV, 256 × 192 matrix, one signal acquired, imaging time of 7 minutes 29 seconds) obtained of the wrist by using a 4-inch solenoid coil and **(e)** 3D spoiled GRE MR image (55/15, 15° flip angle, 1-mm section thickness, 8-cm FOV, 256 × 224 matrix, one signal acquired, imaging time of 6 minutes 38 seconds), obtained at approximately the same level as in **d**, show the normal triangular fibrocartilage (thin arrows), scapholunate ligament (thick arrow), and lunotriquetral ligament (curved arrow).

number of sections increases with increasing TR. The use of a minimum TE for prescription of T1- and proton-density–weighted images is highly advantageous. It not only permits acquistion of more sections (assuming constant TR), but it also accentuates internal structure within those tissues having short T2 times, such as tendons. This is accomplished first, by "broadening the dynamic range" within the tissue, and second, by permitting the acquisition of smaller pixels since there is an improvement in overall S/N if TE is reduced. The pixel size can easily be computed by dividing the FOV (in millimeters) by the imaging matrix. For example, prescription of a 4-cm (40-mm) FOV with a 512 × 256 matrix results in a pixel dimension of 78 × 156 µm (40 mm ÷ 512 pixels = 78 µm in the frequency-encoding direction; 40 mm ÷ 256 pixels = 156 µm in the phase-encoding direction). Imaging time scales linearly with the number of acquisitions, whereas S/N varies as to the square root of the acquisition number. Use of fast (turbo) SE sequences allows one to increase the number of acquisitions while achieving reasonable imaging times. In our experience, blurring becomes unacceptable when small FOVs are used in combination with echo train lengths (ETLs) greater than four (34).

Section thickness contributes the third dimension of an imaging voxel. Reduction in section thickness lessens partial volume effect that may otherwise compromise diagnostic accuracy, but also decreases the S/N. Smaller thicknesses are achievable by using a 3D as compared with a 2D technique, as lesser demands are placed on the gradients. Furthermore, S/N with the 3D technique is often superior to that with a 2D technique because phase encoding is performed in two directions and S/N scales as the square root of the number of phase-encoding steps. Newer platforms will allow prescription of thinner sections with use of both 2D and 3D sequences.

The receiver bandwidth (sampling frequency) is an important parameter that is often overlooked. The S/N is inversely proportional to the square root of the receiver bandwidth; as a result, reduction of this parameter may substantially increase S/N. Small bandwidths can, and should, be used with lower field strengths to increase S/N. There are two potential problems that may be encountered. First, a marked reduction in receiver bandwidth may result in unsightly or even diagnostically detrimental chemical shift artifact (Fig 7). For example, at 1.5 T, the Larmor frequency is approximately 63 MHz; fat and water are out of phase by 3.5 parts per million, and, therefore, the difference in precessional frequency between fat and water protons is 63 MHz × 0.0000035 = 220 Hz. With use of a 32-kHz bandwidth and 256

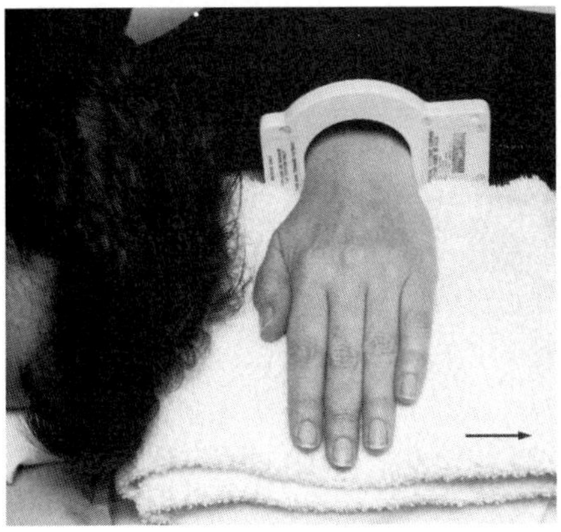

a.

Figure 4. Planar coil used as a "bracelet" coil. **(a)** Three-inch planar coil used to image the wrist with patient positioning identical to that used for the solenoid coil. For patients with larger wrists, a 5-inch planar coil may be used with a short length of polyvinyl chloride, or PVC, pipe interposed between the inner diameter of the coil and the wrist and with sponges for improved stabilization. Arrows indicate the direction of B_0. **(b)** GRE MR image (600/17, 30° flip angle, 3-mm section thickness, 8-cm FOV, 256 × 224 matrix, two signals acquired, imaging time of 4 minutes 32 seconds) obtained of the wrist with use of this coil. Note the radial-sided triangular fibrocartilage defect (arrow).

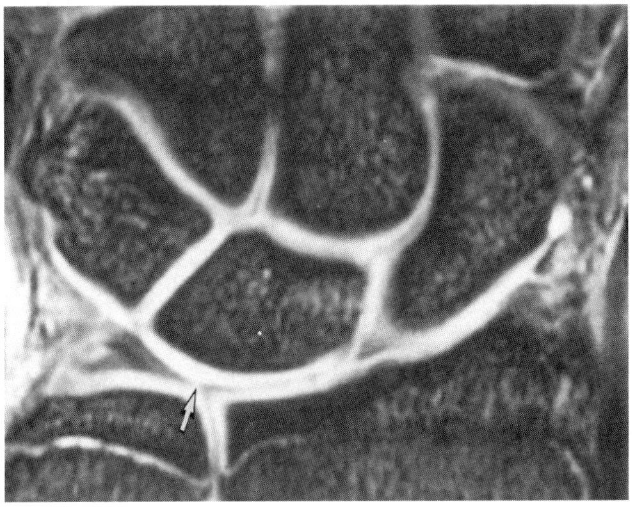

b.

frequency-encoding steps, each pixel is 32,000 ÷ 256 = 125 Hz wide; with an 8-kHz bandwidth and 256 frequency-encoding steps, each pixel is 31 Hz wide. Assuming a 12-cm FOV, with the 32-kHz bandwidth, the chemical shift = 220 Hz ÷ 125 Hz per pixel = 1.8 pixels; with the 8-kHz bandwidth, the chemical shift = 220 Hz ÷ 31 Hz per pixel = 7 pixels! The former translates into 1 mm, whereas the latter translates into 4 mm. At 0.5 T, the Larmor frequency, number of Hertz per pixel at constant receiver bandwidth, and resultant chemical shift artifact are one-third of those values listed at 1.5 T. Chemical shift artifact at high field strengths can be partly circumvented by employing chemical shift saturation techniques (see below) and prescribing a bandwidth no lower than approximately 10–11 kHz. The second potential problem associated with reduction in receiver bandwidth is that of increased sampling time with resultant increase in TE and decrease in image coverage.

It is useful to consider the following simple equation: imaging time = TR × number of signals acquired × number of phase-encoding steps. (For fast SE sequences, this product is divided by the echo train number [ETL], which indicates the number of phase encodes performed per TR period.) On the basis of the imaging time equation, it is apparent that improvement in spatial resolution is most expeditiously achieved by prescribing smaller FOVs, as opposed to larger imaging matrices. Simply put, a decrease in FOV is "free," but an increase in matrix may be "costly." For example, the identical in-plane pixel size of 312 × 417 µm can be achieved by using either an 8-cm FOV with a 256 × 192 matrix or a 16-cm FOV with a 512 × 384 matrix; the latter, however, requires twice the imaging time because the number of phase-encoding steps has been doubled. When imaging an asymmetric anatomic region, one may choose to employ a rectangular FOV, to reduce imaging time. This option maintains the spatial resolution in the phase-encoding direction by reducing the number of phase-encoding steps with concomitant reduction in the FOV in the phase-encoding direction alone. It should only be employed if there is an adequate S/N, since this ratio is proportional to the square root of the number of phase-encoding steps.

Fat-suppression techniques, which include STIR and chemical shift presaturation, are commonly used to improve lesion conspicuity. In our institution, chemical shift presaturation is preferred because S/N and image coverage per unit time are superior to that achievable with conventional or fast SE inversion-recovery techniques. If homogeneous and robust fat suppression cannot be achieved with the former technique, either because of unfavorable anatomic geometry or field heterogeneity, we will then prescribe the fast SE inversion-recovery sequence.

The spatial resolution necessary for diagnosis is difficult to establish but is obviously dependent on both the dimensions of the size of the structure of interest and inherent contrast resolution. In the clinical scenario, in-plane resolution of approximately 300 µm or less has been reported by numerous authors (18–23,27–32,35,36). With a 4-inch solenoid coil, Erickson et al (19), Oneson et al (20,21), Timins et al (22), and Hinke et al (23) achieved approximately 312 × 312–417-µm in-plane pixel dimensions in studies of the foot, wrist, and thumb (8-cm FOV, 256 × 192–256 matrix, and 2.5–3.0-mm section thickness). Totterman and Miller (35) achieved 312 × 312-µm resolution in their studies of the wrist by using a homemade coil and 3D GRE technique (8-cm FOV, 256 × 256 matrix, and 1-mm partition [section] thickness). Waldschmidt et al (36), using a simple 3-inch planar coil, achieved 156 × 312-µm pixel dimensions in studies of the patellar cartilage performed on volunteers (8-cm FOV, 512 × 256 matrix, 3-mm section thickness). Drape et al (27–29) and Goettmann et al (30) reported 117 × 334-µm (3-cm FOV, 256 × 128 matrix, and 3-mm section thickness) and 70 × 140-µm (1.8-cm FOV, 256 × 128 matrix, and 2–3-mm section thickness) pixel dimensions in studies of the nail apparatus performed with use of 3-cm local coils in conjunction with a local gradient coil. Richard et al (31,32) achieved 70 × 390-µm pixel dimensions in the imaging of skin by using a 3-cm coil also in concert with a local gradient coil (1.8 × 5-cm FOV and 3-mm section thickness). Maurer et al (18) achieved 100 × 100-µm pixel dimensions in the imaging of skin, joints, and tendons by using a 2.5-cm planar coil (2.5 cm FOV, 256 × 256 matrix, and 2-mm section thickness). The weaknesses of such high-resolution techniques are twofold: potentially substantial increases in imaging time (with attendant increased risk of patient motion), and restriction of the technique to very small regions of interest.

MR microscopy.—A particularly exciting branch of MR research is that of "MR microscopy." This work has been performed predominantly on high-field-strength (4.7–9.4 T), small-bore (~15 cm) units in conjunction with solenoid, Helmholtz, or high-temperature superconducting surface coils. Peck et al (37) have shown that microcoils as small as 50 μm in diameter may be feasible. Two main applications have been addressed in the literature—specimen analysis and in vivo small animal research.

Johnson et al (38) believe that MR microscopy has many potential advantages over conventional microscopy. First, MR microscopy is nondestructive. Second, it differentiates tissue structure on the basis of "proton stain," obviating complex histologic staining techniques and tissue dessication. Third, it is inherently 3D, permitting multiplanar evaluation.

Imaging time for specimens has been reported to be as high as 8 hours with use of conventional 2D techniques; this results in 24 × 24-μm in-plane resolution and 250-μm section thickness (39). Use of a 3D technique permits one to obtain much thinner sections and, therefore, to acquire isotropic (cubic), or nearly isotropic, data sets (39–42). Initial imaging times with a 256 × 256 matrix with 256 partitions in the z phase-encoding direction and partial Fourier technique, yielding 70-μm isotropic voxels, were reported to be as high as 13.6 hours (41)! By reducing the number of partitions to 64—which is feasible if a thin specimen section measuring on the order of 5 × 5 × 2 mm is being examined—imaging time may be shortened considerably with concomitant reduction of the voxel size dimension to 20 × 20 × 30 μm (40). More recently, fast SE techniques have been adapted for use in MR microscopy (42). This technique cannot only substantially reduce imaging time, but it also minimizes artifact attributable to susceptibility and diffusion. Two-dimensional 1-mm-thick images with 30–70-μm in-plane spatial resolution may be obtained in 1–2 minutes, and 3D images with 70–117-μm isotropic voxels may be obtained in 4½ hours. Johnson et al (38) predict that 10-μm spatial resolution will soon be attainable.

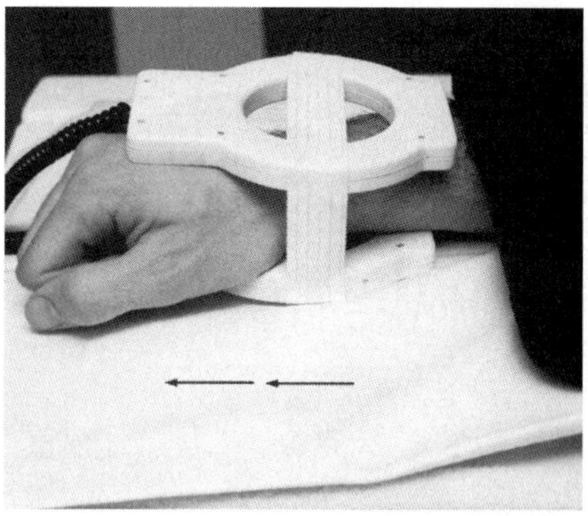

a.

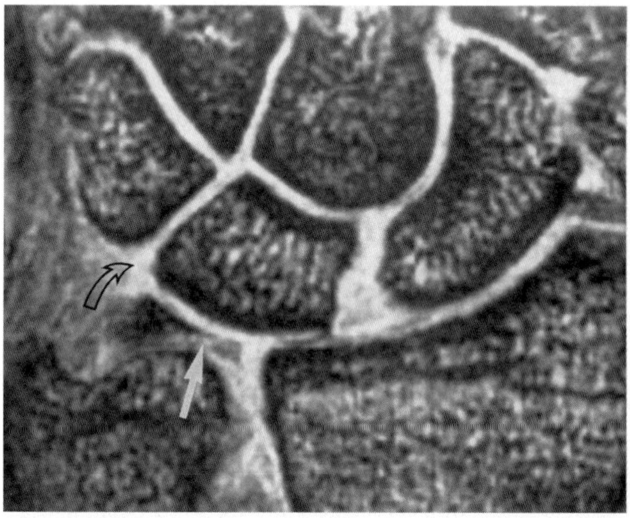

b.

Figure 5. Dual 3-inch loop configuration. **(a)** Two 3-inch loops may be used with phased-array technology or a passive combiner box for evaluation of the wrist with the patient positioned prone and the arm extended overhead. Arrows indicate the direction of B_0. **(b)** Three-dimensional spoiled GRE MR image (69/15, 20° flip angle, 1.3-mm section thickness, 8-cm FOV, 256 × 256 matrix, one signal acquired, imaging time of 9 minutes 29 seconds) obtained of the wrist with use of this setup. Note the triangular fibrocartilage defect (solid arrow) and probable lunotriquetral ligament defect (open arrow).

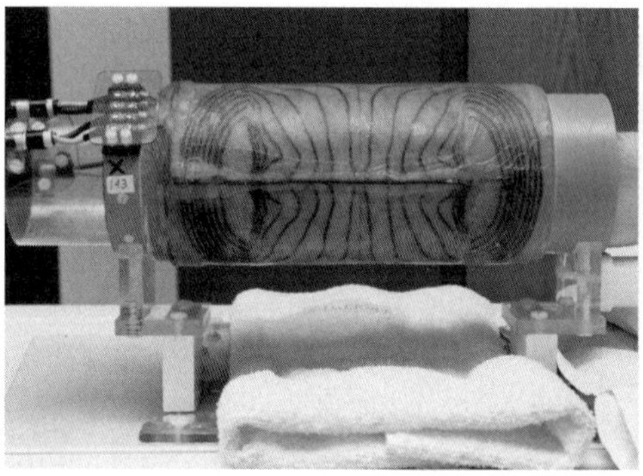

a.

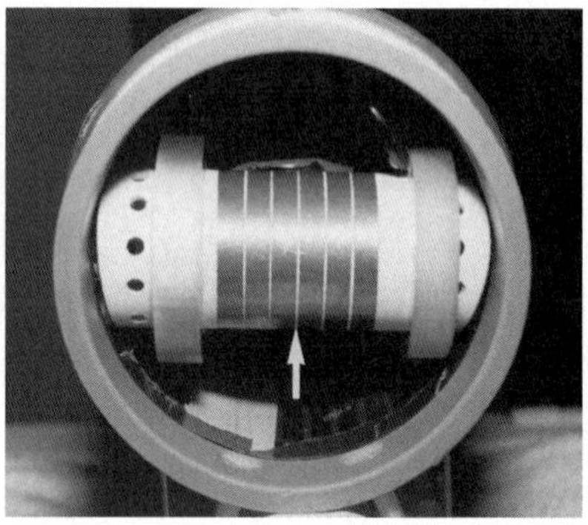

b.

Figure 6. Local gradient coil. **(a)** Note the cylindric coil with exposed wiring. **(b)** End-on view of the local gradient coil shows a small solenoid RF coil (arrow) used to image specimens. In actual use, this coil is placed at the center of the local gradient coil.

MR microscopy has been used to obtain in vivo images of normal and diseased rats with use of both 2D and 3D techniques (43,44). Beckmann et al (43) imaged rat hind paws to monitor the progression of induced arthritic alterations by using 3D technique with 94 × 81 × 60-μm voxels in 55 minutes. Johnson et al (unpublished data, 1997) obtained rat brain and muscle MR angiograms by using 3D techniques with 58–94-μm isotropic voxel dimensions (Fig 8).

Johnson (oral communication, 1997) describes three practical niches for MR microscopy: in the operating room in lieu of frozen sections, in the community instead of hematoxylin-eosin stains, and by molecular biologists for the evaluation of embryos (45). He predicts the first will prove practical since current imaging times of approximately 1 hour or less are comparable to the time required for conventional processing of specimens. The last named application is

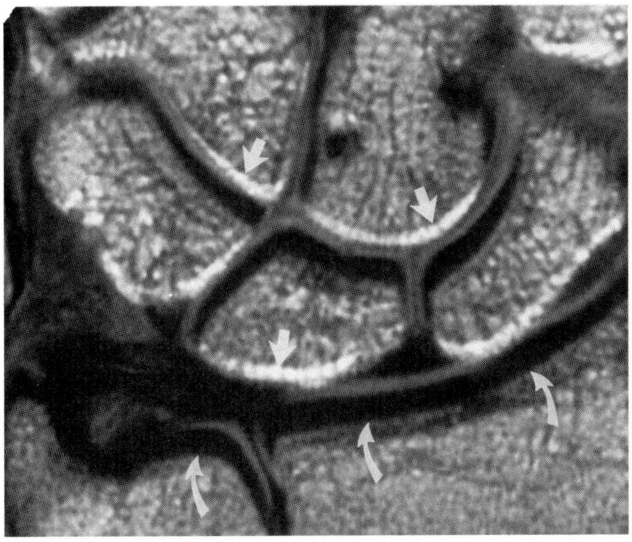

Figure 7. Effect of receiver bandwidth at 1.5 T. MR image of a cadaveric wrist with use of 4-kHz receiver bandwidth shows marked chemical shift artifact manifested by hyperintense margins (straight arrows) and artifactual "thickening" of the cortex (curved arrows). The frequency-encoding direction is oriented from top to bottom, and the phase-encoding direction from right to left.

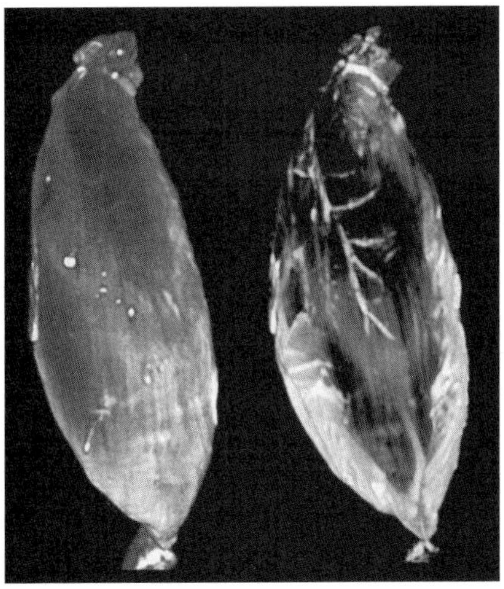

Figure 8. MR microscopy. Long-axis MR images of rat leg muscle obtained at 9.4 T (58 × 58 × 58-µm isotropic voxel size) after the supplying vessel had been isolated and infused with gadolinium in gelatin to provide a vascular stain. The volume-rendered image (left) shows the exterior surface of the muscle bundle; the image on the right has been rendered with transparency so that the internal vasculature is evident. (Images courtesy of Marie Delnomdidieu, SCD, and G. Allan. Johnson, PhD, Duke Center for In-Vivo Microscopy, Durham, NC, a National Institutes of Health Resource [P41O5959].)

already routinely used at his institution. Unfortunately, it is unlikely that interpretation of these images will fall within the province of the radiologist.

US Scanning

Advances in US technology over the past few years have resulted in a remarkable surge in the interest for musculoskeletal sonography. Though this modality has been used for the diagnosis of musculoskeletal abnormalities for more than a decade, in the United States—with the exception of a few "elite" centers—its use has been limited because of the ready availability and imaging capabilities of MR imaging. Efforts toward cost containment coupled with elevation of industry US performance standards have prompted many imagers to reevaluate this incredibly versatile modality. Though its detractors maintain that musculoskeletal US is operator dependent, impressive attendance at musculoskeletal US meetings and the recent highly publicized dead heat in the "head-to-head" competition between US and MR imaging during the 1996 Olympics suggest that more imagers will accept this challenge. Furthermore, musculoskeletal sonography is a dynamic study that permits the imager to examine the area of interest as the patient performs various maneuvers.

Insonation frequency continues to be a critical determinant of spatial resolution. Currently, commercially available units are capable of producing frequencies in the range of 9–13 MHz. Use of broad-bandwidth technology is reported to further enhance spatial resolution. Specialty units used for skin imaging are capable of insonating in the range of 20–100 MHz (46–52). Imaging depth penetration is inversely related to insonation frequency, being limited to 4 cm at 12 MHz, 2 cm at 20 MHz, 1.7 mm at 40 MHz, and 1 mm at 92 MHz.

Spatial resolution is somewhat harder to establish for US equipment than for the equipment of other imaging modalities. Axial resolution is the ability to separate two objects lying in tandem along the axis of the beam and is given by the following equation: AR = (PW × SS)/2, where AR = axial resolution, PW = pulse width, and SS = speed of sound. Pulse width equals the wavelength (which is inversely proportional to insonation frequency) times the number of emitted pulses; the average speed of sound in soft tissue is 1,540 m/sec. Lateral resolution is the ability to separate two adjacent objects and is dependent on the wavelength, depth of scanning, and aperture size according to the following equation: LR = (D × WL)/A, where LR = lateral resolution, D = depth, WL = wavelength, and A = aperture. Multiple focal zones are produced by varying the aperture width in relation to depth, providing more uniform resolution. To compensate, there may be a concomitant reduction in frame rate. Commercially available probes with insonation frequencies of 9–13 MHz achieve in-plane resolution in the range of 200–450 µm and section thicknesses on the order of 0.5–1.0 mm. Use of 20-MHz frequency permits in-plane resolution of 70–80 × 70–200 µm; 40-MHz frequency, 30 × 94 µm; and 92-MHz frequency, 21 × 45 µm (47,52). Stiller et al (51) claim that individual cells may be resolved by using transducers in the range of 300–600 MHz.

Dynamic range is analogous to the selectable image "window" used for displaying MR and CT images. As one expands the dynamic range, the images appear smoother and flatter, but by the same token, one may appreciate subtler internal detail. Choice of dynamic range is often subjective, related to both operator preference as well as the specific anatomic region and diagnostic question.

Elective reduction of frame rate increases the number of data lines obtained and improves lateral resolution. This is a viable option in musculoskeletal imaging, in which patient motion is not a problem.

As stated above, MR phased arrays consisting of multiple local coils are used to maintain spatial resolution while extending the extent of coverage. One vendor has recently introduced US software that similarly allows the imager to obtain panoramic, high-resolution images with a handheld transducer without the need for position sensors (extended FOV, SieScape; Siemens Medical Systems, Ultrasound Group, Issaquah, Wash) (Fig 9) (53).

As of this writing, most manufacturers continue to use "one × two arrays," which consist of numerous elements each measuring several millimeters in length. However, a recently released technology using "two × two arrays" that consist of multiple rows of 1,024 elements promises to dramatically improve US imaging (voxel image processing, active matrix arrays; GE Medical Systems, Milwaukee, Wis) (Fig 10). By expanding the aperture in two dimensions, one can shrink the image voxel to provide uniform section thickness and improved resolution. This technology will be a critical component in pushing 3D US to new levels of performance.

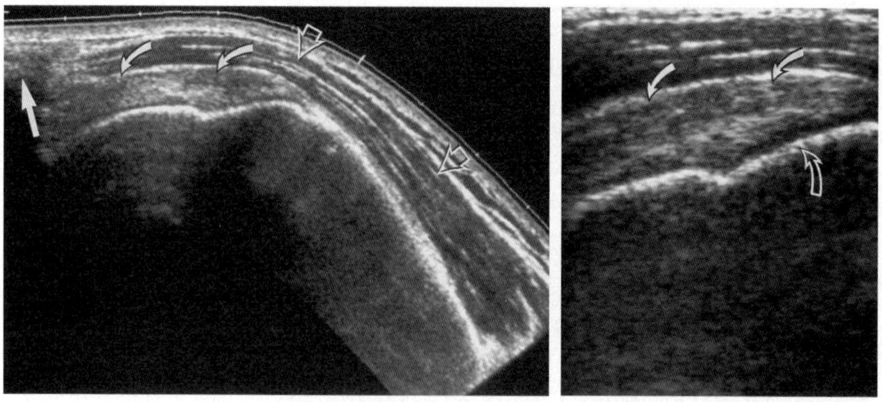

a. b.

Figure 9. Extended-field-of-view US imaging (SieScape, Siemens Medical Systems). **(a)** Oblique coronal US image of the shoulder shows shadowing from the acromion (solid straight arrow), the supraspinatus tendon (curved arrows), and the deltoid muscle (open arrows). **(b)** One of the many frames used to form the composite image shows the supraspinatus tendon (solid arrows) and greater tuberosity (open arrow). These frames may be reviewed retrospectively after the composite image is frozen.

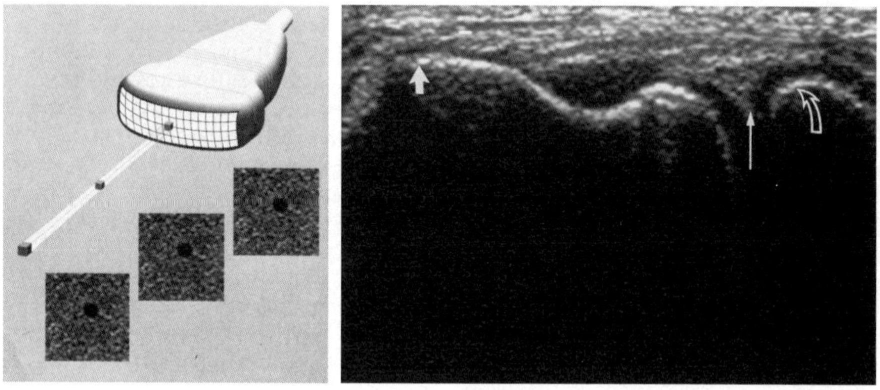

a. b.

Figure 10. Two-dimensional ultrasound array. **(a)** Diagram shows that the transducer elements are arranged both in columns and rows, yielding small voxels of uniform size throughout the image. Note that the cysts are accurately displayed at all depths, as represented in the three insets. (Image courtesy of Kristin LaConte, Ultrasound Division, GE Medical Systems.) **(b)** Coronal US image obtained with 13-MHz insonation frequency shows the normal radiocapitellar meniscus (thin arrow) outlined by fluid. Thick arrow = lateral epicondyle, curved arrow = radial head.

THE TISSUES

Bone

There are two processes of bone histogenesis; these are referred to as intramembranous and endochondral ossification. Intramembranous (mesenchymal) ossification occurs through direct mineralization of vascular connective tissue, whereas endochondral ossification arises within a cartilage model. Intramembranous ossification occurs within the flat bones and contributes width to the shafts of long bones (the periosteal collar), whereas endochondral ossification is responsible for the longitudinal growth of long bones and the formation of the axial skeleton. Both intramembranous and endochondral ossification result in lamellar bone formation.

All bones consist of peripheral cortical (compact) bone and central medullary (trabecular or cancellous) bone (Fig 11). In the case of a long bone, there is an inverse relationship between the quantity of cortical and trabecular bone at any given site. For example, cortical bone is thickest within the diaphysis of long bones, a site where trabecular bone is quite sparse; conversely, cortical bone becomes quite thin in the metaphyseal and epiphyseal regions, sites where trabecular bone is prominent. Cortical bone composes 80% of skeletal bone mass.

Cortical bone.—Cortical bone is composed of osteons (haversian systems)—cylindric units that are oriented roughly parallel to the long axis of the bone. Osteons measure approximately 250 μm in width by 1–5 cm in length and are in turn composed of concentric layers of bony lamellae that measure approximately 2–3 μm in thickness. These lamellae are demarcated by regularly arranged osteocytes. There is a faint "cement line" at the outer margin of each osteon, and the space between adjacent osteons is filled with interstitial lamellae. Circumferential lamellae are formed by the periosteum and, in the diaphysis, are arranged concentrically about the medullary cavity.

The center of each secondary osteon contains the haversian canal, which typically conveys one artery and one vein to the osteonal unit. These canals vary in diameter and area, having a mean diameter of approximately 50–100 μm; those canals closest to the medullary cavity are larger in caliber (1,54,55). Volkmann canals are oriented roughly perpendicular to the long axis of the long bone and carry blood from one osteon to another. Nutrient arteries and emissary veins course through the nutrient foramen into the diaphysis.

The outer surface of cortical bone is lined with periosteum, a dense fibrous connective tissue that is anchored to the cortical bone by means of perforating Sharpey fibers. The innermost layer of the periosteum is the cambium layer, which consists of a layer of osteoblasts. The inner surface of cortical bone is lined by the much thinner endosteum, which also possesses osteogenic capacity.

Medullary bone.—Though trabecular bone constitutes only 20% of skeletal bone mass, it possesses approximately 20 times more surface area per unit volume. Since its cells lie mainly between laminae or on the surface of trabeculae, trabecular bone has a higher rate of metabolic activity than does cortical bone. As stated previously, trabecular bone, in contradistinction to cortical bone, is concentrated at the ends of long tubular bones. Both short bones and flat

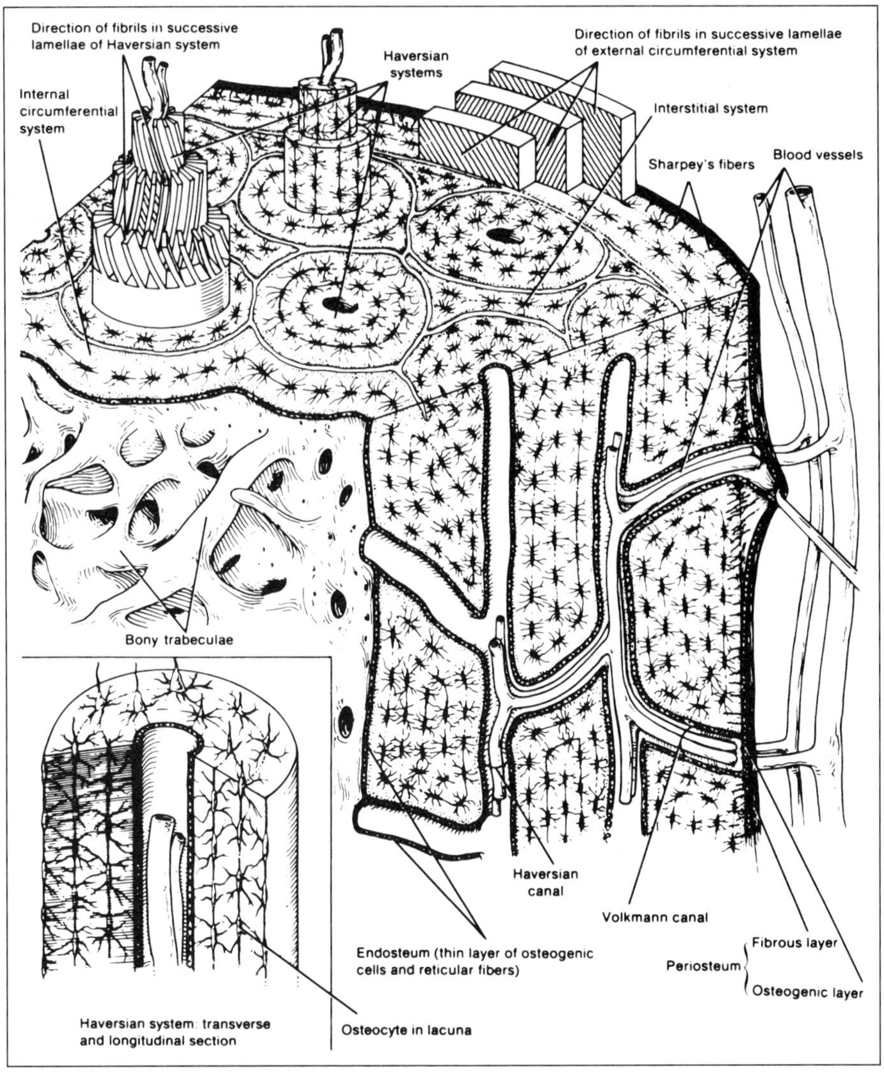

Figure 11. Diagram depicts osseous anatomic structures. (Image courtesy of R. G. Kessel, MD, professor emeritus of biological sciences, University of Iowa, Iowa City.)

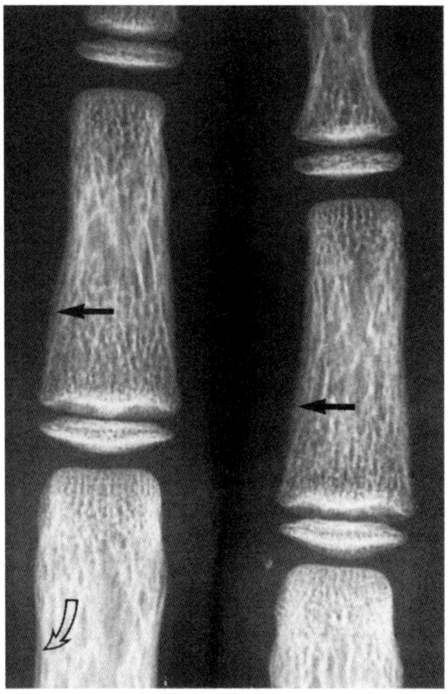

a.

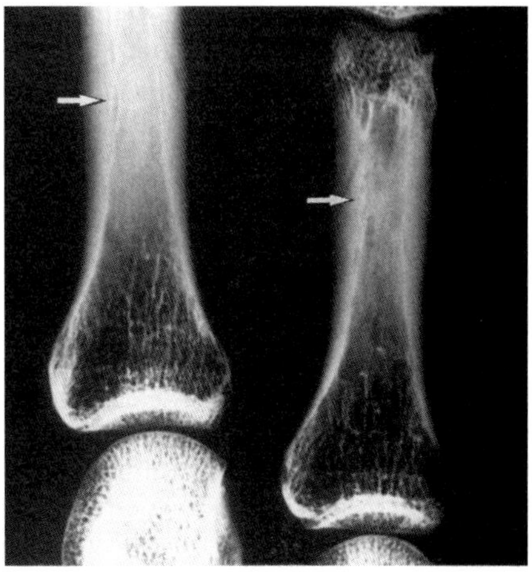

b.

Figure 12. Bone: high-resolution radiography. **(a)** Radiograph of the hand, in a young child with renal osteodystrophy, obtained by using radiographic magnification with a micro–focal spot shows subperiosteal resorption (solid arrows) and cortical tunneling (open arrow). Note excellent trabecular detail. (Reprinted, with permission, from reference 4.) **(b)** Radiograph of an adult hand obtained by using a mammographic unit with a small focal spot shows what may be normal haversian canals (arrows).

bones, however, have much thinner cortices and trabecular bone is more evenly distributed.

Epiphyseal and metaphyseal trabeculae within long bones act to absorb impact loads across synovial joints and, therefore, protect articular cartilage and subchondral bone. Trabecular orientation is a manifestation of the Wolff law, which states that bony structures orient themselves in form and mass to best resist intrinsic forces. In the femur, for example, both compressive and tensile groups are described. Reduced weight bearing causes resorption of these trabeculae, those bearing least weight affected first.

In addition to bone trabeculae, the medullary cavity contains bone marrow. Yellow marrow consists primarily of fat cells and connective tissue, whereas red marrow consists of protein (15%), hematopoietic cells (40%), fat cells (40%), and connective tissue. The distribution of hematopoietic and fatty marrow is dependent on patient age and metabolic state. In the long bones, the epiphysis initially contains hematopoietic marrow, but once ossification of this secondary center occurs, there is conversion to predominantly yellow marrow. Nevertheless, small subchondral rests of hematopoietic marrow frequently persist throughout adulthood.

High-resolution radiography possesses a spatial resolution unmatched by its imaging rivals. Assuming a pixel size of 25–50 µm, this modality can consistently depict cortical cutting cones (sites of haversian canal enlargement by means of osteoclastic activity) in the setting of metabolic disease and may be capable of depicting normal cortical haversian systems (Fig 12). Subchondral and trabecular bone are similarly displayed in stunning detail (Fig 12).

With a minimum pixel size of approximately 400 µm, the spatial resolution of CT is an order of magnitude less than that of radiography (Fig 13). The primary advantage of CT is, instead, its tomographic capability.

Conventional wisdom initially decreed that MR imaging would not enable evaluation of cortical bone. Current MR techniques permit depiction of cortical anatomic features and abnormalities, though in some instances with less detail than that achievable with CT. Cortical bone

Figure 14. Normal osseous anatomic features: MR imaging. **(a)** Axial T1-weighted image (800/46, 2-mm section thickness, 4-cm FOV, 256 × 224 matrix, one signal acquired, imaging time of 3 minutes 9 seconds) obtained of the distal phalanx of the finger with use of a 1-inch solenoid coil shows intracortical vasculature (arrows). **(b)** Coronal T1-weighted MR image (500/35, 2-mm section thickness, 4-cm FOV, 512 × 256 matrix, four signals acquired, imaging time of 8 minutes 36 seconds) obtained of the finger with use of a 1-inch solenoid coil demonstrates exquisite cortical and trabecular anatomic features. In-plane spatial resolution of approximately 80 × 160 µm is substantially superior to that of CT but still less than that of magnification radiography.

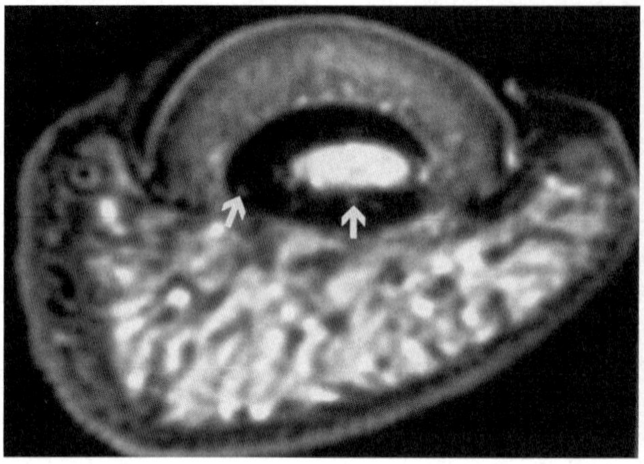

a.

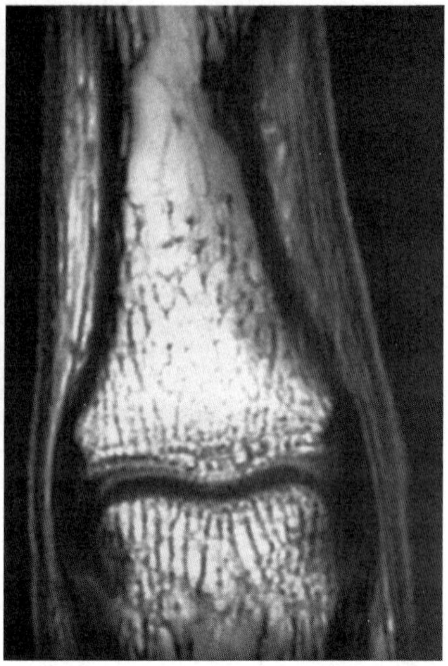

b.

generally appears as a signal void, but both nutrient foramina and even branching intracortical vessels can be frequently visualized (Fig 14a). Normal periosteum remains elusive, but periosteal reaction can be depicted.

Trabeculae are commonly observed by using standard, clinical MR sequences. Fine detail, however, is best demonstrated with a high-resolution technique (Fig 14b). Hematopoietic and fatty marrow can be readily distinguished with use of commercially available sequences. On T1-weighted images, hematopoietic marrow appears relatively hypointense in contrast to hyperintense fatty marrow. The appearance is somewhat similar on T2-weighted images, though the contrast between the two types of marrow is not nearly as great. The addition of fat-suppression renders hematopoietic marrow relatively hyperintense in relation to the suppressed fatty marrow. Islands of hematopoietic marrow often contain central fatty marrow, giving rise to the "bull's-eye" sign described by Schweitzer et al (56). Comparison of images obtained both in-phase (in which the signal intensity of fat and water are additive) and out-of-phase (in which the signal intensities of fat and water subtract) may be helpful to distinguish hematopoietic marrow from infiltrative neoplasm or other marrow packing disorders. These images can be obtained quickly by using GRE sequences with TEs appropriate for the field strength. At 1.5 T, in-phase images can be obtained with TE values that are approximately multiples of 4.2 msec and out-of-phase images can be obtained with TE values of approximately 2.1, or $[2.1 + (n \times 4.2)]$ msec, where n is a positive integer. Ramifying intramedullary vessels are seen routinely, particularly if fat-suppression techniques are used.

With US, the interface between soft tissue and cortical bone is echogenic because of an inherent high acoustical impedance mismatch. Subtle surface irregularities, "pits," erosions, and nutrient foramina can be easily visualized. Van Holsbeeck et al (57) have shown that pitting of the humeral head is often associated with rotator cuff abnormality (Fig 15). Internal cortical structure and underlying trabecular bone, however, remain inaccessible. Because bone is an anisotropic structure, sound velocity depends on whether the insonated beam is parallel or perpendicular to the orientation of the haversian systems (58). Several investigators have employed US in the analysis of bone densitometry (59).

Joint

There are two major categories of joints (arthroses): nonsynovial or "solid" joints (synarthroses) and synovial joints (diarthroses). Nonsynovial joints are those in which adjacent bones are linked by intervening solid connective tissue. These joints may be further divided into fibrous joints and cartilaginous joints. In fibrous joints, adjacent bones may be connected by a sutural ligament (sutures, which unite many of the

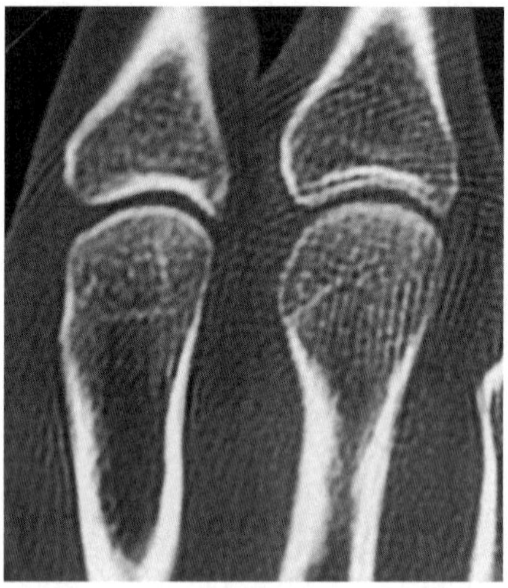

Figure 13. Normal osseous anatomic features: CT scanning. Coronal CT scan (9.6-cm FOV, 1-mm section thickness, 512 × 512 matrix) obtained through the metacarpophalangeal joints with the patient positioned prone, the arm abducted 180°, the elbow flexed 90°, and the thumb facing up. Spatial resolution is approximately an order of magnitude less than that of magnification radiography. Cortical and trabecular detail are clearly inferior to that of magnification radiography.

cranial bones), a collagenous interosseous ligament or membrane (syndesmoses, as in the case of the "fibrous" superior articulation of the sacroiliac joint and the interosseous membrane uniting the midportion of

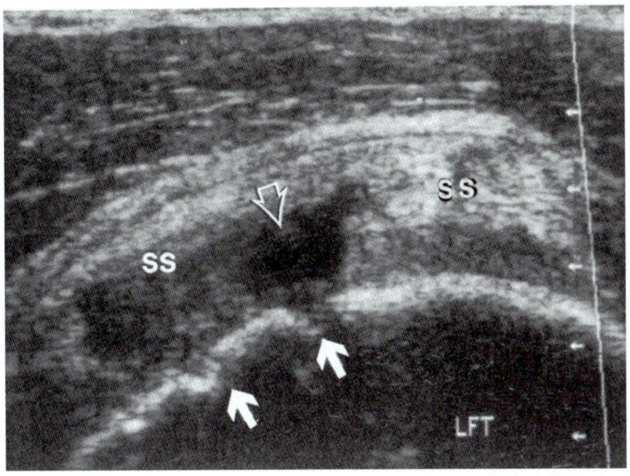

Figure 15. Sagittal US image obtained with 7.5-MHz insonation frequency demonstrates a partial, undersurface supraspinatus (*SS*) tear (open arrow) and associated small humeral cortical "pits" (solid arrows). (Reprinted, with permission, from reference 57.)

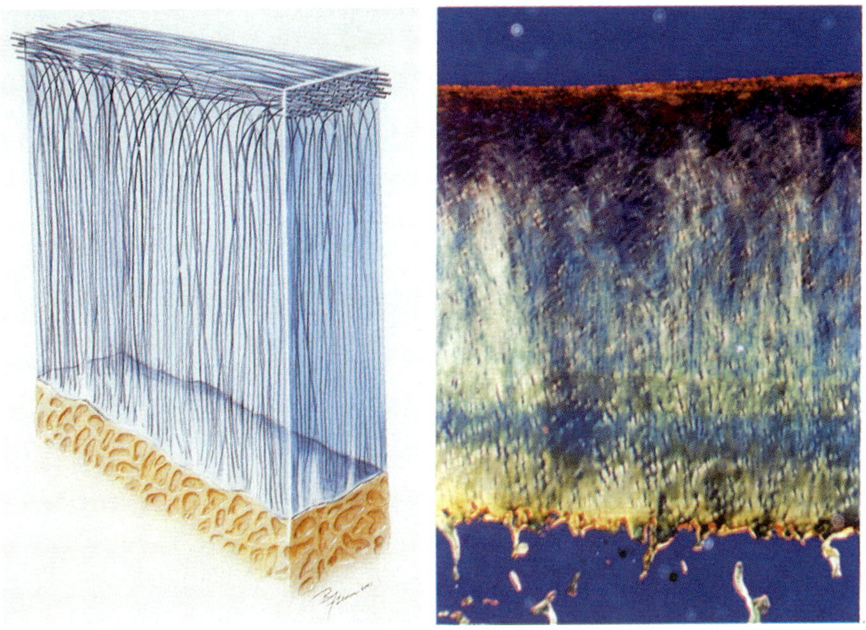

a. b.

Figure 16. Normal hyaline cartilage. **(a)** Sketch depicts the orientation of collagen fibers within hyaline cartilage as perpendicular to subchondral bone within the deep zone, curved within the intermediate zone, and parallel to the surface within the superficial zone. (Reprinted, with permission, from reference 61.) **(b)** Photomicrograph of histologic specimen stained with picrosirius red and viewed with polarized light depicts the superficial zone as orange, intermediate zone as black, and deep radial zone as green. (Original magnification, ×20.)

the radius and ulna), or cartilaginous periodontium (gomphoses, as in the case of the articulation between the teeth and alveolar sockets of the mandible and maxilla). The cartilaginous joints are divided into synchondroses in which adjacent bones are united by hyaline growth cartilage (as in the epiphyseal plates) and symphyses in which a fibrocartilaginous disk is sandwiched between two layers of hyaline growth cartilage (as in the symphysis pubis). The term synostosis refers to a state of rigid bony union that occurs after cessation of growth. This is the normal fate of synchondroses, most sutures, and some symphyses.

The remaining discussion addresses specifically synovial joints, in which adjacent bones are joined by "cavitated connective tissue" with the result being a more complex yet more mobile joint. The nonosseous components of synovial joints include hyaline articular cartilage, the joint capsule, synovium, and synovial fluid. Additional structures found in some synovial joints include an articular disk or meniscus and intraarticular ligaments.

Hyaline cartilage.—Hyaline articular cartilage is a remarkable tissue that has a low coefficient of friction yet is capable of absorbing large compressive forces. The thickness varies, reaching approximately 5–7 mm in large joints. By weight, this tissue is composed of the following: water (65%), chondrocytes (5%), collagen (15%), and proteoglycans (15%). It is nourished almost entirely by synovial fluid, with only the deepest layers *potentially* receiving blood supply from subchondral bone.

Radially oriented chondrocytes are responsible for production of both proteoglycans and collagen. Proteoglycan molecules avidly attract water molecules, and augmented swelling pressure is responsible for "inflation" of cartilage tissue. Application of an external compressive load squeezes water out of the cartilage and into the synovial cavity. Both water and proteoglycan concentrations vary with depth—the former being highest in concentration at the surface, the latter most concentrated in the deeper layers.

Hyaline cartilage is primarily composed of type II collagen fibers, the diameter and concentration of which are also depth dependent. The thin surface collagen fibers act as a filter, preventing entrance of molecules larger than 6 nm. The thicker deep collagen fibers are anchored to the subchondral bone. Collagen is believed to restrict the size and orientation of proteoglycan molecules and provide tensile strength during cartilage "swelling."

Hyaline cartilage has been subdivided into four somewhat arbitrary zones defined by both microanatomic and ultrastructural features. The cartilage arcade model proposed by Benninghoff is useful in the understanding of both cartilage anatomic features and abnormalities (60,61) (Fig 16). The superficial (tangential) zone composes approximately 3%–12% of the overall cartilage thickness, and its collagen fibers are ordered primarily parallel to the articular surface. The intermediate zone is thicker than the superficial zone, and its collagen fibers curve as they course toward the superficial zone, giving the appearance of a more random orientation. The deep radial zone composes over 50% of cartilage thickness. The collagen fibers are thickest in this region and are oriented perpendicular to the subchondral bone. The zone of calcified cartilage is demarcated from the deep radial zone by the undulating tide mark.

Without the aid of intraarticular contrast material, cartilage thickness can only be inferred indirectly with radiography or CT (except in cases of chondrocalcinosis or vacuum

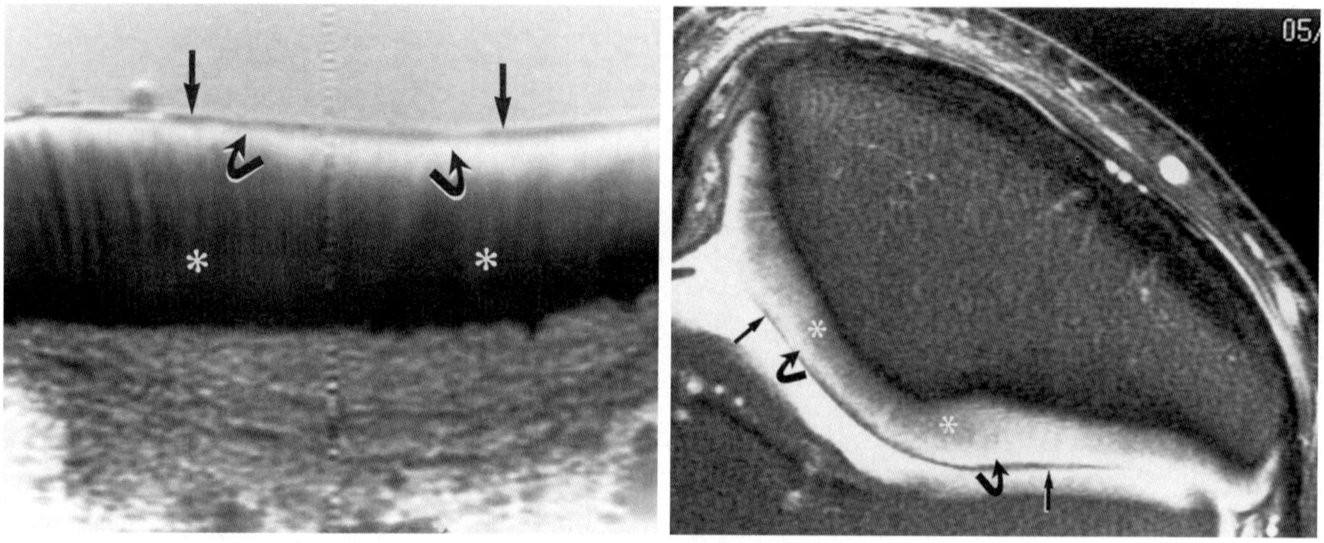

a. b.

Figure 17. Normal hyaline cartilage: MR imaging. **(a)** Axial fat-suppressed proton-density–weighted MR image (2,000/35, 2-mm section thickness, 4-cm FOV, 512 × 256 matrix, four signals acquired, imaging time of 34 minutes 16 seconds) obtained of a patellar specimen with use of a 1-inch solenoid coil shows three laminae: superficial (straight arrows), intermediate (curved arrows), and deep (*). Note parallel, alternating hyperintense and hypointense bands within the deep zone. **(b)** Axial in vivo proton-density–weighted fat-suppressed MR image (2,600/33, 3-mm section thickness, 8-cm FOV, 512 × 256 matrix, three signals acquired, imaging time of 16 minutes 49 seconds) obtained of normal patellar cartilage with use of a 3-inch planar coil shows similar laminar anatomic features: superficial zone (straight arrows), intermediate zone (curved arrows), deep zone (*). Note striations within the deep zone similar to those demonstrated in the specimen.

joint). Early MR studies reported a bilaminar appearance (62,63), but most investigators currently describe a trilaminar appearance (36,64–67). Although to date there is still controversy concerning the thickness and signal intensities of these laminae, investigators are moving closer to a consensus. The histologic superficial zone is likely represented by a hypointense lamina (14,36,61,64,65,68–70). The thickness of this zone appears to be dependent on selection of TE, becoming much more conspicuous as TE is increased (70). The immediately subjacent lamina appears relatively hyperintense and the deepest lamina hypointense. Waldschmidt et al (36,61) further demonstrated the deep lamina to be heterogeneous, manifested by alternating hyperintense and hypointense bands (Fig 17). Rubenstein et al (70) showed two additional deep laminae that they postulate to represent the zones of uncalcified and calcified cartilage.

The signal intensities of these laminae have been variably attributed to water content, proteoglycan concentration, and collagen orientation (36,61,67,70,71). Though this controversy is far from resolved, it is the author's belief that, on the basis of orientation experiments designed to exploit magic angle effects, signal intensity is primarily attributed to collagen orientation (Fig 18).

With US, adult hyaline cartilage appears predominantly hypoechoic in vivo, the surface presumably "silhouetted" by adjacent tissue (Fig 19a). When overlying cuff tissue is absent—such as in the setting of a complete rotator cuff tear—one may visualize the surface as a relatively thin, hyperechoic layer outlined by fluid (Fig 19b). The source of this surface layer, as compared with that demonstrable with MR imaging, has been attributed to an impedance mismatch between fluid and hyaline cartilage (72,73). This occurs because the speed of sound in saline measures 1,531 m/sec, whereas the speed of sound in human cartilage has been reported to be on the order of 1,658–1,750 m/sec (73,74). A second, deeper hyperechoic interface represents either the calcified cartilage–noncalcified cartilage or cartilage–subchondral bone interface (72).

Investigators have examined cartilage specimens with use of frequencies that range from 25 to 100 mHz (72,73,75). Kim et al (72) examined immature porcine hyaline cartilage by using 50-mHz US backscatter microscopy. This "growth cartilage" can be considered analogous to the epiphyseal plate (Fig 20a). Three laminae were observed and consisted of—from superficial to deep—hypoechoic, hyperechoic, and anechoic layers (Fig 20b). Cartilage canals (ie, discrete vascular channels) could be discerned in those specimens obtained from the youngest pigs. It is tempting to speculate that a somewhat similar pattern can be discerned in infants and young children in vivo

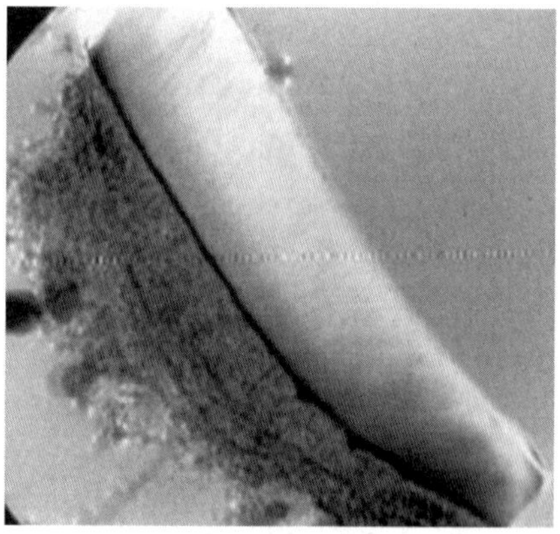

Figure 18. Magic angle effects within hyaline cartilage. Axial MR image (same parameters as Fig 17a) of the same cartilage specimen as in Figure 17a after rotation by approximately 55° shows relatively equivalent signal intensities throughout most of the specimen attributable to T2 augmentation.

with use of clinical equipment (Fig 20c). Agemura et al (75) demonstrated focal variation in propagation speed within the three histologic zones by using adult bovine cartilage specimens. This effect was attributed to collagen orientation, with the highest speeds noted in regions in which fibers are oriented perpendicular to the insonating sound beam (75).

Capsule and synovium.—The fibrous joint capsule is composed of interlacing bundles of collagen fibers and is attached typically near the ends of opposing bones. In the long bones, however, the site of attachment is of-

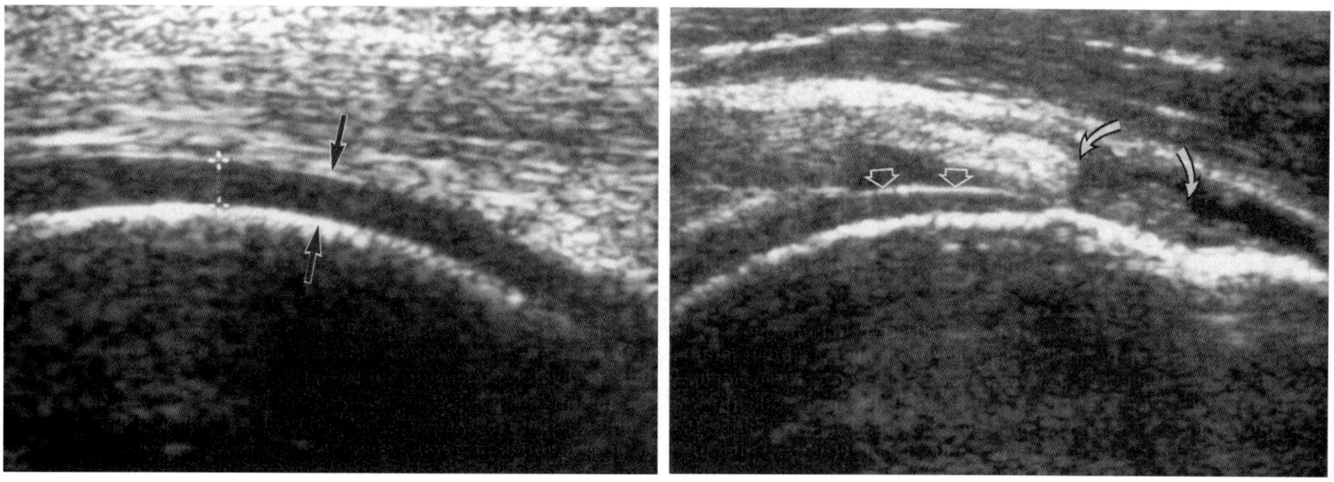

a. b.

Figure 19. Normal hyaline cartilage: US imaging. (a) Sagittal US image of the femoral trochlea shows hypoechoic hyaline cartilage (arrows) that is easily distinguished from underlying hyperechoic cortical bone. An insonation frequency of 9 MHz was used, and cartilage thickness measured 1.7 mm. Note the absence of discrete laminar anatomic features. (b) Oblique coronal US image of the left shoulder with use of 9-MHz insonation frequency. Note the presence of complete tear of the rotator cuff with retraction (solid arrows). In this example, the superficial aspect of the hyaline cartilage appears hyperechoic because of an acoustical impedance mismatch between cartilage and adjacent fluid (open arrows).

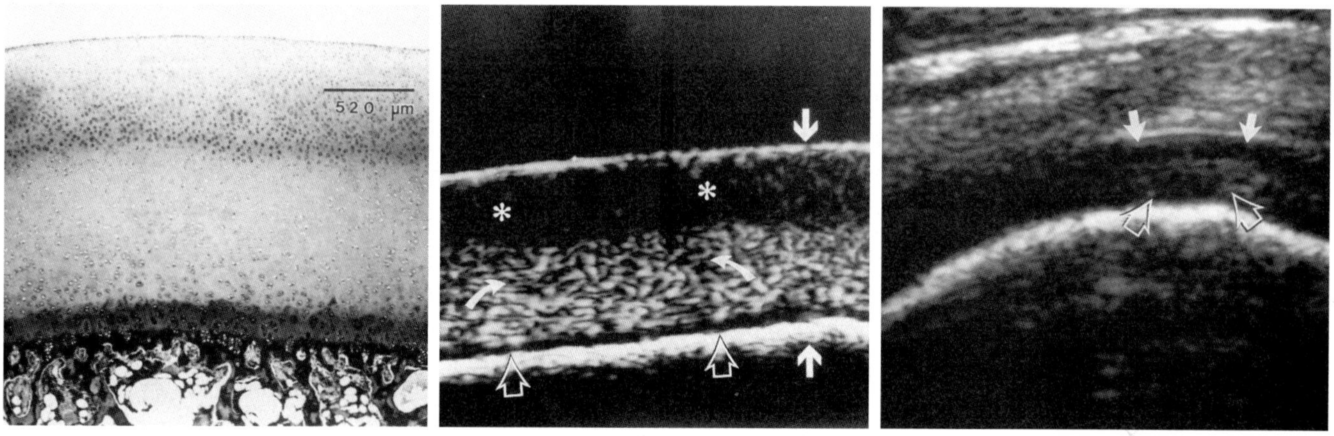

a. b. c.

Figure 20. Normal growth cartilage: US imaging. (a) Histologic image of growth cartilage from a 20-week-old pig. Note zonal anatomic features. (Safranin O stain; original magnification, ×40.) (Reprinted, with permission, from reference 72.) (b) Corresponding in vitro US image obtained by using a 50-MHz transducer shows three zones that appear—from superficial to deep—hypoechoic (*), hyperechoic (curved arrows), and anechoic (open arrows). Two hyperechoic lines (straight solid arrows) represent the water-cartilage interface and either an uncalcified-calcified cartilage or a cartilage–subchondral bone interface. (Reprinted, with permission, from reference 72.) (c) In vivo US image of the humeral growth cartilage obtained in a 6-year-old child with use of 9-MHz insonation frequency. Notice the hypoechoic superficial zone (solid arrows) and the moderately hyperechoic subjacent zone (open arrows). The appearance is similar to that shown in **b**, with the exception that the thin, hypoechoic deep zone is not visualized.

ten quite removed from the articular surface. There may be local thickening of fiber bundles that may be referred to as capsular or intrinsic ligaments (see below). In addition, some are reinforced by the attachments of tendons.

The synovial membrane (synovium) lines the joint space of synovial (diarthrodial) joints. Hyaline and fibrocartilaginous surfaces are devoid of synovial tissue. In addition, there is a transitional zone beginning a few millimeters from the peripheral extent of hyaline articular cartilage that is also devoid of synovium and often referred to as the "bare area." The inner synovial intima is formed by one or two layers of cells, whereas the more peripheral subintimal lamina consists of either loose connective tissue, fibrous tissue, or fat. The synovial membrane associated with these three tissues is therefore described as areolar, fibrous, or adipose. Vascular structures and lymphatics are also located deep to the lining cells.

Normal synovial fluid is clear or pale yellow and has a cell count of approximately 60 per milliliter. This fluid is produced by the synovial membrane, which also removes materials from the articular cavity via the subintimal capillaries and venules. The synovial fluid produces lubrication for the adjacent joint surfaces and is responsible for the nutrition of hyaline cartilage.

Other associated structures.—More complex synovial joints contain an articular disk or meniscus that is situated against the opposing hyaline cartilage surfaces. A disk divides the joint into two separate cavities, as is commonly observed within the sternoclavicular and distal radial ulnar joints. The meniscus, which represents an incomplete disk, is observed routinely in the knee joint and sometimes within the acro-

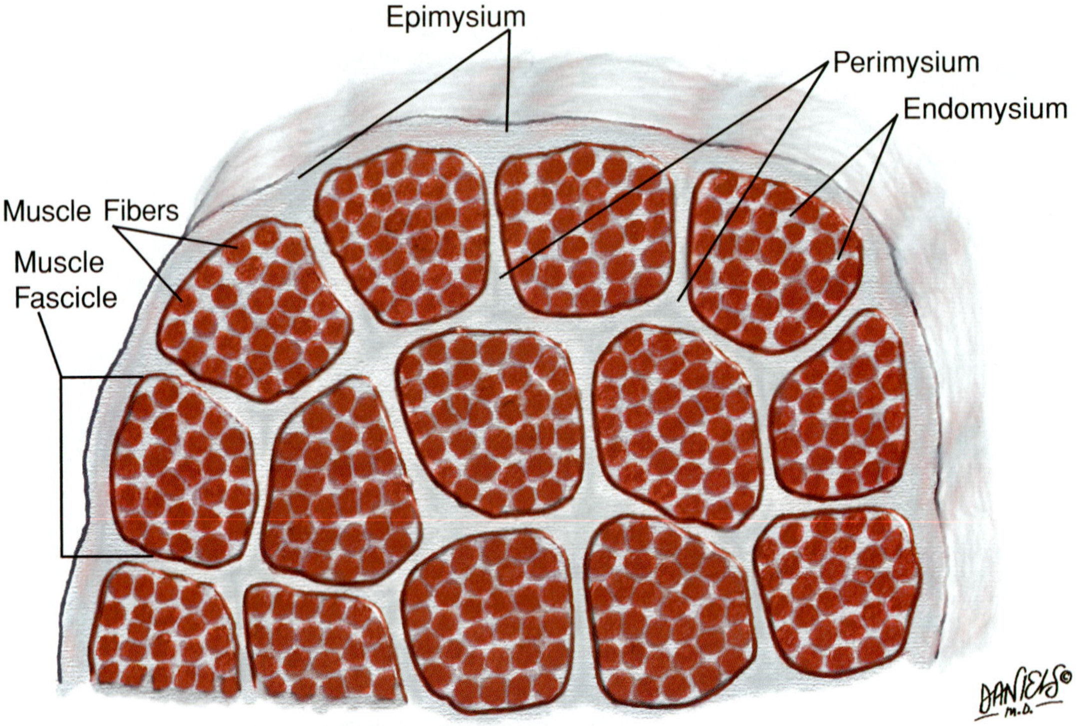

Figure 21. Sketch shows histologic organization of muscle tissue.

mioclavicular joint. These two structures are predominantly found in joints in which the opposing surfaces are relatively incongruous. At histologic examination, these structures consist of fibrocartilage, with the fibrous component usually predominating. They probably function to absorb shock, improve congruity, distribute weight, protect the articular margins, and aid in the spread of lubricating synovial fluid.

Labra are also predominantly fibrous, but unlike menisci, are not truly compressed between articular surfaces. Common examples include the glenoid and acetabular labra, which act both to deepen shallow joint sockets and spread joint lubricant.

Articular disks, menisci, and labra all have similar imaging appearances. These structures appear hypointense on MR images (Fig 3d, 3e) and hyperechoic on US scans (Fig 10b).

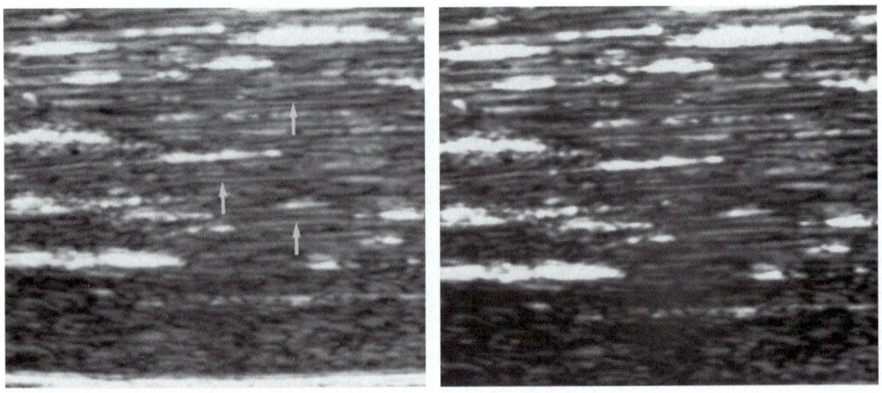

a. b.

Figure 22. Normal muscle anatomic features: US imaging. **(a)** Longitudinal US image of a portion of the biceps muscle obtained by using 9-MHz insonation frequency and 60-dB dynamic range shows innumerable hyperechoic lines consistent with perimysial tissue (arrows). **(b)** At 30 dB, the same region shows greater contrast. Excessive reduction in dynamic range may result in failure to depict subtle interfaces.

Muscles

Skeletal muscle fibers, which are long and cylindrical in structure, represent the cellular unit of muscle. Fibers are grouped together in bundles known as fasciculi and numerous fasciculi unite to form an individual muscle. The fibers vary in length and diameter depending on the muscle; fasciculi likewise may be either coarse (as in the case of large muscles) or very fine (as in the case of small muscles that coordinate precise movement). Individual fibers are separated by endomysium, fasciculi are segregated by the more substantial perimysium, and the entire muscle is surrounded by the epimysium (Fig 21).

Muscles may be categorized on the basis of fascicular orientation, which reflects gross muscle shape and function. A parallel arrangement is seen in quadrilateral muscles (eg, thyrohyoid) and straplike muscles (eg, sternohyoid, sartorius), in which fibers often course nearly the full length of the muscle. A similar arrangement is seen in the rectus abdominis, but in this instance, the muscle is subdivided by tendinous intersections and fibers course only within segments. In fusiform muscles, the fasciculi become nearly parallel in the midportion but converge toward the tendon. An oblique fascicular arrangement is one in which the fascicular orientation is angled in relation to the line of traction. These include triangular (eg, adductor longus), unipennate or semipennate (eg, flexor pollicis longus), bipennate (eg, rectus femoris), and multipennate (eg, deltoid) muscles. Bipennate muscles are those that have a single central tendon, whereas multipennate muscles

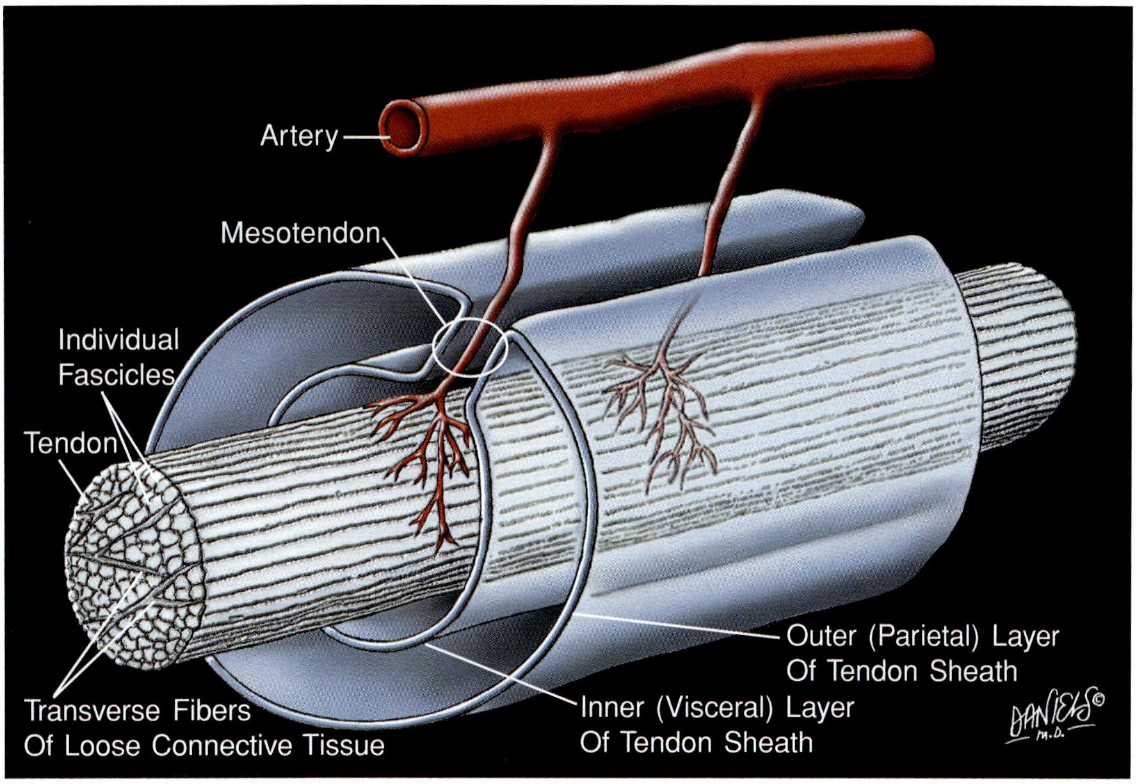

Figure 24. Sketch shows normal tendon and tendon sheath anatomic features. (Modified and reprinted, with permission, from reference 78.)

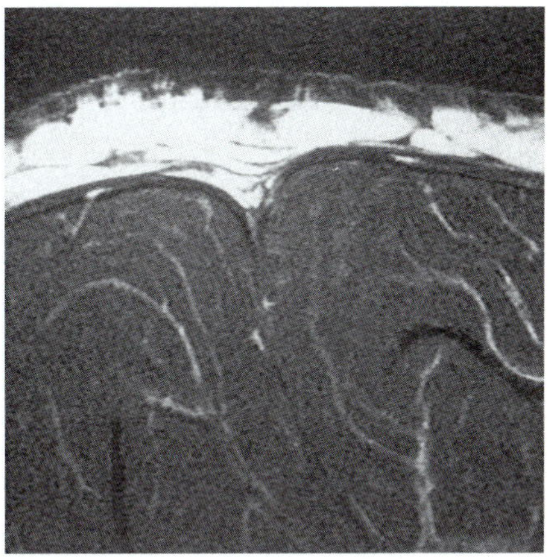

Figure 23. Normal muscle: MR imaging. T1-weighted axial image (500/32, 3-mm section thickness, 4-cm FOV, 512 × 256 matrix, four signals acquired, imaging time of 8 minutes 36 seconds) obtained of leg muscle with use of a 1-inch planar coil. Note that, compared with the US image, the MR image is capable of only demonstrating coarse intramuscular structure, even if a high-resolution technique is used.

possess several tendons coursing through the muscle substance. A spiral arrangement of fascicles is noted in muscles that curve or literally spiral between their origin and insertion (eg, pectoralis major, latissimus, supinator muscles).

US can demonstrate intramuscular structure to the fascicular level. The relatively hypoechoic fasciculi are clearly demarcated by echogenic perimysial septa (76) (Fig 22). MR imaging, by comparison, is able to depict only coarse intramuscular structure (Fig 23).

Tendons

Tendons are critical components of the musculotendinous unit, acting to connect muscle to bone. The tensile strength is reported to be similar to that of bone; a tendon 1 cm^2 in cross section can support 600–1,000 kg (1).

Tendons are composed of 68% water, which is largely contained in an extracellular matrix (77). Collagen composes approximately 70% of the dry weight of the tendon and is represented by the highly ordered, type I variety. Tropocollagen units associate to form fibrils, parallel fibrils unite to form fibers (the basic tendon unit), and fibers are grouped together in fascicles (Fig 24) (78). Collagen fibers are invested by the endotenon, fascicles by the peritenon, and the entire tendon by the epitenon, which is contiguous with both the peritenon and endotenon (77,79). Some tendons possess a paratenon, which invests the epitenon; in these tendons, the paratenon and epitenon may together be referred to as the peritendon. Elastin, which is a minor component of tendon, confers some flexibility.

Collagen fibers and fibrils appear somewhat wavy in the resting state, becoming straight when the tendon is stretched to 4% beyond its resting length (79,80). Tendon fibers are predominantly oriented parallel to one another at light microscopy examination. Jozsa et al (79), using electron microscopy, demonstrated a more complex arrangement. In their work, fibers were also seen to course horizontally and transversely, and the longitudinal fibrils formed spirals. This complex configuration may protect the tendon attachment sites (81).

Synovial tendon sheaths invest tendons that course beneath ligamentous bands and retinacula. They are composed of two layers: an inner visceral layer that is attached by loose connective tissue to the underlying tendon and an external parietal layer that is contiguous with adjacent periosteum or connective tissue. In actuality, the sheath is invaginated by the tendon, so that the visceral and parietal layers are typically connected by a mesotendon that provides a route for the vascular supply (Fig 24). The cells lining the sheath are identical to those that line synovium (82). Those tendons lacking a true sheath, such as the Achilles tendon, are instead invested by a peritenon.

Tendon vascular supply varies as to specific anatomic region and ten-

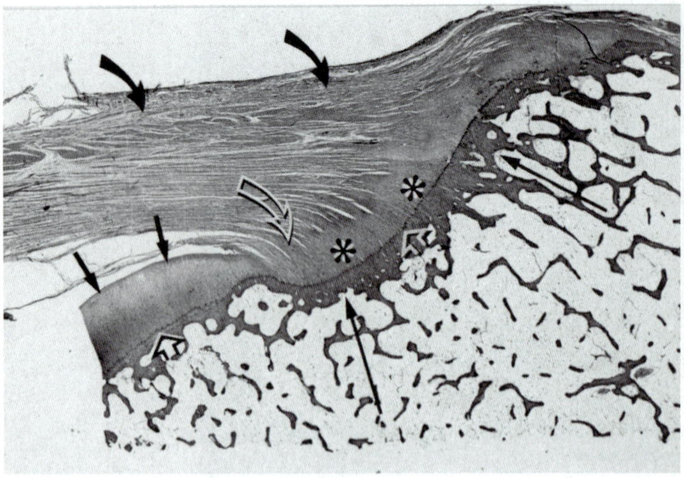

a.

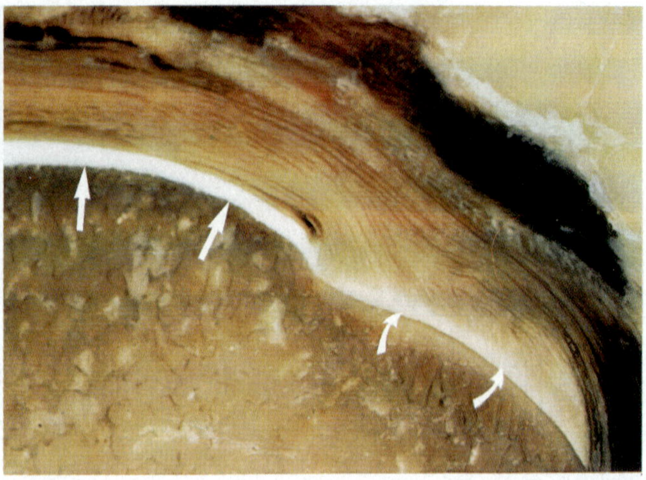

b.

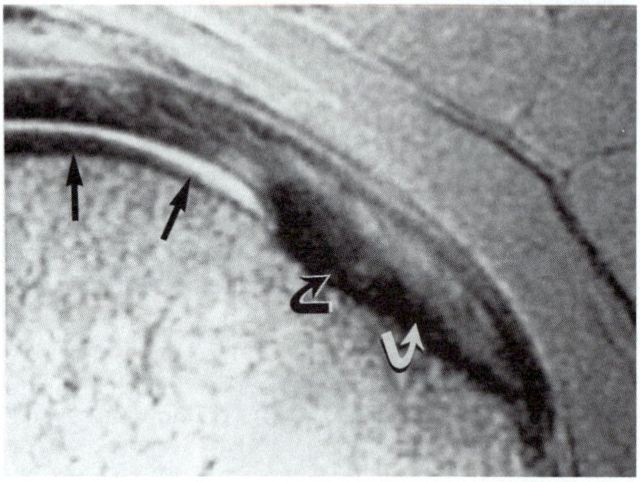

c.

Figure 25. Fibrocartilaginous insertion of tendon-rotator cuff. **(a)** Photomicrograph of a coronal histologic section shows hyaline cartilage (short solid arrows), rotator cuff tendon (curved solid arrows), subchondral bone (long solid arrows), fibrocartilaginous insertion (*), and tidemark (open straight arrows). Note that the hyaline cartilage and fibrocartilage appear similar and that the more proximal cuff fibers curve toward their insertion site (open curved arrow), whereas the more distal fibers insert at a more acute angle. (Hematoxylin-eosin stain; original magnification, ×9.) (Reprinted, with permission, from reference 84.) **(b)** Photograph of coronal cryomicrotome section obtained in a 37-year-old cadaver shows similar findings. Note that the hyaline articular cartilage appears bright white (straight arrows), whereas fibrocartilage has a paler appearance (curved arrows). **(c)** T1-weighted coronal MR image (600/38, 1-mm section thickness, 5-cm FOV, 256 × 256 matrix, four signals acquired, imaging time of 20 minutes 32 seconds) corresponding to **b.** Note that fibrocartilage appears relatively hypointense (curved arrows) as compared with the more heterogeneous hyaline cartilage (straight arrows).

don type. Most "round" tendons derive their blood supply from the paratenon, entering the substance at intervals along the tendon length. "Flat" tendons, such as the rotator cuff constituents, are supplied primarily by vessels coursing longitudinally along the entire length of the tendon (83). In their work on cuff vascularity, Rathbun and Macnab (83) discovered radical differences in the blood supply of the supraspinatus tendon as compared with that of the remaining three cuff constituents (subscapularis, teres minor, and infraspinatus tendon). Unlike the latter tendons, the supraspinatus was found to have a large, relatively avascular zone, which in some specimens was located 1 cm away from the insertion onto the greater tuberosity, whereas in others it extended right to the insertion site. This zone was found in all cadaveric shoulder specimens in their series, the youngest of which were under 20 years of age.

Tendon configurations may be relatively "simple," being derived from one muscle, or relatively "complex," being derived from two or more muscles. Examples of the former include the tibialis posterior, tibialis anterior, and hand flexor tendons, whereas examples of the latter include the Achilles, quadriceps, and the rotator cuff tendons. Sesamoid bones, which may be either osseous or cartilaginous, are found in many tendons that are closely applied to an osseous surface.

Tendon attachments to bone (entheses) can be categorized as fibrous and fibrocartilaginous (84–86). The histologic mode of attachment has been related to tendon mobility, the tendon fiber–to-bone angle, and the presence or absence of an overlying retinaculum. Tendons that have a uniplanar motion and attach to bone at an acute angle—such as the phalanges of the foot—have fibrous attachments. Retinacula redirect the course of underlying tendons, maintaining an acute angle in relation to the bony attachment site; examples include the peroneus brevis, tibialis posterior, and tibialis anterior tendons (86). Those tendons that control motion in more than one plane and insert onto bone nearly perpendicular to the cortex, such as the Achilles

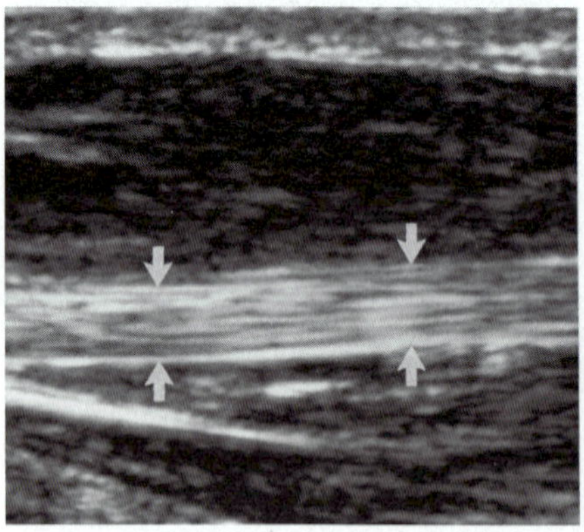

Figure 26. Normal tendon anatomic features: US imaging. Longitudinal US image of the flexor pollicis longus tendon obtained with use of 9-MHz insonation frequency shows numerous echogenic intratendinous interfaces, resulting in a "fibrillar" appearance. The tendon measures approximately 3 mm in diameter (arrows).

and supraspinatus tendons, have thick fibrocartilaginous attachments, which are believed to minimize tendon fraying. The fibrocartilage at these entheses is derived from the embryonic bone rudiment that re-

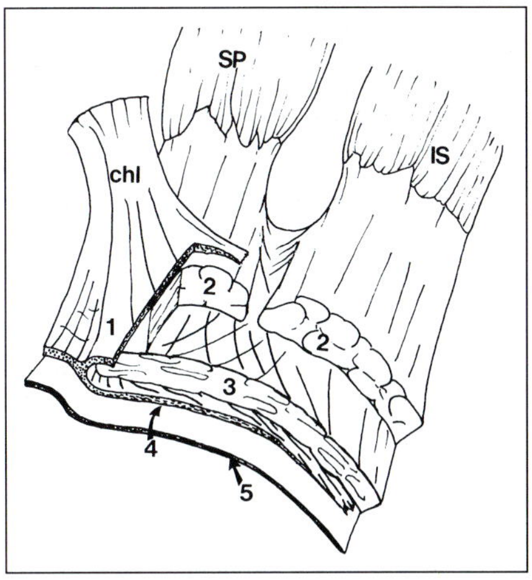

a.

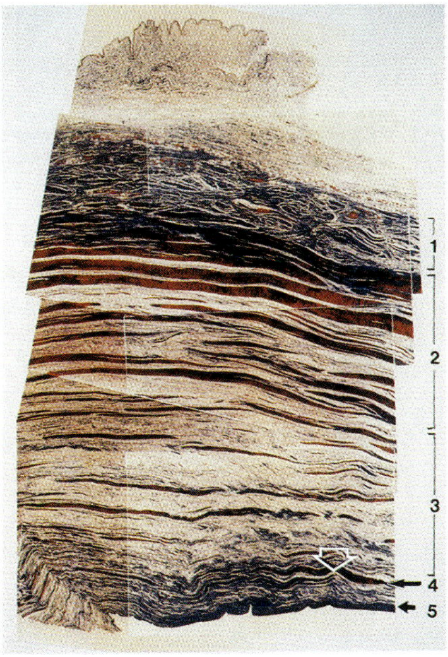

b.

Figure 28. Complex tendon anatomic features: rotator cuff. **(a)** Sketch of the rotator cuff shows the supraspinatus (*SP*), infraspinatus (*IS*), coracohumeral ligament (*chl*), and five layers of the cuff (*1–5*). (Reprinted, with permission, from reference 90.) **(b)** Composite histologic image shows the five cuff layers (*1–5*). (Hematoxylin-eosin stain; original magnification, ×9.) (Reprinted, with permission, from reference 90.)

mains after endochondral ossification has ceased in either epiphyseal or apophyseal centers. The attachment possesses the following four discrete layers, from superficial to deep: tendon, uncalcified fibrocartilage, calcified fibrocartilage, and bone. As in hyaline cartilage, the uncalcified and calcified zones are demarcated by a tidemark (Fig 25).

Both US and MR imaging are capable of showing exquisite intratendinous structure. With the former modality, an echogenic "fibrillar pattern" is routinely observed in all ten-

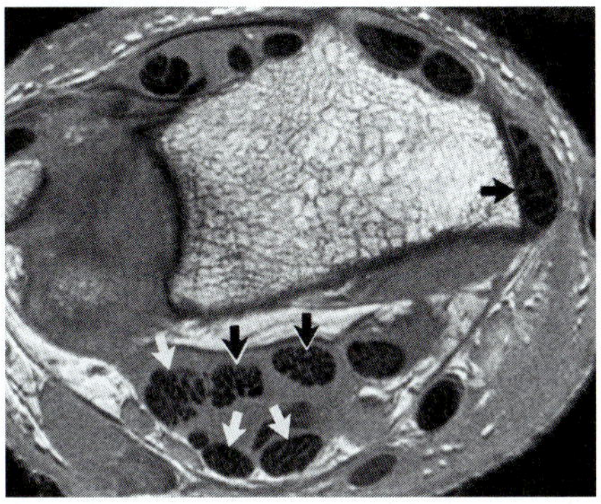

Figure 27. Normal tendon anatomic features: MR imaging. Axial T1-weighted MR image (550/35, 2-mm section thickness, 8-cm FOV, 512 × 512 matrix, two signals acquired, imaging time of 37 minutes 46 seconds) obtained of a cadaveric wrist shows internal interfaces within numerous tendons (arrows). Such interfaces are uncommonly seen on clinical images and are never seen to a degree comparable to this image, or the preceding clinical US images.

dons with use of state-of-the-art equipment (Fig 26). With the latter modality, visualization of structural detail within the predominantly hypointense tendon is dependent both on the size of the tendon being imaged and the technique. Whereas intratendinous structure is easily appreciated within the Achilles tendon by using routine clinical MR parameters, detail is seldom demonstrable in smaller tendons unless high-resolution technique is employed (Fig 27). The choice of TE greatly affects tendon signal intensity and potentially might reveal subtler tendon abnormalities (87).

Two clinically relevant and prototypic "complex" tendons are worthy of more detailed review. The Achilles tendon is the largest tendon in the human body. It arises from the gastrocnemius and soleus aponeuroses and inserts onto the calcaneus. At its cranial end, the gastrocnemius contribution is located within the posterior aspect of the tendon, whereas the soleus contribution is located anteriorly. These contributions then twist as the tendon courses inferiorly, and in the most common anatomic variant, the gastrocnemius contribution is located posterolaterally and the soleus contribution is located predominantly anteriorly (88). Bertolotto et al (89) using 10–15-mHz transducers, showed different intratendinous structural patterns that they attribute to interfaces between these two portions.

The rotator cuff is remarkably complex, composed of capsule, ligaments, and the cuff tendons proper (90). The tendons, which include the supraspinatus, infraspinatus, subscapularis, and teres minor, "splay out and interdigitate to form a common, continuous insertion on the humerus" (90). The fibrocartilaginous insertion site is thickest medially where collagen fibers are oriented nearly perpendicular to bone but becomes gradually thinner proceeding laterally to the edge of the greater tuberosity where fibers are practically parallel to bone. The subscapularis and supraspinatus tendon join to form a sheath that surrounds the biceps tendon at the proximal part of the bicipital groove.

Histologic analysis of the supraspinatus and infraspinatus tendons and adjacent structures reveals a complex composed of five layers (Fig 28) (90). The most superficial layer measures approximately 1 mm thick and is composed of superficial fibers of the coracohumeral ligament. Layer 2 is 3–5 mm thick and is composed of closely packed, parallel supraspinatus and infraspinatus tendon bundles. Layer 3 is approximately 3 mm thick and is composed of smaller tendon fascicles that intersect one another at an angle of roughly 45°. Layer 4 is composed of predominantly extracapsular loose connective tissue that anteriorly becomes continuous with the deep aspect of the coracohumeral ligament. Layer 5 is approximately 1–2 mm thick and is composed of the capsule. The capsule deep to the supraspinatus and infraspinatus tendons is thickened by a strip of tissue that courses perpendicular to the long axis of the tendon fibers. This region is referred to as the "rotator cable"; the reportedly thinner cuff tissue lateral to this region is termed the "rotator crescent" (91). This recent anatomic work has potentially great clinicopathologic relevance. First, rotator cuff tears are frequently manifested by delamination, which may be attributable to the multilayer composition of the cuff. Second, patients who are "cable dominant" (ie, those who possess a well-developed rotator cable) may incur a full-thickness tear of the rotator cuff yet retain much of their range of motion.

Both MR imaging and US are capable of depicting the structural complexity and heterogeneity of the rotator cuff. However, as in the case of "simple" tendons, US better displays the fibrillar nature of the constituent tendons (Figs 29,30). The spatial resolution of US will exceed that of MR unless small surface coils are used

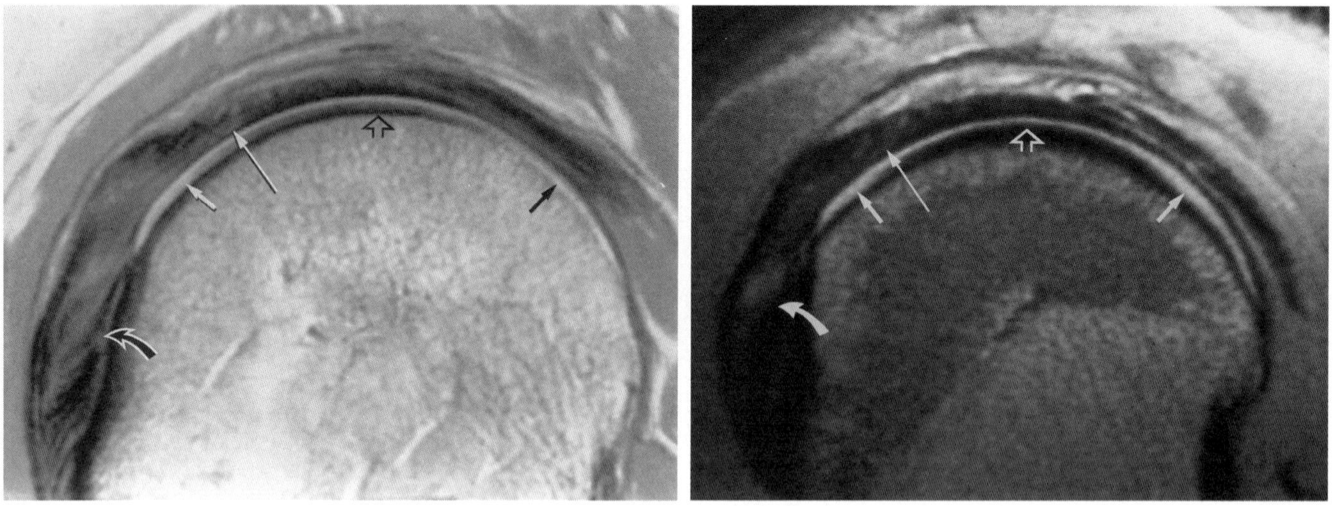

a. b.

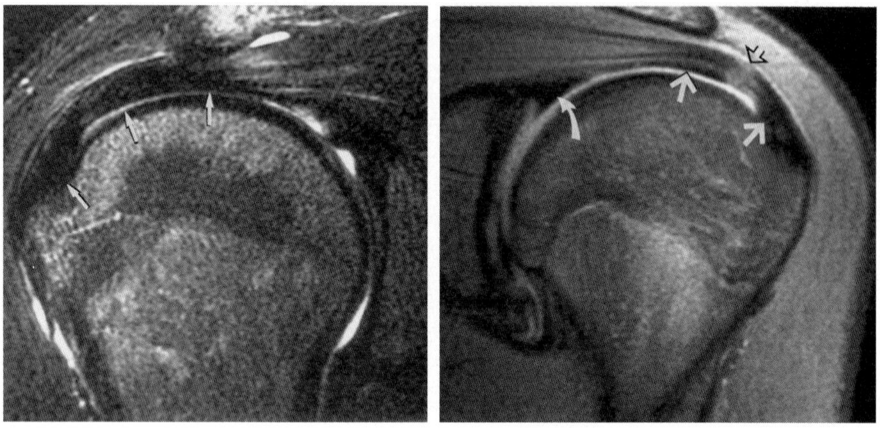

c. d.

Figure 29. Normal rotator cuff: MR imaging. **(a)** Sagittal T1-weighted MR image (600/28, 2-mm section thickness, 6-cm FOV, 256 × 256 matrix, two signals acquired, imaging time of 10 minutes 17 seconds) of the same cadaveric shoulder as in Figure 25c, obtained with anterior oriented to the left, shows heterogeneity within the rotator cuff that may, in part, be attributed to its complex anatomic features as well as magic angle effects. Long solid arrow = dominant supraspinatus contribution, curved solid arrow = subscapularis contribution. In addition, note heterogeneity of the humeral hyaline cartilage attributable to individual laminae at the 12-o'clock position (open arrow), with relative homogeneity of the cartilage at the 2- and 10-o'clock positions attributable to magic angle effects (short solid arrows). **(b)** Sagittal proton-density–weighted fat-suppressed fast SE MR image (1,500/32, 3.5-mm section thickness, 8-cm FOV, 256 × 192 matrix, ETL of two, two signals acquired, imaging time of 4 minutes 51 sections) obtained in vivo in an asymptomatic volunteer with use of a single 3-inch planar coil shows findings analogous to those in the cadaveric specimen (arrows are as described in **a**). **(c)** Coronal T2-weighted image (3,000/105, 3.5-mm section thickness, 6-cm FOV, 256 × 192 matrix, ETL of four, four signals acquired, 12.8-kHz bandwidth, imaging time of 9 minutes 42 seconds) obtained in a different asymptomatic volunteer with use of a 3-inch planar coil shows superior definition of the rotator cuff (arrows) and adjacent tissues. Imaging time using an 8-cm FOV and two signals acquired will be less than 5 minutes (assuming the other parameters to be constant). **(d)** Coronal proton-density–weighted fat-suppressed fast SE MR image (1,500/29, 3.5-mm section thickness, 10-cm FOV, 256 × 192 matrix, two signals acquired, imaging time of 4 minutes 54 seconds) obtained in a patient with use of a 5¼-inch curved planar coil shows the rotator cuff (straight arrows) and superior labrum (curved arrow) to good advantage. Note focal hyperintensity attributable to magic angle effects (open arrow).

and appropriate imaging parameters prescribed.

Their highly ordered collagenous structure renders tendons anisotropic and therefore extremely susceptible to artifact when imaging both with US and MR imaging. The angle between the transducer face and the tendinous surface is absolutely critical; an angle that deviates from the perpendicular will cause the tendon to appear artifactually hypoechoic (Fig 30c) (92). Interestingly, Lehtinen et al (93) have proposed that angulation may be useful to distinguish early tendinitis from artifactual hypoechogenicity. Tendons that course at or near the magic angle of 55° in relation to B_0 become artifactually hyperintense on MR images because of T2 augmentation (Fig 29d) (94–97).

Tendons appear as hyperattenuating structures on CT images and may be initially mistaken for vessels. Though CT has been used in the past for diagnosis of tendinous abnormality, it has been largely supplanted by MR imaging and US.

Ligaments

Ligaments, like tendons, are composed of dense connective tissue. Unlike tendons, however, there is much more variability as to the relative amounts of collagen, elastin, and even fibrocartilage (98–100). There is also variability in blood supply; for example, the anterior cruciate ligament is relatively poorly vascularized as compared with the medial collateral ligament. The functional importance of these differences is a subject of debate.

Anatomically, ligaments may be divided into three types according to location. Capsular ligaments are those that blend with the joint capsule; examples include the deep medial ligamentous component of the medial collateral ligament of the knee, the glenohumeral ligaments of the shoulder, and the anterior talofibular ligament of the ankle. Intraarticular ligaments are those that reside entirely within a joint; the best example is the anterior cruciate ligament of the knee. Extraarticular and extracapsular ligaments are those that reside superficial to the joint proper; an example is the lateral collateral ligament of the knee.

Milz et al (101) have examined cadaveric lateral ankle ligaments by using a 13-mHz insonation frequency.

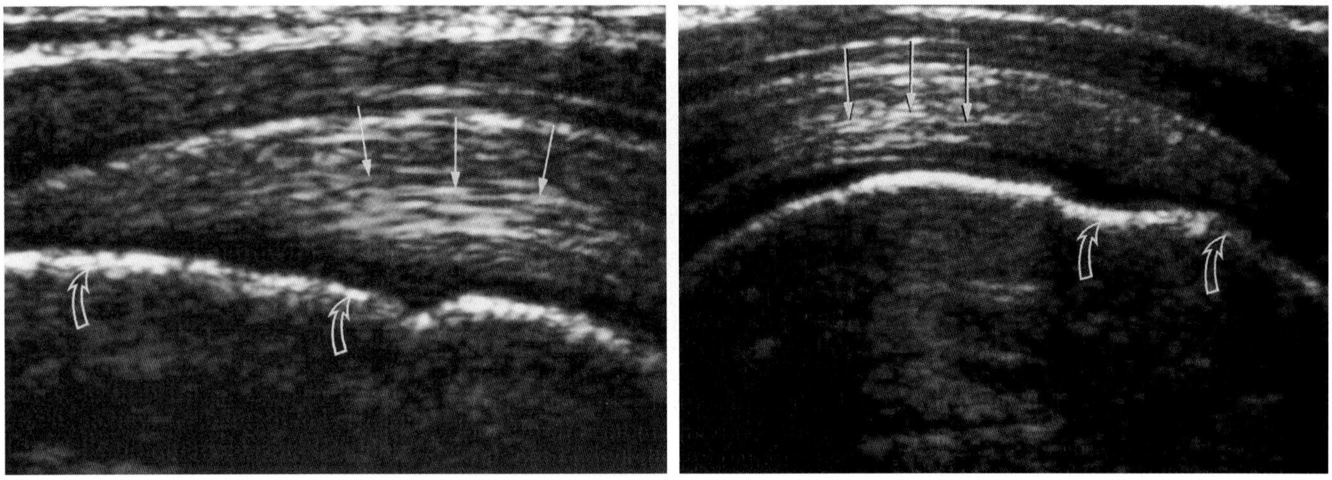

a. b.

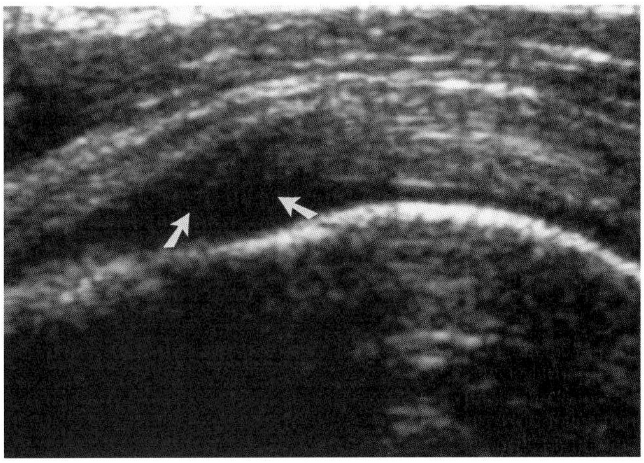

c.

Figure 30. Normal rotator cuff: US imaging. **(a)** Sagittal US image of the rotator cuff, with anterior oriented to the left and obtained with 9-mHz insonation frequency, shows a complex, fibrillar pattern within the echogenic cuff (straight arrows) and the greater tuberosity insertion site (curved arrows). **(b)** Oblique coronal US image of the rotator cuff obtained with 9-MHz insonation frequency shows the fibrillar pattern within the echogenic rotator cuff (straight arrows) and the greater tuberosity insertion site (curved arrows). Note the small imaging FOV in these images obtained with minimum depth. **(c)** Oblique coronal US image obtained with 9-MHz insonation frequency shows an artifactual hypoechoic region (arrows) attributable to tendon anisotropy.

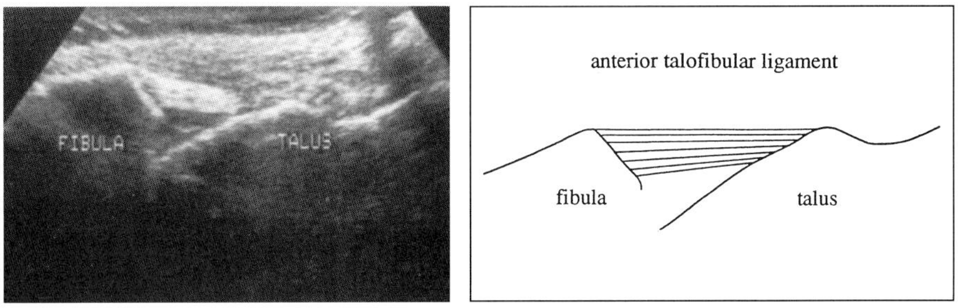

a. b.

Figure 31. Normal ligament: US imaging. **(a)** Axial US image of a cadaveric ankle with use of 13-MHz insonation frequency shows the striated anterior talofibular ligament coursing between the fibula and talus. (Reprinted, with permission, from reference 101.) **(b)** Corresponding sketch of the anterior talofibular ligament. (Reprinted, with permission, from reference 101.)

These investigators found the ligaments to possess anisotropic properties analogous to tendons. When the sound beam was oriented perpendicular to the course of the ligaments, they appeared as markedly hyperechoic, "parallel-layered structures" (Fig 31). As the angle of insonation became more acute, however, the appearance became increasingly hypoechoic.

Ligaments generally appear either striated or homogeneously hypointense on MR images. Examples of the former include the extrinsic radiocarpal, deep deltoid, posterior talofibular, and anterior cruciate ligaments (Fig 32a, 32b). Examples of the latter include the anterior talofibular ligament and superficial deltoid ligaments (Fig 32c). It is reasonable to assume that those of the second group might appear similarly striated provided one could achieve sufficient spatial resolution.

CT portrays ligaments as relatively hyperattenuating structures, similar to tendons. Intraligamentous structure is occasionally seen.

Neurovascular

Vessel.—Three zones are observed in all vessels with the exception of capillaries and sinusoids. The tunica intima, situated adjacent to the lumen, is composed of a single layer of endothelial cells and underlying, longitudinally arranged subendothelial connective tissue. Intimal thickness varies with age, being almost imperceptible in children, more conspicuous in young adults, and quite thick in older adults. The tunica media is fibromuscular in composition and circumferentially oriented. The tunica adventitia is predominantly longitudinally oriented and blends with the surrounding connective tissue. Both the overall and individual tunic thicknesses vary as to the type and location of the vessel. With respect to overall caliber, muscular arteries are thicker than elastic arteries and the latter are similar or thicker than veins.

Three discrete sonographic interfaces are generally described within arteries. These interfaces consist of a thin, echogenic layer that may be attributable to impedance mismatch or the internal elastic membrane rather than the intima per se; a thicker, hypoechoic medial layer; and the echogenic adventitial layer (Fig 33).

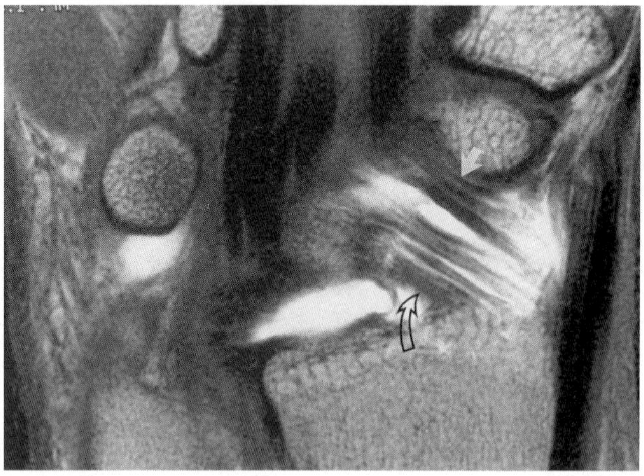

a.

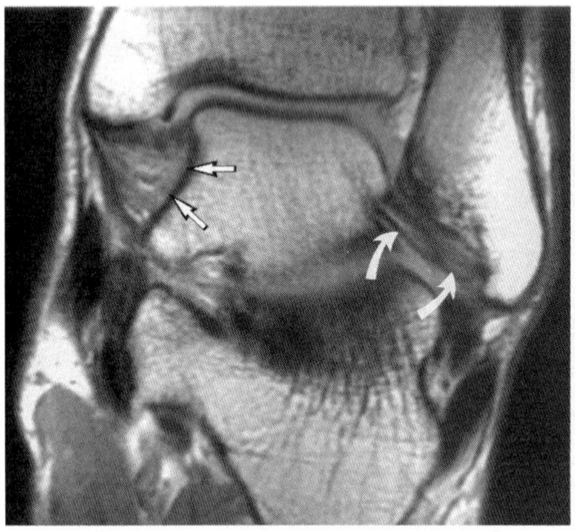

b.

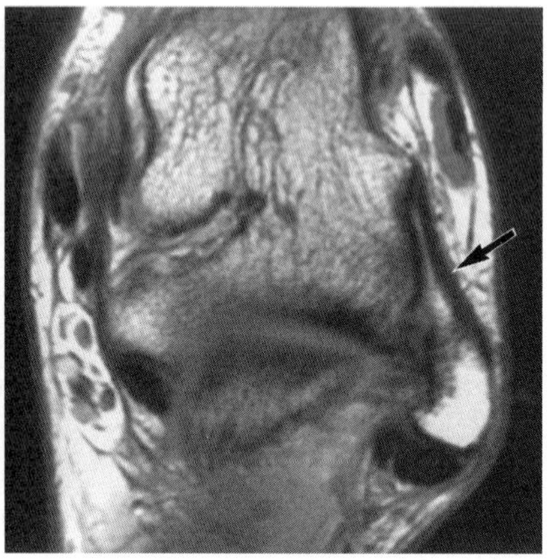

c.

Figure 32. Normal ligaments: MR imaging. **(a)** T1-weighted coronal MR image (500/51, 2-mm section thickness, 8-cm FOV, 512 × 512 matrix, two signals acquired, imaging time of 26 minutes) obtained through the volar aspect of a cadaveric wrist after intraarticular injection of a gadolinium contrast material and with use of a solenoid coil shows striations within the radioscaphocapitate (solid arrow) and long radiolunate (open arrow) ligaments. **(b)** Coronal proton-density–weighted fast SE MR image (1,500/24, 3-mm section thickness, 9-cm FOV, 256 × 256 matrix, two signals acquired, ETL of two, imaging time of 6 minutes 33 seconds) obtained of the ankle in a normal volunteer with use of two 3-inch loops with phased-array technique demonstrates striations within the deep deltoid (straight arrows) and posterior talofibular (curved arrows) ligaments. **(c)** Axial proton-density–weighted fast SE image (1,500/24, 3-mm section thickness, 9-cm FOV, 256 × 256 matrix, ETL of two, two signals acquired, imaging time of 6 minutes 33 seconds) obtained in the same volunteer shows a relatively homogeneous anterior talofibular ligament (arrow).

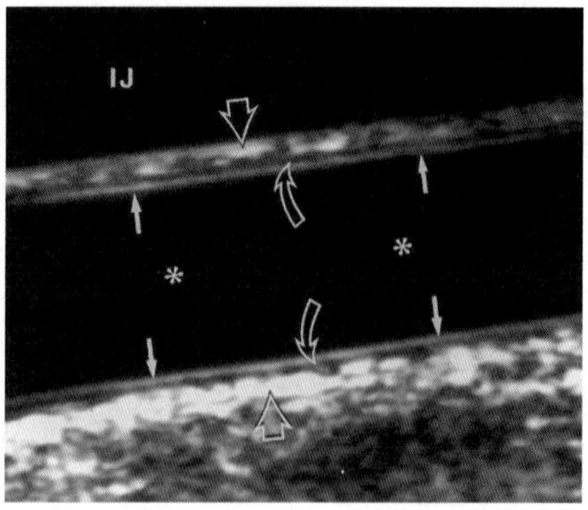

▲
Figure 33. Normal arterial anatomic features: US imaging. Longitudinal US image of the common carotid artery obtained in a 6-year-old child with use of 9-MHz insonation frequency shows the hypoechoic lumen (*), adjacent internal jugular vein (*IJ*), echogenic interface between blood and the inner arterial wall (solid arrows), the hypoechoic tunica media (open curved arrows), and the echogenic tunica adventitia (open straight arrows).

Martin et al (102), in an in vitro investigation of excised human femoral arteries, compared US images (obtained with use of a 42-MHz probe yielding 40 × 280-μm in-plane spatial resolution) with both MR images (obtained with use of a 1.5-T unit, local gradient insert, and small solenoid coil yielding 156 × 156-μm in-plane spatial resolution) and corresponding histologic sections. The sonographically hypoechoic tunica media corresponded to a hyperintense region and the echogenic adventitia to a hypointense region on T2-weighted images (Fig 34). The MR signal intensity of flowing blood is variable and dependent on both flow dynamics and the choice of imaging sequence. MR angiographic techniques can be successfully adapted to imaging of small parts (Fig 35). Both color Doppler and power Doppler imaging are capable of showing submillimeter vessels (103,104).

Nerve.—Peripheral nerve trunks are composed of fasciculi, which are in turn composed of fibers. The trunks are surrounded by epineurium, the fasciculi by perineurium, and the fibers by endoneurium. The size, number, and pattern of fasciculi depend on the individual nerve, distance from site of origin, and the amount of pressure to which the nerve is subjected.

Peripheral nerves exhibit characteristic sonographic features (Fig 36). Silvestri et al (105), using 10–15-MHz insonation frequency, showed linear, parallel hypoechoic regions separated by hyperechoic bands. The former were hypothesized to represent neuronal fascicles and the latter perineurium. A much smaller number of fascicles was demonstrated on US images in comparison to the actual number as established with light microscopy, which was attributed to coalescence of fascicles and/or to some of the fascicles being oriented obliquely in relation to the ultrasound beam.

MR imaging similarly shows internal neural structure, though it too cannot precisely replicate fascicular anatomic features (106,107) (Fig 37). Small neural and perineural masses are demonstrable, a notable example being a Morton (interdigital) neuroma (Fig 38) (19).

Other Tissues

Fascia, aponeuroses, retinacula.—According to the textbook, *Anatomy of the Human Body* by Henry Gray (1), "fascia is a term so vague that it signifies little more than collections of connective tissue large enough to be visible to the unaided eye." Aponeuroses are composed of compact collagen fibers arranged in several layers. The constituent fasciculi are arranged parallel to one another within a given layer but differ in inclination from those in adjacent laminae. Aponeuroses are directly or indirectly attached to muscle. Retinacula represent localized transverse thickenings of the deep fascia that are anchored at both ends to underlying bony prominences. These function to retain un-

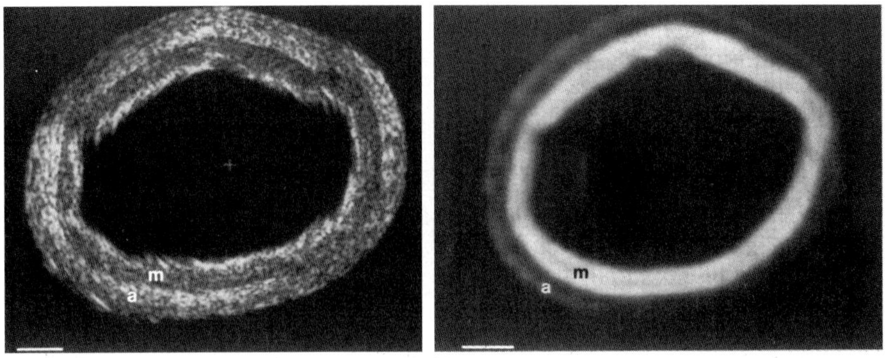

a. b.

Figure 34. Normal arterial anatomic features: high-resolution MR imaging versus US imaging. **(a)** Axial US image of an excised femoral artery obtained with 42-mHz insonation frequency shows the hypoechoic tunica media (*m*) and hyperechoic tunica adventitia (*a*). (Reprinted, with permission, from reference 102.) **(b)** Corresponding T2-weighted axial MR image (2,000/16, 2-mm section thickness, 4-cm FOV, 256 × 256 matrix, imaging time of <10 minutes) obtained of the same vessel with use of a local gradient coil with a 42-mm solenoid coil shows the hyperintense tunica media (*m*) and the hypointense tunica adventitia (*a*). (Reprinted, with permission, from reference 102.)

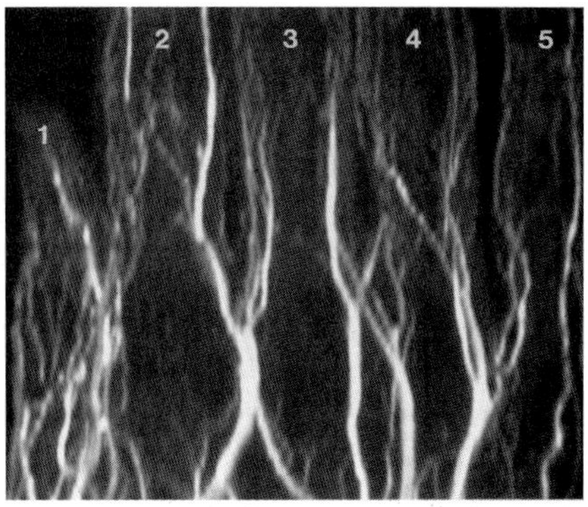

Figure 35. Small parts: MR angiography. Collapsed coronal, reformatted maximum intensity projection image of the hand from a patient with vascular disease (axial source images: 39/8.7, 64 1.5-mm sections, 10-cm FOV, 256 × 192 matrix, one signal acquired, imaging time of 9 minutes 45 seconds) obtained with a solenoid coil shows arterial vessels. Numbers *1–5* indicate the digits, beginning with the thumb.

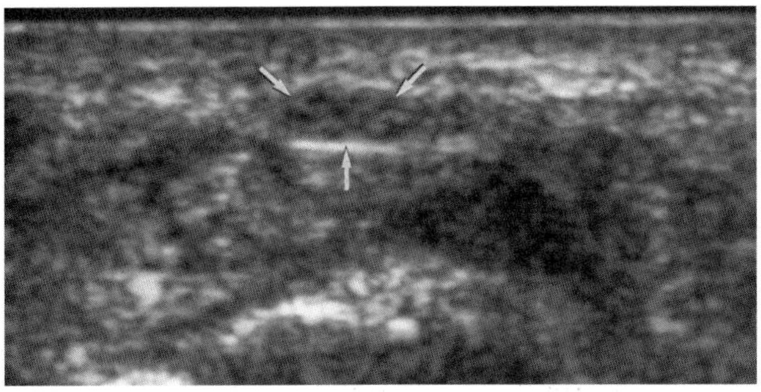

◀**Figure 36.** Normal neural tissue: US imaging. Axial US image of the wrist with 9-MHz insonation frequency shows normal median nerve that displays distinct heterogeneity (arrows). This has been likened to the appearance of the normal ovary.

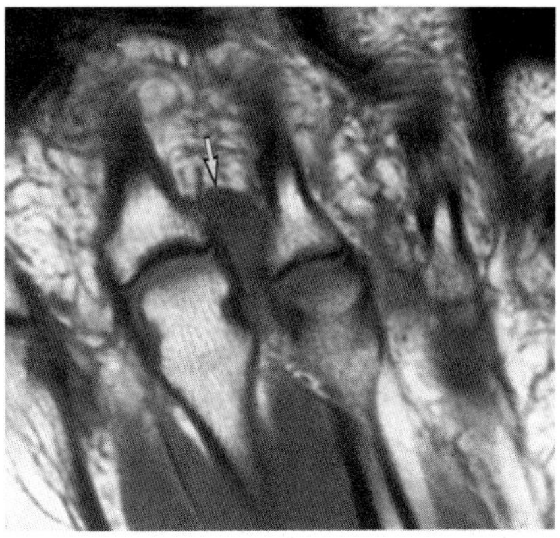

Figure 38. Morton interdigital neuroma: MR imaging. Axial T1-weighted image of the forefoot (500/27, 3-mm section thickness, 8-cm FOV, 256 × 256 matrix, two signals acquired, imaging time of 8 minutes 44 seconds) obtained of a forefoot with use of a 4-inch solenoid coil shows a neuroma at the second web space (arrow); the neuroma measured a few millimeters in diameter.

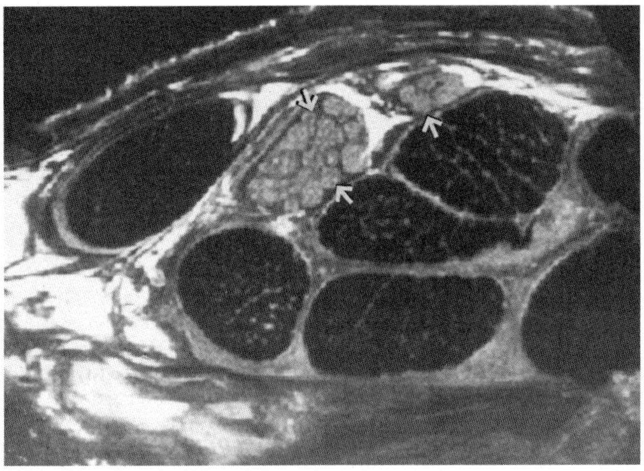

Figure 37. Normal neural tissue: MR imaging. Axial T1-weighted image (500/28, 1-mm section thickness, 3-cm FOV, 320 × 320 matrix, 12 signals acquired, imaging time of 32 minutes) obtained of a cadaveric wrist with use of a 33-mm solenoid coil on a 3-T MR unit shows the internal anatomic features of the median nerve. Numerous neural bundles, representing fascicles or groups of fascicles, are depicted (arrows). This "fascicular" appearance can be seen (though with less detail) on high-resolution clinical MR images. (Reprinted, with permission, from reference 107.)

derlying tendons, thereby preventing bowstring deformity during normal activity. Fascia, aponeuroses, and retinacula appear hypointense with all MR sequences unless oriented at or near the magic angle, hyperechoic with US, and hyperattenuating with CT.

Skin.—Skin composes approximately 8% of the total body mass. It consists of 70% water and varies in thickness from 1.5 to 4.0 mm. The two major categories of skin are thick (hairless) skin, which is found on the palms, soles of the feet, and on the flexor aspects of digits, and thin (hairy) skin, which covers the great majority of the body.

The two chief layers are the epidermis and dermis, which are distinct from the underlying hypodermis (Fig 39). The epidermis is further divided into the superficial stratum corneum and the deeper germinative zone, the latter consisting of the stratum basale, stratum spinosum, and the stratum granulosum. The stratum corneum, which is composed of closely packed layers of flattened, dead cells, is most developed in thick skin. The collagen-rich dermis consists of two layers, the papillary and reticular dermis. The former is located immediately deep to the epidermis, its papillary surface interdigitating with the base of the epidermis. The latter is the thicker of the two layers, and its collagen fibers are also thicker than those in the papillary layer. Additional structures of interest include hair follicles, sebaceous glands, arrector pili muscles, and sweat glands. While all of these structures can be found in hairy skin, only the last named is observed in thick, hairless skin.

Numerous investigators have studied the in vivo MR characteristics of normal skin (16,18,26,31,32, 108). All investigators employed small RF coils; some investigators also used local gradient coils to further improve spatial resolution and decrease the TE (26,31,32). The epidermis appears relatively hyperintense, the dermis hypointense, and the largely fatty subcutaneous hypodermis hyperintense (Fig 40). Since the epidermis and dermis have similar water content, Richard et al (32) believe the contrast in signal intensity is attributable to differences in proton density. The signal intensity of the upper dermis changes with aging, presumably due to an increase in water content and concomitant decrease in collagen and proteoglycan content. The thickened stratum corneum can be discerned as a discrete layer on both the palm and heel but cannot be visualized on thin, hairy skin. Cutaneous appendages appear as intermediate-signal-intensity inclusions within the dermis.

Normal skin has been studied with sonography with use of transducers ranging from 20 to 100 MHz (46–52). Reported in-plane resolution ranges from 80 (axial) × 200 (lateral) μm with 20-MHz insonation frequency to 17 (axial) × 33 (lateral) μm with 68-MHz insonation frequency. The depth of field, as expected, is markedly limited at such high frequencies, reported at 1 mm or less. At 20 MHz, the echogenic dermis can be distinguished from the hypoechoic subcutaneous fat, and pilosebaceous units are recognizable, whereas the epidermis can only be visualized on the palm and sole. At 40 MHz, the epidermis becomes visible on thin, hairy skin. Different epidermal strata may be resolved on thick skin when operating at frequencies above 40 MHz. An interesting finding in aged skin is the subepidermal low-echogenic band, or SLEB, which has been attributed to increased water content (48).

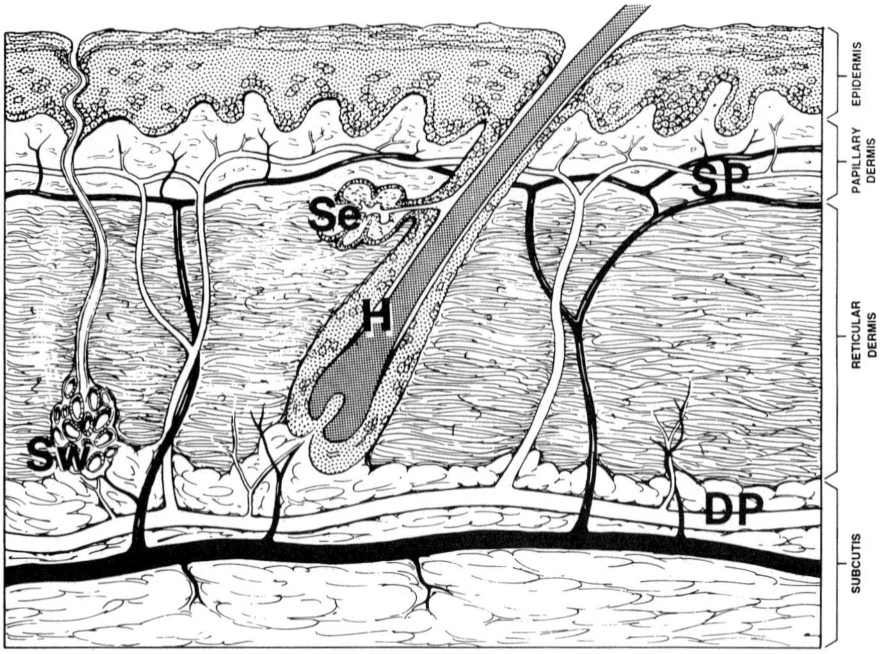

Figure 39. Sketch shows normal skin anatomic features. *DP* = deep vascular plexus, *H* = hair follicle, *Se* = sebaceous gland, *SP* = superficial vascular plexus, *Sw* = sweat gland. (Reprinted, with permission, from reference 47.)

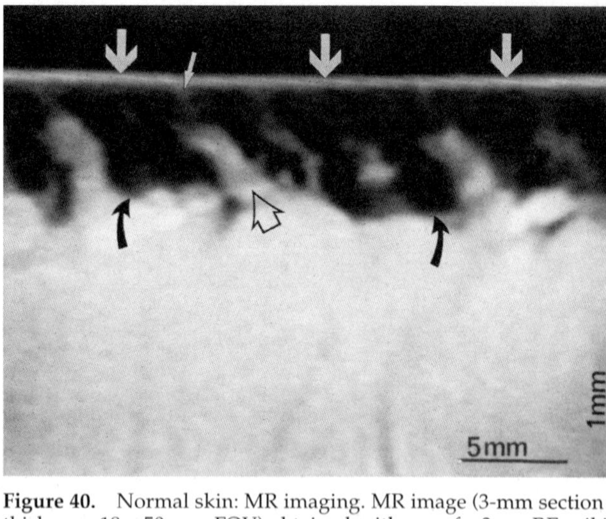

Figure 40. Normal skin: MR imaging. MR image (3-mm section thickness, 18 × 50-mm FOV) obtained with use of a 3-cm RF coil in combination with a local gradient coil shows normal skin anatomic features. The epidermis (large white arrows) appears hyperintense, and the dermis (curved arrows) appears hypointense. Cutaneous appendage (small white arrow) and hypodermal invagination (open arrow) are depicted. (Reprinted, with permission, from reference 31.) Compare this image with Figure 1, which was obtained at 0.5 T.

Nails.—The nail apparatus includes the nail plate, nail folds, epidermis, germinative matrix, and dermis (Fig 41) (27–30). The nail plate is similar to the stratum corneum of skin. The proximal nail fold overlies the root of the nail plate and the lateral folds overly its sides. The undersurface of the nail plate is lined by squamous epithelium, which is continuous with that of the proximal nail fold and thickens at the nail root to form the germinative matrix. Deep to the epidermis is the highly vascularized dermis, which can be subdivided into the papillary and reticular dermis. The latter contain numerous (93–501 per square centimeter) glomus bodies, which represent arteriovenous shunts measuring on the order of 300 μm long. These remarkable structures consist of an afferent arteriole,

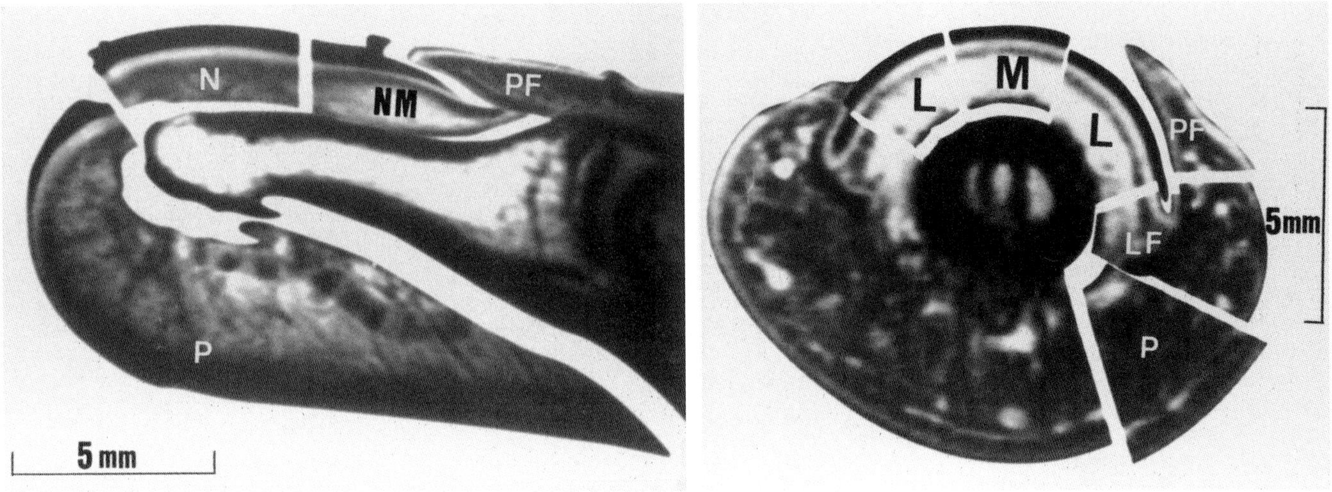

a. b.

Figure 41. Normal nail apparatus: MR imaging. **(a)** Longitudinal MR image of the fingertip obtained with a 3-cm-diameter RF coil with a local gradient coil. *N* = nail bed, *NM* = nail matrix, *P* = pulp, *PF* = proximal fold. (Reprinted, with permission, from reference 29.) **(b)** Axial MR image of the fingertip with use of the same coil setup. *L* = lateral, *LF* = lateral fold, *M* = median, *P* = pulp, *PF* = proximal fold. (Reprinted, with permission, from reference 29.)

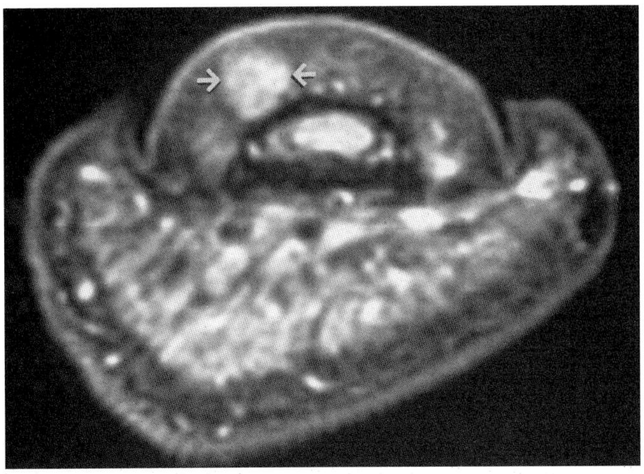

Figure 42. Glomus tumor. Contrast-enhanced axial T1-weighted MR image (800/46, 2-mm section thickness, 4-cm FOV, 256 × 224 matrix, one signal acquired, imaging time of 3 minutes 9 seconds) obtained of the fingertip with use of a 1-inch solenoid coil shows a 2.3-mm glomus tumor (arrows).

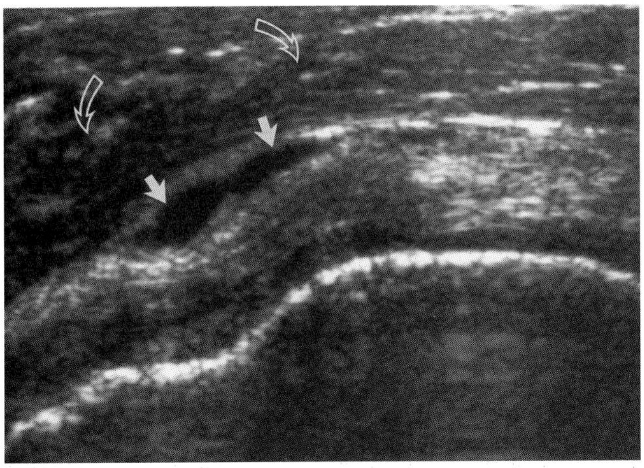

Figure 43. Sagittal US image of the shoulder with anterior oriented to the left obtained with 9-MHz insonation frequency shows fluid within the subacromial-subdeltoid bursa (solid arrows). Open arrows indicate deltoid muscle.

an anastomotic vessel known as the Sucquet-Hoyer canal, a primary collecting vein, intraglomerular reticulum, and a capsular portion. The dermis is adherent to the underlying periosteum of the distal phalanx.

Drape et al (27–29) and Goettmann et al (30) have provided tremendous insights into the MR imaging anatomic features of the normal and diseased nail apparatus by using the local gradient coil/small RF coil configuration described previously. The nail plate appears hypointense, its surface detectable only by covering it with a thin layer of paraffin. The epidermis appears relatively hyperintense, in continuity with the matrix epithelium, whereas the dermis of the nail bed appears of intermediate signal intensity. Glomus bodies appear as punctate, hyperintense foci on both T2- and contrast material–enhanced T1-weighted images. There is a hyperintense region within the dermis located just beneath the germinative matrix ("subnail matrix") that corresponds to the lunula—the familiar convex, white region seen at the proximal aspect of some, but not all, nails (27). At histologic examination, though this region is very vascular and exhibits considerable enhancement after the administration of intravenous contrast material, it is nearly devoid of glomus bodies. Glomus tumors as small as 2 mm may be detected by using a high-resolution MR technique (Fig 42).

Jemec and Serup (109) and Fornage et al (47) have used high-resolution US to study the nail plate.

Bursae.—Bursae occur in regions where moving structures are tightly opposed. Subcutaneous bursae are flattened, synovial-lined sacs tethered by dermis and periosteum; these bursae function to separate skin and bone. Other bursae are situated between adjacent tendons (subtendinous), between tendons and bones or ligaments, between muscle and bone (submuscular synovial), between aponeuroses and bone (subfascial), or between ligaments (interligamentous).

Distended, fluid-filled bursae are easily visualized with either US or MR imaging (110) (Fig 43). Collapsed bursae may appear simply as interfaces with the adjacent soft tissues.

CONCLUSION

Advances in imaging technology have enabled depiction of musculoskeletal structures to a level undreamed of only 10 years ago. In this article, four imaging modalities capable of depicting high-resolution musculoskeletal anatomic features were reviewed. The "functional physics" of each modality was presented with the aim of suggesting ways to improve image quality. The discussions of anatomic and histologic features, though not without controversy, provide a relative sense of constancy in comparison to the vicissitudes of modern imaging technology. The (current) imaging characteristics of these tissues has been discussed with special emphasis on MR imaging and US—two modalities that, while considered complementary in the past, are becoming more competitive. ■

Acknowledgments: The contributions of those who helped me on this project are gratefully acknowledged. David Daniels, MD, and Robert Fenn of Medical Center Graphics both provided their excellent artwork. Donald Jacobson, PhD, provided much needed help in the radiographic and CT physics sections and obtained the radiograph of the normal hand. Robert Prost, BS, carefully reviewed the MR physics section. G. Allan Johnson, PhD, provided valuable insight into the field of MR microscopy and reviewed this section of the text. Gordon Brandt, MD, David Gustafson, PhD, and Paul Jones, PhD, of Siemens Medical Systems, and Kris LaConte, Patricia Schubert, and Michael Hall, of GE Medical Systems provided help in the general US physics section as well as additional insights regarding the latest US technologic breakthroughs. W. Dennis Foley reviewed the ultrasound physics text. Lloyd Estkowski, RTR, David Horzewski, RTR, and Yonker Wang, MD, PhD, performed MR imaging on specimens and in healthy volunteers. Beth Beck, RTR, coordinated the setup of the "models" for the surface coil photography. Gail Akre, RTR, performed the CT of the normal hand. Marilyn Burns provided excellent secretarial assistance. The staff of Medical Center Graphics provided the high-quality photographs. Those in the musculoskeletal section at Henry Ford Hospital—Marnix van Holsbeeck, MD, J. Antonio Bouffard, MD, Joseph Craig, MD, and Kahlil Shirazi, MD—inspired me to explore the possibilities of musculoskeletal US despite my strong bias for MR imaging. Marie Delnomdedieu and G. Allan Johnson, PhD (of the Duke Center for In-Vivo Microscopy, a National Institutes of Health resource [P4105959]), Stephanie Richard, MD, Jean-Luc Drape, MD, Jane Hawnaur, MRCP, FRCR, J. Buckland-Wright, PhD, M. Benjamin, and Paul Babyn, MD, supplied prints for reproduction. Stanley S. Siegelman, MD, provided me with the opportunity to write this article. Last, I would like to thank my comrades in the musculoskeletal section, Michael Timins, MD, and Guillermo F. Carrera, MD, for providing hard-copy images for reproduction and for reviewing the manuscript.

References

1. Gray H; Williams PL, Warwick R, Dyson M, et al, eds. Anatomy of the human body. 37th ed. Edinburgh, Scotland: Churchill Livingstone, 1989.
2. Netter FH. The CIBA collection of medical illustrations: musculoskeletal system. I. Anatomy, physiology, and metabolic disorders. Summit, NJ: CIBA-GEIGY, 1987.
3. Takahashi S, Sakuma S. Magnification radiography. Berlin, Germany: Springer-Verlag, 1975.
4. Buckland-Wright JC, Bradshaw CR. Clinical applications of high-definition microfocal radiography. Br J Radiol 1989; 62:209–217.
5. Buckland-Wright JC, Macfarlane DG, Lynch JA, Jasani MK, Bradshaw CR. Joint space width measures cartilage thickness in osteoarthritis of the knee: high resolution plain film and double contrast macroradiographic investigation. Ann Rheum Dis 1995; 54:263–268.
6. Buckland-Wright JC, Macfarlane DG, Lynch JA, Clark B. Quantitative microfocal radiographic assessment of progression in osteoarthritis of the hand. Arthritis Rheum 1990; 33:57–65.
7. Buckland-Wright JC, Carmichael I, Walker SR. Quantitative microfocal radiography accurately detects joint changes in rheumatoid arthritis. Ann Rheum Dis 1986; 45:379–383.
8. Doi K, Genant HK, Rossmann K. Comparison of image quality obtained with optical and radiographic magnification techniques in fine-detail skeletal radiography: effect of object thickness. Radiology 1976; 118:189–195.
9. Genant HK, Doi K, Mall JC. Optical versus radiographic magnification for fine-detail skeletal radiography. Invest Radiol 1975; 10:160–172.
10. Wou PCS, Lima E, Turner C, Rigden S, Buckland-Wright JC. Short communication: quantitative macroradiography with biochemical correlation of children with renal osteodystrophy. Br J Radiol 1993; 66:743–747.
11. Murphey MD. Digital skeletal radiography: spatial resolution requirements for detection of subperiosteal resorption. AJR 1989; 152:541–546.
12. Muller R, Hildebrand T, Ruegsegger P. Non-invasive bone biopsy: a new method to analyse and display the three-dimensional structure of trabecular bone. Phys Med Biol 1994; 39:145–164.
13. Bonse U, Busch F, Gunnewig O. 3D computed x-ray tomography of human cancellous bone at 8 micron spatial and 10^{-4} energy resolution. Bone Miner 1994; 25:25–38.
14. Cole PR, Jasani MK, Wood B, Freemont AJ, Morris GA. High resolution, high field magnetic resonance imaging of joints: unexpected features in proton images of cartilage. Br J Radiol 1990; 63:907–909.
15. Shellock FG, Schaefer DJ, Kanal E. Physiologic responses to an MR imaging procedure performed at a specific absorption rate of 6.0 W/kg. Radiology 1994; 192:865–868.
16. Hawnaur JM. Skin: MR imaging findings at middle field strength. Radiology 1997; 201:868–872.
17. Kneeland JB, Hyde JS. High-resolution MR imaging with local coils. Radiology 1989; 171:1–7.
18. Maurer J, Requardt H, Muller F, et al. Indications for the application of a high resolution coil in MR tomography. Fortschr Rontgenstr 1994; 160:353–360.
19. Erickson SJ, Canale PB, Carrera GF, et al. Interdigital (Morton) neuroma: high-resolution MR imaging with a solenoid coil. Radiology 1991; 181:833–836.
20. Oneson SR, Scales LM, Erickson SJ,Timins ME. MR imaging of the painful wrist. RadioGraphics 1996; 16:997–1008.
21. Oneson SR, Scales LM, Timins ME, Erickson SJ, Chamoy L. MR imaging interpretation of the Palmer classification of triangular fibrocartilage complex lesions. RadioGraphics 1996; 16:97–106.
22. Timins ME, O'Connell SE, Erickson SJ, Oneson SR. MR imaging of the wrist: normal findings that may simulate disease. RadioGraphics 1996; 16:987–995.
23. Hinke DH, Erickson,SJ, Chamoy L, Timins ME. Ulnar collateral ligament of the thumb: findings in cadavers, volunteers, and patients with ligamentous injury (gamekeeper's thumb). AJR 1994; 163:1431–1434.
24. Szeglowski SD, Hornak JP. Asymmetric single-turn solenoid for MRI of the wrist. Magn Reson Med 1993; 30:750–753.
25. Totterman SM, Heberger R, Miller R, Rubens DJ, Blebea JS. Two-piece wrist surface coil. AJR 1991; 156:343–344.
26. Bittoun J, Saint-Jalmes H, Querleux BG, et al. In vivo high-resolution MR imaging of the skin in a whole-body system at 1.5 T. Radiology 1990; 176:457–460.
27. Drape JL, Wolfram-Gabel W, Idy-Peretti I, et al. The lunula: a magnetic resonance imaging approach to the subnail matrix area. J Invest Dermatol 1996; 106:1081–1085.
28. Drape JL, Idy-Peretti I, Goettmann S, et al. MR imaging of digital mucoid cysts. Radiology 1996; 200:531–536.
29. Drape JL, Idy-Peretti I, Goettmann S, et al. Subungual glomus tumors: evaluation with MR imaging. Radiology 1995; 195:507–515.
30. Goettmann S, Drape JL, Idy-Peretti I, et al. Magnetic resonance imaging: a new tool in the diagnosis of tumours of the nail apparatus. Br J Dermatol 1994; 130:701–710.
31. Richard S, Querleux B, Bittoun J, et al. Characterization of the skin in vivo by high resolution magnetic resonance imaging: water behavior and age-related effects. J Invest Dermatol 1993; 100:705–709.
32. Richard S, Querleux B, Bittoun J, et al. In vivo proton relaxation times analysis of the skin layers by magnetic resonance imaging. J Invest Dermatol 1991; 97:120–125.
33. Seo GS, Aoki J, Moriya H, et al. Hyaline cartilage: in vivo assessment with magnetization transfer imaging. Radiology 1996; 201:525–530.
34. Rilling WS, Prost RW, Erickson SJ, et al. High resolution fast spin echo imaging: artifact assessment and optimization of acquistion parameters (abstr). Presented at the 93rd Annual Meeting of the American Roentgen Ray Society, San Francisco, Calif, April 1993.
35. Totterman SM, Miller RJ. Scapholunate ligament: normal MR appearance on three-dimensional gradient-recalled-echo images. Radiology 1996; 200:237–241.
36. Waldschmidt JG, Rilling RJ, Kajdacsy-Balla AA, et al. High resolution MR im-

aging of hyaline cartilage: normal anatomy, diagnostic pitfalls, and pathology (abstr). Radiology 1996; 201(P):535.
37. Peck TL, Magin RL, Lauterbur PC. Design and analysis of microcoils for NMR microscopy. J Magn Reson 1995; 108:114–124.
38. Johnson GA, Benveniste H, Black RD, et al. Histology by magnetic resonance microscopy. Magn Reson Q 1993; 9:1–30.
39. Kapadia RD, High WB, Soulleveld HA, Bertolini D, Sarkar SK. Magnetic resonance microscopy in rat skeletal research. Magn Reson Med 1993; 30:247–250.
40. Banson ML, Cofer GP, Black R, Johnson GA. A probe for specimen magnetic resonance microscopy. Invest Radiol 1992; 27:157–164.
41. Suddarth SA, Johnson GA. Three-dimensional MR microscopy with large arrays. Magn Reson Med 1991; 18:132–141.
42. Zhou X, Cofer GP, Suddarth SA, Johnson GA. High-field MR microscopy using fast spin-echoes. Magn Reson Med 1993; 30:60–67.
43. Beckmann N, Bruttel K, Mir A, Rudin M. Noninvasive 3D MR microscopy as a tool in pharmacological research: application to a model of rheumatoid arthritis. Magn Reson Imaging 1995; 13:1013–1017.
44. Rudin M. MR microscopy on rats in vivo at 4.7 T using surface coils. Magn Reson Med 1987; 5:443–448.
45. Smith BR, Johnson GA, Groman EV, Linney EA. Magnetic resonance microscopy of mouse embryos. Proc Natl Acad Sci USA 1994; 91:3530–3533.
46. Dummer W, Blaheta HJ, Bastian BC, Schenk T, Brocker EV, Remy W. Preoperative characterization of pigmented skin lesions by epiluminescence microscopy and high-frequency ultrasound. Arch Dermatol 1995; 131:279–285.
47. Fornage BD, McGavran MH, Duvic M, Waldron CA. Imaging of the skin with 20-MHz US. Radiology 1993; 189:69–76.
48. Gniadecka M, Gniadecki R, Serup J, Sondergaard J. Ultrasound structure and digital image analysis of the subepidermal low echogenic band in aged human skin: diurnal changes and interindividual variability. J Invest Dermatol 1994; 102:362–365.
49. Gupta AK, Turnbull DH, Foster FS, et al. High frequency 40-MHz ultrasound: a possible noninvasive method for the assessment of the boundary of basal cell carcinomas. Dermatol Surg 1996; 22:131–136.
50. Harland CC, Bamber JC, Gusterson BA, Mortimer PS. High frequency, high resolution B-scan ultrasound in the assessment of skin tumours. Br J Dermatol 1993; 128:525–532.
51. Stiller MJ, Gropper CA, Shupack JL, Lizzi F, Driller J, Rorke M. Diagnostic ultrasound in dermatology: current uses and future potential. Cutis 1994; 53:44–48.
52. Turnbull DH, Starkoski BG, Harasiewicz KA, et al. A 40–100 MHz B-scan ultrasound backscatter microscope for skin imaging. Ultrasound Med Biol 1995; 21:79–88.
53. Weng L, Tirumalai AP, Lowery CM, et al. US extended–field-of-view imaging technology. Radiology 1997; 203:877–880.
54. Black J, Mattson R, Korostoff E. Haversian osteons: size, distribution, internal structure, and orientation. J Biomed Mater Res 1974; 8:299–319.
55. Georgia R, Albu I, Sicoe M, Georoceanu M. Comparative aspects of the density and diameter of Haversian canals in the diaphyseal compact bone of man and dog. Morphol Embryol 1982; 28:11–14.
56. Schweitzer ME, Levine C, Mitchell DG, Gannon FN, Gomella LG. Bull's eyes and halos: useful MR discriminators of osseous metastases. Radiology 1993; 188:249–252.
57. Van Holsbeeck MT, Kolowich PA, Eyler WR, et al. Ultrasound depiction of partial-thickness tears of the rotator cuff. Radiology 1995; 197:443–446.
58. Kann P, Schulz U, Nink M, Pfutzner A, Schrezenmeir J, Beyer J. Architecture in cortical bone and ultrasound transmission velocity. Clin Rheumatol 1993; 12:364–367.
59. Antich PP, Pak CY, Gonzales J, Anderson J, Sakhaee K, Rubin C. Measurement of intrinsic bone quality in vivo by reflection ultrasound: correction of impaired quality with slow-release sodium fluoride and calcium citrate. J Bone Miner Res 1993; 8:301–311.
60. Benninghoff A. Form und bau der gelenkknorpel in ihren beziehungen zur funktion. Anat Enthicklungsgesch 1925; 76:43.
61. Waldschmidt JG, Rilling RJ, Kajdacsy-Balla AA, Boynton MD, Erickson SJ. In vitro and in vivo MR imaging of hyaline cartilage: zonal anatomy, imaging pitfalls, and pathologic conditions. RadioGraphics 1997; 17:1387–1402.
62. Conway WF, Hayes CW, Laughran T. Cross-sectional imaging of the patellofemoral joint and surrounding structures. RadioGraphics 1991; 11:195–207.
63. Hayes CW, Sawyer RW, Conway WF. Patellar cartilage lesions: in vitro detection and staging with MR imaging and pathologic correlation. Radiology 1990; 176:479–483.
64. Modl JM, Sether LA, Haughton VM, Kneeland JB. Articular cartilage: correlation of histologic zones with signal intensity at MR imaging. Radiology 1991; 181:853–855.
65. Monson NL, Haughton VM, Modl JM, Sether LA, Ho KC. Normal and degenerating articular cartilage: in vitro correlation of MR imaging and histologic findings. J Magn Reson Imaging 1992; 2:41–45.
66. Recht MP, Resnick D. MR imaging of articular cartilage: current status and future directions. AJR 1994; 163:283–290.
67. Rubenstein JD, Kim JK, Morava-Protzner I, Stanchev PL, Henkelman MR. Effects of collagen orientation on MR imaging characteristics of bovine articular cartilage. Radiology 1993; 188:219–226.
68. Fry ME, Jacoby RK, Hutton CW, et al. High-resolution magnetic resonance imaging of the interphalangeal joints of the hand. Skeletal Radiol 1991; 20:273–277.
69. Hodgson RJ, Barry MA, Carpenter TA, Hall LD, Hazleman BL, Tyler JA. Magnetic resonance imaging protocol optimization for evaluation of hyaline cartilage in the distal interphalangeal joint of fingers. Invest Radiol 1995; 30:522–531.
70. Rubenstein JD, Kim JK, Henkelman RM. Effects of compression and recovery of bovine articular cartilage: appearance on MR images. Radiology 1996; 201:843–850.
71. Paul PK, Jasani MK, Sebok D, Rakhit A, Dunton AW, Douglas FL. Variation in MR signal intensity across normal human knee cartilage. J Magn Reson Imaging 1993; 3:569–574.
72. Kim HK, Babyn PS, Harasiewicz KA, Gahunia HK, Pritzker KP, Foster FS. Imaging of immature articular cartilage using ultrasound backscatter microscopy at 50 MHz. J Orthop Res 1995; 13:963–970.
73. Myers SL, Dines K, Brandt DA, Brandt KD, Albrecht ME. Experimental assessment by high frequency ultrasound of articular cartilage thickness and osteoarthritic changes. J Rheumatol 1995; 22:109–116.
74. Aissen A, McCune WJ, MacGuire A. Sonographic evalulation of the cartilage of the knee. Radiology 1984; 153:781–784.
75. Agemura DH, O'Brien WD Jr, Olerud JE, Chun LE, Eyre DE. Ultrasonic propagation properties of articular cartilage at 100 MHz. J Acoust Soc Am 1990; 87:1786–1791.
76. Lund PJ, Nisbet JK, Valencia FG, Ruth JT. Current sonographic applications in orthopedics. AJR 1996; 166:889–895.
77. O'Brien M. Functional anatomy and physiology of tendons. Clin Sports Med 1992; 11:505–520.
78. Resnick D. Diagnosis of bone joint disorders. 3rd Ed. Philadelphia, Pa: Saunders, 1995.
79. Jozsa L, Kannus P, Balint JB, Reffy A. Three-dimensional ultrastructure of human tendons. Acta Anat 1991; 142:306–312.
80. Renstrom P, Johnson RJ. Overuse injuries in sports: a review. Sports Med 1985; 2:316–333.
81. Stolinski C. Disposition of collagen fibrils in human tendons. J Anat 1995; 186:577–583.
82. Schmidt D, Mackay B. Ultrastructure of human tendon sheath and synovium: implications for tumor histogenesis. Ultrastruct Pathol 1982; 3:269–283.
83. Rathbun JB, Macnab I. The microvascular pattern of the rotator cuff. J Bone Joint Surg [Br] 1970; 52:540–553.
84. Benjamin M, Evans EJ, Copp L. The histology of tendon attachments to bone in man. J Anat 1986; 149:89–100.
85. Evans EJ, Benjamin M, Pemberton DJ. Fibrocartilage in the attachment zones of the quadriceps tendon and patellar ligament of man. J Anat 1990; 171:155–162.
86. Frowen P, Benjamin M. Variations in the quality of uncalcified fibrocartilage at the insertions of the extrinsic calf muscles in the foot. J Anat 1995; 186:417–421.
87. Koblik PD, Freeman DM. Short echo time magnetic resonance imaging of tendon. Invest Radiol 1993; 28:1095–1100.
88. Minne J, Depreux, Fontaine. Structure du tendon d'Achille: importance de ses constituants. C R Ass an Atomistes 1953; 33:663–666.
89. Bertolotto M, Perrone R, Martinoli C, et al. High resolution ultrasound anatomy of normal Achilles tendon. Br J Radiol 1995; 68:986–991.
90. Clark JM, Harryman DT III. Tendons, ligaments, and capsule of the rotator cuff: gross and microscopic anatomy. J Bone Joint Surg [Am] 1992; 74:713–725.
91. Burkhart SS, Esch JC, Jolson RS. The rotator crescent and rotator cable: an anatomic description of the shoulder's "suspension bridge." Arthroscopy 1993; 9:611–616.
92. Fornage BD. The hypoechoic normal tendon: a pitfall. J Ultrasound Med 1987; 6:19–22.
93. Lehtinen A, Bondestam S, Taavitsainen M. Use of angulation in the detection of tendinitis with US. Eur J Radiol 1994; 18:175–179.
94. Berendsen HJ, Migchelsen C. Hydration structure of fibrous macromolecules. Ann NY Acad Sci 1965; 125:365–379.
95. Erickson SJ, Prost RW, Timins ME. The "magic angle" effect: background physics and clinical relevance. Radiology 1993;

188:23–25.
96. Erickson SJ, Cox IH, Hyde JS, Carrera GF, Strandt JA, Estkowski LD. Effect of tendon orientation on MR imaging signal intensity: a manifestation of the "magic angle" phenomenon. Radiology 1991; 181:389–392.
97. Fullerton GD, Cameron IL, Ord VA. Orientation of tendons in the magnetic field and its effect on T2 relaxation times. Radiology 1985; 155:433–435.
98. Johnston RB, Seiler JG, Miller EJ, Drvaric DM. The intrinsic and extrinsic ligaments of the wrist: a correlation of collagen typing and histologic appearance. J Hand Surg [Br] 1995; 20:750–754.
99. Lyon RM, Akeson WH, Amiel D, Kitabayashi LR, Woo SL. Ultrastructural differences between the cells of the medical collateral and the anterior cruciate ligaments. Clin Orthop 1991; 272:279–286.
100. Serafini-Fracassini A, Field JM, Smith JW, Stephens WG. The ultrastructure and mechanics of elastic ligaments. J Ultrastruct Res 1977; 58:244–251.
101. Milz P, Milz S, Putz R, Reiser M. 13 MHz high-frequency sonography of the lateral ankle joint ligaments and the tibiofibular syndesmosis in anatomic specimens. J Ultrasound Med 1996; 15:277–284.
102. Martin AJ, Ryan LK, Gotlieb AI, Henkelman RM, Foster FS. Arterial imaging: comparison of high resolution US and MR imaging with histologic correlation. RadioGraphics 1997; 17:189–202.
103. Newman JS, Adler RS, Rubin JM. Power Doppler sonography: use of measuring alterations in muscle blood volume after exercise. AJR 1997; 168:1525–1530.
104. Newman JS, Laing TJ, McCarthy CJ, Adler RS. Power Doppler sonography of synovitis: assessment of therapeutic response—preliminary observations. Radiology 1996; 198:582–584.
105. Silvestri E, Martinoli C, Derchi LE, Bertolotto M, Chiaramondia M, Rosenberg I. Echotexture of peripheral nerves: correlation between US and histologic findings and criteria to differentiate tendons. Radiology 1995; 197:291–296.
106. Blake LC, Robertson WD, Hayes CE. Sacral plexus: optimal imaging planes for MR assessment. Radiology 1996; 199:767–772.
107. Ikeda K, Haughton VM, Ho K, Nowicki BH. Correlative MR: anatomic study of the median nerve. AJR 1996; 167:1233–1236.
108. Hyde JS, Jesmanowicz A, Kneeland JB. Surface coil for MR imaging of the skin. Magn Reson Med 1987; 5:456–461.
109. Jemec GB, Serup J. Ultrasound structure of the human nail plate. Arch Dermatol 1989; 125:643–646.
110. Van Holsbeeck M, Strouse PJ. Sonography of the shoulder: evaluation of the subacromial-subdeltoid bursa. AJR 1993; 160:561–564.

Susan D. Wall, MD • J. Michael Howe, MSLS • Rajiv Sawhney, MD

Human Immunodeficiency Virus Infection and Hepatitis: Biosafety in Radiology[1]

THE risk of occupational acquisition of the human immunodeficiency virus (HIV), hepatitis B virus (HBV), or hepatitis C virus (HCV) is introduced when exposure to bloodborne pathogens occurs in the health care setting. This is especially important for radiologists who perform diagnostic or therapeutic procedures involving needles or other sharp instruments and possibly get splashed with blood. The risk of HIV seroconversion per sharp injury with infected blood is low (average, 0.3%), but the risk of developing the acquired immunodeficiency syndrome (AIDS) is high once infection occurs. Recent data indicate exposure to a high volume of blood or high concentration of virus increases the risk, but postexposure prophylaxis with nucleoside analogs decreases the risk by 79%. HBV is even more prevalent and more infectious than HIV, and exposure results in seroconversion in 12%–30% of those who have not been immunized. HCV is less infectious than HBV, but the risk of chronic hepatitis is greater, and 10%–12% of patients infected will eventually have cirrhosis or hepatocellular carcinoma. Protection against transmission of HIV, HBV, or HCV is enhanced with the use of universal precautions including specific behaviors to reduce the risk of injury with sharp instruments and splashing with blood.

Index terms: Acquired immunodeficiency syndrome (AIDS) • Hepatitis, 761.291 • Radiology and radiologists • State-of-art reviews

Radiology 1997; 205:619–628

[1] From the Department of Radiology (S.D.W., R.S.) and the AIDS Information Center (J.M.H.), University of California—San Francisco, San Francisco Veterans Administration Medical Center, 4150 Clement St, San Francisco, CA 94121. Received May 5, 1997; accepted and revision requested June 19; revision received August 13. **Address reprint requests to** S.D.W.

Occupational exposure to bloodborne pathogens introduces an important threat to health care workers (1–3). This is especially true for radiologists who perform invasive procedures and for those at risk of being splashed with blood or bloody body fluid (4,5). The AIDS epidemic has heightened the awareness of the potential for transmission of infectious disease in the health care setting. In addition, while the risk of occupational transmission of HIV is important, there is an even greater risk of transmission of HBV and HCV (6,7). In this article, we present the data to date regarding the risk of occupational acquisition of these viruses, and we provide guidelines for reducing that risk in the radiology department. Additionally, we discuss current recommendations regarding postexposure prophylaxis for both HIV infection and hepatitis.

HIV INFECTION RISK

Since the recognition of the first cases of AIDS in 1981, HIV infection continues to be a serious problem in the United States. There are approximately 650,000–900,000 U.S. residents infected with HIV, and about 41,000 new infections occur each year (8). Individuals infected today with HIV live longer after infection than those infected in the early years of the epidemic because of the use of combination therapy including nucleoside analogs (zidovudine [ZDV; formerly known as AZT, aziothymidine, or Retrovir] and lamivudine [3TC]) that inhibit viral replication and protease inhibitors (indinavir) that can reduce HIV viral titers and improve depressed CD4 lymphocyte counts. Therefore, the period between initial infection with HIV and clinical manifestation of AIDS likely will be extended beyond the current mean of 11 years. Many HIV-positive individuals will seek medical care and require radiologic procedures for non–AIDS-related conditions over the next decade, even in communities without a large population of persons at high risk for HIV disease. In addition, when patients are ill with AIDS, the majority will be examined in the radiology department. Therefore, there will continue to be an increase in the number of HIV-positive patients needing health care involving diagnostic and therapeutic radiologic procedures. Consequently, the risk of occupational exposure to HIV for health care workers who work in a department of radiology will persist for the foreseeable future. Although the data indicate the risk of occupational infection with HIV to be low, the risk for acquiring AIDS is high once infection occurs. For all of these reasons, protection against transmission of HIV in the health care setting is critically important.

Two types of data provide useful information regarding the risk of occupational acquisition of HIV disease: anecdotal case reports and prospective cohort studies. Each type provides important but very different information. Anecdotal case reports document the existence of risk and provide some information regarding the mode of transmission. In the United States, 52 definite and 111

Abbreviations: AIDS = acquired immunodeficiency syndrome, CDC = Centers for Disease Control and Prevention, HBV = hepatitis B virus, HCV = hepatitis C virus, HIV = human immunodeficiency virus, OSHA = Occupational Safety and Health Administration, 3TC = lamivudine, ZDV = zidovudine.

probable cases of occupational HIV acquisition have been reported by the Centers for Disease Control and Prevention (CDC) following thorough evaluation (9). Most investigators agree, however, that underreporting by health care workers is prevalent. Almost all of the documented cases (47 of 52, 90%) involved exposure to infected blood or blood-contaminated body fluid. Three involved exposure to highly concentrated virus in research laboratories, one involved exposure to visibly bloody fluid, and one involved exposure to an unspecified fluid. None involved exposure to body fluid not contaminated with blood. In the majority of the documented cases (45 of 52, 87%), infection resulted from being stuck with a needle or from percutaneous injury with a sharp object. Of the remaining seven cases, five can be attributed to mucocutaneous exposure, one to both percutaneous and mucocutaneous exposure, and one to an unknown mode of exposure. It is clear from these data that injury from a needle or sharp object involving infected blood poses the single greatest risk to health care workers for occupational transmission of HIV. This is especially important for radiologists (and radiology nurses and technologists) who perform diagnostic and therapeutic procedures involving needles and/or vascular access, and it is notable that often they do so in darkened rooms.

The anecdotal case reports, however, do not allow for an estimation of the magnitude of risk. For that, the other type of data—prospective cohort studies—is required. These studies provide a numerator (number of health care workers seroconverted) and a denominator (number of discrete exposures to HIV-infected blood). Twenty-five such studies since 1983 documented the average risk of HIV transmission following a single percutaneous exposure to infected blood to be 0.3% (21 infections per 6,498 exposures) (6,10,11). Hence, for some exposures the risk is less than 0.3%, and for others it is greater.

A recent study by the CDC addressed exposure characteristics that affect the magnitude of risk (12). Performing a retrospective case-control study, the authors compared the details of exposure and of postexposure care of 31 health care workers who seroconverted to HIV-positive and of 679 who did not. This study documented an increased risk when exposure involved a deep percutaneous injury (subsequently described as one that bleeds spontaneously), visible blood on the sharp device causing the injury, a device that had been used for venous or arterial access, or a source patient in the terminal stages of disease (death occurring within 60 days) (Table 1). Three of these characteristics are related to the volume of blood and one is related to the concentration of virus (which is highest during early and terminal stages of disease) (12). The average risk associated with mucous membrane exposure (approximately 0.1%) and intact skin exposure (less than 0.1%) probably also are increased with a high volume of blood and a high viral titer (13). It should be noted that prolonged exposure to nonintact skin has been documented to result in seroconversion on the basis of prior anecdotal case reports.

Table 1
Factors Affecting Occupational Transmission of HIV

Factor	Adjusted Odds Ratio
Deep injury (intramuscular, spontaneous bleeding)	16.1
Source patient terminally ill	6.4
Visible blood on sharp device	5.2
Sharp device used for vascular access	5.1
Postexposure prophylactic zidovudine used	0.2

Note.–All data significant at $P < .01$.
Source.–Adapted from Table 1 in reference 13.

HEPATITIS RISK

Although overshadowed by publicity about HIV disease, HBV remains the most common important blood-borne pathogen to infect health care workers. HBV is a DNA virus that does not itself destroy hepatocytes. Rather, cellular injury occurs due to an intense immune response. Many infected health care workers have no symptoms (14). Most HBV-infected patients recover fully, but in 10%–25% chronic infection occurs, which leads to death from cirrhosis in 10%–15% or hepatocellular carcinoma in 10% (7,15). In the United States, infection generally occurs by means of percutaneous or sexual exposure, while in Asia maternal-fetal contact is the predominant mode of transmission.

HBV poses a considerably greater risk to health care workers than does HIV because HBV is both more prevalent and more infectious. Prevalence of HBV in the United States overall is 0.1%–0.5%, but it is considerably greater in high-risk populations such as those who are recipients of blood products, intravenous drug users, homosexually active men, health care workers, and clients or staff of institutions for the developmentally disabled (16). It is more infectious than HIV because of a higher concentration of circulating virus. One milliliter of HIV-positive blood contains approximately 10^1–10^4 viral particles, but the same volume of HBV-positive blood contains as many as 10^{13} viral particles (17). Also, HBV survives in dry blood for up to a week, whereas HIV is easy to kill with virucidal hospital disinfectant or a dilute (1:10 or 1:100) solution of household bleach. Consequently, there is substantial risk of transmission of HBV whenever parenteral exposure involving contaminated blood occurs. Reports from the CDC and others indicate that without immunoprophylaxis, approximately 12% of percutaneous exposures to HBV surface antigen–positive blood will lead to seroconversion, and this increases to 30% when the source patient is positive for HBV envelope antigen (7). However, transmission of HBV after percutaneous exposure is rare among persons who have been successfully immunized.

Immunization programs against HBV have been only partially successful. The prevalence of HBV in serum of health care workers has decreased since the development of the recombinant DNA vaccine, but it remains two to four times higher than that in blood donor control subjects (18). In one recent study at a large inner-city teaching hospital, 23% of health care workers were unvaccinated (19). Hence, nonparticipation by employers, individual health care workers, or both is one reason for incomplete immunization. Another reason is that vaccine failure can occur in as many as 12% of cases, even when the suspension is delivered properly (20,21). Proper delivery involves intramuscular injection into the deltoid (not gluteal) muscle that is repeated at 1 month and again at 6 months. A protective titer (>10 mIU/mL) results in 88% of individuals. Nonresponse corresponds to patient characteristics of older age, obesity, and smoking. If titers are not at the protective level after completion of a proper immunization series, a repeat booster should be given. If this fails to stimulate an adequate antibody response, consideration should be

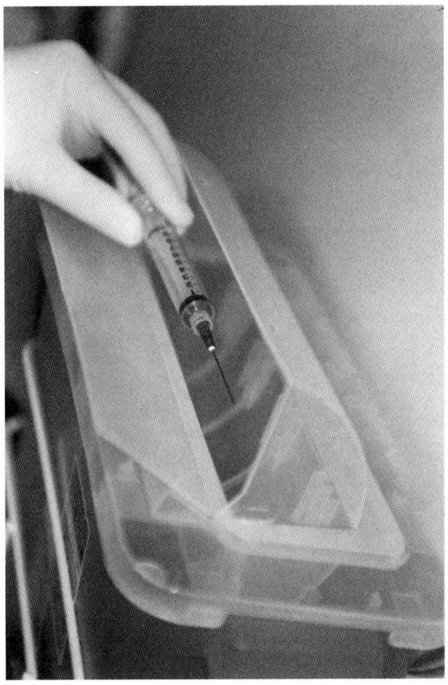

Figure 1. Wall-mounted disposal system for sharp objects (Sage Products, Crystal Lake, Ill). This container allows the needle and syringe to be disposed of without separation, and the curved container lid prevents extension of the sharp object through the opening.

given to vaccination with polyvalent serum–derived vaccine depending on the risk of exposure. Unfortunately, each year approximately 8,700 health care workers contract hepatitis B, and annually there are as many as 130–190 deaths from HBV that are attributed to occupational infection (22). For all these reasons, experts in hepatology call for universal vaccination against HBV; in some states infants and prepubescent teenagers are being vaccinated. Certainly, protection against exposure to infected blood in the health care setting is important. Furthermore, it should be noted that the federal Occupational Safety and Health Administration (OSHA) requires the provision of free immunization against HBV within 2 weeks to new employees in the health care setting.

Recombinant DNA HBV vaccine is safe, free of side effects, and nonallergenic. Pregnancy is not a contraindication. Although some reports advocate a booster every 3 years, long-term follow-up has shown that once a protective titer against HBV has been achieved, protection can last for at least 9 years. Physicians are responsible not only for their own safety in the health care setting, but also for that of those who work with them. As it may be very difficult for each employee to get to the personnel health department to have his or her HBV titer checked, department chairpersons should assume responsibility for ensuring employees are tested. This can be accomplished simply by assigning 1 day for a departmental nurse to draw a blood sample from each employee, which can then be delivered to the laboratory for HBV titers. (Repeat this in 1–2 weeks for any absent employees.) Anyone without a protective titer should follow the guidelines above. If a nonprotected health care worker should sustain percutaneous exposure to HBV, hepatitis B immunoglobulin and the vaccine should be administered together as soon as possible after exposure.

HCV was discovered in 1989. It is believed to be responsible for the majority of non-A, non-B hepatitis infections that stem from transfusions with contaminated blood or blood products. A conservative estimate of prevalence of HCV carriers in the United States is 0.6%. Approximately 160,000 new cases are reported each year. Transmission is similar to that of HBV, but enzyme immunoassay evidence of seroconversion can occur as early as 4–6 weeks after exposure compared with an average of 6–9 weeks for HBV seroconversion. The risk of chronic disease once HCV infection occurs is much greater than that with HBV. With the use of polymerase chain reaction testing for HCV RNA, at least 85% of all persons with acute HCV infection can be shown to remain chronically infected. Liver enzyme levels remain elevated and chronic liver disease develops in approximately 70% (23). Ten percent to 20% of these carriers will subsequently develop cirrhosis, and a smaller percentage will develop hepatocellular carcinoma (24). However, data are limited about HCV transmission by means of percutaneous exposure. Reports have shown the risk of seroconversion in health care workers who have sustained percutaneous exposure to HCV-infected blood to be as high as 6%–10% (25). This represents a risk that is 10–33 times greater than the transmission risk of HIV and 10–20 times less than that of HBV. This is consistent with the circulating viral titer of HCV, which is between that of HIV and that of HBV. Because immunoglobulin is derived from plasma that has been screened for anti-HCV antibodies, there is no evidence to support its use as postexposure prophylaxis (25). There is no available vaccine against HCV (26).

PRECAUTIONS FOR RADIOLOGY PERSONNEL

Precaution against transmission of HIV, HBV, HCV, and any other blood-borne infectious organisms does not necessitate extraordinary measures, nor does it preclude touching patients or treating them with proper respect. It simply calls for good common sense to protect against injury from sharp objects and from splashing blood. For example, barrier precautions need not be worn during routine fluoroscopic gastrointestinal studies, but they should be used while examining a patient with a history of hematemesis or hematochezia. The suggestions noted below should be practiced routinely, as it is not possible to know the antibody status of all patients, and if that information is available it cannot be relied on to be accurate because there is a period between infection and the development of detectable antibodies.

DO NOT RECAP NEEDLES. This is the single most important behavior that all health care workers should practice. The recapping of needles or their improper disposal has been the cause of the majority of needle-stick injuries. All needles (with syringe attached) and other sharp instruments should be disposed of directly into a readily available, puncture-resistant container (Fig 1). Particular care in interventional radiology must be taken when a sharp stylet must be resheathed or a Seldinger-type needle must be reassembled for a second pass to access a bile duct or an artery.

The word "sharp" should be stated clearly whenever a sharp instrument is set down. Sharp instruments should never be handed from one person to another. Rather, one person should place the instrument on the immediate sterile work area (patient's drapes), say "sharp," and withdraw the hand before another person reaches for the instrument.

Puncture-resistant containers stabilized with a wide base to prevent spillage (Fig 2a) should be available in every room. Set in a rack with wheels as shown, the container (Sage Products) is easily positioned so that disposal of sharp objects directly by the radiologist precludes additional handling by an assistant. The container should have a wide opening (Fig 2b), so disposal can be accomplished while sterile technique is maintained. The container should be emptied routinely when it is when one-half to two-thirds full; this reduces the risk of injury to the next person disposing of sharp objects and to housekeeping personnel.

If a reusable sharp instrument must be retained on the angiography or interventional table (ie, for percutaneous transhepatic cholangiography), prepare a controlled protected environment with a long metal container and a lid placed consistently at the back of the table (Fig 3). Leaving sharp instruments exposed on the tray, covered by a towel, or stuck into a sponge box increases risk of accidental stick. Sutures should be placed with a hemostat and not by hand. In fact, the hemostat should be used to cover the suture needle tip while tying, and the needle should be cut and disposed of as soon as it is no longer needed. Glass syringes should never be used. During angioplasty procedures this dictates use of a special plastic syringe and tubing (CO-Set closed inject delivery system; Baxter, Irvine, Calif) that does not absorb nitroglycerine, as most plastic syringes do. Polycarbonate syringes (Schneider/Namic, Glens Falls, NY) are less prone to breakage during forceful balloon inflation for percutaneous transluminal angioplasty procedures. Gauze should be used (with double-gloved hands—see below) when opening an ampule of lidocaine, which frequently is included in the commercially prepared procedure trays that often are used for minor procedures. Adequate lighting is mandatory for any procedure involving sharp instruments, and this requires a special effort in radiology.

Use of gloves will decrease by more than 50% the volume of blood transferred to the skin when needlestick injury occurs, and they should be worn whenever needles are used (27). Use of double gloves further protects against percutaneous injury, and this is important when considering the overall 10% rate of occult glove perforation in interventional radiology procedures (28). Indeed, occult perforations increase from 7% for short interventional procedures to 23% for those extending beyond 2 hours. In addition, it has been found that 1% of unused gloves have occult perforations (28). Therefore, it is wise to consider routine double gloving (with exceptions in cases in which the minor tactile reduction might increase risk to the patient or operator) and a change of both inner and outer gloves for prolonged or excessively bloody procedures.

Protective garb should be used during any procedure in which exposure to blood or bloody body fluid might occur either because of the use of sharp instruments or because of the potential for splashing. During angiography and other interventional procedures, this garb includes a fluid-impermeable disposable gown, gloves, hat, mask (that covers the ears), boots, and a transparent plastic face shield (Fig 4). Glasses provide less protection to the eyes against splashing fluid than does a face shield, especially those shields that are attached to the top of the mask (Fig 4b) (Fluid Shield; Technol Medical Products, Fort Worth, Tex) as opposed to those that rest on the forehead and are open below, the direction from which splashing fluid would originate. All personnel (technologists, nurses, observers) within splashable distance during a procedure should cover their mucous membranes including ears, eyes, nose, and mouth. The hat and mask with face shield shown in Figure 4b are optimal, and they provide more protection than do protective eyeglasses alone.

Communication among physicians, technologists, and nurses involved in a procedure is now more important

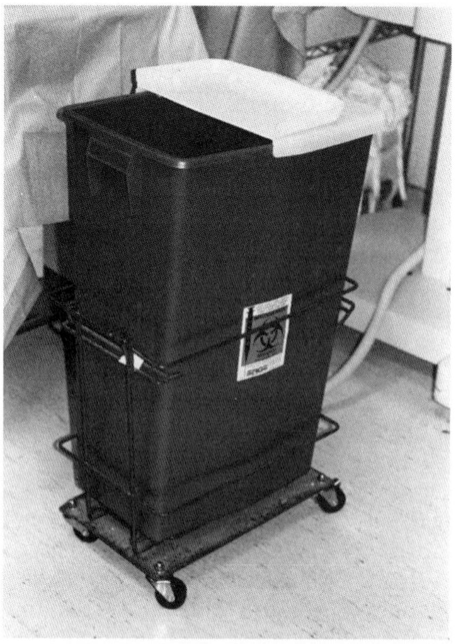

a.

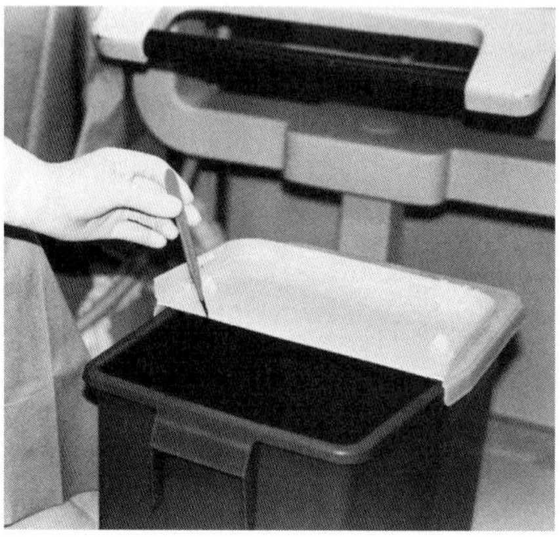

b.

Figure 2. Container for disposing of sharp objects. **(a)** Set on a rack with wheels, this puncture-resistant container (Sage Products) is stable, is easily movable, and can be made accessible for immediate disposal of sharp objects by the radiologist. **(b)** It has a wide opening that allows for disposal of sharp objects directly by the radiologist while sterile technique is maintained. It is never allowed to be more than one-half to two-thirds full.

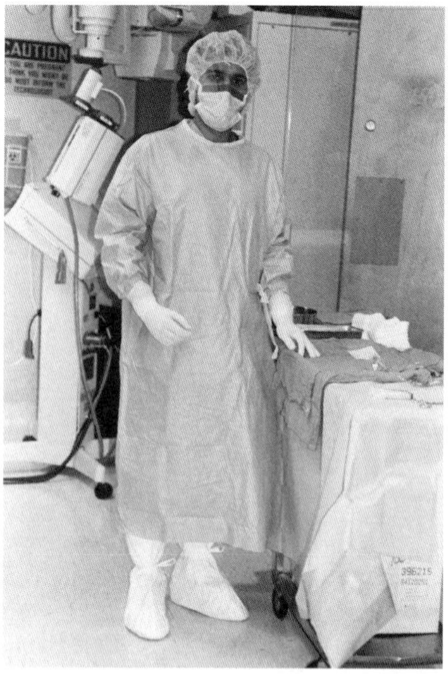

a.

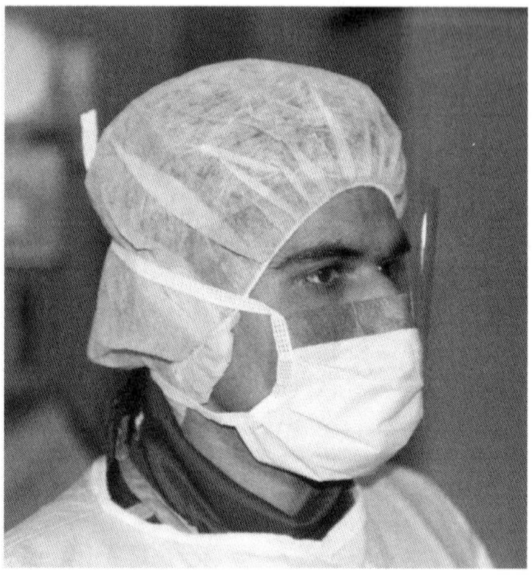

b.

Figure 4. Routine angiography attire. **(a)** Routine barrier precautions during angiography include fluid-impermeable gown, gloves, hat, mask with face shield, and boots. **(b)** The face shield extends upward from the mask, preventing fluid from being splashed into the eyes but without impairing visibility. Ears are covered by the hat, and the mask covers the mouth and nose.

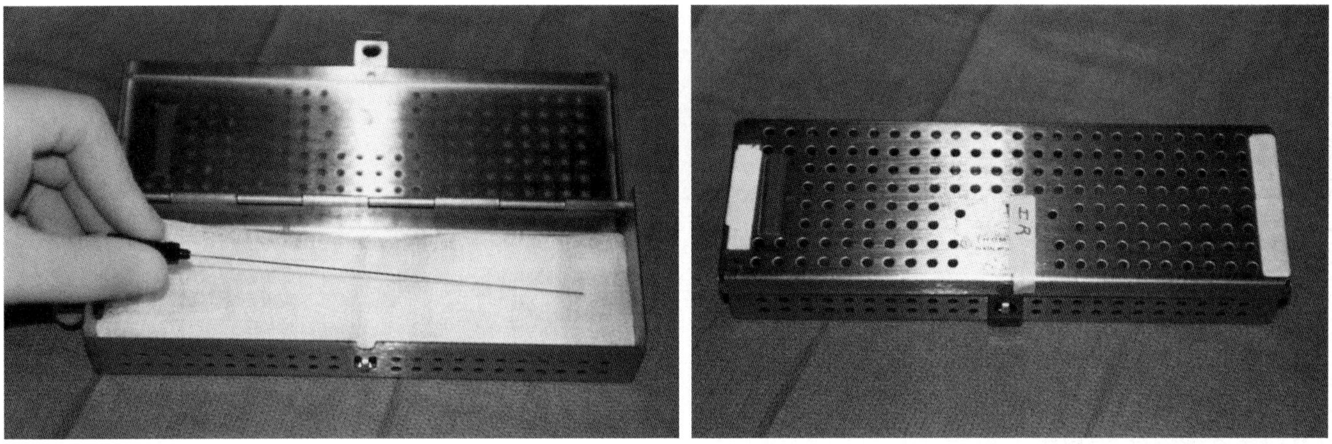

a. b.

Figure 3. Metal tray for sharp objects. **(a)** The stylet of a biliary access needle is placed in a metal tray until access is achieved so as not to leave it exposed on the table or on the patient's drapes. **(b)** The metal top is attached by hinges and covers the tray whenever a stylet has been placed into it. All other sharp objects are disposed of immediately after use and not kept on the tray.

than ever before. The patient should be informed that the staff will be speaking to each other regarding the procedure while it is being performed. In addition, all persons involved should speak freely to each other in order not to make surprise movements and to avoid accidents with sharp objects. OSHA requires that employers minimize the need for mouth-to-mouth resuscitation by making mouthpieces and other ventilation devices immediately available. Therefore, they should be stocked in each room in a radiology department.

Sterile plastic covering of the image intensifier and nonsterile covers on the x-ray tube and foot pedal make cleanup of equipment easy, and it prevents blood contamination of areas that can be difficult to disinfect. The angiographic table and equipment that have been contaminated with body fluids are cleaned with virucidal solution after every procedure. Universal precautions dictate that this be done routinely, not just for blood from patients with a known infectious disease.

Numerous products to improve safety with sharp objects and to protect against splashing of fluids are now available or in development. Indeed, more than 450 patent applications have been filed in the past 5 years. Generally, these products are more expensive than traditional products, and few have been evaluated in a controlled manner to determine cost versus benefit or risk versus benefit for health care workers and patients. However, some have gained acceptance and appear efficacious. For example, needle devices that contain the arterial blood within a clear plastic vacuum side arm provide protection against splashing during double-wall arterial access (Fig 5) (SOS Pulse-Vu needle; Angiodynamics). The hemostatic diaphragm that prevents arterial spray of blood when access is achieved introduces only a slight change in tactile sensation of the guide wire. It is especially useful in angiography performed in inner-city trauma patients because these patients often are young with easily accessible arteries and frequently are at risk for bloodborne infectious disease. Plastic syringes for local anesthesia can be adapted with a retractable plastic sleeve that allows their reuse and safe retention on the interventional table (Fig 6) (Monoject; Sherwood Medical). Intravenous access devices should have a retractable needle to avoid the risk of injury while a catheter is placed in a newly acquired access site. OSHA, in its "Occupational Exposure to Bloodborne Pathogens: Final Rule" report, advised against the use of needles in intravenous catheter connections, and so "piggybacking" of intravenous medications and fluids should be performed with needleless devices (Fig 7) (Access Pin with Safesite valve; B. Braun Medical) (29). A "closed" angiographic flush system prevents the risk that someone—either the radiologist during the procedure or assistants cleaning after the procedure—will be splashed with blood because the fluid was disposed of into a bowl (Fig 8). Such a system allows for the aspiration of a heparin and saline solution used for flushing or of contrast material, as well as the disposal of body fluids into a closed container. It should be used for drainage procedures regardless of the body fluid aspirated. Use of bowls increases the risk of splashing, and they should be omitted from the interventional procedure table. Commercial bowls with absorbent material and plastic covers with an access site for emptying a syringe are less safe in our experience than the "closed" angiographic flush system shown in Figure 7. This is so because of the potential to overfill the bowl and to spill during emptying (the lid has a perforated opening) and because they present a greater risk for housekeeping personnel.

The physician performing the procedure is responsible for the safety of not only the patient but also all the team members. As such, it is important throughout and especially at the completion of the procedure to be certain that all bloody fluid is disposed of in a closed system and all sharp objects have been removed from the table. This ensures that technologists and housekeeping personnel are not exposed to potential splashing or sharp injury in the process of cleaning. All team members must be vigilant regarding their own habits, as well as the habits of others, in order to prevent violations of proper infectious disease control and to optimize the safety of all.

IF EXPOSURE OCCURS

If splashing with blood or bloody body fluid should occur, wash the exposed skin immediately with soap and water (a virucidal agent is not recommended), and profusely flush exposed mucous membranes with water or saline. Change out of blood-soaked clothes. Clean counter sur-

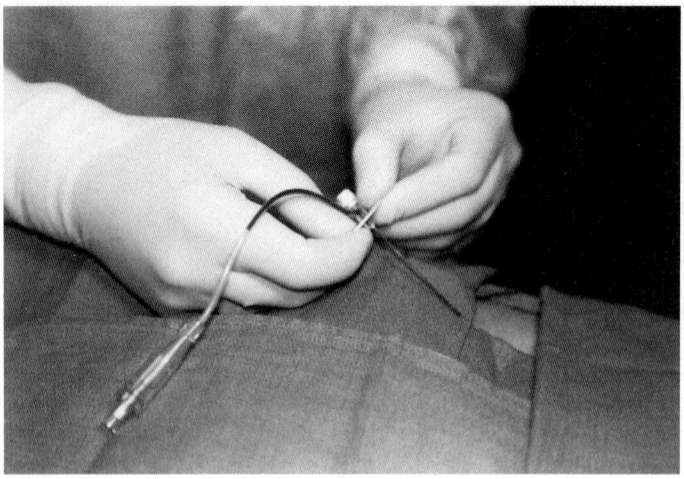

5.

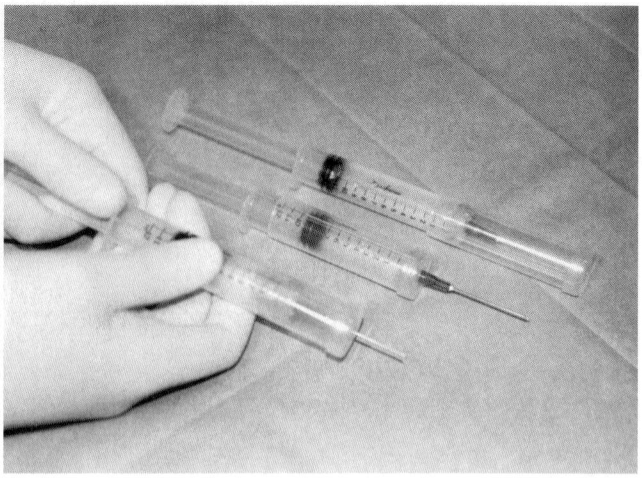

6.

Figures 5–7. **(5)** Vascular access without arterial spray. This Seldinger-style, double-wall needle (SOS Pulse-Vu needle; Angiodynamics, Glens Falls, NY) contains the arterial blood within a clear plastic vacuum side arm by means of a hemostatic valve that prevents arterial spray of blood. **(6)** Plastic needle sheath. This plastic syringe filled with local anesthetic has been adapted with a retractable plastic sleeve (Monoject; Sherwood Medical, St Louis, Mo) that allows its reuse and safe retention on the interventional procedure tray. **(7)** Needleless intravenous catheter connector. OSHA's advice against the use of needles in intravenous catheters was based on an evaluation by the U.S. Food and Drug Administration, so a needleless device (Access Pin with Safestie valve, B. Braun Medical, Bethlehem, Pa) should be used to "piggy-back" infusion catheters.

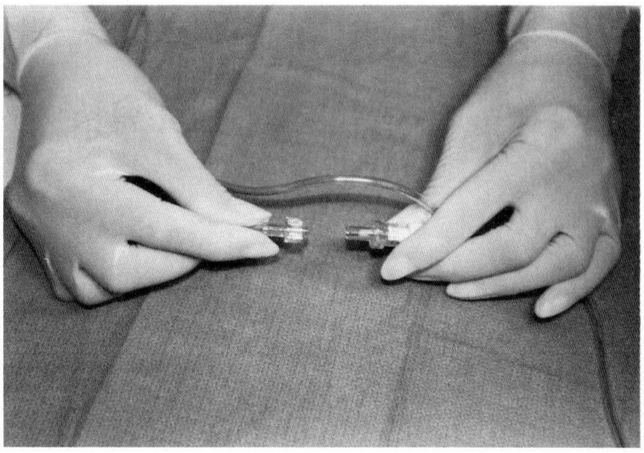

7.

faces and contaminated equipment with household bleach (5% sodium hypochlorite) diluted 1:10 or 1:100 or with hospital virucidal disinfectant. If injury from a sharp object occurs, observe for spontaneous bleeding. Immediately contact the "hot line–on call" infectious disease consultant. Such a position exists for 24-hour immediate consultation at each of the four hospitals of the University of California, San Francisco (30), and at other institutions that have a well-developed response to OSHA's mandate for follow-up of health care worker exposure to blood. Patient history should be reviewed, and HBV, HCV, and HIV serostatus should be obtained. If this information is unknown, some states require patient permission to test the source patient for HIV status. In our experience, however, this information is usually always provided. The exposure characteristics should be reviewed and the health care worker should be advised regarding recommendations for HIV postexposure prophylaxis (Table 2). If in doubt about postexposure prophylaxis, antiretroviral nucleosides ZDV and 3TC should be administered as soon as possible (preferably within 1–2 hours). This can be discontinued if expert consultation later advises against its use. A protease inhibitor (indinavir) should be included if the source patient is in the terminal stage of AIDS (determined on the basis of high viral titers) or has been taking both ZDV and 3TC (because of a possible resistant strain). Radiologists should be aware that the viral inoculum is 100 times greater when injury occurs with an 18-gauge hollow needle contaminated with blood from a patient with symptomatic AIDS than that from a suture needle exposed to blood from an asymptomatic HIV-positive person (24). The health care worker should submit a blood sample for baseline HIV testing and for analysis of HBV titer. If a full course of HBV vaccine had not been administered previously or if a protective titer (>10 mIU/mL) had not been achieved, HBV serum immunoglobulin should be given within 24 hours if the source patient is HBV positive, and the recombinant DNA vaccine should be administered.

Of importance, the CDC study that identified exposure factors that increased the risk of occupational transmission of HIV also documented a 79% reduced risk of seroconversion when ZDV was used as postexposure prophylaxis following injury with a sharp object contaminated with HIV-positive blood (13). Previously, ZDV administration following occupational exposure was controversial, and it has not been approved by the U.S. Food and Drug Administration for use as postexposure prophylaxis. However, even without a randomized, controlled trial to confirm the CDC data, antiretroviral treatment is now considered the standard of care and is recommended by the U.S. Public Health Service in the event of a parenteral occupational exposure and some splash exposures to HIV (Table 2) (6,31–33). Administration of antiretroviral prophylaxis should begin as soon as possible following exposure (within 1–2 hours) because of a limited window of opportunity to intervene before viral dissemination occurs (6). Viruses inoculated percutaneously are initially taken up by cutaneous dendritic cells that then present antigens to T lymphocytes and other immune effector cells. Transmission to local lymph nodes occurs prior to systemic dissemination, neither of which occur instantaneously. Hence, a limited interval ex-

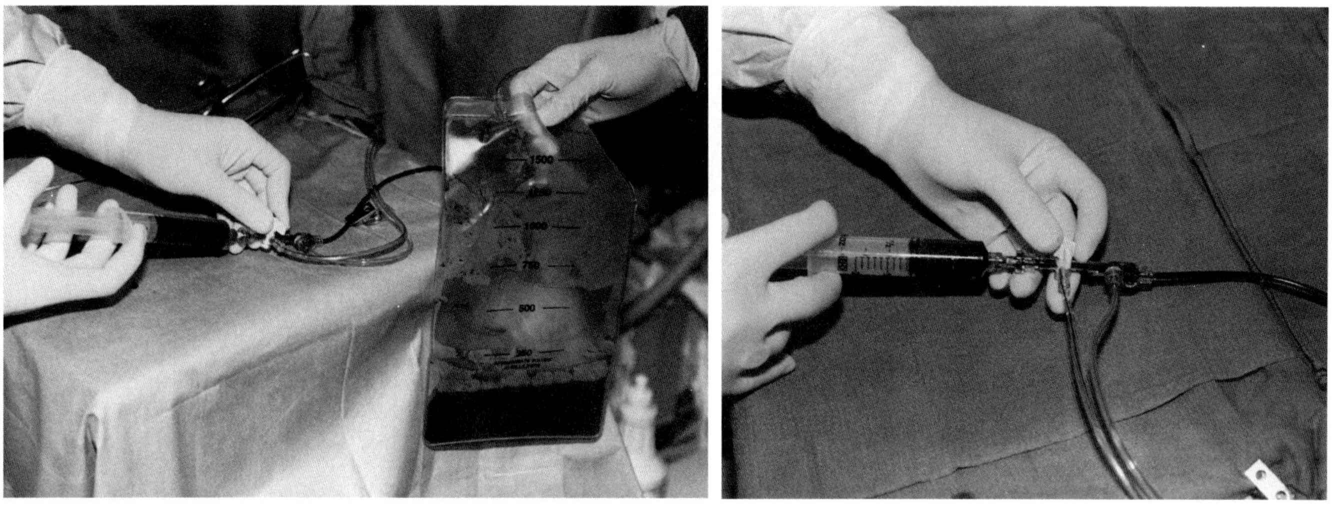

a. b.

Figure 8. Closed flush system. **(a)** A closed flush system (Angiofill II fluid managment system; AngioDynamics, Queensbury, NY) provides for a protected disposal of blood or body fluid via tubing into a plastic bag. **(b)** A one-way valve allows for aspiration of a heparin and saline solution or of contrast material, as well as the closed disposal of blood or drainage fluid.

Table 2
HIV Postexposure Prophylaxis

	Source Patient HIV Positive		
Exposure	Asymptomatic, Known Low Titer	AIDS, Symptomatic	Terminal AIDS or Acute Seroconversion, Known High Titer
Percutaneous injury			
Superficial	Offer	Recommend	Strongly encourage
Visibly bloody vascular access device	Recommend	Recommend	Strongly encourage
Deep injury (intramuscular, spontaneous bleeding)	Recommend	Strongly encourage	Strongly encourage
Mucosal splash			
Small volume and brief	Offer	Offer	Offer
Large volume or prolonged	Offer	Recommend	Recommend
Large volume and prolonged	Recommend	Recommend	Strongly encourage
Cutaneous splash			
Small volume and brief	Offer if nonintact skin	Offer if nonintact skin	Offer if nonintact skin
Large volume or prolonged	Offer; recommend if nonintact skin	Offer; recommend if nonintact skin	Offer; recommend if nonintact skin
Large volume and prolonged	Offer; recommend if nonintact skin	Recommend; especially if nonintact skin	Recommend; especially if nonintact skin

Source.–Adapted from Table 3 in reference 6.

ists during which sufficient interruption of viral replication and assistance to the host immune response might eradicate the virus inoculum (6).

ZDV prophylaxis is not 100% efficacious, however (10). To our knowledge, there have been 11 failures among exposed health care workers in spite of proper administration of ZDV. For this reason, and because of growing viral resistance to ZDV with its increasingly widespread use, combination therapy with two nucleosides (ZDV and 3TC) is used when postexposure prophylaxis is recommended (34) (Table 2). Furthermore, there is evidence of a synergistic effect when two-drug antiretroviral therapy is used (31). Finally, a protease inhibitor (indinavir, IDV) is added if the injury involved a high volume of blood and/or a high titer of virus (terminal illness in source patient) or when a resistant strain is likely because the source patient has been taking ZDV and 3TC.

The currently recommended dosage of ZDV is 1,200 mg/d for 3 days then 1,000 mg/d for 25 days and is tolerated adequately by most health care workers. Previously, higher doses resulted in a high rate of poor tolerance (50%–75%) largely due to gastrointestinal symptoms, headache, and fatigue (1,10). Rarely, 3TC (administered as 150 mg twice a day) can cause pancreatitis. Indinavir toxicity includes gastrointestinal symptoms, and after prolonged use 10% of patients will develop mild hyperbilirubinemia and 4% will develop kidney stones (0.8% in the first 4 weeks). The latter risk can be limited by drinking at least 1.5 L of fluid a day (31). If indinavir therapy is used (recommended dose is 800 mg three times a day), the package insert should be read carefully because certain other drugs such as nonsedating antihistamines are contraindicated. Data are limited regarding fetal safety with antiretroviral therapy in the first trimester of pregnancy. Drug toxicity monitoring should include a complete blood cell count and renal and liver function tests at baseline and every 2 weeks with a 1-month follow-up. All health care workers who receive postexposure prophylaxis are encouraged to enroll in an anonymous registry developed by the CDC, Glaxo Wellcome, and Merck to monitor toxicity and efficacy (telephone 888-737-4448, 888-PEP-4HIV).

The importance of counseling the exposed health care worker cannot be overstated. Exposure to HIV, HBV, or HCV is a frightening experience. In the event of exposure to HIV, health care workers should be reminded that most occupational exposures do not result in seroconversion, and that they have a 99.7% chance of not becoming HIV positive. These odds are even more favorable with the use of postexposure prophylaxis. However, a mixed message is given when the health care worker is counseled to avoid possible secondary transmission through unsafe sex or pregnancy during the window period of possible seroconversion. Baseline HIV serostatus testing should be repeated at 6 weeks, 3 months, and 6 months. To our knowledge, in only one reported case did seroconversion occur more than 6 months after exposure, and this occurred in a nurse exposed and infected simultaneously with HIV and HCV seroconverting at 8–9½ months to HIV-positive and 10½-13½ months to HCV-positive (35). This case is of some additional interest because of the onset at 8 months of fulminant hepatitis leading to death at 28 months after exposure.

Most health care workers in whom seroconversion occurs have sustained a flulike illness that usually manifests 2–4 weeks after exposure. Symptoms include a maculopapular rash, fever, headache, and malaise, and sometimes lymphadenopathy is noted at physical examination. Occasionally odynophagia is present, and endoscopy or barium radiography reveals an isolated giant (>2 cm) ulcer in the middle or distal esophagus with surrounding mucosa that is normal. These signs and symptoms of HIV seroconversion illness remit spontaneously, but health care workers should be advised to seek medical care and return for repeat HIV testing if they should occur.

PHYSICIAN-TO-PATIENT TRANSMISSION

As of January 1, 1995, information about investigations of 64 health care workers infected with HIV had been reported to the CDC. The CDC published data that indicate the risk of HIV transmission from an infected health care worker to a patient is too small to measure (36). No radiologists were involved in the study. The investigation reviewed HIV test results of 22,171 patients of 51 health care workers infected with HIV. For 37 of the 51 health care workers, no seropositive patients were reported among 13,063 patients. For the remaining 14 health care workers, 113 seropositive patients were reported among 9,108 patients, but epidemiologic and laboratory follow-up did not show any health care worker to have been a source of HIV transmission for any of the patients tested. The authors conclude that the risk of transmission of HIV from a health care worker to a patient is immeasurably small, and that retrospective notification of a patient regarding the health care worker's serostatus need not be done routinely. Other investigators agree and conclude that the estimated risk of HIV transmission from physician to patient during invasive radiologic procedures is so low that universal practice restrictions on HIV-positive interventional radiologists are not warranted (37).

Until recently there had been only a single report of HIV transmission from a health care provider (dentist) to a patient since the AIDS epidemic began in 1981. That case continues to generate controversy and conflicting conclusions regarding the mode or even the actuality of transmission from the health care provider (38,39). The fact that a second case was reported only recently in spite of very careful scrutiny for many years further supports the low (indeed immeasurable) risk of clinician transmission to patient (40). The second case, reported in January 1997, involved an orthopedic surgeon who transmitted HIV to one patient 2 years prior to the surgeon becoming ill with AIDS (41). He was not known to be HIV seropositive at the time of the transmission. The procedure was prolonged (10 hours), and there was a known sharp injury to the surgeon that could have exposed his blood to the patient. David Bell, MD, chief of the CDC hospital infections program, has indicated no plans to change the CDC recommendations regarding the practice of HIV-positive health care workers (noted below) (40).

The unusual cluster of six HIV cases involving the Florida dentist resulted in a CDC revision of the guidelines for managing infection in health care providers even though they had not done so previously with 350 recognized nosocomial cases of HBV transmission during invasive procedures from 34 infected health care providers (42). A recent nosocomial outbreak of HBV from a cardiothoracic surgeon and an outbreak of HCV from a cardiac surgeon have been reported (43,44). All of the health care providers involved in HBV transmission who have been tested had HBV envelope antigen, a marker of a high viral titer (45). In spite of these cases, many consider the current CDC recommendations to be overly conservative because they require that patients of a health care provider infected with HIV or HBV (but not HCV) be notified prior to certain procedures. These include "exposure-prone procedures" such as those that involve proximity of a physician's finger and needle tip in a body cavity where visualization is restricted. Experts agree that such notification essentially brings to an end the practice of a surgeon or an interventional radiologist. The work by Hansen and McIntire (37) document the very low risk of physician transmission of HIV to patient. In addition, it provides important objective data to support individual practice decisions regarding the performance of invasive procedures by radiologists, as well as the notification of their positive HIV status during the patient's informed consent process where allowed by state law or hospital policy.

SUMMARY

Radiologists frequently perform invasive diagnostic and therapeutic procedures involving needles and/or vascular access, and often they do so in darkened rooms. Therefore, they are at risk of exposure to blood-borne pathogens. The risk of HIV infection with a single sharp injury is low (0.3%), and on average 99.7% of exposures will not result in infection. However, this seroconversion rate is increased when a high volume of blood or a high concentration of virus is inoculated, and it is decreased by 79% when postexposure prophylaxis is used.

An estimated 800,000 needle-stick injuries and other injuries from sharp objects to health care workers occur annually in the United States (25). Approximately 16,000 of these involve HIV-contaminated blood, and even more are contaminated with HBV or HCV (46). Needle-stick injury therefore poses the single greatest risk to health care workers regarding occupational transmission of HIV.

Because most patients in the radiology department have an unknown HIV or hepatitis serostatus, all patients should be regarded as potentially infectious, and precautions should be universal. In fact, the 1991 OSHA ruling made compliance with the CDC Universal Precautions Guidelines the enforceable national standard. Real-time oral communication among all members of the radiology team and scrupulous attention to safe technique are absolutely essential.

Radiologists are not in agreement regarding the use of precautions against injury with a sharp object and splashing (47–50). Many have adapted some of their habits to conform well to the CDC and OSHA guidelines regarding universal precautions, but some remain skeptical regarding the risk of exposure to themselves. Consequently, in some areas resistance to the above recommendations persists. However, the data to date provide a compelling argument for protection against occupational exposure to blood either by percutaneous sharp injury or splashing on mucous membranes or interrupted skin.

A number of resources were made available in early 1997 for easy access to the most current data regarding occupational transmission of HIV or hepatitis. For instance, the CDC has a World Wide Web site (*http://www.cdc.gov*) and a facsimile information service through the Hospital Infections Program directory (telephone 404-332-4565). Also, the National AIDS Clearinghouse can be reached by telephone (800-458-5231), as can the HIV/AIDS Treatment Information Service (800-448-0440). The postexposure prophylaxis protocol used at the University of California, San Francisco, can be reviewed by visiting its World Wide Web site at *http://epi-center.ucsf.edu*. And up-to-date information is available to both Veterans Administration and other health care staff worldwide by J. Michael Howe, MSLS, of the AIDS Information Center, a service of the VA HIV/AIDS National Training Program, located at the Veterans Administration Medical Center, San Francisco, University of California, San Francisco (*hivinfo@itsa.ucsf.edu*). ■

Acknowledgments: The authors thank Theresa L. Wright, MD, and Peter C. Jensen, MD, for their helpful review of the manuscript, as well as Aija Krusa for her invaluable assistance with manuscript preparation.

References

1. Gerberding JL. Management of occupational exposures to blood-borne viruses. N Engl J Med 1995; 332:444–451.
2. Sepkowitz KA. Occupationally acquired infections in health care workers. II. Ann Intern Med 1996; 125:917–928.
3. Gerberding JL. Incidence and prevalence of human immunodeficiency virus, hepatitis C virus, and cytomegalovirus among health care personnel at risk for blood exposure: final report from a longitudinal study. J Infect Dis 1994; 170:1410–1417.
4. McWilliams RG, Blanshard KS. The risk of blood splash contamination during angiography. Clin Radiol 1994; 49:59–60.
5. Hansen ME, Miller GL III, Redman HC, McIntire DD. Needle-stick injuries and blood contacts during invasive radiologic procedures: frequency and risk factors. AJR 1993; 160:1119–1122.
6. Gerberbering JL. Prophylaxis for occupational exposure to HIV. Ann Intern Med 1996; 125:497–501.
7. Zuckerman AJ. Occupational exposure to hepatitis B virus and human immunodeficiency virus: a comparative risk analysis. Am J Infect Control 1995; 23:286–289.
8. Holmberg SD. The estimated prevalence and incidence of HIV in 96 large U.S. metropolitan areas. Am J Pub Health 1996; 85:642–654.
9. Centers for Disease Control and Prevention. HIV/AIDS surveillance report: U.S. HIV and AIDS cases reported through December 1996. Vol 8, no. 2. Atlanta, Ga: Centers for Disease Control and Prevention, 1997; 20–21.
10. Tokars JI, Marcus R, Culver DH, et al. Surveillance of HIV infection and zidovudine use among health care workers after occupational exposure to HIV-infected blood. Ann Intern Med 1993; 118:913–919.
11. Henderson DK. HIV-1 in the health care setting. In: Mandell GL, Bennet JE, Dolin R, eds. Principles and practices of infectious diseases. 4th ed. New York, NY: Churchill Livingston, 1995; 2632–2656.
12. Saag MS, Crain MJ, Decker WD, et al. High-level viremia in adults and children infected with human immunodeficiency virus: relation to disease stage and CDC4+ lymphocyte levels. J Infect Dis 1991; 164:72–80.
13. Centers for Disease Control and Prevention. Case-control study of HIV seroconversion in health-care workers after 12/22/95 percutaneous exposure to HIV-infected blood: France, United Kingdom, and United States, January 1988–August 1994. MMWR 1995; 44:929–933.
14. Denes AE, Smith JL, Maynard JE, Doto IL, Berquist KR, Finkel AJ. Hepatitis B infection in physicians: results of a nationwide seroepidemiologic survey. JAMA 1978; 239:210–212.
15. Mast EE, Alter MJ. Prevention of hepatitis B virus infection among health care. In: Ellis RW, ed. Hepatitis B vaccines in clinical practice. New York, NY: Dekker, 1993; 295–307.
16. Robert LM, Chamberland ME, Cleveland JL. Investigations of patients of health care workers infected with HIV: the Centers for Disease Control and Prevention database. Ann Intern Med 1995; 122:653–657.
17. Sattar SA, Springthrope VS. Survival and disinfectant in activation of the human immunodeficiency virus: a critical review. Rev Infect Dis 1991; 13:430–447.
18. Gibas A, Blewett DR, Schoenfeld DA, Dienstag JL. Prevalence and incidence of viral hepatitis in health workers in the prehepatitis B vaccination era. Am J Epidemiol 1992; 136:603–610.
19. Thomas DL, Factor SH, Kelen GD, Washington AS, Taylor E Jr, Quinn TC. Viral hepatitis in health care personnel at The Johns Hopkins Hospital: the seroprevalence of and risk factors for hepatitis B virus and hepatitis C virus infection. Arch Intern Med 1993; 153:1705–1712.
20. Roome AJ, Walsh SJ, Cartter ML, Hadler JL. Hepatitis B vaccine responsiveness in Connecticut public safety personnel. JAMA 1993; 270:2931–2934.
21. Wood RC, MacDonald KL, White KE, Hedberg CW, Hanson M, Osterholm MT. Risk factors for lack of detectable antibody following hepatitis B vaccination of Minnesota health care workers. JAMA 1993; 270:2935–2939.
22. Centers for Disease Control and Prevention. Recommendations for preventing transmission of immunodeficiency virus and hepatitis B virus to patients during exposure-prone invasive procedures. MMWR 1991; 40:1–9.
23. Centers for Disease Control and Prevention. Recommendations for follow-up of health-care workers after occupational exposure to hepatitis C virus. MMWR 1997; 45:603–606.
24. Choo QL, Kuo G, Weiner AJ. Isolation of a DNA clone derived from a blood-borne non-A, non-B viral hepatitis genome. Science 1989; 244:359–362.
25. Tereskerz T, Pearson R. Universal precautions: still missing the point on needlesticks. Infect Control Hosp Epidemiol 1991; 12:211–213.
26. Pugliese G, Favero MS. HIV postexposure prophylaxis recommendations. Infect Control Hosp Epidemiol 1996; 17:476–477.
27. Mast ST, Woolwine JD, Gerberding JL. Efficacy of gloves in reducing blood volumes transferred during simulated needlestick injury. J Infect Dis 1993; 168:1589–1592.
28. Hansen ME, McIntire DD, Miller GL III. Occult glove perforations: frequency during interventional radiologic procedures. AJR 1992; 59:131–135.
29. Occupational Health and Safety Administration, Department of Labor. Occupational exposure to bloodborne pathogens: final rule (29 CFR 1910.1030). Federal Register December 6, 1991; 56(235):64060.
30. Gerberding JL. Postexposure prophylaxis for human immunodeficiency virus at San Francisco General Hospital. Am J Med 1997; 102:85–89.
31. Centers for Disease Control and Prevention. Update: provisional public health service recommendation for chemoprophylaxis after occupational exposure to HIV. MMWR 1996; 45:468–472.
32. Carpenter CC, Fischl MA, Hammer SM, et al. Antiretroviral therapy for HIV infection in 1996: recommendations of an international panel. JAMA 1996; 276:146–154.
33. Katz MH, Gerberding JL. Postexposure treatment of people exposed to the human immunodeficiency virus through sexual contact or injection-drug use. N Engl J Med 1997; 336:1097–1100.
34. Bell DM, Gerberding JL. Human immunodeficiency virus postexposure management of healthcare worker: report of a workshop. Am J Med 1997; 102:1–3.
35. Ridzon R, Gallagher K, Ciesielski C, et al. Simultaneous transmission of human immunodeficiency virus and hepatitis C virus from a needle-stick injury. N Engl J Med 1997; 336:919–922.
36. Roberts LM, Chamberland ME, Cleveland JL, et al. Investigation of patients of

health care workers infected with HIV: the Centers for Disease Control and Prevention database. Ann Intern Med 1995; 122:653–657.
37. Hansen ME, McIntire DD. HIV transmission during invasive radiologic procedures: estimate based on computer modeling. AJR 1996; 166:263–267.
38. Barr S. The 1990 Florida dental investigation: is the case really closed? Ann Intern Med 1996; 124:250–254.
39. Brown D. The 1990 Florida dental investigation: theory and fact. Ann Intern Med 1996; 124:255–256.
40. Anonymous. CDC: French HIV surgical case will not affect US policy on infected providers. Hosp Infect Control 1997; 24: 33–36.
41. Dorozynski A. French patient contracts AIDS from surgeon. Br Med J 1997; 314: 250.
42. Bell DM, Shapiro CN, Gooch BF. Preventing HIV transmission to patients during invasive procedures. J Pub Health Dent 1993; 53:170–173.
43. Harpaz R, Von Seidlein L, Averhoff FM, et al. Transmission of hepatitis B virus to multiple patients from a surgeon without evidence of inadequate infection control. N Engl J Med 1996; 334:549–554.
44. Esteban JI, Gomez J, Martell M, et al. Transmission of hepatitis C virus by a cardiac surgeon. N Engl J Med 1996; 334:555–560.
45. Gerberding JL. The infected health care provider (editorial). N Engl J Med 1996; 334:394–395.
46. Hansen ME, McIntire DD, Miller GL III, Redman HC. Use of universal precautions in interventional radiology: results of a national survey. Am J Infect Control 1994; 22:1–5.
47. Hansen ME, Miller GL III, Redman HC, McIntire DD. HIV and interventional radiology: a national survey of physician attitudes and behaviors. JVIR 1993; 4:229–236.
48. Wall SD, Olcott EW, Gerberding JL. AIDS risk and risk reduction in the radiology department. AJR 1991; 157:911–917.
49. Williams DM, Marx MV, Korobkin M. AIDS risk and risk reduction in the radiology department (commentary). AJR 1991; 157:919–921.
50. Hall FM. Double gloving during interventional procedures (letter). AJR 1993; 161:678.

Suresh K. Mukherji, MD • Harold R. Pillsbury, MD • Mauricio Castillo, MD

Imaging Squamous Cell Carcinomas of the Upper Aerodigestive Tract: What Clinicians Need to Know[1]

THE development of modern imaging techniques has substantially altered the treatment and management of malignancies of the upper aerodigestive tract. Important decisions that were once made during surgery are now made in advance of surgery by using information from computed tomography (CT) and magnetic resonance (MR) imaging. Imaging helps determine tumor resectability and the extent of surrounding tissue that must be resected to ensure adequate surgical margins. Because it improves the accuracy of staging, pretreatment imaging is accepted as an important adjunct to physical examination in patients with malignancies of the upper aerodigestive tract (1–8).

Detailed counseling is important for patients with head and neck malignancies, because surgical treatment of tumors in this region of the body results in anatomic alterations that can cause important lifestyle changes. Properly performed imaging provides detailed information about the extent and depth of tumors, information that often cannot be ascertained by means of physical examination alone. Although mucosal spread is better detected by means of direct visualization, deep extension is better evaluated by using cross-sectional imaging rather than endoscopy. Pretreatment imaging provides information that may determine whether patients are candidates for organ preservation therapy, either surgery or radiation therapy.

Because of advancements in head and neck imaging, some otolaryngologists or radiation oncologists may not be aware of its effect on the treatment and management of squamous cell carcinomas (SCCs) of the upper aerodigestive tract. Similarly, some radiologists may not be familiar with the specific information that must be conveyed to the referring clinician.

The intent of this article is to provide guidelines on specific information that must be transmitted to the referring otolaryngologist or radiation oncologist and that will alter the care of patients with SCC of the upper aerodigestive tract. The terminology used in this article is standard and used by referring clinicians. Knowledge of this terminology and treatment options is essential. This article is not intended to provide an in-depth discussion of the controversies surrounding the benefits and pitfalls of various cross-sectional imaging modalities used for head and neck imaging (9–12). Evaluation of cervical lymph nodes for metastases from SCC will also not be addressed, since other, excellent articles discuss the role of imaging in that situation (13–17). The focus of this text is to provide guidelines on the information that imaging can provide that will directly affect the treatment and care of patients with head and neck cancer.

IMAGING STRATEGIES

CT Technique

Axial images are obtained with the patient supine. The head is carefully aligned in the cephalocaudal axis. Malposition may result in an appearance that simulates disease or abnormality. Direct coronal and axial scanning should be performed in any patient suspected of having a nasopharyngeal, palatal, or skull base carcinoma. The optimal field of view varies between 14 and 18 cm; the final field of view is dependent on the size of the patient. The maximal section thickness should not exceed 3 mm. Contiguous sections should be obtained through the primary site, while an intersection gap of 2 mm can be used to image the remainder of the neck.

All studies performed to evaluate neoplasms should include the intravenous administration of contrast material. Intravenous contrast material helps increase the conspicuity of the primary tumor and is essential for evaluating cervical nodal metastases. Bolus administration is the preferred technique. We prefer spiral CT, as this technique reduces both motion artifact and contrast material load compared with standard dynamic CT (18,19). Proper gantry angle is essential in the oropharynx and oral cavity to avoid dental-related artifacts. The gantry angle should be changed to avoid artifacts from dental amalgam, thereby optimizing visualization of the oral tongue and tongue base. Sections parallel to the ramus of the mandible should be obtained from the top of the mandibular alveolar ridge to the hyoid bone. If the larynx and hypopharynx must be studied in detail, sections must be parallel to the true vocal cords (TVC) for that portion of the study. The plane of the hyoid bone is similar to that of the laryngeal ventricle and may be used to approximate the angle of the TVC. In addition to the soft-tissue window settings, all images should be reconstructed with bone algorithms, which are helpful for detection of bone and cartilage invasion.

Index terms: Head and neck neoplasms, CT, 26.1211, 27.1211 • Head and neck neoplasms, diagnosis, 26.37, 27.37 • Head and neck neoplasms, MR, 26.1214, 27.1214 • Larynx, CT, 271.1211 • Larynx, MR, 271.1214 • Larynx, neoplasms, 271.37 • Mouth, neoplasms, 262.37 • Nasopharynx, neoplasms, 263.37 • Pharynx, CT, 263.1211 • Pharynx, neoplasms, 263.37 • State-of-art reviews • Tongue, neoplasms, 262.37

Radiology 1997; 205:629–646

[1] From the Department of Radiology (S.K.M., M.C.) and the Division of Otolaryngology Head and Neck Surgery (S.K.M., H.R.P.), University of North Carolina School of Medicine, 3324 Infirmary CB 7510, Chapel Hill, NC 27599-7510. Received June 6, 1997; accepted and revision requested July 22; revision received August 6. **Address reprint requests to** S.K.M.

Abbreviations: SCC = squamous cell carcinoma, TVC = true vocal cords.

MR Imaging Technique

Images of the nasopharynx and oropharynx are obtained with a standard head coil. Depending on the body habitus of the patient, the floor of the mouth can often be imaged with this coil. Images of the neck are obtained with a neck coil. Knowledge of the site of the primary tumor permits a focused study that eliminates unnecessary imaging, thus reducing overall imaging time. Shorter imaging time also reduces the likelihood that images will be degraded by motion.

MR imaging studies of the oropharynx, hypopharynx, and oral cavity should be performed in both the axial and coronal planes. The ideal section thickness is 4 mm or less. The optimal field of view for the axial views is 16–18 cm for T1-weighted sequences and 18–20 cm for T2-weighted sequences. This slightly larger field of view with the T2-weighted sequences results in a better signal-to-noise ratio.

T1-weighted coronal images obtained without contrast material should be acquired in patients with nasopharyngeal carcinoma to evaluate for evidence of skull base invasion. Intravenous paramagnetic contrast material should be routinely used in patients with SCC of the upper aerodigestive tract. We suggest that T1-weighted images be obtained before and after the use of intravenous paramagnetic contrast material. A nonenhanced T1-weighted sequence should be performed in the same plane prior to contrast material administration so high-signal-intensity fat or proteinaceous fluid will not be confused with enhancement. Contrast-enhanced T1-weighted images are necessary to evaluate for perineural spread and tumor extension into the cavernous sinus. Fat-saturation imaging permits better identification of the tumor margins because it helps separate the enhancing tumor margins from background fat (20). This is especially important for oral cavity and oropharyngeal cancers when one is attempting to determine their relationship to the lingual septum and neurovascular bundle (20,21).

In the past, one of the major drawbacks of performing MR imaging for the evaluation of patients with squamous cell carcinoma of the extracranial head and neck has been motion artifact. Tumors that involve the upper aerodigestive tract often partially obstruct the airway. The resulting dyspnea is worsened by the fact that many of these patients have underlying chronic obstructive pulmonary disease due to a long smoking history. Recent developments in fast MR imaging techniques permit rapid image acquisition that reduces motion artifacts encountered in this patient population (20,22–24). Continued developments in this area may permit MR imaging to provide studies that are of consistently higher quality due to a reduction in patient motion than have been previously possible (20,22–24).

Figure 1. Nasopharynx. TNM classification and guidelines for the information that must be conveyed to the referring clinician when evaluating imaging studies obtained in patients with nasopharyngeal carcinoma.

TNM Staging

- TIS Carcinoma in situ
- T1 Tumor confined to the nasopharynx
- T2 Tumor extends to soft tissues of oropharynx and/or nasal fossa
  - T2a without parapharyngeal extension
  - T2b with parapharyngeal extension
- T3 Tumor invades bony structures and/or paranasal sinuses
- T4 Tumor with intracranial extension and/or involvement of cranial infratemporal fossa, hypopharynx, or orbit

Imaging Checklist

- Detailed assessment of the spread pattern of tumor with an emphasis on the deep and superior extension
- Skull base erosion
- Involvement of the mandibular division of the fifth cranial nerve
- Cavernous sinus involvement

TUMOR LOCATIONS

Nasopharynx (Figs 1, 2)

SCC accounts for 70% of superficial malignancies in the nasopharynx (Figs 1, 2) (25,26). Lymphomas account for approximately 20%, and the remaining 10% consist of a variety of lesions including adenocarcinoma, rhabdomyosarcoma, adenoid cystic carcinoma, melanoma, plasma cell myeloma, fibrosarcoma, and carcinosarcoma (26).

The World Health Organization has classified nasopharyngeal carcinoma into three types based on histopathologic charcateristics: SCC (type 1), nonkeratinizing carcinoma (type 2), and undifferentiated carcinoma (type 3) (25). Type 1 tumors are keratinized lesions similar to SCCs found in the remainder of the upper aerodigestive tract. Type 2 lesions have little or no keratin production and, because of their resemblance to urinary tract tumors, are sometimes referred to as transitional cell carcinomas. Type 3 carcinomas often resemble large cell lymphomas and constitute a diverse group of malignancies that include lymphoepitheliomas and spindle cell and clear cell varieties of SCC (27). Whereas World Health Organization type I and type II nasopharyngeal carcinomas are primarily cancers of adults, the undifferentiated type III nasopharyngeal carcinomas have a distinct bimodal age distribution (26).

Several factors have been linked to an increased likelihood of developing SCC of the nasopharynx. Immunoglobulin A antibodies against Epstein-Barr virus have been associated with the undifferentiated form of this tumor. Human leukocyte antigen A2 and human leukocyte antigen B-Sin histocompatibility loci have been identified as possible markers for genetic susceptibility to SCC among the Chinese population (28). The incidence appears to decrease among Chinese subjects born in North America, although the rate is still seven times higher than that in native Americans (29). Other risk factors include ingestion of nitrosamines (present in dry-salted fish), inhalation of polycyclic hydrocarbons, poor living conditions, and chronic sinonasal infections (26).

Deep fascial planes are conduits for tumor spread. Other potential pathways for growth include muscle bundles, neurovascular bundles, the mucosa, and the submucosa. Spread of tumor may be altered by normal structures that are resistant to invasion. In the nasopharynx, these include the cartilaginous portion of the eustachian tube and the pharyngobasilar fascia (visceral fascia) (30,31). Thus, early lesions located in the fossa of Rosenmüller are limited to the visceral space by the surrounding visceral fascia.

Progressive growth of nasopharyngeal carcinomas results in extension of these tumors anteriorly, inferiorly, lat-

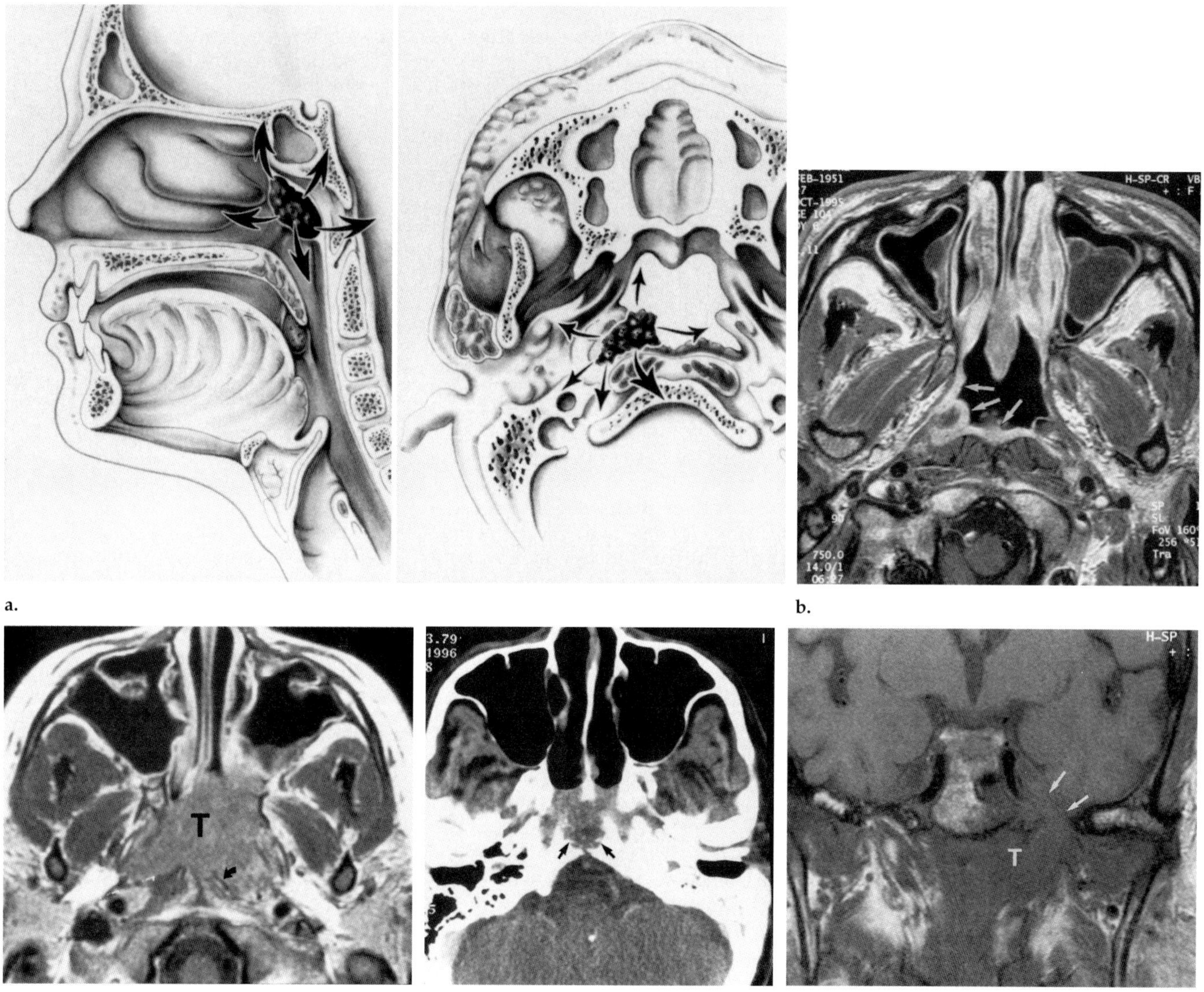

a. b. c. d. e.

Figure 2. Nasopharyngeal carcinoma. **(a)** Schematic illustrations demonstrate the potential pathways of spread for nasopharyngeal carcinomas. **(b)** Axial contrast material–enhanced T1-weighted (750/14 [repetition time msec/echo time msec], two signals acquired) MR image demonstrates a low-volume nasopharyngeal carcinoma that involves the mucosa, overlies the torus tubarius, and extends posteriorly to involve the fossa of Rosenmuller (arrows). The small size of this tumor gives this a favorable appearance for treatment with high-dose brachytherapy alone. **(c)** Axial contrast-enhanced T1-weighted MR image (450/20) shows a large nasopharyngeal carcinoma situated primarily within the visceral space. The tumor (*T*) extends deep to invade the longus coli of the neck (arrow). The large bulk of the tumor give this lesion an unfavorable imaging appearance for treatment with high-dose brachytherapy alone. **(d)** Axial contrast-enhanced CT scan shows a nasopharyngeal carcinoma that has eroded the clivus (arrows). This bone erosion is clinically occult and causes the tumor stage to be moved up to T3. These imaging findings necessitated that this tumor be treated with chemotherapy and concominant three-dimensional conformal radiation therapy with a skull base boost. **(e)** Coronal noncontrast T1-weighted (695/15) MR image obtained in a patient with an advanced nasopharyngeal carcinoma (*T*) shows perineural extension along the third division of cranial nerve V into the cavernous sinus (T4) (arrows). This spread into the cavernous sinus was clinically occult and necessitated three-dimensional conformal treatment planning to encompass the cavernous sinus and skull base.

erally, and superiorly. Lateral extension into the deep structures of the nasopharynx is facilitated by the sinus of Morgagni, a natural fascial defect that allows the passage into the cartilaginous portion of the eustachian tube and the levator veli palatini muscle (25,30). This natural defect, situated in the superior portion of the lateral wall of the nasopharynx, provides access for advanced tumor to extend into the masticator and the pre- and poststyloid parapharyngeal spaces. Once in these areas, tumors may involve the levator veli palatini muscle and the tensor muscle of the velum palatinum and the third division of the fifth cranial nerve and may encase the neurovascular structures of the post–styloid-parapharyngeal space. Advanced lesions may invade the skull base, and the most common sites of erosion are the petroclinoid fissure and foramen lacerum. This is attributed to the proximity of the fossa of Rosenmüller to the petroclinoid fissure. Aggressive lesions may extend directly into the foramen lacerum and encase the internal carotid artery, then gaining access into the cavernous sinus. Nasopharyngeal carcinomas may also involve the cavernous sinus through retrograde spread along the mandibular division of the fifth cranial nerve (31).

Anterior extension into the posterior nasal cavity can be visualized by means of direct endoscopy. However, continued extension into the pterygopalatine fossa is best detected with imaging. Inferior extension along the lateral pharyngeal walls and anterior and posterior tonsillar pillars is seen in nearly one-third of patients (25). This form of spread is often submucosal and may be clinically occult. Diagnosis of inferior extension based solely on findings at clinical examination may, in fact, be involvement of the retropharyngeal lymph nodes and not direct tumor invasion.

The standard treatment for nasopharyngeal carcinoma is radiation therapy. The role of surgery is limited to biopsy and preliminary staging. The American Joint Committee on Cancer TNM staging system for nasopharyngeal carcinoma is based primarily on findings from endoscopic examination with emphasis on anterior and inferior tumor extension. However, clinical evaluation of nasopharyngeal carcinoma may result in a gross underestimation of lesion size and extent. Deep and superior tumor spread is better evaluated with cross-sectional imaging studies than with endoscopy (32).

The standard treatment for nasopharyngeal carcinomas is aimed at the site of the primary tumors and at the lymph nodes (25). Superficial tumors limited to the mucosal space without invasion of the deep fascial and muscular planes may be treated with high-dose brachytherapy. The imaging appearance that favors use of localized high-dose brachytherapy is that of a superficial carcinoma that can be encompassed within 2 cm of the brachytherapy applicator. Presence of deep extension into the masticator and parapharyngeal space, as identified at CT or MR imaging, contraindicates treatment with high-dose brachytherapy. Anterior extension into the posterior nasal cavity or pterygopalatine fossa necessitates conformal therapy such as shaped three-field technique (opposed lateral fields and a single anterior field).

Invasion of the skull base and cranial nerves causes a nasopharyngeal carcinoma to be upstaged (to T4) (32). Cavernous sinus involvement may result from (*a*) direct skull base invasion, (*b*) retrograde spread of tumor along the mandibular division of the trigeminal nerve, (*c*) extension into the foramen lacerum with continued antegrade spread along the internal carotid artery, or (*d*) retrograde spread along the maxillary division of the trigeminal nerve following involvement of the pterygopalatine fossa. Imaging evidence of cavernous sinus invasion necessitates that the superior border of the radiation port be raised to include the floor of the anterior and middle cranial fossae. Advanced local and regional disease such as skull base erosion and cavernous sinus invasion may indicate the need for concomitant chemotherapy (21).

CT and MR imaging are complementary modalities for evaluating nasopharyngeal carcinoma. CT is more sensitive for detection of early cortical destruction, whereas MR imaging best demonstrates soft-tissue extension into the cavernous sinus (11,12,33–36). Patients with nasopharyngeal carcinoma that was detected initially with MR imaging and that extends to the skull base without invasion of the cavernous sinus or clivus should undergo coronal CT (with 1–2-mm-thick contiguous sections) reconstructed with bone algorithms for detection of early cortical erosion (35). Similarly, a nasopharyngeal carcinoma that extends to the skull base should be evaluated with MR imaging to determine the superior extent of the tumor (11), specifically whether there is skull base or cavernous sinus involvement via the petroclival fissure or foramen lacerum, or retrograde perineural spread along the mandibular or maxillary divisions of the trigeminal nerve (12,34–36).

Involvement of high posterior cervical lymph nodes is common in cases of advanced nasopharyngeal carcinoma. These nodes may be treated with electron-beam radiation therapy. However, the strength of the electron-beam therapy depends on the extent of nodal disease and its relationship to the spinal cord. In these patients, cross-sectional imaging plays an essential role in (*a*) determining the depth of the deep margin of the involved posterior lymph node from the skin surface and (*b*) determining the distance between the deep margin of the involved posterior lymph node and the spinal cord.

Oropharynx (Fig 3)

The oropharynx consists of (*a*) the pharyngeal wall situated between the nasopharynx and the pharyngoepiglottic fold, (*b*) the soft palate, (*c*) the tonsillar region, and (*d*) the tongue base (Fig 3). The anterior margin of the oropharynx is formed by a plane that joins the posterior border of the soft palate, the anterior tonsillar pillars, and the circumvallate papillae. The superior border of the ororpharynx is located at the soft palate and the ridge of pharyngeal musculature that opposes the soft palate when the soft palate is elevated (Passavant ridge). The oropharynx is bordered inferiorly by the vallecula. The posterior border of the oropharynx is formed by the posterior pharyngeal wall. The lateral margin consists of the tonsillar region. The tonsillar region consists of the anterior tonsillar pillar (palatoglossus muscle), posterior tonsillar pillar (palatopharyngeus muscle), and the lymphoid tissue-containing fossa situated between these two pillars, termed the palatine (faucial) tonsil (37,38).

The majority of tumors involving the oropharynx are SCCs; other, less common, lesions include lymphoma, minor salivary gland tumors, and rare mesenchymal lesions (21). The spread pattern, lymphatic drainage, and surgical approach for oropharyngeal tumors varies with the specific site of origin (21,37,38).

The classification of the American Joint Committee on Cancer for oropharyngeal SCC is based primarily on the ability of the examining physician to obtain a gross estimate of the size of the tumor at endoscopy (32) (Fig 3). However, the extent of the tumor is often underestimated at physical examination because these lesions tend to spread submucosally (37) (Fig 4).

The most commonly performed surgical procedure for treatment of tongue base carcinomas (Fig 4) is a partial glossectomy. This procedure requires preservation of one lingual artery and one hypoglossal nerve. Either CT or MR imaging may be preoperatively used to evaluate patients with tongue base carcinoma. Information that will directly affect the surgical approach is whether the tumor involves the ipsilateral neurovascular bundle, whether there is submucosal involvement in adjacent areas including the floor of the mouth, and whether the tumor crosses the midline. If the tumor crosses the midline, its relation to the contralateral lingual neurovascular bundle must be determined. Spread of tumor across the midline and in proximity to the opposite lingual neurovascular bundle precludes a partial glossectomy and necessitates a total glossectomy. At many institutions, this radical form of resection is often considered an unacceptable alternative.

Treatment of tonsillar (Fig 5) and soft-palate (Fig 6) carcinomas depends on lesion size and involvement of surrounding structures. In these tumors, bone erosion is an unusual finding and is present only in advanced soft-palate carcinomas that have involved the hard palate. Detailed imaging of the soft-tissue extent of tonsillar and soft-palate carcinomas provides information that may affect their surgical resection. Although CT is commonly used to evaluate the primary lesion, the extent of these tumors is better assessed with MR imaging. Early tumors, localized in the tonsillar fossa or soft palate, may undergo a wide local excision through an intraoral approach. Advanced tumors, which may extend submucosally through the superior constrictor muscle and invade

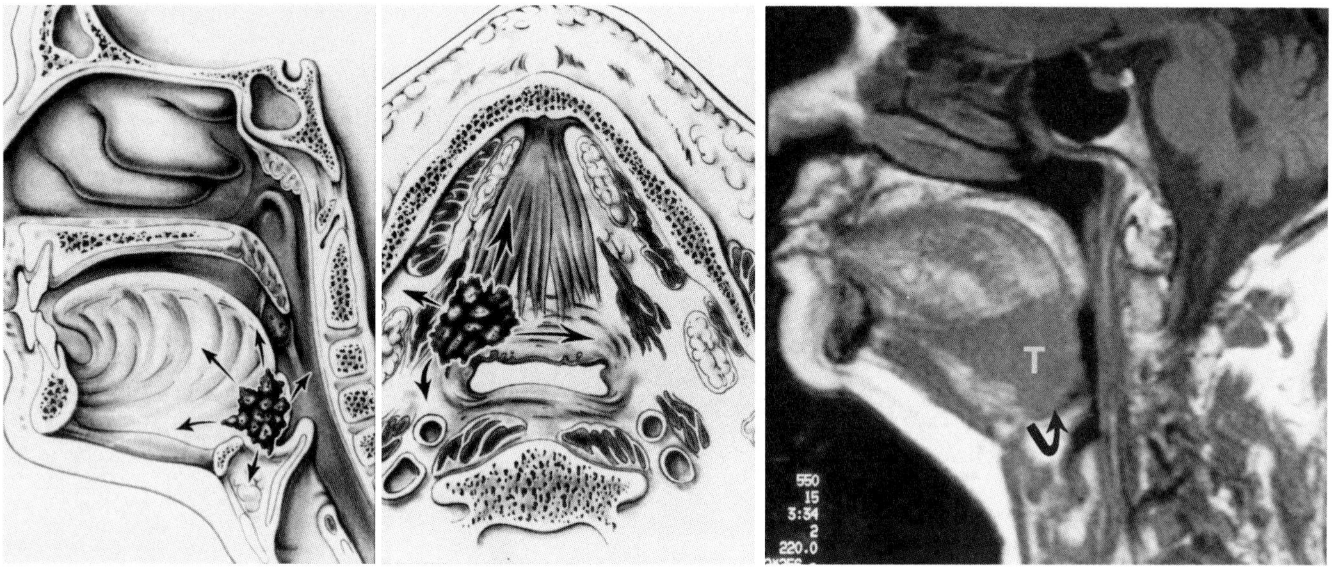

a. b.

Figure 4. Tongue base carcinoma. **(a)** Schematic illustrations demonstrate the potential pathways of spread for a tongue base carcinoma. **(b)** Sagittal T1-weighted (550/15) MR image demonstrates an SCC involving the tongue base (*T*). The lesion extends inferiorly to the root of the tongue and involves the vallecula. The surgical management of a tumor with this type of spread pattern would include total glossectomy. This patient was treated with radiation therapy and concomitant chemotherapy.

TNM Staging

TIS	Carcinoma in situ
T1	Tumor 2 cm or less in greatest dimension
T2	Tumor more than 2 cm but not more than 4 cm in greatest dimension
T3	Tumor more than 4 cm in greatest dimension
T4	Tumor invades adjacent structures (eg, pterygoid muscle[s], mandible, hard palate, deep muscle of tongue, larynx)

Imaging Checklist

Tongue base carcinoma

- Extension to floor of mouth and surrounding structures
- Relationship to ipsilateral lingual neurovascular bundle
- Extension across midline and relationship to contralateral neurovascular bundle

Tonsil, soft-palate, or posterior pharyngeal wall carcinoma

- Detailed evaluation of submucosal extension into the soft tissues of the neck (pre- and poststyloid parapharyngeal space, nasopharynx)
- Tongue base invasion
- Encasement of carotid artery
- Bone erosion
- Pre-vertebral muscle invasion

Figure 3. Oropharynx. TMN classification and guidelines for the information that must be conveyed to the referring clinician when evaluating imaging studies obtained in patients with squamous cell carcinoma of the oropharynx.

the parapharyngeal and masticator spaces, require resection of portions of the tongue base, mandible, and maxilla. Progressive growth of these tumors may result in encasement of the internal carotid artery (Fig 5c) or extension superiorly along the fascial and muscle planes into the skull base. This deep submucosal extension cannot usually be identified with endoscopy (37). At many institutions, imaging evidence of encasement of the internal carotid artery or bulk disease that abuts the skull base precludes surgery.

Oral Cavity (Fig 7)

The oral cavity comprises the lip, upper and lower gingiva, buccal mucosa, hard palate, floor of the mouth, and oral (anterior two-thirds) tongue. As with oropharyngeal carcinomas, it is important to know the subsite of the primary oral cavity tumor prior to interpretation of images, since the spread patterns and treatment options vary depending on location (Fig 7).

Lip cancer.—Early lesions are difficult to differentiate from the normal obicularis oris muscle. The lesions that require imaging are advanced, infiltrative tumors whose margins cannot be identified at clinical inspection. The information that must be ascertained for advanced lesions is their full extent and the presence of bone erosion. Subtle bone erosion usually occurs along the buccal surface of the mandibular or maxillary alveolar ridge and is best detected with CT. Conventional CT may be supplemented by using dental CT software or dental occlusive radiographs. The presence of bone erosion causes these lesions to be changed to stage T4, thereby contraindicating treatment with wide local excision and necessitating resection with either a partial mandibulectomy or maxillectomy (28).

Floor of the mouth carcinoma.—The American Joint Committee on Cancer staging classification provides little guidance for the surgical treatment of SCC arising in the floor of the mouth (32) (Fig 8). The surgical approach for these carcinomas is based on extent of tumor as determined with physical examination and imaging. The specific issues that must be assessed on imaging studies and that will affect the surgical treatment are bone erosion and degree of submucosal extension.

Low-volume superficial lesions are often not seen on imaging studies. These lesions are resected by means of wide local excision through a transoral approach. Floor of mouth carcinomas may extend laterally to invade the mandible or submucosally along the muscle and fascial planes to invade the adjacent lingual neurovascular bundle or tongue base (38,39). Tumors that extend along the mylohyoid or hyoglossus muscles require a combined transoral and cervical approach to ensure adequate resection.

The relationship of a floor of mouth cancer with the midline lingual septum and with the contralateral lingual neurovascular bundle must be determined before surgery. Tumors that show invasion of the ipsilateral and contralateral neurovascular bundles require a total glossectomy. While this procedure technically can be performed, the morbidity associated with it is believed to be unacceptable at most institutions and dictates that these patients be offered other treatment alternatives.

Bone erosion by a floor of mouth carcinoma causes the lesion stage to be changed to T4 (32). The type of resection is based on the amount of erosion as detected at preoperative imaging. Lateral floor of mouth tumors that are clinically fixed to the mandible should be imaged with thin-section CT (contiguous 1–2-mm-thick sections) reconstructed with a bone algorithm. Tumors with bone erosion limited to the lingual cortex of the mandible may be treated with a marginal mandibulectomy, thereby preserving the continuity of the mandible. However, tumors that invade the lingual cortex and extend into the marrow necessitate treatment with segmental mandibulectomy followed by reconstruction.

Floor of mouth tumors may extend posteriorly to the tongue base and may occasionally extend over the free margin of the mylohyoid muscle into the soft tissues of the neck. These tumors are stage T4 lesions that necessitate mandibulotomy, in addition to a combined transoral and cervical approach.

Oral tongue carcinoma.—The majority of SCCs in the oral tongue arise from its lateral borders and undersurface (Fig 9). These tumors remain localized to the oral tongue until they become very large (40). Tumors that arise from the anterior and middle third of the tongue tend to spread to the floor of the mouth and to the root of the tongue. Tumors that arise from the posterior third of the oral tongue may extend to the tongue base and spread in a pattern similar to that of tongue base cancers (38,40).

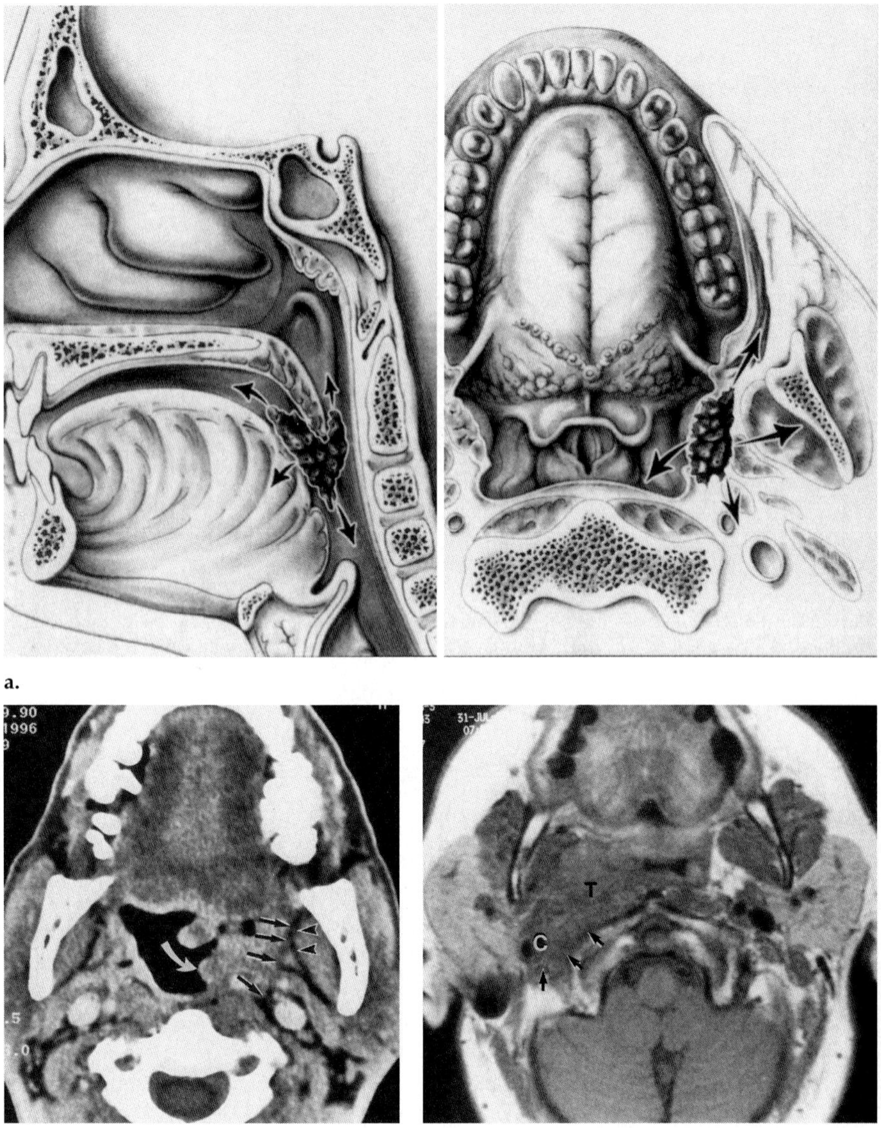

Figure 5. Tonsillar carcinoma. **(a)** Schematic illustrations demonstrate the potential pathways of spread for a tonsillar carcinoma. **(b)** Axial contrast-enhanced CT scan obtained through the tonsil shows a tumor arising from the left tonsil (curved arrow). The tumor is localized to the visceral space and does not cross the midline or extend deeply to involve the parapharyngeal space. Straight arrows = lateral margin of tumor, arrowheads = parapharyngeal space. These imaging findings indicated that this patient's tumor could be resected with a partial pharyngectomy. **(c)** Noncontrast axial T1-weighted (660/15, two signals acquired) MR image of a tonsillar carcinoma (*T*) shows the lesion to extend deeply into the pre- and poststyloid parapharyngeal space. The tumor invades the long mucles of the neck and encases the carotid artery (*C*) and jugular vein (arrows). Deep muscle invasion and carotid encasement classify these tumors as unresectable at most institutions.

The surgical options for carcinomas that arise from the oral tongue are wide local excision, partial glossectomy, or total glossectomy. Low-volume superficial lesions that have no imaging findings indicative of perineural or vascular invasion may be adequately treated with wide local excision or localized radiation therapy. Advanced lesions that do not cross the midline may be adequately treated with a partial glossectomy.

Bone erosion is seen only with advanced tongue carcinomas (40). Lateral tumors that extend inferiorly into the floor of the mouth spread in a pattern similar to that of floor of mouth tumors. Infiltrative oral tongue tumors that invade the floor of the mouth require removal of the involved structures in addition to a partial glossectomy. The presence and extent of bone erosion as identified at CT determine the type of mandibulectomy. Tumors that cross the midline and have

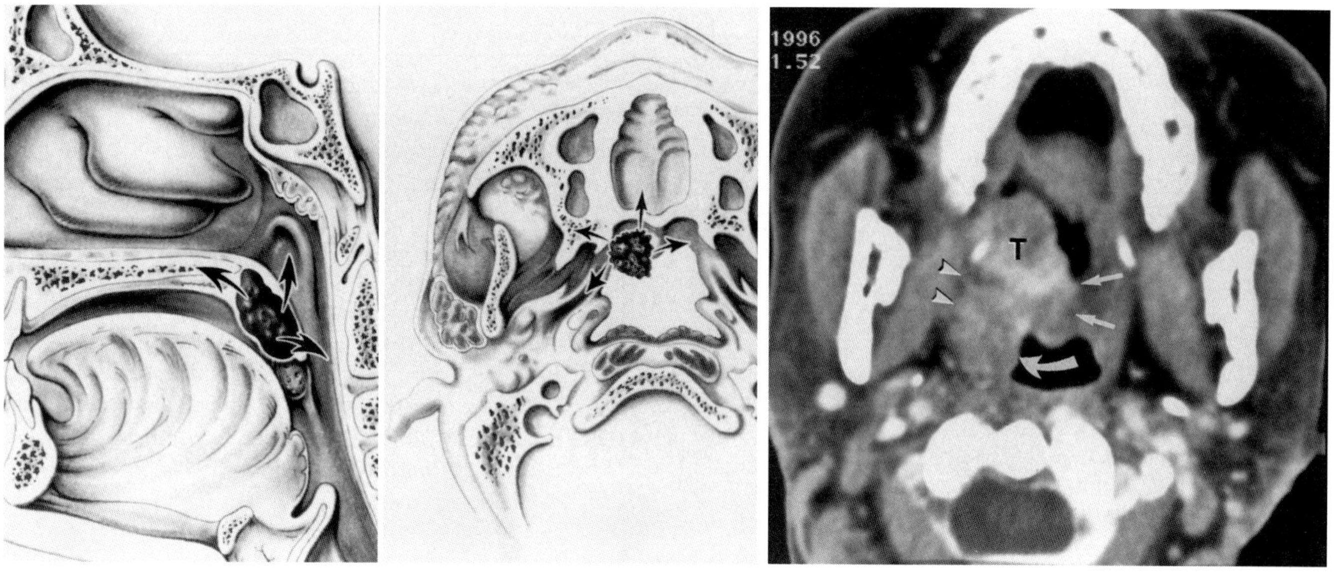

a. b.

Figure 6. Soft-palate carcinoma. **(a)** Schematic illustrations demonstrate the potential pathways of spread for a soft-palate carcinoma. **(b)** Axial contrast-enhanced CT scan through the soft palate shows an extensive carcinoma involving the soft palate (*T*), which spreads posteriorly to involve the tonsil (curved arrow). The lesion extends medially along the soft palate and crosses the midline (straight arrows). The tumor extends deeply through the superior constrictor muscle to involve the parapharyngeal space (arrowheads). This deep extension into the parapharyngeal space was clinically occult and precluded treatment with intraoral excision and necessitated a mandibulotomy and partial pharyngectomy.

imaging findings indicative of invasion of the contralateral lingual neurovascular bundle require a total glossectomy for curative resection or nonsurgical organ preservation therapy.

Buccal carcinoma.—The buccal mucosa covers the lips and cheeks. It is continuous with the gingiva of the buccal surface of the maxillary and mandibular alveolar ridges and with the retromolar trigone (40). Buccal carcinomas most commonly originate along the lateral walls and are usually low-grade carcinomas (Fig 10). Early buccal carcinomas are difficult to visualize and may be indistinguishable from the obicularis oris muscle. The most common spread patterns for buccal cancers are lateral submucosal extension along the buccinator muscle to the pterygomandibular raphe and erosion of underlying bone.

Low-volume lesions that are limited to the buccal mucosa may be resected through a transoral wide local excision. Tumors that extend submucosally to the pterygomandibular raphe require an extensive resection. Buccal carcinomas that erode the underlying bone require a segmental mandibulectomy or partial maxillectomy (40).

Gingiva and hard-palate carcinoma.—The gingiva is the mucous membrane covering the floor of the mouth, the mandible, and the maxilla. The upper gingiva is continuous with the mucosa of the hard palate. Primary SCC of the hard palate is rare. SCC involving the hard palate usually results from extension of a primary gingival SCC (40) (Fig 11). Primary malignant tumors of the hard palate are usually minor salivary gland carcinomas; the most common is adenoid cystic and mucoepidermoid types.

Tumors arising from the gingiva have well-defined spread patterns that directly affect their surgical management. Advanced tumors that involve the mucosal surface of the hard palate may erode into the bony hard palate and eventually into the nasal cavity. Tumors arising from the lower gingiva may erode the underlying lingual cortex of the mandible or extend posteriorly into the floor of the mouth.

On the basis of cross-sectional imaging findings, the extent of gingival and hard-palate tumors is often underestimated (38,40). Therefore, the extent of such tumors is often better assessed at endoscopy. CT is ideal to evaluate bone erosion. The amount of bone erosion determines the type of surgical resection. Low-volume, superficial tumors that do not erode the underlying bone may be excised through an intraoral wide local excision. Slow-growing lesions arising from the lower gingiva may result in saucerization of the mandibular cortex with preservation of the medullary cavity. Tumors that demonstrate this type of bone erosion may be successfully treated with a marginal mandibulectomy. Invasion of the medullary cavity necessitates a segmental mandibulectomy. This type of bone erosion usually occurs from involvement of the occlusal surface and is more common in edentulous patients. Bone erosion of the maxillary alveolar ridge by upper gingival carcinomas necessitates a partial maxillectomy.

Patients with carcinomas that involve the hard palate must be evaluated for bone erosion and perineural invasion. Thin-sectional coronal CT (1–2-mm-thick contiguous sections) is ideal to identify erosion of the hard palate. Bone erosion dictates the need for resection through a partial maxillectomy rather than a wide local excision. Perineural extension via the greater and lesser palatine nerves into the pterygopalatine fossa is a common pathway for tumor spread in adenoid cystic carcinomas. MR imaging should be performed to evaluate the pterygopalatine fossa and foramen rotundum in all patients with adenoid cystic carcinoma. Because of its rich neurovascular plexus, involvement of the pterygopalatine fossa complicates resection and often necessitates a total maxillectomy in order to gain adequate access to this region.

Retromolar trigone carcinoma.—The retromolar trigone is a small triangle-shaped area posterior to the last molars (40). Because of their unique location, SCCs that arise in the retromolar trigone have complex spread patterns (38,40) (Fig 12). The pterygomandibular raphe is a band of connective tissue situated beneath the mucosal surface of the retromolar trigone. The pterygomandibular raphe attaches superiorly at the hook of the hamulus of the medial pterygoid plate and inferiorly to the posterior aspect of the mylohyoid line of the mandible. The pterygomandibular raphe forms a junction between the oral cavity, oropharynx, and nasopharynx and serves as a common insertion point for the buccinator muscle, the obicularis oris muscle, and the superior constrictor muscle. Thus, tumors that arise in the retromolar trigone may grow anteriorly along the obicularis oris or buccinator muscles into the buccal region and thus mimic a buccal carcinoma. Alternatively, these tumors may grow posteriorly along the superior constrictor muscle into the tonsil. Superior growth along the pterygomandibular raphe allows for access to the skull base and nasopharynx, whereas inferior growth results in invasion of the floor of the mouth.

Low-volume, superficial lesions arising in the retromolar trigone may be excised with a transoral approach. Tumors that at imaging show extension along the muscle planes into adjacent regions cannot undergo transoral resection.

Because of the proximity between the maxillary tuberosity and the anterior aspect of the ascending ramus of the mandible, early retromolar trigone tumors may erode bone. Bone erosion is usually clinically occult and seen only at imaging. Bone erosion renders these lesions as stage T4 and necessitates a partial mandibulectomy or maxillectomy.

Larynx

The larynx is divided into the supraglottis, glottis, and subglottis (41,42). The supraglottic larynx is located above the TVC and extends from the tongue base and valleculae to the laryngeal ventricle. The contents of the supraglottic larynx are the epiglottis, aryepiglottic folds, false vocal cords, laryngeal ventricle, and the arytenoid processes of the arytenoid cartilages. The epiglottis attaches inferiorly to the thyroid cartilage via the thyroepiglottic ligament and anteriorly to the hyoid bone via the thyrohyoid ligament. The superior portion of the epiglottis, which is situated posterior to the hyoid bone and vallecula, is called the "free margin." The aryepiglottic folds are formed by mucosal reflections extending from the inferior and lateral aspects of the epiglottis to the arytenoid processes of the arytenoid cartilages. The false vocal cords are the inferior continuation of the aryepiglottic folds and form the superior border of the laryngeal ventricle (2,3). The glottic larynx consists of the TVC and anterior and posterior commissure. The ante-

Figure 7. Oral cavity. TMN classification and guidelines for the information that must be conveyed to the referring clinician when evaluating imaging studies obtained in patients with squamous cell carcinoma arising in the various subsites of the oral cavity.

TNM Staging

TX	Primary tumor cannot be assessed
T0	No evidence of primary tumor
Tis	Carcinoma in situ
T1	Tumor 2 cm or less in greatest dimension
T2	Tumor more than 2 cm but not more than 4 cm in greatest diameter
T3	Tumor more than 4 cm in greatest dimension
T4 (lip)	Tumor invades adjacent structures (eg, through cortical bone, skin of face, inferior alveolar nerve, floor of mouth)
T4 (oral cavity)	Tumor invades adjacent structures (eg, through cortical bone, into deep [extrinsic] muscle of tongue, maxillary sinus, skin; superficial erosion alone of bone/tooth socket by gingival primary is not sufficient to classify as T4)

Imaging Checklist

Lip carcinoma

- Bone erosion
- Soft-tissue invasion

Floor of mouth carcinoma

- Extent of bone erosion
- Deep invasion along the mylohyoid and hyoglossus muscles
- Relationship to ipsilateral lingual neurovascular bundle
- Extension across midline and relationship to contralateral neurovascular bundle
- Tongue base invasion
- Extension into the soft tissues of the neck

Oral tongue carcinoma

- Invasion of ipsilateral lingual neurovascular bundle
- Extension across midline and relationship to contralateral neurovascular bundle
- Invasion of the floor of the mouth and associated bone erosion

Buccal carcinoma

- Submucosal extension
- Bone erosion

Gingiva and hard-palate carcinoma

- Bone erosion
- Perineural invasion of the incisive canal and greater and lesser palatine foramen

Retromolar trigone carcinoma

- Bone erosion
- Submucosal spread
- Perineural invasion

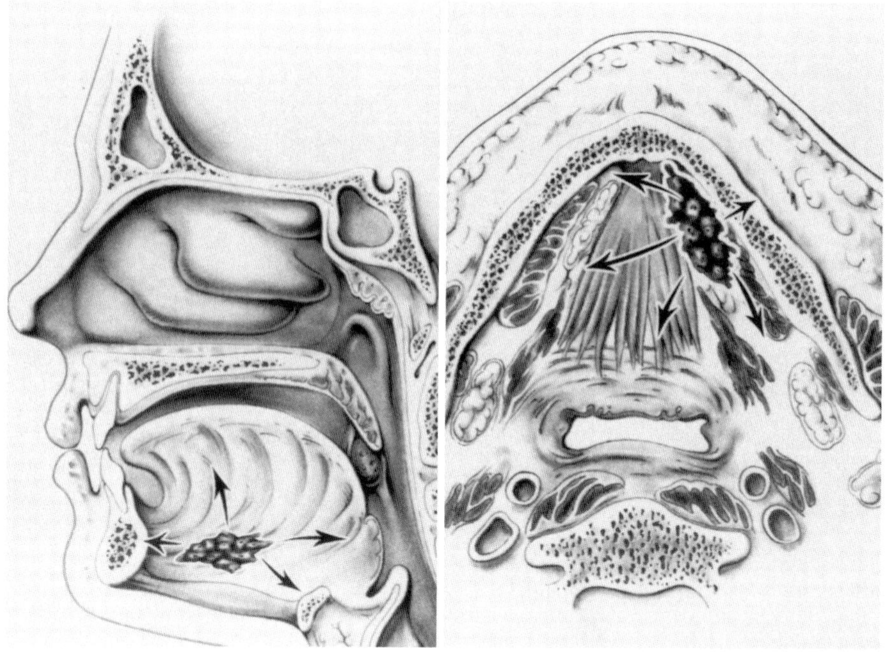

a.

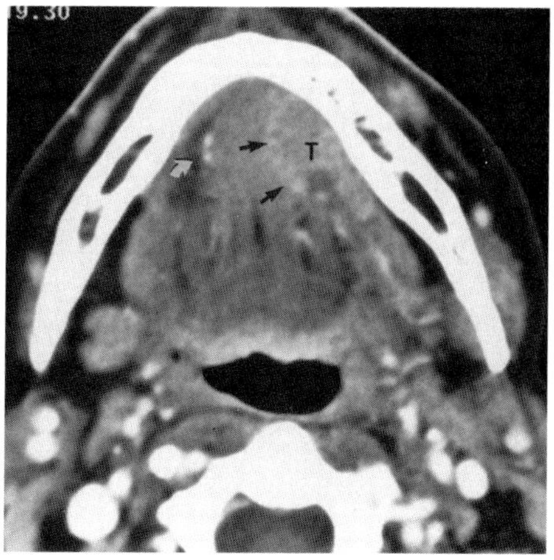

b.

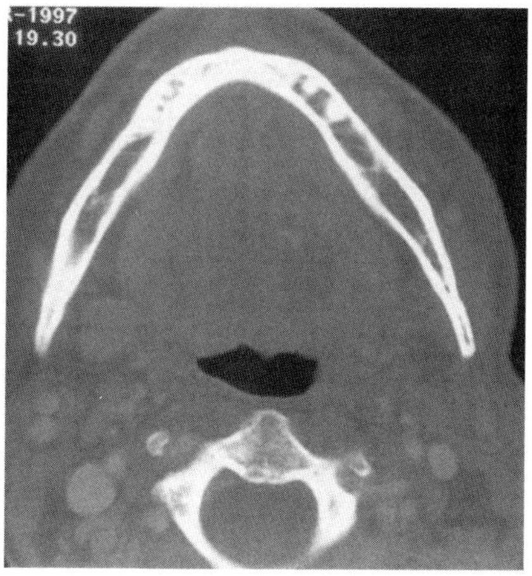

c.

Figure 8. Floor of mouth carcinoma. **(a)** Schematic illustrations demonstrate the potential pathways of spread for a floor of mouth carcinoma. **(b)** Axial contrast-enhanced CT scan shows an anterior floor of mouth carcinoma (*T*), which invades the normal low attenuation surrounding the lingual artery (straight arrows). This finding is highly suggestive of invasion of the lingual neurovascular bundle. (Compare to normal uninvolved side [curved arrow].) The lesion is delimited medially by the lingual septum and involves the contralateral lingual neurovascular bundle. At clinical examination, the tumor was fixed to the mandible. However, the study reconstructed with bone algorithm **(c)** shows no erosion of the lingual cortex of the mandible. The absence of bone erosion allowed this patient to be treated with an intraoral approach and marginal mandibulectomy.

rior commissure is the laryngeal mucosa that covers anterior portions of the TVC where they abut the laryngeal surface of the thyroid cartilage in the midline glottis (43). The posterior commissure is the midline laryngeal mucosal surface situated between the attachment of the TVC to the arytenoid cartilages (44). The subglottic larynx extends from the undersurface of the TVC to the base of the cricoid cartilage (41,42). Treatment of laryngeal carcinomas depends on the location and extent of the primary tumor.

Supraglottis (Figs 13, 14).—Laryngeal organ preservation surgery is precision surgery performed with the intent of conserving the voice while successfully resecting the primary tumor. The most commonly performed laryngeal conservation technique for supraglottic carcinomas is the supraglottic laryngectomy. This technique is used to treat tumors arising from the laryngeal surface of the epiglottis, false vocal cord, or aryepiglottic fold. This surgery entails resection of the false vocal cords, aryepiglottic folds, epiglottis, preepiglottic space, superior half of the thyroid cartilage, and hyoid bone. The inferior margin of a standard supraglottic laryngectomy is the laryngeal ventricle. Certain institutions may elect to perform an extended supraglottic laryngectomy to treat those tumors that involve portions of the arytenoid cartilage (45).

Early low-volume tumors situated along the free margin of the epiglottis may be successfully treated with local resection (45–47). These early lesions are often not detected on imaging studies. The role of imaging in these small tumors is to exclude submucosal extension that may not be identified at endoscopy.

When imaging is performed to evaluate supraglottic carcinomas, one should attempt to determine which patients are candidates for a supraglottic laryngectomy. Imaging findings that contraindicate a supraglottic laryngectomy are presence of transglottic extension, cartilage invasion, and exolaryngeal tumor spread.

Cartilage invasion may be detected with both CT and MR imaging and is more common in glottic tumors than supraglotttic carcinomas. Replacement of the high-signal-intensity marrow within the cartilage on T1-weighted MR images without contrast material or increased signal intensity on T2-weighted images is suggestive but not pathognomonic for cartilage invasion from adjacent tumor. Reports of studies in which both modalities were directly compared show MR to be more sensitive but less specific than CT for detection of cartilage invasion; however, MR is less specific than CT (6).

Because the inferior margin of a standard supraglottic laryngectomy is the laryngeal ventricle, supraglottic carcinomas that extend inferiorly to cross the ventricle (transglottic) and involve the TVC cannot be adequately treated with this approach. (It should be noted that the term "transglottic" may also be used to describe TVC carcinomas that extend superiorly to cross the laryngeal ventricle, thereby entering the supraglottic larynx.) Cartilage invasion and exolaryngeal tumor spread preclude a supraglottic laryngectomy. Despite the fact that some modifications of the supraglottic laryngectomy allow for resection of portions of the thyroid and arytenoid cartilages, the presence of cartilage invasion generally precludes its use. Other factors that contraindicate supraglottic laryngectomy—such as mucosal involvement of the pyriform sinus, vocal cord fixation, and proximity of the tumor to the circumvallate papillae—are difficult to assess with imaging and are better evaluated at endoscopy.

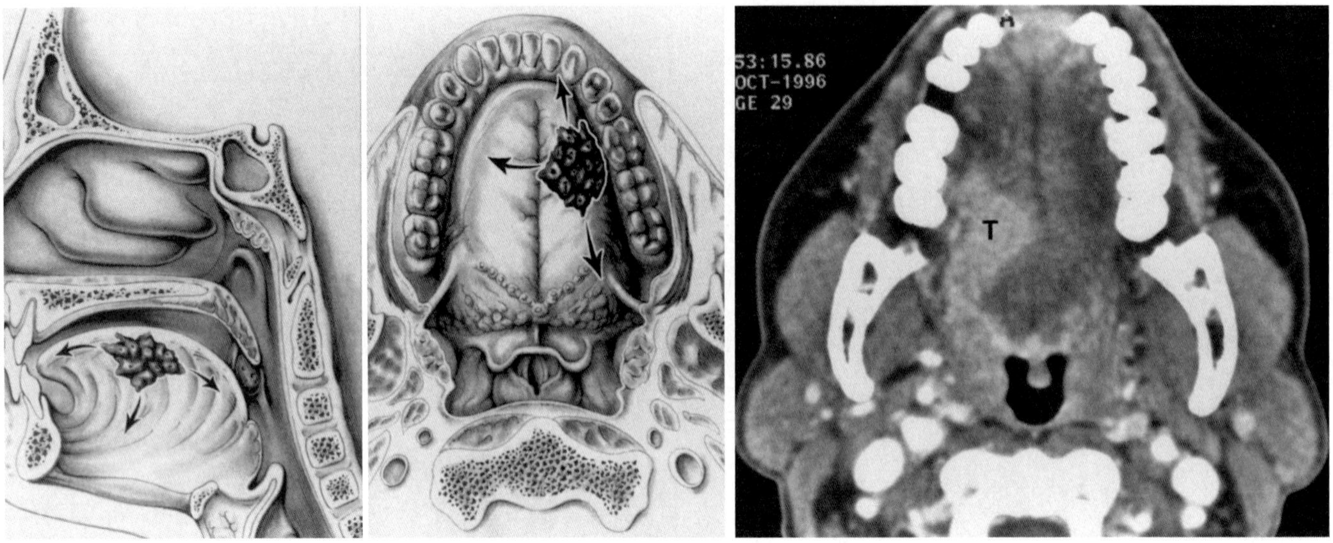

a. b.

Figure 9. Oral tongue carcinoma. **(a)** Schematic illustrations demonstrate the potential pathways of spread for an oral tongue carcinoma. **(b)** Contrast-enhanced CT scan of an oral tongue carcinoma illustrates an SCC (*T*) that does not cross the midline or invade the tongue base. These findings permitted resection with a hemiglossectomy.

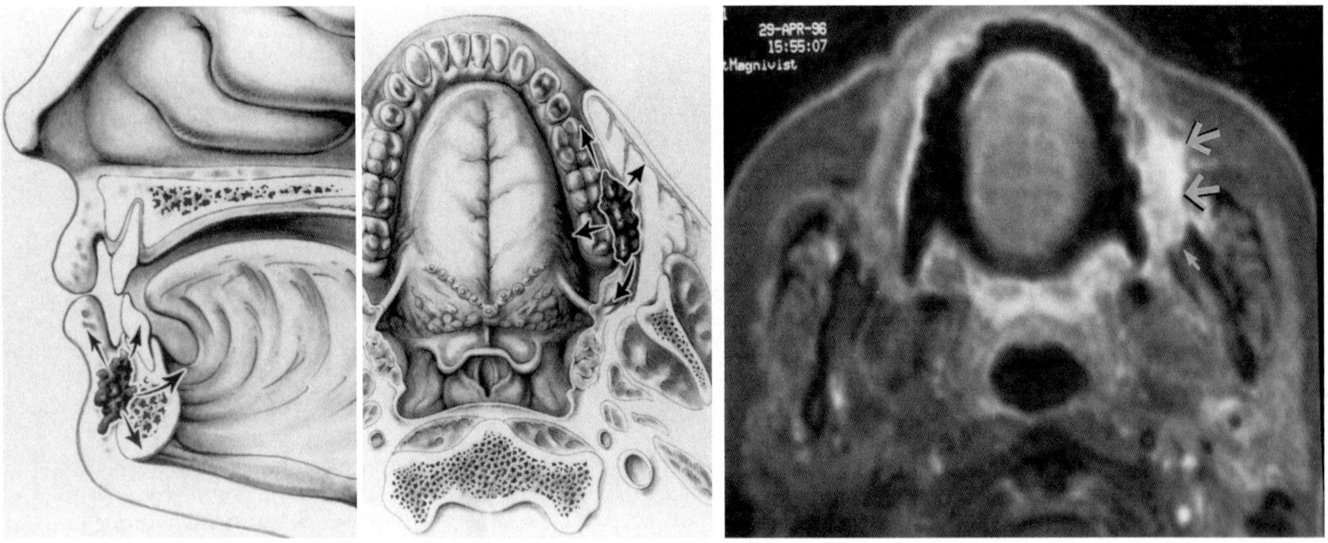

a. b.

Figure 10. Buccal carcinoma. **(a)** Schematic illustrations demonstrate the potential pathways of spread for a buccal carcinoma. **(b)** Axial fat-suppressed, gadolinium-enhanced (gadopentetate dimeglumine), T1-weighted (605/15, two signals acquired) MR image shows a buccal carcinoma (large arrows) that extends posteriorly along the buccinator muscle. There is erosion of the anterior portion of the ramus of the mandible (small arrow). Intially, this disease was staged as T1. The bone erosion caused the stage to be changed to T4 and necessitated a hemimandibulectomy and partial maxillectomy for cure.

Recently, other forms of organ preservation surgery have become more commonly used for the treatment of supraglottic carcinoma (48). One of the most frequently used procedures is the supracricoid laryngectomy with crichohyoidopexy (48). This technique permits resection of advanced supraglottic carcinomas (T3 or T4) that cross the laryngeal ventricle and are therefore unresectable with a standard supraglottic laryngectomy. This procedure also permits the reconstruction of a neolarynx that maintains physiologic function (respiratory, phonatory, sphincteric) (49,50). Supracricoid laryngectomy with cricohyoidopexy is suitable for supraglottic carcinoma (*a*) extending into the laryngeal ventricle, (*b*) invading the glottis and the anterior commissure with or without impaired mobility of the TVC and (*c*) in selected cases with small areas of thyroid cartilage invasion (T4) (48,49, 51). This technique removes both TVC and false vocal cords and the paraglottic spaces, thyroid cartilage, epiglottis, and the preepiglottic space (48). The cricoid cartilage, hyoid bone, and at least one arytenoid cartilage are spared (48). The contraindications for performing this procedure are subglottic extension greater then 7 mm with cricoid cartilage invasion, arytenoid cartilage fixation, or massive invasion into the preepiglottic space (48). However, some investigators suggest that isolated preepiglottic space invasion is not a contraindication, as the entire preepiglottic space is entirely removed during a standard supracricoid laryngectomy with cricohyoidopexy (48).

Patients with transglottic supraglottic carcinomas who have imaging findings of extensive subglottic extension that precludes treatment with

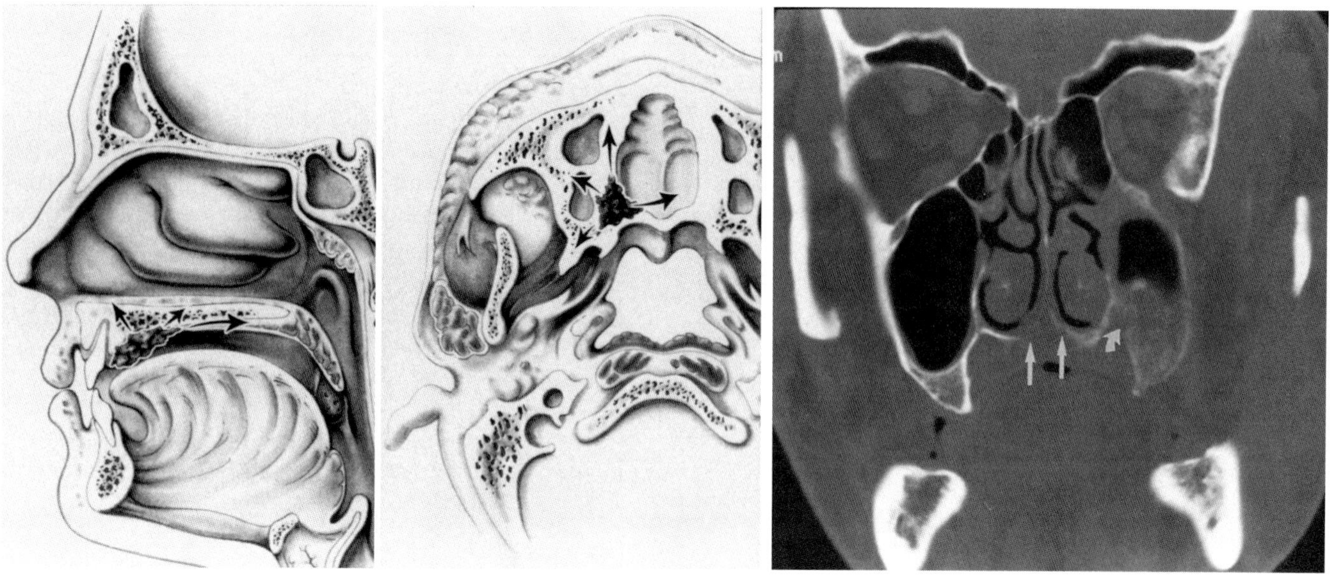

a. b.

Figure 11. Hard-palate carcinoma. **(a)** Schematic illustrations demonstrate the potential pathways of spread for a hard-palate carcinoma. **(b)** Coronal CT scan obtained in a patient with a hard-palate carcinoma demonstrates extensive bone erosion of the hard palate (straight arrows) and medial wall of the maxillary sinus (curved arrow). These findings preclude surgical treatment with wide local excision and necessitate treatment with an extended maxillectomy.

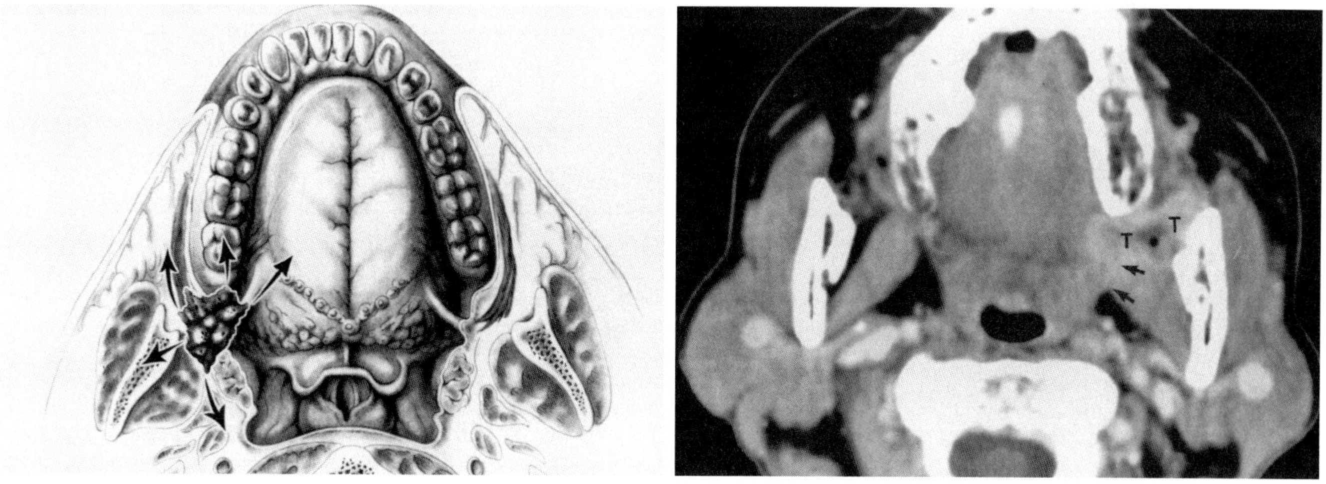

a. b.

Figure 12. Retromolar trigone carcinoma. **(a)** Schematic illustrations demonstrate the potential pathways of spread for a retromolar trigone carcinoma. **(b)** Axial contrast-enhanced CT scan from a patient with a retromolar trigone carcinoma illustrates an aggressive tumor (*T*) arising posterior to the maxillary tuberosity. The lesion extends anterolaterally along the buccinator muscle and posteriorly to involve the fat located between the mandible and the medial pterygoid muscle (pteryomandibular space). The tumor also involves the pterygomandibular raphe and extends posteromedially along the superior constrictor muscle (arrows). This deep extension and proximity to the mandible and maxilla precluded wide local excision and necessitated a partial mandibulectomy and maxillectomy.

a supraglottic or supracricoid laryngectomy may be candidates for a near total laryngectomy (48,52). This technique allows partial removal of the involved cricoid cartilage and tracheal rings. This procedure may be extended superiorly and laterally and allow resection of the hypopharynx in addition to the supraglottic larynx. This technique allows some phonation but requires permanent tracheostomy (48,52).

A growing number of patients with supraglottic carcinomas are being treated nonsurgically. Radiation therapy allows for preservation of laryngeal function. Although voice preservation may be obtained with a standard supraglottic laryngectomy, voice quality is generally better in patients treated with radiation therapy. Patients who refuse surgery or who are poor surgical candidates may also be treated with radiation therapy.

The results of primary radiation therapy for supraglottic carcinomas have been variable; primary control rates ranged from 70% to 90% for stage T1 and T2 lesions but were less than 40% for stage T3 and T4 lesions (53,54). The selection criteria for treatment with definitive radiation therapy have been based primarily on the T stage as assessed with clinical examination and the willingness of the patient to return for frequent follow-up visits. Pretreatment CT imaging is predictive of local control in patients treated with definitive radiation therapy. Specifically, tumor volume, preepiglottic spread, and cartilage invasion help predict the likelihood of cure for supraglottic cancers treated with radiation therapy alone. There is a strong correlation between tumor volume and local control. Recent studies have identified a linear relationship between likelihood of local control and tumor size (55). Tumors with volumes of less than 6 cm^3 have an 89% likelihood of local control, while tumors with volumes greater than 6 cm^3 have a 52% chance that control of the primary site will be achieved with radiation therapy alone (55).

Preepiglottic space tumor invasion causes the stage of supraglottic carcinomas to be changed to T3. This criterion is difficult to identify at clinical examination and can be identified with CT or noncontrast sagittal T1-weighted MR imaging. There is no relationship between preepiglottic space involvement and local control. However, the likelihood of preserving laryngeal function after radiation therapy depends on the extent of preepiglottic space invasion. Patients with tumors invading less than 25% of the preepiglottic space have a significantly higher likelihood of maintaining a functional larynx after radiation therapy than those with tumors with more than 75% preepiglottic space invasion (55).

The presence of cartilage invasion at pretreatment imaging correlates with an increased incidence of treatment failure (56,57). Although radiation therapy may cure early cartilage invasion (58), patients with imaging evidence of cartilage invasion should be considered at high risk for failure and warrant close follow-up.

Ongoing investigations are now concentrating on serial tumor volumes (as seen on imaging studies) as a means of predicting which advanced supraglottic carcinomas may be successfully treated with laryngeal preservation protocols that use combined chemotherapy and radiation therapy. It has been shown that a greater than 50% reduction in tumor size as determined at clinical examination after an initial course of chemotherapy is predictive of laryngeal carcinomas that may be controlled with definitive radiation therapy (59). It remains to be seen if changes in image-based tumor volume measurements that occur as a result of induction chemotherapy will be able to identify patients who are suitable candidates for nonsurgical organ preservation treatment.

Glottis (Figs 15, 16).—Laryngeal conservation surgery for glottic carcinomas attempts to preserve voice yet resect the primary lesion. Tumors of the true vocal cord that are clinically staged as T2 lesions may have imaging evidence of cartilage invasion, which upstages these tumors to T4. These tumors often involve the anterior commissure and invade the laryngeal surface of the thyroid cartilage at the insertion of the Broyle ligament (44).

Figure 13. Supraglottis. TMN classification and guidelines for the information that must be conveyed to the referring clinician (surgeons and radiation oncologists) when evaluating imaging studies obtained in patients with SCC of the supraglottic larynx.

TNM Staging

TIS	Carcinoma in situ
T1	Tumor confined to one subsite of supraglottis with normal vocal cord mobility
T2	Tumor invades mucosa of more than one adjacent subsite of supraglottis or glottis or region outside the supraglottis (eg, mucosa of base of tongue, vallecula, medial wall of pyriform sinus without fixation of the larynx
T3	Tumor limited to larynx with vocal cord fixation and/or invades any of the following: postcricoid area, preepiglottic space tissues
T4	Tumor extends through the thyroid cartilage, and/or extends into soft tissues of the neck, thyroid, and/or esophagus

Imaging Checklist

Surgery

- Cartilage invasion
- Exolaryngeal spread
- Transglottic extension
- Pyrifrom sinus invasion

Radiation therapy

- Tumor volume
- Cartilage invasion
- Preepiglottic invasion

Specific issues that must be addressed when evaluating glottic carcinomas in patients who elect to be treated surgically are listed in Figure 16. Low-volume tumors limited to the midportion of the TVC and that do not involve the anterior commissure or ipsilateral cricoarytenoid joint may be treated with laser cordectomy. The most commonly performed partial laryngectomy procedure to treat TVC tumors is a vertical hemilaryngectomy. The standard hemilaryngectomy involves resection of the affected TVC, ipsilateral false vocal cord, and adjacent thyroid cartilage. Modifications of hemilaryngectomy allow for resection of more advanced tumors. An extended vertical hemilaryngectomy may be performed to treat tumors that involve the arytenoid cartilage or cross the anterior commissure to involve the anterior one-third of the contralateral TVC. A supracricoid (subtotal) laryngectomy may be used to treat stage T1 and T2 glottic tumors that invade the paraglottic space or cross the anterior commissure to involve the contralateral TVC. This procedure includes resection of the supraglottis, glottis, and thyroid cartilage. Tumors that cannot be successfully resected with conservation surgery require a total laryngectomy (60).

Imaging to evaluate TVC carcinomas should be performed to determine which patients are suitable candidates for a voice-sparing laryngectomy (41,42). Early tumors that invade the anterior commissure, posterior commissure, or paraglottic fat obviate resection with cordectomy. Imaging findings that contraindicate a vertical hemilaryngectomy are cartilage invasion, transglottic extension to involve the false vocal cord, extension across the anterior commissure with involvement of more than one-third of the contralateral TVC, extension into the posterior commissure, and subglottic extension greater than 10 mm anteriorly or greater than 5 mm posteriorly (41). A supracricoid laryngectomy resects the supraglottic and glottic larynx and may be used to treat advanced glottic carcinomas that cannot be treated with a hemilaryngectomy. However, subglottic extension prevents a supracricoid laryngectomy from being performed subsequently and necessitates total laryngectomy for cure.

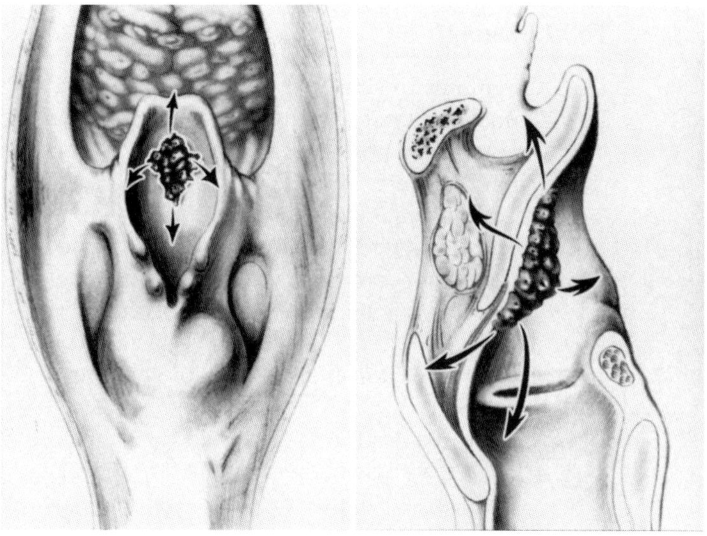

a.

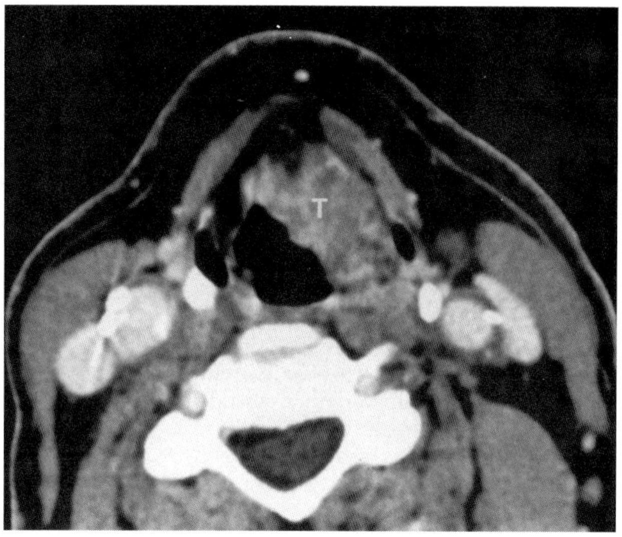

b.

Figure 14. Supraglottic carcinoma. **(a)** Schematic illustrations demonstrate the potential pathways of spread for a supraglottic carcinoma. **(b)** Contrast-enhanced CT scan of a supraglottic carcinoma shows a high-volume (more than 8 cm^3) supraglottic carcinoma (*T*). This tumor was staged clinically as T2, and the patient was initially thought to be a candidate for supraglottic laryngectomy. **(c)** Contrast-enhanced CT scan obtained through the TVC from the same patient in **b** shows transglottic extension along the anterior aspect of the left TVC (arrow). This extension was submucosal and contraindicated supraglottic laryngectomy. This patient was subsequently treated with total laryngectomy.

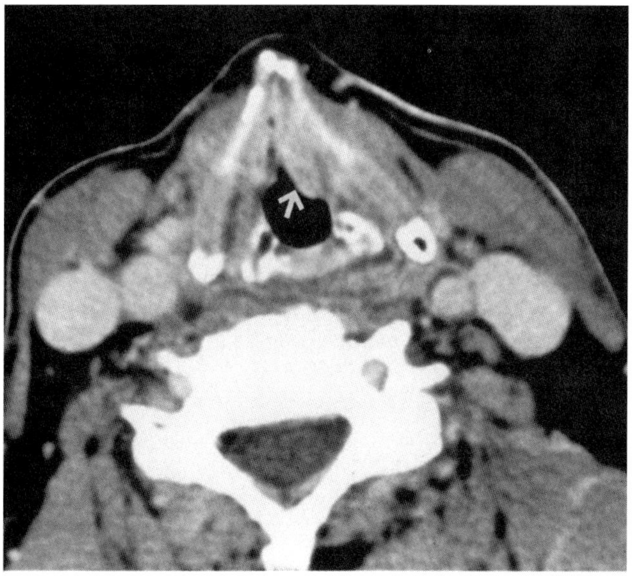

c.

Supracricoid laryngectomy with cricohyoidoepiglottopexy has gained acceptance as a form of organ preservation surgery for patients with advanced glottic carcinoma. Some authors suggest that this procedure is the treatment of choice for patients with advanced glottic carcinomas who wish to be treated with organ preservation surgery (48,61–63). The most important difference between the supracricoid laryngectomy with cricohyoidopexy (supraglottic carcinomas) and the supracricoid laryngectomy with cricohyoidoepiglottopexy (glottic carcinomas) is as follows. The supracricoid laryngectomy with cricohyoidopexy (supraglottic carcinomas) entails completely resecting the epiglottis whereas the supracricoid laryngectomy with cricohyoidoepiglottopexy (glottic carcinomas) spares the suprahyoid portion of the epiglottis (48). The contraindications for performing a supracricoid laryngectomy with cricohyoidoepiglottopexy for the treatment of glottic carcinomas are subglottic extension greater than 7 mm with cricoid cartilage invasion or arytenoid cartilage fixation (48). Invasion of the preepiglottic space is a contraindication for supracricoid laryngectomy with cricohyoidoepiglottopexy. When present, the epiglottis cannot be spared and glottic carcinomas with this spread pattern require resection with supracricoid laryngectomy with cricohyoidopexy (48).

Patients with glottic carcinomas that have imaging findings of extensive subglottic extension that preclude treatment with a vertical or supracricoid laryngectomy may be candidates for a glottosubglottic laryngectomy (48,64,65). This technique permits partial removal of the cricoid cartilage and tracheal rings but, similar to the near total laryngectomy, requires permanent tracheostomy (48,64,65).

Radiation therapy has gained acceptance as an effective treatment for stage T1 and T2 TVC carcinomas. Reported local control rates are lower for stage T3 carcinoma of the TVC. Pretreatment CT enables patients to be identified who can be successfully treated with definitive radiation therapy. Investigators have recently developed risk profiles based on pretreatment CT findings that appear to be effective predictors of local control in patients with TVC carcinomas. This risk profile is based on tumor volume and the status of the laryngeal cartilages (66–68). Imaging evidence of cartilage invasion (stage T4) significantly reduces the likelihood of local control and may preclude treatment with radiation therapy (56,57).

There are three separate risk groups based on pretreatment CT findings. The ideal CT profile for glottic carcinoma is a volume of more than 3.5 cm^3 with either no cartilage sclerosis or sclerosis of a single laryngeal cartilage. Tumors with this favorable CT profile have a 90% chance of being locally controlled with radiation therapy alone. The moderate-risk group consists of patients with low tumor volume (less than 3.5 cm^3) and sclerosis of two laryngeal cartilages or patients with a tumor volume greater than 3.5 cm^3 with either no cartilage sclerosis or single cartilage sclerosis. Patients with this moderate-risk profile have a 40%–50% chance that their disease will be controlled with radiation therapy. The high-risk group consists of patients who have a high tumor volume (more than 3.5 cm^3) and combined sclerosis of the ipsilateral arytenoid and adjacent cricoid cartilage. Patients in this group have less than a 20% chance that local control will be achieved if they are treated with definitive radiation therapy (66,69).

Patients in the moderate- and high-risk groups who elect to be treated with definitive radiation therapy are considered at higher risk for treatment failure at the primary site and warrant close clinical and imaging follow-up. Because these patients are closely monitored, they may demonstrate a higher overall local control rate with salvage surgery, since local recurrences may be identified at an earlier stage. We currently recommend that a repeat imaging study be performed 3–4 months after completion of radiation therapy to evaluate the response of glottic and supraglottic tumors. Complete resolution of a tumor on this imaging study compared with the pretreatment study indicates local control, while less than 50% tumor shrinkage indicates treatment failure. Tumors that have a 50%–75% reduction in size are indeterminate and warrant further studies to determine stability (70,71).

Stratification of patients into high- and low-risk groups for failure at the primary site with radiation therapy alone has the potential to improve local control rates for a selective group of patients. This approach also may reduce the morbidity of treatment by causing high-risk patients to undergo surgical resection, since salvage surgery is associated with a higher risk of complications. Volume data analysis may also be used to determine which larger volume tumors should be treated with chemotherapy before radiation therapy in an attempt to preserve laryngeal function (66,72). A quantitative volume reduction of 50% or more following neoadjuvant therapy is generally accepted as an indication to proceed with high-dose radiation therapy. Patients whose tumors do not respond to the initial trial of chemotherapy may be offered surgical cure (72).

Subglottis.—Primary subglottic tumors are less common than glottic or supraglottic carcinomas (Fig 17). Early lesions may be treated with radiation therapy. Advanced tumors involving the undersurface of the TVC are usually treated with a total laryngectomy. Because the cricoid cartilage is the foundation of the larynx, a voice-sparing laryngectomy with a partial cricoidectomy is not a feasible option for treating low-volume tumors. The role of imaging is to evaluate for cartilage invasion, to demonstrate the inferior extent of tumor, and to help identify the extent of tracheal resection necessary for adequate margins (44).

Figure 15. Glottis. TMN classification and guidelines for the information that must be conveyed to the referring clinician (surgeons and radiation oncologists) when evaluating imaging studies obtained in patients with SCC of the glottic larynx.

TNM Staging

TIS	Carcinoma in situ
T1	Tumor limited to vocal cord(s) (may involve anterior or posterior commissures) with normal mobility
T1a	Tumor limited to one vocal cord
T1b	Tumor involves both vocal cords
T2	Tumor extends to supraglottis and/or subglottis and/or with impaired vocal cord mobility
T3	Tumor limited to the larynx with vocal cord fixation
T4	Tumor invades through thyroid cartilage and/or to other tissues beyond the larynx (eg, trachea, soft tissues of neck, including thyroid, pharynx)

Imaging Checklist

Surgery

- Transglottic extension
- Subglottic extension and relationship to cricoid cartilage
- Cartilage invasion
- Involvement of the anterior commissure
- Involvement of the cricoarytenoid joint
- Extension to the posterior commissure
- Deep invasion of the paraglottic fat

Radiation therapy

- Tumor volume
- Cartilage sclerosis
- Cartilage invasion

Hypopharynx

The hypopharynx (laryngopharynx) is the portion of the upper aerodigestive tract that extends from the hyoid bone superiorly and extends inferiorly to the inferior aspect of the cricoid cartilage (32,73) (Figs 18, 19). Above the hyoid bone is the oropharynx. Below the cricoid cartilage, the hypopharynx becomes the cervical esophagus. Most authors divide the hypopharynx into three regions: the posterior pharyngeal wall, the pyriform sinuses, and the postcricoid region (32,73,74). Some authors also refer to a fourth, or "marginal," area that consists of the lateral pharyngeal wall. The posterior wall of the hypopharynx starts at the level of the valleculae (74). Above this, the posterior wall is continuous with the posterior wall of the oropharynx and extends inferiorly to the level of the postcricoid region. The pyriform sinus is a lateral recess created by the aryepiglottic fold. There are two pyriform sinuses, each with an anterior wall, a medial wall, and a lateral wall (73). The lowest part of each pyriform sinus is called the apex, which lies at the level of the TVC. The paired aryepiglottic folds make up the medial walls of the pyriform sinuses. The two pyriform sinuses merge posteriorly at the level of the cricoid cartilage to form the postcricoid region. The postcricoid region, also called the pharyngoesophageal junction, is the portion of the hypopharynx situated posterior to the cricoid cartilage (32,73,74). This portion of the pharynx allows for passage of food from the pyriform sinus into the cervical esophagus. The postcricoid hypopharynx abuts the posterior ring of the cricoid cartilage and the arytenoid cartilages (73). The anterior wall

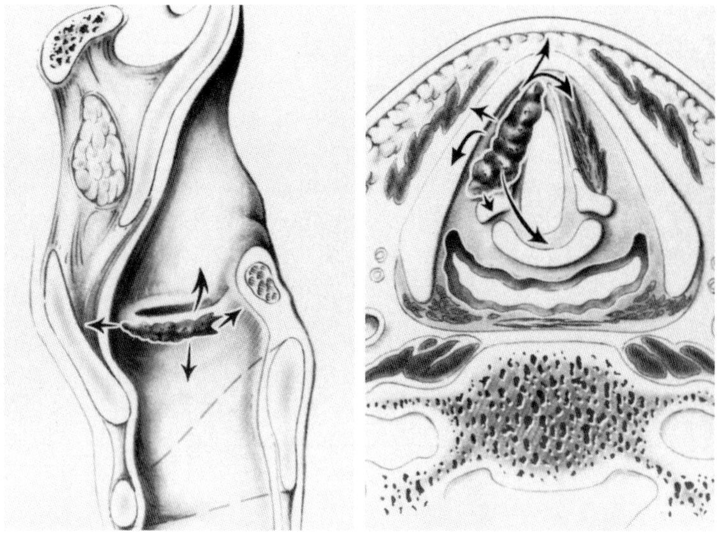

a.

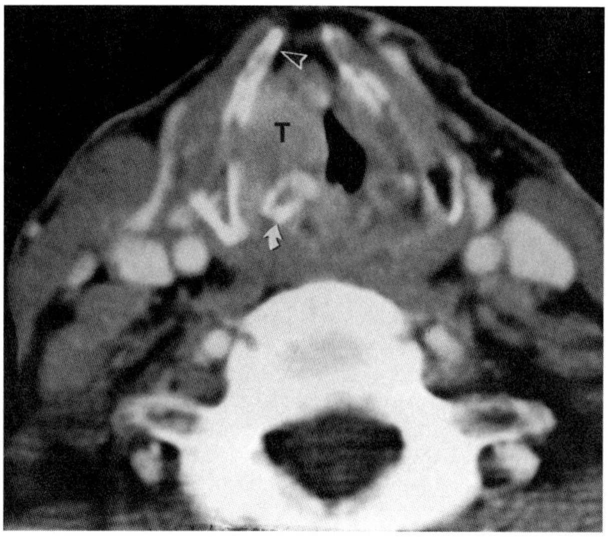

b.

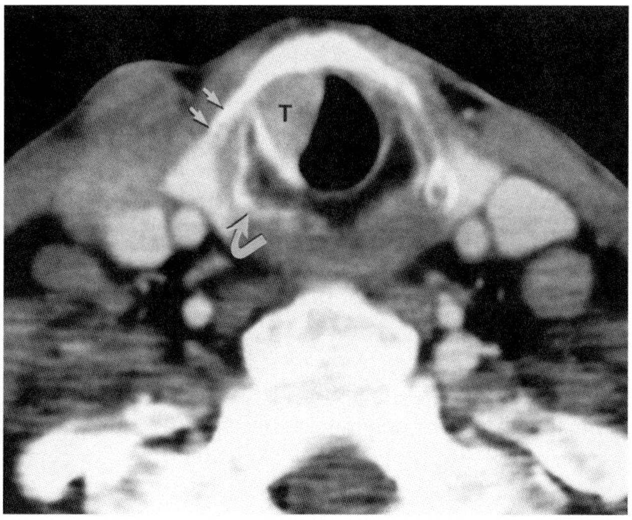

c.

Figure 16. Glottic carcinoma. **(a)** Schematic illustrations demonstrate the potential pathways of spread for a glottic carcinoma. **(b)** Contrast-enhanced CT scan obtained through the TVC shows a high-volume (more than 3.5 cm^3) tumor arising from the right TVC (*T*) with sclerosis of the adjacent arytenoid cartilage (arrow) and subtle sclerosis of the anterior aspect of the right thyroid cartilage (arrowhead). **(c)** Contrast-enhanced CT scan obtained through the subglottis of the same patient as in **b** shows bulk subglottic extension (*T*) and sclerosis of the right half of the cricoid cartilage (curved arrow) and right half of the thyroid cartilage (straight arrows). The high volume and multiple sclerotic cartilages preclude treatment with definitive radiation therapy. The subglottic extension contraindicates treatment with partial laryngectomy (hemilaryngectomy, supracricoid laryngectomy). This patient was treated with total laryngectomy.

of the postcricoid region is also the posterior wall of the lower larynx. This common wall is sometimes referred to as the "party wall." The transition from the postcricoid region can be separated from the cervical esophagus by noticing the transition from the relatively flat postcricoid region to the rounded appearance of the cervical esophagus.

Hypopharyngeal carcinomas may be treated surgically or with definitive radiation therapy. Surgical treatment options include transoral wide local excision, partial laryngopharyngectomy, or total laryngopharyngectomy. The American Joint Committee on Cancer staging system has little influence on the surgical treatment of hypopharyngeal carcinomas. Tumors confined to the lateral pharyngeal wall have the same stage regardless of the size and type of resection necessary for adequate treatment (73). The extent of disease is often underestimated at endoscopy because of the tendency of hypopharyngeal carcinomas to spread submucosally. Submucosal extension is better evaluated with imaging. Failure to identify the extent of disease results in an inadequate resection.

The specific issues that must be addressed when evaluating hypopharyngeal carcinomas are whether the tumor crosses the midline, whether the tumor extends into the apex of the pyriform sinus, whether cartilage erosion is present, whether inferior tumor extension is present, and whether the prevertebral muscles have been invaded.

Low-volume superficial lesions located in the superior aspect of the hypopharynx may be resected with a transoral wide local excision. Lesions of similar size situated inferiorly may require a midline mandibulolabial approach and a transhyoid or lateral pharyngotomy. Advanced lesions involving the lateral or posterior pharyngeal wall but not crossing the midline may be treated with a partial laryngopharyngectomy. Advanced tumors that cross the midline require a total laryngopharyngectomy.

Tumor involvement of the apex of the pyriform sinus is an important factor in carcinomas that arise in this location that are to be treated surgically. The apex of the pyriform sinus is located at the level of the TVC. Because of its proximity to the cricoarytenoid joint, tumors that involve the apex are highly likely to invade the larynx and erode cartilage (73). Anterior spread of these tumors results in invasion of the cricoarytenoid joint and muscles, thyroarytenoid joint, and paraglottic fat. Because of these factors, pyriform sinus carcinomas that involve the apex are treated with total laryngopharyngectomy, whereas tumors that spare the apex may be treated with partial laryngopharyngectomy.

The inferior margin of a tumor and its relationship to the esophageal inlet also must be addressed. Invasion of the postcricoid region with extension into the cervical esophagus requires an esophagectomy in addition to a total laryngopharyngectomy. Invasion of the fascia and fixation to the underlying anterior longitudinal ligament is unusual in hypopharyngeal carcinomas. Deep spread into the prevertebral musculature contraindicates surgical resection (73).

Radiation therapy has been shown to be a useful alternative for treating stage T1 and T2 pyriform sinus carcinomas. Because of the deficiencies of the American Joint Committee on Cancer system to portray these lesions accurately, the reported control rates vary (32). Recent investigations have shown that pretreatment CT may be used to identify patients who can be treated with radiation therapy alone. Tumor volume and apical involvement are two important risk factors in patients who are candidates for treatment with radiation therapy alone. The local control rate for tumors with total volumes of less than 6.5 cm^3 is 90%, whereas the local control rate for lesions with volumes of more than 6.5 cm^3 is 25% (1). Tumors with minimal (defined as apical involvement less than 10 mm in largest dimension) or no apical involvement have an 89% chance of local control, while tumors with bulk apical disease (defined as apical tumor involvement greater than 10 mm in largest dimension) have a 25% chance of cure when treated with definitive radiation therapy. Data suggest that the favorable CT profile for a pyriform sinus tumor curable with radiation therapy is a volume of less than 6.5 cm^3 and minimal or no apical disease (1). Patients who fit this profile have a local control rate of over 90% when treated with radiation therapy alone (1). An unfavorable CT profile is a volume of more than 6.5 cm^3 or bulk apical disease. Patients in this category are at higher risk for treatment failure and warrant close follow-up. High-volume tumors and bulk apical disease may be best treated with surgery or combined chemotherapy and hyperfractionated radiation therapy. In this group of patients, CT may help identify advanced tumors that are amenable to organ preservation by treatment with combined chemotherapy and radiation therapy. Recent studies have shown induction chemotherapy to be predictive of patients with pyriform sinus cancers that may be treated with definitive radiation therapy (75). Patients with a complete response based on clinical observation after three cycles of chemotherapy are considered suitable candidates for nonsurgical organ preservation treatment with radiation therapy. However, patients with a partial response are treated surgically (75). It may be possible that image-based tumor volume measurements that quantify the degree of tumor shrinkage from induction chemotherapy may identify a cohort of patients in whom local control could still be achieved with nonsurgical laryngeal preservation treatment.

In conclusion, modern imaging plays an important role in the management of malignancies of the upper aerodigestive tract. Radiologic evaluation ensures accurate staging and provides essential information about the tumor extent that directly affects the surgical approach necessary for curative resection. Recent findings also suggest that imaging will play an essential role for both identifying and monitoring patients who are candidates for both surgical and nonsurgical organ preservation treatment. ■

Figure 17. Subglottis. TMN classification and guidelines for the information that must be conveyed to the referring clinician when evaluating imaging studies obtained in patients with SCC of the subglottic larynx.

TNM Staging

TIS	Carcinoma in situ
T1	Tumor limited to the subglottis
T2	Tumor extends to vocal cord(s) with normal or impaired mobility
T3	Tumor limited to larynx with vocal cord fixation
T4	Tumor invades through cricoid or thyroid cartilage and/or extends to other tissues beyond the larynx (eg, trachea, soft tissues of neck, including thyroid, esophagus)

Imaging Checklist

- Inferior extent
- Cartilage invasion

Figure 18. Hypopharynx. TMN classification and guidelines for the information that must be conveyed to the referring clinician (surgeons and radiation oncologists) when evaluating imaging studies obtained in patients with SCC of the hypopharynx.

TNM Staging

Tis	Carcinoma in situ
T1	Tumor limited to one subsite of hypopharynx and 2 cm or less in greatest dimension
T2	Tumor involves more than one subsite of hypopharynx or an adjacent site, or measures more than 2 cm but not more than 4 cm in greatest diameter without fixation of hemilarynx
T3	Tumor measures more than 4 cm in greatest dimension or with fixation of hemilarynx
T4	Tumor invades adjacent structures (eg, thyroid/cricoid cartilage, carotid artery, soft tissues of neck, prevertebral facial muscles, thyroid, and/or esophagus)

Imaging Checklist

Surgery

- Midline extension
- Apical involvement
- Extension into the esophageal inlet
- Cartilage invasion
- Anterior extension into paraglottic space
- Exolaryngeal spread
- Prevertebral muscle invasion

Radiation therapy

- Tumor volume
- Apical involvement
- Cartilage invasion

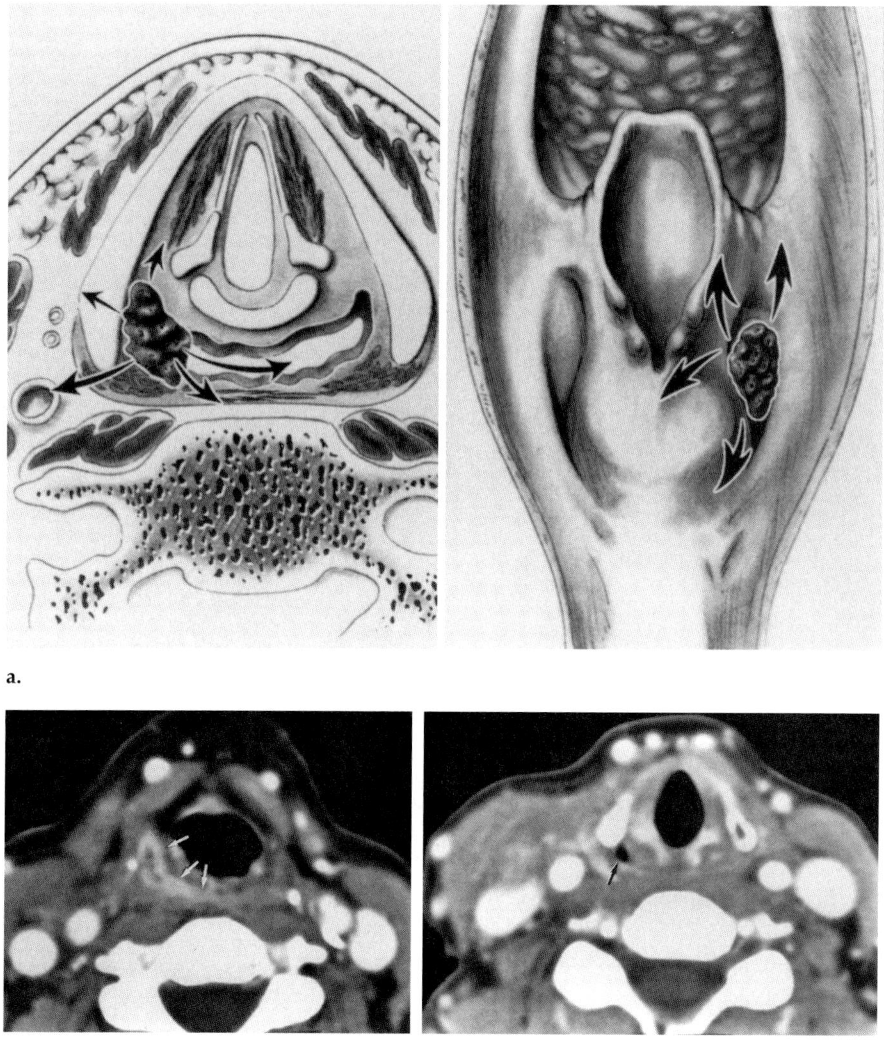

a.

b. c.

Figure 19. Pyriform sinus carcinoma. **(a)** Schematic illustrations demonstrate the potential pathways of spread for a pyriform sinus carcinoma. **(b)** Contrast-enhanced CT scan obtained in a patient with a low-volume (less than 6 cm^3) pyriform sinus carcinoma arising from the right pyriform sinus (arrows). The tumor extends to the midline, thereby precluding treatment with wide local excision or partial pharyngectomy. **(c)** CT scan obtained at the level of the TVC in same patient as in **b** shows no evidence of bulk apical disease (arrow). The low volume and lack of bulk apical disease give this tumor a favorable CT appearance for treatment with definitive radiation therapy.

Acknowledgment: We thank Neil McKinney for the schematic illustrations used in this article.

References

1. Pameijar FA, Mancuso AA, Mendenhall WM, Parsons JT, Mukherji SK, Kubilis PS. Evaluation of pretreatment computed tomography as a predictor of local control in T1/T2 pyriform sinus carcinoma treated with definitive radiotherapy. Head Neck (in press).
2. Charlin B, Brazeau-Lamontagne L, Guerrier B, Leduc C. Assessment of laryngeal cancer versus endoscopy. J Otolaryngol 1989; 18:283–288.
3. Katsantonis GP, Archer CR, Rosenblum BN, Yeager VL, Friedman WH. The degree to which accuracy of preoperative staging of laryngeal carcinoma has been enhanced by computed tomography. Otolaryngol Head Neck Surg 1986; 95:52–62.
4. Sulfaro S, Barzan L, Quertin F, et al. T staging of laryngohypopharygeal carcinoma. Arch Otolaryngol Head Neck Surg 1989; 115:613–620.
5. Munoz A, Ramos A, Ferrando J, et al. Laryngeal carcinoma: sclerotic appearance of the cricoid and arytenoid cartilage—CT pathologic correlation. Radiology 1993; 189:433–437.
6. Becker M, Zbaren P, Laeng H, Stoupis C, Porcellini B, Vock P. Neoplastic invasion of the laryngeal cartilage: comparison of MR imaging and CT with histopathologic correlation. Radiology 1995; 194:661–669.
7. Saleh EM, Mancuso AA, Stringer SP. Relative roles of computed tomography and endoscopy for determining the inferior extent of pyriform sinus carcinoma: correlative histopathologic study. Head Neck 1993; 15:44–52.
8. Marks JE, Kurnik B, Powers WE, Ogura JH. Carcinoma of the pyriform sinus: an analysis of treatment results and patterns of failure. Cancer 1978; 41:1008–1015.
9. Lufkin RB, Hanafee WN, Wortham D, Hoover L. Larynx and hypopharynx: MR imaging with surface coil. Radiology 1986; 158:747–754.
10. Castelijns JA, Gerritsen GJ, Kaiser MC, et al. Invasion of laryngeal cartilage by cancer: comparison of CT and MR imaging. Radiology 1988; 167:199–206. [Erratum: Radiology 1988; 168:582.]
11. Teresi LM, Lufkin RB, Vinuela F, et al. MR imaging of the nasopharynx and the middle cranial fossa. II. Malignant tumors. Radiology 1987; 164:817–821.
12. Chong VFH, Fan YF. Detection of recurrent nasopharyngeal carcinoma: MR imaging versus CT. Radiology 1997; 202:463–470.
13. Som PM. Lymph nodes. In: Som PM, Curtin H, eds. Head and neck imaging. 3rd ed. New York, NY: Mosby, 1996; 772–793.
14. Som PM. Update on imaging metastatic lymph cervical lymph nodes: criteria and differential diagnosis. AJR 1992; 158:961–969.
15. Mancuso AA, Maceri D, Rice D, et al. CT of cervical lymph node cancer. AJR 1981; 136:381–385.
16. Mancuso AA, Harnsberger HR, Muraki AS, et al. Computed tomography of cervical and retropharyngeal lymph nodes: normal anatomy, variants of normal, and applications in staging head and neck cancer. II. Pathology. Radiology 1983; 148:715–723.
17. Yousem D, Som PM, Hackney DB, et al. Central nodal necrosis and extracapsular neoplastic spread in cervical lymph nodes: MR imaging versus CT. Radiology 1992; 182:753–759.
18. Suojanen JS, Mukherji SK, Whippold FJ. Spiral CT of the larynx. AJNR 1994; 15: 1579–1582.
19. Mukherji SK, Castillo M, et al. Comparison of dynamic and spiral CT for imaging of the glottic larynx. J Comput Assist Tomogr 1995; 19:899–904.
20. Escott EJ, Rao VM, Guitterrez JE. Comparison of dynamic contrast-enhanced gradient-echo and spin-echo sequences in MR of head and neck neoplasms. AJNR 1997; 18:1411–1419.
21. Mukherji SK, Weissman JL, Holliday R. The pharynx. In: Som PM, Curtin H, eds. Head and neck imaging. 3rd ed. New York, NY: Mosby, 1996; 437–488.
22. Takashima S, Noguchi Y, Okumura T, Hideharu A, Tetsuro K. Dynamic MR imaging in the head and neck. Radiology 1993; 189:813–821.
23. Ross MR, Schomer DF, Chappell P, Enzmann DR. MR imaging of head and neck tumors: comparison of T1-weighted contrast-enahnced fat-suppressed images with conventional T2-weighted and fast spin-echo T2-weighted images. AJR 1994; 163:173–178.
24. Mukherji SK, Tart RP, McGorray S, Belden C, Fitzsimmons J, Guy J, Mancuso AA. Fat-suppressed MR of the orbit and cavernous sinus: comparison of fast spin echo and conventional spin echo. AJNR 1994; 15:1707–1714.
25. Mendenhall WM, Million RR, Mancuso AA, Stringer SP. Nasopharynx. In: Million RR, Cassisi NJ, eds. Management of head and neck cancer: a multidisciplinary approach. Philadelphia, Pa: Lippincott, 1994; 599–626.
26. Neel HB, Slavitt DH. Nasopharyngeal cancer. In: Bailey BJ, ed. Head and neck surgery: otolaryngology. Philadelphia, Pa: Lippincott, 1993; 1257–1260.
27. Shanmugaratnam K, Sobin LH. Histologic typing of upper respiratory tract tumors. In: International histologic classification of tumors, no. 19. Geneva, Switzerland: World Health Organization, 1978.
28. Simons MJ, Wee GB, Day NE, Morris PJ, Shanmugaratnam K, De-The GB. Immu-

nogenetic aspects of nasopharyngeal carcinoma. I. Differences in HLA antigen profiles between patients and control groups. Int J Cancer 1974; 13:122–124.
29. Dickson RI. Nasopharyngeal carcinomas: an evaluation of 209 patients. Laryngoscope 1981; 91:333–334.
30. Lederman M. Cancer of the nasopharynx: its natural history and treatment. Springfield, Ill: Thomas, 1961; 1–50.
31. Mancuso AA, Hanafee WN. Nasopharynx and parapharyngeal space. In: Computed tomography and magnetic resonance imaging of the head and neck. 2nd ed. Baltimore, Md: Williams & Wilkins, 1985; 428–498.
32. American Joint Committee on Cancer; Fleming ID, Cooper JS, Henson DE, et al, eds. AJCC cancer staging manual. 5th ed. Philadelphia, Pa: Lippincott-Raven, 1997; 21–47.
33. Olmi P, Fallai C, Colagrande C, Giannardi G. Staging and follow-up of nasopharyngeal carcinoma: magnetic resonance imaging versus computerized tomography. Int J Radiat Biol Phys 1995; 32:795–800.
34. Chong VFH, Fan YF. Skull base erosion in nasopharyngeal carcinoma: detection by CT and MRI. Clin Radiol 1996; 51:625–631.
35. Chong VFH, Fan YF, Khoo JBK. Nasopharyngeal carcinoma with intracranial spread: CT and MR characteristics. J Comput Assist Tomogr 1996; 20:563–569.
36. Sham JST, Cheung YK, Choy D, Chan FL, Leong L. Nasopharyngeal carcinoma: CT evaluation of patterns of tumor spread. AJNR 1991; 12:265–270.
37. Million RA, Cassisi NJ, Mancuso AA. Oropharynx. In: Million RR, Cassisi NJ, eds. Management of head and neck cancer: a multidisciplinary approach. Philadelphia, Pa: Lippincott, 1994; 401–431.
38. Mancuso AA, Hanafee WN. Oral cavity and oropharynx including tongue base, floor of mouth and mandible. In: Computed tomography and magnetic resonance imaging of the head and neck. 2nd ed. Baltimore, Md: Williams & Wilkins, 1985; 358–427.
39. Mukherji SK, Weeks S, Castillo M, Krishnan LA. Squamous cell carcinomas that arise in the oral cavity and tongue base: can CT help predict perineural or vascular invasion? Radiology 1996; 198:157–162.
40. Million RA, Cassisi, NJ, Mancuso AA. Oral cavity. In: Million RR, Cassisi NJ, eds. Management of head and neck cancer: a multidisciplinary approach. Philadelphia, Pa: Lippincott, 1994; 599–626.
41. Curtin HD. Larynx. In: Som PM, Curtin HD. Head and neck imaging. 3rd ed. St Louis, Mo: Mosby–Year Book, 1995; 612–707.
42. Mancuso AA, Hanafee WN. Larynx and hypopharynx. In: Computed tomography and magnetic resonance imaging of the head and neck. 2nd ed. Baltimore, Md: Williams & Wilkins, 1985; 241–357.
43. Kallmes DF, Phillips CD. The normal anterior commissure of the glottis. AJR 1997; 168:1317–1319.
44. Million RR, Cassisi NJ, Mancuso AA. Larynx. In: Million RR, Cassisi NJ, eds. Management of head and neck cancer: a multidisciplinary approach. Philadelphia, Pa: Lippincott, 1994; 431–497.
45. Boyd JH, Johnson JT, Curtin HD. Carcinoma of the supraglottic larynx. Rochester, Minn: Custom Printing, 1993; 12–67.
46. Jackson C, Jackson CL. Cancer of the larynx. Philadelphia, Pa: Saunders, 1939; 52.
47. Zeitels SM, Vaughn CW, Domanowski GF. Endoscopic management of early supraglottic cancer. Ann Otol Rhinol Laryngol 1990; 99:951–956.
48. Maroldi R, Battaglia G, Nicolai P, et al. CT appearance of the larynx after conservative and radical surgery for carcinomas. Eur Radiol 1997; 7:418–431.
49. Chevalier D, Piquet JJ. Subtotal laryngectomy with cricohyoidpexy for supraglottic carcinoma: review of 61 cases. Am J Surg 1994; 168:472–473.
50. Laccourreye H, Laccourreye O, Weinstein G, Menard M, Brasnu D. Supracricoid laryngectomy with cricohyoidoepiglottopexy: a partial laryngeal procedure for glottic carcinoma. Ann Otol Rhinol Laryngol 1990; 99:421–427.
51. Laccourreye H, Laccourreye O, Weinstein G, Menard M, Brasnu D. Supracricoid laryngectomy with cricohyoidpexy: a partial laryngeal procedure for selected supraglottic and transglottic carcinomas. Laryngoscope 1990; 100:735–741.
52. Pearson BW. Subtotal laryngectomy. Laryngoscope 1981; 91:1904–1911.
53. Mendenhall WM, Million RR, Cassisi NJ. Squamous cell carcinoma of the supraglottic larynx treated with radical irradiation: analysis of treatment parameters and results. Int J Radiat Oncol Biol Phys 1984; 10:2223–2230.
54. Freeman DE, Mancuso AA, Parsons JT, et al. Irradiation alone for supraglottic carcinoma: can CT findings predict treatment results? Int J Radiat Oncol Biol Phys 1990; 19:485–490.
55. Mancuso AA, Mukherji SK, Mendenhall WM, Kotzur I, Freeman D. Value of pretreatment CT as a predictor of outcome in supraglottic cancer treated with radiation therapy alone (abstr). Radiology 1994; 193(P):262.
56. Castelijns JA, Van den Brekel MW, Smit EM, et al. Predictive value of MR imaging-dependent and non–MR imaging–dependent parameters for recurrence of laryngeal cancer after radiation therapy. Radiology 1995; 196:735–739.
57. Castelijns JA, Van den Brekel MW, Tobi H, et al. Laryngeal carcinoma after radiation therapy: correlation of abnormal MR imaging signal patterns in laryngeal cartilage with the risk of recurrence. Radiology 1996; 198:151–155.
58. Million RR. The myth regarding bone or cartilage involvement by cancer and the likelihood of cure by radiotherapy. Head Neck 1989; 11:30–40.
59. Wolf GT, Hong WK, Fischer SG. Neoadjuvant chemotherapy for organ preservation: current status. In: Shah JP, Johnson JT, eds. Head and neck cancer: proceedings of the fourth international conference on head and neck cancer, Toronto, July 28–August 1, 1996. Arlington, Va: The Society of Head and Neck Surgeons, 1996; 89–97.
60. Leach JL, Schaefer SD. Diagnosis and treatment of cancer of the glottis and subglottis. Rochester, Minn: Custom Printing, 1993; 12–72.
61. Labayle J, Bismuth R. La laryngectomie totale avec reconstitution. Ann Otolaryngol Chir Cervicofac 1971; 88:219–228.
62. Piquet JJ, Desaulty A, Decroix G. La crico-hyoido-epiglotto-pexie: technique operatoire et resultats fonctionnels. Ann Otolaryngol Chir Cervicofac 1974; 91:681–686.
63. Charlin B, Guerrier B, Balmigere G. Subtotal laryngectomy with cricohyoidopexy. Head Neck Surg 1988; (suppl 1):17–24.
64. Bartual Vicens R, Bartual Pastor J, Otero Gomex Q. Sobre la laringectomia total reconstructiva. Acta Otolaringol Esp 1973; 24:1–16.
65. Serafini I. Laringectomia glotticosottoglottica. In: Carlon G, ed. Il carcinoma dellalaringe dalla patologia alla clinica. Piccin Padova 1990; 289–293.
66. Pameijar FA, Mancuso AA, Mendenhall WM, Parsons JT, Kubilis PS. Can pretreatment computed tomography predict local control in T3 squamous cell carcinomas of the glottic larynx treated with definitive radiotherapy. Int J Radiat Oncol Biol Phys (in press).
67. Lee WR, Mancuso AA, Saleh EM, et al. Can pre-treatment computed tomography findings predict local control in T3 squamous cell carcinomas of the glottic larynx treated with radiotherapy alone? Int J Radiat Oncol Biol Phys 1993; 25:683–687.
68. Mukherji SK, Mancuso AA, Mendenhall WM, Kotzur IM, Fein D. Can pre-treatment computed tomography predict local control in T2 glottic carcinomas treated with radiation therapy alone? AJNR 1995; 16:655–662.
69. Mendenhall WM, Parsons JT, Mancuso AA, Pameijer FJ, Stringer SP, Cassisi NJ. Definitive radiotherapy for T3 squamous cell carcinoma of the glottic larynx. J Clin Oncol 1997; 15:2394–2404.
70. Mukherji SK, Mancuso AA, Kotzur I, et al. Radiologic appearance of the irradiated larynx. I. Expected changes. Radiology 1994; 193:141–148.
71. Mukherji SK, Mancuso AA, Kotzur I, et al. Radiologic appearance of the irradiated larynx. II. Primary site response. Radiology 1994; 193:149–154.
72. Induction chemotherapy plus radiation compared with surgery plus radiation in patients with advanced laryngeal cancer: The Department of Veterans Affairs Laryngeal Cancer Study Group. New Engl J Med 1991; 1685–1690.
73. Million RR, Cassisi NJ, Mancuso AA. Hypopharynx: pharyngeal walls, pyriform sinus, postcricoid pharynx. In: Million RR, Cassisi NJ, eds. Management of head and neck cancer: a multidisciplinary approach. Philadelphia, Pa: Lippincott, 1994; 505–532.
74. Barnes L, Gnepp DR. Diseases of the larynx, hypopharynx, and esophagus. In: Barnes L, ed. Surgical pathology of the head and neck. New York, NY: Dekker, 1985; 141–226.
75. Lefebvre JL, Chevalier D, Luboinki B, Kirkpatrick A, Collette L, Sahmoud T. Larynx preservation in puriform sinus cancer: preliminary results of a European organization for research and treatment of cancer phase III trial. J Natl Cancer Inst 1996; 88:890–899.

Editor's Page

Valediction: Sweet Sorrow

PARTING

This is the final issue of my 12-year period as Editor of *Radiology*. I will be saddened not to be serving in 1998. I shall miss the intellectual stimulation and the sense of mission. My sorrow is tempered by a lingering joy that comes from a conviction that the peer review process for scientific manuscripts, which I have served, is a bastion of honor in contemporary society.

THE MOTHPROOF CLOSET

Skepticism and cynicism are rife in our society. We have become accustomed to dealing with mistrust, doubt, and a sneering disbelief in the integrity of our major institutions including the government, the legal profession, and the media. Some years ago, I read a particularly cutting comment, "We live in a society where in the mothproof closet dwells the moth." In other words, our problems often extend to the very essence of our institutions. Thus, dishonesty, unfairness, and callousness are magnified because they are found where integrity, impartiality, and compassion have been proclaimed. However, on the basis of my long experience working directly with the process of reviewing and selecting scientific manuscripts for publication, I am proud to declare that the system works extremely well!

There have been sporadic reports with pointed criticisms of the review process, but I have never encountered truly negative judgments from individuals who were directly involved with the process. My own perception is that the vast majority of reviewers are extremely fair and objective with a clear knowledge that they are part of a mission to serve the discipline of radiology. There are rare incidents of rivalry between competing factions and the promotion of self-interest, but the Editor is available to supervise the process and to counter undesirable influences. The use of a computer tracking system greatly facilitates matters, and reviewers' performance can be carefully monitored (1).

THE REVIEW PROCESS

Radiology enjoys the services of a corps of over a thousand unpaid reviewers. Using guidelines set by the Editor, reviewers read papers diligently. They judge for accuracy, appropriateness of references, and quality of illustrations. Most important, they determine if conclusions are well documented by data in the manuscript. Even when a paper is judged to be of insufficient merit to justify publication, helpful suggestions are offered for revising and improving the quality of the work. Reviews generally consist of a 2–4-page typed document. Active reviewers receive a new manuscript every 2½–3 weeks. They devote several hours a week throughout the year to the review process. Authors receive three detailed reviews and a definitive decision on the acceptance of their paper generally within 6 weeks and invariably within 8 weeks from the date of submission. Reviewers receive the comments of the other two reviewers and a copy of the Editor's letter to the author.

QUID PRO QUO

The Golden Rule.—The system of reviewing scientific manuscripts works because there is an effective process of quid pro quo at work. Referees are willing to devote their precious time on a regular basis because of rich, nonmonetary rewards. Most reviewers are also authors submitting manuscripts to the Journal. We conducted a survey of the 940 individuals who had reviewed manuscripts for *Radiology* over a 4-year period from 1986 to 1990. We found that 85% of the reviewers had submitted at least one of their own manuscripts, that over 50% of the reviewers had submitted five or more manuscripts, and that 26% of the reviewers had submitted nine or more manuscripts. Thus, the reviewers and the authors are essentially the same group. Individuals reason that their efforts to provide careful, detailed, and helpful critiques are worthwhile because the system offers similar, timely evaluations of their own submissions. It is an example of the Golden Rule at work.

Assistant professors.—Younger reviewers, often assistant professors who completed their fellowship training 1–3 years earlier, make up a group that declares reviewing is particularly rewarding. Their energy and enthusiasm make them our finest referees. They more than compensate for a relative lack of experience by a particularly careful study of manuscripts. I have received scores of letters from such individuals thanking me for the honor and privilege of reviewing for the Journal and informing me that the process of reviewing had greatly increased their own skills at planning studies, establishing standards, analyzing scientific data, and preparing their own scientific manuscripts. Several dozen of these young reviewers have avowed that their association with the Journal has been the single most satisfying, valuable, and rewarding experience in their academic careers.

Index terms: Editor's Page • Radiology (journal)
Radiology 1997; 205:647–648

Noblesse oblige.—A coterie of experienced senior individuals is also devoted to the review process. They enjoy serving through a sense of duty, a feeling that they wish to support the discipline of radiology. I have been chided on several occasions for a failure to keep them occupied with an adequate number of manuscripts to review.

MISSION ACCOMPLISHED?

In an editorial in the January 1986 issue of *Radiology* (2), I set out the objectives for authors, reviewers, and readers under my editorship. We would avoid arbitrary standards, nurture young reviewers, promote the concept of reviewing as a formal scholarly activity, and provide an appropriate balance of materials for the radiologist in clinical practice. Our goals for the sort of scientific articles we wish to publish were more formally defined in 1989 (3).

An important issue was not addressed in the initial stated plans. Would we effect an improvement in the quality of the science in our published works? Editors must set high standards and campaign for better education of clinical scientists in their discipline. We presented an article in 1988 stressing adequate preparation, the need to establish definite diagnostic criteria, proper gathering and analysis of data, and the avoidance of bias (4). We have lobbied with radiology research funding groups that more effort should be spent "getting ready to begin;" that young investigators should be supported in formal training in clinical epidemiology before embarking on complicated research projects. An appreciable number of radiologists have taken such training, and they have helped raise the standards in their parent institutions. I communicated regularly with our reviewers to indicate selected items to be emphasized in their reviews. One example is the need for data on interobserver variation whenever diagnostic criteria are vague or complicated or subjective. An additional recurrent problem has been a failure to define adequately the patient population. This matter has been addressed in a tutorial in this issue (5).

THE WHITE STALLION

Searching for an additional metaphor, I turn to the forefront of contemporary culture: the cinema. We recall that Ronald Reagan made reference to the plots of John Wayne movies to document his principles and to support his positions on several key national issues. Robert Bolt, the screenwriter for one of my favorite motion pictures, *Lawrence of Arabia*, provided a wonderful interlude for the Arab chieftain, portrayed by Anthony Quinn. Battle weary and yearning to withdraw from the attacks on desert railways, the Quinn character muses, "I must find something honorable." Shortly thereafter he liberates a brilliant white stallion and leads the animal off into the sunset. We can view scientific journals as the white stallion in our current battle-weary medical community.

DEEP GRATITUDE

I leave with a deep sense of indebtedness to the hundreds of individuals who have worked so tirelessly and so effectively for the Journal these past dozen years. I have attempted to recognize the most faithful by means of vignettes citing prolific reviewers (6,7), letters of recommendation to promotion committees, Editor's Recognition Awards, and appointments to the *Radiology* Editorial Board. However, these measures still fall short of a proper expression of gratitude. There is also no adequate means for me to convey sufficient praise and thanks to the wonderful support provided by our Deputy Editors and by the *Radiology* staff in Baltimore, Md, and Oak Brook, Ill. I can only leave my dedicated supporters with an invocation: Together we have ridden the noble steed. There are no moths in our closet!

Finally, to my friend and able successor, Tony Proto, I counsel:

Beware,
The Journal is an insistent mistress
Demanding intense devotion
Striving, as in my case,
To capture heart and soul.

Stanley S. Siegelman, MD
Editor

References

1. Siegelman SS. Assassins and zealots: variations in peer review—special report. Radiology 1991; 178:637–642.
2. Siegelman SS. *Radiology* 1986. Radiology 1986; 158:265–266.
3. Siegelman SS. *Radiology* statement of purpose 1990. Radiology 1989; 173:467–468.
4. Siegelman SS. Advice to authors. Radiology 1988; 166:278–280.
5. Eng J, Siegelman SS. Improving radiology research methods: what is being asked and who is being studied? Radiology 1997; 205:651–655.
6. Siegelman SS. *Radiology*'s most prolific reviewers. Radiology 1989; 173:217–218.
7. Siegelman SS. *Radiology*'s most prolific reviewers. Radiology 1994; 190:311–312.

Joseph F. Polak, MD, MPH

Duplex Sonography: Can It Be Used to Evaluate Carotid Artery Stents?[1]

The article by Robbin et al is timely (1). Carotid artery stent placement is being proposed as an alternative to carotid endarterectomy for the treatment of carotid artery disease. Since duplex sonography is believed to be an efficacious method of monitoring the therapeutic success of carotid artery surgery, it would seem likely that carotid artery ultrasound (US) may have a role in the evaluation of the efficacy of carotid artery stent placement.

The data in the study of Robbin et al (1) can be better understood by looking at the diagnostic accuracy of duplex US for the detection of disease in native carotid arteries and for following up recurrent carotid artery lesions after carotid endarterectomy. In addition, it seems necessary to examine how the data presented by Robbin et al can give a measure of the accuracy of duplex US in patients who have undergone placement of a carotid artery stent.

The diagnostic accuracy of carotid artery US for the detection of carotid artery disease has been studied in many individual laboratories and more recently in the context of large trials of carotid artery surgery. Carotid artery US is well recognized as an efficacious method of evaluating the carotid arteries before surgery (2). Carotid artery US has played different roles in two large trials that compared medically treated patients with patients who underwent carotid artery surgery: the Asymptomatic Carotid Atherosclerosis Study (ACAS) and the North American Symptomatic Carotid Endarterectomy Trial (NASCET). Carotid artery US was critical in the work-up and selection process of patients enrolled in the ACAS (3). The performance of carotid artery US as a screening test, however, was dismal in the NASCET (4,5). Of the many possible explanations for the latter, the most likely is simply poor quality-control procedures. Laboratories that participated in the NASCET failed to control for the marked variability in the way that carotid artery US measurements were performed. In support of this explanation are data from the ACAS that show excellent diagnostic specificity and strong positive predictive value for detection of internal carotid artery stenoses of at least 60% (6). Findings in the ACAS and other studies have shown that the peak-systolic velocity in the internal carotid artery is a robust parameter for measuring the severity of carotid artery stenosis (7,8).

With use of an appropriate peak-systolic value as the cutoff point, Doppler sonography has been shown to be cost-effective when combined with magnetic resonance angiography for the detection of patients with symptomatic (≥ 70%) (9) or asymptomatic (≥ 60%) (10) stenosis in the internal carotid artery. It is therefore surprising that the accuracy of peak-systolic velocity seems poor for the detection of significant carotid artery stenosis after stent placement.

Acquisition of data on the time course for recurrence of carotid artery stenosis after surgery, as evaluated with US, would cast some light on what to expect after placement of a carotid artery stent. These data may help understand whether detection of recurrent stenosis is critical in patients who have undergone placement of a carotid artery stent. On the basis of findings in the literature about carotid endarterectomy, recurrent stenosis appears to be asymptomatic, with an incidence of 8.8%–19.0% (11–13). Cases in which recurrent stenosis is symptomatic are relatively uncommon, with an incidence less than 3%–4% (14). Recurrent carotid artery stenosis may actually be an indicator of good outcome, as patients with recurrent stenosis seem to do better than patients without recurrent stenosis (15). Data from the carotid endarterectomy literature suggest that the rate of lesion recurrence after placement of a carotid artery stent should be low. This is consistent with the findings reported by Robbin et al: two occlusions and three significant (≥ 50%) stenoses, for a rate of recurrent stenosis of five (2.9%) of 170 stenoses (1). Data for carotid endarterectomy also indicate that most recurrent lesions detected with carotid artery US are not associated with cerebrovascular symptoms. This was also observed by Robbin et al, although the number of significant stenoses detected with arteriography was small.

In the study of Robbin et al, cases of recurrent stenosis were used as outcomes and the sensitivity of carotid artery US for the detection of stenosis in a carotid artery stent was evaluated. There were few cases of recurrent stenosis; therefore, it is not possible to give an accurate estimate of the sensitivity of velocity criteria at Doppler US in patients with recurrent stenosis after placement of a carotid artery stent. In a previous report from the same institution, Yadav et al reported four cases of recurrent stenosis in the first 107 cases of placement of a carotid artery stent (126 vessels) (16). Presumably, some of these patients did not undergo carotid artery US and their data are not included in the current analysis. Findings in the study of Robbin et al, however, give the reader important information about what to expect when Doppler velocity parameters are applied to the detection of recurrent stenosis after placement of a carotid artery stent. Specificity with the peak-systolic velocity parameters was good, and the negative predictive value was high (Tables 1, 2). The sensitivity of Doppler velocity parameters cannot be accurately estimated, however, as stenosis recurred (≥ 60%) in only one case. By increasing the velocity cutoff point, the specificity and positive predictive value should increase and the sensitivity should decrease. The effect on sensitivity cannot be seen in their study, however, as the number of positive outcomes is small. This expected increase in specificity is seen, however, when the peak-systolic velocity cutoff is increased from 1.25 to 1.7 m/sec (Tables 1, 2).

Index terms: Carotid arteries, flow dynamics, 172.91 • Carotid arteries, stenosis or obstruction, 172.76 • Carotid arteries, US, 172.12983 • Editorials

Radiology 1997; 205:649–650

[1] From the Department of Radiology, Harvard Medical School, Brigham and Women's Hospital, 75 Francis St, Boston, MA 02115. Received September 17, 1997; accepted September 18. **Address reprint requests to** the author.

See also the article by Robbin et al (pp 748–756) in this issue.

One question remains: What should be done when findings at Doppler US are abnormal and no significant stenosis is seen at arteriography? The peak-systolic velocity was above 1.7 m/sec in four cases, but findings at arteriography were positive in only one case. Is it possible that significant stenoses were missed at arteriography? This possibility is difficult to study objectively. On the basis of objective outcomes, these patients remain asymptomatic and are unlikely to undergo an additional interventional procedure. In a recently published series (13), recurrent stenosis was studied in patients after carotid endarterectomy. On the basis of Doppler peak-systolic velocity above 1.25 m/sec, the recurrence rate was 19% (13). This is higher than the rate of 10.7% (18 of 168 patients) reported with the same cutoff point to define recurrent stenosis after placement of a carotid artery stent (1). The presence of mildly elevated Doppler velocities may therefore represent a ubiquitous finding in many patients after placement of a carotid artery stent.

In conclusion, the article by Robbin et al is timely (1). Their data suggest that the presence of a carotid artery stent does not affect the ability to perform an adequate duplex US examination. They also found that the rate of recurrent stenosis is low, within the range reported after carotid endarterectomy. Their data also suggest that the velocity cutoff points routinely used to help detect significant stenosis in native carotid arteries (17) are likely too low to be useful in follow-up after placement of a carotid artery stent. Determination of the sensitivity of Doppler sonography for the detection of recurrent stenosis after placement of a carotid artery stent will have to wait for results in a larger single-center series or in a multicenter study with sufficient positive outcomes at arteriography. ■

Table 1
Accuracy with Peak-Systolic Velocity Cutoff of 1.25 m/sec

	Findings at Angiography		
Findings at Duplex US	Positive	Negative	Total
Positive	1	17	18
Negative	0	150	150
Total	1	167	168

Note.—Data are number of patients. Findings reflect recurrent stenosis after placement of a carotid artery stent (excluding total occlusion): sensitivity, 100% (1/1 [estimates are inaccurate]); specificity, 89.8% (150/167); positive predictive value, 5.5% (1/18 [wide confidence intervals]); negative predictive value, 100% (150/150).

Table 2
Accuracy with Peak-Systolic Velocity Cutoff of 1.7 m/sec

	Findings at Angiography		
Findings at Duplex US	Positive	Negative	Total
Positive	1	3	4
Negative	0	164	164
Total	1	167	168

Note.—Data are number of patients. Findings reflect recurrent stenosis after placement of a carotid artery stent (excluding total occlusion): sensitivity, 100% (1/1 [estimates are inaccurate]); specificity, 98.2% (164/167); positive predictive value, 25% (1/4 [extremely wide confidence intervals]); negative predictive value, 100% (164/164).

References

1. Robbin ML, Lockhart ME, Weber TM, et al. Carotid artery stents: early and intermediate follow-up with Doppler US. Radiology 1997; 205:748–756.
2. Carroll B. Carotid sonography: state of the art. Radiology 1991; 178:303–313.
3. Executive Committee for the Asymptomatic Carotid Atherosclerosis Study. Endarterectomy for asymptomatic carotid artery stenosis. JAMA 1995; 273:1421–1428.
4. North American Symptomatic Carotid Endarterectomy Trial Collaborators. Beneficial effect of carotid endarterectomy in symptomatic patients with high-grade stenosis. N Engl J Med 1991; 325:445–453.
5. Eliasziw M, Rankin RN, Fox I, et al. Accuracy and prognostic consequences of ultrasonography in identifying severe carotid artery stenosis. Stroke 1995; 26:1747–1752.
6. Howard G, Baker W, Chambless L, et al. An approach for the use of Doppler ultrasound as a screening tool for hemodynamically significant stenosis (despite heterogeneity of Doppler performance): a multicenter experience. Stroke 1996; 27:1951–1957.
7. Hunink MGM, Polak JF, Barlan MM, O'Leary DH. Detection and quantification of carotid artery stenosis: efficacy of various Doppler velocity parameters. AJR 1993; 160:619–625.
8. Schwartz S, Chambless L, Baker WH, Broderick J, Howard G, for the Asymptomatic Carotid Atherosclerosis Study Investigators. Consistency of Doppler parameters in predicting arteriographically confirmed carotid stenosis. Stroke 1997; 28:343–347.
9. Kent KC, Kuntz KM, Patel MR, et al. Perioperative strategies for carotid endarterectomy: an analysis of morbidity and cost-effectiveness in symptomatic patients. JAMA 1995; 274:888–893.
10. Patel MR, Kuntz KM, Klufas RA, et al. Preoperative assessment of the carotid bifurcation: can magnetic resonance angiography and duplex ultrasonography replace contrast arteriography? Stroke 1995; 26:1753–1758.
11. Turnipseed W, Berkoff H, Crummy A. Postoperative occlusion after carotid endarterectomy. Arch Surg 1980; 115:573–574.
12. Zierler R, Bandyk D, Thiele B, Strandness DE Jr. Carotid artery stenosis following endarterectomy. Arch Surg 1982; 117:408–415.
13. Golledge J, Cuming R, Ellis M, Davies A, Greenhalgh R. Duplex imaging findings predict stenosis after carotid endarterectomy. J Vasc Surg 1997; 26:43–48.
14. Callow A. Recurrent stenosis after carotid endarterectomy. Arch Surg 1982; 117:1082–1085.
15. Bernstein E, Torem S, Dilley R. Does carotid restenosis predict an increased risk of late symptoms, stroke, or death? Ann Surg 1990; 212:629–636.
16. Yadav J, Roubin G, Iyer S, et al. Elective stenting of the extracranial carotid arteries. Circulation 1997; 95:376–381.
17. Polak JF, Dobkin GR, O'Leary DH, Wang AM, Cutler AS. Internal carotid artery stenosis: accuracy and reproducibility of color-Doppler–assisted duplex imaging. Radiology 1989; 173:793–798.

John Eng, MD • Stanley S. Siegelman, MD

Improving Radiology Research Methods: What Is Being Asked and Who Is Being Studied?[1]

PEER reviewers like to read well-written research reports and recommend them for publication. An author, however, may find this assertion difficult to appreciate when a manuscript is returned with a long list of "suggested" revisions, especially since these comments are typically weighted toward criticism rather than praise. Most of these comments can be roughly divided into two categories: (*a*) comments concerning the form of presentation and (*b*) comments concerning the study design and methods.

Problems with the form of presentation may be annoying, but they are seldom the primary reason for manuscript rejection. It is relatively easy to address presentation problems, even at such a late stage as manuscript review. By applying appropriate guidelines and principles (1), the manuscript can be revised to meet the expectations of a journal's readers.

Usually mixed into the comments about presentation are comments in the second category: those concerning study design and methods. Sometimes, these comments can be adequately addressed by clarifying a particular point. More often, however, these comments highlight major weaknesses in the study and may be the reason for downgrading a manuscript's priority for publication. The most important problems of this type involve poorly formed research questions and inadequately defined study populations. Both have a substantial influence on the manuscript review process. For example, a research article addressing a good question by using straightforward methods will almost always be published, whereas an article reporting on brilliant methods applied to a poorly formed research question is in serious danger of rejection. Furthermore, important issues involving the study population are often overlooked; currently, the greatest problem found in manuscripts submitted to *Radiology* is the failure to define the study population adequately.

Unlike problems with presentation, those involving study design and methods are difficult to address retroactively, if at all. Instead, these problems are best addressed while the study is being planned, long before the eventual drafting of a manuscript. It has been said that the best time to write the Materials and Methods section of an article is when the study is being planned. It forces the researcher to think completely through the methods and allows mentors and collaborators to provide meaningful comments. Supervision by a knowledgeable mentor is the best way to prevent methodologic problems; however, such mentors are often unavailable. As a supplement to good mentorship, we offer the following guidelines.

THE RESEARCH QUESTION

Rigorous research begins with a properly posed research question. Some experienced clinical researchers assert that creating, refining, and succinctly stating a research question is the most important intellectual activity in academic research and is the most important single determinant of success. A properly posed research question has three key characteristics: (*a*) importance, (*b*) novelty, and (*c*) answerability. To illustrate these characteristics, suppose a newly developed imaging modality M is particularly good at providing morphologic or functional information associated with disease D. An initial research question might be: "*What is the value of imaging modality M in diagnosing (or ruling out) disease D?*"

This type of question is common in radiology research. Let us examine this question in terms of the three characteristics mentioned.

Importance

The research question given above is a good one only if disease D represents an important health problem with substantial morbidity or sequelae if it is undiagnosed. Some less obvious reasons why the proposed research question would be unimportant are as follows: a very accurate diagnosis of disease D can already be made with a different modality, the diagnosis of disease D can be made from clinical findings that do not involve imaging (eg, results of physical examination and laboratory tests), or patients in whom disease D is diagnosed without imaging receive the same treatment (eg, surgery) regardless of the radiologic findings. These issues demonstrate the differences between "diagnostic accuracy efficacy" (which includes sensitivity and specificity) and "diagnostic thinking efficacy" (which includes the effect of a test on pretest probability), two of the six levels in the technology as-

Index terms: Radiology and radiologists, research • Radiology (journal) • Special reports

Radiology 1997; 205:651–655

[1] From the Department of Radiology, The Johns Hopkins Hospital, Central Radiology Bldg, Rm 117, 600 N Wolfe St, Baltimore, MD 21287 (J.E.); and the Editorial Office, *Radiology*, Baltimore, Md (S.S.S.). Received May 28, 1997; revision requested July 9; revision received August 5; accepted August 6. J.E. was a Robert Wood Johnson Clinical Scholar during manuscript preparation. **Address reprint requests to** J.E.

Abbreviations: AIDS = acquired immunodeficiency syndrome, PCP = *Pneumocystis carinii* pneumonia.

sessment model defined by Fryback and Thornbury (2). Notice that the importance of the research question may be based more on the clinical context of disease D than on the quality of images from modality M.

Important research questions come in many forms, and the research question we propose in this example, which involves a specific disease and imaging modality, is only one type. Other potentially important research questions involve the comparison of two (or more) imaging modalities for the same disease or the consideration of outcomes other than the familiar ones of sensitivity, specificity, and accuracy. Some important alternative outcomes include cost, cost-effectiveness, and patient-centered outcomes such as morbidity, quality of life, and patient preferences.

In clinical research circles, the question of importance is sometimes known as the "so what?" criterion. Imagine that the proposed study is successfully performed and positive findings are reported. Would our understanding of the natural cause or natural history of the disease be improved? What difficult clinical problem would these results help solve? How would these results change the clinical practice of radiologists or referring physicians? Would the study's results help other researchers trying to determine the appropriate clinical role of a radiology test? In other words, "so what?"

Novelty

If the research question is answered, the result should be new information. What does the research add to the body of scientific knowledge? The desire for new information, however, does not always require a completely original research question (3). Perhaps there are very few studies in the literature that examine the same important research question, so a well-designed follow-up study is warranted. Is the proposed study design better than that of previous studies? Even if there are already many studies in the literature about the application of imaging modality M in the diagnosis of disease D, another study may still be valuable for confirming the results of the earlier studies, especially if the new study addresses weaknesses of previous studies. In performing such a study, there is also the chance that the previous results would be refuted, which would certainly constitute new information. Another opportunity for novel research is the application of imaging modality M in the diagnosis of disease D in a certain subset of patients in whom the diagnosis is otherwise clinically difficult to establish.

Novelty or innovation as a key issue is quite familiar to many "experienced" investigators. A surprising number of manuscripts currently submitted to *Radiology* include the words "new," "novel," or "innovative" in the title. This practice is discouraged (4,5); it is the reviewers and the editor who must judge whether a scientific paper contains new information.

Answerability

To be answerable, a good research question must state the study's major clinical variables in specific terms. In our example, the word "value" is too vague and makes the question unanswerable. We can revise the question and state our idea in more specific terms: *Is imaging modality M a sensitive and specific method for diagnosing (or ruling out) disease D?*

The question is still imprecise because it does not define how high modality M's sensitivity and specificity must be for the question to be answered "yes" versus "no." A stronger question would propose comparing modality M to a standard modality S, as follows: *Is imaging modality M a more sensitive and specific method for diagnosing (or ruling out) disease D than is imaging modality S?*

Radiologic findings, not modalities themselves, are what radiologic diagnoses are based on, so an even stronger research question would focus on the findings, as follows: *Is finding F with imaging modality M more sensitive and specific for diagnosing (or ruling out) disease D than is finding G with imaging modality S?*

The question is still not answerable because the study population has not been identified. We need to specify the group of patients in whom we will answer the question: *Is finding F with imaging modality M more sensitive and specific for diagnosing (or ruling out) disease D than is finding G with imaging modality S in patient population P?*

The definition of the study population is often left out of the design of radiology research, even though it is a primary determinant of the generalizability and ultimate usefulness of the information reported by a research study. It is not sufficient simply to state, "the study population was *N* patients with pathologically confirmed disease D who underwent imaging modality M." The process of adequately defining the study population is discussed next.

DEFINING THE STUDY POPULATION

What is meant by "defining the study population"? It is simply making an explicit statement of how the study participants were chosen from the universe of all possible participants. Let us consider a more concrete example. Suppose we have decided on a research question involving the acquired immunodeficiency syndrome (AIDS) and *Pneumocystis carinii* pneumonia (PCP). Perhaps we are interested in improving the characterization of computed tomographic (CT) findings in PCP.

The first step in defining the study population is to establish the *target population,* the general group of individuals about which the study will provide information. A target population is usually defined by stating the general clinical and demographic characteristics of the individuals of interest (Fig 1). In our example, we could define our target population to be "AIDS patients suspected of having PCP." Our definition would also have to include how the diagnosis of AIDS is being defined and what criteria are used to identify patients who are suspected of having PCP. The latter is particularly important in radiology because diagnostic imaging, unlike drug treatment, is most often applied to patients who are suspected of having a disease and not to those who are known to have it.

The target population is usually stated in somewhat general terms, emphasizing only the most important characteristics of the individuals of interest. Furthermore, the target population is almost always too large to study in its entirety. We cannot, for example, study every patient who has AIDS and is suspected of having PCP. The next step, then, is to define the study's *inclusion criteria,* also known as *selection criteria,* which specify those in the target population who will actually be considered for the study. Individuals satisfying the inclusion criteria are said to be *eligible* for the study. Inclusion criteria typically specify characteristics such as age range, sex, disease type, presenting symptoms, stage and severity of disease, abnormal laboratory tests, and other clinical requirements. The inclusion criteria also typically limit

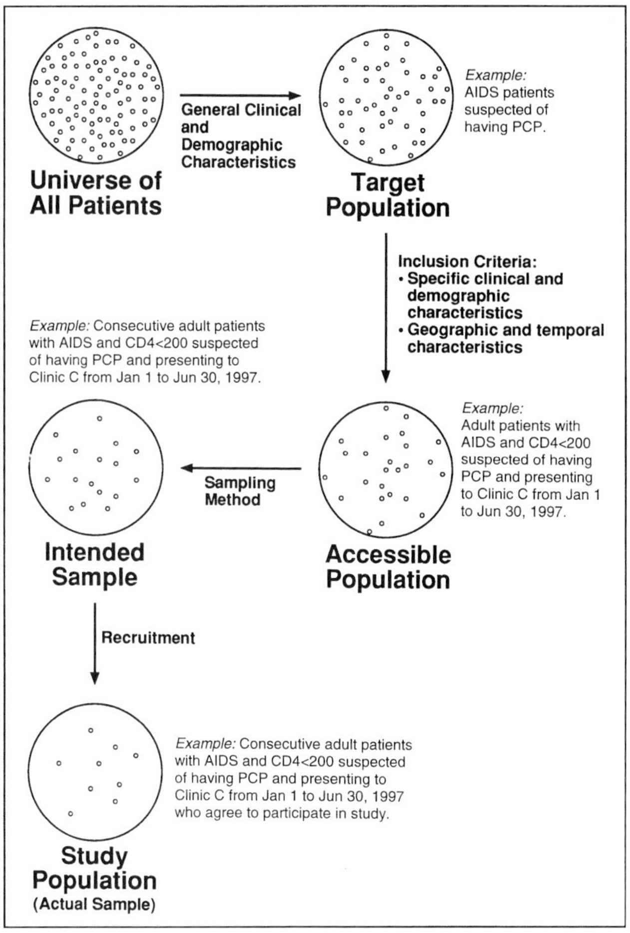

Figure 1. Steps in defining the study population. *CD4<200* = CD4 cell count of less than 200 per cubic millimeter, *Jan* = January, *Jun* = June.

the target population to a specific geographic location and time. The population that results from the application of the inclusion criteria is sometimes called the *accessible population.* In our example, we might define the accessible population to be "adult AIDS patients with a CD4 cell count less than 200 per cubic millimeter who are suspected of having PCP and who are seen in clinic C during the period of January 1 to June 30, 1997."

SAMPLING

It is usually still not feasible to study everyone in the accessible population because it is too large; so, some form of sampling is required (Fig 1). The sampling strategy defines yet another group, the *intended sample.* There are many different types of sampling, ranging from simple random sampling to judgmental sampling ("handpicking"). The most appropriate type of sampling depends on the specific research question. In our example, some form of random sampling is desirable to avoid introducing *selection bias,* a type of error in which a study's outcome is influenced by how the particular subjects were selected rather than by the test or intervention being studied. One appropriate approach is to choose a consecutive sampling strategy in which we enroll the next *N* patients seen in clinic C. (Strictly speaking, a consecutive sample is not a random sample, but an approximation to one.) Random sampling also deals with the problem of *confounding,* a situation in which a study's results are distorted by the presence of secondary factors that influence simultaneously the other variables being studied. Although it is possible to compensate for selection bias and known confounding factors with careful nonrandom sampling, compensation for unknown confounding factors requires a random sampling method. Not all studies require random sampling. Some studies of healthy subjects, for example, may not need a random sample.

Because the clinical research environment is imperfect, not every patient meeting the selection criteria actually participates. A patient may not agree to participate in the study for a number of possible reasons, or there can be logistic problems in recruiting patients for the study. So, the last step in defining the study population is to define a recruitment strategy aimed at maximizing the number of eligible patients who actually participate in the study. Sometimes the researcher has little control over the fraction of eligible patients who are enrolled; however, records should be kept on how many eligible patients do not enroll, and these records should be used to report an enrollment fraction. If a large number of eligible patients do not enroll, then the actual sample may not be representative of the intended sample. One way to handle situations of low enrollment is to perform statistical comparisons of demographic and other characteristics between the actual sample and the group of subjects who did not enroll. The absence of a statistically significant difference can sometimes exclude the presence of large biases within the actual sample.

GENERALIZABILITY

Why are these definition steps important? Because at each step after the definition of the target population, we must ensure that certain patients are not preferentially excluded in ways that could affect the variables we are observing. Stating these definitions enables the reader to judge whether the final actual sample, the study population proper, is truly representative of the target population.

In radiology research, the accessible population is often defined by who undergoes a particular imaging examination. For example, we might propose a study of consecutive AIDS patients with suspected PCP who underwent chest CT. The problem with this approach is that we have excluded all AIDS patients with suspected PCP who did not undergo CT. It is possible that patients who undergo CT tend to be the ones with more advanced disease, which could be associated with different radiologic findings (and outcomes) than those in patients with milder disease. If our diagnostic imaging method performs better in the enrolled patients because they have a different stage of disease than the "average" patient with the disease, then we have introduced *spectrum bias* (6,7).

Ideally, the accessible population should be defined without any imaging requirements. If imaging criteria must be included in the definition of the accessible population, then this situation should be recognized as an automatic source of potential bias in the study. In this case, the inclusion criteria should state how patients were chosen to undergo the imaging examination. The subsequent research report should critically discuss the inclusion criteria and estimate the degree and direction of the potential bias.

Having a representative study population means that findings in the actual sample reasonably apply to the target population as well. This property is called the *generalizability* of the study. In practice, there is often a trade-off between a study design's generalizability and feasibility. We may decide to enroll patients from a tertiary care clinic because it provides closer follow-up than a primary care clinic, even though the spectrum of disease among patients in the primary care clinic is more representative of all patients with the disease. It is also more difficult to control for selection bias, confounding, and random variation in broadly defined, generalizable study populations.

Even the highest standard of clinical research, the randomized controlled clinical trial, is not exempt from the issue of generalizability. These studies typically involve evaluations of drug treatments under strict protocols at academic medical centers. These strict protocols usually involve many specific inclusion and exclusion criteria so that the target populations of these studies are usually small subsets of all patients with the disease being treated. Furthermore, study participants are probably more likely than nonparticipants to receive good ancillary medical care. As with all clinical studies, the evaluation of a randomized clinical trial's generalizability requires a thorough analysis of the inclusion and exclusion criteria.

Figure 2. Summary of advice for planning and reporting on research.

Defining the study population: summary of advice for planning and reporting research.

1. State the general clinical and demographic characteristics of the subjects being studied. This defines the target population.
2. State the specific clinical, demographic, geographic, and temporal characteristics of the subjects being studied. These compose the inclusion (or selection) criteria, and they define the accessible population.
3. State the sampling strategy being used. This defines the intended sample.
4. Avoid incorporating imaging requirements into the inclusion criteria.
5. Account for eligible subjects (those who satisfied the inclusion criteria) who did not enroll in the study.
6. If the sensitivity of a technique is to be determined for a group of subjects with disease, then the study population should include a spectrum of disease severity and comorbid conditions.
7. If the specificity of a technique is to be determined for a group of subjects without disease, then the study population should include a reasonable number of subjects with conditions that may be confused with the disease of interest and cause false-positive diagnoses.
8. In a retrospective study of a series of cases collected without a specific protocol, report the number of cases with a particular diagnosis as a percentage, not as the sensitivity.
9. Include a discussion of the limitations of the study and estimate the magnitude and direction of potential biases.

SOME PROBLEMS WITH THE POPULATION

Having put forth the preceding general principles, we comment on some specific situations involving the study population and patient selection that are commonly identified in the peer review process.

Sensitivity and Specificity

It is difficult to develop a satisfactory study population in a retrospective study because the investigator cannot control the selection criteria or data collection retrospectively. A proper clinical report that presents conclusions about the sensitivity and specificity of a diagnostic technique should satisfy certain criteria. If the term "sensitivity" is used, the reader must be assured that a total spectrum of subjects with disease was studied, including patients in various phases of the illness and those with confounding variables such as obesity, uncooperativeness, or the existence of a second illness (1,6), all of which could make the disease difficult to detect in practice. Similarly, the population of control patients should contain a reasonable number of subjects with conditions likely to challenge the specificity by leading to false-positive diagnoses. Thus, a study of a technique for detecting metastases to the liver should include control subjects with cirrhosis or fatty infiltration of the liver (1). For retrospective studies, the reporting of sensitivity and specificity should be reserved for rigorous studies with meticulous patient selection methods and statistical checks for bias. Otherwise, if one detects a new, potentially important finding in a retrospective study of a series of patients, one should simply report the percentage of patients in whom the new finding was detected, not the sensitivity of the examination.

Illogical Patient Selection

Improper patient selection not infrequently leads to specious conclusions. A common approach in clinical studies is to present a new technique N for evaluating patients suspected of having disease D because the currently available techniques have high specificity but limited sensitivity. This often occurs because the morphologic and functional disturbances consist of mixtures of different features of disease D, which we will call D1 and D2. The established techniques may be extremely accurate in the detection of D1 but insensitive to D2. Thus, lesions manifesting only feature D2 are not detected. A study is done in which technique N helps detect 95% of 40 subjects with disease D. Alas, however, the high sensitivity of technique N is illusory. Patient selection is not carefully outlined in the Materials and Methods section. The Results section reveals that only four subjects had biopsy proof of disease D and that the other 36 subjects were considered to have the disease because they had positive findings with the established imaging techniques. Do you detect the faulty logic? Because the established techniques were used to select patients with disease D, mostly "easy" cases (those with feature D1) were selected for the study. To establish that technique N has added value, one should study subjects suspected of having the disease who have negative findings with established techniques (presumably because of feature D2). The data in the study do not document the added value of technique N because of patient selection bias.

Examples of the phenomenon just illustrated occurred in magnetic resonance (MR) imaging studies in patients with hemangioma of the liver. Because CT had at best an 80% sensitivity in the detection of hemangioma (8), MR imaging was pursued as a possibly more sensitive technique. In many submitted research reports, the study population included a large proportion of patients with diagnostic CT examinations as proof of the existence of hepatic hemangioma. The patient population to be studied should be those suspected to have hemangioma with negative CT findings. We know of no such study.

In making the preceding comments, we do not wish to advocate undue editorial bias against certain types of research studies. A thoughtfully designed, well-executed retrospective study can provide important information and may be the only feasible method in certain situations, such as in the study of a rare disease. Even a descriptive study—one designed to measure the value or distribution of an existing variable rather than an association between variables—can be valuable. No particular study design should be considered inherently better or worse than another. A good study is one in which a good research question is combined with whatever study design is appropriate for answering the question. Since all study designs have their potential weaknesses, the investigator should explicitly consider the sources of bias in any study and attempt to control for them wherever possible.

The design of high-quality research studies requires dedicated mentorship and years of experience. The need for mentorship is not easily outgrown—it is common for even the most experienced researchers to have mentors. Although points concerning the research question and study population (Fig 2) may appear to be matters of common sense, the most experienced researchers continue to emphasize them time and again, and we trust for good reason. When planning a study, appropriate attention to forming the research question and defining the study population enhances the quality of the research and increases the likelihood that the subsequent report will receive a high priority for publication. ■

Acknowledgment: The authors thank Leon Gordis, MD, MPH, DrPH, for helpful discussions and suggestions concerning the manuscript.

References

1. Siegelman SS. Advice to authors. Radiology 1988; 166:278–280.
2. Fryback DG, Thornbury JR. The efficacy of diagnostic imaging. Med Decis Making 1991; 11:88–94.
3. Cummings SR, Browner WS, Hulley SB. Conceiving the research question. In: Hulley SB, Cummings SR, eds. Designing clinical research. Baltimore, Md: Williams & Wilkins, 1988; 12–17.
4. Siegelman SS. Modesty, please (editor's page). Radiology 1993; 186:36.
5. Kaufman L. First new assessment of self-characterization of published work: a unique view obtained with novel methods. Radiology 1992; 183:323–324.
6. Ransohoff DF, Feinstein AR. Problems of spectrum and bias in evaluating the efficacy of diagnostic tests. N Engl J Med 1978; 299:926–930.
7. Begg CB, McNeil BJ. Assessment of radiologic tests: control of bias and other design considerations. Radiology 1988; 167:565–569.
8. Ashida C, Fishman EK, Zerhouni EA, Herlong FH, Siegelman SS. Computed tomography of hepatic cavernous hemangioma. J Comput Assist Tomogr 1987; 11:455–460.

Abstractors of Current Literature 1997

The Abstracts of Current Literature section of *Radiology* is made possible by the efforts of 16 abstractors, who search through 19 medical journals for articles of interest to radiologists. Because of their work, each month this section contains approximately 40 abstracts of journal articles of particular relevance to medical imaging specialists. We extend our appreciation to these abstractors for their contributions to this feature of *Radiology* in 1997.

STANLEY S. SIEGELMAN, MD, *Editor*

Journal of Pediatrics
A'Delbert Bowen, MD
Children's Hospital of Pittsburgh
Pittsburgh, Pa

Archives of Pediatric and Adolescent Medicine
Archives of Disease in Childhood
Paula W. Brill, MD
New York Hospital–Cornell Medical Center
New York, NY

Obstetrics and Gynecology
Jeanne Anne Cullinan, MC
Vanderbilt University Medical Center
Nashville, Tenn

Annals of Thoracic Surgery
Sheila D. Davis, MD
New York Hospital–Cornell Medical Center
New York, NY

Journal of the American College of Surgery
Terry Elwing, MD
University of Missouri
Columbia, Mo

American Journal of Pathology
Arnold C. Friedman, MD
Medical College Hospitals
Philadelphia, Pa

Journal of Urology
Urology
Stanford M. Goldman, MD
University of Texas
Houston, Tex

Annals of Internal Medicine
Janet Kuhlman, MD
University of Wisconsin Medical School
Madison, Wis

Gastroenterology
Duane G. Mezwa, MD
William Beaumont Hospital
Royal Oak, Mich

Journal of Vascular Surgery
Daniel Picus, MD
Mallinckrodt Institute of Radiology
St Louis, Mo

American Journal of Cardiology
Patricia A. Randall, MD
SUNY Health Science Center
Syracuse, NY

Arthritis & Rheumatism
David Sartoris, MD
University of California Medical Center
San Diego, Calif

Journal of Bone and Joint Surgery
William W. Scott, Jr, MD
The Johns Hopkins Hospital
Baltimore, Md

Thorax
David L. Spizarny, MD
Henry Ford Hospital
Detroit, Mich

American Heart Journal
Journal of Thoracic and Cardiovascular Surgery
Robert M. Steiner, MD
Thomas Jefferson University Hospital
Philadelphia, Pa

Pediatrics
Beverly P. Wood, MD
Children's Hospital Los Angeles
Los Angeles, Calif

Noriyuki Kato, MD • Michael D. Dake, MD • D. Craig Miller, MD • Charles P. Semba, MD
R. Scott Mitchell, MD • Mahmood K. Razavi, MD • Stephen T. Kee, MD

Traumatic Thoracic Aortic Aneurysm: Treatment with Endovascular Stent-Grafts[1]

PURPOSE: To demonstrate the feasibility and safety of endovascular stent-graft placement for treatment of traumatic aortic aneurysm.

MATERIALS AND METHODS: Ten patients with traumatic aortic aneurysm were treated with endovascular stent-grafts. Three patients had an acute traumatic aneurysm; seven had a chronic aneurysm. Stent-grafts were constructed from modified Z-stents covered with woven polyester or expanded polytetrafluoroethylene graft material and were deployed through a 20–24-F delivery sheath in an exposed artery located remotely from the lesion.

RESULTS: Stent-graft placement and thrombosis of the aneurysmal sac were successful in all patients. Major complications were encountered in three patients after endovascular treatment. One patient had a perigraft leak; complete thrombosis of the aneurysmal sac was achieved after coil embolization of the leak. Transposition of the left subclavian artery was necessary to relieve left arm ischemia in another patient. In the third patient, stent placement in the left main stem bronchus was needed to relieve left lung atelectasis. All patients were alive and without complications during the follow-up period (mean, 15 months).

CONCLUSION: Transluminal placement of endovascular stent-grafts is a technically feasible method for treatment of traumatic thoracic aortic aneurysm and may be an effective alternative to open-chest surgery.

Thoracic aortic injury is a potential life-threatening complication of chest trauma. Regardless of whether the injury is caused by means of nonpenetrating or penetrating trauma, approximately 80%–90% of those affected die at the scene or at an emergency room. Therefore, only approximately 10%–20% of patients with thoracic aortic injuries survive the immediate injury (1–3). Surgical repair is the standard method of treatment; however, surgery is often complicated because of nonaortic injuries (2,4). The few patients who survive the immediate injury often develop a chronic aortic aneurysm with a high attendant risk of fatal rupture (5,6). Traditionally, chronic traumatic aortic aneurysms are also surgically repaired, although the operation is associated with many major and minor complications (7). Since Parodi et al (8) described their first clinical experience with the use of a stent-graft to treat an abdominal aortic aneurysm, endoluminal stent-graft placement is emerging as an alternative to traditional surgery when patients with aneurysmal or occlusive disease have important coexistent morbidities (8–17). There is still controversy about how to manage both acute and chronic aortic injuries (1–6). We describe our experience using endoluminal placement of stent-grafts to treat traumatic descending thoracic aortic aneurysm in 10 cases. The purpose of our study was to demonstrate the feasibility and safety of the endoluminal treatment in patients with a thoracic aortic aneurysm.

MATERIALS AND METHODS

Patient Selection

From July 1992 through December 1996, 97 patients underwent repair of a descending thoracic aortic aneurysm with the use of stent-grafts. Ten patients (10%) had a traumatic injury that involved the descending thoracic aorta (Table 1). The cause of the aneurysm was determined on the basis of the patient's history, including any physical trauma, and examination of past and current imaging studies. Chest radiographs, computed tomographic (CT) scans of the chest, and aortographic images were obtained in each patient. Aortic injuries were classified in two groups, acute and chronic. Those patients in whom the interval between injury and treatment was 1 month or less were designated as having an acute injury, and those in whom the interval was more than 1 month were classified as having a chronic injury. In two cases of chronic injury, the diagnosis was determined exclusively on the basis of imaging findings because the patients did not remember any history of severe chest trauma. In both of these patients, a radiographic appearance typical of a chronic traumatic aneurysm was noted, without evidence from the patient's history or imaging results that suggested another origin. Accordingly, on the basis of this criterion, three patients were included in the acute group (injury-to-treatment interval, 17–28 days; mean, 24 days), and seven were included in the chronic group (injury-to-treatment interval, 2 months to 50 years; mean, 21 years). In all patients with chronic injury, the decision to proceed with aneurysm repair was made when expansion of the aneurysm was confirmed with the results of serial imaging studies.

The cause of aortic injury was a motor vehicle accident in two acute and four

Index terms: Aneurysm, aortic, 563.732 • Aorta, grafts and prostheses • Aorta, interventional procedure, 563.1269

Radiology 1997; 205:657–662

[1] From the Division of Cardiovascular-Interventional Radiology, Stanford University Medical Center, Stanford Vascular Center, H-3647, 300 Pasteur Dr, Stanford, CA 94305-5105. Received February 26, 1997; revision requested March 31; revision received and accepted August 15. **Address reprint requests to** M.D.D.

Table 1
Patient Characteristics

Patient	Age (y)	Sex	Mechanism of Injury	Interval between Injury and Treatment	Indication	Location at Aortic Injury	Diameter of Aneurysm (cm)
1	35	M	Motor vehicle accident	28 d	Previous surgery	Isthmus	4.5
2	35	F	Gunshot	17 d	Previous surgery	Distal descending thoracic aorta	5.0
3	60	M	Motor vehicle accident	42 y	Preference	Isthmus	7.0
4	39	M	Motor vehicle accident	12 y	Preference	Isthmus	8.0
5	67	F	Motor vehicle accident	2 mo	Preference	Isthmus	6.5
6	69	F	Unknown	Unknown	Severe chronic pulmonary disease	Isthmus through proximal descending thoracic aorta	9.0
7	71	M	Motor vehicle accident	27 d	Diffuse coronary artery disease	Isthmus through proximal descending thoracic aorta	5.0
8	66	M	Motor vehicle accident	4 mo	Respiratory failure	Isthmus	5.0
9	70	M	Fall	50–60 y	Coexisting thoracic and abdominal aortic aneurysms; desire for simultaneous treatment	Isthmus	5.0
10	47	F	Unknown	Unknown	Preference	Isthmus through proximal descending thoracic aorta	7.0

chronic cases, a fall from a height of 20 feet (6 m) in one chronic case, gunshot in one acute case, and unknown in the two chronic cases already mentioned. The patients were aged 35–71 years (mean, 56 years). Six were men and four were women. Indications for the stent-graft procedure in the acute patient group included no surgical access due to previous thoracic intervention in one patient, abdominal intervention with pancreatic fistula in one patient, and severe coronary artery disease in one patient. Indications in the chronic group were no surgical access due to previous surgery in one patient, respiratory failure in two patients, and patient preference in four patients. The investigational review board approved our study, and complete, informed consent was obtained from all patients.

Stent-Graft Details

The dimensions used for custom fabrication of stent-grafts were determined on the basis of contrast material–enhanced spiral CT and arteriographic images. Stent-grafts were constructed from a series of modified Z-stents (Cook, Bloomington, Ind) covered with woven polyester vascular graft material (Meadox Medicals, Oakland, NJ) (9). Expanded polytetrafluoroethylene (Impra, Tempe, Ariz) was used instead of woven polyester in one case when no woven polyester graft of appropriate size was available. Each stent body was 2.0 or 2.5 cm in length, and individual stents were connected to each other by using 2-0 polypropylene sutures (Ethicon, Sommerville, NJ). The diameter of the stent was 10%–15% larger than the diameter of proximal and distal portions of the aneurysm neck. The polyester graft material was used after the crimps were hand ironed over a cylindric mandrel. Ten-millimeter-diameter expanded polytetrafluoroethylene graft material was used in one device after it was dilated to the appropriate size with a series of sequentially larger angioplasty balloons. Grafts were attached to the stents by using interrupted 5-0 or 6-0 polypropylene sutures (Ethicon) at each end. All stent-grafts were made by hand and were individually designed for each patient. It took approximately 2–3 hours to construct each stent-graft. Gas sterilization of the stent-grafts was performed by using ethylene oxide. The sterilization cycle was 28 hours in total: 4 hours for ethylene oxide gas exposure, and 24 hours for aeration. Therefore, 30–31 hours are necessary to prepare for a stent-graft procedure.

Technique

Nine of 10 procedures were performed in the operating room after the patient had received general anesthesia and intubation had been performed. One stent-graft placement was performed in the angiography suite because high-quality fluoroscopic imaging was mandatory to deploy the stent-graft precisely above the celiac artery. Cardiopulmonary bypass equipment was available to support an emergent open-chest surgical procedure.

Transesophageal ultrasonography was used to identify the true neck of the aneurysm with precision and to avoid the pitfall of misinterpretation of an aortic segment with arteriographically inapparent mural thrombus as a desired target for the anchoring of the stent-graft. Surgical exposure of the common femoral artery, common iliac artery, or abdominal aorta was used to obtain vascular access. A 10-mm-diameter side limb of polyester graft was attached to an iliac artery or to an aorta in three patients to facilitate introduction of the device. Direct access via a femoral artery or the infrarenal aorta was performed in the other patients. The stent-graft was loaded into a loading cartridge with the same diameter as the delivery sheath.

Initially, a complete arteriographic evaluation of the lesion was performed by using a 5-F pigtail angiographic catheter (Mallinckrodt, St Louis, Mo) introduced through a 5-F sheath (USCI, Billerica, Mass) by using direct arterial access or a side-limb graft. Arteriographic images were obtained with a bedside C-arm angiographic unit (OEC; Diasonics, Salt Lake City, Utah) capable of digital acquisition and subtraction playback functions, including roadmapping guidance, or a conventional stationary angiographic unit (Multistar; Siemens Medical Systems, Erlangen, Germany).

After identification of the most appropriate angiographic projection to best display the involved aortic segment and its proximal and distal uninvolved necks, the 5-F sheath and catheter were exchanged for a 18–24-F delivery sheath (Cook) over a 260-cm-long 0.035-inch-diameter stiff guide wire (Medi-tech/Boston Scientific, Watertown, Mass). Heparin (150–200 U per kilogram body weight) was administrated intravenously immediately after the delivery sheath was inserted. Before insertion, the delivery sheath and dilator were softened by means of submersion into a basin of sterile, hot saline to facilitate passage through a tortuous iliac artery or aorta. Subsequently, the delivery sheath and dilator were advanced until the tip of the sheath was positioned just proximal to the aortic aneurysm. The stent-graft was then advanced from the loading cartridge through the delivery sheath by means of a blunt polyethylene pusher, which was constructed by cutting off the tapered end of an appropriately sized dilator. The stent-graft was deployed by pulling back the sheath while the pusher was firmly held stationary in position. This allowed the self-expanding device to deploy at the target position. Additional technical aspects of the stent-graft deployment procedure have been previously described (9–13).

Arteriography was performed after stent-graft deployment in all cases (completion arteriography). If any additional stent-graft was necessary to ensure complete isolation and sealing off of the aneurysm, the stent-graft was deployed at the same session with a single administra-

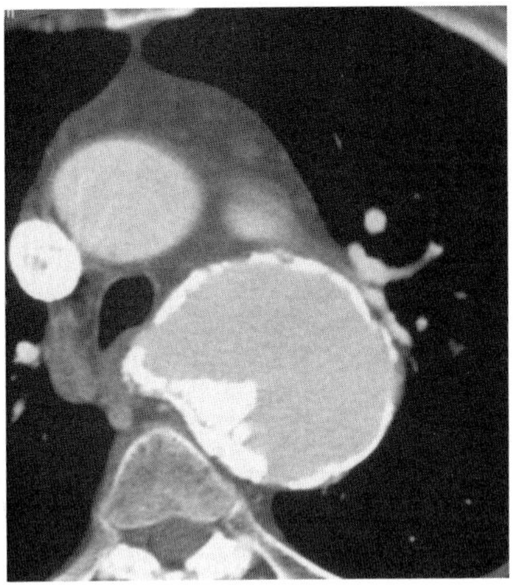

a.

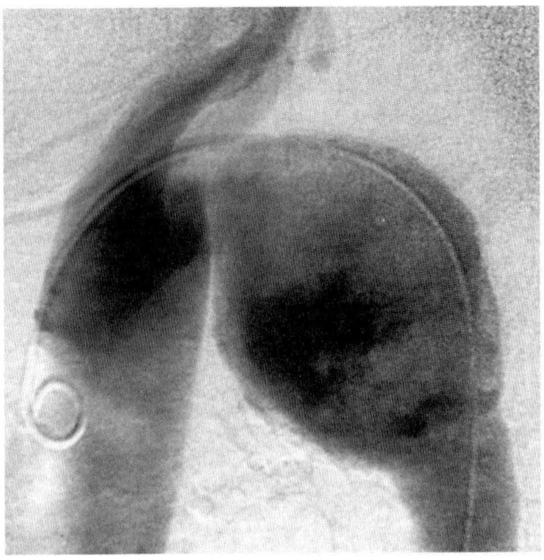

b.

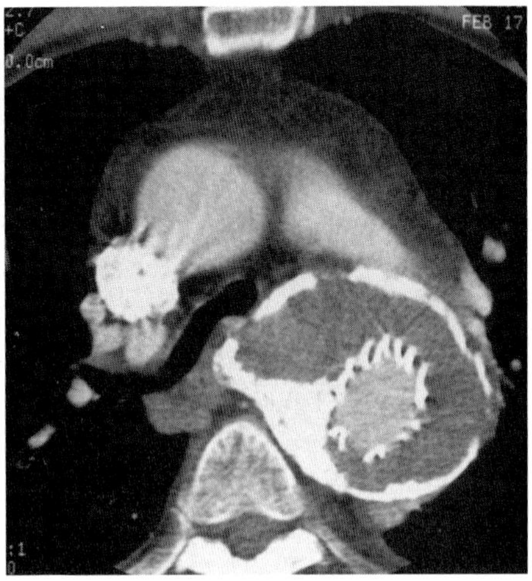

c.

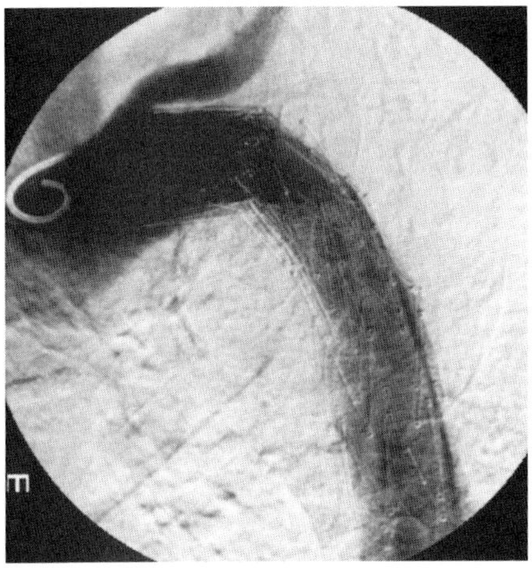

d.

Thoracic aortic aneurysm in a 60-year-old man. This patient had been involved in a motor vehicle accident 42 years before treatment. Aneurysm enlargement up to 8.0 cm in diameter was noted during follow-up. This patient was a candidate for surgery, but he preferred to undergo endoluminal treatment. **(a)** Thoracic contrast-enhanced spiral CT scan shows a huge aneurysm with enormous calcification in the aneurysm wall. **(b)** Left oblique arteriogram shows the typical configuration of the chronic traumatic aneurysm. Follow-up **(c)** contrast-enhanced spiral CT scan and **(d)** arteriogram obtained after stent-graft placement show the absence of aneurysm filling.

tion of general anesthesia and intubation. After completion arteriography, the access site was repaired, and the effect of the heparin was reversed with an intravenous dose of protamine sulfate. No further anticoagulation therapy was provided.

Follow-up Protocol

Follow-up imaging, including contrast-enhanced spiral CT and conventional arteriography, was routinely performed before the patient was discharged. If a perigraft leak was identified, balloon dilation or coil embolization of tracts was performed as soon as possible. After the patient was discharged, contrast-enhanced spiral CT was performed at 6 months and annually, and arteriography was performed 12 months after the procedure.

RESULTS

In nine of 10 patients, the aneurysm was located at the aortic isthmus or at the proximal descending thoracic segment that extends from the isthmus. In one patient with a gunshot injury, a pseudoaneurysm was identified just above the celiac artery. The diameter of the aneurysm was 4.5–9.0 cm (mean, 6.2 cm). All chronic aneurysms that were diagnosed many years after a traumatic injury had a conspicuous, heavily calcified peripheral rim.

Stent-graft placement was technically successful in all patients without any immediate complications (Figure, Table 2). The dimensions of stent-grafts were 24–36 mm in diameter (mean, 28 mm) and 4.0–14.0 cm in length (mean, 9.2 cm). Only one stent-graft was used in nine patients; two stent-grafts were needed to bridge the aneurysmal sac completely in one patient. Selection of the access site for stent-graft introduction was dependent on the diameter and tortuosity of femoral and iliac arteries. A common femoral artery approach was used in six patients. The distal infrarenal abdominal aorta was directly used in one patient. In two patients, a 10-mm side-limb graft attached to the lower abdominal aorta was used as an access conduit. Similarly, a side-limb graft attached to the common iliac artery provided the access in one patient.

Thrombosis of the aneurysmal sac was obtained after stent-graft deployment in all patients.

There were three major complications. In one patient, a perigraft leak was noted on a follow-up contrast-enhanced spiral CT scan obtained before the patient was discharged from the hospital. The tract that led to the aneurysmal sac originated at the distal end of the stent-graft, which was located along the lesser curvature of the distal aortic arch. In an attempt to obliterate the perigraft tract, we initially dilated the stent-graft by using a 25-mm-diameter valvuloplasty balloon; however, this failed to eliminate the leak. Subsequently, we embolized the tract with microcoils placed by way of a coaxially introduced microcatheter located in the perigraft fistula. A follow-up contrast-enhanced CT scan obtained 2 days after coil embolization showed no leak.

Mild numbness and pallor of the left hand were evident 14 hours after stent-graft placement in one patient. In this case, the stent-graft was deployed in the distal aortic arch just across the most distal aspect of the left subclavian artery origin. At fluoroscopy, blood flow through the left subclavian artery did not appear to be impeded, and there was no pressure gradient across the left subclavian artery origin. It was noted during the early postoperative period that the left upper extremity was asymmetrically cool, with a diminished radial pulse. These findings were associated with digital paresthesia. Thoracic aortographic findings allowed confirmation of thrombosis of the left subclavian artery. Subsequently, after 6 hours of transcatheter regional thrombolysis, only partial left subclavian artery recanalization was evident. Although the ischemia did not appear to be limb threatening, surgical transposition of the left subclavian artery to the left carotid artery was performed because of the neurologic findings and the presence of residual thrombus. After

Table 2
Results of Stent-Graft Placement for Treatment of Traumatic Thoracic Aortic Aneurysm

Patient	Stent-Graft Size*	No. of Stent- Grafts	Access Site	Delivery Sheath Size (F)	Thrombosis of Aneurysmal Sac	Complications
1	24.0 × 8.0	1	Femoral artery	24	Yes	None
2	24.0 × 7.5	1	Femoral artery	18	Yes	None
3	28.0 × 12.5, 30.0 × 7.5	2	Femoral artery	22	Yes	None
4	28.0 × 14.0	1	Femoral artery	24	Yes	None
5	30.0 × 4.0	1	Abdominal aorta	24	Yes	Left subclavian artery ischemia, necessitating transposition
6	30.0 × 10.0	1	Side-limb graft to common iliac artery	24	Yes	Left subclavian artery closure and airway collapse, necessitating stent placement
7	34.0 × 10.0	1	Femoral artery	24	Yes	None
8	32.0 × 6.0	1	Femoral artery	24	Yes, after coil embolization of perigraft leak	Perigraft leak
9	36.0 × 7.5	1	Side-limb graft to abdominal aorta	24	Yes	None
10	25.0 × 5.0	1	Side-limb graft to abdominal aorta	20	Yes	None

* Size is reported as diameter in millimeters × length in centimeters.

the operation, the patient recovered uneventfully without any clinical sequelae.

In another case, the left subclavian artery was inadvertently partially covered by the stent-graft, which was placed several millimeters higher than desired. The patient, however, did not develop any symptoms related to the left subclavian artery occlusion. In this case, a spiral CT scan obtained before the stent-graft procedure showed marked aneurysmal compression of the left main stem bronchus. Immediately after the procedure, collapse of the left lung was noted on a chest radiograph obtained while the patient was in the intensive care unit. It was thought that the left lung atelectasis was due to further compression of the bronchus by means of the aneurysm and was exacerbated because of intubation, general anesthesia, and associated increased secretion. In an effort to restore airway patency rapidly and avoid potential complications related to prolonged atelectasis, a Palmaz stent (P308; Cordis, Miami Lakes, Fla) was placed in the compressed left main stem bronchus. After bronchial stent placement, the left lung atelectasis was completely resolved on radiographs obtained within 12 hours. Two days after the procedure, thrombosis of the aneurysmal sac was confirmed with follow-up CT findings. The patient was discharged on the 3rd postoperative day.

No other major or minor complications were observed, including paraplegia, infection, embolization, renal or respiratory failure, or myocardial infarction. There were no procedure-related deaths. During the follow-up (range, 1–20 months; mean, 15 months), all patients were alive without any complications, including aneurysm expansion or rupture.

DISCUSSION

Thoracic aortic injury is an uncommon entity that represents one of the most catastrophic complications of chest trauma. Approximately 90% of nonpenetrating thoracic aortic injuries are caused by a deceleration injury, most commonly a motor vehicle accident (1,2). Similarly, in our study, six of the seven cases of nonpenetrating injury for which the mechanism of injury was confidently established were the result of a motor vehicle accident.

Parmley et al (2) reported that only 38 (13.8%) of 275 individuals with blunt aortic injuries survived long enough to reach a hospital for treatment, and more than 30% of the individuals in this group die within 24 hours. On the basis of these and similar results from other studies, there is no doubt that immediate diagnosis and treatment is mandatory to reduce mortality. Duhaylongsod et al (18) categorized acute traumatic aortic injuries into an "early type," which usually results in death at the scene of the accident or within 24 hours, and a "late type," which follows a more protracted course. They stated that patients with a "late type" injury may remain hemodynamically stable, and aortic repair can be delayed, provided that increased aortic wall tension and elevated systolic ejection fraction are avoided. Actually, the cases of acute injury in our study could not be categorized as "early type" according to the classification of Duhaylongsod et al. Owing to hemodynamic instability, however, any further delay in aortic repair was deemed to be unacceptable (2,5).

The mortality rate associated with emergent surgery for treatment of acute aortic injury is 15%–29%, according to the results of contemporary studies (4,19–22). The relatively high surgical mortality rate is due partially to the frequency of coexisting serious nonaortic injuries. However, the high rate is also attributed to considerable surgical morbidity that accompanies open thoracotomy and emergent surgical repair in victims of serious generalized trauma.

Penetrating injuries to the thoracic aorta are as lethal as or more lethal than nonpenetrating injuries. Cornwell et al (3) reported an overall mortality rate of 85% in patients with a gunshot wound to the thoracic aorta. They concluded that only prevention can make a difference. As such, it is conceivable that an effective, less invasive alternative to conventional surgery could potentially benefit patients with acute nonpenetrating or acute penetrating aortic injuries.

The diagnosis of a traumatic aortic aneurysm is determined on the basis of imaging results and the patient's history (2,4). A chest radiograph often shows widening of the mediastinum, and CT findings may provide some clues to the diagnosis. A chronic traumatic aortic aneurysm may expand slowly, sometimes over several decades, and it is common that the diagnosis of these aneurysms is made incidentally (6,7). In such cases, the findings on imaging studies may provide the only clues about the cause of the aneurysm because patients may forget a remote episode of chest trauma. In our series, two patients did not remember a history of trauma; however, the appearance of the aneurysms on the imaging studies strongly suggested a traumatic origin. The aneurysms were located at the isthmus, a segment involved in more than 90% of traumatic aortic aneurysm cases (19). Also, in both cases, the lesion had a circumferential, heavily calcified aneurysmal wall, which is one of the most typical morphologic characteristics of chronic traumatic aortic aneurysm (23). There were no coexisting findings suggestive of another aneurysm cause, including atherosclerosis, dissection, or infection.

Because chronic traumatic aneurysms are not uniformly stable, they are usually repaired electively (2,5,6,23,24). Alternatively, after surviving the immediate injuries, patients could be medically treated in a manner similar to that with which patients with acute type B aortic dissection are treated (25). Bennett and Cherry (23), however, reported that only 43 (41%) of 105 chronic aortic aneurysm cases were stable without eventual development of symptoms or enlargement. In fact, radiographically proved enlargement was noted in 21% of cases. Finkelmeier et al (6) reported that 20 of 60 patients with untreated chronic aortic aneurysm died of complications attributed to the aortic lesion, and 15 of 20 deaths were due to aneurysm rupture. In all of the chronic cases in our series, the decision to proceed with aneurysm repair was made when aneurysm expansion was confirmed at follow-up imaging.

Open-chest surgery for repair of chronic traumatic aneurysm results in a mortality rate of 5%–18%, due mainly to bleeding, heart failure, or renal failure, and a morbidity rate of 11%–50% related to bleeding, heart failure, renal failure, and spinal cord injury (6,7,26). In addition, surgical repair of a chronic aneurysm is associated with a rate of minor complications as high as 52.9%, including Horner syndrome and vocal cord paralysis, due to the unique location of the aneurysm (7). It is well known that patients who undergo successful surgery and have no other serious injuries can live without adverse sequelae because they are often young and otherwise healthy (27). Therefore, several kinds of less invasive and potentially safer methods of treatment have been tried (6).

Placement of endovascular stent-grafts for the treatment of abdominal aortic aneurysm was clinically initiated by Parodi et al (8) in 1992. Since then, several investigators (9–17) have accumulated substantial clinical experience with different stent-graft devices used for a variety of vascular applications. In terms of acute aortic injury, Williams et al (28) used Z-stents covered with polytetrafluoroethylene in a canine model in which an acute aortic rupture was artificially created and concluded that stent-graft treatment of aortic rupture was feasible. Since 1992, in our experience with stent-grafts for the treatment of thoracic aortic aneurysm, the aneurysm in 10 (10%) of 97 patients had a traumatic origin. In our series, there were contraindications to conventional surgery in more than half of these patients, including all patients with an acute injury.

One advantage of the stent-graft procedure over conventional surgery is the absence of aortic clamping that may contribute to major complications, including paraplegia. It remains debatable whether cross-clamping time alone can predict the relative risk of paraplegia; however, it is indisputable that cross clamping is associated with a risk of paraplegia (18). By comparing endovascular and open surgical procedures, Dake et al (9) commented that stent-graft placement eliminates the opportunity to reimplant intercostal arteries to a vascular graft; consequently, stent-graft placement may expose the patient to a higher risk of paraplegia. The risk of paraplegia may not be increased, however, in cases of nonpenetrating thoracic aortic aneurysm, because the lesion is most often located at the isthmus and does not involve segments with branches to the spinal cord. The fact that there were no instances of paraplegia in the patients in our series is in accordance with this presumption.

In addition, endoluminal repair of a thoracic aneurysm by using stent-grafts can eliminate thoracotomy; thoracotomy may cause respiratory problems, especially in patients with preexisting compromised pulmonary function. We did not experience any other major coexistent morbidities in our series, including complications such as myocardial infarct, heart failure, renal failure, distal embolization, or infection; however, the number of patients in our series was limited. Indeed, if a stent-graft procedure can reduce perioperative morbidity, it may lead to a reduction in the cost of hospitalization.

On the basis of our experience, endoluminal repair of traumatic aneurysms by using stent-grafts appears to be promising; however, several limitations remain to be overcome. The concept of stent-graft treatment of aneurysmal disease is based on the ability of the device to successfully bridge the aneurysmal sac and isolate it from the circulation by forming a tight seal between graft material and the aortic wall at the proximal and distal portions of the aneurysm neck. Therefore, sufficiently long proximal and distal neck portions of normal caliber are necessary to anchor the stent-graft and form a complete seal (9,29).

Seventy percent to ninety percent of nonpenetrating injuries to the thoracic aorta involve the proximal descending segment, and most affect the isthmus (2). It may be difficult to treat aneurysms in this location with stent-grafts because the aneurysm frequently originates just beyond the left subclavian artery, leaving an insufficiently long proximal portion of the neck between the subclavian artery and the aneurysm. In our series, the left subclavian artery was inadvertently covered with stent-grafts in two patients. In both cases, the aneurysm was located within 12 mm of the left subclavian artery, and the stent-graft was not precisely deployed within the short proximal portion of the neck. Either antecedent creation of a left carotid–to–subclavian arterial bypass graft or surgical transposition of the left subclavian artery to the left carotid artery before stent-graft placement may avoid such complications in cases with a proximal part of the neck that is less than 20 mm in length. Alternatively, a more desirable approach is technical improvement of the deployment mechanism to allow the precise placement that is needed in cases with a sharply defined target.

Also of concern is the longitudinal flexibility of the stent-graft design used in this series. Our stent-graft is semirigid and is not flexible enough to conform to the curve of the distal arch and/or proximal descending aorta in all cases. The inability to hug the curved aortic contour securely may cause a perigraft leak. We encountered one case of perigraft leak in this series; this leak was repaired with coil embolization of the perigraft tract. In our overall thoracic stent-graft experience since 1992 (30), there have been 10 cases of perigraft leak, which were successfully treated by means of coil embolization. Although follow-up in our series was of short duration (mean, 15 months at the time this article was written), coil embolization appears to be a feasible and durable method for treatment of perigraft leak. Recently, we used stent-grafts constructed of 2-cm-long stent bodies to increase the longitudinal flexibility when placement in the aortic arch was intended.

Currently, stent-grafts are not commercially available for general use in the United States. Consequently, each device must be individually designed and custom fabricated by hand to meet specifications derived on the basis of imaging studies. As such, at least 30 hours are needed to prepare an aortic stent-graft fully, as was described in the Materials and Methods section. In emergency cases, without an available and sufficient inventory of sterilized devices, a requisite 30-hour delay is unacceptable and severely diminishes the attractiveness of endovascular treatment.

The delivery sheaths we used are big and relatively stiff. Consequently, there were some cases in which iliac or aortic access was necessary because the common femoral, external iliac, or common iliac arteries were not large enough to accommodate the delivery system. Even when common femoral artery access is possible, an arteriotomy is necessary to allow introduction of the delivery sheath and the dilator. In some anatomic situations, the large delivery sheath is almost occlusive in the arteries that lead to the aorta. To prevent thrombus formation in these arteries, as well as in the lumen of the sheath, anticoagulation with heparin is necessary during the procedure. This is a potential disadvantage, because patients with acute traumatic aortic injuries often have coexisting severe nonaortic injuries with a risk of bleeding. Future technical developments will, we hope, yield improved stent-graft designs, more sophisticated delivery systems, and a degree of overall miniaturization that will address some of the current limitations.

Our limited experience demonstrates the feasibility and safety of endovascular stent-graft treatment in patients with a traumatic thoracic aortic aneurysm. Improved emergency medical transport systems are resulting in an increase in the number of patients with a thoracic aortic injury who reach the hospital. In the past, these patients would have died at the scene, without any available treatment. These patients are potential beneficiaries of a less invasive endovascular procedure. Similarly, stent-graft placement may be performed with less risk than open-chest repair in patients with a chronic traumatic aneurysm who have a severe coexisting medical disease that limits surgical options. Further long-term follow-up is mandatory, however, before this alternative method can be confidently recommended and its use widely adopted. ■

References

1. Strassmann G. Traumatic rupture of the aorta. Am Heart J 1947; 33:508–515.
2. Parmley LF, Mattingly TW, Manion WC, Jahnke EJ. Nonpenetrating traumatic injury of the aorta. Circulation 1958; 17:1086–1101.
3. Cornwell EE, Kennedy F, Berne TV, Asensio JA, Demetriades D. Gunshot wounds to the thoracic aorta in the 90s: only prevention will make a difference. Am Surg 1995; 61:721–723.
4. Turney SZ, Attar S, Ayella R, Cowley RA, McLaughlin J. Traumatic rupture of the aorta: a five-year experience. J Thorac Cardiovasc Surg 1976; 72:727–732.
5. Spencer FC, Guerin PF, Blake HA, Bahnson HT. Report of fifteen patients with traumatic aneurysm of thoracic aorta. J Thorac Cardiovasc Surg 1961; 41:1–22.
6. Finkelmeier BA, Mentzer RM, Kaiser DL, Tegtmeyer CJ, Nolan SP. Chronic traumatic thoracic aneurysm. J Thorac Cardiovasc Surg 1982; 84:257–266.
7. Bacharach JM, Garratt KN, Rooke TW. Chronic traumatic thoracic aneurysm: report of two cases with the question of timing for surgical intervention. J Vasc Surg 1993; 17:780–783.
8. Parodi JC, Palmaz JC, Barone HD. Transfemoral intraluminal graft implantation for abdominal aortic aneurysms. Ann Vasc Surg 1991; 5:491–499.
9. Dake MD, Miller DC, Semba CP, Mitchell RS, Walker PJ, Liddell RP. Transluminal placement of endovascular stent-grafts for the treatment of descending thoracic aortic aneurysms. N Engl J Med 1994; 331:1729–1734.
10. Razavi MK, Dake MD, Semba CP, Nyman URO, Liddell RP. Percutaneous endoluminal placement of stent-grafts for the treatment of isolated iliac artery aneurysms. Radiology 1995; 197:801–804.
11. Mitchell RS, Dake MD, Semba CP, et al. Endovascular stent-graft repair of thoracic aortic aneurysms. J Thorac Cardiovasc Surg 1996; 111:1054–1062.
12. Fann JI, Dake MD, Semba CP, Liddell RP, Pfeffer TA, Miller DC. Endovascular stent-grafting after arch aneurysm repair using the "elephant trunk". Ann Thorac Surg 1995; 60:1102–1105.
13. Semba CP, Kato N, Kee ST, et al. Acute rupture of the descending thoracic aorta: repair using endovascular stent-grafts. JVIR 1997; 8:337–342.
14. Marin ML, Veith FJ, Cynamon J, et al. Initial experience with transluminally placed endovascular grafts for the treatment of complex vascular lesions. Ann Surg 1995; 222:449–469.
15. Chuter TAM, Green RM, Ouriel K, Fiore WM, DeWeese JA. Transfemoral endovascular aortic graft placement. J Vasc Surg 1993; 18:185–197.
16. May J, White GH, Yu W, et al. Early experience with the Sydney and EVT prostheses for endoluminal treatment of abdominal aortic aneurysms. J Endovasc Surg 1995; 2:240–247.
17. Moore WS, Vescera CL. Repair of abdominal aortic aneurysm by transfemoral endovascular graft placement. Ann Surg 1994; 220:331–341.
18. Duhaylongsod FG, Glower DD, Wolfe WG. Acute traumatic aortic aneurysm: the Duke experience from 1970 to 1990. J Vasc Surg 1992; 15:331–343.
19. Turney SZ. Blunt trauma of the thoracic aorta and its branches. Semin Thorac Cardiovasc Surg 1992; 4:209–216.
20. Cowley RA, Turney SZ, Hankins JR, Rodriguez A, Attar S, Shanskar BS. Rupture of thoracic aorta caused by blunt trauma. J Thorac Cardiovasc Surg 1990; 100:652–661.
21. Verdant A, Page A, Cossette R, Dontigny L, Page P, Maillot R. Surgery of the descending thoracic aorta: spinal cord protection with the Gott shunt. Ann Thorac Surg 1988; 46:147–154.
22. Mattox KL, Holzman M, Pickard LR, Beall AC, DeBakey ME. Clamp/repair: a safe technique for treatment of blunt injury to the descending thoracic aorta. Ann Thorac Surg 1985; 40:456–463.
23. Bennett DE, Cherry JK. The natural history of traumatic aneurysms of the aorta. Surgery 1967; 61:516–523.
24. Groves LK. Traumatic aneurysm of the thoracic aorta. N Engl J Med 1964; 270:220–224.
25. Walker WA, Pate JW. Medical management of acute traumatic rupture of the aorta. Ann Thorac Surg 1990; 50:965–967.
26. Nagel CB, Williams GR. Method of repair in the surgical treatment of aneurysms of the descending thoracic aorta. Am J Surg 1966; 112:709–715.
27. DeBakey ME, Cooley DA, Crawford ES, Morris GC. Aneurysms of the thoracic aorta: analysis of 179 patients treated by resection. J Thorac Surg 1958; 36:393–420.
28. Williams DM, Andrews JC, Chee SS, Marx MV, Abrams GD. Canine model of acute aortic rupture: treatment with percutaneous delivery of a covered Z stent—work in progress. JVIR 1994; 5:797–803.
29. Chuter TAM, Green RM, Ouriel K, DeWeese JA. Infrarenal aortic aneurysm structure: implications for transfemoral repair. J Vasc Surg 1994; 20:44–50.
30. Kato N, Semba CP, Dake MD. Embolization of peri-graft leaks following endovascular stent-grafting of aortic aneurysms. JVIR 1996; 7:805–811.

Eric Therasse, MD • Manon Choinière, PhD • Gilles Soulez, MD • Vincent L. Oliva, MD
Pierre Rousseau, MD • François Fugère, MD • Daniel Boudreault, MD
Jean R. Cusson, MD, PhD

Percutaneous Biliary Drainage: Clinical Trial of Analgesia with Interpleural Block[1]

PURPOSE: **To determine the analgesic efficacy and safety of interpleural block for percutaneous biliary drainage.**

MATERIALS AND METHODS: **In this double-blind study, 34 age- and sex-matched patients who were to undergo percutaneous biliary drainage because of malignant biliary obstruction were randomly assigned to the true-block group (30 mL 0.5% bupivacaine block) or placebo-block group; all had access to a patient-controlled analgesia (fentanyl) pump. Self medication, pain reports, blood pressure, heart rate, and oxygen saturation were monitored during and until 8 hours after drainage. The McGill Pain Questionnaire was administered 1 hour after biliary drainage.**

RESULTS: **Patients in the placebo group self administered statistically significantly more fentanyl than did patients in the true-block group (P = .008). Peak pain scores (10-point scale) and McGill Pain Questionnaire scores were statistically significantly higher for the placebo group patients (P = .017 and P = .001, respectively). There were no differences between groups in terms of blood pressure, heart rate, and oxygen saturation. Two patients had pneumothorax caused by the interpleural block.**

CONCLUSION: **Interpleural block was effective in decreasing pain and opioid requirements during and after percutaneous biliary drainage and did not compromise the cardiopulmonary status of the patient. However, the rate of pneumothorax was higher than previously reported.**

Percutaneous biliary drainage (PBD) frequently is performed in patients who are severely debilitated because of neoplastic disease. These interventions may be lengthy and painful, necessitating effective analgesia that will not compromise the cardiorespiratory status of the patient (1,2). Unfortunately, close patient monitoring by an anesthesiologist, as is necessary when general or epidural anesthesia is used, is usually not available in the angiographic suite. At our hospital, as at many other centers, an anesthesiologist is sometimes present at PBD procedures in the angiographic room (for patients with unstable cardiopulmonary status), but anesthesiologists are too busy to work in the angiographic suite on a regular basis. General anesthesia also carries risks that are sometimes prohibitive—especially for a percutaneous procedure, one of the advantages of which is precisely to lower the anesthetic risks associated with more aggressive surgical interventions. Celiac block has already been proposed as an analgesic method for PBD (3). Unfortunately, this technique was proved to be ineffective in a randomized double-blind clinical trial (4).

To provide analgesia during PBD, the interventional radiologist most often relies on ad hoc intravenous administration of opioids and benzodiazepines, as clinically needed during the procedure (5). Although sufficient in some cases, intravenous sedation is often inadequate and is not tailored to specific situations; sometimes, large doses of opioids, which may cause respiratory depression, are needed. Intravenous sedation can therefore lead to inadequate analgesia and an unstable cardiorespiratory status in the patient that distracts the interventionalist during the procedure (1). In this setting, other analgesic methods that can safely provide adequate pain relief during PBD must be investigated.

Interpleural block (IPB)—administration of a local anesthetic drug in the pleural space—produces regional analgesia of the ipsilateral hemithorax and upper hemiabdomen. The analgesic efficacy of IPB has been demonstrated for surgical interventions (6,7) and for postoperative pain (8–11). Results of a nonrandomized, uncontrolled study (2) have shown IPB to be a promising method for PBD analgesia. However, these results were based on a small sample size, and the data were not collected with a double-blind procedure. Further research is clearly needed to assess the usefulness of IPB in interventional radiology. Our hypothesis was that, in comparison with a placebo, IPB could decrease both pain and opioid requirements

Index terms: Anesthesia • Bile ducts, interventional procedure, 76.1263 • Bile ducts, neoplasms, 76.32 • Bile ducts, percutaneous drainage, 76.1263 • Bile ducts, stenosis or obstruction, 76.32, 76.33 • Efficacy study

Abbreviations: IPB = interpleural block, PBD = percutaneous biliary drainage, PCA = patient-controlled analgesia, VAS = visual analogue scale.

Radiology 1997; 205:663–668

[1] From the Departments of Radiology (E.T., G.S., V.L.O.), Anesthesiology (M.C., P.R., F.F., D.B.), and Clinical Pharmacology (J.R.C.), University of Montreal Medical Center, Pavillon Hotel-Dieu, 3840 St Urbain St, Montreal, Quebec, Canada H2W 1T8. Received May 27, 1997; revision requested July 8; revision received August 4; accepted August 5. Supported by grant no. 941308 from the Fonds de la Recherche en Santé du Québec. **Address reprint requests to** E.T.

during PBD. The purpose of this study, therefore, was to evaluate the analgesic efficacy and safety of IPB during PBD.

Table 1
Characteristics of Patients and PBDs

Characteristic	Group 1	Group 2	*P* value
Patients			
Sex (M/F)*	9/8	9/8	>.99
Mean age (y)†	69.0 ± 10.2	65.1 ± 11.3	.30
Body mass index†	25.3 ± 2.8	25.1 ± 6.6	.92
PBD			
Procedure time (min)†	62.3 ± 42.8	71.8 ± 45.9	.55
Largest PBD catheter size†	8.4 F ± 1.4	8.2 F ± 0.9	.74
Left lobe access/right lobe access‡	3/12	6/16	.71
Level of difficulty§	1.40 ± 0.63	1.50 ± 0.63	.66

Note.—Group 1 patients received PCA and true IPB; group 2 patients received PCA and a placebo IPB.
* Data are number of patients.
† Data are means ± 1 standard deviation.
‡ Data are number of accesses.
§ Data are the mean difficulty ± 1 standard deviation, as subjectively scored with a three-point scale (1 = easy, 2 = intermediate, 3 = difficult).

MATERIALS AND METHODS

The 34 participants were recruited from the population of consecutive patients who needed PBD because of malignant biliary obstruction. Those excluded were patients who (*a*) had pulmonary fibrosis or infection, (*b*) required regular administration of opioids during the 48 hours before PBD, or (*c*) were not able to meet the study requirements because of mental instability or language difficulty. Approval of this study was obtained from the ethics committee of our institution. Many patients had previously undergone endoscopic retrograde cholangiopancreatography, and cholangiography or endoscopic stent placement were not possible. Scheduled PBD procedures included "a priori" right external or external-internal biliary drainage, with or without stent placement.

All patients in the study were provided with a patient-controlled analgesia (PCA) pump and were randomly assigned to receive either the true IPB (group 1) or a placebo IPB (group 2). Assignment to groups was achieved with the aid of a table of random numbers. The study was conducted in a double-blind manner such that the patient, the interventionalist, the staff, and the research nurse who collected the data were unaware of group assignment. Only the anesthesiologist who performed the IPB knew the patient's group assignment.

All eligible patients who agreed to participate in the study provided written, informed consent after the goals and steps of the study were explained. The research nurse then instructed them in the use of PCA pump, and the anesthesiologist verified that all instructions were well understood when the patient was provided with the pump.

All IPBs were performed by one of six anesthesiologists (including P.R., F.F., D.B.), who used the following standardized procedure (8) throughout the course of the study. The IPB was performed on the right side with standard hemodynamic monitoring (arterial blood pressure, pulse rate, oxygen saturation, and cardioscopy) in the recovery room. The patient was placed in the left lateral decubitus position. After administration of asepsis and local anesthesia (5 mL of 1% lidocaine [Xylocaine; Astra Pharma, Mississauga, Ontario, Canada]), a 17-gauge Tuohy needle (Sims A. Smithe Industries Medical Systems, Keene, NH) was inserted in the right seventh intercostal space, 10 cm from the spinous process of the dorsal column (12). A small, 20-gauge catheter (Concord Portex; Sims A. Smithe Industries Medical Systems) was threaded through the needle into the pleural space located posteriorly between the two pleura at the T7-T8 intercostal space. The needle was then removed and the patient assumed the dorsal decubitus position. A chest radiograph was obtained to rule out the presence of pneumothorax. Thirty milliliters of 0.5% bupivacaine (Marcaine; Sanofi-Winthrop, Markham, Ontario, Canada) with a 1/200,000-concentration of epinephrine was injected through the interpleural catheter. Because the IPB takes approximately 30 minutes to have an effect, the patient was sent to the angiographic suite at least 30 minutes after performance of the IPB. To ensure that the study remained double-blinded, patients in group 2 (placebo) were treated the same (instructions, positioning, asepsis, etc) as patients in group 1 (IPB), except that the former received only local skin anesthesia (5 mL of 1% lidocaine, same as group 1 patients) at the expected site of interpleural catheter placement. A sham catheter was also taped on the back of these patients to mimic a functional interpleural catheter. Material expense for the IPB, including the cost of the epidural tray and local anesthetic, was less than $15.00.

Opioid analgesia was initiated immediately before transhepatic puncture by means of intravenous injection of a loading dose of 1.5 µg of fentanyl per kilogram body weight (µg/kg) administered by the research nurse in the angiographic suite. The patients were provided with a PCA pump (Graseby 3300; Minogue Medical, Montreal, Quebec, Canada), which was programmed to deliver fentanyl at the patient's request. The pump was set with a 3-minute lockout. Even though the pump did not inject medication more often than every 3 minutes, it recorded the number of times the patient pushed the button. During PBD, the PCA boluses were set at 0.3 µg/kg of fentanyl. Once the procedure was completed, PCA was continued for 8 hours (0.2 µg/kg, with a 6-minute lockout interval); afterward, conventional on-demand analgesia was substituted. If pain control was inadequate, the interventionalist asked the anesthesiologist to increase the PCA fentanyl dose. No sedative or analgesic medication other than that from the PCA pump was used during the study. The decision to provide the patient with oxygen was left to the discretion of the interventionalist, whose decision was based on continuous-pulse oxygen saturation monitoring. Although we routinely provide oxygen to patients who receive intravenous sedation, some patients in this study with high oxygen saturation did not receive oxygen; these patients reported almost no pain and made little use of opioids. The interpleural catheter was withdrawn after PBD, and a chest radiograph was obtained to rule out the presence of a pneumothorax.

All PBDs were performed with the same technique, with standard hemodynamic monitoring, by one of four equally skilled interventionalists (including E.T., G.S., V.L.O.). Arterial blood pressure, pulse rate, oxygen saturation, cardioscopy, and breathing pace were evaluated by the research nurse before PBD (before the administration of the fentanyl loading dose) and every 15 minutes during the procedure. The duration of the PBD procedure was recorded. Vital signs were evaluated every 60 minutes for 8 hours after the end of the procedure.

All patients were asked to rate their pain level by using a 10-cm-long visual analogue scale (VAS), on which the left and the right boundaries were, respectively, "no pain" and "unbearable pain." This validated scale (13) does not necessitate written intervention from the patient and was administered with the same frequency as the monitoring of vital signs. On each occasion, the patient rated the intensity of the current pain (prospective pain evaluation). One hour after the end of PBD, the patients were asked to describe the overall pain they felt during the procedure by using the McGill Pain Questionnaire (14) and to provide two additional VAS ratings to describe pain intensity at its worst and overall during the procedure (retrospective pain evaluation). The same VAS measurements were also completed by the interventionalist who performed the PBD. In addition, the interventionalist evaluated pain relief provided by means of the method of analgesia on another VAS ("no pain relief" to "complete pain relief").

The research nurse monitored the vital signs and simultaneously assessed the patient's degree of sedation by using a four-point scale (0 = wide awake and alert, 1 =

Table 2
Evaluation of Pain during PBD and after PBD

Pain Score	Group 1*	Group 2*	*P* Value† Between Groups	*P* Value† Between Times
	Prospective Pain Evaluation			
Mean score				
During PBD‡	1.03 ± 1.16	2.69 ± 2.26	.005	.07
After PBD‡	0.91 ± 0.99	1.71 ± 0.80		
Peak score				
During PBD‡	2.36 ± 2.61	4.68 ± 2.98	.017	.17
After PBD‡	2.19 ± 1.98	3.30 ± 1.88		
	Retrospective Pain Evaluation during PBD			
Patient evaluation				
Worst‡	3.88 ± 2.96	6.77 ± 2.64	.008	NA
Overall‡	2.41 ± 2.32	3.70 ± 1.87	.100	NA
McGill Pain Questionnaire	12.25 ± 12.67	27.10 ± 8.76	.001	NA
Interventionalist evaluation				
Worst‡	3.51 ± 2.17	5.42 ± 2.00	.020	NA
Overall‡	1.51 ± 1.39	2.82 ± 1.48	.020	NA

* Group 1 received PCA and true IPB; group 2 received PCA and placebo IPB. Data are mean scores ± 1 standard deviation.
† NA = not applicable.
‡ Data are from the VAS.

drowsy on occasion but easily aroused, 2 = somnolent but easily aroused, 3 = somnolent and difficult to arouse). Side effects of the analgesic medication were noted, along with the treatment required (15).

All medications delivered and all attempts by the patient to receive medication from the PCA pump were recorded during and until 8 hours after the end of PBD. After the procedure, the interventionalist assessed the overall level of difficulty of the PBD procedure, on a three-point scale (1 = easy, 2 = moderately difficult, 3 = difficult).

Before the start of the study, we estimated that a sampling size of 17 patients per group would ensure that the statistical power to detect group differences was beyond .80 for a statistical significance threshold set at .05, given that expected differences would be large enough to be clinically meaningful (16,17). Calculation of the sample size was obtained by assuming that the intergroup mean differences for the VAS pain scores and the analgesic consumption (through the PCA pump) were at least 50%, given that the standard deviations were approximately 50% of the mean (large size effect) (16).

Group comparability with regard to demographic and medical variables were analyzed by using Student *t* tests for continuous data and χ^2 analyses for categorical data. Outcome measurements that were collected on more than one occasion were averaged (eg, pain scores) or cumulated (eg, medication data) and were analyzed with two-way analyses of variance with repeated measures on one factor (during and after PBD). For each measurement, parametric (Student *t* test) and nonparametric (χ^2 test) tests were performed, as applicable. For all analyses, a *P* value of less than .05 was considered to indicate a statistically significant difference.

RESULTS

Demographic characteristics of the patients in both groups and details of the PBDs are presented in Table 1. There were no statistically significant differences between the two groups. Nine patients underwent a left bile duct access only (n = 4) or in association with a right bile duct access (n = 5). Five of the 17 patients in group 2 underwent bilateral PBD. Two patients in group 1 underwent transhepatic cholangiography only and did not undergo PBD because biliary disease was too advanced. Results in these two patients contributed to the safety data about IPB but did not contribute to the analysis of pain measurement and opioid consumption.

Pain scores during and after PBD are listed in Table 2. For all measurements, the patients in the IPB group reported statistically significantly less pain than those in the placebo group. This was true both during and after the IPB. The intergroup differences for the peak pain intensity were 2.3 and 1.1 points on the 10-point VAS during PBD and 8 hours after PBD, respectively. In both groups, reported pain intensity increased during PBD and decreased afterward, although this difference was not statistically significant (P = .07). Interestingly, reported pain intensity for group 1 patients during PBD was even lower than reported pain intensity for group 2 patients after the procedure. The retrospective mean VAS score for the pain at its worst during the procedure was 2.89 points higher in group 2 than in group 1 (P = .008). Four patients, all in the IPB group, reported that they did not feel any pain during the procedure. The mean pain intensity score obtained with the McGill Pain Questionnaire was more than twice as high for group 2 patients than for group 1 patients (P = .001). The interventionalist-measured patient pain intensity was also statistically significantly higher for patients in the placebo group than for those in the IPB group. When the interventionalists rated the overall pain relief patients in each treatment group experienced, a mean difference of 3.1 on the VAS was found in favor of the patients in group 1 (mean ± 1 standard deviation, 7.4 ± 2.1 for group 1 vs 4.3 ± 2.6 for group 2; P = .001).

Analgesic medication in patients in both groups is shown in Table 3. On average, patients in group 1 self-administered approximately half the fentanyl dose needed by group 2 patients during and until 8 hours after PBD. Only three patients required an increase in self-administered fentanyl dosage (from 0.3 to 1.0 µg/kg) because of inadequate pain control, and all of these patients were in the placebo group. During and after PBD, unsuccessful PCA demands were two to three times higher in the placebo group than in IPB group; this difference was statistically significant (P = .047) when the number of unsuccessful PCA demands were considered in relation to the duration of the procedure (dose per hour). In both groups, the PCA fentanyl delivered and the number of unsuccessful PCA demands per hour were statistically significantly higher during the PBD than during the 8-hour follow-up.

Vital signs and side effects noted before, during, and after PBD are reported in Table 4. There were no statistically significant differences in mean heart rate, systolic blood pressure, mean level of sedation, oxygen saturation, and respiratory frequency between patients in groups 1 and 2, and there was no case of respiratory depression (respiratory rate below 10 breaths per minute or oxygen saturation of less than 90%). After PBD, systolic blood pressure and oxygen saturation decreased slightly (but statistically significantly) in patients in both groups, and the worst degree of sedation increased slightly. No patient had bile collections, pleural effusion, or marked hemobilia related to PBD. Three patients in group 1 reported slight transient thoracic pain after IPB: In two patients, the pain was right sided; in one patient, the pain was left sided although IPB was administered on the right side. In all cases, the thoracic pain disappeared within 1 hour and was not related to a pneumothorax. Two patients in group 1 experienced a right-sided pneumothorax. The pneumothorax in one patient did not produce symptoms, but in one patient, the pneumothorax enlarged progressively and drainage with a chest tube was necessary a few hours after PBD. There were no other complications or side effects, and toxicity due to local anesthetic did not occur.

Table 3
Analgesic Medication Needed during PBD and after PBD

Pain Score	Group 1*	Group 2*	*P* Value: Between Groups	*P* Value: Between Times
	Successful Delivery of PCA Fentanyl			
Total doses				
During PBD (μg)	86.40 ± 95.30	198.20 ± 170.90	.008	.2400
8 h after PBD (μg)	127.00 ± 89.30	220.20 ± 97.40		
Doses per hour[†]				
During PBD (μg)	76.70 ± 70.80	181.90 ± 134.40	.006	<.0001
After PBD (μg)	15.90 ± 11.20	27.50 ± 12.20		
	Unsuccessful Demands for PCA Fentanyl			
Total no. of demands				
During PBD	9.50 ± 15.20	17.50 ± 16.60	.100	.1300
8 h after PBD	4.40 ± 4.60	14.20 ± 22.10		
No. of demands per hour[†]				
During PBD	8.00 ± 10.98	19.10 ± 23.50	.047	<.0001
8 h after PBD	0.55 ± 0.57	1.78 ± 2.76		

* Group 1 received PCA and true IPB; group 2 received PCA and placebo IPB. Data are means ± 1 standard deviation.
[†] Square root transformation was performed with these data to homogenize the variance.

DISCUSSION

Our results clearly demonstrate that IPB substantially reduces pain intensity and opioid drug requirement during and after PBD. IPB also produces few side effects and does not compromise the cardiorespiratory status of the patient, which is particularly important in those who are severely weakened because of neoplastic disease.

Measurements of the peak VAS pain scores during the procedure, as well as the retrospective measurements of pain "at its worst," are probably the most appropriate measurements to evaluate intermittent and sudden painful experiences during PBD. Indeed, pain stimuli are low between dilations and catheter insertions, which is one reason why intravenous sedation is not appropriate for PBD. Indeed, during these procedures, large doses of analgesic drugs are needed to relieve important, sharp, and transient painful stimuli. These stimuli then quickly disappear, and the unopposed effects of opioids may lead to respiratory depression. In addition, there are limitations to the use of increased opioid doses to increase the analgesic effect of intravenous sedation; these limitations are well demonstrated by the fact that although opioid administration was higher in group 2 patients, analgesia was better in group 1 patients (especially for "peak" and "at its worst" pain measurements).

There is no perfect analgesic method to treat PBD-induced pain. Celiac block has proved to be ineffective as an analgesic method for PBD (4). General and epidural anesthesia induce hemodynamic changes (mainly peripheral vasodilatation) that necessitate monitoring by an anesthesiologist who may not always be available in the angiographic suite. General anesthesia is also associated with additional risks in patients with a poor cardiorespiratory status. Although complications were reported (1) to be more common with intravenous sedation than with epidural anesthesia, the latter necessitates the presence of an anesthesiologist in the angiographic room. Conversely, IPB does not necessitate continuous monitoring by an anesthesiologist. Therefore, IPB can easily be performed at a remote area, and the patient can be sent to the angiographic suite for PBD when the interventionalist is ready, which avoids schedule disturbances.

At our hospital, IPB was usually set up the day before the scheduled PBD. For some emergency cases, the anesthesiologist performed the IPB in the recovery room, between other anesthetic procedures in the operating room. However, as at many institutions, an anesthesiologist was not always available on short notice. Although IPB is relatively easy to perform for those with experience with epidural anesthesia (because the needle placement technique is similar), radiologists who do not perform IPB on a regular basis could easily puncture the visceral pleura and produce a pneumothorax. Anesthesiologists are also better trained to treat the patient if anesthetic toxicity supervenes after inadvertent intravascular injection of the local anesthetic. For these reasons, radiologists at our institution prefer not to perform the IPB themselves.

The exact mechanism of action of IPB has not been clearly established. A likely explanation, demonstrated with dermatome testing (11), is retrograde diffusion of the drug through the parietal pleura, which causes intercostal nerve blocks. The hemithorax analgesia provided by IPB extends from the sternal notch to the pubic symphysis and appears ideal for painful unilateral procedures (such as PBD) that mainly involve the flank and upper quadrant ipsilateral to the block (2). One would therefore expect IPB to be efficient for reduction of PBD-induced pain no matter where the PBD puncture is performed on the side of the IPB, although a correlation between IPB analgesia and PBD puncture site has not been specifically evaluated.

IPB has yielded good results for various surgical interventions (6,7) and for postoperative pain control (8–11). The advantages of IPB are technical simplicity, absence of cardiorespiratory depression, and less-demanding monitoring. IPB is currently performed with 0.5% bupivacaine, 30 mL of which correspond to the highest dose that has been safely used for this method of analgesia (18). We chose this dose so that it could not be argued that the amount of drug was insufficient if IPB proved to be ineffective.

PCA is designed to accommodate the wide range of analgesic needs that can be anticipated for management of acute postoperative pain. The PCA pump is programmed not to exceed a maximum preestablished dose per period of time. Before a painful procedure, the directions for use of the pump are given to the patient so that adequate analgesia can be obtained without unwanted drowsiness. PCA is currently used for postoperative pain control (19,20). Results of many studies (19–24) with various populations have demonstrated the safety and effi-

Table 4
Vital Signs and Side Effects

Measurement	Group 1*	Group 2*	P Value: Between Groups	P Value: Between Times†
Mean heart rate (beats per minute)				
Before PBD	75.40 ± 14.80	76.40 ± 8.00	.99	.310
During PBD	77.00 ± 17.30	76.60 ± 9.90		
After PBD	80.40 ± 16.70	79.00 ± 16.70		
Systolic blood pressure (mm Hg)				
Before PBD	125.40 ± 19.40	117.60 ± 14.20	.54	.001
During PBD	93.90 ± 4.90	94.50 ± 1.30		
After PBD	131.70 ± 28.20	122.40 ± 16.60		
Lowest value of oxygen saturation (%)				
Before PBD	93.90 ± 4.90	94.50 ± 1.30	.41	.002
During PBD	91.10 ± 3.40	92.20 ± 2.50		
Lowest respiratory frequency after PBD (breaths per minute)	18.90 ± 4.50	17.20 ± 2.60	.22	NA
Degree of sedation				
During PBD‡	0.29 ± 0.47	0.27 ± 0.46	.46	.001
After PBD‡	0.93 ± 0.27	0.80 ± 0.41		

* Group 1 patients received PCA and true IPB; group 2 patients received PCA and placebo IPB. Data are means ± 1 standard deviation.
† NA = not applicable.
‡ Data are based on the highest score on the three-point scale used to determine degree of sedation.

cacy of PCA. In our study, the PCA drug dosage was chosen on the basis of results from clinical studies and pharmacokinetic data (4,21,22,25,26). Fentanyl was preferred to morphine because a fast-acting drug with a short half-life seemed more appropriate to treat sudden and intermittent pain stimuli during PBD. Furthermore, PCA combined with pain intensity measurements may serve as a dependent variable to evaluate other analgesic methods by comparing the rate of use of the PCA pump with or without the other investigated mode of analgesia (23,24,27). In our study, the use of PCA in both groups (associated with pain score measurement) allowed the evaluation of analgesia and elimination of the potential bias of an external assessment by the interventionalist (27,28). The statistically significant decrease in fentanyl needed by patients in the IPB group compared with those in placebo group indicates a strong analgesic effect provided by IPB both during and for 8 hours after PBD.

The VAS is one of the most commonly used methods for the assessment of pain intensity. The patient indicates pain intensity on a 10-cm-long line with extremities identified as "no pain" and "unbearable pain", and the distance is measured in millimeters (13,29). Although the pain VAS measures only one dimension of a painful stimulus (intensity), the McGill Pain Questionnaire allows evaluation of other aspects of a painful experience. This questionnaire comprises a list of adjectives to measure the different dimensions of pain, and scores are calculated on the basis of the words the patient chooses to describe the painful experience (14).

Measurements of procedure-related alterations in blood pressure and heart rate are a way to evaluate the physiologic response to pain. Because both parameters typically increase in response to the stress of pain, their measurements provide an indirect means for assessment of the pain level. In our study, these physiologic parameters did not differ statistically significantly between groups. This is probably due to the fact that the vital signs were recorded every 15 minutes and not continuously. Continuous monitoring might have better demonstrated transient heart rate and blood pressure modifications in relation to intermittent pain stimuli during PBD.

Reported complications of IPB include pneumothorax, hemothorax, and local anesthetic toxicity (30). The frequency of pneumothorax appears to be related to the technique used and to the anesthesiologist's experience and appears to be fairly low (2%) (30). However, the number of cases of pneumothorax were rather high in the present study. Although all IPBs were performed with a standardized procedure, the anesthesiologists who performed the IPB had various levels of experience with this method. Low levels of experience with the technique may explain, in part, the higher rate of pneumothorax. Indeed, the first pneumothorax encountered in this study (which necessitated drainage with a chest tube) occurred in the first patient who underwent IPB. However, the small number IPBs performed in this study are not sufficient to provide reliable data about the exact rate of pneumothorax. Further studies with larger sample sizes are needed to determine the true prevalence and clinical importance of pneumothorax, especially given the high analgesic efficacy of IPB. Also, the catheter placement technique used in this study involved sharp-needle insertion, which could increase the risk of pneumothorax. Development of a blunt-needle insertion technique without catheter positioning could theoretically lower the risk of pneumothorax (31).

Although anesthetic toxicity did not occur in this study, adverse reactions such as arrhythmia, seizure, and hypotension may follow IPB. The interventionalist should avoid excessive use of lidocaine during performance of PBD with IPB because summation of systemic absorption of lidocaine and bupivacaine could result in severe toxicity. However, because IPB does not totally abolish PBD-induced pain, local anesthesia with lidocaine is still necessary in many patients. Although the use of a decreased amount of interpleural bupivacaine during IPB would be a way to decrease the theoretical risk of toxicity, it could also result in decreased efficacy.

One limitation of this study is the evaluation of pain relief provided by IPB in patients in whom left bile duct access for PBD was required. Indeed, unilateral right IPB may not provide the same level of analgesia for right and left bile duct approaches, in which case bilateral IPB may be necessary. Enrollment in this study was based on "a priori" right bile duct access. An unexpected left bile duct access was sometimes necessary after evaluation of the percutaneous transhepatic cholangiograms or for various technical reasons during the procedure. Yet, we were able to demonstrate a strong global analgesic effect of IPB for PBD, although nine patients underwent "a posteriori" left bile duct access alone or in association with a right bile duct approach. By combining right and left bile duct access, all patients underwent successful PBD, with adequate drainage of both liver lobes either externally or internally.

Few patients underwent manipulations with percutaneous instruments larger in diameter than 9 F, and we cannot evaluate the analgesic efficacy of IPB for interventions with larger instruments. However, dilation of the

PBD access site to a larger diameter (12–16 F) is becoming less common. Indeed, such dilation was needed mainly to position percutaneous plastic endoprostheses that have been advantageously replaced by metallic stents that use much smaller introducers.

In conclusion, IPB is an effective method for reduction of both pain intensity and opioid drug requirements during and after PBD. IPB does not compromise the cardiorespiratory status of the patient, and IPB-induced pneumothoraxes did not result in major complications. However, the frequency of pneumothorax was higher than has been previously reported. Although the rate of pneumothorax was high in this series, other therapies such as opioids for sedation also incur risks. Thus, in a population of high-risk patients, the risks associated with IPB may be acceptable. Technical developments in anesthesia should help to prevent pneumothorax in the future, whereas further studies with larger sample sizes are needed to determine the rate and clinical importance of pneumothorax, especially given the high analgesic efficacy of IPB. ■

Acknowledgments: The authors express their gratitude to Hélène Lanctôt, RN, for her invaluable help during the course of this study. Special thanks are also addressed to Marc Dumont, MS, who conducted all the statistical analyses. Finally, Minogue Laboratories and David Bull Laboratories are thanked for having graciously provided the PCA pumps and the prefilled syringes for the study.

References

1. Harshfield DL, Teplick SK, Brandon JC. Pain control during interventional biliary procedures: epidural anesthesia vs i.v. sedation. AJR 1993; 161:1057–1059.
2. Rosenblatt M, Robalino J, Bergman A, Shevde K. Pleural block: technique for regional anesthesia during percutaneous hepatobiliary drainage. Radiology 1989; 172:279–280.
3. Lieberman RP, Nance PN, Cuka DJ. Anterior approach to celiac plexus block during interventional biliary procedures. Radiology 1988; 167:562–564.
4. Savader SJ, Bourke DL, Venbrux AC, et al. Randomized double-blind clinical trial of celiac block for percutaneous biliary drainage. JVIR 1993; 4:539–542.
5. Mueller PR, Wittenberg KH, Kaufman JA, Lee MJ. Pattern of anesthesia and nursing care for interventional radiology procedures: a national survey of physician practices and preferences. Radiology 1997; 202: 339–343.
6. Schlesinger TM, Laurito CE, Baughman VL, Carranza CJ. Interpleural bupivacaine for mammography during needle localization and breast biopsy. Anesth Analg 1989; 68: 394–395.
7. Trivedi N, Robalino J, Shevde K. Interpleural block: a new technique for regional anesthesia during percutaneous nephrostomy and nephrolithotomy. Can J Anaesth 1990; 37:479–481.
8. Reiestad F, Stromskag KE. Intrapleural catheter in the management of post-operative pain: a preliminary report. Reg Anesth 1986; 11:89–91.
9. Covino BG. Interpleural regional analgesia. Anesth Analg 1988; 67:427–429.
10. Kambam JR, Hamdte RE. Intrapleural anesthesia for post-thoracotomy pain relief. Reg Anesth 1987; 12:106–107.
11. Bruce DL, Gerken V. Post cholecystectomy pain relief by intrapleural bupivacaine in patients with cystic fibrosis. Anesth Analg 1987; 66:1187–1189.
12. Ben-David B, Lee E. The falling column: a new technique for interpleural catheter placement. Anesth Analg 1990; 71:212.
13. Choinière M, Ansel R. A visual analogue thermometer for measuring pain intensity. J Pain Symptom Manage 1996; 11:299–311.
14. Melzack R. The McGill Pain Questionnaire: major properties and scoring methods. Pain 1975; 1:277–299.
15. Egbert AM, Parks HL, Short LM, Burnett ML. Randomized trial of postoperative patient-controlled analgesia vs intramuscular narcotics in frail elderly men. Arch Intern Med 1990; 150:1897–1903.
16. Cohen JC. Statistical power analysis for the behavioral sciences. 2nd ed. Hillsdale, NJ: Erlbaum, 1988.
17. Hays WL. Statistics. New York, NY: Holt, Rinehart, & Winston, 1963.
18. Seltzer LI, Larijani EG. Intrapleural bupivacaine: a kinetic and dynamic evaluation. Anesthesiology 1987; 67:790–800.
19. Owen H, Mather LE, Rowley K. The development and clinical use of patient-controlled analgesia. Anaesth Intensive Care 1988; 16:433–447.
20. White PF. Use of patient-controlled analgesia for management of acute pain. JAMA 1988; 259:243.
21. Mather LE, Owen H. The scientific basis of patient-controlled analgesia. Anaesth Intensive Care 1988; 16:427–436.
22. Tamsen A, Hartvig P, Fagerlund C, et al. Patient-controlled analgesic therapy. II. Individual analgesic demand and analgesic plasma concentrations of pethidine in postoperative pain. Clin Pharmacokinet 1982; 7:164–175.
23. Lehmann KA. New development in patient-controlled post-operative analgesia. Ann Med 1995; 27:271–282.
24. Smythe M. Patient controlled analgesia: a review. Pharmacotherapy 1992; 12:132–143.
25. Jaffe JH, Martyn WR. Opioid analgesics and antagonists. In: Gilman AG, Guilman LS, Rall TW, et al, eds. The pharmacological basis of therapeutics. 7th ed. New York, NY: Macmillan, 1985; 491–531.
26. Owen H, Glavin RJ, Reekie RM, et al. Patient-controlled analgesia. Anaesthesia 1986; 41:1230–1235.
27. Silverman DG, O'Connor TZ, Brull SJ. Integrated assessment of pain scores and rescue morphine use during studies of analgesic efficacy. Anesth Analg 1993; 77:168–170.
28. Lehmann KA. Patient-controlled intravenous analgesia for postoperative pain relief. Adv Pain Res Ther 1991; 18:481–506.
29. Huskisson EC. Visual analogue scales. In: Melzack R, ed. Pain measurement and assessment. New York, NY: Raven, 1983; 33–40.
30. Murphy DF. Interpleural analgesia. Br J Anaesth 1993; 71:426–434.
31. Akins EW, Hawkins IF, Mladinich C, Tupler R, Siragusa RJ, Pry R. The blunt needle: a percutaneous access device. AJR 1989; 152:181–182.

George X. Szymski, MD • Alexandra N. Albazzaz, DO • Brian Funaki, MD • Jordan D. Rosenblum, MD
Craig A. Hackworth, MD • Brian W. Zernich, DO • Jeffrey A. Leef, MD

Radiologically Guided Placement of Pull-type Gastrostomy Tubes[1]

PURPOSE: To evaluate percutaneous placement of pull-type gastrostomy tubes that has traditionally necessitated endoscopic guidance.

MATERIALS AND METHODS: From September 1995 through March 1997, 63 pull-type gastrostomy tubes were placed in 64 patients. Retrograde catheterization of the esophagus was performed through the stomach. Then the gastrostomy tube was pulled through from the mouth into the stomach.

RESULTS: Gastrostomy tube placement was successful in 63 (98%) of 64 patients in 65 attempts. One procedure was stopped when the patient reported chest pain after gastric insufflation, and a second placement attempt was initially unsuccessful. Major complications occurred in three (5%) patients: exit site infection necessitating tube removal (n = 2) and prolonged bleeding necessitating transfusion (n = 1). Minor complications occurred in six (9%) patients: failure of placement (n = 2), exit site infection (n = 1), leakage around the tube (n = 1), tube migration (n = 1), and inadvertent tube removal (n = 1). There were no cases of peritonitis, tract disruption, or gastrostomy-related death.

CONCLUSION: Percutaneous placement of a pull-type gastrostomy tube was performed with a minimum risk of tract disruption and peritonitis. The tube was safely and effectively placed by radiologists.

PERCUTANEOUS placement has replaced surgical placement as the most common method of gastrostomy tube deployment (1,2) and was first described by Gauderer et al in 1980 (3). Percutaneous procedures are performed with either a push technique (the gastrostomy tube is "pushed" directly through the abdominal wall after serial dilation) or a pull technique (the tube is "pulled" from the mouth, down the esophagus, and through the abdominal wall). Many variations in both techniques have been described (4–7); radiologists typically place push-type tubes and endoscopists generally place pull-type tubes. Owing to the secure retaining device and large inner lumen of pull-type tubes, surgeons have described their placement during open gastrostomy (8).

In this study, we evaluated placement of large-bore, self-retaining, pull-type gastrostomy tubes with radiologic guidance. This technique combines the advantages of fluoroscopic guidance with the advantages of pull-type gastrostomy tubes, which are typically placed by endoscopists. We initially placed these gastrostomy tubes in only neurologically compromised patients to avoid accidental dislodgement. Owing to the ease of placement and simple construction, however, pull-type tubes have become the device we prefer to place at gastrostomy.

MATERIALS AND METHODS

Between September 1995 and March 1997, a pull-type gastrostomy tube was placed in 64 patients (39 female and 25 male patients, aged 16–96 years [mean, 67 years]) with stroke (n = 32), central nervous system malignancy (n = 10), other neurologic syndromes (n = 14 [including myasthenia gravis [n = 3]; Jakob-Creutzfeldt disease [n = 2]; cerebellar syndrome [n = 2]; Parkinson disease [n = 3]; amyotrophic lateral sclerosis, or ALS, [n = 2]; and neurofibromatosis [n = 2]]), head and neck malignancy (n = 4), or gastric outlet obstruction (n = 4).

During the first 10 months of the study, operator preference generally determined whether the tube would be placed with a pull (n = 21) or push (n = 42) technique. Beginning in July 1996 until the end of the study, 43 of 50 tubes were placed with a pull technique. Pull-type tubes were placed in all uncooperative patients (n = 17) during the entire study to help prevent inadvertent tube removal. Two types of gastrostomy tubes were placed (MIC Removable Pull PEG, Medical Innovations, Draper, Utah [n = 54]; Ponsky "Pull" PEG, Bard, Tewksburg, Mass [n = 9]). Both are 20-F tubes with 13-F inner lumina and have similar mushroom-shaped retaining devices (Fig 1).

Prior to the procedure, patients fasted overnight, if possible, or for a minimum of 6 hours if the procedure needed to be performed the same day. In patients with head and neck malignancies, the most recent computed tomographic examination was reviewed to rule out a completely obstructive lesion. All patients received prophylactic antibiotics intravenously (1 g of ceftizoxime sodium), immediately before the procedure. Additionally, 1 mg of glucagon was administered intravenously to prevent stomach decompression due to peristalsis. Fentanyl citrate and midazolam hydrochloride were administered intravenously to provide sedation. Upper endoscopy bite block (Endo Bite-Block; Encom-

Index terms: Gastrostomy, 72.1269 • Stomach, interventional procedure, 72.1269

Radiology 1997; 205:669–673

[1] From the Department of Radiology, the University of Chicago, MC 2026, 5841 S Maryland Ave, Chicago, IL 60637. From the 1997 RSNA scientific assembly. Received June 3, 1997; revision requested July 8; revision received and accepted August 7. **Address reprint requests to** G.X.S.

pas Unlimited, St Petersburg, Fla) was placed, and Xylocaine 10% oral spray (Astra, Westborough, Mass) was sprayed onto the posterior wall of the oropharynx to reduce the gag reflex.

If a nasogastric tube was in place, it was used to allow insufflation of the stomach. If a nasogastric tube was not in place, orogastric or nasogastric placement of a 5-F end-hole catheter (MPA; Cook, Bloomington, Ind) was performed. The stomach was insufflated until the greater curvature was 4–5 cm below the margin of the 12th rib. The puncture site was located away from the rib margin to help prevent pain from tube movement (9). The middle body of the stomach was located for puncture, the skin was anesthetized with 1% lidocaine, and a 1.5-cm-long incision was made (9). A single-wall puncture of the stomach was performed with a T fastener (Cope gastrointestinal suture anchor set; Cook), and a 145-cm-long (standard-length), 0.035-inch guide wire (LLT; Cook) was advanced into the stomach (Fig 2). A hemostat was clamped onto the suture of the T fastener to provide tension with gravity and hold the stomach to the abdominal wall.

A moderate curve was formed on the dilator of a 30-cm-long, 10-F vascular sheath (Braun, Bethlehem, Pa) to facilitate guidance of the catheter tip toward the gastroesophageal junction. The puncture needle was then removed, and the vascular sheath was advanced over the guide wire and into the stomach (Fig 3). The catheter used for gastric insufflation was left in place to act as a target. The 10-F sheath and dilator were used to direct the guide wire posteriorly and medially toward the gastroesophageal junction (Fig 4). Either the guide wire used in the initial access into the stomach or a hydrophilic guide wire (Roadrunner PC; Cook) was advanced into the esophagus (Fig 5), along with the 10-F sheath (Fig 6).

Once the wire entered the oropharynx, it usually exited the mouth. To facilitate this, a catheter with a gentle curve (RC-1; Cook) was used to guide the wire out of the mouth (Fig 7). Additionally, turning the patient's head to the side or turning the fluoroscope to a lateral position helped advancement of the guide wire out of the mouth. The standard-length guide wire was then exchanged for a 260-cm-long (exchange-length) guide wire, and a snare included in the pull percutaneous endoscopic gastrostomy kit was tightened onto the middle portion of the guide wire. Both were advanced into the sheath and out of the mouth. After the snare exited the mouth, the guide wire was removed.

The gastrostomy tube was attached to the snare by advancing the dilator of the gastrostomy tube completely through the loop of the snare and then passing the opposite end of the gastrostomy tube completely through the wire loop of the gastrostomy tube, forming a secure knot with the two wire loops. The gastrostomy tube was completely lubricated (Surgilube; Fougera, Melville, NY) to facilitate passage through the esophagus and coated with povidone-iodine (Betadine ointment; Purdue Fredrick, Norwalk, Conn) to help prevent site infection. The tube was then pulled down the esophagus and through the abdominal wall. Often, a mild amount of resistance was encountered at the gastroesophageal junction as the retaining device passed this area. The position was confirmed fluoroscopically (Fig 8), and the tube was secured with an external ring. The T fastener was simply released.

After the procedure, intermittent suction was begun in the stomach, and feeding was withheld for 24 hours. Residual stomach volumes were measured during the next 2 days. Tubes placed to treat gastric outlet obstruction were used immediately.

Jejunal extension tubes (wire-guided jejunal feeding or gastric decompression tubes [Bard]) were placed through the pull-type gastrostomy tube in patients at high risk for aspiration. The extension tubes fit into both kinds of pull-type tubes used in this study. If aspiration occurred after placement of a pull-type gastrostomy tube, a jejunal extension tube was placed through the gastrostomy tube without disturbing the original gastrostomy tube tract. Pull-type gastrostomy tubes were not removed or exchanged during the course of the study except in case of infection. Complications were defined as major or minor. Major complications were defined as procedural complications that prolonged hospital stay. Minor complications included self-limited events and placement failures.

Follow-up information was obtained in 60 (94%) patients at 30 days and in 52 (81%) at 60 days. All available charts and records were reviewed (n = 51), and phone interviews were conducted (n = 43) with either the patients or their families. The average follow-up was 4.7 months (range, 1–18 months).

RESULTS

Gastrostomy tube placement was successful in 63 (98%) of 64 patients with 65 attempts. Two attempts were unsuccessful. One procedure was abandoned in a 59-year-old woman after she experienced chest pain during placement. During this procedure, the stomach had been accessed, but the guide wire and a portion of the sheath looped in the peritoneum, which allowed a pneumoperitoneum to develop. The chest pain appeared to have been related to the developing pneumoperitoneum, as no further signs or symptoms of a myocardial infarction ensued. Eventually, the patient underwent surgical placement of a gastrostomy tube. In a different patient, the procedure was abandoned owing to loss of percutaneous access to the stomach and the development of a pneumoperitoneum. The procedure was repeated, and a gastrostomy tube was successfully placed 2 days later. Two of the gastrostomy tubes were removed after they were no longer needed. In 60 patients with follow-up information, the 30-day mortality was 10% (six patients). No deaths were attributed to gastrostomy tube placement.

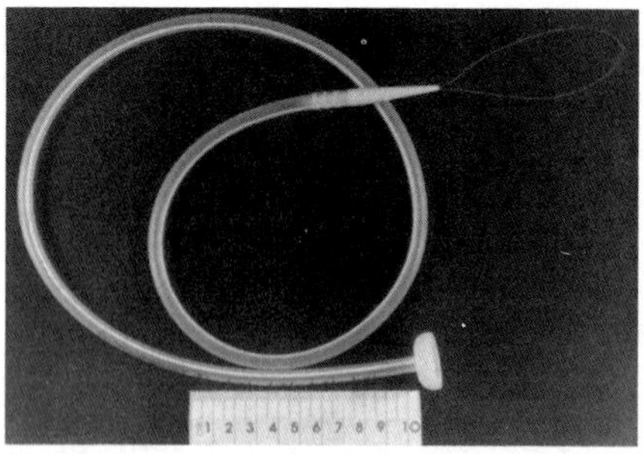

Figure 1. MIC Removable Pull PEG gastrostomy tube. The ruler indicates centimeters.

Major complications occurred in three (5%) patients: exit site infection that necessitated tube removal (n = 2) and prolonged bleeding that necessitated transfusion (n = 1). The site infections occurred 8 and 18 days after initial gastrostomy tube placement and both necessitated surgical débridement and removal of the gastrostomy tube. One of the site infections was necrotizing fasciitis. One patient with leukemia and malnutrition experienced bleeding 4 days after the procedure and underwent transfusion of 2 units of blood; the precise location of the hemorrhage could not be identified, but the bleeding stopped spontaneously.

Minor complications occurred in six (9%) patients: failure of placement (n = 2), exit site infection (n = 1), leakage around the tube (n = 1), tube migration (n = 1), and inadvertent tube removal (n = 1). There were no cases of peritonitis, tract disruption, or gastrostomy-related death. Minor complications included self-limited events in four (6%) of the 64 patients and failures of placement in two (3%). One episode of leakage from the tract was resolved with ostomy care and a slight temporary increase in tension on the gastrostomy tube. A single episode of minor site infection occurred 23 days after catheter placement and was resolved with continued ostomy care. Tube migration into the rectus abdominis muscle occurred 3½ months after gastrostomy tube placement in a 39-year-old woman with gastric obstruction due to metastatic leiomyosarcoma. This occurred after the tract had matured, and a replacement tube was advanced into the stomach without further sequelae. A 79-year-old patient with obstructive gastric carcinoma intentionally pulled his tube out owing to his impaired mental status.

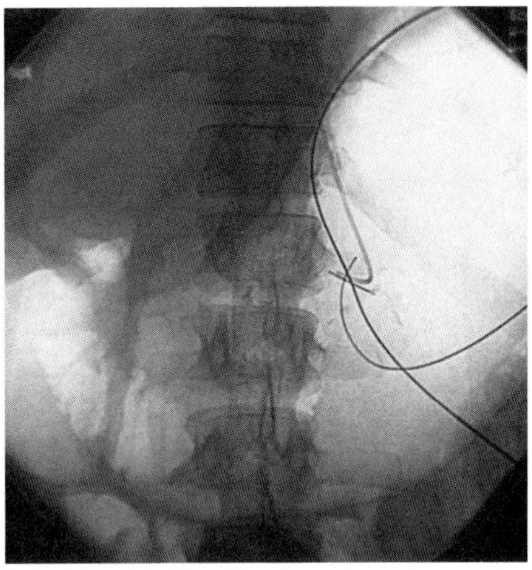

2.

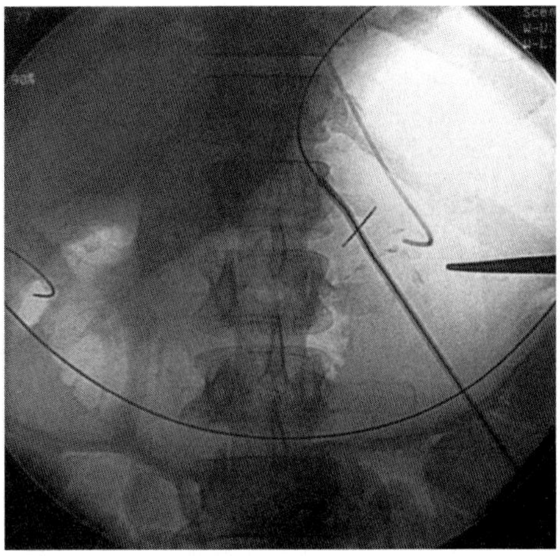

3.

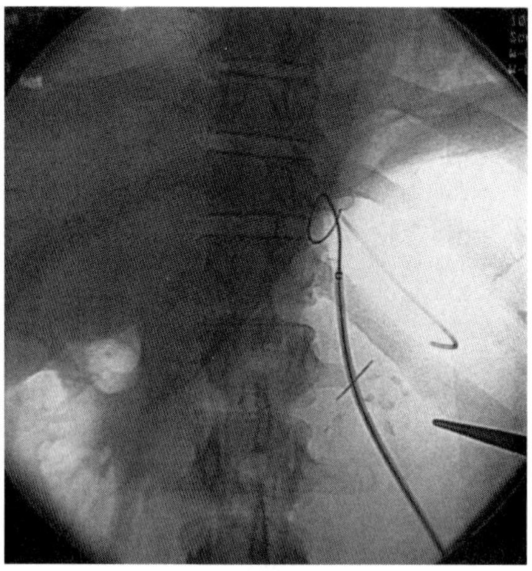

4.

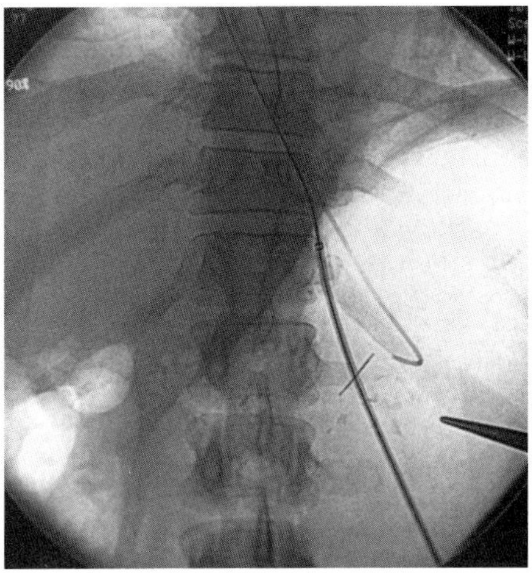

5.

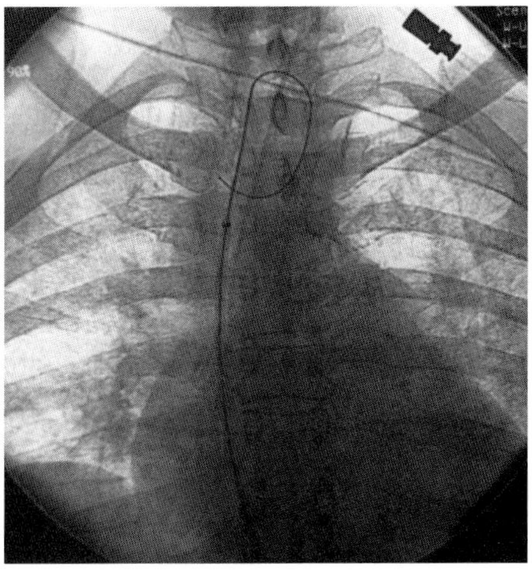

6.

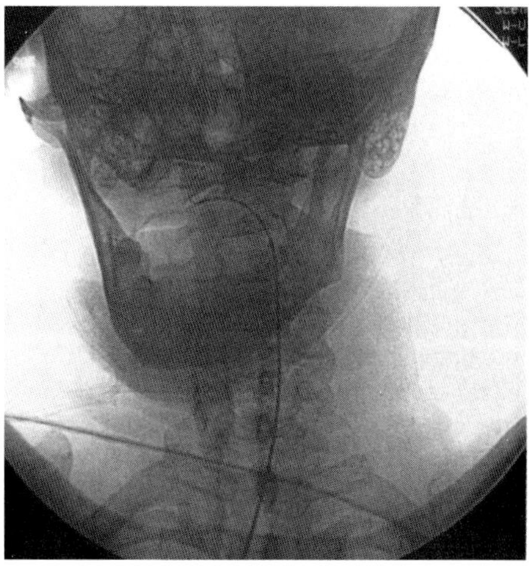

7.

Figures 2–7. Fluoroscopic images depict radiologically guided placement of a pull-type gastrostomy tube in one patient. **(2)** Passage of the guide wire into the stomach. The T fastener is located in the stomach. **(3)** The vascular sheath is advanced into the stomach. **(4)** The guide wire and sheath are advanced toward the gastroesophageal junction. **(5)** The guide wire is advanced into the esophagus. **(6)** The vascular sheath is advanced over the guide wire in the esophagus. **(7)** A catheter is used to help direct the guide wire out of the patient's mouth.

The clinical service physicians opted not to have the tube replaced owing to the patient's poor prognosis. No tube exchanges were necessary during the study period.

Two episodes of delayed aspiration occurred. One episode of massive gastric aspiration occurred 3 days after gastrostomy tube placement after delivery of a large feeding bolus. An episode of aspiration pneumonia occurred 7 days after tube placement and was resolved after treatment with antibiotics.

After gastrostomy tube placement for stomach decompression in one patient, the patient's symptoms did not resolve. The clinical service physicians referred the patient for a surgical gastrostomy. A diagnosis of gastric torsion around the first gastrostomy tube was made by the surgeons at surgery. However, the replacement gastrostomy tube did not help alleviate the patient's symptoms. Eventually, the patient was referred back to the radiology department to undergo exchange of the surgically placed gastrostomy tube for a gastrojejunostomy tube, which helped partially relieve the symptoms.

Seven jejunal extension tubes were placed. In five patients, jejunal extension tubes were placed during the initial gastrostomy tube placement. In three of these patients, the jejunal extension tubes were guided directly into the duodenum. In the other two patients, a loop had to be formed in the stomach fundus before the extension tube would advance easily into the jejunum. The loop configuration did not impede function and allowed use of an alternate technique for placement of the jejunal extension tube (10). In two patients, jejunal extension tubes were placed within 1 month of the initial gastrostomy tube placement, one for symptoms of aspiration and the other for pain with feedings thought to be related to distention of the stomach.

DISCUSSION

Percutaneous, fluoroscopically guided placement of a gastrostomy tube has many advantages compared with endoscopic placement, including a greater success rate (1). Fluoroscopic guidance allows visualization of the stomach, even in very large patients, whereas endoscopic placement is not possible owing to the inability to transilluminate the abdominal wall. Four obese patients in our series were referred by the gastrointestinal clinic physicians after unsuccessful endoscopic placement. We successfully placed gastrostomy tubes in all of these patients. Use of fluoroscopic guidance also decreases the risk of colonic perforation, as the air-filled colon is routinely identified. Alternatively, contrast material can be administered orally the night before the procedure to help visualize the colon (10). Fluoroscopically guided placement of a gastrostomy tube can be performed by only one operator, whereas two operators are necessary in the endoscopic procedure. Although methods can be devised to help limit the number of physicians needed to perform endoscopic placement, the procedure itself is inherently more labor intensive.

Our poor experience with placement of push-type gastrostomy tubes without performing four-point gastropexy procedures prompted us to seek alternate placement techniques. We did not experience the reliability of placement with push-type tubes reported by others (11,12), with major complications in three of four push-type tubes in a single month prior to this study. We then began to perform four-point gastropexy procedures in all patients. This prevented peritonitis but not tube dislodgement. Several push-type gastrostomy tubes dislodged because the retaining balloon ruptured or the thread broke that locked the pigtail loop. Our difficulties were not unique. Early tube dislodgement with push-type tubes was reported in 9.5% of patients in an early review of data in the radiology literature (13). In a later meta-analysis of the data in the literature, only 1.3% of tube dislodgements necessitated fluoroscopic guidance to replace the gastrostomy tube (1). In their own hospital, however, the authors reported a 12% tube dislodgement rate, with 3% of their 33 patients requiring fluoroscopic guidance for the replacement procedure (1). Presumably, most accidental dislodgements necessitate tube replacement without guidance or complication, generally after the tract has matured. Additionally, in some of the earlier series, the higher rate of accidental tube dislodgement may have been a result of use of balloon-retained tubes rather than locking-loop tubes (14).

Pull-type gastrostomy tubes are more secure than the conventional push-type tubes typically placed by radiologists. Typical push-type gastrostomy tubes are held in position with either locking loops or retaining balloons. Both mechanisms can be accidentally released (15–17). In one series, continued problems with the locking loop mechanism on the 12-F Wills-Oglesby tube (Cook) prompted the authors to advocate placement of pull-type gastrostomy tubes as the method of choice, with placement of push-type tubes percutaneously only if all else failed (15). Balloon-retained tubes have problems due to accidental deflation or disruption (8,14,18–20). Additionally, accidents such as injection of a feeding bolus into the balloon port can occur (21). In contrast, the retention device on the pull-type gastrostomy tube cannot be deflated, unlocked, or injected with a feeding bolus. If a peel-away sheath is used (11,22), the tract is overdilated, which further contributes to tube instability. The dilator on a pull-type tube is attached to the tube and is exactly the same size as the tube itself (Fig 1). This design adds to its security and helps limit peritoneal leakage of stomach contents.

Push-type tubes are less durable and more prone to occlusion than pull-type tubes owing to their smaller size. Even the largest 16-F locking-loop tubes are limited by the Luer-Lok mechanism. The inner lumen of the male Luer-Lok adapter measures 5–8 F, which is much smaller than the 13-F inner lumen of the typical pull-type gastrostomy tube. The push-type tube is also longer, and meticulous flushing is generally necessary to maintain patency. Most push-type gastrostomy tubes do not have good long-term patency and necessitate tube exchange more frequently (15,23,24). No pull-type tubes needed to be exchanged during follow-up in our study, with a maximum follow-up of 18 months. This same long-term success with pull-type gastrostomy tubes has been reported by others (13).

If symptoms of gastric aspiration develop, pull-type gastrostomy tubes can be converted to gastrojejunostomy tubes without having to remove the original tube. If aspiration occurs with the typical push-type gastrostomy tube, the entire tube must be removed and replaced over a guide wire. Prior to tract maturation, which necessitates a minimum of 2–4 weeks (13), tube exchange may cause tract disruption and peritonitis. Two episodes of aspiration occurred early in our series and may have been related to unfamiliarity of the nursing staff or resident physicians with gastrostomy tube maintenance. We have since provided specific instructions for proper gastrostomy tube maintenance, use, and evaluation.

Two failures of placement occurred during the initial 15 procedures. Both occurred prior to the routine performance of a single gastropexy procedure to help hold the stomach to the abdominal wall during tube placement. After these two unsuccessful procedures, we began to use T fasteners routinely and have had no additional unsuccessful procedures. Additionally, both failures occurred during attempts to snare a guide wire in the stomach, as previously described in antegrade approaches to gastrostomy tube placement (13,25). Currently, we continue to perform retrograde catheterization of the esophagus and have found that snaring a guide wire in the stomach is rarely necessary to establish access for placement of a pull-type gastrostomy tube.

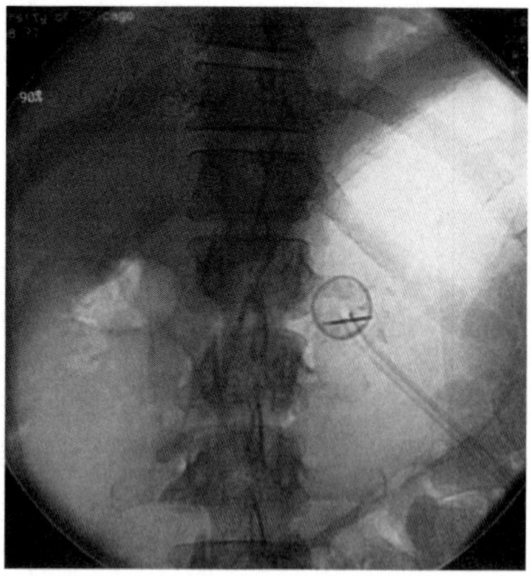

Figure 8. Fluoroscopic image depicts the final position of the gastrostomy tube.

Tube migration into the subcutaneous tissue occurred in one patient with gastric obstruction due to metastatic leiomyosarcoma. This occurred several months after the initial tube placement and may have been related to either the continued growth of the patient's malignancy or to continued tension on the gastrostomy tube (26). A replacement tube was advanced into the stomach through the mature tract. No additional complications were identified.

Disadvantages of pull-type tubes compared with push-type tubes include the higher risk of infection inherent in the placement technique. The incidence of infection in our series (3%) is similar to infection rates reported for endoscopic placement. Although copious amounts of povidone-iodine ointment are used, tube placement is not sterile, since the tube passes through the mouth, esophagus, and stomach. A single episode of necrotizing fasciitis occurred 8 days after tube placement. This complication is described in the gastrointestinal literature (27). Recommended means to prevent this complication include administering intravenous antibiotics, coating the tube with povidone-iodine ointment, and creating a more generous opening at the gastrostomy incision site (9,27). The particular complication in our study may have been related to inadequate incision size. Use of incisions 0.5 cm larger than the tube (12 mm for a 20-F tube) (9), or up to 2 cm, has been advocated (27). A second infection that necessitated surgical débridement of the gastrostomy site occurred 18 days after placement in an obese patient undergoing chemotherapy. The cause of her infection was likely related to the long subcutaneous tract and to her compromised immune status (28).

Another disadvantage of placement of pull-type gastrostomy tubes is the potential to seed metastases from esophageal or oropharyngeal malignancies into the stomach. In patients with high-grade obstructive lesions, placement of pull-type gastrostomy tubes is still possible, as the dilator would pass through the obstruction first and allow passage of the tube. Theoretically, dilation of the lesion in this fashion will promote seeding of the ostomy site. This is a very rare complication (29,30). In our series, this was not a major consideration since the majority of our patients had neurologic abnormalities rather than head and neck malignancies. If the patient is cooperative and able to care for their gastrostomy, however, placement of a push-type tube may be preferable. We believed that the subsequent risk of accidental tube dislodgement was greater than the risk of tract seeding in our patients.

Conscious sedation was used in all our procedures, except in one patient who required general anesthesia for nasogastric tube placement. A pull-type gastrostomy tube can be placed without anesthesia or conscious sedation when necessary in patients who cannot tolerate sedation (25), but it is not recommended unless absolutely necessary. No episodes of aspiration related to procedural sedation occurred. The intravenous sedation necessary in our 10 most recent placements of a pull-type gastrostomy tube consisted of an average of 2 mg (range, 0.5–3.5 mg) of midazolam hydrochloride and an average of 140 µg (range, 25-250 µg) of fentanyl citrate.

The technique for placing a pull-type gastrostomy tube is slightly more time-consuming than that for placing a push-type gastrostomy tube. Access from the mouth is necessary. The average procedure time for our 10 most recent placements of a pull-type gastrostomy tube was 25 minutes (range, 15–40 minutes). The procedure time was considered to start at the time sedation was first administered and end at the time the procedure was complete. This is slightly longer than necessary to perform a four-point gastropexy procedure and place a push-type gastrostomy tube, which previously took us approximately 20 minutes.

In summary, the pull-type gastrostomy tubes typically placed by endoscopists were safely and effectively placed by radiologists, and some of the complications that can occur with the push-type tubes were minimized. The risk of infection was lower with the push-type tube, but the pull-type tube is secure, which minimizes the risk of tract disruption and subsequent peritonitis or peritoneal injection of a feeding bolus. Additionally, the pull-type tube is inherently simpler in design, less prone to mechanical malfunction, and less likely to obstruct. Performance of a prospective randomized trial would help define the relative merits of each type of gastrostomy tube more clearly. ■

References

1. Wollman B, D'Agostino HB, Walus-Wigle JR, Easter DW, Beale A. Radiologic, endoscopic, and surgical gastrostomy: an institutional evaluation and meta-analysis of the literature. Radiology 1995; 197:699–704.
2. Jarnagin WR, Duh QY, Mulvihill SJ, Ridge JA, Schrock TR, Way LW. The efficacy and limitations of percutaneous endoscopic gastrostomy. Arch Surg 1992; 127:261–264.
3. Gauderer MW, Ponsky JL, Izant RL Jr. Gastrostomy without laparotomy: a percutaneous endoscopic technique. J Pediatr Surg 1980; 15:872–875.
4. Sacks BA, Vine HS, Palestrant AM, Ellison HP, Shropshire D, Lowe R. A nonoperative technique for establishment of a gastrostomy in the dog. Invest Radiol 1983; 18:485–487.
5. Preshaw RM. A percutaneous method for inserting a feeding gastrostomy tube. Surg Gynecol Obstet 1981; 152:658–660.
6. Lechner G, Waneck R, Schiessel R. Transcutaneous gastrostomy by the Seldinger method under local anesthesia. ROFO 1981; 135:104–105.
7. Russell TR, Brotman M, Norris F. Percutaneous gastrostomy: a new simplified and cost effective technique. Am J Surg 1984; 148:132–137.
8. Delicata RJ, Carey PD, Rees BI. A simplified and safe method of open gastrostomy. J R Coll Surg Edinb 1996; 51:124–125.
9. Grant JP. Percutaneous endoscopic gastrostomy: initial placement by a single endoscopic technique and long-term follow-up. Ann Surg 1993; 217:168–174.
10. Darcy MD. Radiologic percutaneous transgastric jejunostomy. Semin Intervent Radiol 1996; 13:299–307.
11. Deutsch LS, Kannegieter L, Vanson DT, Miller DP, Brandon JC. Simplified percutaneous gastrostomy. Radiology 1992; 184:181–183.
12. O'Donovan NA, Heelan JA. Percutaneous gastrostomy without gastropexy. Can Assoc Radiol J 1995; 46:194–195.
13. Towbin RB, Ball WS Jr, Bissett GS III. Percutaneous gastrostomy and percutaneous gastrojejunostomy in children: antegrade approach. Radiology 1988; 168:473–476.
14. Hicks ME, Surratt RS, Picus D, Marx MV, Lang EV. Fluoroscopically guided percutaneous gastrostomy and gastroenterostomy: analysis of 158 consecutive cases. AJR 1990; 154:725–728.
15. Elliott LA, Sheridan MB, Denyer M, Chapman AH. PEG: is the E necessary? a comparison of percutaneous and endoscopic gastrostomy. Clin Radiol 1996; 51:341–344.
16. Gauderer MW. Gastrostomy techniques and devices. Surg Clin North Am 1992; 72:1285–1298.
17. Darcy MD. Comparison of radiologic, endoscopic, and surgical enteral access procedures. Semin Intervent Radiol 1996; 13:289–297.
18. Simons ME, Yeung EY, Ho CS. Percutaneous fluoroscopic gastrostomy and transgastric jejunostomy. Semin Intervent Radiol 1996; 13:159–167.
19. Gauderer MW, Stellato TA. Gastrostomies: evolution, techniques, indications and complications. Curr Probl Surg 1986; 23:657–719.
20. Gowen GF. The management of complications of Foley feeding gastrostomies. Am Surg 1988; 54:582–585.
21. Kadakia SC, Cassaday M, Shaffer RT. Comparison of Foley catheter as a replacement gastrostomy tube with commercial replacement gastrostomy tube: a prospective randomized trial. Gastrointest Endosc 1994; 40:188–193.
22. Ryan JM, Hahn PF, Boland GW, McDowell RK, Saini S, Mueller PR. Percutaneous gastrostomy with T-fastener gastropexy: results of 316 consecutive procedures. Radiology 1997; 203:496–500.
23. Meier R, Bauerfeind P, Thumshirn M, Hoffmann R, Gyr K. Percutaneous endoscopic gastrostomy (PEG) for long term nutrition: comparison of 2 different caliber tubes. Schweiz Rundsch Med Prax 1992; 81:1254–1257.
24. McLoughlin RF, Gibney RG. Fluoroscopically guided percutaneous gastrostomy: tube function and malfunction. Abdom Imaging 1994; 19:195–200.
25. Rosenzweig TB, Palestrant AM, Esplin CA, Gilsdorf RB. A method for radiologic-assisted gastrostomy when percutaneous endoscopic gastrostomy is contraindicated. Am J Surg 1994; 168:587–590.
26. van Bergeijk JD, Mulder CJ. Frequent submucosal migration of soft percutaneous endoscopic gastrostomy catheters, and conservative management. Endoscopy 1995; 27:406.
27. Greif JM, Ragland JJ, Ochsner MG, Riding R. Fatal necrotizing fasciitis complicating percutaneous endoscopic gastrostomy. Gastrointest Endosc 1986; 32:292–294.
28. Calton WC, Martindale RG, Gooden SM. Complications of percutaneous endoscopic gastrostomy. Milit Med 1992; 157:358–360.
29. Lee DS, Mohit-Tabatabai MA, Rush BF Jr, Levine C. Stomal seeding of head and neck cancer by percutaneous endoscopic gastrostomy tube placement. Ann Surg Oncol 1995; 2:170–173.
30. Wilson WR, Hariri SM. Experience with percutaneous endoscopic gastrostomy tube placement on an otolaryngology service. Ear Nose Throat J 1995; 74:760–762.

Book Reviewers 1997

The book reviews that appeared among the pages of *Radiology* in 1997 were made possible by the efforts of 49 reviewers who produced more than 87 reviews. Because of their work, each issue of *Radiology* features careful and objective reviews of books on topics of interest to the clinical radiologist or physicist. We extend our thanks to these reviewers for their efforts, with special thanks to Alan E. Oestreich, MD, for handling the reviews of foreign (non-English) books and to Alan D. Steinfeld, MD, for handling the reviews of books on radiation therapy.

—STANLEY S. SIEGELMAN, MD, *Editor*
—HARRY J. GRIFFITHS, MD, *Book Review Editor*

Paul R. Algra, MD, PhD
Alexander A. Bankier, MD
Kevin M. Baskin, MD
Harold D. Batt, MD
Giampiero Beluffi, MD
Leonard Berlin, MD, FACR
Johan G. Blickman, MD, PhD
David G. Bragg, MD
Terry M. Button, PhD
Bernice M. Capusten, MD
Arthur A. Castagno, MD
Robert B. de Costa, MB, BS, DRACR
Linda Dehrer-Wendt, AA, RT(R)
Bernadine Donahue, MD
René P. duCret, MD
John C. Egelhoff, DO
Mary L. Fischer, MD
Thomas J. Gilbert, Jr, MD, MPP
Jim Glockner, MD, PhD
David S. Gooden, PhD, JD
Harry J. Griffiths, MD
James G. Hazel, Jr, MD
Barry D. Herman, MD
Stephen H. Hite, MD
Barry Jesser, RT(R)
Neil D. Johnson, MD
Pam Johnson, BS, RT(R)
Arshad A. Khan, MD
Mitchel M. S. Kim, MD
Kristine M. King, MD
Jay J. Listinsky, MD, PhD
David S. Martin, MD
Thomas C. Matson, MD
Timothy E. Moore, MD
Sundeep M. Nayak, MD
Alan E. Oestreich, MD
Paul N. Olson, MD
Susan Palasis, MD
Stanley L. Parker, MD
Karim Rezai, MD
Patricia A. Skundberg, BAS, RT(R)
S. Horatio Slawson, MD
Philippe Soyer, MD, PhD
Murali Sundaram, MD, FRCP
Michael H. Swirsky, MD
Richard A. Szucs, MD
Joseph H. Tashjian, MD
Jaime Tisnado, MD, FACR, FACC
Beverly P. Wood, MD

Hans-Joachim Wagner, MD • Stefan Müller-Hülsbeck, MD • Michael B. Pitton, MD
Wolfgang Weiss, MD • Marcus Wess, MD

Rapid Thrombectomy with a Hydrodynamic Catheter: Results from a Prospective, Multicenter Trial[1]

PURPOSE: To evaluate efficacy and safety of a hydrodynamic rheolytic thrombectomy device for rapid percutaneous treatment of acute thromboembolic occlusions of native lower-extremity arteries and bypass grafts.

MATERIALS AND METHODS: In 50 patients, thrombectomy was performed with the rheolytic catheter at four centers. Patients had acute occlusions of native lower-extremity arteries (n = 39) or acute thrombosis of lower-limb bypass grafts (n = 11). Estimated occlusion age was 5 days ± 5. Mean thrombus length was 15 cm ± 11. Clinical success was measured on a scale of -3 (deterioration) to +3 (improvement) with established criteria.

RESULTS: With the thrombectomy catheter, the majority of thrombus material was removed and antegrade blood flow was reestablished in 45 (90%) patients. Technical success (residual luminal narrowing <50%) was 52% with use of the device alone. Adjunctive therapy was performed in 45 patients. Clinical improvement after intervention was +3 in 25 (50%) patients, +2 in 10 (20%), +1 in six (12%), and 0 (no improvement) in nine (18%). Clinically unimportant complications related to use of the device were one (2%) distal embolization and two (4%) dissections. Laboratory analysis revealed hemolysis without clinical sequelae. Primary patency rates were 76% after 30 days, 74% after 3 months, and 69% after 1 year.

CONCLUSION: The hydrodynamic catheter appears to be safe and effective for rapid thrombectomy.

Limbs with acute occlusions of peripheral arteries that cause ischemia can be classified into three categories (1): viable limbs, threatened limbs, and irreversibly ischemic limbs. If acute occlusion of the vessels can be compensated by blood flow from collateral vessels, limbs will typically demonstrate signs of incomplete ischemia. In such a clinical situation, local intraarterial thrombolysis has become a well-established method of treatment of thromboembolic occlusions of native lower-limb arteries and infraaortic bypass grafts (2–7).

Patients with symptoms of acutely threatened lower limbs require rapid revascularization and, because intraarterial thrombolysis is usually deemed too time-consuming, success is not always predictable. Thus, surgical intervention is necessary (8).

To overcome the drawbacks associated with local thrombolysis (namely, high costs for patient monitoring in the intensive care unit, long procedure times, and increased morbidity with longer duration of therapy [9]), efforts have been made to develop a percutaneous alternative to the surgical balloon thrombectomy method (10).

To our knowledge, percutaneous aspiration or suction thromboembolectomy is the oldest and clinically most widespread technique (11,12), and it is the only percutaneous thrombectomy technique for which long-term results are available (13). However, the technique is sophisticated, is associated with possible blood loss, is difficult to use for removal of larger thrombi, and necessitates use of a relatively large sheath (8F); thus, suction thromboembolectomy is performed only in specialized centers.

In recent years, various catheters have been introduced for the purpose of percutaneous thrombectomy. Some devices fragmentate thrombi (14,15), some devices macerate and aspirate thrombi (16,17), and other devices fragmentate thrombi with ultrasound (US) assistance and aspirate (18). Clinical application of these systems, however, has been restricted to smaller patient groups and feasibility studies.

The purpose of this study was to evaluate the clinical efficacy and safety of a hydrodynamic catheter in a prospective, multicenter trial for treatment of nonselected acute occlusions of lower-limb native arteries and bypass grafts.

MATERIALS AND METHODS

Study Design

The study protocol was approved by the local Ethics Committee at the principal investigator center (Philipps University Hospital). Patients were considered for inclusion in the study who had acute occlusions of lower-limb arteries or bypass grafts and were referred to the radiology

Index terms: Arteries, extremities, 92.411, 92.442 • Arteries, stenosis or obstruction, 92.411, 92.442 • Arteries, thrombosis, 92.442 • Arteries, transluminal angioplasty, 92.1269, 92.1283 • Thrombectomy, 92.1265, 92.1269, 92.1283

Radiology 1997; 205:675–681

[1] From the Department of Diagnostic Radiology, University Hospital, Philipps University, Baldingerstr, 35033 Marburg, Germany (H.J.W., M.W.); the Department of Diagnostic Radiology, University Hospital, Christian Albrechts University, Kiel, Germany (S.M.H.); the Department of Radiology, University Hospital, Johannes Gutenberg University, Mainz, Germany (M.B.P.); and the Department of Diagnostic Radiology, University Hospital Rechts der Isar, Technical University, Munich, Germany (W.W.). From the 1996 RSNA scientific assembly. Received October 30, 1996; revision requested December 20; revision received July 31, 1997; accepted August 4. **Address reprint requests to** H.J.W.

departments at the participating centers for treatment of these lesions.

Inclusion criteria were (*a*) acute (less than 14 days old) thrombotic or embolic occlusion of a native artery below the aortic bifurcation or (*b*) acute (less than 14 days old) thromboembolic occlusion of a bypass graft below the aortic bifurcation, and (*c*) intraarterial angiographic proof of occlusion.

Exclusion criteria were (*a*) thrombectomy or thrombolysis within 14 days before the procedure, (*b*) contraindication for percutaneous transluminal angioplasty at the site where thrombectomy was performed (eg, arterial pseudoaneurysm or aneurysm), (*c*) contraindication for anticoagulation with heparin, (*d*) contraindication for use of contrast material, (*e*) contraindication for mild hemolysis (eg, severe anemia), (*f*) nonhealed injury (attributable to surgery or trauma) to the target vessel or graft (eg, anastomosis less than 14 days old), (*g*) uncontrollable hemorrhagic diathesis, (*h*) vascular surgery performed in the target vessel or graft within 4 weeks before the procedure, (*i*) no runoff vessel (no perfused tibial artery below the proximal third of the calf), (*j*) lack of compliance with follow-up visits, (*k*) inclusion in other trials, (*l*) age less than 18 years, and (*m*) pregnancy or nursing. All patients were prospectively and consecutively recruited on an intent-to-treat basis. Patients who gave written informed consent were included in the study unless they met any of the exclusion criteria.

Since this feasibility trial was planned to prospectively evaluate procedural efficacy and safety, 50 patients were enrolled at six study centers. The maximum number of patients a single center could recruit for the study was limited to 20. Centers that recruited fewer than three patients were excluded. The study began in March 1995, and patient recruitment was terminated after 50 patients were included in the study. All patients were followed up prospectively for 3 months and after that time by means of retrospective analysis.

Recruitment

From March through December 1995, a total of 50 patients were prospectively and consecutively enrolled in the trial. Four centers recruited patients (one center recruited 19 patients, one center recruited 18, one center recruited 10, and one center recruited three). Two centers did not recruit any patients.

Patients

The 28 men and 22 women in the study population had a mean age of 69 years ± 11 (age range, 44–86 years). Of the 50 patients, 39 (78%) had acute occlusions of native arteries and 11 (22%) had acute occlusions of bypass grafts. In 45 patients, the mean walking distance was 80 m ± 113, measured with the treadmill test (1). The mean ankle-brachial index was 0.33 ± 0.3. According to the suggested standards (1), 24 (48%) limbs were deemed viable and 26 (52%) limbs were deemed threatened. Thirty-eight (76%) patients reported preexisting chronic limb ischemia.

Patients demonstrated the typical risk factors. Thirteen (26%) patients had diabetes, 19 (38%) were tobacco users, 17 (34%) had hypertension, 14 (28%) had hyperlipidemia, 14 (28%) had coronary artery disease, three (6%) had carotid artery disease, four (8%) had impaired renal function, and four (8%) had pulmonary disease. Twenty-eight (56%) patients had more than one risk factor and 14 (28%) patients had more than two risk factors.

Pretreatment angiography revealed two (4%) iliac artery occlusions, 13 (26%) superficial femoral artery occlusions, 22 (44%) popliteal artery occlusions, and two (4%) tibial vessel occlusions. If an occlusion extended over more than one segment, the most proximal vascular segment was used to stratify the patients. Of the 11 (22%) bypass graft occlusions, 10 were femoropopliteal and one was femorotibial; five of these occlusions were in vein grafts and six were in prosthetic grafts. The mean occlusion length was 15 cm ± 11. The estimated occlusion age (determined from patient history) was 5 days ± 5. Table 1 summarizes the pretreatment data of the patients.

Thrombectomy Technique

A pretreatment angiogram was obtained in all patients. For the interventional procedure, a puncture was made at the contralateral common femoral artery in patients with suprainguinal occlusions and at the ipsilateral common femoral artery in patients with infrainguinal occlusions. A 6-F sheath was placed retrograde when the contralateral approach was used and antegrade when the ipsilateral approach was used. A dose of 5,000 IU of heparin was administered immediately after placement of the sheath. Before thrombectomy was performed, it was necessary to determine whether the entire lesion could be crossed with a guide wire and catheter. If this "guide wire test" was not successful, the patient was excluded from the trial and thrombectomy was not performed. When the guide wire was passed through the entire occlusion successfully, the guide wire used for recanalization was exchanged for a stiff 0.018-inch wire (Control wire; SCIMed, Minneapolis, Minn). The thrombectomy catheter (AngioJet; Possis Medical, Minneapolis, Minn) was then advanced over the wire 2 cm above the proximal margin of the occlusion.

The hydrodynamic device consists of a 5-F double-lumen catheter that is 105 cm long and accepts a 0.018-inch guide wire. The smaller lumen of the catheter is used to supply the catheter tip with saline jets. The saline jets that emerge at the tip of the catheter are generated by an external drive unit with a positive-displacement pump that generates pressures up to 10,000 psi (Fig 1). The saline injected into the catheter is supplied by a 1,000-mL plastic bag containing physiologic saline solution to which 5,000 IU of heparin was added. The pump creates a cyclic saline flow of 60 mL/min. The saline jets exit at the tip of the catheter through three radially oriented holes of 25–50 µm in diameter. These jets aid in the formation of a recirculation pattern to fragmentate the thrombotic material. An additional three saline jets are directed retrogradely into the larger exhaust lumen of the catheter. These jets create a so-called "Venturi effect" that aids in evacuation of the macerated thrombus material (Fig 1). The exhaust of the catheter is controlled by a roller pump so that the entire catheter operates in an isovolumic mode. The aspirated effluent material is collected in a bag. After the drive unit is assembled and the disposable pump and catheter are connected, the entire unit can be activated by a foot switch.

When the thrombectomy catheter is 2 cm above the lesion, the drive unit is activated and the catheter is advanced over the guide wire through the entire thrombus. The catheter should be advanced at a constant velocity of 0.5–1.0 cm/sec. When the distal margin of the occlusion has been reached, the procedure can be repeated by pulling the activated catheter back over the guide wire. After the first antegrade and retrograde passage of the thrombectomy catheter, we obtain a control angiogram of the treated segment. This angiogram usually reveals creation of a small channel through the entire lesion.

To enhance the function of the catheter, it is possible to bend the tip of the catheter to a 30° curve. Curving of the catheter allows guidance of the device. After reintroduction of the catheter and advancement over the guide wire to the distal margin of the occlusion, the guide wire can be pulled back into the catheter lumen to increase efficacy of the device further. The catheter is then pulled back through the occlusion in a spiral mode. Pulling of the catheter through the occlusion in this mode allows direction of the saline jets to all parts of the arterial or graft wall and enables evacuation of wall-adherent residual thrombi. The J-shaped catheter can also be advanced in an antegrade fashion to remove further thromboembolic material. Advancement of the J catheter in this fashion must be performed carefully, especially if the catheter is not used over the guide wire because of the potential for dissections and subintimal passage. Retraction of the 0.018-inch guide wire enhances the function of the device because the guide wire obstructs the exhaust lumen partially if it is in place. However, the additional outflow of debris is limited by the external roller pump. Also, sacrificing the guide wire might result in an adverse outcome if the lesion cannot be recanalized a second time.

The amount of thromboembolic material removed with the thrombectomy catheter can be controlled with injection of contrast material through the side port of the sheath. The catheter can be passed through the lesion as often as necessary; however, passage is limited to a total device activation time of 15 minutes or injection of a total amount of 1,000 mL of saline. The reason for these

Table 1
Pretreatment Data in the 50 Patients

Data	Recruited Patients
Mean age (y)	69 ± 11 (44–86)*
Sex (M, F)	28, 22
Ischemia	
Viable lower limbs	24 (48)
Threatened lower limbs	26 (52)
Preexisting chronic limb ischemia	38 (76)
Occluded vascular segment	
Native artery	39 (78)
Iliac arteries	2 (4)
Femoral arteries	13 (26)
Popliteal arteries	22 (44)
Tibial arteries	2 (4)
Bypass graft	11 (22)
Femoropopliteal	10 (20)
Femorotibial	1 (2)
Mean occlusion length (cm)	15 ± 11
Estimated mean age of occlusion (d)	5 ± 5
Mean walking distance (m)	80 ± 113†
Mean ankle-brachial index	0.33 ± 0.3
Risk factors	
Smoking	19 (38)
Diabetes	13 (26)
Hyperlipidemia	14 (28)
Carotid artery disease	3 (6)
Coronary artery disease	14 (28)
Pulmonary disease	4 (8)
Renal insufficiency	4 (8)

Note.—Numbers in parentheses are percentages.
* Indicates age range.
† Walking distance was measured in 45 patients with the treadmill test.

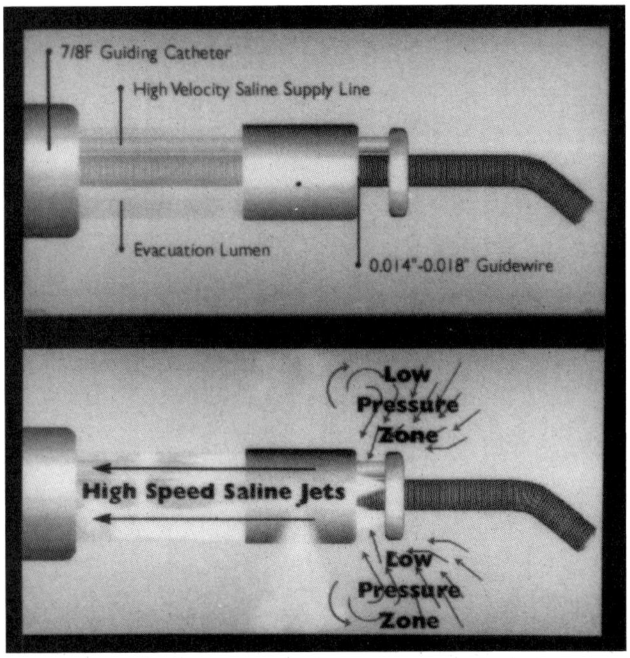

Figure 1. Drawings show the tip of the thrombectomy catheter (upper) and catheter function (lower). Three saline jets are radial to the catheter, and three other jets are directed toward the exhaust lumen to create the Venturi effect for removal of thrombus material. The saline jets create a low-pressure zone inside the vessel; this low-pressure zone creates a 360° Bernoulli effect. The resultant Bernoulli effect attracts thrombi around the tip for rapid removal.

restrictions is the possibility of increased hemolysis with use of a longer activation time.

When the investigator determined that the achieved lumen could not be improved further or that the occlusive material was removed completely, thrombectomy was terminated and a control angiogram was obtained immediately. The angiogram was obtained to demonstrate not only the treated segment but also the entire vessel or vessels from the sheath down to the pedal arch. This angiogram was used to assess the angiographic success with use of the thrombectomy device alone and help detect complications (eg, dissections, distal embolization). Residual stenosis was calculated by measuring the narrowest segment and relating it to a normal reference segment above the formerly occluded vessel segment. The measurements were calibrated with radiopaque centimeter markers that were located underneath the patient.

If the occlusive material had been removed completely with the catheter or the investigator was satisfied with the achieved lumen, intervention was terminated. For this purpose, the sheath was retrieved immediately, and the patient received heparin intravenously (to double the prothrombin time) for the next 3 days.

If residual luminal narrowing was present, each investigator was allowed to perform any adjunctive therapy deemed helpful in achieving final success. The only therapy not allowed was repeated use of the thrombectomy device.

After completion of the procedure, a final angiogram was obtained to document the vascular system from the sheath to the pedal arch. This angiogram was used to assess the final angiographic results and overall angiographic and interventional complications.

Laboratory Tests

To evaluate the hemolytic effect of the thrombectomy device, blood samples were obtained immediately before the procedure, after intervention, and at 24 hours, 30 days, and 3 months after the procedure. Laboratory values determined were hemoglobin, hematocrit, platelet count, plasma-free hemoglobin, haptoglobin, lactate dehydrogenase, blood urea nitrogen, and creatinine.

Definitions

All data were assessed according to the recommendations of the American Heart Association, the Society of Vascular Surgery, and the Society of Cardiovascular and Interventional Radiology (1,19,20). Angiographic success was defined as restoration of blood flow in a formerly occluded vascular or graft segment with residual luminal narrowing of less than 50%. Clinical success was recorded on a scale from -3 (deterioration) to +3 (improvement) according to guidelines proposed by Rutherford and Becker (19).

Follow-up

All patients were examined 24 hours, 30 days, 3 months, and at least 1 year after the thrombectomy procedure. Follow-up included physical examination, treadmill test, pulse status, ankle-brachial index measurement, and color flow duplex sonography of the treated extremity. If results from color flow duplex sonography were uncertain or suggested a hemodynamically significant reobstruction (luminal narrowing >50%), an intraarterial angiogram was obtained. Intraarterial angiography was performed in all patients who showed deterioration of clinical condition.

Statistical Analysis

All analyses were performed on an intention-to-treat basis. The data are expressed as the mean + standard deviation. Homogeneity of variances was proved with the Kolmogoroff-Smirnoff test. For randomly distributed data, the *t* tests were used, and for nonrandomly distributed data, the matched pairs or *U* test were used. A *P* value less than .05 was considered statistically significant. The primary patency, mortality, and limb-salvage rates were determined with Kaplan-Meier analysis.

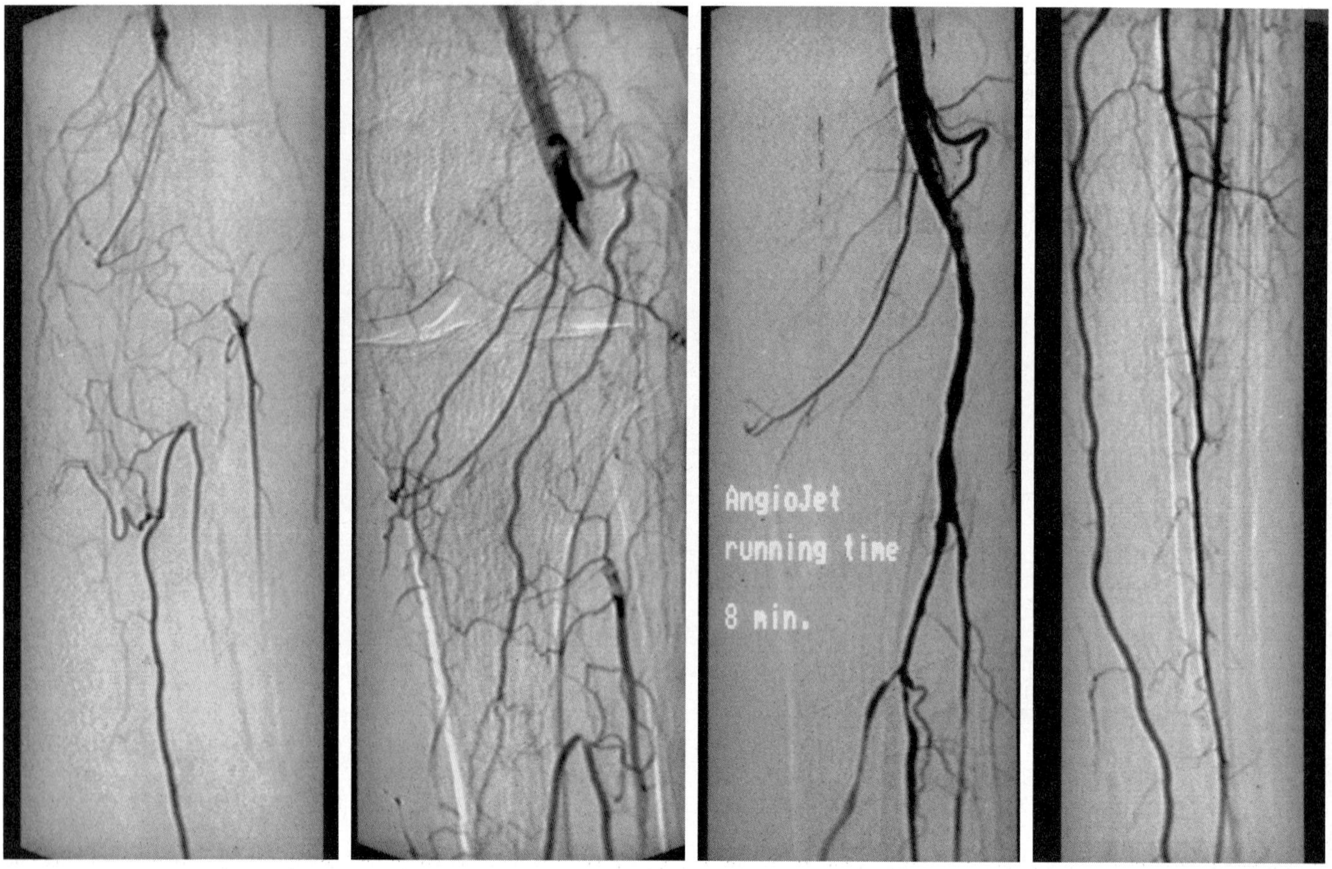

a. b. c. d.

Figure 2. Hydrodynamic thrombectomy of an embolic occlusion of a popliteal artery. **(a)** Angiogram shows complete occlusion of the popliteal artery. **(b)** Magnified angiogram shows the embolus in the popliteal artery extending into the proximal portion of the tibial arteries. **(c)** Angiogram obtained after activation of the thrombectomy device for 8 minutes shows that flow is restored with minimal residual thrombus material at the popliteal arterial wall. No adjunctive treatment was necessary. **(d)** Runoff angiogram shows no evidence of distal embolization.

RESULTS

Treatment Data

None of the patients were withdrawn from the trial because of a failed guide wire test. The 100% success in transversing the guide wire indicated that the clinical diagnosis of an acute thromboembolic occlusion was correct in all patients.

The mean activation time of the thrombectomy device was 7 minutes, 28 seconds ± 4 minutes, 42 seconds. The mean amount of injected saline was 416 mL ± 269 and the mean collected effluent was 428 mL ± 277. These data confirmed the flow rate of 60 mL/min and the isovolumic mode of operation of the device.

With the thrombectomy device, the majority of thrombus material was removed and antegrade blood flow was reestablished through the formerly occluded segment in 45 (90%) of the 50 patients.

The angiographic success (residual luminal narrowing < 50%) with use of the thrombectomy catheter alone was 52%. This result was demonstrated on the angiogram obtained immediately after use of the thrombectomy catheter and before use of any other endovascular technique (Fig 2). However, because residual luminal narrowing was present that was attributable mainly to atherosclerotic plaque material, wall-adherent thrombus, or organized thromboembolic particles, additional treatment was necessary in 45 (90%) patients.

Adjunctive Therapy

Balloon dilation was performed in 31 (62%) patients. The mean length of the treated lesions was 4 cm ± 3. In 15 (30%) patients, local intraarterial thrombolysis was performed with continuous infusion of urokinase (Actosolv; Hoechst, Frankfurt, Germany) (12 patients; mean dose, 1,926,000 IU ± 997,000; mean infusion time, 54 hours ± 23) or continuous infusion of recombinant tissue plasminogen activator (Actilyse; Thomae, Biberach, Germany) (three patients; mean dose, 13 mg ± 15; mean infusion time, 26 hours ± 20). The additional thrombolysis necessitated overnight hospitalization and monitoring in the intensive care unit. Aspiration thrombectomy was performed in nine (18%) patients, necessitating an increase in sheath size from 6F to 8F. Stent implantation was performed in three (6%) patients, and surgical revision was performed of stenosis of an anastomosis in a previously occluded bypass graft in five (10%) patients.

After intervention was complete, angiographic success was achieved in 45 (90%) patients. The mean residual luminal narrowing was 29% ± 26.

Treatment Failure

Treatment failure occurred in five (10%) patients. In one patient, treatment was aborted because of technical problems with the catheter (the drive unit showed the "outflow" alarm, which could not be canceled). In four (8%) patients, treatment was completed but was not technically successful. In all cases of treatment failure, the occlusive material was not removed sufficiently.

Clinical Success

According to the recommended criteria, improvement was categorized

Table 2
Treatment Data and Procedural Success in 50 Occlusions

Treatment Data and Success	Occlusions
Mean activation time	7 min 28 sec ± 4 min 42 sec
Mean injected volume of saline (mL)	416 ± 269
Mean volume of effluent (mL)	428 ± 277
Angiographic success after thrombectomy alone	26 (52)
Additional treatment performed	
Fibrinolysis	15 (30)
Aspiration thrombectomy	9 (18)
Balloon dilation	31 (62)
Stent implantation	3 (6)
None	5 (10)
Angiographic success after termination of the procedure	45 (90)
Clinical success	
+3	25 (50)
+2	10 (20)
+1	6 (12)
0	9 (18)

Note.—Numbers in parentheses are percentages.

Table 3
Complications Related to the Thrombectomy Device, Adjunctive Methods, and Vascular Access Route

Complication	Treated Lower Limbs (n = 50)
None	39 (78)
Distal embolization	3 (4)
Related to thrombectomy	1
Related to balloon dilation	2
Arterial dissection	3 (6)
Related to thrombectomy	2
Related to balloon dilation	1
Perforation of tibial arteries	2 (4)
Hematoma at puncture site	2 (4)
Conservative treatment	1
Surgical revision	1
Retroperitoneal bleeding	1 (2)

Note.—Numbers in parentheses are percentages.

as +3 in 25 (50%) patients, +2 in 10 (20%) patients, and +1 in six (12%) patients. No improvement was noted in nine (18%) patients (category 0). None of the patients demonstrated deterioration of clinical condition after the procedure (categories −1 to −3) (Table 2).

The mean ankle-brachial index increased significantly to 0.77 ± 0.3 the day after intervention ($P < .001$). The mean walking distance increased to 294 m ± 203 ($P < .001$).

Complications

A total of 11 complications occurred in 11 limbs (Table 3). Complications related to use of the thrombectomy device were noted during three procedures: one distal embolization and two dissections. The distal embolization was managed by means of activation of the thrombectomy catheter after its advancement to the embolus. The arterial dissections were deemed hemodynamically insignificant, were not treated specifically, and did not lead to clinical sequelae.

Complications attributable to adjunctive methods and to the vascular access route are listed in Table 3. The two distal embolizations related to percutaneous transluminal angioplasty were treated successfully with percutaneous aspiration embolectomy. The two perforations of tibial arteries sealed spontaneously and were clinically unimportant.

Hemolysis

Table 4 shows the mean ± standard deviations of the data obtained before intervention, after intervention, and during follow-up. The data demonstrated signs of hemolysis with a mean thirty-sixfold increase in the plasma-free hemoglobin level, but only a slight decrease in the haptoglobin level. Clinical signs of hemolysis (macrohematuria the 1st day after intervention) occurred in only one patient. All pathologic values returned to physiologic values within the first 24 hours after the procedure. In two patients, a slight transient impairment of renal function was noticed. The creatinine levels increased to a maximum of 2.1 mg/dL (110 µmol/L) in these patients. None of the patients developed renal failure. The mean serum creatinine level decreased after the procedure, attributable mainly to hydration of the patients with saline solution before and during intervention.

Follow-up

Reocclusions during the first 3 months after thrombectomy occurred in nine patients at 1 (n = 5), 4 (n = 1), 30 (n = 2), and 42 (n = 1) days (Table 5). The primary patency rate was 82% after 24 hours, 76% at 4 weeks, 74% at 3 months, 72% at 6 months, 69% at 1 year, and 69% at 2 years (Fig 3). In cases of rethrombosis, additional percutaneous hydrodynamic thrombectomy was performed in combination with other, suitable endovascular techniques.

Amputations were performed on three lower limbs. One above-the-knee amputation was performed 1 day after thrombectomy and one was performed 17 days after thrombectomy. One below-the-knee amputation was performed after 2 days. Toe amputation was performed in one patient 30 days after the procedure. Amputations were performed only in patients in whom the revascularization procedure failed. None of these patients were deemed suitable candidates for a surgical reconstructive procedure. None of the amputations were a consequence of any complication related to the intervention. The limb-salvage rate was 98% at 24 hours, 94% at 4 weeks, 94% at 3 months, and 94% 1 year after the procedure (Table 5).

None of the patients died within the first 30 days after the procedure. The mortality rate is shown in Table 5.

DISCUSSION

Our multicenter trial demonstrated the efficacy and safety of the hydrodynamic thrombectomy device. The major advantages associated with any percutaneous thrombectomy system are the short period of time needed for revascularization; the possibility of "unmasking" underlying obstructions immediately, making them eligible for treatment; and the avoidance of thrombolytic drugs, which increase the morbidity associated with percutaneous vascular interventions.

As shown in our study, the majority of thromboembolic material was removed with the rapid or rheolytic thrombectomy catheter. However, remaining wall-adherent material necessitated adjunctive use of fibrinolysis or aspiration thrombectomy. The removal of the majority of thrombus material can decrease the time necessary for thrombolysis, thereby reducing the dose of thrombolytic agent, and thus decrease the morbidity associated with fibrinolysis. The additional use of aspiration thromboembolectomy might obviate thrombolysis. However, this technique necessitates use of larger-size sheaths and knowledge of this special technique.

Advantages associated with this particular thrombectomy device compared with those associated with other devices currently under investigation are the small size of the catheter (5F); use of the smaller-size catheter reduces the risk of bleeding at the arterial access site. The small size of the catheter also enables treatment of tibial arteries down to the pedal vessels. This feature is not only helpful in cases of ascending arterial thrombosis in patients with primarily infrapopliteal occlusive disease (eg, patients with diabetes), but also in cases of distal embolization. The device has shown the ability to remove thrombus material in small vessels successfully in our trial and also in preliminary trials in which the device was used in coronary vessels (21).

The results obtained with the device are remarkable for the low rate of induced distal embolization. Throughout our trial, we found distal emboli related to the thrombectomy catheter in only one procedure. Other studies that used hydrodynamic thrombectomy devices reported a rate of 40% for distal thrombus displacement in the first 20 patients treated; this rate of distal displacement led to modification of the technique (22). Use of the Amplatz (Microvena, White Bear Lake, Minn) and Hydrolyser (Cordis Europa, Roden, the Netherlands) thrombectomy devices is recommended along with an inflated cuff positioned distal to the vascular obstruction to prevent embolization (23). Placement of the inflated cuff not only complicates the entire procedure but also increases pain and discomfort to the patient. Reekers et al (22) changed the technique and now recommend treatment of the most distal part of the thrombotic lesion with thrombolysis rather than with the thrombectomy catheter. Use of thrombolysis is, at least in part, a contraindication of the intention of such thrombectomy systems because thrombolysis should not be necessary when these systems are used.

Steerability of the thrombectomy devices is also important. The system can be used over a 0.018-inch guide wire, and the possibility of bending the tip of the catheter makes it steerable without the need of a guide wire. Other systems are more rigid (aspiration thrombectomy catheters, hydrodynamic thrombosuction catheter) or lack a guide wire lumen (Amplatz thrombectomy device). For the purpose of steerability, these systems necessitate use of large-diameter guiding catheters (9F or 10F); use of the larger catheters increases the risk of complications at the vessel entry site. For "cross-over" procedures, the ability to advance the catheter over a guide wire is necessary; otherwise a guiding catheter must be used.

The isovolumic mode of removal of thrombus material with the particular hydrodynamic device seems advantageous, since fluid overload might easily lead to congestive heart failure in these particular patients in whom concomitant cardiac or coronary artery disease is prevalent. The possibility of fluid overload has been reported with use of other hydrodynamic thrombectomy systems (22).

Table 4
Indicators of Hemolysis before and after Thrombectomy

Parameter	Before Thrombectomy	After Thrombectomy: Immediately	24 hours	30 days
Hemoglobin (g/L)	141 ± 18	130 ± 17*	129 ± 18	134 ± 15
Hematocrit (%)	40.6 ± 5.5	37.6 ± 4.5*	36.4 ± 5.2	39.1 ± 4.5
Plasma-free hemoglobin (g/L)	28 ± 14	101 ± 125†	27 ± 16	44 ± 52
Haptoglobin (g/L)	2.5 ± 1.0	2.2 ± 1.0*	1.8 ± 1.0	2.3 ± 0.9
Lactate dehydrogenase (U/L)	224 ± 94	275 ± 146†	264 ± 84	176 ± 38
Creatinine (μmol/L)	110 ± 70	90 ± 50	100 ± 40	110 ± 30
Blood urea nitrogen (mmol/L)	11.8 ± 8.2	10.4 ± 5.0	11.1 ± 6.1	16.8 ± 7.1

* Value was statistically significantly less ($P < .05$; Wilcoxon matched pairs test) than the pretreatment value.
† Value was statistically significantly greater ($P < .05$; Wilcoxon matched pairs test) than the pretreatment value.

Table 5
Follow-up Results

Parameter	After the Procedure: Immediate	24 hours	4 weeks	3 months
Primary patency (%)	92	82*	76*	74*
Ankle-brachial index	0.33 ± 0.3†	0.77 ± 0.3‡	0.87 ± 0.2	0.92 ± 0.1
Walking distance (m)	80 ± 113†	294 ± 203‡	299 ± 233	392 ± 256
Limb salvage	100§	98§	94§	94§
Above-knee amputation‖	0	1	2	2
Below-knee amputation‖	0	0	1	1
Toe amputation‖	0	0	0	1
Mortality (%)	0	0	0	0

* Assessed with color flow Doppler US.
† Pretreatment values.
‡ $P < .001$ compared with pretreatment value.
§ Value is expressed as a percentage.
‖ Cumulated data over the period from intervention through the end of follow-up.

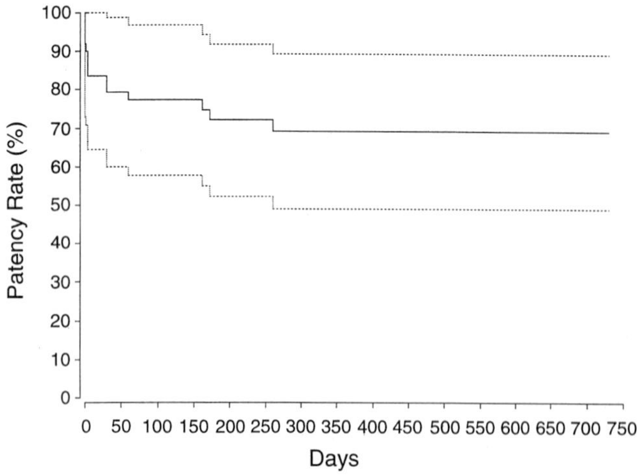

Figure 3. Graph shows follow-up primary patency rates (solid line) determined with Kaplan-Meier analysis. The dotted lines indicate the 95% Hall-Wellner confidence interval.

A disadvantage of the device used in our study is the need for a special drive unit. Use of the drive unit increases the price of the procedure, although a definite price proposal has not yet been made, to our knowledge. Alternative hydrodynamic systems that create lower pressures (about 750 psi) can be used with a conventional angiographic injector (hydrodynamic thrombosuction catheter).

Another disadvantage of the system is the limited capacity in removing wall-adherent thrombus material; this capacity is limited further in cases of organized thrombus material. The removal of soft, fresh thrombus material is not a problem with any of the current thrombectomy devices and has been proved in numerous in vitro studies (14,16,24,25). The clinical problem, however, is that most patients have occlusions that are typically composed of a combination of fresher and older parts. It is easy to debulk the fresh part of the thrombus material; however, problems occur with treatment of older, dehydrated, and especially partially or completely organized thrombotic material. With all thrombectomy devices, removal of organized material is unique in that typically no substantial amount of organized material can be removed (22,23). The only applicable percutaneous thrombectomy device for this particular problem seems to be an aspiration thrombectomy device because it simply removes all material (12). In the case of wall-adherent material, the aspiration thrombectomy device can be used in conjunction with a rotating basket that detaches the material from the arterial wall (13).

The problem of reduced efficacy of thrombectomy systems is also true in cases of embolic occlusions because the occlusive material typically comprises older, organized parts that cannot be removed with simple fragmentation.

Our findings with regard to hemolysis could prove that use of the device produces a slight hemolytic effect, but we did not find this effect to be clinically relevant. Our results are in accordance with those of a trial that concentrated on the hemolytic effect of the Amplatz device (26).

In summary, our feasibility study demonstrated that use of the small-caliber hydrodynamic thrombectomy catheter can effectively and safely replace the time-consuming and cost-intensive method of local intraarterial fibrinolysis. However, a direct comparison of both techniques for the treatment of acute limb ischemia caused by thromboembolic occlusions of native arteries or bypass grafts is necessary. Prospective, randomized trials must be conducted that also include determination of cost-effectiveness. ■

References

1. Rutherford RB, Flanigan DP, Gupta SK, et al. Suggested standards for reports dealing with lower extremity ischemia. J Vasc Surg 1986; 4:80–94.
2. Dotter CT, Roesch J, Seaman AJ. Selective clot lysis with low-dose streptokinase. Radiology 1974; 111:31–37.
3. Katzen BT, Edwards KC, Albert AS, van Breda A. Low-dose direct fibrinolysis in peripheral vascular disease. J Vasc Surg 1984; 1:718–722.
4. Hess H, Mietaschk A, Brückl R. Peripheral arterial occlusions: a 6 year experience with local low dose thrombolytic therapy. Radiology 1987; 163:753–758.
5. McNamara TO, Bomberger RA, Merchant RF. Intra-arterial urokinase as initial therapy for acutely ischemic lower limbs. Circulation 1991; 83(suppl):106–119.
6. Sullivan KL, Gardiner GA, Kandarpa K, et al. Efficacy of thrombolysis in infrainguinal bypass grafts. Circulation 1991; 83(suppl):99–105.
7. Leblang SD, Becker GJ, Benenati JF, Zemel G, Katzen BT, Sallee SS. Low-dose urokinase regimen for the treatment of lower extremity and graft occlusions: experience in 132 cases. JVIR 1992; 3:475–483.
8. Walker WJ, Giddings AEB. A protocol for the safe treatment of acute lower limb ischemia with intra-arterial streptokinase and surgery. Br J Surg 1988; 75:1189–1192.
9. Sullivan KL, Gardiner GA, Shapiro MJ, Bonn J, Levin DC. Acceleration of thrombolysis with a high-dose transthrombus bolus technique. Radiology 1989; 173:805–808.
10. Tawes RL, Harris EJ, Brown WH, et al. Arterial thromboembolism: a 20-year perspective. Arch Surg 1985; 120:595–599.
11. Sniderman KW, Bodner L, Saddekni S, Srur M, Sos TA. Percutaneous embolectomy by transcatheter aspiration. Radiology 1984; 150:357–361.
12. Starck EE, McDermott JC, Crummy AB, Turnipseed WD, Acher CW, Burges JH. Percutaneous aspiration thrombo-embolectomy. Radiology 1985; 156:61–66.
13. Wagner HJ, Starck EE, Reuter P. Longterm results of percutaneous aspiration embolectomy. Cardiovasc Intervent Radiol 1994; 17:241–246.
14. Bildsoe MC, Moradian GP, Hunter DW, Castaneda-Zuniga WR, Amplatz K. Mechanical clot dissolution: new concept. Radiology 1989; 171:231–233.
15. Ritchie JL, Hansen DD, Vracko R, Auth DC. Mechanical thrombolysis: a new rotational catheter approach for acute thrombi. Circulation 1986; 73:1006–1012.
16. Drasler WJ, Jenson ML, Wilson GJ, et al. Rheolytic catheter for percutaneous removal of thrombus. Radiology 1992; 182: 263–267.
17. Reekers JA, Kromhout JG, van der Waal K. Catheter for percutaneous thrombectomy: first clinical experience. Radiology 1993; 188:871–874.
18. Schmitz-Rode T, Günther RW, Müller-Leise C. US-assisted aspiration thromboembolectomy: in vitro investigations. Radiology 1991; 178:677–679.
19. Rutherford RB, Becker GJ. Standards for evaluating and reporting the results of surgical and percutaneous therapy for peripheral arterial disease. Radiology 1991; 181: 277–281.
20. Pentecost MJ, Criqui MH, Dorros G, et al. Guidelines for peripheral percutaneous transluminal angioplasty of the abdominal aorta and lower extremity vessels. Circulation 1994; 89:511–531.
21. Ramee SR, Kuntz RE, Schatz RA, et al. Preliminary experience with the Possis coronary AngioJet rheolytic thrombectomy catheter in the VeGAS I pilot study (abstr). J Endovasc Surg 1995; 2:234.
22. Reekers JA, Kromhout JG, Spithoven HG, Jacobs MJHM, Mali WMPH, Schultze-Kool LJ. Arterial thrombosis below the inguinal ligament: percutaneous treatment with a thrombosuction catheter. Radiology 1996; 198:49–53.
23. Tadavarthy SM, Murray PD, Nazarian GK, Amplatz K. Mechanical thrombectomy with the Amplatz device: human experience. JVIR 1994; 5:715–724.
24. van Ommen V, van der Veen FH, Habets J, Wellens HJ. In vivo evaluation of the hydrolyser hydrodynamic thrombectomy catheter. JVIR 1994; 5:823–826.
25. Schmitz-Rode T, Günther RW. Percutaneous mechanical thrombolysis: a comparative study of various rotational catheter systems. Invest Radiol 1991; 26:557–563.
26. Nazarian GK, Qlan Z, Coleman C, et al. Hemolytic effect of the Amplatz thrombectomy device. JVIR 1994; 5:155–160.

Ziv J. Haskal, MD • Andrew Davis, MD[2] • Ashford McAllister, MD[3] • Emma E. Furth, MD

PTFE-encapsulated Endovascular Stent-Graft for Transjugular Intrahepatic Portosystemic Shunts: Experimental Evaluation[1]

PURPOSE: **To evaluate the safety and efficacy of a stent-graft designed for a transjugular intrahepatic portosystemic shunt (TIPS), assess angiographic and hepatic biologic responses to polytetrafluoroethylene (PTFE)-encapsulated stents, and compare with a bare stent.**

MATERIALS AND METHODS: **Twelve TIPS (eight with flexible PTFE-encapsulated balloon-expandable stent-grafts and four control TIPS with bare Wallstents) were created in 12 pigs. Shunt venography was performed at 1-month intervals and necropsy of graft-containing animals at 1, 2, 3, 4, and 5 months. Control animals were sacrificed at 6 weeks. Detailed histopathologic analyses were performed.**

RESULTS: **The stent-grafts were readily deployed in all cases. Seven of eight graft TIPS remained fully patent during the follow-up period without luminal encroachment. Typical myofibrolasts proliferated on the abluminal surface of the graft, without extension into the lumen. No inflammatory reaction was present. Cellular overgrowth from the hepatic vein occluded the end of one graft at 3 months, partly related to rapid axial growth of that animal. The endoluminal surface of this shunt was otherwise patent. At 4–6 weeks, one control TIPS was occluded and the other three showed 45%–85% stenoses. No bile staining was seen in any case.**

CONCLUSION: **This PTFE-encapsulated stent-graft is biocompatible and safe to place. It markedly improves TIPS patency, providing almost uninterrupted, unimpeded patency in this model.**

Creation of a transjugular intrahepatic portosystemic shunt (TIPS) has proved very effective for treatment of a variety of complications of portal hypertension, including variceal hemorrhage, severe ascites, and Budd-Chiari syndrome. Its conclusive therapeutic role, however, remains clouded by the problem of unpredictable shunt durability. When bare metal stents are used, stenoses of the intraparenchymal shunt tract or outflow hepatic vein lead to recurrent portal hypertension in 25%–75% of patients within 6–12 months of shunt creation (1–4). Although shunt function can be restored in nearly all cases by means of angioplasty or placement of additional stents, this entails expensive and invasive follow-up studies.

The porcine model appears very suitable for studying the histopathologic response to TIPS and methods to modify it. TIPS can be created in pigs by using techniques and equipment identical to those used in humans. While it is possible to embolize the intrahepatic portal vein and create acute presinusoidal portal hypertension in swine, it is presently impossible to maintain elevated portal pressures because of the rapid hepatic regeneration of their livers and natural recanalization of intentionally occluded portal veins (5). Fortunately, shunts lined by conventional noncovered stents promptly develop narrowings despite the absence of portal hypertension. Within a month of the TIPS procedure, most swine develop TIPS stenoses due to myofibroblastic proliferation similar to those seen in human TIPS. To a degree, this has proved an advantage of the normotensive model, as it obviates additional animal procedures designed to create portal hypertension, particularly ones that may affect animal well-being.

Mating a porous metal stent with biocompatible graft material can improve shunt patency by providing a barrier to the proliferative tissue that narrows the shunt lumen. In 1995, Nishimine et al (6) compared 13 bare-stent porcine TIPS with 13 TIPS grafts composed of off-the-shelf polytetrafluoroethylene ([PTFE] IMPRA, Tempe, Ariz) hand-sewn onto a combination of Wallstents (Schneider, Minneapolis, Minn) and Gianturco Z-stents (Cook, Bloomington, Ind). At 4 weeks, one control TIPS was "patent" (defined as <50% stenosis), while nine of 13 grafts demonstrated less than 50% stenosis. By 3 months, six of 13 grafts had less than 50% stenoses. In five cases, hepatic vein stenosis contributed to loss of graft patency.

We looked to expand on these results in our work by helping to design an encapsulated PTFE stent-graft specifi-

Index terms: Grafts, 957.1268 • Hypertension, portal, 957.711 • Interventional procedures, experimental, 957.1268 • Shunts, portosystemic, 957.1268 • Stents and prostheses, 957.1268

Abbreviations: PTFE = polytetrafluoroethylene, TIPS = transjugular intrahepatic portosystemic shunt.

Radiology 1997; 205:682–688

[1] From the Departments of Radiology (Z.J.H., A.D., A.M.) and Pathology (E.E.F.), Hospital of the University of Pennsylvania, 3400 Spruce St, Philadelphia, PA 19104. From the 1996 RSNA scientific assembly. Sponsored by Johnson and Johnson and IMPRA. Received June 3, 1997; revision requested July 22; revision received August 1; accepted August 4. **Address reprint requests to** Z.J.H.
[2] Current address: Radiology Associates of Pensacola Hospital, Fla.
[3] Current address: Columbia Springs Medical Center, Lithia Springs, Ga.

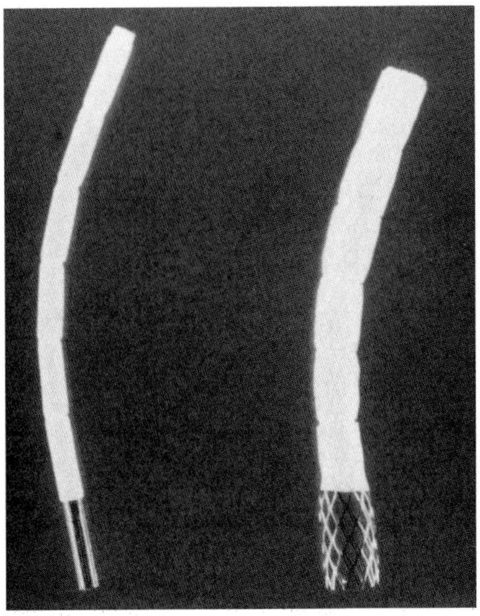

Figure 1. Photograph of the PTFE stent-graft in unexpanded and expanded states.

cally for TIPS. In this study, we had three objectives: to evaluate the safety and efficacy of a stent-graft device created and designed specifically for TIPS, to evaluate the angiographic and hepatic biologic responses to stents completely encapsulated within expanded PTFE, and to compare these with the results from a control population that received a bare stent.

MATERIALS AND METHODS

The experimental protocol was approved by the University Institutional Review Board and Animal Care Committee. We used 12 Hormel pigs (Harlan Sinclair Laboratories, Indianapolis, Ind) with initial weights of 24.3–31.0 kg. All animals were in good physical health at the start of the study. Because domestic swine can grow very rapidly, gaining 5–8 kg per week, this particular breed was chosen for its slower, flatter growth curve.

The animals were sedated by using an initial intramuscular injection of ketamine, xylazine, and atropine. Once the animal was sleepy, an intravenous catheter was inserted into an ear vein. Thiopental sodium was administered intravenously, and the animals were endotracheally intubated. During the procedure, they were maintained under general anesthesia with use of inhaled isoflurane. A single dose of 500 mg of cefazolin was administered intravenously for antibiotic prophylaxis at the start of each procedure.

The technique for creating the intrahepatic shunt was identical to the technique we use for creating TIPS in humans, with the exception of the use of a coaxial 20-gauge "finder" needle (Cook) for portal vein puncture. The latter proved useful in porcine TIPS creation because of the soft, easily disrupted nature of noncirrhotic porcine liver parenchyma. The right (n = 8) or left (n = 4) neck and sternal regions of the animals were shaved and sterilely prepared and draped. Percutaneous access to the external jugular vein was achieved by means of blind venous puncture with use of physical landmarks, sonographic guidance, or fluoroscopic puncture during injection of contrast material through the catheter in the ear vein. No surgical cutdown was performed. A 40-cm-long, curved, 10-F hemostatic sheath (Cook) was advanced into the inferior vena cava. A 5-F curved angiographic catheter was used to locate a suitable hepatic vein, and hand-injected free hepatic venography was performed. Right or left hepatic veins were used, depending on the variant hepatic vein anatomic features of the individual animals. A sheathed, 15-gauge Colapinto needle (Cook) was introduced over a guide wire into this hepatic vein. A 20-gauge, long needle was introduced coaxially through the Colapinto needle. The larger outer needle was rotated to direct the fine needle into the anticipated location of the portal vein. The fine needle was passed into the liver parenchyma and slowly withdrawn while suction was applied with a syringe partly filled with iodinated contrast material (various standard contrast media were used). When blood return was noted in the syringe, contrast material was injected to confirm that the portal vein had been entered. Typically, one to seven needle passes were required. A 0.018-inch nitinol guide wire was advanced into the portal vein. The needles and surrounding sheaths were gently advanced into the portal vein; particular care was taken during this last step because of the propensity of the main portal vein to develop spasm. Because of the relative hypercoagulability of swine, 2,000 U of heparin was injected into the portal vein at this point. Hand-injected portal venography was performed. The intrahepatic tract was dilated to 8 or 10 mm in diameter with an angioplasty balloon. The tract was imaged with venography and its length measured by bending a guide wire across its length. No transhepatic access was needed for localization of the portal vein.

Stent-Graft Description and Deployment

The device consists of six balloon-expandable Palmaz stents (Johnson & Johnson, New Brunswick, NJ) encapsulated within thin-wall, expanded PTFE (IMPRA). The leading, portal-end stent is 3 cm long (model P308M) and half covered by PTFE. The trailing series of 1.2-cm-long stents (model P128M) are completely encapsulated within the uninterrupted length of monolithic PTFE graft. An approximately 2-mm length of PTFE without stent bridges the distance between each individual stent and its neighbor. These graft "hinges" allow the stent-graft to flex (Figs 1, 2) in its unexpanded and expanded states. The device length is cut to match the measured length that will receive the stent by using a sharp scissors or scalpel to cut off individual 1.2-cm-long encapsulated stents at the trailing end of the graft. The PTFE graft material encasing the stents can be expanded to four times its unexpanded diameter without affecting its structural integrity. The internodal distance of the graft material (akin to pore size) is 30 µm. This distance is unaffected by balloon expansion. The water entry pressure of the graft is 9.0 lb per square inch.

In preparation for graft delivery, a 40-cm-long, 14-F hemostatic sheath (Cook) was introduced into the portal vein. In one case, this long sheath was unavailable, so the device was delivered "bare," without incident, through the liver parenchyma. In each case, the graft was manually mounted on an 8-cm-long, 10-mm-diameter PE-MT balloon (Medi-tech/Boston Scientific, Watertown, Mass). The hemostatic valve of the sheath was temporarily opened by using a short, 13-F, Peel-Away introducer (Cook) or short segment of custom sterile polyethylene tubing (similar to the manner in which an uncovered Palmaz stent is introduced into a vascular sheath). The graft was advanced into position over a stiff guide wire so that the bare leading half of the long portal stent was positioned within the lumen of the main portal vein. The stent-graft was fully expanded by inflating the balloon with 6 atm of pressure. During inflation, the leading, bare half of the longer portal stent was first to expand due to the lack of surrounding graft material and liver parenchyma. This anchored the graft within the portal system; the remainder of the graft expanded thereafter (Fig 3). The unencapsulated portion of the portal stent also allowed antegrade intrahepatic portal flow through the open interstices of the stent. All grafts were positioned so that their trailing, graft-encapsulated end extended up to the hepatic vein junction with the vena cava, if not a short distance into the vena cava. In two cases, it was determined that a short additional length of stent-graft was required at the cephalic end of the shunt. In these cases, a shorter, 3-cm-long stent-graft segment (three encapsulated, 1-cm-long stents) was partially overlapped within the initial graft.

Control Group

Four control TIPS were created in four animals. These TIPS were lined with one or two overlapping 10-mm-diameter, 42- or 68-mm-long, off-the-shelf Wallstents. The stents were dilated with 10-mm angioplasty balloons.

After deployment of the control and the graft devices, hand-injected portal venography was performed to assess graft position and shunt. The catheters were removed, and hemostasis was achieved at the external jugular puncture site by using manual compression. The animals were extubated, and they recovered from anesthesia. After one animal early in the study developed apparent symptoms of hepatic encephalopathy (diminished response to stimulation, poor appetite, apparent confusion), it

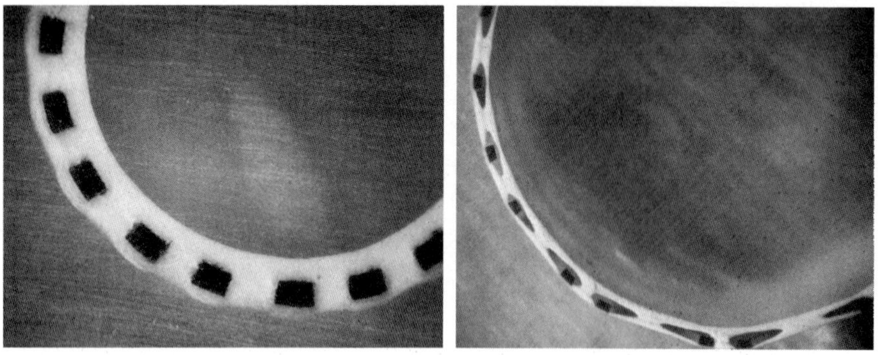

a. b.

Figure 2. Cross-sectional photomicrographs of the stent-grafts in **(a)** unexpanded (original magnification, ×10) and **(b)** expanded (original magnification, ×4) states. The unexpanded view demonstrates the complete encapsulation of the stent struts within the PTFE graft. After expansion, the graft material between the stent interstices is stretched, yet the stent remains encapsulated within PTFE. Small air pockets develop around the stent struts where the graft has been stretched. (Images courtesy of Christopher Banas, IMPRA, Tempe, Ariz.)

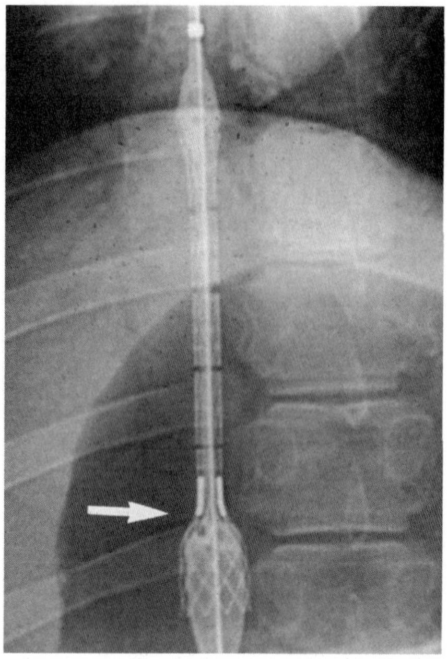

Figure 3. Spot radiograph demonstrates a stent-graft during dilation and deployment. Radiopaque markers indicate the leading edge of the graft material. The leading, partially bare portal stent expands first, anchoring the device within the portal vein (arrow). At 6 atm of inflation pressure, the graft was fully dilated (not shown).

and all subsequent animals were given a custom, low-protein diet. No heparin, oral anticoagulation, antiplatelet therapy, or antibiotics were administered beyond those given during the implant procedure.

Follow-up Shunt Venography

At approximately 1-month intervals, the animals were reanesthetized and percutaneous jugular access was achieved by means of the same or a contralateral vein. A 5-F, curved catheter was used to catheterize the shunts, and portal venography was performed in multiple projections. A final TIPS venogram was obtained before sacrifice. Percentage of shunt stenosis was calculated by measuring the narrowest portions of the shunts with use of a magnifying glass and reticle.

Histopathologic Examination

The original experimental protocol was designed to last 3 months. Two animals with a graft were sacrificed at 1 and 2 months, respectively, for early pathologic examination. Three animals were sacrificed at approximately 3 months. As the uninterrupted patency and lack of stenosis of the stent-grafts became evident, the three remaining animals were allowed to continue to 4, 4, and 5 months before sacrifice. The control group animals ($n = 4$) were sacrificed at 4–6 weeks because of shunt occlusion or almost complete midshunt, parenchymal tract stenoses.

Each animal was euthanized with an intravenous injection of Beuthanasia D solution (Schering-Plough Animal Health, Kenilworth, NJ). The liver, suprahepatic inferior vena cava, and portal vein were immediately removed en bloc. The shunts were gently flushed with saline, and the samples were placed into 10% neutral buffered formalin. Gross examination was performed shortly thereafter. Samples of liver parenchyma from the area of liver drained by the hepatic vein from which the TIPS was created were obtained in several cases. The shunts were cut open longitudinally, and gross observations were recorded and photographs obtained. The stent-graft samples were embedded within methyl methacrylate. Multiple, thin, longitudinal sections were cut along the graft from free portal vein to free suprahepatic inferior vena cava. The individual wires of the Wallstent control specimens were gently dissected free under a microscope. These specimens were sectioned in a manner similar to that of the graft specimens. Both groups were stained with hematoxylin-eosin, trichrome, and bile-specific stains.

RESULTS

All devices proved safe to introduce and accurate to deploy. The control stents and the grafts were delivered and deployed at their intended sites with 100% technical success. There were no complications attributable to either device. Tract measurement indicated that 8-cm-long grafts were required in each case. Thus, two trailing, 1.2-cm-long stents were cut from the graft, resulting in an overall initial length of 7.8 cm. The one episode of moderate hepatic encephalopathy resolved promptly with institution of our custom low-protein animal diet. All subsequent animals were automatically fed this diet after TIPS creation. Although elevated serum ammonia levels were demonstrable in some animals (as high as 95 mmol/L), there were no other detectable incidents of encephalopathy. All animals fed normally and gained weight proportional to their weight and frame.

Follow-up Venography

Stent-grafts.—Seven of eight grafts remained widely patent throughout the duration of the experiment without any venographic evidence of luminal narrowing or encroachment (Fig 4). In each case, there was demonstrable hepatopetal intrahepatic portal flow through the noncovered leading end of the portal vein stent. This confirmed that the bare, intraportal segment of the leading stent remained patent and allowed continued nutrient portal perfusion to the liver segment peripheral to the graft. In two cases, mild stenoses (12% and 15%, respectively) developed within the hepatic vein end of the graft. There was one graft occlusion at 3-month follow-up.

Control group.—At 4–6 weeks, one bare-stent TIPS was occluded. The remaining three control TIPS revealed intraparenchymal shunt stenoses measuring 45%, 65%, and 85%, respectively, at their narrowest portions.

Gross and Histopathologic Examination

Stent-grafts.—The explanted livers appeared normal at gross examination. The bare struts of the leading stents of the grafts were well incorporated within the walls of the patent portal veins. The interstices of the stents appeared free of tissue. The fully encapsulated trailing ends were all attached to the hepatic veins and inferior vena cava. Conversely, the midportions of the grafts were relatively loosely attached within the pa-

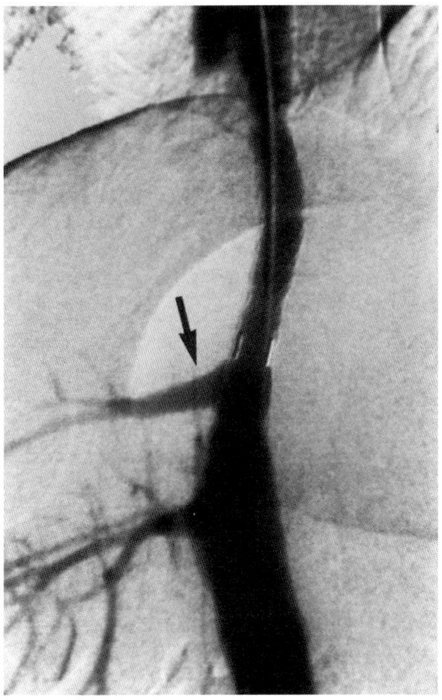

Figure 4. Five-month follow-up venogram demonstrates a fully patent shunt. A peripheral right portal vein branch receives flow through the bare interstices of the leading stent (arrow).

renchymal tract; while the 1-month specimen was anchored at the portal vein end, it appeared entirely unattached to the surrounding liver parenchyma. There were no gross differences between the hepatic lobe bearing the TIPS and the remainder of the liver. Gross examination of the lumina of the patent grafts demonstrated no visible thrombus or tissue accumulation within the graft lumina. There was no gross evidence of bile staining.

In the one case of stent-graft occlusion, the portion of graft that had lain across the hepatic vein ostium at deployment, was, at necropsy, found to lie approximately 1 cm deep within the hepatic vein. Because of the rapid growth of these animals, the hepatic vein (and liver) outgrew the upper end of the graft. A thick rind of fibrous tissue had developed around the graft ostium and grown down approximately 2 cm into the graft. This growth of fibrous tissue extended approximately 2 cm along the luminal surface of the graft toward the portal end, causing the occlusion (Fig 5). Notably, the majority of the graft (ie, the remainder that lay caudal to this tissue downgrowth) was free of stenosis or intraluminal tissue and was remarkable only for a small amount of postmortem thrombus.

There were several consistent features among all the grafts. Hematoxylin-eosin and trichrome stains indicated that a prominent, dense layer of myofibroblasts and collagen matrix had appeared along the abluminal surface of each stent-graft. Comparing 1-, 3-, 4-, and 5-month specimens, this tissue appeared to grow progressively thicker over time (Fig 6). In each case, this circumferential collar of tissue formed the boundary between the graft and the surrounding hepatic parenchyma. Similar tissue was present at the abluminal surfaces of the graft that lay within the hepatic vein. Hematoxylin-eosin, trichrome, and bile-specific stains revealed no evidence of bile staining or bile duct proliferation within the graft lumina, or in the hepatic tissues surrounding them. There was no evidence of noteworthy inflammatory or foreign body response. High-magnification views of the graft itself indicated that at 3 months, scattered collagen-producing fibroblasts were visible within the substance of the PTFE, presumably growing toward the lumen (Fig 7). Within the air pockets created around each stent strut by stretching of the graft were collections of red blood cells and myofibroblasts. In two cases (3- and 4-month explants), layers of collagen tissue grew down along the luminal surface of the graft from the hepatic vein end. These cells quickly tapered off and disappeared approximately 2 cm from the hepatic vein end of the graft (Fig 8). In only one case (a 4-month explant), a short, isolated segment of single-cell endothelium was identified within the lumen of the midportion of the graft (Fig 9).

The leading, partially bare stent at the portal end of the grafts was well incorporated within a thin layer of myofibroblasts and collagen matrix similar to those surrounding the intraparenchymal portions of the stent-graft. This tissue was lined by a single-cell layer of endothelium. Examination of the two cases in which an overlapping graft extension was placed at the hepatic venous end revealed no histologic differences from the single-thickness stent-grafts. In two animals, samples of the hepatic parenchyma that drained into TIPS-bearing veins were examined microscopically. The liver was normal. No findings could be attributed to complete obstruction of the hepatic vein outflow by the graft. In both cases, there was no evidence of congestive hepatopathy (ie, findings that could theoretically lead to partial Budd-Chiari syndrome).

Control group.—The explanted livers appeared normal at gross examination. The stent lumina were lined by a white tissue that was thickest at the middle, intraparenchymal portion of the shunt tract. Microscopic examination revealed a thick layer of myofibroblasts and collagen matrix enveloping the stents and narrowing the shunt lumen. The composition of these cell layers was identical to that seen surrounding the abluminal outer surface of the stent-grafts. No bile staining or bile duct proliferation was visible.

DISCUSSION

To assess the results of the tested device, it is first useful to consider the characteristics of an ideal TIPS stent-graft. These would include device flexibility, easy and trouble-free delivery and deployment, low profile, expansile force sufficient to withstand the recoil of hard cirrhotic liver parenchyma, and ability to be progressively expanded up to 12 mm in luminal diameter. As stent-grafts would be expected to cost more than bare stents, a device whose length is adjustable would obviate multiple overlapping stents. Last, graft biocompatibility and markedly improved, uninterrupted shunt patency are of paramount importance.

This device proved to possess several of these features. It provided some flexibility at the graft hinges, flexing to conform to the curved shunt tracts created within the soft porcine hepatic parenchyma. On the other hand, the intrinsic, high crush resistance of this stent allowed the stent-graft to easily reach and maintain the diameter to which it was balloon-expanded. This lack of recoil represents a theoretic advantage over existing self-expanding stents whose weaker hoop strength may require overdilation and buttressing with overlapping stents to maintain similar lumina. The device length can be customized in each case by cutting off individually encapsulated, 1.2-cm-long stents from the trailing end. In cases in which the graft length is underestimated, a short graft extension (eg, two to three graft-stents long) can be overlapped within the primary graft.

One of the disadvantages of this graft is the apparent need for sheathed delivery. As with Palmaz stents placed in other vascular applications, the safest and most secure method of device delivery is through a sheath or guiding catheter. This prevents the risk of migration of the stent as it is advanced to its intended location. In our application, we placed a 14-F 40-cm-long hemostatic sheath into the portal vein just before graft delivery. We did successfully deliver the graft in one case without a long sheath, though this was not our routine. While sheath placement in and of itself was not a difficult task, it does require the operator to create straighter TIPS tracts that are aimed toward the portal bifurcation. To some degree, this may become a more routine practice, as increasing numbers of TIPS are created in patients with severe ascites and severely shrunken livers. In such cases, one must often aim straight at the portal bifurcation to create the TIPS. In any event, in that delivery of this device limits the locations of potential portal vein puncture, this requirement can make the procedure more difficult for some operators. On the other hand, once delivered into position, the entire device was deployed as simply as a Palmaz stent within an iliac artery—it was highly radiopaque, fully expanded at 6 atm, and underwent little noticeable shortening. The combination of these features allowed very precise positioning.

Venographic follow-up indicated that the device provided exceptional improvement in preventing shunt stenosis (compared with control TIPS). Histologic study of the animals with grafts confirmed the venographic findings (ie, the near absence of any tissue encroachment on shunt lumina). In particular, the parenchymal, intervenous portions of the grafts (ie, the first areas to develop marked stenoses in swine TIPS lined by conventional stents) were free of any luminal tissue growth. Remarkably, the abluminal surfaces of the grafts were surrounded by a thick collar of myofibroblasts and collagen matrix. This tissue appears identical to the tissue enveloping both the bare-stent control TIPS and the human TIPS, except that it was prevented from encroaching on the shunt lumen by the barrier effect of the microporous graft (7,8). Furthermore, no bile staining or duct proliferation was seen in any of our cases. This is in sharp contrast to experience of Saxon et al (9), who, in a report of porcine and human TIPS, suggested that microscopic leaks of bile contributed to loss of shunt patency in a considerable proportion of swine, and by extension, humans.

Similarly, we previously documented venograpically demonstrable bile fistulas in TIPS patients who had repeated shunt thromboses (10). Nine of 200 consecutive patients undergoing prospective shunt venography had demonstrable biliary-to-TIPS fistulas and shunt-related thromboses at rates double that of the larger general cohort of TIPS patients (10). These dramatic cases represented only a small fraction of the overall population that developed shunt stenoses. Furthermore, our explant histologic analyses of human TIPS-containing livers have shown little or no evidence of biliary contribution to TIPS stenosis (7). In our opinion, this problem, while highly visible and prominent, accounts for only a small portion of shunt failures, as most cases require shunt revision for treatment of hepatic vein outflow stenosis. The differences between our experimental results and those of Saxon et al (9) are difficult to explain, but perhaps may be related to their use of a different breed of swine. In practical terms, these distinctions prove unimportant, as stenoses appear to develop in all uncovered porcine TIPS, regardless of the demonstration of bile leaks or duct proliferation.

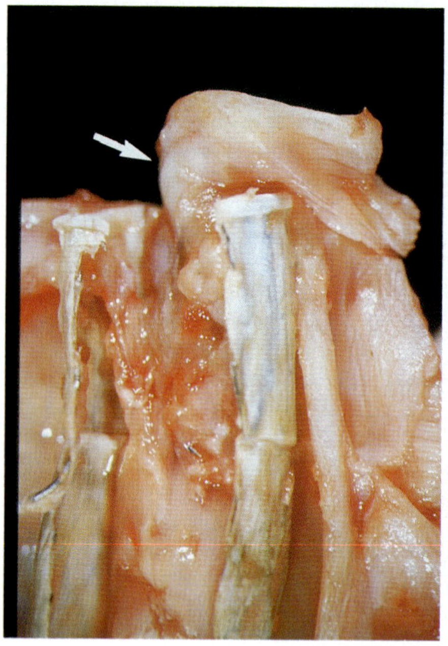

5.

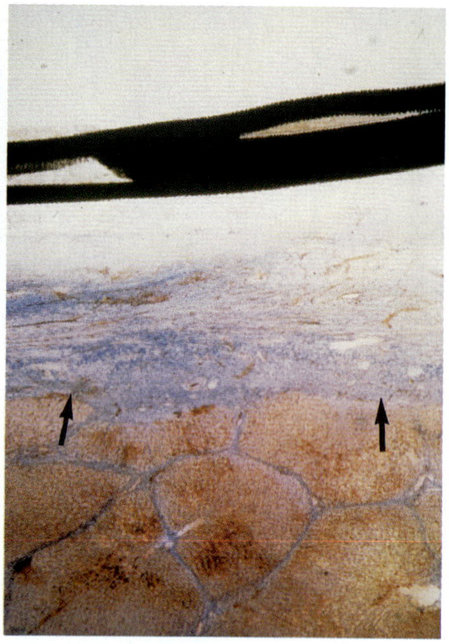

6.

Figures 5, 6. **(5)** Occluded TIPS. Photograph of a gross specimen of the hepatic venous end of a single, occluded stent-graft. A hyperplastic rind of fibroblastic hepatic venous tissue surrounds the upper end of the graft and extends down into the graft (arrow). **(6)** Patent TIPS. Photomicrograph of a longitudinal section of a patent 1-month stent-graft explant from a different animal. The luminal surface is at the top of the figure. The graft is not attached to the liver parenchyma. A thick collar of fibroblasts (arrows) has developed along the abluminal surface of the graft, separating it from the hepatic lobules. (Trichrome stain; original magnification, ×40.)

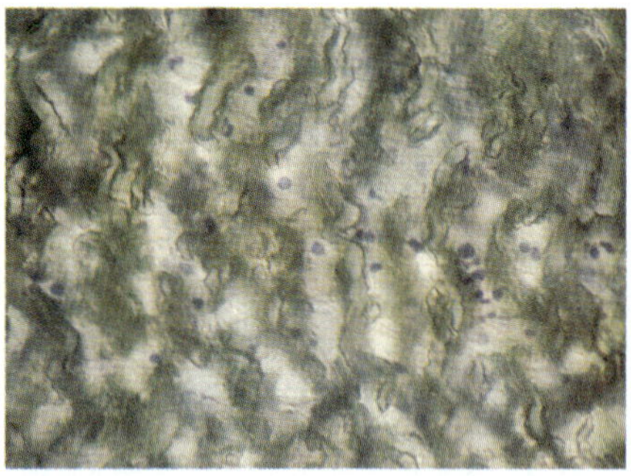

Figure 7. High-power magnification view of the graft from a 3-month explant demonstrates collagen tissue cells within the graft substance. (Trichrome stain; original magnification, ×400.)

Our demonstration of myofibroblast proliferation on the abluminal surfaces of the stent-grafts raises several interesting points. First, it suggests that the fibroblast response to TIPS creation is not necessarily dependent on lumen-borne substances, venous flow, or "jet" phenomena, because the stent-graft effectively separated the TIPS lumen from the reactive liver parenchyma. In our opinion, the parenchymal tissue proliferation is, in part, a healing response to massive local tissue injury that occurs with stretching and tearing of liver parenchyma during tract dilation and stent placement. As fibroblasts are abundant throughout the liver, it is not surprising that they proliferate after angioplasty and stent placement, a natural healing response of hepatic parenchyma. Second, the findings argue that the exclusionary effect of a biocompatible graft is one of the most important characteristics of a TIPS device. This is in contrast to the general objectives of arterial grafts placed within an extra- or endovascular setting. In these cases, an appropriate "healing response" would be charac-

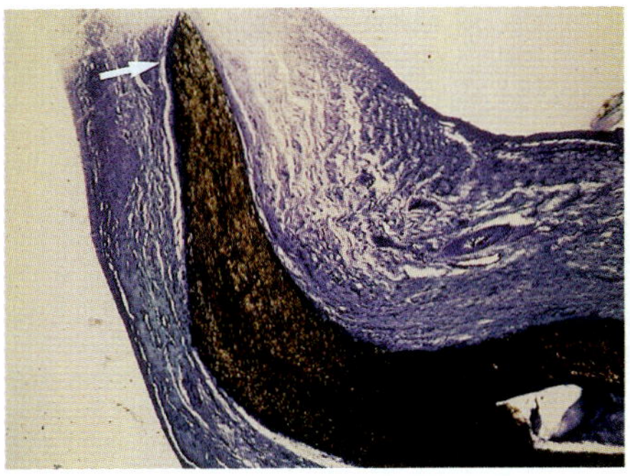

8a.

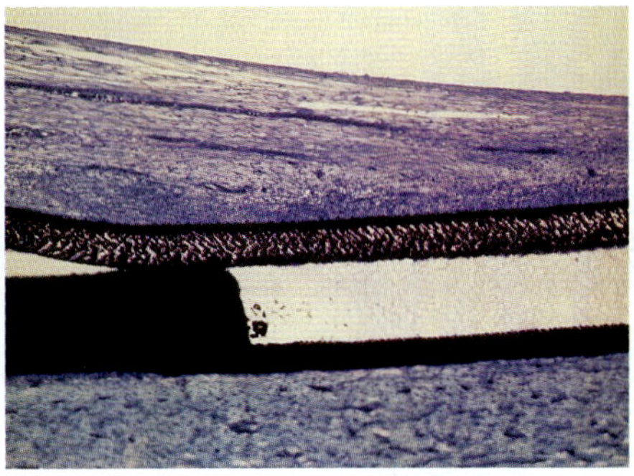

8b.

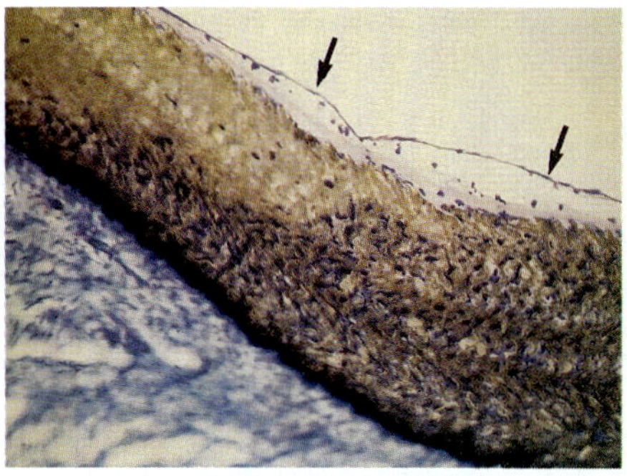

9.

Figures 8, 9. **(8)** Photomicrographs of two adjacent longitudinal sections of a 4-month stent-graft explant. (Trichrome stain; original magnification, ×40.) **(a)** Fibroblast cells from the inferior vena cava have grown over the free hepatic vein end of the graft (arrow) and along the luminal surface of the graft. **(b)** Fibroblast layer thins as it grows toward the midportion of the graft. The portal end is on the right, the caval end on the left. **(9)** Photomicrograph shows an isolated segment of endothelium within the midportion of a 4-month explant (arrows). (Trichrome stain; original magnification, ×40.)

terized by tissue ingrowth and incorporation of grafts within a continuous endothelial layer. In the case of TIPS, we would argue that a suitable "healing response" is reflected by relative absence or minimal tissue proliferation within the shunt lumen, and minimal foreign body giant cell reaction or other evidence of inflammation. This is an important gauge of device efficacy. Graft incorporation and endothelialization are irrelevant to TIPS; only durable, absolute shunt patency, and lack of hemodynamically significant shunt stenosis are important. In fact, it may be argued that limited graft incorporation may prove an advantage to a transplantation surgeon who might more readily dissect around and remove an errant TIPS graft that had extended too cephalad into the suprahepatic inferior vena cava.

One question debated among TIPS investigators and graft manufacturers is whether the trailing hepatic venous end of the device should be bare, to allow inflow from the stent-bearing hepatic vein. In our view, not grafting the entire TIPS length from portal entry site to hepatic vein ostium too narrowly focuses on the problem of parenchymal tract stenosis. This dangerously limits the potential patency of a TIPS stent-graft, as it leaves behind one of the major causes of shunt failure—outflow hepatic vein stenosis. This is, in our experience with human TIPS, the leading site of flow-limiting stenosis that warrants revision, not intraparenchymal tract stenosis. Our animal findings confirmed this problem, as well: Tissue downgrowth into the grafts led to complete shunt occlusion in one case and was microscopically detectable in other cases. In fact, tissue growth extending into the graft lumina from the inferior vena cava may well become the factor that ultimately limits the lumen of human TIPS grafts. In our experience, even a human intrahepatic transcaval portosystemic shunt created by using a gunsight approach (ie, a "TIPS" that entirely avoided the hepatic vein) showed early signs of typical fibroblast proliferation and ingrowth at the inferior vena cava.

One theoretic concern about partially or totally occluding a hepatic vein with a TIPS graft is causing "partial Budd-Chiari" syndrome. This term is somewhat of a misnomer because, unlike true Budd-Chiari syndrome, segmental hepatic vein thrombosis is infrequently associated with any clinical symptomatology (11,12). In fact, one can argue that the moderate to severe hepatic vein stenoses created by current bare-stent TIPS simulate segmental hepatic vein thrombosis by resulting in hepatofugal high-pressure flow within the stenotic outflow hepatic vein. To date, no clinical findings have been associated with this, other than those of recurrent portal hypertension. The promise of improved or uninterrupted TIPS patency may further lessen this risk by durably maintaining low portal and hepatic sinusoid pressures.

The PTFE used in our experiment proved a very suitable material for lining the TIPS. Its biocompatibility might be even better described as "bio-inertness." The material caused minimal or no tissue reaction in this model, and at a 30-µm mean internodal distance, allowed trivial tissue growth across the graft. This is the material that we have since attached to off-the-shelf stents when constructing and implanting our own human TIPS stent-grafts. Our ability to demonstrate nearly endless shunt patency and lack of shunt luminal stenosis with this PTFE-lined TIPS graft, however, does not prove that PTFE is the only suitable graft material for TIPS. Other materials have been tested and others remain to be evaluated. Tanihata et al (13) lined swine TIPS with silicone-impregnated Wallstents. Near 100% early thrombosis occurred, most likely reflecting the intrinsic inflammatory and thrombogenic nature of the silicone material, rather than its impermeability. Recently, we achieved more than 1 year of uninterrupted patency of a TIPS lined with nearly impermeable polyurethane (<7-µm porosity) in a patient with five previous thromboses and a biliary-to-shunt fistula (14). Grafts mated to more conventional materials such as polyethylene terephthalate, polycarbonate urethane, and other graft materials may prove similarly capable of improving TIPS patency. Some of these materials have characteristics that may make them more amenable to combination with metallic stents. Ultimately, though, our results strongly support and validate the concept of a TIPS stent-graft and provide a benchmark against which other such devices and grafts can be measured. ■

Acknowledgment: The authors thank their veterinary technician and anesthetist, Lee Barthel, for her valuable assistance.

References

1. Laberge JM, Somberg KA, Lake JR, et al. 2-year outcome following transjugular intrahepatic portosystemic shunt for variceal bleeding: results in 90 patients. Gastroenterology 1995; 108:1143–1151.
2. Haskal ZJ, Pentecost MJ, Soulen MC, Shlansky-Goldberg RD, Baum RA, Cope C. Transjugular intrahepatic portosystemic shunt stenosis and revision: early and midterm results. AJR 1994; 163:439–444.
3. Hausegger KA, Sternthal HM, Klein GE, Karaic R, Stauber R, Zenker G. Transjugular intrahepatic portosystemic shunt: angiographic follow-up and secondary interventions. Radiology 1994; 191:177–181.

4. Coldwell DM, Ring EJ, Rees CR, et al. Multicenter investigation of the role of transjugular intrahepatic portosystemic shunt in management of portal hypertension. Radiology 1995; 196:335–340.
5. Schenck E, Nelson JA, Starr FL, Coldwell DM. Animal model of portal hypertension with observations regarding the relationship between portal flow and pressure. Invest Radiol 1993; 28:442–445.
6. Nishimine K, Saxon RR, Kichikawa K, et al. Improved transjugular intrahepatic portosystemic shunt patency with PTFE-covered stent-grafts: experimental results in swine. Radiology 1995; 196:341–347.
7. Lehr S, Haskal ZJ, Furth EE, Gannon F. Histopathologic analysis of the biologic response to transjugular intrahepatic portosystemic shunts (TIPS) and proposal of a pathogenetic model (abstr). JVIR 1997; 8: 180.
8. LaBerge JM, Ferrel LD, Ring EJ, Gordon RL. Histopathologic study of stenotic and occluded transjugular intrahepatic portosystemic shunts. JVIR 1993; 4:779–786.
9. Saxon RR, Mendel-Hartvig J, Corless CL, et al. Bile duct injury as a major cause of stenosis and occlusion in transjugular intrahepatic portosystemic shunts: comparative histopathologic analysis in humans and swine. JVIR 1996; 7:487–497.
10. Haskal ZJ, Cope C, Soulen MC, et al. Biliary to transjugular intrahepatic portosystemic shunt fistula: cause of recurrent accelerated shunt occlusion (abstr). Radiology 1995; 197(P):180–181.
11. Beppu M, Fukuzaki T, Mitani K, Fujimoto K, Taniguchi S. Hepatic subsegmentectomy with segmental hepatic vein sacrifice. Arch Surg 1990; 125:1170–1175.
12. Cho KJ, Geisinger KR, Shields JJ, Forrest ME. Collateral channels and histopathology in hepatic vein occlusion. AJR 1982; 139:703–709.
13. Tanihata H, Kubota Y, Uchida BT, Pavcnik D, Saxon RR. Transjugular intrahepatic portosystemic shunt with silicone-covered Wallstents: results in an animal model (abstr). Radiology 1996; 201(P):141.
14. Haskal ZJ, Berkey GS, Furth EE, McAllister A. Experimental and early clinical evaluation of a custom polyurethane thin film coated stent (abstr). Radiology 1996; 201(P):379.

Francesco De Cobelli, MD • Angelo Vanzulli, MD • Sandro Sironi, MD • Renata Mellone, MD
Enzo Angeli, MD • Massimo Venturini, MD • Maria Paola Garancini, MD • Rita Quartagno, MD
Giuseppe Bianchi, MD • Alessandro Del Maschio, MD

Renal Artery Stenosis: Evaluation with Breath-hold, Three-dimensional, Dynamic, Gadolinium-enhanced versus Three-dimensional, Phase-Contrast MR Angiography[1]

PURPOSE: To compare breath-hold, three-dimensional, gadolinium-enhanced magnetic resonance (MR) angiography with three-dimensional, phase-contrast MR angiography in the evaluation of renal artery stenosis.

MATERIALS AND METHODS: Fifty-five consecutive adult patients with clinical suspicion of renovascular disease were prospectively examined with three-dimensional, phase-contrast MR angiography and breath-hold, three-dimensional MR angiography with injection of a standard dose of gadopentetate dimeglumine to evaluate the number of renal arteries and the presence and degree of stenosis. The standard of reference was intraarterial digital subtraction angiography.

RESULTS: Gadolinium-enhanced MR angiography depicted all 105 main renal arteries, whereas phase-contrast MR angiography depicted 104. The number of accessory renal arteries depicted was significantly higher with gadolinium-enhanced (17 of 18) than with phase-contrast (11 of 18) studies ($P = .04$). Both techniques depicted 27 of the 29 stenoses (sensitivity, 93%; $P > .05$). Sensitivities, specificities, and accuracies in the diagnosis of hemodynamically significant stenosis (>50% narrowing) were, respectively, 94%, 96%, and 96% for phase-contrast and 100%, 97%, and 98% for gadolinium-enhanced MR angiography ($P > .05$).

CONCLUSION: Gadolinium-enhanced MR angiography is superior to phase-contrast MR angiography in accessory renal artery depiction. No statistically significant difference in the assessment of stenosis has been found between the two techniques.

INTEREST in the identification of renovascular lesions in patients with hypertension and renal dysfunction has increased because of the availability and effectiveness of treatment with percutaneous transluminal angioplasty, endovascular stent placement, surgical revascularization, or some combination of these (1,2). Magnetic resonance (MR) angiography is performed increasingly often as a noninvasive method of examining patients suspected of having renovascular disease (3–17).

Studies on two- or three-dimensional time-of-flight and phase-contrast MR angiography have been reported on (3–17). Both techniques, however, have drawbacks related to blood inflow and blood motion: reduced sensitivity to in-plane blood flow owing to saturation effects with time-of-flight techniques and increased sensitivity to signal loss from intravoxel spin-phase dispersion owing to turbulent flow with phase-contrast techniques. Moreover, several studies (3–15) in which time-of-flight and phase-contrast MR angiography were used had high sensitivities and specificities for the depiction of proximal lesions but poor sensitivities and specificities for the depiction of accessory renal arteries and for the depiction of the segmental renal arteries. Recently, gadolinium-enhanced MR angiography has been introduced (18–21) for imaging the abdominal aorta and its major branches. By using a short repetition time and a short echo time, this technique may be performed with breath holding (19–21), which allows improved spatial resolution and image quality and shortening of imaging time. This technique is completely independent of flow artifacts and saturation problems.

Breath-hold, three-dimensional, gadolinium-enhanced, fast MR angiography of the renal arteries with a whole-volume body coil after injection of a double or triple dose of gadolinium-based contrast material, which increases cost, has been proposed (19–21). To our knowledge, there have been no prospective evaluations of the phased-array multicoil system in breath-hold, three-dimensional, gadolinium-enhanced, fast MR angiography in the renal arteries. The use of three-dimensional, phase-contrast MR angiography with phased-array multicoils in screening for renal artery stenosis has been described (17). Furthermore, to our knowledge, no dynamic studies with injection of a standard dose of gadolinium-based contrast material in the detection of renal artery stenosis have been reported on.

The aim of our prospective study was to evaluate the accuracy of breath-hold, three-dimensional MR

Index terms: Gadolinium • Magnetic resonance (MR), contrast enhancement, 961.12943 • Magnetic resonance (MR), phase imaging, 961.12942 • Magnetic resonance (MR), three-dimensional, 961.12942 • Magnetic resonance (MR), vascular studies, 961.12942 • Renal arteries, MR, 961.12942 • Renal arteries, stenosis or obstruction, 961.721

Abbreviations: DSA = digital subtraction angiography, MIP = maximum intensity projection, SPGR = spoiled gradient-recalled acquisition in the steady state.

Radiology 1997; 205:689–695

[1] From the Departments of Radiology (F.D.C., A.V., S.S., R.M., E.A., M.V., A.D.M.), Epidemiology (M.P.G.), and Nephrology (R.Q., G.B.), University Hospital, Scientific Institute San Raffaele, Olgettina 60, 20132 Milan, Italy. Received April 21, 1997; revision requested June 16; revision received July 10; accepted July 14. **Address reprint requests to** F.D.C.

Figure 1. Images obtained in a 55-year-old man with two left renal arteries. **(a)** Anteroposterior intraarterial DSA image shows one dominant artery and one inferior accessory artery (arrow). **(b)** Coronal, MIP, phase-contrast MR angiogram (33/6, 20° flip angle) shows both right and left main renal arteries; the inferior polar left renal artery is not evident because the origin of the accessory left renal artery is outside the three-dimensional imaging volume. **(c)** Coronal, MIP, gadolinium-enhanced MR angiogram (7/1.4, 40° flip angle) delineates the accessory left renal artery (long arrow) and shows a false-positive stenosis at the origin of the main left renal artery (short arrow).

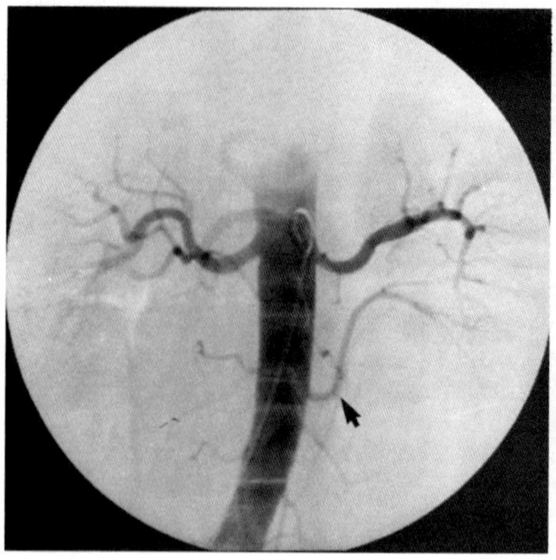

a.

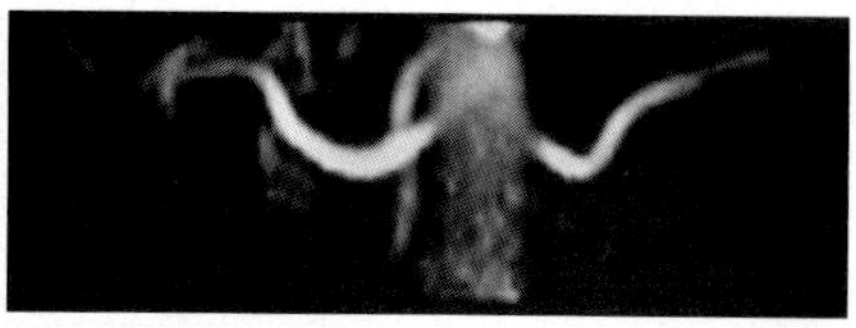

b.

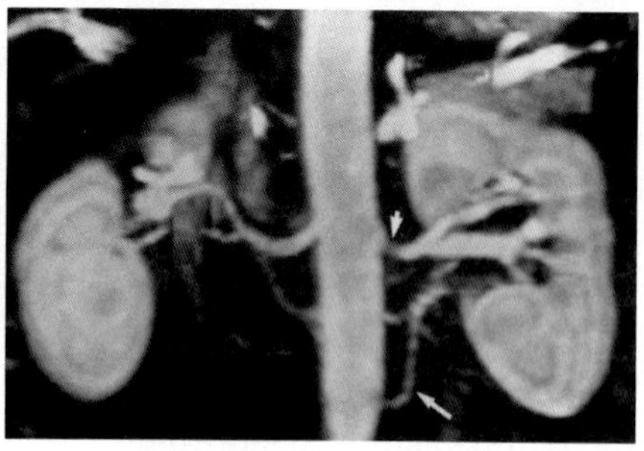

c.

angiography performed with a phased-array multicoil after injection of a standard dose of gadopentetate dimeglumine in the evaluation of renal artery stenosis and to compare the accuracy with that of three-dimensional, phase-contrast MR angiography in the same patients.

MATERIALS AND METHODS

Patients

From April 1996 to January 1997, 55 consecutive patients (29 men, 26 women; age range, 22–75 years; mean age ± standard error, 57 years ± 3) suspected on clinical grounds of having renal artery stenosis were enrolled in the study after they had given informed consent for MR angiography and digital subtraction angiography (DSA). Forty-eight of the 55 patients had hypertension; 11 patients had renal impairment. The mean serum creatinine level was 1.35 mg/dL (120 µmol/L; standard deviation, 1.15 mg/dL [100 µmol/L]; standard error of the mean, 0.22 mg/dL [20 µmol/L]; range, 0.61–6.0 mg/dL [50–530 µmol/L]).

MR Imaging Technique

Images were obtained with a 1.5-T superconducting magnet (Signa Horizon; GE Medical Systems, Milwaukee, Wis) by using an enhanced gradient system with a maximum gradient strength of 23 mT/m and a maximum gradient slew rate of $120\ T \cdot m^{-1} \cdot s^{-1}$. In all patients, version 5.5 operating system software (GE Medical Systems) was used. In all patients, the examination was performed with a phased-array multicoil (four-channel system; Torso-Coil; GE Medical Systems).

To localize the aorta and the ostia of the renal arteries and to evaluate the volume and the morphology of the kidneys, a breath-hold, T1-weighted, fast, multiplanar spoiled gradient-recalled acquisition in the steady state (SPGR) sequence was performed in the coronal and axial planes with the following parameters in all patients: 125/4.2 (repetition time msec/echo time msec), 90° flip angle, 10-mm section thickness, 256 × 192 data matrix (frequency × phase), 40-cm field of view, and one signal acquired. The image acquisition time was 20 seconds for each plane.

After fast, multiplanar, SPGR localizing images were obtained, axial, breath-hold, two-dimensional, phase-contrast images were acquired with different velocity-encoding rates to choose the optimal velocity-encoding rate for renal artery depiction. Imaging parameters were 25/8, 20° flip angle, 256 × 128 matrix, one signal acquired, 10-mm section thickness, 32–36-cm ¾ rectangular field of view (ie, the number of phase-encoding steps was reduced to ¾ of the whole field of view). Flow encoding was performed in all three directions (superoinferior, anteroposterior, and right-left). The acquisition time was 15 seconds for three sections. Flow-encoding velocities of 30, 40, 50, and 60 cm/sec were tried; the velocity with the best arterial depiction was chosen in each patient. In young patients with good cardiac output (24 patients), a velocity-encoding rate of 50 or 60 cm/sec was used; in patients with poor cardiac output, advanced age, and renal impairment (31 patients), the velocity-encoding rate was reduced to 30 or 40 cm/sec.

On the basis of findings of breath-hold, fast, multiplanar SPGR imaging and two-dimensional, phase-contrast imaging, MR angiograms were obtained with a three-dimensional, phase-contrast sequence in the transverse plane with the following parameters: 33/6, 20° flip angle, 16-kHz bandwidth, 2-mm section thickness with no intersection gap and with 28 partitions, 256 × 160 data matrix, 32–36-cm ¾ rectangular field of view, and one signal acquired. To suppress the venous signal from the inferior vena cava, an inferior transverse saturation band was used. The frequency-encoding gradient was from right to left and the velocity-encoding rate was 30–60 cm/sec. Flow encoding was performed in all three directions. The image acquisition time was 8 minutes for each slab.

After three-dimensional, phase-contrast MR angiography, coronal, breath-hold, three-dimensional, fast SPGR sequences were performed before, during, and after injection of gadopentetate dimeglumine (Magnevist; Schering, Berlin, Germany). For breath-hold imaging, the parameters were 7/1.4, 40° flip angle, 32-kHz bandwidth, 2-mm section thickness with no intersection gap and with 28 partitions, 256 × 160–192 data matrix, 40–48-cm ½ rectangular field of view, and one signal acquired. To avoid aliasing of patients' arms with the ½ field of view, the arms were positioned above the head. The imaging time was 21–23 seconds.

The unenhanced images were used as scout views to ensure the proper placement of the imaging volume.

Gadopentetate dimeglumine was injected intravenously through an 18-gauge catheter placed into an antecubital vein. A standard dose of contrast material (0.1 mmol/kg) was administered with a power injector (Spectris MR Injector; MedRad, Pittsburgh, Pa) at 2 mL/sec; this injection was immediately followed by 20 mL of normal saline at 2 mL/sec to complete delivery of the entire dose of contrast material and to flush the vein. Circulation time from the injection site to the renal arteries was calculated with an injection test in an attempt to achieve peak contrast enhancement during acquisition of the central third of k-space lines.

Multiple, sequential, single-level, two-dimensional, fast SPGR sequences were performed during gadopentetate dimeglumine injection every 1.2 seconds for 60 seconds with the following parameters: 7.9/1.3, 20° flip angle, 62.5-kHz bandwidth, 10-mm section thickness, 256 × 160 data matrix, 32–36-cm field of view, and one signal acquired. Image acquisition and the injection of a low dose of gadopentetate dimeglumine (2 mL), which was followed by the physiologic saline flush, were started at the same time; the delay time between the injection and the abdominal enhancement was calculated. To calculate the delay time, we used the following equation: delay time = estimated circulation time − ⅓ acquisition time. For example, in a patient with a circulation time estimated to be 20 seconds, the imaging was started 13 seconds after injection (acquisition time, 21 seconds). This injection technique was used to produce uniform arterial concentration during the central

Correlation between Intraarterial DSA, Phase-Contrast MR Angiographic, and Gadolinium-enhanced MR Angiographic Findings in Evaluating the Degree of Renal Artery Stenosis

MR Angiography	Intraarterial DSA: No Stenosis ($n = 94$)	Mild Stenosis ($n = 11$)	Severe Stenosis ($n = 16$)	Occlusion ($n = 2$)
Phase-contrast technique				
No stenosis	80	2	0	0
Mild stenosis	3	8	1	0
Severe stenosis	3	1	12	0
Occlusion	0	0	3	2
Gadolinium-enhanced technique				
No stenosis	89	2	0	0
Mild stenosis	1	9	0	0
Severe stenosis	3	0	16	0
Occlusion	0	0	0	2

Note.–Data are numbers of vessels.

k-space acquisition and to reduce the superimposition of veins.

The three-dimensional, phase-contrast and three-dimensional, gadolinium-enhanced images were reconstructed by using maximum intensity projection (MIP) techniques after regions of interest, which comprised only the aorta and renal arteries, were drawn. An MIP algorithm was used to provide angiographic projection from any desired viewing angle (usually with angle increments of 15°) around the long axis of the body. Also, multiplanar reconstruction and subvolume MIP images were obtained by reviewing the raw-data images to identify the minimum number of images required to demonstrate the renal arteries. In some cases, reformations were also performed in curved planes. A radiologist (F.D.C. or A.V.) blinded to the results of DSA selected the regions of interest and reconstructed the MIPs. The post-processing time was approximately 20 minutes in each patient.

MR Image Analysis

MR images were prospectively evaluated in conference by two of the authors (F.D.C., A.V.), who were blinded to the angiographic findings. The two readers had to reach a consensus on the following parameters: (*a*) the number of renal arteries depicted, (*b*) the presence of renal artery stenosis, and (*c*) the degree of stenosis. We used the following criteria to grade the stenoses: mild stenosis (<50% narrowing), severe stenosis (50%–99% narrowing), and occlusion (100% narrowing).

On three-dimensional, phase-contrast images, as in previous studies (3–17), absence of stenosis was defined as both a normal-diameter artery and a normal vessel signal. Mild stenosis was defined as a reduction in the arterial diameter without signal loss. Severe stenosis was defined as focal signal loss with distal reconstitution of flow. Vessel occlusion was defined as a complete lack of signal distal to the lesion (12).

On gadolinium-enhanced images, mild stenosis was defined as a reduction (<50%) in the arterial caliber; severe stenosis was defined as a hemodynamically significant reduction (>50%) in the diameter of the artery and normal arterial contrast material enhancement distal to the stenosis. Vessel occlusion was defined as the complete absence of contrast material enhancement.

Intraarterial DSA

All patients underwent intraarterial DSA (with model DVI-S; Philips Medical Systems, Best, The Netherlands) within 1 week of the MR examination. Intraarterial DSA was the standard of reference. DSA was performed by means of catheterization of the suprarenal abdominal aorta through the right or left femoral artery by using a 5-F pigtail catheter. Nonionic contrast material (Iopamiro [iopamidol]; Bracco, Milan, Italy; 300 mg of iodine per milliliter) was injected at 20 mL/sec for 2 seconds; images were obtained in the anteroposterior, left anterior oblique, and right anterior oblique projections. Twenty-eight of the 55 patients underwent selective renal DSA. In all cases, the DSA images were read by one expert interventional vascular radiologist (M.V.) blinded to the MR angiographic results. At substraction angiography, the same grading of renal artery stenosis used at MR imaging was adopted. The arterial stenosis was visually evaluated and graded.

Statistical Analysis

The sensitivity, specificity, accuracy, positive predictive value, and negative predictive value for the depiction of any degree of stenosis and for the depiction of a hemodynamically significant stenosis (>50% narrowing) were calculated for both techniques independently. The sensitivity and specificity for depicting stenosis or occlusion were calculated. Exact two-sided confidence limits for binomial proportions at the 95% level for sensitivity, specificity, accuracy, NPV, and PPV were calculated. To evaluate the differences in the depictions of the renal arteries and of the arterial stenoses on the three-dimensional, phase-contrast images and the gadolinium-enhanced images, the McNemar test was used.

RESULTS

Number of Renal Arteries

Intraarterial DSA revealed 123 renal arteries in the 55 patients. Fifty patients had two kidneys and five patients had a single kidney with one artery for a total of 105 main renal arteries. Multiple renal arteries were detected in 12 patients. DSA showed a total of 18 accessory arteries.

Three-dimensional, phase-contrast images showed 104 of the 105 main renal arteries. The main artery not detected at three-dimensional, phase-contrast MR angiography was outside the imaging volume because it was an artery of a pelvic kidney. Three-dimensional, gadolinium-enhanced MR angiography depicted all 105 main renal arteries seen at intraarterial DSA.

Of the 18 accessory renal arteries depicted at intraarterial DSA, 11 were depicted at phase-contrast MR angiography and 17 at gadolinium-enhanced MR angiography. One of these accessory arteries was missed with both MR angiographic techniques, owing to the small caliber. Of the other six accessory arteries missed at phase-contrast MR angiography, four arteries were outside the imaging volume (Fig 1) and two were too small in caliber to be seen with the technique. The number of accessory renal arteries depicted was significantly higher at gadolinium-enhanced studies than at phase-contrast studies ($P = .04$). No false-positive accessory renal artery was depicted with either technique.

Assessment of the Presence of Stenosis

The findings of both MR angiographic techniques in comparison with those of intraarterial DSA in the depiction of renal artery stenosis are summarized in the Table. Intraarterial DSA showed stenosis in 29 of 123 arteries. In the 29 renal artery stenoses, intraarterial DSA revealed 11 mild stenoses, 16 severe stenoses (Fig 2), and two occlusions. When 115 renal arteries depicted on phase-contrast MR angiograms are considered and the ability to identify the presence of stenosis is evaluated, there were 80 true-negative findings, two false-negative findings, 27 true-positive findings, and six false-positive findings. This yields a sensitivity, a specificity, and an accuracy of 93% (95% confidence intervals: 0.77, 0.99; 0.85, 0.97; and 0.87, 0.97, respectively), a positive predictive value of 82% (95% confidence interval: 0.65, 0.93), and a

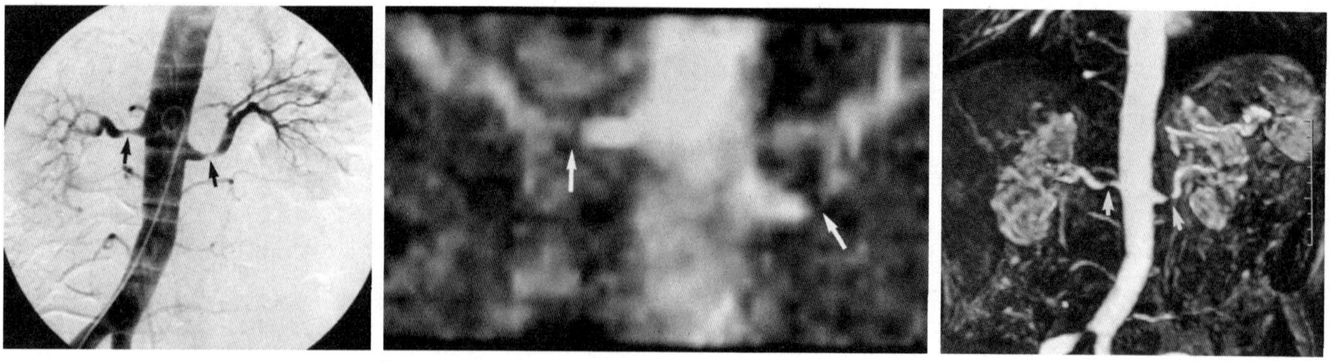

a. b. c.

Figure 2. Images obtained in a 62-year-old man. **(a)** Intraarterial DSA image documents severe bilateral stenoses of the right and left renal arteries (arrows). **(b)** Coronal, MIP, phase-contrast MR angiogram (33/6, 20° flip angle) and **(c)** coronal, gadolinium-enhanced MR angiogram (7/1.4, 40° flip angle) confirm the findings (arrows).

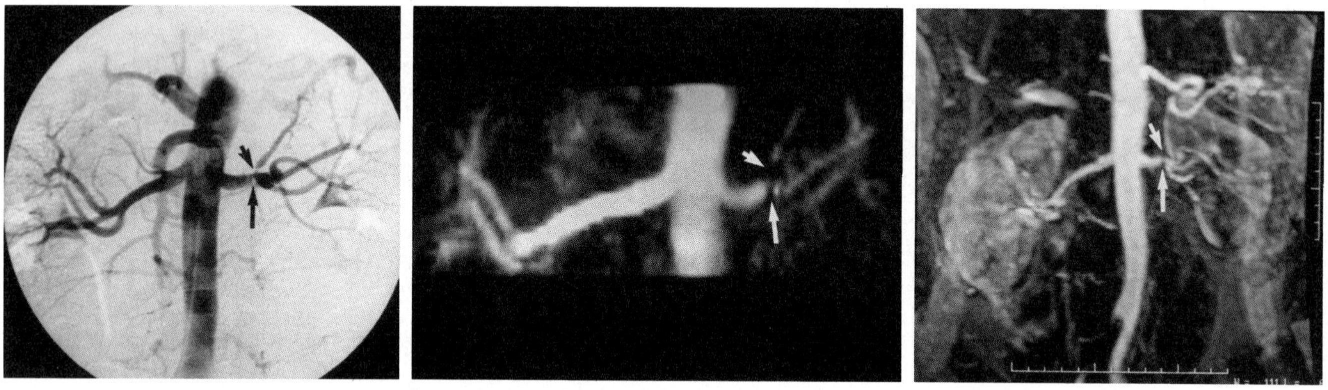

a. b. c.

Figure 3. Images obtained in a 36-year-old woman. **(a)** Anteroposterior intraarterial DSA image shows one fibromuscular dysplasia–induced left renal artery stenosis (long arrow) and one stenosis at one segmental branch of the left artery (short arrow). **(b)** Coronal, MIP, phase-contrast MR angiogram (33/6, 20° flip angle) and **(c)** coronal, MIP, gadolinium-enhanced MR angiogram (7/1.4, 40° flip angle) show the stenoses (long and short arrows).

negative predictive value of 98% (95% confidence interval: 0.91, 1.00). At phase-contrast MR angiography, three normal arteries were graded as mildly stenotic and three normal arteries were graded as severely stenotic. Two mild stenoses were graded as normal arteries.

Gadolinium-enhanced MR angiographic findings in the 122 depicted arteries were true-negative in 89 arteries, false-negative in two arteries, true-positive in 27 arteries, and false-positive in four arteries. These results yielded a sensitivity of 93% (95% confidence interval: 0.77, 0.99), a specificity of 96% (95% confidence interval: 0.89, 0.99), a positive predictive value of 87% (95% confidence interval: 0.70, 0.96), and a negative predictive value of 98% (95% confidence interval: 0.92, 1.00). The accuracy was 95% (95% confidence interval: 0.90, 0.98). At gadolinium-enhanced MR angiography, one normal artery was graded as mildly stenotic and three normal arteries were graded as severely stenotic. Two mild stenoses were graded as normal arteries. No difference between the two techniques ($P > .05$) in the assessment of all stenoses was found.

Twenty-four of the 29 lesions were in the proximal portions of the artery; the remaining five fibromuscular dysplasia–induced stenoses were in the distal portion of the main artery ($n = 3$), in the segmental branches ($n = 1$), or in both the main artery and the segmental branches ($n = 1$) (Fig 3). With regard to only the proximal main artery, both MR angiographic techniques correctly depicted 22 of 24 stenoses; with regard to the distal part of the main artery and the segmental arteries, all stenoses were correctly depicted with both techniques. Phase-contrast MR images showed one false-positive stenosis in the distal part of the main renal artery that was diagnosed as fibromuscular dysplasia (Fig 4).

Assessment of Hemodynamically Significant Stenosis

From a clinical point of view, we can consider together normal vessels and mildly stenotic vessels. In our series, intraarterial DSA revealed 18 vessels with hemodynamically significant stenoses (Fig 2). At phase-contrast MR angiography, which allowed us to distinguish severely stenotic renal arteries from normal or mildly stenotic renal arteries, 93 findings were true-negative, four were false-positive, 17 were true-positive, and one was false-negative; this yielded a sensitivity of 94% (95% confidence interval: 0.73, 1.00), a specificity of 96% (95% confidence interval: 0.90, 0.99), a positive predictive value of 79% (95% confidence interval: 0.58, 0.95), a negative predictive value of 99% (95% confidence interval: 0.94, 1.00), and an overall accuracy of 96% (95% confidence interval: 0.90, 0.99). One severe stenosis was undergraded as mild stenosis. Three normal arteries and one mild stenosis were incorrectly graded as severe stenoses.

For the detection of hemodynamically significant stenosis, findings of gadolinium-enhanced MR angiography were true-negative in 101 arteries, true-positive in 18 arteries, and false-positive in three arteries. There were no false-negative findings. These find-

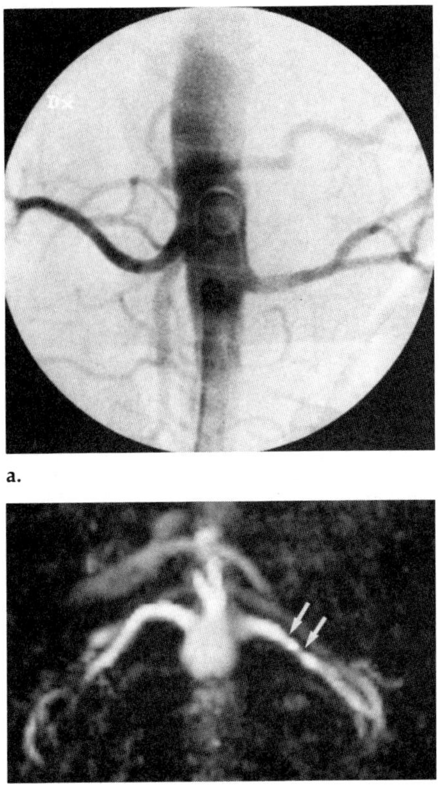

a.

c.

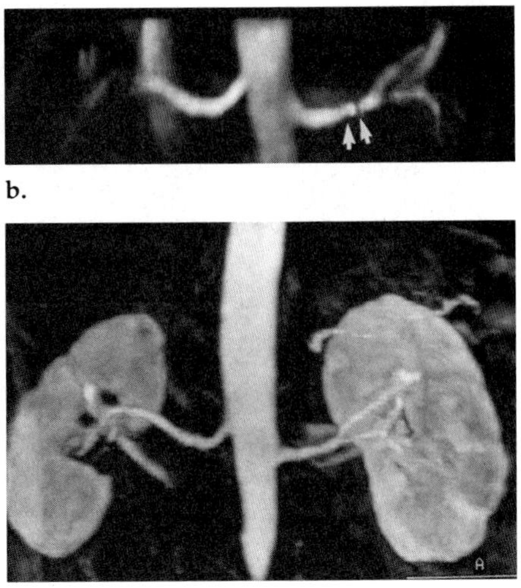

b.

d.

Figure 4. Images obtained in a 31-year-old woman. **(a)** Anteroposterior intraarterial DSA image shows normal, bilateral, single arteries. **(b)** Coronal, three-dimensional, phase-contrast MR angiogram (33/6, 20° flip angle) and **(c)** axial, MIP, phase-contrast MR angiogram (33/6, 20° flip angle) show focal reductions in diameter at the distal portion of the left renal artery (arrows); fibromuscular dysplasia–induced stenoses were incorrectly diagnosed (false-positive findings). **(d)** On the corresponding coronal, MIP, gadolinium-enhanced MR angiogram (7/1.4, 40° flip angle), the stenoses were not evident and this finding was correctly interpreted as negative (true-negative finding).

ings yielded a sensitivity of 100% (95% confidence interval: 0.82, 1.00), a specificity of 97% (95% confidence interval: 0.92, 0.99), a positive predictive value of 86% (95% confidence interval: 0.64, 0.97), and a negative predictive value of 100% (95% confidence interval: 0.96, 1.00). The accuracy was 98% (95% confidence interval: 0.93, 0.99). No difference between the two techniques ($P > .05$) in the assessment of hemodynamically significant stenoses was found.

With both techniques, the two occluded arteries were correctly depicted. In three cases, however, severely stenotic lesions were interpreted as occluded arteries at phase-contrast MR angiography (Fig 5); in these three cases, three-dimensional, gadolinium-enhanced MR angiographic findings were used to correctly classify the grade of the stenosis (Fig 5).

DISCUSSION

Three-dimensional, phase-contrast MR angiography seems to be a useful screening technique in patients suspected to have renal artery stenosis (3–5,10,11,14,16,17,22). Recent articles have reported good sensitivity in the detection of renovascular disease with systolically gated, three-dimensional, phase-contrast MR angiography (16,22) or three-dimensional, phase-contrast MR angiography with a phased-array multicoil (17). However, these techniques still have some limitations in the depiction of accessory renal arteries.

Our findings confirm that one drawback of three-dimensional phase-contrast MR angiography is the poor depiction of accessory renal vessels. In our series, seven of 18 polar arteries were not depicted with three-dimensional, phase-contrast MR angiography. In four cases, the origin of the accessory artery was outside the three-dimensional imaging volume; in three cases, the arteries were of a small caliber. Furthermore, one pelvic main renal artery was not visualized.

As reported in earlier articles (19–21), an important advantage of three-dimensional, dynamic, gadolinium-enhanced MR angiography is the ability to depict accessory renal vessels well, which is mainly because the whole abdominal aorta can be imaged. In our series, all but one accessory artery were prospectively depicted with this technique; the nondepicted artery was of small caliber, and identification was possible on a multiplanar retrospective-reconstruction view. We agree with Holland and colleagues (21) that simple MIP reconstruction is not sufficient for correct accessory renal artery depiction: Small vessels may be obscured by the superimposition of other larger vessels; thus, artery detection requires an accurate evaluation of source images, reformatted images, and multiplanar reconstructions.

Renal artery stenoses were correctly depicted in 27 of 29 cases with both techniques. In two cases, mild stenosis at the origin of the renal artery was not detected with either MR angiographic technique. As previously reported (11,17), a potential pitfall of three-dimensional, phase-contrast MR angiography is the blurring of the renal arteries during imaging, which is performed during shallow respiration. The blurring could mask mild stenosis when not associated with complex flow and intraluminal signal loss.

This also could be true for breath-hold, three-dimensional MR angiography: Respiratory motion due to the inability to hold one's breath for 20 seconds produces blurring artifacts and degrades the image quality; therefore, a mild reduction in the arterial caliber may be missed. Despite these two cases, as emphasized by Holland and colleagues (21), we believe that a breath hold of 20 seconds is reasonable in almost every patient. As previously reported (23), patients with any history of smoking, congestive heart failure, or chronic obstructive pulmonary disease had a mean breath hold of 25 seconds. Our imaging protocol was timed to have the contrast material bolus reach the renal arteries during acquisition of the central third of k-space lines with the techniques to minimize the blurring that can occur if the contrast material bolus is too concentrated in the central lines of k space itself. Before beginning our study, we tested higher rates of contrast material infusion (4–5 mL/sec) to obtain a concentrated bolus during acquisition of the central third of the k-space lines, but this injection protocol produced images degraded by blurring artifacts.

At three-dimensional, phase-contrast MR angiography, one severely stenotic lesion was graded as a mildly stenotic lesion. At fast, three-dimensional, gadolinium-enhanced MR angiography, all 18 severe stenoses were correctly graded. With these results, we can assume that negative findings of a gadolinium-enhanced angiographic study can reliably exclude a hemodynamically significant stenosis. In fact, in our series, MR angiography had 100% sensitivity and negative predictive value in the differentiation of normal or mildly stenotic vessels from hemodynamically significant stenoses. Furthermore, at gadolinium-enhanced MR angiography, correct differentiation between severely stenotic lesions and occluded arteries was always possible, whereas at three-dimensional, phase-contrast MR angiography severe stenoses were seen as occlusion in three cases. This can have a great clinical effect because severe stenoses are suitable for intraarterial DSA and for endovascular treatment, whereas occluded arteries are not.

Three-dimensional, phase-contrast MR angiographic findings were false-positive in six cases for the presence of stenosis and false-positive in four cases for the presence of hemodynamically significant stenosis. In agreement with findings in previous reports (4–8,11,17), some degree of overestimation with three-dimensional, phase-contrast MR angiography can be expected: In fact, signal loss from turbulent flow at the origin of a renal artery can be confused with luminal narrowing; furthermore, signal loss from turbulent flow distal to a stenosis will tend to increase the degree of stenosis. As suggested by de Haan and colleagues (16), the use of cardiac gating may suppress these artifacts, as well as blurring, because of the movement of the vessels during the cardiac cycle; therefore, diastolically gated, three-dimensional, phase-contrast techniques may reduce the number of overestimated lesions and may increase the specificity. However, de Haan and colleagues (16) did not find a statistically significant difference between techniques with cardiac gating and techniques without cardiac gating in the diagnosis of hemodynamically significant stenosis.

Also, at fast, three-dimensional, gadolinium-enhanced MR angiography, we found four false-positive stenoses. These data are in agreement with those of Snidow and colleagues (20), who found six false-positive stenoses in 55 normal main renal arteries with a specificity of 89%.

In our study, we introduced a protocol with injection of a standard dose of gadopentetate dimeglumine and with calculation of the circulation time from the injection site to the renal arteries on the basis of a previous test injection with a small amount of contrast material (2 mL). As reported by Earls and colleagues (24), arterial-phase, dynamic, gadolinium-enhanced MR angiography can be optimized by using a test examination and a power injector. In their work, the success rate in the experimental group of patients who underwent arterial-phase examination was 93% versus a success rate of 61% in the control group of patients who underwent manual injection of gadolinium-based contrast material without a test examination. With our protocol, we had good quality examinations in all patients and we could decrease the amount of gadopentetate dimeglumine (10–20 mL) and thus lower the costs. In fact, our results are comparable to those of Prince and colleagues (19), Snidow and colleagues (20), and Holland and colleagues (21), who administered at least a double or triple dose of contrast material (30–60 mL per patient).

In conclusion, our results suggest that breath-hold, dynamic, three-dimensional, MR angiography with injection of a standard dose of gadolinium-based contrast material is a fast and reliable method of imaging the renal arteries and of assessing renal artery stenosis. Unenhanced, three-dimensional, phase-contrast MR angiography showed lower accuracy in accessory vessel detection but similar results in renal artery stenosis depiction and will remain important because of the cost of contrast material. ■

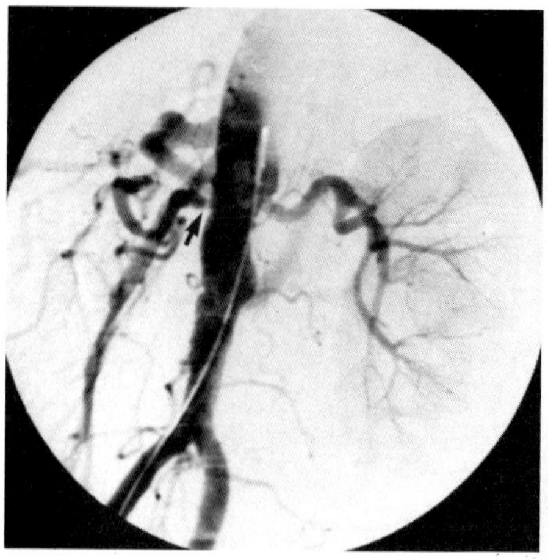

a.

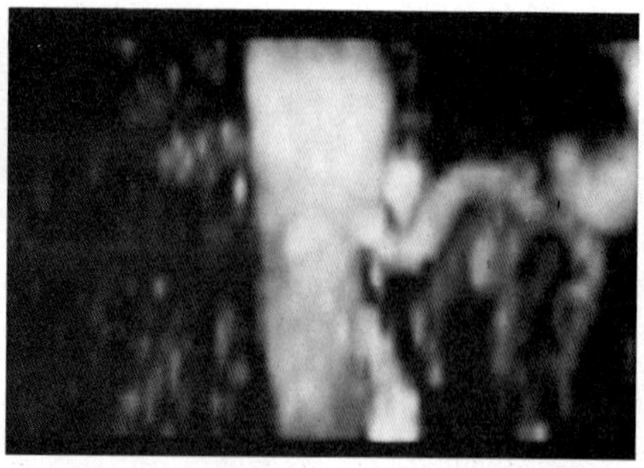

b.

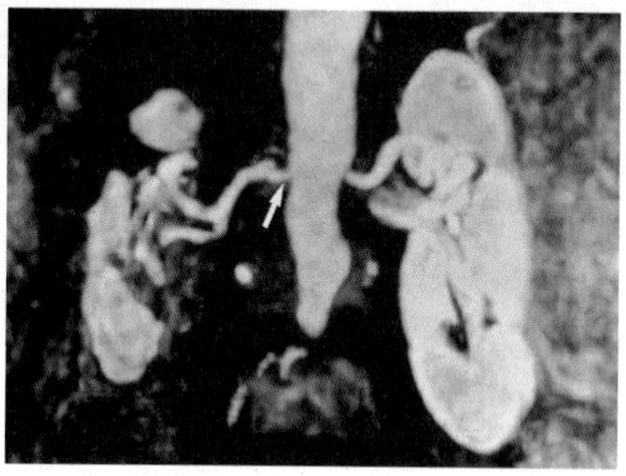

c.

Figure 5. Images obtained in a 67-year-old man. **(a)** Anteroposterior intraarterial DSA image shows one severe stenosis at the origin of the right renal artery (arrow). **(b)** On the coronal, MIP, phase-contrast MR angiogram (33/6, 20° flip angle), the severe stenosis was interpreted as occlusion owing to the complete absence of signal. **(c)** On the coronal, MIP, gadolinium-enhanced MR angiogram (7/1.4, 40° flip angle), the stenosis (arrow) was correctly graded.

References

1. Blum U, Krumme B, Flugel P, et al. Treatment of ostial renal artery stenoses with vascular endoprostheses after unsuccessful balloon angioplasty. N Engl J Med 1997; 336:459–465.
2. Weibull H, Berqvist D, Bergentz SE, Johnsson K, Hulthen L, Manhem P. Percutaneous transluminal renal angioplasty versus surgical reconstruction of atherosclerotic renal artery stenosis: a prospective randomized study. J Vasc Surg 1993; 18:841–852.
3. Gedroyc WM. Magnetic resonance imaging of renal arteries. Urol Clin North Am 1994; 21:201–214.
4. Debatin SF, Spritzer CE, Grist TM, et al. Imaging of renal arteries: value of MR angiography. AJR 1991; 157:981–990.
5. Kim D, Edelman RR, Kent KG, Porter DH, Skillman JJ. Abdominal aorta and renal artery stenosis: evaluation with MR angiography. Radiology 1990; 174:727–731.
6. Kent KG, Kim D, Edelman RR, et al. Magnetic resonance imaging: a reliable test for the evaluation of proximal atherosclerotic renal arterial stenosis. J Vasc Surg 1991; 13:311–818.
7. Squillaci E, Maspes F, Crecco M, Pocek M, Squillaci S, Simonetti G. Magnetic resonance angiography in the evaluation of anatomy and stenosis of the renal arteries. Radiol Med 1992; 84:282–289.
8. Loubeyre P, Revel D, Garcia P, et al. Screening patients for renal artery stenosis: value of three-dimensional time-of-flight MR angiography. AJR 1994; 162:847–852.
9. Carriero A, Magarelli N, D'Ettorre L, Severini S, Tartaro A, Bonomo L. Renal arteries: 3D TOF magnetic resonance angiography before and after Gd-DTPA. Radiol Med 1994; 87:254–259.
10. Zampa V, Mascalchi M, Battolla L, et al. Magnetic resonance angiography of the renal arteries at 0.5T: capabilities and limitations of the 2D phase-contrast technique. Radiol Med 1994; 88:415–419.
11. Grist TM. Magnetic resonance angiography of renal artery stenosis. Am J Kidney Dis 1994; 24:700–712.
12. Hertz SM, Holland GA, Baum RA, Haskal ZJ, Carpenter JP. Evaluation of renal artery stenosis by magnetic resonance angiography. Am J Surg 1994; 168:140–143.
13. Fellner C, Strotzer M, Geissler A, et al. Renal arteries: evaluation with optimized 2D and 3D time-of-flight MR angiography. Radiology 1995; 196:681–687.
14. Loubeyre P, Trolliet P, Cahen R, Grozel F, Labeeuw M, Tran Minh VA. MR angiography of renal artery stenoses: value of the

combination of three-dimensional time-of-flight and three-dimensional phase contrast MR angiography sequences. AJR 1996; 167: 489–494.
15. Borrello JA, Debiao L, Vesely TM, Vining EP, Brown JJ, Haacke EM. Renal arteries: clinical comparison of three-dimensional time-of-flight MR angiographic sequences and radiographic angiography. Radiology 1995; 197:793–799.
16. de Haan MW, Kouwenhoven M, Thelissen GR, et al. Renovascular disease in patients with hypertension: detection with systolic and diastolic gating in three-dimensional, phase-contrast MR angiography. Radiology 1996; 198:449–456.
17. De Cobelli F, Mellone R, Salvioni M, et al. Renal artery stenosis: value of screening with three-dimensional phase-contrast MR angiography with a phased-array multicoil. Radiology 1996; 201:697–703.
18. Prince MR. Gadolinium-enhanced MR aortography. Radiology 1994; 191:155–164.
19. Prince MR, Narasimham DL, Stanley JC, et al. Breath-hold gadolinium-enhanced MR angiography of the abdominal aorta and its major branches. Radiology 1995; 197:785–792.
20. Snidow JJ, Johnson MS, Harris VJ, et al. Three-dimensional gadolinium-enhanced MR angiography for aortoiliac inflow assessment plus renal artery screening in a single breath hold. Radiology 1996; 198: 725–732.
21. Holland GA, Dougherty L, Carpenter JP, et al. Breath-hold ultrafast three-dimensional gadolinium-enhanced MR angiography of the aorta and the renal and other visceral abdominal arteries. AJR 1996; 166: 971–981.
22. Wasser MN, Westenberg J, van der Hulst VPM, et al. Hemodynamic significance of renal artery stenosis: DSA versus systolically gated three-dimensional phase-contrast MR angiography. Radiology 1997; 202: 333–338.
23. Gay SB, Sistrom CL, Holder CA, Suratt PM. Breath-holding capability of adults: implications for spiral computed tomography, fast-acquisition magnetic resonance imaging, and angiography. Invest Radiol 1994; 29:848–851.
24. Earls JP, Rofsky NM, DeCorato DR, Krinsky GA, Weinreb JC. Hepatic arterial-phase dynamic gadolinium-enhanced MR imaging: optimization with a test examination and a power injector. Radiology 1997; 202:268–273.

Research Trainee Prizes from the 1997 RSNA Scientific Assembly and Annual Meeting

In 1994, the RSNA Program Committee, chaired by William M. Thompson, MD, began a new program to recognize the contribution of residents to the RSNA Scientific Assembly and Annual Meeting: the Research Trainee Prize. Each subcommittee of the Program Committee may award one prize each year for the best paper presented by a resident at the RSNA scientific assembly. The Research Trainee Prize consists of $1,000 and a certificate to the individual trainee.

The 1997 Research Trainee Prizes were presented to:

David A. Roberts, MD, PhD
University of Pennsylvania Medical Center
Philadelphia, Pa
"MR Imaging of Human Cerebral Perfusion Using Arterial Spin-tagging: Quantitative Comparison of Results Obtained at 1.5T and 4T" (paper 180)

Arvinder Uppal, MD
Albany Medical Center, Albany, NY
"Clinically Significant Internal Derangement of the Knee: Comparison of Rates of Occurrence at MR Imaging in Patients Referred by Orthopedic versus Non-Orthopedic Specialties" (paper 194)

Jeannette M. Spilde, MD
University of Wisconsin Hospital & Clinics
Madison, Wis
"Evaluation of an Experimental Low-Attenuation Gastrointestinal Contrast Agent for the CT Diagnosis of Intestinal Ischemia and Animal Model" (paper 612)

Babita Jha, MD
Albany Medical College, Albany, NY
"Comparison of Imaging Factors for Tc-99m and In-111 Somatostatin Analogues" (paper 919)

Patricia Tai, MB, BS
London Regional Cancer Centre, London, Ontario, Canada
"Consistency of Target Volume Delineation in Cervical Esophageal Cancer" (paper 1081)

Constantinos T. Sofocleous, MD
St Luke's Roosevelt Hospital, New York, NY
"Initial Clinical Comparison of the Amplatz Thrombectomy Device to the Modified Pulse Spray Pharmacomechanical Thrombolysis in the Treatment of the Thrombosed Hemodialysis Access Graft: Review of 126 Procedures" (paper 1289)

Naoki Takahashi, MD
L.B. Johnson Hospital, Houston, Tex
"Unenhanced Helical CT of Ureterolithiasis: Can CT Predict the Clinical Outcome?" (paper 1544)

Joseph Shemesh, MD • Enrique Z. Fisman, MD • Alexander Tenenbaum, MD, PhD • Sara Apter, MD
Liviu Leibovitch, MD • Samuel Rath, MD • Yacov Itzchak, MD, PhD • Michael Motro, MD

Coronary Artery Calcification in Women with Syndrome X: Usefulness of Double-Helical CT for Detection[1]

PURPOSE: **To determine the usefulness of double-helical computed tomography (CT) for detection of diseased coronary arteries in women with anginal pain, positive exercise stress test results, and angiographically normal coronary arteries (syndrome X).**

MATERIALS AND METHODS: **Double-helical CT of the coronary arteries was performed in 81 consecutive women who were referred for coronary angiography for evaluation of chest pain. Patients were classified into three groups according to stress test and angiographic results: normal (normal exercise test results and angiographically normal coronary arteries), syndrome X (abnormal exercise test results and angiographically normal coronary arteries), and coronary artery disease (at least one diseased vessel seen at angiography).**

RESULTS: **The prevalence of coronary calcification in the syndrome X group was 63% (10 of 16 patients) compared with 96% (45 of 47 patients) in the coronary artery disease group (P = .002) and 22% (four of 18 patients) in the normal group (P = .02). The lowest total coronary calcification score and logarithmic transformed data were found in the normal group (2.9 ± 0.7), statistically significantly higher values were found in the syndrome X group (4.3 ± 1.5), and the highest values were found in the coronary artery disease group (5.1 ± 2.0; for trend, P = .03).**

CONCLUSION: **Double-helical CT may be useful in detection of atherosclerosis in women with syndrome X who demonstrate normal coronary arteries at angiography.**

Syndrome X is defined by the triad of anginal pain, positive exercise stress test results, and angiographically normal coronary arteries (1). The mechanisms responsible for this disorder remain largely speculative. It has been suggested that syndrome X actually includes several heterogeneous clinical entities (2–4). The existence and extent of atherosclerosis of the coronary arterial wall in cases of syndrome X is underestimated substantially with coronary angiography, as demonstrated at intravascular ultrasound (US) performed in small groups of patients (5,6). Intravascular US is obviously of limited clinical use because it is an invasive technique. Fast computed tomographic (CT) techniques such as electron-beam (7) and double-helical (8) CT provide a well-established, noninvasive method for detection of coronary calcification, which is a reliable indicator of advanced atherosclerosis (9,10).

The purpose of this study was to evaluate prospectively the usefulness of double-helical CT in diagnosis of angiographically undetected atherosclerosis in the coronary arterial wall in women with syndrome X.

MATERIALS AND METHODS

Study Population

Of 94 consecutive women who underwent coronary angiography for assessment of chest pain, 81 women (age range, 52–78 years; mean, 64 years) gave informed consent for coronary CT and were included in the study. Double-helical CT was performed within 3 months after angiography (mean, 1.1 months). The patients were classified into three groups according to angiographic and exercise test results. The first group (normal) comprised 18 women with normal exercise test results and angiographically normal coronary arteries, defined as completely patent and a smooth appearance at angiography. The second group (syndrome X) comprised 16 women with abnormal exercise test results and normal coronary arteries. The third group (coronary artery disease) comprised 47 women who had lesions that were depicted in at least one epicardial vessel; 40 of these patients had obstructive lesions (50% stenosis or greater) and seven had nonobstructive lesions (less than 50% stenosis). For each patient, exercise test results and the presence of risk factors for coronary artery disease such as smoking, hypertension, diabetes mellitus, hyperlipidemia, and family history of coronary artery disease were recorded. The mean number of risk factors per patient in each study group was calculated.

Double-Helical CT

Image acquisition.—CT was performed according to a previously described protocol (8) with a commercially available double-helical scanner (CT Twin; Elscint Ltd, Haifa, Israel) and spiral scanning mode (without injection of contrast material). Scanning time was 1 second for two contiguous 2.5-mm sections and 15–22 seconds for the entire zone of interest. CT scans were acquired while the patient performed a single, unforced breath hold. The effective section thickness was 3.2 mm with a reconstruction increment of 3 mm. The total duration of the procedure was 10

Index terms: Arteriosclerosis, 548.76 • Computed tomography (CT), helical, 548.12115 • Coronary vessels, calcification, 548.812 • Coronary vessels, CT, 548.12115 • Syndrome X, 548.812

Radiology 1997; 205:697–700

[1] From the Cardiac Rehabilitation Institute (J.S., E.Z.F., A.T., L.L., M.M.), the Department of Diagnostic Imaging (S.A., Y.I.), and the Heart Institute (S.R.), Chaim Sheba Medical Center, 52621 Tel-Hashomer, Israel; and the Sackler Faculty of Medicine, Tel-Aviv University, Israel (J.S., E.Z.F., A.T., L.L., M.M.). Received April 28, 1997; revision requested June 5; revision received July 7; accepted July 8. **Address reprint requests to** J.S.

minutes. For scoring of calcification, the 20 most cephalic contiguous sections were selected, starting at the level of the first visible coronary artery: the left main coronary artery or the left anterior descending artery. Selection of these sections provided 6-cm coverage of the proximal portion of the coronary arterial tree as measured along the longitudinal axis of the patient.

Determination of coronary artery calcification.—A calcific lesion within a coronary artery was defined as an area of calcification of at least 0.5 mm^2 in which the CT attenuation was above a threshold of 90 HU. Regions of interest were placed around all lesions by an experienced reader (J.S.) and were analyzed automatically by the software of the CT unit. With application of a modification of the scoring method by Agatston et al (7) in which a threshold of 90 HU rather than 130 HU was used, an attenuation factor for each lesion was determined: 1 = 90–199 HU; 2 = 200–299 HU; 3 = 300–399 HU; and 4 = 400 HU or greater. A score for each region of interest was calculated automatically by multiplying the attenuation factor by the area. The total coronary calcification score was the combined sum of the lesion scores for all 20 sections. The reader had no knowledge of patient clinical and angiographic data.

Coronary Angiography

All patients underwent coronary angiography performed in multiple oblique projections with standard techniques. All luminal narrowing in each of the three epicardial coronary arteries was measured and compared with adjacent and apparently uninvolved arterial segments. The angiograms were reviewed independently by two experienced angiographers (A.T., S.R.) who were blinded to the clinical and double-helical CT data.

Stress Test

Exercise testing was performed in all patients with the standard Bruce protocol (11). The test was terminated before the maximal heart rate was reached if the patient demonstrated severe fatigue, angina, depression of the ST segment of 3 mm or greater, systolic blood pressure of 240 mm Hg or greater, diastolic blood pressure of 120 mm Hg or greater, or a decrease in systolic blood pressure. A 12-lead electrocardiogram was obtained and blood pressure was measured before exercise, at each minute interval during the test, and during the 5 minutes of recovery time. Downsloping or horizontal depression of the ST segment of 1 mm or greater that occurred at 60 msec after the J point in at least two consecutive leads were considered a positive test result.

Statistical Analysis

Statistical analysis was performed with SAS software (SAS Institute, Cary, NC) (12). Continuous variables were presented as the mean value ± standard deviation; categorical variables were presented as percentages. The χ^2 test and the Fisher exact test (two-tailed) were used to determine statistically significant differences between proportions. Logarithmic transformation was used to overcome nonsymmetric distribution of the total coronary calcification score. Comparison between groups, including tests for linear trend, was performed with analysis of variance by using the SAS procedure GLM. A P value less than .05 was considered statistically significant.

Table 1
Clinical Characteristics of Patients in the Three Study Groups

Characteristic	Normal* (n = 18)	Syndrome X (n = 16)	Coronary Artery Disease† (n = 47)
Age (y)	63 ± 9.0	64 ± 7.0	64 ± 8.0
Risk factors for coronary artery disease	1.2 ± 0.8	1.1 ± 0.7‡	2.2 ± 1.3

Note.—Numbers are expressed as the mean ± standard deviation.
* For Tables 1–3, indicates women with chest pain, normal exercise test results, and smooth vessels seen at angiography.
† For Tables 1–3, indicates patients with angiographically proved coronary artery disease, including seven patients with vessel stenosis less than 50% and 40 patients with stenosis of 50% or more. Only 45 women with coronary calcification are included in Tables 2 and 3.
‡ P = .67 compared with the normal group and P = .04 for the coronary artery disease group.

RESULTS

The clinical characteristics of the study groups are presented in Table 1. The mean age of the women in the three groups was similar. The mean number of risk factors for coronary artery disease was similar for women in the normal (1.2 ± 0.8) and syndrome X (1.1 ± 0.7) groups (P = .67) and was statistically significantly higher for women in the coronary artery disease group (2.2 ± 1.3, P = .04). Figure 1 shows the prevalence of coronary artery calcification in the study groups. Statistically significant differences were observed among the groups: Women with syndrome X had a prevalence of coronary artery calcification (63%, 10 of 16 women) three times greater than that for women in the normal group (22% [four of 18 women], P = .02) and lower than that in women with angiographically demonstrated coronary artery disease (96% [45 of 47 women], P = .002).

The number of epicardial coronary vessels with calcification was also different among the groups (P = .03 for syndrome X compared with coronary artery disease and P = .10 for syndrome X compared with normal) and the distribution among the women with coronary artery calcification is shown in Table 2. CT measurements obtained in the 59 patients in whom coronary calcification was found are shown in Table 3. The lowest values for total coronary calcification score and logarithmic transformed data were obtained for the normal group (2.9 ± 0.7), statistically significantly higher values were obtained for the syndrome X group (4.3 ± 1.5), and the highest total coronary calcification scores were found in the coronary artery disease group (5.1 ± 2.0; for trend, P = .03).

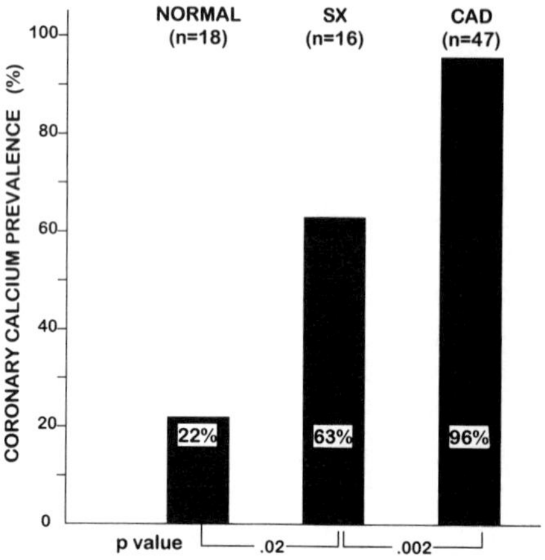

Figure 1. Graph shows the prevalence of coronary calcification in the three study groups. *CAD* = coronary artery disease, *SX* = syndrome X.

Figure 2a demonstrates typical advanced calcification depicted at double-helical CT in a woman with syndrome X despite the angiographically normal coronary arteries depicted in Figure 2b.

DISCUSSION

A cornerstone of syndrome X is the angiographic demonstration of normal coronary arteries in patients with angina and positive stress test results. On an angiogram, however, which is considered a "luminogram," atherosclerotic changes within the arterial wall are underestimated. Therefore, the definition of normality, based solely on angiographic criteria, is far

Table 2
Distribution of Epicardial Coronary Arteries with Calcification among the Study Groups

No. of Calcified Epicardial Vessels	Normal (n = 4)	Syndrome X (n = 10)	Coronary Artery Disease (n = 45)
1	4 (100)	3 (30)	7 (16)
2	0	6 (60)	13 (29)
3	0	1 (10)	25 (55)

Note.—P = .03 for comparison of findings in the syndrome X and coronary artery disease groups, and P = .1 for comparison of results in the syndrome X and normal groups (χ^2 test).

Table 3
CT Measurements among the Women with Coronary Calcification

Measurement	Normal (n = 4)	Syndrome X (n = 10)	Coronary Artery Disease (n = 45)
Total coronary calcium score			
Median	20.3	105.5	265.5
Range	6–34	4–602	1–3,163
Logarithmic transformed data (mean ± standard deviation)	2.9 ± 0.7	4.3 ± 1.5	5.1 ± 2.0

Note.—For trend, P = .03.

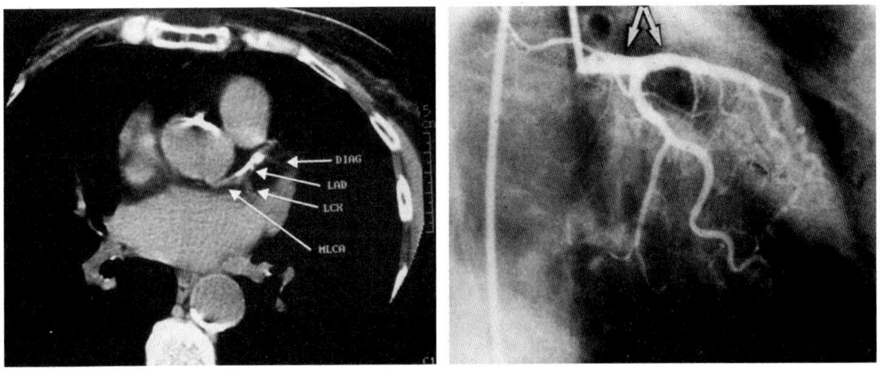

a. b.

Figure 2. **(a)** Double-helical CT scan obtained in a 68-year-old woman with syndrome X shows advanced calcification in the proximal part of the left anterior descending artery (*LAD*) despite a normal appearance at angiography. *Diag* = diagonal branch, *LCX* = left circumflex coronary artery, *MLCA* = main left coronary artery. **(b)** Angiogram shows the segment (between arrows) that corresponds to the calcification detected at double-helical CT.

from ideal: Atheromatosis is primarily a disease of the vascular wall that is visible at angiography only when the disease invades the lumen. Furthermore, the luminal diameter may not be affected, since plaque formation is accompanied by compensatory enlargement (remodulation) of the vessel (13,14). In addition, coronary atherosclerosis remains undetected at angiography if a diffuse process caused a narrowing of the entire vessel lumen (15).

Histopathologic studies have demonstrated that calcific lesions in the coronary artery wall are a specific indicator of atherosclerosis (9,10,16). New-generation fast CT enables accurate detection and measurement of these lesions (7,8).

Our data show that almost two-thirds of the women with syndrome X in our study population had coronary calcification, indicating the presence of an advanced stage of atherosclerosis despite angiographically smooth vessels. Arteries with atherosclerotic changes have been shown to constrict during exercise, while normal coronary arteries dilate (17,18). This mechanism of exercise-induced narrowing of diseased arteries is one of the pathogenic hypotheses that may help explain the occurrence of anginal attacks in the absence of obstructive coronary artery disease in women with syndrome X. This narrowing might be caused by endothelial damage and/or dysfunction, with insufficient production of endothelium-derived relaxing factor (19,20). Morever, since pain may occur without any changes in coronary artery blood flow, it is possible that these patients have an increased perception of pain (21). Other investigators underscore the importance of factors such as small-vessel disease (22), estrogen deficiency (23,24), sympathetic overactivity, and insulin resistance (25).

In our study, we used a noninvasive method to evaluate the arterial wall. The main finding from our study is that advanced calcified atherosclerosis of the coronary arterial wall was present in 63% of the women with syndrome X compared with only 22% of women in the normal group (patients with chest pain, normal exercise stress test results, and normal coronary arteries). These findings are in keeping with those from recent studies of intravascular US in which coronary arterial wall abnormalities were reported to be present in a substantial number of patients with syndrome X. Wiedermann et al (6) used intravascular US to examine 30 patients with syndrome X and found that 18 (60%) of the patients had atherosclerotic changes in the coronary artery wall. They also reported abnormal vasoconstriction with exercise in patients with atheromatous diseased vessels compared with patients with normal walls in whom vasodilation occurred in response to exercise. Using a noninvasive technique, we demonstrated a similar prevalence of abnormal coronary arteries.

One of the clinical applications of examination of coronary vessels with double-helical CT is accurate diagnosis of angiographically normal coronary arteries in elderly women (26). This application for double-helical CT is based on the well-accepted concept (27) that angiographically obstructive disease is very unlikely in the absence of coronary artery calcification. Thus, we recommend that women with anginal chest pain and abnormal exercise stress test results should undergo examination with double-helical CT before a thallium stress test or coronary angiography; use of CT could save unnecessary catheterization whenever coronary artery calcification is absent.

Syndrome X occurs predominantly in postmenopausal women (28). Our study group, biased by the fact that the patients were referred for coronary angiography, comprised women older than 50 years of age, and in this group of patients was a large subset of patients with coronary artery calcification. Further studies should be performed to clarify whether the prevalence of coronary artery calcification is higher also in patients with syndrome X who are younger than 50 years of age. Syndrome X is generally considered a relatively benign clinical entity, is associated with a good prognosis, and only limited therapy is necessary (29,30). However, atherosclerosis of the coronary artery wall may lead to altered endothelial-dependent vasomotion and reduced coronary flow reserve (31). Therefore, we believe that women who have anginal pain, positive exercise stress test results, and normal coronary angiographic findings (but demonstrate coronary calcification at double-helical CT) should receive antiatherosclerotic therapy and probably antiischemic therapy. To what extent the presence of coronary artery calcification changes the prognosis in these patients is another important question that needs investigation.

In conclusion, a substantial number of the women in whom syndrome X was diagnosed exhibited calcified coronary atherosclerosis at double-helical CT despite angiographically smooth vessels. Thus, double-helical CT may be a useful technique for identification of this subset of patients among women with syndrome X. ■

References

1. Kemp HG, Vokonas PS, Cohn PF, Gorlin R. The anginal syndrome associated with normal coronary arteriograms: report of a six year experience. Am J Med 1973; 54:735–742.
2. Cannon RO III, Epstein SE. "Microvascular angina" as a cause of chest pain with angiographically normal coronary arteries. Am J Cardiol 1988; 61:1338–1343.
3. Cannon RO, Camici PG, Epstein SE. Pathophysiological dilemma of syndrome X. Circulation 1992; 85:883–892.
4. Camici PG, Marraccini P, Lorenzoni R, et al. Coronary hemodynamics and myocardial metabolism in patients with syndrome X: response to pacing stress. J Am Coll Cardiol 1991; 17:1461–1470.
5. St Goar FG, Pinto FJ, Alderman EL, et al. Intravascular ultrasound imaging of angiographically normal coronary arteries: an in vivo comparison with quantitative angiography. J Am Coll Cardiol 1991; 18:952–954.
6. Wiedermann JG, Schwartz A, Apfelbaum M. Anatomic and physiologic heterogeneity in patients with syndrome X: an intravascular ultrasound study. J Am Coll Cardiol 1995; 25:1310–1317.
7. Agatston AS, Janowitz WR, Hildner FJ, Zusmer N, Viamonte M, Detrano R. Quantification of coronary artery calcium using ultrafast computed tomography. J Am Cardiol 1990; 15:827–832.
8. Shemesh J, Apter S, Rozenman J, et al. Calcification of coronary arteries: detection and quantification with double-helix CT. Radiology 1995; 197:779–783.
9. Blankenhorn D. Coronary arterial calcification: a review. Am J Med Sci 1961; 242: 1–9.
10. Warburten R, Tampas J, Soule A, Taylor HI.Coronary artery calcification: its relationship to coronary artery stenosis and myocardial infarction. Radiology 1968; 91:109–115.
11. Bruce RA, Hornsten TR. Exercise stress testing in evaluation of patients with ischemic heart disease. Prog Cardiovasc Dis 1969; 11:371–390.
12. SAS Institute. SAS/STAT user's guide, version 6. 4th ed. Cary, NC: SAS Institute, 1990; 2:1072–1126.
13. Glagov S, Weisenberg E, Zarins CK, Stankunacicius K, Kolettis GJ. Compensatory enlargement of various human atherosclerotic arteries. N Engl J Med 1987; 316:1371–1375.
14. White CW, Wright CB, Doty DB, et al. Does visual interpretation of the coronary arteriogram predict the physiological importance of coronary stenosis? N Engl J Med 1984; 310:819–824.
15. De Feyter PJ, Serruys PW, Davis MJ, Richardson P, Lubsen J, Oliver MF. Quantitative coronary angiography to measure progression and regression of coronary atherosclerosis: value, limitation and implication for clinical trials. Circulation 1991; 84:412–423.
16. McCarthy JH, Palmer FJ. Incidence and significance of coronary artery calcification. Br Heart J 1974; 36:499–506.
17. Cox DA, Vita JA, Treasure CB, et al. Atherosclerosis impairs flow-mediated dilatation of coronary arteries in humans. Circulation 1989; 80:458–465.
18. Chesbro JH, Fuster V, Webster MWI. Endothelial injury and coronary vasomotion. J Am Coll Cardiol 1989; 14:1191–1192.
19. Zeiher AM, Drexler H, Wollschlaeger H, Saurbier B, Just H. Coronary vasomotion in response to sympathetic stimulation in humans: importance of the functional integrity of the endothelium. J Am Coll Cardiol 1989; 14:1181–1190.
20. Quyyumi AA, Cannon RO, Panza JA, Diodati JG, Epstein SE. Endothelial dysfunction in patients with chest pain and normal coronary arteries. Circulation 1992; 86: 1864–1871.
21. Chauhan A, Mullins PA, Thuraisingham SI, Taylor G, Petch MC, Scofield PM. Abnormal cardiac pain perception in syndrome X. J Am Coll Cardiol 1994; 24:329–335.
22. Kaski JC, Tousolis D, Galassi AR, et al. Epicardial coronary artery tone and reactivity in patients with normal coronary arteriograms and reduced coronary flow reserve (syndrome X). J Am Coll Cardiol 1991; 18:50–54.
23. Gruchow HW, Anderson AJ, Barboriak JJ, Sobocinski KA. Postmenopausal use of estrogen and occlusion of coronary arteries. Am Heart J 1988; 115:954–963.
24. Rosano GMC, Collins P, Kaski JC, Lindsay DC, Sarrel PM, Poole-Wilson PA. Syndrome X in women is associated with oestrogen deficiency. Eur Heart J 1995; 16:610–614.
25. Dean JD, Jones CJH, Hutchinson SJ, Peters JR, Henderson AH. Hyperinsulinemia and microvascular angina ("syndrome X"). Lancet 1991; 337:456–457.
26. Shemesh J, Tenenbaum A, Fisman EZ, et al. Absence of coronary calcification on double-helical CT scans: predictor of angiographically normal coronary arteries in elderly women? Radiology 1996; 199:665–668.
27. Wexler L, Brundage B, Crouse J, et al. Coronary artery calcification: pathophysiology, epidemiology, imaging methods, and clinical implications—a statement for health professionals from the American Heart Association. Circulation 1996; 94:1175–1192.
28. Kaski JC, Rosano GMC, Collins P, Nihoyannopoulos P, Masseri A, Poole-Wilson PA. Cardiac syndrome X: clinical characteristics and left ventricular function—long-term follow-up study. J Am Coll Cardiol 1995; 25:807–814.
29. Opherk D, Schuler G, Wetterauer K, Manthey J, Schwarz F, Kubler W. Four-year follow-up study in patients with angina pectoris and normal coronary arteriograms ("syndrome X"). Circulation 1989; 80:1610–1616.
30. Radice M, Giudici V, Marinelli G. Long-term follow-up in patients with positive exercise test and angiographically normal coronary arteries. Am J Cardiol 1995; 75: 620–621.
31. Gage JE, Hess OM, Murakami T, et al. Vasoconstriction of stenotic coronary arteries during dynamic exercise in patients with classic angina pectoris: reversibility by nitroglycerin. Circulation 1986; 73:865–876.

Elizabeth G. McFarland, MD • James A. Brink, MD[2] • John Loh, BS • Ge Wang, PhD[3]
Vincent Argiro, PhD[4] • Dennis M. Balfe, MD • Jay P. Heiken, MD • Michael W. Vannier, MD[3]

Visualization of Colorectal Polyps with Spiral CT Colography: Evaluation of Processing Parameters with Perspective Volume Rendering[1]

PURPOSE: To evaluate two key processing steps for detection of colon polyps with spiral computed tomographic (CT) colography with perspective volume rendering (PVR): image reconstruction and opacity assignment of the attenuation data.

MATERIALS AND METHODS: Spiral CT was performed in 10 patients with known polyps confirmed at colonoscopy, and detailed quantitative analyses were performed of data obtained in four. First, anatomic fidelity of three-dimensional (3D) images generated from two-dimensional (2D) source images with *equal* voxel dimensions (87%–90% overlap) was compared with 3D images generated from 2D source images with *unequal* voxel dimensions (0%–80% overlap). Next, the relative dimensions of colorectal polyps to adjacent structures were evaluated for various opacity threshold settings. Then, step and sigmoidal opacity functions were compared with respect to image smoothness and edge sharpness.

RESULTS: PVR images generated after interpolation of image data reconstructed with at least 60% overlap were equivalent in image quality to PVR images generated from source images with equal voxel dimensions. Relative polyp-to–haustral fold dimensions demonstrated substantial distortions with opacity thresholds below −700 HU. The 3D PVR images generated with the sigmoidal opacity function were significantly smoother than those generated with the step opacity function (paired t test, $P < .02$), with small differences noted in edge sharpness.

CONCLUSION: Use of highly overlapping source images (87%–90%) was not necessary to generate 3D PVR images of colorectal polyps. Image artifacts were suppressed with use of an appropriate opacity threshold and a sigmoidal opacity function without substantial loss in edge sharpness.

SPIRAL computed tomographic (CT) colography is a rapidly evolving technology that provides computer-simulated, three-dimensional (3D) endoscopic visualization of the colon mucosa to allow polyp detection (1–9). Noninvasive colon cancer screening with this technique has the potential to increase compliance, reduce costs, and improve diagnostic performance compared with current practice. Prior reports have demonstrated promising preliminary results with use of various two-dimensional (2D) and 3D techniques (1–9).

The ability to acquire thin-section, volumetric data sets with helical CT has led to the expanded use of 3D volume rendering with this application (6–8). Volume rendering is a recent advance that offers distinct advantages over 3D rendering techniques such as maximum intensity projection or shaded surface display (6,11,12). Since volume rendering preserves attenuation information from each voxel in the original data set, this technique is not subject to the potential information loss encountered in maximum intensity projection or to the thresholding errors present in shaded surface display. Although volume rendering is more computationally intensive currently, recent improvements in computer graphics hardware and software enable interactive viewing, formerly practical with only shaded surface display.

For endoscopic visualization of a luminal surface, such as the colon, the additional feature of perspective volume rendering (PVR) is essential. PVR allows distinction between objects of equal size located at different distances from the observer. Rubin et al initially used PVR to help detect polyps in the colon, and they pointed out that multiple processing parameters, each with many degrees of freedom, need to be optimized for clinical application (6). More extensive evaluation of the influence of various 3D processing parameters on image display is necessary to optimize clinical protocols.

The purpose of this study was to evaluate systematically two key steps in the image processing of spiral CT colographic data for polyp detection with use of PVR: (*a*) image reconstruction and (*b*) assignment of opacity for each voxel within the imaging volume. Results were based on qualitative examination of image quality and quantitative measures of polyp-to–haustral fold dimensions, image smoothness, and edge sharpness.

Index terms: Colon, CT, 75.12115 • Colon, neoplasms, 75.311 • Computed tomography (CT), image processing • Computed tomography (CT), three-dimensional • Images, analysis, 75.12115

Abbreviations: FWHM = full width at half maximum, PVR = perspective volume rendering, 3D = three-dimensional, 2D = two-dimensional.

Radiology 1997; 205:701–707

[1] From the Mallinckrodt Institute of Radiology, Washington University School of Medicine, 510 S Kingshighway Blvd, St Louis, MO 63110. Received April 1, 1997; revision requested May 9; revision received August 8; accepted August 11. Supported in part by grants from General Electric and the Association of University Radiologists, the American Cancer Society Institutional Review grant 363804, the Washington University Cancer Center, and the National Institutes of Health grant R29, DK50184. **Address reprint requests to** E.G.M.

V.A. is an officer in Vital Images (Minneapolis, Minn), which develops and markets the VoxelView software used in this study.

[2] Current address: Department of Radiology, Yale University School of Medicine, New Haven, Conn.
[3] Current address: Department of Radiology, University of Iowa, Iowa City.
[4] Current address: Vital Images, Minneapolis, Minn.

MATERIALS AND METHODS

Image Acquisition

After obtaining institutional review board consent, we performed spiral CT in 10 patients (five men and five women; mean age, 63 years) with known colorectal polyps. Patients underwent a standard 24-hour preparation for colonoscopy before the CT examination. The patients were placed supine, and CT examinations of the abdomen and pelvis were performed with spiral CT (Somatom-Plus 4; Siemens Medical Systems, Iselin, NJ) after air insufflation of the colon, with sequential exposures lasting up to 30 seconds (120 kV, 292 mA). Findings were confirmed with colonoscopy performed the same day.

Histographic analyses were performed of the data obtained in all 10 patients, and detailed quantitative analyses were performed of the data obtained in four of the patients. Of the latter patients, two underwent scanning with 5-mm collimation and a pitch of 1, and two with 3-mm collimation and a pitch of 2. These acquisition techniques were chosen to provide sufficient anatomic coverage to image the colon and sufficient longitudinal resolution to help detect clinically relevant polyps 1 cm or more in diameter. Longitudinal resolution is considered adequate when the effective section thickness is less than or equal to the polyp diameter, as long as overlapping images are reconstructed (13,14). The effective section thickness is 5 mm for the acquisition with 5-mm collimation and pitch of 1 and is 3.9 with 3-mm collimation and pitch of 2 (15).

Image Reconstruction

Reconstruction parameters in scans obtained in four patients were chosen to achieve an in-plane voxel dimension of 0.5 mm (zoom, 2.0) and a longitudinal voxel dimension of 0.5 mm (reconstruction interval, 0.5 mm). For scans obtained of each polyp, data from the source images with equal voxel dimensions generated directly from the raw projection data were then selectively loaded to vary the longitudinal dimension. Specifically, data from every other, every fourth, every sixth, and every eighth image were loaded to simulate image reconstruction with longitudinal voxel dimensions of ×2, ×4, ×6, and ×8 in-plane voxel dimensions, respectively. Linear interpolation of these reconstructed image data sets was then performed at the workstation to achieve equal voxel dimensions. Thus, 3D images with equal voxel dimensions generated directly from the raw projection data were compared with those obtained after linear interpolation of source images with unequal voxel dimensions (0%–80% overlap [percentage overlap = EST − reconstruction interval/EST, where EST = effective section thickness]).

3D PVR (VoxelView, version 2.5.2; Vital Images, Minneapolis, Minn) was performed for all images on an independent imaging workstation (Impact; Silicon Graphics, Mountain View, Calif) after linear interpolation of image data. For all images obtained in each patient, an identical view angle, orientation, and position of the colon polyp were prescribed in the orthogonal 2D images to obtain an identical 3D PVR image of the polyp. The full 12-bit range of data were used for this comparison. To properly control other variables, all images were generated with the same step opacity function and standardized beige color map assignment.

All images from the four data sets were reviewed qualitatively at the workstation by two investigators (E.G.M., J.A.B.). Differences in the anatomic detail of polyps and surrounding structures relative to the appearance on images with the highest degree of overlap in each data set were assessed by consensus, with a 4-point scale (1 = no, 2 = mild, 3 = moderate, and 4 = marked degradation).

Opacity Assignment

An important processing step for 3D volume rendering is optimization of the opacity map with which specific levels of opacity are assigned to each attenuation value measured by the CT scanner. The vertical axis of the opacity map represents the scale of opacity values, ranging from 0% to 100% (completely transparent to completely opaque). The opacity assignment is a function common to 3D volume rendering algorithms that greatly influences image display.

First, the histographic distribution of attenuation data was evaluated in all 10 patients. After determining that the frequency distribution of attenuation data across those patients was consistent, we performed selective variation of the opacity threshold with a step function on the 3D PVR images of each of the four polyps generated from source images with equal voxel dimensions (0.5-mm in-plane and longitudinal-plane voxel dimensions), with use of the full 12-bit range of data. The use of a step function set at 100% opacity creates an absolute threshold assignment of the attenuation data, similar to that in shaded surface display. This was done intentionally to restrain the degrees of freedom in this variable, as a first step in determining the optimal opacity threshold. For each polyp, a set of 3D PVR images were generated with use of incremental opacity thresholds ranging from −500 to −900 HU. All images from the four data sets were qualitatively assessed by two investigators (E.G.M., J.A.B.), and differences in image distortion of specific anatomic structures relative to that on the images with the highest threshold value in each data set were assessed by consensus, with a 4-point scale (1 = no, 2 = mild, 3 = moderate, and 4 = marked distortion).

For one image, sufficient surrounding anatomic features of the polyp head, stalk, and haustral folds were present to correlate with an endoscopic image with similar orientation acquired during colonoscopy. In this polyp, relative measures of the width of the colon polyp and a surrounding haustral fold were performed for the various opacity threshold settings, with the standard of reference provided by similar measurements performed on the colonoscopic image of the polyp. The relative ratio of the polyp width to the haustralfold width was used as a comparison rather than an absolute measurement, owing to the lack of an internal measurement standard in both CT colography and fiberoptic colonoscopy. Selective variation of the upper threshold was also performed, and images were inspected visually for image degradation.

After estimating the lower opacity threshold, we then compared the shape of the opacity function between a step function and a sigmoidal function. The sigmoidal function was drawn to be symmetric around this lower threshold, with a half width at 95% maximum of 180 HU. On the basis of the results of the reconstruction analysis, images were used from the two data sets obtained with 5-mm collimation and pitch of 1 (60% overlap) and the two data sets obtained with 3-mm collimation and pitch of 2 (74% overlap). In addition, to increase rendering speed and to employ the results of the threshold experiment, these images were remapped to 8 bits (window, −850 to 275 HU). This permitted exclusion of attenuation values below −850 HU and permitted centering of the opacity curve over the appropriate range of −600 to −700 HU. In these data sets, a step and a sigmoidal opacity function were each applied to generate two different 3D PVR images of the polyp for each data set (total, four pairs).

To quantify image smoothness between the image pairs generated for each data set, a texture analysis method was applied (16). Five identically matched regions of interest representing areas of homogeneous background were identified in each image pair. For each region of interest, neighboring-pixel difference images were computed along the horizontal and vertical axes, respectively. The histograms of these two difference images were then computed, averaged, and normalized (to unit area) for each original rendered image. The histographic mean (texture index) was then computed as a measure of the roughness of the mucosal surface. By definition, the smaller the texture index the more homogeneous and smoother the image.

To quantify differences in edge sharpness between the sigmoidal and step 3D PVR images, the full width at half maximum (FWHM) of the first derivative of the edge attenuation profile was determined to serve as a measure of the edge sharpness (17). A total of five 1-pixel-wide attenuation profiles were measured perpendicular to the edge of the polyp in each 3D PVR image, with use of software in the public domain (Image, version 1.60; National Institutes of Health, Betheseda, Md). The spatial derivatives of the profiles were obtained, and FWHM was determined for each image.

The means of both the texture and edge sharpness analyses were calculated for the

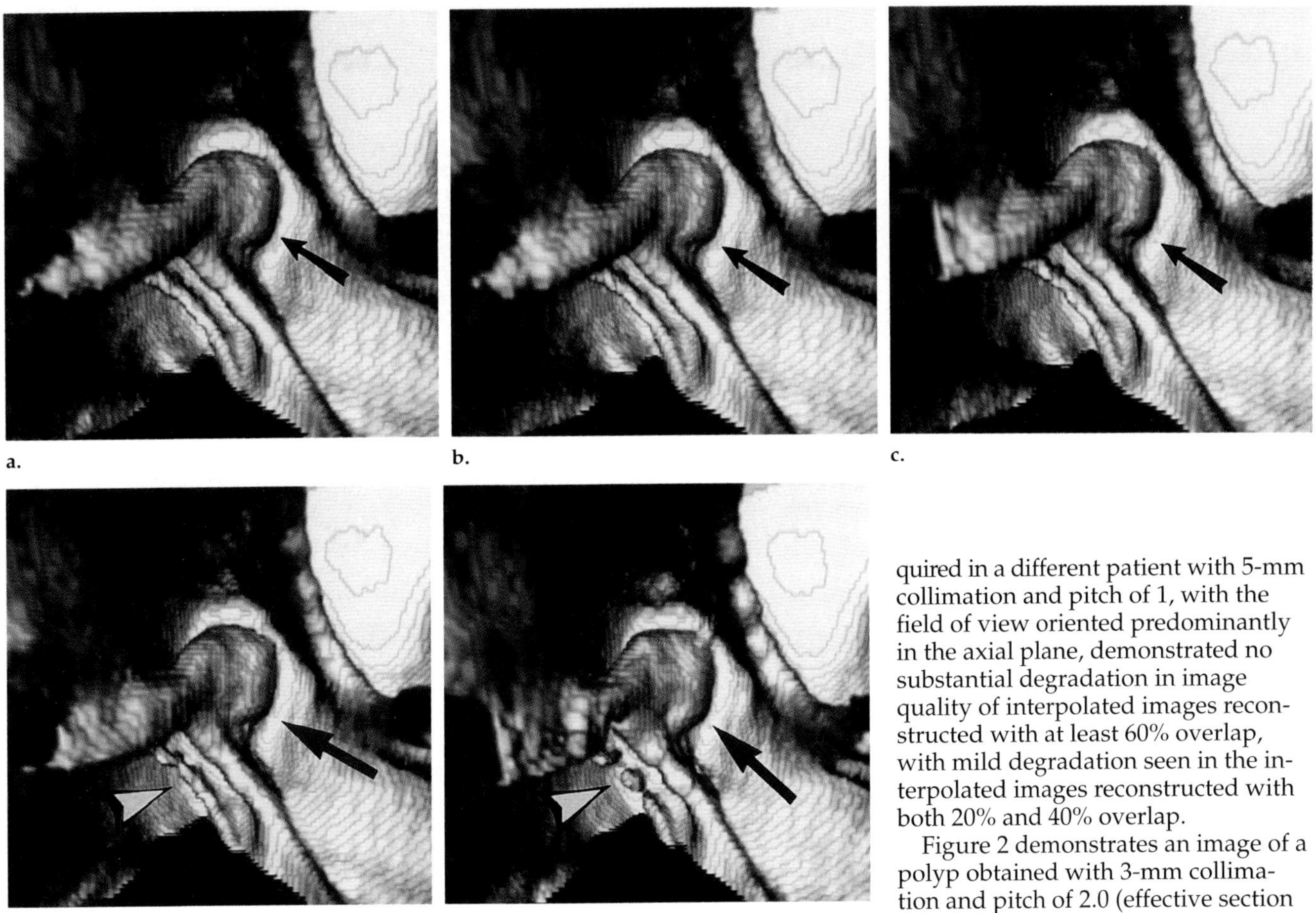

Figure 1. Differences in image quality with variation in longitudinal dimension. 3D PVR images of a polyp (arrow) acquired with 5-mm collimation, pitch of 1, and in-plane voxel dimension of 0.5 mm are shown with variation in reconstruction interval: **(a)** 0.5 mm (90% overlap), **(b)** 1.0 mm (80% overlap), **(c)** 2.0 mm (60% overlap), **(d)** 3.0 mm (40% overlap), **(e)** 4.0 mm (20% overlap). Qualitatively, image quality is maintained between 3D images generated from source images with equal voxel dimension (90% overlap) and interpolated 3D images reconstructed with 80% (in **b**) and 60% (in **c**) overlap. Progressive degradation of a lower haustral fold (arrowhead) is noted in **d** and **e**. All images were generated from full 12-bit range of data, with use of a step opacity function and a standardized beige color map assignment.

five region-of-interest measurements for both the sigmoidal and step images obtained in each patient. The sigmoidal and step image means were compared among the four patients for each analysis, with use of a two-tailed paired t test, with statistical significance accepted at the 5% level.

RESULTS

Image Reconstruction

The 3D PVR images of polyps in four different patients generated from interpolated images with at least 60% overlap were equivalent in quality to those generated from source images with equal voxel dimension (87%–90% overlap). Figures 1 and 2 demonstrate the 3D PVR images of the polyps in two different patients that were obtained with different acquisition parameters and reconstructed with variation in the longitudinal dimension. Figure 1 demonstrates a polyp image obtained with 5-mm collimation and pitch of 1 (effective section thickness, 5.0 mm in FWHM) (15), with the field of view predominantly oriented in the longitudinal plane. The quality of the 3D PVR image generated from a source volume with equal in-plane and longitudinal voxel dimensions (0.5 mm^3, 90% overlap) is similar to that of 3D images generated from interpolated images reconstructed with at least 60% overlap (1.0-mm reconstruction interval, 80% overlap; 2.0-mm reconstruction interval, 60% overlap). Mild degradation was noted in the 3D image generated from images reconstructed with 40% overlap (3.0-mm reconstruction interval), with marked degradation seen in images reconstructed with 20% overlap (4.0-mm reconstruction interval). Images acquired in a different patient with 5-mm collimation and pitch of 1, with the field of view oriented predominantly in the axial plane, demonstrated no substantial degradation in image quality of interpolated images reconstructed with at least 60% overlap, with mild degradation seen in the interpolated images reconstructed with both 20% and 40% overlap.

Figure 2 demonstrates an image of a polyp obtained with 3-mm collimation and pitch of 2.0 (effective section thickness, 3.9 mm) (15), with the field of view oriented predominantly in the longitudinal plane. Image quality of 3D PVR images generated from source images with equal in-plane and longitudinal voxel dimensions (0.5 mm^3, 87% overlap) was similar to that of 3D images generated from the interpolated images reconstructed with 74% overlap (1.0-mm reconstruction interval). Mild irregularities of the haustral folds were noted in the 3D images generated from images reconstructed with 49% overlap (2.0-mm reconstruction interval), with moderate degradation in image quality noted in the 3D images generated from images reconstructed with less overlap (3.0-mm reconstruction interval, 23% overlap; 4.0-mm reconstruction interval, 0% overlap). Images acquired in a different patient with 3-mm collimation and pitch of 2, with field of view oriented predominantly in the axial plane, also demonstrated mild to moderate degradation in the image quality of interpolated images reconstructed with 49% overlap and less.

Opacity Assignment

The frequency distribution of attenuation data in the 10 patients was found to be consistent. The centers of

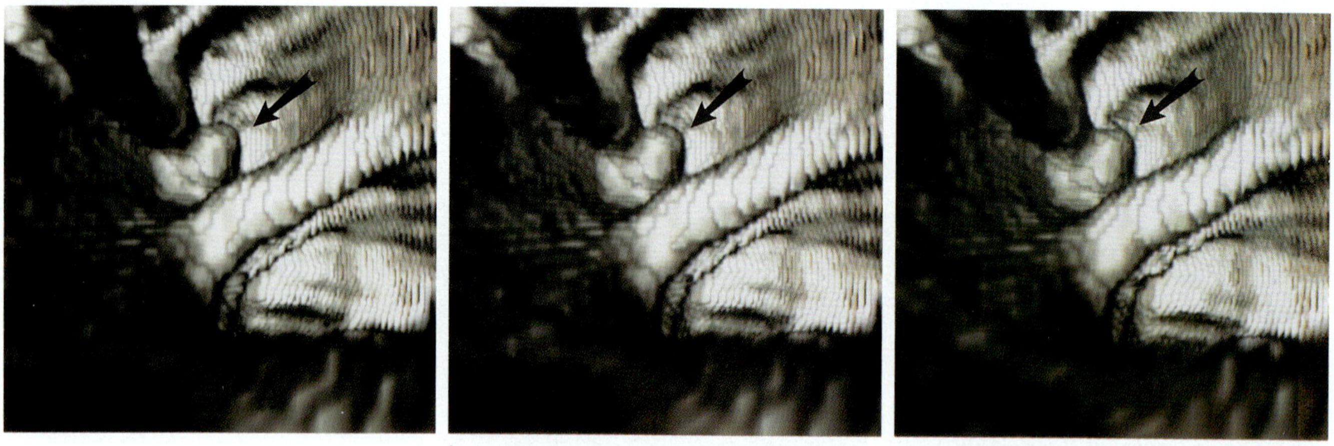

a. b. c.

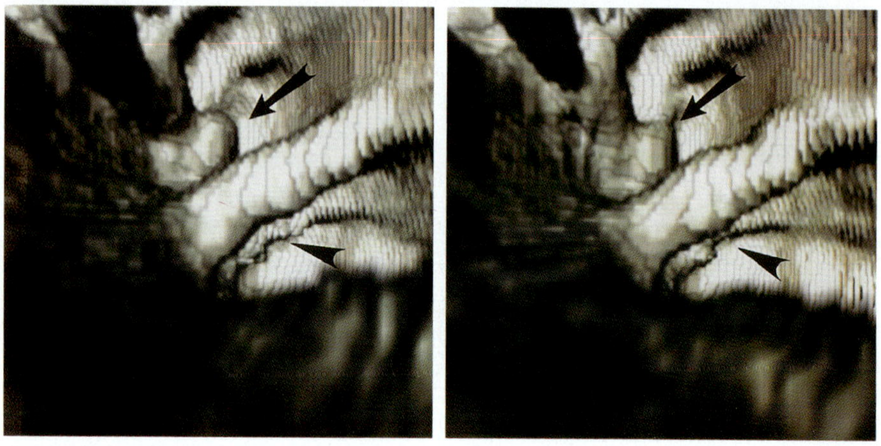

d. e.

Figure 2. Differences in image quality with variation in longitudinal dimension. 3D PVR images of a polyp (arrow) acquired with 3-mm collimation, pitch of 2, and in-plane voxel dimension of 0.5 mm are shown with variation in reconstruction interval: **(a)** 0.5 mm (87% overlap), **(b)** 1.0 mm (74% overlap), **(c)** 2.0 mm (49% overlap), **(d)** 3.0 mm (23% overlap), **(e)** 4.0 mm (0% overlap). Qualitatively, image quality is similar between images generated from source images with equal voxel dimensions (87% overlap [in **a**]) and interpolated images reconstructed with 74% overlap (in **b**). Mild irregularities in the inferior haustral folds (arrowhead) are seen in **c**, with moderate degradation noted in **d** and **e**. All images were generated from full 12-bit range of data with use of a step opacity function and a standardized beige color map assignment.

the two major fat and soft-tissue peaks averaged −109 and 40 HU, respectively, with little variance (standard deviation, 6.8 and 8.0 HU, respectively).

Selective variation in the lower threshold value consistently produced increased distortion of the thinner structures, such as polyp stalks and haustral folds, as the threshold was decreased below −700 HU, owing to volume averaging of these structures with air in the lumen. Specifically, in all four data sets no or subtle distortion was seen in the images obtained with threshold values of −600 to −700 HU, whereas in three of the four data sets moderate and marked distortion was observed in the images obtained with threshold values of −800 and −900 HU, respectively. Figure 3 demonstrates the 3D PVR images of one polyp generated with selective variation in the opacity threshold from −512 to −900 HU compared with the reference colonoscopic image of the polyp. For this polyp, the measured polyp-to–haustral fold ratio from the reference colonoscopic image (ratio, 3.5) was most closely correlated to the images created with opacity threshold values between −512 HU (ratio, 3.7) and −600 HU (ratio, 3.1), with increasing distortion noted in the images generated with opacity threshold values of −700 HU (ratio, 2.6), −812 HU (ratio, 2.6), and −900 HU (ratio, 2.3).

Next, image smoothness and edge sharpness were compared quantitatively between 3D PVR images of polyps generated with step and sigmoidal opacity functions. Results of the texture analysis to quantify image smoothness in four patients showed that the sigmoidal images were significantly smoother (texture index, 2.57 ± 1.98 [mean ± standard deviation]) compared with the step images (texture index, 6.67 ± 3.66, $P < .02$) Figure 4 shows a representative set of sigmoidal and step 3D PVR images of a polyp in one patient. Quantification of the edge sharpness in the four polyps demonstrated a significantly sharper edge with the step function (FWHM mean, 3.22 pixels ± 0.69) compared with the sigmoidal function (FWHM mean, 4.12 pixels ± 0.38; $P < .01$); however, the measured difference in the means of the values in FWHM was less than 1 pixel (mean difference, 0.9 pixel).

Final Image

Figure 5a demonstrates the final image obtained with 5-mm collimation and pitch of 1 with application of all steps evaluated. With use of the interpolated images obtained with 60% overlap and a sigmoidal opacity function centered over a range of −600 to −700 HU, the relative polyp-to–haustral fold ratio was 3.1, similar to the dimensions of the reference colonoscopic image (Fig 3a). Figure 5b demonstrates the corresponding opacity map function.

DISCUSSION

Although recent advances in CT image acquisition and computer graphics have made 3D endoscopic imaging in the colon more feasible, the interaction of the multiple processing parameters that influence 3D display have not been evaluated well, to our knowledge. This study represents a systematic evaluation of two important processing steps for PVR of spiral CT data obtained in colorectal polyps. We found that time-consuming reconstruction of highly overlapping (87%–90% overlap) spiral CT images to pro-

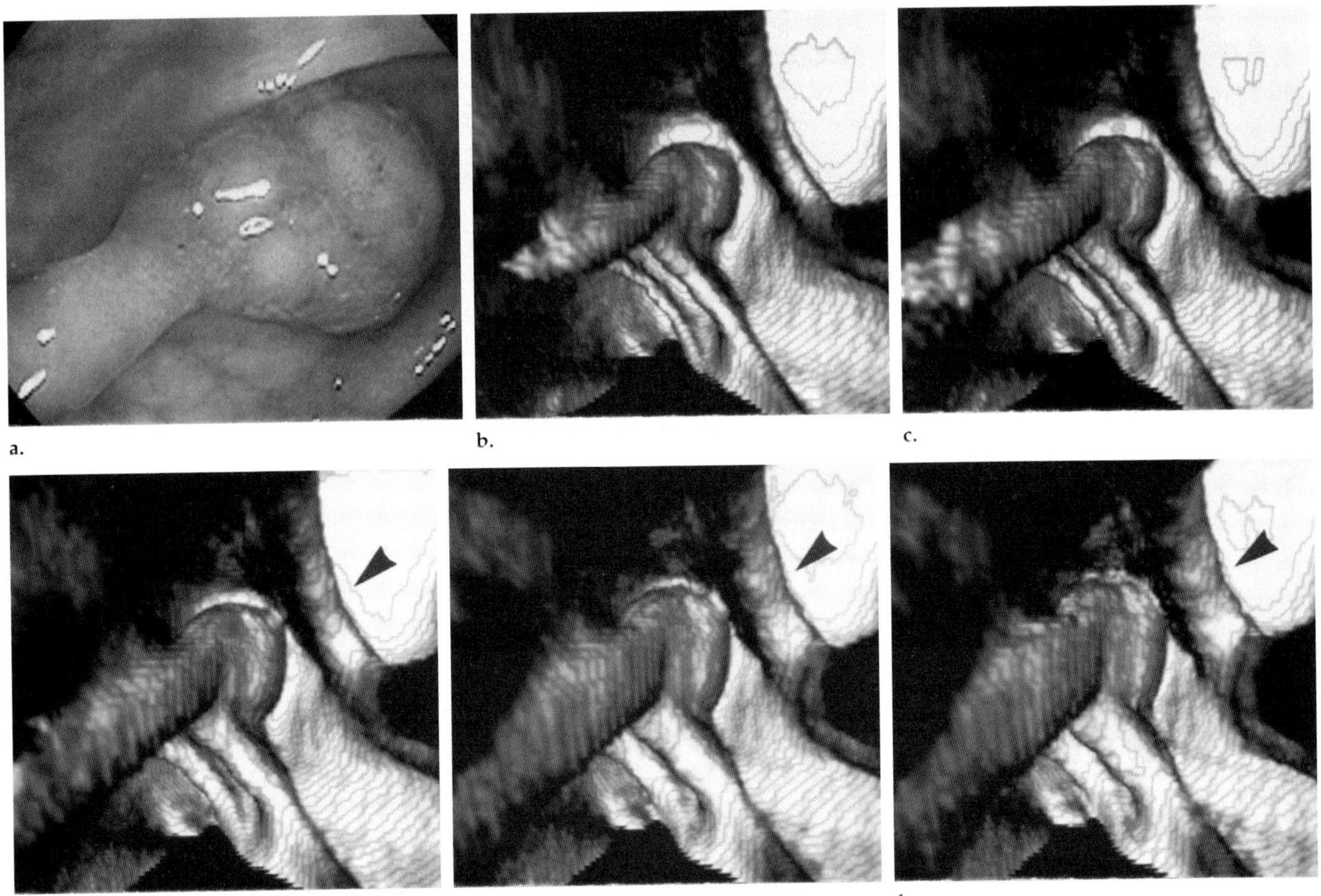

Figure 3. Effect of variation of opacity threshold in 3D PVR images of a polyp acquired from sources images with equal voxel dimensions (5-mm collimation, pitch of 1, 0.5 mm^3, 12-bit range of data, step opacity assignment, gray scale). **(a)** Reference colonoscopic image of the polyp is most closely replicated by the 3D PVR images of the polyp obtained with an opacity threshold between **(b)** −512 HU and **(c)** −600 HU. Increasing distortion of a haustral fold (arrowhead) is shown in images obtained with opacity threshold settings of **(d)** −700 HU, **(e)** −812 HU, and **(f)** −900 HU.

duce source data with equal voxel dimensions is not necessary to depict colorectal polyps with spiral CT PVR, so long as images are reconstructed with at least 60% overlap. Incremental decrease in the lower opacity threshold showed increased distortion of colon structures with values less than −700 HU, which demonstrates the importance of the volume-averaged boundary voxels in 3D PVR images of the colon. Image artifacts may be suppressed with use of a sigmoidal opacity function, in lieu of a step function, with only a small decrement in edge sharpness.

Findings in prior studies have shown that longitudinal resolution can be maintained with spiral CT as long as images are reconstructed with sufficient overlap (13,14). On the basis of both analytic models (13) and physical measurements (14), longitudinal resolution is maximized with reconstruction of approximately five images per nominal section width. For practical clinical application, typically two to four images are reconstructed per nominal section width (18,19). These studies were based on analysis of 2D images reconstructed from raw projection data. In this study, we varied longitudinal voxel dimension and assessed the quality of 3D PVR images for colorectal polyp depiction with spiral CT colography. In addition, we also compared differences in image quality between source images with equal voxel dimensions and source images reconstructed at wider intervals, with intervening data provided by means of linear interpolation of the image data. Consistent with prior results for 2D CT, we determined that image quality was maintained in 3D PVR images of colorectal polyps generated with approximately 40%–60% overlap. We confirmed that the degradation in image quality with sections that overlapped less was worse in images oriented in a longitudinal compared with an axial plane. The ability to reconstruct CT projection data at wider intervals and then perform linear interpolation of the image data at a workstation currently represents a clinical time saving. Although thin-section isotropic spiral CT may be possible in the future (19), dose considerations with this technique will always be a limitation. Low radiation exposure with spiral CT colography will be necessary to meet regulated standards for broad screening protocols.

Determination of the optimal opacity function is another important component of PVR image display. Opacity assignment is a function common to 3D volume rendering algorithms, although its implementation differs across various software programs. With use of the opacity map, specific levels of opacity are assigned to each attenuation value in the image volume. In this study, we first determined that there was a consistent frequency distribution of attenuation data across multiple patients with spiral CT colography. Next we tested the fidelity of image display with use of various opacity thresholds with a step function, and we assessed image distortion as the threshold was lowered. The most accurate relative proportions of polyp to surrounding colonic structures was determined with use of a lower threshold between −500 and −700 HU. There was substantial disproportion of relative polyp-to–haustral fold dimensions as the lower threshold was lowered below −700 HU. When displayed with an opacity threshold of −700 HU or less, thinner structures such as polyp stalks and haustral folds were artificially widened, owing to volume averaging of these structures with air in the lumen.

Our results differ from those of Rubin et al, who found a threshold closer to −980 HU was optimal to display colon anatomic features with 3D PVR (6). This difference most likely reflects the thickness of colon structures that were evaluated in these two studies. We evaluated the thicker structures of polyp heads and adjacent haustral folds and observed distortion of the thinner structures as the threshold was lowered. In the other study, thinner structures such as the distended bowel wall were assessed, and thus partial volume averaging with air had greater impact on the lower threshold used for image display. Although these differences need to be resolved with further study, the impact of the threshold is less important when a more smoothed sigmoidal opacity function and PVR are employed.

The shape of the opacity assignment as a function of CT attenuation was investigated with both step and sigmoidal opacity functions. Theoretically, sigmoidal opacity functions offer the potential to smooth boundaries between areas of low and high opacity by reducing the visible gradient at volume-averaged boundary voxels. In the region of air–soft tissue interfaces of the colon, these boundary voxels are especially important, although owing to scaling factors in Figure 5b this part of the histogram is not clearly depicted. Among numerous nonlinear opacity curves, we chose to investigate a steep sigmoidal curve. We verified that the sigmoidal images were significantly smoother than the step image by means of texture analysis. Edge sharpness would be expected to decrease with a sigmoidal opacity function compared to that with a step function. Although we noted a consistent decrement in edge sharpness with the sigmoidal function, the differences were small and probably not of clinical importance. Thus we conclude that the benefit of artifact suppresssion by means of image smoothing with the sigmoidal function outweighs the measured decrement in edge definition.

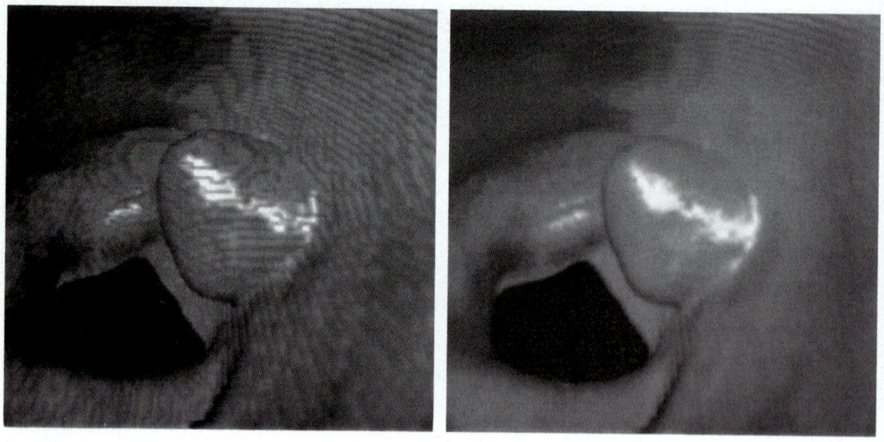

a. b.

Figure 4. Differences in image quality between step and sigmoidal opacity functions. 3D PVR images of a polyp acquired with source images obtained with 60% overlap (5-mm collimation, pitch of 1, remapped to 8-bit range of data, gray scale) generated with **(a)** step opacity function and **(b)** sigmoidal opacity function.

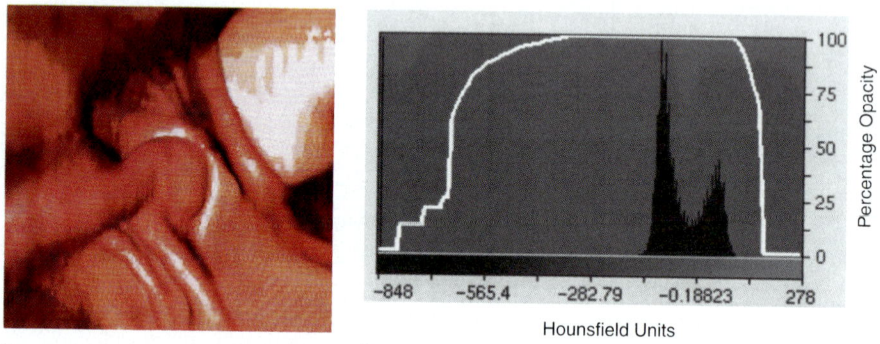

a. b.

Figure 5. Final 3D PVR image of the polyp in Figures 1 and 3 obtained by applying image reconstruction and opacity assignment. **(a)** 3D PVR image generated from source images obtained with 60% overlap (5-mm collimation, pitch of 1, remapped to 8-bit range of data, mucosal red color map) demonstrates similar dimensions to reference colonoscopic image (Fig 3a). **(b)** Corresponding sigmoidal opacity map. The unequal steps in the lower part of the spectrum represent a logarithmic translation of the opacity assignment used in volume rendering.

There are several limitations of this study. First, this analysis was based on a small number of clinical cases. The consistent frequency distribution of the attenuation histogram observed in the colon CT data in these patients, however, would suggest that these results are more widely applicable, but this needs to be verified. Second, variation in image reconstruction was tested in only two image acquisition protocols. The two protocols chosen were based on the criteria of adequate image resolution to detect clinically important colorectal polyps (1 cm or more in diameter) and sufficient anatomic coverage for the colon. These techniques also reflect the range of image acquisition protocols reported previously for spiral CT colography (5,6). Third, determination of the lower opacity threshold needs to be further validated. More rigorous methods could be performed in phantom applications to document changes in absolute measures of specific anatomic structures with variation in the opacity threshold. Although image distortion increased as the opacity threshold was lowered, the clinical importance of these differences needs to be determined. Fourth, variation in the opacity map assignment of the attenuation data was tested with one step and one sigmoidal function. As there are numerous degrees of freedom within this parameter, rigorous systematic variation in the shape of the curves may be warranted.

In summary, PVR techniques provide unique intraluminal visualization of the colon mucosa to allow polyp detection. These techniques have broad applications to other anatomic regions with similar air–soft tissue interfaces, such as tracheobronchial imaging. For clinical application, systematic evaluation of the various processing parameters is necessary to ensure accurate image display. In this study, image reconstruction and opacity map assignment of the attenuation data were evaluated by means of both qualitative and quantitative techniques. Prospective clinical trials are necessary to compare the diagnostic performance of CT with that of endoscopy for the detection of colorectal polyps to determine the clinical usefulness of this noninvasive imaging technique. Use of standardized 3D processing parameters is necessary to achieve more generalizable clinical results in different institutions. ■

Acknowledgment: We thank Thomas K. Pilgrim, PhD, for his statistical guidance in the manuscript.

References

1. Vining DJ, Teigen EL, Stetts D, Vanderwerken B, Kopecky KK, Rex D. Virtual colonoscopy: a 60-second colon examination (abstr). Radiology 1995; 197(P):281.
2. Joffe N, Schwartz RK, Raptopoulos VD, Peppercorn MA, Bitton A. Bowel imaging with volumetric CT: assessing the value of 2D reformations and 3D renderings—work in progress (abstr). Radiology 1995; 197(P): 281.
3. Ogura T, Koizumi K, Sai S, Maruyama M, Terahira T. Three-dimensional CT colonoscopy: comparison with colonoscopy and barium enema examination (abstr). Radiology 1995; 197(P):444.
4. Woodhouse CE, Friedman JL. In vitro air-contrast-enhanced spiral 3D CT (virtual colonoscopy) appearance of colonic lesions (abstr). Radiology 1995; 197(P):500.
5. Hara AK, Johnson CD, Reed JE, et al. Detection of colorectal polyps by computed tomographic colography: feasibility of a novel technique. Gastroenterology 1996; 110:284–290.
6. Rubin GD, Beaulieu CF, Argiro V, et al. Perspective volume rendering of CT and MR images: applications for endoscopic imaging. Radiology 1996; 199:321–330.
7. Hara AK, Johnson CD, Reed JE, Ehman RL, Ilstrup DM. Colorectal polyp detection with CT colography: two- versus three-dimensional techniques—work in progress. Radiology 1996; 200:49–54.
8. Vining DJ. Virtual endoscopy: is it reality? Radiology 1996; 200:30–31.
9. McFarland EG, Wang G, Brink JA, Balfe DM, Heiken JP, Vannier MW. Spiral CT colonography: central axis determination and digital unraveling of the colon. Acad Radiol 1997; 4:367–373.
10. Dachman AH, Lieberman J, Osnis RB, et al. Small simulated polyps in pig colon: sensitivity of CT virtual colography. Radiology 1997; 203:427–430.
11. Johnson PT, Heath DG, Kuszyk BS, Fishman EK. CT angiography with volume rendering: advantages and applications in splanchnic vascular imaging. Radiology 1996; 200:564–568.
12. Rubin GD, Napel S, Leung AN. Volumetric analysis of volumetric data: achieving a paradigm shift. Radiology 1996; 200:312–317.
13. Wang G, Vannier MW. Longitudinal resolution in volumetric x-ray computerized tomography: analytical comparison between conventional and helical computerized tomography. Med Phys 1994; 21:429–433.
14. Kalender WA, Polacin A, Suss C. A comparison of conventional and spiral CT: an experimental study on the detection of spherical lesions. J Comput Assist Tomogr 1994; 18:167–176.
15. Polacin A, Kalender WA, Marchal G. Evaluation of section sensitivity profiles and image noise in spiral CT. Radiology 1992; 185:29–35.
16. Conners RW, Harlow CA. A theoretical comparison of texture algorithms. IEEE Trans Pattern Anal Machine Intelligence 1980; 2:204–222.
17. Brink JA, Heiken JP, Balfe DM, Sagel SS, DiCroce J, Vannier MW. Spiral CT: decreased spatial resolution in vivo due to broadening of section-sensitivity profile. Radiology 1992; 185:469–474.
18. Brink JA. Technical aspects of helical (spiral) CT. Radiol Clin North Am 1995; 33:825–841.
19. Kalender WA. Thin-section three-dimensional spiral CT: is isotropic imaging possible? Radiology 1995; 197:578–580.

Sum & Substance

Whipple's Disease.

George T. Fantry, Stephen P. James. *Dig Dis* 1995; 13:108–118. (G.T.F., Division of Gastroenterology, Rm N3W62, University of Maryland Medical System, 25 S Greene St, Baltimore, MD 21201.)

Whipple disease, first described by George Hoyt Whipple in 1907, is an uncommon systemic bacterial disease that can involve virtually any organ system in the body, which results in a wide variety of symptoms. In most patients, the small intestine is involved, and the chief manifestation is malabsorption. The disease is far more common in men (male:female ratio, 8:1) and usually occurs between the 4th and 6th decades of life (mean age of onset, 50 years). Although there are no specific epidemiologic patterns, the disease, which occurs sporadically, may be more prevalent among individuals who work at farming-related trades.

The bacillus that causes Whipple disease has not been reproducibly cultured. Recently, however, polymerase chain reaction (PCR) techniques have been used to identify genes from the uncultured bacillus. Researchers examined duodenal tissue from five patients with Whipple disease and determined that the bacillus is a gram-positive bacterium closely related to actinobacteria. The organism was designated *Tropheryma whippelii*. Most actinomycetes, including actinobacteria, are aerobic soil organisms. Recently, RNA sequences of *T whippelii* have been found, at analysis with PCR, in peripheral blood mononuclear cells and in pleural effusion cells. These results confirm that the disease is systemic in nature.

This information about the taxonomy of the bacillus does not, however, account for the pathogenesis of Whipple disease. Immunologic deficits are not a hallmark of the disease, and patients apparently do not exhibit increased susceptibility to other infectious agents, nor do they have abnormal humoral immunity. Patients' symptoms are related to extensive infiltration of affected tissues by macrophages and bacilli.

Histopathologically, the appearance of the small bowel mucosa is usually diagnostic: Large foamy macrophages infiltrate the lamina propria and distort the villous architecture. The villi appear blunted and club shaped. Large glycoprotein granules are present in the macrophage cytoplasm. These granules stain positively with the periodic acid–Schiff (PAS) stain and are thought to represent the phagocytosed remnants of the cell wall of the bacilli. In addition, the mucosal and submucosal lymphatic channels are dilated, and fat droplets may be present in the extracellular spaces in the lamina propria; this latter finding indicates that enlarged lymph nodes are obstructing the channels. At electron microscopy, rod-shaped bacillary bodies are visible in the lamina propria; these bodies are 0.25 μm wide and 1.0–2.5 μm long and have a pale central nucleoid. Indicative of the systemic nature of Whipple disease is the fact that similar PAS-positive macrophages and the bacilli have been detected in the liver, heart, lung, and brain, as well as in intestinal tissues.

The most common symptoms in patients with Whipple disease are diarrhea and weight loss, but nonintestinal symptoms are also frequent and may precede the gastrointestinal symptoms by several years. Nonintestinal symptoms include intermittent, migrating arthritis of both large and small joints; arthralgia; low-grade fever; and, rarely, permanent joint deformity. Hyperpigmentation and peripheral lymphadenopathy are present in more than half of the patients with Whipple disease.

Radiologic signs of Whipple disease include marked thickening of the mucosal folds of the proximal portion of the small bowel at barium contrast examination. Paraaortic and retroperitoneal adenopathy have been noted at computed tomography. At endoscopy, the mucosa in the postbulbar duodenum has a characteristic pale, shaggy, yellow appearance, and yellow plaques or areas of erosion may be present.

When a patient is suspected of having Whipple disease, endoscopically guided biopsy of the small bowel mucosa is indicated. Histopathologic findings of lymphatic dilatation and infiltrating PAS-positive macrophages that contain gram-positive, acid-fast–negative bacilli are specific and diagnostic for Whipple disease.

Administration of an appropriate antibiotic therapy regimen has been successful in the treatment of Whipple disease. Because relapses that involve the central nervous system during therapy are a possibility, it is important that the initial treatment include antibiotics that can cross the blood-brain barrier. After 1 year of antibiotic therapy, another biopsy specimen should be obtained from the small bowel mucosa before the end of treatment to confirm the effectiveness of the therapy.

John J. Humpal
RSNA Publications

James H. Oliver III, MD • Richard L. Baron, MD • Michael P. Federle, MD
Brian C. Jones, MD • Reuben Sheng, MD

Hypervascular Liver Metastases: Do Unenhanced and Hepatic Arterial Phase CT Images Affect Tumor Detection?[1]

PURPOSE: **To evaluate the relative roles of unenhanced and hepatic arterial phase (HAP) computed tomographic (CT) imaging in the detection of hypervascular liver metastases.**

MATERIALS AND METHODS: **Eighty-four patients with biopsy-proved liver metastases from hypervascular primary tumors other than hepatocellular carcinoma underwent unenhanced and HAP and portal venous phase (PVP) helical CT studies. Three blinded radiologists evaluated each series of images separately for the number, size, and enhancement characteristics of lesions. Sixty-nine patients had follow-up imaging proof of tumor burden.**

RESULTS: **The three readers detected 381–402 lesions on the PVP images and 397–416 lesions on the unenhanced images. Unenhanced images allowed detection of 72%–80% of the lesions seen on PVP images. They detected 94–137 additional lesions on unenhanced but not PVP images. On the HAP images, 375–395 lesions were identified. HAP images allowed detection of 81%–90% of the lesions seen on PVP images. Forty-five to 78 additional lesions were detected on HAP but not on PVP images. In the 69-patient subset, maximal detection of tumor foci occurred in 94% of patients with unenhanced plus PVP images and in 78% with HAP plus PVP images. Unenhanced plus PVP images allowed detection of 96% of the 322 tumors in the subset population.**

CONCLUSION: **Unenhanced plus PVP CT images allow detection of statistically significantly more hypervascular liver metastases than do HAP plus PVP images or imaging only in the PVP.**

In the recent radiology literature, several studies assessed the value of obtaining helical computed tomographic (CT) images of the liver during both the hepatic arterial phase (HAP) and the portal venous phase (PVP) of contrast enhancement (1–6). Such two-pass techniques, referred to as dual-phase or biphasic helical CT, are now possible due to technical advancements in helical CT scanners. Image acquisition is much faster, and, therefore, the time required to scan the liver is decreased dramatically when using helical CT scanners compared with conventional scanners. The drive to develop and implement HAP imaging has stemmed from the known inability of conventional PVP imaging to enable detection of so-called hypervascular neoplasms in the liver (2,6–9). These tumors include hepatocellular carcinoma (HCC) and metastases from breast carcinoma, melanoma, pancreatic islet cell tumors, thyroid carcinoma, and renal cell carcinoma. Such hypervascular tumors are often less conspicuous or isoattenuating in relation to enhanced liver parenchyma on CT images obtained during the conventional PVP of hepatic enhancement (7,10). While it is now well established that the addition of HAP imaging to conventional PVP imaging greatly increases tumor detection in patients with HCC (1,2,6,11), little is known about the added benefit of biphasic helical CT in patients with hypervascular tumors other than HCC.

We undertook this study to determine whether imaging in the HAP translates into increased tumor detection in patients with hypervascular tumors other than HCC and what the relative roles of unenhanced and HAP imaging are in this subset of patients.

MATERIALS AND METHODS

We reviewed medical, surgical, and radiologic records to identify all patients with a diagnosis of breast carcinoma, neuroendocrine tumor, melanoma, thyroid carcinoma, or renal cell carcinoma who underwent at least one abdominal CT examination at our institution from September 1993 to October 1996. During this period, it was our routine practice to perform unenhanced and biphasic helical CT in all patients known to have or suspected of having hypervascular primary malignancies. Not all patients with hypervascular tumors underwent helical scanning during this period because not all of our CT scanners are helical. Any patients that did not undergo helical scanning were excluded from this study. Eighty-four such patients with biopsy-proved liver metastases from hypervascular nonhepatic primary tumors were identified before initiation of chemotherapy. Hepatic metastases were from breast carcinoma in 26 patients, neuroendocrine tumors in 20 patients, melanoma in 13 patients, renal cell carcinoma in 21 patients, and thyroid carcinoma in four patients. The study population comprised 38 men and 46 women aged 33–81 years (mean, 59 years).

Index terms: Computed tomography (CT), contrast enhancement, 761.12114 • Computed tomography (CT), helical, 761.12115 • Liver, CT, 761.12114, 761.12115 • Liver neoplasms, secondary, 761.332

Abbreviations: HAP = hepatic arterial phase, HCC = hepatocellular carcinoma, PVP = portal venous phase.

Radiology 1997; 205:709–715

[1] From the Department of Radiology, University of Pittsburgh Medical Center, 200 Lothrop St, Pittsburgh, PA 15213-2582. Received April 1, 1997; revision requested June 3; revision received August 4; accepted August 7. **Address reprint requests to** J.H.O.

All examinations were performed with a commercially available helical CT scanner (HiSpeed Advantage; GE Medical Systems, Milwaukee, Wis). All unenhanced scans were obtained incrementally with a 2-second scanning time and 5-mm collimation at 8-mm intervals. Nonhelical scans were used to avoid excessive tube heating that might cause tube-cooling delays during the HAP and PVP phases of the studies. The HAP and PVP images were obtained with helical technique with 7-mm collimation and a 1:1–1:1.5 table pitch. A window width of 150 HU was used for the unenhanced images, whereas a window width of 400 HU was used for the HAP and PVP images. For the contrast material–enhanced portions of the examinations, each patient received 150 mL of either iothalamate meglumine (Conray-60; Mallinckrodt Medical, St Louis, Mo) or ioversol (Optiray 320; Mallinckrodt Medical) intravenously by means of a mechanical power injector (model OP 100; Medrad, Pittsburgh, Pa). Contrast material was injected at rates that ranged from 2.5 to 5.0 mL/sec, with a monophasic rate of injection. The injection rate was 4.0–5.0 mL/sec in 26 patients and was 2.5–3.5 mL/sec in 58 patients. The slower injection rates were often used in patients with poor intravenous access or who had central venous catheters that were not rated for injection rates greater than 3 mL/sec.

After initiating infusion of contrast material, we used scanning delays of 20 seconds (for 4.0–5.0 mL/sec injections) or 28 seconds (for 2.5–3.5 mL/sec injections) before starting to obtain the HAP images. Imaging in the PVP was performed after a scanning delay of 60 seconds (4.0–5.0 mL/sec rate) or 70 seconds (2.5–3.5 mL/sec rate) from initiation of infusion of contrast material. This variation in the length of scanning delays is necessitated by the known relationship between peak hepatic parenchymal enhancement, time to equilibrium, and the rate of infusion of contrast material (12–15).

Each helical acquisition through the liver was accomplished in one or two breath holds. This allowed ample time for patient breathing and required patients to hold their breath for no more than 25 seconds. Two helical acquisitions were rarely required to image the entire liver during either the HAP or the PVP. If necessary, however, patients were allowed a respiration interval of approximately 8 seconds between acquisitions, ensuring that each phase of liver imaging was completed within the necessary time frame.

Studies were evaluated retrospectively by three readers (J.H.O., M.P.F., R.L.B.) blinded to diagnosis, all patient history, and any correlative imaging studies. Each reader interpreted the individual cases separate from the other readers and was blinded to the others' readings. The readers were initially given PVP images only and scored each case for the number of lesions, the size of lesions, and the enhancement characteristics of the lesions. On a different date, the readers evaluated either the unenhanced or the HAP images along with the corresponding PVP images and the score sheets they had filled out previously. This was done because a radiologist in daily practice would not be reading the unenhanced or HAP images without the corresponding PVP images as unopacified vessels on-end may mimic tumors on unenhanced or HAP images. The readers recorded the number of lesions detected on unenhanced or HAP images that were also seen on PVP images, as well as the number of additional lesions seen only on the unenhanced or the HAP images. At a third date, the readers reviewed the remaining images (either unenhanced or HAP), again with the corresponding PVP images and score sheets. For each patient, therefore, three separate readings were performed by each reader.

The readers were not aware of the number of patients with tumors. Sixteen patients without liver metastases were included for evaluation and scoring (in addition to the 84 patients with hypervascular liver metastases), a step that was intended to minimize the readers being overly sensitive to subtle attenuation differences in the liver that could be suggestive of tumor. These patients were not included in the data analysis.

All patients with liver metastases had needle-biopsy proof of the histologic diagnosis of liver metastases. Typically, biopsy was performed of only one lesion. Each patient with multiple lesions was presumed to have multifocal metastases with the same histologic diagnosis as that of the biopsy lesion when the other lesions had the same imaging appearance on unenhanced, HAP, or PVP images as that of the biopsy-proved lesion and did not meet the CT criteria for hemangioma (16,17), cyst (18), or focal fibrosis (19). When any patient had more than 10 lesions, only a maximum of 10 were recorded so that these few patients would not substantially bias the data.

Sixty-nine of the 84 patients with tumor underwent follow-up CT or magnetic resonance (MR) studies to prove total tumor burden by documenting the growth or reduction of each lesion after chemotherapy. Such growth or reduction was determined after the blinded review was completed.

A paired Student t test was used to make paired comparisons of the total number of lesions revealed on unenhanced, HAP, and PVP images. A pair was defined as a reader identifying a lesion with two different imaging techniques, and the t test was conducted across the three readers. A P value of less than .05 was considered to indicate a statistically significant outcome.

Number of Lesions Detected on PVP Only or Combined Images by Readers 1–3

Reader	PVP Images Only	PVP and Unenhanced Images	PVP and HAP Images	Additional Lesions*: Unenhanced Images	Additional Lesions*: HAP Images
1	385	299 (78)	345 (90)	98 (25)	50 (13)
2	381	275 (72)	310 (81)	137 (36)	78 (20)
3	402	322 (80)	330 (82)	94 (23)	45 (11)

Note.—Numbers in parentheses are percentages.
* Number of additional lesions depicted on unenhanced images or HAP images but not on PVP images.

RESULTS

In the 84 patients with biopsy-proved liver metastases from hypervascular primary tumors, the three readers identified 381–402 lesions on the PVP images (Table). The lesions ranged in size from 3 to 140 mm (mean, 21 mm). At a separate sitting, the readers identified a total of 397–416 lesions on the unenhanced images. Interobserver variation was primarily attributable to different readers recording abutting satellite nodules as one lesion or counting each abutting satellite nodule separately. Two hundred seventy-five to 322 (72%–80%) of the lesions seen initially on PVP images were seen on the unenhanced images. In addition, the readers detected 94–137 additional lesions on the unenhanced images that were not seen on the PVP images in 28–40 patients (Fig 1). The average number of lesions seen on PVP images but not seen on unenhanced images was 91; an average of 110 lesions were seen on the unenhanced images but not on the PVP images. Therefore, in the total study population, PVP images revealed fewer lesions than the unenhanced images, although this did not reach statistical significance ($P < .08$). In two (2%) of the 84 patients, the diagnosis of any tumor in the liver was possible only on the unenhanced images. The hypervascular metastatic foci were hypoattenuating relative to the liver parenchyma in 55 of 82 patients. Only those patients with severe diffuse fatty infiltration of the liver (n = 5) had lesions that were hyperattenuating to liver on unenhanced images.

During the evaluation of HAP images, the readers identified a total of 375–395 lesions. Three hundred ten to 345 (81%–90%) of the lesions seen on PVP images were seen on the HAP images. The readers also detected 45–78 additional lesions on HAP images that were not seen on PVP images in 18–26 patients (Fig 2). The average number of lesions seen on PVP images but not on HAP images was 53; an average of 58 lesions were seen on HAP images

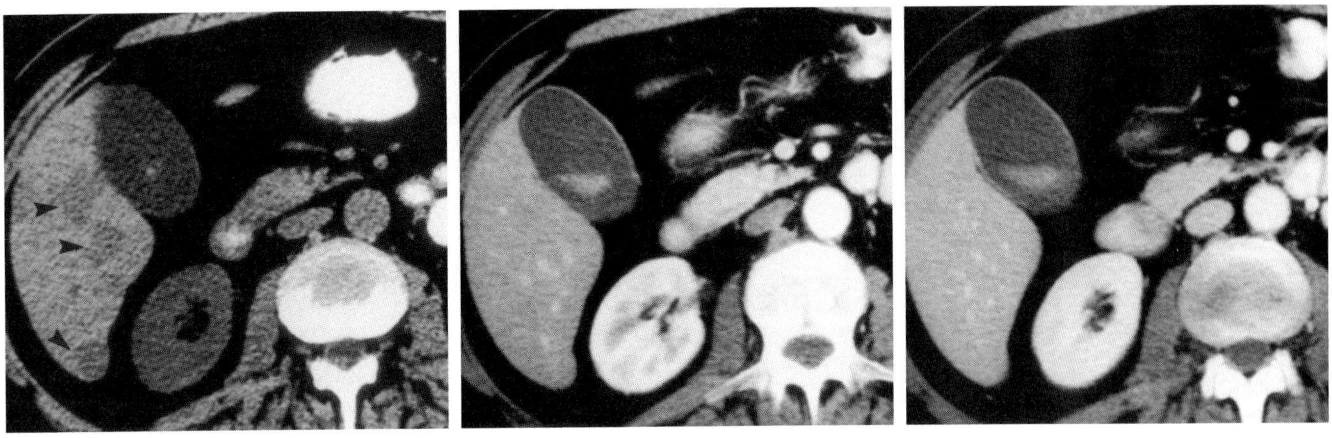

a. b. c.

Figure 1. Liver metastases from thyroid carcinoma. **(a)** Unenhanced image clearly shows several hypoattenuating metastases (arrowheads). Corresponding **(b)** HAP and **(c)** PVP images fail to show any evidence of metastatic disease.

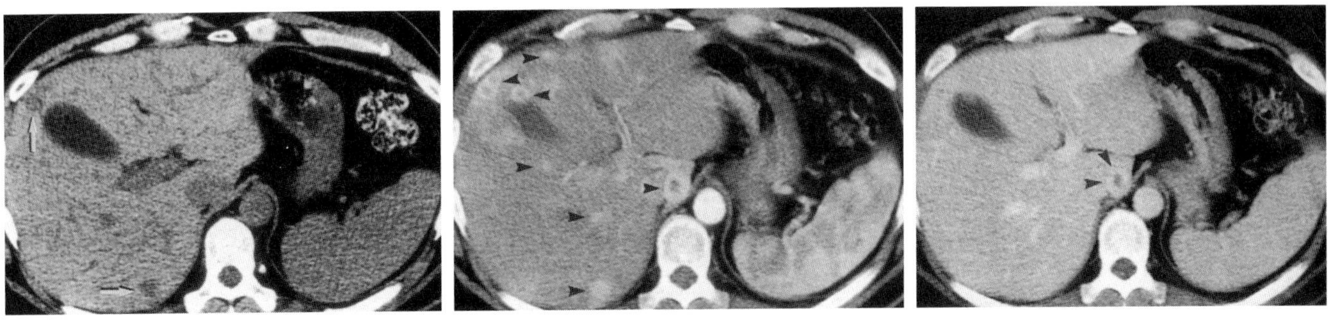

a. b. c.

Figure 2. Thyroid carcinoma metastases in a 43-year-old man. **(a)** Unenhanced image demonstrates two hypoattenuating tumor foci (arrows). **(b)** Corresponding HAP image demonstrates multiple hyperenhancing tumors (arrowheads) that were inapparent on unenhanced and PVP images. **(c)** Corresponding PVP image fails to depict the majority of tumors. The one lesion (arrowheads) that is seen was initially misinterpreted as the inferior vena cava due to its location.

but not on PVP images. Therefore, there was no significant difference in the number of lesions detected on HAP images or PVP images ($P < .88$). In two patients (2%), the diagnosis of any tumor within the liver was possible only on HAP images.

Sixty-nine patients underwent follow-up imaging (CT, CT during arterial portography, CT arteriography, or MR imaging) to confirm the lesions as malignant. In this patient subset, there were 322 proved hepatic metastatic lesions. At the unblinded review of the study examination and all follow-up imaging studies, 247 (77%) of the lesions were identified on the PVP images, 251 (78%) of the lesions were identified on HAP images, and 279 (87%) were identified on the unenhanced images. One hundred three (41%) of the lesions seen on HAP images were predominantly hyperattenuating to liver parenchyma during the HAP; 176 (59%) were homogeneously hypoattenuating (Fig 3) during the HAP. Thirty-four additional lesions not seen on PVP images were seen on HAP images in 16 patients: two of four patients with thyroid carcinoma, six of 16 patients with neuroendocrine tumors, four of 16 patients with renal cell carcinoma, three of 20 patients with breast carcinoma, and one of 13 patients with melanoma. Sixty-three additional lesions not seen on PVP images were seen on unenhanced images in 27 patients: three of four patients with thyroid carcinoma, seven of 16 patients with neuroendocrine tumors, six of 16 patients with renal cell carcinoma, eight of 20 patients with breast carcinoma, and three of 13 patients with melanoma. Of the 34 additional lesions seen on HAP images and the 63 additional lesions seen on the unenhanced images, 22 were seen on both HAP and unenhanced images (Fig 4). Therefore, 75 lesions (23%) that were detected on unenhanced images only, on HAP images only, or with both techniques were not seen on PVP images in 31 (45%) of the 69 patients. In only one patient in this 69-patient subset was the diagnosis of liver metastatic disease revealed only on HAP images. In two patients, the sole evidence of hepatic metastases was seen only on the unenhanced images. Given the fact that all medical centers currently obtain CT images of the liver during the PVP, the addition of unenhanced images resulted in the detection of significantly more hypervascular metastatic lesions than did the addition of HAP images ($P < .004$).

DISCUSSION

CT has become the imaging test of choice for staging tumors in patients with a known primary abdominal malignancy. In addition, until recently, dynamic incremental bolus CT was generally regarded as the optimal noninvasive CT technique for detection of primary or metastatic liver malignancies. This was based on a body of work performed primarily in patients with hypovascular tumors, such as lung and colon carcinoma (20–23). The goal of dynamic incremental bolus CT is to scan during the time of peak hepatic parenchymal enhancement. This peak occurs during the PVP of the contrast enhancement curve, approxi-

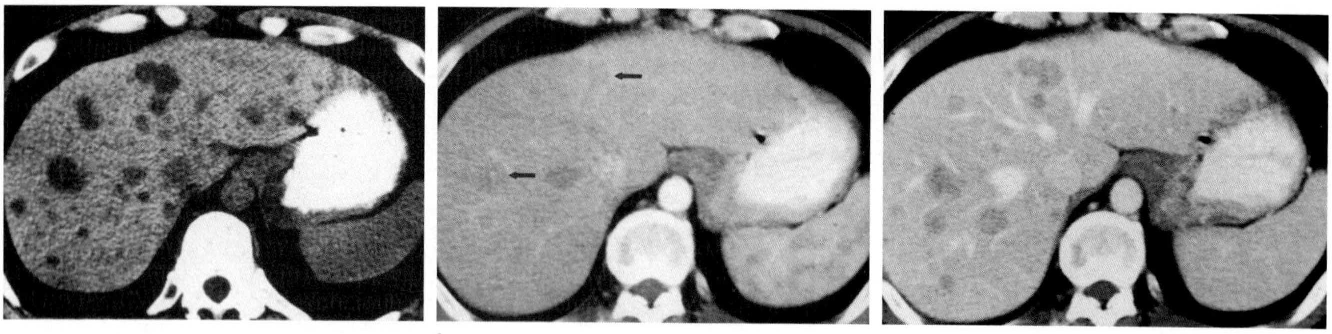

a. b. c.

Figure 3. Pancreatic islet cell tumor metastases to the liver. **(a)** Unenhanced image demonstrates multiple low-attenuation metastases. **(b)** Corresponding HAP image shows that many of the lesions are isoattenuating or hypoattenuating (arrows) to the faintly enhanced liver parenchyma. **(c)** PVP image demonstrates all the tumor foci seen on the unenhanced image.

mately 60–110 seconds after the initiation of the bolus of contrast material depending on the rate of injection and volume of contrast material (14,15). The time of greatest hepatic parenchymal enhancement is also the time of greatest tumor conspicuity in patients with hypovascular liver neoplasms, because these tumors enhance only minimally. As most metastatic neoplasms in the liver are hypovascular, it became convention to image during the PVP.

It has long been known, however, that hypervascular tumors may be isoattenuating, or nearly so, to enhanced liver parenchyma when imaged during the PVP of hepatic enhancement (7,10) (Fig 1). In theory, hypervascular tumors should be more conspicuous during the time that contrast material is being delivered by the hepatic artery but before considerable contrast material is delivered to the hepatic parenchyma via the portal vein. Unfortunately, before the development of helical or electron beam CT technology, it was not possible to image the entire liver during this brief HAP of contrast enhancement. This led some investigators to suggest obtaining unenhanced CT images of the liver as well as the conventional PVP images in an attempt to increase tumor detection rates in patients known to have or suspected of having hypervascular tumors (7).

The issue of the role of unenhanced liver CT imaging remains controversial. Bressler et al (7) reported 11 (39%) of 28 patients with hypervascular liver lesions had tumors that were not apparent on the PVP images but were seen as low-attenuation foci on the unenhanced CT images. That study was performed almost 10 years ago, before the advent of helical CT. Oliver et al (6) reported that, in patients with HCC, unenhanced CT images depicted 17% (47 of 276 tumors) additional tumor foci not seen on PVP images. In 3% of these patients, it was the only CT technique to depict any tumor. Other investigators have questioned whether unenhanced CT images can depict additional tumor nodules in patients with certain hypervascular tumors (8,24). Patten et al (25) contend that even though unenhanced CT images may show additional hypervascular metastatic lesions, PVP images will reveal some evidence of hepatic metastatic disease in most patients.

New developments in CT technology have considerably reduced image acquisition time to the point that the entire liver can be imaged several times during a single CT examination. This ability to scan the liver during different phases of the hepatic parenchymal enhancement curve has led to the biphasic helical CT examination that exploits the dual blood supply to liver parenchyma and the inherent differences in blood supply to liver tumors and the liver parenchyma. Since nearly 100% of the blood supply to liver tumors and only 20%–25% of the blood supply to liver parenchyma is via the hepatic artery, it makes intuitive sense to image early, during the HAP of the enhancement curve, when attempting to identify very vascular tumors within the liver. This HAP occurs approximately 20–45 seconds after the initiation of the intravenous bolus of contrast material. This time period is dependent on circulation times in patients as well as the rate of infusion of contrast material when imaging in this time period. Hypervascular tumors should appear as hyperenhancing masses when compared with the minimally enhanced liver parenchyma during the HAP.

In fact, biphasic helical CT has proved superior to conventional incremental CT, in which images of the liver are only obtained during the PVP of hepatic enhancement, for the detection of HCC tumors (2,6). While HCC is usually a hypervascular tumor, it is unclear how much of the increased detection rates seen in patients with HCC during the HAP are related to the tumor vascularity and how much are related to the fact that the majority of patients with HCC have cirrhosis with concomitant portal venous hypertension and compensatory hepatic artery hypertrophy. While it has been established that the addition of HAP images statistically significantly increases HCC tumor detection over imaging in the PVP only (6), the question remains, Does biphasic helical CT have a role in patients with other types of hypervascular tumors? In addition, does unenhanced CT imaging still have a prominent role in the detection of hypervascular tumors in this era of biphasic helical contrast-enhanced CT studies?

Frederick et al (5) reported on the added benefit of multiphase helical CT in evaluating hepatic metastases in patients with breast carcinoma, but the rate of injection in that study was low (2 mL/sec), which according to the growing clinical experience of many investigators appears to limit the sensitivity of the HAP images. Other studies evaluating the usefulness of biphasic helical CT included patient populations that were composed mainly of patients with HCC and metastases from hypovascular primary tumors such as colon carcinoma, prostate carcinoma, and gastric carcinoma (3,4).

Our study shows that both HAP and unenhanced CT images will depict additional hypervascular tumors within the liver not seen on PVP images. However, unlike previous reports for HCC, unenhanced images depicted statistically significantly more additional lesions than HAP images (28% vs 13% additional lesions, respectively). Unenhanced im-

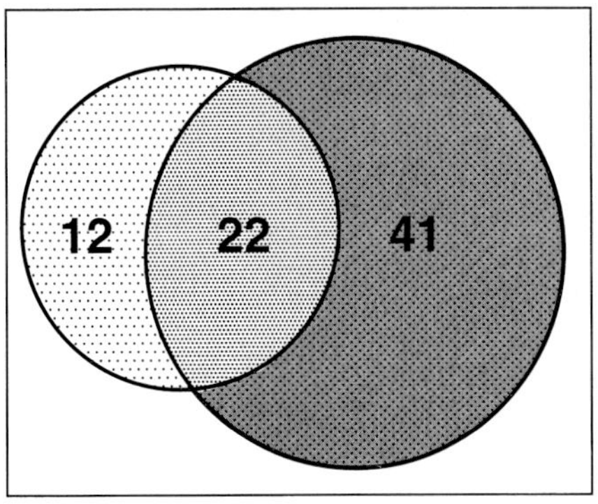

a.

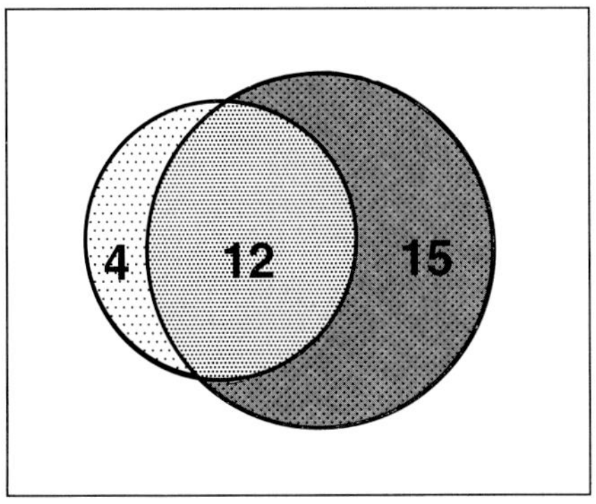

b.

Figure 4. Venn diagrams demonstrate **(a)** the number of additional lesions seen on the HAP images only (light), on the unenhanced images only (dark), and on both images (medium) but that were not seen on the PVP images and **(b)** the number of patients respectively. These data were derived from the subset of 69 patients who had follow-up imaging proof of tumor burden.

ages revealed additional tumor not seen on PVP images in 28–40 patients (33%–48%) (Fig 1).

Within the subset of 69 patients with proof from follow-up CT and/or MR studies that documented total tumor burden, PVP images depicted 77% of the 322 documented tumor foci, missing 75 additional lesions. Unenhanced images depicted 63 (84%) of these 75 lesions. While HAP depicted 34 of the 75 lesions, only 12 of these would have been missed with unenhanced imaging (Fig 3a).

PVP images did not depict the maximal tumor burden in 31 (45%) of the 69 patients with follow-up proof. The addition of unenhanced images to PVP images allowed the maximal depiction of tumor burden in 65 patients (94%). Conversely, HAP and PVP images demonstrated the maximal depiction of total tumor burden in 58 patients (78%) (Fig 3b).

Although all the patients in this study had tumors that are typically considered to be hypervascular, only a minority of the tumors were hyperattenuating to liver parenchyma during the HAP. In the subset of 69 patients with follow-up proof, only 41% of the 322 tumors were hyperattenuating to liver during the HAP. The majority (59%) were hypoattenuating or isoattenuating to liver parenchyma during the HAP. These data were obtained from patients who had not yet undergone chemotherapy. It is our experience, although anecdotal, that once chemotherapy is instituted many tumors that were initially hyperattenuating in the HAP do not enhance to the same degree on follow-up scans. We believe that HAP imaging would be even less effective in patients after chemotherapy. Even though the number of patients with each specific type of tumor is too small to be statistically significant, it is interesting to note that in the subset of 69 patients with proof, 50% of the four patients with thyroid carcinoma had additional tumors identified during the HAP. Additional tumors were detected on the HAP images in 37% of the 16 patients with neuroendocrine tumors, 25% of the 16 patients with renal cell carcinoma, 15% of the 20 patients with breast carcinoma, and 8% of the 13 patients with melanoma. However, only 16% of these additional lesions were seen with HAP only and in only 6% of patients were additional lesions seen with HAP only. While the additional yield of adding HAP images to unenhanced plus PVP images appears to be minimal, in a few cases the HAP results were dramatic (Fig 2). Often, however, the addition of HAP images resulted in increased confidence that a small lesion seen on unenhanced or PVP images was a neoplasm, rather than a small cyst or an area of fibrosis. Seeing positive enhancement within a lesion during the HAP is more specific for neoplasm than is identifying a hypoattenuating lesion that can be difficult to differentiate from a cyst when small. This value of HAP images was not assessed in this study, but certainly adds value to some CT examinations.

Clearly the addition of unenhanced images to PVP images is superior to the combination of HAP plus PVP images when attempting to accurately document hypervascular tumors other than HCC in the liver. These data run counter to those obtained for patients with HCC in whom HAP plus PVP imaging statistically significantly outperformed unenhanced plus PVP imaging (6). We hypothesize that the difference in HAP detection rates for HCC versus other hypervascular tumors may be multifactorial. Perhaps the most important factor is that most patients with HCC have concomitant cirrhosis, whereas those patients with metastatic liver disease do not. Many patients with long-standing cirrhosis develop portal hypertension, which decreases portal venous blood flow to the liver. To compensate, the hepatic arterial blood flow in these patients is increased due to hypertrophy of the hepatic arterial system. This results in patients with cirrhosis having lower peak hepatic parenchymal enhancement during the PVP as well as increased tumoral enhancement during the HAP (due to the dilated hepatic arterial system). These changes would favor detection of hypervascular tumors (such as HCC) during the HAP and decrease the chance of detecting them during the PVP. Therefore, not only is HCC a very vascular tumor, but the changes in blood flow to a cirrhotic liver act synergistically to maximize detection rates of HCC during the HAP.

A second factor to consider is that the unenhanced images are much easier to interpret in patients without cirrhosis. On unenhanced images, the cirrhotic liver is very often quite heterogeneous due to the presence of regenerative nodules and areas of fibrosis. Both of these entities can be hypoattenuating to unenhanced liver parenchyma and frequently cannot be differentiated from tumor on unenhanced images. The fact that most regenerative nodules are isoattenuating or hypoattenuating to liver parenchyma during the PVP does little to help differentiate regenerative nodule from tumor. In these patients, the HAP images often provide the means for separating regenerative nodules from HCC, by showing HAP enhancement in HCC tumors. Most patients with hypervascular metastatic disease in the liver do not have concomitant cirrhosis. Therefore, a hypoattenuating focus in the liver on unenhanced images in a patient without cirrhosis is viewed with much more confidence as representing a neoplasm than it is in a patient with cirrhosis.

Third, many of the so-called hypervascular tumors do not act as such on bolus-enhanced helical CT scans, remaining hypoattenuating to liver parenchyma on both the HAP and PVP images. While most HCC tumors show areas of tumoral enhancement greater than liver parenchymal enhancement during the HAP, the minority of the so-called hypervascular tumors in our study were hyperattenuating to liver in the HAP. Even though certain types of tumors (thyroid, neuroendocrine, and renal) had increased yields on HAP images, many of these tumors

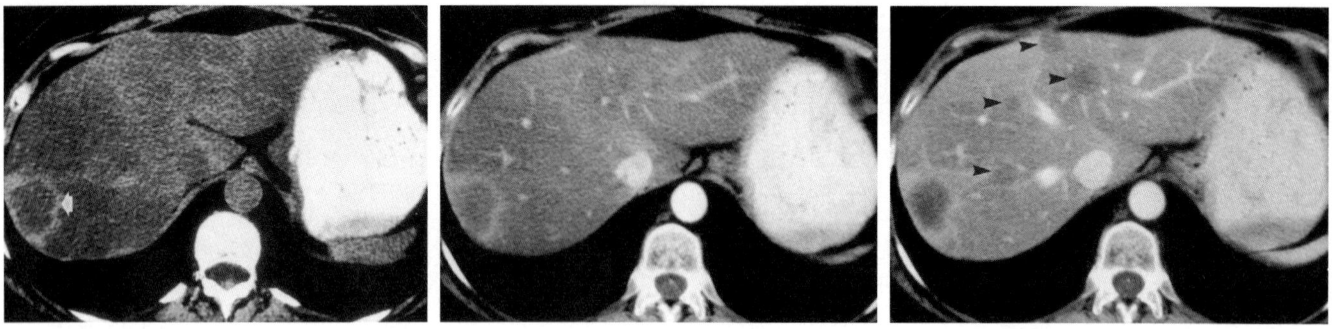

a. b. c.

Figure 5. Breast carcinoma metastases and geographic fatty infiltration of the liver in a 57-year-old woman. **(a)** Unenhanced image demonstrates a suspicious area in the right hepatic lobe (arrow). The remainder of the liver is heterogeneous. **(b)** Corresponding HAP image fails to depict any more definite foci of tumor. **(c)** PVP image at the same level clearly shows several additional tumors (arrowheads) not seen on the unenhanced or HAP images.

were hypoattenuating during the HAP. Among patients with the same type of tumor, the enhancement characteristics during the HAP were unpredictable and varied from patient to patient.

Unenhanced images frequently provided more accurate measurements of individual tumor nodules than did HAP or PVP images because the peripheral margins of hypervascular tumors can often be isoattenuating to adjacent liver parenchyma due to contrast material raising the attenuation value of portions of a lesion to the same degree as that of liver. Unenhanced images also provide more consistent tumor measurements from study to study because both HAP and PVP image appearance and, therefore, tumor size can vary with minor differences in the rate or timing of the bolus of contrast material. While unenhanced images are generally helpful, it is important to remember that in patients with focal, geographic, or diffuse fatty infiltration of the liver it can be difficult to differentiate tumor from areas of fatty infiltration on the unenhanced images only (Fig 5). In fact, in cases of diffuse fatty infiltration, the liver attenuation is decreased so that the normally hypoattenuating metastatic lesions are often isoattenuating and can even be hyperattenuating to the fatty liver parenchyma. This can become more of a problem once systemic chemotherapy is instituted as these patients often develop fatty infiltration of the liver in response to the chemotherapy.

There are several potential limitations of our study that should be put into proper perspective. First, our study was not a prospective study, but rather was a retrospective analysis of a prospectively standardized CT technique for patients known to have or suspected of having metastatic disease to the liver from a hypervascular primary tumor. Thus, there is lack of control over patient selection criteria as to who was referred for CT evaluation. Second, although histologic confirmation of metastatic disease within the liver was obtained in every case, not every tumor nodule underwent biopsy or surgical excision. However, there were a substantial number of patients (69 of the 84 patients) who underwent follow-up correlative imaging studies (CT during arterial portography, CT angiography, biphasic helical CT, and MR imaging) to document total tumor burden. A subset of data from these patients was formed to address this potential limitation, and the results obtained from this subset were very similar to those obtained for the entire study population. Third, our patient population is biased because we practice in a tertiary referral medical center, and, as such, we see a higher percentage of patients with advanced disease than those practicing in a community hospital setting. Therefore, we are uncertain about the influence that unenhanced and/or HAP CT imaging will have on a community medicine–based patient population. Nonetheless, we can only presume that patients with less hepatic metastatic disease will have similar imaging characteristics. We assume our results imply that the ability to detect solitary hepatic lesions should be increased similarly, although we had very few patients with a single lesion. The lack of patients with tumor in liver detected solely with unenhanced or HAP images in large part reflects the advanced stage of tumor in our patients and does not necessarily reflect a low effect in screening patients with lesser tumor involvement.

In conclusion, our data confirm that for evaluating patients known to have or suspected of having hypervascular metastatic disease in the liver, CT imaging in the PVP alone is inadequate to document complete extent of tumor. While both HAP and unenhanced CT images will depict additional foci of hypervascular tumors not seen on PVP images, the combination of unenhanced and PVP CT images appears to be superior to the combination of HAP and PVP images. The value of HAP images in characterizing lesions provides further benefit that was not investigated in this study.

In select cases, HAP imaging can substantially increase hypervascular tumor detection and may be considered in problematic cases. It may be prudent to perform all three phases (unenhanced, HAP, and PVP) during the first CT examination when evaluating a patient known to have or suspected of having hypervascular tumor to optimally screen the liver for metastatic disease and to assess the vascularity of the tumor foci, to determine which sequences should be used for follow-up CT. ■

References

1. Ohashi I, Hanafusa K, Yoshida T. Small hepatocellular carcinomas: two-phase dynamic incremental CT in detection and evaluation. Radiology 1993; 189:851–855.
2. Baron RL, Oliver JH III, Dodd GD III, Nalesnik M, Holbert BL, Carr B. Hepatocellular carcinoma: evaluation with biphasic, contrast-enhanced, helical CT. Radiology 1996; 199:505–511.
3. Bonaldi VM, Bret PM, Reinhold C, Atri M. Helical CT of the liver: value of an early hepatic arterial phase. Radiology 1995; 197: 357–363.
4. Hollett MD, Jeffrey RB Jr, Nino-Murcia M, Jorgensen MJ, Harris DP. Dual-phase helical CT of the liver: value of arterial phase scans in the detection of small (<1.5 cm) malignant hepatic neoplasms. AJR 1995; 164:879–884.
5. Frederick MG, Paulson EK, Nelson RC. Role of triple-phase spiral CT for detecting hepatic metastases in patients with breast carcinoma (abstr). Radiology 1995; 197(P): 139.
6. Oliver JH III, Baron RL, Federle MP, Rockette HE Jr. Detecting hepatocellular carcinoma: value of unenhanced or arterial

phase CT imaging or both used in conjunction with conventional portal venous phase contrast-enhanced CT imaging. AJR 1996; 167:71–77.
7. Bressler EL, Alpern MB, Glazer GM, Francis IR, Ensminger WD. Hypervascular hepatic metastases: CT evaluation. Radiology 1987; 162:49–51.
8. DuBrow RA, David CL, Libshitz HI, et al. Detection of hepatic metastases in breast cancer: the role of nonenhanced and enhanced CT scanning. J Comput Assist Tomogr 1990; 14:366–369.
9. Miller WJ, Baron RL, Dodd GD III, Federle MP. Malignancies in patients with cirrhosis: CT sensitivity and specificity in 200 consecutive transplant patients. Radiology 1994; 193:645–650.
10. Baron RL. Understanding and optimizing use of contrast material for CT of the liver. AJR 1994; 163:323–331.
11. Hwang GJ, Kim MJ, Yoo HS, Lee JT. Nodular hepatocellular carcinomas: detection with arterial-, portal-, and delayed-phase images at spiral CT. Radiology 1997; 202:383–388.
12. Heiken JP, Brink JA, McClennan BL, Sagel SS, Forman HP, DiCroce J. Dynamic contrast-enhanced CT of the liver: comparison of contrast medium injection rates and uniphasic and biphasic injection protocols. Radiology 1993; 187:327–331.
13. Heiken JP, Brink JA, McClennan BL, Sagel SS, Crowe TM, Gaines MV. Dynamic incremental CT: effect of volume and concentration of contrast material and patient weight on hepatic enhancement. Radiology 1995; 195:353–357.
14. Chambers TP, Baron RL, Lush RM. Hepatic CT enhancement. I. Alterations in the volume of contrast material within the same patients. Radiology 1994; 193:513–517.
15. Chambers TP, Baron RL, Lush RM. Hepatic CT enhancement. II. Alterations in contrast material volume and rate of injection within the same patients. Radiology 1994; 193:518–522.
16. Gaa J, Saini S, Ferrucci JT. Perfusion characteristics of hepatic cavernous hemangioma using intravenous CT angiography (IVCTA). Eur J Radiol 1991; 12:228–233.
17. Quinn SF, Benjamin GG. Hepatic cavernous hemangiomas: simple diagnostic sign with dynamic bolus CT. Radiology 1992; 182:545–548.
18. Baron RL, Freeny PC, Moss AA. The liver. In: Moss AA, Gamsu G, Genant HK, eds. Computed tomography of the body with magnetic resonance imaging. 2nd ed. Philadelphia, Pa: Saunders, 1992; 735–821.
19. Ohtomo K, Baron RL, Dodd GD III, et al. Confluent hepatic fibrosis in advanced cirrhosis: appearance at CT. Radiology 1993; 188:31–35.
20. Soyer P, Levesque M, Elias D, Zeitoun G, Roche A. Detection of liver metastases from colorectal cancer: comparison of intraoperative US and CT during arterial portography. Radiology 1992; 183:541–544.
21. Wernecke K, Rummeny E, Bongartz G, et al. Detection of hepatic masses in patients with carcinoma: comparative sensitivities of sonography, CT, and MR imaging. AJR 1991; 157:731–739.
22. Vassiliades VG, Foley WD, Alarcon J, et al. Hepatic metastases: CT versus MR imaging at 1.5 T. Gastrointest Radiol 1991; 16:159–163.
23. Chezmar JL, Rumancik WM, Megibow AJ, Hulnick DH, Nelson RC, Bernardino ME. Liver and abdominal screening in patients with cancer: CT versus MR imaging. Radiology 1988; 168:43–47.
24. Chomyn JJ, Stamm ER, Thickman D. CT of melanoma liver metastases: is the examination without contrast media superfluous? J Comput Assist Tomogr 1992; 16:568–571.
25. Patten RM, Byun JY, Freeny PC. CT of hypervascular hepatic tumors: are unenhanced scans necessary for diagnosis. AJR 1993; 161:979–984.

David A. C. Leggett, MB, BS • Benjamin B. Kelley, MB, BS • Ian H. Bunce, FRACP, FRCPA
Kenneth A. Miles, MD

Colorectal Cancer: Diagnostic Potential of CT Measurements of Hepatic Perfusion and Implications for Contrast Enhancement Protocols[1]

PURPOSE: **To assess changes in hepatic perfusion in patients with colorectal cancer with computed tomography (CT), diagnostic potential of CT perfusion measurements, and implications for design of contrast enhancement protocols.**

MATERIALS AND METHODS: **In 27 patients with colorectal cancer, arterial and portal perfusion were calculated from temporal changes in attenuation after intravenous administration of contrast material.**

RESULTS: **Arterial perfusion greater than 0.25 mL/min/mL was seen in nine (82%) of the 11 patients with overt metastases versus six (38%) of the 16 patients with no overt metastases ($P < .05$). Portal perfusion of 0.25 mL/min/mL or less was found in five (46%) of the patients with overt metastases versus three (19%) of the patients with no overt metastases. Follow-up imaging showed progressive metastatic disease in three patients, all of whom had decreased portal perfusion.**

CONCLUSION: **Increased arterial perfusion appears to be an indicator of liver metastases, whereas reduced portal perfusion may indicate progressive disease. Contrast enhancement protocols that are based on experience with normal livers may not be optimal for patients with metastases.**

Hemodynamic changes have been observed in the livers of patients with hepatic metastases with dynamic colloid scintigraphy (1), Doppler ultrasound (US) (2), and perfusion computed tomography (CT) (3). The fact that such changes may also be observed before detection of metastases on morphologic grounds has led to the concept of occult or micrometastases. Such occult metastases represent a considerable diagnostic challenge because their subsequent appearance after an ostensibly curative resection represents a substantial source of morbidity and mortality.

Nuclear medicine, Doppler US, and perfusion CT have all demonstrated an increase in arterial blood flow or perfusion as a proportion of total liver perfusion in patients with hepatic metastases (1–3). This increase in arterial blood flow results from the fact that metastases derive blood flow almost entirely from the arterial system (4). There is also some evidence of a reduction in portal perfusion resulting from a circulating vasoactive agent that increases splanchnic vascular resistance (5).

Perfusion CT has demonstrated increased arterial perfusion and variable changes in portal perfusion in a small series of patients with liver metastases from various primary tumors (3). To our knowledge, there has been no reported series of CT measurements of hepatic perfusion in patients with a single tumor type.

The purpose of this study was to assess CT measurement of hepatic perfusion in a series of patients with colorectal cancer. This study was performed for two reasons. First, altered perfusion may be an indicator of tumor within the liver. If so, then perfusion changes may have diagnostic potential in detecting occult or micrometastases. Furthermore, normal perfusion in a patient with a focal liver lesion may imply a benign pathologic process. Second, with slip ring CT systems, radiologists can now choose to image the liver in the arterial or portal phases of contrast enhancement or both. The amount of enhancement in each phase depends on liver perfusion. Changes in hepatic perfusion may therefore have implications for the design of contrast enhancement protocols.

MATERIALS AND METHODS

Patients

Twenty-seven consecutive patients with histologically proved colorectal cancer were studied with dynamic CT between March 1996 and January 1997. The 19 men and eight women ranged in age from 41 to 85 years (mean, 69.7 years). Approval was obtained from the Hospital Ethics Committee. Patients were recruited and informed consent was obtained in the radiology department before imaging. All 27 studies were performed at clinically requested, postoperative staging CT.

Index terms: Computed tomography (CT), contrast enhancement, 761.12113, 761.12114, 761.12115 • Computed tomography (CT), helical, 761.12115 • Gastrointestinal tract, neoplasms, 75.32 • Liver neoplasms, secondary, 761.33 • Neoplasms, blood supply, 761.33

Radiology 1997; 205:716–720

[1] From the Centre for Functional Imaging, Wesley Research Institute & Southern X-ray Clinics, 2nd Floor, Day Care Centre, Wesley Hospital, Chasely Street, Auchenflower, Queensland 4066, Australia (D.A.C.L., B.B.K., K.A.M.); and the Wesley Clinic for Haematology and Oncology, Auchenflower, Queensland, Australia (I.H.B.). Received June 9, 1997; revision requested July 8; revision received August 11; accepted August 12. Supported by a grant from the Wesley Research Institute. **Address reprint requests to** D.A.C.L.

Data Acquisition

A single-location dynamic sequence was performed with a spiral CT scanner (CT Twin; Elscint, Haifa, Israel). The section level was preselected from an initial series of images obtained through the liver without contrast enhancement. The level of the section was chosen to include any focal liver lesion or, if no such lesions were identified, then at a representative level of the liver. A section obtained through the midportion of the liver has been found previously to be most effective for minimizing misregistration artifact caused by respiratory motion. If possible, the spleen was included in the section. All patients fasted except for 750–1,000 mL of contrast material (diatrizoate meglumine and diatrizoate sodium, MD-Gastroview; Mallinckrodt Medical, St Louis, Mo) ingested 45–60 minutes before imaging. A 50-mL bolus of iopamidol (Isovue; Bristol-Myers Squibb, Princeton, NJ) (300 mg of iodine per milliliter) was then injected rapidly by hand over no more than 7 seconds at the commencement of the sequence. A section thickness of 10 mm was selected. Data acquisitions of 1-second duration were performed at 0 seconds and at 3, 6, 9, 12, 15, 18, 21, 24, 27, 32, and 37 seconds after commencement of injection of contrast material. The patient was instructed to breathe quietly during the examination. The images were subsequently compressed into a 256 × 256 matrix and transferred to a personal computer for later processing with dedicated software. The perfusion sequence was followed by a conventional contrast-enhanced examination after further administration of contrast material.

Region of Interest Analysis

The first image in the sequence provided baseline attenuation values to be subtracted from subsequent contrast-enhanced attenuation values. Regions of interest were created over the abdominal portion of the aorta, the spleen, and a large area of the liver that was independent of any metastasis that may have been visible on the image. The liver region of interest was made as large as possible (mean, 1,873 pixels; range, 334–5,724 pixels). Time attenuation data from the aortic region of interest were used to determine the peak arterial enhancement. The time of maximum enhancement of the spleen was calculated and used to distinguish between the arterial and portal phases of hepatic perfusion. When the spleen was absent from the section, a region of interest was created over the renal cortex or a region of skeletal muscle, and the time of peak renal or peak muscular enhancement was used to separate the arterial and portal phases of hepatic enhancement. Hepatic arterial and portal perfusion values were calculated with the method described previously by Miles (6) (see Appendix). Hepatic perfusion index values were then calculated for each pixel and displayed as a hepatic perfusion index image. Hepatic perfusion index images were used to determine whether altered perfusion was restricted to the metastases. Arterial perfusion, portal perfusion, and hepatic perfusion index were then calculated and recorded for the large hepatic region of interest.

Data Analysis

Conventional unenhanced and contrast-enhanced images were reviewed by a radiologist and assessed for the presence of focal liver lesions with morphologic criteria consistent with metastases. Any focal lesion that was not clearly benign according to conventional imaging criteria (eg, hepatic cyst) was classified as metastases. Patients were assigned to two groups: those with overt metastases and those without overt metastases.

Arterial and portal perfusion values and the hepatic perfusion index for the liver regions of interest were compared with those reported previously for normal livers. Arterial perfusion values above 0.25 mL/min/mL were considered abnormal; this value was reported as above the upper limit of normal values reported by Miles et al (3) in a series of normal livers. Similarly, portal perfusion values of 0.25 mL/min/mL or below were considered abnormally reduced, also on the basis of values reported in the same series of normal livers.

The numbers of patients with abnormally high arterial or abnormally low portal perfusion in the groups of patients with and those without focal liver lesions were compared with use of the Fisher exact test. A P value less than .05 was considered statistically significant. The median hepatic perfusion index was compared between patients with overt metastases and those without overt metastases by using the Wilcoxon rank sum test.

Follow-up Imaging

Images were reviewed in those patients who had returned for follow-up imaging. The number of patients with portal perfusion less than 0.25 mL/min/mL and progressive disease were compared with the number of patients with portal perfusion less than 0.25 mL/min/mL and no evidence of disease progression by using the Fisher exact test.

RESULTS

Of the 27 patients, 11 had overt metastases and 16 did not have overt metastases. A focal lesion was seen on the section included in the perfusion study in eight of the 11 patients with overt metastases.

Arterial Perfusion

The median value for arterial perfusion was 0.30 mL/min/mL (range, 0.08–0.81 mL/min/mL), compared with a median value of 0.17 mL/min/mL for normal livers reported by Miles et al (3). Of the 27 patients, 15 (56%) had arterial perfusion greater than 0.25 mL/min/mL, comprising nine (82%) of the 11 patients with overt metastases and six (38%) of the 16 patients with no overt metastases. These results provided the optimal threshold value for distinguishing the two groups and were statistically significant ($P < .05$, Fisher exact test).

Portal Perfusion

The median portal perfusion value was 0.38 mL/min/mL (range, 0.05–1.06 mL/min/mL), compared with a median value of 0.34 mL/min/mL reported by Miles et al (3). Of the 27 patients, eight (30%) demonstrated portal perfusion of 0.25 mL/min/mL or less, comprising five (46%) of 11 patients with overt metastases and three (19%) of 16 patients without overt metastases ($P = .14$, not statistically significant).

Hepatic Perfusion Index

The median hepatic perfusion index was 0.48 (range, 0.15–0.89), compared with a median value of 0.33 for normal livers reported by Miles et al (3). The median hepatic perfusion index was higher for patients with overt metastases (0.58) than for those with morphologically normal livers (0.34); however, this difference was not statistically significant ($P = .095$, Wilcoxon rank sum test). On hepatic perfusion index images, abnormal perfusion was demonstrated within and outside of the metastases (Figure).

Follow-up Imaging

Follow-up images were available in eight patients. The median follow-up was 3.5 months (range, 2–7 months). In three patients, progression of metastatic disease was observed. All three patients had a portal perfusion of 0.25 mL/min/mL or less compared with a portal perfusion of 0.25 mL/min/mL or less in only one of five patients with no evidence of progressive disease ($P = .07$, Fisher exact test.) The one patient with low portal perfusion but no overt metastases had an extensive local recurrence of the primary tumor in the pelvis.

DISCUSSION

The fact that small liver tumors are associated with detectable changes in hepatic hemodynamics has been reported previously (1–3). These small metastases may not be detected if conventional imaging techniques such as

CT, US, and magnetic resonance imaging are used. Such lesions have been termed occult or micrometastases. These occult metastases appear in 10%–30% of cases of colorectal cancer in which curative surgery was performed (7) and thus contribute substantially to treatment failure. A tool that can help identify those patients who are at risk of development of occult metastases would have obvious benefits in guiding adjuvant therapy.

Our study has confirmed that altered liver perfusion can be detected with perfusion CT in patients with colorectal cancer. The findings of increased arterial perfusion in patients with overt metastases suggests a role for arterial perfusion measurements as an indicator of metastatic tumor in the liver. This finding is in keeping with the known arterialization of metastases as seen with use of gelatin perfusion and resin techniques. The presence of increased arterial perfusion also has diagnostic potential. With use of conventional structural CT criteria as the standard, arterial perfusion greater than 0.25 mL/min/mL demonstrated a sensitivity of 82% and a specificity of 62% for the detection of metastases. These values of sensitivity and specificity may be artificially low owing to diagnostic errors associated with conventional CT. Further follow-up is necessary to determine whether the patients with apparently false-negative findings truly have metastases rather than other benign focal lesions. Similarly, patients with false-positive findings may in fact have micrometastases that become apparent at follow-up imaging.

Micrometastases have been shown histologically to be associated with overt tumors (8). The concept that increased arterial perfusion indicates micrometastases is supported by demonstration of abnormal perfusion outside overt metastases on hepatic perfusion index images and also by demonstration of increased arterial perfusion in patients with metastases but on CT sections other than that included in the perfusion study. Perfusion CT may also have a role in characterizing focal liver lesions. A finding of increased arterial perfusion in the remaining liver would imply the presence of malignancy, whereas normal perfusion would suggest a benign process.

Portal perfusion changes were variable, increased in some patients and reduced in others. The relevance of our follow-up data is constrained because the follow-up period was short and images were available only in some patients. However, the follow-up data suggest that reduced portal perfusion may indicate progressive disease. A possible reason for reduced portal perfusion is release of a vasoactive agent by the tumor. Release of a vasoactive agent by the tumor may have also been the cause for reduced portal perfusion in the patient with extensive local recurrence of the primary tumor. Alternatively, increased pressure within a liver segment containing enlarging metastases may reduce portal perfusion owing to an impedance effect. This impedance effect has been proposed as a mechanism for sparing of fatty infiltration around hepatic metastases in patients with fatty livers (9).

Increased arterial perfusion as measured at CT has also been demonstrated in cases of hepatic cirrhosis (3). None of our patients had evidence of cirrhotic liver disease, but if cirrhosis was present, increased arterial perfusion could not be considered indicative of malignancy. Portal perfusion is decreased in patients with cirrhosis (3); this finding is in contrast to that in the majority of patients with metastases in whom portal perfusion is normal or increased. However, portal perfusion measurements cannot enable reliable differentiation between malignant disease and cirrhosis, as some patients with malignancy also have decreased portal perfusion. Splenic perfusion measurements may be of value in such patients, as reduced splenic perfusion would imply hepatic cirrhosis (10).

Measurement of the ratio of hepatic arterial blood flow to total hepatic blood flow with Doppler US has been reported as the most sensitive for detection of colorectal liver metastases (2) compared with measurement at CT, US, and laparotomy. Measurement with Doppler US enables effective identification of those patients with colorectal cancer who are at an increased risk of development of hepatic metastases. A recent study has shown that Doppler US measurements correlate more closely with survival than that determined according to the classification of colorectal cancer by Duke (11). However, CT is generally considered more accurate than conventional US in the diagnosis of hepatic metastases. Perfusion CT can be readily incorporated into existing CT protocols, prolonging examination time by only a few minutes. If further research shows diagnostic performance of perfusion CT similar to that of Doppler US, combined conventional and perfusion CT may provide optimal assessment in a single investigation.

CT perfusion measurements provide information that cannot be derived directly from CT with visual impressions of enhancement or from crude measurements alone. This additional information results from the fact that perfusion CT calculations correct for variations in the shape of the contrast material bolus within the aorta that result from differences in cardiac output and central blood volume among individual patients. Furthermore, perfusion is determined by the rate of enhancement, necessitating interpolation between two contrast-enhanced images obtained a few seconds apart. Again, this is a process that cannot be performed readily with visual inspection alone.

Our results are broadly similar to those of Platt et al (12) who reported increased arterial phase enhancement in patients with hepatic metastases. Their measurements of enhancement were related indirectly to perfusion and yielded a sensitivity of 75% for detection of metastases, comparable to our sensitivity of 82%. The control group in that study differed from our group because it comprised patients with no known malignancy. This difference in patient populations would account for the lower specificity in our study, as a proportion of our patients with no visible metastases are likely to have micrometastases and an associated increase in arterial perfusion.

The finding of altered perfusion in the liver in patients with colorectal cancer has implications for contrast enhancement protocols used in conventional CT examinations. The liver demonstrates two phases of enhancement, with contrast material arriving first in the arterial system (arterial phase) and then in the portal vein (portal phase). Since delivery of contrast material is determined by perfusion, the amount of enhancement in each phase will depend on arterial and portal perfusion, respectively. Many studies have used attenuation measurements in normal livers as a model to determine the optimal administration of contrast material during CT. Because perfusion is altered in patients with colorectal cancer, even in the absence of focal liver lesions, normal livers may not be an appropriate model for determining contrast enhancement protocols. The advent of slip ring CT systems has given the radiologist the choice of imaging the liver in the arterial phase, the portal phase, or both. Metastases demon-

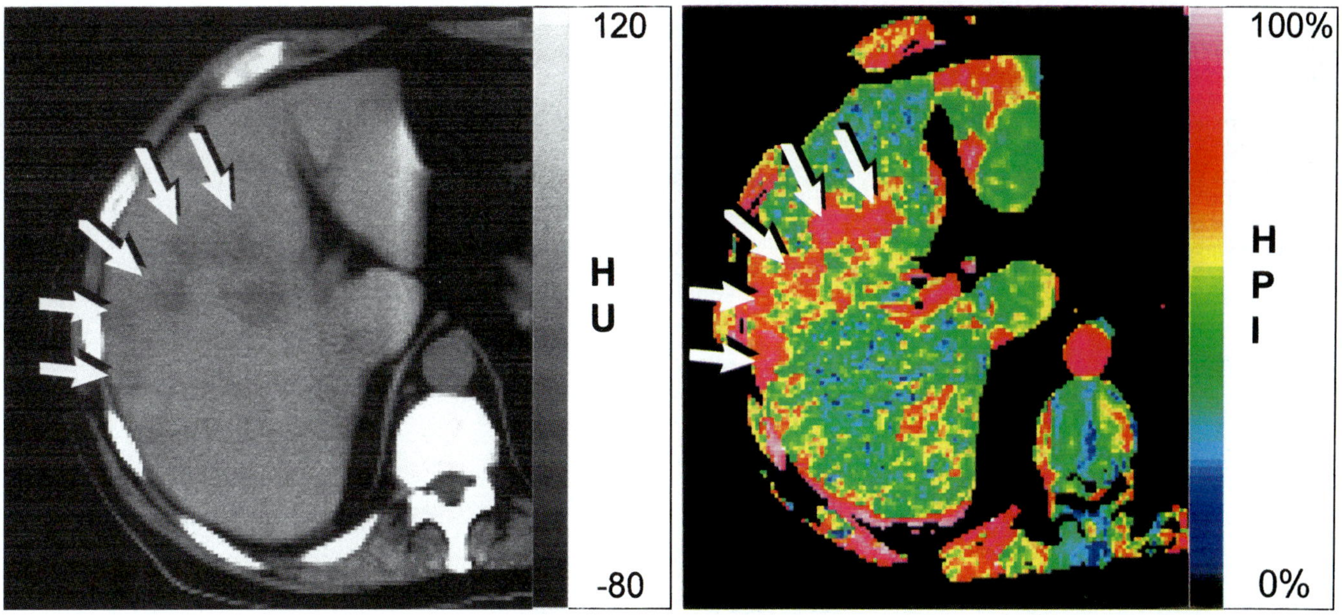

a. b.

(a) Conventional CT scan and **(b)** hepatic perfusion index (*HPI*) image obtained in a patient with multiple overt metastases. The metastases (arrows) demonstrate arterial perfusion close to 100%; however, high hepatic perfusion index values (approximately 50%) are also seen in the intervening liver, implying the presence of micrometastases.

strate increased arterial perfusion but so does the remaining liver, probably because of the presence of micrometastases. This increased perfusion produces enhancement that is greater than normal in the morphologically normal liver surrounding the metastases, thereby reducing the value of arterial phase imaging in the detection of colorectal metastases.

Conversely, metastases have little or no portal perfusion and demonstrate negative contrast compared with portal phase enhancement of the normal liver. Many patients with colorectal cancer demonstrate increased portal perfusion throughout the liver. Increased portal perfusion produces increased portal enhancement, thereby improving visualization of metastases in the portal phase. Thus, portal phase imaging is preferable to arterial phase imaging. However, in patients with decreased portal perfusion, the value of portal phase imaging is reduced, and hence the unpredictable nature of changes in portal perfusion could justify the use of dual-phase imaging.

Colorectal carcinoma is a common malignancy with a high occurrence of secondary hepatic disease. Approximately 20%–25% of patients with colorectal cancer have hepatic metastases at surgery. Assessment of hepatic perfusion with dynamic CT offers potential early detection of secondary disease in the liver in such patients. If CT measurements of hepatic perfusion are subsequently shown to have prognostic importance, then these measurements may be incorporated into existing staging protocols with the possible aim of guiding adjuvant treatment. The prediction of occult metastases has been shown to be feasible with Doppler US. It may be possible to predict occult metastases with perfusion CT and to refine the technique so that the specificity is improved. The presence of high arterial blood flow in the liver (high hepatic perfusion index) in a patient with no morphologic evidence of metastatic disease may indicate an elevated risk of development of secondary disease and thus indicate that more vigilant follow-up or adjuvant chemotherapy is necessary. Similarly, patients with normal hepatic perfusion index values may be at a lower risk of development of secondary disease, and thus the need for adjuvant therapy with associated morbidity could be avoided.

In conclusion, increased arterial perfusion appears to be an indicator of liver metastases, whereas decreased portal perfusion may indicate progressive disease. Contrast enhancement protocols that are based on experience with normal livers may not be optimal for patients with metastases. More patients and follow-up data are necessary in a range of tumor types to confirm the value of perfusion CT. We may be entering a new era in which CT provides physiologic information that may be of greater value than conventional anatomic evaluation alone.

APPENDIX

Measurement of tissue perfusion with dynamic CT necessitates acquisition of a rapid sequence of images without table movement after intravenous administration of a bolus of contrast material. The section level to be studied is chosen from an initial series of conventional unenhanced images. A suitable sequence comprises a baseline unenhanced image (from which initial attenuation values are subtracted from the subsequent changes after injection of contrast material) followed by a series of acquisitions lasting approximately 45 seconds. A short acquisition time (eg, 1 second) and interscan delay (eg, 2 seconds) are used (although the interscan delay can be increased toward the end of the sequence when attenuation values change less rapidly). Perfusion is then calculated from the subsequent temporal changes in contrast enhancement within the organ of interest and aorta.

The amount of contrast enhancement within any organ and the aorta, measured in Hounsfield units, is proportional to the concentration of contrast material and can be displayed as a time-attenuation curve. With use of the indicator dye-dilution theory, it is possible to derive the following general equation for calculation of perfusion, where perfusion is defined as blood flow per unit volume of tissue (6):

$$P = \frac{\text{Slope}_{\text{Max}}}{\text{Attenuation}_{\text{Peak}}}, \qquad \text{(A1)}$$

where P is perfusion in milliliters per minute per milliliter, $\text{Slope}_{\text{Max}}$ is the maximum slope of the tissue time-attenuation curve in Hounsfield units per minute, and $\text{Attenuation}_{\text{Peak}}$ is the peak attenuation in the input vessel in Hounsfield units. This equation applies only if the maximal rate of tissue enhancement occurs before any loss of contrast material from the organ into the venous system. Thus, a short bolus of contrast material is essential to avoid underestimation of perfusion resulting from venous washout. The precise volume of contrast material and rate of injection are not critical to the perfusion calculations but should be chosen so that the injection lasts no longer than 7 seconds, thereby enabling a sufficiently narrow bolus. A 40–50-mL bolus of contrast material with an iodine concentration of 300 mg/mL administered at 7 mL/sec provides a sufficiently short bolus with a concentration of iodine sufficient to maintain an adequate signal-to-noise ratio. A faster injection rate does not produce an improvement in bolus shape owing to the buffering effect of the pulmonary circulation. Use of an 18- or 19-gauge needle or cannula facilitates injection at this rate. It is not essential to standardize the injection rate among patients, as variations in cardiac output and central blood volume will have a greater effect on the final shape of the bolus within the aorta.

Application of the above method to the liver is complicated by the dual blood supply of the liver. The liver demonstrates a characteristic biphasic enhancement pattern. Early enhancement results from contrast material arriving via the hepatic arterial system followed by a second phase when contrast material arrives in the portal vein. The time that peak splenic enhancement occurs is used to separate arterial and portal phases. (When a spleen region is not available [eg, after splenectomy], renal cortex or skeletal muscle can be used as an alternative.) Arterial perfusion is determined by the equation

$$AP = \frac{\text{Slope}_{\text{Max}}}{\text{Enhancement}_{\text{Peak}}}, \qquad (A2)$$

where AP is the arterial perfusion in milliliters per minute per milliliter, $\text{Slope}_{\text{Max}}$ is the maximum slope of the liver time-attenuation curve before splenic enhancement in Hounsfield units per minute, and $\text{Enhancement}_{\text{Peak}}$ is the peak aortic enhancement in Hounsfield units. Portal perfusion is calculated similarly with the equation

$$PP = \frac{\text{Slope}_{\text{Max}}}{\text{Enhancement}_{\text{Peak}}}, \qquad (A3)$$

where PP is the portal perfusion in milliliters per minute per milliliter, $\text{Slope}_{\text{Max}}$ is the maximum slope of the liver time-attenuation curve after splenic enhancement in Hounsfield units per minute, and $\text{Enhancement}_{\text{Peak}}$ is the peak aortic enhancement in Hounsfield units.

The hepatic perfusion index (expressed as a percentage) indicates the proportion of liver perfusion that is arterial and is given by

$$HPI = \frac{AP}{AP + PP} \times 100, \qquad (A4)$$

where HPI is the hepatic perfusion index.

The technique is refined further by a thresholding procedure that eliminates from the analysis any pixels containing fat, air, bone, or intermediate to large blood vessels. All pixels with initial attenuation values below 0 HU or above 300 HU are excluded along with any pixels that change enhancement by more than 100 HU or less than −10 HU. In this way, hepatic vessels are excluded from large hepatic regions of interest. Calculation with use of time-attenuation data from individual pixel positions allows generation of functional images of arterial and portal perfusion and the hepatic perfusion index (3). ■

Acknowledgments: We thank M.P. Hayball, MA, MSc, and the University of Cambridge Department of Radiology for providing the data processing software.

References

1. Leveson SH, Wiggins PA, Giles GR, Parkin A, Robinson PJ. Deranged liver flow patterns in the detection of liver metastases. Br J Surg 1985; 72:128–130.
2. Leen E, Angerson WJ, Wotherspoon H, Moule B, Cook TG, McArdle CS. Detection of colorectal liver metastases: comparison of laparotomy, CT, US, and Doppler perfusion index and evaluation of postoperative follow-up results. Radiology 1995; 195:113–116.
3. Miles KA, Hayball MP, Dixon AK. Functional images of hepatic perfusion obtained with dynamic computed tomography. Radiology 1993; 188:405–411.
4. Ridge JA, Bading JR, Gelbard AS, et al. Perfusion of colorectal liver metastases: relative distribution of hepatic artery and portal vein. Cancer 1987; 59:1547–1553.
5. Leen E, Goldberg JA, Anderson JR, Moule B, Cook TG, McArdle CS. Hepatic perfusion changes in patients with hepatic metastases: comparison with those in patients with cirrhosis. Gut 1993; 34:554–557.
6. Miles KA. Measurement of tissue perfusion using dynamic computed tomography. Br J Radiol 1991; 64:409–412.
7. Takeuchi N, Ramirez JM, Mortensen NJM, Cobb R, Whittlestone T. Intraoperative ultrasonography in the diagnosis of hepatic metastases during surgery for colorectal cancer. Int J Colorectal Dis 1996; 11:92–95.
8. Haugeberg G, Strohmeyer T, Lierse W, Bocker W. The vascularization of liver metastases. Histological investigation of gelatine-injected liver specimens with special regard to the vascularization of micrometastases. J Cancer Res & Clin Oncol 1988; 114:415–419.
9. Itai Y, Maeda M, Echigo J, et al. Hyperattenuating rim on noncontrast CT of the liver: probable peritumoral sparing of fatty infiltration. Clin Radiol 1996; 51:406–410.
10. Miles KA, McPherson SJ, Hayball MP. Transient splenic inhomogeneity at contrast-enhanced CT: mechanism and effect of liver disease. Radiology 1995; 194:91–95.
11. Leen E, Angerson WG, Cooke TG, McArdle CS. Prognostic power of Doppler perfusion index in colorectal cancer: correlation with survival. Ann Surg 1996; 223:199–203.
12. Platt JF, Francis IR, Ellis JH, Reige KA. Liver metastases: early detection based on abnormal contrast material enhancement at dual-phase helical CT. Radiology 1997; 205: 49–53.

Thomas J. Vogl, MD • Andrej Stupavsky, MD • Wassilios Pegios, MD • Renate Hammerstingl, MD
Martin Mack, MD • Thomas Diebold, MD • Klaus-Peter Lodemann, MD
Peter Neuhaus, MD • Roland Felix, MD

Hepatocellular Carcinoma: Evaluation with Dynamic and Static Gadobenate Dimeglumine–enhanced MR Imaging and Histopathologic Correlation[1]

PURPOSE: **To analyze the potential of gadobenate dimeglumine–enhanced magnetic resonance (MR) imaging for the characterization and diagnosis of hepatocellular carcinoma (HCC) by using static and dynamic sequences.**

MATERIALS AND METHODS: **Twenty-eight patients with histopathologically proved HCC were evaluated with T1- and T2-weighted spin-echo and static and dynamic gradient-echo sequences before, during, and after intravenous administration of 0.1 mmol/kg gadobenate dimeglumine (0.5 mol/L).**

RESULTS: **During the perfusion phase of the dynamic sequence, all 16 nodular well-differentiated HCC lesions showed a rapid increase in signal intensity 10–30 seconds after injection followed by a progressive decrease in signal intensity. The nine poorly differentiated HCC lesions showed no rapid increase in signal intensity. All eight large (>3 cm), nodular, well-differentiated HCC lesions showed a hypointense rim before injection and both hypo- and hyperintense rims (double-ring sign) immediately after injection, compared with normal liver parenchyma. About 55 seconds after injection, substantial single-rim enhancement was detected in 21 of the 28 HCC lesions.**

CONCLUSION: **Dynamic gadobenate dimeglumine–enhanced MR imaging allows improved characterization of HCC lesions, which show rapid increase in signal intensity during the early, arterial phase in well-differentiated HCC lesions and a double-ring sign in large well-differentiated nodular HCC lesions.**

Magnetic resonance (MR) imaging with contrast material enhancement has the potential to become the leading imaging modality in evaluation of the liver. Extracellular contrast agents have been shown to be helpful in identifying hypervascular tumor and metastatic disease in this organ (1).

Superparamagnetic iron oxides have undergone the most extensive research to date, with improved lesion detection and differentiation (2). Hepatobiliary agents such as manganese- and gadolinium-based compounds have opened new perspectives in hepatic MR imaging (3–7). Gadobenate dimeglumine (MultiHance; Bracco, Milan, Italy [formerly, gadolinium benzyloxypropionictetraacetic acid or Gd-BOPTA]) is a contrast agent that exhibits high T1 relaxivity. A recently published study showed it to increase the percentage of enhancement of liver parenchyma on gradient-echo (GRE) T1-weighted MR images obtained 40 and 90 minutes after injection, yielding a substantially increased rate of detection of small metastatic lesions (8). In the present phase III study, we analyzed the potential of static and dynamic MR imaging with use of gadobenate dimeglumine for the characterization and diagnosis of hepatocellular carcinomas.

MATERIALS AND METHODS

Gadobenate Dimeglumine

Gadobenate dimeglumine is an octadentate chelate of the paramagnetic ion gadolinium that shows a twofold increase in relaxivity with respect to other gadolinium chelates in a medium containing macromolecules possibly because of weak interactions with the latter and consequent reduced tumbling rate. This agent was shown also to differ from the other currently available gadolinium chelates in that it is not only distributed to the extracellular fluid space, but, thanks to a chain containing a benzene ring on the chelate molecule, it is selectively taken up by hepatocytes and excreted into the bile by the so-called canalicular multispecific organic anion transporter shared with bilirubin (9). In humans, the biliary excretion of the gadobenate ion is low (2%–4% of the injected dose) and much lower than that observed in normal rats, rabbits, and dogs. The contrast enhancement of the signal intensity in the normal liver parenchyma of humans, however, is specific, marked, very prolonged, and dependent on hepatocellular uptake.

Gadobenate dimeglumine therefore belongs to the class of hepatocyte-directed MR contrast agents being developed to improve the accuracy of MR imaging for the detection of liver cancer nodules. Because of the modest biliary excretion, however, the kinetics of the gadobenate ion do not differ substantially from those of the gadolinium chelates available on the market (10,11). Thus, along with the liver-spe-

Index terms: Gadolinium • Liver neoplasms, diagnosis, 761.323 • Liver neoplasms, MR, 761.12141, 761.121412, 761.121415, 761. 12143 • Magnetic resonance (MR), contrast enhancement, 761.12141, 761.12143

Abbreviations: CNR = contrast-to-noise ratio, FLASH = fast low-angle shot, GRE = gradient echo, HCC = hepatocellular carcinoma, ROI = region of interest, SE = spin echo, 2D = two-dimensional.

Radiology 1997; 205:721–728

[1] From the Departments of Radiology (T.J.V., A.S., W.P., R.H., M.M., T.D., R.F.) and Surgery (P.N.), Rudolf Virchow Clinic, Humboldt-University of Berlin, Rudolf Virchow Hospital, Augustenburger Platz 1, D-13353 Berlin, Germany; and Bracco Byk Gulden, Konstanz, Germany (K.P.L.). Received April 21, 1997; revision requested June 5; revision received June 30; accepted July 8. Supported by a grant from Bracco Byk Gulden. **Address reprint requests to** T.J.V.

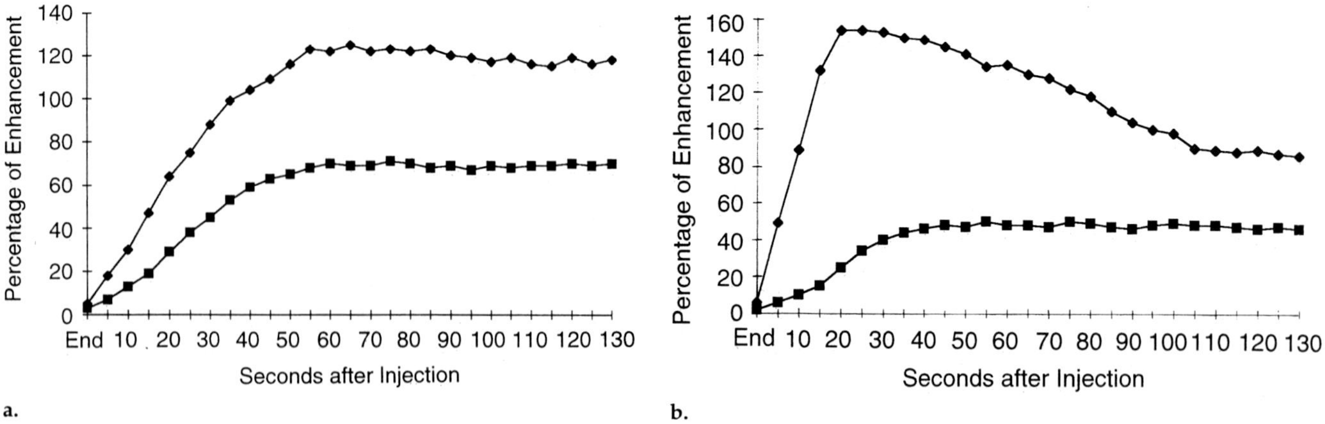

Figure 1. Dynamic evaluation of contrast enhancement of **(a)** noncirrhotic (◆) and cirrhotic (■) liver parenchyma and of **(b)** well-differentiated (◆) and poorly differentiated (■) HCC lesions by using a dynamic T1-weighted FLASH 2D GRE sequence. *End* = end of injection.

cific distribution and enhancement, the kinetics of gadobenate dimeglumine also allow it to be used as an extracellular agent for bolus dynamic MR imaging for the characterization of liver lesions, as well for MR imaging of other organ areas.

Study Design

In this prospective, phase III, double-blinded, randomized trial, 28 patients with known liver lesions were studied by using seven different MR sequence protocols before, during, and after intravenous injection of gadobenate dimeglumine. We used a 1.5-T commercially available unit (Magnetom SP 63; Siemens, Erlangen, Germany) with a conventional body coil. The diagnostic efficacy and safety of gadobenate dimeglumine were evaluated at a dosage of 0.1 mmol per kilogram of body weight (0.5 mol/L). Contrast material was administered as a bolus injection (1 mL/sec) through a 22-gauge cannula, which was placed in the antecubital vein and attached by means of a long connecting tube to a 20-mL syringe to avert having to change the patient's position during the examination. Immediately after bolus injection of the contrast agent, the connecting tube was flushed with 20 cm^3 NaCl 0.9%. In all patients, a follow-up MR imaging study was performed at 6–8 hours with identical pulse sequences.

MR Imaging Technique

The unenhanced examination protocol included conventional T2-weighted (2,000/45–90 [repetition time msec/echo time msec], 8-mm section thickness, no gap, 128 × 256 matrix, two signals acquired) as well as conventional and fat-suppressed T1-weighted (550/15, 8-mm section thickness, no gap, 256 × 256 matrix, four signals acquired) spin-echo (SE) sequences and fast low-angle shot (FLASH) two-dimensional (2D) GRE sequences performed with breath holding (154/6, 70° flip angle) in axial orientation (8-mm section thickness, no gap, 128 × 256 matrix, one signal acquired). The field of view for all sequences was similar (between 350 and 400 mm).

Figure 2. Percentage of enhancement of normal liver parenchyma (gray bar) and cirrhotic liver (white bar) after administration of gadobenate dimeglumine on T1-weighted GRE images. *Late* = 6–8 hours.

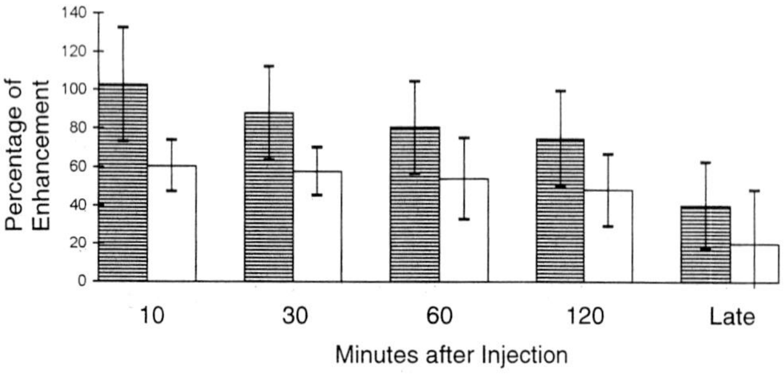

Table 1
Distribution of 104 Liver Lesions Detected on Static Contrast-enhanced Images

Lesion Size	Solitary Lesions: No. of Lesions	Solitary Lesions: No. of Patients	Fewer than 10 Lesions per Patient: No. of Lesions	Fewer than 10 Lesions per Patient: No. of Patients	More than 10 Lesions per Patient: No. of Lesions	More than 10 Lesions per Patient: No. of Patients	All Lesions: No. of Lesions	All Lesions: No. of Patients
<3 cm	6	6	17	9	57	3	80	18
>3 cm	10	10	11	7	3	3	24	20
All	16	16	28	9	60	3	104	28

Table 2
Characteristics of 28 HCC Lesions Visualized on Contrast-enhanced Dynamic T1-weighted GRE Images

Increase in Signal Intensity	Well-differentiated HCC Lesions (n = 19): <3 cm	Well-differentiated HCC Lesions (n = 19): >3 cm	Poorly Differentiated HCC Lesions* (n = 9)
Rapid and high (n = 18)			
Solid	8 nodular	0	0
Double ring	0	8 nodular	0
Multilocular	0	2 diffuse	0
Slow and slight (n = 10)	0	1 diffuse	9 nodular

* All poorly differentiated HCC lesions measured greater than 3 cm.

The dynamic evaluation was performed by using the above-described FLASH 2D GRE sequence with modified parameters (7/3, 15° flip angle) in axial orientation (8-mm section thickness, 128 × 256 matrix, two signals acquired). Dynamic sequences (n = 60) were run immediately after injection. The acquisition time of each sequence was 2.43 seconds followed by an interval of 3 seconds.

At 10, 30, 60, and 120 minutes and at 6–8 hours (to study delayed effects of contrast material) after injection of gadobenate dimeglumine, T1-weighted SE sequences in axial orientation and GRE sequences in axial and sagittal orientations and a fat-

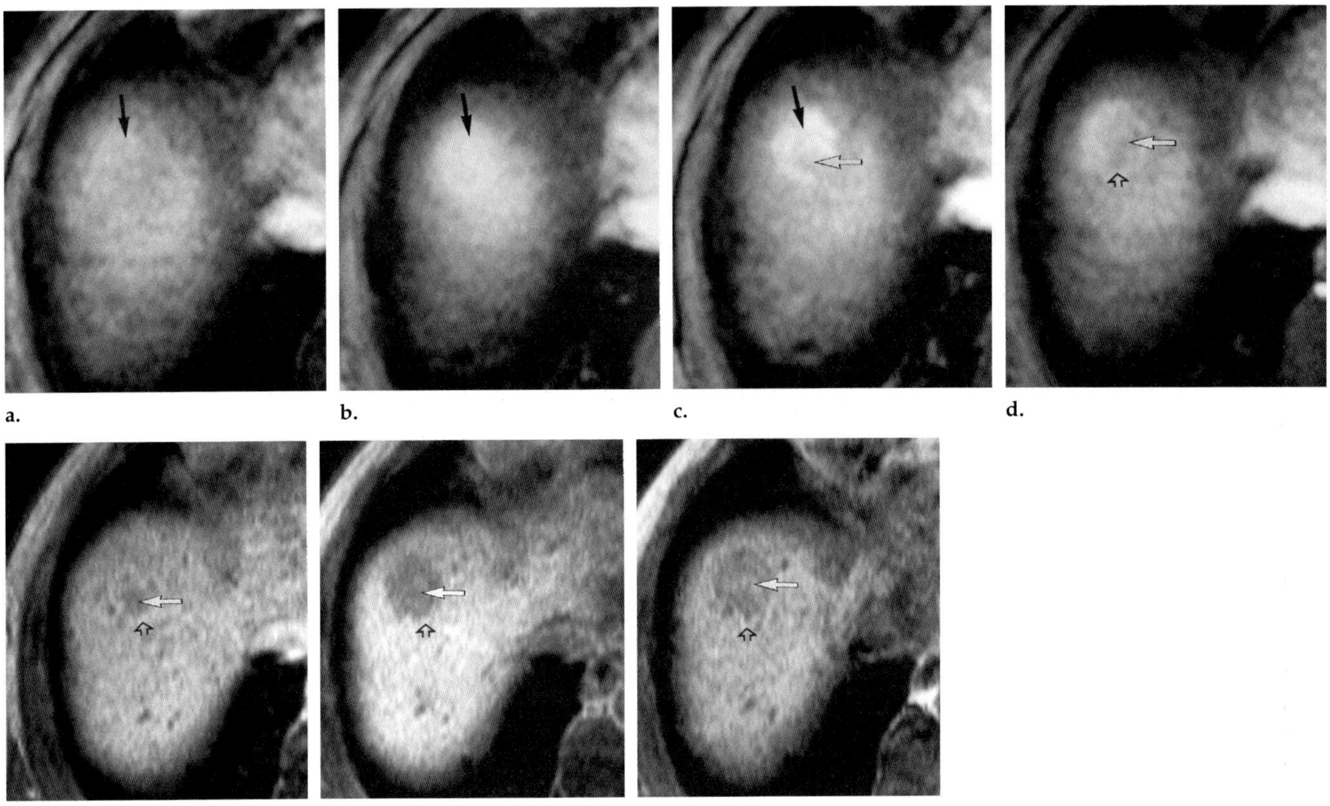

a. b. c. d. e. f. g.

Figure 3. Well-differentiated small HCC lesion in segment VIII. **(a)** Unenhanced dynamic FLASH 2D GRE image (7/5, 15° flip angle) shows that the hyperintense lesion (arrow) can hardly be delineated from the surrounding cirrhotic liver parenchyma. **(b)** Dynamic FLASH 2D GRE image (7/5, 15° flip angle) obtained 30 seconds after injection (arterial phase). During the perfusion phase, the lesion (arrow) enhances considerably. **(c)** Dynamic FLASH 2D GRE image (7/5, 15° flip angle) obtained 40 seconds after injection (venous phase) shows considerably more contrast enhancement of the hypervascularized periphery of the lesion (black arrow) and less enhancement of the central parts (white arrow). **(d)** Dynamic FLASH 2D GRE image (7/5, 15° flip angle) obtained 70 seconds after injection. During the late perfusion phase and the beginning of the distribution phase, the lesion (solid arrow) demonstrates reduced, inhomogeneous signal intensity with respect to the hyperintense outer rim (open arrow). **(e)** Static FLASH 2D GRE image (154/6, 70° flip angle) obtained 10 minutes after injection shows that the lesion is clearly hypointense (solid arrow). There are some inhomogeneities in the center of the tumor. The peripheral rim (open arrow) is hyperintense with respect to normal liver parenchyma and the HCC lesion. **(f)** Static FLASH 2D GRE image (154/6, 70° flip angle) obtained 60 minutes after injection shows that the signal intensity of the tumor and the CNR are substantially changed. The center (solid arrow) of this lesion is hypointense and inhomogeneous. The rim is hardly detectable (open arrow). **(g)** Static FLASH 2D GRE image (154/6, 70° flip angle) obtained 8 hours 20 minutes after injection. The liver parenchyma still shows high signal intensity. A hyperintense outer rim (open arrow) of the HCC lesion (solid arrow), hypointense to the liver, can be delineated.

suppressed T1-weighted sequence (10 and 20 minutes after injection) were performed.

Patients

Patients included in the study had focal suspected primary malignant liver lesions identified by means of clinical investigations (tumor markers) and contrast material–enhanced computed tomography (CT) or MR imaging within the 4 weeks before entering the study. All patients were willing and able to continue study participation through completion of all procedures and observations as required by the trial protocol. The study was approved by the local ethics committee. Fully informed and signed consent was obtained from all patients.

Excluded from the study were patients under 18 years of age; patients who had received any experimental drug within 30 days before entering this study; pregnant or lactating women (women in childbearing age were required to present a negative urine pregnancy test within 72 hours of injection of gadobenate dimeglumine); patients with contraindications to MR imaging, a history of serious adverse events, or allergic reactions after administration of drugs or contrast agents; patients with a transplanted organ; patients with severe liver dysfunction (total bilirubin >5 mg/dL [>85.5 µmol/L] or thromboplastin time <50%), clinically important renal failure (serum creatinine >2 mg/dL [>176.8 µmol/L]), or congestive heart failure (class III or IV according to the classification of the New York Heart Association); patients who had received contrast material during the 24 hours before injection of gadobenate dimeglumine or were scheduled to receive contrast material within 48 hours after; and clinically unstable patients or those with fluctuating laboratory parameters. Patients scheduled for liver biopsy or surgery within the 48-hour follow-up period or within 24 hours before the planned MR examination were also excluded from the study.

Of the 28 patients examined, there were 21 men and seven women who ranged in age from 34 to 73 years (mean age, 59.2 years).

Histopathologic examination revealed hepatocellular carcinoma (HCC) in all 28 patients. Clinical and imaging findings revealed a mild to severe form of cirrhosis in 21 patients.

Histopathologic specimens were obtained by means of resection of tumor in six patients, liver transplantation in five patients, and CT- or ultrasound-guided single biopsy, performed in the areas where the dynamic MR measurements were acquired, in 17 patients.

Image Analysis

Qualitative analysis.—All of the images were interpreted and assessed for character of contrast enhancement; presence or absence of morphologic features such as necrosis (defined as a lesion with high signal intensity on T2-weighted images, low

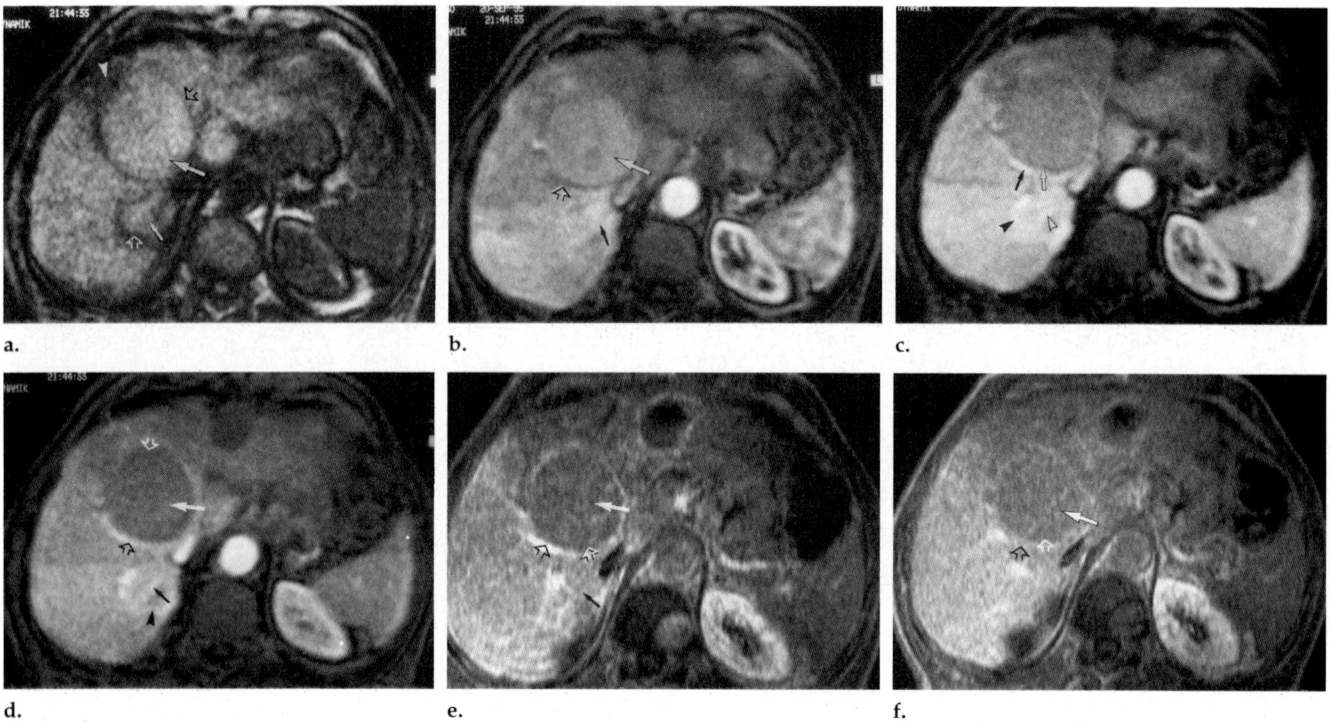

Figure 4. Large, poorly differentiated HCC lesion in segments IV and VIII and a hypervascularized regenerating nodule. **(a)** Unenhanced dynamic FLASH 2D GRE image (7/5, 15° flip angle). The HCC nodule (large white arrow) is of nodular homogeneity and is iso- to hyperintense to liver parenchyma. It is delineated by a markedly hypointense rim (open black arrow) with some inhomogeneous irregularity of the parenchymal bridge (arrowhead) between the HCC lesion and the liver surface. There is a second irregularity in segment VII (small solid white arrow) that is isointense and with a hypointense rim (open white arrow). **(b)** Dynamic FLASH 2D GRE image (7/5, 15° flip angle) obtained 30 seconds after injection. There is no rapid and high increase in signal intensity of the lesion (white arrow) and the rim remains hypointense (open arrow). The liver parenchyma shows inhomogeneous enhancement. Note the discrete hyperintensity of the regenerative nodule in segment VII (black arrow). **(c)** Dynamic FLASH 2D GRE image (7/5, 15° flip angle) obtained 55 seconds after injection. There are two detectable rings around the HCC nodule: an internal, hypointense rim (white arrow) and an outer, hyperintense rim (black arrow). The regenerative nodule (white arrowhead) is hyperintense with discrete rim enhancement (black arrowhead). **(d)** Dynamic FLASH 2D GRE image (7/5, 15° flip angle) obtained 130 seconds after injection. The lesion is completely hypointense (solid white arrow) and surrounded by the hypointense (open white arrow) and hyperintense (open black arrow) rims. Signal intensity of the regenerative node (solid black arrow) and its hyperintense rim (arrowhead) in segment VII remain unchanged. **(e)** Static FLASH 2D GRE image (154/6, 70° flip angle) obtained 10 minutes after injection. The lesion (solid white arrow) is homogeneously hypointense with hypointense inner (open white arrow) and hyperintense outer (open black arrow) rims. The regenerating nodule is inhomogeneously hypointense (solid black arrow). **(f)** Static FLASH 2D GRE image (154/6, 70° flip angle) obtained 60 minutes after injection. Delineation of the HCC nodule (solid arrow) is reduced due to decreasing liver-to-lesion contrast and the lower intensity of the rim (open black arrow). The hypointense inner rim (open white arrow) is hardly detectable.

signal intensity on unenhanced T1-weighted images, and no contrast enhancement), central scar, and/or surrounding capsule; and the form, number, size, and location (hepatic segmental anatomic classification according to Couinaud) of lesions. The enhancement characteristics over time (during the perfusion phase and hepatobiliary phase) were assessed for peripheral and central enhancement patterns. The qualitative analysis was performed by two experienced radiologists (T.J.V., W.P.), and decision was made by consensus. The analyses were cross-referenced with the histopathologic diagnoses.

Quantitative analysis.—For unenhanced and contrast-enhanced (T1-weighted SE and GRE) images, each lesion was evaluated separately for signal intensity in relation to normal liver parenchyma. Signal intensity was read directly from the monitor for lesion, normal liver parenchyma, and spleen or major cirrhotic areas of the livers by using operator-defined regions of interest (ROIs). For lesions with cystic components, care was taken to measure signal intensity only in solid portions of the tumor and outside regions of capsule or scar. Major hepatic and portal vessels were avoided when measuring the signal intensity of normal liver parenchyma. The mean intensities of background noise, including systematic or statistical noise, were measured outside the ROI. ROIs were placed identically on unenhanced and contrast-enhanced images.

A signal-to-noise ratio, SNR, was calculated between the signal intensities of liver tumors and normal background tissue by using the following equation: $SNR = (SI_{lesion} - SI_{noise})/SD_{noise}$, where SI_{lesion} = signal intensity of the lesion, SI_{noise} = signal intensity of the background tissue (measured by placing the ROIs in a position excluding motion artifacts), and SD_{noise} = standard deviation of the signal intensity of the background tissue without artifacts.

The lesion-to-liver contrast-to-noise ratios (CNRs) were determined with the following equation: $CNR = (SI_{lesion} - SI_{liver})/SI_{noise}$, where SI_{lesion} = signal intensity of liver lesion, SI_{liver} = signal intensity of normal liver parenchyma, and SI_{noise} = signal intensity of background tissue (measured by placing the ROIs anterior and posterior to the patient near normal liver parenchyma including motion artifacts).

The degree of contrast enhancement (percentage of enhancement, PE) was described for static and dynamic imaging as follows: $PE = [(SI_{postcontrast} - SI_{precontrast})/SI_{precontrast}] \times 100$, where $SI_{precontrast}$ = signal intensity of tissue on the precontrast image and $SI_{postcontrast}$ = signal intensity on the postcontrast image (gadobenate dimeglumine).

Statistical analysis was carried out for the difference in the CNRs, signal-to-noise ratios, and percentage of enhancement on static unenhanced and gadobenate dimeglumine–enhanced T1-weighted, GRE, and SE images. First, an overall test (Friedman test) was used. If the differences in ratings of sequences were significant, a two-sample Wilcoxon matched-pairs signed-rank test was performed to compare the sequences pairwise. Nonparametric median tests were used because the covariates were not normally distributed. An overall significance level of $\alpha = 5\%$ was stipulated.

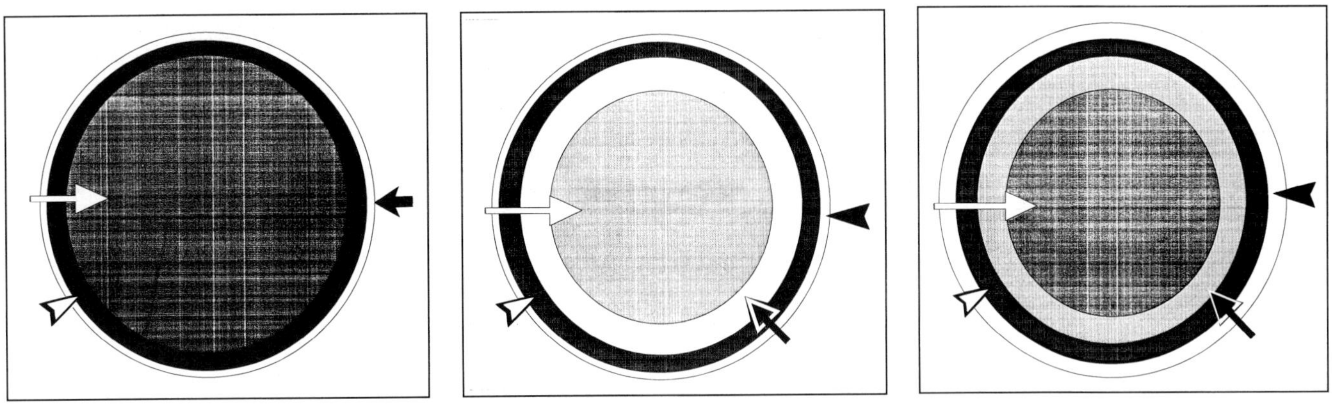

a. b. c.

Figure 5. Schematic diagram of a nodular well-differentiated HCC lesion (>3 cm) with the unenhanced T1-weighted FLASH GRE sequence **(a)** of the dynamic protocol. The central parts of the lesion appear hypointense (white arrow). The arrowhead shows the hypointense internal rim that corresponds to the HCC capsule and parts of the compressed neighboring hepatic parenchyma and surrounding vascular system. The black arrow marks the outer, slightly hyperintense rim, which appears in some large HCC lesions. **(b)** Early perfusion phase 30 seconds ± 10 after intravenous administration of gadobenate dimeglumine. The HCC capsule (white arrowhead) remains hypointense. The peripheral zone (black arrow) of the HCC lesion becomes hyperintense due to early arterial vascularization. This and the hypointense capsule represent the double-ring sign. The central parts of the HCC lesion (white arrow) show a delayed increase in signal intensity. Black arrowhead indicates the outer rim of the tumor (veins, compressed surrounding tissues). **(c)** Late perfusion phase (60 seconds ± 10). The outer rim of the tumor (black arrowhead) reveals marked enhancement with respect to the hypointense capsule (white arrowhead) and peripheral (black arrow) and central (white arrow) tumor parts.

RESULTS

No adverse side effects were observed during or after administration of gadobenate dimeglumine.

Normal Liver Parenchyma versus Liver Cirrhosis

After administration of gadobenate dimeglumine, dynamic T1-weighted GRE images revealed a biphasic contrast effect for the liver, consistent with separate perfusion and distribution phases. During the perfusion phase, a homogeneous increase in the signal intensity of normal liver parenchyma was noted up to 55 seconds after injection (Fig 1a). The peak of signal intensity increase during the perfusion phase showed mean values of maximum percentage of enhancement of 89% ± 29. During the further course of enhancement in dynamic gadobenate dimeglumine–enhanced studies, a plateaulike stabilization of signal intensity was seen at the beginning of the distribution phase. Analysis of the dynamic pattern in patients with liver cirrhosis revealed lower values for percentage of enhancement as compared with noncirrhotic liver parenchyma (Fig 1a).

The mean values of percentage of enhancement in liver tissue after administration of gadobenate dimeglumine on static T1-weighted SE and GRE images obtained at 10, 30, 60, and 120 minutes showed no statistically significant changes, while the 6–8-hour follow-up revealed reduced percentage of enhancement values (Fig 2). We observed different values for percentage of enhancement after administration of gadobenate dimeglumine, depending on the degree of underlying liver disease. For normal liver parenchyma ($n = 7$), a mean percentage of enhancement of 102% ± 30 was calculated for the static T1-weighted sequences performed 10 minutes after injection. In patients with liver cirrhosis ($n = 21$), we observed an inhomogeneous nodular pattern of enhancement with reduced contrast enhancement on the static T1-weighted images: mean percentage of enhancement = 61% ± 13 (Fig 2).

Lesion Detection

T1- and T2-weighted SE and GRE sequences allowed detection of 93 lesions in the 28 patients. Gadobenate dimeglumine–enhanced sequences enabled detection of an additional 11 lesions in five patients. In 25 patients, who had solitary or multiple lesions (two to five lesions per patient), we observed 37 nodular and seven diffuse lesions. In the other three patients, who had multiple lesions, we detected a total of 59 nodular lesions and one diffuse lesion (Table 1). Histopathologic examination revealed HCC in all 28 patients, with well-differentiated HCC in 19 and poorly differentiated HCC in nine patients.

Sixty-three (68%) of 93 lesions (including 37 lesions in two of the three patients with >10 lesions) were hypointense on unenhanced static T1-weighted SE and GRE images. Six lesions in four patients were iso- to hyperintense. Twenty-three lesions in one patient with hemosiderosis and one tumor nodule in a patient with liver cirrhosis were strongly hyperintense on unenhanced T1-weighted SE images.

HCC Lesions

We examined only one histopathologically proved HCC lesion per patient on the dynamic T1-weighted GRE images (Table 2): 16 nodular and three diffuse well-differentiated HCC lesions, and nine nodular poorly differentiated HCC lesions. These 28 HCC lesions showed variable increases in signal intensity, depending on the underlying morphologic condition.

During the arterial part of the perfusion phase of the dynamic sequence (10–50 seconds after injection), we could observe two main groups of HCC lesions (Table 2, Fig 1b): one group with a rapid and high increase in signal intensity associated with hyperintensity to liver parenchyma, with a maximum at 10–30 seconds after injection (Fig 3b); and one group with a slow and only slight increase in signal intensity and hypointense with respect to liver tissue (Fig 4). All lesions in the first group proved to be well-differentiated HCC; none of the poorly differentiated HCC lesions showed the rapid and high increase in signal intensity.

Diffuse well-differentiated HCC lesions ($n = 2$) showed an inhomogeneous, nodular pattern of increase in

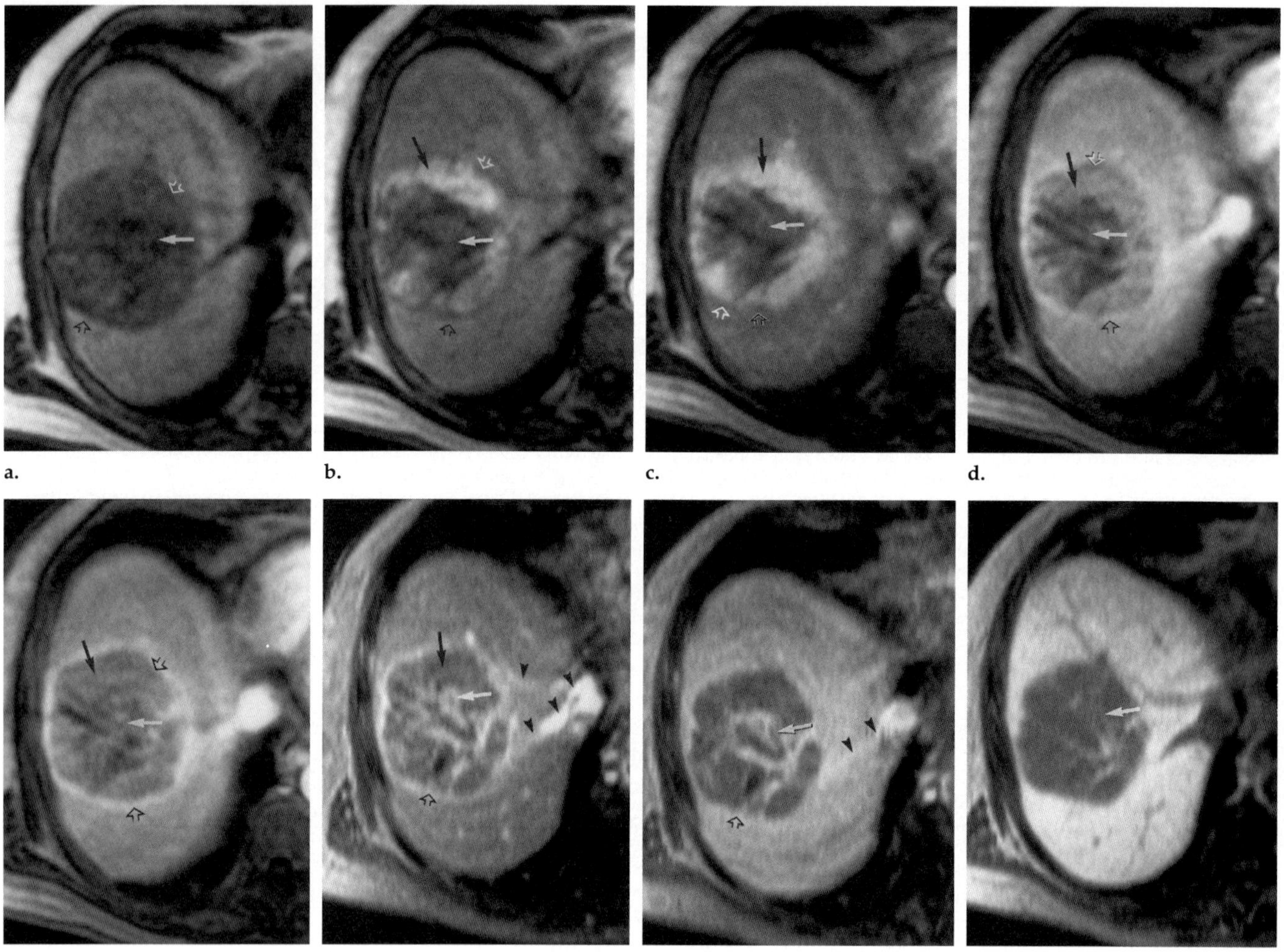

a. b. c. d.

e. f. g. h.

Figure 6. Well-differentiated HCC lesion in segment VIII. **(a)** Unenhanced dynamic FLASH 2D GRE image (7/5, 15° flip angle) shows a hypointense lesion (solid arrow) with a peripheral rim of low signal intensity (open white arrow) and a thin hyperintense outer rim (open black arrow). **(b)** Dynamic FLASH 2D GRE image (7/5, 15° flip angle) obtained 30 seconds after injection of gadobenate dimeglumine (arterial phase). During the perfusion phase, there is considerable inhomogeneous enhancement of the hypervascularized periphery of the lesion (solid black arrow) with minimal enhancement of the center (solid white arrow). The peripheral rim (open white arrow) is hypointense with respect to normal liver parenchyma. The thin hyperintense outer rim (open black arrow) shows no change in signal intensity. The hepatic veins and the inferior vena cava do not enhance. **(c)** Dynamic FLASH 2D GRE image (7/5, 15° flip angle) obtained 40 seconds after injection of gadobenate dimeglumine (venous phase). Ten seconds after obtaining the previous image, the lesion shows a considerably higher degree of enhancement of the hypervascularized periphery (black arrow) with less enhancement of the central parts (solid white arrow). The hypointense internal rim (open white arrow) and hyperintense outer rim (open black arrow) are hardly detectable, with signal intensity similar to that of the peripheral tumor zone. **(d)** Dynamic FLASH 2D GRE image (7/5, 15° flip angle) obtained 70 seconds after injection. During the late perfusion phase and the beginning of the distribution phase, the lesion shows less signal intensity with respect to the hyperintense periphery (solid black arrow). The center of the lesion (white arrow) still shows reduced, inhomogeneous signal intensity. The hypointense inner rim (open white arrow) is not continuously visible. Good delineation of the thin hyperintense outer rim (open black arrow) is noted. **(e)** Dynamic FLASH 2D GRE image (7/5, 15° flip angle) obtained 195 seconds after injection. The lesion demonstrates a more homogeneous signal intensity of the center (white arrow) on this late dynamic image, while the peripheral zone (solid black arrow) shows increased degree of enhancement with exact delineation (open arrows). **(f)** Static FLASH 2D GRE image (154/6, 70° flip angle) obtained 10 minutes after injection shows marked hypointensity (solid black arrow) of the lesion. There are some inhomogeneities and septal enhancements (white arrow) in the center of the tumor. The outer rim (open arrow) is hyperintense with respect to normal liver parenchyma and HCC. The inferior vena cava and hepatic veins (arrowheads) show marked hyperintensity; their connection to the HCC rim is presumed. **(g)** Static FLASH 2D GRE image (154/6, 70° flip angle) obtained 60 minutes after injection. Fifty minutes after the previous image was obtained, there is no noteworthy change in tumor signal intensity and CNR. The center of this lesion (white arrow) demonstrates inhomogeneity and septal enhancements as well. The HCC rim (open arrow) is less enhanced compared with the previous image. The hepatic veins (arrowheads) are also less visible. **(h)** Static FLASH 2D GRE image (154/6, 70° flip angle) obtained 8 hours 20 minutes after injection shows that the liver parenchyma has persistent high signal intensity. The HCC lesion (arrow), hypointense to the liver and without a visible rim, is more homogeneous.

signal intensity that resulted in multilocular rapid increase in signal intensity of the lesion. All eight large (>3 cm in diameter), nodular, well-differentiated HCC lesions showed a hypointense rim before injection of gadobenate dimeglumine, and four of these large HCC lesions showed both an internal hypointense rim and an outer hyperintense rim (Figs 5a, 6a). In the arterial perfusion phase after injection of gadobenate dimeglumine, the hypointense rim showed no noteworthy enhancement. Predominantly, the hyperperfused peripheral part of these large HCC lesions showed rapid and high increase in signal intensity. Central portions of large well-differentiated HCC lesions showed low contrast enhancement (Figs 5b, 6b, 6c), consistent with a lack of vasculariza-

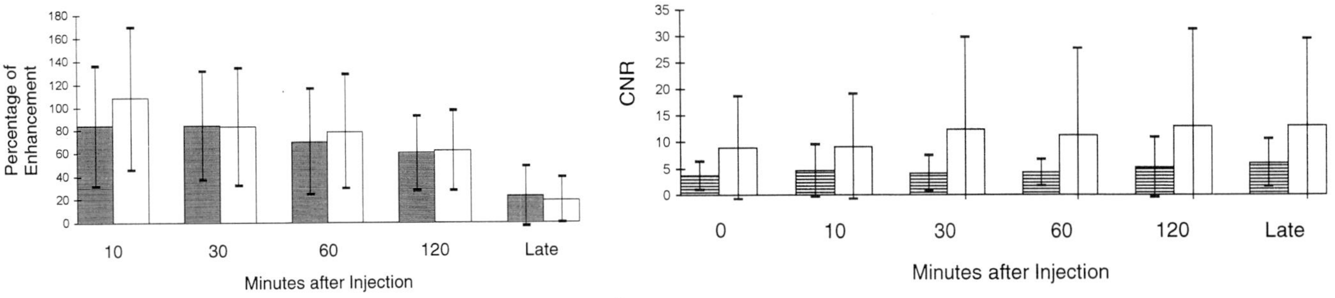

Figure 7. **(a)** Percentage of enhancement (median ± standard deviation) of well-differentiated (gray bar) and poorly differentiated (white bar) HCC lesions on T1-weighted GRE images after injection of gadobenate dimeglumine. *Late* = 6–8 hours. **(b)** Liver-to-lesion CNRs (median ± standard deviation) for well-differentiated (striped bar) and poorly differentiated (white bar) HCC lesions on T1-weighted GRE images obtained before and after injection of gadobenate dimeglumine. *Late* = 6–8 hours.

tion, and inhomogeneous contrast enhancement, presumably due to the hyperenhanced areas (extracellular space). The peripheral rapid and high increase in signal intensity and the surrounding internal hypointense rim were defined as a unique double-ring sign or even as a triple-ring sign, when considering the outer hyperintense rim that appeared in four of the lesions.

During the venous perfusion phase of the dynamic sequence (50–70 seconds), the signal intensity of the HCC lesions decreased. The outer hyperintense rim (surrounding the hypointense tumor capsule) in all HCC lesions became markedly hyperintense possibly due to a direct contact with hepatic veins and the inferior cava (Figs 5c, 6d). This presumed connection could be seen even better in the distribution phase (Fig 6e) of the dynamic sequence or with the static T1-weighted GRE sequences 10 minutes after injection (Fig 6f). Seven lesions had no rim of high signal intensity at the beginning of the venous perfusion phase, including two lesions with no hyperintense rim during the entire dynamic imaging sequence.

The histopathologically proved HCC lesion in one patient with advanced hemosiderosis (23 hyperintense lesions in all) did not show the rapid and high increase in signal intensity, but a rim of hyperintensity was seen on the dynamic enhanced studies.

Independent of the tumor grades, 23 (82%) of the 28 lesions were iso- or hypointense compared with liver parenchyma on dynamic T1-weighted GRE images obtained 3 minutes after injection of contrast material.

With the late static sequences, we noted an unexpectedly high percentage of enhancement of HCC lesions (Fig 7a). T1-weighted GRE images showed distinctly higher mean values of percentage of enhancement as compared with T1-weighted SE images. The HCC lesions showed a wide variation in CNRs after application of gadobenate dimeglumine. The highest overall mean CNR measured for well-differentiated HCC lesions (6% ± 4) and that for poorly differentiated HCC lesions (13% ± 16) were achieved with T1-weighted GRE sequences at 6–8 hours after injection (Fig 7b). Quantitative evaluation of the percentage of enhancement and CNR values revealed no statistically significant differences between well- and poorly differentiated HCC lesions.

DISCUSSION

Consistent with data obtained in the phase I trial (12), we observed a reproducibly increased enhancement of the liver parenchyma on GRE images after intravenous administration of 0.1 mmol per kilogram of body weight gadobenate dimeglumine due to the bilitranslocase-transport mechanism of the contrast agent uptake by the hepatocytes (12,13).

Qualitative and quantitative analysis of normal liver parenchyma after intravenous use of gadobenate dimeglumine revealed a biphasic pattern of contrast enhancement in our series, which also included analysis of the characteristics of gadobenate dimeglumine in a dynamic protocol. The use of the 0.1 mmol/kg gadobenate dimeglumine (0.5 mol/L) yielded the maximum percentage of enhancement during the perfusion phase. We could confirm, as has been reported elsewhere (12), that peak liver signal intensities are seen 10 minutes after injection during the hepatobiliary phase, followed by plateaulike constant signal intensities over approximately 1 hour and a statistically significant enhancement of liver tissue as long as 6–8 hours after application of the contrast agent. Qualitative analysis showed a high degree of enhancement and contrast of the gallbladder and the biliary duct with respect to surrounding liver tissue.

Caudana et al (8) studied the enhancement characteristics of gadobenate dimeglumine 40 and 90 minutes after injection, with best results for the GRE T1-weighted images (mean, 83%), but they failed to observe an increased detection rate of primary cancer nodules. Substantially more small primary HCC nodules were detected on gadobenate dimeglumine–enhanced GRE T1-weighted images than with unenhanced sequences. Consistent with the findings of Caudana et al (8), we observed that primary malignant lesions show a wide variation in CNR. No substantial difference was found in the CNR of HCC lesions before and after administration of gadobenate dimeglumine. This may be a result of the interindividual variability in liver function due to age and type of liver disease (cirrhosis, hepatitis, tumor spread) (14), with reduced contrast material uptake by hepatocytes, and it may be due to the high degree of HCC enhancement (resulting in low CNR), probably because of the retention of some hepatocellular function, pooling of contrast material, and/or the presence of fat or paramagnetic ions (iron, copper) (15,16). Therefore, the nontumorous liver parenchyma showed a function-dependent rise in signal intensity. The early contrast enhancement of the liver parenchyma and histopathologically proved malignant focal lesions occurred during the perfusion phase.

We regularly observed a rapid increase in the enhancement of the well-differentiated HCC lesions immediately after injection of the contrast agent, in the arterial part of the perfusion phase, leading us to a presumption that these lesions are richly arterialized. The rapid increase in signal intensity that we observed in the large (>3 cm) well-differentiated HCC lesions manifested in the periphery of the lesion. This phenomenon was diagnostically relevant. Dynamic sequences with use of gadobenate dimeglumine showed a substantial relation between the rapid and high increase in signal intensity of the perfusion phase in HCC lesions and their morphologic features. We observed no rapid increase in signal intensity in poorly differentiated HCC lesions. Also, we observed peripheral tumor rim enhancement during the venous perfusion phase and, later on, after injection of gadobenate dimeglumine, in both well- and poorly differentiated HCC lesions. Enhancement seen during the venous perfusion phase is generally an indication of venous vascularity and extent of the extracellular spaces, and possibly increased cellular uptake in peritumoral liver tissue. The nonenhancing peripheral rim was defined as a lesion capsule.

It is known that well-differentiated HCC lesions retain some hepatocellular function, with uptake of hepatospecific contrast agents including mangafodipir trisodium (5,17) and gadoxetate disodium (18). Our qualitative and quantitative measurements in well-differentiated HCC lesions substantiate these findings.

Although other groups strongly favor T1-weighted SE and GRE sequences obtained 40 or even 90 minutes after injection of gadobenate dimeglumine, our data show that dynamic imaging helps to overcome some of the problems and that we still have remarkable detection data 120 minutes after injection of gadobenate dimeglumine.

In conclusion, gadobenate dimeglumine–enhanced static and dynamic MR imaging yields an improved detection rate of lesions, and dynamic imaging delivers tumor-specific information for HCC in patients with liver cirrhosis or patients with no underlying liver disease. ■

References

1. Yoshida H, Itai Y, Ohtomo K, Kokubo T, Minami M, Yashiro N. Small hepatocellular carcinoma and cavernous hemangioma: differentiation with dynamic FLASH MR imaging with Gd-DTPA. Radiology 1989; 171:339–342.
2. Bellin MF, Zaim S, Auberton E, et al. Liver metastases: safety and efficacy of detection with superparamagnetic iron oxide in MR imaging. Radiology 1994; 193:657–663.
3. Bernardino ME, Young SW, Lee JKT, Weinreb JC. Hepatic MR imaging with Mn-DPDP: safety, image quality, and sensitivity. Radiology 1992; 183:53–58.
4. Kreft BP, Tanimoto A, Baba Y, Zhao L, Finn JP, Stark DD. Enhanced tumor detection in presence of fatty liver disease: cell-specific contrast agents. JMRI 1994; 4:337–342.
5. Rofsky NM, Weinreb JC, Bernardino ME, Young SW, Lee JK, Noz ME. Hepatocellular tumors: characterization with Mn-DPDP–enhanced MR imaging. Radiology 1993; 188:53–59.
6. Schuman-Gianpieri G, Schmitt-Willich H, Press WR, Negishi C, Weinmann HJ, Speck U. Preclinical evaluation of Gd-EOB-DTPA as a contrast agent in MR imaging of the hepatobiliary system. Radiology 1992; 183: 59–64.
7. Hamm B, Staks T, Muhler A, et al. Phase I clinical evaluation of Gd-EOB-DTPA as a hepatobiliary contrast agent: safety, pharmacokinetics, and MR imaging. Radiology 1995; 195:785–792.
8. Caudana R, Morana G, Pirovano GP, et al. Focal malignant hepatic lesions: MR imaging enhanced with gadolinium benzyloxypropionictetra-acetate (BOPTA)—preliminary results of phase II clinical application. Radiology 1996; 199:513–520.
9. de Haën C, Lorusso V, Tirone P. Hepatic transport of gadobenate dimeglumine in TR-rats. Acad Radiol 1996; 3:S425–S454.
10. Weinmann HJ, Laniado M, Mutzel W. Pharmacokinetics of Gd-BOPTA dimeglumine after intravenous injection into healthy volunteers. Physiol Chem Phys Med NMR 1984; 16:167–172.
11. McLachlan SJ, Eaton S, De Simone DN. Pharmacokinetics behavior of gadoteridol injection. Invest Radiol 1992; 27:S12–S15.
12. Vogl T, Pegios W, McMahon C, et al. Gadobenate dimeglumine: a new contrast agent for MR imaging—preliminary evaluation in healthy volunteers. AJR 1992; 158: 887–892.
13. Cavagna F, Tirone P, Felder E, de Haën C. Hepatobiliary contrast agents for MRI. In: Ferrucci JT, Stark DD, eds. Liver imaging: current trends and new techniques. Boston, Mass: Andover Medical, 1990; 384–393.
14. Schuman-Gianpieri G. Liver contrast media for magnetic resonance imaging: interrelations between pharmacokinetics and imaging. Invest Radiol 1993; 28:753–761.
15. Ebara M, Watanabe S, Kita K, et al. MR imaging of small hepatocellular carcinoma: effect of intratumoral copper content on signal intensity. Radiology 1991; 180:617–621.
16. Kitagawa K, Matsui O, Kadoya M, et al. Hepatocellular carcinomas with excessive copper accumulation: CT and MR findings. Radiology 1991; 180:623–828.
17. Ni Y, Marchal G, Zhang X, et al. The uptake of manganese dipyridoxaldiphosphate by chemically induced hepatocellular carcinoma in rats: a correlation between contrast-media-enhanced magnetic resonance imaging, tumor differentiation and vascularisation. Invest Radiol 1993; 28:520–528.
18. Ni Y, Marchal G, Yu J, Muhler A, Lukito G, Beart AL. Prolonged positive contrast enhancement with Gd-EOB-DTPA in experimental liver tumor: potential value in tissue characterization. JMRI 1994; 4:355–363.

William D. Middleton, MD • Stephanie K. Hiskes, MD • Sharlene A. Teefey, MD • Leslie D. Boucher, MD

Small (1.5 cm or Less) Liver Metastases: US-guided Biopsy[1]

PURPOSE: **To determine the techniques used for and the success of ultrasound (US)-guided biopsy of hepatic metastases 1.5 cm in diameter or smaller.**

MATERIALS AND METHODS: **A computer search of radiology reports identified 29 patients who underwent US-guided biopsy of 30 hepatic masses 1.5 cm in diameter or smaller suspected to be metastases. All 30 lesions were sampled for biopsy with the free-hand technique. Parameters assessed were lesion size and location, needle size, transducer type, number of passes made, cytologic or histologic analysis, and final histologic diagnosis. Biopsies were considered successful if a positive histologic diagnosis of metastasis was made.**

RESULTS: **The mean lesion diameter was 1.3 cm (range, 0.9–1.5 cm). Lesion depth was 3–9 cm (mean, 5 cm). Twenty biopsies were performed with a 22-gauge aspirating needle and analyzed cytologically. An average of 2.7 passes were made per lesion. Phased-array sector transducers were used in 23 lesions. In 28 (93%) lesions and 28 (96%) patients, an adequate specimen was obtained to establish the histologic diagnosis of metastatic disease.**

CONCLUSION: **US appears to be an effective guidance technique for biopsy of small liver metastases.**

Sonography is a well-recognized means of guiding biopsy of liver masses. Reported success rates are 70%–96% (1–9). However, to our knowledge, few studies have been published that correlate the success of the procedure with the size of the lesion. In particular, the ability to confirm the presence of liver metastases in patients with small lesions is poorly documented. Although ultrasound (US) is used routinely to guide biopsy of hepatic lesions at our institution, many clinicians and some radiologists are hesitant to request or recommend US-guided biopsy of a small lesion. The purpose of this study was to determine the techniques used for and the success rate of US-guided biopsies of hepatic metastases 1.5 cm in diameter or smaller.

MATERIALS AND METHODS

A computer search of radiology reports between December 1993 and May 1997 identified by billing code all liver biopsies performed with imaging guidance. A total of 576 liver biopsies were performed during this period; 371 of these were performed with US guidance. The remainder were performed with computed tomographic (CT) ($n = 23$) guidance or fluoroscopic ($n = 182$) guidance. All CT-guided biopsies were for focal liver masses; 177 of the fluoroscopically guided biopsies were of random liver parenchyma. Four fluoroscopically guided biopsies were of bile duct lesions identified on cholangiograms. One of the fluoroscopically guided biopsies was performed in a large focal mass.

Of the 371 liver biopsies performed under sonographic guidance, 247 were biopsies of focal masses and 124 were random biopsies of liver parenchyma. In patients in whom a liver mass was sampled for biopsy with US guidance, radiology reports were reviewed to determine the size of the lesion that was sampled for biopsy. If the size of the lesion was not indicated in the report, the images were reviewed to determine the lesion size. The review identified 30 liver lesions 1.5 cm in diameter or smaller in 29 patients with suspected liver metastases. The 16 men and 13 women ranged in age from 26 to 84 years (mean age, 60 years).

The medical records of the 29 patients were reviewed (S.K.H.) to determine the indication for biopsy and the presence and type of known primary malignancy. US and CT reports and images and the pathology reports were reviewed (S.K.H.) to determine the size of the lesion in which biopsy was performed, the location of the lesion (liver segment and depth from the skin), the appearance and nature of the lesion (solid vs cystic), the type of needle used, the type of transducer used for guidance, the number of passes made, the type of specimen obtained (fine-needle aspiration vs core biopsy), and the final cytologic or histologic diagnosis. Lesions were assumed to be spheric; thus, a single measurement was made with electronic calipers.

All liver biopsies were performed by or with the supervision of an attending radiologist. Different types of commercially available US equipment were used. All procedures were performed with the free-hand technique (ie, needle guides were not used). Patients were given a local anesthetic but were not given a sedative. Needles were advanced into the liver and

Index terms: Liver, biopsy, 761.12985 • Liver neoplasms, secondary, 761.33 • Ultrasound (US), guidance, 761.12985 • Ultrasound (US), utilization, 761.12985

Radiology 1997; 205:729–732

[1] From the Mallinckrodt Institute of Radiology (W.D.M., S.K.H., S.A.T.) and the Department of Pathology (L.D.B.), Washington University School of Medicine, 510 S Kingshighway Blvd, St Louis, MO 63110. Received June 24, 1997; revision requested July 24; revision received August 8; accepted August 11. **Address reprint requests to** W.D.M.

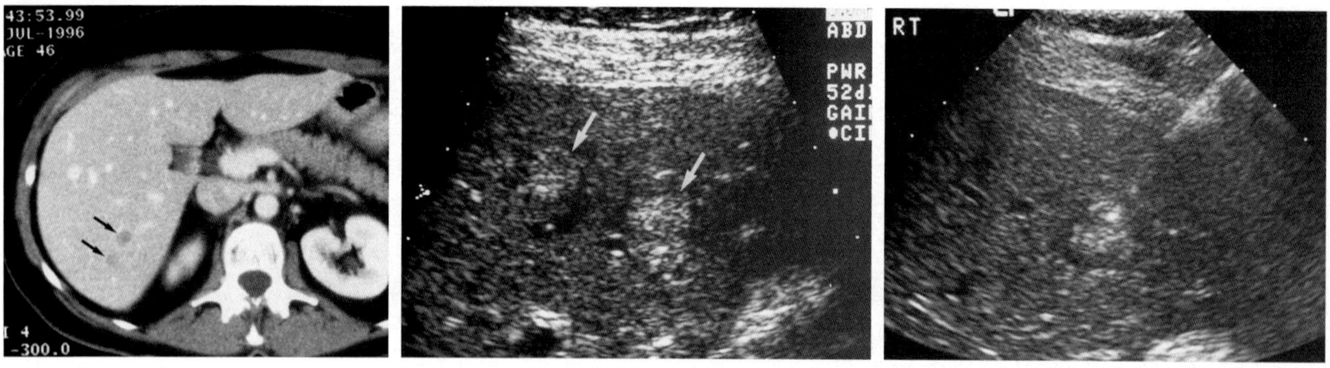

a. b. c.

Figure 1. Bronchogenic carcinoma metastatic to the liver in a 67-year-old woman. **(a)** CT scan obtained with administration of contrast material shows two small, low-attenuation lesions (arrows) in the right lobe of the liver. Several additional lesions of similar size were seen at other levels. **(b)** Transverse sonogram of the liver shows two small hyperechoic lesions (arrows) with faint hypoechoic halos. The larger of these lesions was 1.4 cm in size. **(c)** Transverse sonogram of the liver shows a 22-gauge needle with the tip in the lesion. Cytologic analysis revealed adenocarcinoma.

directed toward the lesion while the patient performed a single breath hold. Patients were required to perform additional breath holds during subsequent needle advancements as fine adjustments were made to the needle trajectory. Fine-needle aspiration was performed with a needle attached to a connecting tube and application of suction with a 30-mL syringe. Fine-needle aspirate specimens were prepared by a cytotechnologist and delivered to the pathology department where a cytopathologist performed an immediate evaluation to determine specimen adequacy. In general, the results of this initial cytologic evaluation were available within 20–25 minutes. Additional specimens were obtained when necessary. Core biopsy specimens were placed in formalin and analyzed by the pathologist the following day.

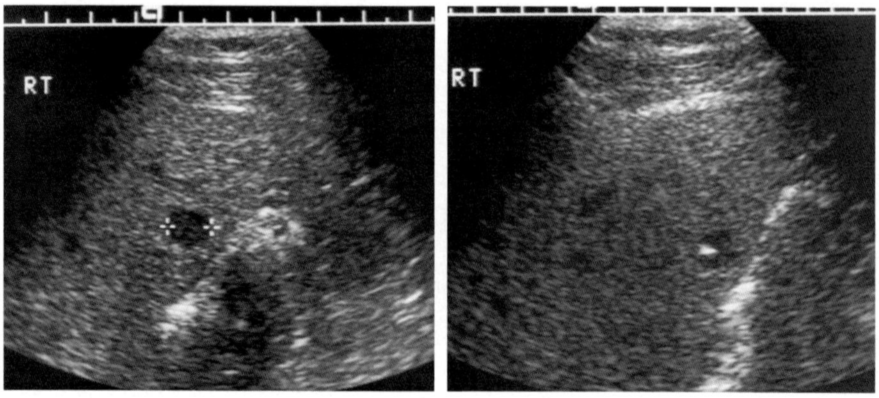

a. b.

Figure 2. Esophageal carcinoma metastatic to the liver in a 52-year-old man. **(a)** Transverse sonogram shows a 9-mm hypoechoic lesion (+ +) corresponding in location to that of an abnormality identified on a positron emission tomographic scan. **(b)** Transverse sonogram shows the tip of a 22-gauge needle in the lesion. Cytologic analysis revealed adenocarcinoma.

RESULTS

Nineteen patients had a known extrahepatic primary malignancy. The location of the primary tumor was the pancreas in five patients, the breast in three, the esophagus in two, the bladder in two, the lymphatic system (lymphoma or leukemia) in two, the lung in one, the cervix in one, the endometrium in one, the testis in one, and the prostate in one. Ten patients had no known primary malignancy. The indication for biopsy of the liver lesions was to confirm the presence of liver metastases in the patients with known primary tumors and to determine the histologic features of liver lesions suspected to be metastases in the patients with no known primary malignancy.

The lesions were 0.9–1.5 cm in diameter (mean diameter, 1.3 cm). The lesion depth was 3–9 cm from the skin surface (mean depth, 5 cm). Of the 30 lesions, eight were located in the right posterior segment, eight were in the right anterior segment, two were in the left medial segment, and 12 were in the left lateral segment. All masses were solid and appeared as target lesions (Fig 1) or as uniformly hypoechoic lesions (Fig 2).

Phased-array sector transducers were used in 23 lesions. Center frequencies in these cases were 7.0 MHz ($n = 2$), 5.0 MHz ($n = 1$), 4.0 MHz ($n = 17$), and 3.5 MHz ($n = 3$). Curved-array transducers were used in seven lesions. Center frequencies in these cases were 5 MHz ($n = 1$) and 4 MHz ($n = 6$).

In 22 lesions, fine-needle aspiration was used successfully to obtain material adequate for a final cytologic diagnosis of metastatic malignancy. In 20 of these 22 lesions, the initial set of aspirates was considered positive by the cytopathologist. In the other two lesions, repeat aspiration was necessary after initial aspiration findings were nondiagnostic. Needle sizes used for aspiration were 23 gauge in one lesion, 22 gauge in 17 lesions, and 20 gauge in four lesions. Four passes were made in two lesions, three passes were made in 14 lesions, two passes were made in four lesions, and one pass was made in two lesions (mean number of needle passes, 2.7).

Core biopsy was performed in six lesions with an automatic spring-loaded needle. In these six lesions, core biopsy was used successfully to obtain adequate tissue for a histopathologic diagnosis of metastatic malignancy. In four of these six lesions, core biopsy was performed initially. In the other two lesions, core specimens were obtained after results from initial fine-needle aspiration biopsy were nondiagnostic. Five of the six lesions were sampled for biopsy with a 20-gauge needle, and one lesion was sampled with a 20-gauge and an 18-gauge needle. One to three needle passes were made (mean number of needle passes, 2.2).

Fine-needle aspiration was nondiagnostic in three lesions in two patients. One patient with Hodgkin disease had a 1.0-cm mass located at a depth of 4 cm in the left lateral segment and a 1.5-cm mass located at a depth of 3 cm in the right anterior segment. In both lesions, findings from fine-needle aspiration performed with a 22-gauge needle were suggestive of recurrent Hodgkin disease. An unequivocal diagnosis was not rendered because classic Reed-Sternberg cells were not present. In this patient, findings from core biopsy performed with a 20-gauge needle of the lesion in the right lobe were positive for Hodgkin disease. The other nondiagnostic fine-needle aspiration findings were in an immunocompromised patient with leukemia, fever, elevated white blood cell count, multiple small liver lesions, and a lung mass. In this patient, a 1.5-cm mass located at a depth of 6 cm in the left lateral segment was aspirated with a 22-gauge needle. This patient was lost to follow-up, and it is uncertain if the liver lesion was attributable to metastatic disease or fungal abscesses. For statistical purposes, all three of these lesions were considered false-negative fine-needle aspiration findings.

Overall, sonographically guided biopsy enabled successful diagnosis of metastatic disease in 28 (93%) of the 30 lesions and in 28 (96%) of the 29 patients. Among the 25 lesions in which fine-needle aspiration was performed, a diagnosis was made in 22 (88%) lesions. A diagnosis was made in all six (100%) lesions in which core biopsy was performed. The final histologic diagnosis was adenocarcinoma in 18 lesions, neuroendocrine tumor in two lesions, lymphoma in two lesions, and various types of cancer in six lesions.

DISCUSSION

Sonography has been used traditionally to guide percutaneous biopsies of large or moderate-sized masses. In 1989, Gazelle and Haaga (10) stated the following in a review article on percutaneous biopsy of abdominal masses.

> For those lesions that are predominantly cystic, larger than 3–5 cm in diameter, and superficially located, sonography is a relatively inexpensive and quick means for localization. For those lesions that are smaller, less superficially located, or lie near other structures, and for many solid lesions, CT is the guidance technique of choice.

Zins et al (9) demonstrated the difficulty associated with biopsy of small liver lesions in an investigation of tract embolization. In that study, 24 focal liver lesions (size range, 0.8–20.0 cm) underwent biopsy with US guidance. The average size of the 18 lesions in which biopsy was performed successfully was 5 cm. The average size of the six lesions in which biopsy results were nondiagnostic was 2.1 cm (range, 1–3 cm). Rosenblatt et al (6) also indicated a potential for false-negative results in lesions smaller than 3 cm in size.

Conversely, there are a few reports that indicate that sonography can be used effectively for biopsy of small abdominal lesions. In 1988, Reading and colleagues (5) reported success with US-guided biopsy of lesions 3 cm or smaller in the abdomen and in superficial structures elsewhere in the body. In that study, the correct histologic diagnosis was made in 115 (91%) of 126 cases. Although success in that study was dependent on the size of the lesion, the rate of correct diagnosis was high even for the smallest lesions. When considering lesions in all locations, the correct diagnosis was made in 19 (79%) of 24 lesions 1.0 cm in size or smaller, in 37 (88%) of 42 lesions of 1.1–2.0 cm, and in 59 (98%) of 60 lesions of 2.1–3.0 cm. In the liver, the correct diagnosis was made in 73 (96%) of 76 lesions. All liver lesions in that study were 3 cm in size or smaller but were not subclassified further.

Our results indicate that US can be effective for guiding biopsy of liver metastases 1.5 cm in diameter or smaller. One advantage of US over CT is that the path of the needle can be observed in real time at US. This continuous feedback allows accurate and rapid reorientation of the needle as it approaches the lesion. Another advantage associated with US-guided biopsy is that the needle can be oriented in nonaxial planes with no difficulty. For these reasons, the majority of biopsies of liver masses are performed at our institution with US guidance. One exception is when the lesion is not visible sonographically. The other occasional exception is when the lesion is visible from only one approach and that approach does not allow safe positioning of the needle.

There are two basic approaches to US-guided biopsy (11,12). We use the free-hand technique, in which the needle and the transducer are held in separate hands and positioned so that the lesion and the needle are visualized simultaneously. An alternative approach is to use needle guides that attach to the transducer and direct the needle in a predetermined direction. The choice of technique depends mainly on the experience and preferences of the individual performing the biopsy. Use of the needle-guide technique ensures that the needle will be directed toward the lesion on the initial pass. In addition, less experience is necessary to master the needle-guide technique than the free-hand technique. However, the lesions that were included in our study had an average diameter similar to that of an "M&M" candy (1.3 cm). With such small lesions, a needle deflection of only 0.6–0.7 cm from the center of the lesion will result in an inadequate sample. Because of the potential for needle deflection and subsequent inadequate sampling, subtle adjustments of the needle path are often necessary when approaching small lesions. We believe that the free-hand technique provides better flexibility in manipulating the needle and transducer once the needle has entered the liver. In addition, the proper initial needle trajectory can be determined with the free-hand technique with real-time observation of the needle used to administer anesthetics as it approaches the liver capsule. Although our data may not be applicable directly to US-guided biopsies performed with needle guides, we suspect that with an experienced operator performing the technique, results from the two techniques would be similar.

An additional choice that must be made when performing a US-guided biopsy of the liver is the type of transducer used to guide the needle. We used many different types of phased-array sector transducers for most of our biopsies. These transducers were chosen because they have a small footprint and provide good acoustic access to the liver from various locations (especially when intercostal and subxyphoid approaches are used). We also frequently used curved-array probes for more superficial lesions. The ability to use any transducer on any unit regardless of the availability of a sterile needle guide is another advantage of the free-hand technique.

Analysis of needle biopsy specimens can be cytologic or histologic. For confirmation of liver metastases, we prefer cytologic analysis of fine-needle aspirates whenever possible. The success of fine-needle aspiration in malignant liver lesions is high regardless of the guidance technique used. The overall sensitivity of fine-needle aspiration for malignant liver lesions has been reported as 84%–94% (13–15), whereas the specificity has been reported as 80%–100% (4,14,15). An advantage of this technique is the use of smaller-gauge needles. We typically use a 22-gauge needle for fine-needle aspiration of liver lesions, as opposed to 20- or 18-gauge needles for core biopsy. In addition, immediate feedback from the cytopathologist is available for fine-needle aspiration specimens. The adequacy of the specimen can then be determined so that additional fine-needle aspiration or core biopsies can be performed if necessary.

The alternative approach is to perform core biopsy initially. The advantage of core biopsy is that additional ancillary studies can be performed on the specimen at a later time if necessary. To a great extent, the approach used depends on the availability and expertise of the pathologists who analyze the specimens.

Our sensitivity of 93% indicates that sonographically guided biopsy enables acquisition of diagnostically adequate material from small liver metastases in various locations. Although we did not analyze our results from lesions larger than 1.5 cm, we doubt that our success is substantially better in those cases. Therefore, we now prefer to perform biopsies in small lesions rather than large lesions if the smaller lesion is in a safer or more accessible location. For instance, we have found that small lesions in the left lobe of the liver can usually be readily sampled for biopsy with a subxyphoid approach. This approach avoids the risk of pneumothorax associated with use of an intercostal approach to perform biopsy of right-lobe lesions of any size.

In analyzing the results of our study, it is important to recognize that the excellent results obtained with liver metastases do not necessarily apply to primary liver tumors, whether they are benign or malignant (16). However, the results of our study indicate that US enables accurate placement of a needle into small liver lesions and acquisition of representative cytologic or histologic material. These results with liver metastases would suggest that any difficulties in making a diagnosis in patients with small primary hepatic tumors is more a limitation of the quantity of material needed for cytologic or histologic analysis than the sampling technique. Also, the majority of biopsies in our study were performed by radiologists with 5–10 years of experience and a special interest in US. As with any procedure-related technique, the results of US-guided biopsies of small liver metastases may not be as good when performed by less experienced radiologists.

One limitation of our study is the method used to identify the study population. The computer search of reports identified patients who had actually undergone a successful or unsuccessful US-guided liver biopsy. However, it was not possible to identify patients who were considered for US-guided biopsy but were not referred for some reason. It is likely that a few patients during this period had small liver lesions and were not referred for US-guided biopsy because the lesion was believed to be particularly difficult to sample for biopsy with sonographic guidance. Therefore, the study group may be biased toward the cases in which lesions were more easily sampled for biopsy with US. We think that this potential bias is small, since only three of the 25 CT-guided liver biopsies performed during this period were in lesions 1.5 cm in diameter or smaller, and none of these lesions proved to be metastases. Thus, there was no apparent trend to refer small liver metastases for CT-guided biopsy. In addition, the inclusion of lesions in all segments and at various depths indicates that we did not routinely refuse to perform biopsy of lesions that were more difficult because of location.

Another unavoidable limitation is that small lesions seen with other techniques but not seen with US were not sampled with US-guided biopsy and were not included in the study. Our results therefore apply to lesions that are visible at sonography and believed to be accessible with US-guided biopsy. During the study period, six patients underwent CT-guided biopsy because they had liver lesions of various sizes that were not visible at sonography. In only one of these six patients was CT-guided biopsy diagnostic of metastatic disease. In another patient, results from CT-guided biopsy suggested metastatic disease but were not conclusive.

In conclusion, we have shown that US guidance is effective for biopsy of small liver metastases. Our experience showed that a diagnosis can be established in 93% of cases in which lesions are 1.5 cm in diameter or smaller. ■

References

1. Chiu KW, Chang-Chien CS, Chen L, Liaw YF. Ultrasonically guided needle aspiration with preparation of cell blocks in the diagnosis of liver tumors. Hepatogastroenterology 1994; 41:30–33.
2. Ferrucci JT Jr, Wittenberg J, Mueller PR, et al. Diagnosis of abdominal malignancy by radiologic fine-needle aspiration biopsy. AJR 1980; 134:323–330.
3. Lees WR, Hall-Craggs MA, Manhire A. Five years' experience of fine-needle aspiration biopsy: 454 consecutive cases. Clin Radiol 1985; 36:517–520.
4. Pinto MM, Avila NA, Heller CI, Criscuolo EM. Fine needle aspiration of the liver. Acta Cytol 1988; 32:15–21.
5. Reading CC, Charboneau JW, James EM, Hurt MR. Sonographically guided percutaneous biopsy of small (3 cm or less) masses. AJR 1988; 151:189–192.
6. Rosenblatt R, Kutcher R, Moussouris HF, Schrieber K, Koss LG. Sonographically guided fine-needle aspiration of liver lesions. JAMA 1982; 248:1639–1641.
7. Schwerk WB, Schmitz-Moormann P. Ultrasonically guided fine-needle biopsies in neoplastic liver disease: cytohistologic diagnoses and echo pattern of lesions. Cancer 1981; 48:1469–1477.
8. Tatsuta M, Yamamoto R, Kasugai H, et al. Cytohistologic diagnosis of neoplasms of the liver by ultrasonically guided fine-needle aspiration biopsy. Cancer 1984; 54: 1682–1686.
9. Zins M, Vilgrain V, Gayno S, et al. US-guided percutaneous liver biopsy with plugging of the needle track: a prospective study in 72 high-risk patients. Radiology 1992; 184:841–843.
10. Gazelle GS, Haaga JR. Guided percutaneous biopsy of intraabdominal lesions. AJR 1989; 153:929–935.
11. Charboneau JW, Reading CC, Welch TJ. CT and sonographically guided needle biopsy: current techniques and new innovations. AJR 1990; 154:1–10.
12. Dodd GD III, Esola CC, Memel DS, et al. Sonography: the undiscovered jewel of interventional radiology. RadioGraphics 1996; 16:1271–1288.
13. Bizjak-Schwarzbarti M. Fine-needle aspiration biopsy in the diagnosis of metastases in the liver. Diagn Cytopathol 1987; 3:278–283.
14. Ho CS, McLoughlin MJ, Tao LC, Blendis L, Evans WK. Guided percutaneous fine-needle aspiration biopsy of the liver. Cancer 1981; 47:1781–1785.
15. Whitlatch S, Nuñez C, Pitlik DA. Fine needle aspiration biopsy of the liver: a study of 102 consecutive cases. Acta Cytol 1984; 28:719–725.
16. Dodd LG, Mooney EE, Layfield LJ, Nelson RC. Fine-needle aspiration of the liver and pancreas: a cytology primer for radiologists. Radiology 1997; 203:1–9.

Kenji Kawamoto, MD • Yoshio Yamada, MD • Takashi Utsunomiya, MD • Hitoshi Okamura, MD
Masanobu Mizuguchi, MD • Makoto Motooka, MD • Nobuaki Hirata, MD • Hideyuki Watanabe, MD
Kenji Sakai, MD • Shinji Kitagawa, MD • Naoko Kinukawa, MS • Kouji Masuda, MD

Gastrointestinal Submucosal Tumors: Evaluation with Endoscopic US[1]

PURPOSE: To describe the endoscopic ultrasound (US) features of benign versus malignant submucosal tumors throughout the gastrointestinal tract.

MATERIALS AND METHODS: One hundred nine patients aged 24–81 years suspected to have submucosal tumors (11 esophageal, 41 stomach, 24 duodenal, and 33 colorectal tumors) at barium studies or endoscopy underwent endoscopic US. The layer of origin, internal echo pattern, and lesion margin were analyzed by means of consensus and independent interpretation by three radiologists.

RESULTS: Endoscopic US findings revealed several distinct patterns among various submucosal tumors. Sixteen (94%) of the 17 homogeneous lesions with histopathologic findings of malignancy were hypoechoic, although 29 (43%) of the 68 homogeneous lesions with histopathologic findings of benignity were similarly hypoechoic. Homogeneous lesions that were anechoic, of intermediate echogenicity, or hyperechoic were almost exclusively benign (39 [98%] of 40). In contrast, 23 (96%) of the 24 malignant lesions were heterogeneous ($n = 7$) or homogeneously hypoechoic ($n = 16$). The sizes of benign and malignant lesions were significantly different ($P < .05$). There was no significant difference in the echo pattern (ie, homogeneous versus heterogeneous), but there was a significant difference in the proportion of hypoechoic versus nonhypoechoic lesions (anechoic, hyperechoic, or of intermediate echogenicity; $P < .001$).

CONCLUSION: The differential diagnosis of gastrointestinal submucosal tumors is assisted with endoscopic US.

The diagnosis of gastrointestinal submucosal tumors with conventional radiography and endoscopy has generally relied on the detection of changes in the gastrointestinal mucosa, that is, on indirect evidence of the presence of a tumor. Detecting such tumors is easy; however, until now, it has been necessary to make a presumptive histopathologic diagnosis on the basis of indirect evidence of the nature of the lesion within the gut wall and its effects outside the gastrointestinal tract.

In contrast, endoscopic ultrasound (US) allows direct evaluation of the tumor, and the extension of the tumor outside the gut wall can be assessed. Accordingly, endoscopic US makes it possible to obtain information that may narrow the differential diagnosis. Moreover, because endoscopic US allows observation of the structure of the gut wall and provides cross-sectional images of the tumor, it enables the differentiation between submucosal tumors and extramural compression. Furthermore, it is also possible to determine tumor size and shape, and to predict the tissue of origin on the basis of the layer in the gut wall and its internal echo pattern.

While several reports on the endoscopic US diagnosis of upper gastrointestinal submucosal tumors have appeared in recent years (1–4), to our knowledge there have been few studies that have compared the endoscopic US findings of lesions in all regions of the gastrointestinal tract, especially the duodenum and large intestine (5,6).

The purpose of this study was to retrospectively compare histopathologic findings and endoscopic US images of submucosal tumors arising throughout the gastrointestinal tract to describe the endoscopic features that help to distinguish between benign and malignant disease.

MATERIALS AND METHODS

Patients

One hundred nine patients (68 men, 41 women; age range, 24–81 years; mean age, 56 years) with a radiographic or endoscopic diagnosis of submucosal tumor underwent endoscopic US at the Department of Radiology, Kyushu University Hospital, Fukuoka, Japan, or at an affiliated institution between August 1988 and August 1996. A histopathologic diagnosis was attained after surgery ($n = 57$), endoscopic resection ($n = 39$), or biopsy ($n = 12$). In one patient, the clinical diagnosis was established after a good response to hormonal replacement therapy. Lesions that caused extramural compression of the gas-

Index terms: Endoscopy, 70.12981 • Gastrointestinal tract, neoplasms, 70.31, 70.32, 70.33 • Gastrointestinal tract, US, 70.12981 • Ultrasound (US), endoscopic, 70.12981

Radiology 1997; 205:733–740

[1] From the Departments of Radiology (K.K., Y.Y., T.U., K.M.) and Medical Information (N.K.), Faculty of Medicine, Kyushu University, Maidashi 3-1-1, Higashi-ku, Fukuoka 812, Japan; the Department of Radiology, Kyushu National Cancer Center, Fukuoka, Japan (H.O.); the Department of Radiology, Saga Medical College, Saga, Japan (M. Mizuguchi); the Department of Radiology, Kitakyushu Medical Center, Kitakyushu, Japan (M. Motooka); the Department of Radiology, Karatsu Red Cross Hospital, Karatsu, Japan (N.H.); the Department of Radiology, University of Occupational Environmental Health, Kitakyushu, Japan (H.W.); the Department of Medicine, Fukuoka Prefecture Kaho Hospital, Fukuoka, Japan (K.S.); and the Department of Radiology, Faculty of Medicine, Fukuoka University, 7-45-1, Nanakuma, Jonan-ku, Fukuoka 814-01, Japan (S.K.). Received January 24, 1997; revision requested March 21; revision received August 11; accepted August 12. **Address reprint requests to** K.K.

trointestinal tract, which can easily be confused with submucosal tumors clinically, were excluded from this study.

There were 102 patients with solitary tumors and seven patients with multiple tumors. Of the seven patients with multiple tumors, five had tumors in the duodenum, one had tumors in the stomach, and one had tumors in the colon. In each instance, multiple lesions in the same patient exhibited similar endoscopic US findings. The lesions were 4–130 mm (mean, 30.3 mm). Eleven lesions were located in the esophagus, 41 in the stomach, 24 in the duodenum, and 33 in the colon. The histopathologic findings of the lesions are shown in Table 1.

Methods

Endoscopic US of the upper gastrointestinal tract and colon was performed with 7.5- or 12.0-MHz radial US endoscopes (model GF-UM3 or UM20 [upper gastrointestinal tract], or model CF-UM3 or UM20 [colon]; Olympus, Tokyo, Japan). The patients received an intramuscular injection of an antispasmodic agent (scopolamine butylbromide [Buscopan; Boehringer Ingerheim, Hyogo, Japan]; 10 mg) at 3 minutes before the examination to suppress peristalsis.

The balloon method was usually used for esophageal observation. In later patients, however, a small-diameter, 12-MHz US probe (UM-2R; Olympus) was passed through the forceps channel of an ordinary endoscope, and the lesion was depicted directly with the water immersion technique.

Intragastric observation was generally done with the water immersion technique and with the patient in the left lateral position. However, lesions proximal to the pyloric ring were sometimes better defined by using the small-diameter probe. Because the duodenum has a narrow lumen, the basic approach was to position the patient to the best advantage and to combine the balloon and water immersion methods. The balloon or water immersion method was used to examine the duodenal bulb with the patient in the right

Table 1
Histopathologic Diagnoses of Submucosal Tumors Examined with Endoscopic US

Histopathologic Diagnosis	Esophagus (n = 11)	Stomach (n = 41)	Duodenum (n = 24)	Colon (n = 33)	Total (N = 109)
Benign lesions	11	29	21	24	85
Granular cell tumor	3	0	0	0	3
Leiomyoma	5	16	1	2	24
Leiomyoblastoma	0	3	1	0	4
Hemangioma	2	0	0	1	3
Lipoma	0	1	1	6	8
Lymphangioma	1	0	1	6	8
Schwannoma	0	2	0	0	2
Gangliocytic paraganglioma	0	0	1	0	1
Heterotopic pancreatic tissue	0	4	1	0	5
Inflammatory fibroid polyp	0	1	0	0	1
Cyst	0	2	8	0	10
Duplication cyst	0	1	1	0	0
Diffuse cystic malformation	0	1	0	0	0
Dilated Brunner gland duct	0	0	7	0	0
Brunner gland hyperplasia	0	0	6	0	6
Adenoma arising from heterotopic gastric mucosa	0	0	1	0	1
Suture granuloma	0	0	0	2	2
Endometriosis	0	0	0	5	5
Unclassified polyp	0	0	0	2	2
Malignant lesions	0	12	3	9	24
Carcinoid	0	2	1	6	9
Leiomyosarcoma	0	8	0	2	10
Malignant lymphoma	0	1	1	1	3
Intramural metastasis	0	1	0	0	1
Early primary carcinoma arising from Brunner gland	0	0	1	0	1

Table 2
Relationship between the Endoscopic US Pattern and Histopathologic Findings (N = 109)

Layer of Origin	Internal Echo Pattern: Homogeneous: Anechoic	Homogeneous: Hypoechoic	Homogeneous: Of Intermediate Echogenicity	Homogeneous: Hyperechoic	Heterogeneous
2–3	...	Carcinoid (n = 9) Leiomyoma (n = 4) Granular cell tumor (n = 3) Hemangioma (n = 1) Inflammatory fibroid polyp (n = 1) Heterotopic pancreatic tissue (n = 1)	...	Brunner gland hyperplasia (n = 6) Unclassified polyp (n = 2)	...
3	Cyst (n = 7) Duplication cyst (n = 1) Lymphangioma (n = 7) Diffuse cystic malformation (n = 1) Hemangioma (n = 1)	Hemangioma (n = 1)	Lipoma (n = 2) Lymphangioma (n = 1) Gangliocytic paraganglioma (n = 1)	Lipoma (n = 6) Suture granuloma (n = 2) Early primary carcinoma (n = 1)	Heterotopic pancreatic tissue (n = 2) Adenoma arising from heterotopic gastric mucosa (n = 1)
4	...	Leiomyoma (n = 8) Leiomyosarcoma (n = 4) Leiomyoblastoma (n = 2) Schwannoma (n = 2)	Leiomyoma (n = 1) Duplication cyst (n = 1)	...	Leiomyoma (n = 11) Leiomyosarcoma (n = 6) Leiomyoblastoma (n = 2)
All layers disrupted	...	Heterotopic pancreatic tissue (n = 1) Malignant lymphoma (n = 3) Endometriosis (n = 5)	...	...	Heterotopic pancreatic tissue (n = 1) Intramural metastasis (n = 1)

lateral position, and the water immersion method was used to examine the second to fourth parts of the duodenum. Before observation of the colon, the patient was given a cathartic (magnesium citrate [34 g; Magcorol P; Horii, Osaka, Japan] or sodium picosulfate [75 mg; Laxoberon; Teijin, Tokyo, Japan]), as is done for routine colonoscopy, and the water immersion technique was generally used. By correctly positioning the patient, infusion of water into the bowel was kept to a minimum.

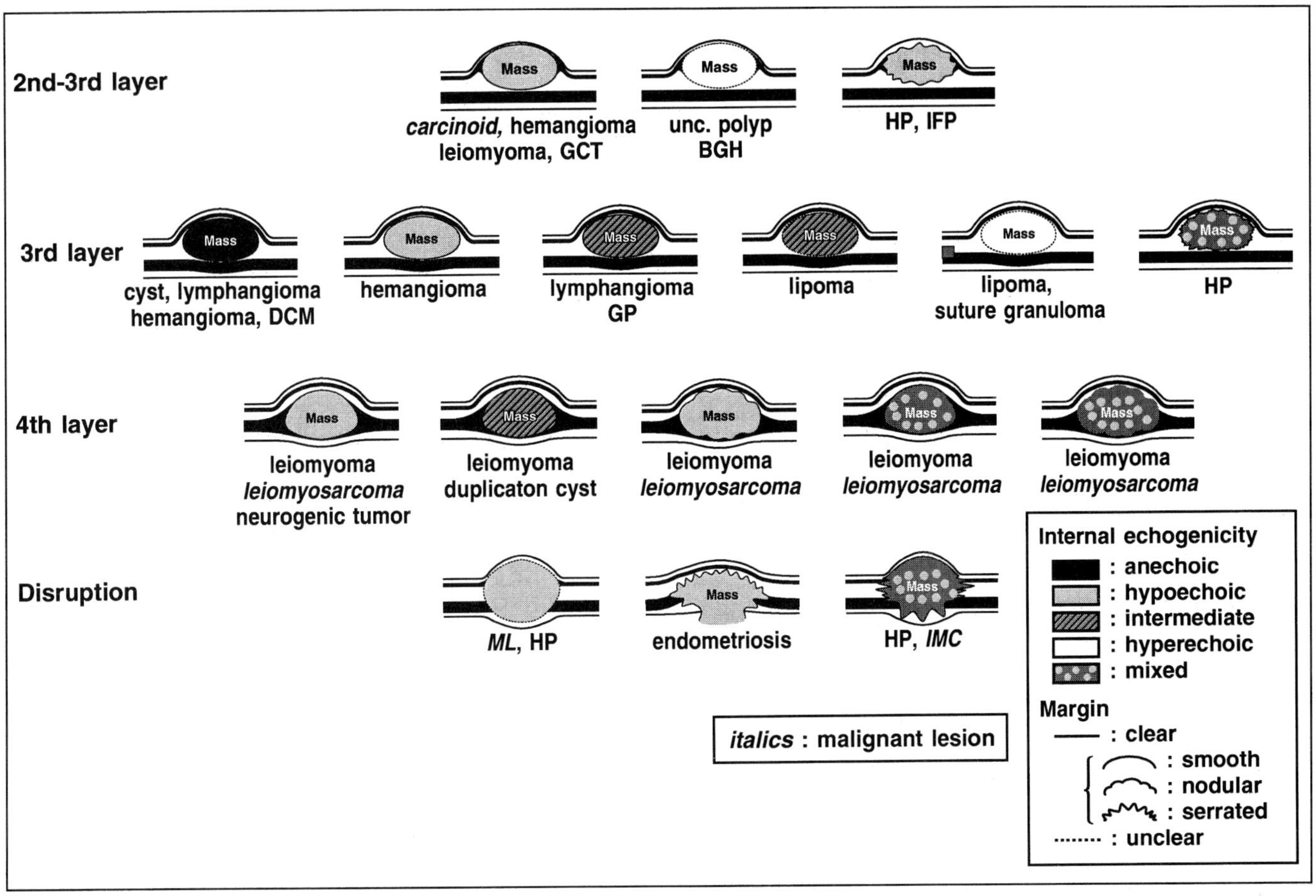

Figure 1. Differential diagnosis of gastrointestinal submucosal tumors with endoscopic US. *BGH* = Brunner gland hyperplasia, *DCM* = diffuse cystic malformation, *GCT* = granular cell tumor, *GP* = gangliocytic paraganglioma, *HP* = heterotopic pancreatic tissue, *IFP* = inflammatory fibroid polyp, *IMC* = intramural metastasis, *ML* = malignant lymphoma.

Table 3
Relationship between Tumor Margin at Endoscopic US and Histopathologic Findings ($N = 109$)

Lesion	Unclear Margins	Clear Margins		
		Smooth	Nodular	Serrated
Benign	Lipoma ($n = 6$) Heterotopic pancreatic tissue ($n = 3$) Brunner gland hyperplasia ($n = 5$) Suture granuloma ($n = 2$) Unclassified polyp ($n = 2$)	Granular cell tumor ($n = 3$) Leiomyoma ($n = 13$) Leiomyoblastoma ($n = 3$) Hemangioma ($n = 3$) Lipoma ($n = 2$) Lymphangioma ($n = 8$) Schwannoma ($n = 2$) Gangliocytic paraganglioma ($n = 1$) Cyst arising from dilated Brunner gland ($n = 7$) Duplication cyst ($n = 2$) Diffuse cystic malformation ($n = 1$) Brunner gland hyperplasia ($n = 1$)	Leiomyoma ($n = 9$) Leiomyoblastoma ($n = 1$)	Leiomyoma ($n = 2$) Heterotopic pancreatic tissue ($n = 2$) Inflammatory fibroid polyp ($n = 1$) Adenoma arising from heterotopic gastric mucosa ($n = 1$) Endometriosis ($n = 5$)
Malignant	Malignant lymphoma ($n = 3$) Early primary carcinoma arising from dilated Brunner gland ($n = 1$)	Carcinoid ($n = 9$) Leiomyosarcoma ($n = 5$)	Leiomyosarcoma ($n = 3$)	Leiomyosarcoma ($n = 2$) Intramural metastasis ($n = 1$)

While observing the lesion in real time, photographs were taken, and the following items were evaluated with agreement among three radiologists (K.K., N.H., and M. Mizuguchi): lesion size, internal echo pattern, layer of origin, and lesion margin. Lesion size was defined as the maximum diameter to the nearest millimeter. The internal echo pattern was classified as homogeneous or heterogeneous. The homogeneous lesions were further subclassified into four categories; anechoic, hypoechoic, of intermediate echogenicity, and hyperechoic. The heterogeneous type was referred to as "mixed." The internal echo pattern of the lesion was compared with the echo patterns of the third and fourth layers of the gut wall. A hyperechoic lesion was defined as having similar echogenicity as the third layer, a hypoechoic lesion as having similar echogenicity as the fourth layer, and an intermediate lesion as having an echogenicity between those of these two layers. An echogenicity the same as that of deaerated water was defined as anechoic.

The layer of origin of the lesion was classified into four categories: second to third, third, fourth, or disruption of the normal architecture. The observers were asked to select one of these four categories (Fig 1); only one option was allowed per lesion. As in earlier reports (7), the entire gastrointestinal tract wall was confirmed to have a five-layered structure. The first, hyperechoic, and innermost layer corresponds to the liquid-mucosa interface. The second, hypoechoic layer is probably produced as the ultrasound beam crosses the deep portion of the mucosa, which includes the muscularis mucosae. The third, hyperechoic layer corresponds to the submucosa and the submucosa–muscularis propria interface. The fourth, hypoechoic layer represents the muscularis propria. The fifth, hyperechoic layer corresponds to the serosa adventitia and the serosa adventitia–peripheral tissue of gut interface.

When attempting to determine the layer of origin, the observers checked for continuity with or disruption of the layers of the adjacent normal gut wall by the lesion. To distinguish between lesions arising from the second to third layers and those arising from the third layer, the presence of fusion between the second layer and the lesion at endoscopic US was used. The margin of the lesion was classified as clear or unclear, and clear margins were subclassified as smooth, nodular, or serrated.

In addition to the consensus assessment, the different parameters (layer of origin, internal echo pattern, and margin) were independently evaluated by three investigators (Y.Y., T.U., K.K.), and the κ coefficient, which is a measure of association, was used to test the degree of agreement.

Histopathologic comparison with the endoscopic US images was done by using hematoxylin-eosin–stained sections of the largest cut surface of the resected specimen. Factors that assisted in distinguishing between benign and malignant submucosal tumors throughout the entire gastrointestinal tract were investigated.

Statistical analysis of the differences between benign and malignant lesions was performed with the Mann-Whitney *U* test for lesion size, and other factors (internal echo pattern and marginal echo pattern) were assessed by using the χ^2 test. A statistical software program (BMDP STATISTICAL PACKAGE; BMDP Statistical Software, Los Angeles, Calif) was used on a workstation (SPARC 20 workstation; Sun Microsystems, Mountain View, Calif). The BMDP 4F and 3S programs were used for the χ^2 test and the Mann-Whitney *U* test, as well as for calculation of the κ statistic (8,9).

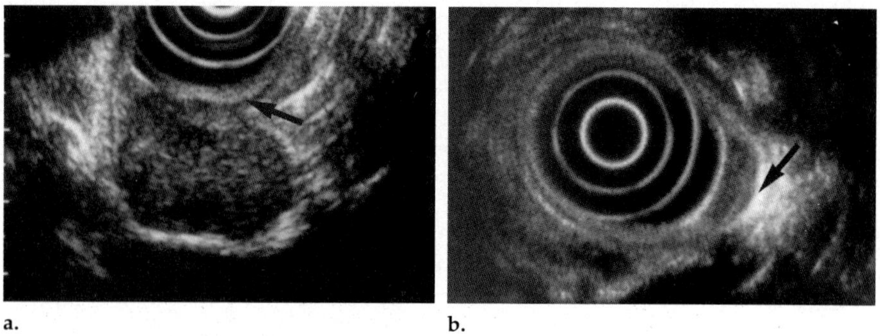

Figure 2. Esophageal submucosal tumors on endoscopic US scans. **(a)** Leiomyoma is shown as a solid mass with mixed, irregular echogenicity that arises from the muscularis propria (arrow). **(b)** Hemangioma is shown as a hypoechoic solid mass in the submucosal layer (arrow).

RESULTS

κ coefficients were calculated for all possible pairs of the three radiologists. The κ coefficients for each pair (K.K. versus Y.Y., Y.Y. versus T.U., and T.U. versus K.K.) were 0.950, 0.950, and 0.925 for layer of origin; 0.960, 0.934, and 0.960 for internal echo pattern; and 0.973, 0.973, and 1.000 for margin type. There was strong agreement between the three radiologists with regard to all of the parameters evaluated.

Table 2 summarizes the relationship among the layer of origin, the internal echo pattern at endoscopic US, and the tumor histopathologic findings. The relationship between the tumor margin and the histopathologic findings is shown in Table 3.

Esophageal Lesions

All of the 11 lesions of the esophagus were benign. Leiomyomas arose in the second to third layers (the muscularis mucosae; $n = 3$) and in the 4th layer (the muscularis propria; $n = 2$) of the esophageal wall and were either hypoechoic ($n = 4$) or mixed ($n = 1$) (Fig 2a). Granular cell tumors ($n = 3$) mainly arose in the second to third layers, and the internal echo pattern was the same as that of leiomyomas (hypoechoic). Two hemangiomas arose in the third layer and were either anechoic ($n = 1$) or exhibited a hypoechoic pattern ($n = 1$) (Fig 2b). Lymphangioma ($n = 1$) arose in the third layer and was of intermediate echogenicity. The margins of all these lesions were smooth, except for two nodular leiomyomas.

Stomach Lesions

Of the 41 lesions of the stomach, 29 were benign and 12 were malignant. Myogenic tumors were the most common ($n = 27$ [66%]), followed by heterotopic pancreatic tissue ($n = 4$ [10%]). Lesions that were located mainly in the second to third layers included two hypoechoic carcinoids (Fig 3a) and one inflammatory fibroid polyp (Fig 3b) with the same internal echo pattern as a carcinoid. However, the inflammatory fibroid polyp differed from the carcinoids with regard to the marginal echo pattern. The margin of the former was serrated, while the margins of the latter were smooth. Diffuse multiple cysts ($n = 1$), lipomas ($n = 1$), and heterotopic pancreatic tissue ($n = 2$) were located in the third layer, but the internal echo pattern of each of these lesions was distinctive (anechoic, hyperechoic, and of mixed echogenicity, respectively).

Lesions that arose in the fourth layer ($n = 30$) were myogenic tumors (leiomyoma [$n = 16$][Fig 3c], leiomyoblastoma [$n = 3$], and leiomyosarcoma [$n = 8$][Fig 3d]), neurogenic tumors ($n = 2$), and a duplication cyst ($n = 1$). Myogenic and neurogenic tumors were equally hypoechoic or showed a mixed pattern.

Lesions that disrupted each layer of the gastric wall were malignant lymphoma ($n = 1$), intramural metastasis ($n = 1$) (Fig 3e), and heterotopic pancreatic tissue ($n = 2$) (Fig 3f). The only poorly defined lesions were heterotopic pancreatic tissue and malignant lymphoma; the other lesions were well defined. Among the well-defined lesions, the only ones with a nodular margin were myogenic tumors ($n = 7$) (Fig 3g). The lesions with a serrated mar-

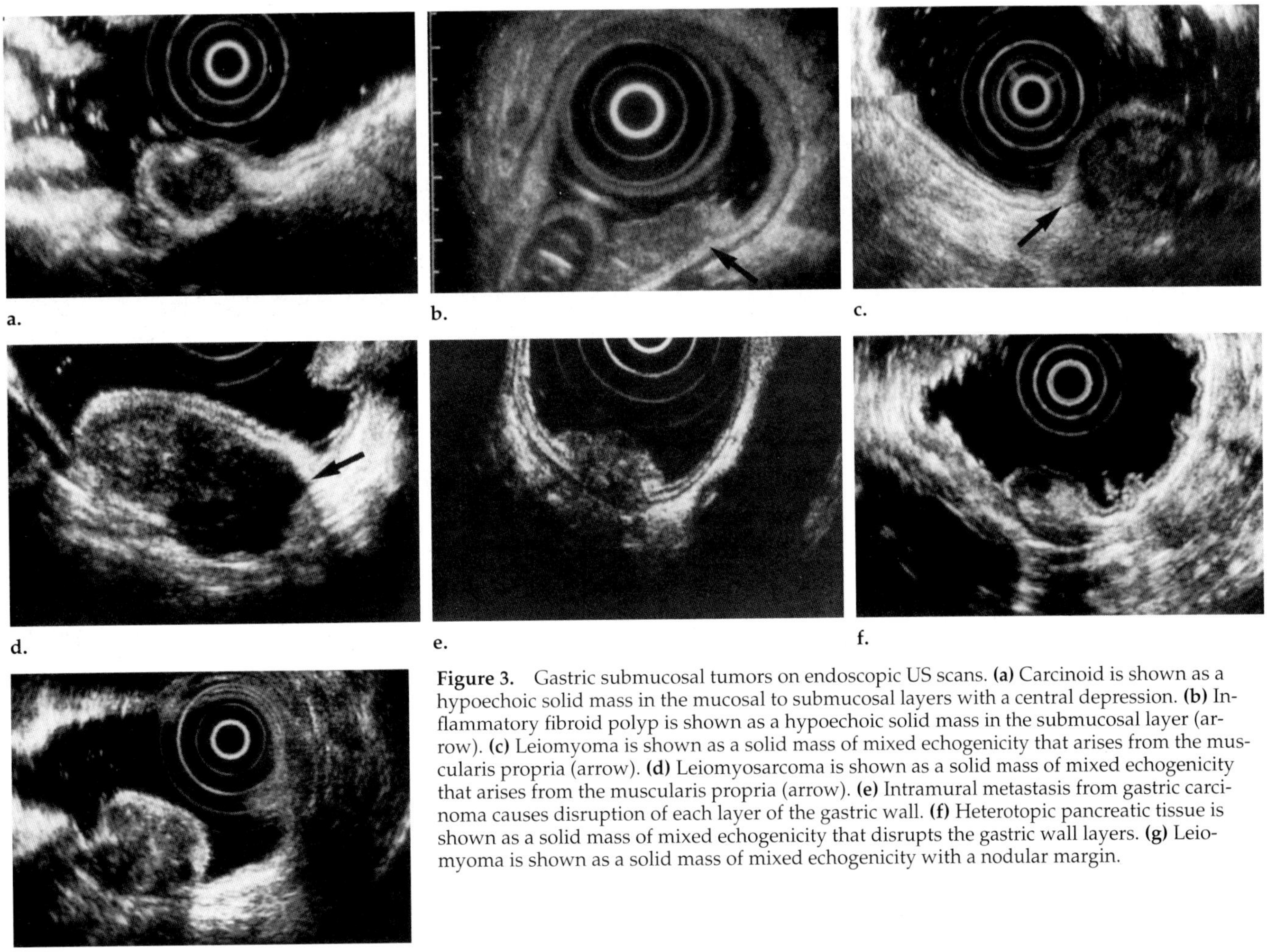

a. b. c. d. e. f. g.

Figure 3. Gastric submucosal tumors on endoscopic US scans. **(a)** Carcinoid is shown as a hypoechoic solid mass in the mucosal to submucosal layers with a central depression. **(b)** Inflammatory fibroid polyp is shown as a hypoechoic solid mass in the submucosal layer (arrow). **(c)** Leiomyoma is shown as a solid mass of mixed echogenicity that arises from the muscularis propria (arrow). **(d)** Leiomyosarcoma is shown as a solid mass of mixed echogenicity that arises from the muscularis propria (arrow). **(e)** Intramural metastasis from gastric carcinoma causes disruption of each layer of the gastric wall. **(f)** Heterotopic pancreatic tissue is shown as a solid mass of mixed echogenicity that disrupts the gastric wall layers. **(g)** Leiomyoma is shown as a solid mass of mixed echogenicity with a nodular margin.

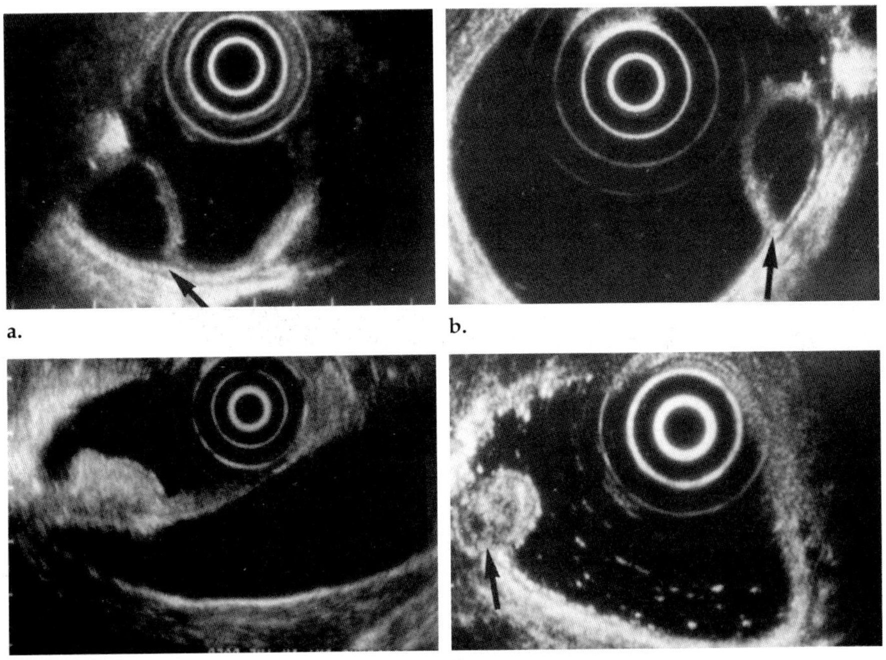

a. b. c. d.

Figure 4. Duodenal submucosal tumors on endoscopic US scans. **(a)** Brunner gland cyst is shown as an anechoic lesion in the submucosal layer (arrow) of the duodenum. **(b)** Lymphangioma is shown as a multilocular anechoic lesion in the submucosal layer (arrow) of the colon. **(c)** Brunner gland hyperplasia is shown as a hyperechoic solid mass in the mucosal to the submucosal layers. **(d)** Lipoma is shown as a hyperechoic solid mass in the submucosal layer (arrow).

gin were myogenic tumors (n = 4), heterotopic pancreatic tissue (n = 1), the inflammatory fibroid polyp (n = 1), and the intramural metastasis (n = 1). Smooth margins were mainly found in myogenic tumors (n = 16).

Duodenal Lesions

Of the 24 lesions of the duodenum, 21 were benign and three were malignant. The internal echo pattern was most commonly anechoic (n = 9 [38%]), followed by hyperechoic (n = 8 [33%]) and hypoechoic (n = 4 [17%]). Among the eight lesions located mainly in the second to third layers, Brunner gland hyperplasia was the most common (n = 6 [75%]), followed by carcinoid (n = 1) and heterotopic pancreatic tissue (n = 1). Among the 13 lesions located in the third layer, cysts were the most frequent (n = 8 [62%]), while the other lesions were lymphangioma (n = 1 [8%]), gangliocytic paraganglioma (n = 1 [8%]), lipoma (n = 1 [8%]), early Brunner gland carcinoma (n = 1 [8%]), and adenoma that possibly arose from heterotopic gastric mucosa ($n = 1$ [8%]). The lesions located in the fourth layer were myogenic tumors (one leiomyoma and one leiomyoblastoma). The only lesion that disrupted all the layers was a malignant lymphoma.

Eight (89%) of the nine anechoic lesions were cysts. Seven of them were histopathologically shown to arise from dilated Brunner glands or ducts (Fig 4a), and one was from a duplication cyst; the ninth anechoic lesion was a lymphangioma (Fig 4b). Among the eight hyperechoic lesions, Brunner gland hyperplasia (Fig 4c) was the most common ($n = 6$ [75%]), followed by lipoma ($n = 1$ [12%]) (Fig 4d) and early Brunner gland carcinoma ($n = 1$ [12%]). The four hypoechoic lesions were carcinoid tumor ($n = 1$ [25%]), heterotopic pancreatic tissue ($n = 1$ [25%]), leiomyoblastoma ($n = 1$ [25%]), and malignant lymphoma ($n = 1$ [25%]). The seven poorly defined lesions were five cases of Brunner gland hyperplasia, one malignant lymphoma, and one early carcinoma that arose from Brunner glands. All of the other 17 lesions had a well-defined margin, which was smooth except in three cases (one leiomyoma with a nodular margin and one case each of heterotopic pancreatic tissue and adenoma that originated from heterotopic gastric mucosa with a serrated margin).

Colorectal Lesions

Of the 33 lesions of the colorectum, 24 were benign and nine were malignant. The internal echo pattern was most commonly hypoechoic ($n = 16$ [48%]), followed by hyperechoic ($n = 9$ [27%]) and anechoic ($n = 6$ [18%]). The lesions located mainly in the second to third layers were carcinoids ($n = 6$), unclassified polyps ($n = 2$), and leiomyoma that originated in the muscularis mucosae ($n = 1$). These lesions were hypoechoic, except for two hyperechoic unclassified polyps. Representative lesions located in the third layer were anechoic lymphangiomas ($n = 6$) (Fig 5a), hyperechoic lipomas ($n = 5$), and suture granulomas ($n = 2$) (Fig 5b). A hypoechoic hemangioma and a lipoma of intermediate echogenicity also were detected. The three lesions located in the fourth layer were myogenic tumors; two were sarcomas. Lesions that disrupted some of the bowel wall layers were endometriosis ($n = 5$) (Fig 5c) and malignant lymphoma ($n = 1$) (Fig 5d). Lesions with a poorly defined margin were lipoma ($n = 6$), suture granuloma ($n = 2$), unclassified polyps ($n = 2$), and malignant lymphoma ($n = 1$). Among the sharply defined lesions, the only nodular ones were myogenic tumors ($n = 3$), and the only serrated ones were endometriosis ($n = 5$). All of the other lesions had smooth margins.

Table 4
Endoscopic US Features of Benign and Malignant Submucosal Tumors

Endoscopic US Feature	Benign Submucosal Tumors ($n = 85$)	Malignant Submucosal Tumors ($n = 24$)	*P* Value
Tumor size (mm)			
Median	22.0	35.5	<.05*
25th percentile	12.0	11.5	
75th percentile	39.0	58.8	
Internal echo pattern (no. of tumors)			
Homogeneous	68	17	>.05†
Hypoechoic	29	16	
Of intermediate echogenicity	6	0	<.001‡
Hyperechoic	16	1	
Anechoic	17	0	
Heterogeneous	17	7	
Marginal echo pattern (no. of tumors)			
Unclear	18	4	>.05§
Clear	67	20	
Smooth	46	14	
Nodular	8	3	>.05‖
Serrated	13	3	

* Mann-Whitney *U* test.
† Homogeneous versus heterogeneous with the χ^2 test.
‡ Low versus intermediate, high, and anechoic with the χ^2 test.
§ Unclear versus clear with the χ^2 test.
‖ Smooth versus serrated with the χ^2 test.

Characteristics of Benignity versus Malignancy

The differential diagnosis of gastrointestinal submucosal tumors with endoscopic US, based on these results, is outlined in Figure 1. Table 4 shows the endoscopic US findings of all submucosal tumors of the gastrointestinal tract divided into benign and malignant conditions. There were 85 benign and 24 malignant lesions. The median, 25th, and 75th percentiles for the sizes of the benign lesions were 22.0 mm, 12.0 mm, and 39.0 mm; those for the sizes of the malignant lesions were 35.5 mm, 11.5 mm, and 58.8 mm. Malignant lesions were significantly larger ($P < .05$, Mann-Whitney *U* test).

Sixteen (94%) of the 17 homogeneous lesions that were histopathologically malignant were hypoechoic; 29 (43%) of the 68 homogeneous lesions that were histopathologically benign were similarly hypoechoic. Homogeneous lesions that were either anechoic, of intermediate echogenicity, or hyperechoic were almost exclusively benign (39 [98%] of 40). In contrast, 23 (96%) of the 24 malignant lesions were either heterogeneous ($n = 7$) or else homogeneous and hypoechoic ($n = 16$).

In addition, there were no malignant lesions that were either anechoic or of intermediate echogenicity, and all of the hyperechoic lesions except one were benign. No significant differences were observed between the two groups in the homogeneity of the internal echo pattern (ie, homogeneous vs heterogeneous); however, there was a significant difference in the echogenicity (ie, hypoechoic versus nonhypoechoic) for the homogeneous lesions ($P < .001$, χ^2 test). In addition, there was no significant difference between the two groups in the echo pattern of the margin (ie, clear vs unclear) or in the shape of the lesions with a clear margin (ie, smooth vs nodular vs serrated).

DISCUSSION

Endoscopic US is being used not only for diagnosing the depth of invasion of gastrointestinal cancer, but also increasingly for qualitatively diagnosing mass lesions covered by normal mucosa (ie, submucosal tumors). A number of studies on gastrointestinal submucosal tumors have already been reported on, but most were limited to lesions of the upper gastrointestinal tract, principally the esophagus and the stomach (1–4,10–14), and there have been few investigations of the duodenum or the lower gastrointestinal tract (5,6). The reason for this is not just that such lesions are less common, but also that the majority are benign tumors and it is difficult to ob-

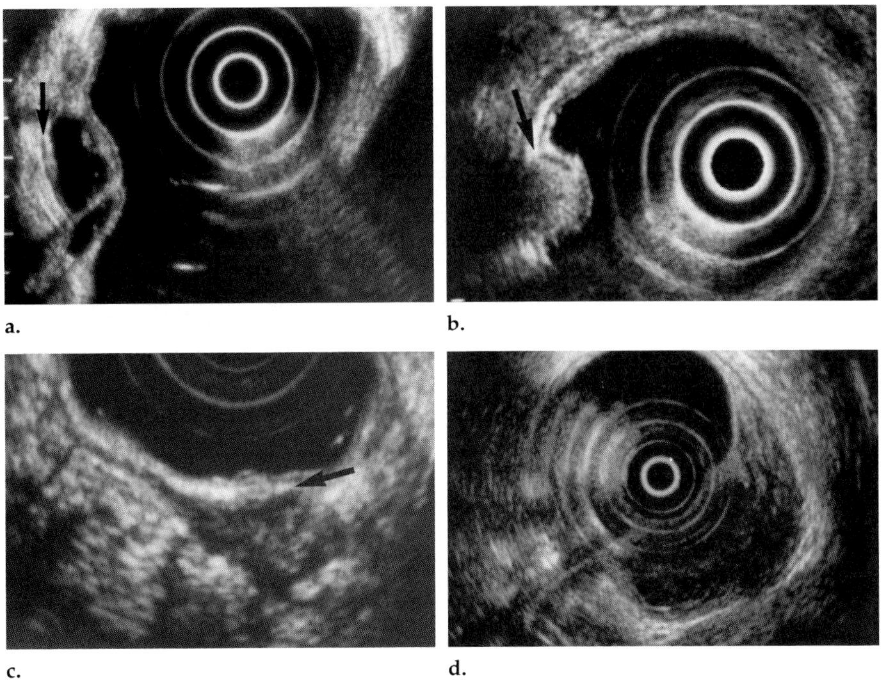

Figure 5. Colonic submucosal tumors on endoscopic US scans. **(a)** Lymphangioma is shown as a multilocular anechoic lesion in the submucosal layer (arrow). **(b)** Suture granuloma is shown as a hyperechoic solid mass with strong echo attenuation in the submucosa (arrow). **(c)** Endometriosis is shown as a hypoechoic lesion with inward growth from the serosa to the submucosa (arrow). **(d)** Malignant lymphoma is shown as a hypoechoic lesion with disruption of each layer of the colonic wall.

tain tissue specimens; it is anatomically difficult to perform endoscopic resection at some sites. Moreover, there have been no studies that have comprehensively compared the endoscopic US findings of submucosal tumors throughout the entire gastrointestinal tract; consequently, there has been no clear assessment of the organ specificity of any of these diseases.

In the present study, we conducted a retrospective comparison of the histopathologic findings and endoscopic US images of submucosal tumors of the esophagus, stomach, duodenum, and colon and rectum. We used endoscopic US to attempt a differential diagnosis, which included distinguishing between benign and malignant disease; we also investigated the special characteristics of submucosal tumors in each part of the gastrointestinal tract.

Endoscopic US Characteristics of Gastrointestinal Submucosal Tumors

Myogenic tumors are representative of submucosal tumors. At endoscopic US, they appear as well-demarcated, hypoechoic lesions with smooth margins that arise in the fourth layer (the muscularis propria) or the second layer (the muscularis mucosae). Myogenic tumors are most commonly found in the stomach, followed by the esophagus; few occur in the large intestine or duodenum. These tumors include leiomyomas, leiomyoblastomas, and leiomyosarcomas, which are reported to be difficult to distinguish from each other (4). In addition, neurogenic tumors can be difficult to differentiate from myogenic tumors. In this study, we encountered two schwannomas of the stomach. Because these were solid, hypoechoic masses that arose in the fourth layer, both were misdiagnosed as myogenic tumors. On the basis of the few cases in the present series, we speculate that the nodular appearance of myogenic tumors may be a factor in differentiating them from schwannomas.

Granular cell tumors are common in the esophagus but uncommon in other parts of the gastrointestinal tract. At endoscopic US, these tumors appeared as hypoechoic solid masses that extended from the lamina propria to the submucosal layer, with features similar to those of leiomyomas that arise in the muscularis mucosae. Tumor cells were observed directly beneath the stratified squamous epithelium at histopathologic examination, and use of the water immersion method of endoscopic US made it possible to confirm that the lesion extended into the lamina propria. Murata and colleagues (15) performed endoscopic US of this lesion by using the balloon method and reported that the echogenicity of the tumor was slightly higher than that of the leiomyoma.

Lipomas were most frequently found in the colon, and, while they were also detected in other parts of the gastrointestinal tract, they were hyperechoic solid tumors with the same echogenicity as the third layer (the submucosa). Because these lesions had the same echogenicity as the submucosa, their margins were unclear (5). Caution in diagnosing is required, however, because in the duodenum it was often difficult to differentiate these lesions from Brunner gland hyperplasia, which shows a similar echogenicity.

Carcinoid is a malignant tumor found throughout the gastrointestinal tract; however, whereas it is most commonly seen in the appendix in western countries, it is seen mainly in the rectum in Japan. Because carcinoid appears as a clearly demarcated hypoechoic mass that arises from the second to third layers (5,16), it is easy to diagnose. Endoscopic US is also very useful for making a prognostic assessment by determining the size, depth of invasion, and lymph node metastasis. Leiomyoma that arises from the muscularis mucosae is difficult to differentiate from carcinoid. Caution also is required because inflammatory fibroid polyps of the stomach show similar endoscopic US features (17). Because the inflammatory fibroid polyp has an irregular base, however, differentiation may be possible by means of very careful interpretation of the endoscopic US findings.

Heterotopic pancreatic tissue was detected in the stomach and duodenum in this study. This lesion was localized in the third layer and appeared as an irregular, solid tumor that was hyperechoic, hypoechoic, of intermediate echogenicity, or of mixed echogenicity with borders that were often indistinct. Cystic change and disruption of the layers were often observed.

Malignant lymphoma and intramural metastasis were hypoechoic lesions with an irregular margin that caused disruption of the layers of the gut wall. This finding may reflect invasive growth to some extent, but it is not specific for malignancy because heterotopic pancreatic tissue and endometriosis also produced a similar appearance of disruption.

Brunner gland hyperplasia and

gangliocytic paraganglioma are representative submucosal tumors that are unique to the duodenum. The former is visualized as a hyperechoic solid mass in the second to third layer. In contrast to the rest of the gastrointestinal tract, the normal wall of the duodenum (especially that of the duodenal bulb) contains intramucosal and submucosal Brunner glands, which Nakata and colleagues (18) have reported are visualized as hyperechoic areas on endoscopic US scans. Gangliocytic paraganglioma, which is a rare lesion of the digestive tract that occurs almost exclusively in the second part of the duodenum, is visualized as a solid mass of intermediate echogenicity in the third layer. This is similar to the findings reported on by Smithline and colleagues (19).

Lymphangiomas are most common in the large intestine, and they form unilocular or multilocular anechoic lesions in the third layer. On the other hand, duodenal cysts also show a similar echo pattern, but almost all of these cysts arise from Brunner glands. Hemangiomas are common in the esophagus and are observed as well-demarcated, hypoechoic, hyperechoic, or anechoic lesions in the third layer.

Intestinal endometriosis disrupts the gut wall layers and is characteristically a hypoechoic lesion that extends from the serosa to the submucosa. This is in contrast with malignant lymphoma, which extends outward. Suture granuloma is a submucosal tumor found in the stump of the appendix after appendectomy. This lesion is visualized as a hyperechoic mass in the third layer and is associated with strong echo attenuation.

Thus, when the endoscopic US findings are identical for several different tumors, such as a lipoma and Brunner gland hyperplasia, a carcinoid and a leiomyoma that arises from the muscularis mucosa, and a cyst that arises from dilated Brunner glands or ducts and a lymphangioma, it should be remembered that the disease may vary with the organ affected. Furthermore, organ-specific diseases, such as granular cell tumor, Brunner gland hyperplasia, suture granuloma, and endometriosis, should always be considered.

Differentiation between Benign and Malignant Lesions by Endoscopic US

Significant differences were observed between the benign and malignant lesions with respect to size ($P < .05$) and echo levels of homogeneous lesions ($P < .01$) among the various factors assessed (size, internal echo pattern, and margin). However, no significant difference was observed between benign and malignant lesions in the homogeneity of the internal echo pattern or the marginal echo pattern. It was surprising that all but one of the lesions that were anechoic, of intermediate echogenicity, or hyperechoic at endoscopic US were benign in this study. However, it was extremely difficult to differentiate between benign and malignant lesions that were hypoechoic or of mixed echogenicity, such as myogenic tumors. For the differential diagnosis of smooth muscle tumors, we have previously reported that the doubling time was useful for estimating the malignant potential and that tumors with a doubling time of 16 months or less should be considered malignant (20). Disruption of the gut wall layers on endoscopic US scans has been suggested to be characteristic of malignant lesions, such as lymphoma or intramural metastasis (21), but it is not specific because some benign lesions such as heterotopic pancreatic tissue or endometriosis also cause the same changes.

In conclusion, the internal echo pattern suggests the histopathologic structure of a lesion or the presence of degeneration, while the layer of origin reflects the site of tumor growth and pattern of invasion. Our results indicate that the differential diagnosis of gastrointestinal submucosal tumors can be facilitated by using endoscopic US to carefully examine the size of the lesion, its echogenicity, its layer of origin, and its margin. ■

Acknowledgments: We gratefully thank Mitsuru Koga, MD, Toru Muranaka, MD, Yukiaki Haraguchi, MD, Toshio Oiwa, MD, Heihachirou Takano, MD, and Nobuo Kojima, MD, for their contribution of some cases and Lawrence D. Buadu, MB, ChB, for his skilled and expeditious editorial assistance in the revision of the manuscript.

References

1. Yasuda K, Nakajima M, Yoshida S, Kiyota K, Kawai K. The diagnosis of submucosal tumors of the stomach by endoscopic ultrasonography. Gastrointest Endosc 1989; 35:10–15.
2. Yasuda K, Cho E, Nakajima M, Kawai K. Diagnosis of submucosal lesions of the upper gastrointestinal tract by endoscopic ultrasonography. Gastrointest Endosc 1990; 36(suppl): 17–20.
3. Tio TL, Tytgat GNJ, den Hartog Jager FCA. Endoscopic ultrasonography for the evaluation of smooth muscle tumors in the upper gastrointestinal tract: an experience with 42 cases. Gastrointest Endosc 1990; 36:342–350.
4. Boyce GA, Sivak MV, Rosch T, et al. Evaluation of submucosal upper gastrointestinal tract lesions by endoscopic ultrasound. Gastrointest Endosc 1991; 37:449–454.
5. Kawamoto K, Ueyama T, Iwashita I, et al. Colonic submucosal tumors: comparison of endoscopic US and target air-enema CT with barium enema study and colonoscopy. Radiology 1994; 192:697–702.
6. Hirata N, Kawamoto K, Ueyama T, et al. Endoscopic ultrasonography in the assessment of colonic wall invasion by adjacent disease. Abdom Imaging 1994; 19:21–26.
7. Aibe T. A study on the structure of layers of the gastrointestinal wall visualized by means of the ultrasonic endoscope. II. The structure of layers of the esophageal wall and colonic wall. Gastroenterol Endosc 1984; 26:1465–1473. [Japanese]
8. Rosner B. Hypothesis testing: categorical data. In: Rosner B, ed. Fundamentals of biostatistics. 4th ed. New York, NY: Wadsworth, 1995; 423–426.
9. Kotz S, Johnson NL, Read CB. In: Encyclopedia of statistical sciences. Vol. 4. New York, NY: Wiley, 1983; 352–354.
10. Caletti G, Zani L, Bolondi L, Brocchi E, Rollo V, Barbara L. Endoscopic ultrasonography in the diagnosis of gastric submucosal tumor. Gastrointest Endosc 1989; 35:413–418.
11. Gordon JS, Rifkin MD, Goldberg BB. Endosonographic evaluation of mural abnormalities of the upper gastrointestinal tract. Gastrointest Endosc 1986; 32:193–198.
12. Yasuda K, Nakajima M, Kawai K. Endoscopic ultrasonography in the diagnosis of submucosal tumor of the upper digestive tract. Scand J Gastroenterol 1986; 21(suppl 123):59–67.
13. Nakayama Y, Asaki S, Ohara S, et al. Diagnosis of submucosal tumors in the upper gastrointestinal tract by endoscopic ultrasonography. II. Prospective differentiation of malignant submucosal tumors. Gastroenterol Endosc 1993; 35:270–278. [Japanese]
14. Mitsunaga A. Diagnosis of submucosal tumors of the upper gastrointestinal tract by endoscopic ultrasonography. Gastroenterol Endosc 1987; 29:3–12. [Japanese]
15. Murata Y, Yoshida M, Akimoto S, Ide H, Suzuki S, Hanyu F. Evaluation of endoscopic ultrasonography for the diagnosis of submucosal tumors of the esophagus. Surg Endosc 1988; 2:51–58.
16. Matsumoto T, Iida M, Suekane H, Tominaga M, Yao T, Fujishima M. Endoscopic ultrasonography in rectal carcinoid tumors: contribution to selection of therapy. Gastrointest Endosc 1991; 37:539–542.
17. Tokumitsu S, Sato H, Kato K, et al. Endoscopic ultrasonographic features of two cases of inflammatory fibroid polyp in the stomach. Prog Gastroenterol Endosc 1991; 38:300–303. [Japanese]
18. Nakata K, Aibe T, Noguchi T, et al. A study of the diagnosis of duodenal ulcer by endoscopic ultrasonography (the first report). Gastroenterol Endosc 1986; 28:1853–1858. [Japanese]
19. Smithline AE, Hawes RH, Kopecky KK, Cummings OW, Kumar S. Gangliocytic paraganglioma, a rare cause of upper gastrointestinal bleeding: endoscopic ultrasound findings presented. Dig Dis Sci 1993; 38:173–177.
20. Ueyama T, Kawamoto K, Iwashita I, et al. Correlation between tumor volume doubling time and histologic findings in gastric smooth muscle tumors: clinical implications of tumor volume doubling time. J Surg Oncol 1995; 60: 12–17.
21. Aibe T, Noguchi T, Nakata K, et al. Advance in the diagnosis of gastric submucosal tumors brought about by endoscopic ultrasonography (EUS). Stomach Intestine 1989; 24:999–1008. [Japanese]

Carlo Procacci, MD • Rossella Graziani, MD • Giuseppe Zamboni, MD • Giorgio Cavallini, MD
Paolo Pederzoli, MD • Alessandro Guarise, MD • Giuseppe Bogina, MD • Carlo Biasiutti, MD
Giovanni Carbognin, MD • Ivo A. Bergamo-Andreis, MD • Gian F. Pistolesi, MD

Cystic Dystrophy of the Duodenal Wall: Radiologic Findings[1]

PURPOSE: **To determine the radiologic characteristics of cystic dystrophy of the duodenal wall.**

MATERIALS AND METHODS: **Ten patients with cystic dystrophy of the duodenal wall and chronic pancreatitis underwent ultrasonography (US) ($n = 10$), computed tomography (CT) ($n = 10$), endoscopic US ($n = 5$), and endoscopic retrograde cholangiopancreatography (ERCP) ($n = 9$). Cystic dystrophy of the duodenal wall was classified as either cystic or solid. The imaging findings were retrospectively analyzed and compared with findings at pancreatoduodenectomy ($n = 10$).**

RESULTS: **The more frequent cystic type ($n = 7$) of cystic dystrophy of the duodenal wall was characterized by the presence of easily recognizable cystic lesions (diameter, more than 1 cm), located within the thickened wall of the second portion of the duodenum. The solid type ($n = 3$) of cystic dystrophy of the duodenal wall demonstrated fibrous thickening of the duodenal wall within which small cysts (diameter, less than 1 cm) were present. The intraduodenal cysts were usually elongated or bilobate with a thick wall. The thickening of the duodenal wall appeared as a solid layer between the duodenal lumen and the pancreas, hypoechoic at US, isoattenuating at unenhanced CT, and hypoattenuating in the early phase (after initiation of infusion of contrast material) and isoattenuating in the late phase (after completion of infusion) at contrast material–enhanced CT. Findings at retrospective analysis of CT and endoscopic US images were characteristic.**

CONCLUSION: **Imaging modalities, notably CT and endoscopic US, helped establish the diagnosis of cystic dystrophy of the duodenal wall.**

Cystic dystrophy of the duodenal wall is a rare lesion that was first described in 1970 by Potet and Duclert (1), to our knowledge, and subsequent contributions were almost all presented in European pathology and gastroenterology literature (2–6). The appearance of the lesion at endoscopic ultrasound (US) (7–10), computed tomography (CT), and magnetic resonance imaging (11) has been described recently. Cystic dystrophy of the duodenal wall may be the only lesion present, but it is usually associated with chronic pancreatitis (3,5,7,11,12). Cystic dystrophy of the duodenal wall may mimic a tumor of the pancreatic head (4,13). We believe that this lesion, whose imaging features need to be better defined, occurs more frequently than is reported in the literature. Cystic dystrophy of the duodenal wall, whose clinical pattern is similar to that of chronic pancreatitis, often recurs even after cystojejunostomy, consequently necessitating pancreatoduodenectomy.

The purpose of this study was to determine the imaging features of cystic dystrophy of the duodenal wall with different modalities.

MATERIALS AND METHODS

After research in our department of pathology, the cases of 10 patients with cystic dystrophy of the duodenal wall and chronic pancreatitis were found. These patients were seen between 1992 and 1996, and each had undergone pancreatoduodenectomy. The imaging findings in these 10 patients were analyzed retrospectively in our department of radiology by three radiologists (C.P., R.G., C.B.), two of whom are experts in pancreatic pathology. The reviewers determined findings by consensus, and they were aware of the clinical pattern and pathologic diagnosis.

The patients were all men, with a mean age at surgery of 41 years (range, 32–59 years). Eight of them were smokers (more than 10 cigarettes per day), and nine had a daily ethanol uptake of more than 80 g. All patients presented with a clinical pattern of chronic pancreatitis with relapsing episodes of abdominal pain, weight loss (four patients), vomiting (three patients) and jaundice (one patient). The mean time between clinical onset of the disease and surgical resection was 4.5 years (range, 1–9 years).

Seven of the 10 patients underwent pancreatoduodenectomy for suspected duodenal or pancreatic neoplasm (three patients) and for cystic dystrophy of the duodenal wall associated with chronic pancreatitis that had been correctly diagnosed at imaging (four patients). In the remaining three patients, pseudocyst alone or with signs of chronic pancreatitis was the initial diagnosis, and they had been followed up conservatively for 1–4 years. During follow-up, two patients underwent pancreato- or cystojejunostomy before they underwent pancreatoduodenectomy. In all three of these patients, surgery was performed to treat persistent or recurring cysts in the duodenal wall with associated pain.

Index terms: Duodenum, cystic dystrophy, 738.3121 • Endoscopic retrograde cholangiopancreatography (ERCP), 77.1222 • Pancreas, CT, 77.12111, 77.12114 • Pancreas, US, 77.12981 • Pancreatitis, 77.291

Abbreviation: ERCP = endoscopic retrograde cholangiopancreatography.

Radiology 1997; 205:741–747

[1] From the Departments of Radiology (C.P., R.G., A.G., C.B., G. Carbognin, I.A.B.A., G.F.P.), Pathology (G.Z., G.B.), Gastroenterology (G. Cavallini), and Endocrine Surgery (P.P.), University Hospital, Policlinico Borgo Roma, 37134 Verona, Italy. Received May 5, 1997; revision requested June 5; final revision received July 29; accepted August 7. **Address reprint requests to** C.P.

On the gross specimen obtained at surgery, disease was confined to the second portion of the duodenum. The duodenal mucosa appeared dome shaped (Fig 1a) in eight cases and normal in two cases. Thickening of the duodenal wall was seen in all the cut specimens and was more evident on the pancreatic side of the supraampullary duodenum. The site of the papilla minor was obstructed in all specimens. In seven cases, the cut specimen showed multiple cysts more than 1 cm in diameter that bulged the mucosal surface of the supraampullary duodenum: We termed this the cystic variant of cystic dystrophy of the duodenal wall (Fig 1b). In three other cases, there was marked thickening of the muscular layer of the duodenal wall within which cysts less than 1 cm in diameter were present: We termed this the solid variant of cystic dystrophy of the duodenal wall (Fig 1c). In seven patients, the thickening of the duodenal wall was associated with fibrosis of the "groove" (ie, the space between the common bile duct, duodenum, and pancreatic head). In all patients the pancreas was fibrotic with calcifications and dilatation of the main pancreatic duct.

At microscopic examination, the inner surface of the cysts was covered with cuboidal epithelium similar to the epithelial lining of the pancreatic ducts (Fig 1d). In four patients the cysts contained calcifications and proteinaceous material. The muscular layer of the duodenal wall was thickened owing to fibrosis and proliferation of smooth muscle. Within the duodenal wall in all cases, exocrine, endocrine, and ductal pancreatic tissue were present that showed histologic changes of chronic pancreatitis such as inter- and intralobular fibrosis and prevailingly lymphoplasma cellular infiltrate. The same changes affected the pancreas.

All US examinations were performed with a convex 3.5- or 5-MHz probe (Esaote Biomedica, Genoa, Italy).

All CT examinations were performed with a conventional scanner (Somatom DR or Somatom HQ; Siemens, Erlangen, Germany). Unenhanced scanning was followed with contrast-enhanced scanning. Iodinated nonionic contrast material was administered intravenously with a power injector as both a 50-mL bolus (2 mL/sec) and a 100-mL infusion (0.8 mL/sec) during data acquisition. First, a set of partially overlapping 8-mm-thick scans (6-mm table movement) were obtained soon after initiation of the infusion of contrast material: This set of images depicted the early phase. Then, additional scans of the pancreatic area were obtained immediately after completion of the infusion: This set of images depicted the late phase.

Endoscopic US (GF-UM 3; Olympus Optical, Hamburg, Germany) was performed in five cases, with variable frequency (7.5–12.0 MHz).

Finally, nine patients underwent endoscopic retrograde cholangiopancreatography (ERCP).

The time lapse between imaging examinations and surgery was not more than 20 days.

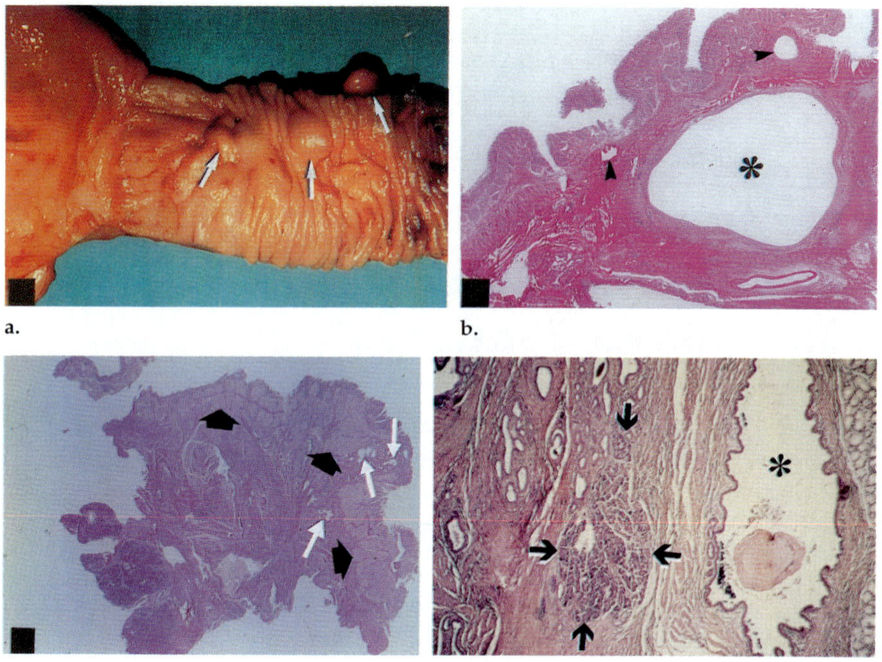

a. b. c. d.

Figure 1. Pathologic features of cystic dystrophy of the duodenal wall. **(a)** Gross specimen of the duodenum after pancreatoduodenectomy: The duodenal mucosa has multiple dome-shaped elevated areas (arrows). **(b)** Histologic slice shows the cystic variant of cystic dystrophy of the duodenal wall, with a large cyst within the duodenal wall (*), as well as other small cysts (arrowheads) within the thickened muscular layer. (Hematoxylin-eosin stain.) **(c)** Histologic slice shows the solid variant of cystic dystrophy of the duodenal wall, with tiny cysts (black arrows) within the markedly thickened and altered muscular layer, as well as hyperplasia of the Brunner glands (white arrows). (Hematoxylin-eosin stain.) **(d)** Histologic slice of the duodenal mucosa and submucosa shows a large cyst with a protein plug (*) and ectopic pancreatic tissue (arrows). (Hematoxylin-eosin stain; original magnification, ×40.)

RESULTS

US Findings

At retrospective review of US scans, a thick hypoechoic layer was seen between the duodenal lumen and the pancreas (Figs 2a, 4a) in five patients (Table 1), and in four of them oblong or bilobate cysts were also present (Fig 2a). Enlargement of the pancreatic head was present in all cases, often associated with the usual features of chronic pancreatitis (ie, dilatation of the main pancreatic duct [seven patients], calcifications [five patients], and pseudocysts [five patients]). The latter were located within the pancreatic head (Fig 2b) or neck. In one patient parenchymal atrophy was present, and in two patients dilatation of the common bile duct was seen.

The prospective diagnosis of cystic dystrophy of the duodenal wall was made on the basis of findings at US (Table 2) in only patients 1 and 2, who were the last patients included in the study (Fig 2a, 2b). Chronic pancreatitis was diagnosed in patients 3–8 with US and was associated with a pseudocyst in five of those six patients (in three of the five patients, cysts were found in the duodenal wall in the cut specimens). In patients 9 and 10, respectively, a presumed diagnosis of a duodenal tumor (remarkable thickening of the wall [Fig 4a]) and a pancreatic tumor (conspicuous enlargement of the pancreatic head) was made.

During retrospective analysis, the initial diagnosis was modified in only patients 3 and 5. Thus, even retrospectively, US allowed the diagnosis of cystic dystrophy of the duodenal wall in only four patients (cystic variant [Table 2]) when it was possible to recognize the thickened duodenal wall that contained variably sized cysts, as well as its overall delimitation from the pancreas.

CT Findings

Retrospective analysis of CT findings (Table 1) showed thickening of the duodenal wall in nine patients and the presence of intramural cysts in seven. The two findings were both demonstrated (Figs 2d–2f, 3, 6) in six patients. In one patient some cysts were recognizable within a duodenal wall that was not noticeably thickened, whereas in the three remaining patients only marked thickening of the duodenal wall (Figs 4b, 5) was

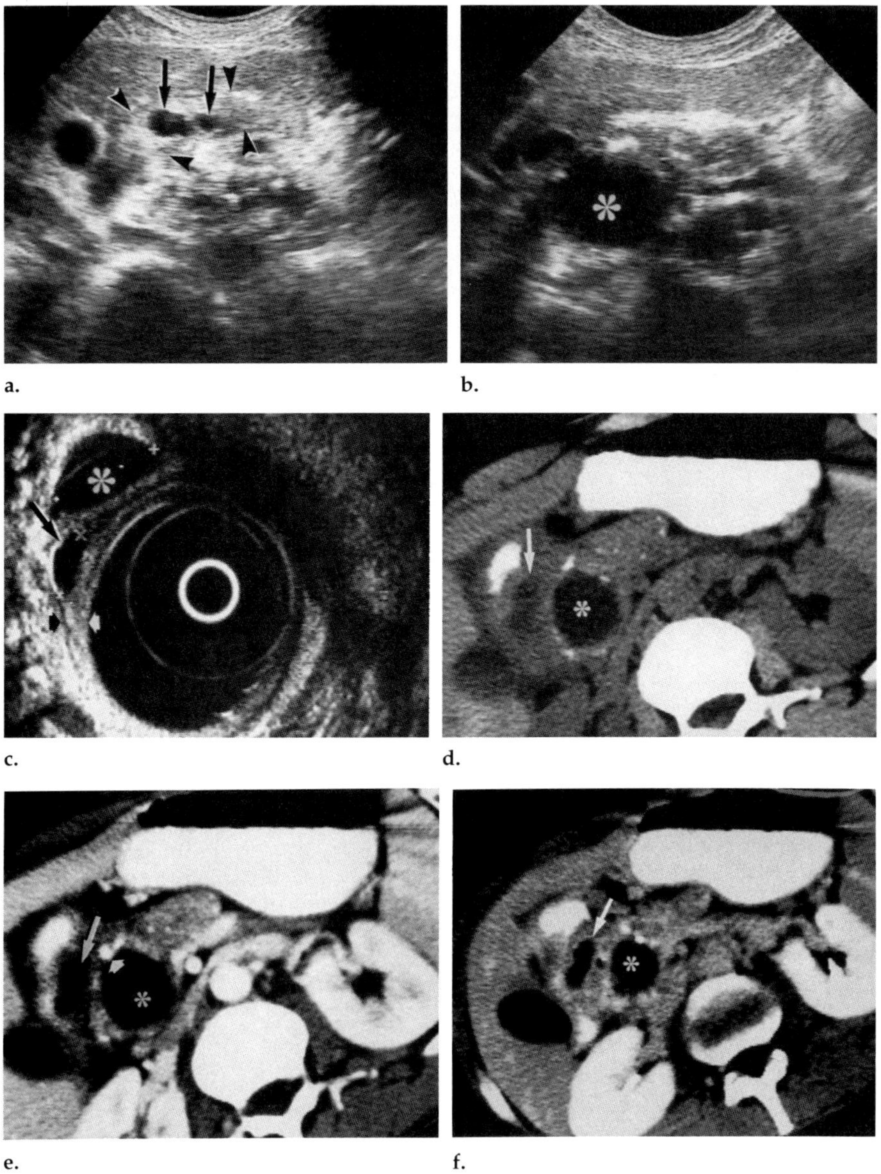

Figure 2. Patient 1. Cystic variant of cystic dystrophy of the duodenal wall. (a) Axial craniocaudal US scan depicts hypoechoic thickening of the duodenal wall (arrowheads), within which a few small cysts are embedded (arrows). (b) Axial craniocaudal US scan depicts a large pseudocyst (*) of the pancreatic head. (c) Endoscopic US scan shows improved demonstration of duodenal wall thickening (short arrows), the intramural cyst (long arrow), and the pseudocyst of the pancreatic head (*). The white circle indicates the endoscope. The cursors indicate the size of the intramural cyst. (d) Unenhanced axial CT scan demonstrates solid tissue, which is isoattenuating to the pancreatic parenchyma, interposed between the duodenal lumen and the pancreatic head. A cyst is embedded (arrow) within the solid tissue. Tiny calcifications and a large pseudocyst (*) are present in the pancreatic head. (e) Early phase contrast-enhanced CT scan depicts the thickened duodenal wall as hypoattenuating to the pancreas and shows improved demonstration of the cyst (long arrow) within it. The gastroduodenal artery (short arrow) is displaced to the left. * indicates the pseudocyst of the pancreatic head. (f) On the late phase contrast-enhanced CT scan, the fibrous tissue cannot be differentiated from the pancreatic head, whereas the intramural cyst (arrow) is better demonstrated. * indicates the pseudocyst of the pancreatic head.

present. The duodenal cyst was almost always elongated (Figs 2d–f, 3) or bilobate (Fig 6b) with a thick fibrous wall. The thickening of the duodenal wall, with or without cysts, appeared as a solid layer between the duodenal lumen and the pancreas, isoattenuating relative to the gland on the unenhanced scan (Figs 2d, 3a, 5a). On the contrast-enhanced scan, the layer became hypoattenuating in the early phase (Figs 2e; 3b; 5b, 5c) and isoattenuating in the late phase (Figs 2f, 3c, 5d). In addition, CT showed a few findings suggestive of but not diagnostic for cystic dystrophy of the duodenal wall; in particular, in four patients the gastroduodenal artery, located between the duodenum and the pancreatic head, was displaced from the duodenal lumen by the interposition of the intramural lesion (Figs 2e, 5b). The stomach was dilated in three patients, owing to compression of the duodenum by the lesion.

The pancreatic head was enlarged in seven patients, the main pancreatic duct was dilated (Fig 5) in five, pancreatic calcifications were recognized in five (Figs 2d–2f, 3, 6c, 6d), and a pseudocyst was seen in four (Fig 2d–f). Parenchymal atrophy was present in one patient, and slight dilatation of the biliary tree was present in three patients.

CT examinations in addition to that performed just before pancreatoduodenectomy were available in three patients, for a range of 1–4 years. In the two patients with the longest follow-up, the pancreas appeared normal in the first two examinations (Fig 6a, 6b). Pancreato- or cystojejunostomy had been performed twice in each of these two patients between the first and last CT examinations, which allowed assessment of the fast, steady worsening of the pancreatic condition: Gradual dilatation of the main pancreatic duct and the development of gross calcifications (Fig 6c, 6d) were seen.

Cystic dystrophy of the duodenal wall was diagnosed prospectively with CT (Figs 2d–2f, 3) in patients 1–4 (Table 2), whose cases were studied most recently. Chronic pancreatitis with the possible coexistence of a duodenal duplication cyst was diagnosed in patients 5 and 6. Diagnoses in other cases included cystic tumor of the pancreas (patient 7), chronic pancreatitis (patient 8), pancreatic tumor (patient 9), and duodenal tumor (patient 10).

The diagnosis of cystic dystrophy of the duodenal wall (cystic) was achieved retrospectively in seven cases on the basis of specific findings (thickening of the duodenal wall and intramural cysts [Fig 6c, 6d]) and nonspecific findings (displacement of the gastroduodenal artery). In an additional case (solid variant), the presence on early phase images of a thick fibrous layer between the duodenal lumen and the pancreas that was hypoattenuating relative to the pancreatic head (Fig 5) led to suspicion for cystic dystrophy of the duodenal wall. In the two remaining cases the lesion appeared as a neoplasm of either the duodenal wall (Fig 4b) or the pancreatic head.

Endoscopic US Findings

Endoscopic US was performed in five patients; in four of them (Table 1) thickening of the second portion of

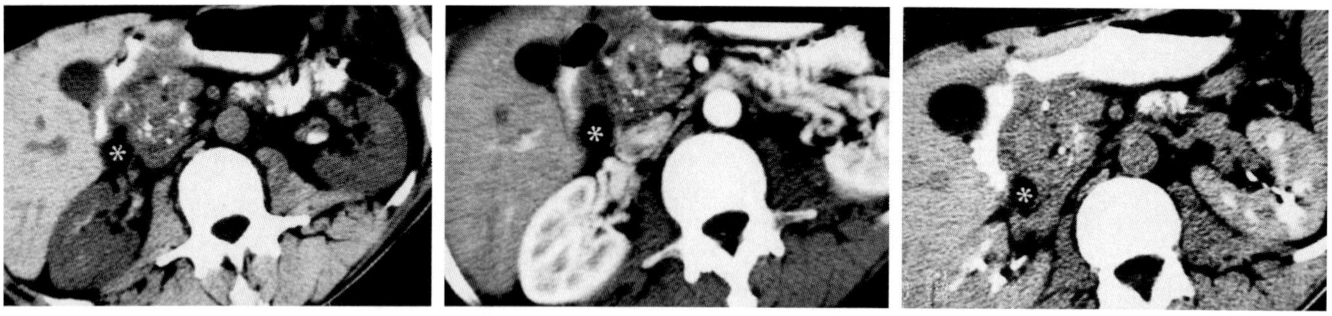

a. b. c.

Figure 3. Patient 2. Cystic variant of cystic dystrophy of the duodenal wall. **(a)** Unenhanced CT scan depicts thickening of the duodenal wall, within which a small cyst (*) is embedded. Small calcifications within the pancreatic head. **(b)** Early phase contrast-enhanced CT scan depicts duodenal wall thickening as hypoattenuating to the pancreatic head. * = small cyst. **(c)** Late phase contrast-enhanced CT scan depicts duodenal wall thickening as again isoattenuating to the pancreatic head. The small cyst (*) is better demonstrated.

the duodenum was depicted on the pancreatic side. In two of the four patients, two and three intramural cysts with a minimum diameter of 8 mm, respectively, were also depicted (Fig 2c). In the same four patients, enlargement of the pancreatic head was seen in two patients, calcifications in three, and pseudocysts in two. In the fifth case only enlargement of the pancreatic head and dilatation of the main pancreatic duct were seen, without apparent duodenal wall changes.

The diagnosis of cystic dystrophy of the duodenal wall (Table 2) was made prospectively in patients 1 and 4 on the basis of identification of cysts embedded within the thickened duodenal wall on the pancreatic side (Fig 2c).

The diagnosis of this lesion was made retrospectively in patients 3 and 5 on the basis of thickening of the duodenal wall (even though no cysts were identified), which can be considered a specific sign for cystic dystrophy of the duodenal wall.

Table 1
Imaging Findings in Retrospective Analysis of Cases of Cystic Dystrophy of the Duodenal Wall

Finding	At US (n = 10)	At CT (n = 10)	At Endoscopic US (n = 5)
Specific			
Duodenal wall thickness	5	9	4
Duodenal cysts	4	7	2
Nonspecific			
Gastroduodenal artery displacement	0	4	0
Stomach dilatation	0	3	0
Associated			
Enlargement of pancreatic head	10	7	3
Atrophy of pancreatic body and tail	1	1	0
Main pancreatic duct dilatation	7	5	1
Calcifications	5	5	3
Pseudocysts	5	4	2
Biliary tract dilatation	2	3	0
Erroneous			
Duodenal duplication cyst	0	0	0
Duodenal tumor	1	1	0
Solid pancreatic tumor	1	1	0
Cystic pancreatic tumor	0	0	0

Note.—Data are number of cases.

Findings at ERCP

ERCP was performed in nine patients. During the endoscopic phase, dome-shaped mucosa was seen in the second duodenal portion in two patients and the finding was confirmed in the subsequent pathologic examination. A nonspecific indentation on the duodenal bulb and hypertrophy of the duodenal plicae were demonstrated in another two patients. The main pancreatic duct was opacified in all patients and showed signs of pancreatitis in eight cases (dilatation in six patients, parietal irregularities in two patients, and communicating pseudocysts in one patient). The duct was regular in the remaining patient.

The diagnosis of cystic dystrophy of the duodenal wall could not be made prospectively or retrospectively in any patient who underwent ERCP. At retrospective analysis in two cases, only the endoscopic demonstration of a dome-shaped mucosal wall in the second duodenal portion indicated this condition. In eight cases, the retrospective diagnosis of chronic pancreatitis was possible.

DISCUSSION

To our knowledge, cystic dystrophy of the duodenal wall was first described in 1970 (1) and has been discussed subsequently almost exclusively in the European literature (2,5–8,14). The lesion is characterized by the presence of cysts within the duodenal wall that originate from ectopic pancreatic tissue. The cysts are usually located in the thickened submucosal or muscular layer, their inner surface is lined with cuboid epithelium similar to that lining pancreatic ducts, and they are embedded with fibrosis and ectopic pancreatic tissue with signs of chronic pancreatitis. Depending on the size of the cysts, the lesion may more frequently show a cystic pattern (lesion diameter, more than 1 cm) or, less frequently, a solid pattern (lesion diameter, less than 1 cm).

This lesion can be induced by inflammation of ectopic pancreatic tissue within the duodenal wall, secondary to obstruction of pancreatic excretory ducts (2,8). The cause of these changes is not known. In previous observations, cystic dystrophy of the duodenal wall was associated with the presence of a normal pancreas or chronic pancreatitis (1,2,4,7,9,11). In our study, chronic pancreatitis was present at surgery in all cases. In two cases in which previous CT examinations were available, however, only cystic dystrophy of the duodenal wall was initially present.

A similar mechanism is considered

Table 2
Imaging Findings and Diagnosis in Cases of Cystic Dystrophy of the Duodenal Wall

Patient No./Age (y)/Sex and Finding	Variant of Cystic Dystrophy	Findings at US (n = 10)		Findings at CT (n = 10)		Findings at Endoscopic US (n = 5)	
		Prospective	Retrospective	Prospective	Retrospective	Prospective	Retrospective
1/36/M	Cystic						
Specific		DC, DWT	DC, DWT	DC, DWT	DC, DWT	DC, DWT	DC, DWT
Nonspecific				GDAD, SD	GDAD, SD		
Associated		BTD, C, EPH, P	BTD, C, EPH, P	BTD, C, EPH, P	BTD, C, EPH, P	C, EPH, P	C, EPH, P
Erroneous							
Diagnosis		CDDW + CP	CDDW + CP	CDDW + CP	CDDW + CP	CDDW + CP	CDDW + CP
2/42/M	Cystic						
Specific		DC, DWT	DC, DWT	DC, DWT	DC, DWT		
Nonspecific				GDAD, SD	GDAD, SD		
Associated		C, EPH, MPDD	C, EPH, MPDD	C, MPDD	C, MPDD		
Erroneous							
Diagnosis		CDDW + CP	CDDW + CP	CDDW + CP	CDDW + CP		
3/32/M	Cystic						
Specific			DC, DWT	DC, DWT	DC, DWT	DWT	DWT
Nonspecific				GDAD	GDAD		
Associated		EPH, MPDD, P	EPH, MPDD	BTD, MPDD	BTD, MPDD	EPH	EPH
Erroneous							
Diagnosis		P + CP	CDDW + CP*	CDDW + CP	CDDW + CP	CP	CDDW + CP*
4/48/M	Cystic						
Specific				DC, DWT	DC, DWT	DC, DWT	DC, DWT
Nonspecific				SD	SD		
Associated		C, EPH, MPDD, P	C, EPH, MPDD, P	C, EPH, P	C, EPH, P	C, P	C, P
Erroneous							
Diagnosis		P + CP	P + CP	CDDW + CP	CDDW + CP	CDDW + CP	CDDW + CP
5/38/M	Cystic						
Specific			DC		DC, DWT	DWT	DWT
Nonspecific							
Associated		C, EPH, MPDD, P	C, EPH, MPDD, P	C, EPH, P	C, EPH, P	C	C
Erroneous				DDC			
Diagnosis		P + CP	CDDW + CP*	DDC + CP	CDDW + CP*	CP	CDDW + CP*
6/40/M	Cystic						
Specific		DWT	DWT		DC, DWT		
Nonspecific							
Associated		C, EPH, P	C, EPH, P	BTD, C	BTD, C		
Erroneous				DDC			
Diagnosis		P + CP	P + CP	DDC + CP	CDDW + CP*		
7/32/M	Cystic						
Specific					DC		
Nonspecific							
Associated		EPH, P	EPH, P	EPH	EPH, P		
Erroneous				CPT			
Diagnosis		P + CP	P + CP	CPT	CDDW + CP*		
8/42/M	Solid						
Specific					DWT		
Nonspecific					GDAD		
Associated		EPH, MPDD	EPH, MPDD	EPH, MPDD	EPH, MPDD	EPH, MPDD	EPH, MPDD
Erroneous							
Diagnosis		CP	CP	CP	CDDW + CP*	CP	CP
9/59/M	Solid						
Specific				DWT	DWT		
Nonspecific							
Associated		A, EPH, MPDD	A, EPH, MPDD	A, EPH, MPDD	A, EPH, MPDD		
Erroneous		SPT	SPT	SPT	SPT		
Diagnosis		SPT	SPT	SPT	SPT		
10/44/M	Solid						
Specific		DWT	DWT	DWT	DWT		
Nonspecific							
Associated		BTD, EPH, MPDD	BTD, EPH, MPDD	EPH, MPDD	EPH, MPDD		
Erroneous		DT	DT	DT	DT		
Diagnosis		DT	DT	DT	DT		

Note.—A = atrophy of pancreatic body and tail, BTD = biliary tract dilatation, C = calcifications, CDDW = cystic dystrophy of the duodenal wall, CP = chronic pancreatitis, CPT = cystic pancreatic tumor, DC = duodenal cyst, DDC = duodenal duplication cyst, DT = duodenal tumor, DWT = duodenal wall thickening, EPH = enlargement of pancreatic head, GDAD = gastroduodenal artery displacement, MPDD = main pancreatic duct dilatation, P = pseudocyst, SD = stomach dilatation, SPT = solid pancreatic tumor.
* Modified diagnosis.

to be the cause of another pathologic entity, "groove" pancreatitis (15–17). This lesion is a form of segmental pancreatitis that affects the groove between the head of the pancreas, the duodenum, and the common bile duct and that sometimes masquerades clinically as pancreatic head carcinoma (17). The macro- and microscopic features of groove pancreatitis reported in the literature (15–19) are very similar to those reported for cystic dystrophy of the duodenal wall. Fléjou et al (2), who described what may be the largest series of cases of cystic dystrophy of the duodenal wall, stated that the lesion patterns are similar to those of groove pancreatitis. They therefore hypothesized that many of these cases represented cystic dystrophy in an enterotropic pancreas. It is possible in the past, as a few authors have stated (2,12,13), that a few cases of cystic dystrophy of the duodenal wall were incorrectly interpreted as a duodenal duplication cyst. In the past we studied duodenal duplication cysts (20); the symptoms and pathologic features in some of those seven patients were similar to those of the patients with cystic dystrophy of the duodenal wall in the present study. In the earlier study, we may have committed a diagnostic error due to the lack of knowledge about cystic dystrophy of the duodenal wall and to the fact that all those lesions were treated with only pancreato- or cystojejunostomy.

In the cystic variant of cystic dystrophy of the duodenal wall, the cysts are easily demonstrated with both US and CT between the duodenum and the pancreatic head and, more rarely, located on the opposite side (1,2,6,7,11). Contrary to a pseudocyst, the lesion of the cystic variant is more frequently elongated or bilobate. CT easily demonstrates the deep location of the cysts within the duodenal wall, as well as the eventual narrowing of the duodenal lumen itself. The fibrous layer, in which the duodenal cysts are embedded, appears hypoechoic to the pancreas at US; the layer is isoattenuating to the pancreas on unenhanced CT scans, becomes hypoattenuating on early phase CT images, and presumably becomes even more hypoattenuating on arterial phase spiral CT scans. As Itoh et al (18) pointed out in cases of groove pancreatitis, this behavior is due to decreased vascularization of the fibrous tissue. The difference in enhancement between lesions of cystic dystrophy of the duodenal wall and the pancreas is more evident when the pancreas is normal or faintly involved. Nevertheless, this difference is also recognizable when advanced chronic pancreatitis is present. In the late phase (portal phase with spiral CT), the fibrous layer of the duodenal wall is again isoattenuating to the pancreas. On the basis of these findings, CT findings are better than US findings to help delimitation of cystic dystrophy of the duodenal wall from the pancreas. When located between the duodenum and the pancreas, the gastroduodenal artery appears displaced from the duodenal lumen owing to the presence of cystic dystrophy of the duodenal wall. Also when it is recognizable, the common bile duct should appear separate from the duodenum. Again, these appearances are more easily determined with CT. The pancreas may appear normal or to have the features of chronic pancreatitis, with dilatation of the main pancreatic duct and calcifications.

If this lesion is suspected on the basis of findings at US and CT, the diagnosis can be confirmed with endoscopic US which, when successful, allows the most thorough analysis of the duodenal wall (2,7,8,11). In the endoscopic phase at endoscopic US, the duodenal mucosa may appear dome shaped, owing to the presence of cystic lesions. Endoscopic US allows detection of the cysts by demonstrating their lack of relation to the pancreas or their location within the submucosal or muscular layer of the

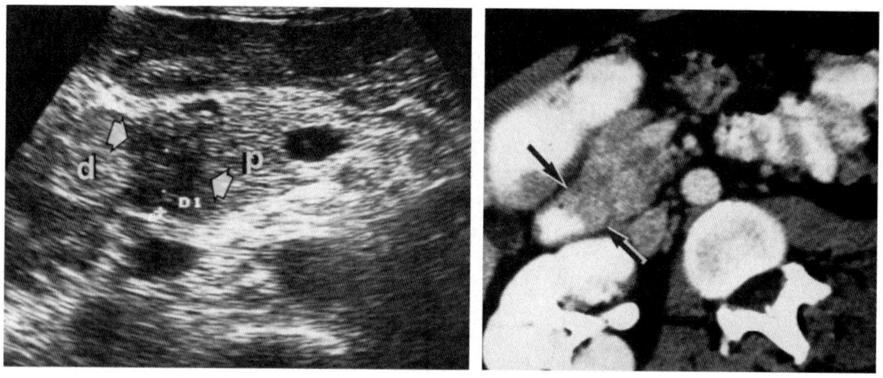

a. b.

Figure 4. Patient 10. Solid variant of cystic dystrophy of the duodenal wall. **(a)** Axial US scan depicts thick hypoechoic tissue (arrows) interposed between the duodenum (*d*) and the pancreatic head (*p*). No cysts are demonstrated. The cursor indicates measurement of the thick tissue. *D1* indicates distance 1 in the measurement system of our US equipment. **(b)** Axial CT scan depicts wall thickening of the second duodenal portion on the pancreatic side (arrows), without cysts.

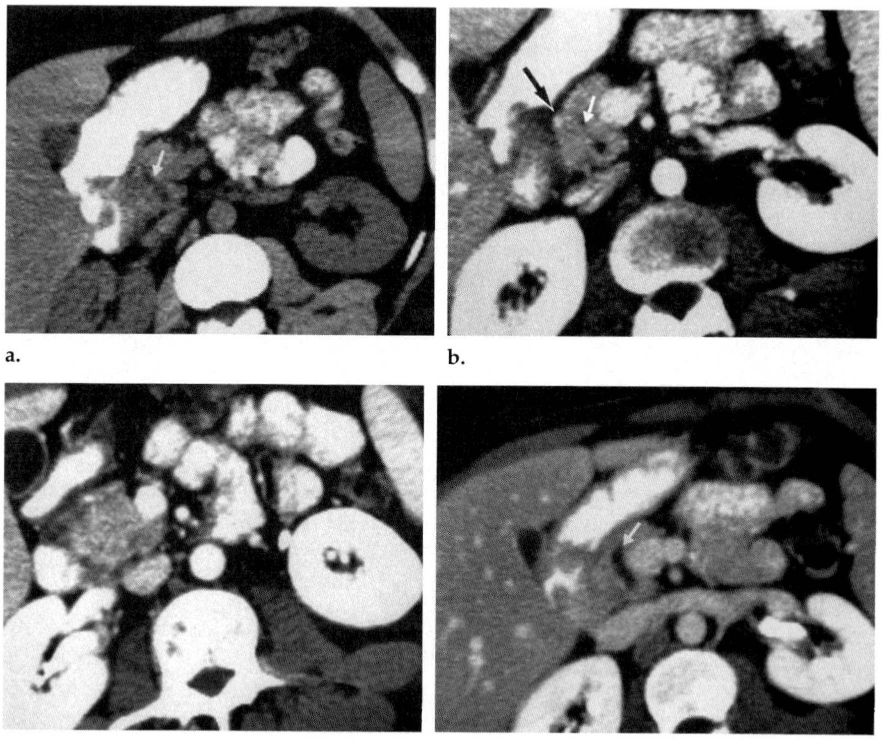

a. b. c. d.

Figure 5. Patient 8. Solid variant of cystic dystrophy of the duodenal wall. **(a)** Unenhanced CT scan depicts thick tissue interposed between the duodenal lumen and the pancreatic head. **(b, c)** Early phase contrast-enhanced CT scans depict the tissue as hypoattenuating to the pancreas and the gastroduodenal artery as medially displaced (black arrow in **b**). **(d)** Late phase contrast-enhanced CT scan depicts the tissue as isoattenuating to the pancreas. White arrow on **a** , **b**, and **d** indicates the dilated main pancreatic duct.

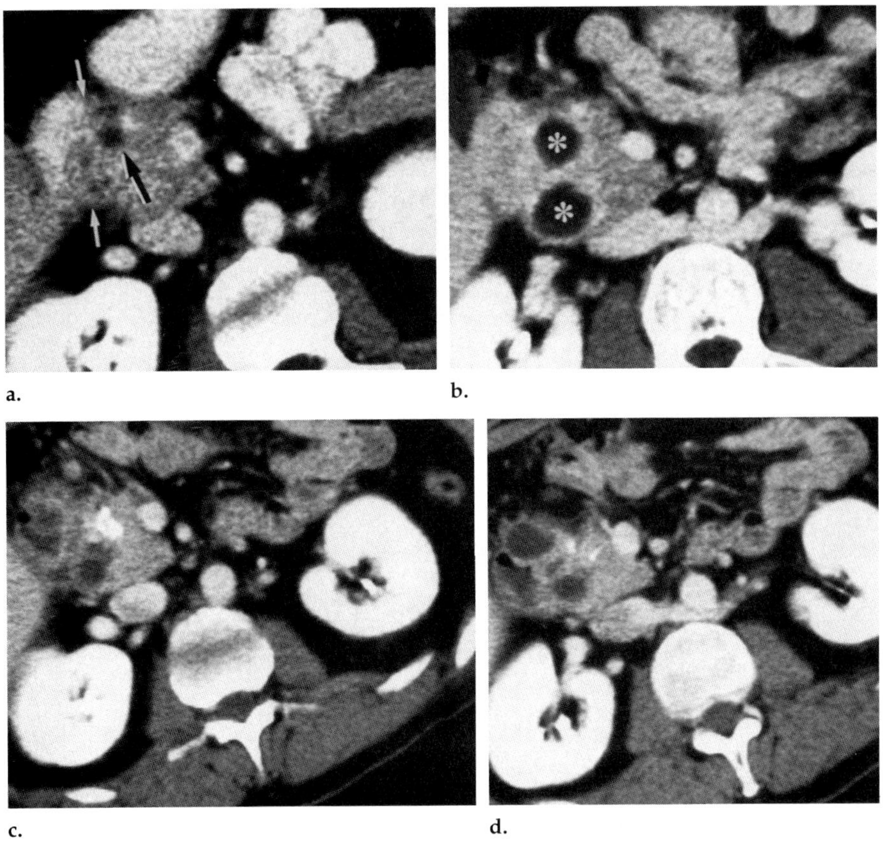

Figure 6. Patient 6. Cystic variant of cystic dystrophy of the duodenal wall. Assessment of evolution with CT. **(a)** Late phase contrast-enhanced CT scan obtained at the time of onset of clinical symptoms depicts the pancreatic head as regular, with thickening of the second duodenal portion (white arrows), within which a tiny cyst is embedded (black arrow). **(b)** Late phase contrast-enhanced CT scan obtained 8 months later depicts a notable increase in the size of the duodenal cysts (*), which are surrounded by a thick layer of fibrous tissue. The pancreas is still normal. **(c, d)** Late phase contrast-enhanced CT scans obtained 3 years later, after unsuccessful pancreato- and cystojejunostomy, show their persistence as well as the appearance of gross calcifications within the pancreatic head.

duodenal wall. The role of ERCP is secondary in the diagnosis of this lesion because it can demonstrate the eventual coexistence of chronic pancreatitis (2,6,10,11).

The solid variant of cystic dystrophy of the duodenal wall is depicted as thickening of the duodenal wall with microcysts embedded within. Diagnosis with US and CT is difficult, as only thickening of the duodenal wall can be identified, which is sometimes not distinguishable from the pancreatic head; thus, a wrong diagnosis of either pancreatic or duodenal neoplasm is possible. In such cases only performance of a precisely timed contrast-enhanced CT examination, especially with spiral technique, may allow differentiation between the fibrous layer of the duodenal wall and the pancreatic head and, thus, acquisition of the correct diagnosis. The solid variant of cystic dystrophy of the duodenal wall can be differentiated from ductal adenocarcinoma, which is also hypoattenuating to the pancreas in the arterial phase, as a result of the oblong morphology of the lesion, which is situated deep in the duodenal wall and does not necessarily involve biliary obstruction. Findings at endoscopic US may help confirm the diagnosis of cystic dystrophy of the duodenal wall more easily by demonstrating the parietal thickening as well as, sometimes, tiny intramural cysts less than 1 cm in diameter that are not identifiable with other imaging modalities (8). ■

Acknowledgment: The authors thank Eileen R. Smith, who assisted us in correcting the manuscript for this article.

References

1. Potet F, Duclert N. Dystrophie kystique sur pancréas aberrant de la paroi duodénale. Arch Fr Mal Appl Dig 1970; 59:223–238.
2. Fléjou JF, Potet F, Molas G, Bernardes P, Amouyal P, Fékété F. Cystic dystrophy of the gastric and duodenal wall developing in heterotopic pancreas: an unrecognised entity. Gut 1993; 34:343–347.
3. Vankemmel M, Paris JC, Houcke M, Laurent JC, Burzynski A. Kystes para-duodénaux juxta-vatériens et pancréatite chronique. Med Chir Dig 1975; 4:181–185.
4. Léger L, Louvel A, Chiche B, Michali P. Les hétérotopies pancréatiques: a propos de 8 nouveaux cas. J Chir 1979; 116:553–560.
5. Martin E, Marche C. Kystes para-vatériens et pancréatites chroniques: 17 cas. Arch Fr Mal Appl Dig 1969; 58:825–827.
6. Eloit S, Charles JF, L'Heveder G, Balouet G, Leroy JP. Dystrophie kystique sur pancréas aberrant. Sem Hôp Paris 1987; 63: 2545–2549.
7. Andrieu J, Palazzo L, Chikli F, Doll J, Chome J. Dystrophie kystique sur pancréas aberrant: apport de l'écho-endoscopie. Gastroenterol Clin Biol 1989; 13: 630–633.
8. Colardelle P, Chochon M, Larvol L, Palazzo L, Fléjou JF, Andrieu J. Dystrophie kystique sur pancréas aberrant antro-bulbaire. Gastroenterol Clin Biol 1994; 18:277–280.
9. Palazzo L, Roseau G, Chaussade S, et al. Dystrophie kystique sur pancréas aberrant de la paroi duodénale (DKPA) associée à la pancréatite chronique calcifiante alcoolique (PCCA): une affection fréquente et méconnue (abstr). Gastroenterol Clin Biol 1992; 16(suppl 2):A141.
10. Visset J, Jais F, Le Bodic MF, et al. Dystrophie kystique sur pancréas aberrant de la paroi duodénale: problèmes diagnostiques et thérapeutiques. Chirurgie 1992; 118:634–636.
11. Godlewsky G, Nguyen Trong A, Ribard D, Maubon A, Pignodel C, Joujoux JM. Dystrophie kystique sur pancréas aberrant: apport de la TDM et de l'IRM. J Chir 1993; 130:403–407.
12. Holstege A, Barner S, Brambs HJ, Wenz W, Gerok W, Farthmann EH. Relapsing pancreatitis associated with duodenal wall cysts: diagnostic approach and treatment. Gastroenterology 1985; 88:814–819.
13. Molas G, Kharsa G, Potet F. Dystrophies kystiques sur pancréas aberrants de la paroi duodenale (abstr). Gastroenterol Clin Biol 1988; 12(suppl 2):A245.
14. Murat J, Gignoux M, Lesbros F. Dystrophie kystique sur pancréas aberrant du bulbe duodénal. Ann Chir 1971; 25:1203–1208.
15. Becker V, Mischke U. Groove pancreatitis. Int J Pancreatol 1991; 10:173–182.
16. Stolte M, Weiss W, Volkholz H, Rösch W. A special form of segmental pancreatitis: "groove pancreatitis". Hepatogastroenterology 1982; 29:198–208.
17. Yamaguchi K, Tanaka M. Groove pancreatitis masquerading as pancreatic carcinoma. Am J Surg 1992; 163:312–318.
18. Itoh S, Yamakawa K, Shimamoto K, Endo T, Ishigaki T. CT findings in groove pancreatitis: correlation with histopathological findings. J Comput Assist Tomogr 1994; 18: 911–915.
19. Toppino M, Campra D, Maramotti M, Regge D, Fronda GR, Recchia S. La "groove pancreatitis": descrizione di un caso di pancreatite cronica focale. Minerva Gastroenterol Dietologica 1995; 41:181–185.
20. Procacci C, Portuese A, Fugazzola C, et al. Duodenal duplication in the adult: its relationship with pancreatitis. Gastrointest Radiol 1988; 13:315–322.

(Preview of) "A Modest Proposal"

As of the present year, *2025*, radiologists can take great pride in their ability to image any part of the human anatomy, including abnormalities that occur in a number of diseases. All body regions can now be scanned, reconstructed as two- or three-dimensional images, and viewed from practically any perspective. We can call up these images using portable microcomputers and view them on high-luminance screens that are contained in our briefcase workstations. We also have the ability to project the images by satellite to any location in the world where the information might be needed for consultation or on-site patient treatment. If problems still remain in the application of modern imaging techniques to human disease, they are primarily within the realm of archiving and displaying the *enormous quantity* of imaging data now available to us. In an effort to compress this incredible amount of data into a form that can be visualized, stored, and transmitted easily for many different clinical applications, I would like to make the following proposal.

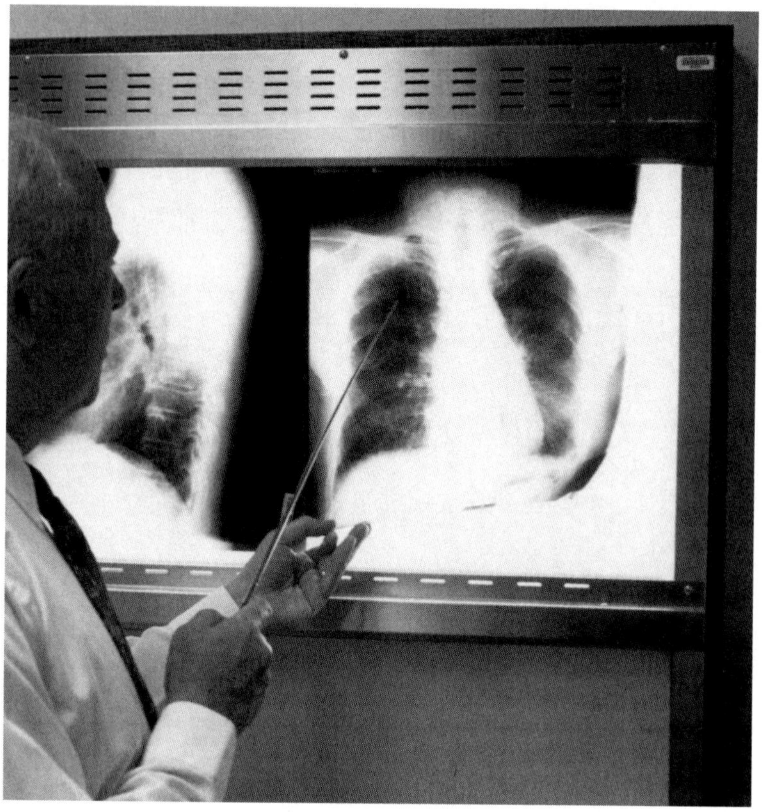

Projectional image of a patient's chest, imprinted on "film" that is displayed on an illuminated "view box."

For most of the 20th century, our antecedents in radiology recorded images of the body by using a medium called "film," which was a transparent Mylar or polyester sheet covered with a silver halide compound. These images were, in effect, planar projections of volumetric data from individual body regions that were imprinted on a hard-copy transparency ("film"). The films were stored in paper jackets that constituted a historical record of all the imaging procedures on a given patient. I would like to propose that we begin to use such thin films again to record and retrieve the tremendous amounts of anatomic and functional data that we now have at our disposal from patient imaging studies. We would have to recall the stored data from distributed electronic archives and from multiple image acquisition sites in order to print the films, but we might then be able to manage many patient problems on the basis of these projectional images alone. Each image on film contains a tremendous amount of compressed visual data, and it can be viewed and compared side by side with historical images on film from the same patients. A simple light source ("light box" or "view box") is needed to view each film transparency, which in turn could reduce our need for high-resolution diagnostic workstations (Figure). If we could train physicians and staff to carry these films to operating rooms and to other patient care and consultation sites, traffic on our currently overworked data networks might be eased and the image display format for many patient studies would be simplified. Because of the portability of films and their ease of packaging, it is conceivable that we might also reinstitute the use of overnight mail to transfer some of these projectional images from institution to institution, or that we might even give them directly *to patients!*

I believe this innovation (the use of projectional images on film to archive and display some of our radiologic information) could have a highly beneficial effect on daily clinical operations and on our ability to serve our patients and clinicians better. However, radiologists will have to relearn the subtleties of interpreting the highly compressed information that is contained within this unique display modality. The diagnostic information required for many patient care decisions is indeed there (ie, on the film), but we must learn how to get at it! I commend this novel solution to you for further discussion as a possible step forward to enrich our armamentarium of image archiving and display methods.

Courtesy of Richard J. Steckel, MD, Los Angeles, Calif

Michelle L. Robbin, MD • Mark E. Lockhart, MD • Therese M. Weber, MD
Jiri J. Vitek, MD • J. Kevin Smith, MD, PhD • Jay Yadav, MD • Atul Mathur, MD
Sriram S. Iyer, MD • Gary S. Roubin, MD, PhD

Carotid Artery Stents: Early and Intermediate Follow-up with Doppler US[1]

PURPOSE: To determine whether ultrasound (US) is a sensitive follow-up method after placement of a carotid artery stent for the detection of significant stenosis, occlusion, and other complications at early and intermediate follow-up.

MATERIALS AND METHODS: Doppler US examinations were performed after stent placement in 170 carotid arteries in 119 patients with angiographic correlation. Prospective diagnostic US criteria for stenosis were peak-systolic velocity greater than 1.25 m/sec, internal carotid artery (ICA) to common carotid artery (CCA) peak-systolic velocity ratio of greater than or equal to 3:1, and intrastent doubling of peak-systolic velocity. Retrospective criteria for stenosis were also applied: peak-systolic velocity greater than 1.7 m/sec, ICA end-diastolic velocity greater than 0.4 m/sec, ICA/CCA peak-systolic velocity ratio greater than 2.0, and ICA/CCA end-diastolic velocity ratio greater than 2.4.

RESULTS: Eighty-seven immediate and 83 intermediate (average, 7.3 months) follow-up US examinations were performed. Two stent occlusions were detected. One or more prospective US criteria were abnormal in 26 arteries with a stent. One or more retrospective criteria were positive in 47 arteries. Angiography showed corresponding findings, with only one significant stenosis (63%) in the ICA stents. Moderate collapse of a CCA stent was depicted at US.

CONCLUSION: Only one significant recurrent stenosis was detected, and no significant stenoses were missed at US. US successfully depicted carotid artery stent occlusion and a moderate stent collapse. Sensitivity in the detection of intrastent stenosis is promising. Further study to refine US criteria in a study with longer term follow-up is needed owing to the lack of significant recurrent stenosis in the intermediate follow-up group.

STROKE is the third largest cause of mortality and the leading cause of serious long-term disability in the United States. The benefit of surgical management of carotid artery stenosis has been demonstrated in two important studies. The North American Symptomatic Carotid Endarterectomy Trial (NASCET) is the benchmark study on the use of carotid endarterectomy in North America. Findings in the NASCET study demonstrated the strong benefit of performance of endarterectomy in appropriate symptomatic patients with carotid artery stenosis of greater than or equal to 70% (1,2). Subsequently, findings in the Asymptomatic Carotid Atherosclerosis Study (ACAS) were that asymptomatic patients with a stenosis of greater than or equal to 60% benefit from performance of endarterectomy (3).

Percutaneous placement of a carotid artery stent is currently being evaluated for the treatment of extracranial carotid artery stenosis. A multidisciplinary team at our institution is investigating placement of carotid artery stents in both symptomatic and asymptomatic patients with extracranial carotid artery stenosis. This prospective study protocol includes baseline, postplacement, and 6-month angiographic and US follow-up (4).

Although findings at angiography are considered the standard of reference for vascular evaluation, it is an invasive and expensive procedure. Color Doppler US is noninvasive, rapid, and relatively inexpensive and should be an excellent modality for the assessment of results after placement of a carotid artery stent. Prior criteria established for grading carotid artery stenosis (5–10) are based on evaluation of the native carotid artery bulb. In recent studies, the NASCET method has been used to calculate stenosis, with peak-systolic flow velocity in the distal internal carotid artery (ICA) as the denominator to determine the percentage stenosis. In the study of Moneta et al (11), the spectral Doppler criteria included peak-systolic velocity of 2.60 m/sec and end-diastolic velocity of 0.7 m/sec for stenosis of 60% or more, with a maximum accuracy of 90%. Criteria in the study of Carpenter et al (12) included peak-systolic velocity greater than 1.70 m/sec and end-diastolic velocity greater than 0.4 m/sec, with an accuracy of greater than 86%. To our knowledge, however, the various existing US criteria have not been studied in carotid arteries in which a stent has been placed. Thus, we found no established US criteria with which to evaluate stenosis in a carotid artery stent.

The objective of this investigation

Index terms: Carotid arteries, flow dynamics, 172.91 • Carotid arteries, stenosis or obstruction, 172.76 • Carotid arteries, US, 172.12983

Abbreviations: ACAS = Asymptomatic Carotid Atherosclerosis Study, CCA = common carotid artery, ICA = internal carotid artery, NASCET = North American Symptomatic Carotid Endarterectomy Trial.

Radiology 1997; 205:749–756

[1] From the Department of Radiology (M.L.R., M.E.L., T.M.W., J.J.V., J.K.S., G.S.R.) and the Division of Cardiovascular Diseases (A.M., S.S.I., G.S.R.), the University of Alabama at Birmingham, 619 S 19th St, New Hillman Bldg 623, Birmingham, AL 35233-1924; and the Atlanta Cardiology Group, Atlanta, Ga (J.Y.). Received February 3, 1997; revision requested March 19; revision received July 2; accepted August 18. **Address reprint requests to** M.L.R.

See also the editorial by Polak (pp 649–650) in this issue.

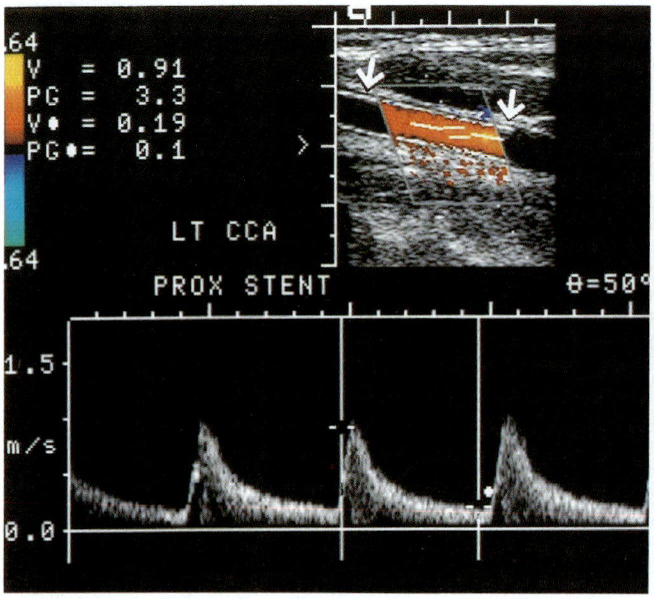

1.

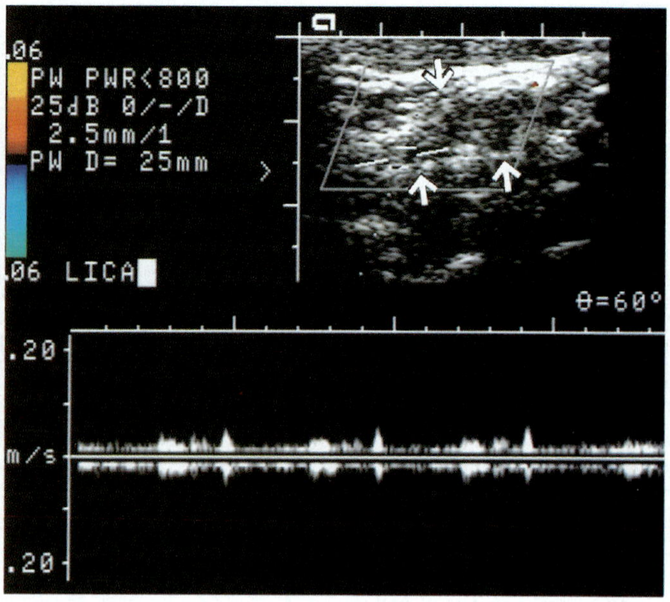

2.

Figures 1, 2. **(1)** Longitudinal duplex Doppler US scan in a normal Wallstent in the CCA. The echogenic margin of the stent is clearly seen (arrows). **(2)** Longitudinal duplex Doppler US scan in an occluded stent between the CCA and the external carotid artery (arrows). No flow was shown within the distal stent.

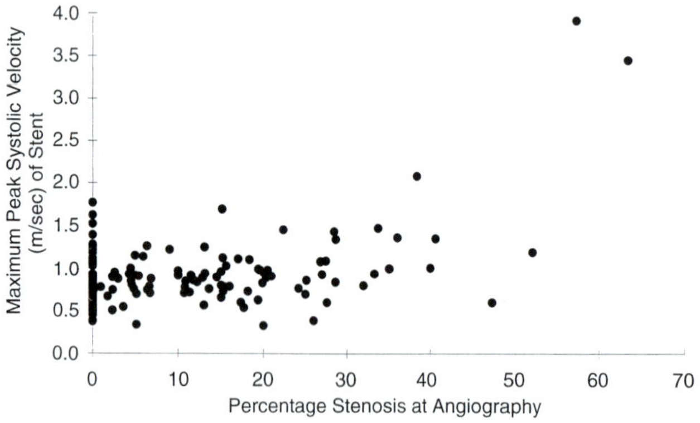

Figure 3. Graph shows ICA/CCA-stent peak-systolic velocity at US relative to the percentage stenosis shown at angiography in all patients who underwent both examinations.

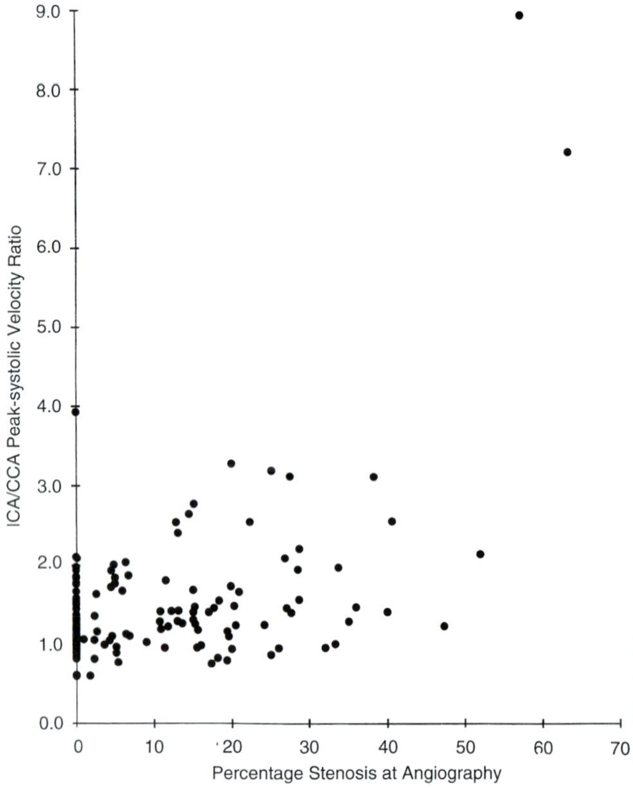

Figure 4. Graph shows ICA/CCA-stent peak-systolic velocity ratio at US relative to the percentage stenosis shown at angiography in all patients who underwent both examinations.

was to evaluate US as a replacement for angiography in the routine follow-up of patients after placement of a carotid artery stent. This study was designed to test the hypothesis that color Doppler US performed after placement of a carotid artery stent is sensitive in the detection of stenosis, occlusion, and other complications.

MATERIALS AND METHODS

Patient Population

Between September 8, 1994, and March 20, 1997, 271 patients (200 men and 71 women, aged 36–88 years [mean, 69 years]) underwent carotid artery angioplasty and placement of a carotid artery stent at our institution according to a prospectively defined protocol approved by our institutional review board (4). The patients generally had a high surgical risk for endarterectomy and significant stenosis at the carotid artery bifurcation. Carotid artery US examinations were added to the protocol in March 1995. The number of patients who underwent carotid artery US after stent placement slowly increased as scheduling difficulties with other tests were overcome.

From this patient pool, an unselected group of 119 patients (87 men and 32 women, aged 35–88 years [mean, 69 years]) underwent US examination in 170 carotid arteries with stents. Of 170 arteries studied, 167 involved stents placed in the ICA, including more than 80% with stents that extended across the bifurcation into the com-

Table 1
Results with Prospective Criteria for Stenosis of Carotid Artery Stent

Criterion	No. of Positive Examinations	No. of Patients with ≥60% Stenosis at Angiography
Peak-systolic velocity		
>1.25 m/sec	18	1
Intrastent ratio, ≥2.0	8	1
ICA/CCA ratio, >3.0	7	1
No. of positive US criteria		
One or more	26	1
Two or more	5	1
Three	2	1

Table 2
Patient Data with Prospective Criteria

Patient No.	Stent: Side	Stent: Carotid Artery	Percentage Stenosis at Angiography	Peak-Systolic Velocity: Stent	Peak-Systolic Velocity: ICA/CCA Ratio	Peak-Systolic Velocity: Intrastent Ratio	No. of Positive US Criteria
1	Left	Internal	22	1.45	2.54	1.04	1
9	Right	Internal	0	1.18	3.93	1.40	1
20	Right	Internal	0	0.55	1.67	2.04	1
22	Right	Internal	20	0.95	3.28	1.79	1
26	Left	Internal	38	2.08	3.10	3.25	3
31	Right	Internal	25	0.86	3.19	2.15	2
33	Left	Internal	27	1.09	3.11	1.95	1
35	Right	Internal	36	1.36	1.46	1.43	1
37	Left	Internal	41	1.35	2.55	1.80	1
53	Left	Internal	57	3.92	8.91	1.13	2
60	Left	Internal	0	1.39	1.76	1.48	1
73	Left	Internal	34	1.47	1.96	2.10	2
74	Right	Common	0	1.62	Not applicable	1.69	1
79	Left	Internal	0	1.26	1.26	1.24	1
82	Left	Internal	17	0.60	0.76	2.14	1
83	Right	Internal	15	1.69	2.77	1.00	1
86	Left	Internal	0	1.26	2.10	1.27	1
88	Left	Internal	6	1.26	2.03	1.00	1
88	Right	Internal	0	1.52	1.85	1.00	1
89	Left	Internal	5	0.91	0.78	2.33	1
96	Right	Internal	0	1.77	0.93	1.81	1
96	Left	Internal	0	1.28	0.95	1.02	1
97	Left	Internal	0	0.73	1.38	2.28	1
102	Right	Internal	29	1.34	2.20	1.60	1
102	Left	Internal	28	1.43	1.93	1.55	1
105	Right	Internal	63	3.45	7.19	4.73	3

mon carotid artery (CCA). A stent in only the CCA was placed in two patients. In one patient with an occluded ICA after endarterectomy, a stent was placed across a high-grade stenosis at the origin of the external carotid artery.

Follow-up US was performed immediately after placement of the stent in 87 arteries in 75 of the 119 patients, in 83 (95%) within 24 hours, and in 87 within 5 days of stent placement. Intermediate 6-month (mean, 7.3 months; range, 1–22 months) follow-up US examinations were performed in 83 arteries in 65 patients who agreed to also undergo follow-up angiography. Some of these patients underwent more than one intermediate follow-up US examination because they had also undergone placement of a stent in the contralateral carotid artery or because of clinical suspicion for recurrent stenosis. An additional 16 patients underwent 6-month follow-up US but declined to also undergo follow-up angiography and, therefore, were not included in the study.

Methods

Duplex US was performed in the carotid artery (128XP or Sequoia; Acuson, Mountain View, Calif) by qualified sonographers under direct supervision of a staff radiologist in a laboratory accredited by the Intersocietal Commission for the Accreditation of Vascular Laboratories and the American College of Radiology. Examinations were scheduled before and within 24 hours after percutaneous transluminal angioplasty and stent placement in the carotid artery. Follow-up examinations were scheduled at 6 months or earlier if there was a concern for recurrent stenosis. Each examination included standard evaluation of the CCA, ICA, external carotid artery, and vertebral artery. Data were collected prospectively. The sonographer and staff radiologist were blinded to the angiographic results. Carotid artery stents were evaluated immediately proximal to the stent; within the proximal, middle, and distal stent; and within the distal ICA. The highest peak-systolic and end-diastolic velocities were recorded at each location. The transducer angle was maintained at less than or equal to 60° for all velocity measurements. Standard transverse and longitudinal color and gray-scale images were obtained in all examinations.

Carotid artery stent placement was performed according to a technical protocol that has been previously described (4). One or more balloon-expandable (Palmaz medium stent; Johnson & Johnson Interventional Systems–Cordis, Warren, NJ) or self-expanding (Wallstent; Schneider, Minneapolis, Minn) stents were placed in the large majority of patients. A different balloon-expandable stent (Cook, Bloomington, Ind) was placed in a small number of patients. The current protocol calls for use of only the Wallstent.

Findings at angiography performed immediately after stent placement and at 6-month follow-up were used as the standard of reference in this study. Stenosis was measured on the basis of the NASCET criteria (1,2). Quantitative angiography was performed with an on-line automatic edge-detection system (Integris; Phillips Medical Systems North America, Shelton, Conn) in at least two orthogonal views. Minimum luminal diameter was measured at the narrowest site in the segment of the carotid artery with the stent and compared with the reference diameter in a nontapering segment of the ICA immediately distal to the segment with the stent. The measurements of stenosis severity were made on the projection that showed the more severe stenosis. The percentage stenosis was calculated automatically and recorded prospectively. For the purposes of this analysis, hemodynamically significant stenoses were defined as those with greater than or equal to 60% diameter reduction, as in carotid arteries without a stent (13).

Data Analysis

Three prospective US criteria were expected to be highly sensitive for detection of stenosis in the carotid artery stent. If any of these three measurements was positive, findings in the examination were considered positive. The prospective criteria included the following: (*a*) Strandness criterion (5): peak-systolic velocity greater than 1.25 m/sec. Note that this criterion is for a stenosis greater than or equal to 60% based on the percentage stenosis of the ICA compared with the carotid artery bulb. (*b*) ICA/CCA peak-systolic velocity ratio greater than 3:1. (*c*) Doubling or greater of the peak-systolic velocity within the stent.

Retrospectively, the criteria of Carpenter et al (12) (which are based on the NASCET method of determining the percentage stenosis by comparison with the diameter in the distal ICA) were applied to the data to

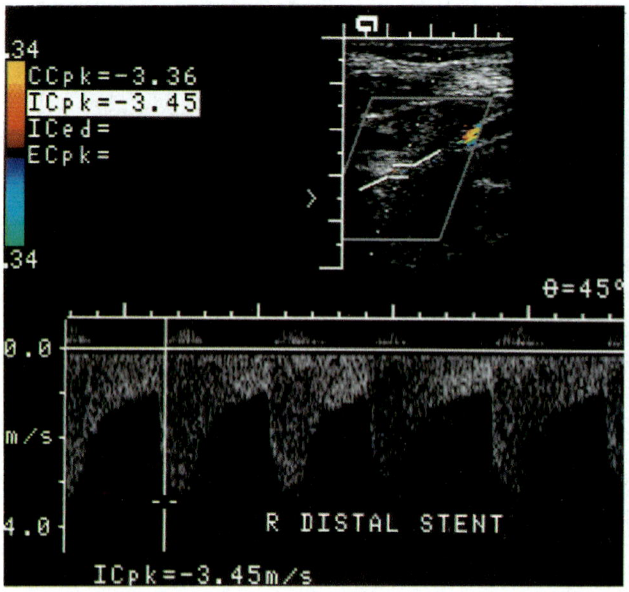

a.

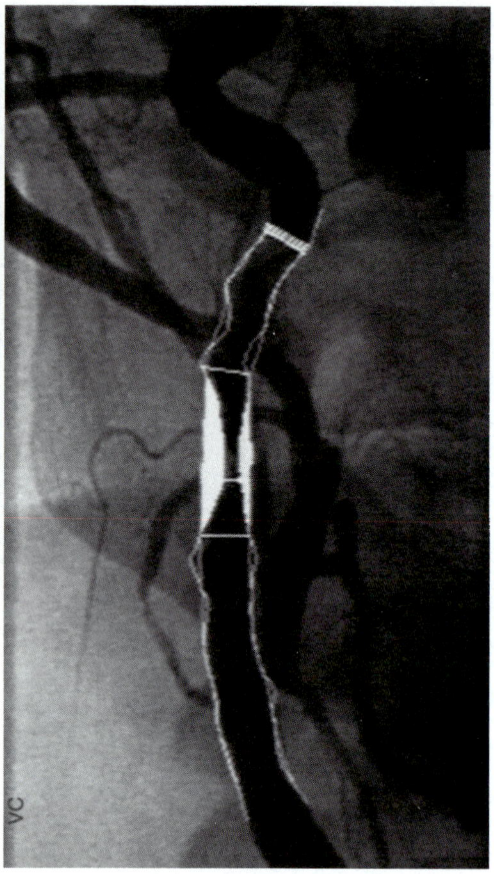

b.

Figure 5. Patient 105. (a) Longitudinal duplex Doppler US scan shows distal stent stenosis with peak-systolic velocity of 3.45 m/sec. **(b)** Carotid angiogram shows an asymmetric stenosis within the stent that was calculated to be a 63% diameter reduction at angiography.

attempt to decrease the high number of false-positive results obtained with the prospective criteria. The retrospective US criteria included the following: (*a*) ICA peak-systolic velocity greater than 1.7 m/sec. (*b*) ICA end-diastolic velocity greater than 0.4 m/sec. (*c*) ICA/CCA peak-systolic velocity ratio greater than 2.0. (*d*) ICA/CCA end-diastolic velocity ratio greater than 2.4. If any of the four measurements was positive, findings in the examination were considered positive.

The US findings were then compared with the angiographic results. Angiograms obtained in the patients with positive prospective and retrospective US findings were further analyzed to determine if there were additional anatomic factors other than stenosis that contributed to the abnormal US results. Diffuse stent narrowing was defined as consistent diameter reduction along the segment with the stent. Focal stent stenosis was defined as diameter reduction over a segment length less than or equal to 10 mm.

RESULTS

An US scan with normal findings in a carotid artery stent that extends from the CCA into the ICA is shown in Figure 1. ICA stents were usually well visualized, with occasional shadowing from calcified plaques between the stent wall and intima. No noticeable shadowing or artifact was noted from the stent material itself. All three types of stent were well seen and had a similar appearance at US. Thus, individual images of the different types of stent are not included in this article.

Two arteries with stents were occluded as depicted at follow-up US. One stent placed early in the series occluded within several hours after placement. Immediate follow-up US was ordered because of the patient's deteriorating clinical symptoms, and findings confirmed the only case of acute ICA stent thrombosis. The only stent placed between the CCA and the external carotid artery (the patient's ICA occluded after prior surgery) was found to be occluded at 6-month follow-up US (Fig 2). In the evaluation of occlusion, there were no false-positive or false-negative findings in the immediate or 6-month follow-up US examinations.

Figure 3 shows a graph of the stent peak-systolic velocity with respect to the percentage stenosis determined at angiography. Figure 4 shows a graph of the maximum ICA/CCA stent peak-systolic velocity ratio with respect to the percentage stenosis determined at angiography.

Prospective Criteria

In the 119 patients who underwent both follow-up US and follow-up angiography, 26 of the 170 arteries with stents met the prospective US criteria (Tables 1, 2). The maximum stenosis within a patent stent was determined as 63% at angiography (Fig 5). Arteries in two patients fulfilled all three prospective criteria, one with 63% stenosis and one with 38% stenosis.

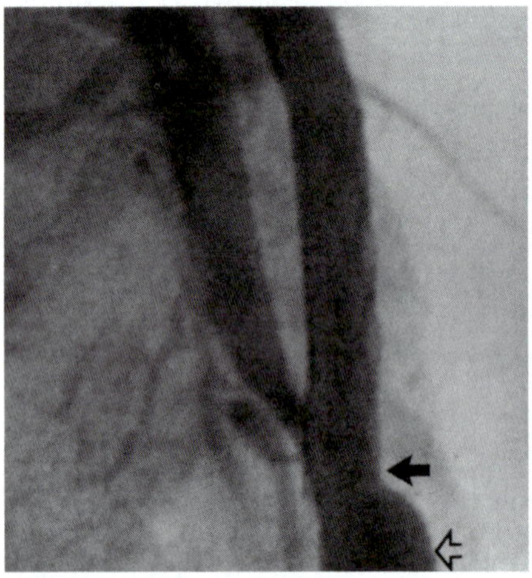

Figure 6. Patient 60. Carotid angiogram shows the stent to be widely patent. Note the marked caliber difference between the CCA (open arrow) and the proximal ICA (solid arrow).

The peak-systolic velocity was greater than 1.25 m/sec in 18 of these 26 patent stents, which met the abnormal US criteria. Seventeen of these 18

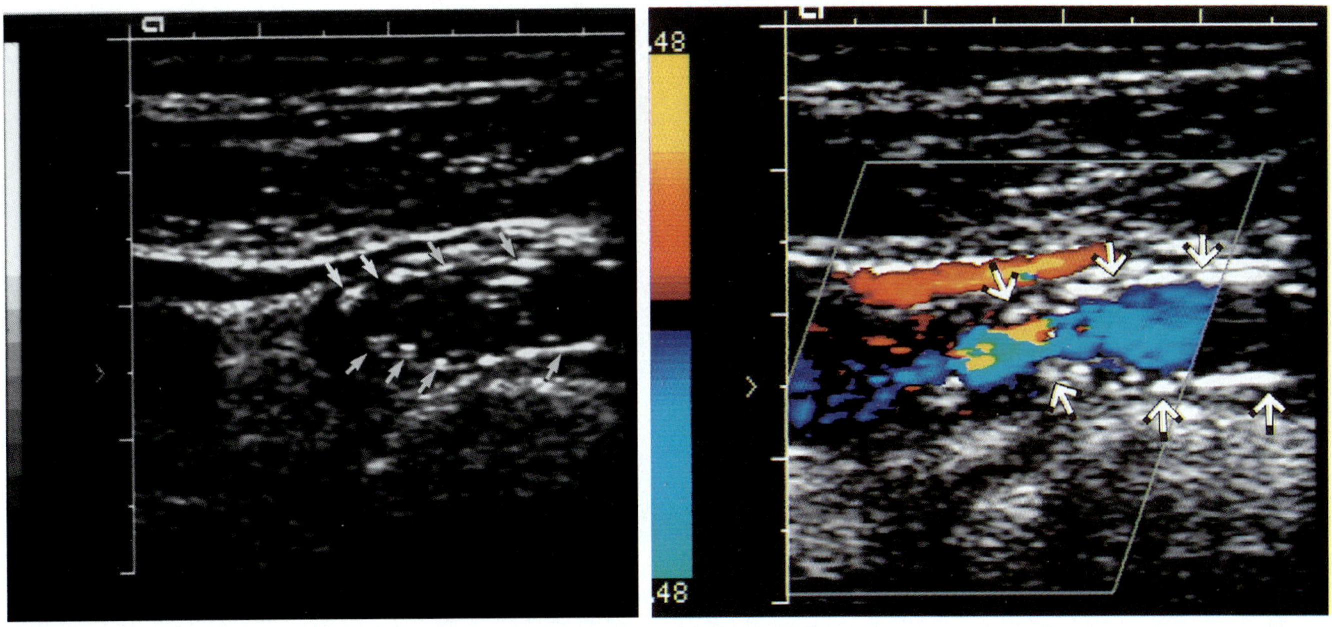

a. b.

Figure 7. Patient 74. (a) Gray-scale US scan shows partial collapse of distal CCA stent, which is shown as a thin discontinuous white line (arrows). (b) Color Doppler US scan shows increased peak-systolic velocity with turbulent flow and aliasing within the distal portion of the ICA stent (arrows), which is consistent with a focal stent collapse.

stents demonstrated non–hemodynamically significant (<60% stenosis) diffuse or focal narrowing or, in one case, collapse. In the remaining stent, findings were abnormal at follow-up US performed within 24 hours of stent placement. At immediate follow-up, this stent was widely patent, but there was a large difference between the diameter of the normal CCA and that of the proximal ICA (Fig 6). Another of the 26 stents showed moderate distal collapse at both color and gray-scale US (Fig 7) without recurrent stenosis within the stent. Distal stent collapse was confirmed with biplane fluoroscopy.

The maximum peak-systolic velocity seen in any stent was 3.92 m/sec, with an angiographically determined stenosis of 57%. In seven patients, the ICA/CCA peak-systolic velocity ratio was greater than 3.0. In these seven patients, either focal or diffuse narrowing was seen in the segment with the stent. In the arteries with 57% and 63% stenosis, the ICA/CCA peak-systolic velocity ratios were elevated (≥7.0) compared with those in the other arteries with stents.

Within eight stents, the peak-systolic velocity at least doubled. Interestingly, the stent in patient 31 did not have a peak-systolic velocity greater than 1.25 m/sec (and therefore was not judged to have a hemodynamically significant stenosis), but the peak-systolic velocity doubled, from 0.40 m/sec within the proximal stent to a maximum 0.86 m/sec at the middle of the stent. Angiographic correlation showed focal 25% narrowing within the middle of the stent (Fig 8), at the site of previous angioplasty.

Retrospective Criteria

In four patients, the peak-systolic velocity was greater than 1.70 m/sec (Table 3).

DISCUSSION

Angiography is currently employed to help assess recurrent stenosis in carotid artery stents. US, a noninvasive low-cost method of screening, may be a valid alternative.

One of the most important roles of US in the evaluation of carotid artery stents is the detection of occlusion. The two cases of stent occlusion in this patient series were correctly identified with US. It is possible that a small residual amount of flow in the stent may not be detected at US, similar to the carotid artery without a stent. In the case of acute stent thrombosis, the patient would likely be brought back to the angiography suite to try to reopen the stent. If an asymptomatic, long-term occlusion (as in our patient with chronic occlusion) is found at US, performance of angiography may be prudent to exclude a residual trickle of flow. If residual flow is found at angiography, use of percutaneous angioplasty techniques may still be possible.

Performance of accurate US analysis of the degree of stenosis is problematic. The presence of residual calcific plaque between the stent and vessel lumen sometimes makes visual analysis of the degree of stent stenosis impossible as the stenosis cannot always be clearly seen. Therefore, as in the carotid artery without a stent, indirect assessment of the degree of stenosis is necessary.

No single set of US criteria for the detection of ICA stenosis is currently used across the country. Previous criteria for relatively broad ranges of stenoses (5,9,10,14–16) were developed on the basis of angiographic measurements of the stenosis present in the ICA relative to the bulb diameter. The NASCET criteria, on the other hand, rely on angiographic measurements of the ICA stenosis relative to the diameter of the distal ICA, distal to any dilatation that may have developed after stent placement. In the NASCET study, stenoses of greater than or equal to 70% were studied. In the ACAS, stenoses of greater than or equal to 60% were studied. In an attempt to meet these new standards, results of many studies with US-angiographic correlation have been published, with varying criteria (12,17).

In this prospective study, we chose to maximize sensitivity, as the clinical consequences in this population of a missed stenosis are far more severe

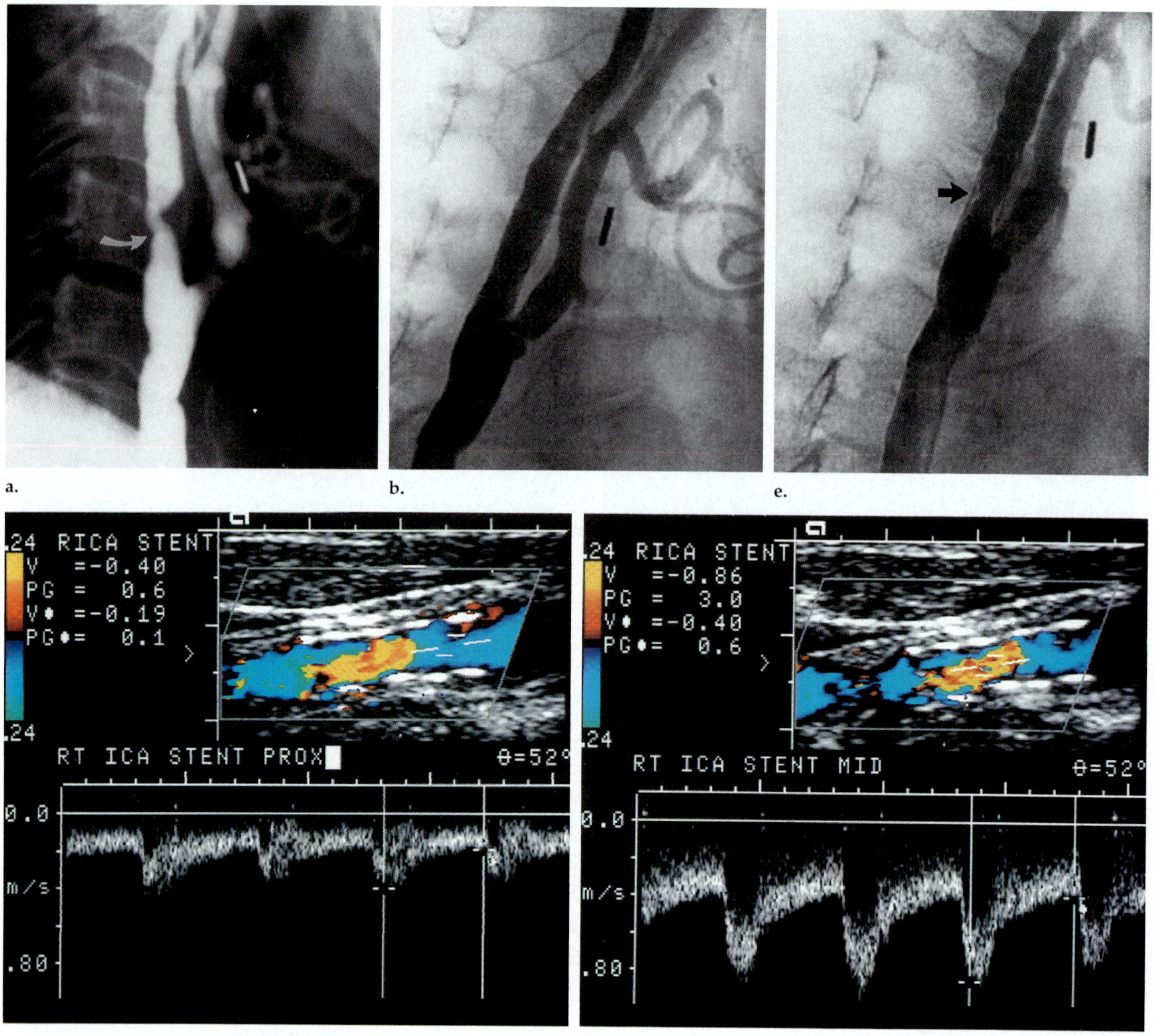

Figure 8. Patient 31. **(a)** Carotid angiogram in the ICA shows stenosis of the proximal ICA prior to stent placement (arrow). **(b)** Carotid angiogram after angioplasty and stent placement shows no significant stenosis. **(c)** Duplex Doppler US scan obtained in the proximal portion of the ICA stent at 6-month follow-up shows a peak-systolic velocity of 0.40 m/sec. **(d)** Duplex Doppler US scan obtained in the midportion of the ICA stent at 6-month follow-up shows a peak-systolic velocity of 0.86 m/sec, which represents a doubling of the peak-systolic velocity. **(e)** Carotid angiogram obtained at 6-month follow-up shows a symmetric stenosis within the ICA stent at the site of initial stenosis, probably secondary to intimal hyperplasia. Note that there is no stent deformation at the site (arrow).

than the consequences of undergoing angiography with negative findings. Use of a peak-systolic velocity of 1.25 m/sec was expected to overestimate the degree of stenosis present in this series, as it did. Fortunately for the patients in this study, in only one patient was the stenosis greater than or equal to 60% at early or intermediate follow-up US and angiography. Unfortunately, reliable criteria for the detection of stent stenosis cannot be determined on the basis of findings in this patient group.

In the patients with angiographic correlation, use of the retrospective criterion of Carpenter et al (12) of ICA peak-systolic velocity greater than 1.7 m/sec would have helped identify only four arteries as potentially stenotic (rather than 18 with the criterion of ICA peak-systolic velocity greater than 1.25 m/sec) and increased the specificity without decreasing the sensitivity. Use of the retrospective criterion of ICA end-diastolic velocity greater than 0.4 m/sec would have identified 15 stenotic arteries, with only one true-positive recurrent carotid artery stenosis. In this study, with only one stenosis greater than or equal to 60%, meaningful sensitivity and specificity values cannot be calculated. Further study in more stenotic stents is needed to determine an appropriate peak-systolic velocity cutoff value for stenosis detection.

The prospective and retrospective criteria were met for ICA/CCA peak-systolic ratios greater than 2:1 or 3:1 in 19 and seven patients, respectively. The hemodynamic effects of the irregularity of the stent itself may cause blood flow disturbance or turbulence. The increase in peak-systolic velocity in the stent should be due to only narrowing (18). In an atherosclerotic carotid artery, however, compliance dif-

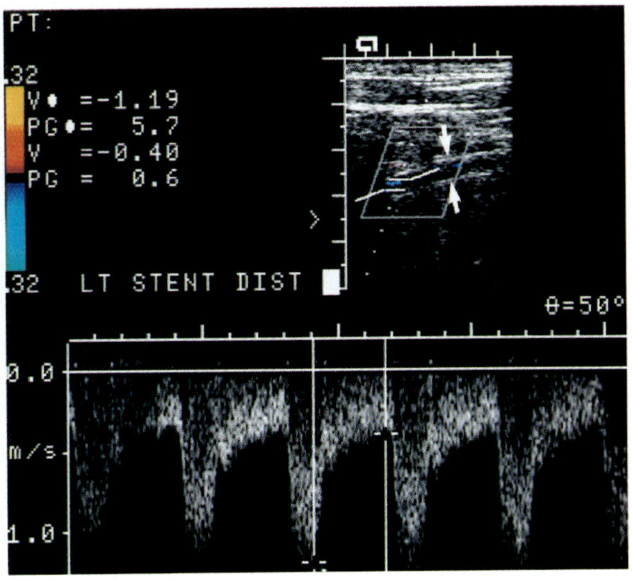

a.

Figure 9. **(a)** Longitudinal duplex Doppler US scan shows distal ICA stenosis with a peak-systolic velocity of 1.19 m/sec and end-diastolic velocity of 0.4 m/sec. Stent borders are indicated by arrows. **(b)** Correlative carotid angiogram shows a long stenosis (52%) in the ICA stent. Stent borders are indicated by arrows.

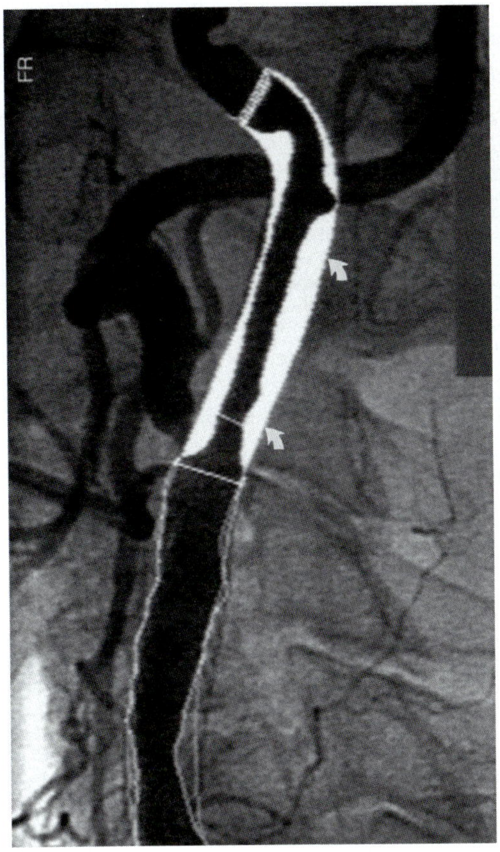

b.

Table 3
Results with Retrospective Criteria for Stenosis of Carotid Artery Stent

Criterion	No. of Positive Examinations	No. of Patients with ≥60% Stenosis at Angiography
Peak-systolic velocity		
>1.7	4	1
ICA/CCA ratio, >2.0	19	1
End-diastolic velocity		
ICA, >0.4	15	1
ICA/CCA ratio, >2.4	37	1
No. of positive US criteria		
One or more	47	1
Two or more	19	1
Three or more	6	1
Four	3	1

ferences between the stent and the vascular wall may cause the peak-systolic velocity within the stent to increase. Another possible source of increased velocity within the stent is effective partial stenosis of the external carotid artery (as a result of the stent crossing the origin of the external carotid artery), which results in shunting of additional blood flow into the ICA. The ICA/CCA peak-systolic velocity ratio was greater than or equal to 7 in the two arteries with the highest percentage stenosis (57% and 63%). The ICA/CCA peak-systolic velocity ratio may prove to be a useful criterion, but more US data obtained in stenotic stents are needed.

A potential pitfall in the carotid artery stent, as in the native carotid artery, is the presence of a long stenosis. In a long stenosis, the increase in peak-systolic velocity may be lower than expected because of high resistance within that long arterial segment. Figure 9 shows a 52% long-segment ICA stenosis with a peak-systolic velocity of 1.19 m/sec and end-diastolic velocity of 0.4 m/sec. Further long-term experience with stents is necessary to determine if US depiction of long stenoses from intimal hyperplasia will be difficult.

Large changes in diameter due to the location of a stent may also cause an increase in velocities without a stenosis present. Normally, the decrease in diameter from the bulb to the ICA is gradual. Significant caliber changes may be present when the stent is placed from the ICA into the CCA. An example of this is seen in the stent placed in patient 60 (Fig 6), in which the immediate follow-up maximum peak-systolic velocity was 1.39 m/sec even though visually at US the stent appeared to be widely patent. There was at least a 50% decrease in the caliber of the stent placed primarily in the ICA compared with the diameters of the bulb and distal CCA. The NASCET criteria ignore anatomic factors that may cause an increase in stent peak-systolic velocity (such as normal changes in arterial caliber from the CCA to the ICA) by measuring only the visualized degree of reduction in diameter of the ICA segment with the stent compared with the diameter of the distal nontapering ICA.

Findings at early follow-up US in the carotid artery stent helped confirm the presence of acute stent occlusion, which was suspected clinically. Immediate follow-up US also helped provide a useful baseline with which to assess changes at the 6-month follow-up.

Another important function of follow-up US may be to help detect stent collapse, which is usually treated with repeat angioplasty of the stent, to prevent potential clot formation between the stent and intima. The occurrence of collapsed carotid artery stents is likely to decrease as self-expanding, elastic stents are used instead of balloon-expandable stents.

The possible failure of digital subtraction angiography to depict stenoses seen at Doppler US is well known (19). In this study, at least two views were always obtained of the carotid artery bifurcation. Under- or overestimation of the percentage stenosis is possible if quantitative techniques alone are relied on, as edge-detection techniques used in the computer analysis programs do not always depict the vessel wall accurately. In this study, however, each image was analyzed by the attending angiographer, and a manual override was performed if necessary to increase the accuracy of the estimation of stenosis.

In summary, the most important result of this study is that no stent occlusion or significant stent stenosis was missed with US in a large group of patients. Sensitivity of the test, however, could not be truly evaluated as only three cases of stenosis greater than or equal to 50% and two occlusions were present in the group. Thus, the prospective and retrospective criteria could not be fully evaluated.

US promises to be a sensitive, noninvasive, inexpensive way to screen for complications after stent placement, as well as to provide baseline data regarding elevations in peak-systolic velocity due to anatomy. By using US as a follow-up screening test, angiography could be reserved for those patients in whom a complication is suspected at US. Further study with long-term follow-up should enable refinement of the US criteria for the detection of stenosis in carotid artery stents. ■

Acknowledgments: The authors thank Camilio Gomez, MD, for allowing his patients to be a part of this study. The authors appreciate the efforts of Lincoln Berland, MD, Jay Listinsky, MD, Desiree Morgan, MD, and Luke Baker, MD, in interpreting findings in some of these US examinations. The authors also thank sonographers Michael Clements, BS, RT, RDMS, RVT, Tamara Jones, RT, RDMS, RVT, Al Hester, RT, RDMS, RVT, Pam McEachern, RT, RDMS, and Lori Perkins, BS, RT, RDMS. The authors appreciate the comments of Lincoln Berland, MD, in reviewing this manuscript and the secretarial assistance of Deonne Willis.

References

1. North American Symptomatic Carotid Endarterectomy Trial (NASCET) Steering Committee. North American Symptomatic Carotid Endarterectomy Trial: methods, patient characteristics, and progress. Stroke 1991; 22:711–720.
2. North American Symptomatic Carotid Endarterectomy Trial Collaborators. Beneficial effect of carotid endarterectomy in symptomatic patients with high grade carotid stenosis. N Engl J Med 1991; 325:445–453.
3. Anonymous. Carotid endarterectomy for patients with asymptomatic internal carotid artery stenosis. Stroke 1994; 25:2523–2524.
4. Yadav J, Roubin GS. Elective stenting of the extra cranial carotid arteries: immediate and late outcome. Circulation 1997; 95:376–381.
5. Strandness DE Jr. Duplex scanning in vascular disorders. New York, NY: Raven, 1990; 92–120.
6. Phillips DJ, Green FM. Flow velocity patterns in the carotid bifurcations of young, presumed normal subjects. Ultrasound Med 1983; 9:39–49.
7. Neale ML, Chambers JL, Kelly A, et al. Reappraisal of duplex criteria to assess significant carotid stenosis with special reference to reports from the North American Symptomatic Carotid Endarterectomy Trial and the European Carotid Surgery Trial. J Vasc Surg 1994; 20:642–649.
8. Carroll BA. Carotid sonography: state of the art. Radiology 1991; 178:303–313.
9. Bluth El, Stavros AT, Marich KW, Wetzner SM, Aufrichtig D, Baker JO. Carotid duplex sonography: a multicenter recommendation for standardized imaging and Doppler criteria. RadioGraphics 1988; 8: 487–506.
10. Withers CE, Gosink BB, Keightley AM, et al. Duplex carotid sonography: peak systolic velocity in quantifying internal carotid artery stenosis. J Ultrasound Med 1990; 9: 345–349.
11. Moneta GL, Edwards JM, Papanicolaou G, et al. Screening for asymptomatic internal carotid artery stenosis: duplex criteria for discriminating 60% to 99% stenosis. J Vasc Surg 1995; 21:989–994.
12. Carpenter JP, Lexa FJ, Davis JT. Determination of sixty percent or greater carotid artery stenosis by duplex Doppler ultrasonography. J Vasc Surg 1995; 22:697–705.
13. Polak Jr. Peripheral vascular sonography. Baltimore, Md: Williams & Wilkins, 1992; 41.
14. Carroll BA. Duplex sonography in patients with hemispheric symptoms. J Ultrasound Med 1989; 8:535–540.
15. Branas CC, Weingarten MS, Czeredarczuk M, Schafer PF. Examination of carotid arteries with quantitative color Doppler flow imaging. J Ultrasound Med 1994; 13:121–127.
16. Zwiebel WJ, ed. Color-duplex features of normal and abnormal carotid arteries. In: Introduction to vascular ultrasonography. Philadelphia, Pa: Saunders, 1992; 123–131.
17. Huston J, Lewis BD, Wiebers DO, Meyer FB, Riederer SJ, Weaver AL. Carotid artery: prospective blinded comparison of two-dimensional time-of-flight MR angiography with conventional angiography and duplex US. Radiology 1993; 186:339–344.
18. Kremkau FW. Diagnostic ultrasound: principles and instruments. Philadelphia, Pa: Saunders, 1993; 192–193.
19. Fontenelle LJ, Simper SC, Hanson TL. Carotid duplex scan versus angiography in evaluation of carotid artery disease. Am Surg 1994; 60:864–868.

Jonathan M. Rubin, MD, PhD • Ronald O. Bude, MD • J. Brian Fowlkes, PhD
R. Steven Spratt, PhD • Paul L. Carson, PhD • Ronald S. Adler, PhD, MD

Normalizing Fractional Moving Blood Volume Estimates with Power Doppler US: Defining a Stable Intravascular Point with the Cumulative Power Distribution Function[1]

PURPOSE: **To normalize the power Doppler ultrasound (US) signal to the expected signal from 100% blood in the calculation of a fractional moving blood volume estimate.**

MATERIALS AND METHODS: **To locate the signal from flowing blood with a consistent backscatter coefficient, the authors estimated the knee of the cumulative Doppler power distribution function. They used a flow-tube phantom to test the use of this knee to locate a radial position that would fall into a region of high shear stress and minimal rouleaux formation. They also studied how well the method normalized fractional moving blood volume estimates of the right renal cortex in a volunteer when simulating different body habitus and in a group of six healthy volunteers to estimate variability.**

RESULTS: **Over five flow velocities and over undersaturated to severely oversaturated receiver gains, the calculated flow-tube area was a mean 89% ± 7 (± standard deviation) of a standard. In humans, the technique normalized the fractional moving blood volume estimates over an 8-dB receiver gain variation; the mean ± standard deviation of fractional moving blood volume estimates for the six volunteers was 37.6% ± 3.6.**

CONCLUSION: **Vascularity estimates with power Doppler US are feasible with a normalization scheme based on the cumulative Doppler power distribution function.**

Although of substantial interest, ultrasound (US) Doppler vascularity measurements have been used on a variable basis in several organ systems (1–4). They have generally, but not exclusively, been based on the counting of color pixels in standard color Doppler US scans and have been used clinically most frequently to assess tumor vascularity in the breast and prostate (5–13). The choice of these organs is informative, because it reveals one of the greatest shortcomings of US vascularity assessments: their depth dependence. In all of the examples in which quantitation has been used, either the target is superficial or the transducer has been positioned very closely to the area of interest. This is because vascularity is assessed by counting the number of color pixels in a given region, and anything that alters color pixel count will affect a vascularity assessment. Unfortunately, the density of blood vessels, the quantity one wishes to measure, is only one of the factors that influences the color pixel count. Major contributors to this measurement are attenuation, aperture size, or any other property that alters the strength of the backscattered echoes. Given identical tissue samples, their vascularity at US will change the deeper in the body they are located. The closer a tissue is to the transducer, the more vascular it will appear. For example, flow in ovaries may be very hard to detect transabdominally and yet very easily seen transvaginally. The vascularity detection improvement is due primarily to a reduced attenuation path in the latter, which yields some combination of higher signal and which allows the use of higher frequency transducers (14). Because of this very definite attenuation effect, vascularity measurements with US are tricky to make and interpret.

A potential solution to this problem does exist. If one can identify an object of known vascularity or blood volume, one can use the Doppler power in that object to normalize the values in the surrounding tissue (15–17). If the tissues of interest are near enough to the known object, the fraction of the Doppler power in the surrounding tissue relative to the standard can be used as a vascularity estimate. This process effectively compensates for any attenuation or transducer beam profile effects. Because blood vessels contain 100% blood, objects of known vascularity exist throughout the body and could be used to normalize vascularity measurements. We will call such measurements fractional moving blood volume estimates (17).

There is one problem, however, that has to be overcome before this method can be applied. The problem arises because the backscattered signal from blood is variable owing mostly to the degree of rouleaux formation (18–22). The reason for this is that rouleaux

Index terms: Blood, flow dynamics, 9*.12983[2] • Blood vessels, US, 9*.12983 • Ultrasound (US), power Doppler studies, 9*.12983 • Ultrasound (US), technology, 9*.12983

Radiology 1997; 205:757–765

[1] From the Department of Radiology, University of Michigan Hospitals, 1500 E Medical Center Dr, Ann Arbor, MI 48109 (J.M.R., R.O.B., J.B.F., P.L.C., R.S.A.); and Diasonics, Santa Clara, Calif (R.S.S.). Received May 19, 1997; revision requested July 8; revision received August 12; accepted August 13. Supported in part by a grant from Diasonics, U.S. Public Health Service grant RO1CA55076 from the National Cancer Institute, and the U.S. Army Medical Research Materiel Command contract DAMD17-94-J-4144. **Address reprint requests to** J.M.R.

[2] 9* indicates vascular system, location unspecified.

effectively increases the size of the scattering units in blood. Clumps of red blood cells will backscatter more ultrasound energy than will individual cells, which makes areas of vessels with more rouleaux have stronger Doppler signals than those with less. This effect is most pronounced when comparing the Doppler power in the center of large blood vessels with the Doppler power in the edges. There is typically much more signal amplitude in the center of the vessels owing to increased rouleaux formation (23). The higher shear rate and shear stress near the vessel wall apply more force to separate rouleaux clumps of red cells. The magnitude of the shear rate, which is directly proportional to the shear stress, depends on the velocity profile (24). For a parabolic flow profile, the shear rate and, thus, the shear stress are directly proportional to the radius (20). Hence, for a 1-cm-diameter vessel, the shear rate at the wall will be 10 times that 0.5 mm from the center of the vessel. For near plug flow, the shear rate at the wall can be arbitrarily high. Because of this variation in the appearance of blood flow, one cannot just identify a blood vessel, obtain a normalization value, and calculate a fractional moving blood volume estimate at a given depth. A more sophisticated technique is required.

It is known that smaller vessels have greater shear than do larger vessels for a given mean velocity (25). Because we would like to normalize vascularity by the power that corresponds to 100% blood in tissue, where the blood vessels are small, a value outside the region of high rouleaux would be appropriate. Because of a condition of no slippage at the wall or boundary, there is no flow immediately adjacent to the wall of a vessel. Hence, the "correct" normalizing value lies somewhere between the high value in the center of a vessel and the zero value at the wall.

To perform a fractional moving blood volume estimate, we first calculate a cumulative Doppler power distribution function over the region of interest (see below). We then identify the knee of the cumulative Doppler power distribution function. This knee is used in an algorithm to define a boundary point within highly vascular areas in which we will search for a normalization value. The knee of this distribution is a reasonable choice for segmenting a population into two groups, which is similar to what is done in segmenting populations in receiver operating characteristic analysis (26,27). Once the normalization value is measured, we use that value to determine the fractional moving blood volume estimate in tissue.

We performed this study to normalize the power Doppler US signal to the expected signal from 100% blood in the calculation of a fractional moving blood volume estimate. We used this technique to compensate for depth, attenuation, receiver gain, and machine variability. Ultimately, we believe that the results strongly suggest that this technique could be generally used to assess vascularity in tissues.

MATERIALS AND METHODS

Definition

The cumulative Doppler power distribution function is the integral of the histogram of the Doppler powers within a region of interest (28). It is defined in a discrete sense as

$$N(p) = \sum_{i=0}^{i=p} n(i),$$

where $n(i)$ is the number of pixels with the ith power value and $N(p)$ is the total number of pixels with power values less than or equal to p; that is, $i \leq p$. Because this is an integral of the histogram, the cumulative Doppler power distribution function has some nice random noise–suppressing properties that make it an interesting candidate for finding a normalization value. In a cumulative distribution, fluctuations are referenced to the entire display range, whereas with a standard histogram, being the derivative of the cumulative distribution, fluctuations are seen relative to locally changing values for which any variation is a much larger percentage.

Phantom Studies

We designed a flow-tube experiment to evaluate the boundary-detection properties of the cumulative Doppler power distribution function. The tube consisted of an elongated balloon of 5.5 mm in diameter in a fluid bath. The balloon was draped across a sound-absorbing pad to suppress reverberations. Flow in the balloon was generated by using a pulsatile pump (Harvard Apparatus, South Natick, Mass) with a 70% duty cycle and 50 strokes per minute. Before reaching the balloon, the fluid passed through a long segment of compliant gum rubber tubing that made the flow nonpulsatile. Degassed water that contained corn starch particles (0.5 g per liter of water) as scatterers was run through the balloon. To simulate real flow-containing tissue, we put cross-linked dextran beads (Sephadex particles; Sigma Chemical, St Louis, Mo; 20–80 μm diameter at concentrations of 0.0373–0.2372 g/L, depending on the background Doppler power level) into the bath outside the balloon. By stirring the bath, we could introduce a Doppler shift in the medium and generate Doppler power in the background similar to the effect of tissue that contains flowing blood. The quantities of cross-linked dextran beads and corn starch were selected so that the tube always visually had more power than the water bath at each flow setting, thus simulating a vessel surrounded by flowing blood within perfused tissue. We made three measurements at each flow rate investigated (Table 1). These three measurements were made with low gain to simulate a weak signal deep in tissue, optimal gain (see below) to simulate tissue that was superficial enough or vascular enough to supply sufficient signal, and high gain in which the signal in the tube was saturated to simulate bad technique or the presence of contrast agents.

To define the gain settings for the flow-tube measurements in testing the cumulative Doppler power distribution function algorithm, we had to define what low gain, optimal gain, and high gain would be. We used VST US scanners (Diasonics, Santa Clara, Calif) to make the measurements. We used a 10-MHz linear-array transducer (Diasonics) with a 6.0-MHz Doppler frequency. The angle of the scanhead to the tube was 22° to generate a Doppler angle. We measured signal strength and saturation level by assigning a green-tag value to Doppler power measurements. Each green-tag step defined by the manufacturer corresponded to 0.4 dB. We set the saturation level such that the highest green-tagged pixels in the flow tube were within three click steps of the highest decibel level, 24 dB. This corresponded to having the highest pixel values in the flow tube be no more than 23.2 dB on the 24-dB scale, which represents the

Table 1
Raw Data from the 15 Flow Experiments

Run	Mean Flow Velocity (cm/sec)	Pulse Repetition Frequency (Hz)	Receiver Gain Setting (dB)	Fractional Area*
1	17	1,250	79	0.849
2	17	1,250	86	0.972
3	17	1,250	92	0.875
4	35	2,250	80	0.941
5	35	2,250	85	0.893
6	35	2,250	90	1.03
7	51	2,750	84	0.894
8	51	2,750	89	0.889
9	51	2,750	94	0.93
10	60	3,500	84	0.704
11	60	3,500	89	0.917
12	60	3,500	94	0.885
13	79	4,500	84	0.903
14	79	4,500	89	0.897
15	79	4,500	94	0.886

* Fractional area is the area of the tube calculated by using the knee of the cumulative distribution over the image divided by the area subjectively determined by tracing the outline of the tube.

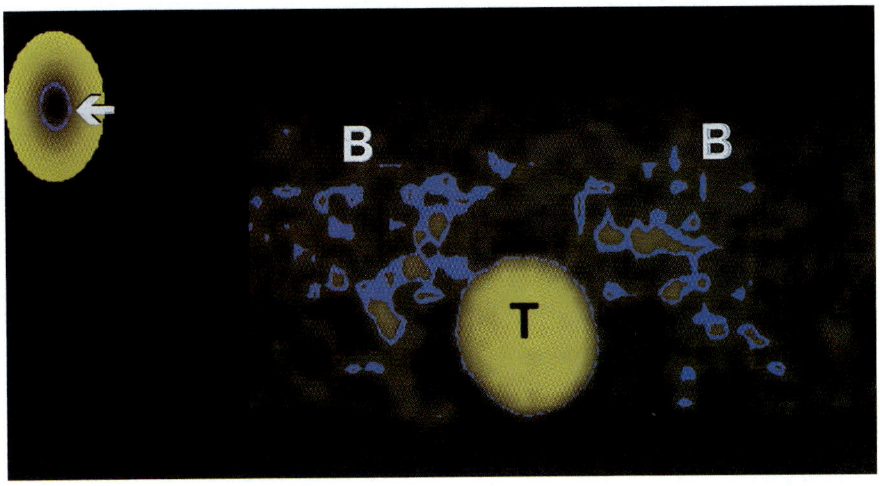

Figure 1. Cross-sectional US image of corn-starch–containing flow tube (*T*) in a water bath (*B*) that contains cross-linked dextran beads. The water bath was manually stirred to generate a Doppler signal, represented in yellow, and simulated viable, blood-perfused tissue. The tube, which represents a blood vessel, corresponds to 100% blood and, hence, has more Doppler power than the water bath, which simulates less vascular tissue. This is demonstrated as a tube brighter than the water bath in power mode. The outer margin of the blue outline of the flow tube marks the boundary of the tube, as calculated by using the automated boundary detector. The blue line is actually thicker than the true boundary threshold for purposes of display. The blue pixels equal the set of all pixels in the image, such that threshold ≤ pixel value ≤ threshold + 0.9 dB. Note that there are regions in the water bath that also either are surrounded by blue or are blue. These correspond to potential areas of 100% blood in tissue. The black area behind the tube and water bath is the top of the sound-absorbing rubber pad. Also note that there is a blue ring in the color wheel in the upper left-hand corner (arrow). The area of the wheel that is located between the blue ring and the outer edge represents the portion of the entire power dynamic range that is assigned to 100% blood in this particular trial.

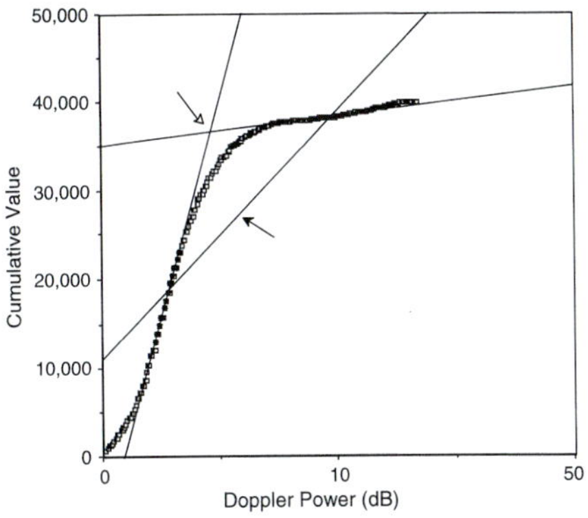

Figure 2. Cumulative distribution for one of the phantom flow experiments. The plot shows the three best-fit lines used in the two-tangent technique. The global best-fit line (solid arrow) intersects the distribution at two points. A tangent line is defined at each intersection point, and the intersection of the tangents (open arrow) defines the position of the knee. This technique clearly underestimates the position of the knee. This particular plot was for one of the undersaturated experiments, which is why it does not extend to 24 dB.

dynamic range of the power-mode signal. When the Doppler gain was set such that the pixels with the highest power in the image fell into this range, the settings were considered optimally saturated. We then set the saturation limit in a range that was clearly undersaturated (5–7 dB), below the optimally saturated setting, and finally set a range in which the Doppler power in the tube was clearly oversaturated (5–7 dB above optimal saturation). A representative image from each flow run was stored digitally to the hard disk on the scanner and transferred to an image analysis program (AVS; Advanced Visual Systems, Waltham, Mass) for analysis.

The boundary of 100% blood as seen with the ultrasound beam in the flow tube was identified by using a cumulative distribution based on the entire data set and was compared to an observer-traced perimeter of the tube, which was considered the standard of reference (Fig 1). To define the region over which the cumulative distribution was taken, an observer first traced the entire area of the stored image of the tube and the water bath, with the exclusion of the sound-absorbing rubber pad. The pad was excluded because, having no "flow," it would bias the measurement by introducing a structure that was much different from the paradigm of interest, that is, blood vessels and background tissue with flow. A cumulative distribution was calculated on the basis of the power values within this enclosed region. The knee or point of maximum curvature of the distribution was then subjectively selected on the cumulative distribution curve for each flow measurement. We used the visual estimate of the knee of the distribution for this calculation because it was deemed to be the best estimator of that point. To compensate for variability, we selected a range of about ±1 dB about the selected threshold and calculated the areas within these limits. Of course, this method of detecting the threshold would not work in practice; therefore, we developed techniques for automating the location of the knee (see below). For this part of the study, however, it was thought that our best estimate of the knee, the visual estimate, was the most appropriate to use.

An observer then traced the tube as a standard of reference for comparison with the cumulative distribution-selected boundary. The tube was traced three times at each flow setting, the area calculated with each traced perimeter, and a mean area calculated for the tube. The mean areas for the cumulative distribution–detected region and for the manually traced region were then compared.

Automated Distribution Determination

To implement a fractional blood volume measurement in vivo and to make more objective measurements, we wanted to use automation to calculate the position of the knee of the distribution. We used two techniques, each of which was initiated in the same way. A best-fit line was first plotted through the distribution by using a standard least-squares technique. For the first technique, the points of intersection of the line with the distribution were located, and tangent lines parallel to the cumulative distribution curve were drawn at the points of intersection. The intersection of these two tangent lines defined the knee of the cumulative distribution. The points of intersection were determined by taking the difference between the cumulative distribution value and the calculated estimate, which was accomplished by using the best-fit line for each successive power value. For those points at which the sign of the difference changes, there must be an intersection between the best-fit line and the distribution between that point and its neighbor, either one of which could be defined as the intersection for the purposes defined here. The tangent lines were empirically defined over 21 point regions, the intersection point ± 10 points (Fig 2). (Further details are in the Appendix.)

The second method begins as the first, with fitting of the cumulative distribution with a best-fit straight line. The distribution is then rotated about the best-fit line so that the line falls onto the abscissa. On the basis of the shape of the cumulative distribution, this function should have a negative curvature and there should therefore be a global maximum. A global maximum could then easily be identified and corresponded to the knee. To account for noise about the global maximum, a region of ±10 points around this initially identified global maximum was selected and fitted with a second-order polynomial. The power value that corresponds to the peak of this polynomial could also represent the knee of the distribution. Although not identical, this technique is similar to other methods in which second-order polynomials are used to search for maxima (29).

The tangent method and then the curve-fitting method, that is, the initial rotated peak and then the second-order polynomial–fitted peak, were then each compared to the subjective standard of reference for finding the knees of the cumulative distributions for the tube-flow data by taking a mean absolute difference between the measurements.

Human Studies

The human studies were divided into two phases. The first consisted of the acquisition of multiple scans in one healthy volunteer at different gain settings to simulate different body habitus, while the second consisted of the acquisition of multiple scans in six healthy volunteers to investigate variability.

In the first phase, the right kidney of a single healthy male volunteer (age, 49 years; weight, 76 kg; height, 173 cm) was scanned on five different occasions. The studies were performed by using a 3.5-MHz curved linear scanhead with a pulse repetition frequency of 1,000, a color Doppler frequency of 2.5 MHz, and an ensemble length of 10. The receiver gain was successively increased from 102 dB to 112 dB in 2-dB steps. Over this range, the images clearly progressed from highly undersaturated to highly oversaturated. This manifested as a lack of flow detection at the 102-dB setting and as a very bright ballooned color display at the 112-dB setting. Again, this range was used to simulate scanning a deep structure without the use of contrast agents. The typical optimal setting for power Doppler, that is, when the noise floor just begins to break through the uniform color background (29), was at about 105–107 dB . During each sampling, the kidney was scanned longitudinally at each gain setting by using a region of interest defined by the machine's color box that included as much of the near-field cortex of the kidney as possible and at least half of the renal sinus. Because of the curvilinear shape of the color box implemented with this probe, some liver and perinephric fat were also included in the region of interest. The image of the cortex chosen for analysis at any given scanning setting was the one that subjectively had the most visible blood flow. The first cumulative distribution was taken over the entire color box, and the knee of the distribution was automatically calculated with both the tangent and the curve-fitting techniques described above. A green tag was assigned to all power values equal to or greater than the value identified as the knee of the distribution. The technique that helped identify a knee that resulted in assigning the greatest fraction of the color dynamic range to potentially 100% blood, that is, that resulted in green tagging of the most pixels, was then used in the next stage of the algorithm.

A second cumulative distribution was then taken over only those points selected in the first run. The knee of this second distribution was then identified by using the two techniques described above, and the value that assigned the largest fraction of the dynamic range to green was again used as the normalization value. This value became the normalization value for the fractional moving blood volume estimation, or, equivalently, the lowest Doppler power that corresponded to 100% blood. This process is demonstrated in Figure 3.

A region of cortex in which the fractional moving blood volume was to be estimated was then traced within the color box by using the machine's tracker ball. Other than the selection of the size and location of the color box itself, this was the only portion of the examination in which there was operator interaction. A fractional moving blood volume estimate was calculated from this region. The means and standard deviations of the selected initial green-tag level were plotted as a function of receiver gain to show the effect of attenuation and, potentially, body habitus on the normalization level. Further, a mean value and a standard deviation of the fractional moving blood volume estimate as a function of receiver gain were plotted over the five measurements.

The second phase comprised examinations of six healthy volunteers (one man, five women; mean age ± standard deviation, 34 years ± 6 years; age range, 27–41 years; mean weight, 78 kg ± 22; weight range, 57–116 kg; mean height, 173 cm ± 11; height range, 160–188 cm) by one examiner (J.M.R.). Each volunteer underwent scanning on 3 different days without preparation, for purposes of practicality. The volunteers were examined by using the same machines described above, with optimization of the setting for power Doppler in the usual manner, that is, the gain was increased sequentially until the noise floor just broke through the uniform background (30). Once the receiver gain was set, the same process for determining the fractional moving blood volume estimate in the single volunteer was used. The means and standard deviations for the fractional moving blood volume estimates for each of the volunteers were plotted.

RESULTS

Flow Experiment

The experimental flow runs are given in Table 1. The area of the tube detected by using the knee of the cumulative distribution was 89% ± 7 of the subjective boundary. It must be said that at the highly saturated settings, the difference between the boundary and the background scatterers in the medium was hard to see, and the knee of the distribution was often thought to be a better marker of the boundary than the standard of reference. Furthermore, it is obvious that there was blooming of the flow tube with increasing gain, which made the detected boundary move outward. This corresponded to a larger tube area for any given velocity (Table 1) and is to be expected with higher levels of saturation. This would manifest in vivo as enlargement of blood vessels with increasing gain.

We then compared the different knee-detecting techniques to see how well they identified the knee compared with the subjectively chosen location (Table 2). It is clear that the tangent method underestimates the subjectively designated position of the knee, thereby assigning more power values to 100% blood. The mean absolute difference between the two tangents and the knee was 0.91 dB. The second-order polynomial–fitting technique more closely approximated the subjectively selected knee: 0.33 dB for the peak value and 0.30 dB for the second-order polynomial–fitted peak.

Human Studies

The segmentation values of vascular structures from the less vascular background were plotted as a function of receiver gain (Fig 4). The plot shows a monotonic decline in the normalization level as a function of receiver gain. The slope is significantly different from zero (95% confidence interval: −0.996, −0.694). This result is what would be expected if the knee of the cumulative distribution were compensating for overlying attenuation and depth of the organ, that is, body habitus. The weaker the flow signal in general, the greater the portion of the dynamic range that may be assigned to 100% blood. Furthermore, despite this change in normalization level with gain, the ultimate fractional moving blood volume estimate is largely independent of receiver gain (Fig 5). This is based on taking a linear regression and determining the slope over the 8-dB highest dynamic range measurements, 104–112 dB, which is 0.00624 (95% confidence interval: −0.00067, 0.01315). Thus, zero is included in the 95% confidence limits. The addition of the lowest dynamic range measurement, 102 dB, produces a significant positive trend in the data, with a slope of 0.00798 (95% confidence interval: 0.00198, 0.01400). Finally, scans obtained in the six volunteers show the means ± standard deviations of the fractional moving blood volume estimates one might expect with this technique (Fig 6). The standard deviation for any single individual can be up to ±0.1. This corresponds to approximately a 30% variation relative to the mean value. However, the mean of the means ± the standard deviation of the means for the six volunteers' fractional moving blood volume estimates is 37.6% ± 3.6.

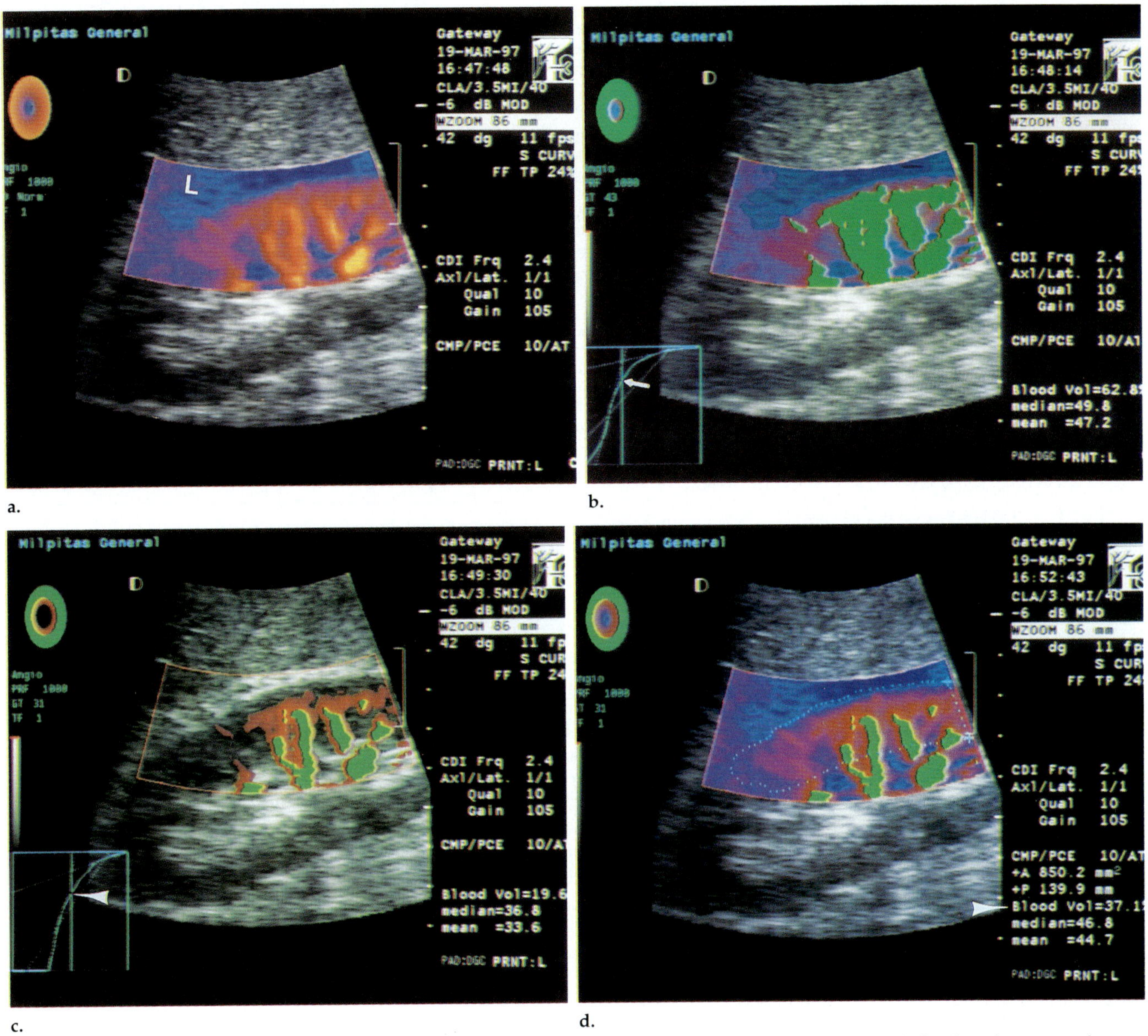

Figure 3. **(a)** Longitudinal US image of the renal cortex with near-field hilar vessels in a 49-year-old volunteer. The brighter the orange, the higher the Doppler power. Blue represents the noise floor or the lowest Doppler power displayed. Notice the large blue area in the near field, which corresponds to liver (*L*). **(b)** Same longitudinal US image as **a** after the first cumulative distribution has been taken over the entire color box in **a.** The green-tagged pixels correspond to those that could represent 100% blood on the basis of the knee of the cumulative distribution plot for the region of interest, shown in the lower left-hand corner. This curve is typical of the initial in vivo distributions in this study. The calculated position of the knee is marked with an arrow. All pixels with power values equal to or greater than the knee are green. (The highlighted pixels adjacent to the green-tagged regions are artifacts of photography and are not included in the green-tagged region.) **(c)** Same longitudinal US image as **b** after the second cumulative distribution has been taken over only those pixels labeled green in **b.** A second group of pixels, a subset of those in **b,** is labeled green and represents the final pixels determined to contain 100% blood. They were selected on the basis of the cumulative distribution plot, shown in the lower left-hand corner. The calculated position of the knee (arrowhead) corresponds to the lowest Doppler power that represents 100% blood; hence, this value is used to normalize all the tissue values in the image. Note that the second distribution demonstrates a much truer vascular geometry because it has segmented high-shear-rate from low-shear-rate blood flow within large vessels. Small vessels in tissue will not show up owing to high shear and partial volume averaging with tissue, that is, a fractional moving blood volume estimate of less than 100%. (The highlighted pixels adjacent to the green-tagged regions are artifacts of photography and are not included in the green-tagged region.) **(d)** Same longitudinal US image as **c** with the region of the cortex to be measured enclosed by the dotted line. The fractional moving blood volume estimate was calculated over that entire region and is normalized by the value selected in **c.** The fractional moving blood volume estimate in this case was 37.1% (arrowhead). (Again, the highlighted pixels adjacent to the green-tagged regions are artifacts of photography and are not included in the green-tagged region.)

DISCUSSION

The ultimate aim of many flow imaging techniques is to image vascularity or perfusion, and US is no exception. The opportunity for US to display vascularity has never been better. With contrast agents on the horizon and power Doppler, it is now possible for US to directly display the amount of moving blood in tissue, because, unlike standard mean-frequency color Doppler, the power in the Doppler signal is a reflection of the vascular blood volume of the tissue sample (20–22,31). Furthermore, power Doppler has the potential to overcome a major limitation of US vascularity measurements. By normalizing power Doppler signals in tissue against a blood vessel that is in or near a region being evaluated, it is possible to compensate for the distance between the transducer and the region of interest, the attenuation coefficient of the overlying tissue, and the available imaging aperture, among other things (32).

The problem with this strategy is that the amplitude of the Doppler shift signal is highly dependent on rouleaux formation (18–22), which makes it impossible to merely select any point within a large vessel for normalization. However, by selecting a normalization value from the region of high shear near the vessel wall, the effects of rouleaux can presumably be minimized. This creates a situation that approximates that in small vessels in tissue where the shear is high and rouleaux is low (25).

Hence, a normalization technique must allow detection of blood vessels and identification of a position in the vessels to use for normalizing. The flow phantom study shows that the cumulative distribution can find blood vessels. In fact, it can optimally find them to within about 0.3 dB relative to the observer. In the clinical portion of the study, we typically used the tangent estimate, the poorer of the two estimating techniques, because it tended to overestimate the number of pixels that may contain 100% blood and thus increased the number of points included in the distribution. However, even by using an optimal technique such as the subjective method in the flow phantom, regions still are selected in the "hypovascular" tissue bath that were identified as flow-containing (Fig 1). Findings in the right kidneys studied were similar. This is not surprising and would be expected, at least in the first distribution, given the presence of small blood vessels inside tissue, which are analogous to the random high signals in the water bath.

We used a continuous-flow phantom, even though flow in vivo can clearly be pulsatile. We decided to do this because power Doppler is generally highly frame averaged in vivo. This has the effect of averaging out the pulsatility in the sampling. Hence, the nonpulsatile phantom would in some sense be an estimate of what happens in this first approximation. Yet, pulsatility will change the velocity distribution in a vessel, which will change the power distribution on the basis of the shear rate effects, as described above. This may require further study.

After determining the knee of the first distribution, we used a second distribution to find the normalization value in vivo. The reason for this is that, as in the flow phantom, the first distribution essentially located the wall or the neighborhood just outside of the walls of blood vessels that would be used for normalization. We needed to find a value inside the vessels to use as a standard in normalization. Thus, the second distribution over only the vessels accomplished this.

If we had not included a second distribution, we would have had the problem of distinguishing an organ of normal vascularity that is located deep in the body from a superficial organ with low vascularity. The reason for this is that the first distribution only basically locates the walls of large vessels, as shown above. It will find the walls whether an organ is deep and normal or superficial and hypovascular. Because we use an approximation of the knee as the threshold and this knee is defined relative to the parenchymal, hypovascular tissue, dividing this threshold into the tissue value will give a similar ratio in both cases. The distinction between a deep organ and a superficial one does not lie in the vessel boundaries but is in the Doppler power of the blood. For identical vessels, the more superficial, the more power the blood will have. This requires that a second distribution be taken over the vessels themselves to actually find a normalization value representative of the blood in the vessels. This value is a function of the vessel depth. We could have just identified the vessels manually or by using some other technique and performed a distribution over the vessels only. Then we would have needed only one distribution. The first distribution lets us automate the method.

There obviously have to be at least two points of negative curvature to find two knees in our process, and it makes sense that there should be at least two. The first knee separates the hypovascular parenchyma from the blood vessels, and the second knee separates the high-rouleaux central portions of blood vessels from the high-shear margins of the vessels. There will always be more points in the first distribution, because it includes the vessels and the hypovascular tissue, and, given a large enough region of interest, the first knee will dominate and will be the one selected with our method. Once the vessels have been segmented out, the method detects the second knee. If the number of points included in this second distribution is small, it may limit the ability to accurately detect a knee in some circumstances. We did not encounter this problem in this study; however, this may require a change in strategy when very small regions are being measured. This effect can be seen in Figure 3b and 3c: The knee is well defined in Figure 3b but is not as well defined, although present, in Figure 3c.

It is clear in this study that we have not determined where that precise site in the vessel is or what the true normalization value should be. However, we have done the next best thing; that is, we have identified a method that compensates for the rouleaux and at-

Table 2

Comparison of Methods for Locating the Knee Position of the Cumulative Distribution for the Flow-Tube Experiments

Run	Subjective Knee Position (dB)	Knee Position: Two-Tangent Model (dB)	Knee Position: Rotated Curve Peak (dB)	Knee Position: Second-Order Polynomial Fitted Peak (dB)
1	6.09	4.69	5.53	5.44
2	9.09	8.06	8.72	8.53
3	10.31	9.19	9.94	9.94
4	5.16	4.41	5.44	5.25
5	7.50	6.38	7.50	7.13
6	9.09	7.50	9.19	8.91
7	6.47	5.81	6.19	6.28
8	8.72	9.28	9.47	9.38
9	9.00	7.78	8.91	8.72
10	8.72	8.34	8.25	8.16
11	7.78	7.03	8.34	7.88
12	9.66	9.28	9.47	9.47
13	5.72	5.16	5.81	5.72
14	6.75	5.91	6.94	6.75
15	9.84	8.63	9.19	9.56

Note.—The subjective knee position is the standard of reference.

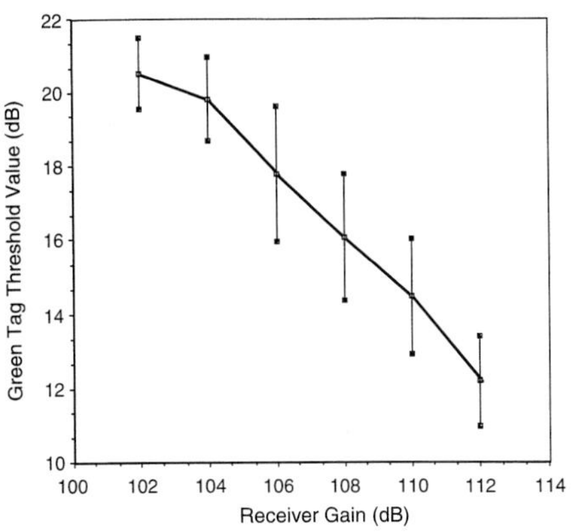

4.

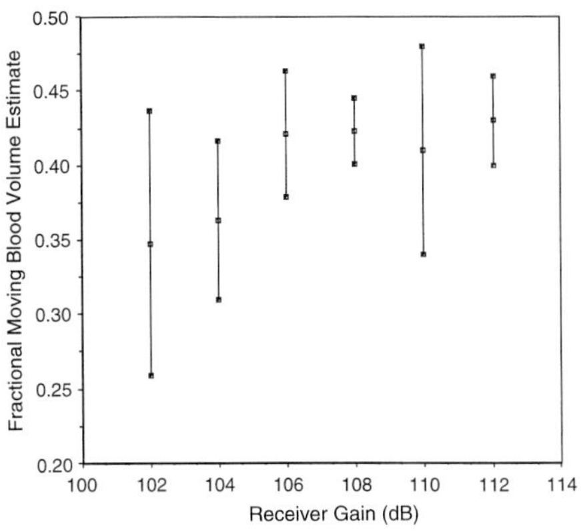

5.

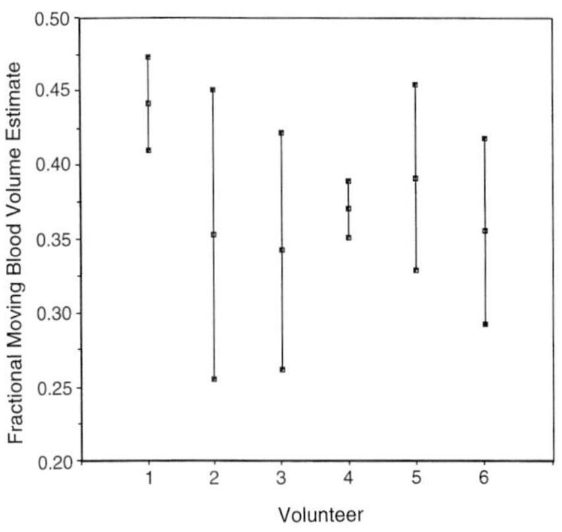

6.

Figures 4–6. **(4)** Green-tag threshold for the first cumulative distribution as a function of the receiver gain. These values represent the threshold for those pixels that may contain 100% blood. Only those pixels with higher power values than the threshold will be considered as possibly containing 100% blood in the algorithm used. The points are bounded above and below by ±1 standard deviation. Notice that the slope is negative, which means that the lower the gain, which corresponds to weak signal or large amounts of attenuation, the more dynamic the range that may be assigned to blood. **(5)** Fractional moving blood volume estimates as a function of receiver gain in the single volunteer. The points represent means ± 1 standard deviation. **(6)** Fractional moving blood volume estimates in the six volunteers. The points represent means ± 1 standard deviation.

tenuation problem in a general way. First, we have shown that the plot of the initial normalization value with receiver gain showed a continuous compensation for different amounts of signal by setting the normalization value to different fractions of the usable color dynamic range (Fig 4). This change in normalization compensated for the varying amounts of backscattered signal received at the different receiver gains, which corresponded to increasing amounts of attenuation, increasing depth, decreasing amounts of available transducer aperture, or a combination of these. The slope of the regression line through the data defined in Figure 4 shows a clear trend, with a 95% confidence interval that did not intersect zero. Thus, there was a distinct and significant decrease in the proportion of the color dynamic range that was assigned to 100% blood as the signal strengthened, or, conversely, the weaker the signal, the more of the dynamic range that was assigned to 100% blood.

This result makes sense if one considers that, if there were no detectable flow, flowing blood would look like everything else, and the entire dynamic range would look as if it contained 100% blood. The same problem would also occur in highly oversaturated images, where the gain is so high that everything, including noise, is enhanced to look like blood. This would have created a jump at the high receiver gain end of the curve if we had gone high enough. However, at that point, everything would be saturated and it would be impossible to distinguish blood vessels from less vascular surrounding tissue. This is unlikely to happen in practice because the user would immediately recognize it and turn the gain down, as occurs in blooming with contrast agents (33,34). However, the differential blooming effect of power Doppler is an advantage here, where, unlike in mean frequency color US, the display increase corresponds to the amount of signal present. Hence, vessels will still look brighter than background tissue, even with blooming (33,34), and our results suggest that as long as tissue can be distinguished from large blood vessels, the fractional moving blood volume estimate method could work in principle.

Second, once depth dependence of the transducer beam profile and attenuation are compensated for, the measurement of the same tissue region should be identical if the normalization method is working. Figure 5 shows this to largely be the case. The slope of the regression line through the data that describe the fractional moving blood volume estimates for gain settings of 104–112 dB was not different from zero to within 95% confidence (35). Hence, when there was sufficient signal to detect, the method compensated for the attenuation and transducer effects, as one would hope. However, when the data included the 102-dB values, there was a significant trend. In addition, the variability in the 102-dB measurement was higher than that in any of the others. The implication here is that when there is very little flow to detect, the method undercompensates and results become more variable. This suggests that when the signal is weak and is harder to detect, the method tends to locate a normalization value within the high-rouleaux portion of the flow stream and would, in a sense, overcompensate for the lost signal in the cortex, where the rouleaux effects are small. This would give a low estimate because the method would be comparing high-rouleaux areas in vessels to low-rouleaux areas in tissue. At some attenuation level, the Doppler signal will be too weak to measure, and any normalization technique will fail. One compensating fact is that when the signal gets very weak, it is still possible to compare the measurement to itself (17). Hence, the normalization from day to day may make it possible to evaluate relative flow changes in the same organ, even if the attenuation is high.

Finally, the evaluation of the volunteers without preparation estimated the potential variability in the method under scanning conditions. Clearly, one would like a technique with little or no variability at all; yet, in some cases the standard deviation in the measurements was up to 10%, which produced a variability relative to the local mean of approximately 30% from day to day, even when the signal was optimized. In these studies, there was no control for hydration, time of day, or fasting; all of which could have influenced the variability. Furthermore, given the single-volunteer studies, where the variance was smaller, it may be reasonable to presume that the variability is the true variation in the blood flow to the renal cortex. It is clear to anyone who does US that there are regions of the cortex with more flow than others; so, when performing scanning in the same person on different days it is possible to obtain different results.

Will such variability preclude using this test? We do not think so. First, the mean values are very close among all the individuals, which suggests that a mean value may be usable in any given case. Thus, taking the mean of several measurements may give very reasonable results. This is exactly what is done presently with all resistive index measurements. Second, there can be equally wide variability among results of other parametric tests, such as resistive indices, pulsatility indices, acceleration, and acceleration times (36–38). Each of these has found use in the medical community. Finally, there are ways to improve the collection on the horizon, that is, three-dimensional imaging (16). This method would be perfectly integrated into a three-dimensional acquisition system. The segmentation would be used in the same way, but the sampling would be more robust. Given the large set of flows that would be sampled in the cortex in three dimensions, the flow variation in an organ would likely decrease.

Besides the limitations described above, there are others. As mentioned above, we have not defined the absolute fractional blood volume in the kidney. Although the mean values obtained are within or close to the published normal levels in the kidney (39–41), we do not know if those numbers measured here are in fact absolute fractional blood volume estimates. This may be true, but it will likely have little effect on the clinical application of such a measure as this. There are plenty of "indices" that relate to physiologic parameters of interest but may not directly measure them, such as the resistive index (42,43). Also, there are clearly flows that will not be included in this measurement. Capillary flow, for instance, is too slow to measure by using present Doppler techniques. Thus, these vessels will not be included in any vascularity estimate derived with our method. Of course, capillaries will not contribute to any US color Doppler vascularity measure, in neither mean-frequency color-flow nor power mode. In addition, vascularity assessments by using color Doppler techniques cannot be easily normalized, unlike ours. Hence, we believe that our method should surpass these.

In conclusion, we have defined a method for normalizing the power Doppler fractional moving blood volume estimate by using properties of the cumulative Doppler power distribution. The technique is almost completely nonsubjective and could easily be automated. The method works in phantom studies to find blood vessel boundaries, can be normalized for depth, gives constant measurements for the same flow situation largely independently of body habitus, and gives reasonable mean fractional moving blood volume estimates in healthy volunteers with a variability similar to that of other functional parametric indices. Further studies in pathologic cases are needed to define its usefulness.

APPENDIX

Quantitatively, the definition of the intersection points and tangent lines looks like this: $P'(x) = Ax + B$, which is the form of the best-fit line for a given distribution, where $P'(x)$ is the estimated cumulative value for a given x, the Doppler power, and A and B are constants. If $P(x)$ is the true distribution of the data, then $P(x) - P'(x)$ will be zero at the points of intersection of the true distribution and the best-fit line. Because this is real data, we cannot rely on the actual points of intersection being in the data set. Hence, one can identify the point in the data set closest to the intersection as being the one where there is a sign change. For example, an intersection would lie immediately between points x_i and $x_i + 1$ if $P(x_i) - P'(x_i) < 0$ and $P(x_i + 1) - P'(x_i + 1) > 0$. As a first approximation, one could choose either x_i or $x_i + 1$ as the intersection. Because we are interested only in a set of points centered at either x_i or $x_i + 1$ to define a tangent, it does not really matter which point we pick. Choosing either one of these points at each intersection, we empirically selected a 21-point region of interest centered about each selected point, for example, $x_i \pm 10$ points, and fitted a line through each group of 21 points. We selected a 21-point region because that worked well empirically. This local, fitted line is the local tangent.

The final complication is that it is possible that there could be more than two intersections of the global best-fit line with the distribution. To get around this possibility, we progressively identified each point of intersection of the best-fit line with the cumulative distribution by moving from the origin toward increasing abscissa values, that is, Doppler power. We then selected the first pair of tangent lines in which the difference between their slopes was negative, that is, in which their slopes were decreasing or the curvature was negative. For example, if T is a tangent line and i is a set of abscissa values of intersection points that range sequentially from 1 to n, then $T(i)$ is the line tangent to the cumulative distribution at i. If slope $T(i)$ is the slope of tangent line $T(i)$ and if $T(i)$ and $T(i + 1)$ are the first pair of tangent lines encountered when moving toward the right from the origin whose difference in slopes is negative (slope $T(i + 1)$ − slope $T(i) < 0$), then the intersection of $T(i)$ and $T(i + 1)$ is the chosen point for the knee. ■

References

1. Tanaka S, Kitamura T, Fujita M, et al. Color Doppler flow imaging of liver tumors. AJR 1990; 154:509–514.
2. Shiamato K, Sadayuke S, Ishigaki T, et al. Intratumoral blood flow: evaluation with color Doppler echography. Radiology 1987; 165:683–685.
3. Bourne T, Campbell S, Steer C, et al. Transvaginal colour flow imaging: a possible new screening technique for ovarian cancer. Br Med J 1989; 299:1367–1370.
4. Luker GD, Siegel MJ. Pediatric testicular tumors: evaluation with gray-scale and color Doppler US. Radiology 1994; 191:561–564.
5. Adler DD, Carson PL, Rubin JM, Quinn-Reid D. Doppler US color flow imaging in the study of breast cancer: preliminary findings. Ultrasound Med Biol 1990; 16: 553–559.
6. Sohn CH, Stolz W, Grischke EM, et al. Die dopplersonographische untersuchung von mammatumoren mit hilfe der farbdoppler-sonographie, der duplex sonographie und des CW-Dopplers. Zentralbl Gynakol 1992; 114:249–253. [German]
7. Dixon JM, Walsh J, Paterson D, Chetty U. Colour Doppler ultrasonography studies of benign and malignant breast lesions. Br J Surg 1992; 79:259–260.
8. Cosgrove DO, Bamber JC, Davey JB, McKinna JA, Sinnett HD. Color Doppler signals from breast tumors: work in progress. Radiology 1990; 176:175–180.
9. Cosgrove DO, Kedar RP, Bamber JC, et al. Breast diseases: color Doppler US in differential diagnosis. Radiology 1993; 189:99–104.
10. Kedar RP, Cosgrove DO, Bamber JC, Bell DS. Automated quantification of color Doppler signals: a preliminary study in breast tumors. Radiology 1995; 197:39–43.
11. Rifkin MD, Sudakoff GS, Alexander AA. Prostate: techniques, results, and potential applications of color Doppler US scanning. Radiology 1993; 186:509–513.
12. Newman JS, Bree RL, Rubin JM. Prostate cancer: diagnosis with color Doppler sonography with histologic correlation of each biopsy site. Radiology 1995; 195:86–90.
13. Carson PL, Moskalik AP, Govil A, et al. The 3D and 2D color flow display of breast masses. Ultrasound Med Biol 1997; 23: 837–849.
14. Shung KK, Sigelmann RA, Reid JM. Scattering of ultrasound by blood. IEEE Trans Biomed Eng 1976; 23:460–467.
15. Hottenger CF, Meindl JD. Blood flow measurement using the attenuation-compensated flowmeter. Ultrason Imaging 1979; 1:1–15.
16. Carson PL, Li X, Pallister J, Moskalik A, Rubin JM, Fowlkes JB. Approximate quantification of detected fractional blood volume in the breast by 3D color flow and Doppler signal amplitude imaging. In: Levy M, McAvoy BR, eds. 1993 ultrasonics symposium proceedings. Institute for Electrical and Electronics Engineers catalog no. 93CH3301-9. Piscataway, NJ: Institute for Electrical and Electronics Engineers, 1993; 1023–1026.
17. Rubin JM, Adler RS, Fowlkes JB, et al. Fractional moving blood volume: estimation with power Doppler US. Radiology 1995; 197:183–190.
18. Sigel B, Machi JJ, Beitler JC, Justin JR. Red cell aggregation as a cause of blood-flow echogenicity. Radiology 1983; 148:799–802.
19. Machi JJ, Sigel B, Beitler JC, Coelho JCU,

Justin JR. Relation of in vivo blood flow to ultrasound echogenicity. JCU 1983; 11:3–10.
20. Shung KK, Cloutier G, Lim CC. The effects of hematocrit, shear rate, and turbulence on ultrasound Doppler spectrum from blood. IEEE Trans Biomed Eng 1992; 39:462–469.
21. Shung KK. In vitro experiment results on ultrasonic scattering in biological tissues. In: Shung KK, Thieme GA, eds. Ultrasonic scattering in biological tissues. Boca Raton, Fla: CRC Press, 1993; 291–312.
22. Shung KK, Kuo IY, Cloutier G. Ultrasound scattering properties of blood. In: Roelandt J, Gussenhoven EJ, Bom N, eds. Intravascular ultrasound. Dordrecht, the Netherlands: Kluwer Academic, 1993; 119–139.
23. Yuan YW, Shung KK. Ultrasonic backscatter from flowing whole blood. I. Dependence on shear rate and hematocrit. J Acoust Soc Am 1988; 84:52–58.
24. Feynman RP, Leighton RB, Sands M. The Feynman lectures on physics. Vol 2. Reading, Mass: Addison-Wesley, 1964; 41–2.
25. Whitmore RL. The flow fluids. In: Whitmore RL, ed. Rheology of the circulation. Oxford, England: Pergamon, 1968; 37–46.
26. Metz CE. Basic principles of ROC analysis. Semin Nucl Med 1978; 8:283–298.
27. Halperin EJ, Albert M, Krieger AM, Metz CE, Maidment AD. Comparison of receiver operating characteristic curves on the basis of optimal operating points. Acad Radiol 1996; 3:245–253.
28. Papoulis A. Probability, random variables, and stochastic processes. New York, NY: McGraw-Hill, 1965; 92–94.
29. Press WH, Flannery BP, Teukolsky SA, Vetterling WT. Numerical recipes in C: the art of scientific computing. Cambridge, England: Cambridge University Press, 1988; 299–302.
30. Rubin JM, Bude RO, Carson PL, Bree RL, Adler RS. Power Doppler US: a potentially useful alternative to mean frequency-based color Doppler US. Radiology 1994; 190:853–856.
31. Meyerowitz CB, Fleischer AC, Pickens DR, et al. Quantification of tumor vascularity and flow with amplitude color Doppler sonography in an experimental model: preliminary results. J Ultrasound Med 1996; 15:827–834.
32. Goldstein A. Physics of ultrasound. In: Rumack CM, Wilson SR, Charboneau JW, eds. Diagnostic ultrasound. St. Louis, Mo: Mosby–Year Book, 1991; 2–18.
33. Murphy KJ, Bude RO, Dickinson LD, Rubin JM. Use of intravenous contrast in transcranial sonography: preliminary observations. Acad Radiol 1997; 4:577–582.
34. Burns PN. Harmonic imaging with ultrasound contrast agents. Clin Radiol 1996; 51(suppl):50–55.
35. Metz CE. Quantification of failure to demonstrate statistical significance: the usefulness of confidence intervals. Invest Radiol 1993; 28:59–63.
36. Kliewer MA, Tupler RH, Carroll BA, et al. Renal artery stenosis: analysis of Doppler waveform parameters and tardus-parvus pattern. Radiology 1993; 189:779–787.
37. Keogan MT, Kliewer MA, Hertzberg BS, DeLong DM, Tupler RH, Carroll BA. Renal resistive indexes: variability in Doppler US measurement in a healthy population. Radiology 1996; 199:165–169.
38. Paulson EK, Kliewer MA, Frederick MG, Keogan MT, Delong DM, Nelson RC. Hepatic artery: variability in measurement of resistive index and systolic acceleration time in healthy volunteers. Radiology 1996; 200:725–729.
39. Selkurt EE. The renal circulation. In: Hamilton WF, Dow P, eds. Handbook of physiology, circulation. Vol 2, section 2. Washington, DC: American Physiological Society, 1963:1471.
40. Ladefoged J, Pedersen F. Renal blood flow, circulation times and vascular volume in normal man measured by the intraarterial injection: external counting technique. Acta Physiol Scand 1967; 69:220–229.
41. Wiencek JG, Feinstein SB, Walker R, Aronson S. Pitfalls in quantitative contrast echocardiography: the steps to quantitation of perfusion. J Am Soc Echocardiogr 1993; 6:395–416.
42. Bude RO, Rubin JM, Platt JF, Fechner KP, Adler RS. Pulsus tardus: its cause and potential limitations in detection of arterial stenosis. Radiology 1994; 190:779–784.
43. Halpern EJ, Deane CR, Needleman L, Merton DA, East SA. Normal renal artery spectral Doppler waveform: a closer look. Radiology 1995; 196:667–673.

Turkey Lionfish

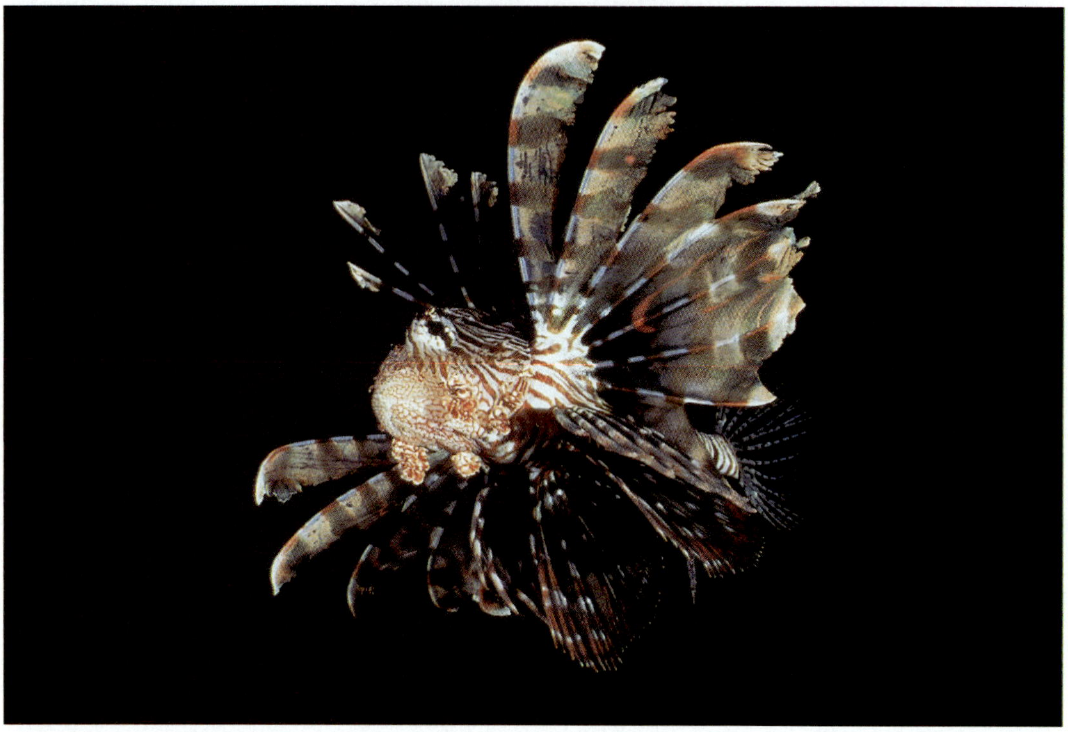

Pterois volitans, turkey lionfish. This member of the scorpion fish family possesses highly venomous, needle-sharp spines that produce agonizing wounds. Red Sea, Egypt.

Flying Gurnard

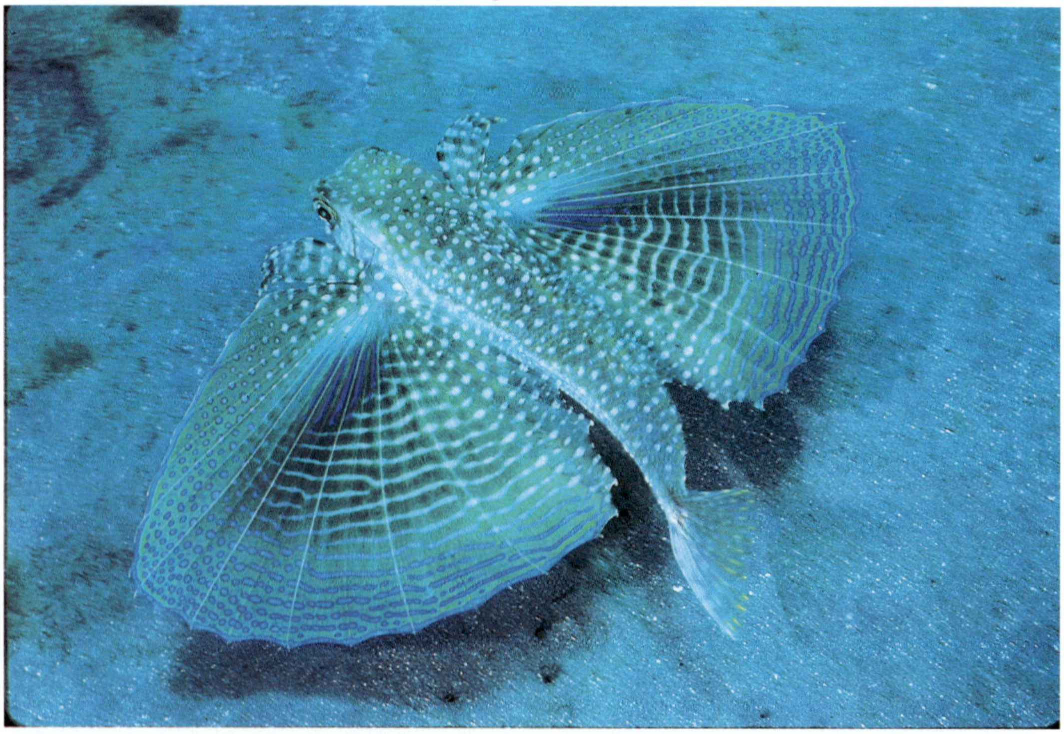

Dactylopterus volitans, flying gurnard. This bottom-dwelling fish can "walk" on modified ventral fins. When alarmed, it spreads its huge pectoral fins like wings and "glides" away to safety. Dominica, British West Indies.

Photographs by David Hall, MD, Woodstock, NY

Peter L. Choyke, MD • McClellan M. Walther, MD • Joseph R. Wagner, MD
Walter Rayford, MD • John C. Lyne, MD • W. Marston Linehan, MD

Renal Cancer: Preoperative Evaluation with Dual-Phase Three-dimensional MR Angiography[1]

PURPOSE: To evaluate the use of dual-phase three-dimensional magnetic resonance (MR) angiography in the preoperative staging of renal cancer.

MATERIALS AND METHODS: MR angiography was performed in 18 patients before performance of partial (n = 7), radical (n = 10), or laparoscopic (n = 1) nephrectomy to treat renal cancer. Dynamic, three-dimensional MR angiograms were obtained with gadoteridol enhancement, breath holding, and a three-dimensional spoiled gradient-echo sequence. Images were obtained at 15-second intervals to achieve opacification of arteries and veins. Source, maximum intensity projection, and multiplanar reconstruction images were evaluated. Imaging results were compared with surgical findings.

RESULTS: Renal arterial phase MR angiograms depicted 30 of 31 (97%) surgically confirmed renal arteries, with one false-positive result (an artery that arose from an early-branching single main renal artery, interpreted as a separate accessory artery). Renal venous phase MR angiograms depicted all seven instances of renal vein involvement, including extension to the inferior vena cava in two patients. Collateral vessels around the tumor, including prominent gonadal veins in three patients, were demonstrated. Additional findings included adenopathy and adrenal and pulmonary metastases.

CONCLUSION: Dual-phase MR angiography of the kidney may be a useful technique in depicting renal vessels before nephrectomy.

Magnetic resonance (MR) imaging has become an important technique for the staging of renal cancers. The ability to detect thrombi in the renal vein and in the inferior vena cava has been demonstrated by using flow saturation (black blood) and time-of-flight (bright blood) techniques (1–4). These techniques are generally satisfactory but can be limited because of flow artifacts. Moreover, they provide little information about the arterial supply to the kidney.

The increasing use of nephron-sparing surgery and laparoscopic surgery for renal cancer has placed more demands on the preoperative imaging work-up of kidney tumors (5–7). Knowledge of arterial anatomy assists surgeons in the planning of the procedure and helps to decrease morbidity (5–7). However, many physicians are reluctant to use conventional angiography on a routine basis because it is invasive, is expensive, and exposes the patient to the risk of nephrotoxicity due to contrast media. Recent advances in the use of three-dimensional (3D) spoiled gradient-echo acquisitions combined with the bolus administration of gadolinium chelates have provided not only a noninvasive alternative to conventional angiography but also the simultaneous depiction of both arterial and venous anatomy (8–12).

Our purpose was to evaluate the use of dual-phase 3D MR angiography of the kidneys in patients who are to undergo partial, radical, or laparoscopic nephrectomy for renal cell carcinoma. This technique allows the demonstration of both the arterial and the venous anatomy in a time-efficient manner and provides additional staging information, such as adrenal and lymph node involvement.

MATERIALS AND METHODS

Eighteen consecutive patients who were to undergo partial, radical, or laparoscopic nephrectomy because of renal cell carcinoma underwent MR imaging before surgery. All patients had undergone computed tomography (CT) with contrast material enhancement of the chest and abdomen at the initial work-up. Seven patients underwent partial nephrectomy because of renal cancer, and the remainder underwent radical (n = 10) or laparoscopic (n = 1) nephrectomy.

The MR imaging protocol was as follows: All images were obtained with a 1.5-T MR imaging unit (Echospeed; GE Medical Systems, Milwaukee, Wis) that was operating with 5.5-level software. The peak gradient strength was 23 mT/m, and the maximal slew rate was 120 $T \cdot m^{-1} \cdot sec^{-1}$. A 20–22-gauge intravenous catheter was placed in an arm vein before the patient was positioned for imaging. The catheter was attached to a dual-headed power injector (Spectris; Medrad, Pittsburgh, Pa). A keep-vein-open drip of normal saline was begun before injection of the contrast material. The following precontrast MR images were

Index terms: Kidney, MR, 81.121411, 81.121412, 81.121415, 81.12142, 81.12143 • Kidney neoplasms, staging, 81.324 • Magnetic resonance (MR), vascular studies • Renal arteries, MR, 961.129412, 961.12942 • Renal veins, MR, 966.129412, 966.12942

Abbreviations: MIP = maximum intensity projection, 3D = three dimensional.

Radiology 1997; 205:767–771

[1] From the Department of Diagnostic Radiology, Warren Grant Magnuson Clinical Center (P.L.C.); and the Urologic Oncology Branch, Division of Clinical Sciences, National Cancer Institute (M.M.W., J.R.W., W.R., J.C.L., W.M.L.), National Institutes of Health, Bldg 10, Rm 1C660, 10 Center Dr, MSC 1182, Bethesda, MD 20892-1182. Received June 17, 1997; revision requested July 14; revision received August 8; accepted August 11. **Address reprint requests to** P.L.C.

acquired: T1-weighted spin-echo axial images (400–450/8 [repetition time msec/echo time msec], 7-mm section thickness, 192 × 256 matrix, two signals acquired, superior and inferior saturation) and fast spin-echo fat-suppressed T2-weighted images (4,000–6,000 [respiration triggered]/102 [effective], 7-mm section thickness, echo train of 12, 192 × 256 matrix, two signals acquired). Precontrast MR imaging was performed through the liver to exclude metastases. A breath-hold spoiled gradient-echo MR image with fat suppression (34.0/1.9, 30° flip angle, 128 × 256 matrix, one signal acquired) was obtained through the inferior vena cava and renal veins.

After precontrast imaging, postcontrast breath-hold 3D MR imaging was performed. The injector was set at a rate of 3 mL/sec for a total of 40 mL of gadoteridol (ProHance; Bracco Diagnostics, Princeton, NJ), followed by a 20-mL flush of normal saline at a rate of 2 mL/sec. Before administration of contrast material, localizing images were obtained with a 3D spoiled gradient-echo, time-of-flight sequence with 28 sections in the coronal plane (8.2/1.4, 45° flip angle, 35–42-cm field of view, 32-kHz bandwidth, 256 × 128 matrix, one signal acquired). Each section was 2.5–3.0 mm in thickness, depending on the size of the patient. The section thickness was selected to encompass the renal hilum posteriorly and the left renal vein anteriorly. The contrast material injection was initiated approximately 5–7 seconds before the onset of imaging. The total breath-hold time was 34 seconds. The first pass of the contrast media was considered to be the renal arterial phase. This sequence was repeated four times, with a 15-second interimaging delay. These images were termed renal venous phase images. T1-weighted spin-echo fat-suppressed axial MR images (450/8, 192 × 256 matrix, two signals acquired) were obtained through the kidneys after MR angiography had been performed. Approximately 1 hour of MR imaging room time was needed to acquire the images in each patient.

MR images were evaluated by a single radiologist (P.L.C.), who used an Advantage Windows workstation (GE Medical Systems). Maximum intensity projection (MIP) and multiplanar reconstruction images were generated in the axial and sagittal planes through the renal arteries and veins.

All patients underwent renal surgery by way of a flank incision ($n = 17$) or laparoscopically ($n = 1$) within 5 days of the acquisition of the MR angiogram. Seven patients underwent partial nephrectomy because of von Hippel–Lindau disease ($n = 6$) or recurrent renal cancer ($n = 1$). The surgeon assessed the number of renal arteries by carefully dissecting each vessel. In the case of complete nephrectomy, each vessel was tied and suture ligatures were applied before the vessel was divided. In the case of partial nephrectomy, each artery that originated in the aorta and could be traced to the kidney or tumor was noted. Only clinically important vessels were reported; minor tributaries were not documented. The patency of renal veins was assessed by palpating the renal vein and the inferior vena cava. Tumor thrombus was milked back into the renal vein, which was then tied and divided. Venous collateral vessels were dissected, tied with suture ligatures, and divided. All information was recorded on the surgical note. This information was compared with the results of MR angiography. Only the side that was exposed during surgery was evaluated in terms of the number of renal arteries because none of these patients underwent surgical exploration with a midline incision. Sensitivity and positive predictive value for arterial number and venous thrombus were obtained.

Table 1
Results of CT and MR Imaging in 18 Patients with Renal Carcinoma

			MR Images				
			Precontrast			Postcontrast	
Finding	No. of Observations	CT Scans	T1-weighted	T2-weighted	Spoiled Gradient-Echo	T1-weighted	3D Time-of-Flight
Adenopathy	8	7	7	7	3	8	5
Renal vein thrombus	7	5	6	4	7	5	7
Inferior vena cava thrombus	2	2	2	2	2	2	2
Adrenal metastases	4	4	4	3	3	4	3
Liver metastases	3	3	3	3	0	3	3
Vertebral metastases	1	0	0	0	0	0	1
Extensive collateral vessels	4	2	0	0	1	2	4
Renal arteries	31	12	10	6	4	12	30

Table 2
Identification of Renal Arteries on Arterial Phase MR Images

No. of Renal Arteries per Kidney	No. of Patients
1	12
2	4
3	2

RESULTS

Dual-phase MR angiography was successful in all 18 patients. There were eight right-sided and 10 left-sided renal tumors. A comparison of CT and MR imaging results is provided in Table 1.

Renal Arteries

Renal arteries were identified on all arterial phase images. The number of renal arteries varied between one and three (Table 2; Figs 1, 2). Because only the side on which surgery was performed was evaluated, contralateral arteries detected at MR angiography were not confirmed and were not included in sensitivity determinations. Of the 31 renal arteries identified at surgery, 30 were detected at MR angiography (sensitivity, 97%). A third renal artery that arose from the iliac artery in an ectopic kidney was overlooked at MR angiography. Also, one false-positive MR angiogram was obtained (positive predictive value, 97%). In this case, a second renal artery detected at MR angiography proved to arise from an early-branching single main renal artery. This error did not pose a surgical problem because the anatomy was easily identified at surgery.

On the MIP images, it was often difficult to distinguish between a lumbar artery and a renal artery. Axial reformatted images clarified this by demonstrating that the lumbar arteries coursed posteriorly around the vertebral bodies, whereas the renal arteries continued laterally. Another problem was that early bifurcation of a single renal artery was difficult to distinguish from two separate renal arteries that arose independently (Fig 2). This pitfall was not clinically important because it was easily recognized by the surgeon.

Venous contamination (ie, early filling of the left renal vein) was generally not a serious problem in the interpretation of renal arterial anatomy (Fig 1). The type of venous contamination that caused the greatest difficulty at interpretation was superimposition of the left renal vein over the left renal artery, which occurred in five cases; by using multiplanar reconstructions, however, the renal vein was edited from the image, which permitted clear depiction of the arteries.

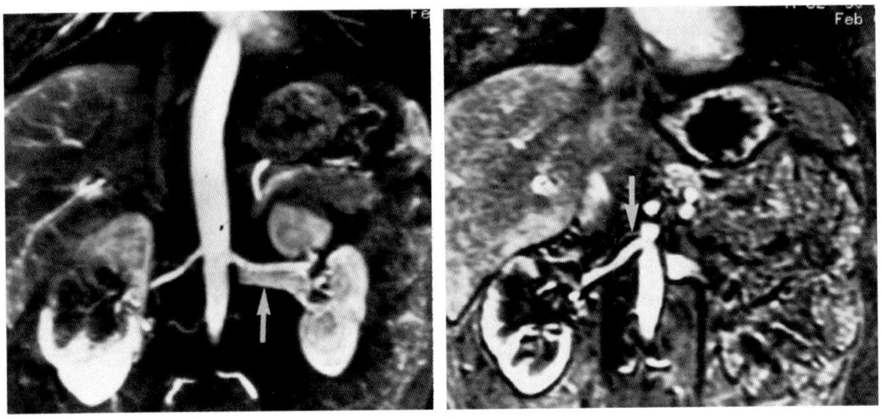

a. b.

Figure 1. Early phase MR angiogram (8.4/1.4) demonstrates the value of the evaluation of the source coronal images, as well as the MIP images. **(a)** MIP image demonstrates what appears to be a single renal artery supplying each kidney. Some early venous drainage is present in the left renal vein (arrow). There is a poorly enhancing tumor in the right upper pole. **(b)** Source coronal MR angiogram demonstrates a small accessory right renal artery (arrow), which was not seen on the MIP image.

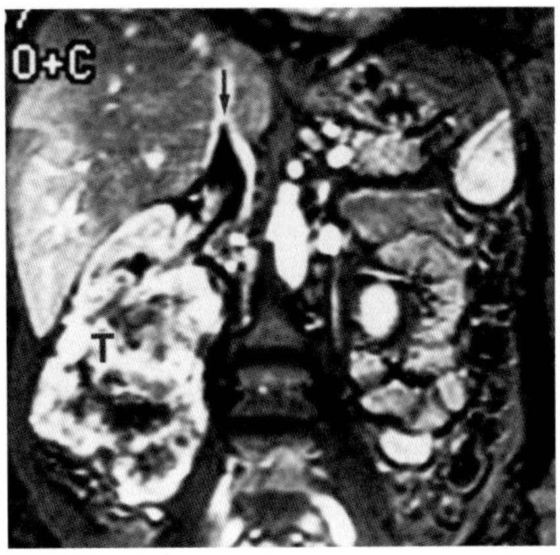

Figure 4. Delayed source coronal MR angiogram (8.4/1.4) demonstrates low-signal-intensity thrombus in the right renal vein and inferior vena cava (arrow). Note that the superior extent of the thrombus is well depicted on this coronal image. *T* = tumor.

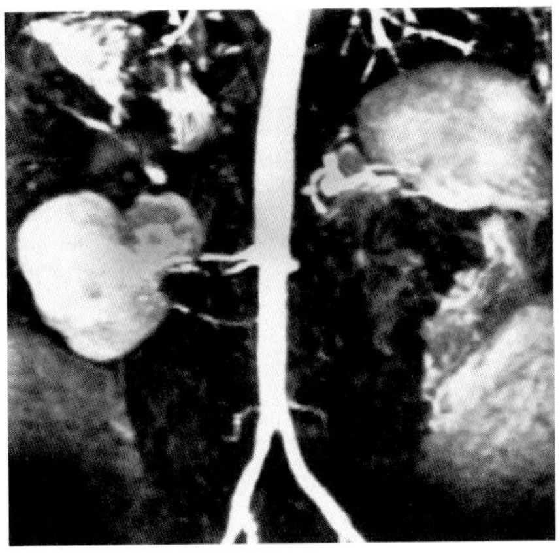

2.

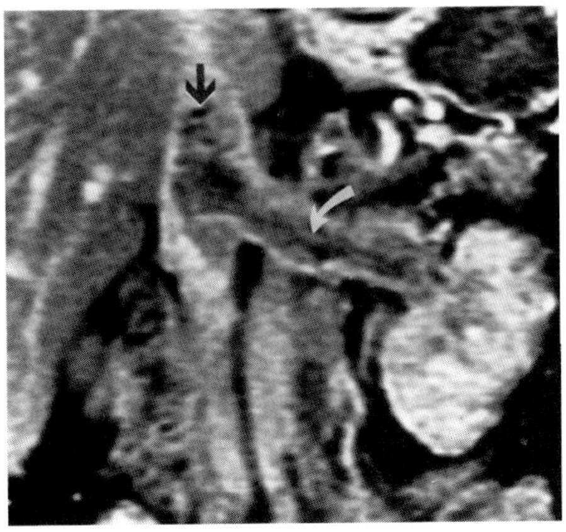

3.

Figures 2, 3. **(2)** Source coronal MR angiogram (8.4/1.4) demonstrates three renal arteries to the right kidney, which contains a renal cancer. The patient had previously undergone left nephrectomy. Note that it can be difficult to distinguish between an early-branching single renal artery and two separate renal arteries. The vessels appear to be incomplete because this plane of section did not encompass all parts of the renal arteries. **(3)** Delayed source coronal MR angiogram (8.4/1.4) demonstrates low-signal-intensity thrombus in the left renal vein and extending into the intrahepatic inferior vena cava. Note the tumoral enhancement in most of the thrombus (curved arrow). The small focus of low signal intensity (straight arrow) likely represents a flow void within a tumor vessel.

Renal Veins

Venous phase images demonstrated normal renal veins and a normal inferior vena cava in 11 patients. Renal vein thrombus was seen in seven patients, and extension of the inferior vena cava was seen in two of these patients. These findings were confirmed at surgery and resulted in 100% sensitivity and 100% specificity. Peak opacification of renal veins occurred by the third postcontrast imaging run, approximately 90 seconds after initiation of the contrast material injection (Figs 3, 4). In several instances, even more delayed (fourth and fifth imaging runs) were necessary to opacify the entire inferior vena cava. All thrombi contained a mixture of tumor (enhancing) and bland (nonenhancing thrombus) components. Bland thrombus was more readily depicted than tumor thrombus. Bland thrombus was lower in signal intensity compared with tumor thrombus, which was enhanced and was thus more difficult to distinguish from the normally enhancing lumen of the inferior vena cava (Fig 4).

The inferior vena cava was not well depicted on the MIP images because it was hypointense relative to the arteries. Instead, multiplanar reconstruction images in the coronal and axial planes were most helpful for identification of thrombus in the renal vein and inferior vena cava. The coronal plane images proved to be the most reliable for detection of thrombus in the right renal vein. The reformatted axial and source coronal images were the best to use for detection of thrombus in the left renal vein. Reformatted oblique views allowed depiction of the entire left renal vein from the renal hilum to the inferior vena cava.

Delayed scans (third to fifth imaging run) were best for detecting thrombus in the inferior vena cava because of the delay in filling of the infrarenal inferior vena cava. Because thrombus in the inferior vena cava can extend inferiorly, we waited until the entire inferior vena cava was opacified before ending the imaging.

Venous Collaterals

In addition to the main renal artery and venous anatomy, dual-phase MR angiography also allowed detection of the collateral venous circulation. Prominent gonadal veins were identified in three patients (Fig 5). Extensive pericapsular veins were identified in all tumors in the patients who were to undergo radical nephrectomy (Fig 5). Identification of these collateral vessels was considered to be helpful to the surgeons in the planning of their approach.

Other Findings

Delayed images were also useful for the identification of additional sites of disease. Additional findings included ipsilateral adrenal metastases in two patients, extensive nodal disease (Fig 6) in three patients, and pulmonary metastases in four patients, although these findings were usually present on

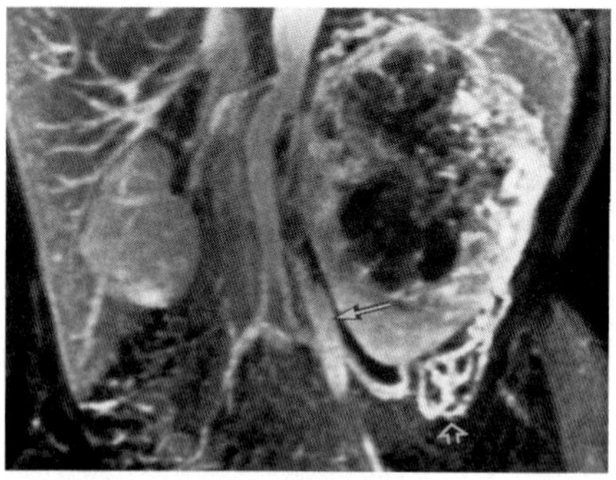

Figure 5. Delayed MIP image demonstrates extensive venous collaterals (open arrow) around a large left renal cancer. A large gonadal vein (arrow) is also seen.

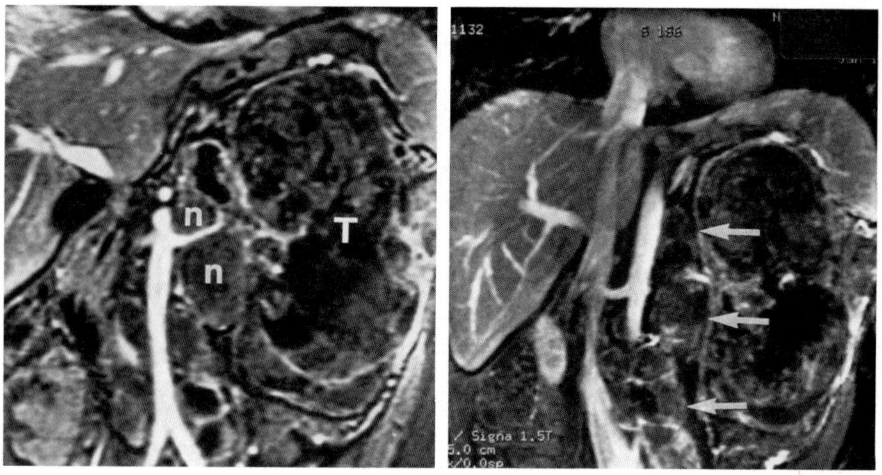

a. b.

Figure 6. MR images demonstrate extensive lymphadenopathy arising from large left-sided renal cancer. **(a)** Early phase source coronal MR angiogram (8.4/1.4) obtained during the arterial phase demonstrates that the renal artery is encased and narrowed because of extensive lymphadenopathy. *n* = lymph node, *T* = tumor. **(b)** Delayed source coronal MR angiogram (8.4/1.4) demonstrates extensive adenopathy displacing the inferior vena cava. Arrows = lymph nodes.

CT scans and on images obtained with other MR imaging pulse sequences (Table 1).

DISCUSSION

Gadolinium-enhanced MR arteriography has provided a dramatic improvement in noninvasive vascular imaging of abdominal vessels (8–11). This technique provides sufficient detail for reliable detection of major branch vessels of the abdominal aorta and has been used for the evaluation of atherosclerotic disease and aneurysms of the aorta (8–14). Gadolinium-enhanced arteriography has also been specifically applied to renovascular imaging, including detection of renal artery stenosis and identification of accessory renal arteries before donor nephrectomy (15,16). In this study, we demonstrated that gadolinium-enhanced MR angiography can be useful for the assessment of renal arteries before surgery for kidney cancer.

Typically, venous contamination is considered to be an undesirable artifact on MR angiograms because it may interfere with the identification of renal arteries. However, delayed gadolinium-enhanced MR angiograms can provide useful information in the evaluation of patients with renal cancer because this technique allows one to assess renal vein and inferior vena cava involvement. Our results confirm that this technique is a useful adjunct to conventional nonenhanced gradient-echo MR imaging for the assessment of renal vein patency.

The technique of dual-phase gadolinium-enhanced MR angiography has several advantages. First, it provides the surgeon with a reliable depiction of the arterial anatomy. This is of particular importance during a partial nephrectomy, because the surgeon must perform the resection with controlled ischemia, and during laparoscopic surgery, at which there is a limited field of view. Gadolinium-enhanced MR angiography allows assessment of venous invasion, although it is equivalent to breath-hold gradient-echo and spin-echo MR imaging with spatial presaturation pulses. MR angiography can also be used to distinguish between bland and malignant thrombus on the basis of the degree of enhancement of the thrombus. Finally, this technique demonstrates the collateral vasculature, including the pericapsular venous supply and prominent gonadal veins.

Disadvantages of MR angiography include the necessity for a relatively lengthy (34-second) breath hold, which not all patients can perform. It is our practice to train the patient to extend the duration of the breath hold by first taking three consecutive deep breaths. Moreover, we instruct the patient to let the air out slowly if he or she cannot hold the breath for the duration of the entire acquisition. Software, which was not available during this study, will speed the acquisition of the entire sequence (17). Centric k-space sampling (central lines of k space will be filled early in the sequence rather than sequentially) will also permit shorter breath holds (18,19). Faster imaging may also allow the assessment of intrarenal vessels.

Another limitation of the current technique is that venous contamination of the arterial phase occurred in about a third of the patients. In no case did it interfere with the ability to detect the renal arteries. Limited multiplanar reconstructions through the renal arteries eliminated any artifact from the overlying left renal vein. The increased speed of imaging combined with automated detection of bolus arrival will improve the arterial acquisition by reducing the amount of venous contamination (18,19). Bolus timing or automatic bolus detection may also permit the use of lower doses of contrast agents, which will make the study more cost effective (18–20).

Although 3D MIP reconstructions are attractive, they do not always contain as much information as the source images: With the MIP algorithm, smaller vessels "drop out" and are not depicted. We therefore routinely evaluate both the source coronal images and the reformatted axial images with electronic workstations. Source images provide a better assessment of the inferior vena cava and renal veins than the MIP images because of the lower signal intensity of the veins compared with the arteries. The MIP program we use, which is the standard algorithm for this MR imager, relies on high-contrast structures to decrease background noise. Unfortunately, the result is that fainter, thinner vessels are impossible to see on MIP images. Variable-thickness slabs of source images with and without MIP images may provide a better assessment of smaller vessels than either source images or full MIP images. Axial reconstructions from the 3D data set were useful for the differentiation of lumbar arteries from renal arteries and were most helpful for the assessment of the left renal vein for thrombus. With a four-window electronic display, the

MIP image and reformatted axial, sagittal, and coronal source images can be displayed simultaneously and cross referenced by using standard software. A complete review of the imaging study with the surgeon took 10 minutes.

Our current renal cancer staging protocol includes acquisition of T1- and T2-weighted images of the liver to exclude metastases and of a breath-hold gradient-echo image to evaluate the renal veins and inferior vena cava, followed by multiphase 3D MR angiography. CT adequately depicts adrenal and lymph node pathologic conditions, but with MR imaging the status of the renal vein and inferior vena cava can be clarified. MR angiography provides an added dimension by depicting the arterial anatomy, venous collaterals, and status of the renal veins and inferior vena cava.

In summary, dual-phase renal MR angiography for renal cancers is a relatively simple and accurate method for the comprehensive vascular assessment of the renal arteries, veins, and collaterals. Improvements in this technology will lead to even higher quality images with decreases in both acquisition time and contrast agent dose. ■

Acknowledgment: The authors thank Barbara McCoy for manuscript preparation.

References

1. Semelka RC, Shoenut JP, Magro CM, et al. Renal cancer staging: comparison of contrast-enhanced CT and gadolinium-enhanced fat-suppressed spin-echo and gradient-echo MR imaging. JMRI 1993; 3: 597–602.
2. Horan JJ, Roberston CN, Choyke PL, et al. The detection of renal carcinoma extension into the renal vein and inferior vena cava: a prospective comparison of venacavography and MRI. J Urol 1989; 142:943–948.
3. Roubidoux MA, Dunnick NR, Sostman HD, Leder RA. Renal carcinoma: detection of venous extension with gradient-echo MR imaging. Radiology 1992; 182: 269–272.
4. Myeneni L, Hricak H, Carroll PR. Magnetic resonance imaging of renal carcinoma with extension into the vena cava: staging accuracy and recent advances. Br J Urol 1991; 68:571–578.
5. Polascik TJ, Pound CR, Meng MV, Partin AW, Marshall FF. Partial nephrectomy technique, complications and pathological findings. J Urol 1995; 154:1312–1318.
6. Walther MM, Choyke PL, Weiss G, et al. Parenchymal sparing surgery in patients with hereditary renal cell carcinoma. J Urol 1995; 153:913–916.
7. Butler BP, Novick AC, Miller DP, Campbell SA, Licht MR. Management of small unilateral renal cell carcinomas: radical versus nephron-sparing surgery. Urology 1995; 45:34–40.
8. Prince MR, Yucel EK, Kaufman JA, Harrison DC, Geller SC. Dynamic gadolinium-enhanced three-dimensional abdominal MR arteriography. JMRI 1993; 3:877–881
9. Prince MR. Gadolinium-enhanced MR aortography. Radiology 1994; 191:155–164.
10. Shetty AN, Shirkhoda A, Bis KG, Alcantara A. Contrast enhanced three-dimensional MR angiography in a single breath-hold: a novel technique. AJR 1995; 165:1290–1292.
11. Leung DA, McKinnon GC, Davis CP, Pfammatter T, Krestin GP, Debatin JF. Breath-hold contrast-enhanced, three-dimensional MR angiography. Radiology 1996; 200:569–571.
12. Prince MR, Narasimham DL, Stanley JC, et al. Breath-hold gadolinium-enhanced MR angiography of the abdominal aorta and its major branches. Radiology 1995; 197:785–792.
13. Laissy JP, Soyer P, Tebboune D, Tiah D, Hvass U, Menu Y. Abdominal aortic aneurysms: assessment with gadolinium-enhanced time-of-flight coronal MR angiography (MRA). Eur J Radiol 1995; 20:1–8.
14. Petersen MJ, Cambria RP, Kaufman JA, et al. Magnetic resonance angiography in the preoperative evaluation of abdominal aortic aneurysms. J Vasc Surg 1995; 21:891–898.
15. Siegelman ES, Gilfeather M, Holland GA, et al. Breath-hold ultrafast three-dimensional gadolinium-enhanced MR angiography of the renovascular system. AJR 1997; 168:1035–1040.
16. Snidow JJ, Johnson MS, Harris VJ, et al. Three-dimensional gadolinium-enhanced MR angiography for aortoiliac inflow assessment plus renal artery screening in a single breath hold. Radiology 1996; 198: 725–732.
17. Korosec FR, Frayne R, Grist TM, Mistretta CA. Time resolved contrast-enhanced 3D MR angiography. Magn Reson Med 1996; 36:345–351.
18. Prince MR, Chenevert TL, Foo TKF, Londy FJ, Ward JS, Maki JH. Contrast-enhanced abdominal MR angiography: optimization of imaging delay time by automating the detection of contrast material arrival in the aorta. Radiology 1997; 203:109–114.
19. Foo TKF, Sarantathan M, Prince MR, Chenevert TL. Automated detection of bolus arrival and initiation of data acquisition in fast, three-dimensional, gadolinium-enhanced MR angiography. Radiology 1997; 203:275–280.
20. Earls JP, Rofsky NM, DeCorato DR, Krinsky GA, Weinreb JC. Breath-hold single-dose gadolinium-enhanced three-dimensional MR aortography: usefulness of a timing examination and MR power injector. Radiology 1996; 201:705–710.

Book Review

Genitourinary Radiology: The Requisites

Ronald J. Zagoria, MD, and Glenn A. Tung, MD

St Louis, Mo: Mosby–Year Book, 1997. ISBN 0-8016-7482-4. Cloth, $74.95; pp 418; 593 figures; tables; text boxes.

This book is the latest in the Requisite series from Mosby–Year Book. The books in the series are intended to provide core material in major subspecialty areas of radiology. This text is divided into 10 chapters with abundant images and diagrams. Text boxes highlight important points and differential diagnoses. The book includes intravenous urography and other conventional contrast material–enhanced studies as well as ultrasonography (US), computed tomography (CT), and magnetic resonance (MR) imaging.

The first chapter is an introduction to radiologic methods of evaluating the genitourinary tract. The chapter begins with a discussion of iodinated contrast media and the treatment of reactions to contrast media. The remainder of the chapter summarizes imaging methods used in evaluation of the genitourinary tract, including conventional contrast-enhanced studies, US, CT, MR imaging, angiography, and nuclear medicine. Also included is a helpful series of appendixes with suggested imaging protocols. The final chapter provides an introduction to percutaneous interventional urinary tract procedures and interventions in female and male infertility as well as percutaneous transluminal angioplasty.

Chapters 2–9 are arranged by anatomic part. Chapter 2 reviews anatomy and congenital abnormalities of the kidney and retroperitoneum. Chapter 3 on renal masses uses the "balls vs beans" approach to discuss solitary and infiltrative renal masses. This chapter also includes a section on syndromes associated with renal cysts and tumors and a discussion of the indeterminate renal mass. Chapter 4 on diffuse parenchymal abnormality of the kidney reviews the causes of renal atrophy and enlargement as well as medullary and cortical nephrocalcinosis. The renal sinus, pelvocalyceal system, and ureters are the subject of chapter 5, which employs a number of urograms and nice schematic diagrams to illustrate intrinsic and extrinsic disorders of the collecting system and ureter. Chapter 6 on the lower urinary tract covers disorders of the bladder and urethra, including neoplasms, infection, and trauma, as well as neuromuscular disorders of the lower urinary tract. The chapters on the female and male genital tracts each begin with a brief review of embryology, anatomy, and physiology. Chapter 7 on the female genital tract discusses congenital anomalies, pelvic pain, ovarian cyst, infertility, and gynecologic tumors. The male genital tract is the subject of chapter 8, in which a problem-oriented approach is used to address such topics as scrotal pain, prostatic nodules or enlargement, and erectile dysfunction. Chapter 9 on the adrenal glands reviews benign and malignant adrenal masses and discusses selected clinical problems in adrenal imaging such as the incidental adrenal mass and localization of pheochromocytomas.

This book is a well-written and -organized review of the essentials of contemporary genitourinary radiology. Each chapter contains high-quality images and diagrams that illustrate the various disorders under discussion. The text boxes are helpful to reinforce the major points and differential diagnoses. The inclusion of chapters on the female and male genital tracts sets this book apart from other introductory textbooks of uroradiology that do not cover the genital tracts. The chapter on interventional procedures is a nice introduction, but those who are looking for a more in-depth discussion will want to consult a book on interventional radiology, which is a subspecialty in its own right.

The authors have accomplished their goal of producing a succinct and well-written textbook of the fundamentals of genitourinary imaging. The book is affordable, especially considering the many images, and a good value. I would recommend this book to radiology residents seeking an introduction to the subject at the beginning of their training or a review for board examinations. I have received favorable comments from residents who have seen or read the book. It will also prove useful to residents in other specialties such as urology or gynecology and the general radiologist looking for a concise review of contemporary genitourinary imaging and a quick reference book.

Reviewed by Richard A. Szucs, MD

Deborah Levine, MD • Carol A. Hulka, MD • Jack Ludmir, MD • Wei Li, MD
Robert R. Edelman, MD

Placenta Accreta: Evaluation with Color Doppler US, Power Doppler US, and MR Imaging[1]

PURPOSE: **To determine the value of transabdominal ultrasound (US), transvaginal US, color Doppler US, power Doppler US, and magnetic resonance (MR) imaging in the diagnosis of placenta accreta.**

MATERIALS AND METHODS: **Nineteen patients in the third trimester of pregnancy who were at risk for placenta accreta underwent color Doppler and power Doppler US; 18 patients also underwent MR imaging. Images were interpreted prospectively for signs of accreta by two reviewers. The reviewers' confidence in their diagnosis was graded on a five-point scale.**

RESULTS: **Outcomes at delivery were as follows: normal placenta (n = 11), hysterectomy owing to uncontrollable bleeding (n = 1), and placenta accreta (n = 7). Five cases of lower-uterine-segment placenta accreta were diagnosed with a high level of confidence with vaginal and power Doppler US. In one patient with a posterior placenta who had previously undergone myomectomy, MR imaging enabled the diagnosis of placenta accreta, which was not well depicted at US.**

CONCLUSION: **In patients with a history of uterine scars, vaginal US with power Doppler US performed well in the evaluation of lower-uterine-segment placenta accreta. MR imaging depicts posterior placenta accreta.**

PLACENTA accreta, including its variants placenta increta and placenta percreta, is a placental disorder that may result in substantial intrapartum morbidity and mortality. Hysterectomy for placenta accreta frequently is necessary because of uncontrollable bleeding. Abnormalities in the placental attachment may result in the attachment of the placenta directly onto the myometrium (placenta accreta), extension more deeply into the myometrium (placenta increta), or invasion into or through the uterine serosa (placenta percreta). These conditions are rare in otherwise uncomplicated pregnancies but occur in 5% of patients with placenta previa (1). Clarke and colleagues (1) found that uterine scarring from cesarean section increases the prevalence of placenta previa from 0.26% with an unscarred uterus to 0.65% after one cesarean section and to as much as 10% after four or more cesarean sections. The frequency of placenta accreta in the presence of placenta previa increases from 24% after one cesarean section to 67% after four or more cesarean sections (1).

The gray-scale ultrasound (US) findings of placenta accreta and its variants have been previously described and include loss of the normal hypoechoic retroplacental myometrial zone, thinning or disruption of the hyperechoic uterine serosa–bladder interface, presence of focal exophytic masses, and lacunar flow within the placenta (2–6).

Doppler US has been suggested to aid in the diagnosis of placenta accreta because it highlights areas of increased vascularity with dilated blood vessels that cross the placenta and uterine wall (7–11) and demonstrates a transition between the retroplacental hypoechoic zone with normal Doppler signal and the absence of both the Doppler signal and the myometrial zone (12). None of these studies, however, has prospectively compared gray-scale and Doppler US findings to determine whether the use of Doppler adds to the diagnostic accuracy in these cases. In addition, to our knowledge, the use of power Doppler US has not been described in the diagnosis of placenta accreta.

Three case reports have described the use of magnetic resonance (MR) imaging in the evaluation of placenta accreta (13–15). To our knowledge, however, the accuracy of this method in the diagnosis of accreta has not been assessed.

The purpose of this study was to compare the accuracies of transabdominal and transvaginal gray-scale US with those of traditional color Doppler US, power Doppler US, and MR imaging in the characterization of placenta accreta.

MATERIALS AND METHODS

Between May 17, 1995, and April 8, 1997, 19 patients underwent US evaluation because they had a high risk of placenta accreta. MR imaging was performed in 18

Index terms: Placenta, abnormalities, 857.824 • Pregnancy, MR, 85.1214 • Pregnancy, US, 85.1298, 85.12983, 85.12989

Abbreviation: RARE = rapid acquisition with relaxation enhancement.

Radiology 1997; 205:773–776

[1] From the Departments of Radiology (D.L., C.A.H., W.L., R.R.E.) and Obstetrics and Gynecology (J.L.), Beth Israel Deaconess Medical Center, 330 Brookline Ave, CC483F, Boston, MA 02215. From the 1996 RSNA scientific assembly. Received June 2, 1997; revision requested July 8; revision received July 25; accepted August 4. **Address reprint requests to** D.L.

Summary of Patient History, Reviewer Diagnoses, and Outcome

Gestational Age (wk)	Prior Surgery*	Placental Location†	Placenta Previa	Reviewer 1 Diagnoses‡		Reviewer 2 Diagnoses‡		Mode of Delivery*	Placenta
				US	MR Imaging	US	MR Imaging		
26	CS	A	Yes	4	4	3	3	CS§	Normal‖
26	CS	A	No	1	1	1	1	CS	Normal
27	CS	A, P	Yes	4	4	4	4	CS§	Accreta
28	CS	A	Yes	1	2	1	3	CS	Normal
29	CS	A, P	Yes	1	1	2	3	CS	Normal
30	CS	A, P	Yes	5	5	4	2	CS	Accreta
32	CS	A	Yes	5	NA	5	NA	CS§	Percreta
32	CS	A	No	1	1	1	1	CS	Normal
32	CS	P	Yes	1	1	1	2	CS	Normal
33	CS	A	Yes	5	5	4	4	CS§	Accreta
33	CS	A	Yes	4	4	3	4	CS	Accreta
33	CS	A, P	Yes	1	2	1	2	CS	Normal
34	CS	A	No	1	1	1	1	Vaginal	Normal
34	CS	A	No	4	4	4	4	CS	Accreta
34	Myomectomy	A	No	1	1	1	1	CS	Normal
35	Myomectomy	P	No	3	4	3	3	CS	Accreta
36	Myomectomy	Fundal	No	1	3	2	3	CS	Normal
38	CS	A	Yes	1	1	1	1	CS	Normal
39	CS	A	No	1	1	1	1	CS	Normal

* CS = cesarean section.
† A = anterior, P = posterior.
‡ Scoring system was as follows: 1 = definitely normal, 2 = probably normal, 3 = indeterminate, 4 = probably abnormal, 5 = definitely abnormal. NA = not applicable; MR imaging was not performed.
§ Hysterectomy was performed.
‖ In this case, no placenta accreta was seen at surgery; however, bleeding could not be controlled, and a hysterectomy was performed.

patients. One patient had a cerebral aneurysm clip and thus could not undergo MR imaging. Sixteen patients had previously undergone cesarean section, 11 of whom had anterior placentas with placenta previa and five of whom had anterior placentas over the region of the scar. Three patients had previously undergone myomectomy, and the placenta was located over the region of myomectomy. Gestational ages ranged from 26 to 37 weeks (mean, 32.1 weeks). This study was approved by the internal review board of our institution. Written informed consent was obtained from all patients before imaging with Doppler US and MR imaging.

All patients underwent routine obstetric US in addition to evaluation of the placenta. All US scans and MR images were obtained by one of the authors (D.L.). All US scans were obtained with commercially available real-time equipment by using 3.5- or 5-MHz linear or sector transducers transabdominally and 7- or 5-MHz sector transducers transvaginally (models 128 or 128XP, Acuson, Mountain View, Calif; and models HDI or UM9, ATL, Bothell, Wash). To evaluate the placenta, transabdominal images were obtained with emphasis on the myometrial zone. Color Doppler and power Doppler US scans of the most suspicious regions were obtained. Doppler power settings were at the level approved for fetal use. If the region of concern was in the lower uterine segment, transvaginal US was performed, with gray-scale, color, and power Doppler US performed in the most suspicious regions. A small amount of fluid in the urinary bladder aided the evaluation of the uterine and bladder serosa; therefore, all endovaginal scans were obtained with a partially full bladder.

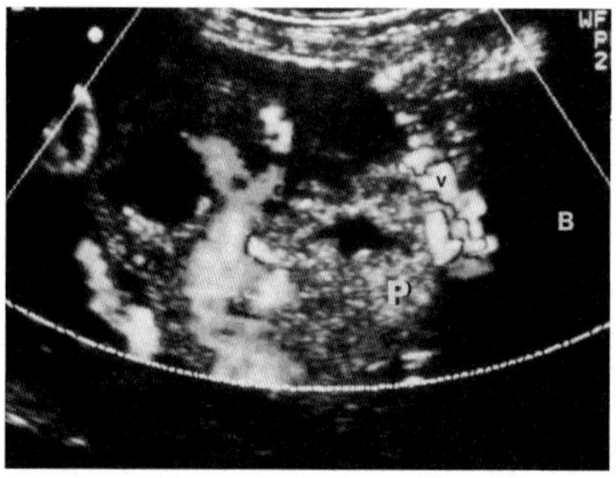

Figure 1. Placenta percreta diagnosed with transabdominal US. Vessels (*v*) extend from the placenta (*P*) to the bladder (*B*).

MR imaging was performed with a 1.5-T superconductive system (Vision; Siemens, Erlangen, Germany) by using a four-element body phased-array coil ($n = 17$) or a body coil ($n = 1$). The minimum rise time was 600 μsec (for a 25-mT peak gradient amplitude). The whole-body specific absorption rate was kept to less than 3.0 W/kg. Patients were supine, with their feet entering the magnet bore first to minimize feelings of claustrophobia. A scout view was obtained, and placental images were obtained in the sagittal, coronal, and axial planes with respect to the uterus. The first three patients underwent imaging with a turbo spin-echo technique (3,000/138 [repetition time msec/echo time msec], one acquisition, 5-mm section thickness, 22.5 × 30-cm field of view, 116 × 256 acquisition matrix, 16-second imaging time); subsequent patients underwent imaging with the half-Fourier single-shot rapid acquisition with relaxation enhancement (RARE) imaging technique (echo spacing of 4.2

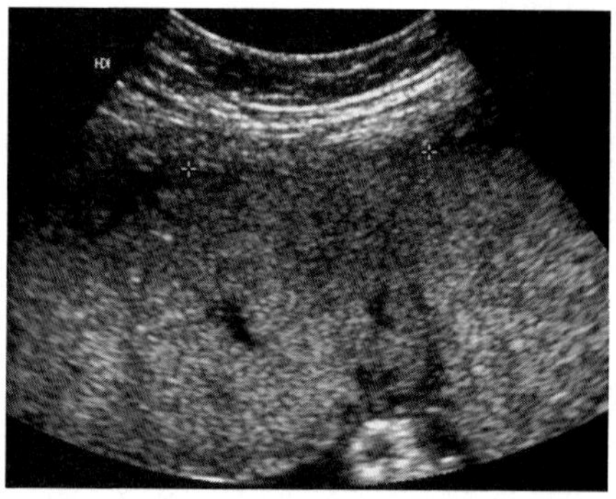

Figure 2. Placenta accreta diagnosed with transabdominal US. Sagittal US scan obtained over the region of the cesarean section scar shows a loss of the myometrial zone, with a subtle bulge of placenta in the region of accreta (calipers).

msec, single shot/60 msec, echo train length of 72, one acquisition, 5-mm section thickness, 26 × 35-cm field of view, 128 × 256 acquisition matrix, and 19-second imaging time). A refocusing flip angle of 130° instead of 180° was used to minimize the amount of radio-frequency power deposition. In four patients, a smaller field of view (26 × 26 cm) and thin sections (2.8–4 mm) were used to provide improved placental and myometrial detail.

At present, there is no evidence to suggest that short-term exposure to electromagnetic fields harms the developing fetus (16–20). Because of potential unknown effects of the electromagnetic field, however, the duration of exposure was limited. Our current examination time is less than 20 minutes.

All US and MR images were interpreted

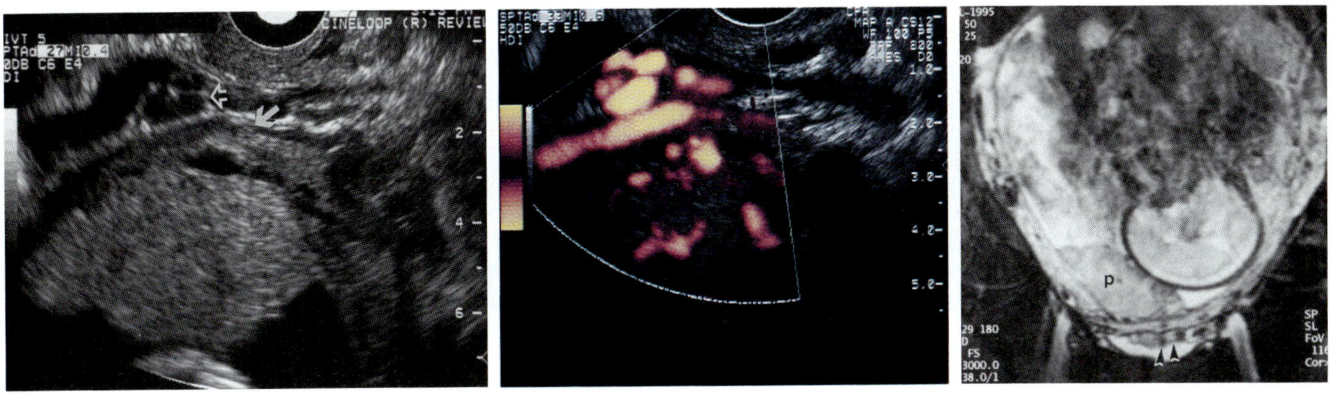

a. b. c.

Figure 3. Placenta accreta diagnosed with transvaginal US. **(a)** Sagittal transvaginal gray-scale US scan shows a thin myometrial zone with a small region of placental tissue that extends to the serosa (solid arrow). Bladder varices are seen in this region (open arrow). Other sections showed more extensive thinning of the myometrial zone. **(b)** Power Doppler US scan shows no extension of vessels from the placenta to the bladder varices. **(c)** Turbo spin-echo coronal MR image (3,000/138) shows myometrium between the placenta (*p*) and bladder varices (arrowheads).

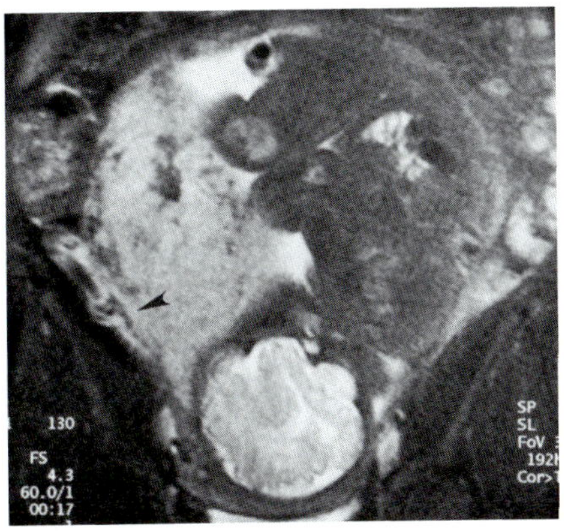

Figure 4. Placenta accreta diagnosed with MR imaging in a patient who had previously undergone posterior myomectomy. Coronal single-shot RARE MR image (single shot/60) shows absent myometrium in a posterolateral location (arrowhead). This region was not well evaluated with US.

at the time of study by the author monitoring the examinations (D.L.). Each modality was scored to indicate whether accreta was demonstrated, and with what confidence, as follows: 1, definitely normal; 2, probably normal; 3, indeterminate; 4, probably abnormal; 5, definitely abnormal. Placenta accreta was diagnosed with the criteria used by Finberg and Williams (3), as follows: loss of the normal retroplacental myometrial zone, thinning or disruption of the uterine serosa–bladder interface, and presence of focal exophytic masses. The obstetrician caring for the patient was notified of the findings.

At the end of the study, all US scans and MR images were reviewed by a second author (C.A.H.) for diagnosis and confidence in diagnosis. MR images were read with knowledge of the results of the US scans because US influences the protocol for the MR studies, and in future clinical practice it is likely that MR images will be read with knowledge of the US results.

Follow-up data were obtained from the obstetricians at the time of delivery and from pathology reports. One patient delivered vaginally, and the remainder delivered by means of cesarean section. The sensitivity and specificity of US and MR imaging were compared, with a positive test result defined as a score of 4 (probably abnormal) or 5 (abnormal). The most confident diagnoses of the two reviewers were used for statistical analysis. The κ statistic was used to compare US findings with the combination of US and MR imaging findings.

RESULTS

A summary of patient history, reviewer diagnoses (most confident diagnosis with any US modality and most confident diagnosis with MR imaging), and outcome is given in the Table.

The clinical outcome and US findings of the first reviewer were as follows: There were 12 nonaccreta placentas at delivery, seven of which were anterior or fundal without previa. In each of these cases, transabdominal US examinations enabled a confident diagnosis without the use of color or power Doppler techniques. In four cases of placenta previa without placenta accreta, transvaginal US allowed for a more confident diagnosis than did transabdominal US in two cases, transvaginal power Doppler US increased the confidence in diagnosis in one case, and there was no difference in confidence in diagnosis with transvaginal or transabdominal US in one case.

One patient with previa but no accreta at cesarean section had uncontrollable bleeding when the placenta was removed, which necessitated hysterectomy. In this case, transabdominal US demonstrated a focal exophytic mass lateral to the cervix. This was better depicted with transvaginal US. Color Doppler US was not helpful, but power Doppler US demonstrated the extension of placental vessels to the periphery of the exophytic component of the placenta. This did not increase the confidence in the diagnosis. MR imaging had similar findings, which were suggestive of placenta accreta. This was a US and MR imaging misdiagnosis of placenta accreta. The focal bulge seen at prenatal imaging was believed to be a thin, but intact, region of myometrium.

Transabdominal and transvaginal US findings were consistent with the histopathologic diagnosis of placenta percreta in one patient in whom vessels were seen that extended from the placenta into the bladder. Color Doppler and power Doppler US demonstrated the marked vascularity of the placenta but did not change the confidence in diagnosis in this case (Fig 1).

Six patients had placenta accreta. In one patient, transabdominal US scans were suspicious for placenta accreta in a location above the field of view of the transvaginal probe (Fig 2). Neither traditional color Doppler US nor power Doppler US increased the confidence in this diagnosis. Findings at transabdominal US (with and without Doppler) were indeterminate in one patient with a posterior placenta and a history of posterior myomectomy; again, this region was outside the field of view of the transvaginal probe. In the remaining four patients (all of whom had placenta previa), findings at transabdominal US (with and without Doppler) were indeterminate, although all four patients had transvaginal US scans that were suspicious for accreta. Color Doppler US did not increase the confidence in diagnosis in these patients. Power Doppler US demonstrated vessels bridging from the placenta to the margin of the uterus in two patients and thus increased the confidence in diagnosis. In addition, bladder varices also were present in one of these patients. Power Doppler US showed that the region of varices was not connected to the region that caused accreta to be suspected (Fig 3). This allowed the patient to be surgically treated for placenta accreta and not for placenta percreta.

One patient had bladder varices without accreta. In this patient, power Doppler US clearly demonstrated that there was no abnormal vasculature between the placenta and the region of bladder varices.

In the six patients with findings suspicious for accreta at transabdominal US, transvaginal US, or both, MR imaging did not increase the level of confidence in diagnosis. In the patient with the posterior placenta and a history of previous posterior myomectomy, MR imaging demonstrated a 4-cm-diameter area of placenta with loss of the myometrium (Fig 4). In the 11 cases judged to be normal with US, MR images were indeterminate in one, probably normal in two, and normal in the remainder.

The second reviewer tended to be less confident in the diagnosis of placenta accreta. This was believed to be secondary to lack of real-time depiction of the placenta-myometrium interface.

The sensitivity and specificity of US in the diagnosis of placenta accreta were 86% (six of seven) and 92% (11 of 12), respectively. The addition of MR imaging to US increased the sensitivity to 100%; however, it should be noted that US was 100% sensitive for the diagnosis of anterior placenta accreta. The weighted κ statistic was 0.92, consistent with almost-perfect agreement, when comparing US with US and MR imaging combined.

DISCUSSION

The prenatal diagnosis of placenta accreta is crucial for appropriate counseling and surgical planning to be performed. All cases of accreta in this study were correctly identified prenatally, patients were appropriately counseled with regard to the possibility of blood loss and need for hysterectomy, and we were prepared for appropriate management at delivery.

Finberg and Williams (3) evaluated patients with placenta previa and a history of one or more cesarean sections. By using criteria of loss of the normal hypoechoic retroplacental myometrial zone, thinning or disruption of the hyperechoic uterine serosa–bladder interface, and the presence of focal exophytic masses, they found that US had a sensitivity of 93% (depicting 14 of 15 cases of placenta accreta) and a specificity of 79% (negative US results in 15 of 19 patients without histopathologic evidence of placenta accreta) in the diagnosis of placenta accreta. Subsequent articles describing the use of color Doppler US and MR imaging in the diagnosis of placenta accreta either have been case reports or have not compared the additional techniques with gray-scale US to determine whether the addition of Doppler techniques is worthwhile.

In this study, we found that gray-scale US was adequate for the evaluation of most placentas. When the retroplacental clear space was normal (>2 mm), Doppler evaluation and MR imaging did not add additional information. When the retroplacental clear space was 2 mm or less, the location of the placenta determined which modality was best suited for the most specific diagnosis. For patients with an anterior placenta and a suspicious area outside the range of the transvaginal probe, transabdominal US was best.

Of the different techniques, transvaginal US with power Doppler gave the most information in patients with an anterior placenta previa; however, use of power Doppler US did not add additional information in most other cases. MR imaging was best in one patient with a scar in the posterior uterus, because the posterior myometrium was difficult to evaluate with US. This was the only case in which MR imaging added additional information to that available with US. These results suggest that in patients at risk for accreta, MR imaging should be reserved for those with a placenta that is difficult to evaluate with US.

Further studies in which these imaging modalities are used are necessary in obstetric patients at risk for placental disorders to validate our findings. ■

References

1. Clarke SL, Koonings PP, Phelan JP. Placenta previa/accreta and prior cesarean section. Obstet Gynecol 1985; 66:89–92.
2. Guy G, Peisner DB, Timor-Tritsch IE. Ultrasonographic evaluation of uteroplacental blood flow patterns of abnormally located and adherent placentas. Am J Obstet Gynecol 1990; 163:723–727.
3. Finberg H, Williams J. Placenta accreta: prospective sonographic diagnosis in patients with placenta previa and prior cesarean section. J Ultrasound Med 1992; 11:333–343.
4. de Mendonca L. Sonographic diagnosis of placenta accreta. J Ultrasound Med 1988; 7:211–215.
5. Tabsh K, Brinkman C, King W. Ultrasound diagnosis of placenta increta. JCU 1982; 10:288–290.
6. Pasto M, Kurtz A, Rifkin M, Cole-Beuglet C, Wapner R, Goldberg B. Ultrasonographic findings in placenta increta. J Ultrasound Med 1983; 2:155–159.
7. Megier P, Desroches A. Prenatal color Doppler diagnosis of placenta previa accreta. Ultrasound Obstet Gynecol 1994; 4:437–438.
8. Lerner J, Deane S, Timor-Tritsch IE. Characterization of placenta accreta using transvaginal sonography and color Doppler imaging. Ultrasound Obstet Gynecol 1995; 5:198–201.
9. Chou M, Ho E, Lu F, Lee Y. Prenatal diagnosis of placenta previa/accreta with color Doppler ultrasound. Ultrasound Obstet Gynecol 1992; 2:293–296.
10. Jauniaux E, Toplis P, Nicolaides K. Sonographic diagnosis of a non-previa placenta accreta. Ultrasound Obstet Gynecol 1996; 7:58–60.
11. Rosemond R, Kepple D. Transvaginal color Doppler sonography in the prenatal diagnosis of placenta accreta. Obstet Gynecol 1992; 80:508–510.
12. Hoffman-Tretin J, Koenigsberg M, Rabin A, Anyaegbunam A. Placenta accreta: additional sonographic observations. J Ultrasound Med 1992; 11:29–34.
13. Thorp J, Councell R, Sandridge D, Wiest H. Antepartum diagnosis of placenta previa percreta by magnetic resonance imaging. Obstet Gynecol 1992; 80:506–508.
14. Leaphart W, Schapiro H, Broome J, Welander C, Bernstein I. Placenta previa percreta with bladder invasion. Obstet Gynecol 1997; 89:834–835.
15. Bakri Y, Sundin T, Mansi M, Jaroudi K. Placenta percreta with bladder invasion: report of three cases. Am J Perinatol 1993; 10:468–470.
16. Schwartz J, Crooks L. NMR imaging produces no observable mutations or cytotoxicity in mammalian cells. AJR 1982; 139:583–585.
17. Reid A, Smith F, Hutchinson J. Nuclear magnetic resonance imaging and its safety implications: follow-up of 181 patients. Br J Radiol 1982; 55:784–786.
18. Kanal E, Gillen J, Evans J, Savitz D, Shellock F. Survey of reproductive health among female MR workers. Radiology 1993; 187:395–399.
19. Baker P, Johnson I, Harvey P, Mansfield P. 3 year follow-up of children imaged in utero using echo planar magnetic resonance. Am J Obstet Gynecol 1994; 170:32–33.
20. Wolff S, Crooks L, Brown P, Howard R, Painter R. Tests for DNA and chromosomal damage induced by nuclear magnetic resonance imaging. Radiology 1980; 136:707–710.

Vassilios Raptopoulos, MD • Paula Touliopoulos, MD[2] • Qing F. Lei, MD[3]
Thomas G. Vrachliotis, MD[4] • Sandy C. Marks, Jr, DDS, PhD

Medial Border of the Perirenal Space: CT and Anatomic Correlation[1]

PURPOSE: To explore the mode of spread of disease between the perirenal space and the perivascular central retroperitoneum and to determine the anatomy along the medial border of the perirenal space.

MATERIALS AND METHODS: Anatomic dissection, injection of latex, and observation of cross sections of the abdomen were performed in nine cadavers. Attention was paid to the juncture of the central prevertebral, perivascular, and extraperitoneal regions, and the perirenal space. Anatomic findings were correlated with observations made at computed tomography (CT) in 82 patients with retroperitoneal hemorrhage (n = 24), inflammation (n = 37), and neoplasia (n = 21) involving the perirenal spaces or the central retroperitoneum.

RESULTS: Along most of the length of each kidney, no apparent fascia separates the perirenal space from the central retroperitoneum. At this location, septa between fat lobules form a fenestrated multitier barrier. These septa were imperceptible on CT scans obtained in healthy individuals. After injection of latex in cadavers, this potential barrier was seen. In the clinical study, spread of disease was allowed in only 38 (30%) of 128 instances of potential spread. Spread was facilitated along the renal vessels and the interlobular septa.

CONCLUSION: Beyond the kidneys, the renal fascia is closed, forming a cone superiorly and an inverted cone inferiorly. A network of interlobular septa acted as a barrier or pathway to the free spread of disease from the perirenal space to the central retroperitoneum or from the central retroperitoneum to the perirenal space.

The division of the retroperitoneum into distinct anatomic compartments has been useful in understanding the mode of spread and containment of various diseases (1–3). In the axial plane, the retroperitoneum is divided into three distinct compartments by the anterior and posterior renal fasciae: the anterior pararenal, the perirenal, and the posterior pararenal spaces (1–7). These three compartments have been described and labeled. The central retroperitoneum, anterior to the lumbar spine, however, is not referred to as a distinct compartment, despite the fact that it contains vital structures such as the abdominal aorta and inferior vena cava and is frequently occupied by serious disease, such as abdominal lymphoma or ruptured abdominal aortic aneurysm.

In conventional anatomy, the anterior renal fascia blends with the connective tissues of the central prevertebral space around the great vessels, whereas the posterior renal fascia is attached to the ipsilateral psoas muscle. This leaves an opening between the perirenal space and the central perivascular space that allows communication between the right and left perirenal spaces (1,2,4,5,8,9). This concept has changed little in the past 100 years (4) (Fig 1). Clinical observations at computed tomography (CT) performed in patients with various retroperitoneal diseases, however, showed infrequent or decreased spread of disease between the perirenal space and the central retroperitoneum. Furthermore, spread of disease from one perirenal space to the other via the central retroperitoneum is a rare occurrence (10–12).

Our objective in this study was to explore the mode of spread of disease between the perirenal space and the central retroperitoneum. We tested the hypothesis that there is a relatively strong barrier at the medial border of the perirenal space, and our goal was to determine whether this barrier is anatomic or functional. Accordingly, we determined the anatomy along the medial border of the perirenal space in both healthy patients and those with disease.

MATERIALS AND METHODS

Anatomic dissection in the abdomen was performed in nine cadavers at the University of Massachusetts Medical School. The transition from the central retroperitoneum to the right and left perirenal spaces was studied with three different methods: conventional dissection (n = 2), dissection after injection of colored latex into the perirenal space (n = 2) or central retroperitoneum (n = 2), and dissection of cadaveric cross sections of the abdomen

Index terms: Kidney, anatomy, 81.92 • Retroperitoneal space, 87.92 • Retroperitoneal space, CT, 87.12115

Radiology 1997; 205:777–784

[1] From the Department of Radiology, Beth Israel Deaconess Medical Center and Harvard Medical School, 330 Brookline Ave, Boston, MA 02215 (V.R., T.G.V.); and the Department of Cell Biology, University of Massachusetts Medical School, Worcester (V.R., P.T., Q.F.L., S.C.M.). Received March 11, 1997; revision requested May 12; final revision received and accepted August 7. Q.F.L. supported by a fellowship from West China University Medical Center. **Address reprint requests to** V.R.
[2] Current address: Department of Radiology, Good Samaritan Hospital, Phoenix, Ariz.
[3] Current address: Department of Anatomy, West China University of Medical Sciences, Chengdu, Sichuan, People's Republic of China.
[4] Current address: Department of Radiology, Ohio State University Medical Center, Columbus.

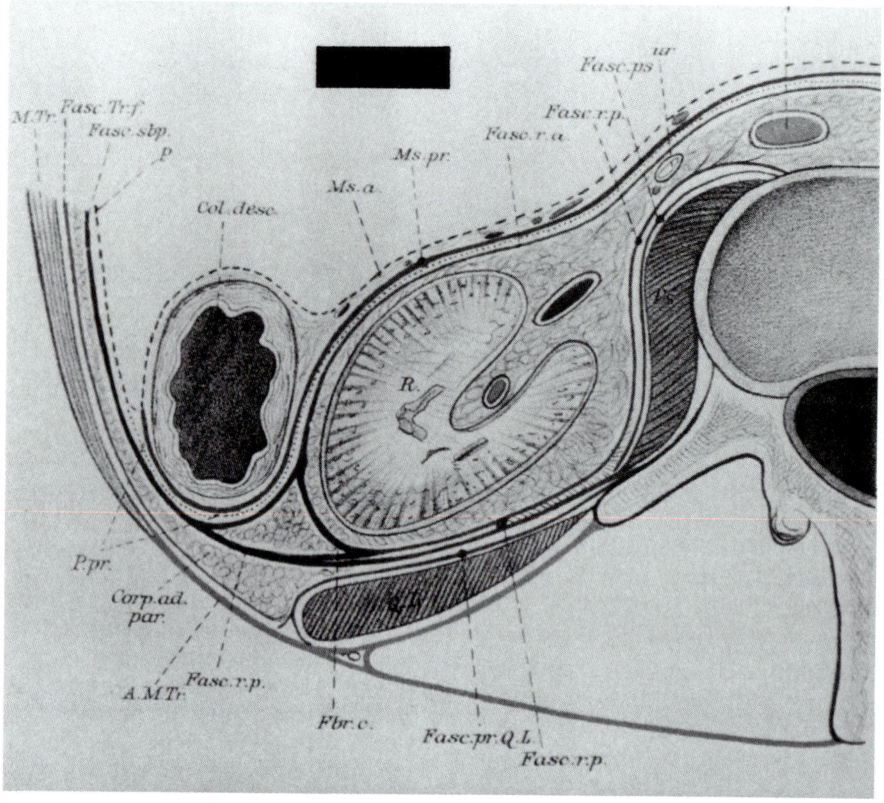

Figure 1. Drawing by Greota (4) of the left cross section at the level of the renal hilum (seen from above) shows the relationship of the posterior renal fascia (*Fasc.r.p.*) and psoas muscle. Anterior renal fascia (*Fasc.r.a.*) extends anteriorly to the renal vein (ureter [*ur*]) and aorta (*A*). Gerota did not draw a distinct divider between the central retroperitoneum and the perirenal space. *A.M.Tr.* = aponeurosis propria musculi transverse abdominus, *Col.desc.* = descending colon, *Corp.ad.par.* = corpus adiposum pararenale, *Fasc.pr.Q.L.* = fascia propria quadratus lumborum, *Fasc.ps* = fascia psoas major, *Fasc.sbp.* = fascia subperitonaeali, *Fasc.Tr.f.* = fascia transversalis tibrosa, *Fbr.c.* = fibrous capsule, *M.Tr.* = muscle transversus, *Ms.a.* = mesocolon anterior, *Ms.pr.* = mesocolon posterior, *P* = peritonaeum, *P.pr.* = peritonaeum parietale, *R* = kidney.

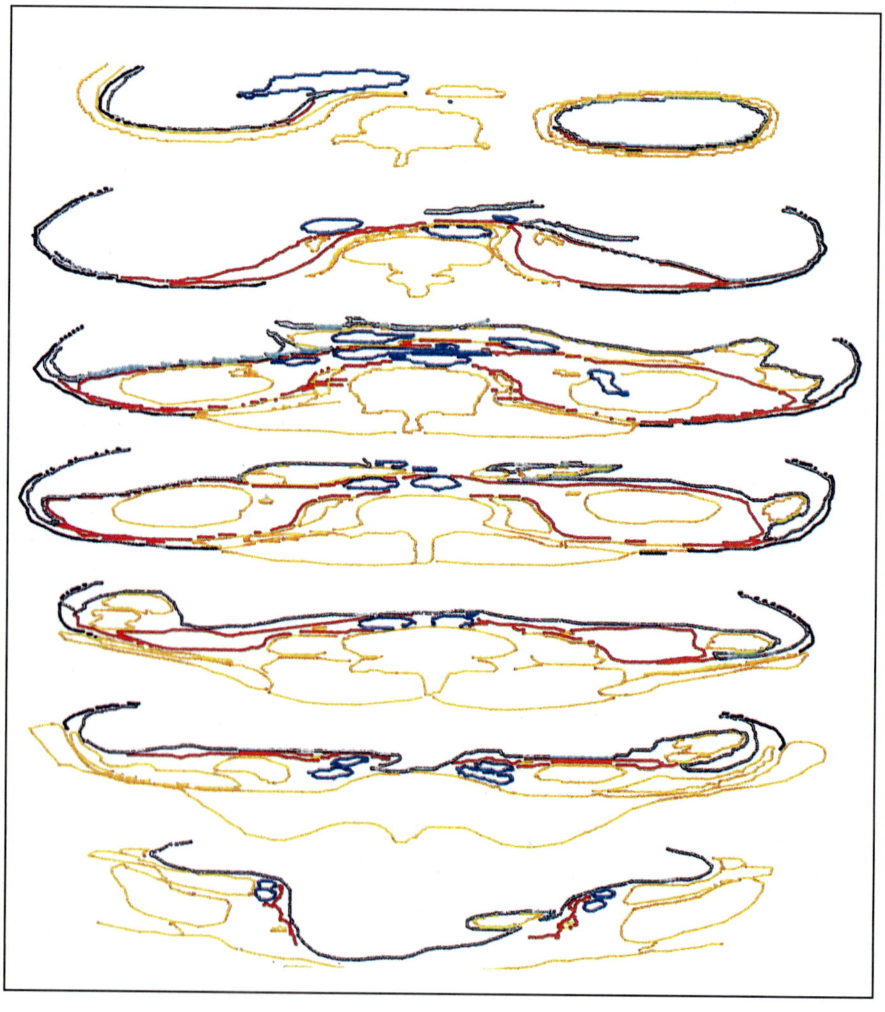

Figure 2. Computer-generated drawing shows tracings on a cadaveric cross section with three-dimensional reformations. Various colors depict major dividers, including parietal peritoneum (green); renal fascia (red); great vessels (blue); and kidneys, muscles, and spine (yellow). The tracings have been rotated on their x axes and stacked to provide a three-dimensional conception of the relations of fasciae with the imaginary body in a semiupright position. A 72° angle was depicted to avoid overlapping of individual tracings. The anterior and posterior renal fasciae (red) join medially above and below the kidneys, whereas they leave an opening along most of the kidneys (yellow). The posterior fascia is attached to the psoas muscle, and the anterior fascia extends over the aorta and vena cava. A shaded surface display could provide a three-dimensional model to better illustrate these fascial relationships. This could not be obtained, however, because of the large gaps between the cross-sectional levels traced, as determined on the basis of the section thickness (3–5 cm).

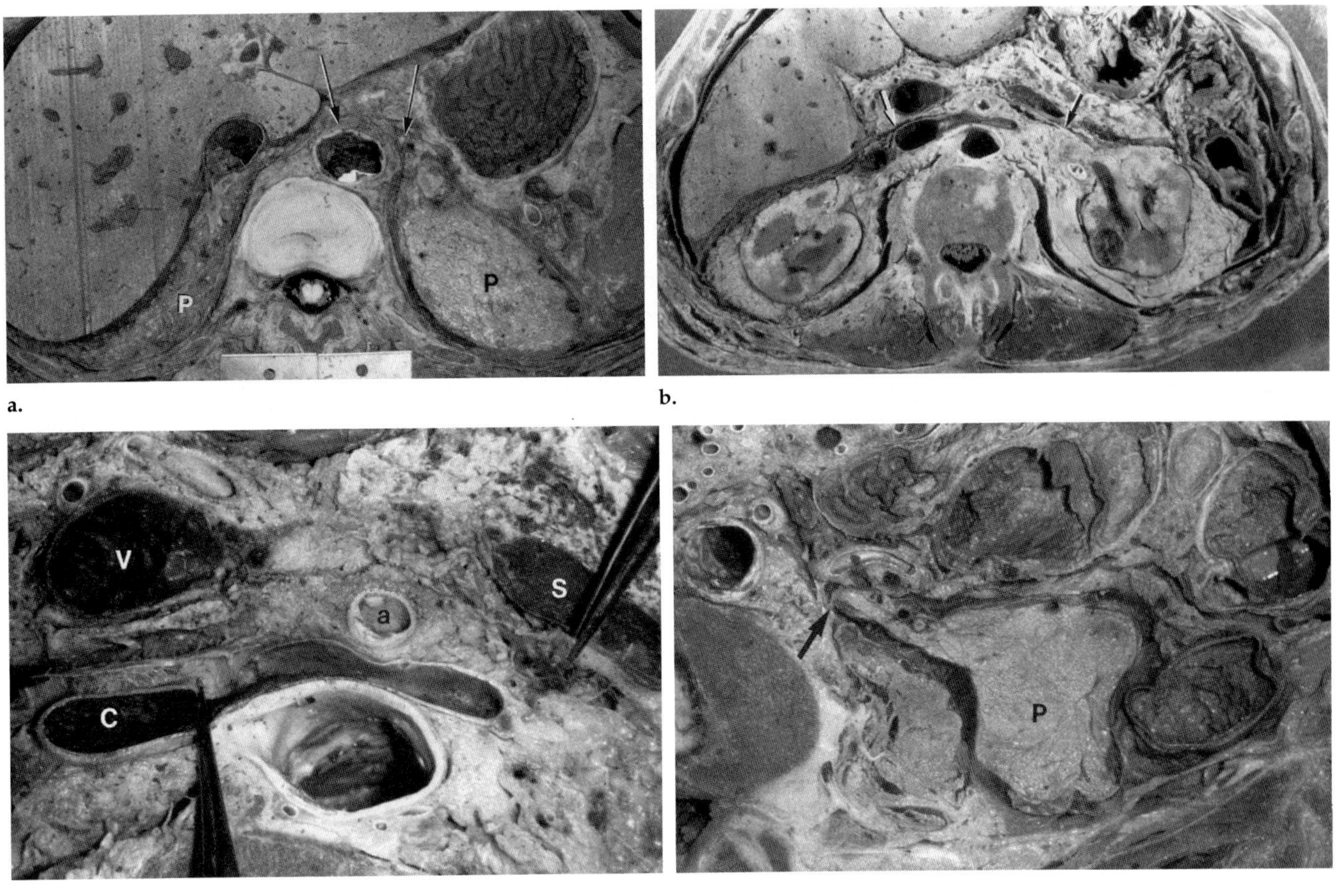

Figure 3. The renal fasciae on cadaveric cross sections. **(a)** Superiorly, each perirenal space (*P*) is closed by medial merging of the anterior and posterior renal fasciae. **(b)** At the level of the left renal hilum, the right and left posterior renal fasciae are attached on the ipsilateral psoas muscle. Anteriorly, each renal fascia extends anterior to the aorta and inferior to the vena cava (arrows). **(c)** Close-up of image in **b** shows detail of the anterior extent of the renal fasciae. Left anterior renal fascia (held by surgical clamp) extends behind the splenic vein (*s*) but in front of the superior mesenteric artery (*a*) to the posterior border of the superior mesenteric vein (*v*). Right anterior renal fascia (held by another surgical clamp) extends in front of the inferior vena cava (*c*), to which it is strongly attached. Medially, neither anterior renal fascia joins with the ipsilateral posterior fascia, whereas there is no distinct border between the central retroperitoneum and either perirenal space. **(d)** Close-up at level caudal to the lower pole of the left kidney shows that the renal fascia completely envelops the fat-filled perirenal space (*P*), which closes medially (arrow).

Table 1
Spread of Disease between Central Retroperitoneum and Perirenal Space

	Spread			
Disease	None	Partial	Free	Total
Hemorrhage	21 (55)	7 (19)	10 (26)	38
Inflammation	45 (80)	8 (14)	3 (5)	56
Neoplasia	24 (71)	0	10 (29)	34
Total	90 (70)	15 (12)	23 (18)	128

Note.—Data are number of instances of potential spread in 82 patients. Numbers in parentheses are percentages.

($n = 3$). The relationships of the fasciae were noted and photographed, and resistance to separation with gentle blunt dissection was noted. The two cadavers in which conventional dissection was performed were embalmed, and the other seven cadavers were not. None of the cadavers had any abdominal scars, and the causes of death were attributed to natural extraabdominal conditions. In one unembalmed cadaver, however, extensive retroperitoneal hemorrhage secondary to unsuspected rupture of an abdominal aortic aneurysm was found. No abdominal abnormalities were detected in the other eight cadavers.

Anatomic Study

Conventional dissection.—Two unembalmed cadavers were frozen (−50°F), and their torsos were transected at the transverse plane at about the middle renal level. Afterward the hemitorsos were thawed, and anatomic dissection was performed.

Latex injection followed by dissection.—Injection of liquid colored latex was performed with a technique described previously (3,7,13,14). Briefly, four unembalmed cadavers were frozen (−50°F), and their torsos were sectioned in the transverse plane at the middle renal level. After the torsos had thawed, a 5% barium sulfate mixture of colored liquid latex (Connecticut Valley Biological Supply, Southampton, Mass) was injected in the perirenal space of two cadavers and in the central retroperitoneum of the other two cadavers. The injection site for the perirenal space was chosen as the midpoint between the anteromedial curve of the kidney and the anterior renal fascia. The injection in the central retroperitoneum was anterolateral to the aorta (at the 2 or 10 o'clock position). Latex was injected in both the caudal and cephalad cadaveric hemitorsos. The liquid latex mixture was injected with a 50-mL syringe and a 12-cm-long, 14-gauge needle. Surface spread was avoided by injecting through a 12-gauge hole in a clear plastic plate that was tightly pressed on the surface of the specimen. The injected latex was solidified in situ by injecting 10–50 mL of 10% acetic acid. About 100–

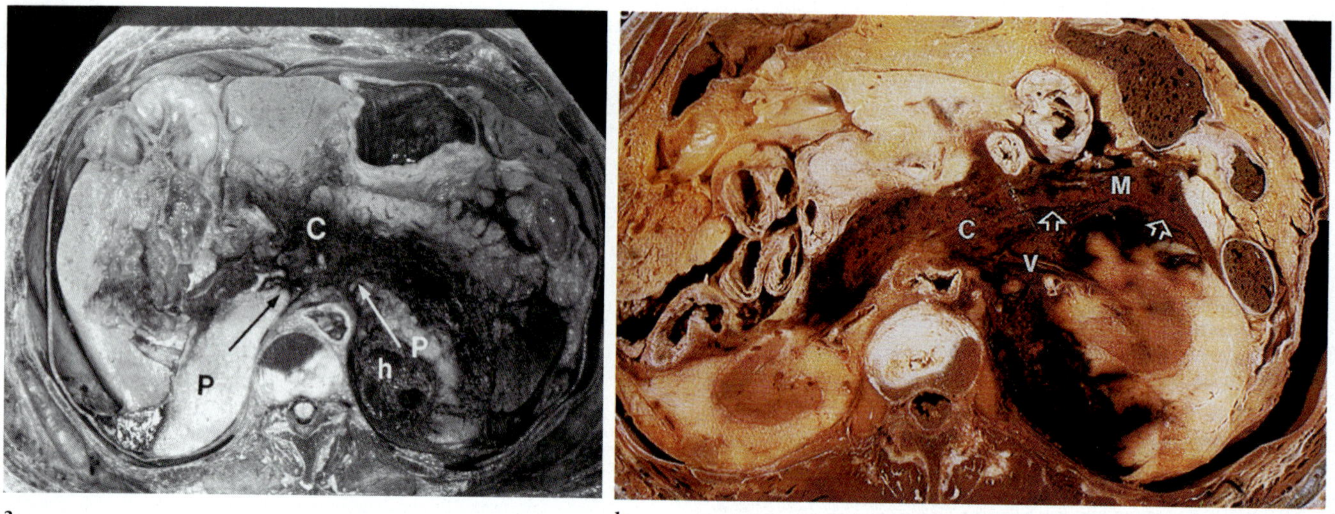

a. b.

Figure 4. Cross sections of cadaver with ruptured abdominal aneurysm. **(a)** Cephalic to upper pole of kidney. Blood centrally (*C*), anterior to the aorta and diaphragmatic crura, represents superior spread from hemorrhage in the preaortic and mesenteric regions. Anterior and posterior fasciae join medially (arrows) and enclose the perirenal spaces (*P*) bilaterally. Hemorrhage (*h*) in the left perirenal space extends from inferior preaortic spread of disease into the perirenal space rather than from spread in the superior central retroperitoneum (*C*). Asymmetric and nonpredictable spread of hemorrhage along the fat of the perirenal spaces is due to the presence of the barrier of multitier interlobular septa. **(b)** At the level of the left renal vein (*V*), hemorrhage extends from the central retroperitoneum (*C*) into the left perirenal space but barely into the right perirenal space. No distinct fascial barrier can be identified between the perirenal and central retroperitoneum. From there, hemorrhage extends superiorly and inferiorly **(a, c)**. Blood in the left perirenal space is contained laterally by the barrier of multitier interlobular septa. On the left, the anterior renal fascia (open arrows) provides a distinct border that separates the spread of blood in the perirenal space from the spread of hemorrhage into the retromesenteric region of the descending colon mesentery (*M*) in the anterior pararenal space. **(c)** Close-up of section caudal to **b**, below the lower pole of the kidney, shows portion of aortic aneurysm (*A*) and retroperitoneal hemorrhage. The renal fascia separates (open arrows) the perirenal space (*P*) from the central retroperitoneal collection (*C*). Hemorrhage (*H*) in the perirenal space extends inferiorly from lateral spread of hemorrhage at the level of the renal vessels.

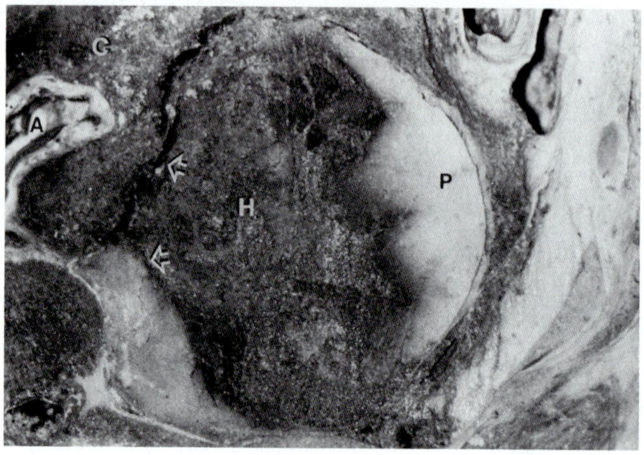

c.

150 mL of the latex was injected in each site according to the size of the cadaver and the resistance felt during injection. The injection of 10% acetic acid immediately followed the latex injection. This amount and sequence of injections was previously shown to be adequate to help determine retroperitoneal spread (3,13). The cadaveric cross sections were then refrozen. Anatomic dissection was performed at a later date, after rethawing.

Cadaveric cross sections.—The posterior abdominal fasciae (including the posterior parietal peritoneum, anterior and posterior renal fasciae) were also examined in cross sections of three unembalmed cadavers. In one cadaver, fortuitous hemorrhage from an unsuspected ruptured aortic aneurysm was found. The cadavers were frozen to −50°C, and the abdomens were transected at 3–5-cm intervals. The resultant 3–5-cm-thick slices were photographed on both the cephalic and caudal surfaces, and the posterior fasciae were traced on transparent films placed directly on the specimen. These transparencies were then retraced with a computer program (PCED; Jandel Scientific, Corte Madera, Calif), and the computer traces were reassembled into a single computer-generated image that portrayed the three-dimensional topography of the fascial planes (Fig 2). The sections were subsequently thawed and dissected.

Anatomic dissection and observation were performed by three investigators

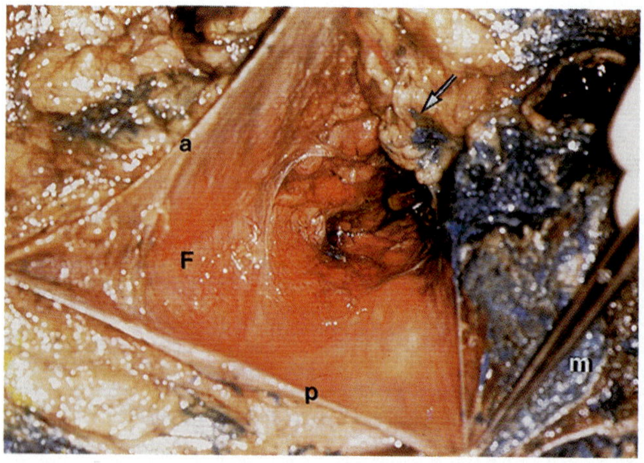

Figure 5. Close-up of cadaveric hemitorso transected at about the level of the renal hilum, seen from above after the right kidney and perirenal fat were removed. Glistening anterior (*a*) and posterior (*p*) renal fasciae (*F*) remain. Blue latex was injected into the central retroperitoneum posteriorly with a portion distributed into the psoas muscle (*m*). No fascia separates the perirenal space from the central retroperitoneum. Fat lobules and interlobular septa, which are partially stained blue, protrude in the perirenal space (arrow). Inferiorly, the anterior and posterior fasciae join to form an inverted cone.

(V.R., Q.F.L., S.C.M.) by consensus. The anatomic slides were reviewed by four observers (V.R., P.T., Q.F.L., S.C.M.) by consensus.

Clinical Study and CT Correlation

To provide CT correlation of cadaveric findings, the CT scans were reviewed of 111 consecutive patients with retroperitoneal disease seen at Beth Israel Hospital. The scans of 82 of those patients were selected on the basis of the presence of CT abnormalities in the central retroperitoneum or in either the right or left perirenal space. The extent and distribution of these CT abnormalities in these compartments and the appearance of the interposed renal fasciae and interlobular septa were noted. Assessments were made by two observers (V.R., T.G.V.) by consensus.

Among the 82 patients, 24 had presumed retroperitoneal hemorrhage, 37 had inflammation, and 21 had neoplastic conditions. Among the 24 patients with presumed retroperitoneal hemorrhage, 18 had a ruptured abdominal aortic aneurysm and six had spontaneous hemorrhage from renal carcinoma. Among the 37 patients with inflammation, 25 had pancreatitis with retroperitoneal spread, nine had renal inflammation or abscess with perirenal spread, and three had urinoma secondary to obstructing ureteral stones. Among the 21 patients with neoplastic conditions, 10 had renal carcinoma, two had non-Hodgkin lymphoma that involved the perirenal space, and seven had retroperitoneal spread of pancreatic cancer.

Among the 82 patients, potential for spread of disease (ie, disease present on either side of the border between the central retroperitoneum and either perirenal space) was noted in 128 instances (hemorrhage in 38 instances, inflammation in 56, and neoplasia in 34). The presumed diagnoses were based on clinical evidence. The presumed origin of disease was based on both clinical and CT findings. For instance, in a patient with renal cell carcinoma, the origin of disease was presumed to be in the ipsilateral perirenal space with potential for spread into the central retroperitoneum. Conversely, in a patient with pancreatitis, the origin of disease was considered to be in the central retroperitoneum with potential for spread into the perirenal space. If disease extended toward both renal hila, on either side of the retroperitoneal great vessels, potential for bilateral spread was considered. Although concurrent origins of disease in more than one compartment were theoretically possible (eg, multifocal hemorrhage in a patient with bleeding diathesis), such cases ($n = 8$) were excluded, on the basis of clinical judgment. Patients with Hodgkin disease and retroperitoneal lymphadenopathy and patients with retroperitoneal trauma or previous surgery were not included in the study.

The degree of severity of disease in each compartment was graded on a scale from 0 to 4 as follows: 0 = normal; 1 = linear strands; 2 = mixed, mostly linear strands and less homogeneous pattern; 3 = mixed, less linear and mostly homogeneous pattern; and 4 = homogeneous pattern. Distention of a space by disease was not considered in the grading of severity. Such appearance was generally present in cases of homogeneous involvement (score, 4), and its inclusion would create additional variables at the high end of the scale, which would create some imbalance. Assessment was performed separately for each right and left perirenal space and the central retroperitoneum. The difference in the appearance of involvement in neighboring spaces was calculated on a five-point scale and was considered as indicative of barrier (B): $B = S_O - S_S$, where S_O = grade at space of origin, and S_S = grade at space of spread. Complete permeability (no bar-

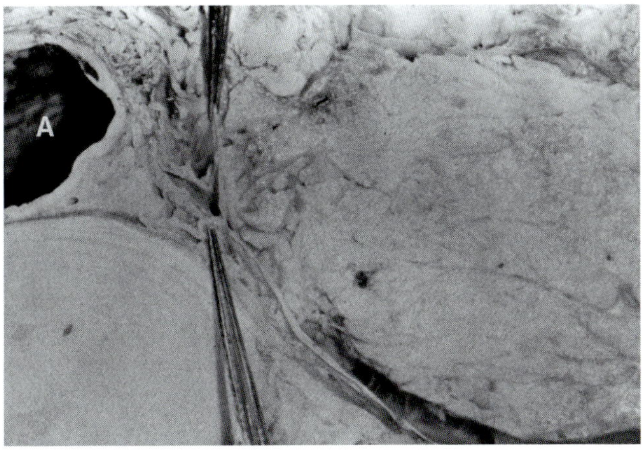

Figure 6. Specimen from axial cadaveric cross section shows a network of thick interlobular septa (two are held by surgical clamps) that surround the aorta (*A*). These septa form a variable barrier to spread of disease, and numerous septa with variable orientation produce a multitier barrier.

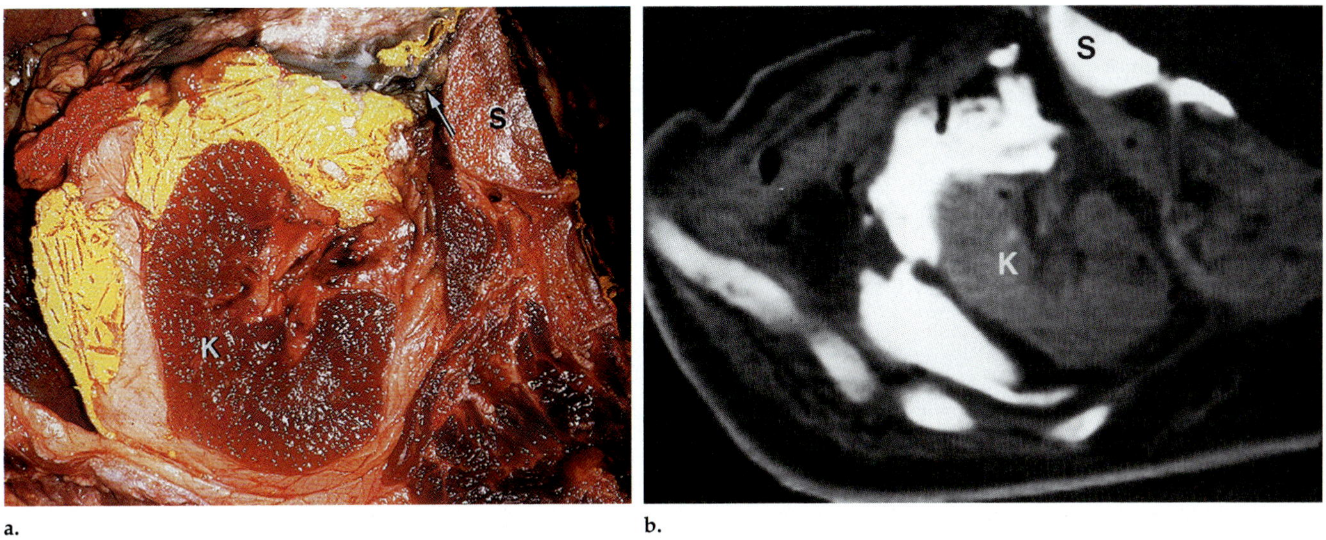

Figure 7. Yellow latex was mixed with 5% barium emulsion and injected into the right perirenal space. **(a)** Spread within the perirenal space, lateral to the kidney (*K*), is confined by interlobular septa, and only a droplet spreads medially, along the right renal vein (arrow) in front of spine (*S*). **(b)** CT scan in a hemitorso shows interlobular septa that confine perirenal spread of the barium-latex mixture in a pattern not uncommonly seen on CT scans obtained in patients with retroperitoneal disease. *K* = kidney, *S* = spine.

Figure 8. Close-up of cadaveric cross section with yellow latex injected into the perirenal space, anterior to the kidney. The latex is dispersed in a lacy pattern along and between interlobular septa. It reaches both the kidney (arrow) and the anterior renal fascia (*F*) but does not extend to the aorta (*A*). No distinct fascia limits the spread of latex to the central retroperitoneum.

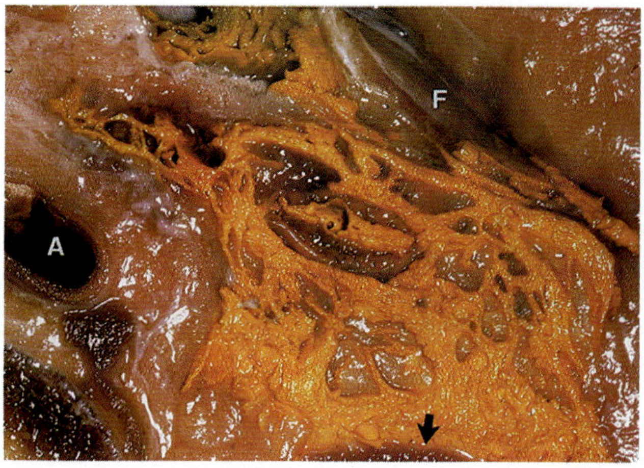

rier) was considered when disease severity was graded similarly in two neighboring compartments (B = 0). Complete barrier (no spread) was considered when $S_S = 0$ ($B = S_O$) and incomplete barrier (partial spread) when $S_O > S_S$.

Statistical Analysis

For nominal measurements, such as the presence or absence of spread of disease to either side of a potential barrier, the tables for χ^2 analysis of contingency were used. For differences in ordinal scale measurements, such as the grade for the severity of disease or the grade for the barrier to disease spread from one space to the other, the Wilcoxon signed-rank test was used. For comparison of spread or barrier between the left and right sides, the Mann-Whitney rank-sum test was used. A *P* value less than .05 was considered to indicate a statistically significant difference.

RESULTS

Anatomic Study

Conventional dissection.—The posterior renal fascia was seen to attach onto the psoas muscle (Fig 3a, 3b).

Centrally, the anterior renal fascia joined with the posterior renal fascia superiorly and inferiorly but not in the middle (Figs 2–4). Superiorly, the anterior and posterior renal fasciae join and attach to the crux of the ipsilateral hemidiaphragm (Fig 4a). Thus, the renal fasciae form a cone that contains part of the upper half of the ipsilateral kidney, adrenal gland, and perirenal fat.

Inferiorly, a slightly different process occurs. The two fasciae merge medially into a single fascia (Figs 1, 3c, 4c, 5). This single fascia extends medially and attaches at the aorta and vena cava or at the iliac vessels. On each side, the renal fasciae form an inverted cone that contains the lower pole of the ipsilateral kidney, ureter, and perirenal fat (13).

In the middle, and for a varying craniocaudal extent, the perirenal space remains "open" medially along most of the length of each kidney and in communication with the central retroperitoneum (Figs 2, 3b, 4b). Interlobular septa are present, however, that form an incomplete and variable connection between the anterior and posterior renal fascia (Fig 6). Although we did not survey these septa specifically, in our experience they are often imperceptible on CT scans obtained in healthy individuals, and they are analogous to the bridging septa described by Kunin (15) that divide the perirenal space into multiple subcompartments (Fig 7).

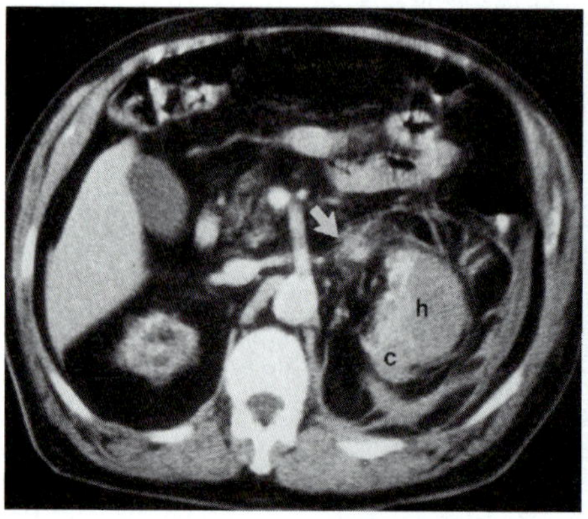

9.

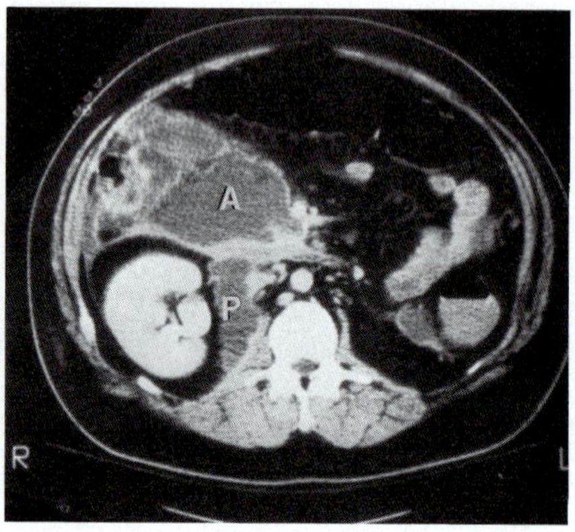

10.

Figures 9, 10. **(9)** Spontaneous subcapsular and perirenal hematoma in a 62-year-old man with renal cell carcinoma (*c*). CT scan depicts subcapsular hemorrhage (*h*) that compresses the kidney. In the perirenal space, hemorrhage extends along interlobular septa to the renal fascia. Medially, hemorrhage stops abruptly (arrow) and is confined in the perirenal space by thickened interlobular septa. **(10)** Retroperitoneal pancreatic fluid collection in a 29-year-old man with a 2-week history of pancreatitis. CT scan depicts fluid that extends into the anterior pararenal space (*A*) to the ascending colon. Fluid also extends into the medial portion of the perirenal space (*P*). In the perirenal space, spread stops abruptly, despite the absence of an anatomic fascial barrier. A similar barrier is formed medially, at the lateral edge of the inferior vena cava.

Table 2
Spread of Disease between Central Retroperitoneum and Perirenal Space

Grade of Disease	Space of Origin	Space of Spread of Disease 0	1	2	3	4	Total
None	0						0
Strands	1	**12**	**7**				19
Mixed, strands	2	**12**	1	**4**			17
Mixed, homogeneous	3	**30**	5	2	**7**		44
Homogeneous	4	**36**	2	1	4	**5**	48
Total		**90**	15	7	11	5	**128**

Note.—Data are number of instances of potential spread in 82 patients. Vertical boldface column denotes complete barrier (no permeability). Diagonal boldface column denotes no barrier (complete permeability). Numbers in between indicate partial barrier.

Latex injection followed by dissection.—Colored latex was seen to travel along the planes formed by the interlobular septa and by the renal great vessels (Fig 7). The interlobular septa acted as barriers to the free spread of latex from the perirenal space to the central

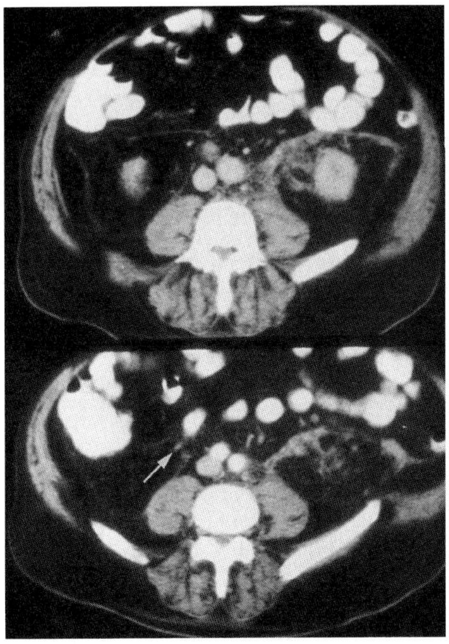

Figure 11. Resolving non-Hodgkin lymphoma in the left perirenal space in a 58-year-old man. Two axial CT scans obtained at the level of the lower pole of the kidney and below show thickening of the interlobular septa and anterior renal fascia. The perirenal space is closed, and strands are seen in the paraaortic region. On the right, nonthickened renal fasciae leave the perirenal space open medially. In the caudal section, the fasciae converge around the ureter (arrow), which closes the perirenal space.

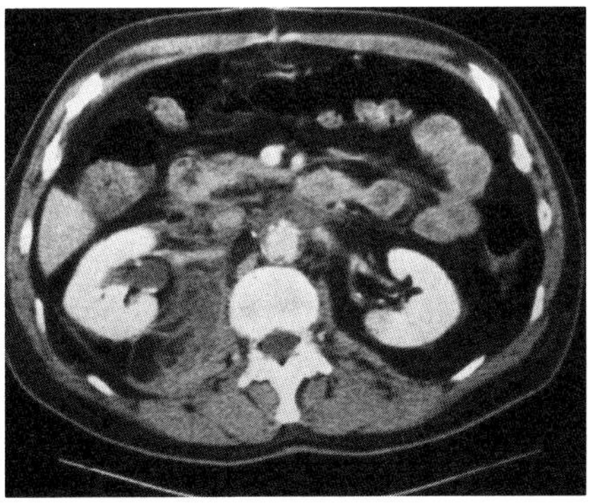

Figure 12. Forniceal rupture with resultant extravasation of urine in a 62-year-old man with right renal colic. Axial CT scan obtained at the level of the renal hilum shows spread of urine into the perirenal space and along interlobular septa. Posterior to the renal artery, there is no spread of disease into the central retroperitoneum. Posterior and anterior to the vena cava, septal thickening indicates a pathway into the periaortic region and a potential pathway from the right to the left perirenal space along the left renal artery. Despite the absence of an anatomic border, there is no spread of urine from the periaortic region into the left perirenal space.

retroperitoneum or from the central retroperitoneum to the perirenal space (Figs 5–8). Thus, we developed the concept of a septal pathway-barrier, which we tested in clinical studies.

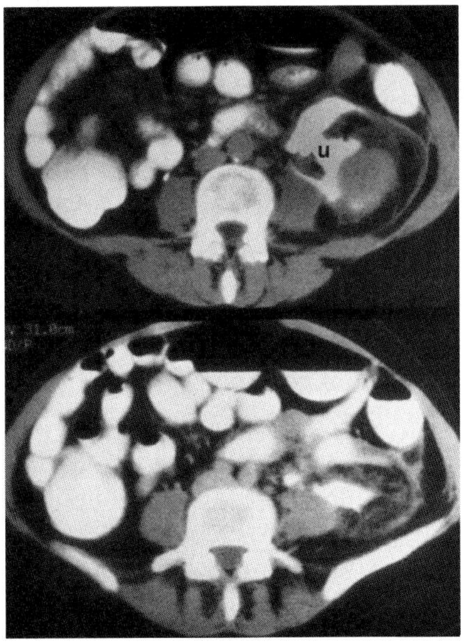

Figure 13. Urinoma (*u*) secondary to ureteral obstruction in a 38-year-old man. Axial CT scans show extravasation of opacified urine into the perirenal space that is confined medially around the ureters by the medial closure of the renal fasciae. There is no spread of opacified urine into the central retroperitoneum.

Clinical Study and CT Correlation

The CT scans obtained in the 82 patients showed 128 instances of potential spread of disease between the central retroperitoneum and either perirenal space. Actual spread was seen, however, in only 38 (30%) instances. Spread of disease occurred in 17 (45%) of the 38 patients with hemorrhage, in 10 (29%) of the 34 patients with neoplasia, and in 11 (20%) of the 56 patients with inflammation (Figs 9–11). The difference in this distribution was statistically significant ($P < .03$). Furthermore, the degree of spread (none [complete barrier, $S_S = 0$], partial [partial barrier, $S_O > S_S$], or free [no barrier, $S_O = S_S$]) differed with the disease category (Table 1). Differences were significant in comparisons among all three disease categories and between each combination of two of the three categories ($P < .003$, Pearson χ^2). In three patients, disease was seen in all three anatomic regions (right and left perirenal spaces and central retroperitoneum).

Differences in the barrier to spread of disease in 128 potential instances were also significant (Table 2). On a scale of 0–4, the median grade of disease at the space of origin (S_O) was 3 (range, 1–4) and at the space of spread (S_S) was 0 (range, 0–4) ($P < .001$). In 90 instances (70%), the barrier was complete ($B = S_O$ or $S_S = 0$). Among the cases in which there was spread of

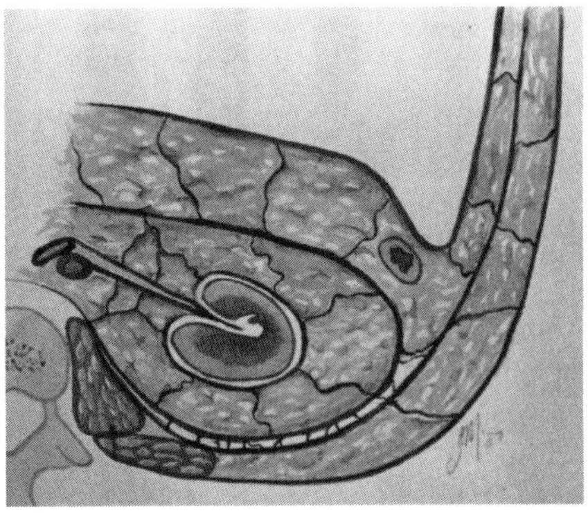

Figure 14. Diagram shows the multitier septal barrier-pathway concept. The parietal peritoneum and fasciae (thick black lines) form the boundaries of the retroperitoneal compartments. Interlobular septa (thin wavy lines) are not consistent and vary from patient to patient, and in our experience, increase in conspicuity at CT with increasing body weight. The interlobular septa act as incomplete barriers inside and between retroperitoneal compartments. Frequently, they may form a multitier septal barrier. Conversely, these septa act as pathways or conduits of disease, giving a lacy appearance to many retroperitoneal diseases.

disease from one of the three regions to another region ($n = 38$), differences in the grade of disease were also significant: The median grade at the space of origin was 3 (range, 1–4) and at the space of spread was 1 (range, 1–4) ($P < .001$). No differences were found, however, in comparisons of the spread of disease between the right or left perirenal space to the central retroperitoneum or from the central retroperitoneum to the right or left perirenal space.

On a scale of 0–4, the average grade of disease at the space of origin was 3.0 ± 1.3 (mean ± standard deviation) and at the space of spread was 1.4 ± 2.32. With the assumption that the grades are intervals (eg, grade 4 is twice as serious as grade 2 or grade 3 is three times as serious as grade 1), a paired *t* test was performed. The average difference (barrier) of 1.6 ± 0.32 (95% confidence interval, 1.06, 2.32) was statistically significant ($P < .001$).

Pathway-Barrier Theory

These results confirm the pathway-barrier theory. In the majority of cases (more than two-thirds of our cases), a complete barrier in spread of disease existed at the border of the perirenal spaces and the central retroperitoneum. In cases of spread of disease, disease was less severe in the space of spread compared with in the space of origin. Disease spread was facilitated along the interlobular septa and the renal vessels (Fig 12). Conversely, roughly parallel septa acted as a multitier barrier to spread of disease. Similarly, within the perirenal space, Kunin (15) already described bridging septa that limit the spread of pus or tamponade within the perirenal space. Craniocaudal spread of disease was also determined by the presence of similar interlobular septa (Figs 4, 13). Understanding of these pathway-barriers is facilitated by considering both the interlobular septa and the fasciae as three-dimensional planes (6) (Fig 5).

DISCUSSION

There is some disagreement and confusion concerning the continuity of the perirenal spaces and the central retroperitoneum. According to Gerota (4), the anterior renal fascia crosses over the aorta and vena cava to the contralateral side (Fig 1). Somogyi et al (8) found such communication of extravasated urine on CT scans obtained after blunt trauma. Experimentally at CT, Kneeland et al (9) found evidence of contralateral spread of water-soluble contrast material injected in the perirenal spaces of cadavers. This communication, however, is not accepted by others (1,12,16). In particular, Meyers (1) and Martin (16) maintain that the anterior renal fascia is fused with the connective tissue around the great vessels and disrupts the communication of the two perirenal spaces.

Our observations support both views. At the level of the renal hilum and along most of the length of the kidneys, the anterior renal fascia extends medially in front of and attaches onto the central great vessels (Fig 3). The width of these vessels does not fill in the central retroperitoneum, however, which allows communication between the two perirenal spaces. On clinical images, however, this communication is not commonly seen, and contralateral spread of disease was seen in only three instances in our series.

Although the connection between the two perirenal spaces is controversial, a distinct border has not been described, to our knowledge. The transition between the central retroperitoneum and either perirenal space is continuous and uninterrupted and our data confirm previous observations of the absence of a separation by a distinct fascial or other landmark throughout most of the length of the kidneys (1,4,8,9,12,16). Superiorly and inferiorly we found a distinct anatomic separation made by the juncture of the anterior and posterior renal fasciae with the perirenal space, which forms a cone superiorly and an inverted cone inferiorly (Figs 3, 5).

In the middle craniocaudal dimension, the anterior and posterior renal fasciae do not join centrally and a barrier is provided by the interlobular septa (Fig 14). These interlobular septa act as either a pathway or an anatomic barrier. Their action is slightly different from that in interfascial spread of disease, in which the renal fascia acts as a conduit for spread of disease from the anterior pararenal space (3). In cases of disease spread, these interlobular septa facilitate spread not only in the perirenal space (15) but also throughout the central retroperitoneum. Conversely, the septa may react and thicken and, thus, act as pathophysiologic barriers. This explains why hemorrhage, which is usually acute and expansive, spreads more readily than other conditions (eg, neoplasm, infection). In 45% of our 38 cases of hemorrhage, spread was seen though the juncture of the perirenal space and central retroperitoneum. Reaction to inflammation and neoplasia produced a more effective barrier, with spread seen in 20% of 56 and 29% of 34 cases, respectively. Once spread occurred, the quantity was reduced more often in cases of inflammation than in cases of hemorrhage. In general, disease spread appeared to be facilitated by reaction (as in inflammation) or dissection (as in hemorrhage) along fascial and septal planes. In contrast, no partial spread was noted in tumors, presumably owing to the destructive power of neoplasia.

This variability in degree of retroperitoneal spread according to underlying disease has also been observed in experimental studies of cadaveric injections and in clinical situations (13,17). This may explain the prompt retroperitoneal distribution of air (the most permeable substance) after presacral insufflation before retroperitoneal pneumography, when gas distributed into the perirenal space allowed visualization of the adrenal glands at plain radiography in the abdomen. It may also help resolve an apparent controversy about the retroperitoneal spread of cadaveric injections: More extensive retroperitoneal spread has been observed of directly injected water-soluble contrast material (9,13) than of the thicker latex solutions (17).

We conclude that multitier interlobular septa along the length of the kidney, at the medial perirenal space, act as a barrier or pathway to restrict the spread of disease from the perirenal space to the central retroperitoneum or from the central retroperitoneum to the perirenal space. ■

References

1. Meyers MA. The extraperitoneal spaces: normal and pathologic anatomy. In: Dynamic radiology of the abdomen: normal and pathologic anatomy. 4th ed. New York, NY: Springer-Verlag, 1994; 219–239.
2. Korobkin M, Silverman PM, Quint LE, Francis IR. CT of the extraperitoneal spaces: normal anatomy and fluid collections. AJR 1992; 159:933–941.
3. Raptopoulos V, Kleinman PK, Marks S Jr, Snyder M, Silverman P. Renal fascial pathway: posterior extension of pancreatic effusions within the anterior pararenal space. Radiology 1986; 158:367–374.
4. Gerota D. Beitrñge zur kenntniss des befestigungsapparates der niere. Arch Anat Physiol Anat Abstr 1895; 19:256–285.
5. Moss AA, Bush WH. The kidneys. In: Moss AA, Gamsu G, Genant HK, eds. Computed tomography of the body. 2nd ed. Vol 3. Philadelphia, Pa: Saunders, 1992; 933–1017.
6. Molmenti EP, Balfe DM, Kanterman RY, Bennet HF. Anatomy of the retroperitoneum: observations of the distribution of pathologic fluid collections. Radiology 1996; 200:95–103.
7. Lei QF, Marks SC Jr, Touliopoulos P, Raptopoulos V. Fascial planes and compartments of the posterior abdomen: the perirenal and pararenal pathways. Clin Anat 1990; 3:1–15.
8. Somogyi J, Cohen WN, Omar MM, Makhuli Z. Communication of right and left perirenal spaces demonstrated by computed tomography. J Comput Assist Tomogr 1979; 3:270–273.
9. Kneeland JB, Augh YH, Rubenstein WA, et al. Perirenal spaces: CT evidence for communication across the midline. Radiology 1987; 164:657–664.
10. Kenney PJ, Panicek DM, Witanowski LS. Computed tomography of ureteral disruption. J Comput Assist Tomogr 1977; 11:480–484.
11. Siegel MJ, Balfe DM. Blunt renal and ureteral trauma in childhood: CT patterns of fluid collections. AJR 1989; 152:1043–1047.
12. Feldberg MAM, Koehler PR, van Waes PFGM. Psoas compartment disease studied by computed tomography. Radiology 1983; 148:505–512.
13. Raptopoulos V, Lei QF, Touliopoulos P, Vrachliotis TG, Marks SC Jr. Why perirenal disease does not extend into the pelvis: the importance of closure of the cone of the renal fascia. AJR 1995; 164:1179–1184.
14. Marks SC Jr, Raptopoulos V, Kleinman P, Snyder M. The anatomical basis for retrorenal extensions of pancreatic effusions: the role of the renal fasciae. Surg Radiogr Anat 1986; 8:89–97.
15. Kunin M. Bridging septa of the perinephric space: anatomic, pathologic, and diagnostic considerations. Radiology 1986; 158: 361–365.
16. Martin CP. Anatomical notes: a note on the renal fascia. J Anat 1942; 77:101–103.
17. Mindell HJ, Mastromatteo JF, Dickey KW, et al. Anatomic communications between the three retroperitoneal spaces: determination by CT-guided injections of contrast material in cadavers. AJR 1995; 164:1173–1178.

Joachim Berkefeld, MD • Johannes Kirchner, MD • Hans Michael Müller, MD
Ullrich Fries, MD • Jürgen Kollath, MD

Balloon Dacryocystoplasty: Indications and Contraindications[1]

PURPOSE: To define the indications and contraindications for balloon dacryocystoplasty.

MATERIALS AND METHODS: Eighty-five patients with severe epiphora due to partial (n = 47) or complete (n = 38) obstruction of the nasolacrimal duct (NLD) were treated with balloon dacryocystoplasty (DCP). Steerable micro–guide wires with flexible tips were used. Success rates of DCP were evaluated clinically and dacryocystographically during the acute phase and at 6- and 12-month follow-up. Failures and recurrences were correlated with clinical and dacryocystographic indications for treatment.

RESULTS: Recanalization was successful in 35 (92%) of 38 patients with isolated focal stenoses (n = 20) or short-distance occlusions (n = 18) of the NLD. Among all 85 patients, recanalization was successful in 25 patients (66%) with complete and 37 patients (79%) with partial obstructions. In the absence of the main predictors for recurrent obstructions (ie, active inflammation, filling defects due to calculi, long-distance occlusions, and posttraumatic lesions), 12-month patency rates were 89% (17 of 19 focal stenoses) and 94% (15 of 16 focal occlusions). Otherwise, reobstruction rate was 46% (12 of 26 cases).

CONCLUSION: Balloon dacryocystoplasty is successful only in select cases. To achieve results comparable to those of operative treatment, the indication should be limited to patients with circumscribed focal stenoses or occlusions of the NLD. Active dacryocystitis, dacryocystolithiasis, and posttraumatic lesions are the main contraindications.

Since 1990, the interventional method of fluoroscopically guided balloon dacryocystoplasty (DCP) for recanalization of obstructed tear ducts has been described (1). In patients with severe epiphora (ie, watering of the eyes), dilation of stenotic lesions of the lacrimal draining system was proposed as an alternative to operative treatment (1–4). Several studies showed the feasibility of the new technique (1–5), which is based on the passage of a guide wire through the lacrimal ducts followed by balloon dilation at the site of obstruction. Technical and clinical success rates between 59% and 90% have been described in the literature (1–6). Lee et al (6)—although leading in the development of tear-duct interventions—were the first to publish rather disappointing results, with technical failure rates of DCP procedures between 29% and 41% and even higher recurrence rates between 45% and 80% in a 2-year follow-up. Consequently, the investigators from that group suggested primary stent placement for tear-duct obstructions instead of balloon dilation (7,8).

Similar to Ilgit et al (2) and Janssen et al (3), we tried to improve the recanalization procedure with the use of flexible, steerable guide wires, instead of stiff instruments, to minimize the trauma to the ductal structures and thus obtain better results.

The purpose of this larger pilot study was a wider clinical application of balloon DCP to discover appropriate indications and contraindications. In particular, we analyzed cases with technical and clinical failures or recurrences to determine possible influencing factors that would enable prediction of a positive or negative outcome after balloon dilation of tear-duct stenoses. Before controlled randomized studies for the comparison between interventional and operative treatment could be started, this step seemed to be necessary.

MATERIALS AND METHODS

Between 1993 and 1996, 85 patients (49 women, 36 men; age range, 21–86 years; mean age, 51 years) were treated with balloon DCP. All patients had severe, grade 4 or 5 epiphora (according to the scale of Munk et al [1]) that necessitated dabbing with a handkerchief more than 10 times a day or caused permanent complaints. In all cases, conservative treatment with decongestant eyedrops, irrigation, and probing had failed.

For diagnostic purposes, digital subtraction dacryocystography (9) with a distention technique (10) was performed. After intubation of the lower canaliculus, a 22-gauge Teflon cannula was advanced into the common canaliculus to minimize reflux. Water-soluble, nonionic contrast material (iopromide, Ultravist 300; Schering, Berlin, Germany) was injected perma-

Index terms: Lacrimal gland and duct, 223.1492 • Lacrimal gland and duct, interventional procedure, 223.126

Abbreviations: DCP = dacryocystoplasty, NLD = nasolacrimal duct.

Radiology 1997; 205:785–790

[1] From the Institute of Neuroradiology (J.B.), Institute of Diagnostic Radiology (J. Kirchner, J. Kollath), and the Clinic of Ophthalmology (H.M.M., U.F.), Johann Wolfgang Goethe University, Schleusenweg 2-16, 60528 Frankfurt am Main, Germany. From the 1996 RSNA scientific assembly. Received May 21, 1997; revision requested June 19; revision received July 28; accepted August 4. **Address reprint requests to** J.B.

nently during the acquisition of the digital subtraction dacryocystographic series (posteroanterior projection; frame rate, one per second). Thus, a widening of the lacrimal draining system could be achieved to distinguish functional narrowings from fixed stenotic lesions. The site of obstruction was described according to anatomic landmarks (Table 1). Short-distance focal obstructions, confined to one anatomic region, were distinguished from long-distance diffuse lesions that covered the entire length of the nasolacrimal duct (NLD) or lacrimal sac. Furthermore, isolated NLD or junctional obstructions were distinguished from multiple lesions with additional stenoses of the canaliculi or the lacrimal sac.

To describe the morphologic results of the DCP procedures, we measured the degree of stenoses in a manner similar to the evaluation of carotid artery stenoses according to the criteria of the North American Symptomatic Carotid Endarterectomy Trial Collaborators, or NASCET (11): The percentage of stenosis was defined in relationship to the diameter of normally distended parts in the midportion of the NLD. The anatomic narrowings at the inlet and outlet of the NLD were not used for reference measurements. Only symptomatic patients with high-grade obstructions with more than 70% narrowing of the luminal diameter or complete obstructions were considered for DCP. Prestenotic dilatation and impairment of flow with reflux of contrast material through the canaliculi were further criteria to assume a severe high-grade stenosis. To avoid the risk of laceration of the small-caliber canaliculi, canalicular stenoses or stenoses in the upper portion of the lacrimal sac were not dilated (1).

Preinterventional dacryocystography showed 47 partial and 38 complete obstructions of the NLD or at the junction between the lacrimal sac and NLD. Most frequently, idiopathic obstructions ($n = 61$) were treated; these obstructions probably represented residuals after dacryocystitis. At the time of DCP, however, no active inflammation was present in these patients.

Despite clinical signs of chronic but still active dacryocystitis, DCP was performed in 13 patients in the initial phase of our experience with the idea to improve lacrimal drainage by removing tight stenoses.

Focal lesions at the outlet of the NLD near the valve of Hasner ($n = 6$) were probably related to inborn narrowings. In five cases, obstruction was caused by facial fractures or iatrogenic trauma to the NLD during maxillary sinus surgery.

All DCP procedures were performed on an outpatient basis with topical anesthesia. Two to three proxymetacaine eyedrops (Proparakain-POS 0.5%; Ursapherm, Bübingen, Germany) were applied to the eyelids and 1 mL was injected into the canaliculi. The nasal mucosa was also anesthestized. Our recanalization technique is similar to the approach described by Ilgit et al (2). After widening the puncta, a 22- or 24-gauge Teflon cannula (Terumo, Tokyo, Japan) was introduced into one of the canaliculi, preferably the upper canaliculus. A 0.016-inch steerable micro–guide wire (Stubbie; Target, Fremont, Calif) with a short flexible tip or alternatively a 0.014-inch wire with hydrophilic coating (Transend EX; Medi-tech/Boston Scientific, Watertown, Mass) was advanced through the cannula into the lacrimal sac. Only in cases of failure of the flexible instrument ($n = 12$) did we use the stiffer, ball-tip wire (Cook, Bloomington, Ind) used by Song et al (4). Under fluoroscopic control, the guide wire and cannula were angled upward and pushed forward into the NLD. After passage of the NLD, the curved distal end of the wire was manipulated out of the nasal cavity under lateral fluoroscopic control. A 3-mm percutaneous transluminal angioplasty balloon (Viper; Medi-tech/Boston Scientific) was introduced over the wire from a nasal approach. Dilation with pressures up to 8 atm for 1–2 minutes was performed at the site of obstruction.

After DCP, the patients were treated with decongestant eyedrops (xylometazoline hydrochloride, Otrivin; Dispersa, Germering, Germany) for 5 days (one drop three times per day). In the presence of inflammatory changes, antibiotic eyedrops (gentamicin, Refobacin; Merck, Darmstadt, Germany) were administered four times per day.

For morphologic evaluation of the DCP result, dacryocystograms obtained immediately after balloon dilation were compared with the findings on preinterventional dacryocystograms. Clinical and dacryocystographic reevaluation followed at intervals of 6 and 12 months after the procedure.

For partial and complete obstructions, full success of dacryocystoplasty was defined as less than 30% residual stenosis on distention dacryocystograms after balloon dilation. Partial response was defined as improvement but presence of a residual stenosis of more than 30%. Recurrences were assumed in patients with a restenosis of more than 70% or with reocclusion.

Clinical categories for the evaluation were (*a*) complete disappearance of symptoms, (*b*) minor temporary epiphora grade 1–2 (according to the Munk scale) necessitating dabbing with a handkerchief less than five times a day, (*c*) unchanged symptoms, and (*d*) worsening. Technical, dacryocystographic, and clinical circumstances of cases with technical failures or recurrences were analyzed to determine possible factors influencing the outcome after DCP procedures.

RESULTS

In the 47 patients with partial obstruction, dacryocystography showed clinically relevant (>70%) narrowing of the lumen of the NLD often combined with prestenotic dilatation and impairment of flow. In 23 of these patients, the lower lacrimal sac and the junction between the lacrimal sac and NLD were also involved. Isolated circumscribed NLD or junctional stenoses were found in 20 patients, and 27 patients showed multiple or diffuse lesions. In addition to junctional or NLD stenoses, dacryocystograms in nine patients showed marked presaccal strictures of the canaliculi. In 11 patients, the upper portion of the lacrimal sac was involved. Diffuse stenoses of the lacrimal draining system were present in 13 patients. Intraluminal filling defects at the level of the lacrimal sac or the NLD were visible on the dacryocystograms in nine patients.

Of the 38 patients with complete obstruction, 18 showed short-distance focal occlusions of the distal NLD. A stump of the proximal NLD was still visible. The entire NLD was occluded

Table 1
Dacryocystographic Findings

Site and Morphology of Obstruction	No. of Patients
Partial obstructions of the NLD	47
Focal stenoses of NLD or junction*	20
Multiple or diffuse stenoses of NLD or junction*	13
Additional stenoses	
Upper lacrimal sac	11
Canaliculi	9
Filling defects	9
Complete obstructions of the NLD	38
Short-distance (distal NLD)	18
Long-distance (entire NLD)	20
Additional stenoses	
Upper lacrimal sac	5
Canaliculi	6
Filling defects	5

* Junction = the junction between the lacrimal sac and the NLD.

Table 2
Technical Factors in DCP for Partial and Complete Obstructions

Factor	No. of Patients*
Partial obstructions ($n = 47$)	
Overall technical success	37 (79)
Normal lumen	30
Residual stenosis	7
Technical failures	10 (21)
Causes of technical failures	
Canalicular and saccal strictures	8
Dacryolith	1
Elastic recoil	1
Complete obstructions ($n = 38$)	
Overall technical success	25 (66)
Normal lumen	22
Residual stenosis	3
Technical failures	13 (34)
Causes of technical failures	
Long-distance rigid lesions	7
Short-distance rigid lesions	2
Canalicular and saccal stenoses	4

* Numbers in parentheses are percentages.

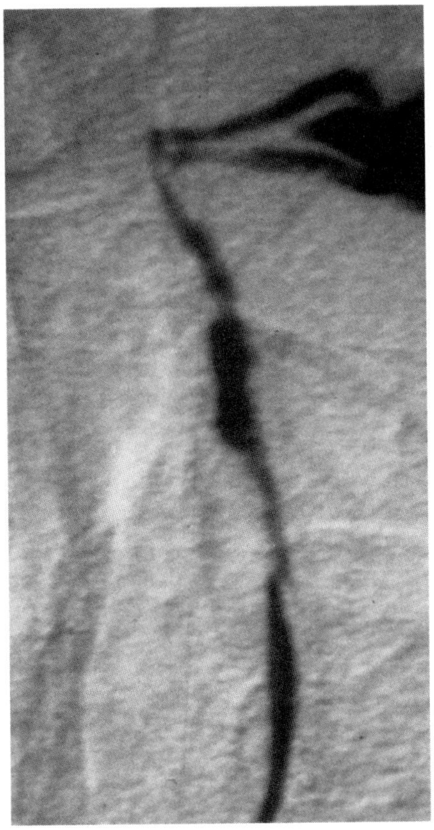

Figure 1. Digital substraction dacryocystogram in a patient with permanent epiphora shows diffuse strictures of the common canaliculus, lacrimal sac, and large parts of the NLD. Recanalization by means of balloon DCP was attempted. The narrow space in the upper saccal region together with an acute angle between canaliculi and lacrimal sac made the passage of flexible and ball-tip guide wires impossible.

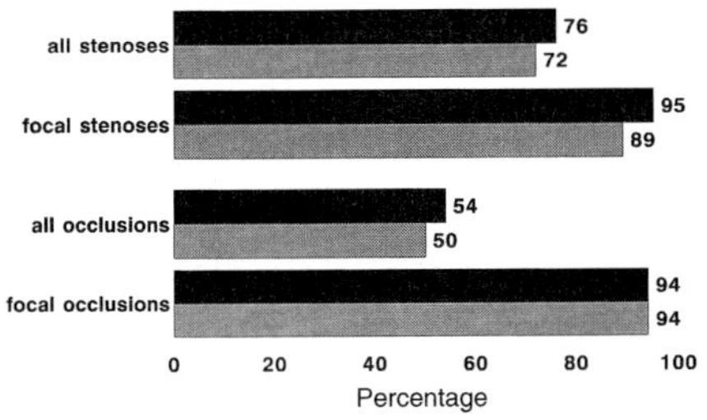

Figure 2. Patency rates (represented by the numbers at the end of the bars) of the lacrimal draining system 6 (black bars) and 12 (gray bars) months after successful DCP in patients with partial (n = 37) or complete (n = 26) obstruction of the NLD. Most of the recurrences occurred during the first 6 months. The results for a mixed spectrum of indications (*all stenosis* or *all occlusions*) are compared with the results in cases of focal lesions in the absence of contraindications such as dacryocystitis, calculi, or traumatic changes.

Table 3
Six-month Patency and Recurrence Rates after DCP for Partial and Complete Obstructions

Characteristic	No. of Patients*
Partial obstructions (n = 37)	
Overall patency	28 (76)
Recurrences	9 (24)
Restenosis	8
Reocclusion	1
Recurrences related to	
Dacryoliths	4
Active dacryocystitis	2
Multiple or diffuse lesions	2
Unclear	1
Complete obstructions (n = 26)	
Overall patency	14 (54)
Recurrences	12 (46)
Reocclusions	10
Restenoses	2
Recurrences related to	
Long-distance lesions	6
Short-distance lesions	1
Bony narrowings	3
Dacryoliths	2

* Numbers in parentheses are percentages.

in the other 20 cases. Canalicular stenoses were demonstrable on dacryocystograms in six patients; five patients had strictures of the upper lacrimal sac. Filling defects in the lumen of the lacrimal sac were visible in five patients (Table 1).

In 47 patients with partial obstructions (Table 2), recanalization was technically successful in 37 patients (79%). After DCP, 32 patients showed a normal luminal diameter or minor (<30%) residual stenosis. Dacryocystographic improvement but residual stenosis up to 50% was visible in five patients. Causes of technical failure were (*a*) stenoses of the presaccal canaliculi or the upper lacrimal sac (n = 8), (*b*) obstruction of the entrance of the NLD by dacryoliths (n = 1), and (*c*) elastic recoil after dilation (n = 1). Figure 1 shows a case of diffuse strictures of the lacrimal draining system including a upper saccal stenosis. Guide-wire placement failed due to the narrow space for manipulation and acute angles between the canaliculi and the lacrimal sac.

Among the 38 patients with complete obstruction (Table 2), recanalization was technically successful in only 25 (66%). A normal lumen or minor (<30%) residual stenoses could be demonstrated in 22 cases and three postinterventional dacryocystograms showed residual stenoses up to 70%. Causes of technical failures were (*a*) the rigidity of the lesion (n = 9) and (*b*) the presence of canalicular and saccal stenoses (n = 4).

In 37 patients with partial obstruction and successful DCP, follow-up dacryocystograms showed long-term patency rates of 76% after 6 months and 73% after 12 months (Fig 2). In focal, circumscribed junctional or NLD stenoses without concomitant dacryocystitis, dacryolithiasis, or bony narrowing (n = 18), 6- and 12-month patency rates were 94% and 89%, respectively. Twenty-six patients with former complete obstruction showed patency rates of 54% after 6 months and 50% after 12 months (Fig 2). In 16 patients with focal short-distance occlusions of the distal portion of the NLD, only one recurrence was observed during the 1st year (patency rate, 94%).

Evaluation of the overall patency rates showed that most of the recurrences occurred during the first 6 months. Therefore, the 6-month results were analyzed in more detail: Of the nine patients with recurrence of partial obstructions (24%), one patient showed worsening of the degree of stenosis on dacryocystograms and showed a complete obstruction of the NLD. The recurrent strictures in the other eight patients were unchanged in comparison to the status before DCP. Probable influencing factors for the occurrence of reobstructions (Table 3) were the presence of filling defects on preinterventional dacryocystograms in four patients. In three of these patients, dacryolithiasis was proved with ultrasound (US) examinations of the lacrimal sac and at surgery (Fig 3).

In two patients with restenoses, recurrent episodes of active dacryocystitis were observed. Another two recurrences were associated with multiple or diffuse strictures. Only one of 18 circumscribed NLD or junctional stenoses showed a reobstuction during the first 6 months after DCP.

After dilation of complete obstructions (Table 3), 12 (46%) of 26 patients showed recurrences with reocclusions (n = 10) and high-grade restenoses (n = 2). Six reocclusions occurred after recanalization of long-distance and rigid lesions that covered the entire NLD. To pass the lesion, forceful advancement of the guide wire was necessary in each of these cases.

Figure 4 shows an example of recurrent obstruction after forceful recanalization. In two patients, a via falsa (ie, a wrong channel outside the anatomic course of the NLD that was created at DCP) was obvious on follow-up dacryocystograms.

Only one reobstruction was observed in 16 recanalized cases with short-distance occlusions of the distal NLD (Fig 5). Of the five patients with bony narrowings due to facial trauma, three had recurrent obstructions during the first 6 months. Proved dacryolithiasis was probably involved in the development of reobstruction in two patients. Additionally, one of them had recurrent episodes of dacryocystitis.

The clinical results generally corresponded to the dacryocystographic findings. After 6 months, 24 (65%) of the 37 patients with partial obstructions were free of epiphora after successful DCP. Six patients (16%) showed a clear improvement with minor temporary complaints. Because of recurrences, the condition of five patients (14%) was unchanged in comparison to their status before DCP, and and the condition of two patients (5%) worsened. Of the 26 patients with complete obstruction, 12 patients (46%) were free from symptoms, two patients (8%) improved, 11 patients (42%) showed no relevant change, and the condition of one patient (4%) worsened.

Except for the case that showed a change from a partial to a complete obstruction, which may be related to the DCP procedure, no side effects with serious clinical consequences occurred. During guide-wire manipulation or balloon inflation, 58 of the 85 patients reported a slight to moderate temporary pain, which was well tolerated. Eight patients complained of severe, less tolerable pain during the procedure; six of them had clinical signs of active or subacute dacryocystitis. Minor bleeding from the nasal cavity or the lacrimal punctum was observed in 24 patients. All pain and bleeding episodes resolved spontaneously at the end of DCP without any further treatment. Thirty-two patients showed a delayed clinical improvement probably due to postprocedural swelling of the ductal mucosa. During the 1st week, they had major residual epiphora, which resolved completely within 5 days.

Among the technical complications, two cases of iatrogenic via falsa that occurred during the recanalization procedure need to be mentioned. After disruption of the bony wall of the ductal lumen, the wrong channel was dilated. One of these patients became free of symptoms, and one had a recurrent occlusion after 4 months. In two patients, fragments of a broken guide wire had to be endoscopically extracted out of the inferior nasal meatus. After attempted DCP, no clinical worsening was observed in patients with technical failures, and operative dacryocystorhinostomy was not impeded.

DISCUSSION

A wide clinical application of DCP in our pilot study and the experiences

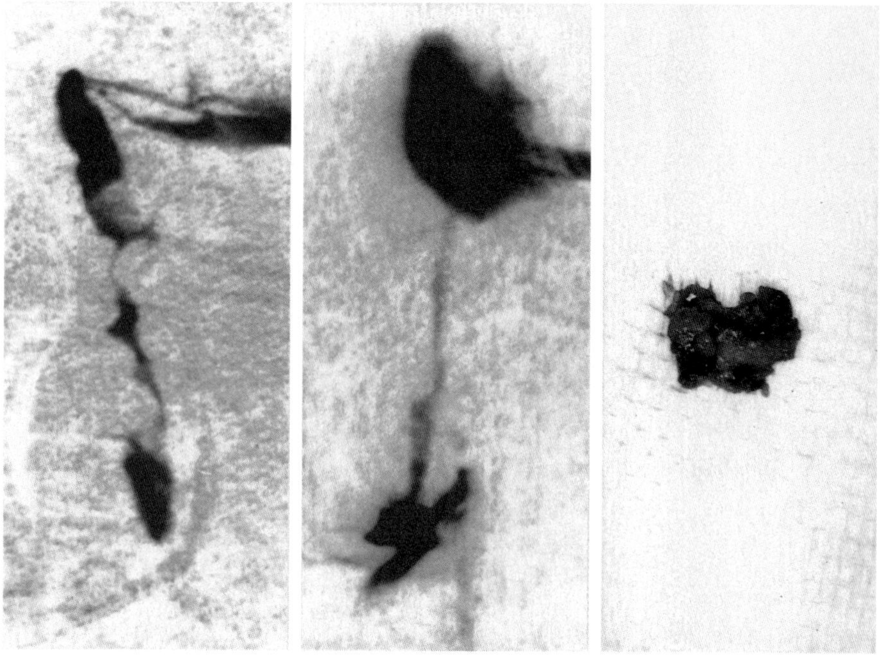

a. b. c.

Figure 3. **(a)** Preinterventional dacryocystogram shows a filling defect in the lower lacrimal sac and diffuse stenosis of the NLD after chronic dacryocystitis. **(b)** After DCP, distention dacryocystogram shows that the ductal lumen has smoother contours, but diffuse narrowing and impairment of flow with massive reflux of contrast material through the canaliculi is still demonstrable. Clinical symptoms did not resolve completely. After a short period with minor complaints, severe grade 5 epiphora recurred within 6 weeks. **(c)** Photograph of a large dacryolith that obstructed the entrance of the NLD; it had been removed surgically.

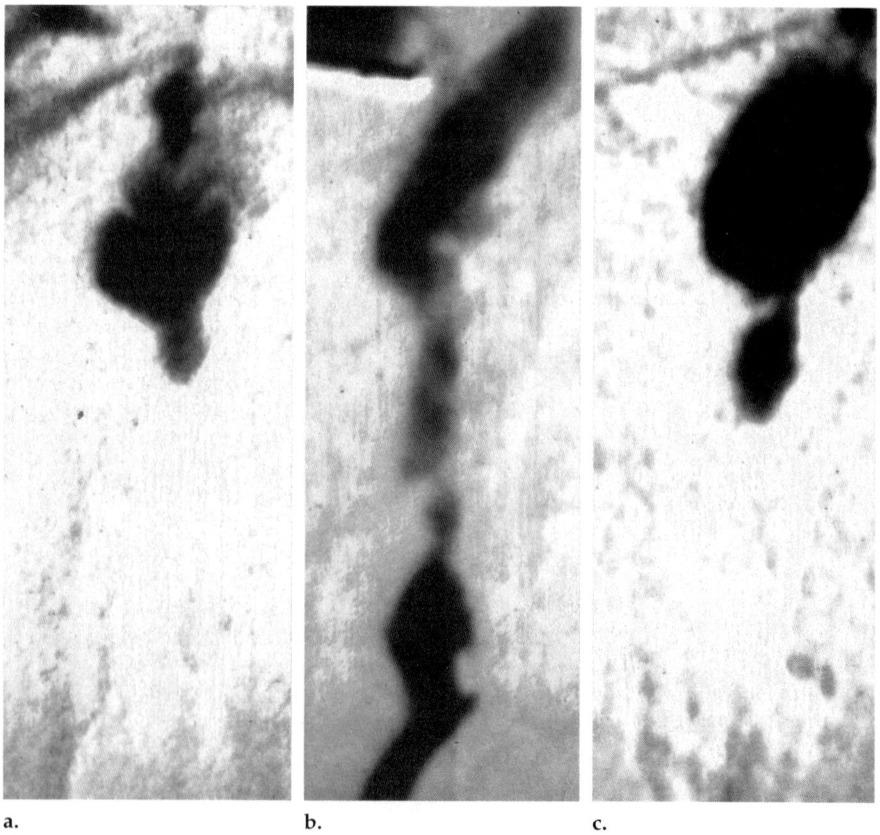

a. b. c.

Figure 4. **(a)** Preinterventional dacryocystogram shows complete chronic obstruction of the NLD. During recanalization, the guide wire had to be advanced forcefully because of high rigidity of the lesion. **(b)** Dacryocystogram obtained after dilation shows that patency of the NLD was reestablished, with a residual stenosis of the distal part. **(c)** Six-month follow-up dacryocystogram shows a reocclusion at the same location.

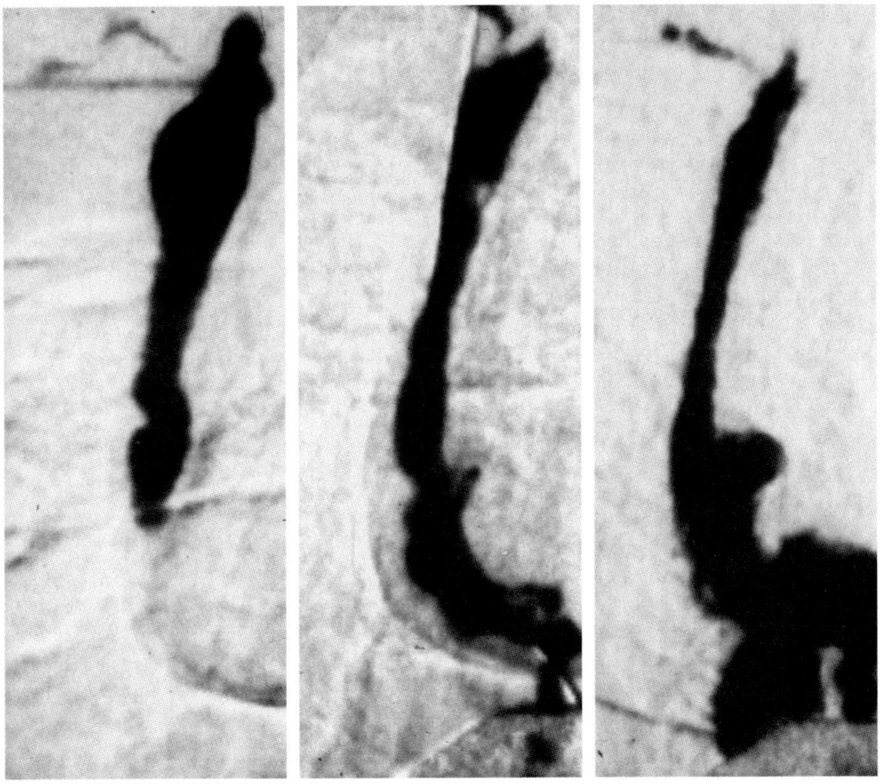

a. b. c.

Figure 5. **(a)** Preinterventional dacryocystogram shows short-distance focal occlusion of the distal NLD at the level of the valve of Hasner in a patient with severe epiphora. **(b)** Dacryocystogram obtained after balloon dilation shows that the lumen is widely patent and a good flow of contrast material through the lacrimal pathways into the inferior nasal meatus can be demonstrated. The patient became free of symptoms. **(c)** Twelve-month follow-up dacryocystogram shows no evidence of recurrence. Likewise, there was no clinical evidence of recurrence at 12-month follow-up.

of other authors (2,6) show that interventional recanalization of tear-duct obstructions has some disadvantages due to technical failures or frequent recurrences. The results of the analysis of the technical part of the procedure indicated two major difficulties in the passage of the lacrimal draining system with catheters and guide wires. First, overcoming presaccal and upper saccal strictures, and second, recanalizing long-distance rigid occlusions that involve the entire length of the NLD.

Strictures of the canaliculi and the upper lacrimal sac can be a serious obstacle for the passage of steerable guide wires. When flexible systems are used, the floppy tip of the wire gets stuck or coiled in the small lumen of the lacrimal sac and cannot be advanced into the NLD. Janssen et al (3) developed a 4.7-F tear-duct catheter for the guidance of wires. In our experience, this device is too large in diameter and may cause laceration of stenotic canaliculi. As a guiding cannula for the wire, we found a 22- or 24-gauge plastic sheath of a catheter needle to be advantageous. Together with flexible 0.016- or 0.014-inch micro–guide wires, these thin-caliber instruments ensure a minimally traumatic approach to the NLD. The relatively stiff, ball-tip wire developed by Song et al (4) can easily be angled to manipulate the tip into the lacrimal sac and the junction between the sac and the NLD. The rigid tip, however, makes the smooth passage of stenotic lesions difficult and may increase the risk of via falsa or ductal wall damage. Goo et al (12) tried to dilate even presaccal obstructions. The experiences are limited, and high recurrence rates up to 60%–70% were reported. The risk of canalicular occlusion caused by laceration or recurrent stenosis seems to be high. Operative reconstruction may be difficult in such cases (13), and at present dilation of canalicular stenoses cannot be recommended.

The rigidity of many complete obstructions of the NLD necessitates stiff instruments, which can be advanced forcefully. The concept of minimal traumatization is not always applicable in these instances. Via falsa or damage of the ductal wall cannot be averted in all cases and may be one cause of unfavorable long-term results in long-distance rigid occlusions of the NLD. Similar to the concept of Ilgit et al (2), we prefer the flexible guide wire as the initial tool for recanalization. In the case of failure, the stiffer, ball-tip wire can be used. One of the disadvantages of the stiffer wire is the straight distal end, which must be extracted out of the nasal cavity with a hook. According to our observations, this part caused more discomfort for the patients than the manipulation with curved steerable wires. In some cases, recanalization of complete obstructions was successful with the help of hydrophilic-coated wires (3). To improve the guidance of soft microwires, thin-lumen tear-duct catheters with straight and angled tips should be designed from a relatively stiff plastic material.

The occurrence of reobstructions seems to be mainly related to one of the following factors: (*a*) recurrent episodes of active dacryocystitis, (*b*) filling defects due to stone formation on the initial dacryocystogram, (*c*) posttraumatic strictures with bony narrowings, or (*d*) long-distance rigid occlusions of the NLD.

Patients with active inflammatory changes should not undergo dilation. Several investigators of studies dealing with DCP agree with this contraindication (1,3,6). Our results indicate that the potential benefit from removal of tight strictures is limited to a short-term period. Active dacryocystitis then seems to be involved in the development of restenoses (Table 3). Clinically, the patients with active dacryocystitis in our study showed no spread of inflammation after DCP. The risk of this kind of complication, however, cannot be denied (14).

Closely related to inflammatory changes is dacryolithiasis, which is frequently a sequelae of chronic infection (15,16). Stones seem to be a common cause of reobstruction after DCP (Table 3). Thus, filling defects indicating dacryolithiasis on dacryocystograms together with corresponding US findings can be regarded as a contraindication for the performance of DCP. Song et al (17) describe an interventional approach for stone removal that may be a perspective for the future.

Posttraumatic stenoses show a poor long-term outcome. Most of the bony narrowings are too rigid for balloon dilation, and permanent impairment of flow may favor secondary inflammatory changes as a cause of reobstruction. Primary operative treatment should be preferred in these cases.

Rigid occlusions involving the entire length of the NLD are frequently seen on dacryocystograms of patients with epiphora. Balloon DCP can be attempted to avert the more invasive operation. Recurrence rates between 45% and 80% show the limited value of balloon dilation (4,6). However, short, distal occlusions in the region of the valve of Hasner with a visible stump of the NLD can be recanalized technically successfully, and these patients may have a favorable long-term prognosis with a patency rate of 94% after 1 year.

The cause of early reobstructions in long-distance occlusions may be the unavoidable traumatization of the ductal wall and reactive mucosal overgrowth.

The results of the studies by Song et al (7,8) show that placement of plastic stents in the tear ducts apparently improves technical success rates and midterm patency rates in cases with complete obstructions. The long-term implantation of NLD stents, however, was associated with recurrence rates between 15% and 64%, depending on the location of the obstruction (18). Stent occlusions due to incrustation with mucoid material have been described; these occlusions require reinterventions for the maintenance of patency. A more serious complication seems to be the overgrowth of the proximal end of the stent by granulation tissue (18). Total obstruction of the lacrimal sac or the common canaliculus with the impossibility of classic operative dacryocystorhinostomy may occur.

Song et al (18) proposed stent extractions in cases with complications and found 73% of the lacrimal draining systems patent after stent removal. Further follow-up, however, showed a 58% reobstruction rate; thus, temporary stent placement does not seem to be a satisfactory therapeutic alternative. The results obtained by Song et al, especially the relatively high rates of stent obstructions, indicate that the implantation of plastic prostheses for predominantly benign stenoses of a small-caliber slow-flow ductal system has limitations and may cause complications that render operative reconstruction of the lacrimal pathways difficult. For these reasons, we maintain a skeptical position concerning tear-duct stent implantation and prefer operative treatment in cases not suitable for DCP.

For external or endoscopic operative dacryocystorhinostomy, technical success rates between 86% and 100% have been described (19,20). In a retrospective analysis of a large series of 1,014 cases, Emmerich et al (20) found a functional long-term success rate of 85% (follow-up range, 1–11 years; mean, 35.6 months). In comparison to balloon DCP, the outcome after operative treatment of postsaccal stenoses seems to be independent from the cause and extension length of stenotic lesions.

With regard to negative side effects, DCP can be regarded as a safe procedure. Serious complications did not occur and are not reported in the literature (1–6). Several patients experienced less tolerable pain under topical anesthesia. Additional local anesthesia with an infratrochlear block may be advantageous to increase the tolerance to the mechanical stress during the procedure (4,21). General anesthesia, which is mostly required for operative dacryocystorhinostomy, is not necessary for balloon DCP.

In conclusion, the analysis of technical failures and long-term results of DCP procedures shows possible predictors of the outcome of the patients. The best prognosis can be expected in patients with focal, partial junctional or NLD obstructions and short-distance occlusions of the distal NLD (with a visible stump of the proximal NLD). With proper indications, clinical long-term success rates of more than 80% can be achieved; thus, surgery or stent placement for many symptomatic lesions can be averted. Active dacryocystitis, dacryolithiasis, or posttraumatic lesions can be regarded as contraindications. Patients with multiple or diffuse stenoses or chronic occlusions of the entire NLD may undergo DCP of postsaccal lesions without negative consequences. A comparison of the technical failure and recurrence rates of DCP with those of operative dacryocystorhinostomy reveals that the latter are less acceptable. ■

References

1. Munk PL, Lin DTC, Morris DC. Epiphora: treatment by means of balloon dilation of the nasolacrimal drainage apparatus. Radiology 1990; 177:687–690.
2. Ilgit ET, Yüksel D, Ünal M, Akpek S, Isik S, Hsanreisoglu B. Transluminal balloon dilation of the lacrimal draining system for the treatment of epiphora. AJR 1995; 165:1517–1524.
3. Janssen AG, Mansour K, Krabbe GJ, van der Veen S, Helder A. Dacryocystoplasty: treatment of epiphora by means of balloon dilation of the obstructed nasolacrimal duct system. Radiology 1994; 193:453–456.
4. Song HY, Ahn HS, Park CK, Kwon SH, Kim CS, Choi KC. Complete obstruction of the nasolacrimal system. I. Treatment with balloon dilation. Radiology 1993; 186:367–371.
5. Kumar EN. Technical note: non-surgical treatment of epiphora by balloon dacryocystoplasty—the technique. Br J Radiol 1995; 68:1116–1118.
6. Lee JM, Song HY, Han YM, et al. Balloon dacryocystoplasty: results in the treatment of complete and partial obstructions of the nasolacrimal system. Radiology 1994; 192: 503–508.
7. Song HY, Jin YH, Kim JH, Sung KB, Han YM, Cho NC. Nasolacrimal duct obstruction treated nonsurgically with the use of plastic stents. Radiology 1994; 190:535–540.
8. Song HY, Jin YH, Kim JH, Huh SJ, Kim YH, Kim TH, Sung KB. Nonsurgical placement of a nasolacrimal polyurethane stent. Radiology 1995; 194:233–237.
9. Galloway JE, Kavic TA, Raflo GT. Digital subtraction macrodaryocystography: a new method of lacrimal system imaging. Ophthalmology 1984; 91:956–962.
10. Iba GB, Hanafee WN. Distension dacryocystography. Radiology 1968; 90:1020–1022
11. Eliasziw M, Smith RF, Singh N, Holdsworth DW, Fox AJ, Barnett HJM. Further comments on the measurement of carotid stenosis from angiograms. Stroke 1994; 25:2445–2449.
12. Goo DE, Song HY, Yoon H, Sung, K. Lacrimal canalicular strictures: safety and effectiveness of balloon dilatation (abstr). Radiology 1996; 201(P):411.
13. Balatsoukas DD, Hintschich CR, Klauss V. Ursachen, operationsmethoden und ergebnisse primär versorgter canaliculus verletzungen. Klin Monatsbl Augenheilk 1992; 200:43–47.
14. Glatt HJ. Dacryocystoplasty: an oculoplastic surgeon's perspective (letter). Radiology 1991; 180:289.
15. Hawes MJ. The dacryolithiasis syndrome. Opthalmic Plast Reconstr Surg 1988; 4:87–90.
16. Herzig S, Hurwitz JJ. Lacrimal sac calculi. Can J Ophthalmol 1979; 14:17–20.
17. Song HY, Jin YH, Lee HK, Sung KB. Nonoperative management of dacryolithiasis. JVIR 1995; 6:647–650.
18. Song HY, Jin YH, Kim JH, et al. Nonsurgical placement of a nasolacrimal polyurethane stent: long-term effectiveness. Radiology 1996; 200:759–763.
19. Sprekelsen MB, Barberan MT. Endoscopic dacryocystorhiostomy: surgical technique and results. Laryngoscope 1996; 106:187–189.
20. Emmerich KH, Busse H, Meyer-Rusenberg HW. Dacryocystorhinostomia externa. Technik Indikationen Ergebnisse Ophthalmologe 1994; 91:395–398.
21. Kratky V, Hurwitz JJ, Ananthanrayan C, Avram DR. Dacryocystorhinostomy in elderly patients: regional anesthesia without cocaine. Can J Ophthalmol 1994; 29:13–16.

Alfred G. Janssen, MD • Khaled Mansour, MD • Johanna J. Bos, MSc

Obstructed Nasolacrimal Duct System in Epiphora: Long-term Results of Dacryocystoplasty by Means of Balloon Dilation[1]

PURPOSE: **To evaluate the long-term results of balloon dacryocystoplasty in the treatment of epiphora due to obstruction of the nasolacrimal ducts.**

MATERIALS AND METHODS: **One hundred eyes in 84 patients with complete or incomplete obstruction of the lacrimal sac and duct were selected for dacryocystoplasty. A catheter with a balloon diameter of 3 mm was used. Follow-up was 5–48 months. No stents were placed. A Kaplan-Meier analysis was used to evaluate patency.**

RESULTS: **The long-term primary patency rate was 70% ± 7 (± standard error). Repeat dacryocystoplasty was successful in 10 of the 11 cases with initial failure or reobstruction during follow-up, which yielded a long-term secondary patency rate of 81% ± 7. There was no association between the length of the obstruction or the duration of symptoms before dacryocystoplasty and the initial and long-term success. Initial and long-term success was statistically significantly higher in dacryocystoplasty for an incomplete obstruction rather than for a complete obstruction.**

CONCLUSION: **The long-term results of dacryocystoplasty, followed if necessary by repeat dacryocystoplasty, are good. Dacryocystoplasty is a safe and simple procedure and could become the treatment of choice for epiphora due to obstruction of the nasolacrimal ducts. Dacryocystorhinostomy is indicated when dacryocystoplasty or repeat dacryocystoplasty fails or when dacryocystoplasty is contraindicated (eg, in anatomic malformations in the lacrimal duct or bony canal).**

EPIPHORA, or tearing, can be caused by reflex hypersecretion of tears owing to infection, irritation of anatomic origin (eg, eyelid malformations, trichiasis), and obstruction of the lacrimal drainage system. Epiphora due to obstruction is generally treated surgically by means of dacryocystorhinostomy. Since 1990, a limited number of publications have reported on the results of dacryocystoplasty, a nonsurgical treatment that involves fluoroscopically guided balloon dilation (1–5). However, only a limited number of cases with limited follow-up have been reported on.

Between September 1992 and September 1996, we performed dacryocystoplasty in 100 eyes in 84 patients. The first objective of this study was to evaluate the long-term primary patency of the nasolacrimal system after dacryocystoplasty. The second objective was to determine whether patency is associated with the duration of the epiphora and the length or severity of the obstruction.

MATERIALS AND METHODS

Patient Selection

Initial selection was done by the referring ophthalmologists (including K.M.), who performed a full ophthalmologic examination to exclude active dacryocystitis and reflex hypersecretion. Subsequently, the nasolacrimal duct system was irrigated with physiologic saline. When the results of this test suggested the presence of an obstruction, patients were referred to the Department of Radiology, De Tjongerschans Hospital, Heerenveen, The Netherlands, for subtraction dacryocystography to establish the type and length of the obstruction. Subtraction dacryocystography was performed with a nonionic, water-soluble contrast medium (iopromide [Ultravist 300 R; Schering, Berlin, Germany]) administered through a small lacrimal catheter inserted into the inferior canaliculus.

If a severe obstruction distal to the canaliculi was found, subtraction dacryocystography was repeated after wedging the superior lacrimal point with a second, nonconducting lacrimal catheter to prevent reflux of contrast medium and to determine whether the obstruction was complete or partial. A total obstruction at any point was considered to be present when, after wedging of the second lacrimal point, dacryocystography showed no passage of contrast medium beyond that point. In cases of total obstruction, dacryocystoplasty entails recanalization by using a guide wire. The obstruction was defined as partial when passage of contrast medium was observed with or without wedging of the second lacrimal point.

Patients were selected for dacryocystoplasty if a complete or partial obstruction was diagnosed at the lacrimal sac, the junction between the lacrimal sac and duct, the duct, or the valve of Hasner, irrespective of the length of the obstruction, the duration of the epiphora, or the patient's age. Exclusion criteria were stenosis at the inferior, superior, or common canaliculus (which, as stressed by Glatt [6], involves a risk of damage to the lacrimal pump); acute dacryocystitis or other specific, acquired nasolacrimal sac and duct obstructions, such as posttraumatic ob-

Index terms: Lacrimal gland and duct, 223.1211, 223.1295, 223.143, 223.1492 • Lacrimal gland and duct, interventional procedure, 223.126

Radiology 1997; 205:791–796

[1] From the Departments of Diagnostic and Interventional Radiology (A.G.J.) and Ophthalmology (K.M.), De Tjongerschans Hospital, Thialfweg 44, 8441 PW Heerenveen, the Netherlands; and the Department of Health Sciences, University of Groningen, Groningen, the Netherlands (J.J.B.). Received April 24, 1997; revision requested May 27; revision received July 21; accepted August 4. **Address reprint requests to** A.G.J.

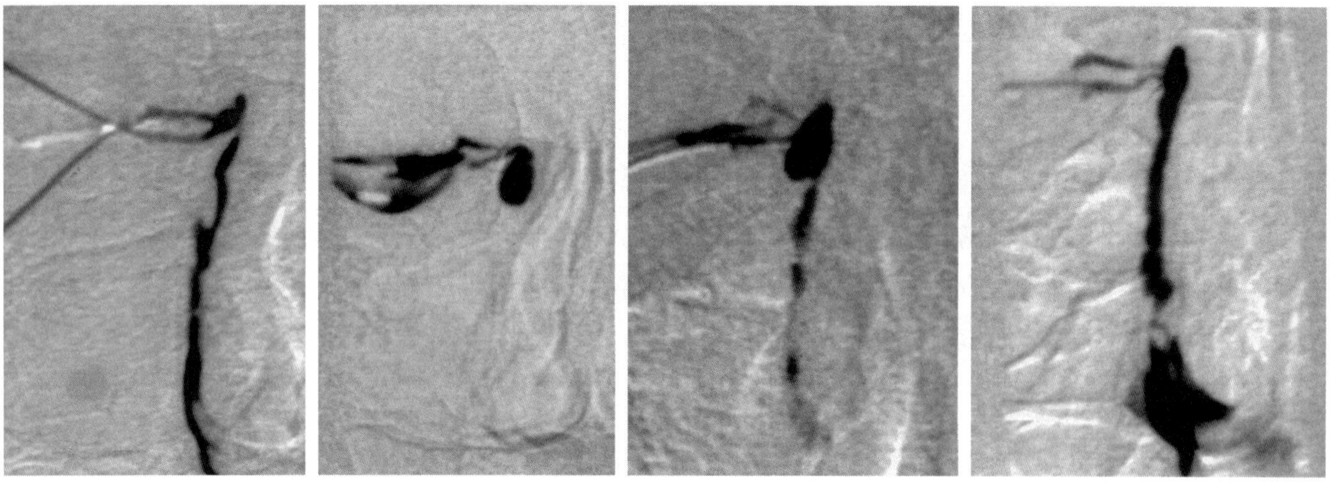

a. b. c. d.

Figure 1. Obstructions selected for dacryocystoplasty. **(a)** Digital subtraction dacryocystographic image shows partial obstruction of the lacrimal sac at the level of the common canaliculus. **(b)** Digital subtraction dacryocystographic image shows complete obstruction at the level of the junction between the lacrimal sac and duct. The lacrimal sac is dilated. **(c)** Digital subtraction dacryocystographic image shows partial obstruction at the level of the junction between the lacrimal sac and nasolacrimal duct and severe stenosis of the lacrimal duct. **(d)** Digital subtraction dacryocystographic image shows partial obstruction at the level of the valve of Hasner. Note the rare absence of the common canaliculus. The canaliculi enter the lacrimal sac separately.

struction of the bony canal; tumors (eg, papilloma, carcinoma); sarcoidosis; or Wegener granulomatosis. If dacryocystographic findings were suggestive of any of these diagnoses or if during dacryocystoplasty the guide wire could not be passed with ease, immediate (preferably by using contrast medium in the lacrimal duct) computed tomography (CT) of the lacrimal duct system was performed. Figure 1 shows some obstructions selected for dacryocystoplasty; Figure 2 shows some obstructions excluded from dacryocystoplasty.

Patient Population

Dacryocystoplasty was performed in 100 eyes (49 left eyes, 51 right eyes) in 84 patients (59 female, 25 male; age range, 1–82 years; mean age, 61.3 years). In 16 patients, dacryocystoplasty was performed in both the left and the right eyes, in one session in some cases. The youngest patient, a 1-year-old girl, had congenital nasolacrimal duct obstruction, which was frequently complicated by infection and did not respond to probing. All other cases of epiphora were idiopathic, that is, were due to primary acquired nasolacrimal duct obstruction. The duration of epiphora varied from 1 to 76 years (mean, 6.0 years).

Epiphora was evaluated subjectively according to the scale of Munk and colleagues (1), which has also been used in other studies (3–5): grade 0 indicates no epiphora; grade 1, occasional epiphora that requires drying or dabbing less than twice a day; grade 2, epiphora that requires drying two to four times a day; grade 3, epiphora that requires drying five to 10 times a day; grade 4, epiphora that requires drying more than 10 times a day; and grade 5, constant tear overflow. All patients had severe epiphora grade 5 (n = 99) or grade 4 (n = 1).

At dacryocystography, complete (n = 27) or partial (n = 73) obstruction was found and the site and length of the obstruction were established. The obstructions were of the lacrimal sac (n = 51), the junction between the lacrimal sac and the duct (n = 62), the lacrimal duct (n = 51), the valve of Hasner (n = 27), and, frequently, a combination of these sites. After the patient had been fully informed of the procedure and informed consent was obtained, dacryocystoplasty was performed in the same session or shortly thereafter.

Technique

Dacryocystoplasty was performed on an outpatient basis after topical anesthesia. Two to four drops of 0.4% oxybuprocaine hydrochloride (Monofree R; Bournonville-Pharma, Almere, The Netherlands) were applied to the conjunctival sac, a small amount of 1% lidocaine (Xylocaine 1%; Astra, Rijswijk, The Netherlands) was mixed with the iopromide used in dacryocystography, and 10% lidocaine (Xylocaine R spray 10%; Astra) was delivered to the nasal mucosa by means of a nebulizer. In the first group of 26 cases, dacryocystoplasty was performed with a nontraumatizing, 0.025-inch guide wire with a flexible curved tip (Terumo, Tokyo, Japan), a small lacrimal catheter (sialography catheter; PBN Medicals, Stenløse, Denmark) and a rigid balloon catheter with a diameter of 4.5 F, a balloon 3 mm in diameter and 2 cm in length, and a tip of 5 mm distal to the balloon (DCDS-100; Cook Europe, Eindhoven, The Netherlands). In some cases, the tip prevented access to an obstruction high in the lacrimal sac.

In the next group of 74 cases, we used a modified method. For dacryocystoplasty, we used a shapable, hydrophilic, coated, 0.025-inch guide wire (NaviGuide; Meditech/Boston Scientific, Maastricht, The Netherlands); a 20-gauge, 51-mm, soft, plastic vascular sheath (Abbocath; Abbott Ireland, Sligo, Republic of Ireland); and a highly flexible, 3.4-F balloon catheter with a balloon diameter of 3 mm and a balloon length of 2 cm (No Tip Bijou 3.0-20; Schneider [Europe], Bülach, Switzerland). This catheter has no tip distal to the balloon; thus, even a stenosis high in the lacrimal sac can be reached.

The guide wire was curved at the tip by hand, and the vascular sheath was curved at the tip over a wire loop by immersing it in hot water (Fig 3). After dilation of the lacrimal point, the vascular sheath was introduced over the wire into the inferior or superior canaliculus and advanced to the common canaliculus. By rotating the sheath, the sharp curve between the common canaliculus and the lacrimal sac was straightened. Under fluoroscopic guidance, the guide wire was gently advanced to the lacrimal sac and duct down to the inferior meatus of the nasal cavity, followed by the sheath. The 0.025-inch wire was removed from the sheath and replaced with a 0.018-inch wire with a flexible curved tip (Terumo). Changing wires is necessary because the balloon catheter is adjusted to a 0.018-inch wire.

At the start of the procedure, we used a 0.025-inch wire because of its good shapability, pushability, and visibility under fluoroscopy. The balloon catheter was passed retrogradely over the wire until the deflated balloon touched the tip of the vascular sheath. The guide wire was clipped on either side of the sheath-catheter combination. With fluoroscopic control, we positioned the balloon catheter at the site of the stenosis by pushing the catheter upward with one hand and pulling the wire and vascular sheath partially out of the canaliculus with the other.

The balloon was inflated twice for 30 seconds. The wire and the balloon catheter

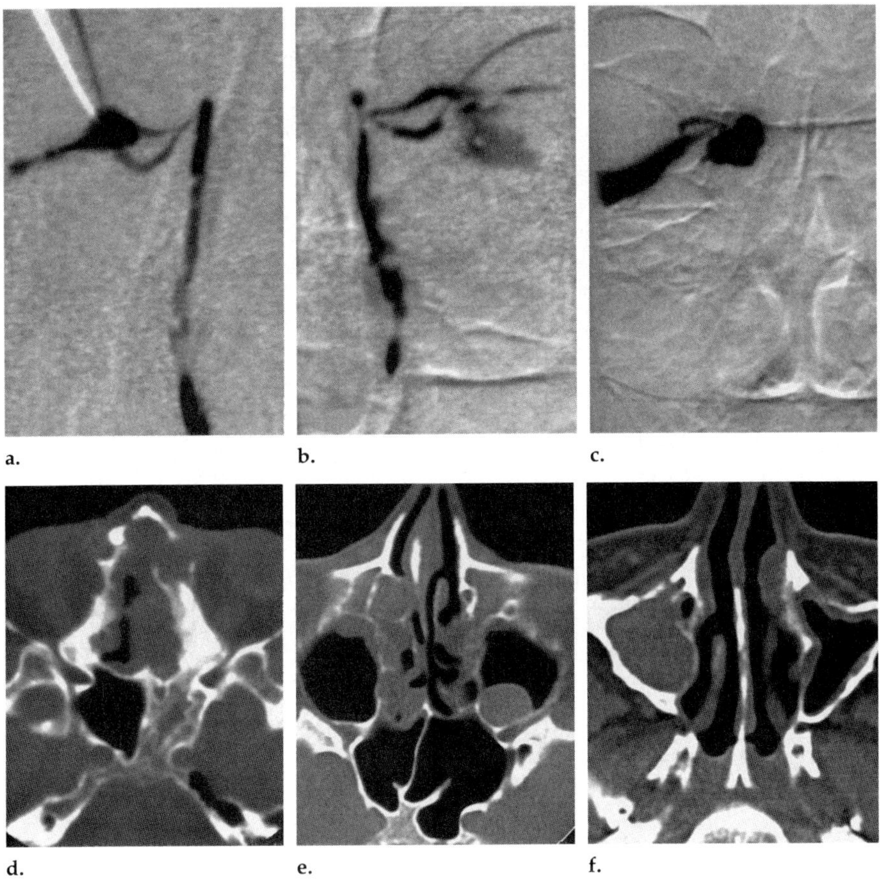

Figure 2. Obstructions not selected for dacryocystoplasty. **(a)** Digital subtraction dacryocystographic image shows partial obstruction of the common canaliculus and the superior canaliculus adjacent to it. **(b)** Digital subtraction dacryocystographic image shows partial obstruction of a lacrimal sac not selected for dacryocystoplasty because of the severe partial obstruction of the common canaliculus and the inferior canaliculus. **(c)** Digital subtraction dacryocystographic image shows complete obstruction of the lacrimal sac in a patient with Wegener granulomatosis. A guide wire could not pass the obstruction. **(d)** CT scan obtained in the same patient as in **c** shows septal destruction and destruction of the bony lacrimal canal on both sides and the formation of granulomas. **(e)** CT scan shows complete obstruction of the lacrimal duct that could not be passed with a guide wire. Note the nasal polyposis. One of the polyps has destroyed the right bony lacrimal canal. **(f)** CT scan shows complete obstruction of the left lacrimal duct as a complication of a Caldwell-Luc operation in which the left bony lacrimal canal was damaged.

were then removed, and the lacrimal system was irrigated with physiologic saline through the vascular sheath. This was followed by irrigation of the lacrimal ducts with 0.5 mL (2 mg) of dexamethasone (prepared according to the formulary of the Dutch Pharmacists). Simultaneously, the vascular sheath was pulled out of the canaliculus.

After the procedure, eye drops (1 mg/mL dexamethasone and 3 mg/mL gentamicin sulfate [Dexamytrex]; Tramedico, Weesp, The Netherlands; one drop six times daily in the involved eye for 1 week) were prescribed.

All patients were followed up with office examination by their ophthalmologist (including K.M.) within 2 months after the procedure. Long-term success was evaluated by interviewing the patients at the end of follow-up, again by using the scale of Munk and colleagues (1). A good result was defined as epiphora grades 0 and 1, and a poor result as epiphora grades 2–5. The follow-up was 5–48 months (mean, 21 months). The procedure caused no complications. During balloon dilation, some of the patients experienced mild pain; however, there was no need for sedation, except in our youngest patient.

Analysis

The nasolacrimal duct system of one eye was used as the unit of analysis, because it is the clinically relevant unit. A Kaplan-Meier analysis was used to evaluate cumulative primary and secondary patency. Univariate analysis of the association between covariates and the initial and long-term success was performed by using the Pearson χ^2 test. A P value of less than .05 was considered to indicate a statistically significant difference.

RESULTS

Long-term primary patency was 70% ± 7 (± standard error), and long-term secondary patency was 81% ± 7. A plateau has not yet been reached, but a tendency can be observed. Primary patency was defined as a good result without further intervention and was evaluated with Kaplan-Meier survival analysis (Fig 4, Table 1). The patency curves originate at a point less than 1; the y intercept represents the probability of immediate clinical success.

Immediate clinical failures occurred in four eyes (in two eyes, epiphora grade 5 remained unchanged; in two eyes, epiphora grade 5 was reduced to grade 3). There were 18 reobstructions during follow-up: eight after treatment of a complete obstruction, and 10 after treatment of a partial obstruction. The obstructions occurred 1–36 months after dacryocystoplasty (mean, 8.1 months; the four initial failures are excluded). Fourteen reobstructions (which includes the four immediate clinical failures) occurred in the 1st year. One year after treatment, another eight reobstructions occurred, bringing the total to 22 reobstructions. All reobstructions originated from epiphora grade 5 and were grade 3 (in six eyes), grade 4 (in two eyes), and grade 5 (in 14 eyes) after dacryocystoplasty.

In addition to the evaluation of cumulative primary and secondary patency, we evaluated whether initial and long-term success rates were associated with the (*a*) duration of symptoms before dacryocystoplasty (ie, ≤1 year [31 eyes] or >1 year [69 eyes]), (*b*) length of obstruction (ie, a short obstruction restricted to one level [38 eyes] or an obstruction extended to two, three, or four levels [62 eyes]), and (*c*) degree of obstruction at dacryocystography (ie, complete obstruction [27 eyes] or partial obstruction [73 eyes]) (Tables 2–7). The analysis demonstrated no relationship between initial or long-term success and the duration of epiphora (Tables 2 and 3) or the length of the obstruction (Tables 4 and 5). Partial and complete obstructions, however, showed a difference in initial and long-term success rates after dacryocystoplasty. Both the initial success and the long-term success were higher in cases with partial obstruction than in cases with complete obstruction (P = .03 and P = .006, respectively) (Tables 6 and 7).

All patients with initial failure or reobstruction during follow-up (22 eyes) were offered repeat dacryocystoplasty. In 11 cases, the patient refused to undergo an additional procedure. In the other 11 cases (two of four eyes with initial failure and nine of 18 eyes with reobstruction during follow-up), repeat dacryocystoplasty was successful in 10 eyes (epiphora grade 0), and epiphora declined from grade 3 to grade 2 in one eye.

DISCUSSION

Traditionally, epiphora due to obstruction of the lacrimal duct has been treated surgically with dacryocystorhinostomy, which involves the removal of bone between the lacrimal sac and nasal mucosa. Subsequently, the lacrimal sac and nasal mucosa are opened and sutured to each other, which results in a bypass of the lacrimal duct. In 1990, Munk and colleagues (1) developed a nonsurgical alternative. They performed dacryocystoplasty with balloon dilation of the nasolacrimal drainage apparatus. A balloon catheter was passed retrogradely over a guide wire that had been inserted antegradely into the lacrimal duct.

Different authors have reported varying results of dacryocystoplasty in series that usually involve a limited number of patients and limited follow-up. A few studies with larger numbers of patients and longer follow-up have been reported on. In 1994, Lee and colleagues (3) published the results of dacryocystoplasty in 81 eyes with a maximum follow-up of 30 months. They found an overall cumulative patency rate of 23%. In 1995, Ilgit and colleagues (5) reported the results of dacryocystoplasty in 80 eyes with a maximum follow-up of 18 months. Their overall initial success rate was 69%. However, restenosis occurred in 26% during follow-up. In our study, we had a primary patency rate of 70% after dacryocystoplasty in 100 eyes with a follow-up of 5–48 months.

The differences in results can probably be explained by differences in patient selection and different dacryocystoplasty techniques. The results reported by Lee and colleagues (3) may have been negatively affected by the inclusion of eight patients with posttrauma obstruction and possible deformation of the bony lacrimal canal and 13 patients with stenosis of the common canaliculus. Ilgit and colleagues (5) also included 13 patients with stenosis of the common canaliculus, which was dilated by using a 2-mm balloon. We did include patients with posttrauma obstruction, but only after we performed CT of the lacrimal duct system to evaluate the bony lacrimal canal. We excluded patients with an obstruction at the common canaliculus.

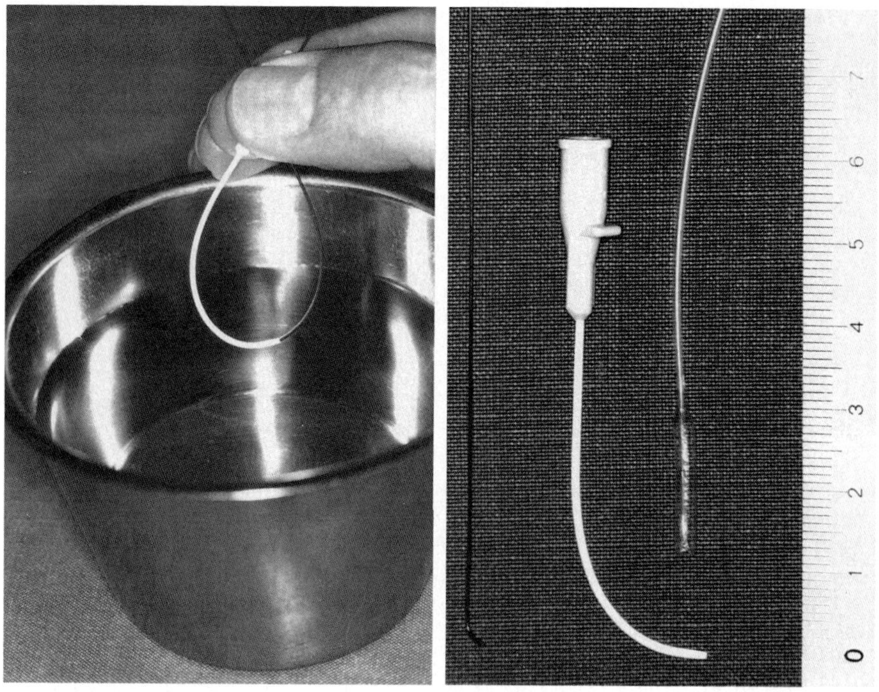

Figure 3. (a) By immersing it in hot water, the 20-gauge vascular sheath curves at the tip over a wire loop. (b) Curve at the tip of the guide wire is shaped by hand at the most distal 3 mm of the wire. Note the curved vascular sheath and the inflated balloon located at the tip of the catheter. Scale is in centimeters.

Ilgit and colleagues (5) included six patients with a reobstruction after dacryocystorhinostomy. In these patients, dacryocystoplasty involved dilation of the opening between the lacrimal sac and the nose. We treated one patient with a reobstruction after dacryocystorhinostomy. Dacryocystography and CT of the lacrimal duct system showed that the opening made during surgery was completely closed and the continuity of mucosa and bone completely restored. In this patient, dacryocystoplasty of the original obstruction of the nasolacrimal duct was successful.

CT of the lacrimal duct system can be very helpful in patient selection, because it shows both facial skeletal bone and adjacent soft tissues (7,8). We performed conventional axial CT immediately after dacryocystography with administration of the residual, water-soluble iopromide that is left in the nasolacrimal duct system. CT of the lacrimal duct system is indicated in patients with posttrauma obstruction (9), patients with previous dacryocystorhinostomy failure (10), or if the guide wire cannot be passed with ease during dacryocystoplasty.

Another explanation of the differences in results can be the use of different techniques. We used nonmetal,

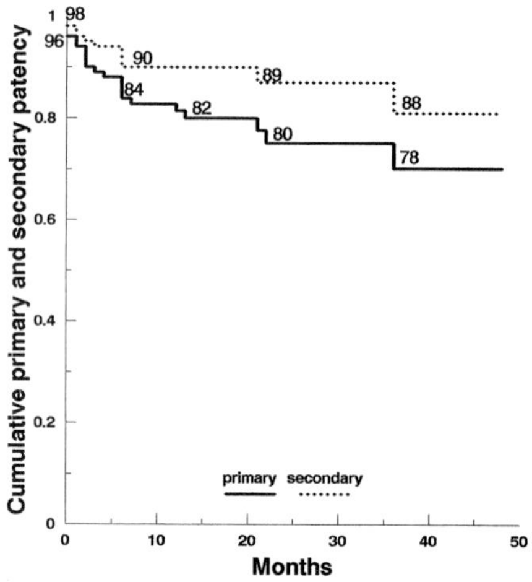

Figure 4. Primary and secondary patency rates after dacryocystoplasty in 100 eyes.

atraumatic guide wires, which did not cause false passage. Lee and colleagues (3) reported false passage in three eyes and Ilgit and colleagues (5) reported false passage in seven eyes. Ilgit and colleagues (5) used balloon catheters with a diameter of 4 mm. Lee and colleagues (3) used balloons with diameters of 4–5 mm, and both Lee and Ilgit inflated the balloon for at least 5 minutes. We inflated a balloon 3 mm in diameter for 30 seconds. The time is sufficient to tear the fibrotic component of the obstruction, and the diameter prevents damage to the lac-

Table 1
Life-Table Analysis of Primary Patency and Secondary Patency after Dacryocystoplasty in 100 Eyes

Outcome	Interval (mo)	No. at Risk	Failures	Cumulative Patency (%)	Standard Error (%)
Primary patency	0–0*	96	4	96	2
	0–1	94	2	94	2
	1–2	90	4	90	3
	2–3	89	1	89	3
	3–4	88	1	88	3
	4–6	84	4	84	4
	6–12	83	1	83	4
	12–13	82	1	81	4
	13–21	81	1	80	4
	21–22	80	1	78	5
	22–36	79	1	75	5
	36–48	78	1	70	7
Secondary patency†	0–0	98	2	98	1
	0–1	96	2	96	2
	1–2	95	1	95	2
	2–6	94	1	94	2
	6–21	90	4	90	3
	21–36	89	1	87	4
	36–48	88	1	81	7

Note.—Success in eyes without reobstruction at 48 months is likely to extend beyond this period.
* Four eyes had initial failure.
† In 11 of 22 cases (four initial failures and 18 reobstructions during follow-up), repeat dacryocystoplasty was performed.

Table 6
Association between Initial Success and Obstruction

Obstruction	Initial Success	Initial Failure	Total
Complete	24	3	27
Partial	72	1	73
Total	96	4	100

Table 7
Association between Long-term Success and Obstruction

Obstruction	Long-term Success	Long-term Failure*	Total
Complete	16	11	27
Partial	62	11	73
Total	78	22	100

* Four initial failures and 18 reobstructions.

Table 2
Association between Initial Success and Duration of Symptoms

Duration of Symptoms	Initial Success	Initial Failure	Total
≤1 y	29	2	31
>1 y	67	2	69
Total	96	4	100

Table 4
Association between Initial Success and Length of Obstruction

Length of Obstruction	Initial Success	Initial Failure	Total
One level	38	0	38
Two to four levels	58	4	62
Total	96	4	100

Table 3
Association between Long-term Success and Duration of Symptoms

Duration of Symptoms	Long-term Success	Long-term Failure*	Total
≤1 y	26	5	31
>1 y	52	17	69
Total	78	22	100

* Four initial failures and 18 reobstructions.

Table 5
Association between Long-term Success and Length of Obstruction

Length of Obstruction	Long-term Success	Long-term Failure*	Total
One level	30	8	38
Two to four levels	48	14	62
Total	78	22	100

* Four initial failures and 18 reobstructions.

rimal duct, assuming that the bony canal in adults is 4–6 mm (11). CT of the lacrimal duct system in the patients in our study revealed that the minimum diameter of the bony canal can be 2.5–4.0 mm. Unlike Lee and colleagues (3) and Ilgit and colleagues (5), we used a catheter with the balloon placed at the catheter tip. As a result, the tip of the catheter did not need to be passed into the common canaliculus in cases with an obstruction high up in the lacrimal sac.

Analysis of the association between (*a*) the dacryocystoplasty results and (*b*) the duration of epiphora or the length of the obstruction demonstrated surprising results. Ilgit and colleagues (5) concluded that their lower overall success rate compared with that reported by Lee and colleagues can partly be attributed to the different times between treatment and the onset of complaints (for Lee and colleagues, a mean of 7.5 years; for Ilgit and colleagues, a mean of 3.4 years). However, we did not find any statistically significant difference in the initial or long-term success rate between patients with epiphora for 1 year or less and those with epiphora for more than 1 year. Also, we did not find a statistically significant difference in the initial or long-term success rate between patients with a short obstruction and patients with an extended obstruction of the lacrimal duct.

A less surprising outcome of our study was the statistically significant difference in the initial or long-term success rate between partial obstructions and complete obstructions. Complete obstructions require recanalization with the guide wire. Similar differences were reported by Lee and colleagues (3) and Ilgit and colleagues (5), despite their different definitions of "complete obstruction." Their approach in defining a complete obstruction is more functional than ours, which means that in their study an obstruction may be considered complete even when the passage of contrast medium is possible.

Although dacryocystoplasty is increasingly being performed to treat epiphora due to lacrimal obstruction, little is known about the underlying mechanism of the procedure. Linberg and McCormick (12) studied pathologic changes in the membranous nasolacrimal duct in patients with acquired nasolacrimal duct obstruction and found a loose structure of connective tissue around the stratified columnar epithelium of the lacrimal duct. Within this structure, a venous plexus, collections of lymphocytes, and some fibrous tissue were found. In patients with acquired obstruction, (*a*) vascular congestion, (*b*) lymphocytic infiltration, and (*c*) edema cause compression of the duct. This stenosis results in the pooling of tears and infection. Infection increases inflammatory edema and, eventually, gives rise to fibrosis. At the same time, infection might cause reflex hypersecretion of tears. This vicious cycle was also mentioned by Duke-Elder (13).

Hurwitz (14) assumed that in the early stages of obstruction, when fibrosis is still limited, steroid treatment might reverse the process. After dacryocystoplasty, we flushed the lacrimal system with physiologic saline and dexamethasone. Eye drops that contain dexamethasone and gentamicin were prescribed for 1 week. Apart from balloon dilation, this might be an essential factor with respect to the success of the procedure.

Dalgleish (15) flushed the lacrimal duct system in a large series of asymptomatic patients and found obstruction in 9%–10% of patients aged 40 years or older. At the age of 90 years, 35%–40% of patients had obstructions. These patients were asymptomatic because tear production decreases with age. The success of dacryocystoplasty does not necessarily have to be the result of long-term patency of the nasolacrimal duct itself. In some cases, it may be caused by breaking the vicious cycle of obstruction and infection. To test this hypothesis, further study of the lacrimal duct system in patients who are asymptomatic after dacryocystoplasty or dacryocystorhinostomy is necessary.

Currently, epiphora due to obstruction of the lacrimal sac and duct is treated surgically with dacryocystorhinostomy. According to Hurwitz (16), the indications for dacryocystorhinostomy include epiphora due to acquired obstruction within the nasolacrimal sac and duct, a mucocele of the lacrimal sac, chronic dacryocystitis or conjunctivitis due to lacrimal sac obstruction, lacrimal sac infection that must be relieved before intraocular surgery, and congenital nasolacrimal duct obstruction that cannot be cured by probing. Contraindications for dacryocystorhinostomy include acute dacryocystitis and tumor of the lacrimal sac. In fact, these are the same indications and contraindications that we consider appropriate for dacryocystoplasty. In experienced hands, dacryocystorhinostomy has a success rate of 90% (17). Possible complications of dacryocystorhinostomy include orbital emphysema, hemorrhage, infection, or even cerebrospinal fluid leakage (16). In our series, no complications occurred.

The long-term primary patency rate of dacryocystoplasty in our series of 100 obstructed lacrimal duct systems is 70% ± 7. The results of repeat dacryocystoplasty after re-obstruction are good. Repeat dacryocystoplasty was performed in 11 patients, with a successful outcome in 10 patients. We achieved an overall long-term patency rate of 81% ± 7. These results are promising. Dacryocystoplasty appears to be a simple, safe procedure performed with local anesthesia and on an outpatient basis. Compared with dacryocystorhinostomy, dacryocystoplasty is a less invasive and lower cost procedure.

We believe that dacryocystoplasty may become the treatment of choice for epiphora due to obstruction of the nasolacrimal duct system at the saccular or subsaccular level. Dacryocystorhinostomy should be kept in reserve in case of failure of dacryocystoplasty and repeat dacryocystoplasty. In our opinion, dacryocystorhinostomy will continue to be the treatment of choice in cases of posttraumatic or congenital obstruction of the bony canal or obstruction of the nasolacrimal duct due to polyps or granuloma. Placement of a stent in the lacrimal duct system, as advocated by Song and colleagues (18,19), is an interesting possibility, but may cause chronic infection and fibrotic reactions in the long run. Our results indicate that a large number of patients who receive a stent as initial therapy of obstruction of the lacrimal duct system may not require a stent. This suggests that the indications for stent placement should be reconsidered. ■

Acknowledgments: We thank Mereke L. B. Gorsira, BA, for correcting the manuscript and Ad J. Petersen for his help with the photographs.

References

1. Munk PL, Lin DTC, Morris DC. Epiphora: treatment by means of dacryocystoplasty with balloon dilation of the nasolacrimal drainage apparatus. Radiology 1990; 177: 687–690.
2. Song HY, Ahn HS, Park CK, Kwon SH, Kim CS, Choi KC. Complete obstruction of the nasolacrimal system. I. Treatment with balloon dilation. Radiology 1993; 186:367–371.
3. Lee JM, Song HY, Han YM, et al. Balloon dacryocystoplasty: results in the treatment of complete and partial obstructions of the nasolacrimal system. Radiology 1994; 192: 503–508.
4. Janssen AG, Mansour K, Krabbe GJ, van der Veen S, Helder AH. Dacryocystoplasty: treatment of epiphora by means of balloon dilation of the obstructed nasolacrimal duct system. Radiology 1994; 193:453–456.
5. Ilgit ET, Yüksel D, Unal M, Akpek S, Ilsik S, Hasanreisoglu B. Transluminal balloon dilation of the lacrimal drainage system for the treatment of epiphora. AJR 1995; 165: 1517–1524.
6. Glatt HJ. Dacryocystoplasty: an oculoplastic surgeon's perspective (letter). Radiology 1991; 180:289.
7. Zinreich SJ, Miller NR, Freeman LN, Glorioso LW, Rosenbaum AE. Computed tomographic dacryocystography using topical contrast media for lacrimal system visualization. Orbit 1990; 9:79–87.
8. Moran CC, Buckwalter K, Caldemeyer KS. Helical CT with topical water-soluble contrast media for imaging of the lacrimal drainage apparatus. AJR 1995; 164:995–996.
9. Glatt HJ. Evaluation of lacrimal obstruction secondary to facial fractures using computed tomography or computed tomographic dacryocystography. Ophthalmic Plast Reconstr Surg 1996; 12:284–293.
10. Glatt HJ, Chan AC, Barrett L. Evaluation of dacryocystorhinostomy failure with computed tomography and computed tomographic dacryocystography. Am J Ophthalmol 1991; 112:431–436.
11. Duke-Elder S, ed. Textbook of ophthalmology. Vol 1, The development, form and function of the visual apparatus. London, England: Kimpton, 1946; 235.
12. Linberg JV, McCormick SA. Primary acquired nasolacrimal duct obstruction: a clinicopathologic report and biopsy technique. Ophthalmology 1986; 93:1055–1063.
13. Duke-Elder S, ed. Textbook of ophthalmology. Vol 5, The ocular adnexa. London, England: Kimpton, 1952; 5302.
14. Hurwitz JJ. Diseases of the sac and duct. In: Hurwitz JJ. The lacrimal system. Philadelphia, Pa: Lippincott-Raven, 1996; 117–118.
15. Dalgleish R. Idiopathic acquired lacrimal drainage obstruction. Br J Ophthalmol 1967; 51:463.
16. Hurwitz JJ. Dacryocystorhinostomy. In: Hurwitz JJ. The lacrimal system. Philadelphia, Pa: Lippincott-Raven, 1996; 261–290.
17. Hurwitz JJ, Rutherford S. Computerized survey of lacrimal surgery patients. Ophthalmology 1986; 93:14–19.
18. Song HY, Ahn HS, Park CK, Kwon SH, Kim CS, Choi KC. Complete obstruction of the nasolacrimal system. II. Treatment with metallic stents. Radiology 1993; 186:372–376.
19. Song HY, Jin YH, Kim JH, Sung KB, Han YM, Cho NC. Nasolacrimal duct obstructions treated nonsurgically with use of plastic stents. Radiology 1994; 190:535–539.

Roland R. Lee, MD • Mark W. Becher, MD • Mark L. Benson, MD • Daniele Rigamonti, MD

Brain Capillary Telangiectasia: MR Imaging Appearance and Clinicohistopathologic Findings[1]

PURPOSE: To demonstrate the clinical and magnetic resonance (MR) imaging findings of brain capillary telangiectasia and compare them with postmortem specimens.

MATERIALS AND METHODS: MR images obtained in and clinical histories of 18 adult patients with a presumed diagnosis of capillary telangiectasia examined within 3 years were retrospectively reviewed. All patients had undergone MR imaging with conventional T1- and T2-weighted spin-echo sequences and gadolinium-enhanced T1-weighted and susceptibility-sensitive gradient-echo (GRE) sequences. No biopsies had been performed. Fourteen patients had undergone clinical and MR imaging follow-up (median, 11 months). Postmortem tissues from three cases of histopathologically confirmed capillary telangiectasia were imaged.

RESULTS: All lesions were small, homogeneously enhancing, and hypo- to isointense on T1-weighted images and iso- to slightly hyperintense on proton-density– and T2-weighted images. None was hypointense on proton-density– or T2-weighted images. All lesions showed marked GRE signal loss. None had changed at follow-up. Two patients had multiple classic cerebral cavernous angiomas. The three specimens showed no abnormal susceptibility and contained no hemosiderin at tissue analysis.

CONCLUSION: Capillary telangiectasia has mild contrast material enhancement but is otherwise undetectable on conventional MR images. It lacks the "hemosiderin rim" of cavernous angioma and demonstrates increased susceptibility only on GRE images, likely owing to blood oxygen-level–dependent contrast. GRE is essential in diagnosing brain capillary telangiectasia, which could otherwise be misdiagnosed as neoplasia, subacute infarction, or demyelination.

THERE are four major vascular malformations of the central nervous system: parenchymal arteriovenous malformation (AVM), venous angioma, cavernous angioma, and capillary telangiectasia (1). The magnetic resonance (MR) imaging characteristics of AVMs, venous angiomas, and classic cavernous angiomas are well documented (2–4). The MR imaging appearance of capillary telangiectasia has not been as widely appreciated. We performed this study to demonstrate the clinical and MR imaging findings of brain capillary telangiectasia and to compare them with findings in postmortem specimens.

MATERIALS AND METHODS

Patients

MR images and clinical findings in 18 patients (eight men, 10 women; age range, 18–77 years; median age, 48 years; mean age, 45 years) with presumed radiologic diagnosis of capillary telangiectasia who underwent imaging at our institution in 1993–1996 were retrospectively reviewed by two board-certified neuroradiologists (R.R.L., M.L.B.); the MR imaging characteristics, diagnosis at presentation, clinical history, and laboratory findings were tabulated. The MR imaging findings were tabulated separately by each radiologist; there were no differences in their readings. Minimal disagreements (such as measurements, which differed by at most 1–2 mm) were resolved by means of consensus.

All patients underwent conventional MR imaging on a 1.5-T imager (Signa 4X or 5X, GE Medical Systems, Milwaukee, Wis; or Magnetom, Siemens Medical Systems, Iselin, NJ) with 5-mm, contiguous, axial sections obtained by using a spin-echo T1-weighted sequence (450–650/11–20 [repetition time msec/echo time msec]), conventional double-echo proton-density– and spin-echo T2-weighted sequences (2,500–3,000/20–34, 100), a T1-weighted sequence after the intravenous administration of 0.1 mmol/kg gadopentetate dimeglumine (Magnevist; Berlex Laboratories, Wayne, NJ), and a gradient-echo (GRE) sequence sensitive for susceptibility (5) (500–800/25–35, 20° flip angle, 3–5-mm section thickness). For all sequences, a 24-cm field of view and a 256 × 192 matrix were used.

In all patients, the proton-density– and T2-weighted sequences were performed before the intravenous administration of gadopentetate dimeglumine. In 14 patients, the GRE sequence was performed before gadopentetate dimeglumine administration, because the lesions had been seen at previously performed contrast material–enhanced MR imaging or computed tomography (CT). In four patients, the gadopentetate dimeglumine was administered before the GRE sequence: In two, it was given 6 hours before; in two, it was given about 15 minutes before.

Two patients also underwent fast spin-

Index terms: Angioma, central nervous system, 10.3149, 17.1494 • Brain, MR, 10.12141 • Cerebral blood vessels, abnormalities, 17.1494, 17.3149 • Magnetic resonance (MR), tissue characterization, 10.12141 • Telangiectasia, 17.1494

Abbreviations: AVM = arteriovenous malformation, BOLD = blood oxygen–level dependent, GRE = gradient echo.

Radiology 1997; 205:797–805

[1] From the Neuroradiology Division, Department of Radiology and Radiological Science (R.R.L., M.L.B.); the Neuropathology Division, Department of Pathology (M.W.B.); and the Department of Neurosurgery (D.R.), The Johns Hopkins University School of Medicine, Baltimore, Md; and the Division of Neuroradiology, Department of Radiology, University of New Mexico, Albuquerque (R.R.L.). Received July 9, 1996; revision requested August 7; revision received and accepted August 7, 1997. **Address reprint requests to** R.R.L., Department of Radiology, Veterans Affairs Medical Center (114M), 2100 Ridgecrest Dr SE, Bldg 49A, Albuquerque, NM 87108.

Table 1
Clinical Findings and Laboratory Results

Patient No./ Sex/Age (y)	Clinical Presentation	Physical Examination Findings	Associated Diagnoses	Laboratory Results and Imaging Findings
1/F/34	Nystagmus, dysequilibrium, ataxia	NA	Oculopalatal myoclonus syndrome	Normal cerebrospinal fluid, normal positron emission tomographic scan, electronystagmographic findings of nystagmus
2/F/77	Left tinnitus	Decreased pinprick sensation in left side of face	Rheumatoid arthritis	Rheumatoid factor negative, positive findings for antinuclear antibody, normal immune complexes
3/F/47	Migraines since puberty	Normal	NA	NA
4/F/61	Diplopia, right ptosis	Diplopia, ptosis	Large right parasellar meningioma	NA
5/F/39	Paresthesia in all four limbs, numb tongue	Decreased pinprick sensation in four limbs	NA	No peripheral neuropathy, normal vitamin B_{12} level, normal vitamin E level, negative results of heavy metal screening
6/M/42	Slurred speech, facial droop	NA	Bell palsy	NA
7/F/67	Left-sided weakness, hyperreflexia	NA	Dermatomyositis	NA
8/M/31	AIDS*, transient aphasia, hand numbness	No fixed focal deficit	AIDS* (two CD4 cells per cubic millimeter)	CSF† normal (three times)
9/M/20	Seizure disorder	Normal	Multiple cerebral cavernomas	Electroencephalographic findings: occasional sharp waves in right temporal lobe
10/M/33	Headache, chills, nausea, 103°F‡ temperature	No focal neurologic deficit	HIV-positive§ (318 CD4 cells per cubic millimeter)	CSF† protein level, 1.77 g/L; otherwise normal
11/M/31	Dizziness, vertigo, nausea, vomiting, right-sided facial weakness	Ataxia, right-sided facial weakness	Multiple cerebral cavernomas	NA
12/F/49	Headaches	Normal	NA	Thyroid test results normal
13/M/57	Follow-up right parietal astrocytoma	Left hand weak, clumsy; seizures	Right parietal anaplastic astrocytoma	NA
14/M/49	Leg weakness, fatigue, headache, blurred vision	Mild bilateral leg weakness	NA	NA
15/F/55	Hearing loss greater in right ear than in left ear, tinnitus	Normal	Hypertension	NA
16/M/55	Dizziness, dysequilibrium	Ataxia	Hypertension, diabetes mellitus	Bright olivary nuclei in the medulla oblongata on T2-weighted MR images
17/F/49	Migraines since age 17 y	Normal	NA	Cerebral angiographic findings normal, normal cerebrospinal fluid
18/F/18	Migraines	NA	NA	NA

Note.—NA = Not available.
* AIDS = acquired immunodeficiency syndrome.
† CSF = cerebrospinal fluid.
‡ 39.4°C.
§ HIV = human immunodeficiency virus.

echo T2-weighted imaging (4,000/102) in addition to conventional spin-echo T2-weighted imaging.

Seven of the patients were referred from outside institutions, which included three major academic medical centers. In none of the MR imaging examinations performed outside our institution was a susceptibility-sensitive GRE sequence used. The initial radiologic diagnosis in five of the seven patients was neoplasm (astrocytoma), multiple sclerosis, or infarction. Vascular malformation was suggested in two patients.

Because of the mild symptoms associated with these lesions and their location in the pons, which made them unamenable to biopsy in the face of such mild symptoms, biopsy was performed in none of these lesions. Given the mild symptoms and presumptive diagnosis of capillary telangiectasia, no direct treatment of any of these lesions was performed. One of the patients died (of unrelated causes) during the 3 years of this study; however, permission for autopsy or limited necropsy was denied.

MR imaging and clinical follow-up findings were obtained in 14 of the 18 patients. The duration of follow-up was 3–82 months (median, 11 months; mean, 23 months).

Neurohistopathologic Specimens

Four nonarterial vascular malformations (three capillary telangiectasia cases and one cavernous angioma) were identified as part of routine postmortem neurohistopathologic evaluations of central nervous system tissue from four different adults. The cavernous angioma was from the cerebrum (anterior temporal lobe); the three capillary telangiectasia lesions were from the cerebrum (superior frontal gyrus), cerebellar vermis, and basis pontis. Only one patient had exhibited neurologic symptoms (seizure disorder) that may have been related to the lesion (temporal lobe cavernous angioma). None of these specimens was from any of the 18 patients discussed above.

In two of these four patient samples, MR imaging had been performed while the patient was alive (5-mm unenhanced T1- and T2-weighted sequences only). No abnormality had been demonstrated on MR images obtained in the patient with the superior frontal gyrus lesion (capillary telangiectasia). However, in the other patient, the anterior temporal lobe lesion exhibited typical cavernous angioma features, with a hypointense peripheral hemosiderin rim that surrounded a heterogeneous central region on T2-weighted images.

All four specimens were fixed in 10% neutral buffered formalin for 2 weeks before dissection. Histopathologic preparations were made from each lesion, and the adjacent serial tissue slab was left intact for specimen imaging.

Table 2
Imaging Characteristics of Lesions

Patient No./Sex/Age (y)	Sequence					Size (mm)	Location	CT Findings	Follow-up Imaging	Associated Vascular Malformations
	GRE	T1-weighted	Proton-Density-weighted	T2-weighted	T1-weighted Gadolinium-enhanced					
1/F/34	Slightly hypointense	Isointense	Slightly hyperintense	Slightly hyperintense	Slightly hyperintense	9	Right side of medulla	NA	4 y 6 mo	NA
2/F/77	Very hypointense	Slightly hypointense	Slightly hyperintense	Slightly hyperintense	Slightly hyperintense	9	Ventral middle part of pons	Unenhanced: lesion missed	4 y 1 mo	NA
3/F/47	Very hypointense	Slightly hypointense	Slightly hyperintense	Slightly hyperintense	Slightly hyperintense	9	Left lower part of pons	NA	4 mo	NA
4/F/61	Slightly hypointense	Isointense	Isointense	Isointense	Slightly hyperintense	7	Left parasagittal part of pons	NA	2 y 1 mo	NA
5/F/39	Slightly hypointense	Isointense	Slightly hyperintense	Slightly hyperintense	Slightly hyperintense	8	Left parasagittal part of pons	NA	3 y 9 mo	NA
6/M/42	Slightly hypointense	Isointense	Slightly hyperintense	Slightly hyperintense	Slightly hyperintense	4	Dorsal middle part of pons	NA	NA	NA
7/F/67	Very hypointense	Slightly hypointense	Slightly hyperintense	Isointense	Very hyperintense	20	Entire right side of pons, dorsal left side of pons	Unenhanced: lesion missed	10 mo	Contiguous small anterior vein
8/M/31	Slightly hypointense	Isointense	Slightly hyperintense	Slightly hyperintense	Slightly hyperintense	13	Dorsal right side of pons	Unenhanced: lesion missed	7 mo	Contiguous small posterior vein, large, right-sided cerebellar peduncular venous angioma
9/M/20	Very hypointense	Slightly hypointense	Slightly hyperintense	Isointense	Slightly hyperintense	6	Left middle part of pons	NA	NA	Multiple cerebral cavernous angiomas
10/M/33	Slightly hypointense	Isointense	Isointense	Isointense	Slightly hyperintense	9	Ventral right part of pons	Contrast-enhanced: lesion depicted	NA	NA
11/M/31	Both lesions slightly hypointense	Both lesions isointense	Both lesions isointense	Both lesions isointense	Both lesions slightly hyperintense	5, 3	Lower middle part of pons, lower left side of pons	NA	12 mo	Multiple cerebral cavernous angiomas
12/F/49	Slightly hypointense	Isointense	Isointense	Slightly hyperintense	Slightly hyperintense	5	Ventral left side of pons	NA	NA	NA
13/M/57	Slightly hypointense	Isointense	Isointense	Isointense	Slightly hyperintense	4	Left middle part of pons	Unenhanced: lesion missed	5 mo	NA
14/M/49	Slightly hypointense	Isointense	Isointense	Isointense	Slightly hyperintense	14	Left middle part of pons	NA	5 mo	NA
15/F/55	Slightly hypointense	Isointense	Isointense	Isointense	Slightly hyperintense	8	Left middle part of pons	NA	8 mo	NA
16/M/55	Slightly hypointense	Isointense	Isointense	Isointense	Slightly hyperintense	8	Left middle part of pons	NA	1 y 2 mo	Small draining vein in left side of pons, small right frontal venous angioma
17/F/49	Very hypointense	Isointense	Slightly hyperintense	Isointense	Very hyperintense	7	Right temporal tip	Contrast-enhanced: lesion depicted	6 y 10 mo	NA
18/F/18	Very hypointense	Slightly hypointense	Isointense	Isointense	Very hyperintense	12	Right caudate nucleus	NA	3 mo	NA

Note.—NA = not available.

These four postmortem specimens were separately submerged in a water bath and imaged with a 1.5-T MR imager (Signa 5.5; GE Medical Systems) by using T1-weighted (500/11–13), conventional proton-density– and T2-weighted (2,500/17, 100), and GRE (500/30, 20° flip angle) sequences performed in the anatomically axial plane. Because the piece of pons tissue was only 2–3 mm thick and the other pieces were fragments of about 5 mm thick, to improve the signal-to-noise ratio, imaging was performed with the water bath (which contained the sample at the bottom) on top of a 3-inch surface coil, instead of inside a head coil. To reduce the partial-volume effect, 1.4–2.0-mm sections were obtained through the lesions. Whole-brain imaging was not performed, because the existence of the vascular malformations was not ascertained until after the brains had been cut. Contrast material enhancement could not be performed in these postmortem tissue samples.

The specimens were examined histologically and pathologically, and findings were correlated with the MR imaging findings.

RESULTS

Patient Data

Eighteen patients presented with minor neurologic symptoms ranging from headaches or migraines (five patients), dysequilibrium or dizziness (three patients), tinnitus (two patients), facial weakness (two patients), and limb weakness (two patients) to slurred speech (one patient) and transient aphasia (one patient). Four patients presented with symptoms directly related to known diagnoses: tumor (two patients), infection (one patient), and multiple cavernomas (one patient); capillary telangiectasia in these patients was asymptomatic and was an incidental finding. Seven patients had normal findings of clinical examination. Ataxia and facial palsy were found in two patients. Oculopalatal myoclonus, facial anesthesia, and hearing loss were found in one patient each.

Four patients had undergone documented cerebrospinal fluid analysis; in all four, the cerebrospinal fluid was normal, except for an elevated protein level in one patient with the human immunodeficiency virus, or HIV.

Table 1 summarizes the clinical features and laboratory results available in each patient.

MR imaging findings (and CT findings, when available) in each patient are summarized in Table 2. Of the 19 lesions, 16 were located in the pons, one was in the temporal lobe, one was in the medulla, and one was in the caudate nucleus. They were 3–20 mm in diameter (median, 8 mm; mean, 8.4 mm). All lesions of interest were solitary, except for in patient 11, who had two pontine capillary telangiectasia lesions. As detailed in Table 2 and illustrated in Figures 1 and 2, all capillary telangiectasia lesions had similar appearances: They were almost undetectable on unenhanced T1-, proton-density–, and T2-weighted images. Some were slightly hyperintense on proton-density and T2-weighted images, but none was hypointense. All showed pronounced loss of signal intensity on the GRE images, and all demonstrated mild contrast material enhancement on T1-weighted images.

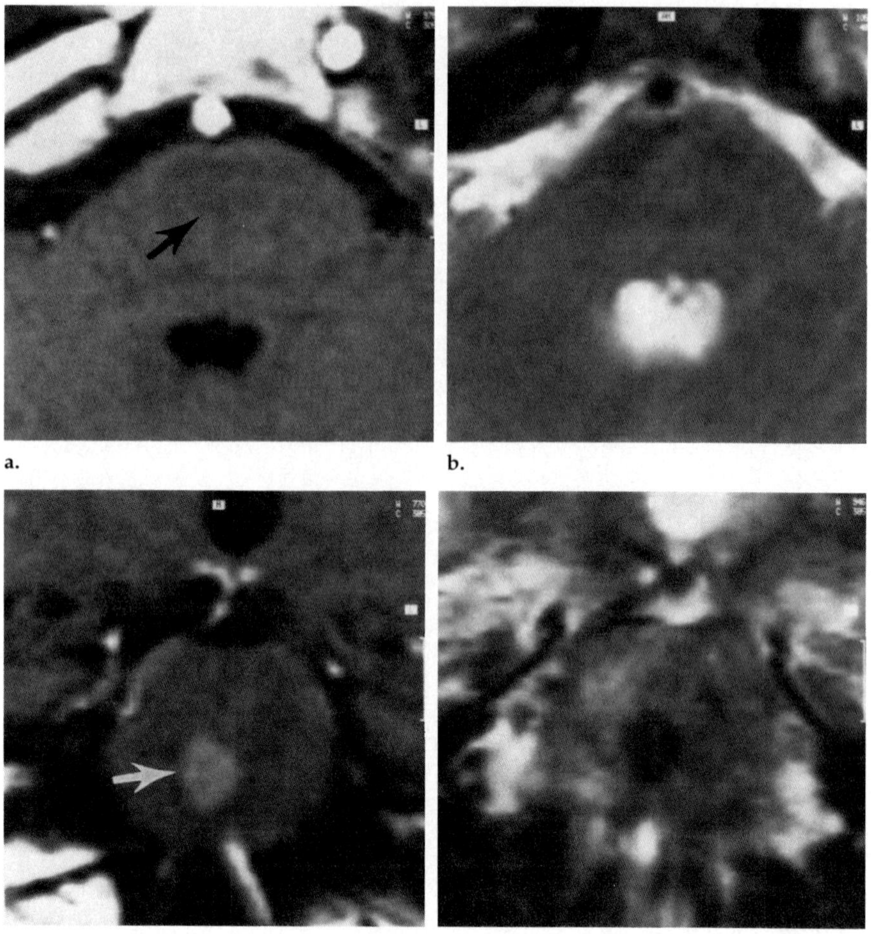

c. d.

Figure 1. Patient 2. Typical appearance of capillary telangiectasia in the pons. **(a)** Axial T1-weighted image (500/22) shows subtle T1 prolongation in the ventral middle part of the pons (arrow). **(b)** Axial T2-weighted image (2,500/80) correspondingly shows a subtle hyperintense lesion. No hypointense signal is present. **(c)** Coronal gadolinium-enhanced T1-weighted image (500/22) shows a well-circumscribed, enhancing, round lesion in the ventral middle part of the pons (arrow). **(d)** Coronal GRE image (800/35, 20° flip angle) shows corresponding, marked, susceptibility-related signal intensity loss, presumably from a blood oxygen-level–dependent (BOLD) effect due to deoxyhemoglobin.

MR imaging and clinical follow-up findings were obtained in 14 of the 18 patients. In all patients, the MR imaging appearance of each lesion was completely unchanged on each follow-up image. Clinically, all patients remained stable, except for patient 1, who has had gradually worsening leg weakness and ataxia over the 5 years of follow-up in spite of seven completely unchanged MR images obtained over this period.

Of interest is that the contrast material–enhancing capillary telangiectasia lesion in patient 17 was visible in retrospect on her initial contrast-enhanced CT scan (but was not detectable on the precontrast CT scan obtained concurrently) and had not changed in size during 7 years. Patient 10 had undergone contrast-enhanced CT 2 days before MR imaging; the capillary telangiectasia had been seen prospectively, which prompted the performance of MR imaging. These lesions were not detectable on unenhanced CT scans in six patients, which included patients 10 and 17.

As detailed in the last column of Table 2, five patients had associated vascular malformations, which in-

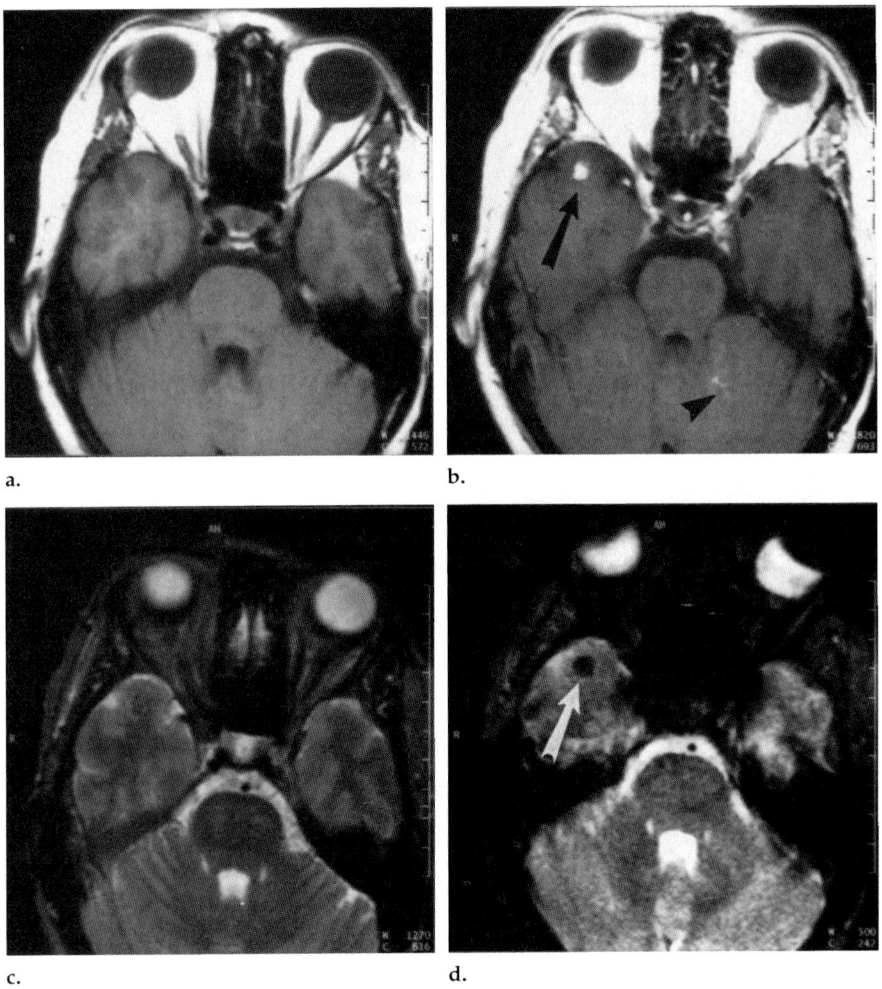

Figure 2. Patient 17. Capillary telangiectasia in the right temporal tip. **(a)** Axial T1-weighted image (600/15) is unremarkable, although in retrospect the right temporal tip lesion may be subtly detected. **(b)** Axial gadolinium-enhanced T1-weighted image (600/15) clearly demonstrates the enhancing, round, 7-mm lesion (arrow). Note the brushlike appearance of the anterior border of the lesion. A tiny left vermian venous angioma is incidentally noted (arrowhead). **(c)** Axial T2-weighted image (2,500/80) shows no definite abnormality. In particular, no hypointense signal is seen. **(d)** Axial GRE image (850/35, 10° flip angle) shows markedly increased susceptibility blooming (arrow) of the capillary telangiectasia lesion that corresponds to the region of enhancement.

cluded venous angiomas and multiple cavernomas.

Specimen Neurohistopathologic Examination

The superior frontal gyrus, cerebellar vermis, and basis pontis lesions had similar gross and microscopic appearances. They were small collections of tiny, red-brown dots without disruption or discoloration of the parenchyma (Fig 3a). Microscopically, they were composed of numerous thin-walled, ectatic individual vessels among normal neuropil elements (Fig 4). The majority of vessels had capillary-type walls. One lesion in the cerebellar vermis also contained a population of venous-type channels, although a dominant draining vein suggestive of a venous angioma was not evident. Many vessels contained red blood cells with adjacent tissue that lacked calcification, extraluminal hemorrhage, or hemosiderin-laden macrophages. These lesions are consistent with capillary telangiectasia.

The anterior temporal lobe specimen had the classic gross and histologic appearance of a cavernous angioma. Grossly, there was a readily identifiable mass of red-brown tissue and vascular material with brown discoloration and compression of the surrounding neuropil. The central aspect of the lesion was a complex network of cavernous channels and hyalinized vessels without arterial features or intervening neuropil. Focal calcifications were present, and the surrounding parenchyma was markedly gliotic with numerous hemosiderin-laden macrophages.

Specimen MR Imaging

Of the three specimens, only one (the superior frontal gyrus lesion) had capillary telangiectasia that was definitely perceptible on the thin-section, specimen T1-weighted images. The T1-weighted images demonstrated areas with minimal loss of T1 signal, which corresponded to the dilated vascular cavities. Also, in only this specimen was capillary telangiectasia perceptible on conventional T2-weighted images, which demonstrated some T2 prolongation. Lesions in the other two specimens were not obviously visible on conventional T1- and T2-weighted spin-echo images, which is in agreement with typical in vivo MR images (Table 2, Fig 3b).

None of the capillary telangiectasia specimens exhibited any increased susceptibility on the GRE images, which reflects the histopathologic lack of hemosiderin or calcification (Fig 3c). In contrast, the cavernous angioma tissue specimen demonstrated loss of T1 and T2 signal peripherally and exhibited the classic in vivo MR imaging appearance of a marked peripheral ring of susceptibility "blooming" on the GRE images obtained both while the patient was alive and in the necropsy tissue specimen. This blooming corresponded to the histopathologically demonstrated hemosiderin rim.

DISCUSSION

Of the four generally recognized intracranial parenchymal vascular malformations, three are readily detected radiologically: AVMs, venous angiomas, and cavernous angiomas have a characteristic MR imaging appearance, and AVMs and venous angiomas also have a characteristic angiographic appearance (1). The angiographically occult vascular malformations are generally accepted to comprise the histopathologically defined entities of capillary telangiectasia and cavernous angioma (6–11). Both capillary telangiectasia and cavernous angioma are found widely distributed in the central nervous system, although capillary telangiectasia is most commonly found in the basis pontis (8–11).

Capillary telangiectasia lesions are small, usually less than 2.0 cm in diameter, and appear as numerous, minute red-brown circles and lines in otherwise undistorted parenchyma. They are most commonly, but not exclusively, located in the pons (12), and

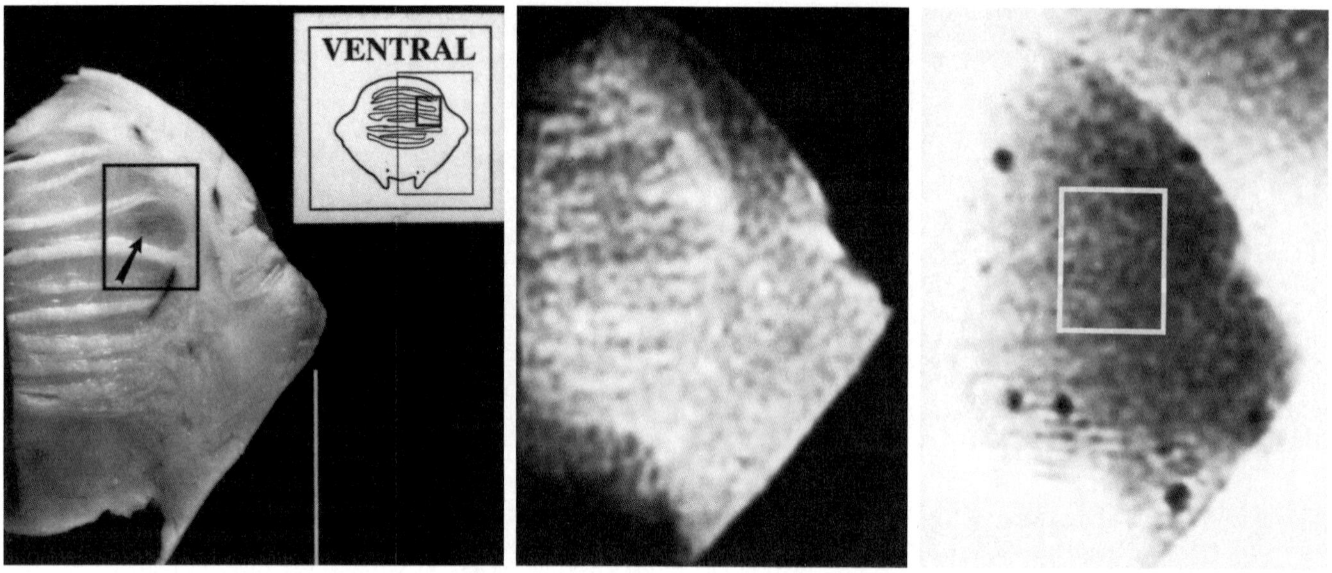

a. b. c.

Figure 3. Capillary telangiectasia specimen images. **(a)** Axial hemisection of the pons with capillary telangiectasia in the lateral basis pontis gray matter (boxed region). Inset diagram shows orientation of the pons specimen. The lesion (arrow) consists of a slight blush of fine vessels and does not distort the gross architecture. Bar = 1.0 cm. **(b)** Conventional T1-weighted image (500/13, 1.0-mm section thickness) of the tissue specimen in a water bath shows no definite lesion. **(c)** Susceptibility-sensitive GRE image (500/30, 20° flip angle, 1.4-mm section thickness) of the specimen in a water bath. No area of abnormal susceptibility dephasing that corresponds to the histopathologically demonstrated lesion is shown on this image, which reflects the histopathologically confirmed absence of hemosiderin-laden macrophages. The expected BOLD signal intensity loss is, however, also absent, likely owing to postfixation alteration of the red blood cell metabolic state (ie, the deoxyhemoglobin state no longer obtains in this postfixation tissue specimen). (The small black dots of susceptibility dephasing represent tiny air bubbles adherent to the specimen surface.) The box in **a** and **c** marks the area shown in Figure 4.

Figure 4. Neurohistopathologic features of capillary telangiectasia. **(a)** Gross detail of the boxed region in Figure 3 shows small ectatic vascular structures (arrows) in the basis pontis gray matter. Bar = 1.0 mm. **(b)** High magnification of this region reveals irregular, dilated vascular channels with capillary-type walls within normal neuropil. Note the intact pontine neurons and lack of astrocytosis or hemosiderin-laden macrophages. (Hematoxylin-eosin stain; original magnification, ×200.) Bar = 50 μm.

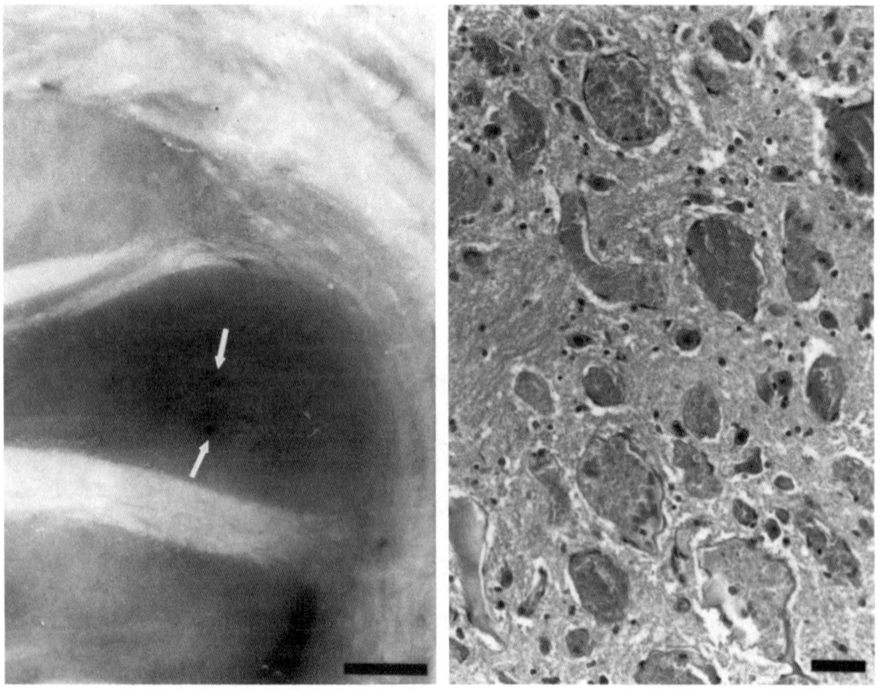

a. b.

their estimated prevalence at autopsy is 0.4% (13). In their review, McCormick and colleagues (14) found 38 capillary telangiectasia lesions in the posterior fossa, mostly in the pons, and 22 in the supratentorial compartment.

Microscopically, they are composed of ectatic individual vessels with thin, capillary-type walls that course among normal architectural elements without adjacent gliosis or hemosiderin deposition (1,8–10). Although radiologically distinct from venous angioma, capillary telangiectasia is difficult, and sometimes impossible, to distinguish microscopically from venous angioma if the characteristic larger-diameter draining vein of the latter is not included in the sample (1).

Cavernous angiomas are grossly recognizable lesions composed of a central core of spongy blood-filled vascular channels with compression and hemosiderin staining of the surrounding parenchyma. The vascular channels of cavernous angiomas are variable, but the characteristic lesion is a collection of tightly packed complex vessels with interconnected cavernous formations that have incomplete septa-like walls, hyalinization, and calcification (1,8–10). As opposed to the other vascular malformations, which typically are composed of abnormal vessels that interrupt normal parenchyma, cavernous angiomas markedly distort normal architectural structures and contain only small islands of residual neuropil. The pa-

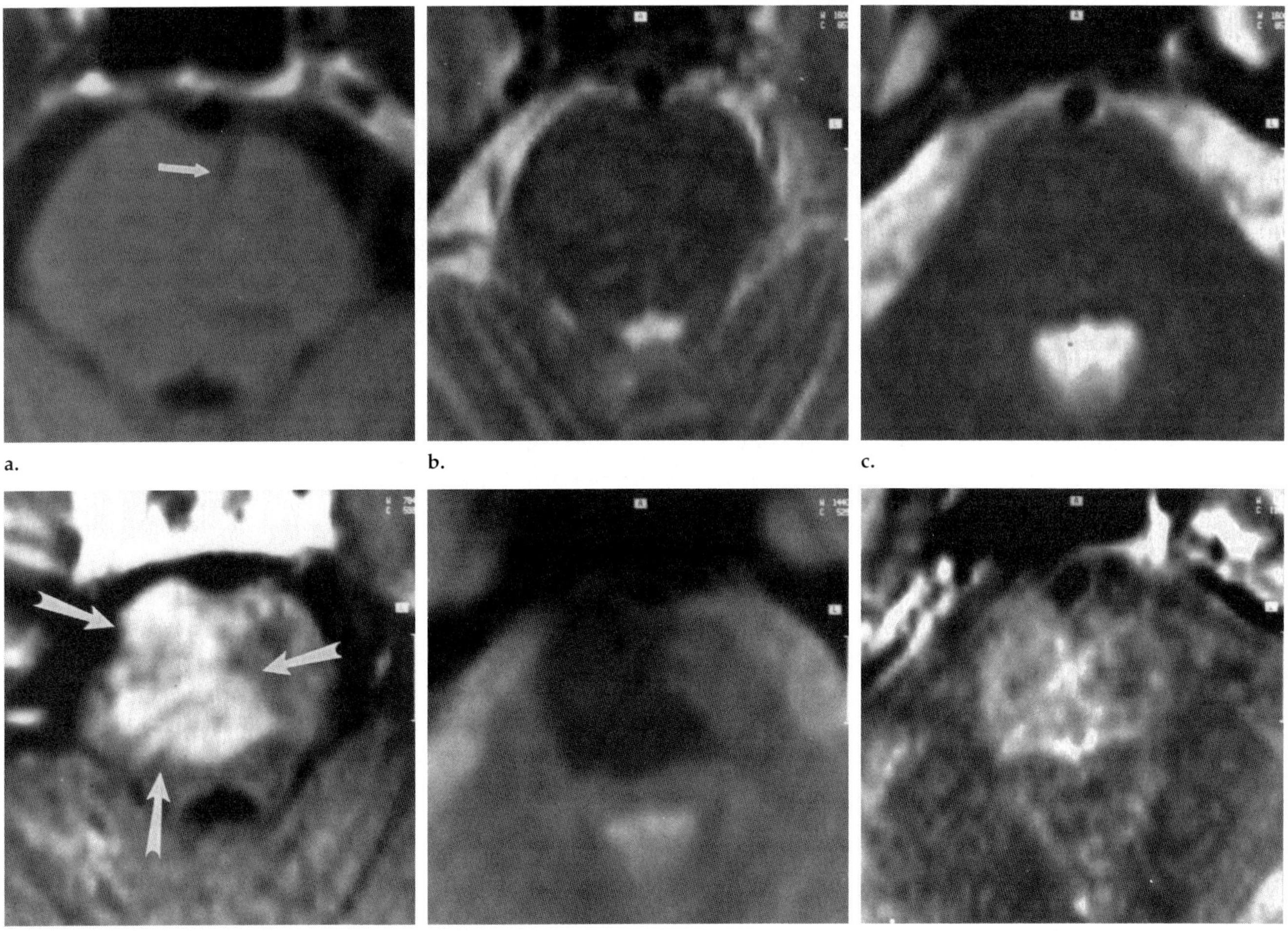

a. b. c. d. e. f.

Figure 5. Patient 7. Large capillary telangiectasia lesion. **(a)** Axial T1-weighted (700/15) and **(b, c)** consecutive axial 5-mm T2-weighted (2,500/80) images demonstrate no abnormality, except for a possible small draining vein in the ventral left part of the pons (arrow in **a**). In particular, no hypointense or hyperintense signal is seen on the T2-weighted images. **(d)** Gadolinium-enhanced T1-weighted image (600/15) shows a large region of enhancement (arrows) that involves the entire right side of the pons and extends into the posterior left side of the pons. **(e)** Susceptibility-sensitive GRE image (500/20, 20° flip angle) shows markedly increased susceptibility dephasing that corresponds to the region of enhancement in **d.** **(f)** Proton-density–weighted image (2,500/20) shows subtle T2 prolongation that corresponds to this same distribution. The reason that the lesion is invisible in **b** and **c** is that the mild T2 prolongation evidenced here is counteracted by the T2 shortening (presumably owing to the BOLD effect of deoxyhemoglobin in capillary telangiectasia) in **e**.

renchyma that surrounds cavernous angiomas is compressed and has extensive astrocytosis and numerous hemosiderin-laden macrophages and may contain calcified capillary networks.

The diagnosis of these occult vascular malformations (cavernous angioma and capillary telangiectasia) is greatly facilitated by MR imaging. The diagnosis cannot be made angiographically. CT diagnosis of cavernous angioma is often difficult, and CT diagnosis of capillary telangiectasia is generally not possible (1,4,7).

However, cavernous angioma has a well-known classic appearance on MR images (4). Its hallmark is a surrounding hypointense hemosiderin ring with an internal "popcorn" appearance on T2-weighted images. The presence of hemosiderin is well documented in histopathologic specimens (1,4,11,15); this was corroborated in the tissue specimen examined in this study.

The MR imaging appearance of capillary telangiectasia is not well known. Although no histopathologic material was obtained from any of the cases in this series, there is strong circumstantial evidence that the imaged lesions represent capillary telangiectasia: (*a*) All lesions had a similar appearance at all MR imaging sequences, which indicates that they likely represent a single diagnostic entity. (*b*) They corresponded in location and size to the histopathologically well-documented entity. (*c*) The lesions for the most part caused minimal symptoms and were isolated, which is in keeping with the known characteristics of capillary telangiectasia. (*d*) The MR imaging appearance of the three histopathologically confirmed specimens on T1-, T2-, and proton-density–weighted images corresponded to the in vivo appearance of the lesions in the 18 patients and was markedly different from the appearance of the cavernomas. (*e*) The normal laboratory values and stable imaging and clinical follow-up findings for up to several years in these patients are consistent with a benign, incidental, vascular lesion rather than entities that have a similar appearance with conventional MR imaging sequences (such as multiple sclerosis, subacute stroke, or tumor).

As illustrated here, capillary telangiectasia lesions have a typical MR appearance. They are small, enhancing lesions that are usually located in the pons and that are often undetectable on conventional T1- and T2-weighted images. They demonstrate susceptibility dephasing on GRE images.

A recent article by Barr and colleagues (16) described similar MR imaging findings in 12 patients, but only seven of those patients had confirmatory GRE sequences performed, and no histopathologic material was examined.

The MR imaging characteristics of capillary telangiectasia may be understood by analyzing tissue composition. Their mild enhancement with contrast material is explained by their being composed of ectatic blood vessels. Their imaging characteristics on GRE and T2-weighted images may also be explained by their composition as follows: The observed susceptibility dephasing could theoretically be caused by air, calcium, melanin, hemosiderin, ferritin, or deoxyhemoglobin (5). However, capillary telangiectasia as described in the pathology literature and in the three specimens examined in this study does not contain air, calcium, melanin, hemosiderin-laden macrophages, or ferritin (1,8–10). (Absence of calcification in these lesions is also supported by the undetectability at unenhanced CT of all lesions in this study that were imaged with CT.) This leaves only deoxyhemoglobin as a plausible source of the observed susceptibility dephasing. This agrees with the observed histopathologic composition of capillary telangiectasia lesions, which are composed of ectatic vessels that contain static blood whose hemoglobin presumably desaturates to the deoxyhemoglobin state.

It is plausible that the hemoglobin in these lesions is only partially desaturated to deoxyhemoglobin. Because the amount of susceptibility-induced dephasing in MR imaging is dependent on the oxygenation level of the hemoglobin (17,18), the paramagnetic effect of the deoxyhemoglobin in capillary telangiectasia would be mild, which would explain why capillary telangiectasia demonstrates signal intensity loss on GRE but not on T2-weighted images. Cavernomas, on the other hand, contain numerous hemosiderin-laden macrophages and often are calcified; hence, they show marked signal intensity loss on T2-weighted and GRE images (4). The above argument is plausible (and is supported by the MR imaging characteristics of the histopathologic specimens) but is not definitely proved, because direct in vivo sampling of the lesions was not performed. The BOLD effect was not demonstrated in the capillary telangiectasia tissue specimens, presumably owing to alterations in the red blood cells and their oxygenation state after histochemical fixation.

Fast spin-echo imaging was not used in this study (except as an adjunctive sequence in two patients in whom no susceptibility was shown with those fast spin-echo sequences) but is well documented to be less sensitive to susceptibility than conventional spin-echo imaging owing to short interecho spacing times (19,20). Hence, fast spin-echo imaging (which is being used increasingly in neuroimaging owing to its short total imaging time) would also fail to demonstrate the characteristic blooming in these lesions on long–repetition time, long–echo time images.

One pitfall to diagnosis is the smallness of these lesions. Once detected at conventional spin-echo imaging, a GRE sequence is imperative to demonstrate mild susceptibility blooming to establish the diagnosis of capillary telangiectasia. However, if the section thickness used is too large (such as in conventional brain axial sections, eg, 5 mm with a 2-mm gap), the lesion may be missed, and the diagnosis of benign capillary telangiectasia would not be made. (In fact, such an error was initially made in patient 16 after 5-mm GRE images showed no abnormal susceptibility, but this was rectified after the patient returned and 3-mm GRE images were obtained that did demonstrate abnormal susceptibility.) Hence, a directed thin-section (3 mm with a 0.5-mm gap or contiguous 3-mm sections) GRE sequence in the axial (and coronal) planes may be necessary to demonstrate the increased susceptibility and make the diagnosis.

Barr and colleagues (16) described an irregular or brushlike border of this lesion. Eleven of our 18 lesions had portions of their borders that had this appearance after contrast material administration (such as the anterior margin of the lesion in Fig 2b). Also, our findings on GRE images agree with the findings Barr and colleagues (16) reported for selected patients who underwent imaging with a similar pulse sequence.

Our patients with capillary telangiectasia presented with a varied assortment of mild neurologic symptoms, and several lesions were discovered only incidentally. The differential diagnosis of enhancing lesions in the pons includes neoplasms such as astrocytoma or lymphoma, subacute infarction, active demyelination, or acute inflammatory processes such as acute disseminated encephalomyelitis, or ADEM, in addition to capillary telangiectasia. In this differential diagnosis, generally only capillary telangiectasia lesions contain blood products, so only these would demonstrate increased susceptibility on GRE images; thus, GRE images are key to establishing the correct diagnosis.

Conversely, given the microscopic composition of dilated sacs of blood in capillary telangiectasia, a lack of susceptibility renders that diagnosis unlikely, which leaves the differential diagnosis of demyelination, ischemia, neoplasm, or acute inflammatory process.

The implications of an incorrect diagnosis are profound, because of the different prognoses of these other diagnoses and their psychological effect on the patient and his or her family. Even if the management for these other diagnoses would still be "watchful waiting," we strongly believe that it is important to suggest the correct diagnosis of benign (incidental) capillary telangiectasia and avoid an erroneous and potentially psychologically devastating diagnosis of multiple sclerosis, brain stem stroke, or lymphoma.

The distinction between the different nonarterial vascular histopathologic entities (venous angioma, cavernous angioma, and capillary telangiectasia) at times may be difficult. A given lesion may contain features that are usually associated with another type of lesion. The most common occurrence is the association of a cavernous malformation and features of capillary telangiectasia, both in the vicinity and at a distance (7,21,22). As detailed in Table 2, two of our patients (patients 9 and 11) had multiple classic cerebral cavernomas in addition to pontine capillary telangiectasia, and one of these patients (patient 11) was the only patient in our series to have more than one capillary telangiectasia lesion. The coexistence of pontine capillary telangiectasia with multiple cavernomas supports the concept that these entities may be related as two ends of a spectrum, as proposed earlier by Rigamonti and colleagues (21), rather than the hypothesis that they are two completely different coexistent lesions in these patients. These patients are being followed up at yearly intervals to evaluate whether the pontine capillary telangiectasia lesions will in time evolve into classic cavernomas.

Cavernous malformations are associated with venous malformations in 10%–15% of cases (23). Less well known but of theoretic importance is the observation that capillary telangiectasia is associated at times with enlarged venous structures (16,24). In our series, three of the lesions (in patients 7, 8, and 16) had associated small linear structures that have the appearance of draining veins (Fig 5), but these did not exhibit the prominent size and contrast material enhancement typical of classic venous angiomas (3). However, this does suggest the possibility of a developmental spectrum that relates capillary telangiectasia and venous angioma, especially because these entities cannot be histopathologically distinguished from each other, unless a draining vein is seen (1).

More studies are necessary to understand the importance of these combination lesions; however, as a group, nonarterial vascular malformations are most commonly either asymptomatic incidental postmortem findings or causally related to seizure disorders (especially cavernomas) (15).

The importance of a clearer understanding of the pathogenetic relationship, if any, between the different vascular lesions is related to our present inability to clearly understand the natural history of these lesions. So far, no lesions identified as solitary classic capillary telangiectasia lesions in this series have hemorrhaged, but more long-term follow-up is necessary to assess their natural history. Our ability to predict the chance of bleeding (or repeat bleeding), and therefore to counsel our patients, is at present limited by our incomplete understanding of the nature of the histopathologic spectrum of these nonarterial vascular malformations.

In conclusion, capillary telangiectasia lesions are not uncommon; they are vascular lesions composed of dilated capillaries, usually located in the pons, that have a characteristic MR imaging appearance that correlates with their microscopic tissue composition: (*a*) Being vascular lesions, they mildly enhance with gadopentetate dimeglumine. (*b*) Lacking hemosiderin, they are not hypointense on conventional or fast spin-echo T2-weighted images and may be undetectable on conventional unenhanced T1- and T2-weighted images. (*c*) Because they are composed of sacs of stagnant blood that has presumably partially converted to deoxyhemoglobin, they exhibit susceptibility dephasing, which is evident only on GRE (T2*-weighted) images. This dephasing is probably due to the BOLD effect.

Classic capillary telangiectasia lesions are distinguishable from cavernous angiomas at MR imaging. This is because the latter, which contain hemosiderin-laden macrophages, contain regions that are hypointense on T2-weighted images, whereas capillary telangiectasia lesions do not contain hemosiderin and are not hypointense on T2-weighted images.

The GRE (T2*-weighted) sequence is essential in diagnosing capillary telangiectasia lesions. Without it, their mild gadopentetate dimeglumine enhancement and subtle hyperintense or isointense signal on conventional T2-weighted MR images is nonspecific and could suggest the diagnoses of neoplasm (eg, lymphoma), multiple sclerosis, and subacute infarction, all of which may have a poorer prognosis and are more psychologically devastating to the patient than a diagnosis of capillary telangiectasia, a presumably benign (often incidental) cryptic vascular malformation. The presence of susceptibility makes the diagnosis of multiple sclerosis, neoplasm, or subacute infarction unlikely.

Patients with capillary telangiectasia generally present with mild symptoms such as headache, vertigo, or mild facial weakness or may be asymptomatic.

The coexistence of pontine capillary telangiectasia and multiple classic-appearing cerebral cavernomas lends support to the hypothesis that capillary telangiectasia and cavernous angioma may represent two ends of a spectrum of angiographically occult vascular malformations.

The presence of a small draining vein associated with some capillary telangiectasia lesions suggests that there may also be a spectrum between capillary telangiectasia and venous angioma. ■

Acknowledgments: We thank Robert M. Elfont, MD, Richard F. Lewis, MD, David S. Zee, MD, Clifford T. Solomon, MD, and William R. Tyor, MD, for referring patients to us, and we thank Mary T. Lally, RT, Cheryl L. Moser, RT, and Hugh B. Wall, RT, for technical assistance.

References

1. Challa VR, Moody DM, Brown WR. Vascular malformations of the central nervous system. J Neuropathol Exp Neurol 1995; 54:609–621.
2. Graves VB, Duff TA. Intracranial arteriovenous malformations: current imaging and treatment. Invest Radiol 1990; 25:952–960.
3. Truwit CL. Venous angioma of the brain: history, significance, and imaging findings. AJR 1992; 159:1299–1307.
4. Gomori JM, Grossman RI, Goldberg HI, Hackney DB, Zimmerman RA, Bilaniuk LT. Occult cerebral vascular malformations: high-field MR imaging. Radiology 1986; 158:707–713.
5. Atlas SW, Mark AS, Grossman RI, Gomori JM. Intracranial hemorrhage: gradient-echo MR imaging at 1.5T. Radiology 1988; 168:803–807.
6. Robinson JR, Awad IA, Masaryk TJ, Estes ML. Pathological heterogeneity of angiographically occult vascular malformations of the brain. Neurosurgery 1993; 33:547–555.
7. Awad IA, Robinson JR, Mohanty S, Estes ML. Mixed vascular malformations of the brain: clinical and pathogenetic considerations. Neurosurgery 1993; 33:179–188.
8. Burger PC, Scheithauer BW, Vogel FS. Surgical pathology of the nervous system and its coverings. 3rd ed. New York, NY: Churchill Livingstone, 1991; 439–443.
9. Russell DS, Rubinstein LJ. Pathology of tumours of the nervous system. 5th ed. Baltimore, Md: Williams & Wilkins, 1989; 735–736.
10. Jellinger K. Vascular malformations of the central nervous system: a morphological overview. Neurosurg Rev 1986; 9:177–216.
11. McCormick WF. The pathology of vascular ("arteriovenous") malformations. J Neurosurg 1966; 24:807–816.
12. White RJ, Wood MW, Kernohan JW. A study of fifty intracranial vascular tumors found incidentally at autopsy. J Neuropathol Exp Neurol 1958; 17:392–398.
13. Sarwar M, McCormick WF. Intracerebral venous angioma: case report and review. Arch Neurol 1978; 35:323–325.
14. McCormick WF, Hardman JM, Boulter TR. Vascular malformations ("angiomas") of the brain with special reference to those occurring in the posterior fossa. J Neurosurg 1968; 28:241–251.
15. Simard JM, Garcia-Bengochea F, Ballinger Jr WE, Mickle JP, Quisling RG. Cavernous angioma: a review of 126 collected and 12 new clinical cases. Neurosurgery 1986; 18: 162–172.
16. Barr RM, Dillon WP, Wilson CB. Slow-flow vascular malformations of the pons: capillary telangiectasias? AJNR 1996; 17:71–78.
17. Ogawa S, Lee TM, Kay AR, Tank DW. Brain magnetic resonance imaging with contrast dependent on blood oxygenation. Proc Natl Acad Sci 1990; 87:9868–9872.
18. Ogawa S, Lee TM, Nayak AS, Glynn P. Oxygenation-sensitive contrast in magnetic resonance image of rodent brain at high magnetic fields. Magn Reson Med 1990; 14:68–78.
19. Jones KM, Mulkern RV, Schwartz RB, Oshio K, Barnes PD, Jolesz FA. Fast spin-echo MR imaging of the brain and spine: current concepts. AJR 1992; 158:1313–1320.
20. Mulkern RV, Wong STS, Winalski C, Jolesz FA. Contrast manipulation and artifact assessment of 2D and 3D RARE sequences. Magn Reson Imaging 1990; 8:557–566.
21. Rigamonti D, Johnson PC, Spetzler RF, et al. Cavernous malformations and capillary telangiectasia: a spectrum within a single pathological entity. Neurosurgery 1991; 28:60–64.
22. Sasaki O, Tanaka R, Koike T, Koide A, Koizumi T, Ogawa H. Excision of cavernous angioma with preservation of coexisting venous angioma. J Neurosurg 1991; 75:461–464.
23. Rigamonti D, Spetzler RF. The association of venous and cavernous malformations: report of four cases and discussion of the pathophysiological, diagnostic, and therapeutic implications. Acta Neurochir (Wien) 1988; 92:100–105.
24. Blackwood W. Two cases of benign cerebral telangiectasis. J Pathol Bacteriol 1941; 52:209–212.

Ray's Days

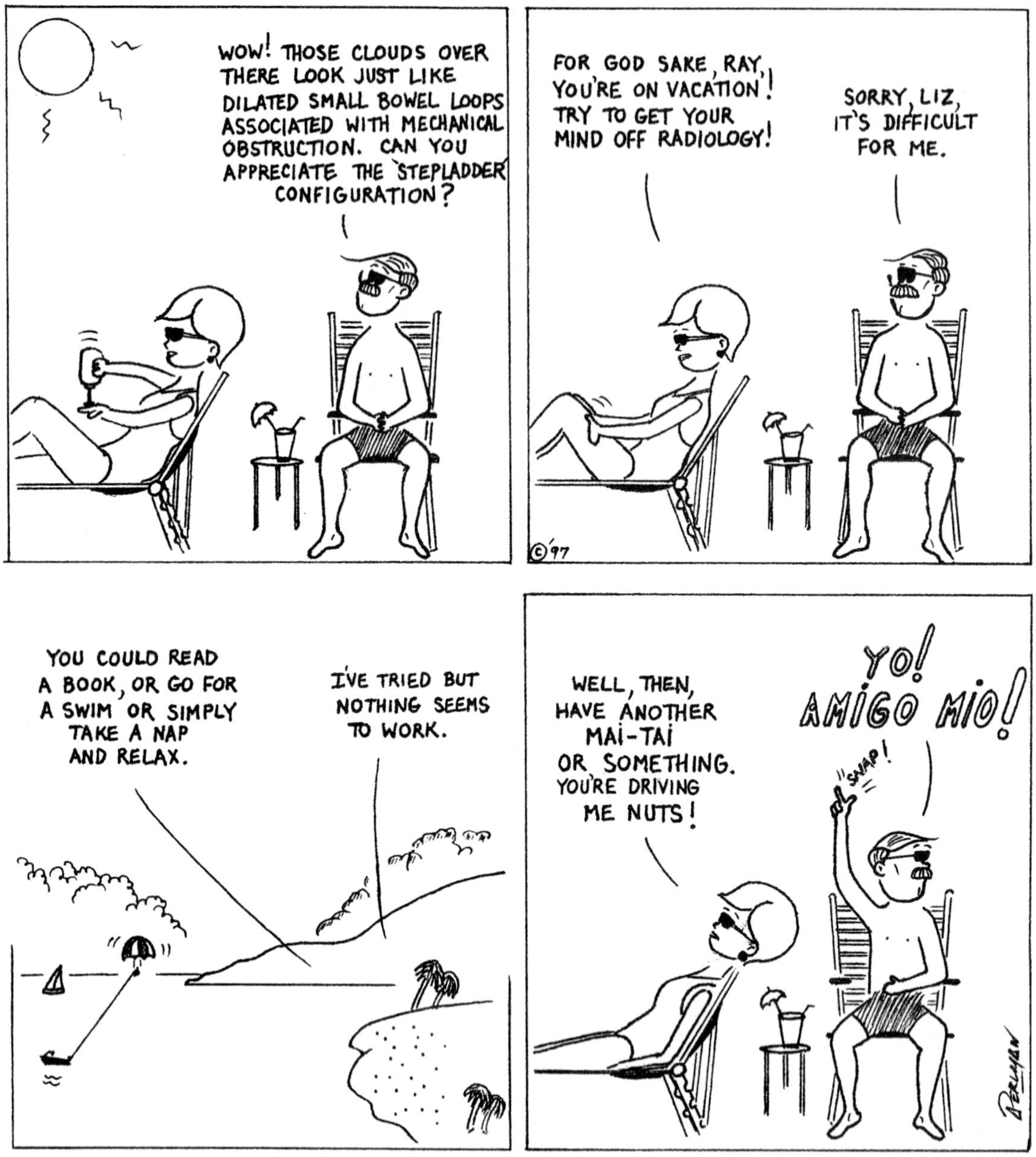

Steven J. Perlman, MD, Cincinnati, Ohio

Allen B. Oser, MD • Christopher J. Moran, MD • Bruce A. Kaufman, MD • Tae S. Park, MD

Intracranial Tumor in Children: MR Imaging Findings within 24 Hours of Craniotomy[1]

PURPOSE: **To evaluate whether very early magnetic resonance (MR) imaging enables distinction of residual tumor from benign postoperative change in children.**

MATERIALS AND METHODS: **Forty-six postoperative MR examinations were performed in 43 children with intracranial tumors within 24 hours of the completion of surgery during a 2-year period. These examinations were categorized according to whether residual tumor could be definitely identified or excluded, or whether the diagnosis was uncertain.**

RESULTS: **Contrast enhancement occurred in 33 of 46 MR examinations performed within 24 hours of surgery. In 18 instances, this was associated with obvious residual tumor. In 15 patients, only small amounts of linear or patchy enhancement were seen. Of these, seven patients (46%) were disease-free for an average of 4.5 years. Assessment for postoperative enhancement was hampered in seven patients because of the presence of methemoglobin in the tumor bed. Contrast enhancement was not observed in two patients before surgery.**

CONCLUSION: **Surgically induced, MR-detectable contrast enhancement and extracellular methemoglobin formation occurs within 24 hours of the completion of intracranial surgery. This can interfere with the detection of small amounts of residual tumor.**

THE identification of suspected or unsuspected residual tumor in the bed of a resected intracranial tumor has important therapeutic implications. Decisions regarding early reoperation and/or therapeutic protocols depend in part on the presence and volume of residual tumor. In some instances, overall survival has been linked to the amount of postoperative residual volume (1).

Central nervous system imaging with computed tomography (CT) (2–6) and magnetic resonance (MR) imaging (7–13) in the postoperative period has been extensively evaluated. A common problem with postoperative imaging has been the inability to enable distinction of postoperative changes (hemorrhage and contrast material enhancement) from residual tumor. In theory, if the imaging study could be performed soon enough after the surgical procedure, the postoperative enhancement may not have developed, and the presence of enhancing tissue should indicate residual tumor (4). Blood at the operative site is a further confounding factor, on both CT and MR images. Since the detection of blood on routine MR images requires the development of blood breakdown products, very early imaging may precede this transformation.

The purpose of this study was to evaluate prospectively the usefulness of MR imaging performed within 24 hours of surgery for the detection of residual tumor in pediatric patients undergoing craniotomy for brain tumor.

MATERIALS AND METHODS

All patients undergoing craniotomy for tumor resection between May 1992 and May 1994 were eligible for study with MR imaging within 24 hours of completion of surgery. Fifty-two procedures were eligible for the study. All examinations were performed with appropriate patient monitoring and sedation. MR imaging was performed with a 1.5-T commercially available MR imager (Magnetom; Siemens, Erlangen, Germany). Unenhanced imaging sequences consisted of T1-weighted spin-echo (600/14 [repetition time msec/echo time msec], two signals acquired) and/or magnetization-prepared rapid gradient-echo (10/4, 10° flip angle, one signal acquired) sequences. Proton-density– and T2-weighted spin-echo sequences (3,500/19–93, one signal acquired) were also performed but were not specifically evaluated in this study. After intravenous administration of 0.1 mmol/kg gadopentetate dimeglumine (Magnevist; Berlex Laboratories, Wayne, NJ), T1-weighted spin-echo sequences (600/22, two signals acquired) were performed in at least two imaging planes, with imaging completed within 10–15 minutes after injection.

Of the 52 eligible intracranial procedures, 46 postoperative MR examinations in 43 patients were performed according to protocol within 24 hours of completion of surgery. The exclusions included five instances in which a postoperative MR examination was not performed within 24 hours because of clinical instability (two cases),

Index terms: Brain, surgery, 13.456, 15.456 • Brain neoplasms, in infants and children, 10.30 • Brain neoplasms, MR, 13.12143, 15.12143 • Magnetic resonance (MR), contrast enhancement, 13.12143, 15.12143 • Magnetic resonance (MR), in infants and children

Radiology 1997; 205:807–812

[1] From the Section of Neuroradiology, Mallinckrodt Institute of Radiology, Washington University School of Medicine, St Louis, Mo (A.B.O., C.J.M.), and the Department of Neurosurgery, Washington University School of Medicine, St Louis Children's Hospital, Mo (B.A.K., T.S.P.). From the 1995 RSNA scientific assembly. Received March 31, 1997; revision requested May 13; revision received July 17; accepted July 23. **Address reprint requests to** A.B.O., Neuroradiology Section, Department of Radiology, University of Alabama at Birmingham, 619 S 19th St, Birmingham, AL 35223.

patient refusal (one case), or for unknown reasons (two cases) and one case in which a preoperative examination performed at an outside hospital was unavailable for analysis. Three patients had two eligible surgeries during the study period and were thus included twice. As a result, the analysis was based on 46 examinations performed in 43 patients (28 boys, 15 girls; age range, 1.0–19.1 years; mean age, 8.2 years).

All patients were evaluated with unenhanced and enhanced MR imaging before surgery. On average, preoperative examinations were performed 7 days before surgery, with a range of 1–42 days.

Careful supervision and selective use of parenteral sedatives resulted in technically successful procedures in all 46 examinations. No patient had any postoperative complication that could be linked to performance of early MR imaging.

The variety of tumor types seen in this study reflects the usual distribution seen in pediatric populations. Supratentorial tumors (25 patients) included astrocytoma ($n = 8$), oligodendrogliomas ($n = 2$), primitive neuroectodermal tumor ($n = 2$), craniopharyngioma ($n = 2$), choroid plexus papilloma ($n = 2$), pineal tumor ($n = 2$), and several others ($n = 7$). Infratentorial tumors (18 patients) included medulloblastoma ($n = 7$), ependymoma ($n = 5$), astrocytoma ($n = 4$), choroid plexus papilloma ($n = 1$), and hemangioblastoma ($n = 1$).

For the purposes of this study, the immediate preoperative and postoperative examinations were reviewed by two neuroradiologists (C.J.M., A.B.O.) without knowledge of the pathologic diagnosis or patient outcome, and agreement was reached by consensus. The preoperative examinations were analyzed for tumor location, enhancement, and hemorrhage. Postoperative examinations were evaluated in conjunction with the preoperative examinations for definite residual tumor mass, for the presence of blood breakdown products (as indicated by hyperintensity on the T1-weighted images), and for contrast material enhancement.

The postoperative examinations were categorized into one of the following four groups (Table 1): Category 1 consisted of obvious residual tumor mass as well as definite contrast enhancement in the tumor and tumor bed (which are, in general, inseparable) (Fig 1). Category 2 consisted of obvious postoperative enhancement at the tumor bed without the presence of definite residual tumor mass (Fig 2). Category 3 consisted of the absence of both contrast enhancement and residual tumor mass at the tumor bed (Fig 3). Category 4 consisted of an examination in which residual tumor mass and enhancement were either obscured by the presence of hemorrhage at the operative site or were unable to be accurately assessed because of the lack of preoperative enhancement of the tumor (Fig 4). These categories were designed to help determine whether there was evidence of residual tumor on the postoperative MR images. When postoperative enhancement was detected, an attempt was made to classify the pattern of enhancement as masslike, nodular, or linear.

Table 1
Categories of Postoperative Findings

Category	Mass	Enhancement	Hemorrhage	MR Evidence of Residual Tumor	Comments
1	Yes	Yes	Yes/no	Definitely yes	Residual mass on postoperative MR images matches the preoperative appearance
2	No	Yes	Yes	Unsure	Small amounts of linear or patchy enhancement at tumor bed
3	No	No	No	Definitely not	No tumor bed enhancement or visually detectable residual mass
4	No	Unsure	Yes/no	Unsure	Presence of hemorrhage in the tumor bed might be obscuring small residual tumor, or tumor did not enhance before surgery, so residual, if any, not likely to enhance

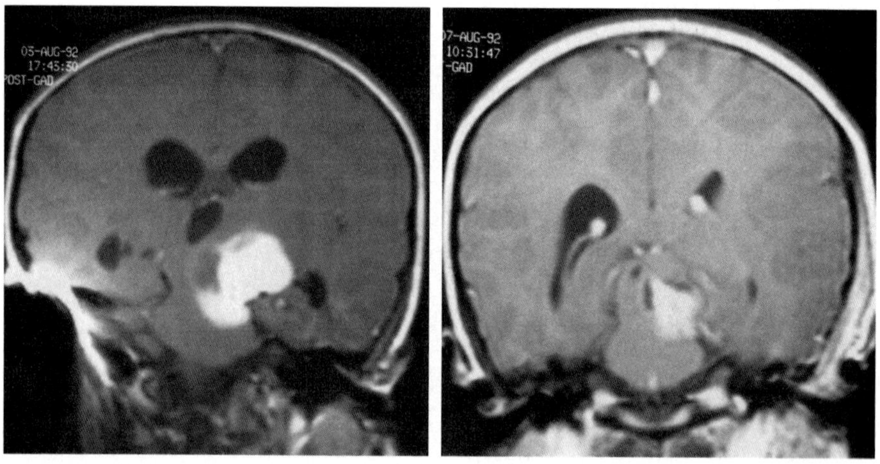

a. b.

Figure 1. Category 1 postoperative findings (definite postoperative mass and enhancement) in a 6-year-old boy. **(a)** Preoperative MR image shows an enhancing juvenile pilocytic astrocytoma in the left aspect of the midbrain. **(b)** Postoperative MR image demonstrates an obvious residual enhancing mass. The location of the tumor allowed only subtotal resection.

Postoperative follow-up consisted of standard clinical and imaging approaches. Postoperative adjuvant radiation and/or chemotherapy was used in many cases. Cases were categorized on the basis of outcome as disease-free, stable disease, progressive disease, or regressing disease (Table 2).

RESULTS

Of the 46 postoperative MR examinations performed within 24 hours of the completion of surgery, 33 (72%) showed contrast enhancement in the tumor bed. There were 18 with obvious residual mass, which matched the tumor mass seen on the preoperative examination (category 1). Fifteen cases showed definite contrast enhancement but no definite mass (category 2). There were four cases in which neither residual mass nor any postoperative enhancement was observed (category 3). In nine cases, the assessment of postoperative residual enhancing tumor was not considered possible (category 4). This was due to either the presence of blood breakdown products, presumably methemoglobin which obscured visualization of possibly enhancing tissue (seven cases), or the absence of contrast enhancement in the tumor preoperatively (two cases).

A prior procedure had been performed in 19 patients. This included 11 patients who underwent a prior partial surgical resection, two who

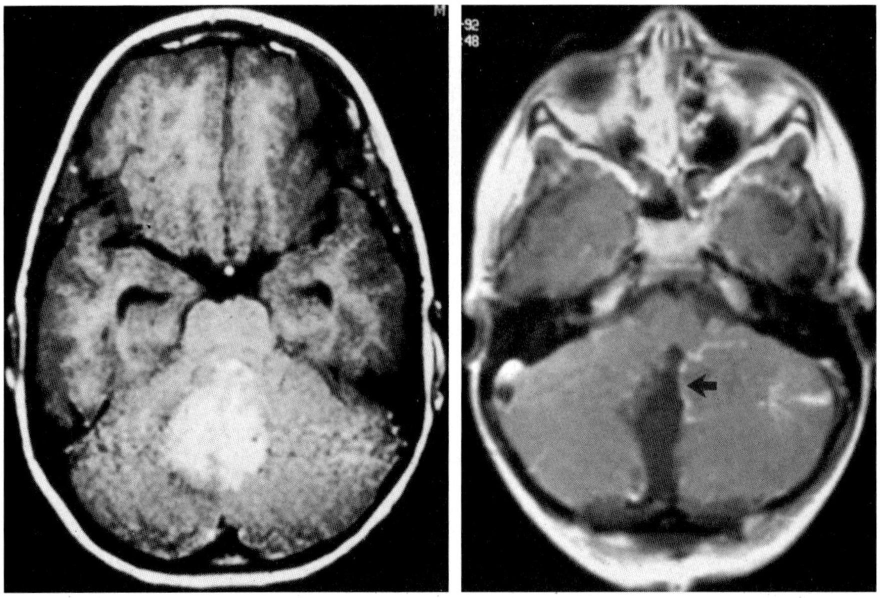

a. b.

Figure 2. Category 2 postoperative findings (postoperative enhancement at operative site without residual mass) in a 5-year-old boy. **(a)** Preoperative MR image shows a medulloblastoma. The patient underwent a total gross resection. **(b)** Immediate postoperative MR image shows linear enhancement (arrow) along the medial aspect of the left side of the resection bed. A venous malformation is seen in the left cerebellar hemisphere. This patient later died of local and distant recurrence.

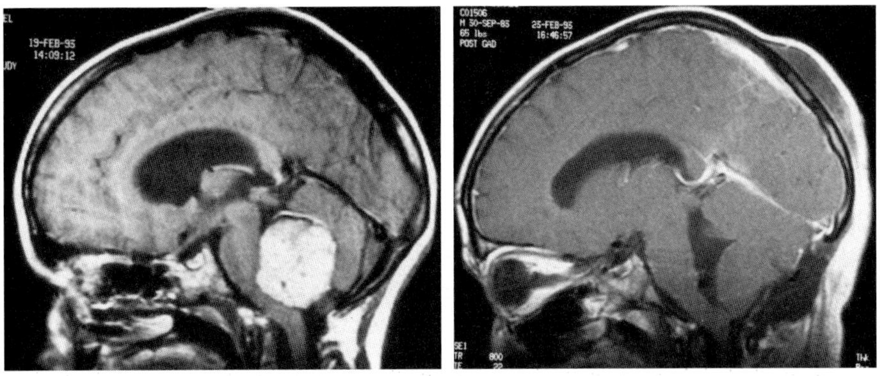

a. b.

Figure 3. Category 3 postoperative findings (no postoperative enhancement or mass) in a 10-year-old boy with a choroid plexus papilloma. **(a)** Preoperative MR image shows a large enhancing mass filling the fourth ventricle. **(b)** Immediate postoperative MR image shows that there is no contrast enhancement or methemoglobin in the surgical bed. This patient has had no evidence of tumor recurrence after 4 years.

underwent prior stereotactic needle biopsy, and six who underwent ventriculostomy placement without biopsy. Of the patients who had undergone a prior procedure, 12 patients (63%) had obvious residual tumor mass.

There has been an average of 3.6 years of clinical follow-up. The average follow-up in patients who died was 0.9 year. Excluding deaths, the average follow-up was 4.4 years.

Postoperative radiation therapy and/or chemotherapy was used after 26 (57%) of the 46 imaging studies. Of 18 category 1 cases, six (33%) received radiation therapy, one (6%) received chemotherapy, four (22%) received both radiation and chemotherapy, and seven (39%) received neither. In category 2 (n = 15), three (20%) received radiation therapy, one (7%) received chemotherapy, eight (53%) received both radiation and chemotherapy, and three (20%) received neither. None of the category 3 cases received either chemotherapy or radiation therapy. In category 4 (n = 9), three (33%) received chemotherapy and six (67%) received neither.

Nine of the 43 patients (11 examinations) included in this study died. Four of these examinations demonstrated obvious residual tumor after surgery (category 1). However, six of these examinations, in six separate patients, demonstrated no evidence of residual mass on the postoperative MR images, although there was some contrast enhancement in the tumor bed (category 2). All of these patients demonstrated progressive disease at follow-up neuroimaging, with the exception of one patient who died from causes not associated with tumor recurrence or spread. One additional patient has demonstrated progressive disease, but is still alive. Four patients were followed elsewhere, and their records were not accessible.

Among the other patients, the clinical outcome in the follow-up period has in general been good or excellent. Twenty-one patients were free of disease by clinical and radiologic parameters. Nine patients (10 examinations) had follow-up imaging evidence of stable tumor, as evidenced by residual enhancing mass that did not change in size over the follow-up period.

Of the 18 cases with a definite postoperative mass (category 1), three patients were disease-free at the most recent follow-up. These patients had postoperative regression of the residual tumor as a result of adjunctive treatment. Nine patients showed either stable or regressing tumors. In four cases, the residual tumor showed progression, and these patients have died.

Of the 15 patients with tumor bed enhancement without mass (category 2), seven were disease-free at the most recent follow-up. In seven cases, there was progression of disease, with regrowth of tumor at the primary site. All of these patients with tumor recurrence have died. One patient died from complications of endocrine dysfunction after resection of a craniopharyngioma. No correlation between the patterns of enhancement and the follow-up status of the patients was seen.

In all four of the patients who had no residual enhancing tumor (category 3), there has been no evidence of recurrent disease.

Of the seven patients in whom postoperative hemorrhage or lack of preoperative enhancement made assessment of postoperative residual impossible (category 4), six patients remained disease-free at follow-up. One patient continued to have a small area of contrast enhancement that became apparent on further follow-up examinations. This patient showed no evidence of tumor growth on additional follow-up MR images.

DISCUSSION

To our knowledge, this is the first large series of children studied with

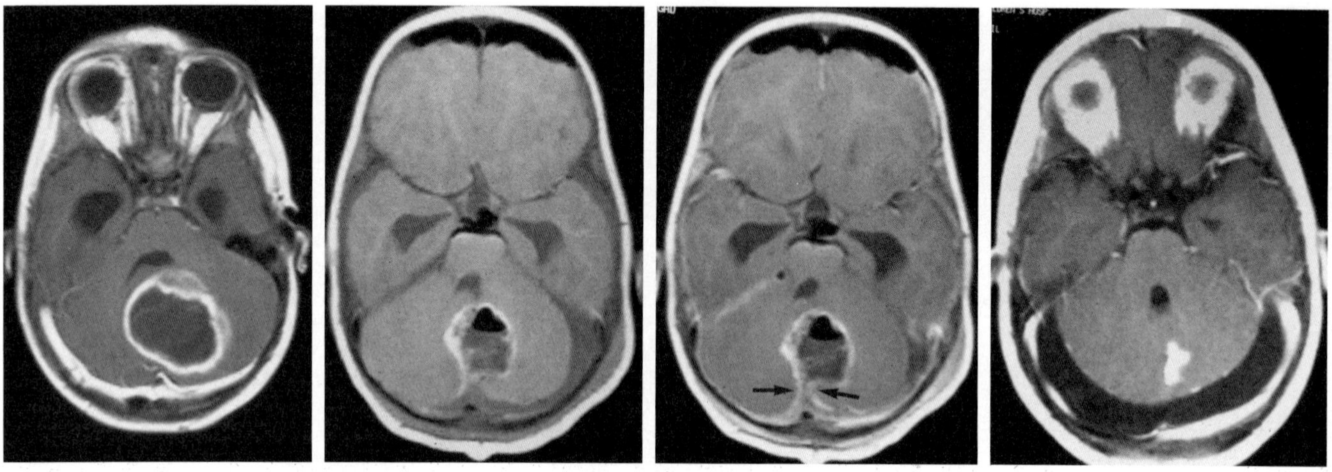

Figure 4. Category 4 postoperative findings (unable to assess for postoperative residual) in a 1-year-old girl. **(a)** Preoperative MR image shows a cystic astrocytoma with an enhancing rim. **(b)** Postoperative unenhanced MR image demonstrates methemoglobin in the entire surgical bed. **(c)** After intravenous administration of gadopentetate dimeglumine, MR image shows superimposed enhancement is detectable only at the incision site in the cerebellum (arrows). **(d)** MR image obtained 6 weeks later shows an enhancing mass at the tumor resection site. At biopsy, this proved to be residual tumor. This small residual enhancing mass was likely present in the immediate postoperative period but was obscured by methemoglobin. After reoperation, the patient has remained disease-free for 3 years.

MR imaging within the first 24 hours after craniotomy for resection of intracranial neoplasms. Our purpose was to establish whether an imaging examination could be performed before the development of surgery-related contrast enhancement and blood breakdown product formation, both of which may obscure visualization of residual tumor. Contrast enhancement at this early stage could in theory provide the best possible immediate evaluation for postoperative residual tumor.

Contrast enhancement was observed in 33 (72%) of the 46 MR examinations. In 18 cases, this enhancement was clearly associated with residual tumor mass that had enhanced preoperatively. All of these tumors were of such size and/or location that a gross total resection was not feasible.

The distinction between enhancement of a residual mass and enhancement without a residual mass could be made easily. Fifteen cases (33%) demonstrated contrast enhancement in the tumor bed without evidence of residual mass. These cases represent false-positive results for testing the hypothesis that *any* enhancement seen on postoperative MR images within 24 hours represents residual tumor. To determine whether this enhancement represented small amounts of residual tumor or whether it was simply a result of postoperative pathophysiologic factors (see below), clinical and imaging follow-up was necessary since immediate reoperation was not performed. The first subsequent postoperative MR examination was not specifically used in this regard because of the wide range of time intervals between the immediate examination (within 24 hours) and the first subsequent examination.

In our series, seven of these 15 patients with enhancement without gross residual mass were disease-free by MR imaging and clinical criteria at the most recent follow-up. Seven patients developed MR imaging and clinical evidence of progressive disease. Six of these patients are now deceased. (One additional death was unrelated to tumor recurrence.) Furthermore, there were intermediate examinations in four cases that did not demonstrate contrast enhancement in the tumor bed. We think that in most, if not all, of the cases of contrast enhancement after apparent total gross resection, the contrast enhancement is due to postoperative pathophysiologic factors and not due to small amounts of tumor left behind by the surgeon. Since 80% of these patients received adjuvant therapy (radiation and/or chemotherapy) after surgery, small amounts of residual tumor responsible for the postoperative enhancement may have been eradicated or suppressed by these additional treatments.

Although benign postoperative enhancement has been previously detected as early as 3 days after surgery with CT and MR imaging (2,4,5,8,12,14–17), most previous reports found no early enhancement. Forsting et al (8) found no "benign enhancement [on postoperative MR images] related to surgical trauma" during the first 4 days after surgery for malignant glioma. More recent, very early postoperative enhancement has been reported. Enhancement of the resected brain surface on MR images obtained within 24 hours of surgery occurred in seven (64%) of 11 adults undergoing nonneoplastic cortical resection (13). Contrast enhancement occurred on 10 (37%) of 27 very early (24-hour) CT scans obtained in a population similar to that in the current report (6).

Our study, as well as the other more recent reports (6,13), represents a break from the older findings. According to their findings of the absence of very early enhancement, generally less than 72 hours, most of these earlier reports suggest that if MR imaging were to take place early enough, the processes responsible for the repair function may not have had enough time to produce detectable contrast enhancement (2,8,18). A so-called "diagnostic window" for residual tumor during the first few days after resection had been suggested (2,12,16,19,20). We believe that our results contradict the possibility of a useful diagnostic window during which postoperative residual tumor can be completely excluded. In addition, assessment of the pattern of postoperative enhancement provided no additional contribution in the assessment for residual tumor, despite the observations of others (9,21).

In our series, there were nine examinations in which an assessment for residual tumor on the basis of the finding of postoperative contrast enhancement could not be made. In general, this determination was made on the basis of the presence of enough

Table 2
Clinical Categories on the Basis of Outcome

Clinical Category	Description
Disease free	No evidence of disease at imaging, combined with surgical impression regarding extent of resection (total); imaging remains without evidence of recurrence
Stable disease	Known residual either per operative note (eg, "small amount left on brain stem") or per imaging, with no clinical or radiologic change over time
Progressive disease	Known residual disease seen to increase in size and/or scope over time; typically seen progressing per imaging rather than per clinical indications
Regressing disease	Known residual disease (per operative report and confirmed with imaging) that regresses with time or treatment

methemoglobin such that it was considered possible that small amounts of contrast enhancement could be obscured (Fig 4). In two cases, the lack of enhancement before surgery made the use of postoperative enhancement impossible to assess for residual tumor.

Contrast enhancement in postoperative tissues in the brain has several possible origins: neovascularity, blood-brain barrier breakdown, surgical technique, and direct extravasation of contrast material from injured tissue (22–28). Jeffries et al (2) demonstrated the presence of postoperative neovascularity at 4 days in an experimental model and suggested that postoperative enhancement is due to a higher concentration of these new blood vessels. Enzman et al (14) also found vascular proliferation as early as 4 days after experimental brain injury. On the other hand, experimental studies have shown that the blood-brain barrier is disrupted as early as 3 hours after experimental mechanical injury to the brain (28–30).

The time interval between the intravenous administration of contrast material and image acquisition may be important with respect to the physiologic mechanisms of enhancement (8). If the primary mechanism of very early enhancement is leakage of contrast material through surgically damaged tissue (rather than tumor vascularity), dynamic imaging during the injection of contrast material may improve the specificity of the examination for residual tumor. Tumor enhancement may thus predominate over nonneoplastic enhancement under these conditions. Our protocol used our standard postcontrast timing, with postcontrast imaging performed immediately after, but not during, injection of contrast material.

The surgical injury of blood vessels results in red cell extravasation, which may continue in very tiny amounts despite excellent hemostasis. While not clinically important, the small amount of extravasated blood at the surgical site is often easily identified on both CT scans and MR images. On CT scans, detection of blood is straightforward (6). Studies have shown that hemorrhage is detected on CT scans obtained within 24 hours of surgery and can be seen on scans obtained up to several days or weeks after surgery (6). Since MR detection usually requires the time-dependent transformation of hemoglobin into deoxyhemoglobin and methemoglobin (31), very early MR imaging may not be subject to the problem of residual enhancing tumor obscuration in the same manner as CT. However, methemoglobin was identified in 20 (43%) of our very early postoperative MR examinations.

Although it was initially thought that the time course of degradation of blood products to MR-detectable extracellular methemoglobin (hyperintense on T1-weighted images) might increase the sensitivity of very early MR imaging for the detection of residual tumor, it has been shown by others that there is an accelerated development of methemoglobin in patients who have undergone neurosurgery (8,16). This rapid transformation into methemoglobin has been postulated to be the result of the use of hydrogen peroxide as a hemostatic and cleansing agent during surgery (8,32). However, our neurosurgeons do not use this or other oxidizing agents.

In most of these cases with methemoglobin present, superimposed contrast enhancement contributed additional information and enabled proper categorization. There were seven patients in whom the presence of methemoglobin in the tumor bed impeded evaluation for small amounts of contrast enhancement. In one case, a small amount of residual enhancing astrocytoma obscured on the postoperative examinations was proved on subsequent studies (Fig 4).

In our series, early postoperative MR examinations demonstrated conclusive evidence of either the presence or absence of residual tumor in 22 examinations (48%). For these patients, the postoperative MR study was critical in determination of early postoperative prognosis and protocols. In the other 24 examinations (52%), the question of residual tumor was unresolved, due either to the small amounts of contrast enhancement in the tumor bed or methemoglobin obscuring the tumor bed. This creates some ambiguity in postoperative decision making, although in practice most of these patients were considered to have had a gross total resection until clinical and MR imaging follow-up proved otherwise. The interpretation of any postoperative image, whether in clinical practice or as part of a research protocol, requires caution if the only finding is minimal enhancement. This is especially important when this image is used to plan treatment or assess the effectiveness of treatment.

Additional efforts on the part of the staff and patients were often necessary to adhere to this time schedule. Our results do not warrant additional sociologic and financial costs. At present, we obtain postoperative MR images in the first few days after surgery, when convenient, before discharge from the hospital. ■

References

1. Wood JR, Green SB, Shapiro WR. The prognostic importance of tumor size in malignant gliomas: a computed tomographic scan study by the Brain Tumor Cooperative Group. J Clin Oncol 1988; 6:338–343.
2. Jeffries BF, Kishore PRS, Singh KS, Ghatak NR, Krempa J. Contrast enhancement in the postoperative brain. Radiology 1981; 139:409–413.
3. Krishna Rao CVG, Kishore PRS, Bartlett J, Brennan TG. Computed tomography in the postoperative patient. Neuroradiology 1980; 19:257–263.
4. Cairncross JG, Pexman JHW, Rathbone MP, Delmaestro RF. Postoperative contrast enhancement in patients with brain tumor. Ann Neurol 1985; 17:570–572.
5. Steinbok P, Poskitt K, Cochrane DD, Flodmark OO. Early computed tomographic scanning after resection of brain tumors in children. Childs Nerv Syst 1991; 7:16–20.
6. Kaufman BA, Moran CJ, Park TS. Computer tomographic scanning within 24 hours for a tumor in children. Pediatr Neurosurg 1995; 22:74–80.
7. Forsting M, Albert FK, Kunze S. Early postoperative CT and MRI in gliablastoma. Neuroradiology 1991; 33(suppl):25–27.
8. Forsting M, Albert FK, Kunze S, Adams HP, Zenner D, Sartor K. Extirpation of glioblastomas: MR and CT follow-up of residual tumor and regrowth. AJNR 1993; 14:77–87.
9. Bird CR, Drayer BP, Medina M, Rekate HL, Flom RA, Hodak JA. Gd-DTPA-enhanced MR imaging in pediatric patients after brain tumor resection. Radiology 1988; 169:123–126.
10. Burke JW, Podrasky AE, Bradley WJ. Meninges: benign postoperative enhancement on MR images. Radiology 1990; 174:99–102.
11. Dickman CA, Rekate HL, Bird CR, Drayer BP, Medina M. Unenhanced and gadolinium-DTPA-enhanced MR imaging in post-

operative evaluation in pediatric brain tumors. J Neurosurg 1989; 71:49–53.
12. Laohaprasit V, Silbergeld DL, Ojemann GA, Eskridge JM, Winn HR. Postoperative CT contrast enhancement following lobectomy for epilepsy. J Neurosurg 1990; 73:392–395.
13. Henegar MM, Moran CJ, Silbergeld DL. Early postoperative magnetic resonance imaging following nonneoplastic cortical resection. J Neurosurg 1996; 84:174–179.
14. Enzman DR, Britt RH, Yeager AS. Experimental brain abscess evolution: computed tomographic and neuropathologic correlation. Radiology 1979; 133:113–122.
15. Wakai S, Andoh Y, Ochiai C, Inoh S, Nagai M. Postoperative contrast enhancement in brain tumors and intracerebral hematomas: CT study. J Comput Assist Tomogr 1990; 14:267–271.
16. Albert FA, Forsting M, Sartor K, Adams HP, Kunze S. Early postoperative magnetic resonance imaging after resection of malignant glioma: objective evaluation of residual tumor and its influence on regrowth and prognosis. Neurosurgery 1994; 34:45–60.
17. Lanzieri CF, Larkins M, Mancall A, et al. Cranial postoperative site: MR imaging appearance. AJNR 1988; 9:27–34.
18. Sze G. New applications of MR contrast agents in neuroradiology. Neuroradiology 1990; 32:421–438.
19. Ciric I, Ammirati M, Vick N, Mikhael M. Supratentorial gliomas: surgical considerations and immediate postoperative results. Neurosurgery 1987; 21:21–26.
20. Cairncross JG, Pexman JHW, Rathbone MP, DelMaestro RF. Postoperative contrast enhancement in patients with brain tumor. Ann Neurol 1985; 17:570–572.
21. Nicoletti GF, Barone F, Passanisi M, Mancuso P, Albanese V. Linear contrast enhancement at the operative site on early post-operative CT after removal of brain tumors. J Neurosurg Sci 1994; 38:131–135.
22. Zagzag D, Goldenberg M, Brem S. Angiogensis and blood-brain barrier breakdown modulate CT contrast enhancement: an experiment in a rabbit brain-tumor model. AJNR 1989; 10:529–534.
23. Gado MH, Phelps ME, Coleman RE. An extravascular component of contrast enhancement in cranial computed tomography. Radiology 1975; 117:589–593.
24. Elster AD, Jackels SC, Allen NS, Marrache RC. Europium-DTPA: a gadolinium analogue traceable by flourescence microscopy. AJNR 1989; 10:1137–1144.
25. Elster AD, DiPersio DA. Cranial postoperative site: assessment with contrast-enhanced MR imaging. Radiology 1990; 174: 93–98.
26. Cloughesy TF, Black KL. Pharmacological blood-brain barrier modification for selective drug delivery. J Neurooncol 1995; 26: 125–132.
27. Baldwin SA, Fugaccia I, Brown DR, Brown LA, Scheff SW. Blood-brain barrier breach following cortical contusion in the rat. J Neurosurg 1996; 85:476–481.
28. Roman-Goldstein SM, Barnett PA, McCormick CI, Ball MJ, Ramsey F, Neuwelt EA. Effects of gadopentetate dimeglumine administration after osmotic blood-brain barrier disruption: toxicity and MR imaging findings. AJNR 1991; 12:885–890.
29. Hirano A, Becker NH, Zimmerman HM. Pathological alterations in the cerebral endothelial cell barrier to peroxidase. Arch Neurol 1969; 20:300–308.
30. Okudera H, Kyoshima K, Kobayashi S, Sugita K. Intraoperative CT scan findings during resection of gilial tumours. Neural Res 1994; 16:265–267.
31. DiChiro G, Brooks RA, Girton ME, et al. Sequential MR studies of intracerebral hematomas in monkeys. AJNR 1986; 7:193–199.
32. Meyding-Lamade U, Forsting M, Albert F, Kunze S, Sartor K. Accelerated methaemoglobin formation: potential pitfall in early postoperative MRI. Neuroradiology 1993; 35:178–180.

Barbara S. Hertzberg, MD • Mark A. Kliewer, MD • James D. Bowie, MD

Fetal Cerebral Ventriculomegaly: Misidentification of the True Medial Boundary of the Ventricle at US[1]

PURPOSE: **To investigate the implications of mistaking the medial surface of the cerebral hemisphere for the medial wall of the lateral ventricle at antenatal ultrasonography (US) and to identify US clues that might help avoid this interpretive error.**

MATERIALS AND METHODS: **In 50 second- and third-trimester fetuses, a directed attempt was made to demonstrate the medial surface of the cerebral hemisphere and the medial wall of the lateral ventricle on images that depicted the lateral wall of the ventricle. In each fetus, measurements of the diameter of the false ventricular atrium were compared with the true diameter of the lateral ventricle to assess the potential magnitude of error.**

RESULTS: **The average diameter measured with the medial surface of the cerebral hemisphere was 10.7 mm, compared with the true mean ventricular diameter of 6.2 mm. This value was greater than or equal to 10 mm (the generally accepted upper limit of normal for the ventricular diameter) in all 15 third-trimester fetuses and in 16 (46%) of 35 second-trimester fetuses. The parietal occipital fissure was demonstrated along the medial surface of the cerebral hemisphere in 36 (72%) of 50 fetuses, and the medial surface of the cerebral hemisphere could be traced posteriorly around the occipital lobe in 45 (90%).**

CONCLUSION: **When ventriculomegaly is suspected, the examiner should make a direct attempt to find the medial wall of the ventricle and distinguish it from the medial boundary of the cerebral hemisphere. Correct identification of the anatomic interfaces is facilitated by demonstrating that the cerebral interface contains the parietal occipital fissure and can be traced posteriorly around the occipital lobe.**

Accurate measurement of the cerebral ventricles is perhaps the single most important task in ultrasound (US) evaluation of the fetal central nervous system (1,2). Enlarged or misshapen ventricles are important markers for both central nervous system abnormality and more global fetal disorders. Even minimal degrees of ventriculomegaly have been associated with an increased incidence of adverse outcomes (3–7). Misdiagnosis of ventricular dilatation in normal fetuses, however, results in serious costs to the parents, who must endure needless worry, and to the health care system, which must provide a course of unnecessary counseling and additional, potentially harmful testing.

Confusion about the landmarks of the ventricles has increased since assessment of the ventricles has become a routine component of the obstetrical US examination. A range of pitfalls in the identification and assessment of cerebral ventriculomegaly have been previously described (1,8–11). These descriptions emphasize the importance of locating the lateral wall of the ventricle within the background of the hypoechoic brain. In our experience, however, the mistaken identification of the medial surface of the cerebral hemisphere for the medial wall of the lateral ventricle has been the source of much confusion and misdiagnosis during both the second and third trimesters of pregnancy, yet this pitfall has not been emphasized in the literature, to our knowledge. This recurrent problem has been the impetus for many of the referrals we receive from outside institutions to evaluate suspected hydrocephalus. We undertook this study to describe and define the origins of this pitfall, to ascertain the potential magnitude of the mismeasurement, and to identify US clues that might help prevent misidentification of ventriculomegaly that results from imaging the medial surface of the hemisphere.

MATERIALS AND METHODS

Fifty fetuses ranging in gestational age from 15 weeks 6 days to 36 weeks 1 day underwent prospective US performed by one of three experienced sonologists (B.S.H., M.A.K., J.D.B.). Indications for US included gestational age, fetal anatomy, size-date discrepancy, fetal growth, advanced maternal age, low α-fetoprotein, suspected preterm labor, and prior preterm delivery. Criteria for inclusion in the study group included a normal fetal anatomic survey with depiction of the intracranial structures routinely seen at US, such as the thalami, cisterna magna, and cerebellum. If routine intracranial anatomy could not be clearly depicted because of maternal obesity or fetal position, the fetus was not included in the study. Consecutive fetuses were selected for inclusion in the study on days when one of the authors was working in the obstetrical US service, during times when performance of the study would not cause undue patient backlog.

In each fetus in the study, an attempt was made to obtain three axial images that demonstrated the following combinations of anatomic features in the cerebral hemisphere farthest from the transducer: *(a)* reflections from the medial surface of the cerebral hemisphere and the lateral wall of the lateral ventricle (Figure, part a), *(b)* reflections

Index terms: Brain, US, 16.1298 • Fetus, central nervous system, 161.92, 856.92

Radiology 1997; 205:813–816

[1] From the Department of Radiology, Duke University Medical Center, Rm 2534, Blue Zone S, Durham, NC 27710. Received June 13, 1997; revision requested July 24; revision received August 6; accepted August 7. **Address reprint requests to** B.S.H.

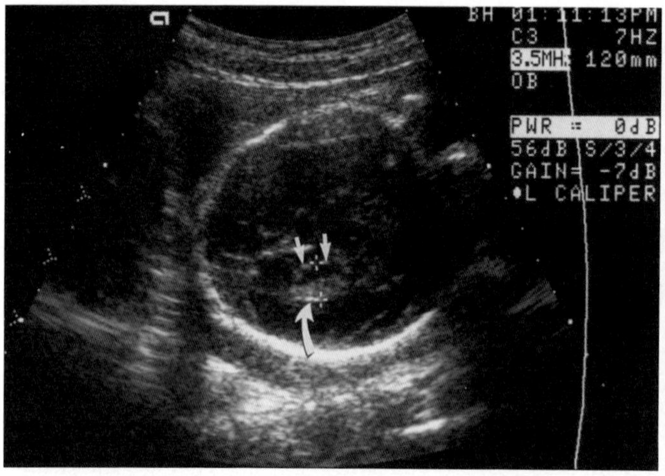

a.

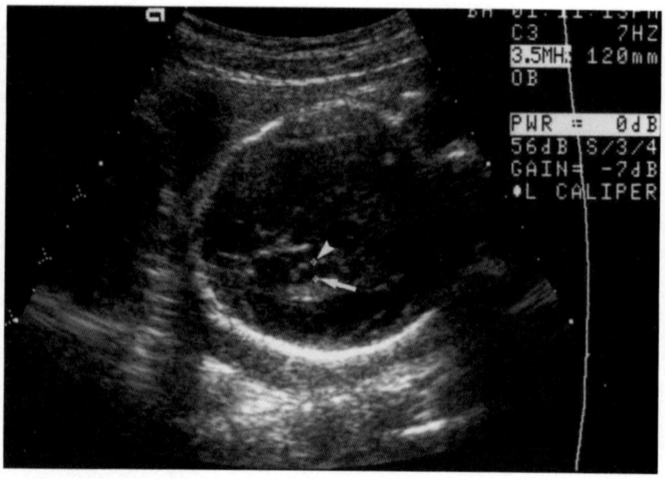

b.

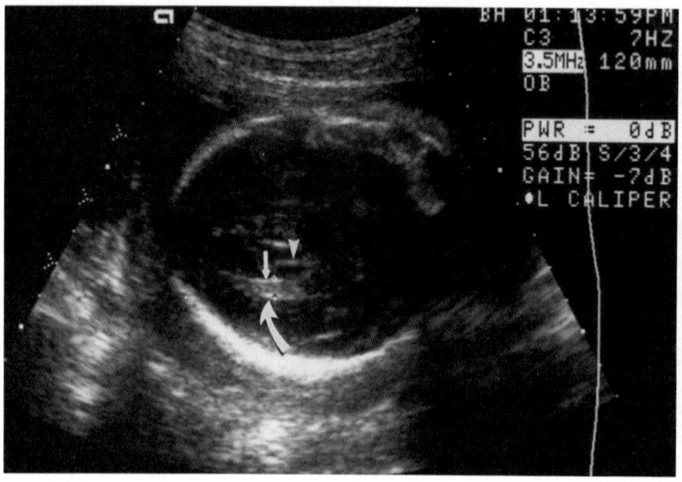

c.

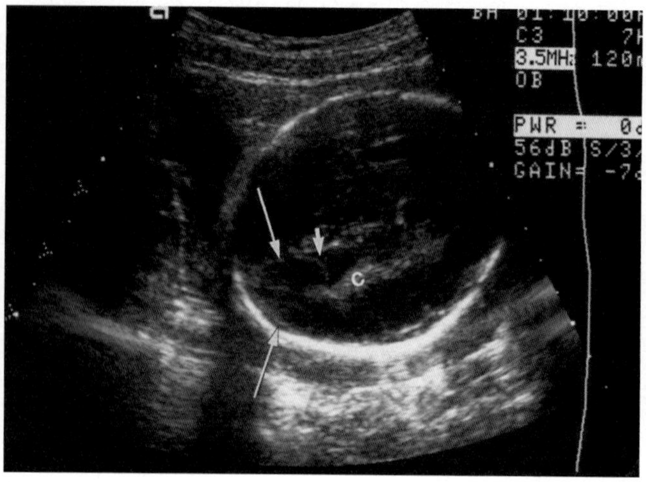

d.

US images of a fetal head at 26 weeks 5 days gestation. **(a)** Image depicts an echo arising from the medial surface of the cerebral hemisphere (straight arrows) and an echo arising from the lateral wall of lateral ventricle (curved arrow). Electronic calipers measure the diameter (10.1 mm) of the pseudoventricle created if the cerebral hemisphere interface is used for measurement instead of the medial wall of ventricle. **(b)** Image shows placement of electronic calipers to measure the distance between the medial surface of the choroid plexus (arrow) and the medial surface of the cerebral hemisphere (arrowhead). This space, which measures 4.6 mm, corresponds to the choroid plexus–ventricular wall separation. The space will be erroneously perceived as enlarged if the medial surface of the cerebral hemisphere is misidentified as the medial wall of the ventricle. **(c)** In this image, electronic calipers positioned on the reflection from the true medial wall of the lateral ventricle (straight arrow) and the lateral wall of the lateral ventricle (curved arrow) measure the true diameter (6.1 mm) of the ventricle. Echo arising from the medial surface of the cerebral hemisphere (arrowhead) is also seen, which allows comparison of the true lateral ventricle and the pseudoventricle that will be perceived if the medial surface of the cerebral hemisphere is mistaken for the medial wall of the ventricle. **(d)** Image depicts the parietal occipital fissure as a V-shaped indentation (short arrow) in the interface from the medial surface of the cerebral hemisphere. The cerebral hemisphere interface (long arrows) is followed posteriorly around the occipital lobe. C = choroid plexus.

from the medial and lateral walls of the lateral ventricle (Figure, part b), and *(c)* reflections from the medial surface of the cerebral hemisphere and the medial wall of the lateral ventricle. To assess the magnitude of the measurement error that results from misidentification of the medial surface of the cerebral hemisphere for the medial wall of the lateral ventricle, the following measurements were obtained with electronic calipers: *(a)* the distance between the medial surface of the cerebral hemisphere and the lateral wall of the lateral ventricle (Figure, part a) and *(b)* the distance between the medial surface of the choroid plexus and the medial surface of the cerebral hemisphere (Figure, part b). The true diameter of the lateral ventricle was obtained by measuring the distance between the medial and lateral walls of the ventricle at the level of the atrium (Figure, part c). In addition, the space was measured between the medial surface of the choroid plexus and the medial wall of the ventricle. Finally, when the echo arising from the medial surface of the cerebral hemisphere was seen, an attempt was made to trace this interface posteriorly around the occipital lobe and to demonstrate a V-shaped indentation in the interface that corresponded to the parieto-occipital fissure (12) (Figure, part d).

US examinations were performed (XP, Acuson, Mountain View, Calif; HDI 3000, ATL Ultrasound, Bothell, Wash) with transabdominal vector and curvilinear transducers that ranged in frequency from 2.5 to 5.0 MHz. The transducer frequency and configuration were selected to optimize depiction of intracranial structures.

RESULTS

The medial surface of the cerebral hemisphere could be demonstrated on axial images obtained in all 50 fetuses when it was intentionally sought. In the majority (47 [94%] of 50 fetuses), both the medial wall of the cerebral hemisphere and the medial wall of the lateral ventricle could also be demonstrated on the same image.

The mean distance from the medial surface of the cerebral hemisphere to the lateral wall of the lateral ventricle was 10.7 mm (range, 6.6–17.9 mm). This value represents the width of the pseudoventricle created by misidentification of the medial surface of the cerebral hemisphere as the medial wall of the lateral ventricle. In 31 (62%) of 50 fetuses, the value was at least 10 mm, the generally accepted upper limit of normal, but in 30 (60%) of the fetuses, the extent of apparent ventriculomegaly was mild (<15 mm). In comparison, the mean true ventricular diameter (distance from the medial wall of the lateral ventricle to the lateral wall of the lateral ventricle) was 6.2 mm (range, 3.1–8.6 mm).

The mean separation between the medial surface of the choroid plexus and the medial surface of the cerebral hemisphere (the spurious measure of the separation of the choroid plexus from the ventricular wall) was 5.2 mm (range, 1.1–10.3 mm). In comparison, the mean distance from the medial wall of the ventricle to the choroid plexus (the true choroid plexus–ventricular wall separation) was 1.0 mm (range, 0–5.1 mm).

A V-shaped indentation in the reflection from the medial surface of the cerebral hemisphere was found in 36 (72%) of 50 fetuses. When demonstrated, this finding helped identify the interface of the medial surface of the cerebral hemisphere and helped distinguish it from the medial wall of the lateral ventricle. Moreover, in 45 (90%) of the 50 fetuses, the medial wall of the cerebral hemisphere could be followed posteriorly around the occipital lobe.

The width of the pseudoventricle created by misidentification of the echo from the medial surface of the hemisphere as the medial wall of the ventricle increased with increasing gestational age. This pseudoventricle had a mean width of 9.7 mm in second-trimester fetuses and of 13.1 mm in third-trimester fetuses. A value at least 10 mm was obtained in all 15 third-trimester fetuses but in only 16 (46%) of the 35 second-trimester fetuses. Likewise, the apparent fluid-filled space between the medial surface of the choroid plexus and the medial surface of the cerebral hemisphere was also larger for third-trimester fetuses (mean, 8.0 mm) than for second-trimester fetuses (mean, 3.9 mm).

DISCUSSION

Assessment of the cerebral ventricles is of pivotal importance for patient counseling and treatment. Several previously described pitfalls have the potential to create a spurious appearance of ventriculomegaly (1,8–11). For example, ventricular size can be overestimated by measuring in an off-axis image plane of section, positioning the calipers perpendicular to the midline rather than perpendicular to the long axis of the ventricle, or positioning the calipers on the outer surface of the ventricular wall (8). Further, the white matter of the normal fetal brain is relatively echopenic, so the appearance of the brain that surrounds the lateral ventricle can simulate that of fluid in a dilated ventricle (9–11). Some investigators have advocated locating the middle cerebral artery to aid identification of the true margin of the brain (9).

A more definitive and straightforward approach derives from careful consideration of the orientation of the choroid plexus within the ventricle (1,10). If the ventricle is dilated, the gravity-dependent choroid plexus dangles toward the lateral wall of the lateral ventricle. In comparison, in a normal-sized ventricle, the choroid plexus has a more horizontal orientation and is close to the lateral wall of the lateral ventricle. These landmarks are well defined and relatively easy to depict, so the identification of the lateral wall of the lateral ventricle should be unambiguous in most cases.

Unfortunately, no such obvious US landmark has been described to help distinguish the medial surface of the cerebral hemisphere from the medial wall of the lateral ventricle. In both the fetus erroneously identified as having ventricular dilatation (owing to imaging the medial surface of the cerebral hemisphere) and the fetus with true mild ventricular dilatation, the choroid plexus appears to be separated from the perceived medial wall of the ventricle by a fluid-filled space. Indeed, the separation of the choroid plexus from the medial ventricular wall is considered one of the earliest signs of ventriculomegaly.

When ventriculomegaly is suspected, the examiner should make a specific effort to find the medial wall of the ventricle. In the course of this study, we were able to identify other US markers that could help map this anatomic landscape. In the majority of fetuses, a slight adjustment in transducer orientation helped depict a prominent V-shaped indentation in the interface of the medial surface of the cerebral hemisphere but not in the medial wall of the lateral ventricle. This prominent indentation corresponds to the parietal occipital fissure (12). Also helpful is demonstration that the reflection from the medial wall of the hemisphere continues posteriorly as it courses around the occipital lobe. Finally, with concerted effort, both the medial wall of the hemisphere and the medial wall of the lateral ventricle can be demonstrated in most fetuses, which would definitively eliminate any potential confusion of these two structures.

With use of the standard of 10 mm as the upper normal limit for the ventricular atrial diameter (1,2,13–16), misidentification of the medial boundary of the cerebrum as the medial wall of the ventricle would have led to an erroneous diagnosis of ventriculomegaly in 62% of fetuses. The error rate was substantially greater for third-trimester fetuses than for second-trimester fetuses, as might be expected considering the relative stability in the size of the ventricular atrium throughout the second and third trimesters (13) compared with that of the enlarging, growing brain around it. Though misidentification of the medial surface of the cerebral hemisphere as the medial wall of the ventricle would frequently have resulted in an erroneous diagnosis of ventriculomegaly, the enlargement would have been classified as mild (<15 mm) in all but one late third-trimester fetus.

Although we did not specifically test this hypothesis, we suspect that the medial surface of the cerebral hemisphere is more likely to be mistaken for the medial wall of the ventricle when the fetal head is imaged under the technically difficult circumstances produced by suboptimal maternal body habitus and fetal position. In such cases, anatomic landmarks are obscure, and confident identification of the ventricular wall may be challenging. It is precisely in these cases, however, that the examiner needs to be most alert to this pitfall. By being cognizant of the potential for this pitfall that simulates mild ventriculomegaly, the sonologist should be able to make the key observations necessary to prevent a potentially serious misdiagnosis of ventriculomegaly. ■

Acknowledgment: We thank Susan Murray for assisting in the preparation of the manuscript for this article.

References

1. Filly RA, Goldstein RB, Callen PW. Fetal ventricle: importance in routine obstetric sonography. Radiology 1991; 181:1–7.
2. Filly RA, Cardoza JD, Goldstein RB, Barkovich AJ. Detection of fetal central nervous system anomalies: a practical level of effort for a routine sonogram. Radiology 1989; 172:403–408.
3. Goldstein RB, La Pidus AS, Filly RA, Cardoza JD. Mild lateral cerebral ventricular dilatation in utero: clinical significance and prognosis. Radiology 1990; 176:237–242.
4. Mahony BS, Nyberg DA, Hirsch JH, Petty CN, Hendricks SK, Mack LA. Mild idiopathic lateral cerebral ventricular dilatation

in utero: sonographic evaluation. Radiology 1988; 169:715–721.
5. Bromley B, Frigoletto FD Jr, Benacerraf BR. Mild fetal lateral cerebral ventriculomegaly: clinical course and outcome. Am J Obstet Gynecol 1991; 164:863–867.
6. Patel MD, Filly AL, Hersh DR, Goldstein RB. Isolated mild fetal cerebral ventriculomegaly: clinical course and outcome. Radiology 1994; 192:759–764.
7. Achiron R, Schimmel M, Achiron A, Mashtach S. Fetal mild idiopathic lateral ventriculomegaly: is there a correlation with fetal trisomy? Ultrasound Obstet Gynecol 1993; 3:89–92.
8. Heiserman J, Filly RA, Goldstein RB. Effect of measurement errors on sonographic evaluation of ventriculomegaly. J Ultrasound Med 1991; 10:121–124.
9. Case KJ, Hirsch J, Case MJ. Simulation of significant pathology by normal hypoechoic white matter in cranial ultrasound. JCU 1983; 11:281–285.
10. Cardoza JD, Filly RA, Podrasky AE. The dangling choroid plexus: a sonographic observation of value in excluding ventriculomegaly. AJR 1988; 151:767–770.
11. Chin DH, Callen PW, Filly RA. The lateral cerebral ventricle in early second trimester. Radiology 1983; 148:529–531.
12. Patriquin H, Fontaine S, Michaud J, Lafortune M, Boisvert J. Development of the fetal brain in the second trimester: an anatomic and ultrasonographic demonstration. Can Assoc Radiol J 1992; 43:131–137.
13. Cardoza JD, Goldstein RB, Filly RA. Exclusion of fetal ventriculomegaly with a single measurement: the width of the lateral ventricular atrium. Radiology 1988; 169:711–714.
14. Filly RA, Goldstein RB. The fetal ventricular atrium: fourth down and 10 mm to go. Radiology 1994: 193:315–317.
15. Farrell TA, Hertzberg BS, Kliewer MA, Harris L, Paine SS. Fetal lateral ventricles: reassessment of normal values for atrial diameter at US. Radiology 1994; 193:409–411.
16. Alagappan R, Browning PD, Laorr A, McGahan JP. Distal lateral ventricular atrium: reevaluation of normal range. Radiology 1994; 193:405–408.

Lane F. Donnelly, MD • Lance A. Klosterman, BA

Pneumonia in Children: Decreased Parenchymal Contrast Enhancement—CT Sign of Intense Illness and Impending Cavitary Necrosis[1]

PURPOSE: To determine if computed tomographic (CT) findings of decreased contrast material enhancement are predictive of more intense illness and of the development of cavitary necrosis in children with pneumonia.

MATERIALS AND METHODS: Contrast-enhanced CT scans in 44 children with pneumonia who did not respond appropriately to therapy were compared with precontrast CT scans to evaluate enhancement of consolidated lung parenchyma. Enhancement was correlated with admission to the intensive care unit, length of hospital stay, cavitary necrosis in the lung at follow-up CT, and frequency of lung resection.

RESULTS: Parenchymal enhancement was decreased in 21 children; pneumonia was enhanced in the other 23 children. Decreased enhancement was associated with increased admission to intensive care (14 of 21 [67%] vs five of 23 [22%] children; $P = .0026$), increased length of hospital stay (15 vs 10 days; $P = .0615$), increased frequency of cavitary necrosis at follow-up CT (seven of seven [100%] vs none of three children; $P = .0086$), and increased frequency of resection (two of 21 [10%] vs none of 23 children). At histopathologic examination, diffuse cavitary necrosis was present in resected lobes in two patients.

CONCLUSION: Decreased parenchymal enhancement at CT is a predictor of more intense illness and may herald the development of cavitary necrosis in children with pneumonia.

When children with pneumonia do not respond appropriately to surgical or medical treatment, computed tomography (CT) is often performed to evaluate for pleural complications such as empyema or lung parenchymal complications such as abscess or necrosis. We have noted great variability in the degree of contrast material enhancement at CT in patients with consolidated pneumonia (Figs 1–3). Because of the marked inflammation associated with pneumonia, we propose that pneumonia without necrotic complications shows contrast enhancement and that decreased enhancement is a CT sign of ischemia or infarct and is associated with a worse clinical outcome. The purpose of this study was to determine if there is an association between the presence of decreased parenchymal contrast enhancement on CT scans and an increased frequency of cavitary necrosis and more intense illness than are seen in children with pneumonia that is enhanced on CT scans.

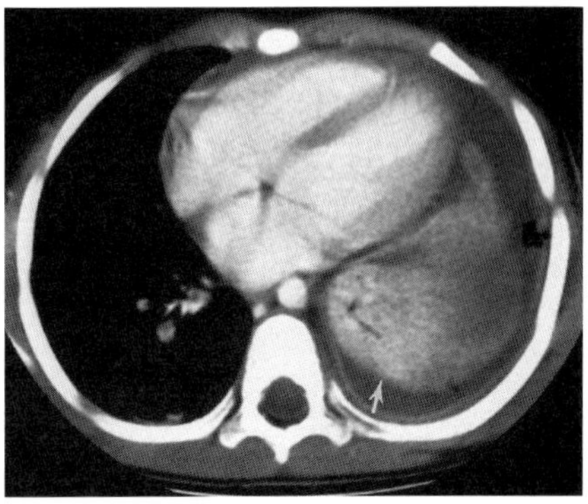

Figure 1. Contrast-enhanced CT scan shows enhancing, consolidated lung (arrow) without evidence of parenchymal complications in a 4-year-old girl with left lower lobe pneumonia.

MATERIALS AND METHODS

The medical records and CT scans of all ($n = 44$) children, aged 0.5–18.0 years (mean, 6.7 years), who underwent CT to evaluate for pleural or parenchymal complications of pneumonia from November 1995 through February 1997 were retrospectively reviewed. The patients included 21 boys and 23 girls. Only previously healthy children with community-acquired pneumonia were included in the study. All children underwent CT because of persistent or progressive illness (fever, respiratory distress, sepsis) despite therapy with antibiotic medications. Some children also had parapneumonic effusions that were evaluated with CT because they did not respond appropriately to drainage.

CT was performed (HiSpeed Advantage; GE Medical Systems, Milwaukee, Wis) before and after intravenous administration of contrast material. In all patients, three initial precontrast axial CT scans were obtained at three levels in the chest with 10-mm section thickness; at least one scan was obtained at the level of maximum lung opacification. Postcontrast scanning was performed with a spiral technique. Section thickness, which depended on patient size, was 7–10 mm, and a single breath-hold technique was used when pa-

Index terms: Children, respiratory system, 60.211 • Computed tomography (CT), helical, 60.12112, 60.12115 • Computed tomography (CT), in infants and children, 60.12111, 60.12112, 60.12115 • Lung, CT, 60.12111, 60.12112, 60.12115 • Lung, infection, 60.211

Abbreviation: ICU = intensive care unit.

Radiology 1997; 205:817–820

[1] From the Department of Radiology, Section of Pediatric Radiology, Duke University Medical Center, Box 3808, Durham, NC 27710 (L.F.D.); the Department of Radiology, Children's Hospital Medical Center, Cincinnati, Ohio (L.A.K.); and the University of Cincinnati, Ohio (L.A.K.). Received June 6, 1997; revision requested July 9; revision received July 21; accepted July 23. **Address reprint requests to** L.F.D.

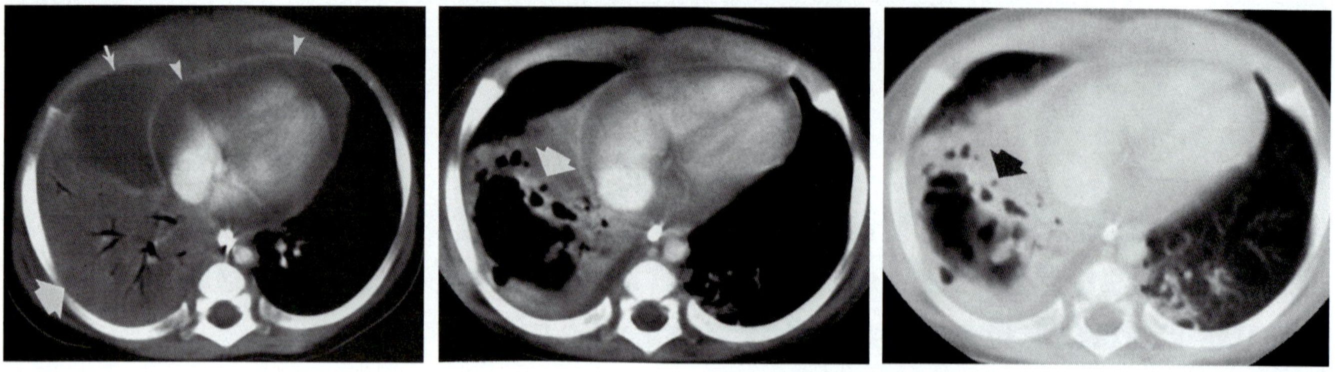

a. b. c.

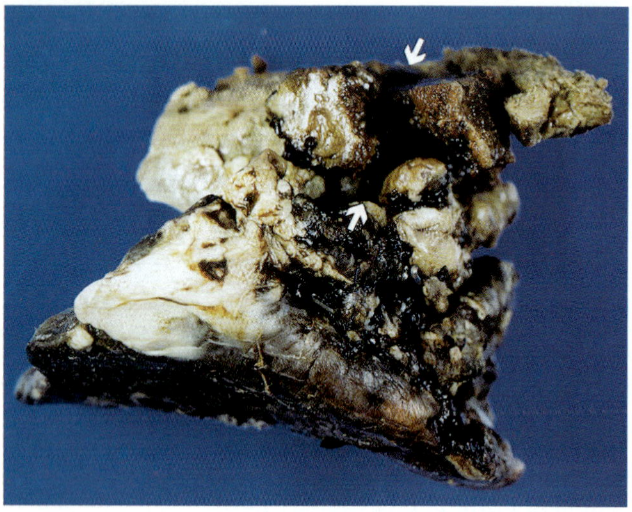

d.

Figure 2. Decreased parenchymal enhancement and subsequent cavitary necrosis in a 6-month-old girl with right lower lobe pneumonia. **(a)** Contrast-enhanced CT scan shows decreased enhancement of the consolidated right lower lobe pneumonia (large arrow). Also present are purulent pericardial effusions (arrowheads) and a right pleural effusion (small arrow). **(b, c)** Contrast-enhanced follow-up CT scans obtained 5 days later with **(b)** lung and **(c)** mediastinal window settings show development of cavitary necrosis of the right lower lobe (arrow). The pericardial and pleural fluid have been drained. **(d)** Pathologic specimen obtained at surgical resection of the right lower lobe shows diffuse necrosis of consolidated pneumonia and a large central cavity (arrows).

tients were able to cooperate. Standard protocols for intravenous administration of CT contrast material in pediatric patients were used in all cases: 2 mL of nonionic contrast material per kilogram of body weight (maximum of 100 mL) were injected by hand, and scanning began immediately after the injection was completed. All scans included in the study demonstrated optimal enhancement.

All patients in this study had pneumonia that occupied all or most (more than 75%) of a lobe, and the lungs did not exhibit volume loss. Lung areas that did exhibit CT signs of volume loss (asymmetric vascular or bronchial crowding, displacement of fissures, linear or triangular shape) were considered to be indicative of atelectasis, and patients with these findings were not included in the pneumonia study group.

Lung parenchyma that was consolidated due to pneumonia was evaluated for degree of enhancement. Consolidated parenchyma was defined as "enhancing" if most of the consolidated lung showed high attenuation (Fig 1), as well as increased attenuation compared with that on the precontrast image. Decreased parenchymal enhancement was considered to be present when most (more than 75%) of the consolidated lung showed diffuse or patchy low attenuation on postcontrast images (Figs 2, 3) and when there were no differences in the appearance of low-attenuating areas when pre- and postcontrast images were compared.

Another CT finding we considered was loss of definition of the border between consolidated lung and adjacent pleural fluid. This was termed "loss of the lung-pleural margin" (Fig 4).

In children who continued to fail to respond to management of their pneumonia, a second follow-up CT scan was sometimes obtained. In patients who underwent chest CT more than once, the follow-up scans were reviewed for development of cavitary necrosis. Cavitary necrosis was defined as a combination of the loss of normal parenchymal lung architecture, a decrease in parenchymal enhancement, and the development of multiple thin-walled cavities filled with fluid or air and without an enhancing border (Figs 2, 3). Areas of cavitary necrosis were differentiated from clearing aerated lung by the loss of normal lung bronchial and arterial architecture and by the presence of cavities, both of which are seen only in cases of necrosis. In resected lobes, pathologic specimens were reviewed for the presence of necrosis.

Chest CT scans were interpreted by the authors, and conclusions were reached by means of consensus. The reviewers were blinded to the clinical data during review.

Medical records were reviewed to determine whether patients were admitted to the intensive care unit (ICU), the number of days of hospitalization, and the frequency of surgical resection of affected lobes. Imaging findings, such as decreased enhancement, were not used in the decision to admit a patient to the ICU; these decisions were based on the clinical condition of the patient.

The ability to predict, on the basis of decreased enhancement on CT scans, increases in the frequency of admission to the ICU, in the mean number of days of hospital stay, in the frequency of lung resection, and in the frequency of cavitary necrosis on follow-up CT scans were analyzed statistically with the Student t test.

RESULTS

Enhancement of consolidated lung parenchyma was seen on CT scans in 23 patients; decreased enhancement was seen on scans in 21 patients. In all cases of decreased enhancement, the lack of enhancement was diffuse throughout the opacified lobe and ranged in quality from homogeneous low attenuation to patchy, heterogeneous low attenuation.

The relationship between decreased parenchymal enhancement and other clinical and CT findings is summarized in the Table. Children with pneumonia that demonstrated decreased enhancement on CT scans had a statistically significantly higher frequency of admission to the ICU (14 of 21 [67%] vs five of 23 [22%] patients; $P = .0026$) and longer average hospital stay (14.8 vs 10.0 days; $P = .0615$).

Ten children underwent follow-up CT (two children underwent follow-up CT three times each). There was a higher frequency of follow-up CT in patients with decreased enhancement than in those without

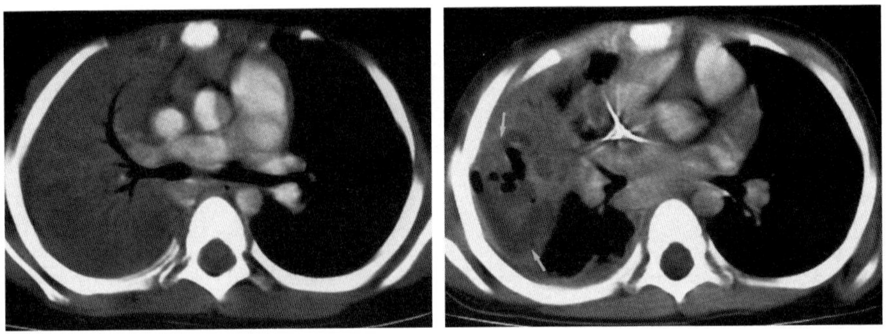

a. b.

Figure 3. Contrast-enhanced CT scans show decreased parenchymal enhancement and subsequent cavitary necrosis in a 4-year-old girl. **(a)** Initial CT scan shows decreased parenchymal enhancement of a right upper lobe pneumonia. **(b)** Follow-up CT scan obtained 5 days later shows development of cavitary necrosis (arrows) of the right upper lobe.

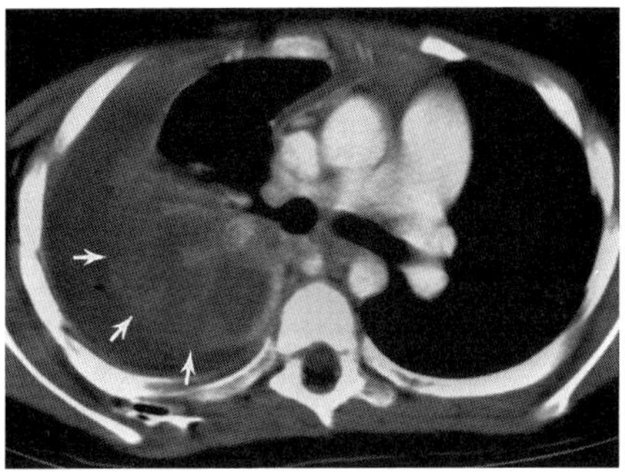

Figure 4. Contrast-enhanced CT scan shows loss of the lung-pleural margin in a 10-year-old girl with right upper lobe pneumonia. There is lack of definition of the border (arrows) between the right pleural effusion and the consolidated posterior segment of the right upper lobe. The consolidated lung also shows decreased enhancement.

(seven of 21 [33%] vs three of 23 [13%]). In patients who underwent follow-up CT, all seven (100%) with lung consolidation that demonstrated decreased parenchymal enhancement on initial CT scans showed cavitary necrosis on follow-up scans, compared with none (0%) of three whose initial scans demonstrated enhanced parenchyma (P = .0086) (Figs 2, 3).

Two patients underwent surgical lobectomy because of progressive and uncontrollable sepsis. Initial CT scans in both demonstrated decreased enhancement, and follow-up CT scans demonstrated cavitary necrosis. Pathologic specimens of resected lobes in both patients demonstrated diffuse cavitary necrosis of the consolidated lung (Fig 2d). Twenty-two of the 23 patients in the enhancing-pneumonia group and 14 of the 21 patients in the decreased-enhancement group required drainage or thoracoscopic débridement owing to parapneumonic effusions.

All 44 children eventually recovered from their illness. One child who underwent lobectomy had necrosis of several toes, which was related to hypotension and treatment with vasopressors, but all other children had no long-term sequelae.

Loss of the lung-pleural margin was seen in 12 of the 21 patients whose scans also demonstrated decreased enhancement (Fig 4). This finding was not present on any scans that showed enhancing parenchyma. This subgroup of 12 patients had a high rate of admission to the ICU (nine of 12 [75%]) and a longer mean hospital stay (15.7 days). The two patients who required surgical lung resection and all seven patients whose follow-up CT scans showed cavitary necrosis were in this subgroup of 12 patients.

DISCUSSION

Complications of childhood pneumonia include parenchymal complications such as necrosis or parapneumonic effusions such as empyema (1–4). When children do not respond appropriately to medical or surgical treatment of pneumonia, we often perform CT to determine the presence of these pleural or parenchymal complications. CT findings have been shown to be accurate for the identification of lung abscess, the differentiation of peripheral lung abscess from empyema, the detection of parapneumonic effusions, the depiction of multiple loculations of parapneumonic effusions, the identification of bronchopleural fistulas, and the identification of malpositioned chest tubes or of failure of lung reexpansion after chest-tube placement, both of which help to indicate when chest-tube drainage therapy will be unsuccessful (5–11).

It has been reported (12–15) that areas of atelectasis demonstrate marked enhancement on contrast-enhanced CT scans. There was initial enthusiasm that, in adults, when lung was collapsed secondary to an obstructing neoplasm, the degree of enhancement could be used for accurate differentiation of enhancing atelectasis from adjacent, nonenhancing neoplasm (12,13). The accuracy of this finding, however, has been debated (14,15). Though we could find no documentation in the literature, it is a common radiology teaching that opacification secondary to atelectasis enhances and that opacification due to pneumonia does not. In this study, the pneumonia in more than half the patients showed diffuse enhancement. All patients with volume loss, which is suggestive of atelectasis, were excluded from the study. Because uncomplicated pneumonias enhance, we have not found enhancement to be a reliable way to differentiate atelectasis from pneumonia.

The pulmonary parenchymal complications of pneumonia represent a spectrum of entities, including pneumatocele, lung abscess, cavitary necrosis, and pulmonary gangrene (16). The name given to the suppurative process depends on the severity and distribution of the process and the temporal relationship with disease resolution. Cavitary necrosis, or necrotizing pneumonitis, is characterized by a dominant area of necrosis with a variable number of thin-walled cavities (16). Lung abscess is characterized by a dominant focus of suppuration surrounded by a well-defined fibrous wall (16). Pneumatoceles may sometimes represent a later stage of resolving or healing necrosis.

CT findings of lung abscess and necrosis have been reported (16), but to our knowledge, the importance of the degree of enhancement of lung parenchyma consolidated due to pneumonia on contrast-enhanced CT scans has not been determined. Pneumonia not complicated by necrosis enhances on contrast-enhanced CT scans. This enhancement is not surprising given the degree of inflammation associated with pneumonia. All the parameters we evaluated—admission to the ICU, mean length of hospital stay, lung resection, and development of cavitary necrosis at follow-up CT—were increased in children whose pneumonia showed decreased enhancement compared with those whose pneumonia showed enhancement, with admission to the ICU (P = .0026) and development of cavitary necrosis at follow-up (P = .0086) being the most statistically significant. Therefore, decreased parenchymal enhancement on CT scans is a predictor of illness that is more intense than that encountered when the finding is parenchymal enhance-

Relationship between Decreased Parenchymal Contrast Enhancement and Other Parameters

Parameter	Decreased Parenchymal Enhancement	Parenchymal Enhancement
No. of patients admitted to ICU*	14/21 (67)	5/23 (22)
Mean no. of days in hospital†	14.8	10.0
No. of patients who underwent lung resection	2/21 (10)	0/23 (0)
Cavitary necrosis findings at follow-up CT‡	7/7 (100)	0/3 (0)

Note.—Data are number of patients in whom parameter is applicable/total number of patients with the CT finding, unless otherwise indicated. Values in parentheses are percentages.

* Difference between groups was statistically significant (P = .0026).

† Difference between groups was statistically significant (P = .00615).

‡ Difference between groups was statistically significant (P = .0086).

ment and may herald the development of cavitary necrosis, possibly related to ischemia and infarct. The additional CT finding of loss of the lung-pleural margin or of an ill-defined border between consolidated lung and adjacent pleural fluid also may be seen in conjunction with decreased enhancement.

The difference in length of hospital stay between patients with enhancing pneumonia and those with nonenhancing pneumonia was not statistically significant (P = .0615). All children in this study were referred for CT because of inappropriate response to therapy. Twenty-two of the 23 patients in the enhancing-pneumonia group had complications related to parapneumonic effusions, which was higher than the percentage of children in the decreased-enhancement group (14 of 21). This increased frequency of parapneumonic effusion in the enhancing-pneumonia group was most likely related to selection bias based on referral patterns for CT. Possibly, the decreased-enhancement group was not responding to treatment and was referred for CT because of parenchymal complications related to necrosis, and the enhancing-pneumonia group was refractory to therapy because of pleural complications. Because parapneumonic effusions contribute to a longer hospital stay, this may explain why there was not a greater difference in length of hospital stay between the two groups.

Cavitary necrosis or necrotizing pneumonia is a complication of severe pneumonia (1,17–26) and was uncommon even during the preantibiotic era (1,17,22–26). Most reports have been of adults. In children, among whom *Streptococcus pneumoniae* is the most frequent bacterial cause of lobar pneumonia, complication due to cavitary necrosis has been only sparsely reported (1,17). The mechanism of pneumonia with necrotic complications is related to thrombotic occlusion of alveolar capillaries secondary to adjacent inflammation, resulting in ischemia and, eventually, necrosis of the lung parenchyma (17). This pathophysiologic mechanism may explain the findings seen on contrast-enhanced CT scans. The decreased enhancement may be related to developing ischemia and infarct and, thus, appears earlier than the development of cavities and the destruction of architecture seen on the CT scans in patients with cavitary necrosis.

It must be stressed that the prognosis associated with pneumonia complicated by cavitary necrosis in children is not the same as that in adults, in whom the outcome is poor, the mortality rate is high (26), and early surgical removal of gangrenous lung has been advocated (17–26). Most children in this series, however, eventually recovered without surgical intervention. Therefore, decreased enhancement of lung parenchyma seen on CT scans is associated with a prolonged, intense illness but is not indicative of a surgical emergency.

In summary, decreased enhancement of consolidated pneumonia on contrast-enhanced CT scans is associated with intense illness and may herald the development of cavitary necrosis, possibly related to ischemia. CT scans that demonstrate this finding in children may indicate intensive surveillance and aggressive medical or surgical therapy. ■

References

1. Kerem E, Bar BZ, Rudenski A, Katz S, Kleid D, Branski D. Bacteremia necrotizing pneumococcal pneumonia in children. Am J Respir Crit Care Med 1994; 149:242–244.
2. Alexander JC Jr, Wolfe WG. Lung abscess and empyema of the thorax. Surg Clin North Am 1980; 60:835–849.
3. Jacobs NM, Lerdkachornduk S, Metzger WI. Pneumococcal bacteremia in infants and children: a ten-year experience at the Cook County Hospital with special reference to the pneumococcal serotypes isolated. Pediatrics 1979; 64:296–300.
4. MacFarlane JT, Finch RG, Ward MG, Macrae AD. Hospital study of community acquired pneumonia. Lancet 1982; 2:25–28.
5. Stern EJ, Sun H, Haramati LB. Peripheral bronchopleural fistulas: CT imaging features. AJR 1996; 167:117–120.
6. Pugatch RD, Sprin PW. Radiology of the pleura. Clin Chest Med 1985; 6:17–32.
7. Himelman RB, Callen PW. The prognostic value of loculations in parapneumonic pleural effusion. Chest 1986; 90:852–856.
8. Waite RJ, Carbonneau RJ, Balikian JP, Umali CB, Pezzella AT, Nash G. Parietal pleural changes in empyema: appearances at CT. Radiology 1990; 175:145–150.
9. Müller NL. Imaging of pleura. Radiology 1993; 186:297–309.
10. Stark DD, Federle MP, Goodman PC, Podrasky AE, Webb WR. Differentiating lung abscess and empyema: radiography and computed tomography. AJR 1983; 141: 163–167.
11. Baber CD, Hedlund LW, Oddson TA, Putman CE. Differentiating empyemas and peripheral pulmonary abscess: the value of computed tomography. Radiology 1980; 135:755–758.
12. Naidich DP, McCauley DI, Khouri NF, Leitman BS, Hulnick DH, Siegelman SS. Computed tomography of lobar collapse. I. Endobronchial obstruction. J Comput Assist Tomogr 1983; 7:745–757.
13. Naidich DP, McCauley DI, Khouri NF, Leitman BS, Hulnick DH, Siegelman SS. Computed tomography of lobar collapse. II. Collapse in the absence of endobronchial obstruction. J Comput Assist Tomogr 1983; 7:758–767.
14. Khoury MB, Godwin JD, Halvorsen RA, Putman CE. CT of obstructive lobar collapse. Invest Radiol 1985; 20:708–716.
15. Davies SG, Turner MJ. Enhancement of collapsed lung: a potential pitfall in CT interpretation. Clin Radiol 1990; 42:192–194.
16. Naidich DP, Zerhouni EA, Siegelman SS. Computed tomography and magnetic resonance of the thorax. 2nd ed. New York, NY: Raven, 1991; 423–426.
17. Yangco B, Derensinski S. Necrotizing or cavitary pneumonia due to streptococcus pneumonia: report of four cases and review of the literature. Medicine 1980; 59:449–457.
18. Danner PK, McFarland DR, Felson B. Massive pulmonary gangrene. AJR 1968; 103:548–554.
19. Gutman E, Pongdee O, Park YS. Massive pulmonary gangrene. Radiology 1973; 107: 293–294.
20. Knight L, Fraser RG, Robson HG. Massive pulmonary gangrene: a severe complication of Klebsiella pneumonia. Can Med Assoc J 1975; 112:196–198.
21. O'Reilly GV, Dee PM, Otteni GV. Gangrene of the lung: successful medical management of three patients. Radiology 1978; 126:575–579.
22. Massachusetts General Hospital Case Records, case 22-1973. N Engl J Med 1973; 288: 1173–1180.
23. Torres A, Agusti GA, Rodriguez-Roisin R, Etopa R, Agusti-Vidal A. Cavitation in bacteremic pneumococcal pneumonia. Am Rev Respir Dis 1984; 130:533–534.
24. Isaacs RD. Necrotizing pneumonia in bacteremic pneumococcal infection. Br J Dis Chest 1986; 80:295–296.
25. Kissner DG, Lawrence WD, Keshishian M. Pneumococcal lung abscess. Am J Med 1988; 84:793–794.
26. Leatherman JW, Iber C, Davis SF. Cavitation in bacteremic pneumococcal pneumonia: causal role of mixed infection with anaerobic bacteria. Am Rev Respir Dis 1984; 129:317–321.

Michael A. DiPietro, MD • Caroline E. Blane, MD • J. Michael Zerin, MD

Vesicoureteral Reflux in Older Children: Concordance of US and Voiding Cystourethrographic Findings[1]

PURPOSE: **To determine if a negative renal sonogram is reliably predictive of the absence of vesicoureteral reflux at voiding cystourethrography (VCUG) in children aged 5 years or older.**

MATERIALS AND METHODS: **Imaging studies in 70 children aged 5 years or older who underwent renal ultrasound (US) and VCUG on the same day were reviewed. These children had initially undergone evaluation because of a urinary tract infection.**

RESULTS: **Five of 70 children had abnormal sonograms; two (40%) of the five had reflux at VCUG. One had mild pelvicalyceal dilatation, and one had a small kidney. The other three (without reflux) had a pelvic kidney, a calyceal diverticulum, or a renal stone. Of 65 children with a negative sonogram, 19 (29%) had reflux at VCUG; 46 (71%) did not. Altogether, of the 70 children, 21 had reflux, 19 (90%) of whom had no sonographic abnormality.**

CONCLUSION: **Children with abnormal screening renal sonograms often have vesicoureteral reflux, but a normal sonogram does not reliably exclude the condition even in children aged 5 years or older. Therefore, VCUG must be performed even in older children, regardless of US findings, if clinical decisions are influenced by documentation of the presence of VUR.**

In young children, especially those less than 1 year of age, there is a risk of renal scarring in cases of urinary tract infection (UTI) in conjunction with vesicoureteral reflux (VUR) (1–3). Therefore, voiding cystourethrography (VCUG) or radionuclide cystography are recommended as essential imaging studies to detect VUR in young children known to have a UTI (4). This may or may not be true, however, in older children who first present with a UTI. Some clinicians believe that VUR rarely leads to renal scarring in older children (aged 5–7 years and older) with a UTI and normal kidneys depicted at imaging (1). Thus, the imaging evaluation for UTI in older children is sometimes limited to the kidneys (renal sonogram), and if the kidneys are shown to be normal, no further evaluation (ie, VCUG) for VUR is performed. The rationale is that most renal damage related to infection and VUR is thought to occur early in life; therefore, if there is no evidence of previous damage to the kidneys at ultrasonography (US), VUR is thought to be either unlikely or unimportant and need not be evaluated.

To investigate this premise would be beyond the scope of this article. Thus, we addressed the simple question of whether a negative renal sonogram is predictive of the absence of VUR in older children by determining the concordance of US and VCUG findings (ie, findings of VUR) in older children with a UTI.

MATERIALS AND METHODS

A database of over 5,000 consecutive genitourinary tract imaging studies obtained at our institution, including renal US scans, VCUG images, and intravenous pyelograms, was examined, and 493 children who underwent VCUG and renal US on the same day were identified. In this group, 216 children were aged 5 years or older at the time of imaging; 103 of the children were evaluated for the first time, and 70 of these 103 children were evaluated because of a UTI. These latter 70 children (64 girls, six boys), aged 5–15 years (mean, 7.3 years), constituted the study sample.

In almost all cases, US and VCUG were performed within 1 or 2 hours of each other, with US before VCUG. Cases were categorized according to the attending radiologist's interpretation at the time of examination. Recorded US abnormalities were not limited to dilatation of the collecting system and parenchymal thinning but included any abnormality such as ectopia and nephrolithiasis.

RESULTS

The 70 children were assigned to two groups on the basis of the US findings (Figure): Sonograms were normal in 65 children and abnormal in five children. In the latter group, three

Index terms: Bladder, radiography, 83.1231 • Genitourinary system, diseases, 81.21, 82.214, 82.85 • Genitourinary system, US, 81.12981, 82.12981 , 83.12981 • Ureter, reflux, 82.1231, 82.85 • Urography, 82.122, 82.1232, 82.1233 • Voiding cystourethrography, 83.1231

Abbreviations: UTI = urinary tract infection, VCUG = voiding cystourethrography, VUR = vesicoureteral reflux.

Radiology 1997; 205:821–822

[1] From the Department of Pediatric Radiology, F3503, University of Michigan Hospitals, 1500 E Medical Center Dr, Ann Arbor, MI 48109-0252. From the 1994 RSNA scientific assembly. Received April 24, 1997; revision requested May 15; revision received and accepted August 4. **Address reprint requests to** M.A.D.

(60%) normal and two (40%) positive VCUG studies were obtained. The three children in whom normal VCUG studies were obtained included a 6-year-old girl with a unilateral pelvic kidney; a 6-year-old girl with a solitary tiny cyst or calyceal diverticulum; and a 9-year-old boy with a single, tiny echogenic focus (possibly a renal stone) that disappeared and has been absent at follow-up US for 4 years. The two children in whom positive VCUG studies were obtained included a 6-year-old girl with mild pelvicalyceal dilatation at US and ipsilateral grade 2 VUR and a 7-year-old boy with a small right kidney (more than 2 standard deviations smaller than the mean for his age) and no collecting-system dilatation at US but with ipsilateral grade 5 VUR at VCUG. Incidentally, the contralateral kidney in this latter child was normal at US, with grade 3 VUR.

Of the 65 children in whom negative renal sonograms were obtained, 46 (including three boys) (71%) had a negative VCUG study, but 19 (including one boy) (29%) had VUR at VCUG. There were eight kidneys associated with grade 1 VUR, 15 associated with grade 2 VUR, and two associated with grade 3 VUR. Six children had bilateral VUR. One of the children with grade 3 VUR and a negative sonogram was 5 years old at the time of initial examination; she is currently healthy at 2-year follow-up and no longer receives antimicrobial prophylaxis. The second child with grade 3 VUR was 7 years old at the time of the initial examinations; she developed a scar on her right kidney, which was noted 1 year later at both US and intravenous pyelography while she underwent continuous treatment with antimicrobial prophylaxis. She then underwent bilateral ureteral reimplantation.

DISCUSSION

The detection of VUR is considered to be important for the long-term prevention of renal scarring (1). Although the authors of a prospective, blinded study (5) reported that intravenous pyelography could be replaced with renal US by using a combination of US and VCUG (5), they did not advocate the replacement of VCUG with US. Whereas the older child has been considered to be at lower risk for the development of scars, most clinicians would still treat severe VUR (grade 3 or higher) in an older child with antimicrobial prophylaxis (1).

The possibility of the replacement of VCUG with screening US, particularly in older children, is appealing. Clinicians may be reluctant to order VCUG in such children because of the need for catheter placement in the bladder. Although such an intervention performed by experienced personnel with aseptic technique is safe and is usually well tolerated, in some cases there is still parental and patient anxiety associated with the procedure.

It has been previously shown (6) in patients of a broad range of ages that US is not a reliable screening technique for VUR. The aim of the present study was specifically to determine in older children whether a negative renal sonogram was predictive of negative VCUG findings. A negative sonogram was obtained in 65 (93%) of 70 patients, and in this group of 65 children, 19 (29%) had unilateral or bilateral VUR. A negative renal sonogram was obtained in two of the three children with grade 3 or higher VUR. Two (40%) of five children in whom abnormal sonograms were obtained had VUR, whereas 19 of the 65 children (29%) in whom normal sonograms were obtained had VUR.

If one were to consider only two of the five cases of abnormal US findings (pelvicalyceal dilatation, small kidney) as suggestive of VUR and the other three (cyst or diverticulum, pelvic kidney, possible tiny stone) as "negative," there would be two patients with positive US findings, both (100%) with VUR, and 68 patients with negative US findings, 19 (28%) with VUR. The conclusion can be stated quite simply: If one needs to identify children with VUR, negative US findings are not sufficient; one must perform VCUG.

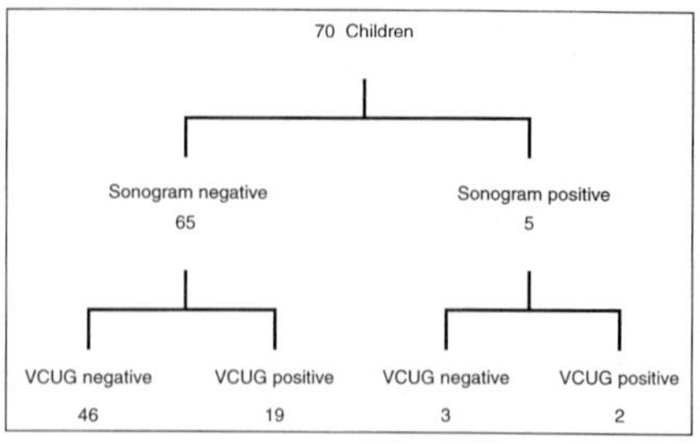

Schematic shows the assignment to two groups of the 70 children in the study group. The children, who were first evaluated because of a UTI, were assigned on the basis of US findings.

In this older-age group with UTI at initial presentation, VUR would have gone undetected in 90% of the children if VCUG had been performed only when the renal sonogram was abnormal. If the diagnosis and characterization of reflux is important to the management of VUR, VCUG is the reliable way to evaluate the patient. The more important questions about the need to detect VUR and the risk of scarring in this older-age group remain unanswered and are beyond the scope of this article. ■

References

1. Gordon I. Urinary tract infection in paediatrics: the role of diagnostic imaging. Br J Radiol 1990; 63:507–511.
2. Ransley PG. Vesicoureteric reflux: continuing surgical dilemma. Urology 1978; 12:246–255.
3. Bloom DA, Bennett CJ. Nonoperative management of vesicoureteral reflux. Semin Urol 1986; 4:74–81.
4. Blickman JG, Taylor GA, Lebowitz RL. Voiding cystourethrography: the initial radiologic study in children with urinary tract infection. Radiology 1985; 156:659–662.
5. Alon U, Pery M, Davidai G, Berant M. Ultrasonography in the radiologic evaluation of children with urinary tract infection. Pediatrics 1986; 78:58–64.
6. Blane CE, DiPietro MA, Zerin JM, Sedman AB, Bloom DA. Renal sonography is not a reliable screening examination for vesicoureteral reflux. J Urol 1993; 150:752–755.

Kari Richter, MD • Sylvia Helen Heywang-Köbrunner, MD • Klaus-Jürgen Winzer, MD
Karl-Jürgen Schmitt, PhD • Heinz Prihoda • Hans D. Frohberg, MD • Hans Guski, MD
Peter Gregor • Jens-Uwe Blohmer, MD • Franz Fobbe, MD • Karin Döinghaus, MD
Gisela Löhr, MD • Bernd Hamm, MD

Detection of Malignant and Benign Breast Lesions with an Automated US System: Results in 120 Cases[1]

PURPOSE: To evaluate clinically an automated ultrasound (US) system for detecting benign and malignant breast lesions.

MATERIALS AND METHODS: A prototype automated US system was used to examine 119 patients: 38 patients with 39 proved malignant breast lesions (7–50 mm), 41 patients with 41 proved benign breast lesions (8–40 mm), and 40 patients without breast lesions. The device yields a three-dimensional set of B-mode scans and reconstructed US images comparable to mammograms. All patients had undergone mammography. Four radiologists who had not performed the examinations independently assessed the mammograms and US images to detect benign and malignant breast lesions.

RESULTS: Each of the four readers did not recognize one to three detectable malignant lesions on mammograms, one to two detectable malignant lesions on US images, two to four detectable benign lesions on mammograms, and five to seven detectable benign lesions on US images. All readers identified the 39 cancers with at least one of the modalities. The 40 cases without lesions were diagnosed correctly more frequently on the US images by three readers and on the mammograms by one reader.

CONCLUSION: Depiction of breast lesions at automated US is reproducible. Automated US is complementary to mammography.

Mammography is the only imaging modality accepted as a screening procedure for detecting presymptomatic breast cancers with a documented reduction in the mortality rate (1–3). However, despite technical advances in mammography and the special training of examiners, up to 50% of cancers diagnosed at screening and so-called interval cancers are retrospectively identified on previously obtained mammograms (4). However, carcinomas that are large enough to be palpated may not be depicted at mammography (5,6).

Because ultrasound (US) and mammography are complementary modalities and the former can be used to differentiate lesions (7), we performed patient examinations with an experimental compression system that compresses the breast as in mammography and that allows systematic manual scanning of the breast through an upper compression plate (8). The lower compression plate is displayed as a bright line when the transducer is perpendicular to the upper plate. This line changes in appearance under lesions, which affect the returned ultrasound signal (8). The system was further improved and automated and now allows US breast examinations to be performed alone or in conjunction with mammography without decompression of the breast (8,9).

The system provides not only an automatically acquired set of three-dimensional B-mode scans, but also two automatically reconstructed survey images of the breast that can be read as mammograms are read. These images are based on the reconstruction of the lower compression plate and how it changes on all the B-mode scans (9). The idea of the combined examination is to detect lesions on the reconstructed US images and mammograms and then to differentiate them on the mammograms and set of B-mode scans (9).

The method is being clinically evaluated with a prototype designed for clinical trials (9). In the prospective study discussed here, mammograms and automatically acquired US images were interpreted by four blinded readers (S.H.H.K., F.F., K.D., G.L.) from different centers who were not involved in the examination of the patients, as is the usual procedure for comparing diagnostic images (10). The aim of the study was to evaluate clinically an automated US system for detecting benign and malignant breast lesions, in part by determining the

Index terms: Breast neoplasms, diagnosis, 00.30 • Breast neoplasms, radiography, 00.11 • Breast neoplasms, US, 00.12987, 00.12989 • Ultrasound (US), comparative studies, 00.12987, 00.12989 • Ultrasound (US), maximum intensity projection, 00.12989 • Ultrasound (US), three-dimensional, 00.12987, 00.12989

Abbreviation: MIP = maximum intensity projection.

Radiology 1997; 205:823–830

[1] From the Departments of Radiology (K.R., H.D.F., P.G., B.H.), Surgery (K.J.W.), Pathology (H.G.), and Gynecology (J.U.B.), Charité Medical School, Humboldt University of Berlin, Schumannstrasse 20/21, D-10117 Berlin, Germany; the Department of Diagnostic Radiology, University of Halle, Halle, Germany (S.H.H.K.); the Medical Engineering Group, Siemens Medical Systems, Erlangen, Germany (K.J.S., H.P.); the Department of Radiology, Auguste Viktoria Hospital, Berlin, Germany (K.R., F.F.); the Department of Gynecological Radiology, University of Erlangen, Erlangen, Germany (K.D.); and the Department of Diagnostic Radiology, Krankenhaus am Urban, Berlin, Germany (G.L.). Received March 17, 1997; revision requested May 12; revision received July 14; accepted July 21. **Address reprint requests to** K.R.

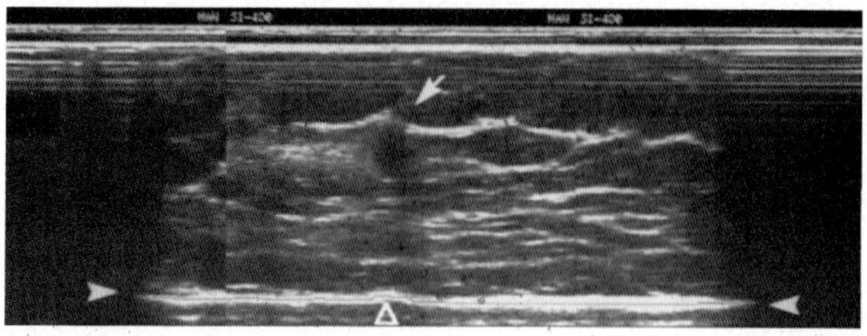

a.

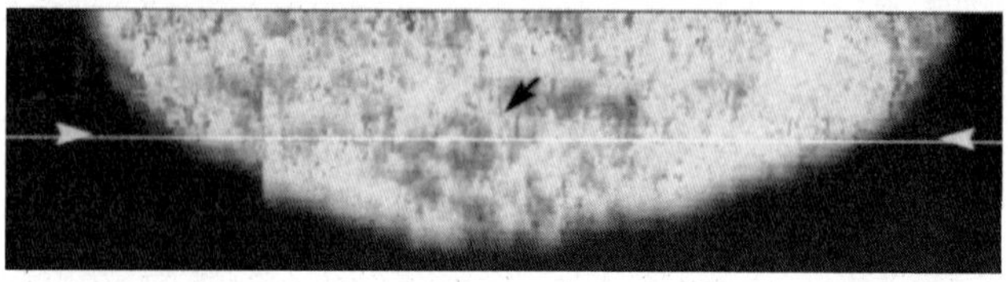

b.

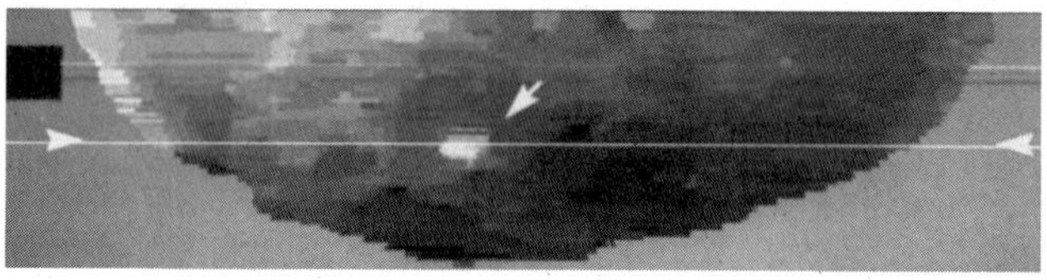

c.

Figure 1. Craniocaudal projections of a nonpalpable carcinoma (maximal histopathologic size, 16 mm) in the left breast in a 58-year-old woman as seen on the evaluation screen. **(a)** B-mode scan of the carcinoma (arrow) shows the lower compression plate as a hyperreflexive line (solid arrowheads) at the bottom of the screen. A black line that follows the course of the reference line shows where the system has automatically determined the line position, which is displayed in shades of gray on the reconstructed images. The reference line is elevated below the carcinoma (open arrowhead) owing to increased sound velocity within the lesion. **(b)** MIP image reconstructed from all B-mode scans displays the brightnes of the reference line as a measure of sound absorption in the breast. The carcinoma is seen as a round area surrounded by a gray halo owing to lateral refractive shadows that surround the lesion on all sides (arrow). The image cursor is a white line (arrowheads) that shows the position of the selected B-mode scan (**a**) within the three-dimensional data set. **(c)** US line map displays the height of the reference line as a measure of sound velocity, which is displayed in shades of gray. Because elevations are encoded in white, as lesions appear on mammograms, the carcinoma is displayed as a white region (arrow). The white line (arrowheads) again corresponds to the image cursor, which is moved simultaneously with the cursor on the MIP image to show the changes in both sound velocity and sound absorption in identical locations expected in the presence of a lesion. Note, the reconstructed images are distorted by a factor of 1:0.7 (distance from outer breast to inner breast:distance from chest wall to nipple). This deficit will be eliminated with further development of the device.

reproducibility of findings, and thus to determine whether it is worthwhile to perfect this technique further.

MATERIALS AND METHODS

Automated Breast US Prototype

The compressed breast is positioned as in mammography and is scanned automatically by a motor-driven, 5-MHz transducer (Sonoline SI 400; Siemens Medical Systems, Erlangen, Germany), which, because of the narrow acoustic window, has to move in three parallel paths to cover the entire upper compression plate (15 × 24 mm, 8-mm-thick Plexiglas) in 90 seconds. This procedure yields a complete three-dimensional set of B-mode scans. The individual images obtained per path while the transducer is moved toward the patient (which results in a total of 600 images) are used to compose 160 B-mode scans of unusually large breadth that represent the three paths of the transducer and display the entire width of the breast. The scanning unit is attached to a normal mammography system (Mammomat 300; Siemens Medical Systems, Solna, Sweden) instead of the usual upper compression plate.

After spatially correct storage of the B-mode scans, the reconstructed survey images are generated by means of postprocessing of the original scans. The lower compression plate (conventional film-cassette holder of the mammography system) is depicted on the individual B-mode scans as a straight hyperreflexive line, because the echoes are reflected by this structure. Under normal tissue, this line is straight and of homogeneous brightness. Under lesions, this line might show changes in brightness as a result of sound attenuation or amplification relative to that of the surrounding normal tissue. A higher sound velocity within a lesion will result in an apparent elevation of the line because the sound impulse passes through the lesion faster (8,9). This line is used as a reference to indicate the presence of a lesion in the breast tissue by displaying the combined acoustic properties of the entire thickness of the part of the breast superficial to it.

This information is automatically extracted from each of the B-mode scans by means of postprocessing. The line position and brightness are displayed in shades of gray on separate reconstructed images: The line position is shown on a US line map and the brightness is displayed on a US maximum intensity projection (MIP) image. The screening images presented for analysis are made by combining the reference lines from all the B-mode scans through the entire breast: The US maps reflect variations in sound velocity and the US MIP images reflect variations in sound amplitude within the tissue (Fig 1). Both reconstructions are displayed on a computer screen. Individual images from the set of B-mode scans can be opened and displayed with the reconstructed images. Thus, it is possible to directly assess and characterize a lesion that has caused a circumscribed disruption on the reconstructed images (Fig 1).

US coupling gel (Sonavelle; Elefant-Chemie Breuhan, Hannover, Germany) is used to ensure adequate contact between the transducer, the upper compression plate, and the breast. The parts of the breast that are not in direct contact with the plates are not depicted because of intervening air. The method has been described in detail before (9).

Patient Examination

After informed consent had been obtained, all consecutive preoperative patients and all consecutive patients undergoing follow-up because of imaging findings of a benign lesion but without histopathologic confirmation were examined with the prototype. The breasts of all patients were examined in the same position at US as they had been at mammography, with craniocaudal and mediolateral oblique (45°) projections and with identical parameter settings. In all consecutive preoperative patients, mammography was performed independently of US, because the diagnostic work-up had been completed before surgery, and recently obtained, meaningful mammograms were available in all patients.

From June 10, 1996, to September 27, 1996, 194 patients were examined; a total of 87 proved cases (82 cases with histopathologic proof, five cases with cytologic proof) in 86 patients were available. All mammograms were independently evaluated by a second radiologist (H.D.F.) with respect to lesion visibility. Lesion visibility on the automatically acquired US images was assessed by the primary examiner (K.R.).

Thirty-nine malignant and 41 benign lesions in 79 patients (one patient had bilateral breast cancer) were included in the study (Table 1). Forty patients who had no lesions were the control subjects in the study. The age of the control subjects (average age, 53.5 years; age range, 31–76 years) was in the same range as that of the patients with benign or malignant lesions. For comparison, images were chosen from those obtained in the group of women not included in the study in whom no histopathologic results were available or who were not scheduled for histopathologic confirmation; the images had been obtained in the breast opposite the breast with the lesion and showed only normal tissue and no lesion. Another prerequisite for healthy control subjects was that mam-

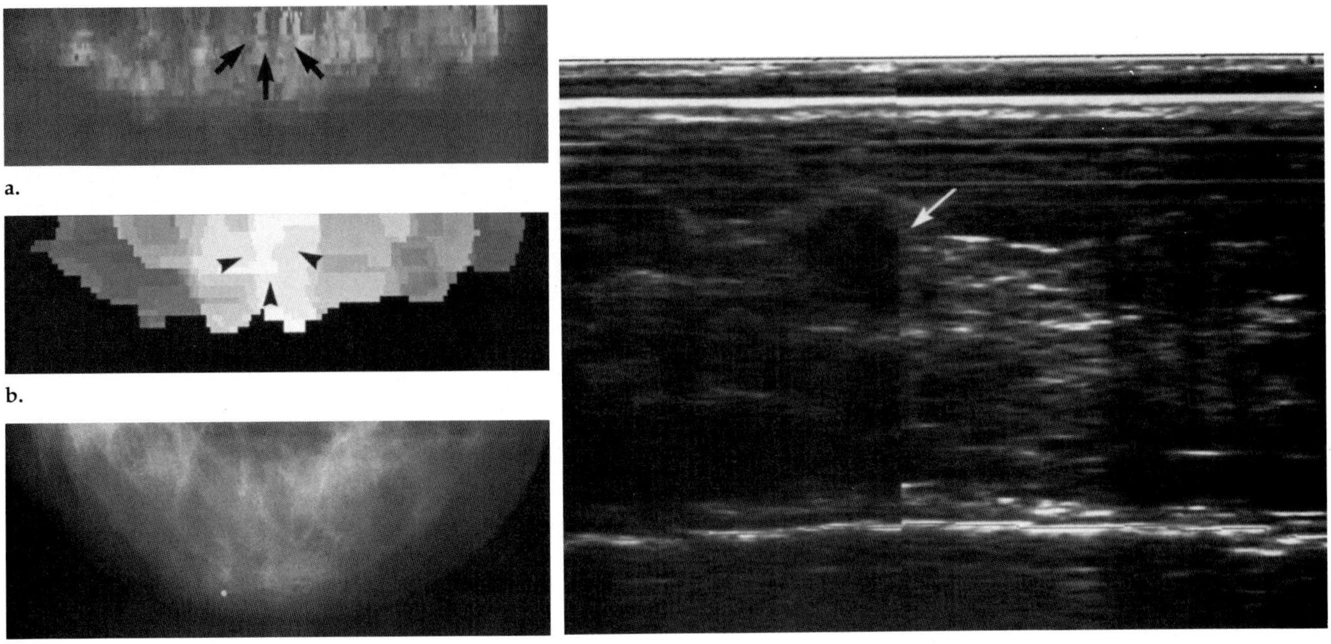

Figure 2. Craniocaudal projections of a palpable, mammographically occult, invasive ductal carcinoma (maximal histopathologic size, 15 mm) in the right breast of a 51-year-old woman. The carcinoma was recognized on the automated US images by all readers (on the MIP image and map and the B-mode scan by two readers, on the map and B-mode scan by two readers). **(a)** MIP image without the image cursor shows the carcinoma (arrows) as a circumscribed region with sound attenuation and amplification. **(b)** Line map without the image cursor shows the lesion (arrowheads) as the brightest region on the image. **(c)** Corresponding B-mode scan shows the lesion (arrow). **(d)** Mammogram does not show the carcinoma in the dense tissue.

mograms with unchanged findings had to be available for at least 2 years. These criteria were met by all 40 control subjects.

Seven cases in seven patients were excluded because they did not meet the inclusion criteria. Because the healthy control subjects were artificially chosen, the readers had to assess only images that showed either a distinct lesion or normal tissue. For this reason, six large, diffuse carcinomas that were identified only as asymmetries in comparison with the opposite breast had to be excluded from the study. One case of an occult lesion had to be excluded after a postoperative control mammogram showed that the lesion had not been removed.

A recent mammogram was available in all 120 cases. The maximal interval between mammography and US was 4 weeks.

Lesion and Patient Characteristics

Of the 39 cancers, 38 were visible on mammograms and 36 were visible on US images. Of the 41 benign lesions, 40 were visible on mammograms and 35 were visible on US images. Each of the 80 lesions was detected with at least one of the two modalities.

Of the 36 sonographically visible carcinomas, 14 (39%) were not palpable and 14 (39%) were 7–15 mm. In the carcinoma group, 10 (26%) of the 38 patients were 50 years of age or younger and 26 (68%) were 60 years of age or younger.

Three asymptomatic, sonographically occult carcinomas were detected on mammograms only because microcalcifications were present. These were noninvasive, intraductal, diffusely growing carcinomas whose size could not be determined histopathologically (the radiologically determined extents of the microcalcifications were 18, 20, and 50 mm). The one carcinoma detected only at US was a palpable lesion with a histopathologically determined size of 15 mm (Fig 2). Of the six benign lesions not visible at US, four consisted of suspicious microcalcifications identifiable only with mammography. Histopathologic findings proved that these four lesions were benign (fibrocystic disease). Two cases of histopathologically proved fibrosis appeared on mammograms as focal lesions without correlates on US images. The size of 21 of the 41 benign lesions could not be determined histopathologically (Table 1), because the radiologically detected foci had no histopathologic correlates or because only cytologic results were available (in the case of punctured cysts).

Selection and Qualifications of the Readers

The readers were four radiologists with experience in mammography and breast US (S.H.H.K., F.F., K.D., G.L.). They were chosen from four different centers to ensure independent assessment and lack of knowledge of the cases in the study. Two of the readers had special experience in breast imaging; the other two had many years of experience in diagnostic radiology without special emphasis on breast imaging. None of the readers had had any practical experience with the automated US method, although one of them had good, theoretic knowledge of the method.

After agreeing to participate in the study, the readers received written information about the principles of automated US and the design and purpose of the clinical study. Immediately before the reading sessions, the readers were introduced to the interpretation of automated US images with examples of benign and malignant lesions (n = 12) and of cases without lesions (n = 3) that were not included in the study. The aim of this introduction was to show the readers how to identify bright areas on the sound velocity images (line maps) (Figs 1c, 2b) and bright or dark areas on the sound absorption images (MIP images) (Figs 1b, 2a) as signs of lesions. They were not supposed to differentiate between lesions and normal tissue (asymmetric distribution of the corpus mammae or pectoral muscle) or artifacts (reconstruction errors, interfering air, etc) on the reconstructed images.

For assessment of the B-mode scans, the readers were instructed to pay attention to changes in the brightness and elevation of the reference line (Figs 1a, 2c) to facilitate the identification of lesions above this line. The readers were asked not to characterize the lesion on the B-mode scan, because only one scan was available to them with no possibility of dynamic assessment.

No instructions were given with regard to the interpretation of mammograms. The instruction took 35–60 minutes per reader.

Blinded Reading and Documentation of Results

The readers assessed mammograms and automated US images that showed the lesion or normal tissue in identical projections. Because the problem of simultaneous projection of several planes remains to be solved for automated US, only one projection was presented; the projection was identical for mammography and US. US images and mammograms were separately and randomly ordered and were interpreted independently of each other. The mammograms were interpreted in the usual way with a light box. A bright lamp and magnifying glass were allowed as aids.

The reconstructed US images (line map, US MIP image) (Fig 1b, 1c) were prepared without an image cursor (Fig 2a, 2b), and all cases were stored in a personal computer, from which they could easily be retrieved for inspection. The two US reconstructed survey images (MIP images and maps) (Fig 2a, 2b) and a B-mode scan, which could not be assigned to any particular region of the reconstructed survey images without the image cursor, were presented. The B-mode scan showed the lesion in the study cases and the normal tissue in the control cases.

For all images (mammogram, line map, MIP image, B-mode scan), an identically numbered hard copy was available on which the readers marked areas where they identified a lesion. The time required by the readers for interpretation of the images and documentation of their findings was registered separately for mammography and US.

Table 1
Patient and Lesion Characteristics

Characteristic	Malignant Lesions (n = 39)*	Benign Lesions (n = 41)†
Patient age (y)		
Average	57.2	46.7
Range	42–75	20–75
Lesion at clinical presentation (no. of lesions)		
Occult	13 (33)	22 (54)
Palpable	24 (62)	16 (39)
Other symptoms	2 (5)	3 (7)
Lesion size (largest diameter)		
≤10 mm (no. of lesions)	4 (10)	6 (15)
11–15 mm (no. of lesions)	11 (28)	5 (12)
16–20 mm (no. of lesions)	8 (21)	5 (12)
>20 mm (no. of lesions)	12 (31)	4 (10)
Not measurable (no. of lesions)	4 (10)	21 (51)
Average size (mm)	19.9	16.5
Size range (mm)	7–50	8–40

Note.—The number in parentheses is the percentage.

* Histopathologic diagnoses: invasive ductal carcinoma, 17 lesions; invasive ductal and intraductal carcinoma, 15 lesions; ductal carcinoma in situ, three lesions; tubular carcinoma, one lesion; lobular carcinoma, one lesion; medullary carcinoma, one lesion; and cystadenocarcinoma, one lesion. There were six cases of multicentric carcinoma and one case of bilateral carcinoma.

† Histopathologic diagnoses: fibrocystic disease, 16 lesions; fibroadenoma, 12 lesions; cyst, six lesions; papilloma, two lesions; postoperative scar, one lesion; benign fibromatosis, one lesion; radial scar, one lesion; fat necrosis, one lesion; and hamartoma, one lesion.

Table 2
Detection of Malignant Lesions (n = 39) on Mammograms and US Images

Images	Reader 1	Reader 2	Reader 3	Reader 4
Mammograms				
Lesions detected	37	37	37	35
Detectable lesions missed	1	1	1	3
US images				
Lesions detected on MIP images	25	28	30	24
Lesions detected on maps	25	26	31	27
Lesions detected on MIP images or maps	31	34	33	28
Lesions detected on B-mode scans	33	28	29	34
Lesions detected on MIP images or maps and B-mode scans	30	27	28	27
Lesions detected on any US image	34	35	34	35
Detectable lesions missed	2	1	2	1

Note.—One carcinoma not visible on the mammograms and three intraductal carcinomas not visible on the US images were excluded.

Analysis of Results

The hard copies on which the readers had marked their findings were analyzed to determine on which images (mammograms, line maps, MIP images, B-mode scans) the readers had identified a lesion. The original interpretation of the images in combination with the histopathologic findings served as a standard. In addition, false-positive and false-negative findings were counted. A suspicious region marked on the reconstructed images (line maps and MIP images) was differentiated on the basis of the primary data according to whether it was an artifact, an additional lesion (in cases with multiple lesions), or a normal structure. After completion of the reading session, the readers were asked to spontaneously comment on the method without knowledge of their results.

RESULTS

Time Required for Image Interpretation and Documentation of Findings

The average time for interpretation and documentation was 45, 53, 60, and 83 seconds per case for mammography (one image read) compared to 69, 96, 99, and 126 seconds per case for US (three images read). The reader with comprehensive theoretic knowledge of automated US was fastest in interpreting the US images. For this reader, the average time required per case remained constant throughout the reading session, whereas the other three readers became faster during the reading session (from an average time of 108–174 seconds initially to an average of 66–99 seconds at the end of the reading).

Detection of Malignant Lesions

The results of the mammographic readings in malignant lesions are summarized in Table 2. A total of four detectable cancers (three were 20 mm and one was 39 mm) were missed by some readers. Two of these were missed by two of the four readers; the other two were each missed by only one reader. Thus, all detectable cancers were identified by at least two readers.

The results of the US readings also are summarized in Table 2. The two reconstructed images (MIP images and maps) were nearly identical with respect to the identification of malignant lesions; reading both reconstructed images together increased the number of cancers detected. One 15-mm detectable cancer was missed by all readers both on the reconstructed images and on the B-mode scan (Fig 3). Another 11-mm cancer was identified on only the B-mode scan by all readers. None of the cancers was found on only the reconstructed images by all readers. In all other instances of missed malignant lesions, the lesions were detected by at least one of the other readers on one or several US images. The smallest cancer of the study (histopathologic size, 7 × 5 mm) was identified by all readers on the reconstructed images and on the B-mode scan. The reader

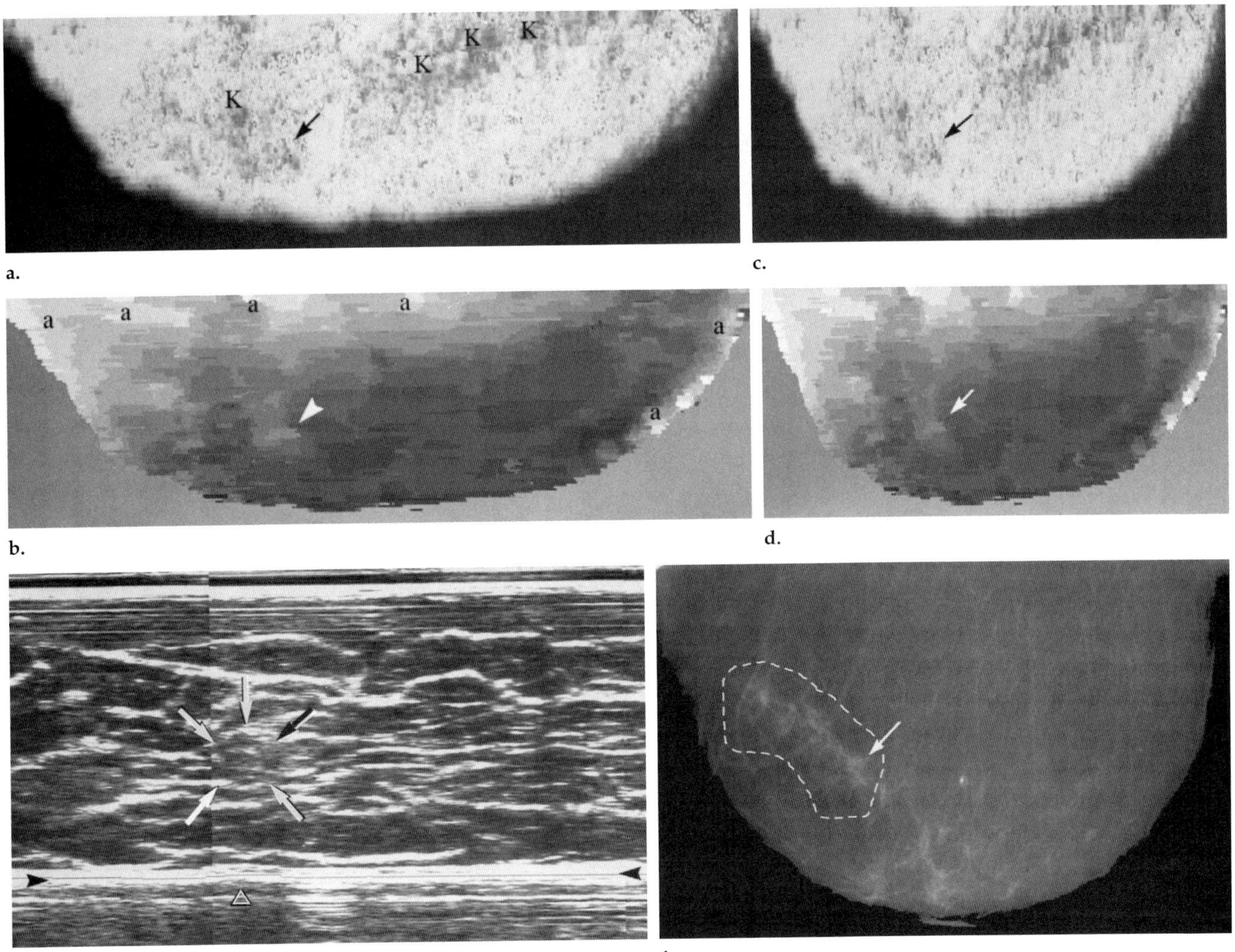

a. c. b. d. e. f.

Figure 3. Craniocaudal projections of a nonpalpable, invasive ductal carcinoma (maximal histopathologic size, 15 mm) in the left breast of a 60-year-old woman. The carcinoma was missed on the automated US images by all readers. **(a)** MIP image shows the carcinoma as a discrete area of sound attenuation (arrow) that is not set off from a region of coupling artifacts (*K*). **(b)** Line map shows brightening in the same region (arrowhead); however, owing to the nonparallel compression plates, this area appears to be contiguous with adjacent normal tissue and is therefore not recognizable as a circumscribed structure. The white regions (*a*) are reconstruction artifacts that make the whole image appear blurred. Because the original display of the reconstructed images used in the study is distorted by a factor of 1:0.7 (distance from outer breast to inner breast:distance from chest wall to nipple), the projection makes the lesion appear oval even though it is round; this contributes to the poor visibility of the lesion. **(c)** MIP image and **(d)** line map of **a** and **b** on a scale of 1:1 (incorrect measure was corrected by using a special external computer program) show the carcinoma (arrow), which is more conspicuous because the actual shape of the lesion is depicted. **(e)** B-mode scan shows the carcinoma (arrows), which is difficult to identify. However, the reference line (solid arrowheads) is elevated below the lesion (open arrowhead). **(f)** Mammogram shows the carcinoma (arrow), but it is poorly demarcated from the surrounding mastopathic structures. All readers therefore marked the entire area (dotted line), which was rated as correct lesion identification.

with theoretic knowledge of the method detected the most sonographically visible cancers (34 of 36 cancers) on one or both reconstructed images; another reader detected the most on the B-mode scans (likewise, 34 of 36 cancers). On all three US images taken together, two readers missed two detectable cancers and the other two readers missed one detectable cancer (histopathologic sizes, 15, 20, and 39 mm).

Combination of Mammography and US

The mammographically occult cancer (Fig 2) was identified by all readers on the reconstructed images and on the B-mode scan; likewise, the three sonographically occult carcinomas were identified on the mammograms by all readers. In all other cases in which the readers did not detect cancer on the mammograms, all readers identified cancer on at least one of the US images. The one carcinoma all four readers did not identify on the US images (Fig 3) was detected on the mammogram by all four of them (Fig 3f). The two readers who each failed to identify one cancer detected by the three other readers on the US images detected these lesions on the corresponding mammograms. Two readers identified all 39 carcinomas on a mammogram, on a reconstructed US image, or both; the other two readers detected 38 carcinomas on a mammogram, on a reconstructed US image, or both and identified one cancer on only the B-mode scan.

Detection of Benign Lesions by the Readers

The results of the mammographic readings in benign lesions are summarized in Table 3. All visible benign lesions were identified by at least one of the readers.

The results of the US readings also

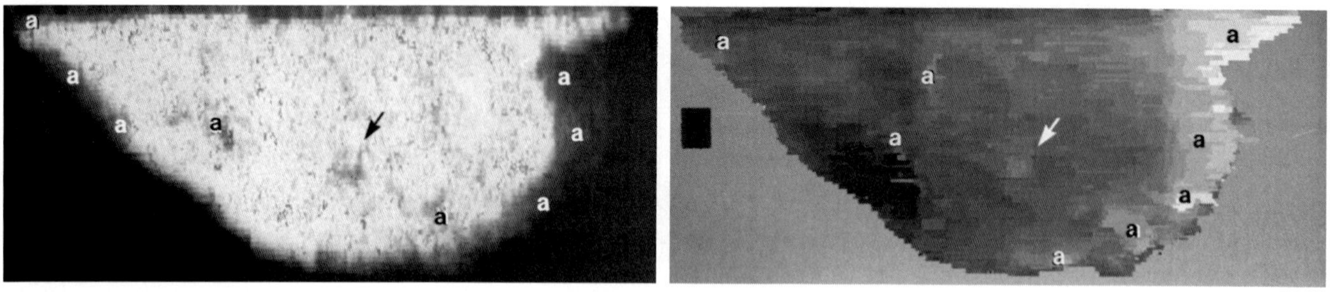

a. b.

Figure 4. Mediolateral projections of histopathologically proved, 7 × 7-mm invasive ductal carcinoma in the left breast in a 67-year-old woman as seen on the evaluation screen. This was the second smallest malignant lesion in the study. **(a)** Mediolateral MIP image and **(b)** mediolateral line map. **a** depicts the cancer as a round structure surrounded by a dark halo (refractive shadowing, arrow). **b** depicts the lesion as a round, brighter region in the same location (arrow). No overlying artifacts (*a*) interfere with the depiction of the lesion. The surrounding normal tissue is homogeneously gray owing to perfectly parallel compression plates. This cancer was detected by all readers. The image quality is much better than it is in Figure 3, although the difference in gray shades between the lesion and surrounding tissue is the same and the projection is much smaller.

are summarized in Table 3. All readers identified more benign processes on the line maps than on the MIP images, and the detection rate was highest for all four readers when these two images were read together. Only one detectable lesion (atypical proliferating mastopathy of histopathologically indeterminable size) was missed on all US images by all readers. One cyst and one 10-mm fibroadenoma were identified only on the reconstructed images by all four readers; another cyst and an 18-mm fibroadenoma were detected only on the B-mode scan by all four readers. All other lesions identified on only the reconstructed images or on only the B-mode scans by individual readers were of various types. The highest number of lesions on one or more of the US images was detected by a reader without prior knowledge of the method.

Table 3
Detection of Benign Lesions (n = 41) on Mammograms and US Images

Images	Reader 1	Reader 2	Reader 3	Reader 4
Mammograms				
Lesions detected	38	38	36	37
Detectable lesions missed	2	2	4	3
US images				
Lesions detected on MIP images	15	14	13	18
Lesions detected on maps	19	20	22	19
Lesions detected on MIP images or maps	22	22	25	23
Lesions detected on B-mode scans	22	17	13	26
Lesions detected on MIP images or maps and B-mode scans	16	11	9	19
Lesions detected on any US image	28	28	29	30
Detectable lesions missed	7	7	6	5

Note.—One lesion not visible on the mammograms and six lesions not visible on the US images were excluded.

Combination of Mammography and US

The mammographically occult lesion was detected on both reconstructed images and on the B-mode scan by all four readers. In all other cases in which individual readers did not detect a lesion on the mammogram, they did identify the lesion on at least one of the US images; only one lesion was missed by one of the readers on both the mammogram and the US images. All readers identified the sonographically occult lesions on the mammograms. The one sonographically visible lesion missed on the US images by all four readers was identified on the mammogram by all of them. All other lesions missed on the US images by individual readers were identified by them on the mammograms. All 41 benign lesions were identified on the mammograms, on a reconstructed US image, or on both by two readers; one reader identified one lesion on the B-mode scan only, and one reader missed one lesion on all images.

Results in the 40 Cases without Lesions

Marking a region on the MIP or map alone was not interpreted as detection of a nonexistent lesion; this was regarded as a false-positive finding only if the area also was marked on the corresponding B-mode scan. With these conditions, more individuals were determined to be healthy by three readers with US than with mammography; the opposite was true in one reader (Table 4). The two readers with special experience in breast imaging classified more cases as healthy on both mammograms and US images than did the other two readers without special experience. All four readers marked an average of 1.2 normal structures per case on MIP images and maps. Only when the corresponding B-mode scan was available was it possible to decide whether the readers erroneously identified a lesion. It was not possible to decide this when the readers marked a region for which no B-mode scan was available. Thus, the number merely indicates the average number of B-mode scans the readers would have retrieved and assessed for each projection.

Marking of Regions on MIP Images and Maps: False-Positive Findings in the 80 Benign or Malignant Lesions

The readers' findings in the cases with lesions were evaluated in the same way as their findings in the cases without lesions. All marked regions on the mammograms, MIP images, maps, and B-mode scans were recorded and matched. In contrast to the rate of false-positive findings in the 40 healthy control cases, the average rate of false-positive findings was lower on mammograms (26 findings in 20 women) and on B-mode scans (23 findings in 17 women). The average number of marked normal structures for all readers and all cases was

Table 4
Mammographic and US Findings in 40 Healthy Control Subjects

Images	Reader 1	Reader 2	Reader 3	Reader 4
Mammograms				
No lesions	22	30	33	18
False-positive findings	31 (in 18 women)	12 (in 10 women)	9 (in 7 women)	26 (in 22 women)
US images				
MIP images				
Normal structures	50	36	58	45
Average no. of structures per case	1.25	0.9	1.45	1.1
Artifacts	45	55	126	37
Maps				
Normal structures	31	45	66	49
Average no. of structures per case	0.8	1.1	1.7	1.1
Artifacts	28	45	91	34
B-mode scans				
No lesions	12	35	37	22
False-positive findings	43 (in 28 women)	5 (in 5 women)	3 (in 3 women)	17 (in 17 women)

likewise lower on the MIP images and maps (0.9 structures per case and 0.7 structures per case, respectively).

Most Important Comments of the Readers

The most important comments of the readers follow. Lesions are detectable on the map and the corresponding B-mode scan after assessment of just a few images (according to two readers). In unclear cases, lesion detection might be improved with better-quality B-mode scans (according to two readers) or with a higher transducer frequency (according to one reader). Differentiation of artifacts from normal tissue might also be possible on MIP images and maps alone without retrieving the corresponding B-mode scans (according to two readers).

DISCUSSION

As long as there is evidence that not all carcinomas are detectable with mammography (4–6), improvement is necessary. The US technique presented here allows automated generation of reconstructed US images of the breast and provides all original data as a three-dimensional set of B-mode scans. The latter can be obtained without a physician and without the influence of individual factors, as with mammography. As with mammograms, these US images allow comparison of the right and left breasts and can be compared with previously obtained images (9). US does not compete with mammography but supplements it. Concurrent examination with mammography and US yields diagnostic information on all areas of the breast in one session. In contrast with conventional US, which is performed with the patient in the supine position, suspicious regions on the mammograms as well as on the reconstructed US images can be reproducibly, spatially matched by retrieving the corresponding B-mode scans. This is the only way to clearly assign a mammographically occult lesion to a correlate on US images (11).

In terms of detectability, the lesions included in the study showed a random bias in favor of mammography; a lower percentage of malignant lesions were detected with US alone. Thus, even if all lesions had been successfully identified with both methods, mammography should have depicted more lesions.

The interpretation of the findings of the combined procedure at present is as follows: Once an abnormality is identified on identical projections of US MIP images, line maps, and mammograms, the examiner retrieves the corresponding B-mode scan for further differentiation. A lesion is assumed to be the cause of the identified abnormality only if it is present on the B-mode scan. If the corresponding B-mode scan does not depict a lesion, the projection on the reconstructed images is interpreted as normal tissue, unless it is an artifact. Small, diffuse cancers are not identifiable as a mass by the pathologist during the macroscopic analysis but only by means of microscopy and are identified mammographically only because of suspicious microcalcifications; thus, a normal US image does not exclude malignancy (8,9).

With the condition that a lesion had to be identified on at least one of the reconstructed images and on the corresponding B-mode scan for definitive diagnosis, the readers detected 27–30 (75%–83%) of the 36 visible cancers on US images. The use of the mammogram as the reconstructed survey image for retrieving the corresponding B-mode scan increased the detection rate to 30–33 (83%–92%) of the 36 cancers. Comparison with the detection rate on mammograms alone (35–37 [92%–97%] of 38 cancers) reveals a poorer result for combined mammography and US. This unexpected decrease is due to the identification of some lesions on the reconstructed US images, mammograms, or both but not on the corresponding B-mode scans. These lesions therefore had to be interpreted as normal tissue according to the above definition.

Under the study conditions, the readers could not combine their mammographic and US findings, as would be the case in routine application of the two methods. However, because only one visible malignant lesion was missed on all US images by all readers (Fig 3), while all other malignant lesions were correctly identified on the B-mode scans by at least some of the readers, it may be concluded that these lesions were visible in principle and might have been identified by all readers after some training. This assumption is supported by the fact that one reader identified 34 of the 36 detectable cancers on the reconstructed images and another detected 34 of the 36 detectable cancers on the B-mode scans.

Furthermore, none of the cancers was identified only on the mammograms, reconstructed images, or both but not on the B-mode scans by all four readers. Misdetection is thus due to individual factors, as suggested by the readers' spontaneous comments on the unusually poor quality of the B-mode scans. The poor quality of the B-mode scans in turn is due to the use of a 5-MHz transducer instead of a 7.5-MHz transducer, which is routinely used in US examinations of the breast.

When the data for all lesions are analyzed together, the rate of detection of malignant lesions is 100% (39 of 39 lesions) for combined mammography and US for all readers, with the condition that each lesion was identified on at least one of the images.

Comparison of automated US and mammography yielded the following results for benign lesions: The readers identified nine to 19 (26%–54%) of the 35 visible lesions on the reconstructed US images and the B-mode scans. The detection rate increased to 13–25 (37%–71%) of the 35 lesions when the mammogram was added in retrieving the corresponding B-mode scan. On the assumption that lesion identification on only one of the US images is sufficient, the readers detected only 28–30 (80%–86%) of the 35 visible benign lesions compared to detection of 36–38 (90%–95%) of 40 lesions on mammograms.

Thus, the results of the US method are poorer for benign lesions than for malignant lesions. However, the detection rate for benign lesions was as high as 40–41 (98%–100%) of 41 lesions when combining mammography and US, with the condition that the lesions were identified on at least one of the US images. For both benign and malignant lesions, our results show that mammography and US are complementary modalities; as expected, this does hold for those lesions that were objectively depicted by means of only one of the two modalities. Furthermore, by identifying the lesion with the complementary method, three of the four readers compensated for misdetection of both benign and malignant lesions owing to individual factors. Only one reader missed one benign lesion with both imaging modalities.

The relatively poorer detection of benign lesions on the reconstructed US images was not unexpected, because some benign lesions do not produce a change in sound parameters and are thus seen only on B-mode scans (8,9). However, it remains unclear why the percentage of benign lesions identified by the readers on the B-mode scans is lower than the percentage of malignant lesions detected, even in those cases in which lesions were identified on the reconstructed images as a change in sound parameters. This is an important observation because the detection with conventional US of previously unknown, mammographically occult, solid focal lesions with histopathologic findings of benignity is a problem in the use of US as a screening method (12).

The findings in patients with benign lesions and healthy control subjects suggest that this problem is unlikely to occur in the same way with automated US. However, it is necessary to determine whether this conclusion is also justified with optimal-quality B-mode scans.

The present financial situation and the worldwide explosion of public health spending have prompted us to compare automated US and mammography in a blind study at an early point to decide whether it is worthwhile to further pursue this modality. However, this early comparison also involves certain conditions that have to be taken into consideration when interpreting the findings. The prototype was originally developed to determine whether it is possible to detect breast lesions on the reconstructed US images. Only after affirmation of this was it planned to improve the prototype by solving recent technical problems (reduction of coupling artifacts, coupling of the entire breast, parallel-plane arrangement of the upper and lower compression plates, etc) and to improve lesion detection by producing better-quality images (Figs 3a–3d, 4).

We deliberately used a 5-MHz, linear-array transducer instead of a 7.5-MHz transducer despite the known loss in B-mode image quality. The former was chosen because of the wider acoustic window, which enabled us to restrict the number of scanning paths for this first application. Despite the limitations, our results show that this US technique supplements mammography, that image interpretation within a reasonable time is possible after an extremely short training period, and that the diagnoses of the original examiner can be reproduced by independent radiologists. A definitive assessment of the diagnostic value of this procedure is not possible on the basis of the findings presented here. Further technical improvement of the method for clinical evaluation and application in a screening population looks promising. ■

References

1. Shapiro S. Periodic breast cancer screening in seven foreign countries. Cancer 1992; 69:1919–1924.
2. Verbeek ALM, Hendriks JH, Holland M, Mravunac F, Sturmans NE, Day NE. Reduction of breast cancer mortality through mass screening with modern mammography. Lancet 1984; 1:1222–1224.
3. McLelland R. Earlier detection of breast cancer: an overview. In: Brünner S, Langfeldt B, eds. Recent results in cancer research: advances in breast cancer detection. Vol 119. Berlin, Germany: Springer Verlag, 1990; 10–17.
4. Ciatto S, Roselli Del Turco M, Zappa M. The detectability of breast cancer by screening mammography. Br J Cancer 1995; 71: 337–339.
5. Jackson PV. The current role of ultrasonography in breast imaging. Radiol Clin North Am 1995; 33:1161–1170.
6. Sickles EA. Imaging technique other than mammography for detection and diagnosis of breast cancer. In: Brünner S, Langfeldt B, eds. Advances in breast cancer detection. Vol 119. Berlin, Germany: Springer Verlag, 1990; 127–135.
7. Stavros AT, Thickman D, Rapp CL, et al. Solid breast nodules: use of sonography to distinguish between benign and malignant lesions. Radiology 1995; 196:123–134.
8. Richter K. Technique for detecting and evaluating breast lesions. J Ultrasound Med 1994; 13:797–802.
9. Richter K, Prihoda H, Heywang-Köbrunner SH, et al. Description and first clinical use of a new system for combined mammography and automated clinical amplitude/velocity reconstructive imaging (CARI) breast sonography. Invest Radiol 1997; 32:19–28.
10. Bassett LW, Bunnell DH, Jahanshahi R, Gold RH, Arndt RD, Linsman J. Breast cancer detection: one versus two views. Radiology 1987; 165:95–97.
11. Conway WF, Hayes CW, Brewer WH. Occult breast masses: use of a mammographic localizing grid for US evaluation. Radiology 1991; 181:143–146.
12. Fung HM, Jackson FI. Clinically and mammographically occult breast lesions demonstrated by ultrasound. J R Soc Med 1990; 83:696–702.

Jaime Feu, MD • Francisco Tresserra, PhD • Rafael Fábregas, MD • Beatriz Navarro, MD
Pedro J. Grases, PhD • Joan Carles Suris, MPH • Alfonso Fernández-Cíd, PhD • Xavier Alegret, PhD

Metastatic Breast Carcinoma in Axillary Lymph Nodes: In Vitro US Detection[1]

PURPOSE: **To establish the ultrasonographic (US) characteristics of benign versus metastatic lymph nodes.**

MATERIALS AND METHODS: **One hundred fifty-eight axillary lymph nodes in 40 patients (age range, 31–73 years) surgically treated for breast cancer have been studied in vitro with a 7.5-MHz US probe in a water bath. The long-to-short axis ratio and the hilar and cortical characteristics were evaluated; the US findings were correlated with the histopathologic findings. To estimate the long-to-short axis ratio, all lymph nodes were measured.**

RESULTS: **Of the 158 lymph nodes, 45 showed histopathologic evidence of metastasis; 38 of the 45 revealed US signs of malignancy. The signs that caused malignancy to be suspected were a long-to-short axis ratio of less than 1.5, absence of a hilus, and disruption of the cortical zone. The most specific sign for the diagnosis of metastasis was absence of the hilus. The increase in the long-to-short axis ratio was the finding that caused the most false-negative interpretations. Signs of malignancy were more accurate in lymph nodes 10 mm or larger than they were in lymph nodes smaller than 10 mm.**

CONCLUSION: **Findings of in vitro US studies of axillary adenopathy provide the basis for the evaluation of lymph node metastasis in vivo before surgery, especially in those lymph nodes 10 mm or larger.**

LYMPH node involvement, tumor size, and systemic metastasis are the most important prognostic factors for breast cancer (1,2). Clinical examination has been the method used the most to determine the involvement of axillary lymph nodes; however, other techniques also have proved useful. Ultrasonography (US) is innocuous with a high sensitivity and specificity in the detection of lymph node metastasis (3–9), which can be confirmed with fine-needle aspiration of the suspicious lymph node (6,10). In vitro US of lymph nodes already has been performed to attain a better understanding of the changes seen with in vivo studies (11,12). This prospective in vitro study of US in axillary lymph nodes in patients with breast cancer has been performed to establish which US characteristics indicate malignancy.

MATERIALS AND METHODS

Forty consecutive patients (age range, 31–73 years; mean age, 48 years) with breast cancer who underwent axillary lymph node dissection composed this study. In fresh, axillary specimens, 158 lymph nodes were palpated and randomly dissected by the pathologist (F.T. or P.J.G.); this preserved some perilymphatic adipose tissue. The intact lymph nodes were attached to a cork base with two needles. They were submerged in a water bath on this support and individually examined by the same examiner (J.F.) with a 7.5-MHz US probe (model SSA-270A, Toshiba, Tokyo, Japan; and Logiq 500 MD, GE Medical Systems, Milwaukee, Wis). The median lymph node size was 12 mm, the mean was 13.01 mm, and the range was 4–30 mm.

The variables considered were as follows: the ratio of the long axis to the short axis, which indicates the shape of the node (round if the ratio is 1.5 or less and oval if the ratio is greater than 1.5); the presence or absence of the hilus (or the hyperechoic central zone of the node); and the preservation or disruption of the cortex (hypoechoic peripheral band). Hypo- or hyperechoic areas were compared with the US signal in the small amount of adipose tissue that surrounds the lymph node. A long-to-short axis ratio of less than 1.5, absence of hilus, and cortical disruption were considered signs of malignancy. At least one of these signs was required for a US diagnosis of malignancy. With each variable taken into account, a US diagnosis was given.

After the US study, each lymph node was sectioned in the most important plane evaluated with US, fixed in 10% formalin, embedded in paraffin, cut into 5–7-μm sections, and stained by using conventional methods (standard hematoxylin-eosin staining). At histopathologic examination, the presence of metastasis, capsular rupture, and other morphologic characteristics of the cortex and medulla were coded. Histopathologic findings were correlated with those obtained with the US study.

All data were filed by using a database (DBASE III+; Ashton-Tate, Torrance, Calif); statistical analysis was performed with conventional software (EPIINFO 6.0, World Health Organization, Geneva, Switzerland; or SPSS 6.0.1, SPSS, Chicago, Ill). To compare the values of each variable, the Fisher exact test and the nonparametric Kruskal-

Index terms: Breast neoplasms, metastases, 00.31 • Lymphatic system, neoplasms, 99.33 • Lymphatic system, US, 99.1298

Abbreviation: PPV = positive predictive value.

Radiology 1997; 205:831–835

[1] From the Departments of Radiology (J.F., B.N., X.A.), Pathology (F.T., P.J.G.), Obstetrics and Gynecology (R.F., A.F.C.), and Epidemiology (J.C.S.), Institut Universitari Dexeus, Paseo de la Bonanova 67-69, 08019 Barcelona, Spain. Received June 11, 1997; revision requested July 22; revision received August 11; accepted August 12. **Address reprint requests to** J.F.

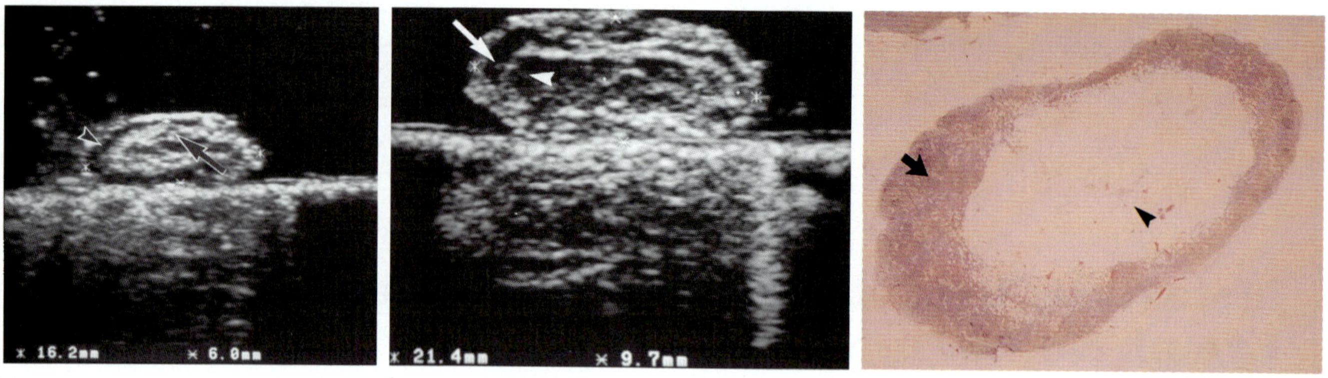

a. b. c.

Figure 1. **(a)** US scan obtained in a 53-year-old woman shows the usual appearance of benign lymph nodes with a hyperechoic hilus (arrow) and hypoechoic cortex (arrowhead). **(b)** US scan obtained in a 47-year-old woman shows the frequent appearance of fatty replacement of the hilus (arrowhead) as a hypoechoic area with a hypoechoic cortex (arrow). **(c)** Histopathologic slice from the cortical zone in the same patient in whom **b** was obtained shows lymphoid tissue (arrow) and fatty replacement of the medulla (arrowhead). (Hematoxylin-eosin stain; original magnification, ×6.)

Wallis test for numeric variables were applied. The sensitivity, specificity, positive predictive value (PPV), negative predictive value, and accuracy were determined by using standard methods. The results were expressed with a 95% confidence interval. The multivariate analysis was performed according to a nonconditional logistic regression. A difference was regarded as significant if *P* was less than .05.

RESULTS

The most common histopathologic diagnosis was infiltrating ductal carcinoma (n = 37), followed by infiltrating papillary carcinoma (n = 1), infiltrating lobular carcinoma (n = 1), and high-grade intraductal carcinoma (n = 1). The mean size of the tumors was 1.88 cm (range, 0.3–4.0 cm). A total of 584 lymph nodes were dissected in the 40 lymphadenectomies performed; 158 (27%) of the 584 lymph nodes randomly detected were studied in vitro with US. Forty-five (28%) of the 158 lymph nodes examined showed histopathologic evidence of metastasis. No abnormality other than sinus histiocytosis could be identified. The mean size of the US-examined lymph nodes was 13 mm (range, 4–30 mm); there was no relationship between nodal size and the presence of metastasis.

Statistically significant differences were found when the results of each of the three variables considered (the long-to-short axis ratio, the presence of the hilus, and the cortical shape) were compared in histopathologically proved benign and malignant lymph nodes (Table 1). Nonpathologic lymph nodes were usually seen at US with a flattened, hyperechoic hilus and a hypoechoic cortex, although sometimes the central zone was also hypoechoic (Fig 1).

The long-to-short axis ratio was considered as pathologic when it was 1.5 or less. This sign was found at US in 37 lymph nodes. Twenty (54%) of the 37 lymph nodes were histopathologically malignant; however, 25 (56%) of the 45 malignant lymph nodes showed a long-to-short axis ratio of more than 1.5.

The hyperechoic central zone of the lymph node (hilus) was absent in 35 cases. In these cases, the central zone appeared as a hypoechoic zone indistinguishable from the cortex; 27 (77%) of the 35 cases were malignant (Fig 2). One hundred five (93%) of the 113 benign lymph nodes showed a preserved hilus that was hyper- or hypoechoic but that was clearly distinguishable from the cortex, frequently by a thin, hyperechoic transition line (T line) (Fig 3). Of the 18 cases in which the hilus was preserved and showed histopathologic evidence of malignancy, 11 (61%) were micrometastases or eccentric metastases; of the remaining seven, five were metastases that were centrally located but that had a high desmoplastic stromal reaction that mimicked a preserved hilus.

The cortex was disrupted (focal or segmentary enlargement of the hypoechoic peripheric zone) in 44 cases, 32 (73%) of which were histopathologically malignant (Fig 4). One hundred one (89%) of the 113 benign lymph nodes were proved to have a preserved cortical shape. Twelve cases with disruption of the cortex, depicted as hypoechoic nodules that simulated eccentric metastatic involvement, proved to be histopathologically nodular areas in which a higher density of lymph tissue was demonstrated. Capsular rupture was present histopathologically in 25 malignant lymph nodes. US depicted this finding as subtle focal or diffuse cortical spiculation in 12 cases; in 11 (92%) of these cases, US showed histopathologically proved capsular rupture. In one case, a nodular hypoechoic zone was seen at the periphery of the node; this proved to be a fibrous nodule that had prompted a false-positive diagnosis.

Table 1
US Signs of Benign and Malignant Lymph Nodes

Sign	Benign (n = 113)	Malignant (n = 45)	*P* Value
Long-to-short axis ratio			
>1.5 (n = 121)	96 (79)	25 (21)	<.001
≤1.5 (n = 37)	17 (46)	20 (54)	
Hilus			
Present (n = 123)	105 (85)	18 (15)	<.001
Absent (n = 35)	8 (23)	27 (77)	
Cortex			
Preserved (n = 114)	101 (89)	13 (11)	<.001
Disrupted (n = 44)	12 (27)	32 (73)	

Note.—Numbers in parentheses are percentages.

When one or more of these variables of malignancy was seen, the US scan was considered to show a metastatic node. US findings suggested metastatic involvement in 56 cases, 38 (68%) of which were histopathologically verified. In 95 (84%) of the 113 cases, the US appearance and histopathologic findings indicated the nodes were benign. There were seven false-negative and 18 false-positive findings. The sensitivity was 84% (38 of 45; 95% confidence interval: 70, 93), the specificity was 84% (95 of 113; 95%

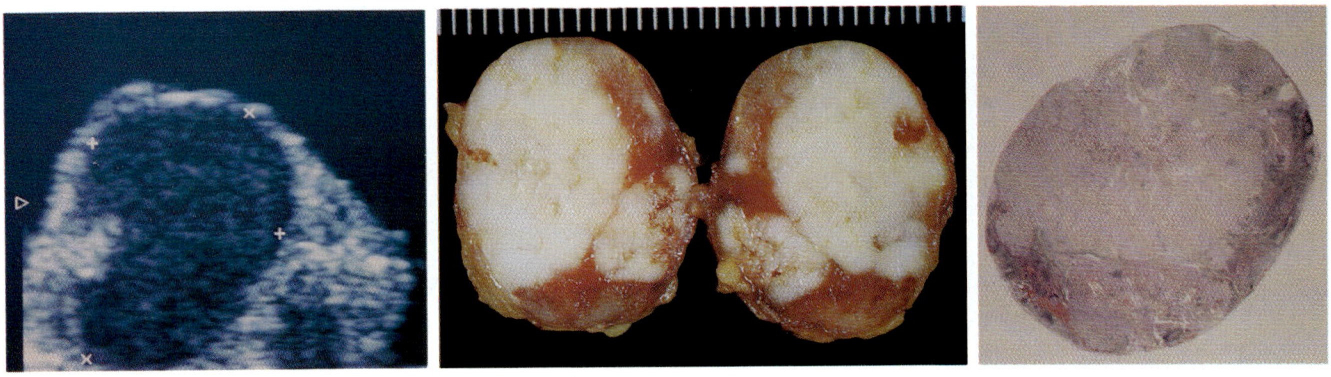

a. b. c.

Figure 2. **(a)** US scan obtained in a 46-year-old woman shows the absence of hilus as a hypoechoic central zone indistinguishable from the cortex. **(b)** Photograph shows that grossly the lymph node is replaced by a white firm tissue. **(c)** Histopathologic slice shows that the structure is totally involved with neoplastic proliferation. (Hematoxylin-eosin stain; original magnification, ×6.)

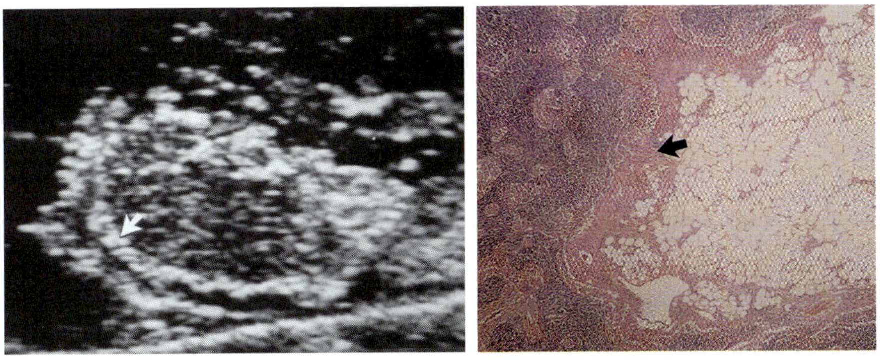

a. b.

Figure 3. **(a)** US scan of a benign node in a 67-year-old woman shows that the cortical zone is separated by a thin, hyperechoic line (T line; arrow), as is usual. **(b)** Histopathologic slice shows that the line is composed of fibrovascular tissue (arrow). (Hematoxylin-eosin stain; original magnification, ×120.)

confidence interval: 76, 90), the PPV was 68% (38 of 56; 95% confidence interval: 54, 79), the negative predictive value was 93% (95 of 102; 95% confidence interval: 86, 97), and the accuracy was 84% (133 of 158; 95% confidence interval, 77, 90). The most specific sign for the detection of metastasis was the absence of the hilus; the least specific US sign was the long-to-short axis ratio, the increase in which resulted in more false-negative diagnoses of metastatic involvement. The multivariate analysis results revealed that characteristics of the hilus and cortex were the only independent variables.

The percentages of false-positive and false-negative findings were higher in those lymph nodes smaller than 10 mm. For that reason, the lymph nodes were separated into two groups: those smaller than 10 mm (33 benign and 12 malignant nodes) and those 10 mm or larger (80 benign and 33 malignant nodes). The statistical results are shown in Table 2. The PPV and specificity of each criterion for the diagnosis of malignancy were higher in lymph nodes 10 mm or larger; however, the sensitivity was higher in those smaller than 10 mm.

When the morphologic features of each lymph node were correlated with the US image, the hilus was the more variable zone. In benign nodes, it usually was hyperechoic, although it could be hypoechoic when there was adipose infiltration. When there was increased vascularization, however, the hilus was hyperechoic. The hypoechoic hilus in those nodes with adipose infiltration was usually distinguished from the cortex by means of a continuous hyperechoic transition line that histopathologically corresponded to fibrovascular tissue that delineated the fat from the lymphatic tissue. When the central zone of the lymph node was composed of sinuses and variable amounts of lymphoid tissue but no adipose tissue, it was also seen as a hypoechoic zone if the number of blood vessels was low (Fig 5) or as a hyperechoic zone if the number of blood vessels was high (Fig 6). The echogenicity seemed to depend more on the number of vessels than on the size of the vessels. Hyperechoic findings at US were related to a higher number of vascular walls.

DISCUSSION

The axillary lymph node status is, in the absence of distant metastasis, the single most important factor predictive of survival in breast cancer (1,2). Axillary lymph node dissection is performed as part of the surgical treatment of breast cancer, mainly for staging and planning adjuvant therapy according to the number of metastatic lymph nodes (13). For this reason, an innocuous, nonsurgical procedure that allows the determination of lymph node status can be useful. US has been proved to have higher sensitivity (62%–72%) and specificity (69%–95%) than clinical examination and other imaging techniques (3–9).

Lymph nodes have a cortex that contains most of the lymphatic tissue (primary or secondary follicles and paracortex) and a central zone or medulla that contains the sinuses, lymphoid tissue, and variable amounts of fat and vessels. The hilus harbors vascular structures and varies in size (14). At US, two zones can be depicted: the periphery or cortex is hypoechoic and the central zone or hilus is usually hyperechoic (3,8,11,12,15).

The signs used the most in vivo to detect lymph node metastasis are lymph node enlargement, variation in shape, and loss of hyperechoic hilus (3). In vitro study findings reveal that the round shape (expressed as a long-to-short axis ratio of less than 2), the hypoechoic hilar zone, and the thickening of the cortex are the most important signs of malignancy (11,12). The mass effect of metastatic tissue that infiltrates a lymph node causes

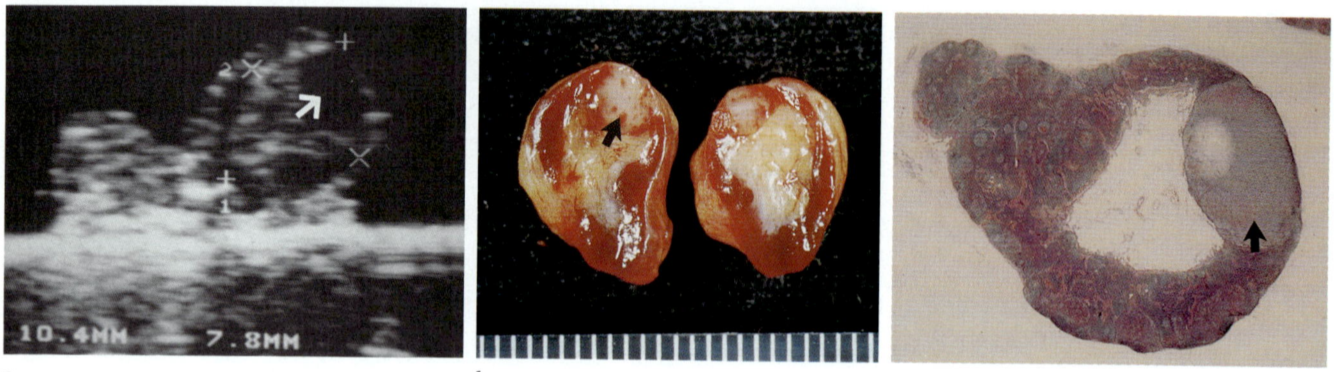

a. b. c.

Figure 4. **(a)** US scan of cortical disruption in a 53-year-old woman shows a hypoechoic nodular area (arrow). **(b)** Photograph shows grossly a white, firm nodule at the periphery (arrow). **(c)** Histopathologic slice shows that this area is composed of metastatic tissue (arrow). (Hematoxylin-eosin stain; original magnification, ×6.)

Table 2
Sensitivity, Specificity, PPV, Negative Predictive Value, and Accuracy of US in Lymph Nodes Smaller than 10 mm or at Least 10 mm

Statistic	Long-to-Short Axis Ratio <1.5		Hilus Absent		Disrupted Cortex		US Diagnostic of Metastasis	
	Nodes <10 mm (*n* = 45)	Nodes ≥10 mm (*n* = 113)	Nodes <10 mm (*n* = 45)	Nodes ≥10 mm (*n* = 113)	Nodes <10 mm (*n* = 45)	Nodes ≥10 mm (*n* = 113)	Nodes <10 mm (*n* = 45)	Nodes ≥10 mm (*n* = 113)
Sensitivity (%)	50 (22, 78)	42 (26, 61)	67 (35, 89)	58 (40, 74)	75 (43, 93)	70 (51, 84)	83 (51, 97)	85 (67, 94)
Specificity (%)	54 (37, 72)	98 (90, 100)	79 (61, 90)	99 (92, 100)	88 (71, 96)	90 (81, 95)	73 (54, 86)	89 (79, 94)
PPV (%)	29 (12, 52)	88 (60, 98)	53 (27, 78)	95 (73, 100)	69 (39, 90)	74 (55, 88)	53 (30, 75)	76 (58, 88)
NPV* (%)	75 (53, 89)	80 (71, 88)	87 (68, 96)	85 (76, 91)	91 (74, 98)	88 (78, 94)	92 (73, 99)	93 (85, 98)
Accuracy (%)	53 (37, 69)	81 (72, 88)	76 (60, 88)	86 (79, 93)	84 (70, 94)	84 (75, 91)	76 (60, 88)	88 (80, 94)

Note.—Numbers in parentheses are the confidence intervals. Of the 45 lymph nodes smaller than 10 mm, 33 were benign and 12 were malignant. Of the 113 lymph nodes 10 mm or larger, 80 were benign and 33 were malignant.
*NPV = negative predictive value.

the node to be round (11). Establishment of a long-to-short axis ratio of less than 2 as a sign of malignancy has a PPV of 82% (11); in our study, the PPV of US when this ratio was considered was 38% (30 of 79) in the whole series and 51% (22 of 43) in those nodes 10 mm or larger. The difference between this result and those of other authors (11) must be due to the large number of histopathologically benign lymph nodes smaller than 10 mm (33 [73%] of 45) in our series; these nodes usually are round. If a long-to-short axis ratio of 1.5 is considered as the cutoff, the PPV increases to 54% (20 of 37) in the whole series and to 88% (14 of 16) in nodes 10 mm or larger. This ratio was the sign that caused the most false-positive findings. The majority of nodes smaller than 10 mm were round, which indicates that nodal shape or size is not a reliable sign of malignancy.

The hilar zone can express a variety of US characteristics, depending on the structures located there. The absence of hilus has been proved to be a strong criterion for malignancy (3,11,12). In our study, it is indeed the sign with the highest PPV in nodes 10 mm or larger. The absence of hilus also causes false-positive diagnoses, especially in those cases with scanty vessels and large amounts of lymphatic tissue. Patients with lymphoma, sinus histiocytosis or other reactive changes, fibrosis, or hematomas show an absence of hilus that can cause an erroneous diagnosis of metastasis (8,11,12,16). Metastasis also is erroneously diagnosed in patients with variants of the normal anatomy of the axilla that can be confused in vivo with abnormal lymph nodes (17). In the present study, sinus histiocytosis was detected in about 40% of lymph nodes; none of them had a false-positive diagnosis. In some cases, the presence of desmoplastic tumoral reaction in the central zone of the node was seen as a hyperechoic

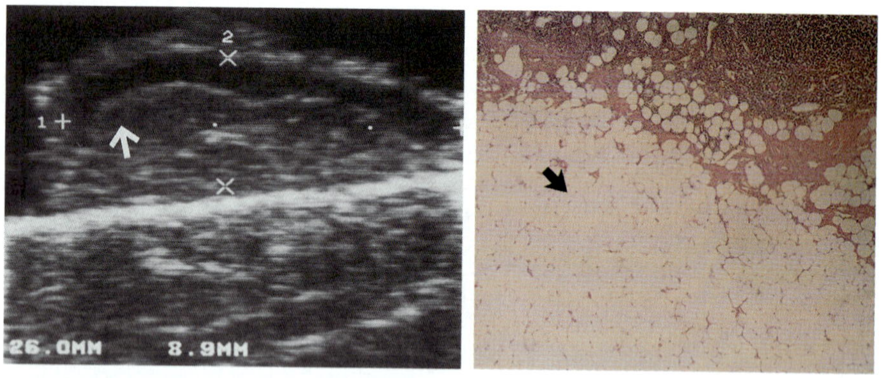

a. b.

Figure 5. **(a)** US scan obtained in a 31-year-old woman shows a hypoechoic hilus (arrow) that corresponds to **(b)** adipose tissue in the medulla with minimal vascularization (arrow) in a histopathologic slice. (Hematoxylin-eosin stain; original magnification, ×120.)

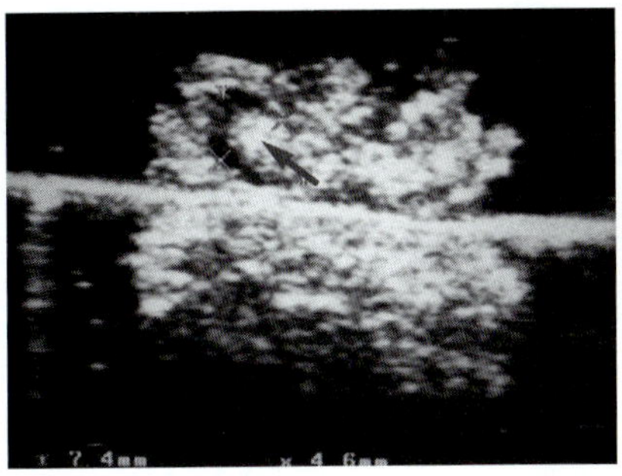

a.

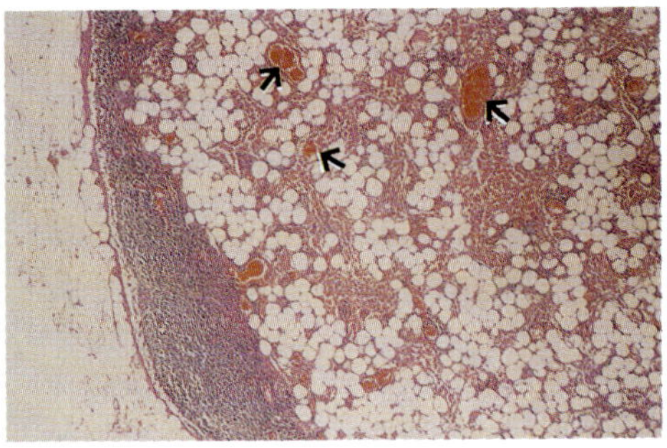

b.

Figure 6. **(a)** US scan obtained in a 49-year-old woman shows a hyperechoic hilus (arrow) that corresponds to **(b)** adipose tissue in the medulla with increased vascularization (arrows) in a histopathologic slice. (Hematoxylin-eosin stain; original magnification, ×120.)

area discernible from the cortex and was erroneously diagnosed as a benign lesion at US. Also, at US, the increase in medullary vascularization produced a hyperechoic area that is independent of other tissues found at the zone (fatty or lymphoid). A higher number of vascular structures correlated with a more hyperechoic signal.

Some authors have related the echogenicity of the hilus with the abundance of fluid-filled sinuses (3,12). We have observed that nodes with few large vessels in the hilus are more hypoechoic than nodes with numerous small vessels in this zone, which suggests that the vascular wall is per se the factor that caused the hyperechoic area. In those cases with adipose involution of the medulla and with minimal vascularization, the hilus appears as a hypoechoic zone that can be erroneously diagnosed. Frequently, however, there is a hyperechoic line (T line) that differentiates the hilus from the cortex, which indicates benignity.

The cortex is composed mainly of lymphoid tissue without sinuses and appears as a hypoechoic zone. Changes in the thickness or shape usually denote metastasis but sometimes can be due to an increase in the density of lymphoid tissue. The reactive nodal changes begin in the cortex, where lymphoid proliferation increases the size of the cortex (3), but metastasis also reaches the cortical zone of the lymph node via afferent lymphatic vessels; hence, diagnosis can be confusing and can be false-positive.

Irregularities and spiculations at the margin of a hypoechoic node have been considered signs of perinodal fat involvement (18). When this feature is detected, it has high specificity; however, the majority of lymph nodes with capsular rupture do not show this sign.

US-guided fine-needle aspiration is useful in diagnosing malignancy (6,10) and can be especially sensitive in axillary lymph nodes smaller than 10 mm in which US alone cannot provide an accurate diagnosis, as has been demonstrated in vitro. Studies performed with power Doppler in vivo provide more details in the detection of lymph node metastasis and can be useful in those nodes smaller than 10 mm (19,20).

In vitro US has proved to be an accurate way to detect lymph node metastasis, especially in nodes 10 mm or larger in which the absence of hilus, cortical disruption, or both indicate the presence of metastasis more than does size or shape. Whereas preoperative axillary US may not replace axillary dissection in many patients because of the need for quantitative assessment of nodal status for adjuvant chemotherapy (13), it may be better than axillary dissection in the determination of which patients need dissection. ■

References

1. Fisher B, Bauer M, Wickerham DL, Redmond CK, Fisher ER. Relation of number of positive axillary nodes to the prognosis of patients with primary breast cancer: an NSABP update. Cancer 1983; 28:282–291.
2. Wilking N, Rutqvist LE, Cartensen J, Mattsson A, Skoog L, participating members of the Stockholm Breast Cancer Study Group. Prognostic significance of axillary nodal status in primary breast cancer in relation to the number of resected nodes. Acta Oncol 1992; 31:29–35.
3. Vassallo P, Wernecke K, Roos N, Peters PE. Differentiation of benign from malignant superficial lymphadenopathy: the role of high-resolution US. Radiology 1992; 183: 215–220.
4. Kauczor HU, Voges EM, Wieland-Schneider C, Mitze M, Thelen M. Value of routine abdominal and lymph node sonography in the follow-up of breast cancer patients. Eur J Radiol 1994; 18:104–108.
5. Vaidya JS, Vyas JJ, Thakur MH, Khandelwal KC, Mittra I. Role of ultrasonography to detect axillary node involvement in operable breast cancer. Eur J Surg Oncol 1996; 22:140–143.
6. Meterissian S, Fornage BD, Singletary SE. Clinically occult breast carcinoma: diagnostic approaches and role of axillary node dissection. Ann Surg Oncol 1995; 2:314–318.
7. Tate JJT, Lewis V, Archer T, Guyer PG, Royle GT, Taylos I. Ultrasound detection of axillary lymph node metastases in breast cancer. Eur J Surg Oncol 1989; 15:139–141.
8. Pamilo M, Soiva M, Lavast EM. Real-time ultrasound, axillary mammography, and clinical examination in the detection of axillary lymph node metastases in breast cancer patients. J Ultrasound Med 1989; 8:115–120.
9. Bruneton JN, Caramella E, Héry M, Aubanel D, Manzino JJ, Picard JL. Axillary lymph node metastases in breast cancer: preoperative detection with US. Radiology 1986; 158:325–326.
10. Fornage BD. Interventional ultrasound of the breast. In: McGahan JP, ed. Interventional ultrasound. Baltimore, Md: Williams & Wilkins, 1990; 71–83.
11. Vassallo P, Edel G, Roos N, Naguib A, Peters PE. In-vitro high-resolution ultrasonography of benign and malignant lymph nodes: a sonographic-pathologic correlation. Invest Radiol 1993; 28:698–705.
12. Rubaltelli L, Proto E, Salmaso R, Bortoletto P, Candiani F, Cagol P. Sonography of abnormal lymph nodes in vitro: correlation of sonographic and histologic findings. AJR 1990; 155:1241–1244.
13. Bryan RM, Mercer RJ, Bennett RC, Rennie GC. Prognostic factors in breast cancer and the development of a prognostic index. Br J Surg 1986; 73:267–271.
14. Van der Valk P, Meijer CJ. The histology of reactive lymph nodes. Am J Surg Pathol 1987; 11:866–882.
15. Yang WT, Ahuja A, Tang A, Suen M, King W, Metreweli C. Ultrasonographic demonstration of normal axillary lymph nodes: a learning curve. J Ultrasound Med 1995; 14:823–827.
16. Bruneton JN, Maestro C, Marcy PY, Padovani B. Echographie des ganglions superficiels. J Radiol 1994; 75:373–381. [French]
17. Moriggi B, Steinechner M. Ultrasonoanatomy for evaluation of the local lymphatic groups of the mamma. Surg Radiol Anat 1994; 16:77–85.
18. Dershaw DD, Selland DG, Tan LK, Morris EA, Abramson AF, Liberman L. Spiculated axillary adenopathy. Radiology 1996; 201:439–442.
19. Draghi F, Campani R. Power Doppler in breast diseases: preliminary results. Radiol Med 1996; 91:577–580.
20. Walsh JS, Dixon JM, Chetty U, Paterson D. Colour Doppler studies of axillary node metastases in breast carcinoma. Clin Radiol 1994; 49:189–191.

Carol A. Hulka, MD • Whitney B. Edmister, SB • Barbara L. Smith, MD, PhD • Lujian Tan, MD
Dennis C. Sgroi, MD • Terrance Campbell, RT • Daniel B. Kopans, MD • Robert M. Weisskoff, PhD

Dynamic Echo-Planar Imaging of the Breast: Experience in Diagnosing Breast Carcinoma and Correlation with Tumor Angiogenesis[1]

PURPOSE: To correlate quantitative echo-planar magnetic resonance (MR) imaging measures of gadopentetate dimeglumine tumor uptake with histologic diagnoses and microvessel density (MVD) and to compare dynamic echo-planar imaging of breast lesions with conventional dynamic MR imaging techniques.

MATERIALS AND METHODS: The study group comprised 63 patients (aged 13–70 years) with 71 breast lesions who underwent conventional and echo-planar MR imaging. The T1 values, change in gadopentetate dimeglumine concentration, and extraction-flow products were calculated with the echo-planar imaging data and were correlated with histologic findings and MVD estimates. Extraction-flow product data normalized to pectoral muscle gadopentetate dimeglumine concentration in invasive cancers was also correlated with MVD.

RESULTS: On average, cancer T1 values were shorter than benign values, but there was substantial overlap between the two groups. Cancers had higher extraction-flow products than benign lesions ($P < .001$). Sensitivity, specificity, positive predictive value, and negative predictive value were 83%, 79%, 67%, and 90%, respectively. Receiver operating characteristic analysis showed improved performance with extraction-flow products than with percentages of signal intensity change. Among the invasive cancers, there was no significant correlation between extraction-flow product and MVD.

CONCLUSION: The T1 value remains important in more precise quantitative estimation of gadopentetate dimeglumine uptake in breast tumors, which helps improve the specificity of dynamic imaging. Tumor MVD affects the contrast medium enhancement of breast lesions, but other factors contribute.

THE need for improved imaging techniques for the diagnosis of breast cancer has resulted in widespread interest in magnetic resonance (MR) imaging of the breast in recent years. Although screening mammography remains the primary tool for early detection, the role of MR imaging of the breast will likely increase in problem-solving situations.

Contrast medium enhancement is essential for differentiating between a breast lesion and normal breast tissue (1–4). Improved depiction of a lesion is also attained with fat-suppression or subtraction techniques, although the latter may be limited by patient motion (5–8). Patterns of dynamic enhancement of breast lesions with conventional and echo-planar imaging techniques have been described by many groups (9–16). Although dynamic MR imaging shows high sensitivity in the diagnosis of invasive carcinoma, overlap in benign and malignant enhancement patterns persists, especially with conventional dynamic techniques. Our early work showed the physiologic modeling of breast cancer enhancement and demonstrated that echo-planar imaging could improve the specificity, compared with the specificity of conventional dynamic techniques, in a small group of patients (14). Other investigators have shown improved specificity over that of previously described conventional techniques when examining predominantly morphologic enhancement patterns such as rim enhancement in malignant lesions (12,17).

Part of the underlying physiology of rapid early gadopentetate dimeglumine uptake by carcinomas is presumably related to tumor angiogenesis, as cancers recruit neovessels to promote further tumor growth. The severity of tumor angiogenesis may correlate with patient morbidity and mortality, according to work by Folkman and Weidner and Folkman and colleagues (18–21). These researchers established a method of measuring tumor microvessel density (MVD) by means of immunohistochemical staining with antibodies to factor VIII and by determining vessel counts. The correlation of MR tumor enhancement patterns with similar histologic measures of tumor MVD has resulted in mixed reports (14,16,22). The mechanism of gadopentetate dimeglumine uptake in tumor tissue is related to a variety of factors, which include MVD, size of the abnormal tumor vessels, and the permeability of those vessels (23–25).

The purpose of this study was to

Index terms: Breast neoplasms, diagnosis, 00.30 • Breast neoplasms, MR, 00.121416 • Gadolinium • Magnetic resonance (MR), contrast enhancement, 00.12143 • Neoplasms, blood supply, 94.30

Abbreviations: DCIS = ductal carcinoma in situ, MVD = microvessel density, ROC = receiver operating characteristic, TI = inversion time.

Radiology 1997; 205:837–842

[1] From the Department of Radiology, Beth Israel Deaconess Medical Center and Harvard Medical School, 330 Brookline Ave, Boston, MA 02215 (C.A.H.); the Department of Radiology and the Nuclear Magnetic Resonance Center (W.B.E., T.C., D.B.K., R.M.W.) and the Departments of Surgery (B.L.S., L.T.) and Pathology (D.C.S.), Massachusetts General Hospital and Harvard Medical School, Boston, Mass. Received May 14, 1997; revision requested July 9; revision received August 13; accepted August 15. Supported by grants from the Massachusetts Department of Public Health, National Institutes of Health grant RO1CA 66072, and a grant from the American Cancer Society. **Address reprint requests to** C.A.H.

correlate quantitative echo-planar measures of gadopentetate dimeglumine tumor uptake with histologic diagnoses and with MVD and to compare dynamic echo-planar imaging of breast lesions with conventional dynamic MR imaging.

MATERIALS AND METHODS

MR Imaging Technique

Between March 1993 and July 1996, patients with breast lesions detected with mammography or physical examination were asked to participate in our MR imaging protocol before surgical excision. Seventy-eight consecutive patients (mean age, 47 years; age range, 13–70 years) provided informed consent and composed the study population. Of these 78 patients, six declined to undergo surgery. The echo-planar imaging data were not usable in four patients owing to hardware failure during imaging. Five patients underwent surgery at outside institutions and were lost to follow-up. Thus, 63 patients with 71 breast lesions (six patients had two lesions and one patient had three lesions) form our study group for the correlation of dynamic echo-planar imaging data with histologic diagnoses. Of these 63 patients, six had histologic samples that were inadequate or showed poor immunohistochemical staining for MVD correlation, in spite of multiple attempts to stain. Thus, correlation of MR data with the MVD data was available in 57 patients.

MR imaging was performed with a 1.5-T MR imager (Signa; GE Medical Systems, Milwaukee, Wis) retrofitted for echo-planar imaging (Advanced Systems, Wilmington, Mass) and with a dedicated breast receiver coil (GE Medical Systems). A power injector (MedRad, Pittsburgh, Pa) filled with gadopentetate dimeglumine (Magnevist; Berlex Laboratories, Wayne, NJ; 0.1 mmol/kg) was used for antecubital venous injection during imaging (3.5 mL/sec).

In both breasts, sagittal, gradient-echo, localizing imaging (33/5 [repetition time msec/echo time msec]) was performed, followed by axial, fast spin-echo, T2-weighted imaging (3,300/30,90 [effective]). Echo-planar imaging–based automatic shimming to maximize field homogeneity across both breasts (26) was followed by three-dimensional, fat-suppressed, gradient-echo imaging in the axial plane (25/6, 30° flip angle). The field of view (28–35 cm) and section thickness (2.2–2.7 mm) varied with patient size. The initial matrix was 256 × 256, with later imaging at 512 × 256. We used a binomial fat-suppression technique, similar to the rotating delivery of excitation off resonance, or RODEO, technique described by Pierce and colleagues (6). T1 values were measured by using echo-planar imaging with an inversion-recovery technique that covered both breasts with 14–20 sections at 3 × 3 × 7-mm resolution (40 × 40-cm field of view with a 128 × 128 matrix) and 6,000/30/60–1,465 (repetition time msec/echo time msec/inversion time [TI] msec; TI in steps of 150 msec from 60 to 1,465 msec). We then varied the TI (125–185 msec) to choose the most effective TI for suppressing fat during dynamic echo-planar imaging. With dynamic imaging, we acquired 40 total images at 6-second intervals before (five images), during, and for approximately 3 minutes after bolus injection of contrast medium (0.1 mmol/kg at 3.5 mL/sec). Multiple levels were imaged simultaneously to cover both breasts. Immediately after dynamic imaging, postinjection, conventional, three-dimensional, gradient-echo images were obtained in approximately 6 minutes with identical parameters as for pre-injection volumetric imaging.

Image Analysis

At the time of image analysis, the radiologist (C.A.H.) correlated the postinjection, three-dimensional, axial images with the mammograms that showed the abnormality or the physical examination findings to ensure that the lesion to be removed was the same as the lesion studied with echo-planar imaging. With the postinjection, three-dimensional, axial images used as anatomic maps, regions of interest that represented the areas of highest enhancement were selected for analysis of the echo-planar imaging data. First, the TI data were converted into T1 maps of the breast. By using these T1 maps, the signal intensity changes were converted during the dynamic imaging to changes in 1/T1 (as this change reflects effective gadopentetate dimeglumine concentration), and a simple kinetic model was used to estimate the extraction-flow product (milliliters of blood per grams of tissue per minute), as described earlier (14).

Comparison of Dynamic Echo-Planar Imaging Data with Dynamic Conventional Imaging Data

One common method of displaying signal intensity changes over time with conventional dynamic imaging has been to calculate the percentage of enhancement over time (2,13,15,16). To demonstrate the effect of the varying baseline T1 values on the percentage of enhancement over time, we estimated the signal intensities by combining the measured T1 values with the R1(t) data computed by using the equation described in our earlier work (14). Receiver operating characteristic (ROC) curves were calculated for each method and were compared by using the CLABROC program (Metz CE, Herman B, Shen JH, Kronnan HS, Wang PL, University of Chicago, Chicago, Ill, 1993), with a binomial distribution assumed. By using a two-tailed multivariate z score test, differences between areas were tested.

Histologic and Microvessel Staining Analysis

Patients underwent mastectomy or excisional biopsy, which allowed histologic diagnosis after MR imaging. Immunohistochemical staining of the paraffin-embedded, formalin-fixed surgical specimens was performed by using factor VIII antibody, according to methods described by Weidner and colleagues (18–20). For each specimen, the areas with the highest MVD were chosen for vessel counting. Individual microvessels were counted in these areas on a ×200 field (×20 objective lens and ×10 ocular lens; 0.7386 mm^2 per field). An independent, blinded reader (D.C.S.) counted the MVDs, which were used for the statistical analyses.

The T1 values for benign diagnoses were compared with those for malignant diagnoses by using the Student t test. The extraction-flow products for benign diagnoses similarly were compared with those for malignant diagnoses.

In the group of diagnoses that also had vessel staining data, the MVD estimates for benign and malignant diagnoses were correlated. The extraction-flow product data were correlated with the MVD estimates by using the Pearson correlation coefficient. Of the 71 lesions, 57 were stained and counted. Fourteen specimens were not available either owing to unavailability of the specimen or poor quality of the stain. Thus, echo-planar imaging data were correlated with MVD data in 57 lesions.

In addition, we investigated a method of normalizing the arterial input function in patients with cancer to assess for improved correlation between extraction-flow product and MVD estimates in these patients. We measured the peak concentration of gadopentetate dimeglumine in the pectoral muscle as an indicator of the overall magnitude of the arterial input function, with the assumption that the physiology of the pectoral muscle is comparable from patient to patient. The extraction-flow product normalized to the peak concentration of gadopentetate dimeglumine in the pectoral muscle was then correlated to the MVD by using the Pearson correlation coefficient to assess for improvement in this subgroup's correlation. Because of partial voluming effects at the current voxel size, ductal carcinoma in situ (DCIS) was excluded from this analysis.

RESULTS

Histologic Diagnoses

Of the 63 patients with 71 lesions, 21 patients had a histologic diagnosis of carcinoma. Fourteen patients had 16 invasive carcinomas: 10 patients had 12 invasive ductal carcinomas (two patients with two separate lesions diagnosed as invasive ductal carcinoma) (Fig 1), and four patients had infiltrating lobular carcinoma. In seven patients, eight lesions were diagnosed as DCIS (one patient had two lesions in distinctly different quadrants). The remaining 42 patients with 47 lesions had benign diagnoses: 14 fibroadenomas (two patients with two fibroadenomas each and one fibroadenoma excised in one of the patients

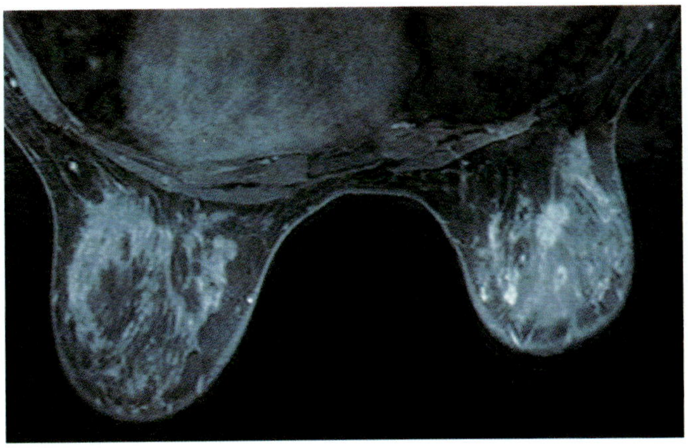

a.

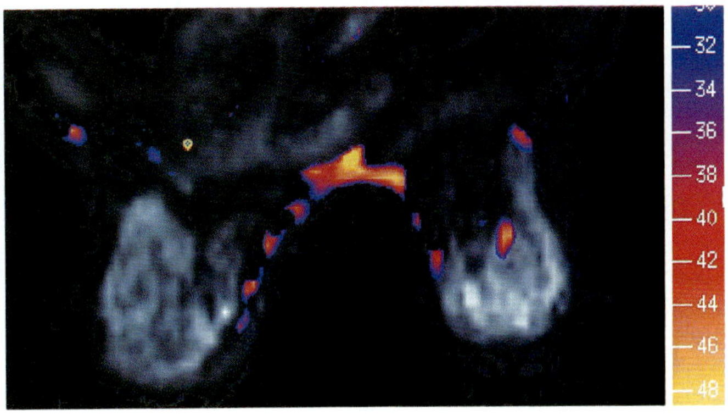

b.

Figure 1. **(a)** Postcontrast, conventional, three-dimensional, gradient-echo, axial MR image (25/6, 30° flip angle) obtained with fat suppression in a 46-year-old woman shows a spiculated, enhancing mass in the right breast. Histologic examination of the excised lesion revealed invasive ductal carcinoma. **(b)** Echo-planar image (6,000/30/170) in the same plane shows the same lesion, which is color coded for the extraction-flow product. The extraction-flow product of this lesion is 46 mL · 100 g^{-1} · min^{-1}, as indicated on the color scale. The high extraction-flow products in the sternum and medial aspects of both breasts represent enhancing bone marrow and intramammary vessels, respectively.

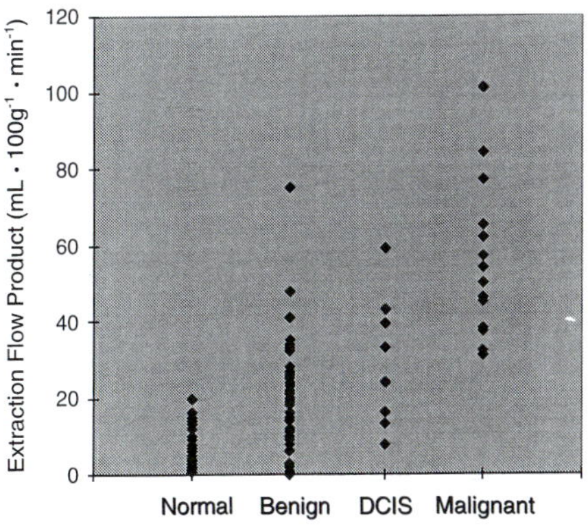

Figure 2. Extraction-flow product versus diagnostic category of breast lesions. Some overlap exists between benign and malignant diagnoses, although most of the lower extraction-flow products in the malignant group are DCIS.

with DCIS), eight fibrocystic changes, four radial scars, four epithelial hyperplasia cases, two epithelial hyperplasia cases with fibrocystic change, two hamartomas, two sclerosing adenosis cases with epithelial hyperplasia, two sclerosing adenosis cases, one papilloma (in the other breast in one of the patients with epithelial hyperplasia with fibrocystic change), one sternalis muscle, one pseudovascular hyperplasia case, one chronic hematoma, one nodular adenosis case, one suture granuloma with fibrocystic change, one neuroma with fibrocystic change, one dermatic lymphadenitis case (in the other breast in the patient with the neuroma), and one lobular carcinoma in situ.

The mean size of all breast lesions was 2.2 cm (range, 0.8–15.0 cm). The mean size of all cancers was 2.0 cm (range, 1.0–5.0 cm); the mean size of all benign lesions was 2.3 cm (range, 0.8–15 cm). In this series, no cancers other than those detected mammographically or at physical examination were identified by means of MR imaging.

MR Data Analyses

As in our earlier small series, the T1 values for cancers were shorter (mean ± standard deviation, 783 msec ± 255) than those for benign lesions (mean, 901 msec ± 367), although the difference was not statistically significant (P = .18).

Analysis of the extraction-flow products of lesions showed statistically significant differences between all cancers (mean, 45 mL · 100 g^{-1} · min^{-1} ± 22) and all benign lesions (mean, 21 mL · 100 g^{-1} · min^{-1} ± 16; $P < .001$) (Fig 2). There was some overlap in these values, as three fibroadenomas had high extraction-flow products of 41, 48, and 75 mL · 100 g^{-1} · min^{-1}, five DCIS lesions had low extraction-flow products of 8, 13, 16, and 24 mL · 100 g^{-1} · min^{-1}, and a reactive lymph node had a high extraction-flow product of 75 mL · 100 g^{-1} · min^{-1}. The extraction-flow products for normal parenchyma (mean, 6.9 mL · 100 g^{-1} · min^{-1}; range, 1–20 mL · 100 g^{-1} · min^{-1}) remained clearly lower than the extraction-flow products for benign lesions ($P < .01$).

The sensitivity and specificity for diagnosing breast cancer with extraction-flow products of greater than 31 mL · 100 g^{-1} · min^{-1} were 83% (20 of 24) and 79% (37 of 47), respectively. This extraction-flow product represents the lowest value in invasive cancers in this study. The positive and negative predictive values were 67% (20 of 30) and 90% (37 of 41), respectively. The percentage of enhancement in each lesion was calculated from our data for the ROC analyses of the extraction-flow product compared with the percentage of signal intensity change. The ROC analysis of the extraction-flow product shows a clear improvement in diagnosing breast cancer, compared with the ROC analysis of the percentage of signal intensity change ($P < .001$) (Fig 3).

MVD Analysis

The mean MVD estimate for malignant lesions of 78 vessels ± 43 in a ×200 high-power field was statistically significantly higher than the mean MVD estimate for benign lesions, which was 34 vessels ± 17 in a ×200 high-power field ($P < .01$) (Fig 4). While a positive overall correlation between the extraction-flow product and MVD was found by using the Pearson correlation coefficient (r = .36, $P < .01$), further analysis showed no significant correlation between the extraction-flow product and the MVD in the benign and the cancer subgroups (P = .4 and .8, respectively) (Fig 5).

Some of the patients with invasive cancers diagnosed who also underwent MVD analysis were excluded from the arterial input analysis owing to excessive motion for pectoral muscle analysis, poor fat suppression, or incomplete dynamic data. For the nine cancers studied, the mean peak gadopentetate dimeglumine concentrations in the pectoral muscles were 0.2 mmol/L ± 0.05 (range, 0.15–0.29 mmol/L). In this group, the correlation coefficient between the extraction-flow product and the MVD was .65 and that between the normalized extraction-flow product and the MVD was .73, showing slight but not statistically significant improvement.

DISCUSSION

These results confirm our early findings that the use of a quantitative measure of early gadopentetate dimeglumine uptake, such as the extraction-flow product, gives improved specificity and sensitivity over the percentage of signal intensity change in the diagnosis of carcinoma. Using the breast lesions' underlying T1 values to calculate the extraction-flow product accounts for this improvement. Earlier studies have shown statistically significant differences in the T1 values of tumors and normal breast tissue, which supports our findings that these differences should not be ignored (1). One of the advantages of echo-planar imaging or other fast imaging techniques is the ability to estimate the effects of the underlying T1 values either by measuring T1 directly or by using different repetition times or flip angles to estimate its effect, which can then be used to estimate changes in the gadopentetate dimeglumine concentration more directly. This change in the concentration of gadopentetate dimeglumine was used in our calculation of the extraction-flow products.

These study results also confirm that the most important window for dynamically measuring gadopentetate dimeglumine uptake in tumors is within the first 2 minutes of enhancement if one hopes to distinguish between benign and malignant tumors by using dynamic data. In addition, it supports the concept that studies that focus on morphology are improved by using rapid image acquisition windows, which essentially adds the advantage of the dynamic differentiation (12,27).

The excellent time resolution of echo-planar imaging allows for precise gadopentetate dimeglumine concentration–versus-time curves to understand the dynamic pattern of contrast medium uptake in a variety of tumors. This rapid data collection also offers complete dynamic coverage of both breasts at multiple levels, which allows for the potential evaluation of unsuspected enhancing foci outside of the primary region of interest. Although we measured dynamic data at 6-second intervals for the time course and data analysis, it is clear from these data that less frequent intervals (two to three points within the 1st minute) should be acceptable. In addition, methods of rapid dynamic imaging other than echo-planar imaging may also provide data for the analysis of dynamic behavior.

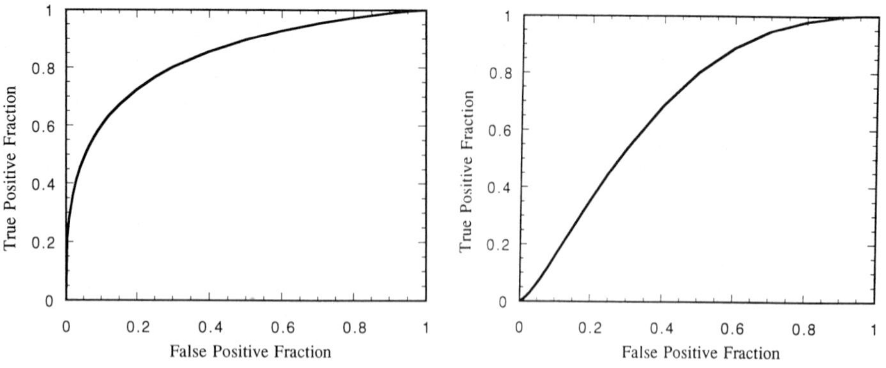

a. b.

Figure 3. **(a)** ROC curve for MR-based extraction-flow products for all breast lesions. **(b)** ROC curve for the same data after analysis for the percentage of change in signal intensity. ROC analysis shows a clear improvement in sensitivity and specificity with the extraction-flow product compared to the percentage of signal intensity change for these data.

The high sensitivity, specificity, and negative predictive value for the diagnosis of breast cancer in this study support the use of MR as an adjunct to mammography in specific situations. Increasing the specificity and negative predictive value of breast MR imaging is important for a variety of reasons. In particular, if MR is used as an adjunct to mammography for screening high-risk patients with dense mammary parenchyma, then the rate of false-positive findings must be low to avoid unnecessary MR-guided biopsy of lesions detected only with MR imaging. Similarly, if MR is used for local staging, a false-positive diagnosis of multicentric disease may result in an unnecessary mastectomy unless MR-guided biopsy is available and accurate.

Because tumor angiogenesis in breast cancer has been reported as predictive of mortality and morbidity and because of the advent of antiangiogenic therapy, an imaging method to predict tumor neovascularity is appealing. However, our initial hypothesis that MVD relates directly to the fast dynamic MR behavior of breast lesions is not fully supported by our study findings. As reported in our earlier article (14), the benign lesions' extraction-flow products and the MVDs were both low and differed significantly from the high extraction-flow products and MVDs in cancers, especially in the invasive cancers. This correlation between general tissue diagnoses (benign versus malignant), MR behavior, and tumor MVD was also reported on recently by Buadu and colleagues (16). However, in our study, further analysis of the data shows that within each diagnostic group (benign lesions, invasive cancers, DCIS, and all cancers), there is no correlation between the MVD estimates and the MR data, which indicates that factors beyond the MVD measured after immunohistochemical staining with factor VIII are involved in the gadopentetate dimeglumine uptake by breast tumors.

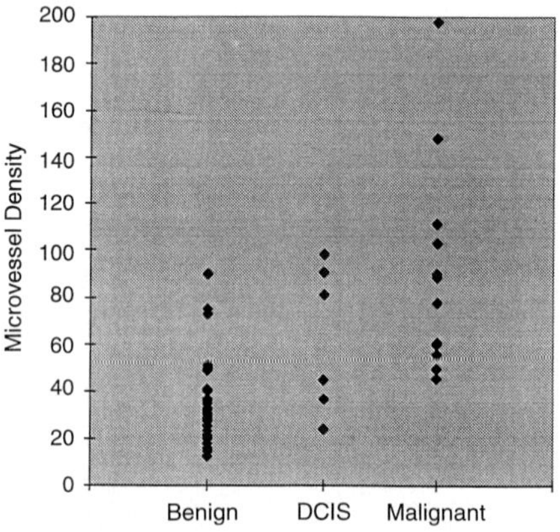

Figure 4. MVD estimate versus diagnostic category of breast lesion. The MVDs in malignant lesions were significantly higher than those in benign lesions ($P < .01$).

The difference between the MR data and MVD estimates within the invasive cancers in this study may be due to a variety of reasons. Certainly, larger populations in the subgroups of cancer and benign diagnoses may show improved correlation, but other factors also explain the lack of correlation in these subgroups. One issue is that a MVD estimate measures a microscopic local peak MVD, while the extraction-flow product estimate is a mean over a much larger volume. While it is reasonable to assume there would be some correlation between the mean and a sampled peak value, the sampling could introduce scatter between these estimates.

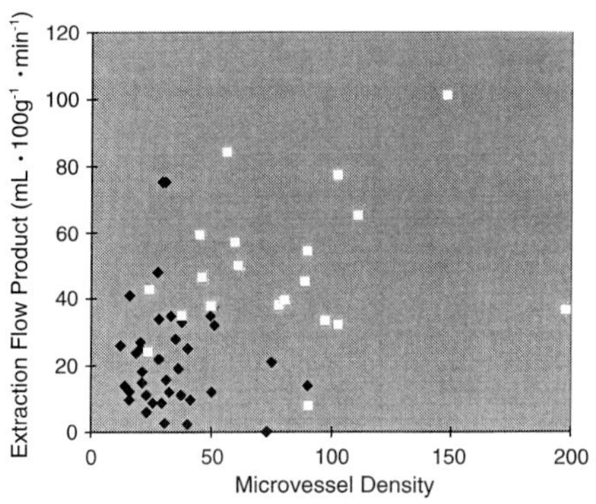

Figure 5. Extraction-flow product versus MVD shows a mild, positive correlation. Within each diagnostic category, however, there is no correlation. Black = benign lesions, white = all malignant lesions.

Another source of error includes potential arterial input variations between patients. To make an initial assessment of this error, we normalized the extraction-flow product to the peak gadopentetate dimeglumine uptake in the pectoral muscle in patients with invasive cancers. The correlation with MVD estimates was not improved statistically significantly. Some values were shifted toward and other values were shifted away from improved correlation. With such a small data set and considerable scatter in both the MVD and the peak gadopentetate dimeglumine uptake in muscle, we cannot draw definitive conclusions with regard to the effect of arterial input variations.

The permeability of malignant tumor vessels owing to their abnormal basement membranes most likely explains the difference between the MR data and the MVD estimates in cancers in this study. Vascular endothelial growth factor is released by tumor cells to induce a hyperpermeable state. This increased permeability allows proteins, which are important for further vascular growth and tumor viability, to diffuse from the vascular lumen. Recently, van Dijke and colleagues (24) addressed the hyperpermeability of tumor vessels in an animal model by using a prototype blood pool MR contrast medium. This group showed a positive correlation between the histologic capillary density and MR imaging findings with a macromolecular contrast medium, which may allow closer estimation of MVD than gadopentetate dimeglumine, as the larger molecule demonstrates a lower permeability through normal vessels than does gadopentetate dimeglumine. Van Dijke and colleagues (24) and Papadimitriou and Woods (28) also reported that increased vessel size and increased density are seen with increased aggressiveness of malignancy. Both an increased vessel permeability and an increased vessel size in malignant tumors likely contribute more to MR contrast medium behavior in breast cancers than just the vessel count, as reflected by the MVD measures.

DCIS continued to show variable enhancement in this study. Studies of MR imaging of DCIS have reported variable sensitivity, ranging from 40% to 100% (27,29). Most recently, Orel and colleagues (27) reported depiction of DCIS with MR imaging in 10 of 13 patients with DCIS by using a two-dimensional, section-selected dynamic technique in some patients and a three-dimensional–volume, whole-breast technique in the remainder. Gilles and colleagues (29) reported enhancement in 34 of 36 patients with DCIS by using early dynamic imaging. This group also reported correlation between tumor angiogenesis and enhancement in these patients. In our study, DCIS enhanced variably, as four lesions showed high extraction-flow products, three showed enhancement similar to that of the surrounding breast parenchyma, and one showed extraction-flow products similar to the majority of benign breast lesions. The variable enhancement of DCIS lowered the sensitivity and specificity of this technique for diagnosing breast cancer in this study. Given the microscopic heterogeneity of DCIS, and noting the generally improved sensitivity for detecting DCIS in the highest-resolution MR studies, we believe the variability in our detection of DCIS is most likely caused by partial volume effects in our large voxels used at present. Comparing techniques between studies is limited, as many studies report morphologic characteristics and this study reports the early fast dynamic behavior. Further larger studies will be necessary for clarification of the behavior of DCIS at MR imaging.

This study focused on fast dynamic data in breast lesions to better define breast lesions' behavior during early contrast medium enhancement and thus to distinguish benign from malignant breast tumors. Recently, the MR morphologic characterization of benign versus malignant breast lesions has been described (12,17,30). Morphologic analysis was not included in this study, as the three-dimensional postcontrast conventional images were obtained at approximately 5 minutes after the injection of gadopentetate dimeglumine to allow 4 minutes of dynamic imaging for full evaluation of the time course data in this study. At 5 minutes after injection, most of the lesions were completely enhanced. Thus, evaluation for rim enhancement and other described features for distinguishing between benign and malignant lesions was not performed. In addition, spatial resolution could be improved by using single breast imaging. The future of breast MR for the evaluation of breast lesions should probably include a combination of early dynamic assessment and morphologic evaluation to increase the specificity of the examination. This combination may be achieved with a compromise, where time resolution is decreased to two to three data points per minute to increase spatial resolution, as indicated earlier in this discussion.

In sum, these study findings demonstrate the importance of measuring a lesions' underlying T1 value when using dynamic MR imaging in the diagnosis of breast cancer. The underlying variability of T1 values, which creates overlap in signal intensity change, is taken into account because the T1 values are used to calculate more precise quantitative estimates of gadopentetate dimeglumine uptake in breast tumors, such as the extraction-flow products used in this study. In addition, dynamic imaging should occur within the first 2 minutes, as the difference between benign and malignant contrast medium dynamics occurs in this time window. Increased MVD contributes to the contrast medium behavior of benign and malignant lesions; however, other factors, such as vessel size and vessel permeability, most likely contribute substantially to gadopentetate dimeglumine uptake in malignant lesions. ■

References

1. Heywang S, Hahn D, Schmidt H, et al. Magnetic resonance imaging of the breast using gadolinium-DTPA. J Comput Assist Tomogr 1986; 10:199–204.
2. Kaiser WA, Zeitler E. MR imaging of the breast: fast imaging sequences with and without Gd-DTPA. Radiology 1989; 170: 681–686.
3. Stack JP, Redmond OM, Codd MB, Dervan PA, Ennis JT. Breast disease: tissue characterization with Gd-DTPA enhancement profiles. Radiology 1990; 174:491–494.
4. Hachiya J, Seki T, Okada M, Nitatori T, Korenaga T, Furuya Y. MR imaging of the breast with Gd-DTPA enhancement: comparison with mammography and ultrasonography. Radiat Med 1991; 9:232–240.
5. Rubens D, Totterman S, Chacko AK, et al. Gadolinium dimeglumine-enhanced chemical-shift MR imaging of the breast. AJR 1991; 157:267–270.
6. Pierce WB, Harms SE, Flamig DP, Griffey RH, Evans WP, Hagans JE. Three-dimensional gadolinium-enhanced MR imaging

of the breast: pulse sequence with fat suppression and magnetization transfer contrast. Radiology 1991; 181:757–763.
7. Harms SE, Flamig DP, Hesley KL, et al. Magnetic resonance imaging of the breast. Magn Reson Q 1992; 8:139–155.
8. Gilles R, Guinebretiere JM, Lucidarme O, et al. Nonpalpable breast tumors: diagnosis with contrast-enhanced subtraction dynamic MR imaging. Radiology 1994; 191: 625–631.
9. Kelcz F, Santyr G, Mongin S, Fairbanks E. Reducing false positive gadolinium enhanced breast MRI results through parameter analysis of the enhancement profile (abstr). In: Proceedings of the 12th Annual Scientific Meeting of the Society of Magnetic Resonance in Medicine. Berkeley, Calif: Society of Magnetic Resonance in Medicine, 1993; 121.
10. Schnall M, Orel S, Muenz L. Analysis of time-intensity curves for enhancing lesions (abstr). In: Proceedings of the 12th Annual Scientific Meeting of the Society of Magnetic Resonance in Medicine. Berkeley, Calif: Society of Magnetic Resonance in Medicine, 1993; 120.
11. Heywang-Kobrunner SH. Contrast-enhanced magnetic resonance imaging of the breast. Invest Radiol 1994; 29:94–104.
12. Orel SG, Schnall MD, LiVolsi VA, Troupin RH. Suspicious breast lesions: MR imaging with radiologic-pathologic correlation. Radiology 1994; 190:485–493.
13. Fobben ES, Rubin CZ, Kalisher L, et al. Breast MR imaging with commercially available techniques: Radiologic-pathologic correlation. Radiology 1995; 196:143–152.
14. Hulka CA, Smith BL, Sgroi DC, et al. Benign and malignant breast lesions: differentiation with echo-planar MR imaging. Radiology 1995; 197:33–38.
15. Stomper PC, Herman S, Klippenstein DL, et al. Suspect breast lesions: Findings at dynamic gadolinium-enhanced MR imaging correlated with mammographic and pathologic features. Radiology 1995; 197: 387–395.
16. Buadu LD, Murakami J, Murayama S, et al. Breast lesions: correlation of contrast medium enhancement patterns on MR images with histopathologic findings and tumor angiogenesis. Radiology 1996; 200:639–649.
17. Gilles R, Guinebretiere JM, Shapeero LG, et al. Assessment of breast cancer recurrence with contrast-enhanced subtraction MR imaging: preliminary results in 26 patients. Radiology 1993; 188:473–478.
18. Folkman J. What is the evidence that tumors are angiogenesis dependent? J Natl Cancer Inst 1990; 82:4–6.
19. Weidner N, Semple J, Welch WR, Folkman J. Tumor angiogenesis and metastasis-correlation in invasive breast carcinoma. N Engl J Med 1991; 324:1–8.
20. Weidner N, Folkman J, Pozza F, et al. Tumor angiogenesis: a new significant and independent prognostic indicator in early-stage breast carcinoma. J Natl Cancer Inst 1992; 84:1875–1887.
21. Folkman J. Clinical applications of research on angiogenesis. N Engl J Med 1995; 333: 1757–1763.
22. Frouge C, Guinebretiere J, Contesso G, et al. Correlation between contrast enhancement on dynamic magnetic resonance imaging of the breast and tumor angiogenesis. Invest Radiol 1994; 29:1043–1049.
23. Larsson HBW, Stubgaard M, Frederikson JL, Jenson M, Henriksen O, Paulson OB. Quantitation of blood-brain barrier defect by magnetic resonance imaging and gadolinium-DTPA in patients with multiple sclerosis and brain tumors. Magn Reson Med 1990; 16:117–131.
24. van Dijke CF, Brasch RD, Roberts TPL, et al. Mammary carcinoma model: correlation of macromolecular contrast-enhanced MR imaging characterizations of tumor microvasculature and histologic capillary density. Radiology 1996; 198:813–818.
25. Dvorak H, Nagy J, Dvorak J, Dvorak A. Identification and characterization of the blood vessels that are leaky to circulating macromolecules. Am J Pathol 1988; 133:95–109.
26. Donahue K, Burstein D, Manning W, Gray M. Studies of Gd-DTPA relaxivity and proton exchange rates in tissue. Magn Reson Med 1994; 32:66–76.
27. Orel SG, Mendonca MH, Reynolds C, et al. MR imaging of ductal carcinoma in situ. Radiology 1997; 202:413–420.
28. Papadimitriou JM, Woods AE. Structural and functional characteristics of the microcirculation in neoplasms. J Pathol 1975; 116: 65–72.
29. Gilles R, Zafrani B, Guinebretiere JM, et al. Ductal carcinoma in situ: MR imaging–histopathologic correlation. Radiology 1995; 196:415–419.
30. Nunes LW, Schnall MD, Orel SG, et al. Breast MR Imaging: interpretation model. Radiology 1997; 202:833–842.

Martine Remy-Jardin, MD, PhD • Jacques Doyen, MD • Jacques Remy, MD
Dominique Artaud, MD • Marc Fribourg, MD • Alain Duhamel, PhD

Functional Anatomy of the Thoracic Outlet: Evaluation with Spiral CT[1]

PURPOSE: To determine the anatomic characteristics of the thoracic outlet before and after dynamically induced modifications.

MATERIALS AND METHODS: Fifty-two volunteers (24 women; 28 men; mean age, 42 years) with no clinical or radiographic indications of thoracic outlet syndrome underwent spiral computed tomography (CT) of the apexes at full inspiration with the arms alongside the body and then with the dominant arm in hyperabduction, with a contralateral rotation of the head.

RESULTS: After elevation of the dominant arm, (*a*) no statistically significant difference was found in median value of the costosubclavian and costoclavicular distances; (*b*) the median distance between the posterior border of the smaller pectoral muscle and the anterosuperior chest wall was 12 mm in all subjects; (*c*) the subclavian artery in 18 (75%) women and in 20 (71%) men and/or the subclavian vein in three (12%) women and in three (11%) men were identified in the costoclavicular space. The median angles of rotation, retraction, and upward displacement of the clavicle were 22°, 32°, and 7°, respectively, in women and 25°, 31°, and 11°, respectively, in men.

CONCLUSION: Spiral CT is expected to be useful for determining the complex pathophysiologic processes that underlie thoracic outlet syndrome.

The neurovascular compression syndromes that occur at the level of the thoracic outlet are usually explained in terms of the natural narrowness of this anatomic region, which can be exaggerated by means of anomalous anatomy and acquired structural lesions.

Three potential sites of neurovascular compression are usually considered in the region of the thoracic outlet. The most proximal is the interscalene triangle, which is a narrow triangular space bounded inferiorly by the first rib and superiorly by the borders of the anterior and middle scalene muscles. As the neurovascular bundle leaves the interscalene triangle, it enters the costoclavicular space, which is bounded superiorly by the clavicle, anteriorly by the subclavius muscle, posteriorly and medially by the first rib and middle scalene muscle, and posteriorly and laterally by the subscapular muscle and scapula. More distally, the neurovascular bundle enters the subcoracoid tunnel and passes beneath the coracoid process, deep to the tendon of the smaller pectoral muscle.

By 1956, this type of compression was considered to be a clinical entity, described as thoracic outlet syndrome (1). Since then, there has been a great deal of controversy about the diagnosis of this syndrome, and therapeutic modalities for treatment of thoracic outlet syndrome remain unresolved. These difficulties are mainly related to the lack of specificity with regard to the clinical presentation of patients with thoracic outlet syndrome, as well as to the lack of objective diagnostic tests, which thus preclude accurate recognition of the component of the neurovascular bundle that is compressed. With an awareness of these limitations, one should not be surprised that the selection of patients for surgical treatment remains "a subjective decision" (2). The popularity of surgery for thoracic outlet syndrome and the difficulties inherent in the lack of specific diagnostic criteria have heightened the controversy about the results of surgery for this condition.

Spiral computed tomography (CT) has become a valuable tool for the diagnosis of several skeletal disorders because it is possible to scan an anatomic region without misregistration and subsequently obtain high-quality reconstructions. Whereas the usefulness of this technique in the evaluation of patients with thoracic outlet syndrome has yet to be demonstrated, the ability to visualize osseous and soft-tissue structures simultaneously should help improve our understanding of these disorders. Nevertheless, a precise knowledge of the functional anatomy of this region is a prerequisite and led us to undertake the present study. The purpose of our study was to analyze the relationships between the neurovascular structures,

Index terms: Arteries, subclavian, 942.12115, 942.92 • Computed tomography (CT), helical, 41.12115 • Thorax, anatomy, 41.92 • Thorax, CT, 41.12111, 41.12115 • Bones, measurement, 41.92 • Bones, CT, 41.12111, 41.12115 • Veins, subclavian, 9462.12115, 9462.12115

Abbreviation: MIP = maximum intensity projection.

Radiology 1997; 205:843–851

[1] From the Department of Radiology, Hôpital Calmette, Blvd Jules Leclerc, 59037 Lille, France. Received June 9, 1997; revision requested July 28; revision received August 13; accepted August 15. **Address reprint requests to** M.R.J.

restraining soft tissues, and bone boundaries of this region before and after postural maneuvers.

MATERIALS AND METHODS

Patients

This prospective study was based on the analysis of CT scans obtained between December 1996 and February 1997. From the daily indications of chest CT scans, 52 patients were selected to undergo spiral CT (without contrast material enhancement) of the thoracic outlet. For the purpose of this anatomic study, patients were included if they (*a*) were physically active; (*b*) had no neck, arm, or shoulder pain; and (*c*) had normal bone structures on standard chest radiographs, with a particular interest in the absence of supernumerary ribs or vertebral anomalies. Patients were excluded if (*a*) the thoracocervicoaxillary anatomy could have been modified by means of (i) lung surgery and/or thoracic radiation treatment or (ii) the concurrent presence of acute or chronic lung infiltration or pleural and/or mediastinal disease; (*b*) clinical features of degenerative or inflammatory musculoskeletal disease were present; (*c*) they had neurologic or vascular symptoms potentially related to a thoracic outlet syndrome; or (*d*) they were physically inactive and prone to muscular atrophy. This protocol was approved by the ethics committee of our institution; informed consent was obtained from each patient.

The study group was composed of 24 women (group 1) and 28 men (group 2), aged 21–69 years (mean, 42 years). The anatomic characteristics of the population are summarized in Table 1. These patients had initially been referred to the radiology department for the following reasons: (*a*) mild form of chronic obstructive lung disease ($n = 25$); (*b*) suspicion for the presence of pulmonary nodules ($n = 14$); and (*c*) suspicion for diffuse infiltrative lung disease, with normal chest radiograph ($n = 13$).

Spiral CT Examination

Data acquisition.—In order to analyze the anatomic characteristics and dynamically induced modifications of the thoracic outlet, each patient underwent two unenhanced spiral CT examinations (Somatom Plus 4A; Siemens Medical Systems, Erlangen, Germany) during the same session. Both examinations were performed with full inspiration while the patient was in the supine position. A first spiral acquisition was obtained with both arms alongside the body and the head located medially (the neutral position) (Fig 1a, 1b). A second spiral CT acquisition was obtained with the patient's dominant arm elevated above the head (approximately 130° of hyperabduction, with external rotation) and contralateral rotation of the head, which remained extended while the contralateral arm was lying alongside the body (the

Table 1
Characteristics of the Study Population

Characteristic	Group 1 (24 women)	Group 2 (28 men)
Median age (y)	42 (24–69)	42 (21–62)
Median height (m)	1.60 (1.46–1.73)	1.77 (1.60–1.83)
Median weight (kg)	62 (43–100)	71 (56–102)
No. of right-handed patients	19	26
No. of left-handed patients	5	2

Note.—Numbers in parentheses are ranges.

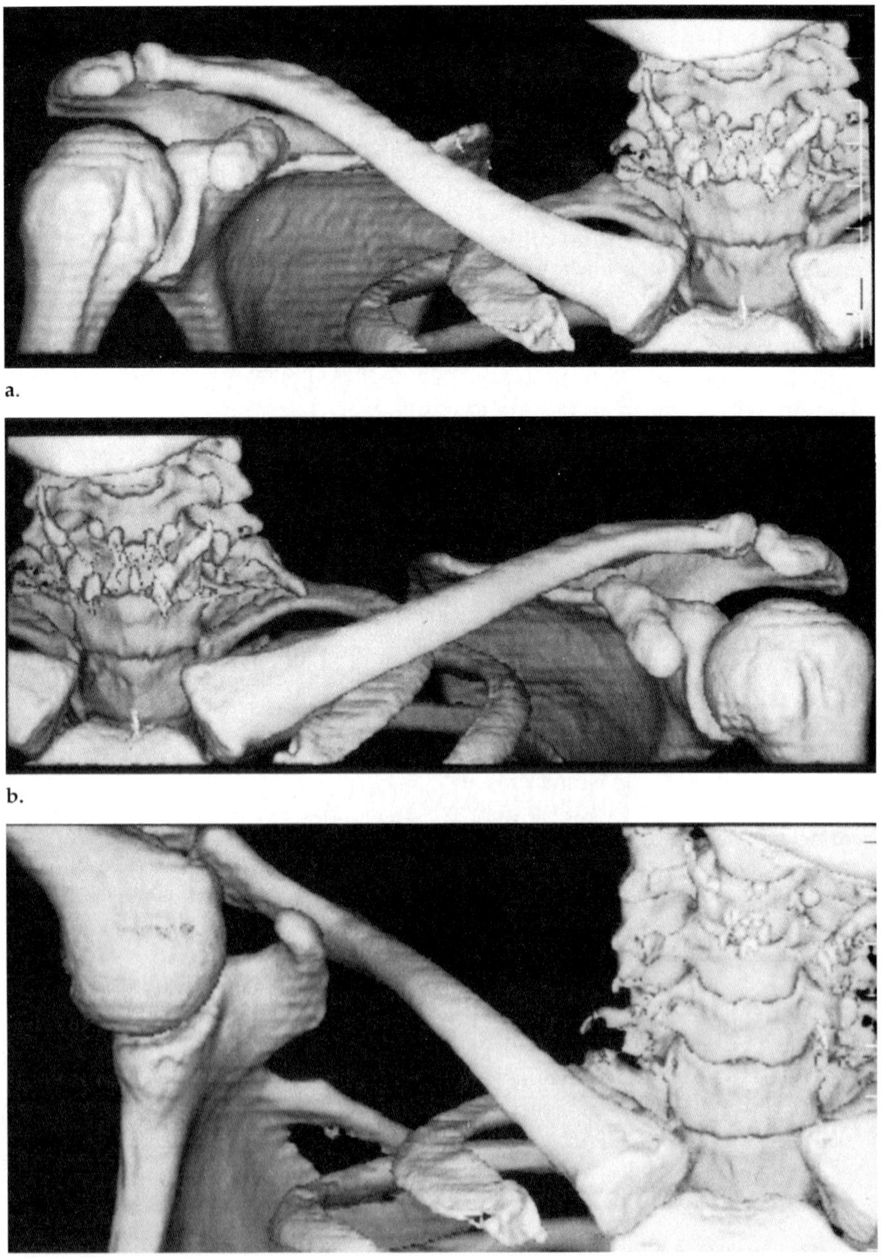

a.
b.
c.

Figure 1. Spiral CT evaluation of the thoracic outlet in a 38-year-old right-handed woman. Three-dimensional anteroposterior shaded-surface displays (threshold, 150 HU) of the **(a)** right and **(b)** left thoracic outlets with the patient in the neutral position show the orientation of the clavicle and the configuration of the costoclavicular space on both sides. **(c)** Three-dimensional anteroposterior shaded-surface display (threshold, 150 HU) of the right thoracic outlet after postural maneuver demonstrates upward displacement and rotation of the clavicle and enlargement of the costoclavicular space.

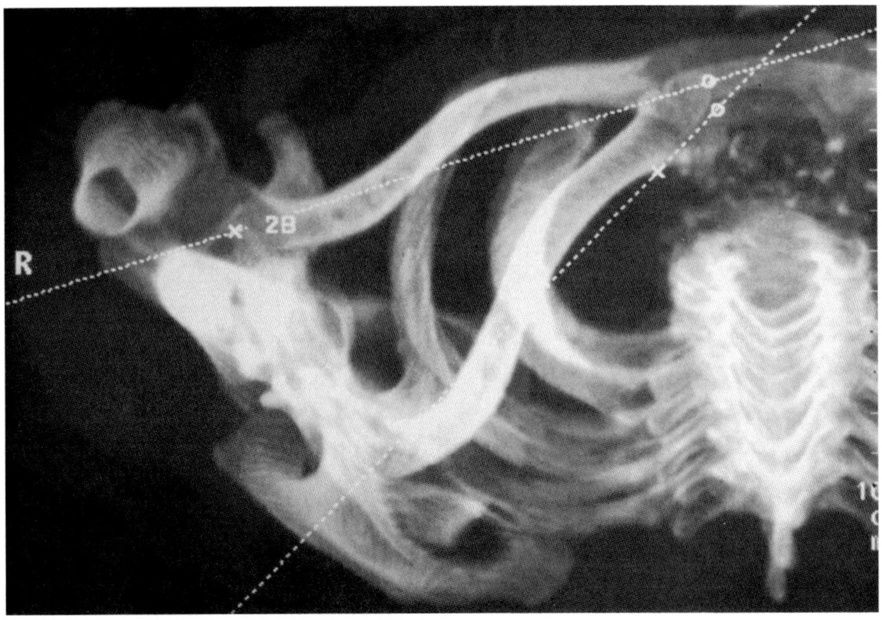

a.

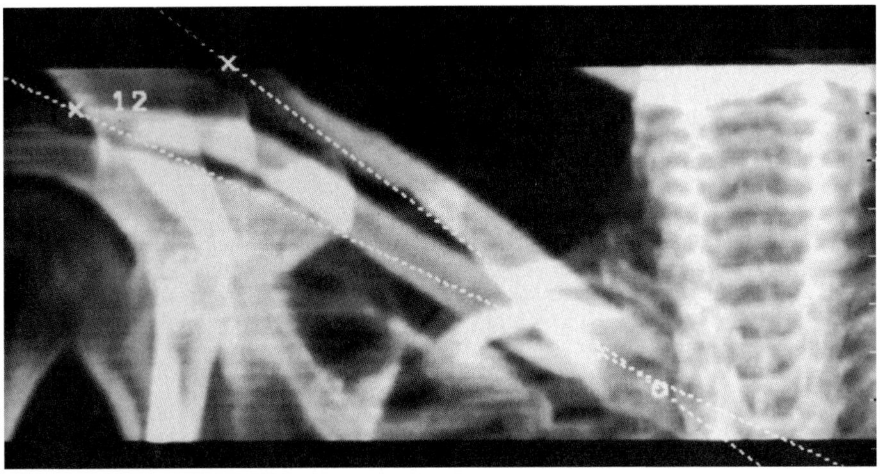

b.

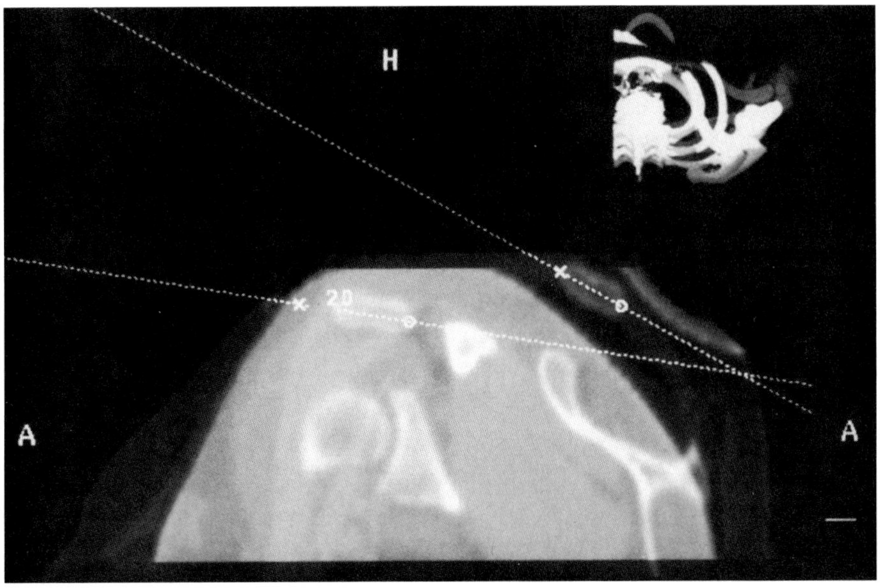

c.

Figure 2. Spiral CT evaluation of the postural displacement of the clavicle in the same patient as in Figure 1. **(a)** Fusion image generated with the horizontal views of the MIP images of the right thoracic outlet before and after postural maneuver enables measurement of the angle of retraction of the clavicle, which, in this case, is 28°. **(b)** Fusion image generated with the anteroposterior views of the MIP images of the right thoracic outlet before and after postural maneuver enables measurement of the angle of upward displacement of the clavicle, which, in this case, is 12°. **(c)** Fusion image generated with the oblique reformations obtained perpendicular to the lateral extremity of the clavicle before and after postural maneuver enables measurement of the angle of rotation of the clavicle, which, in this case, is 20°. *A* = anterior, *H* = horizontal.

Table 2
Orientation of the First Rib

Parameter	Angle between First Rib Axis and Horizontal
Group 1 (24 women)	
Dominant arm in neutral position	29° (7°–43°)
Dominant arm after maneuver	29° (10°–49°)
Contralateral arm in neutral position	30° (6°–49°)
Group 2 (28 men)	
Dominant arm in neutral position	27° (7°–43°)
Dominant arm after maneuver	26° (8°–42°)
Contralateral arm in neutral position	29° (7°–46°)

Note.—Data are medians. Numbers in parentheses are ranges.

postural maneuver) (Fig 1c). This postural maneuver combined the positional characteristics of two maneuvers currently used in the clinical evaluation of thoracic outlet syndrome (2): the maneuver of hyperabduction, with the elbow slightly flexed to maintain external rotation, as used in the Wright maneuver, and the modified Adson maneuver, during which the neck is extended and the head turned toward the unaffected side while the patient is asked to take a deep breath. Usually obtained successively in clinical practice, the characteristics of these basic maneuvers can be summarized as follows (2): (*a*) In the Adson maneuver, the neck is extended and the head is turned *toward* the affected side. With the arms by the side and with deep inspiration, the pulse is obliterated. The test has been considered to be more helpful if the head is turned *away from* the affected side, in which case it is described as the modified Adson maneuver. (*b*) The Wright maneuver is one of hyperabduction, with the elbow slightly flexed to maintain external rotation; the maneuver is positive when the pulse is subsequently obliterated or when the postural maneuver reproduces the clinical symptoms.

For each acquisition, the surveyed volume extended from the fifth thoracic vertebra to the inner extremity of the first rib (mean z-axis coverage, 70 mm; range, 60–80 mm). To include the bone structures of interest, the scanned subvolume was

Table 3
Evaluation of the Costoclavicular Space

Parameter	Group 1 (24 women)			Group 2 (28 men)		
	Dominant Arm in Neutral Position	Dominant Arm after Maneuver	Contralateral Arm in Neutral Position	Dominant Arm in Neutral Position	Dominant Arm after Maneuver	Contralateral Arm in Neutral Position
Smallest distance between clavicle and first rib	3 (1–10)	3 (1–10)*	2 (1–10)	3 (1–9)	7 (1–17)†	2.0 (1.0–6.0)
Largest distance between clavicle and first rib	15 (7–27)	12 (5–32)‡	14 (8–25)	12 (7–25)	12 (5–25)§	12.5 (5.0–22.0)
Distance between subclavius muscle and first rib	8 (1–15)	8 (1–22)‖	8 (2–15)	8 (1–20)	9 (3–13)#	7.0 (1.0–20.0)

Note.—Data are median distances in millimeters. Numbers in parentheses are ranges.
* Mean increase was 4.0 mm; mean decrease was 8.5 mm.
† Mean increase was 6.5 mm; mean decrease was 4.0 mm.
‡ Mean increase was 5.0 mm; mean decrease was 6.5 mm.
§ Mean increase was 5 mm; mean decrease was 7 mm.
‖ Mean increase was 6 mm; mean decrease was 5 mm.
Mean increase was 7.0 mm; mean decrease was 6.5 mm.

selected on the basis of a scout view systematically obtained before each acquisition. For each data acquisition, the scanning parameters were 140 kV, 206 mA, 0.75-second per revolution scanning time, 2-mm collimation, 3 mm per revolution, and pitch of 1.5.

Image reconstruction.—Transverse CT scans of the thoracic outlet in the neutral position and after postural maneuver were reconstructed at 1-mm intervals by using a 180° linear-interpolation algorithm and a standard kernel (370-mm field of view). The images, which were photographed with mediastinal window settings (window width, 350 HU; window level, 50 HU), confirmed the absence of congenital or acquired anomaly of the thoracic outlet in all patients.

For the purpose of the generation of multiplanar and three-dimensional reformations, transverse CT scans of the right and left thoracic outlets were separately reconstructed from each data set (1-mm reconstruction interval, 180° linear-interpolation algorithm, standard kernel, 220-mm field of view). Three series of sagittal reformations were obtained from the medial portion of the upper thoracic vertebrae to the head of the humerus: in the neutral position on both sides and after the postural maneuver on the dominant side. Each series was composed of 17 successive sagittal images, spaced 8–10 mm apart. These images were photographed with mediastinal window settings (window width, 350 HU; window level, 50 HU).

At the level of the dominant arm, three series of fused images were generated to analyze the postural displacement of the clavicle. (*a*) Two cranial-caudal maximum intensity projection (MIP) images were generated from the data set acquired in the neutral position and after postural maneuver; these images were superimposed with the first rib as the fixed structure to allow further measurement of the angle of retraction of the clavicle (Fig 2a). (*b*) Two anteroposterior MIP images were similarly fused to calculate the angle of upward displacement of the clavicle (Fig 2b). (*c*) Two reformations obtained perpendicular to the lateral extremity of the clavicle in both positions were fused to calculate the angle of rotation of the clavicle (Fig 2c). For the planning of adequate planes of reformation, three-dimensional shaded-surface displays of the bone structures in the neutral position and after postural maneuver were systematically reconstructed (threshold, 150 HU); these images also provided an overall view of the bone structures of each thoracic outlet.

Evaluated parameters.—Three parameters were evaluated. The first parameter evaluated was the interscalene triangle. The anatomic situation of the first rib was assessed in the neutral position on both sides and after the postural maneuver of the dominant arm by measuring the angle between the axis of the middle portion of the first rib, that is, the costal shaft (3), and the horizontal. This measurement was obtained on the sagittal reformation that depicted the longest portion of the first rib shaft.

The second parameter was the costoclavicular space. On the sagittal reformations that enabled the concurrent identification of the clavicle and first rib (ie, two to three reformations per patient), the following parameters were recorded in the neutral position for both sides and after the postural maneuver of the dominant arm: (*a*) the minimum distance between the inferior border of the clavicle and the superior margin of the first rib, measured on the reformation that depicted the lower portion of the anterior scalene muscle; (*b*) the maximum distance between the inferior border of the clavicle and the superior margin of the first rib; (*c*) the distance between the inferior border of the subclavius muscle and the superior margin of the first rib; (*d*) the location of the subclavian vessels relative to the narrowest and largest portions of the costoclavicular space and to the costosubclavian space; and (*e*) the location of the subclavius muscle relative to the clavicle. According to the usual anatomic criteria (4), the subclavian artery was defined as the arterial portion that extended from its origin to the outer border of the first rib; from this point to the lower border of the tendon of the teres major muscle, the subclavian artery is known as the axillary artery. Any change larger than 2 mm in the superoinferior distances, measured in both positions, was considered to reflect a postural modification in the costoclavicular space; a difference smaller than 2 mm was considered to be within the range of technically induced errors at manual positioning of the cursor between the two bone structures on the console screen.

The postural changes of the clavicle were analyzed as follows: (*a*) The angle of retraction was measured on the fused cranial-caudal MIP images; the main axis of the clavicle in each position was defined by the line that joined the medial and lateral ends of the clavicle (Fig 2a). (*b*) On the fused anteroposterior MIP images, the main axis of the clavicle in each position enabled calculation of the angle of upward displacement of the clavicle (Fig 2b). (*c*) The angle of rotation of the clavicle was measured on the fused reformations obtained perpendicular to the lateral extremity of the clavicle; the main axis of the clavicle in each position was used to calculate the angle value (Fig 2c).

The third parameter was the subcoracoid tunnel. Owing to the potential neurovascular compression at the level of the subcoracoid tunnel after postural maneuvers, the width of the subcoracoid tunnel was obtained exclusively in this position (and thus, exclusively at the level of the dominant arm). On the sagittal reformation that depicted the anterior end of the coracoid process and the smaller pectoral muscle, the distance between the posterior border of the smaller pectoral muscle and the anterosuperior chest wall was measured at the level of the axillary neurovascular bundle between the axillary vein and artery. The location of the neurovascular bundle relative to the anterior end of the coracoid process was systematically recorded.

Study design.—All reformations were generated by technicians during their daily work-up, and the measurements were obtained at the console after each CT examination by the same radiologist (J.D.). Several weeks after completion of this study, the anatomic characteristics of the thoracic outlet of the entire study group were analyzed at a second interpretation period during which two radiologists (M.R.J., J.R.) used consensus analysis of the location of the

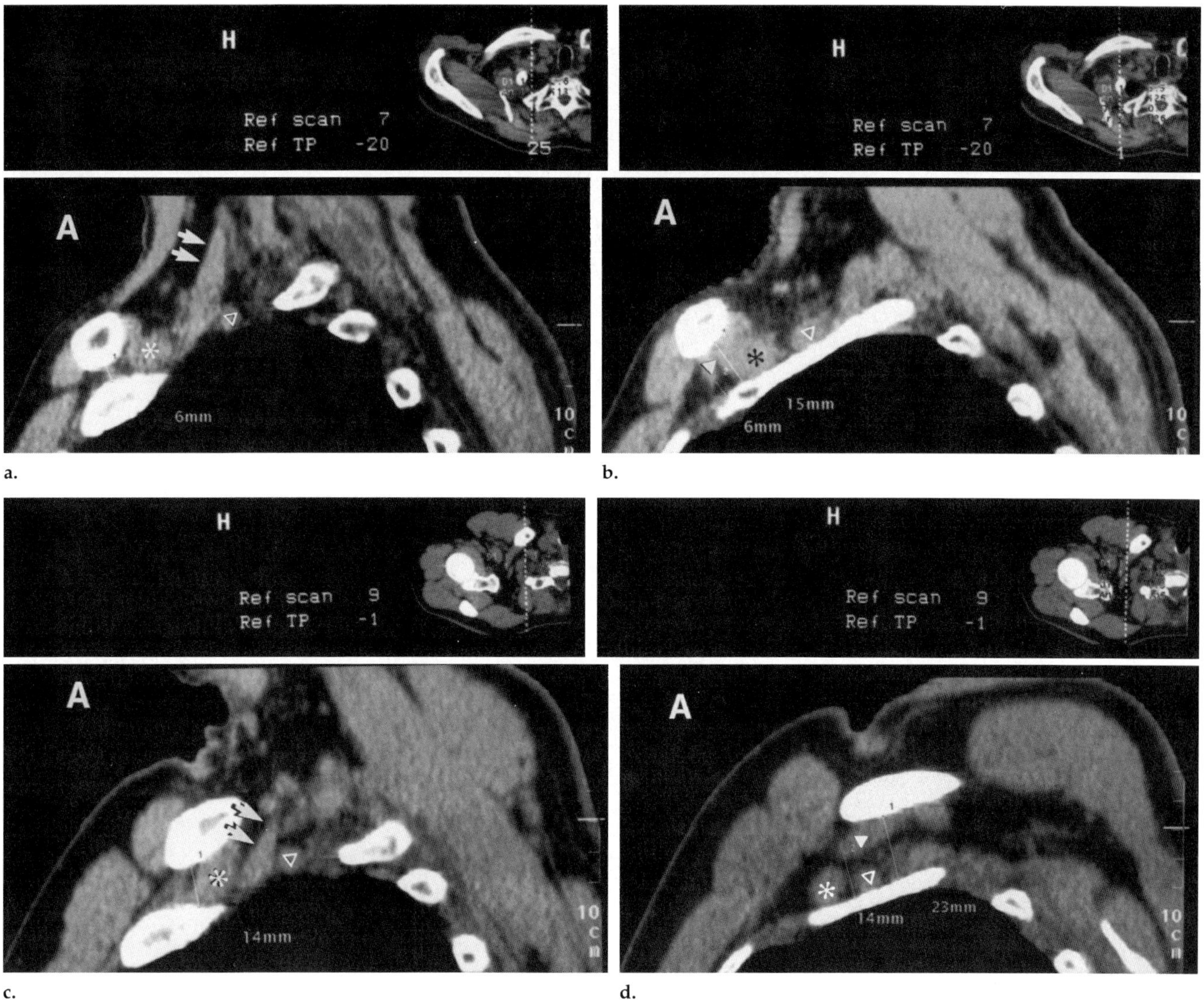

Figure 3. Spiral CT evaluation of the right thoracic outlet in a 45-year-old right-handed man. *A* = anterior, *H* = horizontal. **(a, b)** Sagittal reformation images of the costoclavicular space with the patient in the neutral position illustrate measurements of the **(a)** minimum (6 mm) and **(b)** maximum (15 mm) distances between the inferior border of the clavicle and the superior margin of the first rib. These images also illustrate measurement of the distance between the inferior border of the subclavius muscle and the superior margin of the first rib (ie, 6 mm on **b**). Note the posterior location of the subclavian vein (*) and artery (open triangle) relative to the costoclavicular space and the inferior location of the subclavius muscle (solid triangle in **b**) relative to the clavicular margin. The lower portion of the anterior scalene muscle is clearly depicted (arrows in **a**). **(c, d)** Sagittal reformation images of the costoclavicular space after the postural maneuver demonstrate enlargement of the superoinferior distance measured between the bone structures and/or the subclavian muscle. Note the larger diameter and the anterior location of the subclavian vein (*) relative to the subclavian artery (open triangle), both of which were precisely delineated by means of the surrounding fat planes below the horizontally oriented subclavius muscle (solid triangle in **d**). The lower portion of the anterior scalene muscle (arrows in **c**) is precisely delineated.

bone, vascular, and muscular structures. All comparisons were performed with the Wilcoxon paired-rank test.

RESULTS

Interscalene Triangle

Table 2 lists the results of the evaluation of the interscalene triangle. In group 1 and in group 2, no statistically significant difference was found between the distribution of the angle values of the first rib measured on both sides in the neutral position and after postural maneuver at the level of the dominant arm. After the postural maneuver, (*a*) the median angle was 29° in group 1 patients and 26° in group 2 patients; (*b*) the angle was less than 15° in five (21%) of the 24 women in group 1 and in four (14%) of the 28 men in group 2; (*c*) the angle was greater than 45° in one (4%) patient in group 1 and in no patient in group 2.

Costoclavicular Space

Table 3 lists the results of the evaluation of the costoclavicular space.

Analysis in the neutral position.—No statistically significant differences were observed, in either group of patients, between the distribution of the distances (maximum, minimum, and costosubclavian) measured on both sides (Fig 3a, 3b).

The position of the subclavius muscle relative to the clavicle was analyzed on the sagittal reformations obtained at the level of the largest portion of the costoclavicular space. In the 24 group 1 patients, the location of the subclavius muscle was inferior in 19 (79%) patients and posteroinferior in five (21%) patients; in the 28 group 2 patients, the location of the muscle was inferior in 14 (50%) patients, posteroinferior in 12 (43%) patients, and anteroinferior in two (7%) patients.

The subclavian vein was anterior to the subclavian artery in all patients.

Table 4
Identification of Subclavian Vessels in the Costoclavicular Space

Location and Subclavian Vessel	Group 1 (24 women)			Group 2 (28 men)		
	Dominant Arm in Neutral Position	Dominant Arm after Maneuver	Contralateral Arm in Neutral Position	Dominant Arm in Neutral Position	Dominant Arm after Maneuver	Contralateral Arm in Neutral Position
Narrowest costoclavicular space						
Artery	0 (0)	0 (0)	0 (0)	0 (0)	0 (0)	0 (0)
Vein	0 (0)	0 (0)	0 (0)	0 (0)	0 (0)	0 (0)
Largest costoclavicular space						
Artery	0 (0)	18 (75)	0 (0)	0 (0)	24 (86)	0 (0)
Vein	3 (12)	3 (12)	4 (17)	2 (7)	3 (11)	3 (11)
Costosubclavian space						
Artery	0 (0)	20 (83)	0 (0)	0 (0)	22 (79)	0 (0)
Vein	0 (0)	16 (67)	0 (0)	0 (0)	22 (79)	0 (0)

Note.—Data are number of vessels identified. Numbers in parentheses are percentages.

The subclavian vascular bundle was posterior to the posterior margin of the clavicle and first rib at the level of the narrowest portion of the costoclavicular space on both sides in all patients. At the level of the largest portion of the costoclavicular space, (*a*) the subclavian artery was never identified in the costoclavicular space in all patients and was always located posteriorly, and (*b*) the subclavian vein was identified in the costoclavicular space on the side of the dominant arm in three (12%) patients in group 1 and in two (7%) patients in group 2 and on the contralateral side in four (17%) patients in group 1 and in three (11%) patients in group 2. In the remaining patients, the subclavian vein was located posterior to the costoclavicular space (Table 4).

Analysis after the postural maneuver.—After the postural maneuver, we analyzed modifications in the superoinferior width of the costoclavicular space, in the clavicle and subclavius muscle, and in the location of the subclavian bundle (Fig 3c, 3d).

1. Postural modifications of the superoinferior width of the costoclavicular space. The distribution of the following three measurements was compared before and after the postural maneuver: the minimum and maximum distances between the inferior border of the clavicle and the superior margin of the first rib and the distance between the inferior border of the subclavius muscle and the superior margin of the first rib. The only statistically significant difference we found was in the minimum distance, which was larger in group 2 patients after the postural maneuver.

After the postural maneuver, (*a*) the minimum costoclavicular distance (i) was unchanged in 15 patients in group 1 and in eight patients in group 2, (ii) was increased in seven patients in group 1 and in 18 patients in group 2, and (iii) was decreased in two patients each in group 1 and group 2. (*b*) The maximum costoclavicular distance (i) was unchanged in nine patients in group 1 and in eight patients in group 2, (ii) was increased in four patients in group 1 and in nine patients in group 2, and (iii) was decreased in 11 patients each in group 1 and group 2. (c) The costosubclavian distance (i) was unchanged in 10 patients in group 1 and in 14 patients in group 2, (ii) was increased in five patients in group 1 and in seven patients in group 2, and (iii) was decreased in nine patients in group 1 and in seven patients in group 2.

Table 5
Changes in the Clavicle after Postural Maneuver

Angle Measurement	Group 1 (24 women)	Group 2 (28 men)
Rotation	22° (0° to 65°)	25° (9° to 39°)
Retraction	32° (17° to 40°)	31° (13° to 44°)
Upward displacement	7° (−5° to 24°)	11° (−3° to 25°)

Note.—Numbers in parentheses are ranges.

2. Postural modifications of the clavicle and subclavius muscle. The median values of the angles of rotation, retraction, and upward displacement of the clavicle are summarized in Table 5. The location of the subclavius muscle relative to the inferior border of the clavicle was as follows: (a) in group 1 patients, the location was anteroinferior in 23 (96%) of 24 patients and anterior in one (4%) patient; in group 2 patients, the location was anteroinferior in 26 (93%) of 28 patients, inferior in one (4%) patient, and not analyzable in one (4%) patient owing to the lack of fat planes between the muscular and vascular components of the costoclavicular space.

3. Location of the subclavian vascular bundle (Table 5). Owing to the presence of fat planes, the vascular sections were always clearly visible; the subclavian vein was anterior to the subclavian artery in all patients. The venous sections of the bundle were consistently of greater diameter (average, 12 mm) than the arterial sections (average, 7 mm).

The subclavian vascular bundle was located posterior to the narrowest portion of the costoclavicular space in all patients (Fig 3c). At the level of the largest distance between the inferior border of the clavicle and the superior margin of the first rib, the following vessels were identified within the costoclavicular space: (*a*) the subclavian artery was visible in 18 (75%) patients in group 1 and in 20 (71%) patients in group 2 (Fig 3c); (b) the subclavian vein was visible in three (12%) patients in group 1 and in three (11%) patients in group 2. The vessels identified between the inferior border of the subclavius muscle and the superior margin of the first rib were the subclavian artery in 20 (83%) patients in group 1 and in 22 (79%) patients in group 2 and/or the subclavian vein in 16 (67%) patients in group 1 and in 22 (79%) patients in group 2. After the postural maneuver, the subclavian vein was near the anteroinferior margin of the subclavian muscle in 10 (42%)

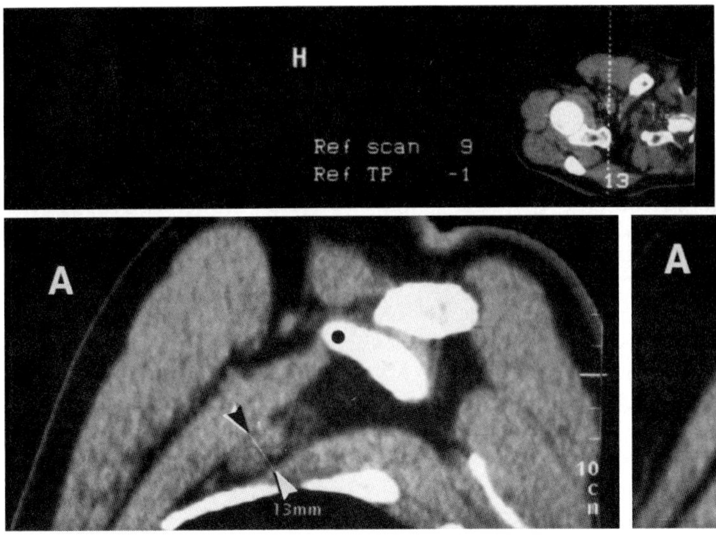

4.

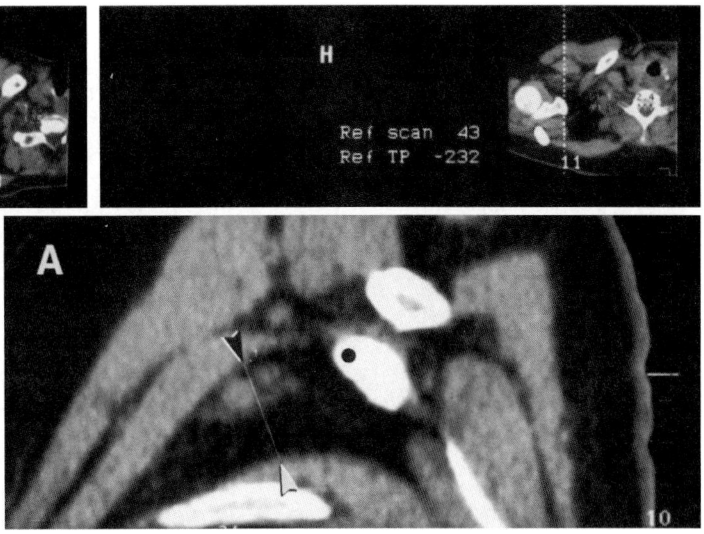

5.

Figures 4, 5. **(4)** Sagittal reformation image obtained at the level of the right subcoracoid tunnel after postural maneuver in a 43-year-old right-handed man. The distance between the posterior margin of the smaller pectoral muscle (black arrowhead) and the anterior margin of the anterior serratus muscle (white arrowhead) is 13 mm. Note that the neurovascular bundle is situated approximately 30 mm inferior to the anterior extremity of the coracoid process (●). *A* = anterior, *H* = horizontal. **(5)** Sagittal reformation image obtained at the level of the right subcoracoid tunnel after the postural maneuver in a 43-year-old right-handed man. The distance between the posterior margin of the smaller pectoral muscle (black arrowhead) and the anterior margin of the anterior serratus muscle (white arrowhead) is 24 mm. Note that the neurovascular bundle is situated approximately 15 mm anterior to the anterior extremity of the coracoid process (●). *A* = anterior, *H* = horizontal.

patients in group 1 and in 11 (39%) patients in group 2.

Subcoracoid Tunnel

After the postural maneuver, the median distance between the posterior border of the smaller pectoral muscle and the anterosuperior chest wall was 12 mm (range, 5–50 mm) in group 1 patients and 12 mm (range, 5–25 mm) in group 2 patients (Fig 4). The anterosuperior chest wall consisted of the anterior border of the anterior serratus muscle in 18 (75%) patients in group 1 and in 21 (75%) patients in group 2 and of the anterior costal margin in six (25%) patients in group 1 and in seven (25%) patients in group 2.

Four patients in group 1 and five patients in group 2 had a distance of less than 10 mm (range, 5–8 mm) at the time of presentation. Three patients in group 1 and one patient in group 2 had a distance of larger than 20 mm (Fig 5) at the time of presentation. The neurovascular bundle was located 20–40 mm below the anterior extremity of the coracoid process in all patients.

DISCUSSION

To our knowledge, the present investigation is the first in vivo anatomic study of the thoracic outlet to provide objective information about the three anatomic parts (interscalene triangle, costoclavicular space, and subcoracoid tunnel) of the outlet before and after a postural maneuver.

At the level of the interscalene triangle, three parameters are known to interfere with the size of this narrow compartment: the level of insertion of the anterior scalene muscle, the degree of obliquity of the middle portion of the first rib, and the width of the anterior and middle scalene muscles (5). Owing to the inability to analyze with confidence the muscular component of the interscalene space on CT scans, we focused our attention on the orientation of the first rib, which influences the orientation of the inferior margin of the interscalene triangle and thus the relationships between the neurovascular structures and the bone boundaries of this narrow space. This in vivo anatomic information was obtained by calculating the angular difference between the main axis of the middle portion of the first rib and the horizontal before (neutral position) and after the postural maneuver.

In patients in both groups, no statistically significant difference was observed between the distribution of the angle values on the dominant and contralateral sides or between the distribution of the angle values before and after postural maneuver of the dominant arm. Whereas the median value of the angles measured after postural maneuver was 29° in group 1 patients and 26° in group 2 patients, a wide range of absolute values was observed in both groups. The angle was less than 15° in five (21%) of 24 patients in group 1 and in four (14%) of 28 patients in group 2, whereas the angle was greater than 45° in one (4%) patient in group 1. These findings are consistent with those of previous anatomic reports (5), according to which there is great variability in the orientation of the middle portion of the first rib.

At the level of the costoclavicular space, our goals were to analyze the anatomic characteristics of the osseous and muscular boundaries of the space and to identify the course of the subclavian vascular bundle in patients before (neutral position) and after the postural maneuver. In group 1 patients in the neutral position, the median values of the narrowest and widest superoinferior costoclavicular distances on the side of the dominant arm were 3 and 15 mm respectively; in group 2 patients, these respective distances were 3 and 12 mm. No statistically significant difference was observed in the distribution of these measurements between the side of the dominant limb and the contralateral side in either group.

It is usually accepted that during hyperabduction and external rotation of the arm, the clavicle tends to be located closer to the superior margin of the first rib (5). Conversely, the only statistically significant modification observed in our study group concerned the distribution of the minimum costoclavicular distance in group 2 patients, which was larger after postural maneuver. In the absence of comparable in vivo data, one may suggest the role of the ipsilateral musculature in men as an explanation of this finding in group 2 patients.

Because the subclavius muscle has also been implicated in the restriction of the available space at the level of the costoclavicular space, we measured the distance between the inferior border of the subclavius muscle and the superior margin of the first rib on both series of sagittal reformations. Despite large variations among individuals, we observed that the median distance, with the patient in the neutral position, varied between 7 and 8 mm, with no statistically significant difference between the dominant and contralateral side. Moreover, we did not observe any statistically significant difference in the distribution of the costosubclavian distances before and after the postural maneuver in either group.

To our knowledge, only limited information is available about the postural changes that occur at the level of the costoclavicular space. In autopsy studies (5), the costosubclavian distance was reported to vary between 10 and 12 mm in the neutral position and between 12 and 15 mm at hyperabduction.

With regard to the relationships between the subclavian and axillary vessels and the thoracic outlet boundaries, we observed marked postural differences at the level of the costoclavicular space. In the neutral position, the subclavian vein was the only vascular structure present at the level of the largest portion of this anatomic compartment: This vessel was located in this space in 12%–17% of patients in group 1 and in 7%–11% of patients in group 2. After the postural maneuver, the subclavian artery was located in the costoclavicular space in 75% of patients in group 1 and in 71% of patients in group 2, which thus enabled demonstration of the posteroanterior displacement of the subclavian vascular bundle.

Owing to the anterior location of the subclavian vein relative to the subclavian artery and the anteroinferior orientation of the subclavius muscle after postural maneuver, it was not surprising to observe close relationships between the subclavian vessels and subclavius muscle after the postural maneuver. The subclavian artery and vein were identified in the costosubclavian space in 20 (83%) and in 16 (67%) patients, respectively, in group 1 and in 22 (79%) patients in group 2. These anatomic findings allow understanding of the potential pathophysiologic importance of the subclavian muscle in vascular compression at the level of the costoclavicular space.

Because the anteroinferior border of the subclavian muscle has been recognized (5) as the fibrous zone responsible for a slight compression of the subclavian vein during hyperabduction, it is of interest to note that after the postural maneuver, the subclavian vein abutted the anteroinferior margin of the subclavian muscle in 10 (42%) of 24 patients in group 1 and in 11 (39%) of 28 patients in group 2.

In addition to the subclavian muscle, the costocoracoid ligament located adjacent to the clavicle has also been implicated in the reduction of the space available to the subclavian vein (6,7), but this anatomic structure could not be specifically evaluated in the present study. At the level of the subcoracoid tunnel, the neurovascular bundle passes beneath the coracoid process deep to the tendon of the smaller pectoral muscle in patients in the neutral position. During hyperabduction, the costocoracoid ligament restricts the space anteriorly, and the vascular bundle is reported (2) to be bowed around the coracoid process. Conversely, we observed that the vascular bundle was located 20–40 mm below the anterior extremity of the coracoid process in all patients.

After the postural maneuver, the median distance between the posterior border of the smaller pectoral muscle and the anterosuperior chest wall was 12 mm in patients in both groups. It is notable that this distance was smaller than 10 mm in nine patients. The subscapular and smaller pectoral muscles enclose the vascular bundle, and compression could occur as a result of hypertrophy of these muscles. The anatomic features described in the present study could help account for the high frequency of false-positive results reported (8–12) in healthy subjects after postural maneuvers.

Because the sternoclavicular joint is considered to be the articulating mechanism of the shoulder girdle with the trunk (13), we evaluated the movements, which are known to occur simultaneously, of the clavicle around three axes: elevation, backward movement, and counterclockwise rotation. The median angle of elevation of the clavicle was 7° in group 1 patients and 11° in group 2 patients; the median angle of retraction was 32° in group 1 patients and 30° in group 2 patients; and the median angle of rotation was 22° in group 1 patients and 25° in group 2 patients.

In an autopsy study, Moseley (13) found that the elevation of the clavicle was 45° from the neutral position, the retraction was 15° beyond the neutral position, and the rotation of the clavicle was 50°. The discrepancies between Moseley's results and ours may be explained in terms of different methodologic approaches. First, Moseley reported autopsy findings, whereas we obtained in vivo measurements. In the living subject, one should consider the role of muscular tone and remember that movements of several anatomic components are known to occur simultaneously, which could account for such differences. In addition, the postural maneuver evaluated in the present study combined deep inspiration, rotation of the head, and hyperabduction, which differs from the simple elevation of the upper limb studied by Moseley. Moreover, Moseley did not make a distinction between the dominant arm and the contralateral side.

Although our results provide objective information about the functional anatomy of the thoracic outlet, the present study has several limitations. First, the analysis of the subclavian vessels was performed with unenhanced CT scans, which hampered precise evaluation at the level of the interscalene triangle. However, presence of fat planes enabled confident analysis of the vascular bundles at the level of the costoclavicular space and subcoracoid tunnel.

Second, the postural maneuver used in the present study was directly influenced by the architecture of the CT unit, in particular, the gantry diameter. According to descriptions (2,14,15) of maneuvers that may compress neurovascular structures at the thoracic outlet, the postural maneuver used in our study can be considered to be a combination of the Wright and Adson maneuvers. However, we should emphasize that we evaluated patients in the supine position, whereas at clinical examination, the patient is in the upright position during the above-mentioned maneuvers. It must also be emphasized that the position of the clavicle is highly dependent on the exact position of the arm. Consequently, because the patient's position could not be completely standardized, slight variations in the clavicular position may have influenced the measurements between the first rib and the clavicle.

Third, in the present study, the functional anatomic evaluation was limited to a single postural maneuver, whereas multiple positional tests are usually performed in succession in clinical practice. This limitation is directly related to the radiation dose inherent to CT, which dictated no more than two acquisitions per patient. By using an anthropomorphic Rando-Alderson phantom, Jurik et al (16) observed that the total effective radiation dose at examination of the sternoclavicular joints and the manubrium of the sternum was lower at spiral CT (0.6 mSv) than at conventional tomography (0.8 mSv). Because spiral CT is diagnostically comparable and in some respects superior to tomography, these authors recommended the use of spiral CT for studies of the sternum. One should underline that the use of a subsecond scanning time in conjunction with a pitch of 1.5, as was used in the present study, allows further reduction in the overall radiation dose.

As regards the various measurements obtained in the present study, these measurements were chosen to be easily reproducible at every examination. However, there is no doubt that other distances could have been evaluated: for example, the distance between the first rib and the clavicle at the level of the subclavian artery. The clinical relevance of these measurements and the need to consider alternative parameters must be further evaluated in a population of patients with thoracic outlet syndrome.

In conclusion, our study highlighted the use of spiral CT to facilitate understanding of the functional anatomy of the thoracic outlet. By integrating transverse CT scans, multiplanar reformations, and rapid three-dimensional displays of contrast-enhanced vascular structures, spiral CT angiography is expected to become an important diagnostic tool for evaluation of thoracic outlet syndrome that will help elucidate the site of vascular obstruction. ■

Acknowledgments: The authors are grateful to our CT technologists, Dominique Dumont, Jean-Pierre Guillot, Olivier Lescieux, Abdel Naili, Bertrand Stock, and Martine Wywijas, who helped generate the multiplanar and three-dimensional reformations and calculate the objective parameters used in the present study.

References

1. Peet RM, Henriksen JD, Anderson TP, et al. Thoracic-outlet syndrome: evaluation of a therapeutic exercise program. Mayo Clin Proc Staff Meet 1956; 31:281–287.
2. Luoma A, Nelems B. Thoracic outlet syndrome: thoracic surgery perspective. Neurosurg Clin North Am 1991; 2:187–226.
3. Gray H. The ribs. In: Williams PL, Warwick R, eds. Anatomy of the human body. 36th ed. New York, NY: Churchill Livingstone, 1980; 289.
4. Gray H. The subclavian system of arteries. In: Williams PL, Warwick R, eds. Anatomy of the human body. 36th ed. New York, NY: Churchill Livingstone, 1980; 692.
5. Mercier CL, Huguet JF. Conception dynamique de la traversée thoracobrachiale. In: Mercier CL, Huguet JF, eds. Les syndromes vasculaires de la traversée thoracobrachiale. Paris, France: Masson, 1976; 7–34.
6. Loewestein PS. Thrombosis of the axillary vein. JAMA 1924; 82:854.
7. McCleery RS, Kesterson JE, Kirtley JA, et al. Subclavius and anterior scalene muscle compression as a cause of intermittent obstruction of the subclavius vein. Ann Surg 1951; 133:588–602.
8. Falconer MA, Weddell G. Costoclavicular compression of the subclavius artery and vein: relation to the scalenus anticus syndrome. Lancet 1983; 2:539–545.
9. Telford ED, Mottershead S. Pressure at the cervicobrachial junction. J Bone Joint Surg 1948; 30:249.
10. Serratrice B, Schiano A. Sur la valeur de certaines manoeuvres d'exploration clinique du hile neurovasculaire du membre supérieur. N Presse Med 1978; 43:3932–3933.
11. Gergoudis R, Barnes RM. Thoracic outlet arterial compression: prevalence in normal persons. Angiology 1980; 31:538–541.
12. Hachulla E, Camilleri G, Fournier C, Vinckier L. Etude clinique, vélocimétrique et radiologique de la traversée thoracobrachiale chez 95 sujets témoins: limites physiologiques et incidences pratiques. Rev Med Int 1990; 11:19–24.
13. Moseley HF. The clavicle: its anatomy and function. Clin Orthop Relat Res 1968; 58:17–27.
14. Pollak EW. Clinical presentation. In: Thoracic outlet syndrome: diagnosis and treatment. Mount Kisko, NY: Futura, 1986; 37–70.
15. Pollak EW. Surgical anatomy of the thoracic outlet syndrome. Surg Gynecol Obstet 1980; 150:97–103.
16. Jurik AG, Lansen LC, Hansen J. Radiation dose by spiral CT and conventional tomography of the sternoclavicular joints and the manubrium sterni. Skeletal Radiol 1996; 25:467–470.

Book Review

Spiral CT of the Chest

Edited by Martine Rémy-Jardin, MD, PhD, and Jacques Rémy, MD

Brooklyn, NY: Springer-Verlag New York, 1996. ISBN 3-540-59185-0. Cloth, $198.00; pp 338; 243 figures; tables.

Dr Rémy-Jardin and Dr Rémy, two internationally known thoracic radiologists with early and extensive experience in spiral computed tomography (CT) of the chest, have assembled a distinguished group of authors to produce this comprehensive book. As stated in the preface, spiral CT of the chest is a changing field in thoracic radiology, and refinements in technique, diagnosis, and application are occurring at a rapid pace. This textbook fulfills the goal of summarizing the current knowledge in a practical format for the practicing radiologist.

Nearly every aspect of the spiral CT examination is covered. Basic knowledge in the performance of the examination—including principles, exposure, techniques of acquisition, injection, and reconstruction—are thoroughly discussed. Subsequent chapters include diseases of various anatomic regions such as focal lung disease and diseases of the lung parenchyma, trachea and bronchi, chest wall, pulmonary vessels, superior vena cava, and thoracic aorta. A special chapter is devoted to pulmonary embolism. Because (*a*) the current trend, in pulmonary embolism, is to perform spiral CT and (*b*) many radiologists perform and interpret this study with difficulty, this textbook is more than worthwhile because of this chapter.

The figures are first-rate. The quality of the appropriately labeled radiographs is excellent. The spiral CT axial images are supplemented with various reconstructions (some in color) and appropriate angiographic images and bronchoscopic photographs. In the preliminary chapters on technique, there are numerous diagrams and tables to supplement the text.

In any multiauthored textbook, there are inevitably some different opinions among authors. One example is whether to scan from the apex of the lung to the base or vice versa. The different authors advocated one of the different methods. Although there is no correct method, a few notes from the editors would have been interesting. In addition, many chapters began with a basic review of the principles and techniques, which were covered more extensively in preceding chapters. On the other hand, in the chapter on the principles of spiral CT, a fair amount of mathematics is presented that is possibly beyond the interest or knowledge of most practicing radiologists. Perhaps a thorough but less technical discussion in the first chapter (without repeated discussion in subsequent chapters) might be considered in future editions.

There are no other textbooks, to my knowledge, that are nearly as comprehensive as this textbook. Technical aspects and medical diseases are well covered. Although the field of spiral CT is changing, this textbook provides the basic framework for anyone, generalist or thoracic radiologist, to practice in this field.

Reviewed by Joseph H. Tashjian, MD

Kenneth D. Hopper, MD • Steven H. King, MS • Mark E. Lobell, MD
Thomas R. TenHave, PhD • Jill S. Weaver, BSRT

The Breast: In-plane X-ray Protection during Diagnostic Thoracic CT—Shielding with Bismuth Radioprotective Garments[1]

PURPOSE: To evaluate the ability of thin overlying bismuth radioprotective shielding to reduce the x-ray dose to radiosensitive superficial organs during diagnostic computed tomography (CT).

MATERIALS AND METHODS: A variety of patient and phantom studies were performed with four thicknesses of bismuth radioprotective latex over the breast. Dose savings were determined with thermoluminescent dosimeters. A prototype and then a final manufactured radioprotective brassiere was constructed and tested for radiation dose savings to the breast during diagnostic chest CT. Preliminary studies were also performed to evaluate shielding of the thyroid, orbit, and testes.

RESULTS: The use of bismuth radioprotective latex saved an average 57% of the radiation dose to the breast from thoracic CT, decreasing the radiation level from an average 2.2 rad (0.022 Gy) to 1.0 rad (0.010 Gy) ($P < .001$). Preliminary tests of shielding other superficial radiosensitive organs frequently included at diagnostic CT (eyes, thyroid gland, and testes) were performed with the same thickness of overlying bismuth radioprotective latex, with similar results. Radiation to the thyroid gland was reduced by 60% (from 0.0573 to 0.0229 Gy) and radiation to the eye and testes was reduced by 40% (from 0.0256 to 0.0154 Gy) and 51% (from 0.0463 to 0.0229 Gy), respectively.

CONCLUSION: The use of in-plane overlying bismuth radioprotective latex manufactured into form-fitting garments did not affect the diagnostic CT image but reduced the amount of radiation to radiosensitive superficial structures.

The increased incidence and awareness of breast cancer have focused attention on predisposing factors including radiation from medical x rays (1,2). We have experimented with the use of thin, in-plane (within the image) radioprotective shielding (bismuth) of the patient's breasts during diagnostic computed tomography (CT). Leaded radioprotective shielding is commonly used in radiologic procedures to block x rays from reaching certain areas, but to our knowledge thin shielding has not been used within the diagnostic portion of an x-ray image. Our goal with this project was to determine if it is possible to decrease radiation exposure during thoracic CT without decreasing image quality in the breast and other commonly scanned superficial radiosensitive organs such as the eye, thyroid, and scrotum.

MATERIALS AND METHODS

Preliminary Studies

Radiation-resistant gloves have been marketed to angiographers in an effort to minimize hand and wrist radiation exposure while they perform cardioangiographic procedures. In these gloves, bismuth or lead is impregnated or coated onto latex. In evaluating these two types of radioprotective material, we found that bismuth provided greater attenuation than did lead, especially at the higher kilovoltage settings used in CT.

Attenuation values for bismuth radioprotective latex (F & L Medical Products, Vandergrift, Pa) were the following: 60 kVp = 32%, half-value layer = 2.3 mm of aluminum; 80 kVp = 25%, half-value layer = 3.3 mm Al; 100 kVp = 18%, half-value layer = 4.3 mm Al; 120 kVp = 14%, half-value layer = 5.6 mm Al. Attenuation values for lead-impregnated latex (International Biomedical, Austin, Tex) were the following: 60 kVp = 34%, half-value layer = 2.2 mm Al; 80 kVp = 30%, half-value layer = 2.8 mm Al; 100 kVp = 24%, half-value layer = 3.6 mm Al; 125 kVp = 20%, half-value layer= −4.4 mm Al.

In addition, the bismuth radioprotective latex was more elastic and moldable to the body's surface than the lead-impregnated latex. For these reasons, we concentrated our study on the bismuth radioprotective latex.

Hereafter, we refer to thickness 1, 2, 3, or 4 of the bismuth radioprotective latex as representing 14%, 28%, 42%, and 56% attenuation values at 120 kV. Each thickness contained 0.85 gm/cm^2 of bismuth and had a lead equivalence of 0.015 mm. All unshielded control radiation measurements were performed in a plane of section with no radioprotective material. Use of the opposite patient or phantom breast as a control while the other breast was shielded would be invalid, as x rays aligned with the shield and control detectors would be attenuated. All patient examinations were performed on either a PQ2000 or PQ5000 CT scanner (Picker International, Highland Heights, Ohio). All phantom studies were performed on the latter. The inherent filtration of the x-ray tubes used during these studies was 1.5–1.8 mm Al at 130 kV.

Initially, thicknesses 1 and 2 of the bismuth were scanned with a standard CT water phantom used for daily calibrations,

Index terms: Breast, CT, 00.1211 • Computed tomography (CT), radiation exposure • Radiations, exposure to patients and personnel

Radiology 1997; 205:853–858

[1] From the Department of Radiology (K.D.H., S.H.K., J.S.W.), the College of Medicine (M.E.L.), and the Center for Biostatistics and Epidemiology (T.R.T.), Penn State University, 500 University Dr, PO Box 850, Hershey, PA 17033. Received January 27, 1997; revision requested March 24; revision received July 7; accepted July 8. **Address reprint requests to** K.D.H.

K.D.H. has filed for patent protection to the U.S. Patent Office for this concept. Patent ownership has been assigned to F&L Medical (Vandergrift, Pa) under a licensing agreement.

with a standard calibration technique (130 kV, 400 mAs). The images were evaluated for any type of artifact on the homogeneous water-phantom image. Scanning was then repeated with a wide variety of clinical techniques with thicknesses 1–4 of the bismuth radioprotective latex. Any fold or crease in the material presented a sharp edge off which beam hardening artifact was created and transmitted through the image. When the material was carefully and smoothly applied over the phantom, however, there was no artifact. We used this information in an application to our institutional review board and obtained approval to begin human testing.

Table 1
Patient Examinations: Absorbed Breast Dose

Shielding	No. of Measurements*	Dose (R): Dose	Dose (R): Standard Deviation	Dose (R): Range	Percentage Change from Control	*P* Value
Thickness 1 (n = 25)						
Maximum	25	3.70	1.40	1.7–7.4	−26.9	.7
Mean	175	2.75	1.37	0.6–7.4	−22.8	.9
Thickness 2 (n = 25)						
Maximum	25	2.84	1.02	1.4–5.5	−43.9	.02
Mean	175	2.14	0.98	0.5–5.5	−39.9	.03
Thickness 3 (n = 10)						
Maximum	10	2.76	0.66	1.5–4.0	−45.5	.02
Mean	70	1.91	0.76	0.8–4.0	−46.3	.001
Thickness 4 (n = 10)						
Maximum	10	2.41	0.71	1.4–3.7	−52.4	.003
Mean	70	1.76	0.64	0.7–3.7	−50.6	.0003
Control (n = 10)						
Maximum	20†	5.06	1.28	3.47–8.53	NA	NA
Mean	140	3.56	1.47	1.09–8.53	NA	NA
Prototype garment						
Thickness 4 (n = 10)						
Maximum	20†	1.39	0.28	NA	NA	<.001
Mean	140	0.96	0.38	0.3–2.3	NA	<.001
Control (n = 10)						
Maximum	20†	2.89	0.96	NA	NA	NA
Mean	140	2.24	0.82	0.6–4.0	NA	NA

Note.—For conversion to SI units, 1 R = 2.58 × 10^{-4} C/kg. NA = not applicable.
* Seven thermoluminescent dosimeters per breast.
† Both breasts.

Human Testing

Initially, 25 adult (18 years or older) female patients were recruited into the study on the basis of the entry criteria: They volunteered, signed a consent form, had both breasts, and were scheduled to undergo medically indicated thoracic CT. Women with childbearing potential were not excluded. A set of seven thermoluminescent dosimeters (TLD 100 lithium floride detectors; Harshaw, Solon, Ohio) were taped on each breast, parallel to the long axis of the patient and medial to the nipple. These detectors are sensitive to 10 mR (25.8 × 10^{-4} C/kg). All detectors came from the same manufactured batch and have a precision of ±15%. This area of the breast was selected because it is relatively flat in the supine patient. Thickness 1 (right breast) or thickness 2 (left breast) of bismuth radioprotective latex was taped over the detectors in 20-cm squares. The scanning protocol and CT technical parameters were not modified in any way because of the patient's inclusion in this study. The detector sets were labeled "right breast" or "left breast" and were returned to the Health Physics Section for dose determination. Each scan was monitored during acquisition to assess any artifact into the diagnostic portion of the image that may have resulted from use of the radioprotective material.

On the basis of results in the first 25 patients, scanning was performed in an additional 10 patients with thickness 3 of bismuth radioprotective latex placed over the right breast and thickness 4 placed over the left breast. To evaluate the unshielded breast dose from our thoracic CT technique, an additional 10 patients were recruited and underwent scanning with detector sets placed on each breast without application of overlying radioprotective material.

On the basis of results in these 45 patients, a garment (brassiere) was manufactured that incorporated the equivalent of four layers of the bismuth radioprotective latex to cover the entire breasts and axilla. An additional 10 patients were then recruited into the study, and scanning was performed with detector sets placed on both breasts just medial to the nipple. For these patients, two other detector sets were placed 1 cm below the brassiere, parallel to and in-line with the other two detector sets. As a result, each breast measurement had its own control.

Phantom Studies

A C-cup brassiere was modified with thickness 2 of the bismuth radioprotective latex sewn inside the right cup and thickness 3 sewn into the left cup. Care was taken during fabrication to ensure there was no overlap or gaps between seams. An anthropomorphic body phantom (Rando; Alderson Research Laboratory, Stamford, Conn) with tissue-equivalent breasts (C cup) (Rando; Phantom Laboratory, Salem, NY) was then scanned with a variety of spiral and conventional techniques with the protective brassiere in place. Thermoluminescent dosimeters were loaded at the base and in the middle portion of the phantom breast to measure absorbed dose. As in the patient studies, detectors (sets of seven) were placed medial to the nipple, and scanning was performed both with and without the brassiere. The scanning parameters selected represent a spectrum of scanning techniques to include varying milliampere and kilovoltage settings and both conventional and spiral (helical) CT.

Preliminary Tests in the Thyroid, Orbit, and Testicle

The anthropomorphic phantom was scanned with superficial detectors taped over the eyes, thyroid, and testes and covered on both sides with thickness 4 of bismuth radioprotective latex. Scanning was performed with standard orbital, cervical spine, or pelvic CT techniques. Specific shapes of the bismuth radioprotective latex were cut and fitted to the eyes, thyroid gland, and testes. A set of four detectors (eight for the testes) were placed underneath the latex on each side. All scanning was repeated with use of unshielded detector sets. These tests were repeated four times for the eyes and thyroid and twice for the testes.

Statistical Analysis

The statistical analysis of significant differences between shielded and unshielded groups for each combination of shield type was performed with a mixed-effects linear model with interactions between shield and shield type and milliampere and kilovoltage settings as covariates. Random effects were included for the subject in the models to account for within-subject correlation. The random-effects variance was allowed to depend on the shield and shield type combination. Bonferroni adjustments were made to *P* values and confidence intervals for shielded and unshielded comparisons within shield type to adjust for multiple comparisons such that the overall probability of a type 1 error was 0.05. Each confidence interval presented in the text and Table 1 was derived by dividing each confidence limit for the raw shielded-to-unshielded difference by the unshielded dose. Few if any departures from normality and constant variance of the residuals under all models were detected with residual diagnoses.

At spiral CT, the x-ray beam crosses the patient's skin surface obliquely, forming a

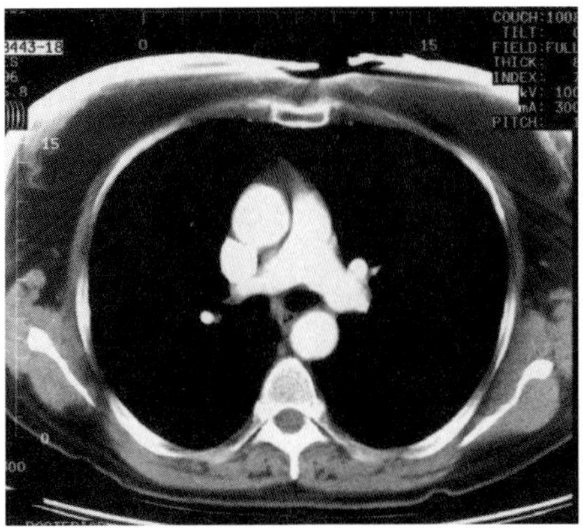

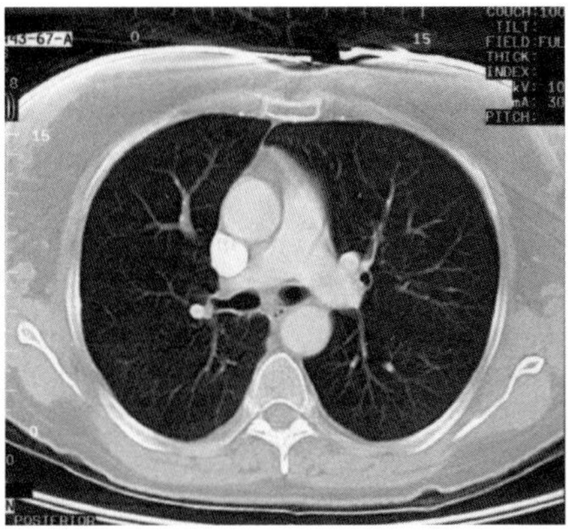

a. b.

(a) Mediastinal (window width, 375 HU; level, 40 HU) and **(b)** lung (window width, 1,800 HU; level, −350 HU) scans were obtained at diagnostic thoracic CT while the patient wore the prototype bismuth radioprotective latex garment. The net effect was to reduce superficial absorbed dose to both breasts by more than one-half. The artifact from this shielding is close to the skin surface and does not project into the diagnostic portions of the image. Both images were obtained in the same section after first a routine reconstruction (once for the mediastinum [standard interpolation and algorithm] and second for the lung parenchyma [extra sharp interpolation and bone algorithm]).

helix. As a result, each superficial point of the patient receives an uneven dose from the x ray, which increased the complexity of our data. For that reason, all data are reported as the mean of all seven detectors, with data from the detector among each set that reported the highest dose, with the percentage change and 95% confidence intervals.

RESULTS

Patient Studies

With use of the maximum dose (among the seven detectors), thickness 1 of bismuth radioprotective latex decreased the breast radiation dose from 5.1 rad (0.051 Gy) to 3.7 rad (0.037 Gy), a difference of −26.9% (95% confidence interval, −1.3%, 0.7% [P = .7]) (Table 1). Use of thickness 2 further decreased the dose to 2.8 rad (0.028 Gy) (−43.9% [95% confidence interval, −1.8%, −0.1%], P = .02), and use of thicknesses 3 and 4 further decreased the dose to 2.8 rad (0.028 Gy) and 2.4 rad (0.024 Gy), respectively. The latter represented a decrease of 52.4% (95% confidence interval, −2.2%, 0.5% [P = .003]) from findings in the unshielded breast. Assessment of the mean absorbed dose in the same patients showed a similar trend. The mean absorbed dose for thickness 4 of the bismuth radioprotective latex was 1.8 rad (0.018 Gy). There was no shielding-related artifact projected into or increased noise within the lung parenchyma or mediastinum in any patient (Figure).

Phantom Studies

Use of the anthropomorphic phantom with its tissue-equivalent breast and the protective brassiere allowed the evaluation of various imaging parameters (milliampere and kilovoltage settings, scan type, and pitch) and their effect on the breast radiation dose. For instance, all patients underwent spiral CT with a pitch of 1.5, 300 mA, and 120 kV. Milliampere settings in patient examinations were varied somewhat, however, on the basis of the patient's size, with a higher milliampere setting used in larger patients. This patient-to-patient variability was eliminated with use of a phantom. In addition, use of the constant-size phantom allowed use of a specially manufactured, well-fitted brassiere.

With standard CT technique (300 mA, 120 kV), the average glandular and superficial breast dose was reduced approximately 1.7 rad (0.017 Gy) (Table 2). For instance, the middle-of-the-breast glandular dose is 5.0 rad (0.05 Gy) for the unshielded breast and 3.0 rad (0.03 Gy) for the breast shielded with thickness 2 of the bismuth radioprotective latex. Use of thickness 3 proportionately decreased the dose further. For instance, the glandular deep breast (chest-wall) dose was decreased from 5.1 rad (0.051 Gy) to 2.8 rad (0.028 Gy) with use of thickness 3.

Modification of the CT technique, as would be expected, resulted in a further decrease in the glandular and superficial breast radiation dose and somewhat reduced the advantages of use of shielding. For instance, a decrease to 110 kV and then to 100 kV (with 300 mA) decreased the middle-of-the-breast glandular dose with use of thickness 2 of bismuth radioprotective latex from 5.0 rad (0.050 Gy) to 2.1 rad (0.021 Gy) and 1.7 rad (0.017 Gy), respectively. A reduction in the kilovoltage setting without use of the protective brassiere resulted in a reduction in the middle-of-the-breast glandular dose to 3.6 rad (0.036 Gy) and 2.5 rad (0.025 Gy), respectively (Table 2).

A decrease in the milliampere setting had an even greater effect. The middle-of-the-breast glandular dose was reduced from 5.0 rad (0.050 Gy) to 3.0 rad (0.030 Gy) with 300 mA and 120 kV and with use of thickness 2 material. A decrease to 200 mA and then to 100 mA further reduced the breast dose to 1.7 rad (0.017 Gy) and 1.2 rad (0.012 Gy), respectively.

In spiral CT, the speed at which the patient moves through the x-ray beam can be varied. When the patient is moved the equivalent of one section per second (assuming 1-second tube rotation), the pitch (patient speed) is 1. If, however, the patient moves through the beam at a rate of more than one section per second, the radiation dose to the patient (and breast) is decreased. For instance, with use of a pitch of 1.5 when the patient moves 1.5 sections per second, the net radiation dose would decrease by one-third. Pitch greater than 1 can be used with breast radioprotective material to further decrease the dose. For instance, a middle-of-the-breast glandular dose that is decreased from 5.00 rad (0.050 Gy) to 3.02 rad (0.0302 Gy) by adding thickness 2 material can be decreased further to 2.18 rad (0.0218 Gy) by using a pitch of 1.5 (Table 2). All of our patient thoracic CT examinations were performed with a pitch of 1.5.

We evaluated the effect of moving the phantom breast closer to the edge of the gantry aperture, by elevating the table 5 or 7.5 cm. Interestingly, with the breasts elevated to touch the gantry (table elevated 7.5 cm) to mimic the position of the breasts in larger women, the breast radiation dose was reduced (Table 2). As CT provides circumferential x rays to the patient (and breast), this reduction is likely a result of the breasts receiving fewer side-to-side x rays.

Patient Studies with the Prototype Brassiere

A prototype brassiere with thickness 4 of the bismuth radioprotective latex was manufactured to fit an average sized breast (C cup). Measurements in these 20 breasts (10 patients) demonstrated a mean reduction in the radiation dose to the breasts from 2.2

Table 2
Phantom Data: Glandular Dose

Position and Technique	Thickness 2 Dose (R) Chest Wall*	Thickness 2 Dose (R) Middle of the Breast*	Thickness 2 Dose (R) Superficial	Thickness 3 Dose (R) Chest Wall*	Thickness 3 Dose (R) Middle of the Breast*	Thickness 3 Dose (R) Superficial
Shielded Breast						
Center chest isocenter in gantry						
300 mA; 120 kV; conventional†	3.14 (0.24)	3.02 (0.22)	3.76 (0.29)	2.77 (0.38)	2.57 (0.16)	3.07 (0.44)
300 mA; 110 kV; spiral; pitch, 1	2.19 (0.31)	2.07 (0.25)	2.55 (0.51)	1.80 (0.15)	1.60 (0.15)	1.88 (0.24)
300 mA; 120 kV; spiral; pitch, 1.5	2.24 (0.77)	2.18 (0.71)	2.01 (0.92)	1.43 (0.27)	1.02 (0.16)	1.61 (0.59)
300 mA; 100 kV; spiral; pitch, 1	1.90 (0.51)	1.73 (0.32)	1.89 (0.35)	1.54 (0.40)	1.73 (0.45)	1.36 (0.22)
200 mA; 120 kV; spiral; pitch, 1	1.74 (0.17)	1.68 (0.37)	2.12 (0.47)	1.76 (0.48)	1.31 (0.14)	1.56 (0.23)
100 mA; 120 kV; spiral; pitch, 1	1.23 (0.32)	1.18 (0.30)	1.05 (0.17)	1.03 (0.24)	0.93 (0.21)	0.82 (0.10)
Center chest elevated above gantry isocenter						
300 mA, 120 kV, conventional						
Isocenter +5 cm	3.60 (1.10)	3.23 (1.03)	3.07 (0.36)	2.65 (0.77)	2.89 (0.67)	2.39 (0.49)
Isocenter +7.5 cm	2.34 (0.50)	2.09 (0.71)	2.57 (0.33)	2.49 (0.54)	1.73 (0.50)	1.99 (0.40)
Unshielded Breast						
Center chest isocenter in gantry						
300 mA; 110 kV; spiral; pitch, 1.0	3.54 (1.19)	3.23 (1.06)	4.21 (0.69)	4.07 (0.67)	4.12 (0.23)	4.32 (0.89)
300 mA; 120 kV; conventional	4.88 (1.37)	5.00 (1.25)	NM	5.09 (1.04)	5.99 (1.59)	NM

Note.—For conversion to SI units, 1 R = 2.58 × 10^{-4} C/kg. Numbers in parentheses are the standard deviation. NM = not measured.
* Glandular dose.
† For equivalent milliampere and kilovolt settings, the radiation dose with a pitch of 1 is equivalent to that at conventional CT.

rad (0.022 Gy) to 1.0 rad (0.010 Gy) (−57.1%, P = .001) (Table 1). Although artifacts were noted in superficial breast tissue, no artifact was seen in the lung parenchyma or mediastinum in any patient as a result of use of the radioprotective garment.

Table 3
Preliminary Data from Other Superficial Radiosensitive Organs

Organ	Thickness 4 Dose (R) Mean	Thickness 4 Dose (R) Standard Deviation	Thickness 4 Dose (R) Maximum
Eye*			
Shielded	1.54	0.16	1.89
Unshielded	2.56	0.26	2.98
Percentage change from control	−39.8		−36.6
Thyroid†			
Shielded	2.29	0.12	2.44
Unshielded	5.73	0.55	6.63
Percentage change from control	−60.0		63.2
Testes‡			
Shielded	2.29	0.19	2.61
Unshielded	4.63	0.51	5.66
Percentage change from control	−50.5		−53.9

Note.—For conversion to SI units, 1 R = 2.58 × 10^{-4} C/kg.
* Orbital CT: 120 kV, 315 mA, 4-mm-thick sections, half field.
† Cervical spine CT: 120 kV, 315 mA, 4-mm-thick sections, full field.
‡ Pelvic CT: 120 kV, 315 mA, 8-mm-thick sections, full field.

Preliminary Tests in the Thyroid, Orbits, and Testicle

Last, we performed preliminary superficial dose measurements with use of radioprotective material to cover other superficial radiosensitive organs (eyes, thyroid, and testes). As in the breast, 40%–60% radiation dose savings were achieved (Table 3). Quantitatively, the greatest dose savings were experienced in the thyroid gland. With use of standard cervical spine CT technique, the mean dose was reduced by more than 3 rad (0.03 Gy) (−60%) with use of thickness 4 of bismuth radioprotective latex. With use of a similar thickness of bismuth radioprotective latex during head or pelvic CT, 40% (from 0.0256 to 0.0154 Gy) and 51% (from 0.0463 to 0.0229 Gy) of the radiation to the eye and testes, respectively, was avoided. Further studies are required to verify these findings.

DISCUSSION

It is an understatement to say that breast cancer is a major national health care concern. In 1994, 180,000 new cases of breast cancer were diagnosed in the United States, and its incidence is increasing (1). While the U.S. female population increased from 104 to 133 million between 1970 and 1994 (+28%), the annual incidence increased from 68,000 to 182,000, an increase of 168%. This disparate increase may be due in part to changing population demographics and increased surveillance (mammography), but other factors must also be at work.

During this same time, explosive advances in radiologic diagnosis have rivaled advances in the initial decades after Roentgen's discovery of the x ray in 1895. Among the many innovations, the development of diagnostic ultrasound, CT, magnetic resonance imaging, and low-dose screen-film mammography has revolutionized our diagnostic approach to medical care.

With these inventions, however, has come increased utilization. Some physicians would argue that many of these diagnostic tests are over used, and clinical acumen has taken a back seat. Regardless, the modern physician is in a position to use an impressive array of diagnostic tests in the evaluation of his or her patients. Fre-

Table 4
Increased Breast Cancer Risk

Average Age (y) at Breast Cancer Occurrence	No. of Cases	Fractional Increase in Breast Cancer Rate over Spontaneous Rate	
		Per 1 R	Per Thoracic CT Examination*
32	27	0.136	0.340 (34.0)
41	80	0.013	0.033 (3.3)
49	85	0.024	0.060 (6.0)
57	13	0.017	0.043 (4.3)

Note.—Data are based on data in reference 2. For conversion to SI units, 1 R = 2.58×10^{-4} C/kg.
* Assumed absorbed breast dose, 2.5 rad (0.025 Gy) per examination. Numbers in parentheses are percentages.

quently, the only restrictions are the physician's judgment and pressures to control costs from third-party payers or managed care providers.

Missing from this equation, though, is an awareness of the radiation dose from many of these radiologic procedures. Thoracic CT is a commonly ordered test, but few requesting physicians are aware that a woman's breast receives 2.0–3.5 rad (0.020–0.035 Gy) of radiation from the examination. In comparison, chest radiography and mammography (3–8) provide approximately 1% and 10% as much dose, respectively. With use of data obtained in A-bomb survivors, Land et al (2) predict that delivery of 1 rad (0.01 Gy) of radiation to the breast of a woman younger than 35 years increases her lifetime breast cancer risk by 13.6%.

The patients included in this study all underwent spiral CT. With this new method, the patient is advanced at an even speed through the x-ray beam while a volume (rather than individual sections) is scanned. The advantages of spiral CT include elimination of section-to-section (breath-to-breath) misregistrations because the entire examination is performed in one patient breath hold. The speed of a spiral examination is also dramatically increased, and the necessary amount of intravenous contrast material is reduced. The routine performance of spiral CT in the chest allows use of a lower milliampere setting and, to some extent, a lower kilovoltage setting, and a greater pitch, all of which reduce the dose to the breast. All the patients in this study underwent scanning in this manner (1.5 pitch, 150–175 mA, 100 kV). The dose savings we report from use of bismuth radioprotective latex shielding are in addition to those afforded with use of these CT technique modifications. Our attempts to further reduce breast dose with use of very low milliampere settings or pitches greater than 1.5 have not been successful because of the unacceptable increase in mediastinal noise and parenchymal blurring. In institutions where conventional CT is performed with higher milliampere and kilovoltage settings or spiral CT is performed with a pitch of 1.0, the radiation dose to the breast and potential dose savings from use of the radioprotective garments would be higher than that reported in our patients.

The breast radiation dose from thoracic CT is dependent on several variables including kilovoltage and milliampere settings (use of higher settings results in increased dose), section thickness (use of thinner sections results in increased dose), number of adjacent sections (acquisition of more sections results in increased dose), and patient size (smaller patients receive an increased dose). Marked variation in radiation dose can be seen in examinations performed with different brands of CT scanners (8–10). At conventional diagnostic chest CT in an average-sized woman, her breasts will receive from 2 rad (0.02 Gy) to 5 rad (0.05 Gy) of absorbed radiation, which is equivalent to the amount of absorbed radiation in 10–25 two-view mammographic examinations and in more than 100 chest radiographs. The seriousness of the dose administered to such a radiosensitive organ should not be understated.

The breast is radiosensitive, or, in other words, the breast is susceptible to cancer induced by radiation. Information on the carcinogenesis of x rays in the breast is inexact, but the breasts of adolescent and young adult women are especially susceptible (1,2,11–14). Although the source of the radiation was mostly not from x rays, the best data acquired to date on the long-term effects of radiation in young female breasts is found in demographic studies of Japanese A-bomb survivors (1,2,14). For instance, delivery of 1 rad (0.01 Gy) of radiation to a woman's breasts before age 35 years fractionally (multiplicatively) increases her risk of breast cancer by 13.6% over the expected spontaneous rate for the general population. Delivery of the same dose after age 35 years fractionally increases a woman's risk of breast cancer by only approximately 2% (Table 4). In long-term follow-up (average, 26 years) of 1,030 patients with scoliosis who had received an average dose of 13 rad (0.13 Gy) of breast radiation from whole-spine radiography during adolescence, Hoffman et al (13) found 11 had developed breast cancers. On the basis of population demographics, however, only six were expected to have developed cancer. Realizing that the average thoracic CT examination delivers 2–5 rad (0.2–0.5 Gy) of absorbed radiation to the female breast, its effect on breast carcinogenesis is obvious in patients older than 35 years of age and especially in patients younger than 35 years.

The primary purpose of thoracic CT is to provide cross-sectional images of the thorax that include the lungs and mediastinum for diagnostic purposes. Unfortunately, the breasts are in the way and receive added dose because of their superficial location. Other superficial radiosensitive organs are likewise needlessly irradiated during radiologic procedures to include the thyroid gland, the lens of the eye, and the testes. Like the breast, these organs are seldom the target of a diagnostic CT examination. Rather, the radiation is incidental, an unwanted by-product.

It is obvious from the data obtained in our study that use of thin layers of radioabsorbent material such as bismuth can provide superficial radiation protection without affecting the quality of the diagnostic CT image. In none of the phantom examinations, even those performed with thickness 4 of the bismuth radioprotective latex, did we see artifact more than 2 cm below the skin surface. In our patient thoracic CT and breast phantom examinations, this artifact was never reflected into the diagnostic portions of the image, specifically the mediastinum and lungs. Results in our other preliminary tests indicate that use of superficial shielding of the eye lens, thyroid, and testes would not affect CT images obtained in the brain, cervical spine, and pelvis, respectively.

Findings in this study demonstrate the potential for use of thinly layered radioprotective garments to significantly reduce superficial absorbed radiation in radiosensitive organs from diagnostic x-ray procedures, especially CT. Whether use of bismuth or lead is optimum will be decided on the basis of ease of manufacturing, versatility, fit, and cost. The optimum amount of bismuth or lead to be used over radiosensitive organs to avoid adversely increasing noise or otherwise affecting image quality must be determined for the eyes, thyroid gland, breast, and testes. The expense of these radioprotective garments may outweigh their advantages.

The results of this study are clear. Use of thinly layered radioprotective material within the plane of a CT image can significantly reduce absorbed radiation dose to superficial radiosensitive organs. Our preliminary results in the breast show a reduction of up to 4 rad (0.04 Gy) with use of these radioprotective garments, depending on the CT technique used. This equates to a savings in that breast of the equivalent of five to 20 two-view mammographic examinations. Use of shielding in the breasts of younger woman may be even more beneficial because of their increased sensitivity.

Thick leaded x-ray shielding has been used to completely block x rays through a given area since shortly after Roentgen's invention of the "invisible light" more than 100 years ago. Findings in our study demonstrate the usefulness of in-plane, thin x-ray shielding to selectively protect superficial radiosensitive organs without affecting the clear CT display of other deeper structures. If such shielding is easy to use and if radioprotective garments can be manufactured inexpensively, the net benefit to patients would be of major importance. ■

References

1. American Cancer Society. Cancer facts and figures. Atlanta, Ga: American Cancer Society, 1994.
2. Land CE, Tokunaga M, Tokuaka S, Nakamura N. Early-onset breast cancer in A-bomb survivors. Lancet 1993; 342:237.
3. Wu X, Gingold EL, Barnes GT, Tucker DM. Normalized average glandular dose in molybdenum target–rhodium filter and rhodium target–rhodium filter mammography. Radiology 1994; 193:83–89.
4. Helvie MA, Chan HP, Adler DD, Boyd PG. Breast thickness in routine mammograms: effect on image quality and radiation dose. AJR 1994; 163:1371–1374.
5. Wu X, Barnes GT, Tucker DM. Spectral dependence of glandular tissue dose in screen-film mammography. Radiology 1991; 179:143–148.
6. Skubic SE, Fatouros PP. Absorbed breast dose: dependence on radiographic modality and technique and breast thickness. Radiology 1986; 161:263–270.
7. Liu B, Goodsitt M, Chan HP. Normalized average glandular dose in magnification mammography. Radiology 1995; 197: 27–32.
8. McCollough CH, Liu HH. Breast dose during electron-beam CT: measurement with film dosimetry. Radiology 1995; 196: 153–157.
9. Evans SH, Davis R, Cooke J, Anderson W. A comparison of radiation doses to the breast in computed tomographic chest examinations for two scanning protocols. Clin Radiol 1989; 40:45–46.
10. Bruggen-Bugaarts BA, Broerse JJ, Lammers JW, Van Waes PF, Geleijns J. Radiation exposure in standard and high-resolution chest CT scans. Chest 1995; 107:113–115.
11. Modan B, Alfandary E, Chetrit A, Katz L. Increased risk of breast cancer after low-dose irradiation. Lancet 1989; 1:629–630.
12. Schüler G, Stoll E. Too little concern for breast cancer risk in radiation protection estimates? Health Phys 1991; 61:405–408.
13. Hoffman DA, Lonstein JE, Morin MM, Visscher W, Harris SH III, Boice JD Jr. Breast cancer in women with scoliosis exposed to multiple diagnostic x rays. J Natl Cancer Inst 1989; 81:1307–1312.
14. Tokunaga M, Land CE, Tokuoka S, Nishimori I, Soda M, Akiba S. Incidence of female breast cancer among atomic bomb survivors, 1950–1985. Radiat Res 1994; 138: 209–223.

Harold L. Kundel, MD • Warren Gefter, MD • Judith Aronchick, MD • Wallace Miller, Jr, MD
Hiroto Hatabu, MD, PhD • Charlene H. Whitfill, MD • Wallace Miller, Sr, MD

Accuracy of Bedside Chest Hard-Copy Screen-Film versus Hard- and Soft-Copy Computed Radiographs in a Medical Intensive Care Unit: Receiver Operating Characteristic Analysis[1]

PURPOSE: **To compare the clinical diagnostic accuracy of hard-copy readings of screen-film bedside chest radiographs and both hard-and soft-copy readings of bedside chest computed radiographs obtained in a medical intensive care unit.**

MATERIALS AND METHODS: **Two samples of 95 cases were assembled from chest images obtained in 541 patients with either screen-film radiography or computed radiography. The cases were stratified according to the clinical problem for which the examination was ordered; the corresponding diagnosis was verified by a panel of two or three radiologists. Four radiologists blindly read the hard-copy images obtained with screen-film or computed radiography. Six months later, the radiologists read the computed radiographs by using an 8-bit, 1,684 × 2,048-pixel display. The data were analyzed by using multireader-multicase receiver operating characteristic (ROC) analysis of variance.**

RESULTS: **No statistically significant differences in the area under the ROC curve were found between any of the methods.**

CONCLUSION: **The results provide some justification for using bedside chest computed radiography and for reading soft-copy images from a high-quality display.**

MOST comparisons of the diagnostic accuracy of screen-film radiography with that of computed radiography have focused on specific abnormalities—either real (1–7) or simulated (8,9). The abnormalities are selected because they represent some fundamental limit on diagnosis; for example, pneumothoraces are limited by edge rendition and nodules by contrast rendition. It is reasoned that if readers can detect subtle pneumothoraces and nodules as well on computed radiographs as on screen-film radiographs, they will do as well or better with other abnormalities. Conversely, if readers cannot detect the limiting abnormalities as well by using computed radiography, then they are at risk of missing similar, subtle abnormalities if they choose to use computed radiography. However, both the images with and the images without specific abnormalities that are used in the test sets are generally highly selected, and, in the absence of a representative sample, it is impossible to extrapolate the results to a clinical population.

This study was performed to compare the clinical diagnostic accuracy of hard-copy readings of screen-film bedside chest radiographs and both hard- and soft-copy readings of bedside chest computed radiographs obtained in a medical intensive care unit (MICU). Receiver operating characteristic (ROC) analysis was performed on stratified random samples of bedside chest radiographs selected during periods when either screen-film radiography or computed radiography was used exclusively for imaging. The reason for requesting the examination was used as an entry criterion to relate the sample to clinical usage rather than to imaging findings. The sample was stratified to include an adequate number of nonroutine cases.

MATERIALS AND METHODS

Study Design

The study was performed in the 12-bed MICU and the 12-bed intermediate medical care unit of the Hospital of the University of Pennsylvania, Philadelphia, as part of a larger study of the effect of a picture archiving and communication system on patient care (10). Data were collected in a sample of 313 patients during February, March, June, and August of 1993—when bedside chest radiographs were obtained by using screen-film radiography—and in a sample of 218 patients during January, March, April, and October of 1994—when bedside chest radiographs were obtained by using computed radiography. Two days selected at random were skipped each week to allow data entry to keep up with data acquisition. At the beginning of each study month, a cohort of five patients was selected randomly from the patients in the

Index terms: Radiography, bedside, 60.11, 60.121 • Radiography, comparative studies, 60.11, 60.121 • Radiography, computer-assisted, 60.121

Abbreviations: ANOVA = analysis of variance, APACHE = Adult Physiology and Chronic Health Evaluation, MICU = medical intensive care unit, MRMC = multireader multicase, ROC = receiver operating characteristic.

Radiology 1997; 205:859–863

[1] From the Department of Radiology, Pendergrass Diagnostic Research Laboratory, University of Pennsylvania Medical School, 308 Stemmler Hall, 36th & Hamilton Walk, Philadelphia, PA 19104-6086. Received October 18, 1996; revision requested January 2, 1997; final revision received July 22; accepted July 23. Supported by grant CA53141 from the National Cancer Institute, U.S. Public Health Service, Department of Health and Human Services. **Address reprint requests to** H.L.K.

MICU. When a patient in the cohort was discharged, the next patient admitted to the unit was added. The clinical and demographic data collected in the cohort patients were more extensive than those collected in the other patients. The data collected included the Adult Physiology and Chronic Health Evaluation (APACHE) III score, which is an index of disease severity at admission (11).

Twice each day, the radiology information system printed a data form for each newly obtained bedside chest radiograph, and a data coordinator used the forms to conduct structured interviews of members of the house staff responsible for individual patients. The reason for requesting the examination was one of the items that was noted. Bedside chest radiographic examinations were divided into routine and nonroutine examinations. Routine examinations, which constitute about 60% of the chest radiographic examinations performed each day, are obtained between 5 and 8 AM to identify unanticipated complications or to follow the progression of known pulmonary disease. Nonroutine examinations are performed whenever needed for the solution of clinical problems. The main reasons for requesting nonroutine examinations were as follows: (*a*) to check the position of a tube or catheter, (*b*) to rule out or follow up on pneumonia, (*c*) to rule out or follow up on congestive heart failure, (*d*) to rule out or follow up on pneumothorax, and (*e*) to rule out or follow up on pleural effusion. Any other reasons were lumped into a miscellaneous category. The reasons for requesting examinations in the cohort patients are shown in Table 1.

Table 1
Distribution of Screen-Film and Computed Radiographic Examinations in the Patient Cohort according to the Reason for Examination

	No. of Examinations	
Reason for Examination	Screen-Film Radiography	Computed Radiography
Routine surveillance	237 (63)	216 (66)
Check tube or catheter	61 (16)	49 (15)
Rule out or follow up on pneumonia	18 (5)	10 (3)
Rule out or follow up on congestive heart failure	9 (2)	6 (2)
Rule out or follow up on pneumothorax	24 (6)	31 (10)
Rule out or follow up on pleural effusion	2 (1)	1 (<1)
Other	27 (7)	12 (4)
Total	378 (100)	325 (100)

Note.—Numbers in parentheses are percentages.

Table 2
Number of Examinations Eligible for Inclusion in the Reader Study and Number of Examinations in Each of the Two Test Samples

	No. of Examinations Eligible for Reader Study		
Reason for Requesting the Examination	Screen-Film Radiography	Computed Radiography	No. of Examinations in Test Samples
Routine surveillance	237	216	35
Check tube or catheter	161	181	15
Rule out or follow up on pneumonia	83	121	15
Rule out or follow up on congestive heart failure	30	33	15
Rule out or follow up on pneumothorax	59	104	15
Rule out or follow up on pleural effusion	12	10	...
Other	140	134	...

Image Acquisition and Display

Screen-film radiographs were exposed without a grid at 76–86 kVp by using Quanta Fast Detail screens and Cronex film (Sterling, Wilmington, Del). Computed radiographic plates (ST-III; Fuji Medical Systems, Stamford, Conn) were exposed by using the same technical factors and were processed and printed with a LINX system (Sterling). The images were preprocessed by using the general chest protocol suggested by Fuji Medical Systems. By using the Fuji notation, the transfer characteristic can be described in terms of the following factors (GA rotational amount, 1.0; GC rotational center, 1.6; GT contrast type, E; GS density shift, −0.1). A single, 28 × 34-cm, hard-copy image was printed on 35 × 43-cm film by using an LP400 laser printer (Sterling). The computed radiographs were archived as 12-bit, 1,684 × 2,048-pixel images on magnetic medium. For the soft-copy portion of the study, the processed images were displayed on a workstation consisting of a host computer (Sun Microsystems, Sunnyvale, Calif), a monochrome monitor (Sun Microsystems) for the mouse-driven user interface, and two display monitors (Megascan; AVP/E Systems, Boston, Mass) with 2,560 × 2,048, 8-bit pixels. The system has a 12-bit frame buffer and a window and level function that converts the images into 8 bits for display. The workstation also supports rove and zoom and gray-scale inversion and high-resolution functions (12). The high-resolution function converts the image that is initially an averaged 842 × 1,024 representation of the original into a full 1,684 × 2,048 representation. The initial image was downgraded in resolution because it could be displayed in 2 seconds, whereas the full-resolution image required 8 seconds. The zoom function uses the full-resolution image.

Selection of Imaging Examinations for Inclusion in the Study

Two image test sets, each consisting of 95 cases, were assembled after all of the patients in the units during the screen-film radiographic and computed radiographic data collection periods had been discharged from the hospital. This allowed the review panel to withdraw records without interfering with patient care. Nonroutine examinations in all patients and routine examinations in cohort patients were eligible for inclusion. A list of examinations according to request categories was made, with the order of the examinations within each category randomized. The list was used to withdraw patient film folders from the film library. When the film library could not locate a film folder, the next examination on the list was chosen. Images were not excluded because of suboptimal radiologic technique.

The number of examinations eligible for the reader study and the number of examinations in the test sets are shown in Table 2 according to the reasons for requesting the examination. Each test set consisted of 95 examinations—35 routine and 60 nonroutine (15 each for tube and catheter checks, pneumonia, congestive heart failure, and pneumothorax). These categories account for 661 of the 703 examinations (94%) in the cohort of the patients in the MICU (Table 1). Patients with pleural effusion were excluded from the sample because they accounted for only three of the 703 examination requests (0.4%) made in the MICU. The remaining 39 examination requests (5.5%) were too heterogeneous to be able to produce a matched test sample in both screen-film and computed radiographic periods. Two images (the test image and the prior image) were included for the routine category and for follow-up because these requests implied a comparison with prior images. One image was selected when the examination was performed to check the position of a catheter or to rule out disease. The number of eligible examinations in the request categories and in the test sets is shown in Table 2.

Verification Panel

After the 190 examinations were selected for inclusion in the reading study,

Table 3
Examples of the Format of the Questions in the Reader Study

Type of Examination	Question
Routine	Compared with that shown on image A, physiology on image B is 1, definitely changed; 2, probably changed; 3, possibly changed; 4, probably unchanged; 5, definitely unchanged. Other findings?
Nonroutine	
Rule out pneumonia	Pneumonia, major atelectasis, or both are 1, definitely present; 2, probably present; 3, possibly present; 4, probably absent; 5, definitely absent. Other findings?
Follow up on congestive heart failure	Compared with image A, the congestive heart failure on image B is 1, definitely changed; 2, probably changed; 3, possibly changed; 4, probably unchanged; 5, definitely unchanged. Other findings?
Check position of new endotracheal tube	The position of the endotracheal tube is 1, definitely incorrect; 2, probably incorrect; 3, possibly incorrect; 4, probably correct; 5, definitely correct. Other findings?

Note.—Image A and image B refer to the prior and current examinations, respectively.

Table 4
Characteristics of the Patient Population from Which the Stratified Sample of Bedside Chest Examinations Was Drawn

Parameter	Examination: Screen-Film Radiography	Computed Radiography
No. of patients	313	228
Ratio of men to women	0.87	0.91
Average age of men (y)	53	54
Average age of women (y)	56	49
Median length of stay (d)	2.8	2.9
Mortality (%)	23	25
Average APACHE III score	58	57

all of the available chest radiographs obtained before and after the test examination were reviewed by a panel of two radiologists who did not participate as readers. The panel determined the "correct" answer to the question implied by the reason for requesting the examination. Was there pneumonia or major atelectasis? Was the tip of a catheter correctly positioned? The panel had the radiology reports and limited clinical information available to them. The panelists made an independent judgment about the test examination and compared it with the report. If both agreed with the report, that was considered to be the truth. If the report was silent or ambiguous, their opinion was the truth. If both disagreed with the report or if they disagreed with each other, they tried to arrive at a consensus by discussion. If they could not arrive at a consensus, a third radiologist gave an independent opinion and the majority decision was final.

Image Reading Test

The hard-copy images were randomized, numbered sequentially, and given in packets of 10 images to four radiologists who were instructed to respond to the question implied by the reason for ordering the examination by using a five-point rating scale. The structure of the response form is shown in Table 3. The radiologists were given the opportunity to indicate if other important findings were present on the images; however, the answers were not used in the analysis. The radiologists were asked to view the images in their usual environment and were not given any time constraints. Six months separated the end of the hard-copy readings and the start of the soft-copy readings.

The soft-copy images were randomized and read by the same four readers from an individual file that was created on the workstation for each reader. It could be accessed only with her or his password, and it displayed the images randomly along with the response format as in Table 3. A mouse-driven cursor was used to enter the rating. As with the hard-copy images, there was no time constraint, and use of the workstation functions (window, level, zoom, inverse) was optional.

Data Reduction

There was one source of ambiguity in scoring the responses that involved a change between the test image and the prior image. A reader could have correctly reported a change but incorrectly reported that disease severity had increased when the panel had determined that it had decreased. Increase or decrease was not included in the responses (Table 3) because increase-decrease disagreement was rare. In an independent study of the MICU cases, we found that in routine cases there was yes-no disagreement but no increase-decrease disagreement in 78 of 416 cases (19%). In the nonroutine cases, there was yes-no disagreement in 27 of 639 cases (4%) and increase-decrease disagreement in three (0.5%).

Data Analysis

The rating scale data were analyzed by using the multireader-multicase (MRMC) ROC analysis of variance (ANOVA) method of Dorfman and colleagues (13). The cases for the comparison of hard-copy and soft-copy computed radiographs were paired (eg, each reader saw the same cases with both displays). Although the diagnostic categories were the same, the individual cases used for the comparison of hard-copy screen-film and computed radiographs were different and, therefore, the cases were unpaired. The public domain MRMC program is designed for paired cases and at present will not handle unpaired cases. To use ANOVA on the screen-film and computed radiographic hard-copy data, Kevin Berbaum, PhD, and Donald Dorfman, PhD, generalized the MRMC program to handle unpaired data by using what is called a split-plot design. The MRMC program uses a jackknife technique to generate ROC area pseudovalues, which are then used in a standard ANOVA. An ANOVA table is generated that includes the variance due to the modality, the readers, and the cases, as well as the interactions. In the split-plot design, readers and cases are random factors and the modality is fixed. The cases are nested within the treatments.

To show the effect of the stratifying variable (reason for examination) on the overall area under the ROC curve (A_z), the MRMC pseudovalues for each request category were averaged to determine a category A_z.

ROC curves for the three conditions were calculated by averaging the confidence ratings of the four readers by using the ROCFIT program (14).

RESULTS

Some of the demographic and medical characteristics of the randomly selected cohort of patients are shown in Table 4. These data and the distribution of examination requests shown in Table 1 indicate that the patient populations in the units during the two study periods were very similar. The distribution of normal and abnormal cases in each request category (as judged by the panel) was also similar ($\chi^2 = 0.8$, 4 *df*).

The mean A_zs for the group and for the individual radiologists are given in Table 5. The difference between screen-film and computed radiographic hard-copy images of −.015 is not statistically significant, with a Satterthwaite approximate F(1,53) of .09. The difference between screen-film and computed radiographic soft-copy images of .010 is not statistically significant, with an F(1,188) of .04. The difference between soft-copy and hard-copy computed radiographs was −.025, with a 95% confidence interval of −.077, .026. The difference is not statistically significant, with an F(1,188) of .91.

The A_z values attributed to each of the request categories are shown in Table 6. The Figure compares the ROC curves for hard-copy screen-film and hard- and soft-copy computed radiographs.

Table 5
A_z Computed with MRMC ANOVA

Reader	Screen-Film Radiography	Computed Radiography: Hard-Copy Images	Computed Radiography: Soft-Copy Images
1	.84	.87	.84
2	.86	.84	.83
3	.85	.93	.86
4	.85	.81	.83
1–4 (mean ± standard deviation)	.85 ± .01	.86 ± .05	.84 ± .01

Table 6
A_z Attributable to Each of the Request Categories

Request Category	Screen-Film Radiography	Computed Radiography
Group average (n = 95)	.84	.85
Routine (n = 35)	.83	.77
Nonroutine		
Congestive heart failure (n = 15)	.87	.88
Pneumothorax (n = 15)	.84	.87
Pneumonia (n = 15)	.81	.96
Tube or catheter check (n = 15)	.91	.87

DISCUSSION

This study differs from other comparisons of screen-film radiography and computed radiography (1–7) because the cases were selected on the basis of preexamination clinical indications rather than postexamination radiologic diagnoses and because the test set is a sample of the MICU population. The request categories provide a way of limiting the range of responses on images, many of which are very complicated. It enabled the use of the ROC analysis by allowing the review panel to characterize each image requested for a specific problem as positive or negative and to characterize the images requested without a specific problem in mind (routine) as changed or unchanged. As a consequence of the method of case selection, some of the biases that are characteristic of laboratory studies are not present. Images were not excluded because they were of poor quality or too easy or difficult to verify. The test sets represent the population in the MICU at the time of their selection, and the results can be interpreted to indicate how expert radiologists perform in average cases rather than how they perform in extreme cases. It has been argued (15) that radiologists add value to the examinations at the extremes. If this is true, then undersampling the most difficult cases will underestimate any real difference in the modalities. Without data about the prevalence of difficult cases, the overall clinical effect cannot be determined. The parallel study of the clinical efficacy of picture archiving and communication systems did not show any detrimental effects after the introduction of computed radiography (10).

The data in Table 6 suggest that there may have been a bias in favor of computed radiography because the pneumothorax and pneumonia cases had higher values for A_z in the computed radiographic sample and the routine cases had lower values. This effect may be due to the sampling of easier cases or to subtle features of pneumothoraces and pneumonia that were missed by either the verification panel or the readers. The most likely explanation is that easier cases were sampled during the computed radiographic period. This problem could have been avoided by obtaining simultaneous computed radiographs and screen-film radiographs in a representative sample of patients; however, the resources to do this were not available to us. The demographic data (Table 4) give us some assurance that the populations were comparable, although this can never be guaranteed.

Most of the statistical methods that have been proposed for comparing two ROC curves are for situations where the same images are read under two conditions (eg, as hard-copy and soft-copy images), and, as a consequence, the readings for individual images are correlated. That is, if a particular image is reported positive with hard-copy display, it is very likely that it will be reported positive with soft-copy display. Hanley and McNeil (16,17) and Metz (14) have proposed methods for comparing ROC curves that account for the correlation between readings of individual cases. These methods cannot be generalized to multiple readers. Swets and Pickett (18) have proposed a general method that can be applied to multiple readers. However, it requires matching cases across modalities and replicate readings. Dorfman and colleagues (13) have used an ANOVA model to generalize the analysis to multiple readers and multiple cases; however, in the public domain version, matching cases across modalities is also required. We have applied a new modification of the MRMC ANOVA to our unpaired data. When this method becomes generally available, it may be useful in comparisons where pairing cases is not possible.

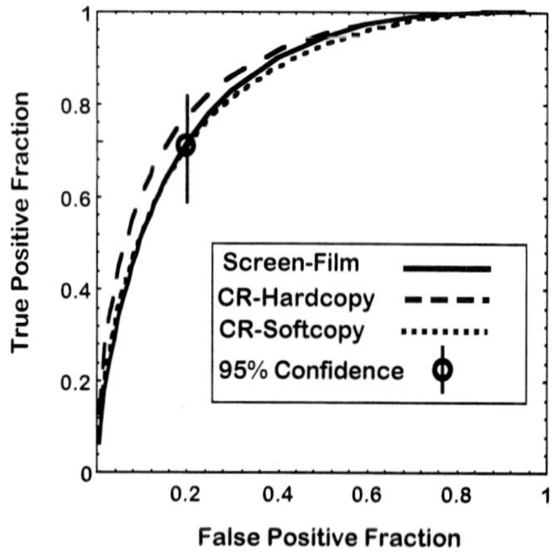

ROC curves for the pooled confidence rating data of the four readers for the three imaging methods used in this study. *CR* = computed radiography.

How positive can we be that the A_z difference of −.025 between hard-copy and soft-copy computed radiographs is due to chance rather than a real difference? The results are based on a sample of four readers and 95 cases. The power calculation of Hanley and McNeil (16,17), assuming a correlation coefficient of .5, shows that about 1,000 cases would be required to be 90% certain that a difference of −.025 was due to chance. This calculation applies to only one reader, and certainly one would not like to generalize results on the basis of one reader, but it is an estimate of an upper limit. When there are multiple readers, the number of cases per reader is smaller, but the computation of power becomes more difficult because it must include estimates of three sources of variance (case, between reader, within reader) and two correlations (case and reader). A simulation was done on the basis of the model of Swets and Pickett (18; equation 5, p 86). ROCFIT (14) was used to estimate the change in case and within-reader variance as the number of cases was increased. The correlation coefficient was set at .5 and the between-reader standard deviation at 0.03 (the average in the present study). This showed that about 800 cases would be necessary for four readers and about 750 for five. A larger sample increases power but also puts a great burden on the readers and especially on the verification panel.

Verification of an unselected clinical sample of cases is a particular problem. Obtaining independent proof for many of the diagnoses made with chest images in an intensive care unit is almost impossible because the chest radiograph is regarded as the clinical standard of reference. This makes the verification panel into a super reader whose diagnosis may be no more reliable than that of the blinded readers. We are currently exploring the use of mixture distribution analysis as a method for comparing screen-film and computed radiographs in a larger but still representative sample, where independent verification may not be necessary (19). ■

Acknowledgments: The authors acknowledge the help of Kevin Berbaum, PhD, and Donald Dorfman, PhD, of the University of Iowa, who did the MRMC split-plot analysis of the unpaired data.

References

1. Fajardo LL, Hillman BJ, Pond GD, Carmody RF, Johnson JE, Ferrell WR. Detection of pneumothorax: comparison of digital and conventional chest imaging. AJR 1989; 152:475–480.
2. Schaefer CM, Greene R, Oestmann JW, et al. Digital storage phosphor imaging versus conventional film radiography in CT documented chest disease. Radiology 1990; 174:207–210.
3. Kehler M, Albrechtsson U, Andresdottir A, Larusdottir H, Lundin A. Accuracy of digital radiography using stimulable phosphor for diagnosis of pneumothorax. Acta Radiol 1990; 31:47–52.
4. Buckley KM, Schaefer CM, Greene R, et al. Detection of bullous lung disease: conventional radiography vs digital storage phosphor radiography. AJR 1991; 156:467–470.
5. Schaefer CM, Greene R, Hall DA, et al. Mediastinal abnormalities: detection with storage phosphor digital radiography. Radiology 1991; 178:169–173.
6. Kehler M, Albrechtsson U, Andresdottir A, et al. Digital luminescence of diagnostic radiography in interstitial lung disease. Acta Radiol 1991; 32:18–23.
7. Thaete FL, Fuhrman CR, Oliver JH, et al. Digital radiography and conventional imaging of the chest: a comparison of observer performance. AJR 1994; 162:575–581.
8. Chakraborty DP, Breatnach ES, Yester MV, Soto B, Barnes GT, Fraser RG. Digital and conventional chest imaging: a modified ROC study of observer performance using simulated nodules. Radiology 1986; 158:35–39.
9. Newell JD, Seeley GW, Hagaman RM, et al. Computed radiographic evaluation of simulated pulmonary nodules: preliminary results. Invest Radiol 1988; 23:267–270.
10. Kundel HL, Seshadri SB, Langlotz CP, et al. Prospective study of a PACS: information flow and clinical action in a medical intensive care unit. Radiology 1996; 199:143–149.
11. Knaus WA, Wagner DP, Draper EA, et al. The APACHE III prognostic system: risk prediction of hospital mortality for critically ill hospitalized adults. Chest 1991; 100:1619–1636.
12. Seshadri SB, Arenson RN, Kundel HL, et al. High-resolution image workstation for intensive care units. RadioGraphics 1994; 14: 863–873.
13. Dorfman DD, Berbaum KS, Metz CE. Receiver operating characteristic analysis: generalization to the population of readers and patients with the jackknife method. Invest Radiol 1992; 27:723–731.
14. Metz CE. Some practical issues of experimental design and data analysis in radiographic ROC studies. Invest Radiol 1989; 24:235–245.
15. Gur D. Operating at the diagnostic margins: image quality considerations. AJR 1993; 160:1341–1342.
16. Hanley JA, McNeil BJ. The meaning and use of the area under a receiver operating characteristic (ROC) curve. Radiology 1982; 143:29–36.
17. Hanley JA, McNeil BJ. A method of comparing the areas under receiver operating characteristic curves derived from the same cases. Radiology 1983; 148:839–843.
18. Swets JA, Pickett RM. Evaluation of diagnostic systems: methods from signal detection theory. New York, NY: Academic Press, 1982; 68–93.
19. Kundel HL, Polansky M. Mixture distribution and receiver operating characteristic analysis of portable chest imaging using screen-film and computed radiography. Acad Radiol 1997; 4:1–7.

Sum & Substance

The Fasciitis-Panniculitis Syndromes: Clinical and Pathologic Features.
Jochanan E. Naschitz, MD, Jochanan H. Boss, MD, Ines Misselevich, MD, Daniel Yeshurun, MD, Itzhak Rosner, MD. *Medicine* 1996; 75:6–16. (J.H.B., Department of Pathology, Bnai-Zion Medical Center, PO Box 4940, Haifa 31048, Israel.)

The fasciitis-panniculitis syndromes encompass a diverse group of clinical entities characterized histologically by fibrous thickening and chronic inflammation of the collagenous subcutaneous septal-fascial-perimysial network. Clinical manifestation includes painful swelling and induration of the skin and underlying soft tissues. Although fasciitis-panniculitis syndromes are confined typically to the forearms and calves, other areas of the body can be involved. The indurated subcutaneous lesions are seen in one of two typical patterns: The first pattern is large circumferential lesions that involve one or more extremities in a sleevelike distribution; the second is plaques that are round, oval or elongated, and single or multiple and involve any region of the body. The clinical course is protracted, but the prognosis is good.

The classic idiopathic fasciitis-panniculitis syndrome, eosinophilic fasciitis, was described 2 decades ago by Shulman, and eosinophilia and polyclonal hypergammaglobulinemia were the hallmarks of the disease. Similar histologic features, however, often without eosinophilia and hypergammaglobulinemia, are also seen in patients with various disorders including morphea profunda, lupus panniculitis, circulatory disorders, toxic oil syndrome, L-tryptophane-induced eosinophilia-myalgia syndrome, graft-versus-host reaction, postirradiation injury, infections, and cancer. The findings are in contrast to those of systemic sclerosis, in which clinical findings, disease course, and histologic features are different. Therefore, the term "fasciitis-panniculitis syndromes" was proposed to categorize these syndromes, which have similar histologic features, and to separate them from systemic sclerosis.

In a recent study of 32 patients with fasciitis-panniculitis syndromes, 14 patients were found to have idiopathic fasciitis-panniculitis syndromes, six patients had fasciitis-panniculitis syndromes secondary to venous, arterial, or lymphatic system disturbances, six patients had a related infectious process, and three patients had fasciitis-panniculitis syndromes associated with cancer; one patient each had local trauma, insect bites, or Sweet syndrome (myeloblastic leukemia complicated by febrile neutrophilic dermatosis and acute sterile myositis). Laboratory findings revealed eosinophilia in only three patients, and hypergammaglobulinemia was seen in only three patients. The interval between the inciting insult and the onset of clinical symptoms in cases of secondary fasciitis-panniculitis syndromes ranged from 2 weeks to 4 months. Diagnosis of fasciitis-panniculitis syndromes may be difficult and may be confused with infection, a soft-tissue neoplasm, deep venous thrombosis, and myxedema. Histopathologically, the outstanding feature in all 32 cases was the partial to subtotal replacement of the subcutaneous fat tissue by fibrotically thickened septa. The thickened septa, which replaced adipose lobules, were composed of edematous or loosely packed to densely compacted collagenous tissue. These thickened septa merged with the expanded and fibrotic muscular fascia.

The initial treatment of fasciitis-panniculitis syndromes is with cimetidine, secondary treatment is with cimetidine and prednisone, and for patients who do not respond to initial or secondary treatment, a combination of cimetidine, prednisone, and methotrexate is used. In the series of 32 patients, those with idiopathic fasciitis-panniculitis syndromes recovered without any of the described late complications, which include muscle atrophy, nerve entrapment, or joint ankylosis. The prognosis of secondary fasciitis-panniculitis syndromes depended in part on the ability to manage the underlying disease.

The fasciitis-panniculitis syndromes describe a group of disorders characterized by induration of the skin caused by chronic inflammation and fibrosis of the subcutaneous septa and muscular fascia. Idiopathic fasciitis, also known as eosinophilic fasciitis, is characterized by eosinophilia and hypergammaglobulinemia. However, fasciitis and panniculitis syndromes associated with a number of clinical disorders have this typical histologic appearance. The concept of the fasciitis-panniculitis syndromes recognizes a stereotypic tissue reaction pattern, highlights the panniculitis in addition to the fasciitis component, and emphasizes the similar response to drug therapy even in different clinical settings.

Loralie D. Ma, MD, PhD
The Johns Hopkins Hospital
Baltimore, Md

Zhiyun Yang, MD • Frederick A. Mann, MD • Louis A. Gilula, MD
Carolyn Haerr, MD • C. Falck Larsen, MD

Scaphopisocapitate Alignment: Criterion to Establish a Neutral Lateral View of the Wrist[1]

PURPOSE: **To determine whether a "true" neutral lateral view of the wrist is necessary for accurate capitolunate angle measurement, to compare two standards of diagnostic adequacy for neutral lateral wrist views (distal radioulnar overlap [RUO] and scaphopisocapitate [SPC] relationship), and to confirm positional reproducibility and measurement precision of the SPC criterion.**

MATERIALS AND METHODS: **Capitolunate angles were measured on neutral lateral and supine pisotriquetral views of 10 normal wrists. Two hundred neutral lateral wrist views were classified by each standard (RUO and SPC) as excellent, acceptable, or unacceptable. In two subgroups, capitolunate angles were measured on the lateral views to determine SPC practicality and sensitivity.**

RESULTS: **Compared with neutral lateral positioning, supinated off-lateral views showed an apparent increase in lunate dorsiflexion of up to 30°. Diagnostically unacceptable, excellent, and acceptable pronosupination was present on 118, 22, and 60 of 200 views by using the RUO criterion and on 40, 79, and 81 of 200 views by using the SPC criterion, respectively. The capitolunate angle did not show a significant difference between each of the two subgroups ($P > .05$).**

CONCLUSION: **A true neutral lateral view of the wrist is necessary for accurate measurement of the capitolunate angle on the basis of a comparison with off-lateral views. SPC relationship provides a diagnostically reproducible standard for a neutral lateral wrist view and should reduce the need for repeat lateral radiographs.**

Carpal collapse and intercarpal instability are important causes of wrist debility and are associated with considerable personal and societal costs. Radiography is an aid to diagnosis and clinical decision making, and confirmation of midcarpal or scapholunate instability guides therapy and enables prediction of outcome (1–5). The standard "true" neutral lateral radiograph of the wrist is the cornerstone for reproducible quantification of intercarpal malalignment and measurement of angular relationships among carpal bones. However, nonstandard positioning (ie, not "true" lateral or posteroanterior radiographs) is known to cause geometric distortion of distal radioulnar and intercarpal relationships that may be erroneously interpreted as malalignment or instability (6–8).

Standard radiographs rely on reproducible positioning on the basis of subjective assessments of physiologically variable external anatomic landmarks at the wrist to obtain lateral radiographs. Traditionally, a true lateral view of the wrist is present when two conditions are met (7,9–11): (*a*) the long axes of the radius and third metacarpal are colinear (neither flexion nor deviations in the sagittal and coronal planes, respectively), and (*b*) there is exact radioulnar overlap (RUO) in which the dorsal cortices of the distal radius and ulna are superimposed (no pronosupination). Unfortunately, reproducible RUO standard neutral lateral radiographs of the wrist may be difficult to obtain in clinical practice (9,12). In fact, exact superimposition of the dorsal cortices of the radius and ulna was present on fewer than 10% of initial lateral wrist radiographs at our institution. Furthermore, an otherwise true RUO standard lateral view of the distal forearm can produce an oblique projection of the carpus and metacarpus for a variety of reasons, including pronosupination at the radiocarpal joint (eg, ulnar translocation in rheumatoid arthritis), developmental dorsal bowing of the distal ulna, or a congenitally prominent dorsal curvature of the distal end of the ulna.

To address these inconsistencies, one of the authors (L.A.G.) suggested a standard for neutral lateral projections of the wrist, on the basis of radiographic anatomic landmarks, according to which palmar radial- and ulnar-sided carpal structures are superimposed. The palmar ulnar-most cortical structure—the palmar surface of the pisiform—was aligned with the most palmar radial-sided carpal structure in the same carpal row—the ventral cortex of the distal scaphoid pole. This resulted in the projectional interposition of the palmar surface of the pisiform between the palmar cortices of the distal scaphoid tubercle and the head of the capitate (the scaphopisocapitate [SPC] relationship).

Given the difficulty in obtaining RUO

Index terms: Wrist, abnormalities, 4331.42, 4332.42, 4336.42 • Wrist, injuries, 4331.42, 4332.42, 4336.42 • Wrist, radiography, 43.11

Abbreviations: RUO = radioulnar overlap, SPC = scaphopisocapitate.

Radiology 1997; 205:865–869

[1] From the Beijing Ji Shui Tan Hospital, China (Z.Y.); the Mallinckrodt Institute of Radiology, Washington University School of Medicine, 510 S Kingshighway Blvd, St Louis, MO 63110 (Z.Y., L.A.G.); University of Washington School of Medicine, Seattle (F.A.M.); the Indianapolis Breast Center, Ind (C.H.); and the Department of Orthopaedic Surgery, Section for Hand Surgery, University Hospital of Copenhagen, Denmark (C.F.L.). Received March 14, 1997; revision requested April 16; revision received August 8; accepted August 11. **Address reprint requests to** L.A.G.

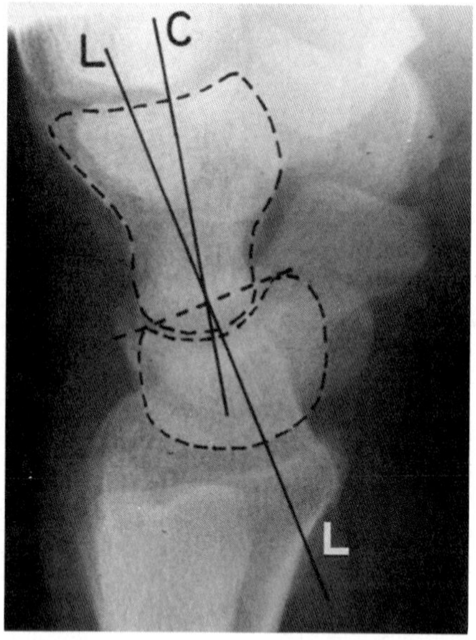

Figure 1. Radiograph of a wrist shows the axial method of measurement. The lunate axis is the line (*L*) drawn perpendicular to the anterior and posterior distal lunate poles or horns. The capitate axis (*C*) is identified by passing a line connecting the center of its head to the center of its distal articular surface. The capitolunate angle is the angle between the two lines.

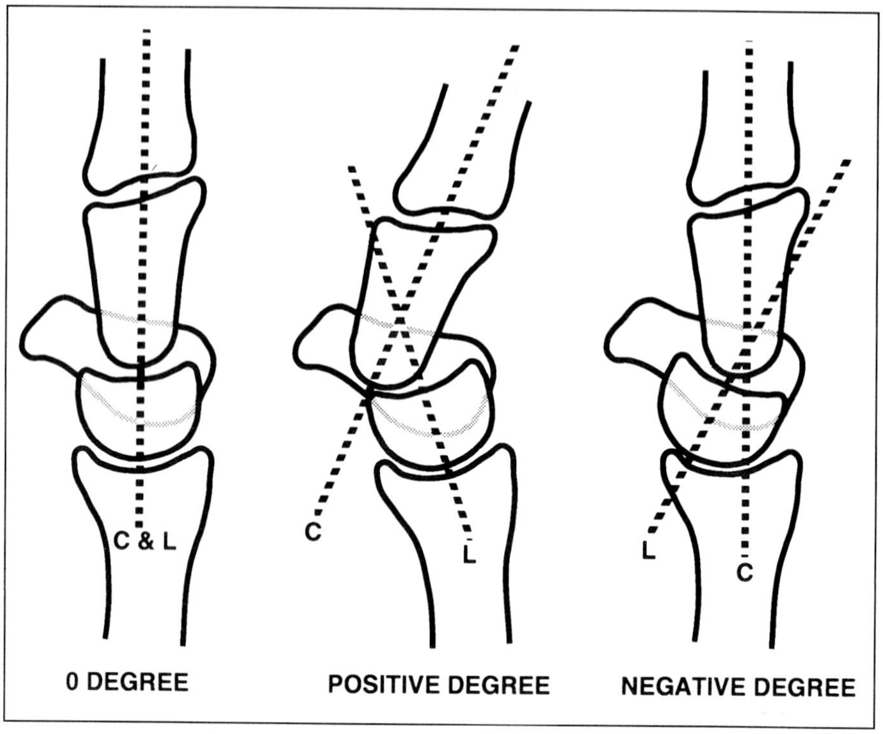

Figure 2. Left: If the lunate (*L*) and capitate (*C*) axes overlapped perfectly or were coaxial, the capitolunate angle was recorded as 0°. Center: If the distal end of the lunate axis was palmar flexed with respect to the capitate axis, the capitolunate angle was recorded as positive. Right: When the distal end of the lunate axis was dorsiflexed with respect to the capitate axis, the angle was recorded as negative.

standard true neutral lateral wrist radiographs and the absence of reported data on the applicability of an intracarpal standard (SPC criterion), we proposed to (*a*) verify whether small variations in pronosupination can lead to apparent (but erroneous) pathologic capitolunate malalignment as reflected by an abnormal capitolunate angle measured on otherwise neutral lateral views of the wrist; (*b*) compare two different standards of diagnostic adequacy for neutral pronosupination on neutral lateral views of the wrist: the RUO standard (ie, overlap of the dorsal cortices of the distal radius and ulna) and the SPC standard (ie, ventral pisiform cortex overlies the interval between the palmar surfaces of the distal scaphoid pole and capitate head); (*c*) determine positional reproducibility and measurement precision of the SPC criterion through measurement of the capitolunate angle in two subgroups; and (*d*) determine whether the capitolunate angles obtained by using these standards differ in a magnitude that might be clinically important.

MATERIALS AND METHODS

Measurement of the Capitolunate Angle

Before final measurements, agreement on methods of measurement was reached between the first (Z.Y.) and senior (L.A.G.) authors. The capitolunate angles were measured with the axial method (2,8,9) (Fig 1). All measurements were made to the nearest 0.5° by using the same commercial goniometer by one musculoskeletal radiologist (Z.Y.). Figure 2 describes the determination of the positive or negative degree of angulation of the capitolunate angle (5,13). One observer (Z.Y.) measured all of the capitolunate angles twice with a ½-year interval between the measurements to calculate intraobserver variability.

Study Populations

To enhance our diagnostic sensitivity, we have routinely obtained a wrist instability series of the historically unaffected and clinically normal wrist as an internal control in patients referred for evaluation of chronic wrist pain or instability. With use of the wrist instability series of the asymptomatic and normal wrists in 10 consecutive patients (five men and five women; age range, 18–55 years; mean age, 29.2 years) referred for chronic wrist pain (group A), the capitolunate angles were measured on both the neutral lateral and pisotriquetral joint (supinated, oblique off-lateral) views.

As part of our routine conventional radiography performed before wrist arthrography, 200 consecutive lateral views of the wrist were obtained between September 1992 and June 1993 with use of a dedicated wrist immobilizer designed by Larsen et al (9) (Fig 3). The immobilizer was used by adjusting screws and Velcro straps about the hand and forearm to stabilize and control the position of the wrist through multiple axes into a "true" lateral position. With this device,

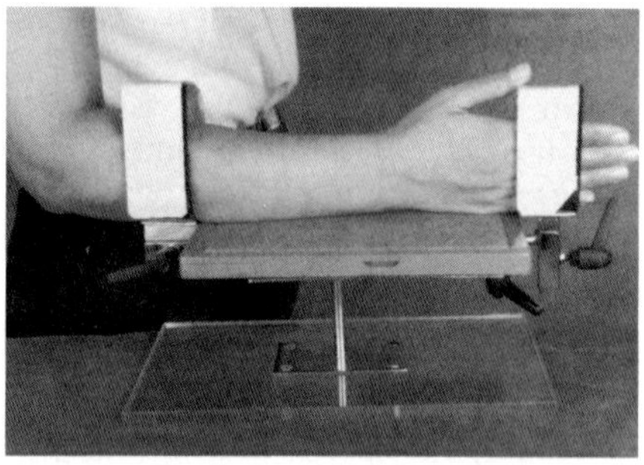

Figure 3. Photograph of the holder designed by Larsen et al (9). The elbow is flexed 90° and is adducted to the side of the patient's body. The third metacarpal shaft is parallel to the long axis of the radius. The ulnar side of the forearm, wrist, and metacarpals lie on a radiographic cassette.

the lateral views for this study were obtained with the patient's arm adducted against the trunk, elbow flexed 90°, forearm held in neutral rotation (no pronation or supination), and the wrist in neutral position (no radial or ulnar deviation, and no palmar or dorsal flexion). All radiographs were obtained with a vertical x-ray beam, at 40-inch tube-film distance, and centered on the distal tip of the radial styloid.

Two groups each with 20 members were selected from the 200 consecutive wrist arthrography cases on the basis of discordant classification between the RUO and SPC criteria. These two groups were designed to test the value of the SPC criterion. One group (group B) was composed

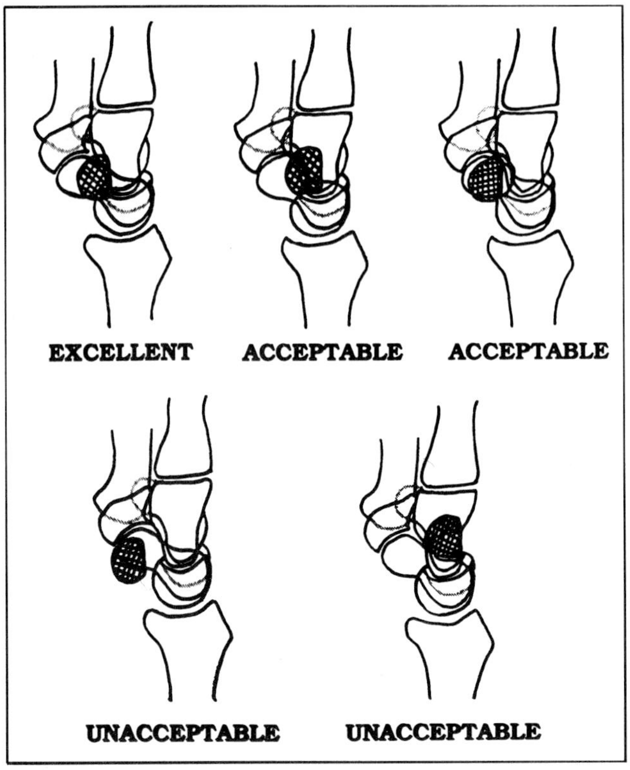

Figure 4. Three classes of the SPC criterion are illustrated. *Excellent* exists when the palmar cortex of the pisiform overlies the central third of the interval between the palmar cortices of the distal scaphoid pole and the capitate head; *acceptable* is present when the palmar cortex of the pisiform projects within the interval between the palmar cortices of the distal scaphoid pole and the capitate head but does not overlap the central third of this interval; and *unacceptable* exists when the palmar cortex of the pisiform projects palmar to the distal scaphoid pole or dorsal to palmar cortex of the capitate head. The pisiform is the area filled with crosshatch marks.

Table 1
Capitolunate Angle on Excellent SPC Lateral and Off-lateral Views in Group A

Patient No.	Lateral View	Off-lateral View	Difference
1	13	14	−1
2	30	5	25
3	25	−4	29
4	15	10	5
5	10	25	−15
6	21	32	−11
7	18	18	0
8	30	12	18
9	20	−7	27
10	20	−10	30
Average	20.3	9.6	10.7

Note.—Data are presented as degrees. Positive numbers refer to palmar flexion of the lunate; negative numbers refer to dorsiflexion (extension) of the lunate on lateral views.

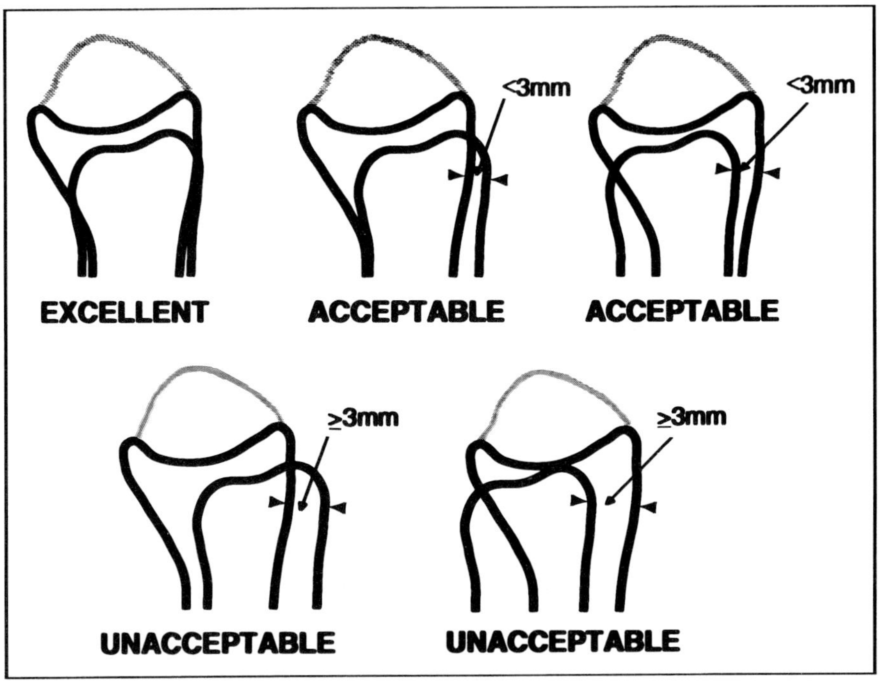

Figure 5. Three classes of the traditional RUO standard are illustrated. *Excellent* exists when the dorsal cortices of the distal radius and ulna are superimposed; *acceptable* is present when there is a less than 3-mm separation between the dorsal cortices of the distal radius and ulna (arrowheads in top row); and *unacceptable* exists when the dorsal cortices of the distal radius and ulna (arrowheads in bottom row) are separated by 3 mm or more.

of 20 excellent SPC relationships: 10 with excellent RUO relationships (subgroup B1; four men, six women; age range, 20–45 years; mean age, 32.6 years) and 10 with unacceptable RUO relationships (subgroup B2; five men, five women; age range, 23–50 years; mean age, 33 years). Capitolunate angles were measured on the lateral views of this group. If a clinical and statistically significant difference existed in the capitolunate angles between subgroups B1 and B2, the SPC criterion was rejected; if no statistically significant difference existed in the capitolunate angles between the subgroups B1 and B2, the SPC criterion was considered adequate for clinical measurements. The other group (group C) was divided into 10 excellent SPC relationships (with excellent RUO at the same time) (subgroup C1; four men, six women; age range, 20–45 years; mean age, 32.6 years) and 10 unacceptable SPC relationships (with unacceptable RUO at the same time) (subgroup C2; five men, five women; age range, 24–53 years; mean age, 34.8 years). Capitolunate angles were also measured on the lateral views of this group. If a statistically significant difference was found in the capitolunate angles between subgroups C1 and C2, the SPC criterion was proved to be adequate for clinical measurements. If no clinical and statistically significant difference was found in the capitolunate angles between subgroups C1 and C2, the SPC criterion was proved to be inadequate for measurements. Here, groups B1 and C1 were the same group of 10 patients because both B1 and C1 required the same conditions.

Definitions and Classifications of "True" Neutral Lateral View

The SPC criterion refers to the relative position of the palmar cortex of the pisiform with respect to the palmar cortices of the head of the capitate and the distal pole of the scaphoid. Figure 4 gives the definitions for three classes of the SPC criterion.

Figure 5 gives the definitions for three classes of the "traditional" RUO standard.

Statistical Methods

A Student *t* test was used to determine the statistical significance of differences found between the capitolunate angles in each of the study groups (neutral lateral vs pisotriquetral oblique off-lateral views of group A and the two subgroups of groups B and C), with α = .05. The variability of measurements was analyzed by means of the paired *t* test between both measurements of each group.

RESULTS

The average difference between capitolunate angles measured on neutral versus oblique off-lateral views was 11° ($P < .05$) with a range from −1° to 30° in an individual patient (Table 1). The apparent change of capitolunate angle found on the off-lateral views manifested as an increase in dorsiflexion ("pseudodorsiflexion") of the lunate (Fig 6).

With use of the forearm and wrist immobilizer developed by Larsen et al (9) (Fig 2), diagnostically unacceptable, excellent, and acceptable pronosupination was present on 118, 22, and 60 of 200 views with the RUO standard, and on 40, 79, and 81 of 200 views with the SPC standard, respectively (Table 2).

Capitolunate angles differed between the SPC excellent subgroups (B1 and B2) and between the SPC excellent versus SPC unacceptable subgroups (C1 and C2) by 1.3° and 0°, respectively ($P > .05$) (Table 3).

The intraobserver variation from both measurements for all of the groups showed no significant difference ($P > .05$).

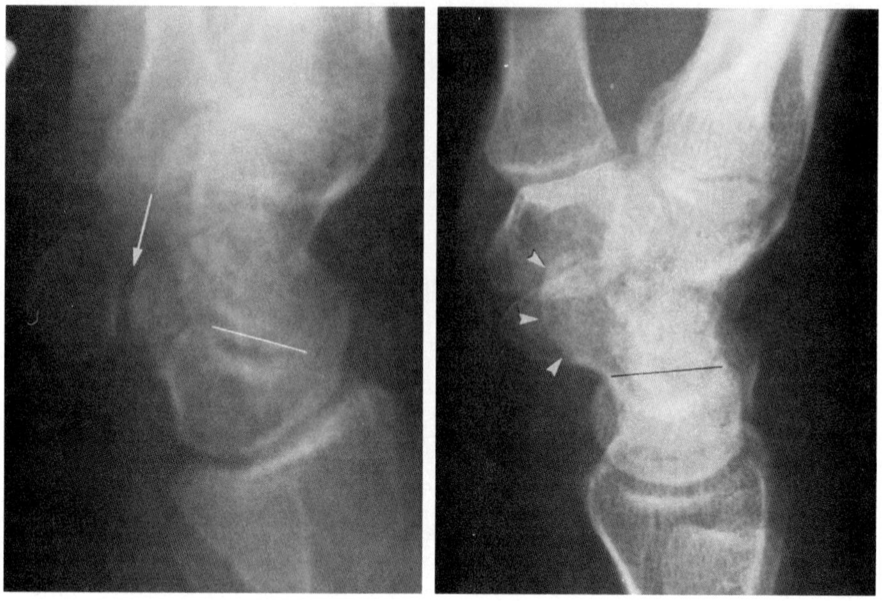

a. b.

Figure 6. Lunate shows an apparent increased dorsiflexion on the off-lateral view **(a)** where the pisotriquetral joint is profiled (arrow); this is not present on the excellent SPC lateral view **(b)** in the same patient. Arrowheads in **b** point to the ventral cortex of the pisiform. White and black lines join the dorsal and ventral distal poles of the lunate and thus identify the inclincation of the distal surface of the lunate.

Table 2
Relationship between SPC and Traditional RUO Criteria on 200 Lateral Views

	SPC Relationship			
RUO	Excellent	Acceptable	Unacceptable	All
Excellent	14	6	2	22
Acceptable	24	29	7	60
Unacceptable	41	46	31	118
All	79	81	40	200

DISCUSSION

A true lateral radiograph is necessary to provide accurate measurement of intercarpal angles, to make accurate assessment of carpal bone alignment and evaluation of the slope of the distal radius (6,14). Variation of carpal bone angles that exceeds 5° on lateral radiographs of the wrists in the same person can be considered clinically important (10). In our study, the patient's asymptomatic, normal wrist was used as the control case, and an average difference of 11° was seen between the capitolunate angles measured between the true and off-lateral views in the same asymptomatic wrist. The largest apparent change (in the same person) between true and off-lateral views was 30° (Table 1, patient 10). This emphasizes the importance of obtaining a true lateral view when evaluating carpal bone alignment.

In this study, a criterion to assess the diagnostic adequacy of a neutral lateral wrist radiograph, the SPC relationship, was introduced and evaluated by comparing it with the widely used RUO standard. Using the principle commonly employed in the osseous pelvis to recognize alignment, in which a posterior structure (coccyx) is aligned with an anterior structure (symphysis pubis), we identified similar opposite-sided structures in the wrist. An ulnar-sided structure (pisiform) that could be routinely seen was used to overlay a radial-sided structure (distal scaphoid pole). It has been our experience that these landmarks are visible on almost all adequately exposed lateral views of the wrist. Moreover, since pronosupination between the forearm and wrist may be induced at physical examination in individuals with ligamentously lax wrist (physiologic or pathologic), the SPC relationship may be a more appropriate identifier for carpal bone alignment. The RUO relationship may be a better standard with which to recognize alignment of the forearm at the distal radioulnar joint.

In our practice, disagreement between the RUO and SPC criteria occurs often. This study demonstrates that a diagnostic SPC relationship was more than twice as commonly obtained as was a diagnostic RUO relationship when a wrist holder was used. This verifies the ease of obtaining diagnostic lateral wrist radiographs when the SPC standard is used for quality control. No statistically significant difference existed in the capitolunate angle between the RUO-excellent and RUO-unacceptable lateral views when both had excellent lateral positioning judged according to the SPC standard. These results demonstrate that if a diagnostic SPC relationship is met, even when the traditional RUO criterion is nondiagnostic, the lateral view is a true lateral of the carpal bones that can be used to evaluate intercarpal angles. Recogni-

Table 3
Capitolunate Angles in Groups B and C

Group*	Criteria	No. of Cases	Capitolunate Angle: Mean†	Range†	Standard Deviation
B1	SPC, excellent; RUO, excellent	10	13.8	8 to 27	5.85
B2	SPC, excellent; RUO, unacceptable	10	15.1	5 to 23	8.12
C1	SPC, excellent; RUO, excellent	10	13.8	8 to 27	5.85
C2	SPC, unacceptable; RUO, unacceptable	10	13.9	−3 to 25	9.73

* Groups B1 and C1 were the same group of 10 patients because both groups required the same conditions.
† The differences in mean angles between groups B1 and B2 ($P = .35$) and between groups C1 and C2 ($P = .49$) were not significant. Data are presented as degrees.

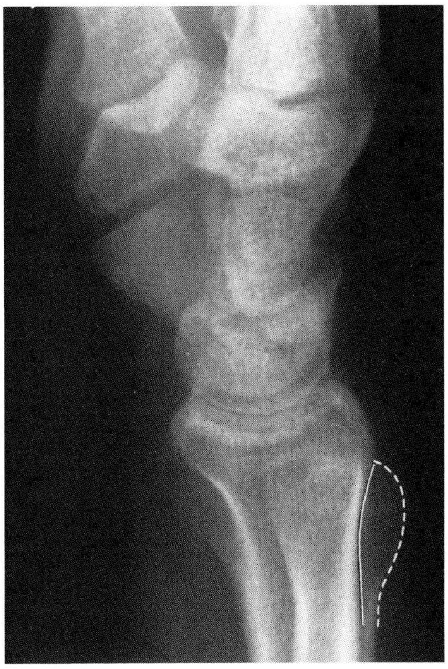

Figure 7. On this excellent SPC lateral view, the distal ulnar cortex is too bowed or too prominent dorsally for routine use of the RUO criterion. (The dashed line traces the dorsal surface of the ulna, and the solid line traces the dorsal surface of the radius.)

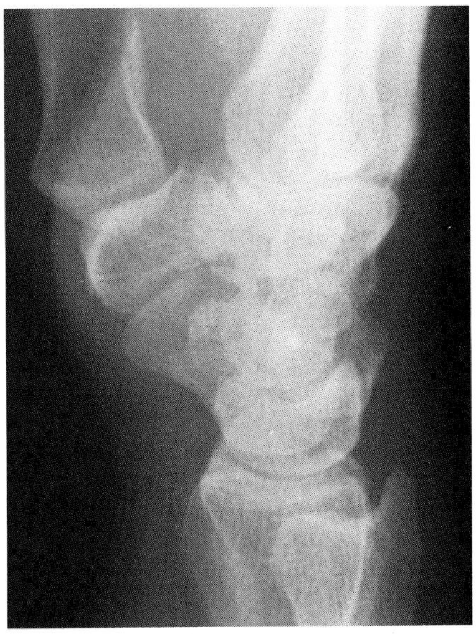

Figure 8. On this lateral view, a nondiagnostic traditional RUO criterion is present as evidenced by the dorsal cortex of the ulna being more than 3 mm dorsal to the dorsal cortex of the distal radius in the presence of an excellent SPC relationship.

tion and utilization of the SPC relationship by physician and technologist should reduce the need for repeat neutral lateral radiographs of the wrist.

Several reasons can be identified to explain why the lateral radiograph may be nondiagnostic (unacceptable positioning) on the basis of the RUO criterion, especially for intercarpal alignment. Evaluation of cases in this study showed that some distal forearm anatomic variances and different projections of the distal forearm made it difficult to judge the traditional RUO criterion as being met. Such situations existed when the distal dorsal convexity of the radius or ulna was too prominent or the distal ulna was too bowed (Fig 7), when the ulna was much shorter than the radius (this makes the convexity of the distal ulna overlie the narrower portion of the distal radius), and when there were multiple dorsal cortical surfaces of the radius making it difficult to know which surface of the distal radius should be used for the RUO determination. Additionally, use of the RUO relationship with subluxation of the distal radioulnar joint would affect, or make very difficult, judgment about adequacy of the true lateral view. In most RUO-unacceptable cases, however, the SPC relationship remained diagnostic (Fig 8).

Because no statistically significant difference existed in the capitolunate angle in the subgroups of SPC-excellent versus SPC-unacceptable views, the SPC criterion was recognized arbitrarily as a means to identify a diagnostic lateral view of carpal bones. It should be recognized that more obliquity of the wrist to produce a much more unacceptable SPC relationship as seen on the pisotriquetral off-lateral view (group A) does result in abnormal capitolunate angles.

We conclude that (*a*) a true neutral lateral view of the wrist is necessary for accurate measurement of carpal alignment as tested by the capitolunate angle on the basis of the off-lateral view in our study; (*b*) an acceptable or excellent SPC relationship provides a diagnostically reproducible standard for neutral lateral views of the wrist and is unaffected by normal distal forearm anatomic and positional variations; and (*c*) utilization of the SPC relationship by both technologists and physicians should reduce the need for repeat lateral radiographs. ■

References

1. Glickel SZ, Millender LH. Ligamentous reconstruction for chronic intercarpal instability. J Hand Surg [Am] 1984; 9:514–525.
2. Gilula LA, Weeks PM. Post-traumatic ligamentous instabilities of the wrist. Radiology 1978; 129:631–651.
3. Trumble TE, Bour CJ, Smith RJ, Glisson RR. Kinematics of the ulnar carpus related to the volar intercalated segment instability pattern. J Hand Surg [Am] 1990; 15:384–392.
4. Taleisnik J, Watson HK, Conn F. Midcarpal instability caused by malunited fractures of the distal radius. J Hand Surg [Am] 1984; 9:350–357.
5. Linscheid RL, Dobyns JH, Beabout JW, Bryan RS. Traumatic instability of the wrist. J Bone Joint Surg [Am] 1972; 54:1612–1632.
6. Larsen CF, Lindequist S, Bellstrom T. Lack of correlation between ulnar variance and carpal bone angles on lateral radiographs in normal wrists. Acta Radiol 1992; 33:275–276.
7. Taleisnik J. The bones of the wrist. In: Taleisnik J, ed. The wrist. New York, NY: Churchill Livingstone, 1985; 1–12.
8. Nakamura R, Hori M, Imamura T, Horii E, Miura T. Method for measurement and evaluation of carpal bone angles. J Hand Surg [Am] 1989; 14:412–416.
9. Larsen CF, Stigsby B, Mathiesen FK, Lindequist S. Radiography of the wrist: a new device for standardized radiographs. Acta Radiol 1990; 31:459–462.
10. Greenspan A. Upper limb II: distal forearm, wrist, and hand. In: Greenspan A, ed. Orthopedic radiology. 2nd ed. New York, NY: Raven, 1992; 6.1–6.5.
11. Bernau A, Berquist TH. Upper extremities. In: Bernau A, Berquist TH, eds. Orthopaedic positioning in diagnostic radiology. Baltimore, Md: Urban & Schwarzenberg, 1983; 110–111.
12. Wicks JE, Beach H. A method for evaluating carpal alignment on lateral radiographs. J Hand Surg [Am] 1985; 10:580–582.
13. Garcia-Elias M, An KN, Amadio PC, Cooney WP, Linscheid RL. Reliability of carpal angle determinations. J Hand Surg 1989; 14:1017–1021.
14. Gilula LA, Totty WG. Wrist trauma: roentgenographic analysis. In: Gilula LA, ed. The traumatized hand and wrist: radiographic and anatomic correlation. Philadelphia, Pa: Saunders 1992; 221–236.

Book Review

Ultrasonografia del Ginocchio in Età Pediatrica [Ultrasound imaging of the pediatric knee]

Domenico Barbuti, MD, and Gianluca Bergami, MD
Naples, Italy: Guido Gnocchi Editore, 1996. ISBN: 88-7947-133-3. Cloth, L.It. 90,000; pp 99; 61 figures.

In this Italian-language monograph, the authors present their experience in a specialized but complicated field: ultrasound (US) imaging of the knee in the pediatric population.

After sonographic anatomic features are presented in a long chapter (with relevant but incomplete information regarding structures shown later in the book), an array of possible, detectable knee conditions is depicted. These conditions include tendon and bursal disorders, osteomyelitis, septic arthritis, hemophilic arthropathy, connective tissue disease, pigmented villonodular synovitis, neoplasia, subluxation, recurvation, slipping patella, ligamentous lesions, osteochrondrosis, and (in a brief presentation) foreign bodies and congenital hypothyroidism.

A highlight is the discussion of sonography in the examination and diagnosis of conditions for which conventional radiography, by comparison, is unsatisfactory: the Osgood-Schlatter lesion, bursitis, connective tissue disease, and slipping patella.

In some cases, the US images are presented beside conventional radiographs or computed tomographic, magnetic resonance, or angiographic images. A rich bibliography and a well-organized subject index complete the book.

Some reproduced images are dark and unclear, and the arrows are not always of the same size and are not uniformly placed. The lack of indicators on images is sometimes discouraging. Use of terminology is not uniform and, hence, confusing. These features detract from the demonstration of the authors' experience.

The authors of *Ultrasonografia del Ginocchio* know their topic well. The textbook is an interesting and valuable reference source for imagers of the child's knee.

Reviewed by Giampiero Beluffi, MD

David M. Panicek, MD • Stephen D. Go, MD • John H. Healey, MD • Denis H. Y. Leung, PhD
Murray F. Brennan, MD • Jonathan J. Lewis, MD, PhD

Soft-Tissue Sarcoma Involving Bone or Neurovascular Structures: MR Imaging Prognostic Factors[1]

PURPOSE: To determine if magnetic resonance (MR) imaging findings of soft-tissue sarcoma involving bone or neurovascular structures allow prediction of local recurrence, distant metastasis, or disease-specific survival.

MATERIALS AND METHODS: Preoperative MR images of 46 patients with soft-tissue sarcoma were reviewed for tumor involving bone or major vessels or nerves. MR imaging findings were correlated with local recurrence, distant metastasis, and disease-specific survival after surgery and chemotherapy and/or radiation therapy. Primary tumors were predominantly in the lower extremity (n = 35 [76%]), deep (n = 44 [96%]), and high-grade (n = 35 [76%]).

RESULTS: On MR images, bone invasion occurred in 12 patients (26%), major-vessel encasement in five patients (11%), and major-nerve encasement in seven patients (15%). In patients with (n = 12) and those without (n = 34) bone invasion, frequencies of disease-related death (in nine [75%] and 12 [35%] patients, respectively) were significantly different (P = .02); frequencies of local recurrence or distant metastasis were not significantly different. In patients with and those without major-vessel or major-nerve encasement, there were no significant differences between frequencies of local recurrence, distant metastasis, or disease-specific survival.

CONCLUSION: In soft-tissue sarcoma, bone invasion on MR images was predictive of decreased disease-specific survival. MR imaging findings of bone or neurovascular involvement otherwise appear to be more important for tailoring surgery than for predicting local recurrence, distant metastasis, or survival.

Local recurrence of soft-tissue sarcomas after surgical excision and radiation therapy occurs in approximately 13%–20% of cases (1–3) and may be associated with subsequent distant metastasis and death (1). In one study (1), metastasis after local recurrence was more common in patients with initial high-grade or deep tumors, and tumor-related death after local recurrence was more common in patients with initial high-grade tumors or tumors larger than 5 cm in diameter. Mandard et al (4) identified several other poor prognostic factors for survival and distant metastasis with univariate analysis: invasive tumor in margins, extracompartmental location, deep tumors, tumor diameter greater than 5 cm, inadequate excision, necrosis, high mitotic count, histologically undifferentiated tumors, and blood vessel invasion. The most important variable for predicting local recurrence with multivariate analysis was the quality of surgery.

Independent, adverse prognostic factors for local recurrence, distant metastasis, and disease-specific survival were identified in a study of 1,041 adult patients with localized soft-tissue sarcoma in an extremity (5). For local recurrence, the adverse factors were age greater than 50 years, presentation with symptoms of locally recurrent disease, microscopic tumor in surgical margins, and histologic subtypes of fibrosarcoma and malignant peripheral nerve tumor. For distant metastasis, adverse factors were intermediate-sized or large tumors, high histologic grade, deep location of tumor, presentation with symptoms of locally recurrent disease, leiomyosarcoma, and nonliposarcoma histologic subtypes. For disease-specific survival, adverse factors were large tumor size, high histologic grade, deep location, presentation with symptoms of locally recurrent disease, histologic subtypes of leiomyosarcoma and malignant peripheral nerve tumor, microscopic tumor in surgical margins, and tumor in the lower extremity.

Hajdu (6) proposed a staging scheme in which three prognostic factors were considered: tumor diameter (<5 cm or >5 cm), tumor grade (low or high), and tumor depth (superficial or deep). With this scheme, prognosis of a small, low-grade, superficial sarcoma was better than that of a large, high-grade, deep sarcoma. The number of unfavorable prognostic variables in a given case determined the stage. For example, the disease-specific survival with stage 0 sarcoma (ie, no unfavorable factors) was 100% and that with stage III sarcoma (with all three unfavorable factors) was 21%.

By demonstrating the local extent of disease, cross-sectional images—particularly computed tomographic and magnetic resonance (MR) images—

Index terms: Histiocytoma, 40.3285 • Leiomyosarcoma, 40.379 • Liposarcoma, 40.371 • Sarcoma, 40.37, 9*[2].33 • Soft tissues, MR, 40.121411, 9*[2].129411 • Soft tissues, neoplasms, 40.37, 9*[2].33 • Synovial sarcoma, 40.374

Radiology 1997; 205:871–875

[1] From the Departments of Radiology (D.M.P., S.D.G.), Surgery (J.H.H., M.F.B., J.J.L.), and Epidemiology and Biostatistics (D.H.Y.L.), Memorial Sloan-Kettering Cancer Center, 1275 York Ave, New York, NY 10021; and Cornell University Medical College, New York, NY. Received April 1, 1997; revision requested May 19; revision received July 2; accepted July 8. This study supported in part by National Institutes of Health, National Cancer Institute grants U01 CA-54046 and CA-47179. **Address reprint requests to** D.M.P.

[2] 9* indicates generalized vein and artery involvement.

serve an important function in the planning of limb-salvaging surgery for soft-tissue sarcomas (7,8). The purpose of this study was to determine if MR imaging findings of soft-tissue sarcoma involving bone or major neurovascular structures allow prediction of local recurrence, distant metastasis, or disease-specific survival.

MATERIALS AND METHODS

All 46 patients with soft-tissue sarcoma who underwent preoperative MR imaging from September 1991 to January 1995 at our institution (a tertiary-care cancer center) and who were prospectively enrolled as part of the multi-institutional study of musculoskeletal tumor staging of the Radiologic Diagnostic Oncology Group (8) composed the current study group. The specific inclusion and exclusion criteria for enrollment in the study of the Radiologic Diagnostic Oncology Group have been reported (8). In our study group, there were 29 men and 17 women. Patient ages ranged from 22 to 79 years (mean, 53 years).

At initial clinical presentation, 38 (83%) patients had localized primary tumor, and eight (17%) had primary and metastatic tumor. Five of the eight patients with metastases at presentation underwent complete resection of those metastases; two of these patients underwent incomplete resection of metastases, and one did not undergo metastasectomy.

The primary lesions of five (11%) patients were smaller than 5 cm in diameter, and the lesions of 41 (89%) patients were larger than 5 cm. The locations of the primary lesions were the following: lower extremity (n = 35 [76%]), upper extremity (n = 5 [11%]), retroperitoneum (n = 3 [7%]), trunk (n = 2 [4%]), and thorax (n = 1 [2%]). Forty-four (96%) tumors were deep, and two (4%) were superficial. Histologic grade was high in 35 (76%) patients and low in 11 (24%) patients. At histologic examination, the following lesions were identified: liposarcoma (n = 11 [24%]), malignant fibrous histiocytoma (n = 8 [17%]), leiomyosarcoma (n = 7 [15%]), synovial sarcoma (n = 5 [11%]), undifferentiated sarcoma (n = 4 [9%]), extraosseous chondrosarcoma (n = 3 [7%]), malignant peripheral nerve tumor (n = 2 [4%]), epithelioid sarcoma (n = 1 [2%]), fibrosarcoma (n = 1 [2%]), extraosseous osteosarcoma (n = 1 [2%]), spindle cell sarcoma (n = 1 [2%]), hemangiopericytoma (n = 1 [2%]), and clear cell sarcoma (n = 1 [2%]).

A surgical margin was considered to be positive if tumor was seen microscopically within one high-power field of the inked margin of the specimen. The margins were positive in 11 (24%) patients, negative in 33 (72%) patients, and unknown in two (4%) patients.

Table 1
Accuracy of MR Imaging for Detection of Bone, Vessel, or Nerve Involvement by Soft-Tissue Sarcoma

MR Imaging Finding	Sensitivity*	Specificity†	Positive Predictive Value	Negative Predictive Value
Bone invasion	91 (11)	94 (35)	83	97
Vessel encasement	40 (5)	93 (41)	40	93
Nerve encasement	40 (5)	88 (41)	29	92

Note.—Numbers are percentages.
* Numbers in parentheses equal the number of true-positive plus false-negative findings.
† Numbers in parentheses equal the number of true-negative plus false-positive findings.

Table 2
Local Recurrence, Distant Metastasis, and Disease-Specific Survival on the Basis of Bone, Vessel, or Nerve Involvement by Soft-Tissue Sarcomas on MR Images

MR Imaging Finding	Local Recurrence	Distant Metastasis	Died of Disease
Bone invasion			
Yes (n = 12)	0 (0)	6 (67)*	9 (75)†
No (n = 34)	7 (21)	18 (53)	12 (35)†
Vessel encasement			
Yes (n = 5)	1 (20)	3 (75)‡	3 (60)
No (n = 41)	6 (15)	21 (54)§	18 (44)
Nerve encasement			
Yes (n = 7)	1 (14)	3 (50)‖	4 (57)
No (n = 39)	6 (15)	21 (57)#	17 (44)

Note.—Numbers are numbers of patients. Numbers in parentheses are percentages.
* n = 9.
† Difference in disease-specific survival was significant (P = .02) between patients with and those without bone invasion. All other comparisons were not significant (P > .05).
‡ n = 4.
§ n = 39.
‖ n = 6.
n = 37.

MR Imaging

MR images were acquired in each case with use of a 1.5-T imager according to the reported protocol (8). In summary, a local coil (or body coil with pelvis or hip lesions) was used to acquire T1-weighted (300–600/10–20 [repetition time msec/echo time msec]) spin-echo axial images of the tumor with 192–256 phase-encoding steps and two signals acquired. Sections were 5 mm thick with a 1-mm intersection gap in lesions smaller than 10 cm in diameter, and 8–10 mm thick with a 1.5-mm intersection gap in lesions larger than 10 cm. Corresponding proton-density– and T2-weighted (2,000–2,500/20, 80) spin-echo axial images were acquired with use of 128 phase-encoding steps and two signals acquired. Coronal and/or sagittal T1-weighted (300–600/10–20) images of the lesion and entire relevant long bone were acquired with the body coil with 5-mm-thick sections with 1-mm intersection gaps. For all MR imaging sequences, the smallest field of view was used that encompassed the region to be imaged and allowed a reasonable number of sections and adequate signal-to-noise ratio.

Superior and inferior presaturation pulses, no phase wrap, and no frequency wrap were selected to reduce artifacts. Fat-saturation pulses and fast spin-echo sequences were not available at the start of the protocol and thus were not employed. None of the patients received gadolinium-based contrast material.

The MR images were analyzed retrospectively by two radiologists (D.M.P., S.D.G.) in conference, and a consensus was reached regarding lesion site and size (in three orthogonal dimensions) and tumor involvement of bone and major nerve or blood vessels. Bone involvement was defined as extension of tumor into bone cortex; periosteal contact alone was not considered sufficient to diagnose bone involvement. Involvement of major nerves or vessels was defined as encasement of those structures with tumor surrounding and contacting at least half the structure's circumference and obliterating the associated fat plane.

The closest distance of the tumor to the major structures was measured in millimeters with use of mechanical calipers.

Surgery

Surgical decisions were made on the basis of tumor location and aggressiveness. Surgery was performed with curative intent and followed with adjuvant chemotherapy and/or radiation therapy. A fat plane between tumor and critical structures was sufficient to exclude invasion or encasement. Bone was resected in those cases in which MR imaging demonstrated gross invasion of bone. Surgical violation of gross tumor was not performed to pre-

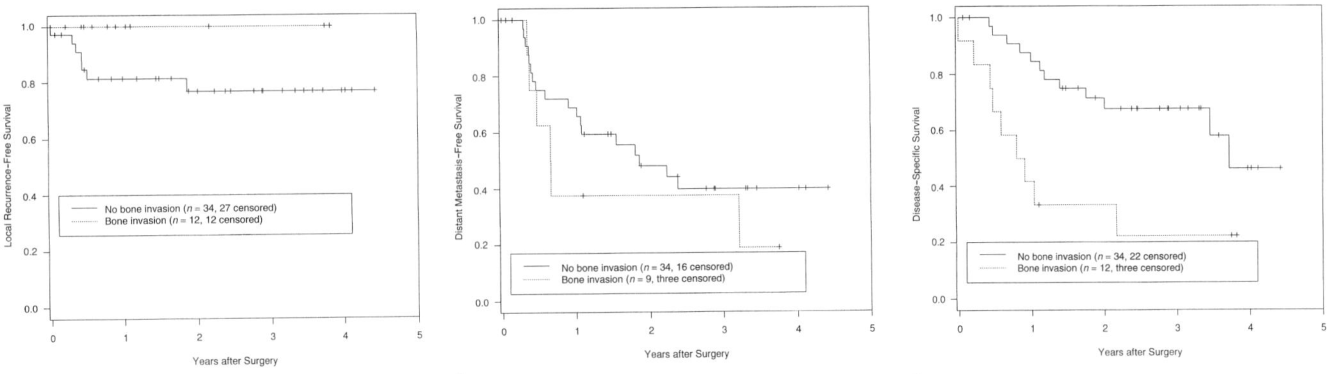

a. b. c.

Figure 1. Kaplan-Meier curves for **(a)** local recurrence–free, **(b)** distant metastasis–free, and **(c)** disease-specific survival on the basis of bone invasion. Three patients with metastases at presentation did not undergo complete resection of those metastases, and these cases were excluded from analysis in **b**.

serve vessels or nerves. Vessels and nerves were preserved if a grossly negative surgical margin could be achieved. Encased vessels or nerves were excised.

Data Analysis

Findings at surgery and pathologic examination of the surgical specimen were used as standards of reference, and the sensitivity, specificity, positive predictive value, and negative predictive value of MR imaging for detecting bone invasion or vessel or nerve encasement were calculated.

The associations between these features and the different end points (ie, local recurrence, distant metastasis, and disease-specific survival) were examined with the Fisher exact test. The rates of occrrence of end-point events were estimated with use of the Kaplan-Meier method and analyzed with use of the log-rank test. Because of the small number of patients, no multivariate analyses were attempted. In all statistical analyses, a two-tailed P value less than .05 was considered statistically significant.

The three cases in which metastases at presentation were not resected were excluded from all analyses of distant metastasis; however, these cases were included in analyses of local recurrence and disease-specific survival.

RESULTS

Surgical Procedures

Forty-three patients underwent limb-salvaging procedures, and three others underwent amputation (below-the-knee amputation, $n = 2$; external hemipelvectomy, $n = 1$). Among those 43 patients who underwent limb-salvaging procedures, subperiosteal resection was performed as part of the resection of the soft-tissue mass in 11 (26%) patients. In the other 32 patients, bone ($n = 11$), major vessel ($n = 3$), or major nerve ($n = 2$) was excised.

Seven patients experienced local recurrence, 24 experienced distant metastasis, and 21 died of disease. One patient died during the initial operation, and another died 41 months after complete resection without documentation of local recurrence or distant metastasis.

MR Imaging

MR images showed bone invasion in 12 (26%) patients, major-vessel encasement in five (11%), and major-nerve encasement in seven (15%). Descriptive statistics regarding the accuracy of the MR imaging findings are presented in Table 1.

Bone invasion.—None of the 12 patients with MR imaging findings of bone invasion experienced local recurrence, but seven (21%) of the 34 patients without bone invasion experienced local recurrence (median time to local recurrence, 5 months) ($P =$ .16) (Table 2). Among patients without metastases at presentation or who underwent complete metastasectomy, distant metastases occurred in six (67%) of nine patients with bone invasion and 18 (53%) of 34 patients without invasion ($P = .70$). Nine (75%) of 12 patients with bone invasion and 12 (35%) of 34 patients without invasion died of disease ($P = .02$).

The rate of local recurrence or distant metastasis in patients with bone invasion was not significantly different from that in patients without ($P =$ .12 and .30 for local recurrence and distant metastasis, respectively). However, the rate of disease-specific survival was lower in patients with bone invasion ($P < .01$).

Kaplan-Meier curves for local recurrence–free, distant metastasis–free, and disease-specific survival regarding bone invasion are shown in Figure 1.

Vessel encasement.—Local recurrence was experienced by one (20%) of five patients with encasement of major vessels (at 4 months) and six (15%) of 41 patients without encasement (median, 5 months) ($P > .90$). Among patients without metastases at presentation or who underwent complete metastasectomy, distant metastasis occurred in three (75%) of four patients with vessel encasement and 21 (54%) of 39 patients without encasement ($P = .60$). Three (60%) of five patients with vessel encasement and 18 (44%) of 41 patients without encasement died of disease ($P = .70$).

The rate of local recurrence, distant metastasis, or disease-specific survival in patients with vessel encasement was not significantly different from that in patients without ($P = .80$, .60, and .60, respectively).

Kaplan-Meier curves for local recurrence–free, distant metastasis–free, and disease-specific survival regarding vessel encasement are shown in Figure 2.

Nerve encasement.—Local recurrence was experienced by one (14%) of seven patients with encasement of major nerves (at 4 months) and six (15%) of 39 patients without encasement ($P > .90$). Among patients without metastases at presentation or who underwent complete metastasectomy, distant metastasis occurred in three (50%) of six patients with nerve encasement and 21 (57%) of 37 patients without encasement ($P =$ .80). Four (57%) of seven patients with nerve encasement and 17 (44%) of 39 patients without encasement died of disease ($P = .70$).

The rate of local recurrence, distant metastasis, or disease-specific survival in patients with nerve encasement was not significantly different from that in patients without ($P = .90$, .80, and .50, respectively).

Kaplan-Meier curves for local recurrence–free, distant metastasis–free,

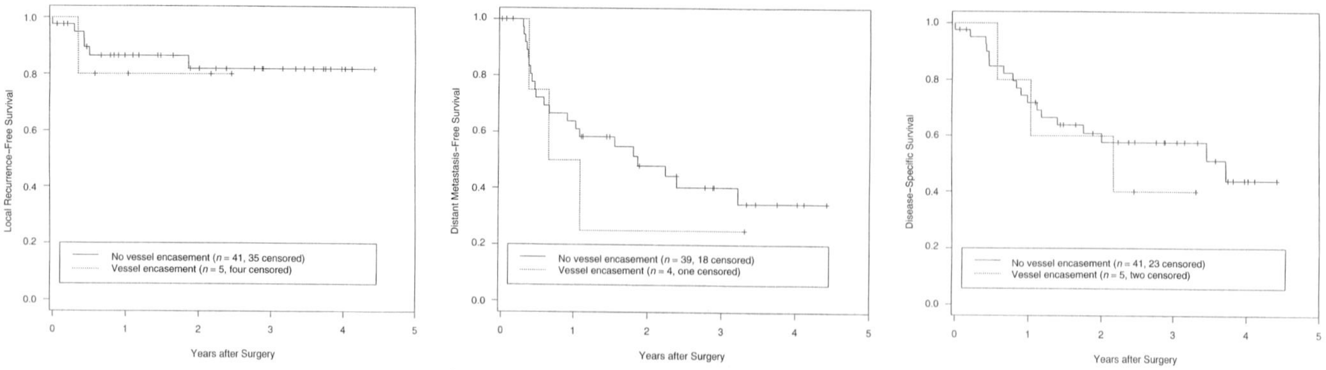

a. b. c.

Figure 2. Kaplan-Meier curves for **(a)** local recurrence–free, **(b)** distant metastasis–free, and **(c)** disease-specific survival on the basis of vessel encasement. Three patients with metastases at presentation did not undergo complete resection of those metastases, and these cases were excluded from analysis in **b**.

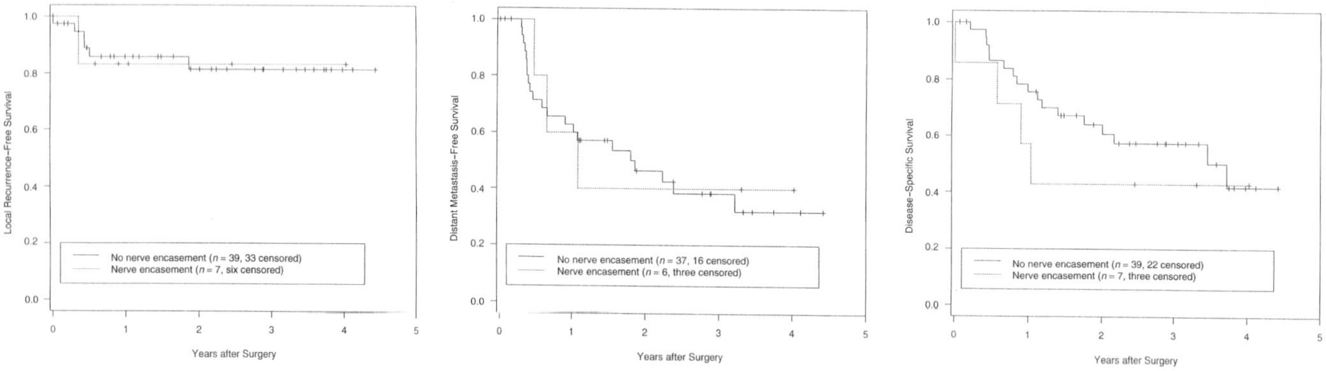

a. b. c.

Figure 3. Kaplan-Meier curves for **(a)** local recurrence–free, **(b)** distant metastasis–free, and **(c)** disease-specific survival on the basis of nerve encasement. Three patients with metastases at presentation did not undergo complete resection of those metastases, and these cases were excluded from analysis in **b**.

and disease-specific survival regarding nerve encasement are shown in Figure 3.

Distance from major structures.—The frequency of local recurrence, distant metastasis, or disease-specific survival associated with lesions more than 1 cm from the nearest bone, vessel, or nerve was not significantly different from that associated with lesions that contacted one (or more) of these structures.

DISCUSSION

Limb-salvaging surgery has become the preferred treatment of soft-tissue (and bone) sarcomas. In most cases, surgical margins and survival with limb-salvaging surgery are comparable to those achieved with amputation, and functional result with limb-salvaging surgery is better than that achieved with amputation. With some distal-extremity lesions, however, amputation and a fitted prosthesis can provide comparable or better functional results (7,9). Limb-salvaging surgery may not be feasible or appropriate if tumor involves critical neurovascular structures or is associated with pathologic fractures. The preoperative evaluation of a patient with soft-tissue sarcoma thus necessitates an accurate assessment of tumor extent. MR imaging can provide such information (8). To our knowledge, however, the prognostic importance of MR imaging findings at local staging with regard to local recurrence, distant metastasis, and disease-specific survival has not been evaluated.

In our study, patients with bone invasion on MR images had a higher frequency and a higher rate of death due to sarcoma than those without bone invasion. However, if we excluded from the analysis of disease-specific survival the three cases in which metastases at presentation were not resected, then analysis with the Fisher exact test or the log-rank test did not show a significant difference in disease-specific survival in those with and those without bone invasion ($P = .17$ and .07, respectively). No statistically significant relationship was evident between MR imaging findings of bone or major neurovascular involvement and local recurrence or distant metastasis. Also, no prognostic significance could be seen with the minimum distance between the tumor and bone or neurovascular structures. These findings, although counterintuitive, may be explainable. First, because of the limited size of our study and the small numbers of patients in some of the patient subsets, the power of the study was small to detect any prognostic factor (if it existed).

Second, the MR imaging findings necessarily influenced the surgical methods employed and thus ultimately altered the likelihood of local disease recurrence. Our surgical strategy involved excision of involved structures. Resection of affected bone yielded negative surgical margins; no patient who underwent this treatment experienced local recurrence—unlike those 34 patients without bone involvement (of whom seven experienced local recurrence). Paradoxically, the requisite resection of involved bone may have enhanced the quality and quantity of locally excised margin and led to the low frequency of local recurrence (none of 12 patients). Thus, the quality and quantity of a surgical margin may influence the local recurrence rate.

The frequency of distant metastasis was unaffected by bone involvement; in our small subset of patients, bone invasion was not associated with a higher frequency of distant metastasis. Biologic aggressiveness of locally invasive tumor was probably different from that of metastatic disease.

Encasement of major nerve or vessel was associated rarely with tumor invasion in these structures. Most nerves and vessels could be preserved if they could be freed at surgery without violating the sarcoma. Adjuvant radiation therapy apparently helped to minimize local recurrence of tumor in patients with preserved major nerves or vessels. We could not address whether resection of neurovascular structures would have reduced the local recurrence rate.

The quality of surgical margins may also influence the local control of sarcomas treated with limb-preserving surgery. The clinical importance of the inflammatory- or reactive-tissue zone around sarcomas is uncertain in the modern era of multiple modality therapy; we did not address this issue. Quantitative methods used to assess changes in inflammatory tissue must be developed for imaging studies and pathologic examination of gross and histologic specimens. In cases in which structures involved with tumor are resected, outcome may be similar to that in cases with no tumor involvement of major structures. Local recurrence might be related to a narrow surgical margin (eg, within 2 mm of tumor); if so, then resection of structures close to the tumor might be worthwhile. Further investigation is needed because our study was not designed to address these issues.

The MR imaging techniques used in our study (between 1991 and 1995) do not represent the current state-of-the-art techniques. For example, high-resolution matrixes, fat-saturation techniques, and gadolinium-based contrast material were not employed. Thus, the prognostic value of MR imaging might have been underestimated, particularly with respect to neurovascular invasion.

The relationship between findings on MR images and those at surgery and pathologic examination was not perfect. The MR imaging findings in some cases were indeterminate for invasion or encasement with tumor (eg, if a structure was contiguous with tumor), and any apparent prognostic value (or lack thereof) of MR imaging would have been affected with classification of those findings as positive or negative. At surgery, major nerves or vessels may have been resected for reasons other than invasion or encasement, and the relationship of those structures to the tumor may not have been assessed by the surgeon (such as during an amputation). Similarly, the completeness of pathologic examination of a specimen can vary depending on tumor size and the complexity or distortion of surrounding anatomic structures. As a result, discrepancies between findings at MR imaging and those at surgical and pathologic examination will occur. The ranges of such discrepancies encountered in our study (Table 1) were similar to those in the 133 patients (of which our patients are a subset) in the project of the Radiologic Diagnostic Oncology Group (8). The relatively low positive predictive values of vessel and nerve involvement are expected consequences of applying an imperfect test (ie, MR imaging) and imperfect interpretation to a population with low frequencies of such involvement.

In soft-tissue sarcoma, MR imaging provides preoperative information about tumor involving bone and neurovascular structures that is indispensable for the planning and success of limb-preserving surgery. In our study, MR imaging findings of bone invasion were predictive of decreased disease-specific survival. MR imaging findings of bone or neurovascular involvement otherwise appear to be more important for tailoring surgery than for predicting local recurrence, distant metastasis, or disease-specific survival. In fact, favorable results that occur with less extensive surgery in less extensive disease may also occur with more extensive surgery in more extensive disease. Further studies with larger numbers of patients in each subset (particularly those with bone invasion or superficial tumors) are needed before firm conclusions can be drawn about the prognostic value of MR imaging in patients with soft-tissue sarcoma. ■

Acknowledgments: We thank Nicole Maurice, MS, and Gina Dimartino, BS, for assistance with data entry.

References

1. Lewis JJ, Leung D, Heslin M, Woodruff JM, Brennan MF. The association of local recurrence with subsequent survival in extremity soft tissue sarcoma. J Clin Oncol 1997; 15:646–652.
2. Suit HD, Proppe KH, Mankin HJ, et al. Radiation therapy and conservative surgery for sarcoma of soft tissue. Prog Clin Cancer 1982; 8:311–318.
3. Eilber FR, Guiliano AE, Huth J, et al. High-grade soft-tissue sarcomas of the extremity: UCLA experience with limb salvage. Prog Clin Biol Res 1985; 201:59–74.
4. Mandard AM, Petiot JF, Marnay J, et al. Prognostic factors in soft tissue sarcomas: a multivariate analysis of 109 cases. Cancer 1989; 63:1437–1451.
5. Pisters PWT, Leung DHY, Woodruff J, Shi W, Brennan MF. Analysis of prognostic factors in 1,041 patients with localized soft tissue sarcomas of the extremities. J Clin Oncol 1996; 14:1679–1689.
6. Hajdu SI. Pathology of soft tissue tumors. 1st ed. Philadelphia, Pa: Lea & Febiger, 1979; 44–47.
7. McDonald DJ. Limb-salvage surgery for treatment of sarcomas of the extremities. AJR 1994; 163:509–513.
8. Panicek DM, Gatsonis C, Rosenthal DI, et al. CT and MR imaging in the local staging of primary malignant musculoskeletal neoplasms: report of the Radiology Diagnostic Oncology Group. Radiology 1997; 202:237–246.
9. Williard WC, Hajdu SI, Casper ES, et al. Comparison of amputation with limb-sparing operations for adult soft tissue sarcoma of the extremity. Ann Surg 1992; 215:269–275.

D. R. Campbell, MD, FRCPC

David B. Fraser, MD President Radiological Society of North America, 1998[1]

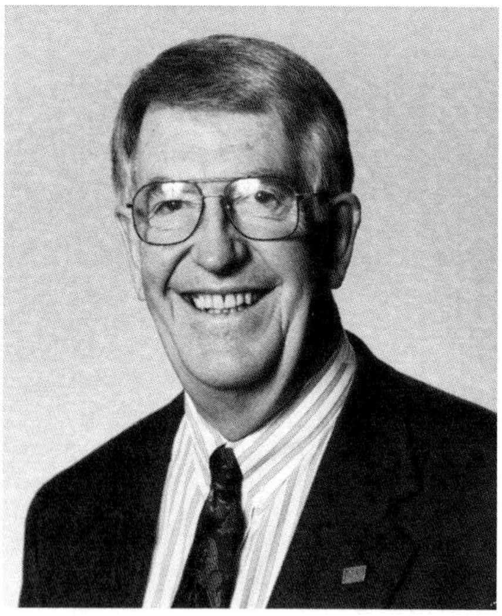

As radiology travels the critical, and frequently changing, pathways leading us to the new millennium, there is a greater need than at any time in the profession's history for patient, prudent, and visionary leadership. The Radiological Society of North America (RSNA) is fortunate to have such a leader for 1998 in the person of David B. Fraser, MD.

Born in Nova Scotia, Dr Fraser took his premedical studies at Dalhousie University from 1950 to 1953. He then studied medicine at the same institution, earning his MD CM in 1958. He entered family practice in Halifax, Nova Scotia, the same year and continued until 1966, after which he entered a residency in diagnostic radiology at Dalhousie. He concluded his residency in 1970 and went on to a fellowship in cardiovascular radiology at Harvard University for 1 year.

He was an associate professor in the Department of Radiology at Dalhousie University and associate radiologist at the Victoria General Hospital in Halifax until 1981, when he became university professor and chairman of the same department.

Dr Fraser continued as professor and head for three full terms, which in itself indicates the high esteem in which he was held by his confreres. In 1995 he began supervision of the complex merger of the radiology departments of the Victoria General Hospital and the Halifax Infirmary into the Imaging Department of the new Queen Elizabeth II Health Sciences Centre. This included opening of an imaging department for a new 420-bed hospital. He is now in his final year as professor and chairman of the amalgamated department and can take pride in the fact that the major problems that arose from the merger will have been overcome before his successor assumes office.

During his career, Dr Fraser has been an active participant in the governance of the university, the hospital, and his professional societies. Within the hospital he has been on numerous committees, including serving as chair of the Credentials Committee, the Executive Committee, and the Clinical Department Heads Planning Committee and as president of the Victoria General Hospital medical staff. At Dalhousie University he was chair of the Medical School Admissions Committee, was directly responsible for establishing radiology research on a permanent footing, and continues to serve as chair of the Board of Directors of the Radiology Research Foundation. His involvement in resident training eventually led to his becoming a member of the Nucleus Committee of the Diagnostic Radiology Specialty Committee of the Royal College of Physicians and Surgeons of Canada. After serving on a number of committees and commissions of the Canadian Association of Radiologists, he was named president of that organization in 1986–1987. He became the second Nova Scotian to hold that office. He served as chair of the Canadian Heads of Academic Radiology and was on the Executive Committee of the International Society of Radiology. He is a Fellow of the American College of Radiology. At the RSNA, he was a member of the Committee on Technical Exhibits and then served as chair of that committee.

But Dr Fraser's contribution to radiology has been much more than this. His primary goal has always been to improve patient care and, in so doing, to increase the credibility of our specialty among our confreres throughout the profession. He is a negotiator and arbiter par excellence. He can arrive at a compromise on virtually any problem. He always insists on hearing all sides of any issue before making a decision. His interpersonal skills and faculty for arbitration have repeatedly served the imaging departments, the hospital administrations and boards, the Canadian Association of Radiologists, the Royal College, and the RSNA. On many occasions, especially recently in this era of cutbacks and health system reform, there were numerous apparently insoluble crises in these organizations that he defused with his calm deliberations.

During these years he has negotiated a long-standing relationship between cardiology and radiology that is unique in Canada. In addition, he has been responsible for guiding his department through an unending sequence of renovations, equipment acquisitions, restraints imposed from all directions, and the most recent amalgamation.

Dr Fraser has been a visiting professor on many occasions and has frequently presented papers—usually in cardiac radiology, in which he found time to continue active practice until close to the end of his administrative terms.

Index terms: Radiological Society of North America • Special communications

Radiology 1997; 205:876–877

[1] From the Radiological Society of North America, 2021 Spring Rd, Suite 600, Oak Brook, IL 60523. **Address reprint requests to** Dr Fraser.

He is a member of the Canadian Medical Association, Canadian Association of Radiologists, Canadian Cardiovascular Society, RSNA, Nova Scotia Medical Society, Nova Scotia Association of Radiologists, Halifax Medical Society, Alpha Omega Alpha Honour Medical Society, Canadian Heads of Academic Radiology, Royal College of Physicians and Surgeons of Canada, and American College of Radiology.

Dr Fraser was elected to the RSNA Board of Directors in 1990, first serving as Liaison Designate for Publications. Following his year as designate, he succeeded Dr O. Wayne Houser as Liaison for Publications. In 1996, he became chairman of the Board and has been president-elect for the past year.

He sleeps only 4 hours a night. The rest of the time he is on the go, either working or exercising—playing badminton or tennis or cycling and, in recent years, playing golf. Over the years, his wife, Jean, has been his constant supporter and is amazing with her willingness to entertain guests on his behalf, often at a moment's notice. Many times she has been asked to prepare a meal for one, two, three, or more guests (or even a whole volleyball team on more than one occasion), sometimes not just to eat but to sleep! The Frasers have raised three fine children, all of whom are married: Elizabeth, Karen, and James, who is also a radiologist at the Queen Elizabeth II Health Sciences Centre. They now have seven grandchildren.

It is with great pride that I present Dr David B. Fraser to the members of the RSNA as its 83rd president. He is the fourth Canadian to hold this position. ■

R. Nick Bryan, MD, PhD
RSNA Board of Directors, Liaison for Publications

Farewell to *Radiology* Editor: Stanley S. Siegelman, MD[1]

DURING the course of his 12-year stewardship of *Radiology*, Stanley Siegelman, MD, took an already impressive journal and raised it to the preeminent position it enjoys today. His work disseminating the startling innovations, rapidly developing technology, advances in diagnosis, and improvements in patient care since 1986 has bolstered radiologists' professional standing in the medical community.

Stanley Siegelman was born in 1932 in New York City. He received his AB degree from Cornell University in 1953 and earned his MD degree from the State University of New York College of Medicine at New York City in 1957. In 1956, he married Doris Franklin, and, together, they had two sons, Evan Siegelman, MD, who practices radiology at the Hospital of the University of Pennsylvania, Philadelphia, Pa, and Bryan Siegelman, DDS, a periodontist who practices in York, Pa.

After an internship at Walter Reed Army Hospital, Washington, DC, from 1957 to 1958, he served as a captain in the Army Medical Corps, Medical Service, at Fort Meade Army Hospital, Fort Meade, Md, from 1958 to 1961. He then pursued his radiology residency training under Harold Jacobson, MD, at Montefiore Hospital and Medical Center, Bronx, NY, from 1961 to 1964, concluding as chief resident in his final year there.

Index terms: Radiology (journal) • Special communication

Radiology 1997; 205:878–879

[1] From the Radiological Society of North America, 2021 Spring Rd, Suite 600, Oak Brook, IL 60523. **Address reprint requests to** the author.

RSNA Past President E. Robert Heitzman, MD, recounts a collaboration with Dr Siegelman on a project for the American College of Radiology early in his career. "His knowledge even then was encyclopedic. Stanley always had the right answer to the question," commented Dr Heitzman. Dr Heitzman later chaired the search committee to replace William R. Eyler, MD, as *Radiology* Editor, and he recalls, "There were about 80 applicants for the position. Stanley Siegelman put his name in, and it went immediately to the top and stayed there. He has moved the journal into the forefront of quality medical journals."

Dr Siegelman stayed at Montefiore for the next 9 years, becoming an assistant professor of radiology and then an associate professor of radiology. In 1973, he moved to the Johns Hopkins Medical Institutions, Baltimore, Md, as a professor of radiology and director of diagnostic radiology. He held the latter post until 1986, when he was appointed Editor of *Radiology*. Dr Siegelman has remarked on his tendency toward a 12-year cycle: He spent 12 years between college, medical school, internship, and army service at Fort Meade; he spent 12 years at Montefiore (including a 3-year residency); he spent 12 years at Johns Hopkins as director of diagnostic radiology; and he spent the past 12 years as Editor of *Radiology*.

Stan Siegelman came to the post of Editor with an impressive background in scientific achievement. His credentials included special expertise in chest, gastrointestinal, genitourinary, musculoskeletal, and cardiovascular imaging, mammography, and particularly computed tomography. At the time of his appointment, he had held consulting positions with eight scientific journals, was the author of eight monographs, and had written over 200 scientific papers. Since becoming Editor, Stan has added to his stature, not only through his editorship but also through his continuing scholarly work. He has continued to publish scientific papers, and he now has over 300 titles to his name. During the course of a productive and prestigious career, Dr Siegelman has given nearly 50 invited lectures, participated in nearly 50 postgraduate courses, and served over 50 visiting professorships.

After settling in as Editor, Dr Siegelman turned his dry wit, quick mind, and scholarly curiosity to a new venue: scholarly publishing. It was not enough that Stan Siegelman edited *Radiology*; he wanted to examine all aspects of publishing a scholarly journal. Using what was then a relatively new tool, he and his staff tracked manuscripts by computer from initial receipt through review, revision, acceptance or rejection, copy editing, and publication. As a result of the statistics compiled by the manuscript tracking program and a careful scoring of both quality and recommendations of reviewers, Dr Siegelman has been able to effect continuous improvement in reviewer quality and reductions in time to decision. Statistics on recommendations of reviewers became the basis of Dr Siegelman's often cited article, "Assassins and Zealots: Variations in Peer Review," which was published in *Radiology* in 1991. In that article, he observed that certain reviewers were very stringent and recommended rejection much more often than the norm, and that another group of reviewers tended to accept a disproportionate number of manuscripts. His continued tracking of the varied standards of individual reviewers allowed him to improve the fairness of the peer review process by considering past reviewer ratings when selecting reviewers for manuscripts and evaluating reviewer recommendations.

In his inaugural editorial, published in the January 1986 issue of *Radiology*, Dr Siegelman acknowledged the accomplishments of his predecessor, Dr William R. Eyler, but promised authors, reviewers, and readers a number of changes. Specifically, he promised that authors would receive a decision on their manuscripts within 7-8 weeks of receipt, that authors whose papers were not accepted would receive constructive criticism, that authors would be given a commitment to publish articles on which revisions were requested, that with the letter of acceptance authors would receive copies of pertinent reviewers' comments and detailed instructions for revisions, that imposition of arbitrary standards would be avoided, and that "*Radiology* would avoid a Procrustean approach to format, style, and subject matter. (Procrustes was the Greek brigand of legend who measured his captives on an iron bed. Victims with dimensions which did not conform were stretched or vital parts were summarily chopped off.)"

Dr Siegelman promised reviewers that *Radiology* would recognize and reward major reviewers to make their efforts more meaningful, that young reviewers would be cultivated, and that efforts would be made to promote the concept of reviewing as an important scholarly activity.

To readers, Dr Siegelman promised that *Radiology* would be directed to the radiologist in clinical practice, that preference would be given to manuscripts that focused on clinical diagnosis while communications describing refinements in techniques and documenting the accuracy of newer imaging modalities would also be published, that original research articles would be supplemented by occasional critical reviews, that a new, solicited "State of the Art" section would appear regularly, that articles would be presented to clarify confusion over the appropriate role of new imaging modalities, and, finally, that a goal would be to maintain an appropriate balance in the number of articles from key areas of interest.

Dr Siegelman implemented several new features during his tenure, all in an effort to add "texture" to the Journal. He created the previously mentioned State of the Art section, which on a recent readership survey was the most widely read section of the Journal. He also instituted companion editorials to accompany and give perspective to important articles; the Devil's Advocate section to provide a forum for other points of view; Sum and Substance articles to provide a quick summary of review articles from other subspecialty journals; the Perspectives and Radiology at Large sections to investigate some of the practical aspects of being a radiologist; Meeting Notes to summarize the RSNA annual meeting; and How I Do It articles to allow experts in specialized procedures to share their knowledge with readers. Dr Siegelman also included Opinions, Editor's Pages, and Interludes to add to the Journal's texture. One of the most important contributions of his tenure may have come from the virtual creation of a new journal. In March 1989, *Radiology* published the first of three supplements that were a collaborative effort of RSNA and the Society of Cardiovascular and Interventional Radiology. Those supplements evolved into the now very well respected *Journal of Vascular and Interventional Radiology*.

Stan Siegelman's reputation for intelligence and efficiency has been long and well established, but recent RSNA Past President Ernest J. Ferris, MD, provides anecdotal proof of both. Dr Ferris writes, "As a visiting professor, I was queried on 12 extraordinarily difficult cases. These cases were one of a kind, and without a built-in computer they bordered on impossible. Nevertheless, perhaps through a stroke of luck, I was able to correctly identify eight out of the 12."

"The presenter then told me that I had done extraordinarily well and received an 80%. I was puzzled because, although math is not my forte, eight out of 12 certainly does not add up to 80%. In response to my query, the presenter indicated that Dr Siegelman had also been presented the same 12 cases and correctly identified 10 out of the 12. Since Dr Siegelman was used as a gold standard (the presenter said he was perfect), 10 out of 12 would be perfect."

Dr Ferris also provides proof that Dr Siegelman's legendary efficiency began early in his career: "As a young resident, I received training from some of the mentors that also taught Stanley Siegelman. Whenever I was presented with a task to do, I did it diligently and performed to the best of my ability either the technical or academic problem that was presented to me. The response I always got from the mentors was that although I had done a good job, Dr Siegelman would have completed it 10 minutes ago."

Further evidence of Dr Siegelman's reputation is provided by two longtime colleagues, David Naidich, MD, and Rogelio Moncada, MD, who write, "Easily overlooked in all his many editorial accomplishments, however, is the true germ of Stan's genius. Stanley Siegelman first and foremost is an extraordinary clinician. From the beginning of his career, those who have known Stan personally or worked beside him know that he is the consummate diagnostician....His reputation as a wizard at differential diagnosis, drawn from an encyclopedic knowledge of the radiologic literature, knows no equal. Through all the years of technological innovation that have so transformed our field, this gift has never left him."

On a personal note, I have had the privilege of working and practicing with Dr Siegelman at Johns Hopkins Hospital for the past 10 years. I have been continuously impressed by his pervasive clinical knowledge and must admit to sneaking many of our toughest neuroradiology cases over to Dr Siegelman for his opinion, as no one knows the whole of imaging literature as well as he does. Dr Siegelman also conveys his knowledge to others as few can; *Radiology's* loss is our department's gain.

In his typically thorough manner, Stan announced his intention to retire 2½ years ago to allow sufficient time for a thorough search for his replacement and an orderly transition between editorial offices. Shortly after he made his announcement, he lost the love of his life, his wife, Doris, to cancer. Everyone who met them at the RSNA meetings during the first 10 years of Stan's editorship knew that they were inseparable. Doris was not only his wife, but was his best friend and collaborator, and she has been missed by all who knew her.

In further recognition of a job well done, the RSNA Board of Directors has granted Dr Siegelman the title of Editor Emeritus of *Radiology*. Stanley Siegelman, you have my thanks, those of the Board of Directors, and those of your many colleagues for your contributions to our Society and our profession. ■

A Note of Thanks

The names that follow in this note of thanks include radiologists, physicists, engineers, statisticians, computer scientists, and members of almost every medical specialty. Each has contributed to the process of reviewing manuscripts for *Radiology*. We hope that the experience has been rewarding for all. The Radiological Society of North America takes this opportunity to recognize these individuals and to express gratitude to them for their most significant contributions.

—Michael A. Sullivan, MD,
RSNA President
—Stanley S. Siegelman, MD,
Editor

Patricia L. Abbitt, MD
Denise R. Aberle, MD
Stacey J. Ackerman, MSE, PhD
Lee P. Adler, MD
Alex M. Aisen, MD
Abass Alavi, MD
Philip O. Alderson, MD
Archie A. Alexander, MD
Michael M. Ambrosino, MD
E. Stephen Amis, Jr, MD
Dee Claire Anderson, MD
James H. Anderson, PhD
Mark William Anderson, MD
James C. Andrews, MD
Jerry S. Apple, MD
Andrew Arai, MD
Ronald L. Arenson, MD
Susan M. Ascher, MD
Frederic B. Askin, MD
Christos A. Athanasoulis, MD
Scott W. Atlas, MD
Mostafa Atri, MD
John H. M. Austin, MD
Mary M. Austin-Seymour, MD
Hector Avram, PhD
Diane S. Babcock, MD
Mark E. Baker, MD
Stephen R. Baker, MD
Robert S. Balaban, PhD
Dennis M. Balfe, MD
William S. Ball, Jr, MD
Emil J. Balthazar, MD
Estelle R. Bank, MD
Marc P. Banner, MD
Peter B. Barker, DPhil
Gary T. Barnes, PhD
Murray G. Baron, MD
Richard L. Baron, MD
Klemens H. Barth, MD
Bruce R. Baumgartner, MD
Norman Joseph Beauchamp, Jr, MD
Thomas J. Beck, ScD
Christoph D. Becker, MD
Gary J. Becker, MD
Joshua A. Becker, MD
John M. Bedwinek, MD
Javier L. Beltran, MD
Beryl R. Benacerraf, MD
Harold F. Bennett, MD, PhD
Carol B. Benson, MD
Walter E. Berdon, MD
Wendie A. Berg, MD, PhD
Colleen J. Bergin, MD
Yahya M. Berkmen, MD
Lincoln L. Berland, MD
Michael A. Bettmann, MD
Gordon H. Beute, MD
C. Roger Bird, MD
Robyn Leah Birdwell, MD
Bernard A. Birnbaum, MD
George S. Bisset III, MD
William C. Black, MD
Duane D. Blatter, MD
Johan G. Blickman, MD, PhD
Russell A. Blinder, MD
Johan L. Bloem, MD
David A. Bluemke, MD, PhD
Joseph Bonn, MD
John M. Boone, PhD
Joseph A. Borrello, MD
Morton A. Bosniak, MD
Jose F. Botet, MD
Paul A. Bottomley, PhD
Robert D. Boutin, MD
James D. Bowie, MD
Lawrence M. Boxt, MD
William G. Bradley, Jr, MD, PhD
Michael N. Brant-Zawadzki, MD
Robert C. Brasch, MD
Ethan M. Braunstein, MD
Robert L. Bree, MD
Robert K. Breger, MD
Steven N. Breiter, MD
Patrice M. Bret, MD
James A. Brink, MD
Alan S. Brody, MD
Jeffrey M. Brody, MD
Douglas L. Brown, MD
Jeffrey J. Brown, MD
Larry R. Brown, MD
Manuel L. Brown, MD
Truman R. Brown, PhD
R. Nick Bryan, MD, PhD
Ronald O. Bude, MD
Peter Buetow, MD
Michael H. Buonocore, MD, PhD
Fred Burbank, MD
D. Lawrence Burk, Jr, MD
David J. Burkart, MD
Patricia E. Burrows, MD
Edwin D. Cacayorin, MD
Ana Cajade-Law, MD
Peter W. Callen, MD
Christopher E. Cann, PhD
Gary R. Caputo, MD
John F. Cardella, MD
Barbara A. Carroll, MD
Paul L. Carson, PhD
William J. Casarella, MD
Philip N. Cascade, MD
Giovanna Casola, MD
Dev P. Chakraborty, PhD
Theodore P. Chambers, MD
Paul J. Chang, MD
Chuslip Charnsangavej, MD
Marvin H. Chasen, MD
Thomas L. Chenevert, PhD
Felix S. Chew, MD
Judith L. Chezmar, MD
Harrell G. Chotas, MS
Peter L. Choyke, MD
Olivier Clement, MD, PhD
Melvin E. Clouse, MD
Richard H. Cohan, MD
Mervyn D. Cohen, MD
Wendy A. Cohen, MD
R. Edward Coleman, MD
Dewey J. Conces, Jr, MD
Thomas E. Conturo, MD
William F. Conway, MD, PhD
Jay S. Cooper, MD
Peter L. Cooperberg, MD
Constantin Cope, MD
Philip Costello, MD
Christopher T. Coughlin, MD
James D. Cox, MD
Jeffrey R. Crass, MD
John J. Cronan, MD
Lawrence E. Crooks, PhD
Joel Cure, MD
Nancy S. Curry, MD
Hugh D. Curtin, MD
Carl J. D'Orsi, MD
Murray K. Dalinka, MD

Michael D. Darcy, MD
Patricia C. Davis, MD
Peter L. Davis, MD
Sheila D. Davis, MD
Edward E. De Lange, MD
Vincent De Maio, MD
Albert De Roos, MD
Arthur A. De Smet, MD
Jorg F. Debatin, MD
Donald Francis Denny, Jr, MD
D. David Dershaw, MD
Terry S. Desser, MD
Beth Deutch, MD
Kevin Dickey, MD
William P. Dillon, MD
Michael A. Dipietro, MD
David G. Disler, MD
W. Thomas Dixon, PhD
Gerald D. Dodd III, MD
Kunio Doi, PhD
Bart L. Dolmatch, MD
Bernadine Donahue, MD
James Donaldson, MD
John L. Doppman, MD
Walter E. Drane, MD
Burton P. Drayer, MD
Andre J. Duerinckx, MD, PhD
Charles Dumoulin, PhD
N. Reed Dunnick, MD
Andrew J. Dwyer, MD
Samuel J. Dwyer III, PhD
James P. Earls, MD
Franklin Earnest, IV, MD
Robert R. Edelman, MD
Richard L. Ehman, MD
G. W. Eklund, MD
Georges Y. El-Khoury, MD
Nancy A. Ellerbroek, MD
James H. Ellis, MD
John Eng, MD
Dieter R. Enzmann, MD
Jonathan I. Epstein, MD
Scott J. Erickson, MD
Rainer Erlemann, MD
David J. Eschelman, MD
Ronald G. Evens, MD
William A. Fajman, MD
Panos P. Fatouros, PhD
Kenneth G. Faulkner, PhD
Peter J. Feczko, MD
Michael P. Federle, MD
Stephen A. Feig, MD
David A. Feinberg, MD, PhD
Frieda Feldman, MD
Merrill I. Feldman, MD, FACR
Brian D. Fellmeth, MD, PhD
Maria del Pilar Fernandez, MD
Sandra K. Fernbach, MD
Ernest J. Ferris, MD
Joseph T. Ferrucci, Jr, MD
Roy A. Filly, MD
Daniel A. Finelli, MD
Hossein Firooznia, MD
Dennis M. Fisher, MD
Elliot K. Fishman, MD
Charles R. Fitz, MD
James L. Fleckenstein, MD
W. Dennis Foley, MD
Thomas K. F. Foo, PhD
John Chetley Ford, PhD
Howard Paul Forman, MD
Bruno D. Fornage, MD
Flemming Forsberg, PhD
Gregory S. Foster, DO
Evan K. Fram, MD
Isaac R. Francis, MD
Joseph A. Frank, MD
Steven David Frankel, MD
James D. Fraser, MD
Carolyn R. Freeman, MB, BS
Patrick C. Freeny, MD
Kirk A. Frey, MD, PhD
Richard M. Friedenberg, MD
Arnold C. Friedman, MD
Paul J. Friedman, MD
J. James Frost, MD, PhD
Carl R. Fuhrman, MD
Ann Fulcher, MD
Ernest V. Garcia, PhD
Geoffrey A. Gardiner, Jr, MD
Brian S. Garra, MD
Spencer B. Gay, MD
Bob W. Gayler, MD
Gregg M. Gaylord, MD
G. Scott Gazelle, MD
Stephen S. Gebarski, MD
Warren B. Gefter, MD
David W. Gelfand, MD
Michael J. Gelfand, MD
Harry K. Genant, MD
Lindell R. Gentry, MD
Ajax E. George, MD
Bernard Ghelman, MD
Rene Gilles, MD
Vicente Gilsanz, MD
Louis A. Gilula, MD
Eric L. Gingold, PhD
Herbert J. Glatt, MD
Harvey S. Glazer, MD
Jerry Glickson, PhD
Claus-C. Gluer, PhD
J. David Godwin, MD
Reginald Goei, MD
Richard H. Gold, MD
Barry B. Goldberg, MD
Henry I. Goldberg, MD
Amy Beth Goldman, MD
Stanford M. Goldman, MD
Ruth B. Goldstein, MD
Antoinette S. Gomes, MD
Charles A. Gooding, MD
Lawrence R. Goodman, MD, FACR
Philip C. Goodman, MD
Mitchell M. Goodsitt, PhD
David P. Gorczyca, MD
Richard M. Gore, MD
Clement J. Grassi, PhD
Joel E. Gray, MD
Reginald E. Greene, MD, PhD
Robert A. Greenes, MD, PhD
Landis K. Griffeth, MD, PhD
N. Thorne Griscom, MD
Stuart A. Groskin, MD
Barry H. Gross, MD
Robert I. Grossman, MD
James F. Gruden, MD
W. Bonner Guilford, MD
Jud W. Gurney, MD
Fernando R. Gutierrez, MD
E. Mark Haacke, PhD
John R. Haaga, MD
David B. Hackney, MD
Francis J. Hahn, MD
Ferris M. Hall, MD
Edward Halperin, MD
Ethan J. Halpern, MD
Ulrike M. Hamper, MD
Steven E. Harms, MD
Kathleen M. Harris, MD
Ziv J. Haskal, MD
Robert R. Hattery, MD
Victor M. Haughton, MD
Randall A. Hawkins, MD, PhD
Curtis W. Hayes, MD
Tamara Miner Haygood, MD, PhD
L. Anne Hayman, MD
Stephen T. Hecht, MD
Jay P. Heiken, MD
E. Robert Heitzman, MD
Clyde A. Helms, MD
Joseph A. Helpern, PhD
Mark A. Helvie, MD
William R. Hendee, PhD
R. Edward Hendrick, PhD
R. Mark Henkelman, PhD
Daniel Henry, MD
Claudia I. Henschke, MD, PhD
Robert J. Herfkens, MD
Peter G. Herman, MD
Marta Hernanz-Schulman, MD
Christian J. Herold, MD
Barbara S. Hertzberg, MD
Richard J. Herzog, MD
Samuel J. Hessel, MD
Sylvia H. Heywang-Kobrunner, MD
Marshall E. Hicks, MD
Charles B. Higgins, MD
Chia-Sing Ho, MB
Juerg Hodler, MD
James C. Hoffman, Jr, MD
Jacqueline Hogge, MD
B. Leonard Holman, MD
Kenneth D. Hopper, MD
Joseph A. Horton, MD
Florence Houn, MD, MPH
David Hovsepian, MD
Hedvig Hricak, MD, PhD
Patricia A. Hudgins, MD
James W. Hugg, PhD
Frans-Jan H. Hulsmans, MD, PhD
David W. Hunter, MD
Robert W. Hurst, MD
David H. Hussey, MD
Nola M. Hylton, PhD
Naiyer Imam, MD
Joseph P. Imperato, MD
Joseph Introcaso, MD
Jeffrey M. Isner, MD
Yuji Itai, MD
Clifford R. Jack, Jr, MD
Valerie P. Jackson, MD
C. Carl Jaffe, MD
Nora A. Janjan, MD
Marcia C. Javitt, MD
R. Brooke Jeffrey, MD
Peter Jezzard, PhD
Blake A. Johnson, MD
Matthew S. Johnson, MD
Pam Johnson, MD
Ferenc A. Jolesz, MD
Bronwyn Jones, FRACP, FRCR
Peter M. Joseph, PhD
R. Gilbert Jost, MD

Saadoon Kadir, MD
Willi A. Kalender, PhD
Lester Kalisher, MD
Emanuel Kanal, MD
Krishna Kandarpa, MD, PhD
Mel L. Kantor, DDS
Phoebe A. Kaplan, MD
David Karasick, MD
Susan V. Kattapuram, MD
Douglas S. Katz, MD
Richard W. Katzberg, MD
Barry T. Katzen, MD
Leon Kaufman, PhD
Rachel B. Kaufmann, PhD
Jeremy J. Kaye, MD
Elias Kazam, MD
Ella A. Kazerooni, MD
Stephen T. Kee, MD
Marc S. Keller, MD
Paul J. Keller, PhD
Elizabeth Kelly-Fry, ScM, EdD
Philip J. Kenney, MD
Mary T. Keogan, MD
Leena Ketonen, MD, PhD
Stephen A. Kieffer, MD
Ruben Kier, MD
Marie Foley Kijewski, ScD
E. Edmund Kim, MD
Carolyn Kimme-Smith, PhD
Gerald A. King, MD
Donald R. Kirks, MD
Lawrence Kleinberg, MD
Mark A. Kliewer, MD
J. Bruce Kneeland, MD
Edmond A. Knopp, MD
Robert E. Koehler, MD
Kelly Koeller, MD
Daniel B. Kopans, MD
Andreas F. Kopp, MD
Melvyn T. Korobkin, MD
David M. Kramer, PhD
Elissa L. Kramer, MD
Sandra Sue Kramer, MD
Gabriel P. Krestin, MD
Irvin I. Kricheff, MD
Kenneth A. Krohn, PhD
Jonathan B. Kruskal, MD, PhD
Janet E. Kuhlman, MD
Alfred B. Kurtz, MD
David C. Kushner, MD
Brian S. Kuszyk, MD
Jeanne M. Laberge, MD
Michel Lafortune, MD
Fred Laine, MD
Faye C. Laing, MD
Lamk M. Lamki, MD
Neela Lamki, MD, FRCP(C)
Erich K. Lang, MD
Philipp Lang, MD
Robert C. Lange, PhD
Curtis P. Langlotz, MD, PhD
Michael Laniado, MD
Richard E. Latchaw, MD
Denis Le Bihan, MD, PhD
Robert L. Lebowitz, MD
Richard A. Leder, MD
Benjamin C. P. Lee, MD
Ding-Jen Lee, MD, PhD
Joseph K. T. Lee, MD
Roland R. Lee, MD
F. T. Lee, Jr, MD
Norman Leeds, MD
Mark H. Leibenhaut, MD
Sher Leiman, MD
Robert E. Lenkinski, PhD
Robert M. Lerner, MD, PhD
Janis Gissel Letourneau, MD
Ann N. Leung, MD
David C. Levin, MD
Marc S. Levine, MD
Robert G. Levitt, MD
Seymour H. Levitt, MD
Howard M. Levy, MD
Lucien M. Levy, MD, PhD
Frank J. Lexa, MD
King C. P. Li, MD, FRCP(C)
Laura Liberman, MD
Herman I. Libshitz, MD
James M. Lieberman, MD
Jonathan M. Links, PhD
Otha W. Linton, MSJ
Jay J. Listinsky, MD, PhD
Andrew W. Litt, MD
Peter J. Littrup, MD
Jay S. Loeffler, MD
Jesus M. Longo, MD
Christine H. Lorenz, PhD
Robert B. Lufkin, MD
Loralie D. Ma, MD, PhD
William J. MacIntyre, PhD
Heber M. MacMahon, MD
Mahmood F. Mafee, MD
Donna Magid, MD
Dean D. T. Maglinte, MD, FACR
B. J. Manaster, MD, PhD
Lawrence G. Manco, MD
Anthony A. Mancuso, MD
Guy Marchal, MD
James E. Marks, MD
Michael P. Marks, MD
Christopher H. Marshall, PhD
Thomas J. Masaryk, MD
Graeme F. Mason, PhD
Vincent P. Mathews, MD
John R. Mathieson, MD
Osamu Matsui, MD
Robert F. Mattrey, MD
Andrew A. Maudsley, PhD
Matthew A. Mauro, MD
John R. Mayo, MD
William W. Mayo-Smith, MD
William H. McAlister, MD
Shirley M. McCarthy, MD, PhD
Thomas R. McCauley, MD
Bruce L. McClennan, MD
Cynthia H. McCollough, PhD
Timothy C. McGowan, MD
Vincent G. M. McDermott, MB
John P. McGahan, MD
Theresa C. McLoud, MD
Elliot R. McVeigh, PhD
L. Santiago Medina, MD
Jon W. Meilstrup, MD
Elias Melhem, MD
Carolyn Cidis Meltzer, MD
Gary L. Merhar, MD
Christopher R. B. Merritt, MD
Dieter Meyerhoff, DR, RER, NAT
Reuben S. Mezrich, MD, PhD
Duane Mezwa, MD
William D. Middleton, MD
Donald L. Miller, MD
John H. Miller, MD
Tom R. Miller, MD, PhD
Wallace T. Miller, MD
Scott A. Mirowitz, MD
Stuart E. Mirvis, MD
Donald G. Mitchell, MD
Julie S. Mitnick, MD
Harold A. Mitty, MD
Michael T. Modic, MD
Paul L. Molina, MD
Rogelio M. Moncada, MD
Barbara S. Monsees, MD
Lee H. Monsein, MD
Elizabeth H. Moore, MD
Sheila G. Moore, MD
Christopher J. Moran, MD
Richard L. Morin, PhD
Thomas W. Morris, PhD
Albert A. Moss, MD
Peter R. Mueller, MD
John P. Mugler III, PhD
Suresh K. Mukherji, MD
Nestor L. Muller, MD, PhD
Peter L. Munk, MD
Mark D. Murphey, MD
Timothy P. Murphy, MD
William A. Murphy, Jr, MD
James B. Naidich, MD
Thomas P. Naidich, MD
Sandy A. Napel, PhD
James A. Nelson, MD
Rendon C. Nelson, MD
Marvin D. Nelson, Jr, MD
Beverley Newman, MD
Geraldine M. Newmark, MD
Edward L. Nickoloff, DSc
John L. Nosher, MD
Robert A. Novelline, MD
David A. Nyberg, MD
James K. O'Donnell, MD
Eric W. Olcott, MD
Roger J. Ordidge, PhD
Susan G. Orel, MD
Douglas A. Ortendahl, PhD
Orlando Ortiz, MD
Zvi H. Oster, MD
David J. Ott, MD
Eric K. Outwater, MD
William E. Palmer, MD
David M. Panicek, MD
Marguerite T. Parisi, MD
Steve H. Parker, MD
Robert W. Parkey, MD
C. Leon Partain, MD, PhD
Cynthia B. Paschal, PhD
Maitray D. Patel, MD
Suresh C. Patel, MD
Mini N. Pathria, MD
Edward F. Patz, Jr, MD
Erik Karl Paulson, MD
William Pavlicek, PhD
Lorie R. Pelc, PhD
Norbert J. Pelc, ScD
David R. Pennes, MD
William H. Perman, PhD
Jerry P. Petasnick, MD
Charles G. Peterfy, MD, PhD
Susan Brothers Peterman, MD, MPH
Roderic I. Pettigrew, MD, PhD
Michael D. Phillips, MD
Theodore L. Phillips, MD

Liane E. Philpotts, MD
Marcelle L. Piccolello, MD
Daniel Picus, MD
Joel F. Platt, MD
Donald B. Plewes, PhD
Rubem Pochaczevsky, MD
Donald A. Podoloff, MD
Joseph F. Polak, MD, MPH
Abraham H. Pollack, MD
Howard M. Pollack, MD
Martin G. Pomper, MD, PhD
Peter Y. Poon, MD
Hollis G. Potter, MD
Thomas R. Pounds, MD
Andrew K. Poznanski, MD
Satish C. Prasad, PhD
Erin Colum Prenger, DO
Steven L. Primack, MD
Martin R. Prince, MD, PhD
Anthony V. Proto, MD
Julien B. C. M. Puylaert, MD, PhD
Robert M. Quencer, MD
Stephen F. Quinn, MD
Douglas J. Quint, MD
Leslie Eisenbud Quint, MD
Nagesh Ragavendra, MD
Philip W. Ralls, MD
Parvati Ramchandani, MD
Patricia A. Randall, MD
Vijay M. Rao, MD
Carl E. Ravin, MD
Murray Rebner, MD
Michael P. Recht, MD
Helen C. Redman, MD
Chet R. Rees, MD
Patrice K. Rehm, MD
Peter Reimer, MD
Caroline Reinhold, MD
James W. Reinig, MD
William R. Reinus, MD
Martine Remy-Jardin, MD, PhD
Donald L. Renfrew, MD
Donald Resnick, MD
Charles Resnik, MD
Handel E. Reynolds, MD
Stephen J. Riederer, PhD
Cameron J. Ritchie, PhD
Douglas D. Robertson, MD, PhD
Neil M. Rofsky, MD
Philip A. Rogoff, MD
Nancy K. Rollins, MD
Pablo R. Ros, MD
Zehava Sadka Rosenberg, MD
C. John Rosenquist, MD
Daniel I. Rosenthal, MD
Jeffrey S. Ross, MD
Henry D. Royal, MD
Stuart A. Royal, MS, MD
Joel D. Rubenstein, MD
Stephen E. Rubesin, MD
Eva Rubin, MD
Geoffrey D. Rubin, MD
Jonathan M. Rubin, MD, PhD
Eric J. Russell, MD
John M. Sabol, PhD
Robert H. Sagerman, MD
Sanjay Saini, MD
Jeet S. Sandhu, MD
Carl M. Sandler, MD
Martin P. Sandler, MD
Cornelia M. Schaefer-Prokop, MD
Barbara Schepps, MD
Steven E. Schild, MD
Robert A. Schmidt, MD
Mark E. Schweitzer, MD
Leanne L. Seeger, MD
Joanna J. Seibert, MD
David J. Seidenwurm, MD
Steven E. Seltzer, MD
Richard C. Semelka, MD
Kitt Shaffer, MD, PhD
Lorraine G. Shapeero, MD
Marcelle J. Shapiro, MD
Patrick F. Sheedy, II, MD
Frank G. Shellock, PhD, FACSM
Sheila Sheth, MD
David S. Shimm, MD
Richard D. Shlansky-Goldberg, MD
William P. Shuman, MD
Gregory T. Sica, MD
Edward A. Sickles, MD
Aslam R. Siddiqui, MD
Barry A. Siegel, MD
Marilyn J. Siegel, MD
Evan S. Siegelman, MD
Edward B. Silberstein, MD
Frederic N. Silverman, MD
Paul M. Silverman, MD
Stuart G. Silverman, MD
William C. Small, MD, PhD
Patricia Smith, MD
Robert C. Smith, MD
Tony P. Smith, MD
Wendy Smoker, MD
Stephen B. Solomon, MD
Peter M. Som, MD
F. Graham Sommer, MD
James A. Sorenson, PhD
H. Dirk Sostman, MD
Michael C. Soulen, MD
Renate L. Soulen, MD
Philippe Soyer, MD, PhD
Robert F. Spataro, MD
Dan Spielman, PhD
Paul W. Spirn, MD
Beverly A. Spirt, MD
Thomas A. Spraggins, PhD
Charles E. Spritzer, MD
Edward V. Staab, MD
Philip Stanley, MD
David D. Stark, MD
Paul Stark, MD
A. Thomas Stavros, MD
Sharon M. Stein, MD
Lynne S. Steinbach, MD
Fred L. Steinberg, MD
Robert M. Steiner, MD
Alan D. Steinfeld, MD, FACR
Carol B. Stelling, MD
David H. Stephens, MD
Eric J. Stern, MD
Randy E. Stevens, MD
Giles W. Stevenson, MD
Paul C. Stomper, MD
Janet Strife, MD
Daniel C. Sullivan, MD
Kevin L. Sullivan, MD
Ronald M. Summers, MD, PhD
Murali Sundaram, MD
Jonathan H. Sunshine, PhD
Joel D. Swartz, MD
Stephen J. Swensen, MD
Gordon Sze, MD
Kenichi Takayasu, MD
Robert D. Tarver, MD
Andrew J. Taylor, MD
George A. Taylor, MD
Kenneth J. W. Taylor, MD, PhD
Sharlene A. Teefey, MD
George Paul Teitelbaum, MD
Clark M. C. Tempany, MD
David I. Thickman, MD
Ruedi F. Thoeni, MD
Frank Deaver Thomas, MD
Stephen R. Thomas, PhD
John R. Thornbury, MD
M. Kristin Thorsen, MD
James H. Thrall, MD
Amy S. Thurmond, MD
Phillip F. J. Tirman, MD
Jaime Tisnado, MD
Barry Toombs, MD
Saara M. S. Totterman, MD, PhD
William G. Totty, MD
Richard B. Towbin, MD
Jeffrey D. Towers, MD
Scott O. Trerotola, MD
Jay S. Tsuruda, MD
David A. Turner, MD
Mary Ann Turner, MD
Robert Turner, PhD
Patrick A. Turski, MD
Diane M. Twickler, MD
Sidney Ulreich, MD
Evan C. Unger, MD
Bruce A. Urban, MD
Arina Van Breda, MD
Marnix T. Van Holsbeeck, MD
Michael W. Vannier, MD
Eric Vansonnenberg, MD
Thomas M. Vesely, MD
David J. Vining, MD
Simon Vinitski, PhD
Robert L. Vogelzang, MD
Thomas J. Vogl, MD
Gustav K. Von Schulthess, MD, PhD
Carl J. Vyborny, MD, PhD
Kay H. Vydareny, MD
Louis K. Wagner, PhD
Richard L. Wahl, MD
Marilyn M. Walkey, MD
James W. Walsh, MD
Arthur C. Waltman, MD
Bruce J. Walz, MD
John C. Wandtke, MD
David M. Warshauer, MD
Peter Nelson Waybill, MD
Richard J. Wechsler, MD
Noah Weg, MD
Janna P. Wehrle, PhD
Jamey Weichert, PhD
Irving N. Weinberg, MD, PhD
Edward Weinberger, MD
Michael W. Weiner, MD
Jeffrey C. Weinreb, MD
Jeffrey P. Weiss, MD
Ralph Weissleder, MD, PhD
Barbara N. Weissman, MD
Jane L. Weissman, MD
Jack L. Westcott, MD
Per-Lennart Westesson, DDS, PhD
Paul S. Wheeler, MD
Charles White, MD

Richard D. White, MD
Susan J. White, MD
Robert I. White, Jr, MD
Alan L. Williams, MD
David M. Williams, MD
John S. Wills, MD
Anthony J. Wilson, MB, CHB
Michael A. Wilson, MD
Helen T. Winer-Muram, MD
Fred Winsberg, MD
Franz J. Wippold, II, MD
Gerhard R. Wittich, MD
Gerald L. Wolf, MD, PhD
Ronald L. Wolf, MD, PhD
Steven D. Wolff, MD, PhD
Samuel M. Wolpert, MD
Beverly P. Wood, MD
Michael L. Wood, PhD
Pamela K. Woodard, MD
John H. Woodring, MD
Kenneth C. Wright, PhD
Martin J. Yaffe, PhD
Wayne F. J. Yakes, MD
Lawrence Yao, MD
Stuart W. Young, MD
David M. Yousem, MD
Kyle Yu, MD
E. Kent Yucel, MD
Heun Yung Yune, MD
J. Michael Zerin, MD
Robert A. Zimmerman, MD
Darryl Zuckerman, MD
Yali Amit, MD
Ty Bae, MS, MD, PhD
Murray Becker, MD, PhD
Clifford Chao, MD
Cecil Charles, MD
Christopher Chong, MD
Patrick M. Colletti, MD
Bradley J. Erickson, MD, PhD
Robert Frost, BS
Mark George, MD
Dr H. A. J. Gielkens
Peter F. Hahn, MD
Larry T. Harashe, MD
Janie Hrung, MD
Revathy B. Iyer, MD
Edmund Kwok, PhD
Mark Langer, MD
Tore Larheim, MD
Weili Lin, MD
Amon Liu, MD
Tom Lue, MD
Andrea Magen, MD
Nancy Major, MD
H. Page McAdams, MD
Luka Milas, MD, PhD
Timothy J. Mosher, MD
P. David Mozley, MD
Mahesh R. Patel, MD
Peter M. T. Pattynama, MD
Mahmood K. Razavi, MD
Beth Schueler, PhD
Dana S. Schwartz, MD
Lynn J. Verbey, PhD
Ken Yamaguchi, MD
Chi-Shing Zee, MD

Abstracts of Current Literature

Thorax

Survival and Prognostic Factors in Resected N2 Non–Small Cell Lung Cancer: A Study of 140 Cases. Johan F. Vansteenkiste, Paul R. De Leyn, Georges J. Deneffe, et al. *Ann Thorac Surg* 1997; 63: 1441–1450. (J.F.V., Respiratory Tumor Unit, Department of Pulmonology, University Hospital Gasthuisberg, Herestraat 49, B-3000 Leuven, Belgium)

Background: The selection of stage IIIA N2 non–small cell lung cancer patients for primary surgical treatment remains controversial. *Methods:* One hundred forty patients with resected non–small cell lung cancer who eventually proved to have pathologic N2 disease were studied with a univariate and multivariate analysis of prognostic factors. *Results:* Nineteen patients had a positive mediastinoscopy; the others had a preoperative N0 or N1 stage. Complete resection rate was 80.7%. Five-year survival was 20.8% (95% confidence interval, 17.2%–24.4%), 32.2% in mediastinoscopy-negative patients. In the univariate analysis, clinical N stage at mediastinoscopy, complete resection, performance status, T stage, number of metastatic levels in adenocarcinoma, and nodal capsule rupture were important factors. In a multivariate model, survival was worse in case of higher T stage (relative risk = 1.43), lower performance status (relative risk = 1.37), involvement of more than one node level (relative risk = 1.68), nonsquamous histology (relative risk = 1.29), and clinical N2 stage (relative risk = 1.43). Long-term survival was unlikely when lactic dehydrogenase or carcinoembryonic antigen levels were elevated. *Conclusion:* In clinical N0 or N1 cancer, complete resection resulted in reasonable survival prospects. In patients with N2 disease discovered at mediastinoscopy surgical treatment was only worthwhile in case of minimal N2. Several unfavorable prognostic factors could be identified in the univariate analysis and confirmed in a multivariate Cox model.
AUTHORS' ABSTRACT

Lymph Node Type as a Prognostic Factor for Survival in T2 N1 M0 Non–Small Cell Lung Carcinoma. Edwin van Velzen, Repke J. Snijder, Aart Brutel de la Rivière, et al. *Ann Thorac Surg* 1997; 63:1436–1440. (Jules M. M. van den Bosch, Department of Pulmonology, Sint Antonius Hospital, PO Box 2500, 3430 EM Nieuwegein, The Netherlands)

Background: Patients with stage II non–small cell lung carcinoma represent a group with varying 5-year survival rates. The influence of specific types of lymph node involvement on survival was investigated. *Methods:* Of 2,009 patients operated on from 1977 through 1993, the cases of 391 patients with pathologic T2 N1 M0 disease were reviewed. The N1 status was refined into lymph node involvement by direct extension or by metastases in lobar or hilar lymph nodes. *Results:* The cumulative 5-year survival rate of all hospital survivors ($n = 369$) was 37.8%. The 5-year survival rate of patients with lobar metastases was superior to that of patients with hilar metastases (57.3% versus 30.3%; $P = .0028$) and that of patients with lymph node involvement by direct extension (57.3% versus 39.1%; $P = .03$). The survival rate did not differ between those with hilar metastases and those with direct extension. Survival was significantly poorer in patients with visceral pleural involvement, in patients with adenocarcinoma, and in patients older than 60 years. Survival was not related to sex, type of resection, central growth, or tumor size. *Conclusion:* Survival differs according to the type of lymph node involvement: Lobar lymph node metastasis seems to be an early stage of the disease, whereas hilar lymph node metastasis represents a more advanced form. However, in T2 N1 M0 disease, other factors besides nodal status also seem to play an important role in postoperative survival.
AUTHORS' ABSTRACT

Factors Influencing Long-Term Survival after Lung Metastasectomy. John H. Robert, Vincenzo Ambrogi, Bernadette Mermillod, et al. *Ann Thorac Surg* 1997; 63:777–784. (J.H.R., Unit of Thoracic Surgery, Hôpital Cantonal Universitaire, CH-1211 Geneva 14, Switzerland)

Background: Disease-free interval, histology of primary tumor, and number and size of metastases resected were studied after resection of pulmonary metastases. *Methods:* Between 1980 and 1993, 276 consecutive patients underwent lung resections for curative removal of metastatic disease. At subsequent relapse, 63 patients had a second-stage metastasectomy, 12 went on to a third phase, and two patients had four stages. *Results:* The primary tumor was sarcoma in 126 cases (46%), teratoma in 88 (32%), carcinoma in 53 (19%), melanoma in five, and miscellaneous in four. Actuarial survival was 64% at 2 Years (95% confidence interval 62%–74%), 48% at 5 years (40%–55%), and 35% at 10 years (23%–44%). *Conclusion:* Survival was not related to disease-free interval. Multivariate analysis showed that nearly all predictive information can be obtained through histologic studies ($P < .0001$); inclusion of the number of metastases resected contributed to a lesser degree ($P = .032$). Short disease-free intervals, numerous lung metastases, or even deposits recurring after a first or second metastasectomy should not preclude patients from operation.
AUTHORS' ABSTRACT

Postpneumonectomy Syndrome with an Ipsilateral Aortic Arch after Left Pneumonectomy. Fared M. Shamji, Jean Deslauriers, Thomas M. Daniel, et al. *Ann Thorac Surg* 1996; 62:1627–1631. (Thomas R. J. Todd, Toronto General Hospital, 10 Eaton-226, 200 Elizabeth St, Toronto, Ontario, Canada M5G 2C4)

Background: Previous reports have described bronchial obstruction after left pneumonectomy (so-called postpneumonectomy syndrome) in the presence of a right aortic arch with the bronchus being compressed between the accenting aorta and thoracic spine. This study reports on four patients with left postpneumonectomy syndrome in the presence of a normally located left aortic arch and ascending thoracic aorta. *Methods:* The case histories of four patients with this syndrome were reviewed, and several features common to all four were noted. In each case, the obstruction was thought to be due to a clockwise rotation of the mediastinum with bronchial compression occurring between the right main pulmonary artery and thoracic spine. *Results:* Three patients were treated by repositioning of the mediastinum, and all three obtained relief of their dyspnea. In these cases, permanent repositioning was ensured by the insertion of a prosthesis filled with saline solution. The fourth patient was successfully treated by resection of a portion of the adjacent thoracic vertebra. *Conclusion:* Postpneumonectomy syndrome can occur after a left pneumonectomy in the absence of a right aortic arch. The authors suggest that mediastinal repositioning with a prosthesis filled with saline solution is simple, is safe, and results in complete relief of preoperative symptoms.
AUTHORS' ABSTRACT

Genitourinary System

Does Resection of Adrenal Metastases from Non–Small Cell Lung Cancer Improve Survival? James D. Luketich, Michael E. Burt. *Ann Thorac Surg* 1996; 62:1614–1616. (M.E.B., Thoracic Surgery, Memorial Sloan-Kettering Cancer Center, 1275 York Ave, New York, NY 10021)

Background: Metastatic non–small cell lung cancer (NSCLC) carries a dismal prognosis, which is minimally affected by chemotherapy. Solitary brain metastases from NSCLC have been resected with 5-year survivals of 10%–30%. The objective of this study was to determine if resection of isolated adrenal metastases improves survival. *Methods:* Isolated adrenal metastases were found in 14 patients with NSCLC. Eight patients had resection after cisplatinum-based chemotherapy, and six received chemotherapy alone. *Results:* Median survival in the surgical group was significantly greater than that in the chemotherapy group (31 versus 8.5 months; $P = .03$). All patients in the chemotherapy group were dead by 22 months. Three-year actuarial survival in the surgical group was 38%. No difference in locoregional stage, size of adrenal metastases, patient

age, or performance status was present between the two groups. *Conclusion:* Long-term disease-free survival is possible after resection of isolated adrenal metastases from NSCLC. Resection of isolated adrenal metastases should be considered if the primary NSCLC is resectable.
AUTHORS' ABSTRACT

Antimitochondrial Antibody (113-1) in the Differential Diagnosis of Granular Renal Cell Tumors. Satish K. Tickoo, Mahul B. Amin, Michael D. Linden, et al. *Am J Surg Pathol* 1997; 21:922–930. (M.B.A., Department of Pathology, Henry Ford Hospital, 2799 W Grand Blvd, Detroit, MI 48202)

Abundant granular eosinophilic cytoplasm is a common feature of renal oncocytoma, chromophobe renal cell carcinoma, eosinophilic variant of papillary renal cell carcinoma, and the granular variant of clear cell renal cell carcinoma (RCC). Each of these entities has a unique architectural pattern and a distinctive molecular or cytogenetic profile. The chief reason for their distinction from one another is the difference in their biologic behavior. Careful and thorough light microscopic examination distinguishes most cases based on individual characteristic architectural and cytomorphologic features. However, precise characterization may be difficult in some cases because of overlapping morphologic features. The authors evaluated the antimitochondrial antibody 113-1 in an attempt to ascertain differences in immunostaining patterns in 57 cases of granular renal tumors, including 20 renal oncocytomas, 15 chromophobe RCCs, 13 granular variants of clear cell RCC, and nine eosinophilic variants of papillary RCC. Distinctive, and nearly exclusive, staining patterns were observed among the groups, with chromophobe RCC showing peripheral accentuation of coarse cytoplasmic granules (15 of 15), renal oncocytoma with diffuse and fine granularity (20 of 20), and granular variant of clear cell RCC with irregular cytoplasmic distribution of coarse granules (11 of 13). Staining was most intense in the eosinophilic variant of papillary RCC and was generally coarsely granular and diffuse. Staining patterns also differed in clear cell areas within chromophobe RCC and the granular variant of clear cell RCC. Although clear cells in the former group showed granular staining with peripheral accentuation, most of the clear cells in the latter lacked any staining. The authors conclude that, in addition to distinct cytoarchitectural features, immunostaining patterns with antimitochondrial antibody 113-1 appear to be a useful discriminatory adjunct in the complex differential diagnosis of granular renal cell tumors.
AUTHORS' ABSTRACT

Three-dimensional Computerized Tomographic Reconstruction of Colovesical Fistulas. Gregory A. Anderson, Ian L. Goldman, Gerald W. Mulligan. *J Urol* 1997; 158: 795–797. (From the Departments of Urology and Radiology, Marshfield Clinic, Wis)

Purpose: Use of three-dimensional tomographic reconstruction in evaluating colovesical fistulas is discussed. *Materials and Methods:* The authors compared three-dimensional computed tomographic (CT) images of colovesical fistulas to conventional CT images. *Results:* Successful surgical repair was facilitated by preoperative radiographic data. *Conclusion:* Three-dimensional CT reconstruction provides superior spatial detail and can clarify complex anatomical relationships preoperatively.
AUTHORS' ABSTRACT

Diagnosis and Management of Ureteroiliac Artery Fistula: Value of Provocative Arteriography Followed by Common Iliac Artery Embolization and Extraanatomic Arterial Bypass Grafting. David R. Vandersteen, Richard R. Saxon, Eugene Fuchs, et al. *J Urol* 1997; 158:754–758. (D.R.V., Mayo Clinic, E-17, 200 First St SW, Rochester, MN 55905)

Purpose: The authors describe an effective multidisciplinary approach to the diagnosis and management of ureteroarterial fistulas that reduces morbidity and mortality. *Materials and Methods:* Five ureteroarterial fistulas in four patients were studied with standard and provocative arteriography (arteriography combined with ureteral manipulation). After establishing the diagnosis, each lesion was treated with percutaneous embolic occlusion of the common iliac artery followed by extraanatomic arterial bypass grafting. All patients had chronic ureteral stenting, prior pelvic irradiation, prior pelvic surgery, and intrapelvic malignancy, and all fistulas presented with urinary tract hemorrhage. *Results:* Standard arteriography was nondiagnostic, but provocative arteriography demonstrated the fistula in each case. Successful embolization of the common iliac artery followed by extraanatomic arterial bypass grafting precluded the need for laparotomy and preserved ipsilateral renal function. *Conclusion:* Provocative arteriography followed by arteriographic common iliac artery embolization and extraanatomic bypass grafting was successful for the diagnosis and treatment of ureteroarterial fistulas. There was no mortality, limb loss, or renal loss.
AUTHORS' ABSTRACT

Cardiovascular System

Treatment of Iatrogenic Femoral Artery Pseudoaneurysm with Percutaneous Thrombin Injection. Chiau-Suong Liau, Feng-Ming Ho, Ming-Fong Chen, et al. *J Vasc Surg* 1997; 26:18–23. (C.S.L., Department of Internal Medicine, National Taiwan University Hospital, No. 7, Chung-Shan S Rd, Taipei, Taiwan, Republic of China)

Purpose: Local compression has been advocated for the treatment of femoral artery pseudoaneurysms. Although it is effective and has a high success rate, this method bears some limitations; among them are prolonged procedure time, discomfort for patients, and recurrence. As a potent thrombosis-inducing agent, thrombin has been used topically, and occasionally intravascularly, for hemostasis. Pseudoaneurysms with a narrow connecting tract to the native artery may be suitable for treatment with thrombin injection to induce intracavitary coagulation. *Methods:* Patients with pseudoaneurysms of the femoral artery were evaluated with ultrasonography (US). Under US guidance, an intravenous catheter was introduced percutaneously into the pseudoaneurysm, with the catheter position confirmed with US. One thousand units of thrombin dissolved in normal saline solution were then injected slowly into the pseudoaneurysm through the catheter to induce thrombosis. The patients were monitored closely for any adverse effects after thrombin injection. *Results:* A total of five patients with femoral artery pseudoaneurysms were treated with direct percutaneous thrombin injection under US guidance. Within seconds of thrombin injection thrombus formation was evident, and blood flow in the pseudoaneurysm soon ceased when the thrombosis extended to the connecting tract. All procedures were uneventful and successful. No recurrence was noted during follow-up periods of 1–28 months. *Conclusion:* The authors' initial experience with the small number of patients demonstrates the simplicity, lack of morbidity, and high success rate for US-guided percutaneous thrombin injection for the treatment of femoral artery pseudoaneurysms.
AUTHORS' ABSTRACT

Cardiac Myxoma: 40 Years' Experience in 63 Patients. Staffan Bjessmo, Torbjörn Ivert. *Ann Thorac Surg* 1997; 63:697–700. (T.I., Department of Thoracic Surgery, Karolinska Hospital, 171 76 Stockholm, Sweden)

Background: Cardiac myxomas were resected in 63 patients, including the first successful procedure in the world. *Methods:* Patient data and data obtained during follow-up of the survivors were reviewed. *Results:* Preoperatively, valve obstruction occurred in 56% and emboli in 32% of the patients. The myxomas were located in the left atrium in 88%, right atrium in 10%, and both atria in one patient (1.6%). One patient died early, and five died late. The 20-year survival rate was 85%. At a median of 13 years (range, 1 month to 42 years) after resection, 26% of the survivors reported having various cardiopulmonary symptoms, 5% had had thromboembolic events, and 69% were asymptomatic. After 2 years, there was a recurrence in a young woman who had had a multifocal myxoma at the time of the primary operation. No other evidence of recurrence was found at autopsy or during repeat echocardiography in the remaining patients during an observation period of 787 patient-years. *Conclusions:* Surgical resection of a single myxoma is a safe and effective treatment, with a low risk of recurrence. After uncomplicated resection, the frequency with which postoperative echocardiography is performed should be limited.
AUTHORS' ABSTRACT

Musculoskeletal

Prognostic Factors in Idiopathic (Primary) Osteomyelofibrosis. Hans Michael Kvasnicka, Juergen Thiele, Cordula Werden, et al. *Cancer* 1997; 80:708–719. (H.M.K. Institute of Pathology, University of Cologne, Joseph-Stelzmann-Str 9, 50924 Cologne, Germany)

Background: Prognostic variables for idiopathic (primary) osteomyelofibrosis (IMF) are ill defined because of the lack of large control studies based on uniform diagnostic criteria. *Methods:* A retrospective clinicopathologic study was performed on 250 consecutively recruited patients (115 men and 135 women) with an established diagnosis of IMF. In contrast to previous studies, the current study cohort encompassed the full spectrum of initial to advanced stages of the disease process according to laboratory data and, particularly, histology. Because of the relatively high patient age at admission (median, 66.5 years), relative survival rates with corresponding life expectancies and disease specific life loss were calculated. Moreover, a classification and regression tree (CART) analysis was performed to segregate the study patients into subgroups with significantly different prognoses. *Results:* Analysis of the life expectancy and the proportion of deaths attributable to IMF showed a global reduction in life expectancy of 31%. Further calculation disclosed a consistently greater impact of disease in older patients. Age, hemoglobin level at admission, and leukocyte and thrombocyte counts remained as the most relevant parameters for prognosis in multivariate consideration (CART analysis) and facilitated a clear-cut separation into three risk groups. The life expectancy of low risk patients was approximately 10 times higher than that of high risk patients (22.07 vs 2.25 years). *Conclusion:* These results are in keeping with the assumption that features signaling bone marrow insufficiency are associated with a worsening of survival. Generalization, indicated by myeloid metaplasia, can occur at every stage, even in so-called hypercellular phases of IMF. Conversely, myelofibrosis alone is not necessarily predictive of poor survival.
AUTHORS' ABSTRACT

Head and Neck

Mediastinal Parathyroid Cysts. Ofer Landau, Dean W. Chamberlain, Renee S. Kennedy, et al. *Ann Thorac Surg* 1997; 63: 951–953. (Shaf Keshavjee, Department of Thoracic Surgery, The Toronto Hospital, 200 Elizabeth St, EN10-224, Toronto, Ontario, Canada M5G 2C4)

Background: Mediastinal parathyroid cysts are a relatively rare clinical entity. The clinical presentation can be quite varied, although most are found incidentally during investigations for esophageal or respiratory symptoms. *Methods:* The authors present a review of the literature and describe two instructive cases showing specific clinical findings. The clinical presentation, radiologic and pathologic findings, and treatment of mediastinal parathyroid cysts are discussed. *Results:* In the first patient, the presenting symptom was increasing hoarseness resulting from paresis of the right recurrent laryngeal nerve. This case illustrates the rare association of a benign mediastinal parathyroid cyst with unilateral vocal cord palsy. The second patient presented with the more classic findings of progressive dyspnea and stridor related to tracheal compression. *Conclusion:* Although mediastinal parathyroid cysts are rare and can have varied presentations, thorough investigation can reveal the underlying cyst. Surgical excision is the treatment of choice and can be expected to produce excellent results.
AUTHORS' ABSTRACT

The Clinicopathological Characteristics of Gonadotroph Cell Adenoma: A Study of 118 Cases. Donald Ming-Tak Ho, Chih-Yi Hsu, Ling-Tan Ting, et al. *Hum Pathol* 1997; 28:905–911. (D.M.H., Department of Pathology and Laboratory Medicine, Veterans General Hospital-Taipei, Taipei 11217, Taiwan, Republic of China)

Gonadotroph cell adenoma was the most common pituitary adenoma, constituting 35% of the pituitary adenomas in our series of 339 patients with surgically removed pituitary adenomas from June 1987 to December 1995. The average age of these patients was 53 years, with a male predominance (1.5:1.0). The most common neurological symptoms were visual symptoms and headache. Amenorrhea and galactorrhea were recorded in 41% and 14%, respectively, of the female patients of reproductive age. Oncocytic change of varying degrees was seen in 69% of the tumors, and the average age of these patients (56 years) was older than that of those who had no such change (47 years) ($P < .005$). Five types of gonadotropin cell adenomas were recognized; they were tumors that contained (*a*) βFSH, βLH, and αSU; (*b*) βFSH and αLH; (*c*) βFSH and αSU; (*d*) βFSH; and (*e*) αSU. The immunostaining of βFSH-containing cells was usually diffuse, whereas staining of βLH- or αSU-containing cells was usually focal. Double immumostaining showed the immunoreactive cells containing one or any combination of the gonadotropin subunits. Increases in serum gonadotropin levels were seen in only 35% of the patients with gonadotropin cell adenoma. There was no correlation between serum hormonal levels and immunostaining results. In the 33 recurrent cases, significant decrease or total absence of immumoreactivity of one or more hormone subunits in subsequent biopsy specimens were seen in three cases.
AUTHORS' ABSTRACT

Pediatrics

Prenatally Detected Posterior Urethral Valves: Qualitative Assessment of Second Trimester Scans and Prediction of Outcome. Kim A. R. Hutton, David F. M. Thomas, Brian W. Davies. *J Urol* 1997; 158: 1022–1025. (From the Department of Paediatric Urology, St James's University Hospital and General Infirmary, Leeds, England)

Purpose: The authors attempted to determine if the degree of second trimester dilatation and/or other qualitative sonographic features of the fetal urinary tract are predictive of postnatal outcome in male neonates with posterior urethral values. *Materials and Methods:* The authors reviewed ultrasound (US) reports and/or hard copy imaging in 17 cases of posterior urethral valves initially detected on second trimester scans (median gestation, 18 weeks; range, 15.0–23.5 weeks). US appearance was categorized according to the pattern and severity of dilatation, cystic change, or echogenicity of the renal cortex and presence of oligohydramnios. Outcome was reviewed at a median follow-up of 5.7 years (range, 4.4–10.0 years). *Results:* In the 17 cases, there was a poor outcome in 10, including death in four and chronic renal failure in six. Seven patients were alive and well with normal renal function at follow-up. The prognosis in cases of moderate or severe upper tract dilatation was poor. Of the nine patients with marked prenatal hydroureteronephrosis, eight (89%) were dead or had chronic renal failure at follow-up. In contrast, only two of the eight patients (25%) with mild upper tract dilatation or dilatation limited to the bladder had chronic renal failure at review ($P = .05$). Three cases of prenatal renal parenchymal change and three of subsequent oligohydramnios had a poor outcome postnatally. *Conclusion:* The prognosis for boys with prenatally detected posterior urethral valves is closely associated with qualitative aspects of second trimester scan findings. This information may be of clinical value in the prenatal counseling of parents.
AUTHORS' ABSTRACT

Changing the Technique of Background Subtraction Alters Calculated Renal Function on Pediatric Mercaptoacetyltriglycine Renography. Hiep T. Nguyen, Gordon R. Gluckman, Barry A. Kogan. *J Urol* 1997; 158:1252–1256. (B.A.K., Department of Urology, University of California School of Medicine, U-575, San Francisco, CA 94143-0738)

Purpose: Although many operative decisions are based on apparent changes in function detected at serial diuretic renography, the reliability of relative renal function data has been questioned. The authors investigated the effect of background subtraction on calculated renal function. *Materials and Methods:* The authors reviewed 23 pediatric mercaptoacetyltriglycine renograms. Regions of interest for background subtraction were redrawn, and relative renal function values were recalculated. *Results:* In patients with left hydronephrosis, left differential renal function was consistently underestimated by 7.3% compared to the superior and 4.7% compared to the average background subtraction technique. In patients with right hydronephrosis, when only lower pole background activity was considered, right differential renal function was

consistently overestimated by 15.8% compared to the superior and 2.4% compared to the average background subtraction technique. In patients younger than 1 year at the time of study, these differences were exaggerated. *Conclusion:* Because of overlapping hepatic background activity, the position of regions of interest for background subtraction may greatly influence calculated renal function. The authors recommend that the preferred method of calculating background subtraction to minimize error be based on a region of interest surrounding the whole kidney. This method is especially pertinent in patients with right hydronephrosis and in those younger than 1 year. Reported relative renal function data should be interpreted with caution.
AUTHORS' ABSTRACT

Evolving Phenotype of Marfan's Syndrome. Karen J. Lipscomb, Jill Clayton-Smith, Rodney Harris. *Arch Dis Child* 1997; 76:41–46. (K.J.L., Department of Cardiology, Manchester Royal Infirmary, Oxford Rd, Manchester M13 9WL, England)

The aim of the study was to examine the evolution of the physical characteristics of Marfan syndrome throughout childhood. Forty children were identified during the development of a regional register for Marfan syndrome. Evolution of the clinical characteristics was determined by repeated evaluation in 10 patients with sporadic Marfan syndrome and in 30 with a family history. Authors of previous reports of children with Marfan syndrome have concentrated on severely affected individuals, including some with neonatal Marfan syndrome, which appears to be a separate condition and was not included in this review. The most frequent musculoskeletal findings at presentation were a combination of tall stature (greater than 97th percentile), limb disproportion, pectus deformity, classic facial features, high arched palate, and arachnodactyly. Pectus deformity and scoliosis tended to become more prominent during the pubertal growth spurt, when many children developed noticeable red striae over the lumbar region and shoulders. Severe cardiovascular abnormalities were not documented as frequently as has been suggested in previous studies, possibly owing to the exclusion of neonatal patients. Fifty-five percent of patients aged younger than 16 years had cardiovascular involvement but remained asymptomatic. Echocardiographic findings of mild aortic root dilatation were found in 17 patients, usually by the age of 9–15 years. This age of onset suggests that absence of aortic root enlargement cannot be used to exclude a diagnosis of the condition in a "marfanoid" child before skeletal growth is complete. Aortic dissection is rare in childhood or adolescence but is well documented in the late teens and early 20s. Assessment of cardiovascular risk cannot be made on the basis of events in preceding generations. Lens dislocation and severe myopia occurred in about 25% of patients. There is considerable intrafamilial phenotypic heterogeneity. Severe aortic complications do not affect all individuals within a given pedigree, and the age at which aortic events occur within a family is variable. Likewise, ocular features do not necessarily "breed true." Musculoskeletal characteristics show intrafamilial variability to a lesser extent. Gene tracking is useful to provide an early diagnosis when skeletal characteristics are absent or minimal when the child is first examined. It is also useful in excluding the diagnosis in a child with a 50% risk of Marfan syndrome. The diagnosis is difficult in children with no family history of the condition, because of the high prevalence of isolated features of Marfan syndrome in the general population. The detection rate of mutations within the fibrillin gene on chromosome 15 is extremely low (10%–20%), and, with one exception, all mutations identified have been unique to a single family. Twenty-five percent of individuals with Marfan syndrome have no family history of the condition. Children who do not fulfill all the clinical criteria but who have at least four skeletal features, especially a pectus deformity, scoliosis, and limb disproportion in association with tall stature, in the absence of overt cardiovascular or ocular manifestations, should undergo periodic reevaluation as more diagnostic features may become apparent with increasing age. Annual slit-lamp examination until the age of 6 years will help in detection of ectopia lentis in most children. Thereafter, visual acuity testing is appropriate. Yearly echocardiographic examination is recommended even in the absence of overt cardiovascular abnormality, because aortic dilatation is clinically silent. By the time of skeletal maturity and the full development of the musculoskeletal phenotype, most affected patients have evidence of cardiovascular abnormality, and the clinical diagnosis is simplified. Some patients do not develop cardiovascular features until adulthood. Therefore, continued echocardiographic surveillance may be appropriate for those patients who do not fulfill the full clinical criteria but have six or more musculoskeletal features in adulthood.
PAULA W. BRILL, MD
New York Hospital–Cornell Medical Center, New York, NY

Mortality, Severe Respiratory Distress Syndrome, and Chronic Lung Disease of the Newborn Are Reduced More after Prophylactic than after Therapeutic Administration of the Surfactant Curosurf. Johannes Egberts, Roland Brand, Herve Waltl, et al. *Pediatrics* 1997; 100:*http://www.pediatrics.org/cgi/content/full/100/1/e4*. (J.E., Department of Obstetrics and Gynecology, Leiden University Hospital, Building 1, P3-P, PO Box 9600, 2300 RC Leiden, The Netherlands)

Prophylactic and rescue treatment with surfactant reduces mortality rate, severity of acute respiratory problems, and the frequency of chronic lung disease in preterm infants. Results of this analysis indicated that prophylactic treatment reduced the mortality rate more effectively than rescue treatment. The combined trials included 345 prophylactically treated infants and 326 enrolled infants who were eligible for rescue therapy if they fulfilled entry criteria for surfactant administration. Analyses were performed to determine whether prophylaxis, when compared with rescue treatment, would result in lower frequency of the following outcome variables: severe respiratory distress syndrome, neonatal mortality, and chronic lung disease of the newborn. The results indicate that the porcine surfactant Curosurf, when administered prophylactically, had marked advantages over rescue therapy in relation to mortality, severity of respiratory distress syndrome, and occurrence of chronic lung disease in the newborn.
BEVERLY P. WOOD, MD
Childrens Hospital, Los Angeles, Calif

Miscellaneous

Lymphocyte-rich Well-differentiated Liposarcoma: Report of Nine Cases. Pedram Argani, Fabio Facchetti, Giorgio Inghirami, et al. *Am J Surg Pathol* 1997; 21:884–895. (Juan Rosai, Department of Pathology, Memorial Sloan-Kettering Cancer Center, 1275 York Ave, New York, NY 10021)

Nine well-differentiated liposarcomas with foci simulating the appearance of malignant lymphoma and other lymphoid disorders are reported. Their clinical presentation and evolution were not significantly different from those of their conventional counterparts lacking a lymphoid infiltrate. Microscopically, these tumors were characterized by areas of ordinary well-differentiated liposarcoma, admixed with discrete nodules comprised of small germinal centers, and separated by an admixture of lymphocytes, spindled stromal cells, collagen, and blood vessels, in which highly atypical tumor cells were embedded. The differential diagnosis included Hodgkin's disease, Castleman's disease, and inflammatory pseudotumor. Immunohistochemical evaluation revealed a predominance of T cells in the lymphocytic population. Molecular genetic studies revealed no evidence of clonal rearrangement of the T cell receptor gene, supporting the interpretation of these lymphocytes as reactive. Awareness of the existence of this variant of inflammatory liposarcoma should prevent its misinterpretation as a primary lymphoproliferative process.
AUTHORS' ABSTRACT